Welcome to...
Fundamentals of Nursing!

2ND EDITION

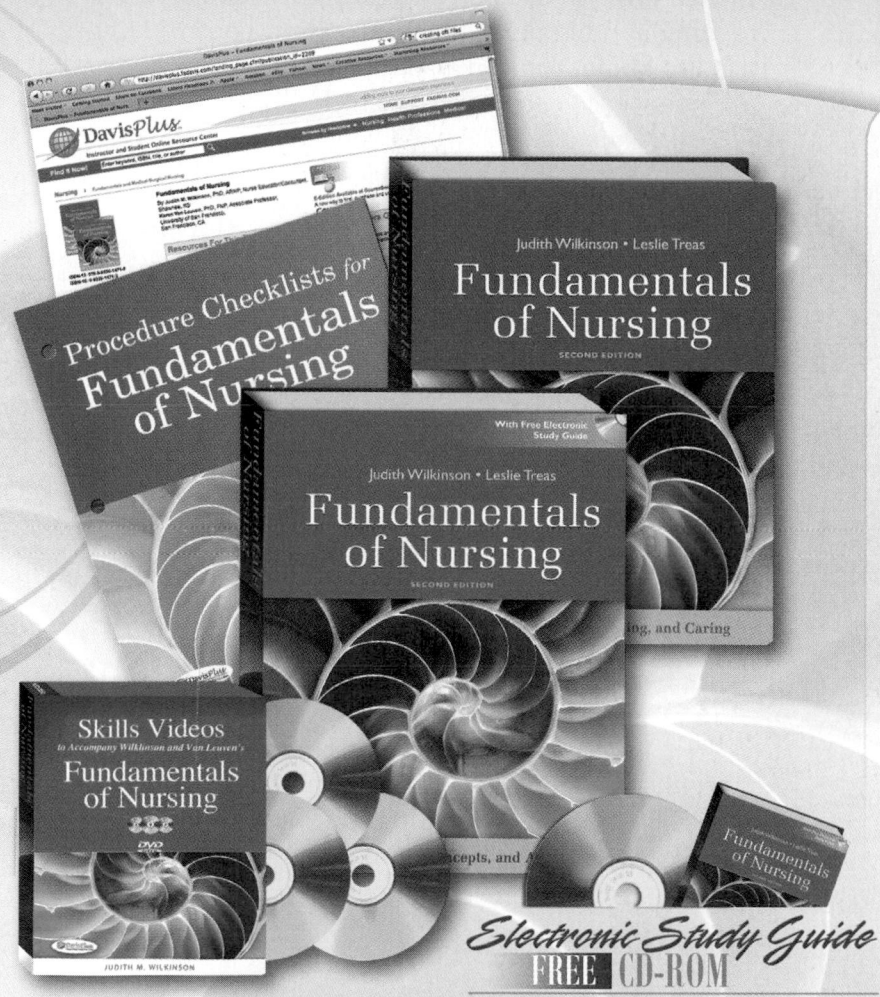

Take advantage of all of the resources this unique, two-volume package offers to make learning easier.

Just read through this guide or listen to "**Getting the Most Out of This Learning Package**" podcast on DavisPlus...

http://davisplus.fadavis.com
Keyword Wilkinson

Your Learning Package features...

✓ The Two-Volume Textbook

✓ The Electronic Study Guide—FREE on the BONUS CD-ROM in Volume 1

✓ Resources Online at DavisPlus...
http://davisplus.fadavis.com
Keyword: Wilkinson

✓ The Skills Videos on DVDs
(purchase separately)

✓ The Procedure Checklist
(purchase separately)

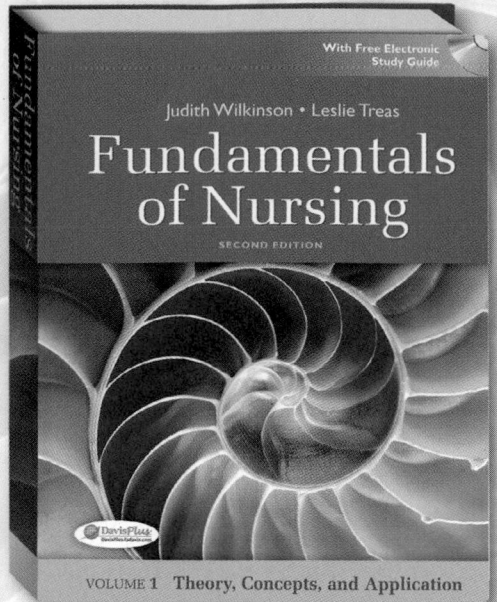

Judith Wilkinson • Leslie Treas

Fundamentals of Nursing

SECOND EDITION

With Free Electronic Study Guide

DavisPlus

VOLUME 1 Theory, Concepts, and Application

VOLUME 1 is your primary classroom/study textbook.

Learning Outcomes guide your
reading and highlight the information you
need to know. You can also refer to them later
to review each chapter's content.

Learning Outcomes

After completing this chapter, you should be able to:

➤ Describe the normal structure and function of the organs in the urinary system.

➤ Describe the processes of urine formation and elimination.

➤ Discuss factors that affect urinary elimination.

➤ Describe the contents of a nursing assessment and physical ___ focused on urinary elimination.

___ pes of urine

___ ntification of

➤ Discuss common elimination problems: urinary tract infection, urinary retention, and urinary incontinence.

➤ Identify nursing diagnoses associated with altered urin elimination.

➤ Describe nursing interventions that promote normal urination.

➤ Provide care for clients experiencing urinary problem

➤ Perform urinary catheterizations following accepted procedures.

➤ Discuss nursing care appropriate for clients who have urinary diversion.

Meet Your Patient

During your assigned clinical experience at University Hospital, the RN asks you to complete the admission process for Marlena, a 55-year-old woman who is complaining of frequent, painful urination. As you interview her, Marlena becomes embarrassed. "I really don't enjoy talking about this," she admits. Then, she asks to use the bathroom. You ask her to give you a midstream clean-catch urine sample while she is in the restroom. When she returns, she gives you a small specimen of pink-colored, strong-smelling urine. "I feel like I have strong urge to go and then I hardly have any urine. It's a little bloody and burns like crazy during my stream," she reports.

You close the door and interview Marlena in private about her usual urination pattern and current symptoms. Your calm approach and straightforward manner put her at ease. She confides that she is sexually active and that her symptoms began after spending the weekend with her new partner. You take her vital signs: oral temperature 99.4°F (37.4°C), radial pulse 88 beats/min, respiratory rate

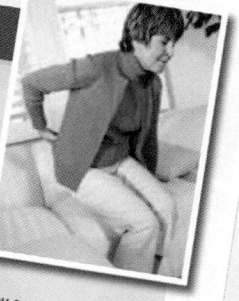

20 breaths/min, and blood pressure 108/72 mm Hg.

After you report your assessment data to the RN, the emergency department (ED) physician asks you to perform a dipstick urinalysis on the urine sample and to send the urine sample to the lab for culture and sensitivity. He asks you: "Well, what do you think we need to do next?" How would you answer his question?

As you gain theoretical and practical knowledge in this chapter, we will return to this case study to discuss how you might answer the physician's question and support Marle ___ 's recovery. You will also have the opportunity to ___ your feelings about giving care that patients may ___ ersonal or even embarrassing.

Meet Your Patient
is a real-life patient scenario
that opens each chapter in
Volume I and continues
throughout the chapter,
helping you apply theory
to practice.

How Does Urinary Elimination Occur?

Where the bladder connects to the urethra is a thickening of smooth muscle, called the **internal urethral sphincter.** When closed, the internal sphincter keeps urine in the bladder from entering the urethra. When the bladder contains 200 to 450 mL of urine (50 to 200 mL in children), the distention activates stretch receptors in the bladder wall. The stretch receptors send sensory impulses to the *voiding reflex center* in the spinal cord, triggering motor impulses that cause the detrusor muscle to contract and the internal sphincter to relax. The internal urethral sphincter is not under voluntary control.

Voiding (also called **urination or micturition**) occurs when contraction of the detrusor muscle pushes stored urine through the relaxed internal urethral sphincter into the urethra. This triggers the conscious urge to void. However, voiding may be voluntarily delayed by inhibiting release of a second, **external urethral sphincter.** When the person is ready to urinate, the brain signals the

Headings in the Form of Questions
help you to organize your thinking. When you review a
chapter for a test, scan the headings and see what you
recall about each of them.

Terms in Boldface Type highlight the
important concepts when they're defined for the
first time. While reviewing the content later, scan
the pages for the bold and italicized words.
If any seem unfamiliar, read the section again.

Knowledge Check Questions

divide the material into small, manageable sections. Perfect for chapter review now and exam prep later.

Critical Thinking Questions

prepare you for the "real world" by providing the practice you need in applying the information you have just learned.

Colorful Icons refer you

to Volume 1, Volume 2, the Electronic Study Guide or Davis*Plus*.

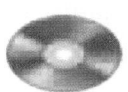 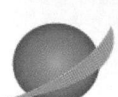 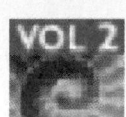

This cross referencing tells you about...

- Additional/enrichment information on the Electronic Study Guide or Davis*Plus*.
- Review material/forms on the Electronic Study Guide or Davis*Plus*.
- Clinical information in Volume 2.

HELPFUL HINT: The sentence before the icon tells you what the material is.

You and **your instructor** will determine when or if you will need to use this material.

Skills/Procedures are introduced in

Volume 1. **Critical Aspect boxes** describe the principles and rationales for the procedure and explain their relevance.

HELPFUL HINT: An icon shows you where in Volume 2 to find the complete, step-by-step procedure you will use in lab to learn and practice the skill.

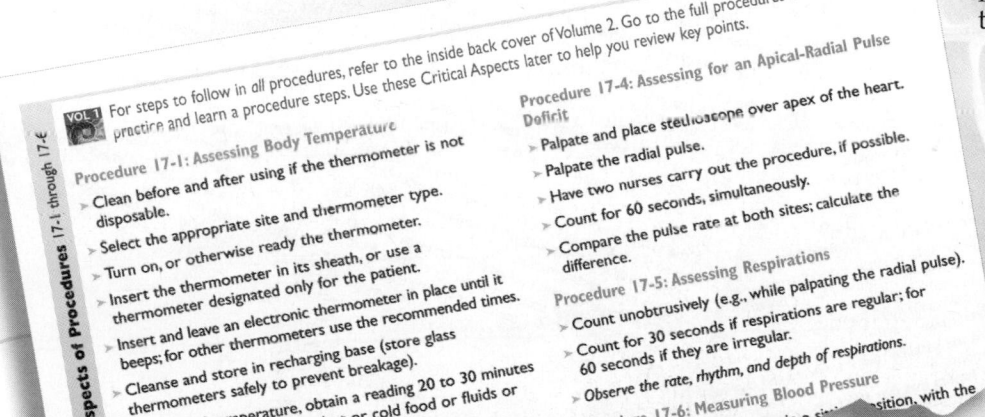

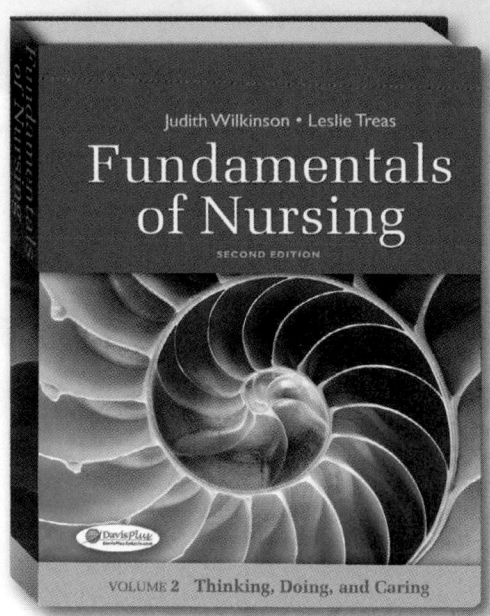

Judith Wilkinson • Leslie Treas

Fundamentals of Nursing

SECOND EDITION

VOLUME 2 Thinking, Doing, and Caring

VOLUME 2 is your primary text for your skills lab and clinical.

THE INFORMATION YOU NEED...

Assessment Guidelines and Tools Boxes provide a quick review of special assessments your patients may need.

Diagnostic Testing Tables
identify the diagnostic tests required by the condition.

Standardized Language Tables (NANDA, NIC and NOC)
are useful for care planning

THE PROCEDURES YOU NEED...

More than 200 Step-by-Step Procedures

HELPFUL HINT: If you find yourself in lab without Volume 2, use the Critical Aspect Boxes in Volume 1 to review the concepts underlying each procedure.

More than 90 Clinical Insight Boxes

present guidelines for clinical care. These guidelines are based more on principles than step-by-step procedures.

Procedure 17-5 **Assessing Respirations**

► For steps to follow in all procedures, refer to the inside back cover of this book.

Critical Aspects

- Count unobtrusively (e.g., while palpating the radial pulse).
- Count for 30 seconds if respirations are regular; for 60 seconds if they are irregular. A 60-second count is recommended for increased accuracy, even for regular respirations.
- Observe the rate, rhythm, and depth of respirations.

Equipment
- A watch with a second hand (or a wall clock)

Delegation
You can delegate the counting of respirations to the nursing assistive personnel (NAP) if you conclude that the patient's condition and the NAP's skills allow. Perform the following assessments, and inform the NAP of any special consider-ations (e.g., the need to keep the patient in a certain posi-tion). Ask the NAP to record and report the respirations to you, and to report immediately if they are not within the normal range for this patient (specify the range).

Pre-Procedure Assessments
- Observe for signs of respiratory distress—brea[...] faster or slower than normal, gasping breaths, [...] confusion, circumoral (around the month) cyanosis. Signs of hypoxemia may indicate that the patient is not ad[...] quately oxygenated.
- Determine the baseline respiratory rate and character of respirations.
- Assess for factors that may affect the respiratory rate (e.g., pain, activity, fever, respiratory disorders).

Procedure Steps
When performing the procedure, al-ways identify your patient according to agency policy and be attentive to stan-dard precautions, hand h[...] safety and n[...]

2. Palpate and count the radial pulse; remember that number. Then [...] your hand on the [...]

Clinical Insights **Caring for a Patient with an Indwelling Catheter**

Clinical Insight 27-1

An indwelling catheter is connected to a drainage tube and collection bag, which constitute a closed system.

Goal 1: Prevent urinary tract infection.

- Do not disconnect the tubing or open the drainage sys-tem (e.g., to obtain specimens or measure the urine). A closed system minimizes the chance for pathogens to enter the system and infect the urinary tract.
- Regularly check connections between the catheter and drainage tubing and the drainage tube and collection bag. Loose connections cause leaks and serve as entry points for pathogens.
- If the system inadvertently becomes disconnected, wipe the ends of both tubes with antiseptic (e.g., alcohol or chlorhexadine-gluconate-alcohol combination product) before reconnecting them.
- If the catheter becomes soiled from drainage or feces, cleanse it w[...] soap and water by cleaning from the [...] the catheter well, and pat it dry. mea[...] [...]es the growth of microb[...]

Goal 2: Maintain free flow of urine.

Maintaining free flow of urine prevents backflow of urine into the bladder, which can cause bladder distention and injury. Stasis of urine also provides a medium for growth of micro-organisms. Note that some of the interventions in this sec-tion are the same as those for preventing infection (goal 1).

- Make sure the tubing and bag remain below the level of the bladder to prevent backflow. Urine drains by gravity in this system.
- If the collecting bag must be higher than the bladder at any time, you must clamp the catheter. Clamping prevents backflow of stagnant urine into the bladder
- Frequently inspect the tubing to ensure that urine flows freely in the tubing. Any kinks, coils, or compression of the catheter or tubing may impede flow and cause backup into the bladder.
- If urine is not flowing, check to be sure the patient [...] lying on the tubing. [...]t allow the collection bag to lie on the fl[...] [...]es the effec[...]

THE EXERCISES AND REVIEW YOU NEED...

Caring for the Garcias

The exercises in the following section allow you to practice the kind of thinking you will use as a full-spectrum nurse. Because these are critical-thinking questions, there is usually no single right answer. We do not provide answers for these questions because it is more important for you to think about the questions than to arrive at the "right" answer. These questions are designed to improve your thinking more than to "cover content." Discuss answers with your peers—discussion can stimulate critical thinking. If you have difficulty with any of these questions, consult with your instructor.

Recall that on Joseph Garcia's preliminary visit to the family medicine center, his blood pressure (BP) was 162/94. On subsequent visits, his BP was 168/100 and 174/98. Mr. Garcia was diagnosed with hypertension and prescribed an antihypertension medication, to be taken each morning. This morning Mr. Garcia presents at the clinic for follow-up. The following information is gathered as he checks in for his visit.

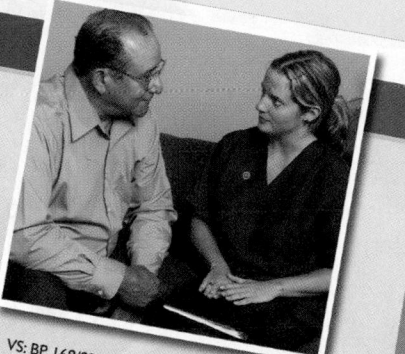

VS: BP, 168/92; pulse, 80; respirations, 20; temperature, 98.4°F (36.9°C)
Weight: 231 lb (105 kg)

Review the preliminary data and the preceding information to answer the following questions:

"Caring for the Garcias"

lets you follow the story of a multi-cultural family and answer questions about their care.

"Applying the Full-Spectrum Nursing Model" Questions

help you develop your clinical reasoning skills by applying the concepts of thinking, doing, and caring.

Critical Thinking and Clinical Reasoning Questions develop the

skills you will use in clinical practice.

"What Are the Main Points in This Chapter?"

Knowledge Maps

are visual summaries of the corresponding material in Volume 1.

Applying the Full-Spectrum Nursing Model

PATIENT SITUATION

A patient in the critical care unit had a stable pulse and BP for the first few days. He has become more ill and now his pulse and BP are weak and difficult to palpate. His last BP reading was abnormally low, so it must be monitored frequently. He is receiving intravenous fluids in both arms.

THINKING

1. *Critical Thinking (Reflecting and deciding what to do).* Which of the patient's vital signs (TPR and BP) might you be able to delegate to nursing assistive personnel?

DOING

2. *Practical Knowledge.* How would you take the patient's blood pressure? Be specific: (a) What site would you use? (b) What equipment would you use?

3. *Nursing Process (Assessment).*
   a. Will you need to validate any of the vital signs you obtain? If so, why?
   b. How could you validate those vital signs?

CARING

4. Assume that you are very busy. How would you demonstrate caring to this patient w are assessing his vital signs (the ones you did not delegate to a NAP)?

Critical Thinking and Clinical Reasoning

1. Recall the clients you encountered at the community health fair (Meet Your Patient, Volume 1). Two-year-old Jason's oral temperature was 102°F (38.9°C); his skin was warm, dry, and flushed. His mother told you that he had been eating poorly and was very irritable. What cues alert you that something is wrong?

2. You have already established (in Volume 1) what, if any, additional information you need to determine the meaning of Jason's temperature elevation.
   a. What theoretical knowledge may account for Jason's temperature?
   b. Are there any actions you should take while meeting with Jason and his mother? If so, what?
   c. What biases do you have that affect your thinking about this situation? (This requires self-knowledge.)

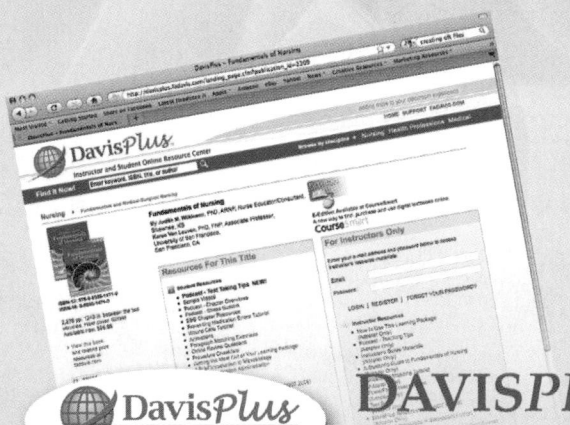
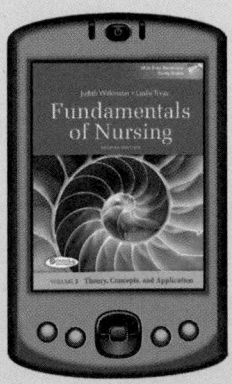
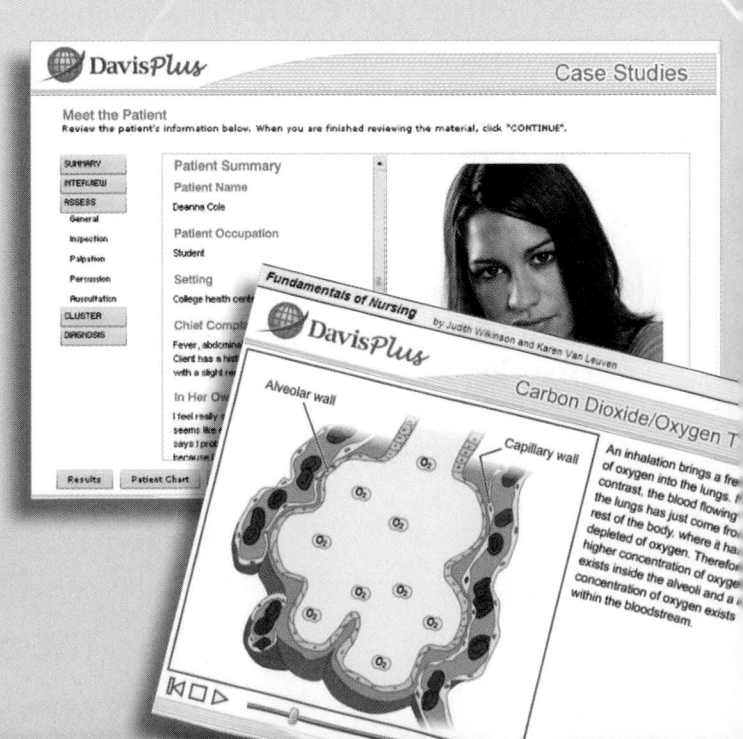

SECOND EDITION

Fundamentals of Nursing

volume 2

Thinking, Doing, and Caring

Judith M. Wilkinson, PhD, ARNP

Leslie S. Treas, PhD, RN, CPNP-PC, NNP-BC

F.A. Davis Company • Philadelphia

F. A. Davis Company
1915 Arch Street
Philadelphia, PA 19103
www.fadavis.com

Printed in the United States of America

Last digit indicates print number: 10 9 8 7 6 5 4 3 2 1

Publisher, Nursing: Lisa B. Deitch
Special Projects Editor: Shirley A. Kuhn
Director of Content Development: Darlene D. Pedersen
Senior Project Editor: Meghan Ziegler
Design and Ilustrations Manager: Carolyn O'Brien

As new scientific information becomes available through basic and clinical research, recommended treatments and drug therapies undergo changes. The author(s) and publisher have done everything possible to make this book accurate, up to date, and in accord with accepted standards at the time of publication. The author(s), editors, and publisher are not responsible for errors or omissions or for consequences from application of the book, and make no warranty, expressed or implied, in regard to the contents of the book. Any practice described in this book should be applied by the reader in accordance with professional standards of care used in regard to the unique circumstances that may apply in each situation. The reader is advised always to check product information (package inserts) for changes and new information regarding dose and contraindications before administering any drug. Caution is especially urged when using new or infrequently ordered drugs.

Library of Congress Cataloging-in-Publication Data

Wilkinson, Judith M., 1939-
   Fundamentals of nursing / Judith M. Wilkinson, Leslie S. Treas. – 2nd ed.
      p. ; cm.
   Includes bibliographical references and index.
   ISBN-13: 978-0-8036-2265-4
   ISBN-10: 0-8036-2265-1
1. Nursing. I. Treas, Leslie S. II. Title.
   [DNLM: 1. Nursing Process. 2. Nursing Care. 3. Nursing Theory. WY 100]
   RT41.W56 2011
   610.73—dc22   2010037617

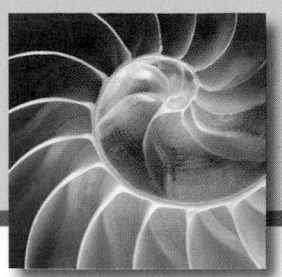

Preface

We chose our book title carefully. We have used the words *theory, concepts, application, thinking, doing, and caring* because we believe that excellent nursing requires an equal mix of knowledge, thought, and action. Nurses use all of these to express caring. It is knowledge and its application—not just the tasks nurses do—that delineate the various levels of nursing. Even so, skillful performance of tasks is essential to full attainment of the nursing role.

We present our material in two volumes to enable students to focus on material suitable for use in specific venues. Volume 2 was designed to be a compact, easy-to-carry reference to use in the skills lab and in clinical. This volume contains practical, "how to" information for safely performing nursing actions and interacting with real patients. Rationales for each action explain the "why behind the what" to help you practice nursing based on concepts rather than cookbook-style steps. Volume 2 offers practice-based forms, assessment questionnaires, and other clinical tips, but it is not limited to skills and procedures. It includes both thinking and doing, the same as does Volume 1; but the emphasis is different in each volume. Volume 2 works seamlessly with Volume 1, the Skills Videos, and the Electronic Study Guide to provide a user-friendly learning experience that will surely stimulate new enthusiasm for learning. For example, throughout Volume 2, students have access to a simulated experience, known as "Caring for the Garcias,"

through which they apply our full-spectrum model of nursing to learn about the nursing role, the healthcare system, and the real-world application of the content in Volume 1.

Other features in each chapter of this volume include critical-thinking activities ("Thinking Critically About...,"); step-by-step procedures and clinical insights (with rationales); exercises to tie the procedures to the skills videos; assessment guidelines and tools; summaries of NANDA/NIC/NOC standardized labels for nursing diagnoses, outcomes, and interventions; a summary of the main points that were covered in Volume 1; and a knowledge map of the main concepts discussed in the chapter. All of these features will be useful during a student's clinical day.

This volume, like Volume 1, will appeal to nontraditional students of the technological generation, encourage independent learning, promote critical thinking, support a variety of learning styles, and assure students that it is possible to achieve excellent nursing despite today's challenges.

We hope you will read the Preface and other introductory material in the front of Volume 1. It explains the philosophical underpinnings for this text and describes in more detail how to use the various pieces of this highly integrated learning package, which is flexible enough to accommodate a variety of teaching styles and curriculums.

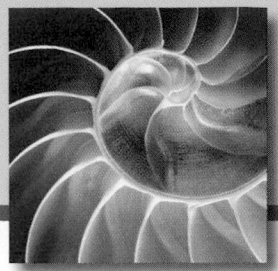

Contents

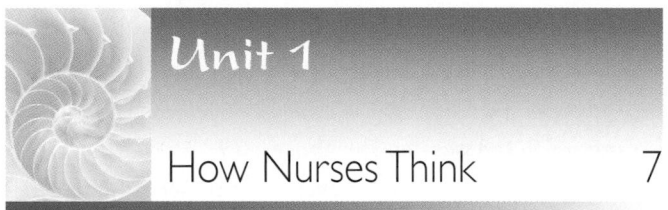
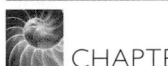
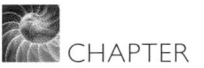
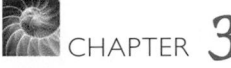
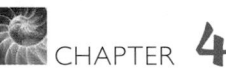
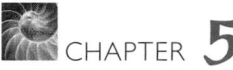

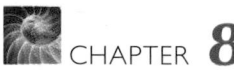
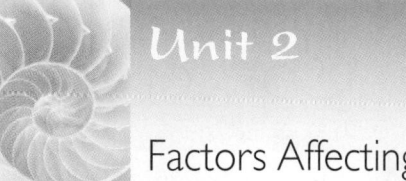

Unit 2

Factors Affecting Health   75

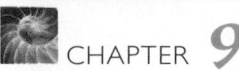
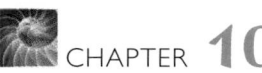

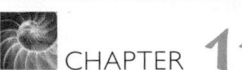
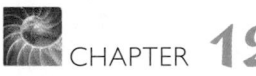
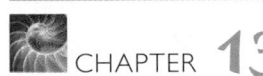
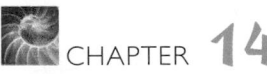

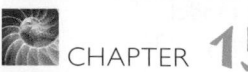

CHAPTER 15

Loss, Grief, & Dying   158

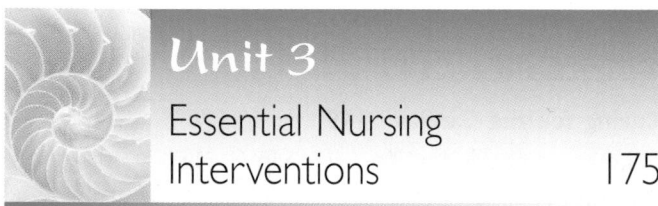

Unit 3
Essential Nursing
Interventions   175

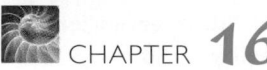

CHAPTER 16

Documenting & Reporting   177

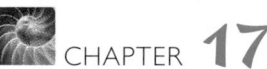

CHAPTER 17

Measuring Vital Signs   192

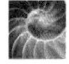

CHAPTER **18**

Communicating & Therapeutic Relationships   220

CHAPTER **19**

Health Assessment: Performing a Physical Examination   230

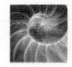

CHAPTER **20**

Promoting Asepsis & Preventing Infection   333

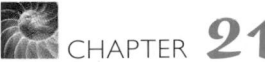

CHAPTER 21

Promoting Safety 366

Caring for the Garcias 366

Practical Knowledge: Knowing Why 367

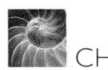

CHAPTER 22

Facilitating Hygiene 384

Caring for the Garcias 384

Practical Knowledge: Knowing How 385

CHAPTER 23

Administering Medication   440

CHAPTER **24**

Teaching Clients   535

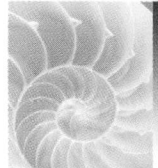

Unit 4

How Nurses Support Physiological Functioning   543

CHAPTER **25**

Stress & Adaptation   545

CHAPTER **26**

Nutrition   556

CHAPTER **27**

Urinary Elimination   603

 CHAPTER **28**

Bowel Elimination   648

CHAPTER **29**

Sensory Perception   687

 CHAPTER **30**

Pain Management   701

 CHAPTER **31**

Activity & Exercise   714

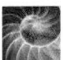

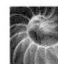

CHAPTER **35**

Oxygenation   833

CHAPTER **36**

Fluids, Electrolytes, & Acid-Base Balance   902

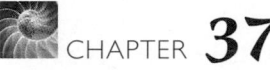

CHAPTER **37**

Perioperative Nursing   954

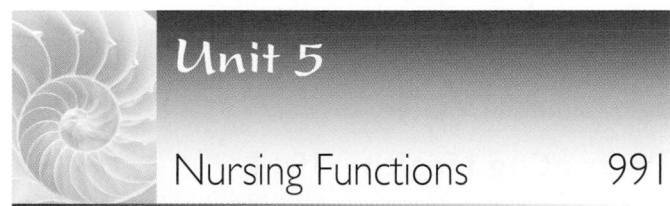

Unit 5

Nursing Functions   991

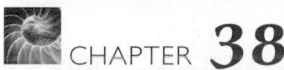

CHAPTER **38**

Leading & Managing   993

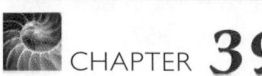

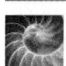
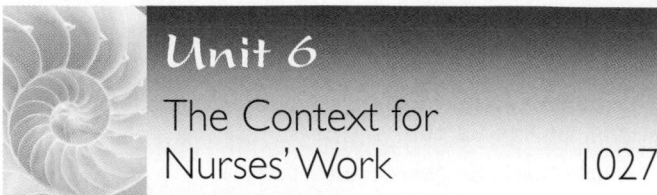

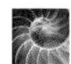

Meet the Garcias

Throughout this text, you will be applying what you have learned as you care for the Garcia family. In Chapter 1, you will meet Joseph Garcia, a construction work supervisor, who arrives at the Family Medicine Center for his first physical exam in 10 years. It is Joe's knee pain that causes him to seek help because it affects his work. But as you will see, Joe will discover he has other serious health problems that require him to be more vigilant about his health. As you read and work through the exercises in "Caring for the Garcias," you will also get to know Joe's wife Flordelisa, his grandchild Bettina, other members of his extended family, and his friends, as they deal with health issues and life changes.

Your experience in caring for the Garcias will show you that patients come to you with symptoms but each person brings unique values, lifestyle, and relationships to the encounter. From the Garcias, you will learn what it means to care for the whole person and how to be a full-spectrum nurse.

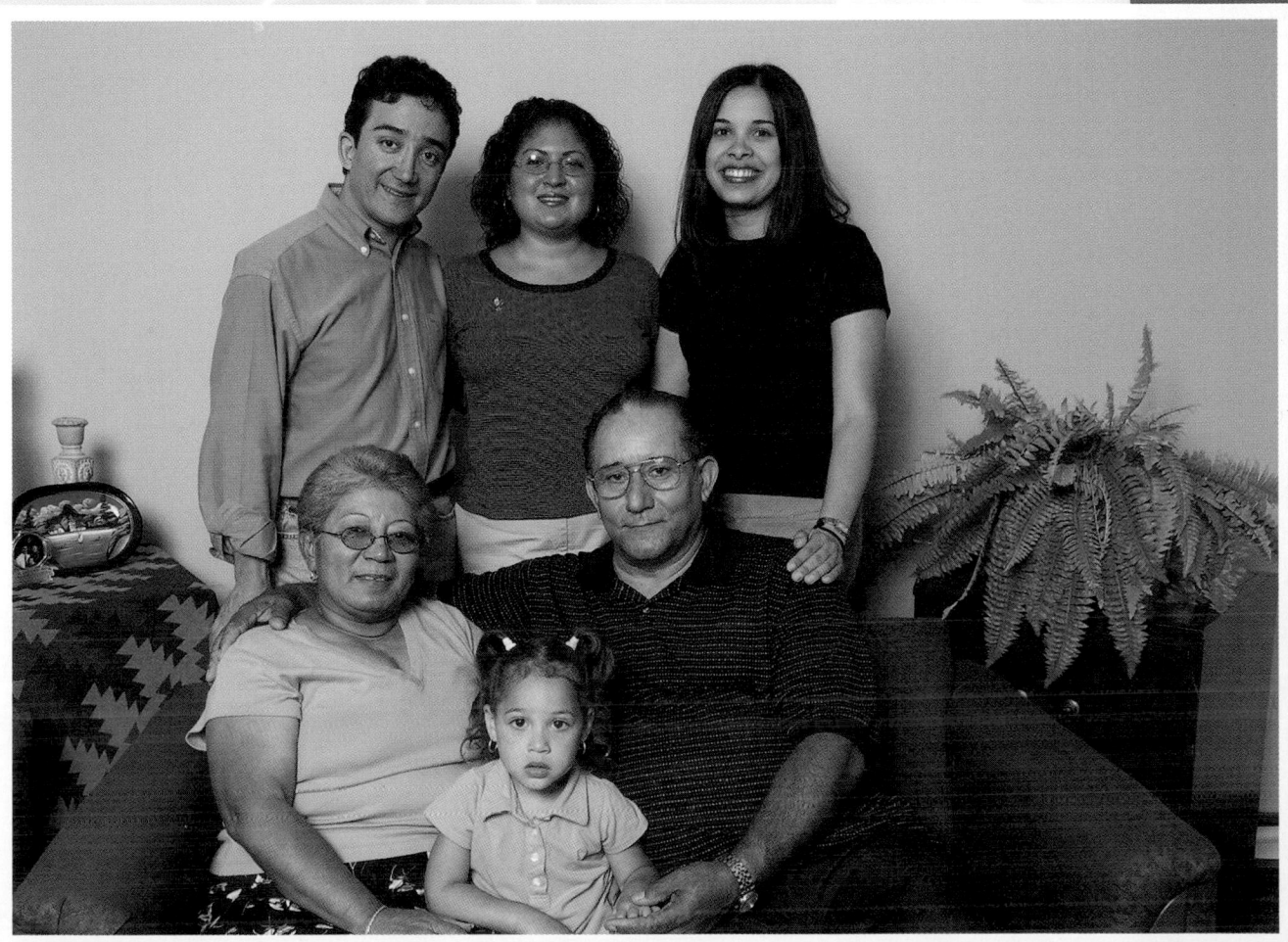

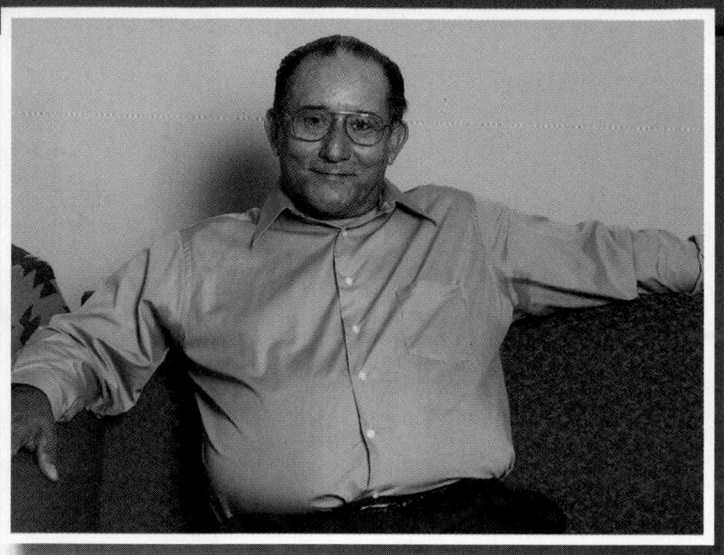

Mr. Joseph Garcia is a new patient at the Family Medicine Center. He arrives at the Center for an appointment for a physical exam and completes the following admission questionnaire.

Name: *Joseph Garcia* DOB: 7 / 12 / 50

Marital Status S (M) W D Partnered

If applicable, spouse/partner name: *Flordelisa*

Occupation: *Construction worker* Spouse/partner occupation: *Daycare teacher*

Does your spouse or partner have any health care problems? If so, please list:

High blood pressure

Do you have children? *Yes* Ages? *30, 27, 22*

Please circle yes or no if you have had the following:

AIDS/HIV +	YES	**(NO)**	Headaches	YES	**(NO)**
Allergies	**(YES)**	NO	Heart Disease	YES	**(NO)**
Anemia	YES	**(NO)**	Hernia	**(YES)**	NO
Anorexia	YES	**(NO)**	Herpes	YES	**(NO)**
Anxiety	YES	**(NO)**	High Cholesterol	YES	**(NO)**
Arthritis	YES	**(NO)**	High Blood Pressure	YES	**(NO)**
Bleeding Disorder	YES	**(NO)**	Kidney Problems	YES	**(NO)**
Breast Problems	YES	**(NO)**	Liver Problems	YES	**(NO)**
Cancer	YES	**(NO)**	Abnormal Mammogram	**(N/A)** YES	NO
Chicken Pox	**(YES)**	NO	Menopause	**(N/A)** YES	NO
Colon Disorder	YES	**(NO)**	Mononucleosis	YES	**(NO)**
COPD/Emphysema	YES	**(NO)**	Multiple Sclerosis	YES	**(NO)**
Depression	YES	**(NO)**	Osteoporosis	YES	**(NO)**
Diabetes	YES	**(NO)**	Pneumonia	YES	**(NO)**
Epilepsy/Seizures	YES	**(NO)**	Polio	YES	**(NO)**
Eye Problems	**(YES)**	NO	Prostate Problems	YES	**(NO)**
Gallbladder Disorder	YES	**(NO)**	Skin Problems	YES	**(NO)**
Stomach Problems/Ulcer	YES	**(NO)**	Stroke	YES	**(NO)**
Gout	YES	**(NO)**	Suicide Attempt	YES	**(NO)**
Gynecological Problems	YES	**(NO)**	Thyroid Problems	YES	**(NO)**
Sexually Transmitted Disease	YES	**(NO)**	Other	YES	**(NO)**

Please list your current medications and dosages. Also list over-the-counter and herbal products you use regularly.

Tylenol Extra Strength 6 per day *Ben-Gay Balm on knees*

MultiVitamin 1 per day

Do you have any allergies to any medications? If YES, please list: None

Please list any surgeries or hospitalizations with the dates:

Tonsils   1956

Hernia repair   1985

When was your last tetanus vaccine?   ????   unknown

Have you had the vaccine for Pneumonia? If yes, when? I don't think so

Have you had the vaccine against hepatitis B?   No   Hepatitis A? No

Have you ever had a sigmoidoscopy or colonoscopy? If YES, when? No

Have you ever had a PSA test to screen for prostate cancer? No

If YES, when?   Has it ever been abnormal?

Any difficulty with achieving or maintaining an erection?   No

Please tell us about yourself.

Do you drink alcohol?   Yes   If yes, what type, how much and how often?

Beer, one or two several times per week

Do you use tobacco? Yes   If yes, how much do you smoke per day? 1 1/2 packs per day

                        At what age did you begin smoking? 16

                        Have you ever tried to quit? yes

                        Would you like to quit? maybe

Do you drink caffeine? Yes   How much per day? 2 cups

Do you use recreational drugs? No   If yes, what type and how often?

Do you exercise?   At work only   Describe the type, frequency, and length of exercise.

Do you have a stressful life? Yes

Is the source of your stress   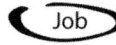 Job   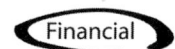 Financial   Family?

Do you use alternative medicine (ex. Chiropractic, acupuncture)? No

Do you have a Living Will or Advance Directive? No

What are your hobbies?   Watching sports on TV, grandkids

Please tell us about your Family History. For any YES answer please indicate your relationship with the person.

Asthma	YES	**NO**		High Blood Pressure	**YES**	NO
Breast Cancer	YES	**NO**		*both parents*		
Cancer *father, prostate*	**YES**	NO		High Cholesterol *mother*	**YES**	NO
Chemical Dependency	YES	**NO**		Kidney Disease	YES	**NO**
Diabetes *mother*	**YES**	NO		Mental Illness	YES	**NO**
Heart Disease *both parents*	**YES**	NO		Osteoporosis	YES	**NO**
Heart Disease Before 55 yo	YES	**NO**		Unusual Disorders	YES	**NO**
				Other		

The Diagnosis

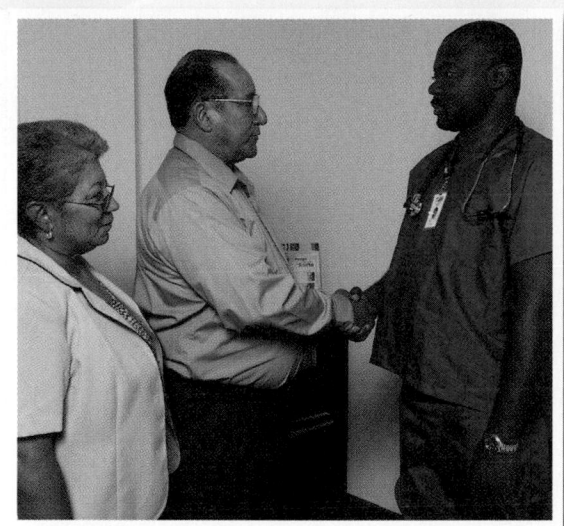

During the visit, the clinic nurse records the following information in Joe's chart.

Height	5 ft 10 in.
Weight	225 lb
BP	162/94 mm Hg
Pulse	84 beats/min
RR	20 breaths/min
Temp	98.2°F oral

Presenting Complaint: Patient states he is here to become established as a patient at the Center and that he has not had a physical exam in over 10 years. Wife accompanies. He is currently experiencing bilateral knee pain that is affecting his work performance. "I supervise construction workers. To check on things, I have to climb up and down ladders, lift things, and crawl around a lot." Has not missed any work but has been using increasing amounts of acetaminophen and ibuprofen "to get through the day." The medications provide only limited relief. States pain occurs daily even if not at work. Describes the pain as "achy" and "dull." Feels best when he is off his feet. Desires pain relief and check-up. Explains that both parents had heart disease. Wife expressing worry that he may be developing heart problems "because he's so tired after work and he gets short of breath easy."

The nurse explains to Joe that he will be seen by the nurse practitioner shortly. She asks Mr. Garcia if he would like his wife to be present for the exam. Mr. Garcia requests that his wife remain in the room.

Jordan Miller, MSN, FNP is on duty at the Center today. Jordan worked as an RN for more than 10 years in the local emergency department and urgent care clinic. He has been a family nurse practitioner (FNP-BC) for more than 5 years. Jordan enters the room and introduces himself to the Garcia couple. To begin the exam, Jordan reviews the information Mr. Garcia supplied on the admission form, and then asks Joe about his family history.

Jordan: "Are your parents still living?"

Joe: "Yes, they're both alive. My father is 80 years old and my mother is 76."

Jordan: "I'd like to hear a little more about your family history. Tell me about your father's cancer. How old was he when he was first diagnosed? Has he had treatment?"

Joe: "He was probably about 60 when he first found out about it. I know he had some kind of surgery and takes medicines but I don't know the details. He seems all right though."

Jordan: "Your father also has high blood pressure and heart disease. Please tell me a little more about that."

Joe: "My father and mother both have high blood pressure and heart disease. They both take medicines for their blood pressure. My father had a small heart attack about 10 years ago. My mother has never had a heart attack that I know of, but she sometimes has chest pain."

Jordan: "Your mother also has diabetes?"

Joe: "She's had that for a long time. My parents joke about that. My father is part Cuban and part Irish. A lot of people in his family, especially on the Cuban side, have diabetes but nobody in my mother's family. Yet my mother is the one with the diabetes!"

Flordelisa: "A lot of people in my family have diabetes too. But so far I'm OK, I think. My family is from Mexico and I know a lot of diabetics back home."

Jordan: "Have you had a health exam lately, Mrs. Garcia?"

Flordelisa: "Not in about a year, but I'm going to schedule an appointment here."

The Garcia couple and Jordan continue to review the health information. After reviewing the history and discussing current complaints, Jordan performs a complete physical exam.

How Nurses Think

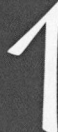

CHAPTER 1

Evolution of Nursing Thought & Action

For a podcast of an overview of this chapter,

 Go to Student Resources, **Podcast – Chapter Overviews, Chapter 1,** on DavisPlus at http://davisplus.fadavis.com/ Wilkinson2

Caring for the Garcias

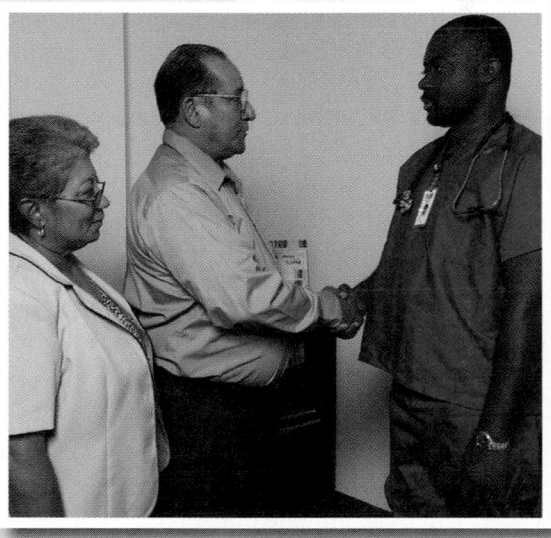

The exercises in the following sections allow you to practice the kind of thinking you will use as a full-spectrum nurse. Because these are critical-thinking questions, there is usually no single right answer. We do not provide answers for these questions because it is more important for you to think about the questions than to arrive at the "right" answer. These questions are designed to improve your thinking more than to "cover content." Discuss answers with your peers—discussion can stimulate critical thinking. If you have difficulty with any of these questions, consult with your instructor.

Review the opening scenario in the front of the book. On the preliminary visit of Joseph Garcia at the Family Medicine Center, he is examined by Jordan Miller, MSN, FNP-BC, an African American man.

A. How would you respond to Mr. Garcia's concerns that he was examined by someone who is "just a nurse"?

B. What factors might be causing Mr. Garcia to question care by "a male nurse"?

THINKING CRITICALLY ABOUT CRITICAL THINKING AND THE NURSING PROCESS

The exercises in the following section allow you to practice the kind of thinking you will use as a full-spectrum nurse. Because these are critical-thinking questions, there is usually no single right answer. We do not provide answers for these questions because it is more important for you to think about the questions than to arrive at the "right" answer. These questions are designed to improve your thinking more than to "cover content." Discuss answers with your peers—discussion can stimulate critical thinking. If you have difficulty with any of these questions, consult with your instructor.

Critical Thinking and Clinical Reasoning

1. At a holiday family gathering, you are at the dinner table with your 60-year-old aunt, your 85-year-old grandmother, and your 15-year-old sister-in-law. Your aunt and grandmother are retired RNs. Your sister-in-law aspires to be a nurse, and you are in school studying to be a nurse.

   a. What factors will influence how each of you views nursing?

   b. Your sister-in-law asks you to define nursing. What would you say?

   c. How could you explain to her how a nurse is different from a nurse's aide or a physician?

2. Review the information on educational pathways into nursing.

   a. What is your personal opinion on the entry-into-practice debate? That is, what minimum level of education should be required to practice nursing?

   b. What reasons can you give to support your opinion?

3. Review the description of the National Student Nurses Association (NSNA). If your program has a local chapter of NSNA, consider attending a meeting or consulting the association web site for more information. Identify at least three potential benefits of joining this organization.

4. For each of the following concepts, use critical thinking to describe how or why it is important to nursing, patient care, or the evolution of nursing thought and action. Note that these are *not* to be merely definitions.

   History of nursing

   The stereotypes of nurses

   The Nightingale era

   Definitions of nursing from the International Council of Nursing (ICN), American Nurses Association (ANA), and the Canadian Nurses Association (CNA)

   Regulation of nursing practice

   Entry into practice debate

   Benner's stages of nursing skill

   Nursing organizations

   The national economy

   Better-informed healthcare consumers

   Use of nursing assistive personnel

   Use of life-extending, high-technology equipment

What Are the Main Points in This Chapter?

➤ Religious organizations and the military have played a major role in the development of nursing and healthcare organizations.

➤ Initially the role of the nurse was limited to bathing, feeding, and supporting the patient; keeping the patient environment clean and orderly; and providing support for the physician.

➤ Contemporary nursing care includes activities that are performed in collaboration with other members of the healthcare team and also independently.

➤ Licensed practical nurses (LPNs or LVNs) are nurses who have successfully completed a practical nursing program and have passed a licensure exam (NCLEX-PN). They are prepared to give direct patient care.

➤ Registered nurses (RNs) are nurses who have successfully completed a registered nurse education program and have passed a licensure exam (NCLEX-RN). There are several types of RN education programs.

➤ Graduate nursing education is designed to prepare the RN for advanced practice, expanded roles, nursing education, or research.

➤ Benner has identified a five-step progression of skill acquisition in nurses: novice, advanced beginner, competence, proficiency, and expert.

➤ Nurse practice acts are laws that regulate nursing practice at the state (and, in Canada, provincial) level.

➤ Nurses engage in health promotion, illness prevention, health restoration, and care of the dying.

➤ Nurses work in a variety of inpatient and outpatient settings, including hospitals, extended care facilities, ambulatory care, and community or home health settings.

➤ The economy, technology, an aging population, increased consumer involvement in health care, the women's movement, and the change in nursing role are forces that have strongly affected nursing.

For practice questions for this chapter,

 Go to **NCLEX-Style Chapter Quiz** on the Student Resource Disk or DavisPlus at http://davisplus.fadavis.com/Wilkinson2

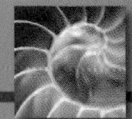 **Knowledge Map**

Factors Affecting the Evolution of Nursing

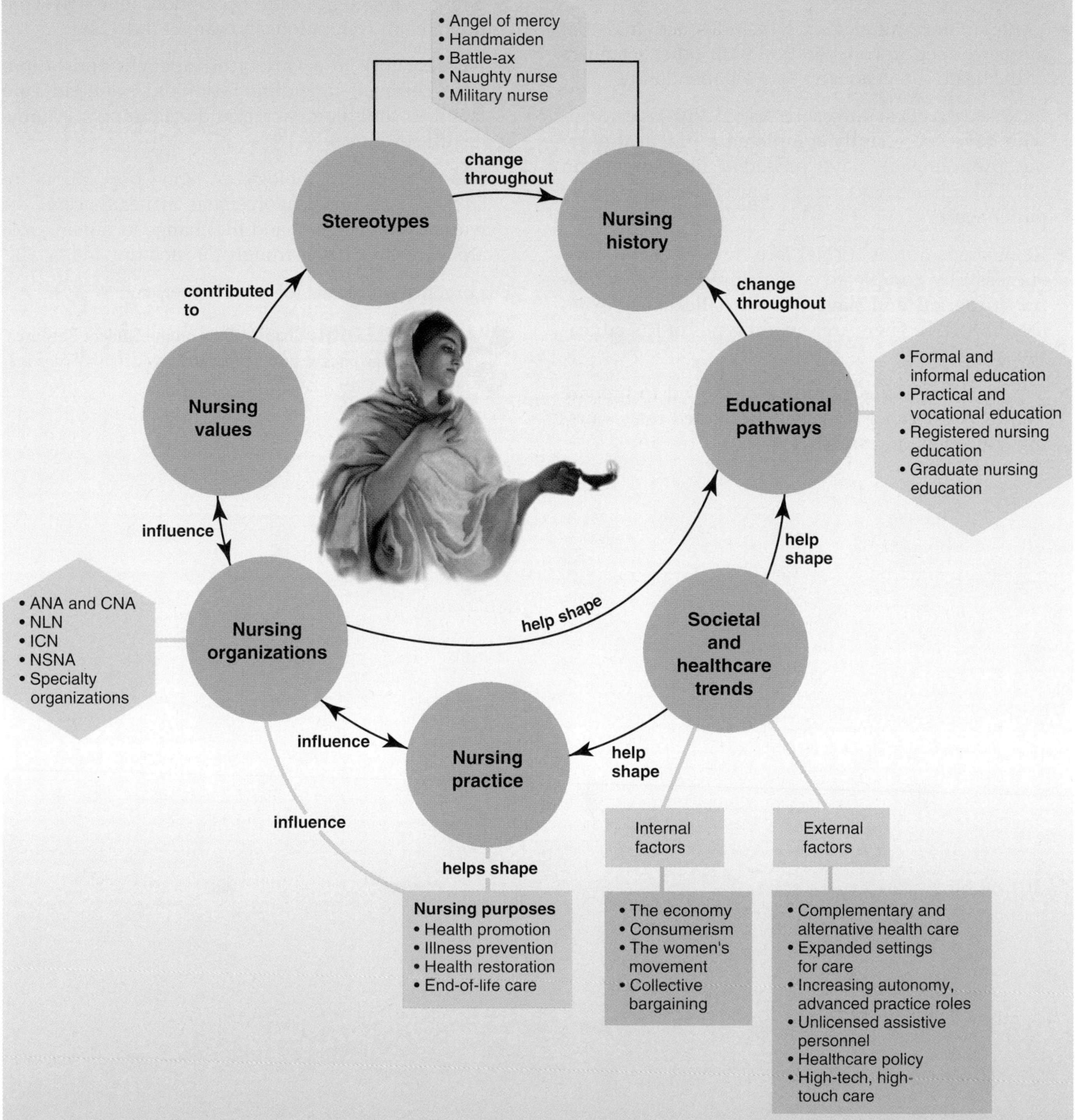

- Angel of mercy
- Handmaiden
- Battle-ax
- Naughty nurse
- Military nurse

Stereotypes

change throughout

Nursing history

contributed to

Nursing values

change throughout

Educational pathways

- Formal and informal education
- Practical and vocational education
- Registered nursing education
- Graduate nursing education

influence

help shape

- ANA and CNA
- NLN
- ICN
- NSNA
- Specialty organizations

Nursing organizations

help shape

Societal and healthcare trends

help shape

influence

Nursing practice

help shape

influence

helps shape

Internal factors

External factors

Nursing purposes
- Health promotion
- Illness prevention
- Health restoration
- End-of-life care

- The economy
- Consumerism
- The women's movement
- Collective bargaining

- Complementary and alternative health care
- Expanded settings for care
- Increasing autonomy, advanced practice roles
- Unlicensed assistive personnel
- Healthcare policy
- High-tech, high-touch care

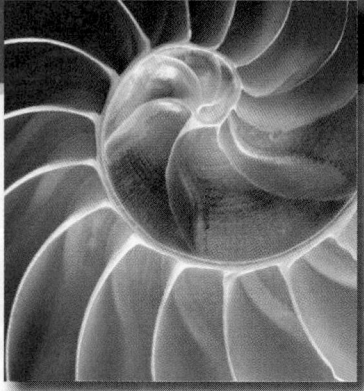

CHAPTER 2

Critical Thinking & Nursing Process

For a podcast of an overview of this chapter,

 Go to Student Resources, **Podcast – Chapter Overviews, Chapter 2,** on DavisPlus at http://davisplus.fadavis.com/Wilkinson2

Caring for the Garcias

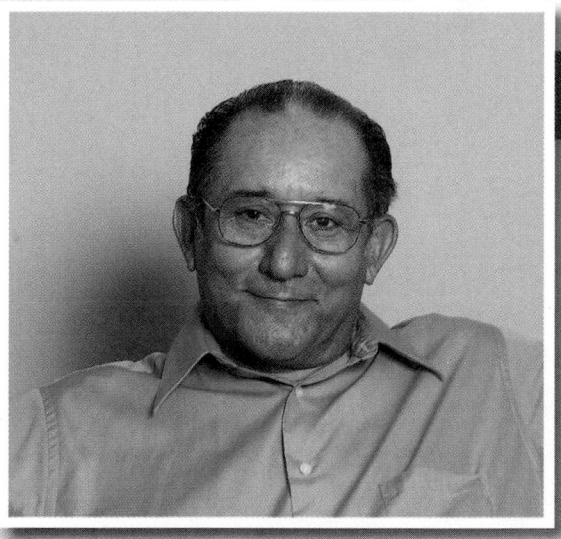

The exercises in this section allow you to practice the kind of thinking you will use as a full-spectrum nurse. Because these are critical-thinking questions, there is usually no single right answer. We do not provide answers for these questions because it is more important for you to think about the questions than to arrive at the "right" answer. These questions are designed to improve your thinking more than to "cover content." Discuss answers with your peers—discussion can stimulate critical thinking. If you have difficulty with any of these questions, consult with your instructor.

Review the opening scenario of Joseph Garcia in the front of this volume. Imagine you are the clinic nurse at the Family Medicine Center. Based on the information presented in the scenario, work through the following questions:

A. Patient Situation
- Why is Mr. Garcia at the clinic?
- What are his wife's concerns?
- Are they similar to or different from his?

B. Critical Thinking
- How do I go about getting the data I need? What sources should I use?
- Are my data congruent?
- What is one possible explanation for what is happening in this situation?

C. Nursing Knowledge
What type of nursing knowledge (theoretical, practical, ethical, or self-knowledge) is needed to answer the following questions?
- What health concerns does Mr. Garcia have that should be addressed by the healthcare team?
- What is the role of Jordan Miller on the health team?
- What role will you play in the care of Mr. Garcia?

(continued on next page)

Caring for the Garcias (continued)

D. **Nursing Process**
- In what phase of the nursing process are you engaged when you are asking Mr. Garcia about the reason for his visit?

- What activities are involved in the diagnosis phase? In planning outcomes? In planning interventions?
- Why would you not, at this point, be using the evaluation phase?

THINKING CRITICALLY ABOUT CRITICAL THINKING AND THE NURSING PROCESS

The exercises in the following sections allow you to practice the kind of thinking you will use as a full-spectrum nurse. Because these are critical-thinking questions, there is usually no single right answer. We do not provide answers for these questions because it is more important for you to think about the questions than to arrive at the "right" answer. These questions are designed to improve your thinking more than to "cover content." Discuss answers with your peers—discussion can stimulate critical thinking. If you have difficulty with any of these questions, consult with your instructor.

 Applying the Full-Spectrum Nursing Model

PATIENT SITUATION

Mrs. Castillo has late-stage cancer and is not expected to live more than a few months. With chemotherapy, she could live perhaps a year or two more. She cannot decide what to do. She knows the chemotherapy will have unpleasant side effects, and be very expensive, and she wants to protect her family from the emotional and financial hardships of a lingering illness. She is showing physical signs of anxiety and distress (e.g., increased heart rate, restlessness, tearfulness). You want to provide support for her decision, whatever it may be.

THINKING

1. *Theoretical Knowledge:* What theoretical knowledge do you need to help Mrs. Castillo?

2. *Critical Thinking (Contextual Awareness):* What details in the scenario represent "patient situation" or "context"?

DOING

3. *Practical Knowledge:*

   a. What practical knowledge do you need to help Mrs. Castillo?

   b. Which skills can you already do, and which ones would you need to learn or review before caring for this patient?

CARING

4. *Ethical Knowledge:* Depending on Mrs. Castillo's decision, can you think of one ethical issue that might arise for you or members of her family later on?

Critical Thinking and Clinical Reasoning

1. At the end of your first nursing class, your instructor gives an overview of a long-term assignment. She informs you that each semester of the program the class is required to complete a project that provides some type of service to the college community or the local community, and that demonstrates the role or importance of nursing. The instructor asks you to begin discussing potential projects and come to class next week prepared to discuss several proposals for your community and the potential benefits of each option. You and several friends gather to talk about the class. "What an odd assignment!" you tell your friends. "How can we possibly do this now? We aren't nurses. We don't have any skills. What could we possibly do?" Your friends echo similar views.

This exercise is designed to help you actually work through the imaginary assignment you have just read. Use the *critical-thinking model* shown in Figure 2-1 and the sample questions in Table 2 2 of Volume 1 to complete the assignment.

 Go to **Chapter 2: Critical Thinking & the Nursing Process.**

    a. *Contextual awareness* is one concept in the critical thinking model. Consider the context in which the assignment was given.

- What, exactly, is this assignment?
- Your instructor is perfectly aware of your knowledge and skill level. Why do you think she would ask students to complete, such an assignment so early in their nursing studies?

    b. To complete this assignment you would need to gather information—to find ways to answer the following questions:

- What will I learn this semester?
- What skills will I have by the time this assignment is due?
- What do nurses do?
- How do nurses interact with the community?
- What does my community need?

You would need to *use credible sources* (another task of critical-thinking thinking) to address these questions.

    c. What sources might you use to answer the first two questions in the bulleted list in (b), preceding?

    d. What are some ways in which you could answer the third and fourth bulleted questions?

    e. What are some ways in which you could obtain information to answer the fifth question?

    f. If you had actually gathered the preceding information, you would then need to consider possible solutions. One way would be to develop a list of community needs, a list of activities nurses engage in, and a list of skills and knowledge you will have at the end of the term. Then look at the overlap between the lists. This should help you to get some ideas for projects. Imagine now that you have a list of possible projects similar to the following:

- Take blood pressures at a neighborhood grocery store for a day.
- Hold a health fair at a neighborhood shopping center.
- Create some materials for teaching about a healthy diet; distribute them at a community event.

Now think critically about this list of projects (this involves *reflective skepticism and exploring and imagining alternatives*). What questions could you ask about each project to help you decide which to actually do?

2. Review the following scenarios. Is critical thinking occurring? If so, which part of the critical-thinking model is the student using, or which critical-thinking skill or attitude from Chapter 2 in Volume 1? If there is no evidence of critical thinking, revise the scenario to include it.

    a. Juan is a first-year nursing student. His clinical rotation is at a skilled nursing facility (SNF). He arrives at the unit at 0700 for the start of the day shift. After hearing the shift change report, he prepares to give his client a bedbath per unit policy.

    b. Lily is teaching her patient, Mr. Johannsen, about the medications he will be taking when he is discharged from the hospital. When Lily reviews the list with him, he says, "That's too many medicines. It's too confusing." Lily devises a schedule and information sheet about the medicines she gives to her client. She reviews the medications and their schedules with Mr. Johannsen and his wife before discharge.

c. Erin is caring for a young man who has had orthopedic surgery after a skiing accident. She is unable to hear his blood pressure when she attempts to take his vital signs. He is alert and able to converse with her. Since she is unable to hear the blood pressure, she records "0" in the client record.

d. As you are walking down the hall on the hospital unit, you hear a patient call out, "Nurse!" When you enter the room, you notice that the bedside is crowded with equipment. The patient is receiving several fluids intravenously, and a unit of blood is hanging from the IV pole. Since you have limited clinical experience you say to the patient, "I'll get you some help."

3. For each of the following concepts, use critical thinking to describe how or why it is important to nursing, patient care, or critical thinking in the nursing process. Note that these are *not* to be merely definitions.

Caring
Critical-thinking skills
Critical-thinking attitudes
Exploring alternatives
The nursing process
Assessment phase
Diagnosis phase

Planning outcomes phase
Planning interventions phase
Implementation phase
Evaluation phase
Theoretical knowledge
Practical knowledge

What Are the Main Points in This Chapter?

➤ Nursing involves thinking, doing, and caring; and all are equally important.

➤ Critical thinking is a combination of reasoned thinking, openness to alternatives, an ability to reflect, and a desire to seek truth.

➤ Critical thinking involves both attitudes and cognitive skills.

➤ Critical thinking attitudes include independent thinking, intellectual curiosity, intellectual humility, intellectual empathy, intellectual courage, intellectual perserverance, and fair-mindedness.

➤ Nurses use critical thinking in all aspects of their practice.

➤ Practical knowledge (knowing what to do and how to do it) and theoretical knowledge (knowing why) are equally important in nursing.

➤ The nursing process is a systematic problem-solving process that guides all nursing actions.

➤ The nursing process consists of six overlapping and interdependent phases: assessment, diagnosis, planning outcomes, planning interventions, implementation, and evaluation.

➤ Critical thinking is used in each phase of the nursing process; it is related to, but not the same as, the nursing process.

➤ Your ability to think critically depends on your theoretical knowledge about critical thinking, your motivation to practice it, and your fund of nursing knowledge.

➤ In full-spectrum nursing the nurse applies thinking, doing, and caring to the patient situation to help effect positive patient outcomes.

For practice questions for this chapter,

 Go to **NCLEX-Style Chapter Quiz,** on the Student Resource Disk or DavisPlus at http://davisplus.fadavis.com/Wilkinson2

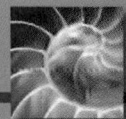

Knowledge Map

Full-Spectrum Nursing

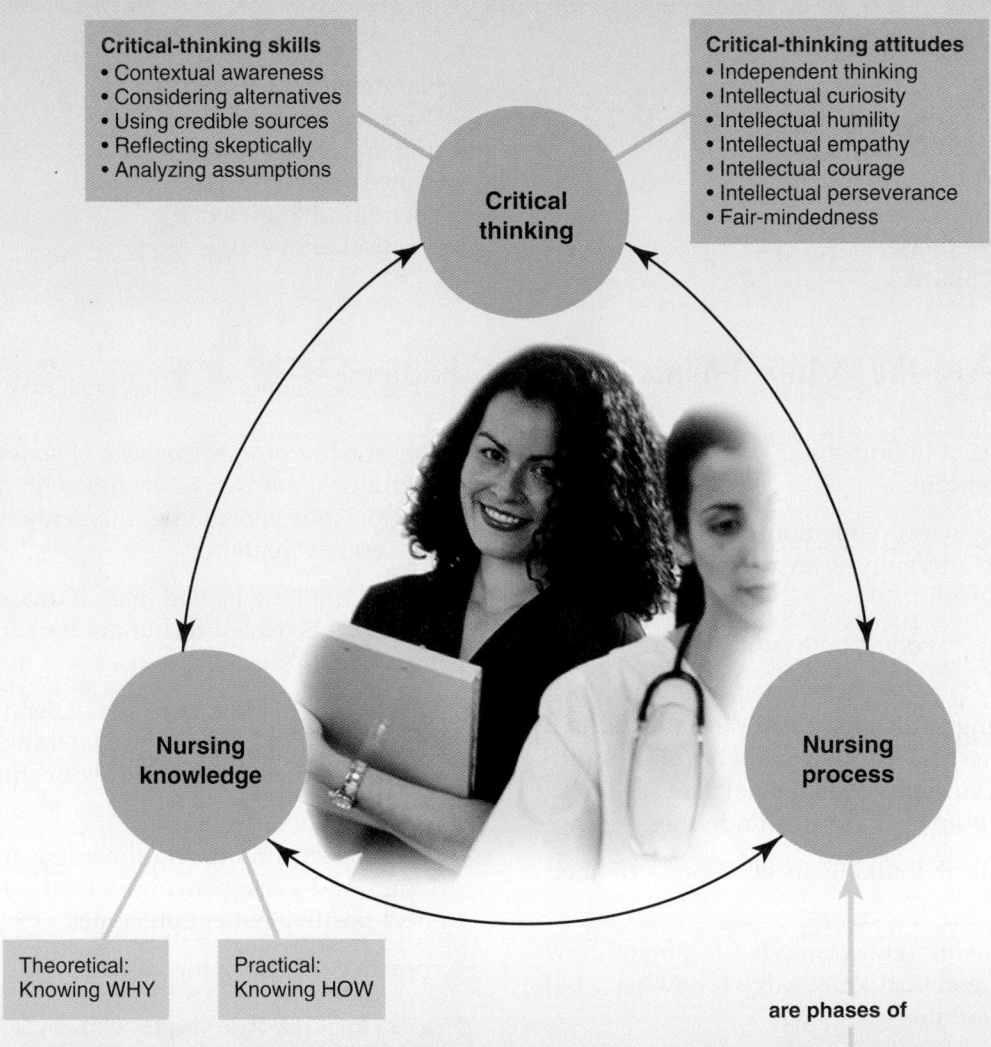

Critical-thinking skills
- Contextual awareness
- Considering alternatives
- Using credible sources
- Reflecting skeptically
- Analyzing assumptions

Critical thinking

Critical-thinking attitudes
- Independent thinking
- Intellectual curiosity
- Intellectual humility
- Intellectual empathy
- Intellectual courage
- Intellectual perseverance
- Fair-mindedness

Nursing knowledge

Nursing process

Theoretical: Knowing WHY

Practical: Knowing HOW

are phases of

- Assessing
- Diagnosing
- Planning outcomes
- Planning interventions
- Implementing
- Evaluating

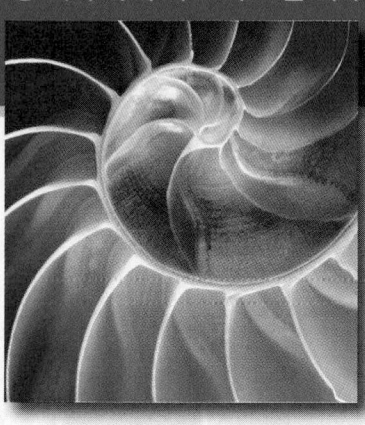

CHAPTER 3

Nursing Process: Assessment

For a podcast of an overview of this chapter,

 Go to Student Resources, **Podcast – Chapter Overviews, Chapter 3,** on DavisPlus at http://davisplus.fadavis.com/ Wilkinson2

Caring for the Garcias

The exercises in the following section allow you to practice the kind of thinking you will use as a full-spectrum nurse. Because these are critical-thinking questions, there is usually no single right answer. We do not provide answers for these questions because it is more important for you to think about the questions than to arrive at the "right" answer. These questions are designed to improve your thinking more than to "cover content." Discuss answers with your peers—discussion can stimulate critical thinking. If you have difficulty with any of these questions, consult with your instructor.

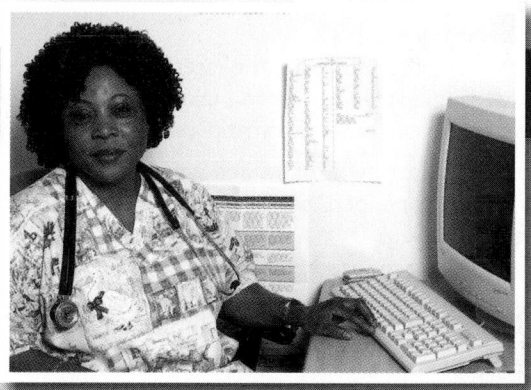

Review the opening scenario of Joseph Garcia in the front of the book. Imagine you are the clinic nurse at the Family Medicine Center.

A. What type of assessment, comprehensive or focused, is being performed at this clinic visit? Explain your thinking.

B. Identify the types of data (e.g., subjective/objective, primary/secondary) that have been gathered so far. Give an example of each type.

C. How might you verify data that Mr. Garcia provided on the intake sheet?

D. Based on what you know about Mr. Garcia, what follow-up assessments would provide useful data to help with the care of Mr. Garcia? Why would you make these assessments?

Practical **Knowledge**
knowing how

In this chapter, practical knowledge involves your skill in using structured and unstructured methods of data collection.

Clinical Insights

Clinical Insight 3-1 ➤ **Preparing for a Patient Interview**

Preparing Yourself

- Be sure you know why you are conducting the interview and how the data will be used. As a student, this may simply mean preparing thoroughly for your clinical assignment.
- Read the patient's chart.

This will give you an idea of where to start with the interview and keep you from covering topics already assessed by other caregivers. Be careful to keep an open mind, though. If you approach an interview with preconceived ideas, you may overlook important data.

- Form some goals for the interview.
- Think of some opening questions.
- Schedule some uninterrupted time for the interview.

Giving the patient your undivided attention builds rapport and helps her to feel freer to share information with you.

- Gather the necessary assessment forms and equipment. You will need a stethoscope, pen, pencil, blood pressure cuff, and thermometer.
- Take a deep breath and compose yourself just before entering the room.

Preparing the Space

- Provide privacy (e.g., ask visitors to wait outside, shut the door). Unless you need information from the visitor (e.g., when the client cannot communicate clearly) you may wish to postpone the interview until it can be done in private.

The presence of even a close family member may inhibit the client in some situations. For example, a wife may not want her husband to know that she had a miscarriage before they were married.

- If others must be present, keep the focus on the client as much as possible.

In some interviews, the client's spouse, family, or partner will offer information that may or may not be pertinent. Focus on the client, but do not ignore the information provided by others.

- Remove distractions (e.g., turn off the television, arrange for someone to watch the children for a while, if they are present).
- Position yourself at the same level as your client, even if the client is in bed. Sit down. Do not hover over the bed.

Preparing the Patient

- Introduce yourself to the patient and others in the room.
- Call the patient by name; ask what name the patient prefers. Don't use endearing terms like "grandma," "dear," and "sweetie."

You may think you are being friendly or expressing your caring, but many people feel belittled by these terms.

- Tell the patient what you will be doing and why. Explain that you will be taking notes and that you will keep all information confidential.
- If you wish to record or videotape the interview, be sure to obtain written permission from the patient.
- Assess readiness to discuss health issues. If the patient indicates that now is not a good time, reschedule (e.g., if the patient has just received some bad news about his condition, or in his personal life, he may need some time to process that information before he can concentrate on interview questions).
- Assess and provide for comfort (e.g., assess and medicate for pain, offer the bedpan, offer a drink of water).
- Assess for anxiety. Be sure the patient is comfortable emotionally as well as physically.

A very anxious person cannot provide good information, so you may need to intervene to relieve anxiety before proceeding.

Clinical Insight 3-2 ➤ **Conducting a Patient Interview**

- Individualize your approach.

Consider the client's age and developmental level. Ask yourself, for example, "What approach is best considering my client's age?" Respect the generational differences of a person older or younger than you.

- Be sensitive to cultural differences (e.g., comfort with eye contact, the need for space).
- Begin with neutral topics, such as the biographical data (e.g., address, contact person, occupation). Ask more personal or sensitive questions after you and the client are more comfortable with each other.

- Use active listening. This is the most important interviewing technique. Focus intently on trying to understand what the client is saying, rather than thinking ahead to what your response to the statement will be. Use the mnemonic FOLK to remember other active listening behaviors:

Face the patient (either sitting or standing).
Open, relaxed posture (arms and legs uncrossed).
Lean toward the patient.
Keep eye contact.

- Do not get caught up in note taking.

Excessive writing interferes with eye contact and may inhibit the client's responses, especially when you are discussing personal issues such as sexuality or drug and alcohol use.

- Pay attention to nonverbal communication.

For example, body language may signal that the person is tired or in pain but is too polite to say so. If the person is fatigued, you may need to end the interview and finish it at another time.

- Use open-ended questions as much as possible, to encourage the client to talk.
- Do not ask too many questions.

Asking too many questions may make you seem merely curious instead of genuinely interested in the client.

- Use neutral statements instead of questions (e.g., instead of "How many children do you have?" say "Tell me about your family").
- Avoid asking "why" (e.g., "Why have you stopped taking your pills?").

"Why" causes some people to become defensive. Parents frequently ask their children, "Why did you do that?" For some people, "why" suggests disapproval.

- Do not use healthcare jargon (e.g., say "I want to take your temperature and blood pressure instead" of "I want to take your vital signs").
- Do not "talk down" to the client (e.g., Don't say, "How often do you go potty?" when interviewing an adult).
- Confirm that clients understand the terminology they use. If a client says, "It's the inflammation that causes me the trouble, you know," you might say, "Tell me where the inflammation is and what happens when you have it."

People may repeat words they hear from care providers without really knowing what the words mean.

- Refocus the client when her story becomes scattered or does not produce useful information. Allow the client to talk about the topics of importance to her, but direct her to topics that need to be covered (e.g., "We haven't talked about your surgery. What do you expect to happen?").
- Curb your curiosity. Do not get caught up in the details of the client's story.

Focus on the information you need to plan care.

- Do not give advice or voice approval or disapproval.

Even if the advice is good (e.g., "It's good that you were firm with your daughter." or "You should take your pills on time."), it may cause the client to be less open with you and interfere with your ability to gather data.

Clinical Insight 3-3 ▶ Closing a Patient Interview

- Prepare the patient for closure. Inform the patient that the interview is nearly finished.
- Summarize the key points of the interview.
- Be sure you have recorded all the important data. Ask the patient, "Is there anything else you would like to tell me?" or "Is there anything else we should talk about?"
- Thank the patient for answering the questions.

- Encourage the patient to keep you informed. For example, you might say, "Please let us know if you think of anything else we should know."
- Tell the patient what to expect next. Let the patient know when you will be leaving, when you will see him again, and what he can expect for the rest of the day (e.g., tests, treatments).
- Ask, "Is there anything I can do for you before I leave?"

Assessment Guidelines and Tools

You can use the forms in this section to make a focused assessment of activities of daily living and to perform a comprehensive patient assessment. If you want to create your own assessment form, you can use an interactive assessment tool,

 Go to **Student Resources, Interactive Assessment Tool,** at http://davisplus.fadavis.com/daviscareplans/index.cfm#Nursing_Diagnosis2

Patient Assessment Tool—Lawton Instrumental Activities of Daily Living (IADL)

Date:_____   Name:_____

Please check the box that most applies for each activity:

Activity	Needs no help (2 pts. each)	Needs some help (1 pt. each)	Unable to do at all (0 pts. each)
1. Using the telephone	___	___	___
2. Getting to places beyond walking distance	___	___	___
3. Grocery shopping	___	___	___
4. Preparing meals	___	___	___
5. Doing housework or handyman work	___	___	___
6. Doing laundry	___	___	___
7. Taking medications	___	___	___
8. Managing money	___	___	___
Total score:___ =	(___ × 2 =)___ +	(___ × 1 =)___ +	0

A patient is awarded 2 points for each area in which he/she can function totally without help, 1 point in those areas that they need some help, and 0 points for those activities that somebody else must do completely for them. The maximum score is 16, minimum score is 0.

Like other evaluations, the IADL scale provides a baseline of data that can be compared with the results of future evaluations. (Note that some activities may be gender specific. Omit these items if the patient does not usually perform those tasks.)

Permission obtained from M. Powell Lawton, Ph.D., Philadelphia Geriatric Center, Philadelphia, PA. May be used freely for patient assessment. Formatted and posted May 25, 1996, to www.acsu.buffalo.edu/~drstall/assessmenttools.html by Robert S. Stall, M.D.

Nursing Admission Data Form

Name: _Ben J. Ivanos_ Age: _24_ Phone #: _618-445-2300_ Date: _05/20/11_ Time: _10:30_

Primary Physician: _Charles Katz_ Phone #: _618-446-8160_

Chief Complaints/Procedure: _ORIF fx (L) leg, Fx (R) femur + (R) ulna_ Height: _5'10"_ Weight (lbs.): _155_

Historian: _Patient_ Temp: _100_ Pulse: _90_ Resp: _16_ BP: _140/82_

Religious Affiliation: _Catholic_ Hospitalized within 30 days: Yes ☒ No ☐

UNABLE TO OBTAIN HISTORY .... ☐	**GASTROINTESTINAL**	Pregnant .... ☐
Reason:_____	Dysphagia .... ☐	Lactating .... ☐
NEUROLOGICAL/SENSORY PERCEPTION	Hiatal Hernia .... ☐	LMP/Date:_____
Glaucoma .... ☐	Liver Disease/Jaundice .... ☐	**VACCINATION/DATE**
Hearing Loss/Deaf .... Right ☐ Left ☐	Pancreatitis .... ☐	Flu:_____ Hepatitis B:_____
Motion Sickness .... ☐	Gall Stones .... ☐	Pneumonia:_____
Paresthesia .... Right ☐ Left ☐	Ostomy .... ☐	**BEHAVIORAL HEALTH**
Fibromyalgia/Migraine .... ☐	Last Bowel Movement: _5/19/05_	Anxiety Disorder .... ☐
Spina Bifida .... ☐	Other:_____	Depression .... ☐
Stroke/CVA/TIA .... ☐	**GENITOURINARY/RENAL**	Suicide (thoughts/attempts) .... ☐
Altered Mental Status .... ☐	Kidney Disease/Urogenital .... ☐	Patient is a Baker Act .... ☐
Other:_____	Prostate Problems .... ☐	Other:_____
CARDIOVASCULAR/HEMATOLOGY	Voiding Problems .... ☐	**CANCER**
Bleeding Problems .... ☐	Other:_____	Type_____ ☐
Blood transfusion in the past 3 months .... ☐	**MUSCULOSKELETAL**	Radioactive Seeds/Implant .... ☐
Chest Pain/Angina .... ☐	Arthritis .... ☐	Date:_____
Heart Attack/Date: .... ☐	Back/Disc Problem .... ☐	Other:_____
Heart Disease .... ☐	Fractures ... _present admission_ ☒	**SOCIAL HISTORY**
High Blood Pressure .... ☐	Other:_____	Tobacco .... ☒
Irregular Beats/Pacemaker/AICD .... ☐	**ENDOCRINE**	Number of years: _3_
Mitral Valve Prolapse .... ☐	Diabetes/type: .... ☐	# of packs per day: _1/2_
Murmur .... ☐	Thyroid Disease .... ☐	Year Quit: _2003_
Peripheral Vascular Disease .... ☐	Other:_____	Would you like smoking cessation info?
Sickle Cell Disease .... ☐	**INFECTIOUS DISEASE**	☒ No ☐ Yes ☐ information provided
Venous Access Device/Type_____ ☐	Fevers .... ☐	Alcohol .... ☒
Other:_____	Hepatitis/type/active .... ☐	Drinks per day: _1_
RESPIRATORY	HIV/AIDS .... ☐	Amount:_____
Asthma .... ☐	Recent Cold .... ☐	Type:_____
Bronchitis _6 months ago_ ☒	Sexually Transmitted Disease/type .... ☐	Recreational Drug .... ☐
COPD/Emphysema .... ☐	Tuberculosis/Active: .... ☐	Amount:_____
Post Nasal Drip/Rhinitis/Sinusitis .... ☒	Other:_____	Type:_____
Pneumonia .... ☐		Year Quit:_____
Tracheostomy .... ☐		Detoxification Protocol Initiated .... ☐
Other:_____		

ALLERGIES & REACTION	None Known ☒	Allergy Bracelet on ☐
Medications: _none_	**Symptoms:**	
		Blood Reaction: ☐
Food/Shellfish/other allergies: _No_		Latex: ☐
Contrast/Dye: _No_		Latex Allergy Protocol Initiated: ☐

PAST HOSPITAL/PROCEDURE (Surgical/Medical/Behavioral Health)	**CURRENT MEDICATIONS** (include ASA/Anticoagulant, over the counter medications, ointments, patches, eye drops, herbal, vitamins and nutritional supplements)			
None	**Medication**	**Dose**	**Frequency**	**Last Dose**
	ASA	"2"	occasionally for HA	
	Food/Drug Interaction information provided ☐			
Initiate Social Service Consult	(Note: Additional medication can be listed on last page)			

ADDRESSOGRAPH

North Broward Hospital District

NURSING ADMISSION DATA

P-10287 · 126005 · (R) 11/02 **Page 1 of 4** 900199

Source: North Broward Hospital District, Ft. Lauderdale, FL.

Nursing Admission Data Form (continued)

PAIN HISTORY

Have you been experiencing pain? ☒ Yes
If yes, when ___Now___ Intensity (0-10): ___10___ Goal (0-10): ___2___
Location: ___Legs and arm, muscles in back___
Radiation: ___No___
Duration: ___Constant___
Quality: ___Sharp, aching___
Aggravating factors ___Movement___

What medications/interventions are effective in relieving your pain?
___Taking PCA Demerol___

Acute Pain Management - It is Your Right brochure provided ☒

PSYCHOSOCIAL ASSESSMENT

☒ Lives alone ☐ Lives with spouse/SO ☐ Nursing Home/ALF
☐ Homeless ☐ Rehab Facility ☐ Other:___
Marital Status ☒ Single ☐ Married ☐ Divorced ☐ Widowed ☐ Separated
Next of Kin: ___Mother, Clara Ivanos___ Phone #: ___618-446-3816___
Supportive Adult: ___ Phone #: ___
Has anybody threatened/hit/abused you within the last year?
☐ Yes (refer to policy RA 004015 mauve manual) ☒ No

EDUCATIONAL LEARNING ASSESSMENT

Learner ☒ Patient ☐ Family ☐ Significant Other
Readiness to learn ☐ Eager to learn ☒ Asks questions
☐ Extremely anxious ☐ Denies need for Education
Knowledge of current health status ☐ No knowledge
☒ Partial understanding ☐ Full understanding
Barriers to learning ☒ Physical ☐ Emotional
☐ Language ☐ Religious ☐ Cultural
☐ Reading Ability ☐ Changes in Short Memory
☐ None
Preferred Learning Method ☒ Reading ☐ Lecture
☒ Video ☒ Demo/Practice
Communication ☒ English ☐ Spanish ☐ Creole
☐ Sign Language ☐ Other:___
Do you have any religious/cultural practices that are important to you or may alter your care or education? ☒ No ☐ Yes ___

☒ Patient Handbook provided ☒ Patient safety information provided
☒ Patient's Bill of Rights and Responsibilities information provided
Other Educational Materials:___

PERSONAL EFFECTS: Do you use the following:

	YES	WITH PT.	FAMILY/SO
Wheelchair	☐	☐	☐
Braces	☐	☐	☐
Cane/Crutches	☐	☐	☐
Walker	☐	☐	☐
Prothesis	☐	☐	☐
Medications	☐	☐	☐
Dentures: (Full)	☐	☐	☐
Upper	☐	☐	☐
Lower	☐	☐	☐
Glasses	☐	☐	☐
Contacts	☒	☒	☐
Hearing Aids	☐	☐	☐
Other:			

Initiate Social Service Consult

ADVANCE DIRECTIVES

Do you have an Advance Directive?
(must check one)
☒ **No** Information provided to patient
☐ **No** Patient elects not to receive information
☐ **Yes** (check advance directive patient states he/she has)
☐ **Living Will** ☐ **Health Care Surrogate** ☐ **State DNAR form**
☐ **Durable Power of Attorney** ☐ **Organ Donation**
(If patient has an Advance Directive, inform patient to provide copy within 24 hours or they may complete a new advance directive or verbalize their wishes)
Do you have a guardian? ☐ Yes name___
(Inform patient to provide guardianship form within 24 hours)
☐ **Patient unable to respond/family not available**

FALL SCREEN: If any of the following are checked, initiate Safety/Protective Intervention Protocol

Inability to understand or follow instructions .... ☐
Impaired mobility, visual impairment, drug therapy, surgical procedure, unsteady gait, incontinence ...... *Casts, Traction* ☒
Unable to use call light .... ☐
Altered mental status ...... *Taking Demerol PCA* ☒
Nocturnal/urgency/frequency in elimination ...... ☐
Dizziness .... ☐
History of falls .... ☐
No Criteria Met .... ☐

NUTRITIONAL SCREEN: If any of the following are checked, enter in the computer request for Nutritional Consult

Nausea/vomiting > 5 days .... ☐
No food/drink for 3 days .... ☐
Recent unexplained weight loss > 10 lbs. .... ☐
Difficulty swallowing/dysphagia .... ☐
Evidence of Stage III - IV pressure ulcer .... ☐
Feeding tube .... ☐
New onset diabetes .... ☐
TPN .... ☐
Pregnant/lactating .... ☐
Surgical patients > 70 years of age .... ☐
Ethnic diet/special needs (include in diet order and order for **Preference consult**) .... ☐
Difficulty chewing (include in diet order and order for **Preference consult**) .... ☐
No Criteria Met .... ☒

FUNCTIONAL SCREEN: If any of the following are checked, please request physician order for physical therapy consult.

New onset of paralysis .... ☐
New onset stroke/CVA .... ☐
New amputation .... ☐
Unsteady gait .... ☐
Decreased mobility ...... *Casts, Tx for Fx* ☒
Dysphagia .... ☐
No Criteria Met .... ☐

Nursing Admission Data Form (continued)

MARK LOCATION
Anterior View / Posterior View / Right Lateral / Left Lateral / Left Foot / Right Foot

* Label Wound Type

WOUND TYPE

P = Pressure ulcer	A = Abrasions
ST = Skin tear	LU = Leg/Foot ulcers
S = Surgical	BR = Bruising
L = Laceration	M = Maceration
B = Burns	O = Other

STAGE
Pressure ulcer only

I: Reddened area, does not resolve with pressure relief.
II: Blister or superficial break in skin.
III: Full thickness wound into subcutaneous tissue.
IV: Full thickness with muscle, bone or tendon tissue exposed.
U = Unable to stage: Necrotic

COLOR WOUND BED

R = Red (new tissue)	Y = Yellow (slough)
P = Pink	B = Black (eschar)

EXUDATE

O = None	SS = Serosanguinous
S = Serous	P = Purulent

ODOR

N = None	S = Slight	F = Foul

SURROUNDING SKIN

OK = Clean & Intact   Ra = Rash
C = Cellulitis (red & tender)
R = Raw & denuded
M = Maceration
I = Induration

Skin Breakdown Present ☐   Consent Obtained ☐   Photograph Taken ☐   Acute/Chronic Wound Flow Sheet Initiated ☐   Swat Consult Initiated ☐

BRADEN SCALE - PRESSURE ULCER RISK ASSESSMENT

	1	2	3	4	Score
SENSORY PERCEPTION Ability to respond meaningfully to pressure-related discomfort	**1. Completely Limited:** Unresponsive (does not moan, flinch, or grasp) to painful stimuli due to diminished level of consciousness or sedation. OR limited ability to feel pain over most of body surface.	**2. Very Limited:** Responds only to painful stimuli. Cannot communicate discomfort except by moaning or restlessness. OR has a sensory impairment which limits the ability to feel pain or discomfort over 1/2 of body.	**3. Slightly Limited:** Responds to verbal commands, but cannot always communicate discomfort or need to be turned. OR has some sensory impairment which limits ability to feel pain or discomfort in 1 or 2 extremities.	**4. No Impairment:** Responds to verbal commands, has no sensory deficit which would limit ability to feel or voice pain or discomfort.	4
MOISTURE Degree to which skin is exposed to moisture	**1. Constantly Moist:** Skin is kept moist almost constantly by perspiration, urine, etc. Dampness is detected every time patient is moved or turned.	**2. Very Moist:** Skin if often, but not always, moist. Linen must be changed at least once a shift.	**3. Occasionally Moist:** Skin is occasionally moist, requiring an extra linen change approximately once a day.	**4. Rarely Moist:** Skin is usually dry, linen only requires changing at routine intervals.	4
ACTIVITY degree of physical activity	**1. Bedfast:** Confined to bed.	**2. Chairfast:** Ability to walk severely limited or non-existent. Cannot bear own weight and/or must be assisted into chair or wheelchair.	**3. Walks Occasionally:** Walks occasionally during day, but for very short distances, with or without assistance. Spends majority of each shift in bed or chair.	**4. Walks Frequently:** Walks outside the room at least twice a day and inside room at least once every 2 hours during waking hours.	1
MOBILITY ability to change and control body position	**1. Completely Immobile:** Does not make even slight changes in body or extremity position without assistance.	**2. Very Limited:** Makes occasional slight changes in body or extremity position but unable to make frequent or significant changes independently.	**3. Slightly Limited:** Makes frequent though slight changes in body or extremity position independently.	**4. No Limitations:** Makes major and frequent changes in position without assistance.	3
NUTRITION usual food intake pattern	**1. Very Poor:** Never eats a complete meal. Rarely eats more than 1/3 of any food offered. Eats 2 servings or less of protein (meat or dairy products) per day. Takes fluids poorly. Does not take a liquid dietary supplement. OR is NPO and/or maintained on clear liquids or IVs for more then 5 days.	**2. Probably Inadequate:** Rarely eats a complete meal and generally eats only about 1/2 of any food offered. Protein intake includes only 3 servings of meat or dairy products per day. Occasionally will take a dietary supplement. OR receives less than optimum amount of liquid diet or tube feeding.	**3. Adequate:** Eats over half of most meals. Eats a total of 4 servings of protein (meat, dairy products) each day. Occasionally will refuse a meal, but will usually take a supplement if offered. OR is on a tube feeding or TPN regimen which probably meets most of nutritionally needs.	**4. Excellent:** Eats most of every meal. Never refuses a meal. Usually eats a total of 4 or more servings of meat and dairy products. Occasionally eats between meals. Does not require supplementation.	4
FRICTION AND SHEAR	**1. Problem:** Requires moderate to maximum assistance in moving. Complete lifting without sliding against sheets is impossible. Frequently slides down in bed or chair, requiring frequent repositioning with maximum assistance. Spasticity contractures or agitation lead to almost constant friction.	**2. Potential Problem:** Moves feebly or requires minimum assistance. During a move skin probably slides to some extent against sheets, chair, restraints, or other devices. Maintains relatively good position in chair or bed most of the time but occasionally slides down.	**3. No Apparent Problem:** Moves in bed and in chair independently and has sufficient muscle strength to lift up completely during move. Maintains good position in bed or chair at all times.		2

RN Signature: _Jm Rhodes RN_   Date: _5/20/11_   TOTAL SCORE: **18**

NOTE: Patients with a total score of 16 or less are considered to be at risk of developing pressure ulcers. Implement Skin Care Protocol. Refer to Surface Bed Decision Tree. (12 or less = high risk)

ANTICIPATED DISCHARGE NEEDS

☒ Transportation   ☐ Placement needed

Medical Equipment: ☐ Oxygen   ☐ CPAP   ☐ Nebulizer   ☐ Blood Glucose Meter   Other: _Crutches, Wheelchair_

Community Services: (Home Health, Reach to Recovery, Meals On Wheels, etc.): _Home Health for f/u on cast care and pain medication. Transportation to physicians office for return visit._

Nurse Signature: _Jm Rhodes RN_	Unit: _3E_	Date: _5/20/11_	Time: _10:45_	
Nurse Signature: _____	Unit: _____	Date: _____	Time: _____	

P-10287 - 126005 - (R) 11/02 **Page 3 of 4**

Nursing Admission Data Form (continued)

OUTPATIENT PRE-ADMISSION NOTE: Date of Call/Visit_____ Date of Surgery:_____ N/A

Autologous Blood ☐   Direct Donor ☐   Confirmed with Blood Bank ☐   # of Units Available___ N/A

Parent Present Induction ☐

Pre-op Work Up:
BGMC ☐   NBMC ☐   IPMC ☐   CSMC ☐
Other:_____

ANESTHESIOLOGIST EVALUATION: ASA class I II III IV   NPO:_____

Anesthesia Plan   Gen ☐   MAC ☐   Regional ☐   Type _____

Airway: _____   Dentition: Good ☐ Fair ☐ Poor ☐   EKG _____

Neck_____   Natural ☐ Caps ☐   CXR ___ N/A

Previous Anesthesia ☐   Dentures/Bridges ☐   H & H _____

Past anesthesia problems_____   Malampati score 1 2 3 4   Platelets _____

OTHER: _____

Comments:_____

Anesthesiologist_____   Date_____   Time_____

INITIAL EVALUATION EXCEEDING 48 HOURS:
No Change in Assessment ☐
Changes in Assessment ☐
Comments:_____
_____
_____
Anesthesiologist:_____
Date/Time: _____

NURSING DIAGNOSIS	NURSING INTERVENTIONS	PLANNED OUTCOME/EVALUATION
Potential/actual knowledge deficit Pre-op preparation/ planned surgical intervention.	☐ Patient/family learning needs/level of understanding assessed. ☐ Clear explanation of pre-operative routine given. ☐ Instructions on turning, coughing, deep breathing, leg exercises given. ☐ Procedure specific instructions _____ ☐ Pain management modalities and scale explained. Modality preference_____ Pain scale goal_____	☐ Patient verbalizes understanding of pre-op preparation, pre-op routine and procedure specific information. ☐ Patient copes with anxiety, shows relaxed affect. ☐ Demonstrates understanding of explanations. ☐ Patient verbalizes understanding of pain management and plan of care. ☐ Needed referrals/arrangements made. ☐ Care individualized to meet patients needs. ☐ Patient verbalizes understanding of discharge plan.
Anxiety *N/A* Psycho/Social	☐ Written copy of pre-op instructions and patient responsibility provided. ☐ Allow to express feelings, ask questions. ☐ Emotional support given. ☐ Sense of wellness promoted. ☐ Cultural/Spiritual Needs: _____ ☐ Discharge planning initiated/home care assessed. ☐ Needs identified/Action:	Standard of Care/Protocol: ☐ Yes R.N. Signature:_____ Date:_____
Actual/Potential Individual Needs Self Care/Discharge Planning		

Nurse Signature: _____   Unit: _____   Date: _____   Time: _____

Nurse Signature: _____   Unit: _____   Date: _____   Time: _____

DATE & TIME	INTERDISCIPLINARY NOTES/ADVANCE DIRECTIVES INFORMATION
5/20/11, 11:00	Healthy young adult, on no meds, admitted via E.D. p̄ motorcycle accident, and reduction and casting of multiple fx ((L) tibia + fibula, (R) femur, and (R) elbow and ulna). Experiencing severe pain r/t fx, bruises and muscle spasms. Plan:
	① Traction per Rx; check weights q̄ 4th
	② Control pain w/PCA Demerol. Assess + instruct prn
	③ Neurovascular + circulatory checks, all extremities, q̄ 2h
	④ Monitor adema of extremities; re-cast after 3 days if edema has subsided.

Nurse Signature: _Jm Rhodes Rn_   Unit: _3E_   Date: _5/20/11_   Time: _11:00_

Nurse Signature: _____   Unit: _____   Date: _____   Time: _____

Current Medications: (Continued)

Medication	Dose	Frequency	Last Dose

THINKING CRITICALLY ABOUT THE NURSING PROCESS: ASSESSMENT

The exercises in the following sections allow you to practice the kind of thinking you will use as a full-spectrum nurse. Because these are critical-thinking questions, there is usually no single right answer. We do not provide answers for these questions because it is more important for you to think about the questions than to arrive at the "right" answer. These questions are designed to improve your thinking more than to "cover content." Discuss answers with your peers—discussion can stimulate critical thinking. If you have difficulty with any of these questions, consult with your instructor.

▨ Applying the Full-Spectrum Nursing Model

PATIENT SITUATION

As the intake nurse in a community-based clinic in Miami, Florida, your role is to complete a comprehensive nursing assessment and initiate a plan of care for the clients. Your first client is a 24-year-old single woman, Sami, who is requesting clinic services for her general healthcare needs. Sami is Cuban American and lives alone in a one-bedroom apartment. She works as a fitness trainer at the local YMCA while attending college part-time. Her family lives in Tampa, Florida. Sami's earnings place her at the poverty level, but she realizes that she must have health care to prevent illness and to detect and receive treatment of illnesses should they arise.

THINKING

1. *Theoretical Knowledge*: To care for Sami, what knowledge would you need that you do not already have? List the URL for at least one online, reputable source for this information.

2. *Critical Thinking*: The nurse asks Sami, "If you can't afford healthcare, couldn't you get a roommate to save some money on rent?" What are some critical thinking questions you should ask yourself when reflecting on this question later?

DOING

3. *Practical Knowledge*: What practical knowledge will you, as the nurse, use in this scenario?

4. *Nursing Process*: What kind of assessment will you make of Sami (e.g., comprehensive, focused, special needs, discharge, etc.)?

CARING

5. *Self-Knowledge*: In what ways are you similar to Sami? In what ways are you different?

▨ Critical Thinking and Clinical Reasoning

1. Recall the definition of subjective data. Make a list of the kinds of patients from whom you might not be able to get subjective data or who might give unreliable data. One example is a baby who cannot talk yet. How many others can you think of?

2. What are some factors that might make it difficult, but not impossible, for a patient to provide you with subjective data? One example is a severely anxious person.

3. For each of the factors in question 2, state what you could do to facilitate collection of reliable subjective data from that person.

4. List your current assessment skills and indicate your comfort level using each skill. Include observation, physical assessment, and interviewing skills. Use a scale of 1–5, with 1 = slightly comfortable; 2 = somewhat comfortable; 3 = moderately comfortable; 4 = fairly comfortable; and 5 = very comfortable.

5. For any skill that you score as 3 or less, write a plan describing what you need to do to move to the higher comfort level.

6. The following are criteria from ANA (2010, in press) professional practice Standard 1. For each of the criteria, write an example of what would constitute evidence (proof) that the standard is being followed in a healthcare agency. The first one is done for you.

   a. "Collects data . . . in a systematic and ongoing process."
      I would look in the care plan for nursing orders that call for some kind of assessment on a scheduled basis. For example, an order might read, "Temperature q4hr" or "Check dressing for drainage once per shift." I would also look at the nursing notes, especially for flow sheets (e.g., vital sign flow sheets, input and output records, neurological checks) to see if assessment findings were recorded at regular intervals. Other evidence would be to observe the nurses doing systematic and ongoing data collection.

   b. "Involves the patient, family/support system, other healthcare providers, and environment, as appropriate, in holistic data collection."

   c. "Prioritizes data-collection activities based on the patient's immediate condition, or anticipated needs . . ."

   d. "Uses appropriate evidence-based assessment techniques and instruments and tools."

   e. "Synthesizes available data, information, and knowledge relevant to the situation to identify patterns and variances."

   f. "Documents relevant data in a retrievable format."

7. Your client, Sami ("Meet Your Patient"), is Cuban American. Having worked with many clients of Cuban heritage and being familiar with nursing literature regarding various cultural patterns, you are aware of the following:

   - Many Hispanic people who live in Miami are bilingual.
   - When communicating, especially with strangers, it is not unusual for Hispanic women not to maintain eye contact. (During the interview, Sami speaks rapidly and does not maintain eye contact with you.)
   - Many people of Cuban descent are Catholic and consider birth control to be taboo.
   - Many Cuban American women do not obtain annual physical examinations (Purnell & Paulanka, 2003).

   a. Looking at the four points from the literature, how is Sami's cultural background similar to or different from your own? Remember that you are looking at cultural patterns, not Sami's individual and personal values and behaviors.

   b. On the basis of your understanding of your own and Sami's culture, what questions might you want to ask Sami to support her reproductive health?

8. What physical examination techniques would you use to:

   a. Assess for a distended bladder?

   b. Get information about a patient's headache?

   c. Obtain data about a patient's ankle edema?

   d. What subjective data could you obtain by using one of the four physical assessment techniques?

9. For each of the following concepts, use critical thinking to describe how or why it is important to nursing, patient care, or assessment. Note that these are *not* to be merely definitions.

Assessment
ANA standards of practice
The Joint Commission
Agency policies
Comprehensive assessments
Focused assessments
Specific special needs assessments:
Pain assessment
Spiritual health assessment

Wellness assessment
The nursing health history
Active listening
Nursing frameworks/models
Validating data
Recording data
Reflecting critically about your
    assessment

What Are the Main Points in This Chapter?

➤ Assessment is a systematic, ongoing process of collecting, categorizing, and recording holistic data about client health status.

➤ Accurate, complete data are essential to effective nursing diagnosis and care planning.

➤ Nursing assessments focus on client responses to illness and stressors rather than on identifying disease processes.

➤ ANA standards of practice state that professional nurses are responsible for assessing clients.

➤ A comprehensive assessment provides information about the client's overall health, whereas a focused assessment provides data about a particular topic, body part, or functional ability.

➤ Special needs assessments provide in-depth information about a particular area of client functioning (e.g., nutrition, pain, lifestyle).

➤ Subjective data can be perceived only by the client; objective data are measurable or observable by the nurse or other healthcare providers.

➤ Nurses obtain data by observing and interviewing patients, and by performing physical assessment.

➤ The formats and frameworks for the nursing health history vary among agencies; however, all have essentially the same components (e.g., chief complaint, family history, review of body systems).

➤ Effective interviews require preparation by the nurse and use of both closed and open-ended questions.

➤ Active listening is one of the most important interviewing techniques.

➤ Validating data helps to ensure that they are accurate, complete, and factual.

➤ Documentation of assessment findings is of critical importance and has professional and legal implications.

➤ When documenting assessments, the nurse should record cues (observations), not inferences (conclusions).

For practice questions for this chapter,

 Go to **NCLEX-Style Chapter Quiz,** on the Student Resource Disk or DavisPlus at http://davisplus.fadavis.com/Wilkinson2

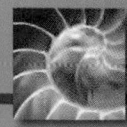

Knowledge Map

Assessment Concepts

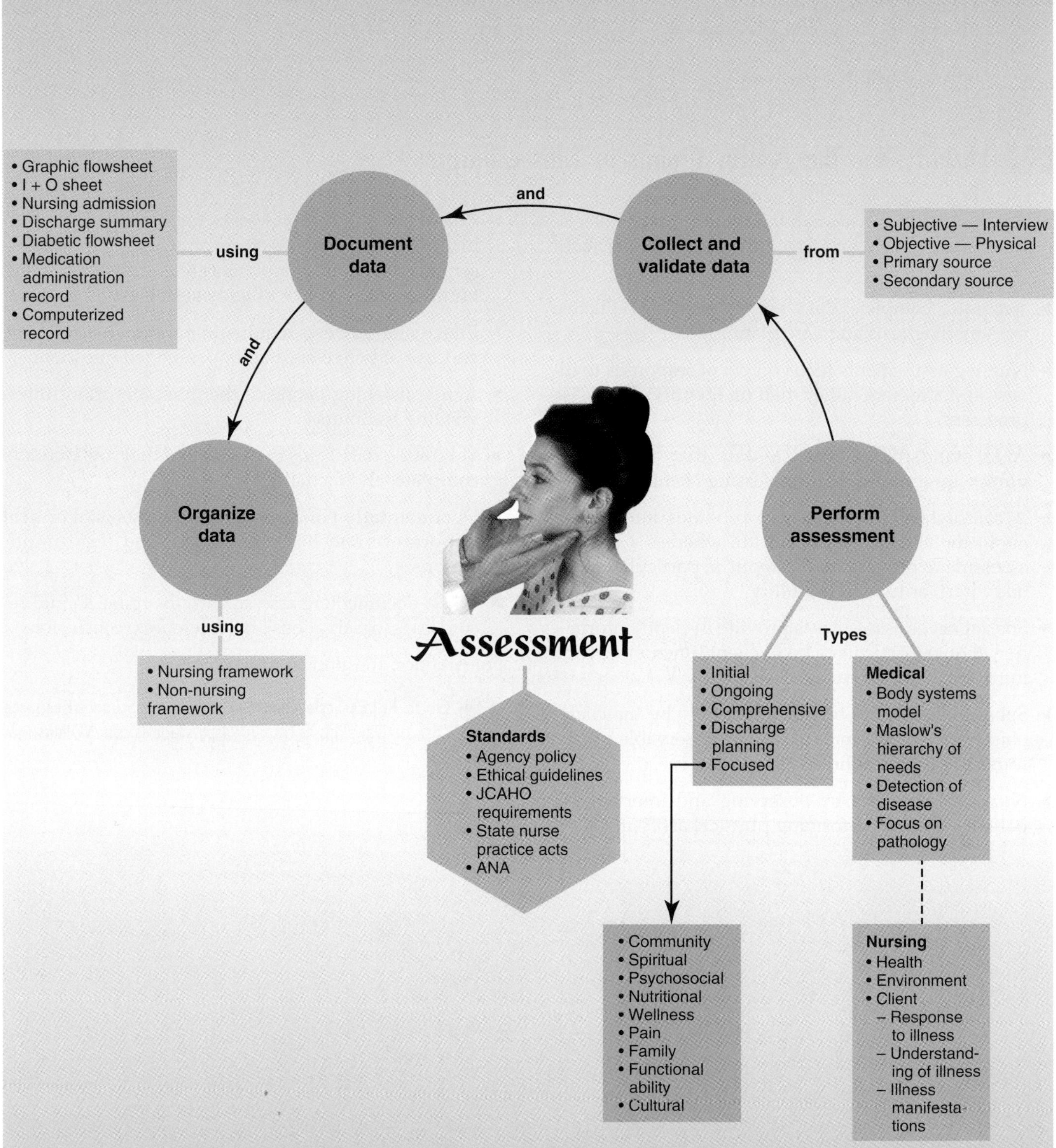

- Graphic flowsheet
- I + O sheet
- Nursing admission
- Discharge summary
- Diabetic flowsheet
- Medication administration record
- Computerized record

using

Document data

and

Collect and validate data

from

- Subjective — Interview
- Objective — Physical
- Primary source
- Secondary source

and

Organize data

using

- Nursing framework
- Non-nursing framework

Assessment

Standards
- Agency policy
- Ethical guidelines
- JCAHO requirements
- State nurse practice acts
- ANA

Perform assessment

Types

- Initial
- Ongoing
- Comprehensive
- Discharge planning
- Focused

Medical
- Body systems model
- Maslow's hierarchy of needs
- Detection of disease
- Focus on pathology

- Community
- Spiritual
- Psychosocial
- Nutritional
- Wellness
- Pain
- Family
- Functional ability
- Cultural

Nursing
- Health
- Environment
- Client
  – Response to illness
  – Understanding of illness
  – Illness manifestations

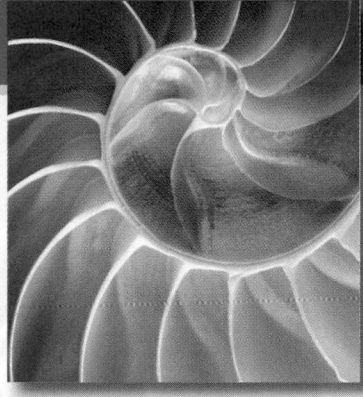

CHAPTER 4

Nursing Process: Diagnosis

For a podcast of an overview of this chapter,

 Go to Student Resources, **Podcast – Chapter Overviews, Chapter 4,** on DavisPlus at http://davisplus.fadavis.com/ Wilkinson2

Caring for the Garcias

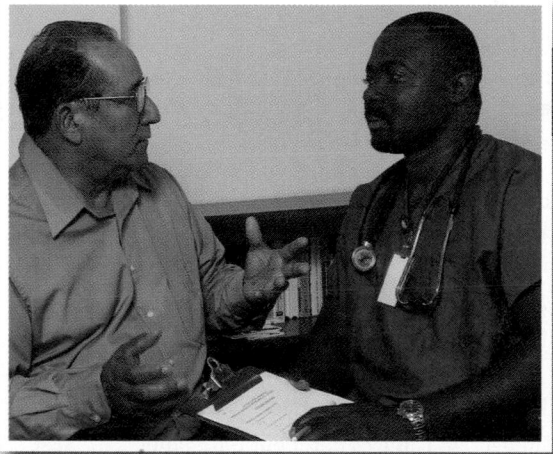

The exercises in this section allow you to practice the kind of thinking you will use as a full-spectrum nurse. Because these are critical-thinking questions, there is usually no single right answer. We do not provide answers for these questions because it is more important for you to think about the questions than to arrive at the "right" answer. These questions are designed to improve your thinking more than to "cover content." Discuss answers with your peers—discussion can stimulate critical thinking. If you have difficulty with any of these questions, consult with your instructor.

Review the opening scenario of Joseph Garcia in the front of this book. After the nurse practitioner completed his interview and physical examination of Mr. Garcia, he listed the following diagnoses on the problem list:

Hypertension
Obesity

Musculoskeletal pain
Tobacco abuse
Family history of prostate cancer
Family history of cardiovascular disease
Family history of diabetes mellitus (DM)

A. What type of problem list does this represent? How is it similar to or different from a problem list that you might generate?

B. Based on the data in the scenario, identify at least one actual, one potential, and one wellness diagnosis for Mr. Garcia. Identify the NANDA-I labels, and describe the cues that support your choices.

C. The nurse has identified a problem of Imbalanced Nutrition: More Than Body Requirements for Mr. Garcia.
  ■ What information do you need in order to determine the etiology of this problem?
  ■ Because you do not have that information, write a two-part diagnostic statement describing Mr. Garcia's nutritional status.

(continued on next page)

Caring for the Garcias (continued)

D. Now rewrite the nutrition statement as a three-part statement, including the phrase "as evidenced by."

E. The nurse has identified Acute Pain (knees) for Mr. Garcia. If the pain were caused by a medical condition, osteoarthritis, how would you write a two-part diagnostic statement to describe this health status?

Practical **Knowledge**
knowing how

In this section, you will find the NANDA-I taxonomy of diagnosis labels and the list of descriptors for NANDA-I nursing diagnoses. Refer to these lists as you develop nursing diagnoses for your patients.

Standardized Language

NANDA International Taxonomy II: Domains, Classes, and Diagnoses (Labels)

This taxonomically organized list represents the NANDA-I-approved nursing diagnoses for clinical use and testing (2009–2011).

Domain 1. Health Promotion

The awareness of well-being or normality of function and the strategies used to maintain control of and enhance that well-being or normality of function

Class 1. Health Awareness Recognition of normal function and well-being

Class 2. Health Management Identifying, controlling, performing, and integrating activities to maintain health and well-being

Approved Diagnoses

00082	Effective Therapeutic Regimen Management (retired diagnosis)
00078	Ineffective Therapeutic Regimen Management
00080	Ineffective Family Therapeutic Regimen Management
00081	Ineffective Community Therapeutic Regimen Management (retired diagnosis)
00099	Ineffective Health Maintenance
00098	Impaired Home Maintenance
00162	Readiness for Enhanced Management of Therapeutic Regimen
00163	Readiness for Enhanced Nutrition
00186	Readiness for Enhanced Immunization Status
00193	Self Neglect

Domain 2. Nutrition

The activities of taking in, assimilating, and using nutrients for the purposes of tissue maintenance, tissue repair, and the production of energy

Class 1. Ingestion Taking food or nutrients into the body

Approved Diagnoses

00107	Ineffective Infant Feeding Pattern
00103	Impaired Swallowing
00002	Imbalanced Nutrition: Less Than Body Requirements
00001	Imbalanced Nutrition: More Than Body Requirements
00003	Risk for Imbalanced Nutrition: More Than Body Requirements

Class 2. Digestion The physical and chemical activities that convert foodstuffs into substances suitable for absorption and assimilation

Class 3. Absorption The act of taking up nutrients through body tissues

Class 4. Metabolism The chemical and physical processes occurring in living organisms and cells for the development and use of protoplasm, production of waste and energy, with the release of energy for all vital processes

Approved Diagnoses

00178	Risk for Impaired Liver Function
00179	Risk for Unstable Blood Glucose Level
00194	Neonatal Jaundice

Class 5. Hydration The taking in and absorption of fluids and electrolytes

Approved Diagnoses

00027	Deficient Fluid Volume
00028	Risk for Deficient Fluid Volume
00026	Excess Fluid Volume
00025	Risk for Imbalanced Fluid Volume
00160	Readiness for Enhanced Fluid Balance
00195	Risk for Electrolyte Imbalance

Domain 3. Elimination and Exchange

Secretion and excretion of waste products from the body

Class 1. Urinary Function The process of secretion, reabsorption, and excretion of urine

Approved Diagnoses

00016	Impaired Urinary Elimination
00023	Urinary Retention
00021	Total Urinary Incontinence (retired diagnosis)

NANDA International Taxonomy II: Domains, Classes, and Diagnoses (Labels)—cont'd

00020	Functional Urinary Incontinence
00017	Stress Urinary Incontinence
00019	Urge Urinary Incontinence
00018	Reflex Urinary Incontinence
00022	Risk for Urge Urinary Incontinence
00166	Readiness for Enhanced Urinary Elimination
00176	Overflow Urinary Incontinence

Class 2. Gastrointestinal Function The process of absorption and excretion of the end products of digestion

Approved Diagnoses

00014	Bowel Incontinence
00013	Diarrhea
00011	Constipation ·
00015	Risk for Constipation
00012	Perceived Constipation
00196	Dysfunctional Gastrointestinal Motility
00197	Risk for Dysfunctional Gastrointestinal Motility

Class 3. Integumentary Function The process of secretion and excretion through the skin

Class 4. Respiratory Function The process of exchange of gases and removal of the end products of metabolism

Approved Diagnoses

00030	Impaired Gas Exchange
00031	Ineffective Airway Clearance
00032	Impaired Spontaneous Ventilation

Domain 4. Activity/Rest

The production, conservation, expenditure, or balance of energy resources

Class 1. Sleep/Rest Slumber, repose, ease, relaxation, or inactivity

Approved Diagnoses

00096	Sleep Deprivation
00165	Readiness for Enhanced Sleep
00095	Insomnia
00198	Disturbed Sleep Pattern

Class 2. Activity/Exercise Moving parts of the body (mobility), doing work, or performing actions often (but not always) against resistance

Approved Diagnoses

00040	Risk for Disuse Syndrome
00085	Impaired Physical Mobility
00091	Impaired Bed Mobility
00089	Impaired Wheelchair Mobility
00090	Impaired Transfer Ability
00088	Impaired Walking
00097	Deficient Diversional Activity
00100	Delayed Surgical Recovery
00168	Sedentary Lifestyle

Class 3. Energy Balance A dynamic state of harmony between intake and expenditure of resources

Approved Diagnoses

00050	Disturbed Energy Field
00093	Fatigue

Class 4. Cardiovascular/Pulmonary Responses Cardiopulmonary mechanisms that support activity/rest

Approved Diagnoses

00029	Decreased Cardiac Output
00033	Impaired Spontaneous Ventilation
00032	Ineffective Breathing Pattern
00092	Activity Intolerance
00094	Risk for Activity Intolerance
00034	Dysfunctional Ventilatory Weaning Response
00200	Risk for Decreased Cardiac Tissue Perfusion
00201	Risk for Ineffective Cerebral Tissue Perfusion
00202	Risk for Ineffective Gastrointestinal Perfusion
00203	Risk for Ineffective Renal Perfusion
00204	Ineffective Peripheral Tissue Perfusion
00205	Risk for Shock
00106	Risk for Bleeding

Class 5. Self-Care Ability to perform activities to care for one's body and bodily functions

Approved Diagnoses

00109	Dressing Self-Care Deficit
00108	Bathing Self-Care Deficit
00102	Feeding Self-Care Deficit
00110	Toileting Self-Care Deficit
00182	Readiness for Enhanced Self-Care

Domain 5. Perception/Cognition

The human information processing system including attention, orientation, sensation, perception, cognition, and communication

Class 1. Attention Mental readiness to notice or observe

Approved Diagnoses

00123	Unilateral Neglect

Class 2. Orientation Awareness of time, place, and person

Approved Diagnoses

00127	Impaired Environmental Interpretation Syndrome
00154	Wandering

Class 3. Sensation/Perception Receiving information through the senses of touch, taste, smell, vision, hearing, and kinesthesia and the comprehension of sense data resulting in naming, associating, and/or pattern recognition

Approved Diagnoses

00122	Disturbed Sensory Perception (specify: Visual, Auditory, Kinesthetic, Gustatory, Tactile, Olfactory)

Class 4. Cognition Use of memory, learning, thinking, problem solving, abstraction, judgment, insight, intellectual capacity, calculation, and language

Continued

NANDA International Taxonomy II: Domains, Classes, and Diagnoses (Labels)—cont'd

Approved Diagnoses

00126   Deficient Knowledge (specify)

00161   Readiness for Enhanced Knowledge (specify)

00128   Acute Confusion

00129   Chronic Confusion

00131   Impaired Memory

00130   Disturbed Thought Processes (a retired diagnosis)

00184   Readiness for Enhanced Decision Making

00173   Risk for Acute Confusion

00199   Ineffective Activity Planning

Class 5. Communication Sending and receiving verbal and nonverbal information

Approved Diagnoses

00051   Impaired Verbal Communication

00157   Readiness for Enhanced Communication

Domain 6. Self-Perception

Awareness about the self

Class 1. Self-Concept The perception(s) about the total self

Approved Diagnoses

00121   Disturbed Personal Identity

00125   Powerlessness

00152   Risk for Powerlessness

00124   Hopelessness

00054   Risk for Loneliness

00167   Readiness for Enhanced Self-Concept

00187   Readiness for Enhanced Power

00174   Readiness for Compromised Human Dignity

00185   Readiness for Enhanced Hope

Class 2. Self-Esteem Assessment of one's own worth, capability, significance, and success

Approved Diagnoses

00119   Chronic Low Self-Esteem

00120   Situational Low Self-Esteem

00153   Risk for Situational Low Self-Esteem

Class 3. Body Image A mental image of one's own body

Approved Diagnoses

00118   Disturbed Body Image

Domain 7. Role Relationships

The positive and negative connections or associations between people or groups of people and the means by which those connections are demonstrated

Class 1. Caregiving Roles Socially expected behavior patterns by persons providing care who are not healthcare professionals

Approved Diagnoses

00061   Caregiver Role Strain

00062   Risk for Caregiver Role Strain

00056   Impaired Parenting

00057   Risk for Impaired Parenting

00164   Readiness for Enhanced Parenting

Class 2. Family Relationships Associations of people who are biologically related or related by choice

Approved Diagnoses

00060   Interrupted Family Processes

00159   Readiness for Enhanced Family Processes

00063   Dysfunctional Family Processes

00058   Risk for Impaired Attachment

Class 3. Role Performance Quality of functioning in socially expected behavior patterns

Approved Diagnoses

00106   Effective Breastfeeding

00104   Ineffective Breastfeeding

00105   Interrupted Breastfeeding

00055   Ineffective Role Performance

00064   Parental Role Conflict

00052   Impaired Social Interaction

00207   Readiness for Enhanced Relationship

Domain 8. Sexuality

Sexual identity, sexual function, and reproduction

Class 1. Sexual Identity The state of being a specific person in regard to sexuality and/or gender

Class 2. Sexual Function The capacity or ability to participate in sexual activities

Approved Diagnoses

00059   Sexual Dysfunction

00065   Ineffective Sexuality Pattern

Class 3. Reproduction Any process by which new individuals (people) are produced

Approved Diagnoses

00208   Readiness for Enhanced Childbearing Process

00209   Risk for Disturbed Maternal/Fetal Dyad

Domain 9. Coping/Stress Tolerance

Contending with life events/life processes

Class 1. Post-Trauma Responses Reactions occurring after physical or psychological trauma

Approved Diagnoses

00114   Relocation Stress Syndrome

00149   Risk for Relocation Stress Syndrome

00142   Rape-Trauma Syndrome

00144   Rape-Trauma Syndrome: Silent Reaction (retired diagnosis)

00143   Rape-Trauma Syndrome: Compound Reaction (retired diagnosis)

00141   Post-Trauma Syndrome

00145   Risk for Post-Trauma Syndrome

NANDA International Taxonomy II: Domains, Classes, and Diagnoses (Labels)—cont'd

Class 2. Coping Responses The process of managing environmental stress

Approved Diagnoses

00148	Fear
00146	Anxiety
00147	Death Anxiety
00137	Chronic Sorrow
00072	Ineffective Denial
00136	Grieving
00135	Complicated Grieving
00069	Ineffective Coping
00073	Disabled Family Coping
00074	Compromised Family Coping
00071	Defensive Coping
00077	Ineffective Community Coping
00158	Readiness for Enhanced Coping (Individual)
00075	Readiness for Enhanced Family Coping
00076	Readiness for Enhanced Community Coping
00172	Risk for Complicated Grieving
00177	Stress Overload
00188	Risk-Prone Health Behavior
00210	Impaired Individual Resilience
00211	Risk for Compromised Resilience
00212	Readiness for Enhanced Resilience

Class 3. Neurobehavioral Stress Behavioral responses reflecting nerve and brain function

Approved Diagnoses

00009	Autonomic Dysreflexia
00010	Risk for Autonomic Dysreflexia
00116	Disorganized Infant Behavior
00115	Risk for Disorganized Infant Behavior
00117	Readiness for Enhanced Organized Infant Behavior
00049	Decreased Intracranial Adaptive Capacity

Domain 10. Life Principles

Principles underlying conduct, thought, and behavior about acts, customs, or institutions viewed as being true or having intrinsic worth

Class 1. Values The identification and ranking of preferred modes of conduct or end states

Approved Diagnoses

00068	Readiness for Enhanced Hope

Class 2. Beliefs Opinions, expectations, or judgments about acts, customs, or institutions viewed as being true or having intrinsic worth

Approved Diagnoses

00068	Readiness for Enhanced Spiritual Well-Being
00185	Readiness for Enhanced Hope

Class 3. Value/Belief/Action Congruence The correspondence or balance achieved between values, beliefs, and actions

Approved Diagnoses

00066	Spiritual Distress
00067	Risk for Spiritual Distress
00083	Decisional Conflict (specify)
00079	Noncompliance (specify)
00170	Risk for Impaired Religiosity
00169	Impaired Religiosity
00171	Readiness for Enhanced Religiosity
00175	Moral Distress
00184	Readiness for Enhanced Decision Making

Domain 11. Safety/Protection

Freedom from danger, physical injury or immune system damage, preservation from loss, and protection of safety and security

Class 1. Infection Host responses following pathogenic invasion

Approved Diagnoses

00004	Risk for Infection
00186	Readiness for Enhanced Immunization Status

Class 2. Physical Injury Bodily harm or hurt

Approved Diagnoses

00045	Impaired Oral Mucous Membrane
00035	Risk for Injury
00087	Risk for Perioperative Positioning Injury
00155	Risk for Falls
00038	Risk for Trauma
00046	Impaired Skin Integrity
00047	Risk for Impaired Skin Integrity
00044	Impaired Tissue Integrity
00048	Impaired Dentition
00036	Risk for Suffocation
00039	Risk for Aspiration
00031	Ineffective Airway Clearance
00086	Risk for Peripheral Neurovascular Dysfunction
00043	Ineffective Protection
00156	Risk for Sudden Infant Death Syndrome
00213	Risk for Vascular Trauma

Class 3. Violence The exertion of excessive force or power so as to cause injury or abuse

Approved Diagnoses

00139	Risk for Self-Mutilation
00151	Self-Mutilation
00138	Risk for Other-Directed Violence
00140	Risk for Self-Directed Violence
00150	Risk for Suicide

Continued

NANDA International Taxonomy II: Domains, Classes, and Diagnoses (Labels)—cont'd

Class 4. Environmental Hazards Sources of danger in the surroundings

Approved Diagnoses

00037   Risk for Poisoning

00180   Risk for Contamination

00181   Contamination

Class 5. Defensive Processes The processes by which the self protects itself from the nonself

Approved Diagnoses

00041   Latex Allergy Response

00042   Risk for Latex Allergy Response

00186   Readiness for Enhanced Immunization Status

Class 6. Thermoregulation The physiologic process of regulating heat and energy within the body for the purposes of protecting the organism

Approved Diagnoses

00005   Risk for Imbalanced Body Temperature

00008   Ineffective Thermoregulation

00006   Hypothermia

00007   Hyperthermia

Domain 12. Comfort

Sense of mental, physical, or social well-being or ease

Class 1. Physical Comfort Sense of well-being or ease and/or freedom from pain

Approved Diagnoses

00132   Acute Pain

00133   Chronic Pain

00134   Nausea

00183   Readiness for Enhanced Comfort

00214   Impaired Comfort

Class 2. Environmental Comfort Sense of well-being or ease in/with one's environment

Approved Diagnoses

00183   Readiness for Enhanced Comfort

00214   Impaired Comfort

Class 3. Social Comfort Sense of well-being or ease with one's social situations

Approved Diagnoses

00053   Social Isolation

00214   Impaired Comfort

Domain 13. Growth/Development

Age-appropriate increases in physical dimensions, maturation of organ systems, and/or progression through the developmental milestones

Class 1. Growth Increases in physical dimensions or maturity of organ systems

Approved Diagnoses

00111   Delayed Growth and Development

00113   Risk for Disproportionate Growth

00101   Adult Failure to Thrive

Class 2. Development Progression or regression through a sequence of recognized milestones in life

Approved Diagnoses

00111   Delayed Growth and Development

00112   Risk for Delayed Development

Source: NANDA International (2009). Nursing Diagnoses: Definitions and Classification 2009–2011.

Descriptors for NANDA-I Nursing Diagnoses

Some NANDA-I labels may include one or more of these descriptors. You may add descriptors to other labels, if necessary, to clarify the diagnostic statement.

Descriptors for the Subject of the Diagnosis (Axis 2)

Individual	A single human being distinct from others, a person
Family	Two or more people having continuous or sustained relationships, perceiving reciprocal obligations, sensing common meaning, and sharing certain obligations toward others; related by blood or choice
Group	A number of people with shared characteristics
Community	A group of people living in the same locale under the same governance. Examples include neighborhoods and cities.

Descriptors for Judgment (Axis 3)

(Suggested; not limited to the following)

Compromised	Damaged, made vulnerable
Complicated	Intricately involved, complex
Decreased	Lessened (in size, amount, or degree)
Defensive	Used or intended to defend or protect
Deficient	Insufficient, inadequate
Delayed	Late, slow, or postponed
Disabled	Limited, handicapped
Disorganized	Not properly arranged or controlled
Disproportionate	Too large or too small in comparison with a norm
Disturbed	Agitated; interrupted, interfered with
Dysfunctional	Not operating normally
Effective	Producing the intended or desired effect

Enhanced	Improved in quality, value, or extent
Excessive	Greater than necessary or desirable
Imbalanced	Out of proportion or balance
Impaired	Damaged, weakened
Ineffective	Not producing the intended or desired effect
Interrupted	Having its continuity broken
Low	Below the norm
Organized	Properly arranged or controlled
Perceived	Observed through the senses
Readiness for	In a suitable state for an activity or situation
Situational	Related to a particular circumstance

Descriptors for Age (Axis 5)

Fetus, neonate, infant, toddler, preschool child, school-age child, adolescent, adult, older adult

Descriptors for Time (Axis 6)

Acute	Lasting less than 6 months
Chronic	Lasting more than 6 months
Intermittent	Stopping or starting again at intervals, periodic, cyclic
Continuous	Uninterrupted, going on without stop

Descriptors for Status of the Diagnosis (Axis 7)

Actual	Existing in fact or reality, existing at the present time.
Health Promotion	Behavior motivated by the desire to increase well-being and actualize human health potential (Pender, Murduagh, & Parsons, 2006, as cited in NANDA-I, 2009)
Risk	Vulnerability, especially as a result of exposure to factors that increase the chance of injury or loss
Wellness	The quality or state of being healthy

Source: NANDA International. (2009). *Nursing diagnoses: Definitions and classification 2009–2011.* Ames, IA: Wiley-Blackwell.

THINKING CRITICALLY ABOUT THE NURSING PROCESS: DIAGNOSIS

The exercises in the following sections allow you to practice the kind of thinking you will use as a full-spectrum nurse. Because these are critical-thinking questions, there is usually no single right answer. We do not provide answers for these questions because it is more important for you to think about the questions than to arrive at the "right" answer. These questions are designed to improve your thinking more than to "cover content." Discuss answers with your peers—discussion can stimulate critical thinking. If you have difficulty with any of these questions, consult with your instructor.

Applying the Full-Spectrum Nursing Model

PATIENT SITUATION

Recall Todd from Volume 1, "Meet Your Patient." You have admitted him from the emergency department (ED). His admitting medical diagnosis is chronic renal failure, and he has a medical history of type 2 diabetes mellitus. Todd is married, 58 years old, and employed. In the past 3 days, he has developed decreased sensation in his bilateral lower extremities with slight mobility impairment.

You will need to ask Todd about his medication regimen, his compliance with his diabetes treatment plan, and the extent to which his family is involved. You will also need to find out what laboratory tests have been completed and how severe his renal dysfunction has become. Your initial impressions about possible problems are:

- Because he has chronic renal failure, you can anticipate a problem with fluid balance.
- He has been admitted to the hospital and is acutely ill, so he may be anxious and fearful.
- He has decreased sensation in his lower extremities, so he may have a mobility or a safety problem.
- He has diabetes, so he is at risk for impaired skin and tissue integrity.
- Because diabetes and renal failure require complex regimens and patient self-care, it is possible that Todd may not be managing his therapy effectively, either because he is not motivated to do so or because he lacks the knowledge to do so.

When Todd and his family arrive on your unit, you begin gathering additional data. Armed with comprehensive data, you then make a list of Todd's health problems, in priority order. These actions illustrate the diagnosis phase of the nursing process phase. The purpose of diagnosing is to identify the client's health status, from which you will create your plan of care.

THINKING

1. *Theoretical Knowledge*: What theoretical knowledge will you need to identify the collaborative problems and nursing diagnoses for Todd?

2. *Critical Thinking (Inquiry Based on Credible Sources)*:

a. What resources would you use to find out more about the pathophysiology of renal failure? How do you know the source is credible?

b. One of your first impressions was that Todd may be anxious and fearful. What data do you need in order to decide whether to write an Anxiety nursing diagnosis? How will you obtain the data?

c. When you are making your assessments of Todd, who is your best source of data? Why?

DOING

3. *Nursing Process (Diagnosis)*:

a. Write one collaborative problem for Todd. If you do not know the potential complications of chronic renal failure, look them up in a medical–surgical or pathophysiology textbook. Also explain why you would not use a nursing diagnosis to describe the problem.

b. After further assessment, you learn that Todd's skin is intact and without redness or lesions. Write a nursing diagnosis (problem and etiology) to describe your concerns about his skin.

c. Based on Maslow's hierarchy of needs, which problem has the highest priority?

CARING

4. *Ethical Knowledge*: The scenario doesn't provide enough information for you to identify the ethical dimensions of Todd's care. However, based on what you already know about him, speculate about some things that might create ethical questions for you.

PATIENT SITUATION

5. *Patient Preferences*: Think critically about the patient's preferences and concerns. Suppose that Todd's main concern is not the same as the high-priority problem you identified. Speculate about some other concerns he might have; what other things might he want to have resolved that could—for him—be more important than his chronic renal failure? Aside from his physical condition, what life concerns do you think Todd might have right now?

Critical Thinking and Clinical Reasoning

1. Sally Jones, a 45-year-old woman, was admitted to your surgical unit directly from the surgical suite. She was in a motorcycle accident this evening. In the emergency department, her blood pressure was falling, and she was bleeding profusely from many sites. She was sent directly to the operating room for a splenectomy, internal fixation of a compound fracture of bilateral femurs, and traumatic amputation of the right hand. During surgery she lost 2000 mL of blood and received 3 units of packed red blood cells (volume = 750 mL) along with 1000 mL of fluid administered intravenously.

     You receive the report on the client at 1900. Sally is receiving IV fluid through several peripheral lines and through a central line (a catheter inserted into a major vein leading to the heart). She has a Foley catheter, which is draining 30 mL of concentrated urine each hour. Sally's vital signs are as follows: temperature, 102.8°F (39.3°C) (rectal); heart rate, 120 beats/ min; respirations, 28 per minute; and blood pressure, 160/86 mm Hg. Her skin is flushed, dry, and warm to the touch. On assessment, you find the following: skin turgor > 3 seconds, dry mucous membranes, and bloodstained dressing on right upper extremity.

     She is complaining of thirst, weakness, and pain at a level of 10 on a scale of 1 to 10 (10 highest). Sally is receiving a continuous infusion of morphine. She refuses to deep-breathe, cough, or attempt to turn. She lies very still and rigid. Sally drifts in and out of sleep but remains asleep for less than 30 minutes each time. She is irritable and restless. She communicates with one-word answers only. Frequently, she displays facial grimaces and becomes increasingly stiff. Her eyes appear dull. She complains of severe pain with any passive or active movements. In answering the following questions, use a nursing diagnosis handbook to look up the NANDA-I defining characteristics, definitions, and so forth, as needed.

   a. Based on the data provided, which of the following NANDA-I labels would you use for Sally? Explain your reasoning.

      Deficient Fluid Volume or Risk for Deficient Fluid Volume

   b. For Sally's diagnosis of Deficient Fluid Volume, what are the cues? What are her related factors?

   c. Using your responses to (a) and (b), write a diagnostic statement that includes problem, etiology, defining characteristics (cues), and the medical condition that the problem is "secondary to."

   d. Think of other explanations for these cues: temperature, 102.8°F (39.3°C); heart rate, 120 beats/min; respirations, 28 per minute; blood pressure, 160/86 mm Hg.

e. Sally certainly has the defining characteristics for the nursing diagnosis Impaired Physical Mobility. If you use this problem label, what would the etiological factors be?

f. Which of those etiological factors could you treat with independent nursing interventions?

g. Sally has the following nursing diagnoses (problem labels only are listed) and collaborative problems:

Deficient Fluid Volume

Acute Pain (abdominal incision, amputation site, fractures)

Risk for Disturbed Body Image

Potential Complication of trauma, surgery, and IV lines: infection

Risk for Ineffective Airway Clearance

- From Sally's perspective, which is probably the highest priority problem?
- Using an urgency (or threat to life) criterion, name Sally's three most important problems and why you consider them most important.

h. Examine your theoretical knowledge. To care for Sally, what additional theoretical knowledge do you need?

i. What practical knowledge will you need to use in her care?

2. You have a homebound client with diabetes who has the beginning of a pressure ulcer. You have been treating the client for Impaired Skin Integrity related to decreased circulation and mobility. However, the client's skin continues to break down.

a. Your client has diabetes mellitus type 2. What type of problem is that (medical, nursing, or collaborative)?

b. What is the client's nursing diagnosis?

c. The client has Impaired Skin Integrity. The break in the body's first line of defense (intact skin) increases the risk for infection. Write a problem statement reflecting that risk nursing diagnosis.

3. For each of the following concepts, use critical thinking to describe how or why it is important to nursing, patient care, or nursing diagnosis. Note that these are *not* to be merely definitions.

The diagnosis step of the nursing process	Collaborative problems
NANDA International	Wellness nursing diagnosis
Patient strengths	Cues
Maslow's hierarchy	Diagnostic label definition
Documenting priorities	Defining characteristics
Nursing diagnoses	Risk factors
Possible nursing diagnoses	Etiological factors

What Are the Main Points in This Chapter?

➤ Nursing diagnosis is the unique obligation of the professional nurse; it cannot be delegated.

➤ An accurate nursing diagnosis is the foundation for the plan of care because it directs the choice of client-centered goals and nursing interventions.

➤ A nursing diagnosis is a statement of health status that nurses can identify, prevent, or treat independently.

➤ A medical diagnosis describes a disease, illness, or injury. A nursing diagnosis, in contrast, more holistically describes human responses to disease, illness, or injury.

➤ Collaborative problems are potential physiological complications of diseases, treatments, or diagnostic studies that nurses monitor and help to prevent but that cannot be treated primarily by independent nursing interventions.

➤ You must determine the "status" of each nursing diagnosis—that is, actual, potential, or possible problem; wellness diagnosis; or syndrome—because each status requires (1) different wording and (2) different nursing interventions.

➤ Diagnostic reasoning involves analyzing and interpreting data, verifying problems with the patient, and prioritizing the problems.

➤ You can never be certain that an inference is accurate, but you can have more confidence in an inference that is well supported by data.

➤ A problem etiology consists of the factors causing or contributing to the problem.

➤ You should involve patients in verifying and prioritizing their problems.

➤ Sound diagnostic reasoning is based on critical thinking and good theoretical and self-knowledge.

➤ A NANDA-I nursing diagnosis consists of a diagnostic label, a definition, defining characteristics, and related or risk factors.

➤ To choose the correct NANDA-I problem label, match the patient's cue clusters to the NANDA-I definition and defining characteristics.

➤ A diagnostic statement consists basically of "problem + etiology"; however, a variety of formats is needed to describe client health status.

➤ In general, the problem side of the diagnostic statement directs the choice of goals; the etiology directs the choice of nursing interventions.

➤ Diagnostic statements should be descriptive, accurate, clear, concise, and nonjudgmental.

➤ One criticism of standardized diagnostic language is that it represents a threat to creative, holistic thinking.

For practice questions for this chapter,

 Go to **NCLEX-Style Chapter Quiz,** on the Student Resource Disk or DavisPlus at http://davisplus.fadavis.com/Wilkinson2

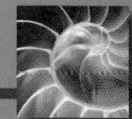

Knowledge Map

Full-Spectrum Nursing

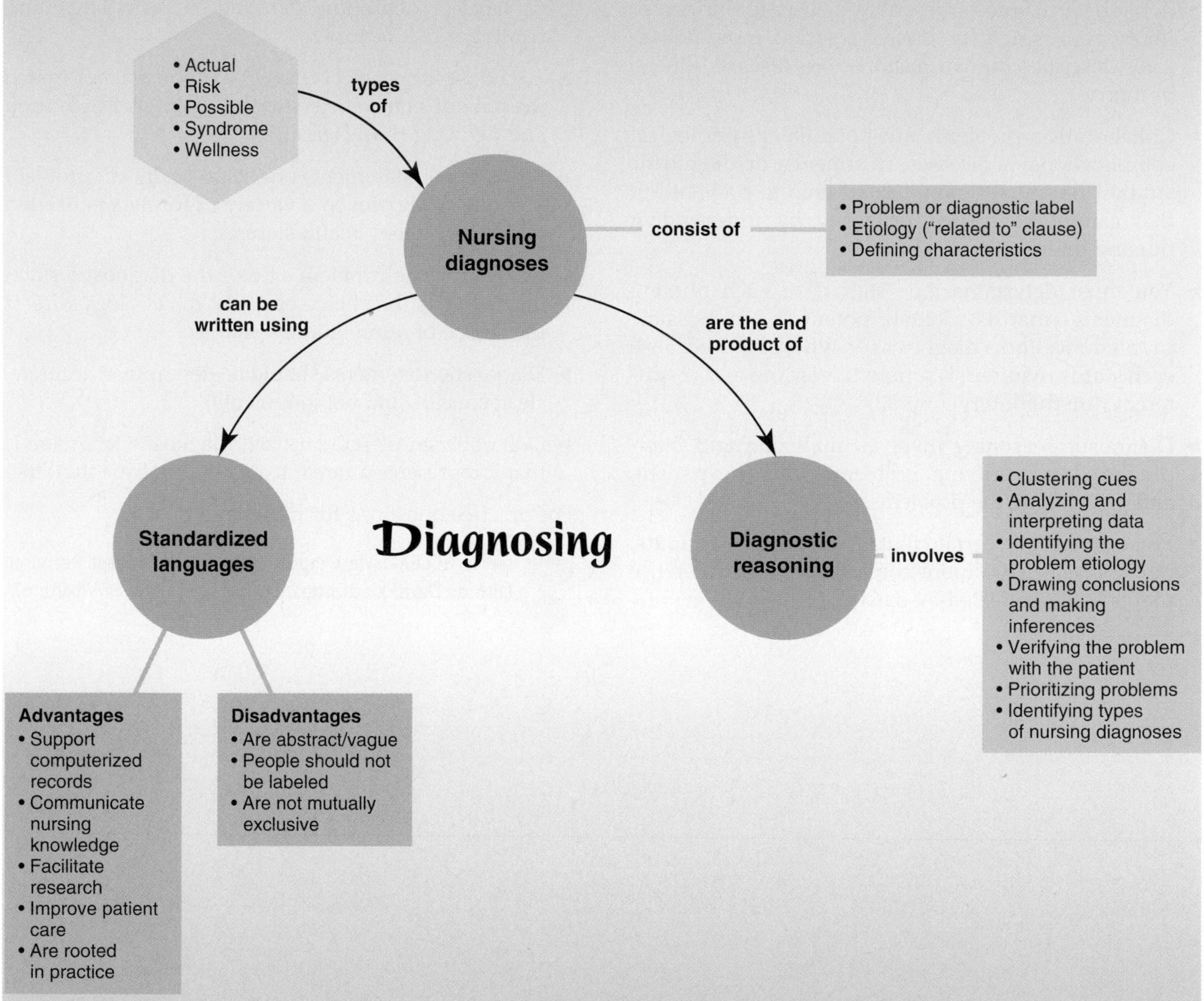

- Actual
- Risk
- Possible
- Syndrome
- Wellness

types of

Nursing diagnoses

consist of

- Problem or diagnostic label
- Etiology ("related to" clause)
- Defining characteristics

can be written using

are the end product of

Diagnosing

Standardized languages

Diagnostic reasoning

involves

- Clustering cues
- Analyzing and interpreting data
- Identifying the problem etiology
- Drawing conclusions and making inferences
- Verifying the problem with the patient
- Prioritizing problems
- Identifying types of nursing diagnoses

Advantages
- Support computerized records
- Communicate nursing knowledge
- Facilitate research
- Improve patient care
- Are rooted in practice

Disadvantages
- Are abstract/vague
- People should not be labeled
- Are not mutually exclusive

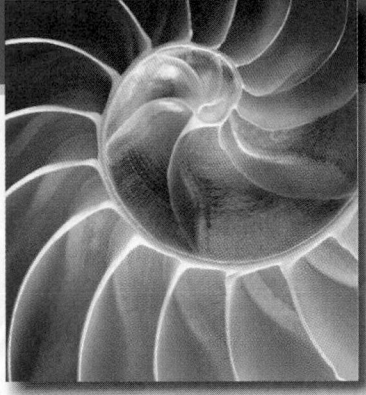

CHAPTER 5

Nursing Process: Planning Outcomes

For a podcast of an overview of this chapter,

 Go to Student Resources, **Podcast – Chapter Overviews, Chapter 5,** on DavisPlus at http://davisplus.fadavis.com/ Wilkinson2

Caring for the Garcias

The exercises in this section allow you to practice the kind of thinking you will use as a full-spectrum nurse. Because these are critical-thinking questions, there is usually no single right answer. We do not provide answers for these questions because it is more important for you to think about the questions than to arrive at the "right" answer. These questions are designed to improve your thinking more than to "cover content." Discuss answers with your peers—discussion can stimulate critical thinking. If you have difficulty with any of these questions, consult with your instructor.

Review the opening scenario of Joseph Garcia in the first pages of this volume. As the clinic nurse, you have written the following nursing diagnostic statement: Imbalanced Nutrition: More Than Body Requirements related to

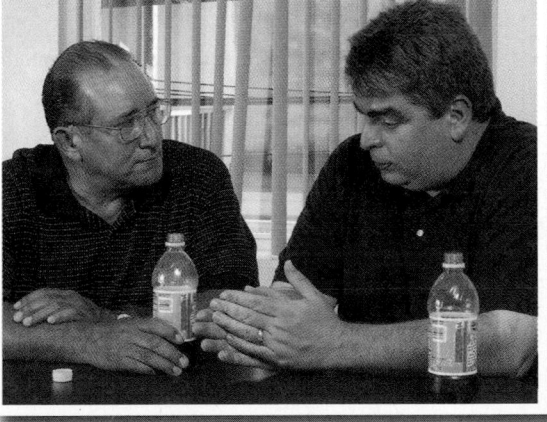

inappropriate food choices and serving size as evidenced by body mass index (BMI) of 32.67.

Write at least two short-term and two long-term goals for Mr. Garcia based on this diagnostic statement. Remember that your goals must be realistic and take into account Mr. Garcia's other health problems.

Practical **Knowledge**
knowing how

Practical knowledge in the planning phase of the nursing process requires you to use a variety of care planning forms. This section includes a discharge planning form, as well as a table of Nursing Outcomes Classification (NOC) measurement scales.

Discharge Planning Form

<table>
<tr>
<td rowspan="3">FOLLOW UP CARE</td>
<td>When to call the doctor; symptom management (pain, nausea); plan for meeting outcomes not met during hospitalization:</td>
</tr>
<tr>
<td>Call your primary physician to find out if an insurance referral form is needed for follow up appointments.
After discharge, you need to call for an appointment to see physician.
Clinic/Physician   Phone #   Date   Time
_____   _____ _____ _____   or ____days _____weeks _____months
_____   _____ _____ _____   or ____days _____weeks _____months
_____   _____ _____ _____   or ____days _____weeks _____months
Plans for follow up Labs/Tests/Treatments
Date   Time   Test/Treatment   Location   Ordered by</td>
</tr>
</table>

PERSONAL CARE	**Bathing:** ❏ No restrictions ❏ Other: _____ **Treatment/Therapy/Wound or Skin Care/ Supplies Needed** 2-Day Supply Sent Home ? ❏ Yes
ACTIVITY/ REHAB	❏ No restrictions ❏ Do not climb stairs ❏ Drive_____ ❏ Return to Work _____ ❏ Do not lift ❏ May lift up to _____lbs ❏ Weight Bearing _____# ❏ Other
DIET	❏ No restrictions ❏ Other: _____ Food/Drug Interactions: ❏ Coumadin ❏ MAO Inhibitors ❏ Other:
MEDICAL EQUIPMENT	❏ 2nd pair of TED hose given
COMMUNITY RESOURCES	**Referral Resource** **Agency** **Phone #** Transportation Arrangements for discharge: ___ Home IV Therapy _____ _____ _____ Home Health _____ _____ Home Oxygen _____ _____ Education/Community Resources:_____ Home PT/OT/Speech _____ _____ _____ Ask-A-Nurse _____ 816-932-0000

Preprinted Discharge Instruction Sheet given to patient   ❏ NA   ❏ Yes
  List Instruction Sheets:

I understand these instructions and agree with this plan of care _____
                                                      Patient/SO Signature

MULTIDISCIPLINARY DISCHARGE INSTRUCTIONS
Shawnee Mission Medical Center
9100 W. 74th Street
Shawnee Mission, Kansas 66204

Form # 60869 Revised: 4/01 PILOT Page 1 of 2

Source: Courtesy of Shawnee Mission Health System, Shawnee Mission, KS

Standardized Language

By combining the following indicators with NOC indicators, you can write observable, concrete, patient outcomes to use in evaluating a patient's response to care.

SCALE NUMBER	1	2	3	4	5*
NOC Measurement Scales					
a	Severely compromised	Substantially compromised	Moderately compromised	Mildly compromised	Not compromised
b	Severe deviation from normal range	Substantial deviation from normal range	Moderate deviation from normal range	Mild deviation from normal range	No deviation from normal range
f	Not adequate	Slightly adequate	Moderately adequate	Substantially adequate	Totally adequate
g	10 and over	7–9	4–6	1–3	None
i	None	Limited	Moderate	Substantial	Extensive
k	Never positive	Rarely positive	Sometimes positive	Often positive	Consistently positive
l	Very weak	Weak	Moderate	Strong	Very strong
m	Never demonstrated	Rarely demonstrated	Sometimes demonstrated	Often demonstrated	Consistently demonstrated
n	Severe	Substantial	Moderate	Mild	None
r	Poor	Fair	Good	Very good	Excellent
s	Not at all satisfied	Somewhat satisfied	Moderately satisfied	Very satisfied	Completely satisfied
u	No knowledge	Limited knowledge	Moderate knowledge	Substantial knowledge	Extensive knowledge

Source: Moorhead, S., Johnson, M., Maas, M., & Swanson, E. (2008). *Nursing outcomes classification (NOC)* (4th ed.). St. Louis, MO: C.V. Mosby, pp. 44–50. Used with permission.

*The scores (1 through 5) are constructed so that 5 is usually the most desirable, and 1 is the least desirable, condition relative to the outcome.

THINKING CRITICALLY ABOUT THE NURSING PROCESS: PLANNING OUTCOMES

The exercises in the following sections allow you to practice the kind of thinking you will use as a full-spectrum nurse. Because these are critical-thinking questions, there is usually no single right answer. We do not provide answers for these questions because it is more important for you to think about the questions than to arrive at the "right" answer.. These questions are designed to improve your thinking more than to "cover content." Discuss answers with your peers—discussion can stimulate critical thinking. If you have difficulty with any of these questions, consult with your instructor.

Applying the Full-Spectrum Nursing Model

PATIENT SITUATION

Ivan Benjamin has just been admitted to an orthopedic unit after an automobile accident. He was driving and has been living at home. Mr. Benjamin is 80 years old. He has these preexisting comorbidities: type 2 diabetes and osteoarthritis. He has casts and traction on both legs and a cast on one arm. He is receiving morphine sulfate intravenously via patient-controlled analgesia (PCA) pump. Imagine that you are an orthopedic nurse and must plan care for Mr. Benjamin. The admitting nurse wrote the following diagnoses and goals on the plan of care.

Nursing Diagnoses	Goals/Expected Outcomes
1. Acute Pain secondary to musculoskeletal trauma (arms, legs, body) and muscle spasms	▪ Demonstrates correct use of PCA pump ▪ Rates pain not higher than 4 on a scale of 1 to 10 at all times
2. Risk for Peripheral Neurovascular Dysfunction secondary to casts/traction	▪ Peripheral pulses palpable ▪ Fingers and toes warm ▪ Fingers and toes without pallor or cyanosis ▪ No edema of fingers and toes ▪ Capillary refill less than 3 seconds

THINKING

1. *Theoretical Knowledge:* What general *theoretical knowledge* will you need to care for this patient? Just identify the topics; limit the answer to about 150 words.

2. *Critical Thinking (Considering Alternatives):* Older adults are especially sensitive to certain medications, including morphine sulfate. What is one thing you could do to ensure Mr. Benjamin's safety while managing his acute pain (there are several; think of just one)?

3. *Critical Thinking (Inquiry):* List at least two more things you need to know about Mr. Benjamin in order to begin his discharge planning.

DOING

4. *Practical Knowledge:* What general *practical knowledge* will you need? What would you do to obtain this knowledge?

5. *Nursing Process:*

   a. *Diagnosis:* What is another nursing diagnosis you might want to assess for Mr. Benjamin?

   b. *Planning Goals:* On the care plan rewrite the goals/expected outcomes for Acute Pain so that they will have all the required components. Assume that today's date is January 4.

CARING

6. *Self-Knowledge:* What *beliefs, values, biases, or emotional responses* might interfere with your ability to provide the best care to Mr. Benjamin?

CONTEXT

7. Think critically about the context. Is there anything in this situation that you have seen before? Identify any familiar elements. For example, you may have an elderly male relative, even if you have never cared for an 80-year-old patient before.

Critical Thinking and Clinical Reasoning

1. Merle Quinn is visiting a family planning clinic, where she has just been informed that she is 6 weeks pregnant. She looks worried and makes the following statements: "This is a shock. I've just started a new business, and I need to work 7 days a week to make it go. . . . I don't know if I am ready to be a mother. . . ." Her husband agrees: "I just don't see how we can afford this. We don't even have any insurance now."

   "Still," Mrs. Quinn says, "I don't see how I could deal with having an abortion. My parents would be devastated. I'm sure they'd never speak to me again." Her husband says, "Not to speak of the fact that the Church forbids it. It would be a sin."

   A week later Mrs. Quinn calls the clinic in tears. She says she has not been able to eat or sleep and that she doesn't know what to do about her pregnancy. "I don't want this baby, but I can't bring myself to have an abortion." The nurse diagnoses Decisional Conflict related to unexpected/unwanted pregnancy and possibly assuming that abortion is her only alternative, as evidenced by statements of indecision, tearfulness, and inability to sleep. She makes an appointment to see Mr. and Mrs. Quinn that same day. Imagine that you are the nurse writing the care plan for the Quinns.

   a. Analyze your assumptions. What values and beliefs do you have that may influence the goals you write for the Quinns? Specifically, how could your values affect the goals you write?

   b. Develop a short-term goal to address the problem clause of this nursing diagnosis. The goal should be one you expect the Quinns to be able to achieve during their appointment that same day.

   c. You also write a goal stating: "By the end of this visit, clients will verbalize and demonstrate decreased anxiety and stress." Which part of the nursing diagnosis does this goal address?

   d. The NOC standardized outcomes "linked" to the NANDA-I diagnosis of Decisional Conflict are the following (definitions are given):

   Decision Making: Ability to choose between two or more alternatives

   Information Processing: Ability to acquire, organize, and use information

   Participation: Health Care Decisions: Personal involvement in selecting and evaluating health care options

   Which of those outcomes is it most important for the Quinns to achieve *today*? Why?

   e. Now imagine that you have written the following individualized goals/outcomes for today's visit with the Quinns:

By the end of this visit, clients will:

1. Verbalize and demonstrate decreased anxiety and stress.

2. Verbalize awareness that they have options for coping with whatever decision they make about the pregnancy.

3. Discuss with the nurse options for continuing or terminating the pregnancy.

4. Verbalize intent to discuss their feelings with family (i.e., their parents).

5. Verbalize intent to discuss feelings with a member of the clergy.

6. Decide whether to continue the pregnancy.

   - Why is outcome 2 so important?
   - What would you have had to assume in order to write outcome 4?
   - What would you have had to assume in order to write outcome 5?
   - Which of the outcomes is/are probably *not* appropriate for today's visit? Why?

2. For each of the following concepts, use critical thinking to describe how or why it is important to nursing, patient care, or the process of planning care. Note that these are *not* to be merely definitions.

Discharge planning
A written, individualized nursing care plan
Standardized care-planning documents (e.g., protocols)
Critical pathways
Computerized care planning
Goals (expected outcomes)
Short-term goals
Long-term goals

Action verbs (in goals)
Essential patient goals
The Nursing Outcomes Classification (NOC)
Aggregate goals
Wellness goals
Concrete, specific goal/outcome statements (as opposed to vague statements)

What Are the Main Points in This Chapter?

➤ During the planning outcomes phase, you will derive goals/expected outcomes from identified nursing diagnoses.

➤ Goals/expected outcomes (1) suggest nursing interventions, (2) serve as criteria for use in the evaluation step of the nursing process, and (3) provide motivation for patients and nurses.

➤ To ensure continuity of care, you should begin discharge planning with the initial patient assessment.

➤ Discharge planning is especially important for older adults and patients with complex needs.

➤ A holistic, individualized patient care plan contains information needed to address (1) basic needs and ADLs, (2) medical and collaborative therapies, (3) nursing diagnoses and collaborative problems, and (4) special teaching and/or discharge needs.

➤ Ideally, a care plan consists of a combination of standardized and individualized goals and interventions.

➤ Standardized approaches to care planning include institutional policies and procedures, protocols, unit standards of care, standardized care plans, critical pathways, and integrated plans of care (IPOCs).

➤ Computerized care planning helps ensure that the nurse considers a variety of interventions and does not overlook common and important interventions; it reduces the time spent on paperwork.

➤ Nursing-sensitive goals (expected outcomes, predicted outcomes, desired outcomes) describe the changes in patient health status that are intended to result from and can be influenced by nursing interventions.

➤ Goals for collaborative problems are usually not nursing sensitive, and should not be included on a nursing care plan.

➤ A goal statement should include a subject, an action verb, a performance criterion, a target time, and special conditions if needed.

➤ For every nursing diagnosis, you must state one "essential" goal-one that, if achieved, would demonstrate problem resolution or improvement.

➤ Among the ANA-recognized standardized vocabularies/taxonomies for describing patient outcomes are NOC, the Omaha System, and the Clinical Care Classification System.

➤ Goals should be concrete, specific, and observable; they should be valued by the patient/family; and they should not conflict with the medical treatment plan.

For practice questions for this chapter,

 Go to **NCLEX-Style Practice Quiz,** on the Student Resource Disk or DavisPlus at http://davisplus.fadavis.com/Wilkinson2

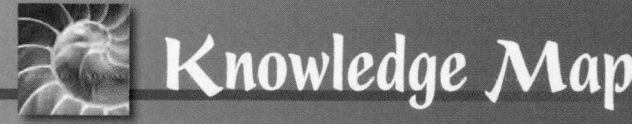

Knowledge Map

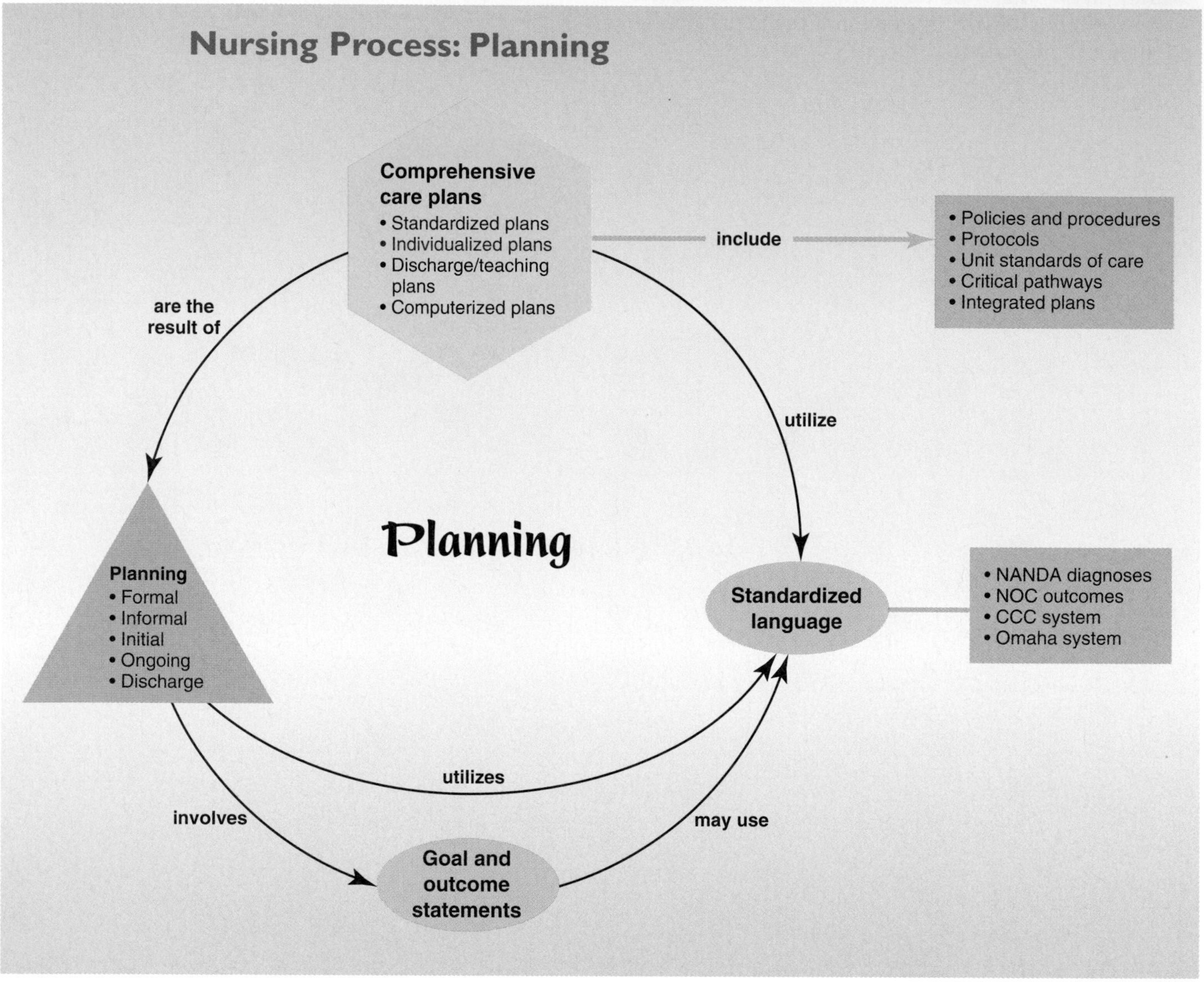

Nursing Process: Planning

Comprehensive care plans
- Standardized plans
- Individualized plans
- Discharge/teaching plans
- Computerized plans

include →

- Policies and procedures
- Protocols
- Unit standards of care
- Critical pathways
- Integrated plans

are the result of

utilize

Planning

Planning
- Formal
- Informal
- Initial
- Ongoing
- Discharge

Standardized language

- NANDA diagnoses
- NOC outcomes
- CCC system
- Omaha system

utilizes

involves

may use

Goal and outcome statements

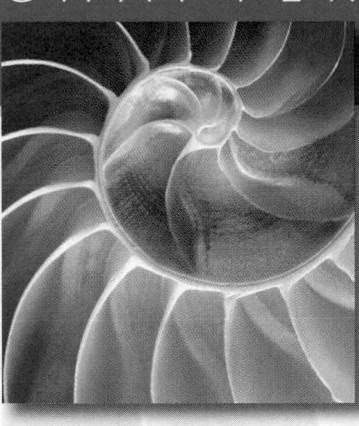

CHAPTER 6

Nursing Process: Planning Interventions

For a podcast of an overview of this chapter,

 Go to Student Resources, **Podcast – Chapter Overviews, Chapter 6,** on DavisPlus at http://davisplus.fadavis.com/ Wilkinson2

Caring for the Garcias

The exercises in the following section allow you to practice the kind of thinking you will use as a full-spectrum nurse. Because these are critical-thinking questions, there is usually no single right answer. We do not provide answers for these questions because it is more important for you to think about the questions than to arrive at the "right" answer. These questions are designed to improve your thinking more than to "cover content." Discuss answers with your peers—discussion can stimulate critical thinking. If you have difficulty with any of these questions, consult with your instructor

Recall that you have written the following nursing diagnosis for Mr. Garcia:

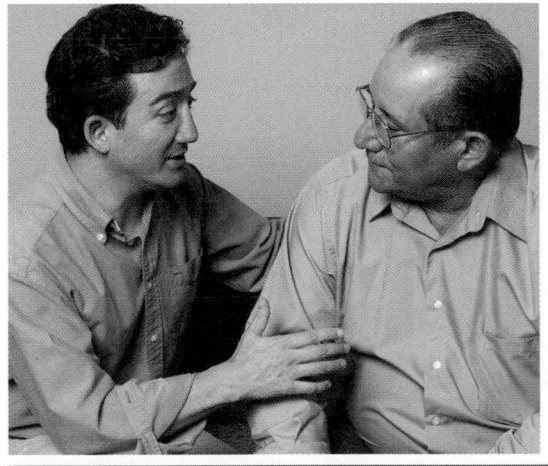

Imbalanced Nutrition: More Than Body Requirements related to inappropriate food choices and serving size, as evidenced by body mass index (BMI) of 32.67.

A. Based on the outcomes you wrote in Chapter 5, identify four possible interventions to address the diagnosis and outcomes.

B. Review the interventions, and identify two that would be most appropriate for the patient given all of the information you have about his health status.

C. Write a nursing order for each of the two interventions you identified above.

THINKING CRITICALLY ABOUT THE NURSING PROCESS: PLANNING INTERVENTIONS

The exercises in the following sections allow you to practice the kind of thinking you will use as a full-spectrum nurse. Because these are critical-thinking questions, there is usually no single right answer. We do not provide answers for these questions because it is more important for you to think about the questions than to arrive at the "right" answer. These questions are designed to improve your thinking more than to "cover content." Discuss answers with your peers—discussion can stimulate critical thinking. If you have difficulty with any of these questions, consult with your instructor.

Applying the Full-Spectrum Nursing Model

Mr. Sanborn is a 65-year-old man who has come to the clinic for a complete physical checkup. He has no health complaints and his physical examination is negative except for a few minor changes associated with aging. During the interview, he tells you that he is gay, and that he has had the same partner for five years. On further questioning, he reveals that he has had numerous sex partners during his lifetime. He says, "I was wondering if I should be tested for HIV" and "Mike, that's my partner, says I ought to get a flu shot and maybe a hepatitis shot. What do you think?"

THINKING

1. *Theoretical Knowledge*: What principles and concepts do you need to know in order to help Mr. Sanborn today?

2. *Inquiry*: Which of those do you already know enough about, and which ones will you have to study further?

DOING

3. *Practical Knowledge*: What psychomotor and communication skills will you need in order to help Mr. Sanborn?

4. *Nursing Process (Assessment)*: What further data do you need about Mr. Sanborn's sexual activity?

5. *Nursing Process (Planning Interventions)*: What is one important nursing intervention for today?

CARING

6. *Self-Knowledge*: How do you feel about same-sex relationships? Would you be able to care for Mr. Sanborn effectively?

7. *Ethical Knowledge*: What does the ANA *Nursing Code of Ethics* say about relationships to patients and the nature of patient health problems. To see the *Nursing Code of Ethics,*

   Go to http://nursingworld.org/ethics/code/protected_nwcoe813.htm

   If you are in Canada, click on "Code of Ethics" when you

   Go to http://www.cna-nurses.ca/cna/default_e.aspx

Critical Thinking and Clinical Reasoning

1. Recall the Quinns from Chapter 5. Merle Quinn is visiting a family planning clinic, where she has just been informed that she is 6 weeks pregnant. She looks worried and makes the following statements: "This is a shock. I've just started a new business and I need to work 7 days a week to make it go. . . . I don't know if I am ready to be a mother. . . ." Her husband agrees: "I just don't see how we can afford this. We don't even have any insurance now."

"Still," Mrs. Quinn says, "I don't see how I could deal with having an abortion. My parents would be devastated. I'm sure they'd never speak to me again." Her husband says, "Not to speak of the fact that the Church forbids it. It would be a sin."

A week later Mrs. Quinn calls the clinic crying. She says she has not been able to eat or sleep and that she doesn't know what to do about her pregnancy. "I don't want this baby, but I can't bring myself to have an abortion." The nurse diagnoses Decisional Conflict related to this unexpected/unwanted pregnancy and inability to accept the only perceived alternative (abortion), as evidenced by statements of indecision, tearfulness, and inability to sleep. The nurse makes an appointment to see Mr. and Mrs. Quinn that same day. Imagine that you are the nurse writing the care plan for the Quinns.

a. *Critical Thinking and Self-Knowledge*: *Analyze your assumptions.* To set aside your assumptions and care for the Quinns, you will need to focus on the Quinns' immediate problem, Decisional Conflict, rather than thinking about what they "ought to do." Remember, the nurse's role is not to make decisions for clients, but to provide information, clarification, and support.

- What questions must you ask in this case to analyze your assumptions?
- What are the answers to those questions?

b. *Critical Thinking and Knowledge of Patient Situation (Context):*

- What is going on in the Quinns' lives that may affect your choice of interventions?
- What is going on with Mrs. Quinn's health status that may affect your choice of interventions?

Now imagine that the nurse has written the following care plan for today's visit with the Quinns:

Outcomes

NOC Outcomes
Decision Making

Participation: Health Care Decisions

Individualized Goals
By the end of this visit, clients will:
1. Verbalize and demonstrate decreased anxiety and stress.
2. Verbalize awareness that they have options for coping with whatever decision they make about the pregnancy.
3. Discuss with the nurse options for continuing or terminating the pregnancy.
4. Verbalize intent to discuss their feelings with family (i.e., their parents).
5. Verbalize intent to discuss feelings with a member of the clergy.

Interventions

NIC Interventions
Decision-Making Support

Family Planning: Contraception

Family Planning: Unplanned Pregnancy

Computer-Generated Nursing Activities
1. Offer emotional support.
2. Inform client(s) of alternative views or solutions.
3. Help to identify advantages and disadvantages of each alternative.
4. Encourage client(s) to explore options, including termination, keeping the infant, or adoption.
5. Provide information as requested by client(s).
6. Serve as liaison between patient and family.
7. Assist in identifying support system.
8. Refer to community agency for counseling, if needed (e.g., family-planning clinic).
9. Discuss factors related to unplanned pregnancy (e.g., no use or misuse of contraceptives).
10. Teach and clarify misinformation about contraceptive use.
11. Teach regarding preparation and procedures.
12. Monitor for complications of procedure.

c. *Nursing Process:* Draw a line through the NIC intervention that, based on its label alone, does *not* appear to be relevant to producing the stated goals. (Note that it also does not appear that it would relieve the problem, reduce the etiology, or relieve Mrs. Quinn's symptoms of anxiety and distress.)

d. *Nursing Process*: Which of the computer-generated activities is/are *not* appropriate for today's visit with the Quinns?

e. *Nursing Process*: For which individualized outcome is there apparently *not* a computer-generated nursing activity?

f. *Critical Thinking*: Look at intervention 6 ("Serve as liaison between patient and family"). What critical-thinking questions should you ask about that intervention with regard to:

- Contextual awareness?
- Credible sources?
- Reflecting skeptically?

g. *Critical Thinking (Prioritizing)*: Which of the computer-generated interventions will you probably need to do first today?

h. *Critical Thinking (Prioritizing)*: Look at computer-generated interventions 2, 3, and 4. Which of these is it most important to do today? Which one could you encourage the Quinns to do during the next week or so? Why?

i. *Nursing Process (Planning Interventions)*: What would you need to do to intervention 1 to turn it into a nursing order that another nurse could use to care for the Quinns?

j. *Nursing Process (Assessment)*: What questions would you need to ask to individualize intervention 1 for the Quinns' care plan?

2. For each of the following concepts, use critical thinking to describe how or why it is important to nursing, patient care, or the process of planning interventions. Note that these are *not* to be merely definitions.

Nursing interventions/strategies/ activities/actions	The nursing diagnosis etiology
Individualized interventions	Client outcomes
Independent interventions	Critical thinking (e.g., contextual awareness, reflecting skeptically)
Collaborative interventions	Computerized care planning program
Dependent interventions	Standardized intervention vocabularies
Theories	Nursing Interventions Classification (NIC)
Research	Wellness interventions
Evidence-based practice	Spiritual care interventions
The patient's problem status	Nursing orders

What Are the Main Points in This Chapter?

➤ Nursing interventions are treatments that nurses perform: (1) in response to nursing diagnoses and (2) for the purpose of achieving client outcomes.

➤ Nursing interventions include such activities as teaching, counseling and emotional support, referral, physical care, and environmental management.

➤ Independent interventions are nurse-initiated treatments—those that nurses perform or delegate based on their knowledge and skills.

➤ Nursing interventions are performed for the purpose of assessing health status, preventing and treating disease/illness, and promoting health.

➤ The RN is responsible for choosing interventions and writing nursing orders; however, the RN can delegate actual performance of some interventions to nursing assistive personnel (NAP) and LPN/LVNs.

➤ Theories influence your perspective: What you notice and identify as a problem, as well as how you define a problem, more or less determines your choice of interventions.

➤ Ideally, a nursing intervention should have a sound basis in research.

➤ When generating interventions, nurses use critical thinking skills such as making interdisciplinary connections, predicting, generalizing, explaining, and making therapeutic judgments.

➤ The American Nurses Association has approved the following three standardized vocabularies for nursing interventions: (1) the Nursing Interventions Classification (NIC), (2) the Omaha System (developed for community health nursing), and (3) the Clinical Care Classification (CCC).

➤ Standardized vocabularies are especially useful in agencies that have computerized care planning systems.

➤ Standardized vocabularies include terminology for describing wellness interventions and spiritual interventions.

➤ Nursing orders, written on the nursing care plan, consist of the detailed instructions for performing nursing interventions.

For practice questions for this chapter,

 Go to **NCLEX-Style Practice Quiz,** on the Student Resource Disk or DavisPlus at http://davisplus.fadavis.com/Wilkinson2

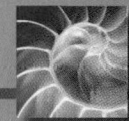

Knowledge Map

Planning Interventions

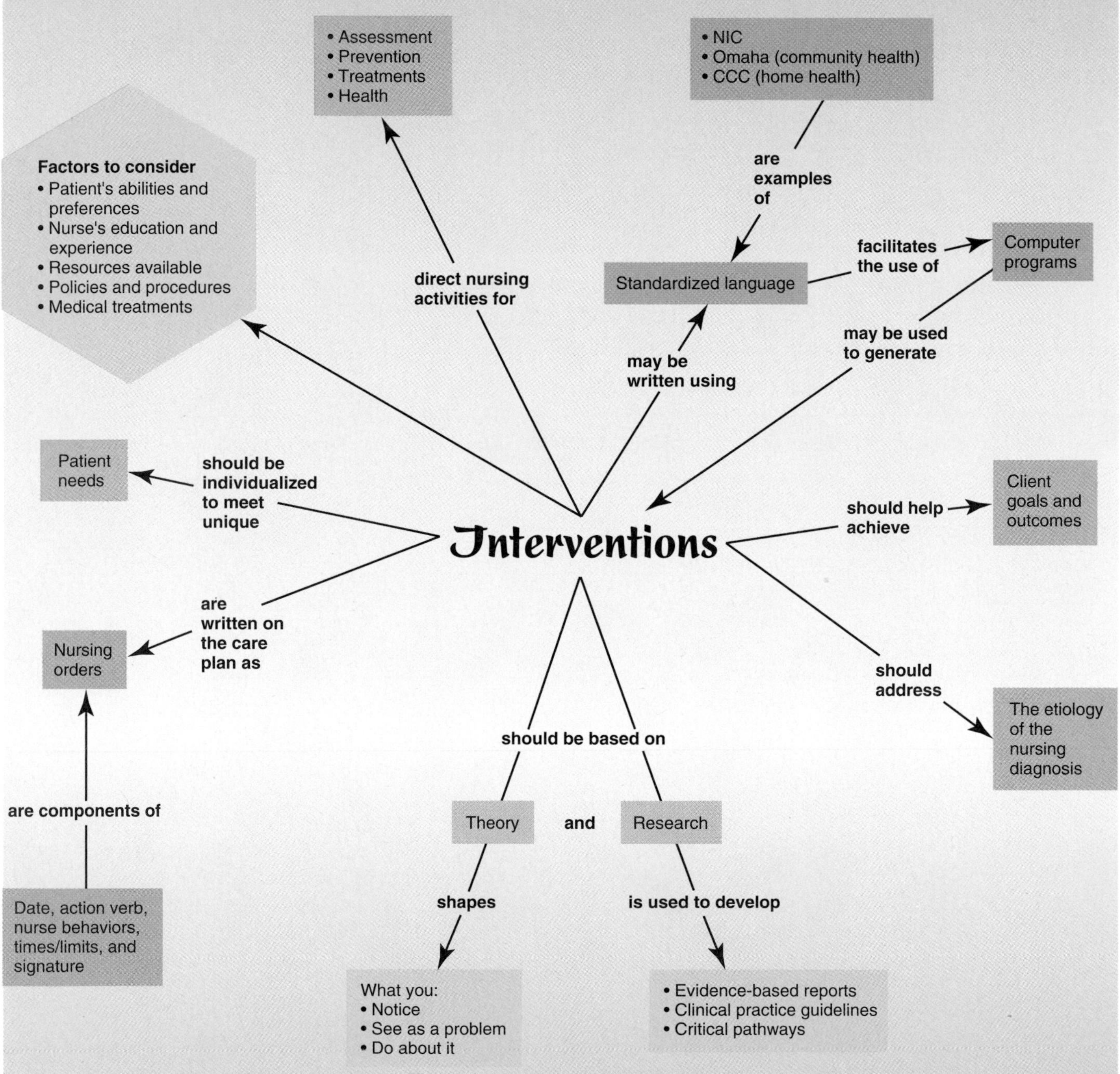

• Assessment
• Prevention
• Treatments
• Health

• NIC
• Omaha (community health)
• CCC (home health)

are examples of

Factors to consider
• Patient's abilities and preferences
• Nurse's education and experience
• Resources available
• Policies and procedures
• Medical treatments

direct nursing activities for

facilitates the use of

Computer programs

Standardized language

may be written using

may be used to generate

Patient needs

should be individualized to meet unique

Interventions

should help achieve

Client goals and outcomes

are written on the care plan as

Nursing orders

should address

The etiology of the nursing diagnosis

are components of

should be based on

Date, action verb, nurse behaviors, times/limits, and signature

Theory   **and**   Research

shapes

is used to develop

What you:
• Notice
• See as a problem
• Do about it

• Evidence-based reports
• Clinical practice guidelines
• Critical pathways

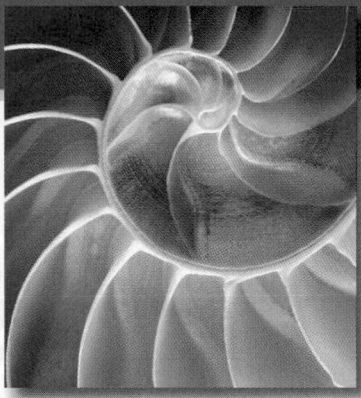

Nursing Process: Implementation & Evaluation

For a podcast of an overview of this chapter,

 Go to Student Resources, **Podcast – Chapter Overviews, Chapter 7,** on DavisPlus at http://davisplus.fadavis.com/ Wilkinson2

Caring for the Garcias

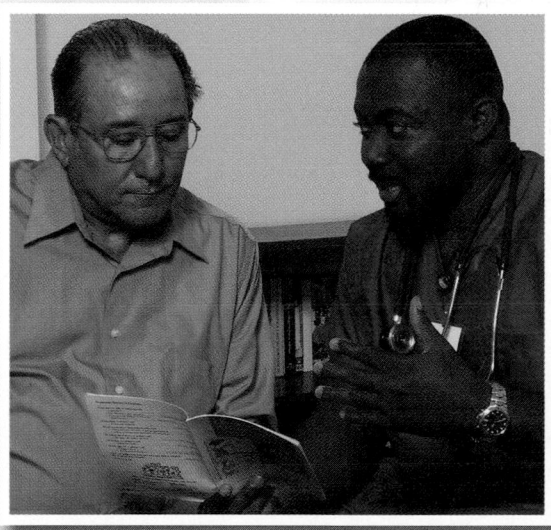

The exercises in the following section allow you to practice the kind of thinking you will use as a full spectrum nurse. Because these are critical-thinking questions, there is usually no single right answer. We do not provide answers for these questions because it is more important for you to think about the questions than to arrive at the "right" answer. These questions are designed to improve your thinking more than to "cover content." Discuss answers with your peers—discussion can stimulate critical thinking. If you have difficulty with any of these questions, consult with your instructor.

The following information is recorded on Mr. Garcia's clinic health record:

> 9/1/11 Imbalanced Nutrition: More Than Body
>   Requirements related to inappropriate food choices
>   and serving size, as evidenced by BMI of 32.67
> *Outcome:* Will lose 5 lb by 10/15/2011
> *Interventions:*

- Collect 3-day nutrition history 9/2/2011 through 9/4/2011.
- Have patient meet with clinic nurse for diet review and nutrition instruction 9/8/2011.
- Provide sample meal plans at 9/8/2011 instruction.
- Phone patient 9/22/2011 to discuss nutrition questions and review progress.
- Have patient return to clinic 10/15/2011 for follow-up visit.

A. What must you do before implementing each nursing intervention?

B. Identify at least two strategies that will help promote Mr. Garcia's participation in and adherence to the plan.

C. How will you determine whether Mr. Garcia has met his goal?

Practical **Knowledge**
knowing how

When implementing and evaluating care, you will need to make good decisions about administering and delegating care. In this section, you will find forms to help you delegate, implement, and evaluate patient care.

Implementation and Evaluation Tools

The first tool in this section (below) is a checklist to help you delegate tasks wisely. It is followed by a Worksheet for Organizing Nursing Care, and then by a delegation grid (also to help you make delegation decisions).

The Worksheet for Organizing Nursing Care allows you to see at a glance the total work you need to accomplish for all your patients. Write on it, in priority order, only the most important things you must accomplish during this one. Room numbers take up less space than names on the form; but do not begin thinking of your patients by room number or diagnosis. They are people, with names. At first, you may also need to make a time-sequenced list, the size of a 3 × 5 card, to help you organize your day. For example, it might read in part:

0700 – Assessments, all patients, begin with Room 310.
0730 – Ambulation: 315, 318
0800 – Change IV, meds 310; check intake
0815 – Meds 315, 318, 319; check intake
0845 – Toilet and bath, 310
and so on.

Worksheet for Organizing Nursing Care

	Patient 1	Patient 2	Patient 3	Patient 4	Patient 5
Room #					
Name pt. prefers					
Admitting diagnosis					
Significant others					
Current health status (received in report). Does the care plan need to be modified?					
Basic care needs: Hygiene Elimination Feeding Dressing Other					
Safety precautions					
Medications					
IVs					
Tests and treatments today					
Prioritized nursing diagnoses					
Interventions that must be done today					
New medical orders to implement					
Teaching and counseling today					

The Five Rights of Delegation—Checklist

Right Task *(Can I delegate it?)*

The task is:

—Delegable for a specific patient.

—Within the nurse's scope of practice.

—Permitted by the state's nurse practice act.

—Permitted by the agency's policies.

Right Circumstance *(Should I delegate it?)*

Consider patient safety:

—Is patient setting appropriate?

—Are adequate resources available?

—Other factors to maintain safety?

Right Person *(Who is best prepared to do it?)*

The right person:

—Is delegating the task (the nurse must be competent to delegate).

—Will be performing the task (the NAP must be competent to do the task).

—Will receive the care (i.e., the severity of the patient's illness is considered).

Right Direction/Communication *(What does the NAP need to know?)*

—The task is described clearly, including its objective, limits, and expectations.

—The delegatee (NAP) understands the communication.

Right Supervision *(How will I follow up?)*

—The nurse monitors, evaluates, and intervenes as needed.

—The nurse obtains feedback from the patient.

—The nurse obtains feedback from the delegatee.

Source: National Council of State Boards of Nursing. (1995). *Delegation: Concepts and decision-making process.* National Council Position Paper. Chicago: Author.

NCSBN Delegation Grid

Elements for review		Client A	Client B	Client C	Client D
Activity/Task Level of client stability	Describe activity/task: Score the client's level of stability: **Client condition:** 0 – Is chronic/stable/predictable 1 – Has minimal potential for change 2 – Has moderate potential for change 3 – Is unstable/acute/strong potential for change				
Level of NAP competence	Score the NAP competence in completing delegated nursing care activities in the defined client population: **NAP is:** 0 – Expert in activities to be delegated, in defined population 1 – Experienced in activities to be delegated, in defined population 2 – Experienced in activities but not in defined population 3 – Novice in performing activities and in defined population				
Level of licensed nurse competence	Score the licensed nurse's competence in relation to both knowledge of providing nursing care to a defined population and competence in implementation of the delegation process: 0 – Expert in the knowledge of nursing needs/activities of defined client population *and* expert in the delegation process 1 – Either expert in knowledge of needs/activities of defined client population and competent in delegation *or* experienced in the needs/activities of defined client population and expert in the delegation process 2 – Experienced in knowledge of needs/activities of defined client population *and* competent in the delegation process 3 – Either experienced in knowledge of needs/activities of defined client population *or* competent in the delegation process 4 – Novice in knowledge of defined population *and* novice in delegation				
Potential for harm	Score the potential level of risk the nursing care activity has for the client *(risk is probability of [the client] suffering harm)*: 0 – None 1 – Low 2 – Medium 3 – High				
Frequency	Score based on how often the NAP has performed the specific nursing care activity: 0 – Performed at least daily 1 – Performed at least weekly 2 – Performed at least monthly 3 – Performed less than monthly 4 – Never performed				
Level of decision making	Score the decision-making needed, related to the specific nursing care activity, client (both cognitive and physical status) and client situation: 0 – Does not require decision making 1 – Minimal level of decision making 2 – Moderate level of decision making 3 – High level of decision making				
Ability for self care	Score the client's level of assistance needed for self-care activities: 0 – No assistance 1 – Limited assistance 2 – Extensive assistance 3 – Total care or constant attendance				
Total Score					

Scoring: A low score on the grid suggests that an activity can be safely delegated. For example if a client's stability is ranked 3 (unstable) and the level of NAP competence is also 3 (novice in the activity), then you probably should *not* delegate to that NAP. Each agency should establish a policy regarding the individual and/or total scores to be considered acceptable for delegating.

Source: Used by permission from the National Council of State Boards of Nursing (NCSBN), Chicago, IL (1997). Retrieved February 1, 2008, from the NCSBN web site (www.ncsbn.org)

Evaluation Checklist

Instructions: Check the appropriate response and follow the associated instructions

Assessment Review

1. Were the assessment data complete and accurate?

___ YES. No action.   ___ NO. Reassess client. Record the new data. Change care plan as indicated

2. Have all data been validated, as needed?

___ YES. No action.   ___ NO. Validate with client (by interview and physical examination), significant others, or other professionals. Record validation (or failure to validate). Change care plan as indicated.

3. Have new data become available that require changes in the plan (e.g., a different problem etiology, new goals/ outcomes, new medical orders)?

___ NO. No action.   ___ YES. Record the new data in the progress notes; redefine problem, goals, nursing orders, as needed.

4. Has the patient's condition changed?

___ NO. No action.   ___ YES. Record data about present health status. Change care plan as indicated.

➤ *Move to a review of the diagnosis step.* ◄

Diagnosis Review

1. Is the diagnosis relevant and related to the data?

___ YES. No action.   ___ NO. Revise the diagnosis.

2. Is the diagnosis well supported by the data?

___ YES. No action.   ___ NO. Collect more data. Support or revise diagnosis.

3. Has the problem status changed (actual, potential, possible)?

___ NO. No action.   ___ YES. Restate the problem.

4. Is the diagnosis stated clearly?

___ YES. No action.   ___ NO. Revise the diagnostic statement.

5. Does the etiology correctly reflect the factors contributing to the problem?

___ YES. No action.   ___ NO. Revise the etiology.

6. Is the problem one that can be treated primarily by nursing actions?

___ YES. No action.   ___ NO. Label as collaborative and consult appropriate health professional.

7. Is the diagnosis specific and individualized to the patient?

___ YES. No action.   ___ NO. Revise diagnosis. Revise outcomes and nursing orders as suggested by the new nursing diagnosis.

8. Does the problem (diagnosis) still exist?

___ YES. No action.   ___ NO. Delete diagnosis and related outcomes and nursing orders.

➤ *Proceed to a review of client goals.* ◄

Planning Review: Outcomes

1. Have nursing diagnoses been added or revised?

___ NO. No action.   ___ YES. Write new outcomes.

2. Are the outcomes realistic in terms of patient abilities and agency resources?

___ YES. No action.   ___ NO. Revise outcomes.

3. Was sufficient time allowed for outcome achievement?

___ YES. No action.   ___ NO. Revise time frame.

4. Do the outcomes address all aspects of the client's problem?

___ YES. No action.   ___ NO. Write additional outcomes.

Evaluation Checklist *(continued)*

Assessment Review

5. Do the expected outcomes, as written, demonstrate resolution of the problem specified in the nursing diagnosis?

___ YES. No action.   ___ NO. Revise outcomes.

6. Have client priorities changed, or has the focus of care changed?

___ NO. No action.   ___ YES. Revise outcomes.

7. Is the client in agreement with the goals?

___ YES. No action.   ___ NO. Get client input. Write outcomes valued by the client.

➤ Proceed to a review of nursing orders. ◄

Planning Review: Nursing Orders

1. Have nursing diagnoses or outcomes been added or revised in previous review steps?

___ NO. No action.   ___ YES. Write new nursing orders.

2. Are the nursing orders clearly related to the stated patient outcomes?

___ YES. No action.   ___ NO. Revise or develop new nursing orders.

3. Is the rationale sufficient to justify the use of the nursing order?

___ YES. No action.   ___ NO. Revise or develop new nursing orders.

4. Are the nursing orders unclear or vague, so that other staff may have had questions about how to implement them?

___ NO. No action.   ___ YES. Revise nursing orders. Add details to make more specific or individualized to the patient.

5. Do the nursing orders include instructions for timing of the activities?

___ YES. No action.   ___ NO. Revise nursing orders: add times, schedules.

6. Was an order clearly and obviously ineffective?

___ NO. No action.   ___ YES. Delete it.

7. Are the orders realistic in terms of staff and other resources?

___ YES. No action.   ___ NO. Revise orders or obtain resources.

8. Have new resources become available that might enable you to change the goals or nursing orders?

___ NO. No action.   ___ YES. Write new goals or nursing orders reflecting the new capabilities.

9. Do the nursing orders address all aspects of the client's health goals?

___ NO. No action.   ___ NO. Add new nursing orders.

➤ Proceed to a review of implementation step ◄

Implementation Review

1. Did the nurse [or NAP] get client input at each step in developing and implementing the plan?

___ YES. No action.   ___ NO. Obtain client input, revise plan and implementation as needed. [Coach NAP or role model, as needed.]

2. Were the nursing interventions acceptable to the patient?

___ YES. No action.   ___ NO. Consult patient; change nursing orders or implementation approach.

3. Did the nurse [NAP] prepare the patient for implementation of the nursing order (e.g., explain what the patient should expect or do)?

___ YES. No action.   ___ NO. Continue same plan, but prepare patient before implementing. Reevaluate.

4. Did the nurse [NAP] have adequate knowledge and skills to perform techniques and procedures correctly?

___ YES. No action.   ___ NO. Continue same plan. Have someone else implement or help the nurse [or NAP] to acquire the needed knowledge or skills. If neither of these is possible, delete nursing order.

(continued)

---

5. Did client or family comply with the therapeutic regimen? Were self-care activities performed correctly?

   ___ YES. No action.

   ___ NO. Reassess motivation, knowledge, and resources. Add outcomes and nursing orders aimed at teaching, motivating, and supporting, patient in carrying out the regimen. Set time for reevaluation.

6. Did other staff members follow the nursing orders?

   ___ YES. No action.

   ___ NO. Implement the omitted nursing orders or ensure that others will do so. Set time for reevaluation. Find out why order was not carried out.

7. Was the plan of care implemented in a manner that communicated caring?

   ___ YES. No action.

   ___ NO. This is a problem that must be addressed by personal and staff development.

After making the necessary revisions to the care plan, implement the new plan and begin the nursing cycle again.

Source: Wilkinson, J. (2007). *Nursing process and critical thinking* (4th ed.). Upper Saddle River, NJ: Prentice Hall, pp. 409–412.

THINKING CRITICALLY ABOUT THE NURSING PROCESS: IMPLEMENTATION & EVALUATION

The exercises in the following sections allow you to practice the kind of thinking you will use as a full-spectrum nurse. Because these are critical-thinking questions, there is usually no single right answer. We do not provide answers for these questions because it is more important for you to think about the questions than to arrive at the "right" answer. These questions are designed to improve your thinking more than to "cover content." Discuss answers with your peers—discussion can stimulate critical thinking. If you have difficulty with any of these questions, consult with your instructor.

Applying the Full-Spectrum Nursing Model

Recall Jeannette Wu from Volume 1. She is a very thin 80-year-old woman who has just been admitted to a skilled nursing facility after fracturing her hip. Her hip was surgically repaired 4 days ago, but because of her overall fragile health and some postsurgery confusion, her recovery is slower than usual. One of her nursing diagnoses is Self-Care Deficit (Bathing/Hygiene, Dressing/Grooming, and Toileting) related to weakness, pain, confusion, and decreased mobility. Her nursing orders include (NIC) Bathing and Self-Care: Activities of Daily Living (ADLs). As the nurse is helping a newly hired nursing assistive personnel (NAP) with Mrs. Wu's bath, she notices a reddened area on Mrs. Wu's sacrum. Realizing that this may be the beginning of a pressure ulcer, the nurse observes carefully and notes a small skin excoriation (abrasion) in the area. She repositions Mrs. Wu to prevent further pressure on her sacrum. After finishing the bath, the nurse records her findings and enters on Mrs. Wu's care plan a nursing diagnosis of Impaired Skin Integrity related to impaired bed mobility and minimal subcutaneous tissue. She writes appropriate nursing orders, including an order to observe skin over bony prominences every 4 hours, and then delegates to the NAP the task of turning and repositioning Mrs. Wu every 2 hours.

THINKING

1. *Theoretical Knowledge*:

   a. What facts and principles do you already know about the causes of pressure ulcers?

   b. Do you have enough information to provide interventions for Mrs. Wu's actual Impaired Skin Integrity? If not, what do you still need to find out?

2. *Critical Thinking (Inquiry)*: What resource would be best to use to find out exactly what is meant by Mrs. Wu's diagnosis of Self-Care Deficit? Why?

DOING

3. *Practical Knowledge*: What do you know about positioning patients? How would you explain to the NAP about how to position Mrs. Wu "to prevent further pressure on her sacrum"?

4. *Nursing Process (Evaluation)*:

   a. To evaluate Mrs. Wu's Impaired Skin Integrity problem, what reassessments would you make?

   b. To evaluate Mrs. Wu's Self-Care Deficit problem, what reassessments would you make? Who can or should make them? How often, or when, would you reassess?

CARING

5. *Self-Knowledge*: How comfortable would you be caring for Mrs. Wu, who is a frail older adult? What is one problem, not described in the scenario, that might arise?

Critical Thinking and Clinical Reasoning

1. You are working a 12-hour shift (1900 to 0700) on a medical unit at a local hospital. You will be caring for six adult patients. Make a list of the theoretical and practical knowledge you need about the patients to begin organizing your work for the shift. You may not yet have enough experience to make a complete list, but speculate about the kinds of information you think you might need. For example, to organize your work, you will need to know whether you have an NAP or LVN/LPN to assist you or whether you are providing total care for the patients.

2. Create a form for organizing your work. You will need to use a separate sheet of paper for this. Be sure it has space for at least six patients. You might begin by making a column for each patient's name and age, for example. Be sure to leave enough room to write the necessary information. For example, you will need more room to write the patients' tests and treatments than for writing in age and gender.

3. Alma Newport, who is 80 years old, has diabetes, severe arthritis, and mild dementia secondary to Alzheimer's disease. She lives alone. She refuses to consider an assisted living facility or nursing home, although her primary provider and children, who live out of town, believe it would be safer for her to do so. On more than one occasion, she has forgotten to turn off a stove burner while cooking, burning the contents of the pan and smoking up the house.

   A home health nurse visits Mrs. Newport once a week. The physician wants Mrs. Newport to check and record her blood sugar levels before each meal. When the nurse asks, she says her blood sugar level is "OK" and shows the nurse the record she has kept, on which she has recorded many extremely low readings (e.g., 17, 20, 80, 24, 17 mg/dL). When the nurse checks Mrs. Newport's blood sugar, she obtains a reading of 210. After calibrating the glucose meter, the nurse writes the following care plan:

   Nursing Diagnosis:
   Deficient Knowledge related to cognitive deficits secondary to dementia

   Desired Outcomes:
   Mrs. Newport will demonstrate correct method for checking her blood sugar by next visit.

   Mrs. Newport will obtain correct readings.

   Nursing Orders:
   Teach correct method of fingerstick and checking blood glucose.

   Evaluate patient's technique at each visit.

   Over the next few weeks, the home health nurse checks Mrs. Newport's log and fingerstick method at each visit. The logs continue to show low readings, and Mrs. Newport remains unable to perform a fingerstick blood glucose test correctly in spite of repeated demonstrations.

   a. Evaluate Mrs. Newport's progress. Has she met, partially met, or not met the desired outcome?

   b. What possible reasons may account for your evaluation (of Mrs. Newport's outcome status)? Hints:
      (1) Use your theoretical knowledge and personal experience with physical changes that occur with aging.
      (2) Use the data you have about Mrs. Newport.
      (3) Use your practical knowledge about nursing diagnoses.

4. A NAP is helping a patient with a shower when her pager goes off. After ensuring the patient's safety, the NAP goes into the hallway and answers her page. You observe that the NAP is still wearing her gloves. How would you handle this situation?

5. For each of the following concepts, use critical thinking to describe how or why it is important to nursing, patient care, or the processes of implementing and evaluating. Note that these are *not* to be merely definitions.

Overlapping (of implementation and other nursing process steps)
Preparing for implementation
Client participation and adherence
Coordination of care
Delegation of care
The "five rights" of delegation

Supervision
Reflecting critically about implementation
Evaluation
Outcomes evaluation
Evaluative statements
Quality assurance programs

What Are the Main Points in This Chapter?

➤ Implementation is the nursing process phase in which you perform or delegate the nursing activities that were planned in preceding steps.

➤ Before performing interventions, you should organize supplies and equipment and ensure the client's readiness.

➤ While implementing care, you will continue to make assessments and evaluate client responses.

➤ Collaboration and coordination of care are important nursing functions.

➤ Delegation is the transfer of responsibility for an action while retaining the accountability for the outcome— this implies that you must supervise those to whom you delegate care.

➤ The "five rights" of delegation are: right task, right circumstance, right person, right direction/ communication, and right supervision.

➤ The final activity in the implementation step is documentation of the care provided. Documenting client responses is actually a part of the evaluation phase; however, you will document both at the same time, often in the same note.

➤ Evaluation is the final step of the nursing process; it is a planned, ongoing, systematic activity in which you use predetermined standards and criteria to make judgments about: (1) patient progress toward health goals; (2) the effectiveness of the nursing care plan; and (3) the overall quality of care on a unit, in an organization, or in a geographical area.

➤ When evaluating client health status, you will compare the client's present data/responses to the desired outcomes (goals) set in the planning outcomes phase.

➤ When evaluating the effectiveness of the nursing care plan, remember that you cannot control all of the variables that influence the success of a nursing activity.

➤ Quality improvement programs are specially designed to promote excellence in nursing; they include structure, process, and outcomes evaluation.

For practice questions for this chapter,

 Go to **NCLEX-Style Chapter Quiz,** on the Student Resource Disk or DavisPlus at http://davisplus.fadavis.com/Wilkinson2

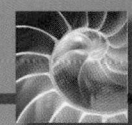

Knowledge Map

Implementation and Evaluation

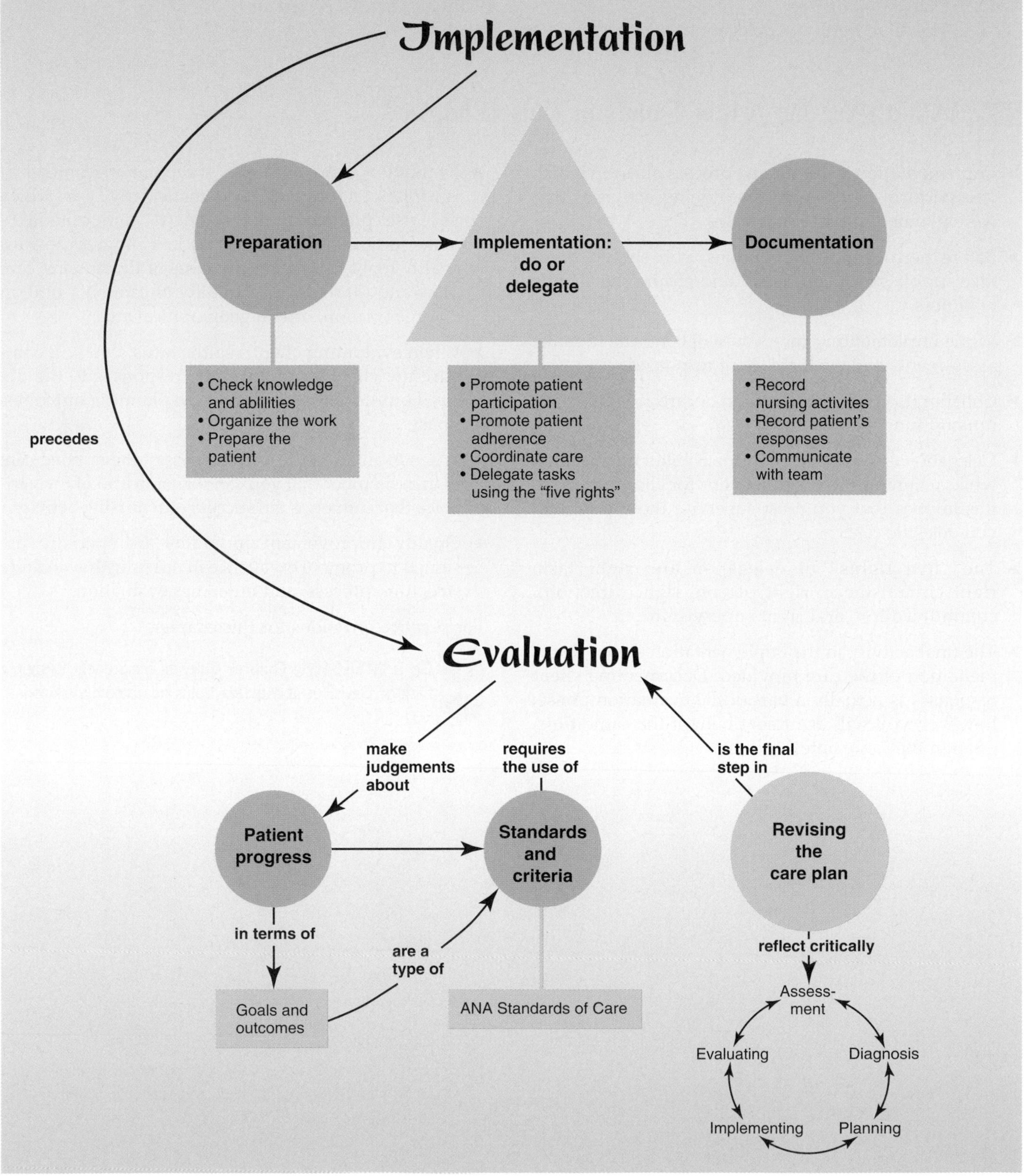

Implementation

Preparation → **Implementation: do or delegate** → **Documentation**

precedes

- Check knowledge and abilities
- Organize the work
- Prepare the patient

- Promote patient participation
- Promote patient adherence
- Coordinate care
- Delegate tasks using the "five rights"

- Record nursing activites
- Record patient's responses
- Communicate with team

Evaluation

make judgements about → **Patient progress**

requires the use of → **Standards and criteria**

is the final step in → **Revising the care plan**

Patient progress → requires the use of → **Standards and criteria**

in terms of → Goals and outcomes

are a type of → Standards and criteria

ANA Standards of Care

reflect critically → Assessment

Assessment → Diagnosis → Planning → Implementing → Evaluating (cycle)

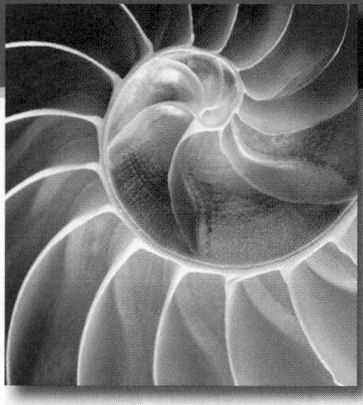

CHAPTER 8

Nursing Theory & Research

For a podcast of an overview of this chapter,

 Go to Student Resources, **Podcast – Chapter Overviews, Chapter 8,** on DavisPlus at http://davisplus.fadavis.com/ Wilkinson2

Caring for the Garcias

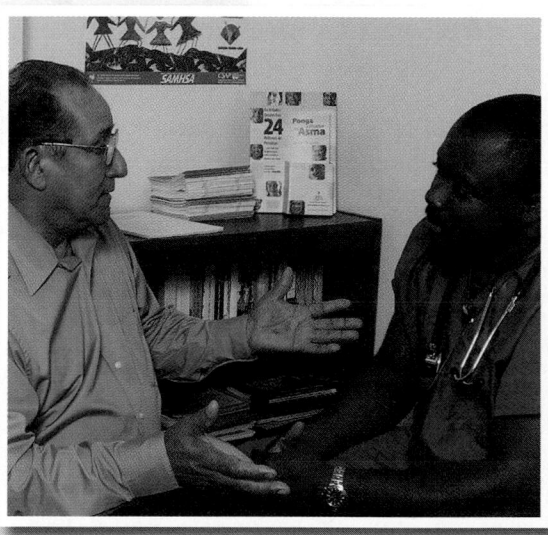

The exercises in the following section allow you to practice the kind of thinking you will use as a full-spectrum nurse. Because these are critical-thinking questions, there is usually no single right answer. We do not provide answers for these questions because it is more important for you to think about the questions than to arrive at the "right" answer. These questions are designed to improve your thinking more than to "cover content." Discuss answers with your peers—discussion can stimulate critical thinking. If you have difficulty with any of these questions, consult with your instructor.

Mr. Garcia arrives at the clinic for a follow-up visit. As you may recall, he has been diagnosed with hypertension. At a previous visit, you wrote a nursing diagnosis of Imbalanced Nutrition: More Than Body Requirements related to inappropriate food choices and serving size, as evidenced by a body mass index (BMI) of 32.67.

Today you have gathered the following intake data:

Blood pressure: 174/96 mm Hg
Heart rate: 88 beats/min
Respiratory rate: 18 breaths/min
Temperature: 98.5°F
Weight: 236 lb

A. What observations can you make about today's data in comparison to his initial visit?

B. As part of the treatment plan for Mr. Garcia, you have been asked to educate him about a diet to assist with weight loss and hypertension management. How would you determine the most appropriate diet to include in your treatment plan?

C. A number of sources recommend the DASH (Dietary Approaches to Stop Hypertension) eating plan. Go to the Internet and search for "Dietary Approaches to Stop Hypertension." Is there sufficient research to support incorporating this information into Mr. Garcia's treatment plan? If so, describe the research, and summarize the DASH eating plan.

69

THINKING CRITICALLY ABOUT NURSING THEORY AND RESEARCH

The exercises in the following sections allow you to practice the kind of thinking you will use as a full-spectrum nurse. Because these are critical-thinking questions, there is usually no single right answer. We do not provide answers for these questions because it is more important for you to think about the questions than to arrive at the "right" answer. These questions are designed to improve your thinking more than to "cover content." Discuss answers with your peers—discussion can stimulate critical thinking. If you have difficulty with any of these questions, consult with your instructor.

Applying the Full-Spectrum Nursing Model

PATIENT SITUATION

You are caring for a 90-year-old patient in a long-term care facility. He is completely dependent for activities of daily living. In addition, he has been unresponsive, cannot swallow safely, and for many months has been receiving fluids and nutrition through a feeding tube. His adult grandson has recently discovered a living will, in which the patient had stated that he does not wish to be kept alive by "artificial means, including being tube fed." The grandson, John, insists that the patient's wishes be honored, but the patient's son (Mr. Lee) threatens a lawsuit if the caregivers discontinue the feedings. They argue loudly, and Mr. Lee yells to his son, "You just want him gone because you're in a hurry to get his money! You know you're getting the major part of it."

THINKING

1. *Theoretical Knowledge*: What facts are important to know in order to decide whether or not to stop the feedings?

2. *Critical Thinking (Analyzing Assumptions)*: Without thinking too carefully about it, what is your first thought about what is causing the disagreement between the Mr. Lee and his son, John? Examine your assumption. How certain are you it is true? What else might be going on in their lives to cause father and son to disagree on this issue?

DOING

3. *Nursing Process (Assessment)*: In order to provide some information about the patient that might be helpful in restoring peace between Mr. Lee and Todd, what patient assessments should you make?

CARING

4. *Ethical Knowledge*: State one ethical issue involved in this case—or one moral problem that it would be present for you if you were involved in it.

Critical Thinking and Clinical Reasoning

1. Recall the scenario about Mr. Wilkey in Volume 1. Imagine you are the charge nurse on the night shift at a long-term care facility. You hear the nursing assistant (NA) and another voice talking loudly down the hall. You immediately go to see what has happened. You are surprised and shocked by what you see. An older patient, Mr. Wilkey, is in bed with another patient, Mrs. Fredrickson, who is crying and shouting, "Get out! Get out!" Mr. Wilkey is tearful and looks frightened. He keeps repeating, "Where is Momma? Where is Momma?" The NA is visibly upset and is grabbing at Mr. Wilkey in an effort to get him out of the bed. Use any nursing theory you wish, or your own idea, and describe each of the following concepts as they apply in this scenario:

   a. Patient (Who is the patient? How do you know?)

   b. Nurse (Who is the nurse? What is she doing that is "nursing"?)

   c. Health (Is the patient healthy? What is the patient's state of health?)

   d. Environment (Where is the nurse–patient encounter occurring?)

2. Recall Maslow's hierarchy of needs. Give one example of a specific nursing intervention a nurse could do to meet each of those needs. If you think the nurse cannot address a need, say why.

   a. Physiological

   b. Safety and security (mental and physical protection)

   c. Love and belonging

   d. Self-esteem (achievement, reputation)

   e. Cognitive needs (knowledge, self-awareness)

   f. Aesthetic needs (beauty, balance, form)

   g. Self-actualization (personal growth, fulfillment)

   h. Transcendence (helping others to self-actualize)

3. You are an emergency department nurse taking care of a 4-year-old child who has had a bike accident. The child has an open abrasion and a few cuts that will require some minor care.

   a. Using Nightingale's theory, what interventions might you use?

   b. Using Watson's theory, what might you do?

   c. Using Henderson's theory, what would be the focus of your interventions?

   d. Choose one of the following theories: Neuman, Orem, or Rogers. Look it up on the URL listed in

 Volume I or on the Student Resource Disk.

   Describe how that theory would direct you in this case.

4. You are working the night shift, and while making your 0200 rounds, you are surprised. As you look into the room of 22-year-old Angela Kindred, you see her mother sitting at her bedside sobbing. Visits are not encouraged at that time of night, and you didn't know Mrs. Kindred was on the floor. Even though Angela's leukemia prognosis is terminal, you understood from the day nurse that the family, as well as Angela, had accepted the inevitable outcome. Explain how you can demonstrate caring to this mother, who will soon lose her beloved daughter. Look at Watson's (1988) ten caring processes below. How can you use them to demonstrate caring to this mother and daughter? Be specific in your answers.

Watson's Ten Caring Processes:

1. Forming a humanistic–altruistic system of values
2. Instilling faith and hope
3. Cultivating sensitivity to self and others
4. Forming helping and trusting relationships
5. Conveying and accepting the expression of positive and negative feelings
6. Systematic use of the scientific problem-solving method that involves caring process

7. Promoting transpersonal teaching–learning
8. Providing for supportive, protective, and corrective mental, physical, sociocultural, and spiritual environment
9. Assisting with gratification of human needs
10. Sensitivity to existential–phenomenological forces

5. You are an emergency department nurse taking care of a 4-year-old child who has had a bike accident. The child has an open abrasion and a few cuts that will require some minor care. However, he is frightened and crying, even though his mother is sitting in the treatment room with him. You ask the mother to hold the child while he is being treated and restrain him, if necessary. In reflecting on this intervention afterward, you decide to find the best evidence for your intervention to be certain you will want to use it in similar situations in the future. Write a PICO question to guide your literature search. Write each part, then write the full statement.

P—

I—

C—

O—

Full statement of the question.

6. Read analytically an article in a research journal. Answer the following questions about the article.

a. What is the article about as a whole? Answer using one sentence.

b. What are the author's main conclusions?

c. Do you think these conclusions are true? If not, why not?

d. Is this article of any significance in nursing? That is how could it be used to improve patient care or nursing education?

7. For each of the following concepts, use critical thinking to describe how or why it is important to nursing, patient care, or nursing theory and research. Note that these are *not* to be merely definitions.

Nursing theory   Nursing research
The science of human caring   Institutional review Board
From novice to expert   Informed consent
Culturally competent care   Research utilization
Evidence-based practice   Analytic reading

What Are the Main Points in This Chapter?

➤ According to Florence Nightingale, nursing theories describe "what is" and "what is not" nursing.

➤ The four basic components of a nursing theory are person, nurse, environment, and health.

➤ A theory is developed by recognizing a need in nursing or by having an idea, using research to determine whether the idea is effective, and then using the research results to define a theory.

➤ Theories help nurses (1) find meaning in their experiences of nursing; (2) organize their thinking around pertinent ideas; and (3) develop new, evidence-based ideas and insights into the work they do.

➤ Nurses use theories as an evidence-based framework for their nursing practice.

➤ Three leaders in nursing caring theories are Dr. Jean Watson, Dr. Patricia Benner, and Dr. Madeleine Leininger.

➤ Nursing research is a systematic, objective process of analyzing phenomena of importance in nursing.

➤ Quantitative research may be generalized to populations similar to the one studied. It has tight controls and large numbers of participants, and the data are statistically analyzed.

➤ Qualitative research tells the lived experience of a person or group of people. It is analyzed by examining the words and actions of a small number of participants.

➤ The research process is a systematic way of organizing, preparing, and presenting research.

➤ Research participants (people in a research study) are protected from harm by specific laws and regulations.

➤ Research reports are critiqued by reading analytically and using preselected criteria.

➤ Nursing research evolved slowly. The advanced education currently available to nurses is propelling research forward.

➤ Evidence-based nursing requires evaluating research to find the best evidence, and then applying it in practice.

➤ The process of finding best evidence consists of: identifying a clinical nursing problem, formulating a searchable question, searching the literature, evaluating the quality of the research, and integrating the research into practice.

➤ The parts of a PICO question are: **P**atient problem, **I**ntervention, **C**omparison intervention, and **O**utcome.

For practice questions for this chapter,

 Go to **NCLEX-Style Chapter Quiz,** on the Student Resource Disk or on DavisPlus at http://davisplus.fadavis.com/Wilkinson2

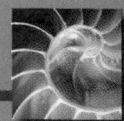 # Knowledge Map

Theory and Research

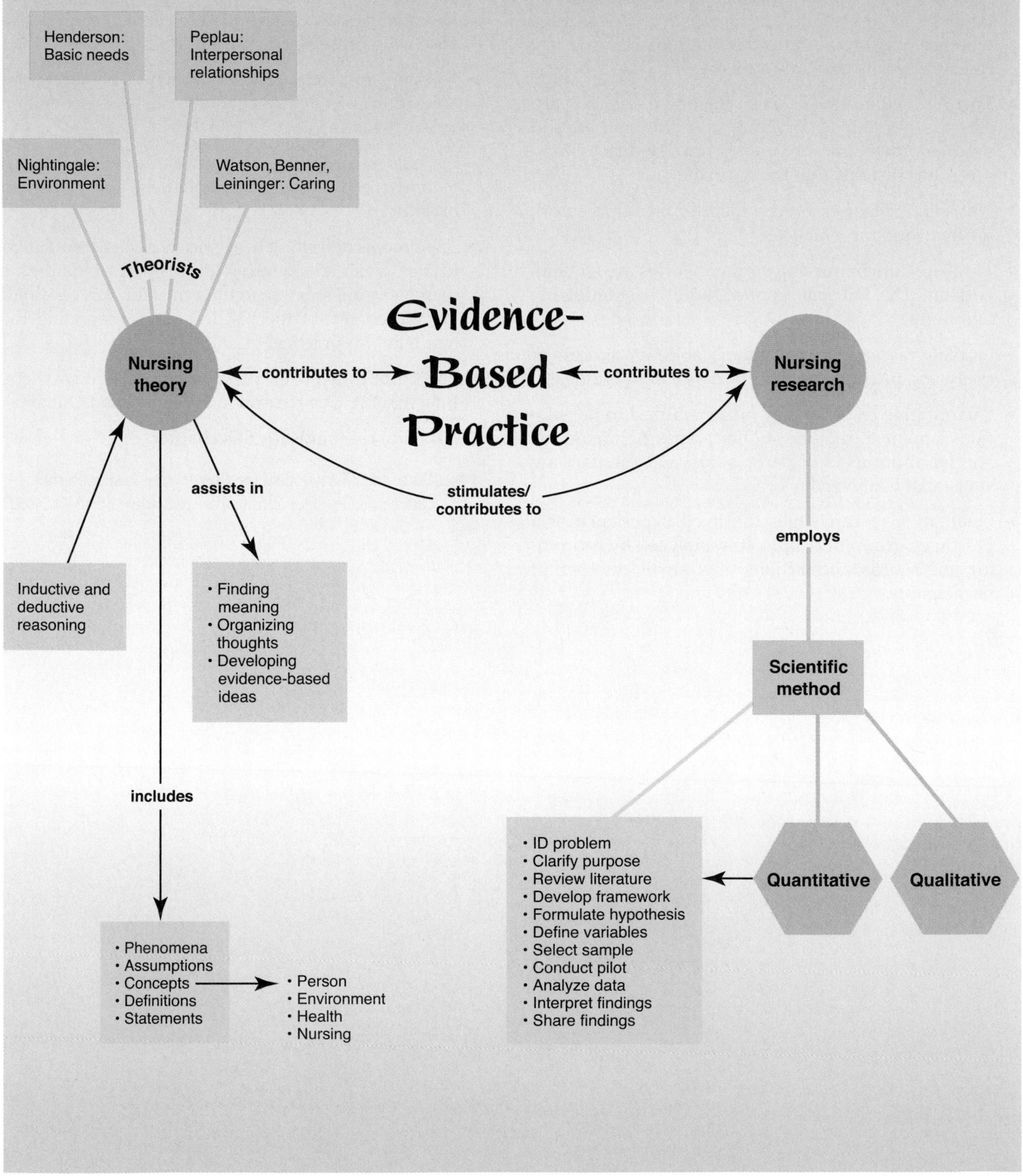

Henderson: Basic needs

Peplau: Interpersonal relationships

Nightingale: Environment

Watson, Benner, Leininger: Caring

Theorists

Nursing theory

→ contributes to →

Evidence-Based Practice

← contributes to ←

Nursing research

assists in

stimulates/ contributes to

employs

Inductive and deductive reasoning

• Finding meaning
• Organizing thoughts
• Developing evidence-based ideas

Scientific method

includes

• Phenomena
• Assumptions
• Concepts
• Definitions
• Statements

• Person
• Environment
• Health
• Nursing

• ID problem
• Clarify purpose
• Review literature
• Develop framework
• Formulate hypothesis
• Define variables
• Select sample
• Conduct pilot
• Analyze data
• Interpret findings
• Share findings

← **Quantitative**

Qualitative

Factors Affecting Health

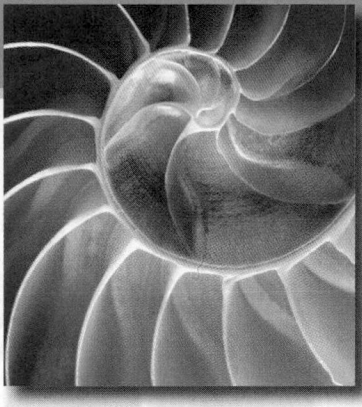

CHAPTER 9

Development Across the Life Span

For a podcast of an overview of this chapter,

 Go to Student Resources, **Podcast – Chapter Overviews, Chapter 9,** on DavisPlus at http://davisplus.fadavis.com/ Wilkinson2

Before working the thinking exercises in this chapter,

 Go to Chapter 9, **Development Through the Life Span— Expanded Discussion,** on the Student Resource Disk or DavisPlus at http://davisplus.fadavis.com/Wilkinson2

Caring for the Garcias

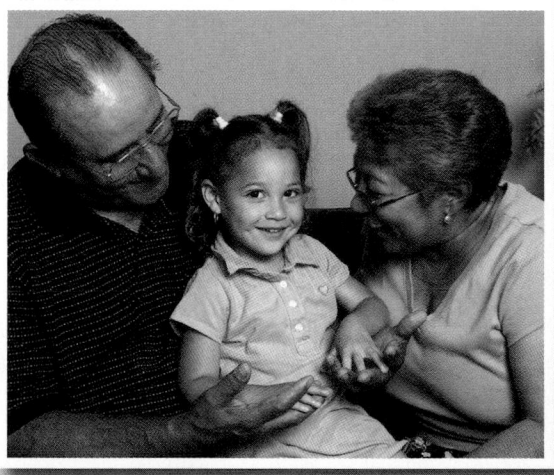

The exercises in the following section allow you to practice the kind of thinking you will use as a full-spectrum nurse. Because these are critical-thinking questions, there is usually no single right answer. We do not provide answers for these questions because it is more important for you to think about the questions than to arrive at the "right" answer. These questions are designed to improve your thinking more than to "cover content." Discuss answers with your peers—discussion can stimulate critical thinking. If you have difficulty with any of these questions, consult with your instructor.

Review the scenario of Joseph Garcia, in the "Meet the Garcias" section before Chapter 1 of this book. Answer the following questions based on that scenario.

A. Evaluate Mr. Garcia's physical health status in comparison to what is expected for someone in his age group.

B. Mr. Garcia and his wife are raising their 3-year-old granddaughter. What effect might this have on Mr. Garcia's ability to accomplish his developmental tasks?

Practical **Knowledge**
knowing how

One important aspect of developmental care across the lifespan is to identify abuse and intervene with patients who are being abused.

Procedures

For a discussion of child and elder abuse and domestic partner violence,

 Go to Chapter 9, **Development Through the Life Span—Expanded Discussion,** on the Student Resource Disk or DavisPlus at http://davisplus.fadavis.com/Wilkinson2

in the following sections:

Part I, Concepts of Development

Part II, Infant Through Middle Age

Part III, Older Adults

Keep in mind that if there is an injury, there is the possibility that it was inflicted. The following flow chart and Procedure 9-1 will aid you in identifying cases of abuse.

Possible Abuse Flow Chart

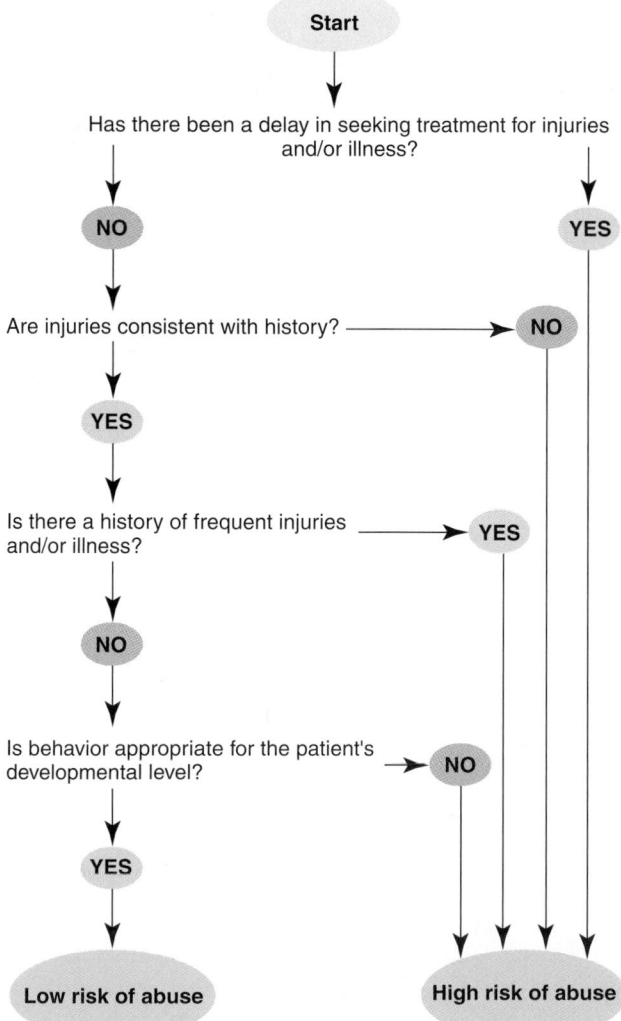

Procedure 9-1 □ **Assessing for Abuse**

➤ For steps to follow in *all* procedures, refer to the Universal Steps for All Procedures found on the inside back cover of Volume 2.

Critical Aspects

- Assess for abuse any time a child or dependent person has an injury.
- Use a nonjudgmental approach; do not make assumptions.
- Remember, the relationship between the suspected abuser and the victim is complex. Love, fear, self-doubt, anger, guilt, and many other emotions are common and can influence the report of the abuse and details implicating the abuser.
- The key to ruling out abuse is to determine whether the injury was intentional or accidental.
- Obtain a focused health history, assessing for physical, sexual, and psychological abuse and neglect.
- Determine whether the caregiver of the suspected victim of abuse has a history of mental health disorder, such as anxiety, depression, or dysfunctional coping.
- Perform a focused physical assessment; ensure the integrity of evidence that may be needed for criminal prosecution.
- For any sexual examination, always have a witness in the room to protect the patient and the examiner.
- Assess whether the injuries are consistent with the history.
- If appropriate, provide the victim with referrals for help in escaping the abusive situation.
- If appropriate, refer the parent, caregiver, or partner involved in abuse to hotlines or agencies focused on stopping the abuse and protecting the victim.
- Report abuse according to agency, state, and federal guidelines.

Pre-Procedure Assessment

- If you suspect sexual abuse, request a forensic nurse or sexual assault nurse examiner (SANE) be present.

A forensic nurse and SANE are specially trained to identify findings that indicate abuse, to support the patient, and to handle the evidence to ensure validity in a court of law.

- Assess for abuse any time a child, dependent person, or spouse has an injury.

Although there is not a strong base of evidence to support screening, The Joint Commission requires that all patients be screened for abuse and domestic violence.

Delegation

Assessment is a nursing responsibility and cannot be delegated.

Procedure Steps

1. When performing the procedure, always identify your patient according to agency policy and be attentive to standard precautions, hand hygiene, patient safety and privacy, body mechanics, and documentation.
Privacy and confidentiality are extremely important for this procedure.

2. Obtain a focused health history.
    a. Collect information from the patient and family members or caregivers separately.
Allows the patient more freedom to express his concerns. An abused person may be afraid to talk with the abuser present. Victims have often been intimidated and will usually support the abuser's version of events. If two adults

accompany a child, it may be that one of them is abusing both the partner and the child. To help rule that out, separate the caregivers to be certain they tell the same story.

    b. Approach the subject in a nonthreatening and caring manner. For example:
    "The law requires us to ask about certain injuries. We are not accusing you of anything. I know you care about your child/parent/spouse and want to do everything possible for her health."
    c. Consider the patient's developmental and cognitive level in assessing whether the story of how the injury occurred is consistent with the injuries.

The patient must be developmentally capable of performing an activity in a situation in which an injury occurred. For example, an infant is not likely to have opened a medication bottle and taken pills; if a child cannot yet walk, it is not likely he reached up to pull a hot pan off the stove.

    d. Observe the patient's behavior. Evaluate whether it is inconsistent with his developmental level.
In the presence of the abuser, it is common for the abuse victim to appear passive and withdrawn and avoid eye contact. The victim may exhibit anxious or fearful behavior; may look to the parent or caregiver before answering questions; may be overly compliant; or may let the abuser answer the questions for him.

(continued on next page)

Procedure 9-1 ■ **Assessing for Abuse** (continued)

e. Ask about the injury or incident. Ask detailed questions about how and when the injury occurred or the illness began:

"When did this injury happen or when did you first begin to feel ill?" "How did you get this injury?" "What happened to you?" "What have you been doing to treat your symptoms since you first became ill?"

A delay of treatment of 12 to 18 hours may indicate abuse (U.S. Department of Justice, 2002). If the details of the history of an injury change during the interview, the likelihood of abuse increases.

f. Ask about past injuries or incidents:

"Have you ever had similar injuries?" "Have you ever required emergency care in the past?"

Abusive behavior typically occurs over and over. If an injury is due to abuse, the patient would most likely have experienced abuse in the past and would have evidence of old injuries.

g. Ask about the patient's usual diet:

"What do you usually eat for breakfast? Lunch? Dinner? What kind of snacks do you have during the day?"

Neglect and/or abuse may be exhibited by an inadequate or inappropriate diet.

h. To assess for sexual abuse:

If a patient is in a potentially abusive situation, the possibility of sexual abuse must be considered.

■ Ask directly whether the patient has been touched inappropriately or forced to have sexual relations.

Whenever possible, question the patient directly so your question will not be misunderstood.

■ Ask whether the patient has genitourinary symptoms: "Have you had any burning or itching when you urinate?

How about any vaginal discharge?"

Genitourinary symptoms in a child may indicate sexual abuse or neglect.

■ Does the child display knowledge or interest in sexual acts inappropriate to his or her age, or even seductive behavior?

■ Does the child appear to avoid another person, or display unusual behavior—either very aggressive or very passive?

■ Does the victim display destructive behaviors, such as alcohol or drug abuse, self-mutilation, or suicide attempts?

■ Is the victim pregnant, particularly if no intimate relationship is known or the victim is very young?

i. To assess for psychological abuse:

■ Ask parents or caregivers, "Are there family members or friends who help you with problems?"

Isolation is a risk factor for abuse. Parents or caregivers may not have the support they need.

■ Ask the patient, "Whom do you talk to when you are having problems?"

An abuser will try to isolate the victim from family and friends over time. Ask questions to determine what the relationship is between the victim and family and friends.

■ Ask, "Tell me how you feel about yourself."

An abuser demeans and degrades the victim so the victim has a low self-worth and feels the "punishment" is deserved; or the victim may desire the attention.

■ Observe if the child acts fearful, shies away from touch, or appears to be afraid to go home.

■ Ask, "Who manages the family finances, and how are

decisions made regarding spending?"

An abuser frequently controls all the finances, and restricts the resources of the victim. Abusers typically seek control of victims by fostering dependency and powerlessness.

3. **Perform a focused physical assessment.**

a. If sexual abuse is suspected from the interview, have a forensic nurse or sexual assault nurse examiner (SANE) present if possible.

For any sexual examination, always have a witness in the room to protect the patient and the examiner.

b. Assess the current injury and look for evidence of previous injuries. Look for the following cues:

■ Bruises that form an outline of a hand, cord loop, buckle, or belt

Observe for signs of physical abuse, especially injuries of different ages, because multiple injuries may show a pattern of abuse. Be careful to assess the bruise accurately. Some home treatments may cause what looks like bruising. For example, moxibustion (includes such things as firmly rubbing a warm spoon down the affected area) is used in some Asian cultures.

■ Injuries that are inconsistent with the history of the injury and are of varying ages (e.g., bruises of different colors, cuts in various stages of healing)

■ Obvious nonaccidental burns, such as burns to both feet and lower legs from immersion in hot water

One method of abuse is to immerse the victim's hands or feet into scalding water. The resulting injury has a well-defined border and usually occurs on both extremities.

■ Circular burns, possibly from cigarettes

Observe for burns all over the body, which will indicate abuse.

■ Bite marks

Bite marks in different areas of the body indicate abuse.

■ Oral ecchymosis or injury from forced oral sex

Forced oral sex will cause injuries to the mouth.

■ Bruising at the crease above the eyelids, tense fontanel if the victim is an infant, hyphema, subconjunctival hemorrhage or retinal bleeding, detached retina, ruptured tympanic membrane

Injuries to the head are common in abuse. Abusive head trauma (ABT, previously referred to as shaken-baby syndrome) is one of the most common and most serious injuries for a young child.

■ Bleeding or bruising of genitalia, poor sphincter tone, encopresis (poor bowel control) and bruises on inner thighs

These signs are indications of sexual abuse.

■ Positive culture for sexually transmitted infection or positive pregnancy test

Sexually transmitted infection, particularly in a child, can indicate sexual abuse.

■ Bruises on wrists and ankles from being restrained

Abused individuals may be tied or locked in a closet or other small space.

■ Refer to the figure for typical features of injuries that may be nonaccidental:
   Injuries to both sides of the body
   Injuries to soft tissue

Accidental injuries are usually over bony prominences. One suspicious pattern is the "swimsuit zone" on the trunk, breast, abdomen, genitalia, and buttocks.

   Injuries in the "triangle of safety": ears, side of face, neck, and top of the shoulders.

Accidental injuries in this area are unusual. ▼

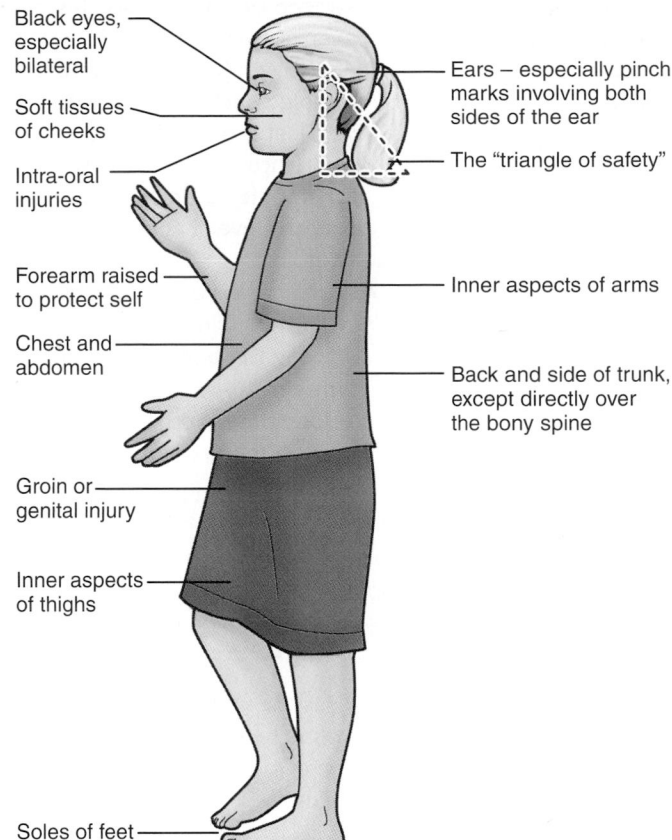

Black eyes, especially bilateral

Soft tissues of cheeks

Intra-oral injuries

Ears – especially pinch marks involving both sides of the ear

The "triangle of safety"

Forearm raised to protect self

Inner aspects of arms

Chest and abdomen

Back and side of trunk, except directly over the bony spine

Groin or genital injury

Inner aspects of thighs

Soles of feet

c. Assess whether injuries are consistent with the history.

If injuries are not consistent with the history, you must assume abuse.

d. Observe for signs of neglect:
   ■ Malnutrition, such as a distended abdomen, or weight markedly below ideal body weight
   ■ Excess body weight for height and age
   ■ Poor hygiene, including oral hygiene
   ■ Ingrown nails
   ■ Untreated sores or pressure sores or other medical conditions
   ■ Matted hair
   ■ Dehydration
   ■ Confusion
   ■ Clothing that is inappropriate for the weather, such as heavy, long-sleeved pants and shirts on hot days

■ Periods of time a young child or frail, older adult is left alone without care or supervision

Signs of neglect occur because of long-term starvation or underfeeding, poor personal care, untreated sores or injuries, and inadequate fluid intake. Neglect *can also* result in childhood obesity as a result of poor quality food, erratic eating patterns, and poor supervision of the diet.

4. If the forensic nurse or primary care provider determines that abuse has occurred, follow legal procedures to ensure that all evidence is secured. If possible, have a forensic nurse and social worker work with the patient.

In situations where violation of the law has occurred, strict procedures are essential to ensure that your findings can be used in a court of law and to protect yourself against legal liability.

(continued on next page)

Procedure 9-1 ▪ Assessing for Abuse (continued)

5. Provide referrals, if appropriate, for the abused person, partner, family member, or caregiver to obtain assistance in escaping the abusive situation and/or stopping the abuse. Resources are available to assist the abused individual and to assist the parent or caregiver to stop the abuse. Be aware of local and national resources.

6. Report concerns regarding abuse according to agency and state guidelines.
Suspected child and elder abuse must be reported to the appropriate agency, according to federal and state laws. Spousal abuse may be mandatory to report, depending on state law. The Joint Commission requires that all cases of possible abuse or neglect are immediately reported in the hospital.

7. Treat physical injuries or refer to the primary care provider for medical care, as needed.
Detection and prevention of abuse require collaborative efforts of the healthcare team.

What if . . .

- **My patient is a child. Are there any special assessments I should make or actions I should take?**

Follow steps 1 through 7, with these modifications:

Note: The interview is important in ruling out sexual abuse in children. Physical findings are often absent, even when the perpetrator admits to penetration of the child's genitalia. Most expert interviewers do not interview children younger than 3 years.

a. To assess for sexual abuse, ask whether the patient has been touched inappropriately:
  - *Child older than 2:* Ask about being touched in "private parts."
  - *Older child:* Ask a question such as, "Sometimes people you know may touch or kiss you in a way that you feel is

strange or wrong. Has this ever happened to you?"
  - *Adolescent:* Ask, "Sometimes people touch you in ways you feel are wrong, This can be frightening, and it is wrong for people to do that to you. Has this ever happened to you?"

b. Ask the parent or caregiver:
  - "Has the child started wetting the bed?" "Or soiling himself?"
  - "Does the child have fears that seem unreasonable?"

Abuse may result in regression to former behaviors. Symptoms of sexual abuse in children may be general and nonspecific, such as sleep disturbances, bedwetting, or excessive fears.

  - "Has the child been masturbating or sexually acting out with other children?"

A child who is sexually abused may exhibit inappropriate sexual behavior.

  - "Has the child ever run away? If she leaves, does she go to someplace safe?" "Is the child/adolescent sexually active?"

An abused child may have feelings of low self worth and may demonstrate risk-taking behavior, such as running away to places that are unsafe.

c. To assess for psychological abuse, ask the parent or caregiver:
  - "Was the child a result of a planned pregnancy? What were the pregnancy, birth, and postpartum period like?"

Risk factors for abuse include an unplanned pregnancy, complications during pregnancy, stressors (e.g., moving, illness, loss of job, divorce), a difficult pregnancy or birth, and lengthy stay in the neonatal intensive care unit.

  - "How would you describe the child now?"

An abusive parent may describe the child as a "problem child" who is always doing something wrong. The opposite is

sometimes seen, when the child is "perfect."

  - "How does the child's behavior compare to that of others in the family?"

Determine whether the parent sees the child differently from siblings. This is a risk factor for abuse.

  - "Has the child experienced physical or emotional problems in the past?"

A history of physical or emotional problems may indicate abuse.

  - "What are your expectations of the child's behavior (e.g., school performance, following instructions, and so forth)?"

The expectations of parents or caregivers who are more at risk to abuse a child may be that the child will "always be a problem" or will be a "perfect" son or daughter.

  - "What form of discipline works best with the child?"

Determine whether the parents or caregivers use physical or emotional punishment that may be abusive or disproportionate for the act or situation.

  - "Do you have any history of depression, anxiety, difficulty coping with situations or everyday life, or other history of mental heath problems?"

Mental health disorders interfere with a person's ability to perceive others and situations in a realistic and appropriate way. When coping is compromised, the risk for abuse escalates.

d. Perform a physical assessment.
  - Signs of physical abuse and neglect in children:
    - Bruises on head, face, ears, buttocks, and lower back that are inconsistent with the history of the injury and are of varying stages of healing (different colors)
    - Hemorrhage of the eye, detached retina, ruptured ear drum

Bruising may occur in different patterns. One pattern is the "swimsuit zone" on the trunk, breast, abdomen, genitalia, and buttocks. Children often have accidental bruises over bony areas, but usually not on the abdomen. Injuries to the head are common in abuse. The abusive head trauma (AHT) syndrome may cause detached retina(s), hemorrhages, and subdural hematomas.

- Signs of sexual abuse in children:
  - Assess for abdominal pain.

Abdominal pain may be a symptom of sexual abuse in children. Signs of sexual abuse may be general and nonspecific in children.

What if. . .

- **My patient is an older adult. Are there any special assessments I should make or actions I should take?**
  - a. Ask the patient and caregiver:
    - "Describe the patient's personal support network. Who visits the patient? How often does the patient have visitors?"

As in spousal abuse, people who victimize older people often isolate the person from any support network.

- "Who is the patient's primary healthcare provider?"

Multiple healthcare providers, or lack of a provider, can be an indication of abuse. The caregiver may bring the patient to a different physician with each injury or illness to avoid discovery.

- "Has the patient ever received the wrong dose of medication?"

Getting the wrong medication or dosage of medication (especially oversedation) may indicate abuse or inability to provide safe care.

- "Who manages the patient's finances?"

Financial abuse is a fairly common form of abuse in this population. Determine who has control of the older person's finances and makes the decisions regarding spending.

- b. Ask the patient:
  - "Do you feel safe in your home?"

The patient who is being abused does not feel safe. Keep in mind that abandonment is a form of abuse.

- "Tell me about your usual day." "Are you able to take care of yourself?" "Who helps you shower and dress?" or "Do you require help with showering or dressing?" "Who is responsible for grocery shopping and cooking in your home?" "How do you get to your appointments or other places you want or need to go?"

To determine the patient's usual level of self-care

  - c. Observe for signs of self neglect.

- **You feel you or the patient is in immediate danger?**

If the patient's or your safety is at risk, immediate intervention is required. You may need to secure the area (e.g., by closing the door), notify the in-house security officer, and then call the police.

Evaluation

- Determine whether abuse may have occurred.
- Ensure that appropriate agencies have been notified of the possible abuse.
- Evaluate whether it is safe to let the patient leave the facility.

Documentation

- Chart all findings factually—do not add any interpretations. For example:

Don't chart:

4-year-old boy admitted with immersion burns to both feet extending to midpoint of shins, such as those found in abuse.

Do chart:

4-year-old boy admitted with first-degree burns to both feet extending to midpoint of shins. Father says, "I put him in the bathtub and didn't realize how hot the water was."

- Follow legal requirements for documenting possible abuse, including disposition of potential evidence.
- If possible, include pictures of the injuries in the charting, using a digital camera.

Photos must be developed in-house because of the requirement to protect confidentiality.

Patient Teaching

- Inform the patient, parent, partner, and/or caregiver of local resources for prevention or intervention in situations of child, spousal, or elder abuse.
- Inform the patient that abuse is suspected. Ask for her perceptions of the situation.
- Emphasize to the patient that her safety is the primary concern.

Home Care

- If potential abuse is identified in the home, follow agency and state legal guidelines.
- If the patient's safety is at risk, immediate intervention is required. You may need to notify the police or call an ambulance.
- If you believe you are at risk for harm (common in abusive situations), leave the setting before notifying the police.

Practice Resources

Dembrow, M., Golden, A., Paulk, D., et al. (2007); The Joint Commission (2008); National Guideline Clearinghouse (2004, 2005a, 2005b); U.S. Department of Justice (2002).

THINKING CRITICALLY ABOUT DEVELOPMENT ACROSS THE LIFE SPAN

The exercises in the following sections allow you to practice the kind of thinking you will use as a full-spectrum nurse. Because these are critical-thinking questions, there is usually no single right answer. We do not provide answers for these questions because it is more important for you to think about the questions than to arrive at the "right" answer. These questions are designed to improve your thinking more than to "cover content." Discuss answers with your peers—discussion can stimulate critical thinking. If you have difficulty with any of these questions, consult with your instructor

Applying the Full-Spectrum Nursing Model

PATIENT SITUATION

Alvin Bell, 82 years old, was just discharged from the hospital following a myocardial infarction (heart attack). On your first home visit to supervise his medication regimen, you notice that the house looks as though it has not been cleaned in weeks. He has what appears to be months' accumulation of newspapers, magazines, and other clutter piled on every flat surface, including the floor. There are dishes piled in the sink, apparently from before his hospitalization. There is hardly any food in the cupboard; when you weigh Mr. Bell, you see that he has lost 3 lb in the 3 days he has been home. He admits he has not been eating: "I'm not hungry, and it's too much trouble." As you talk with him, you learn that his wife died of cancer 7 months ago. He says, "I don't know what to do without her. I hate living alone. There doesn't seem to be much reason for going on." Mr. Bell is alert and oriented, but talks and moves very slowly.

THINKING

1. *Theoretical Knowledge*:

   a. What do you know about depression in older adults? Do you have enough knowledge of that topic to be able to assess whether Mr. Bell is depressed? If not, what resources would you use too find out (list specific resources; that is, give the URL, don't just say "the Internet"; give the name or author of the book, not just "my psych-nursing book").

   b. You will also need to know whether it is normal for appetite to decrease in older adults, and what their calorie needs are compared to other age groups. Where can you go to find this information?

2. *Critical Thinking (Considering Alternatives)*:

   a. As you survey Mr. Bell's overall situation, what is your first impulse for how to improve his situation? What questions come to you?

   b. What community services might be helpful for Mr. Bell?

   c. How would you handle referrals? Would you leave a list of telephone numbers? Would you call the agencies yourself? Explain your thinking.

DOING

3. *Practical Knowledge*: In your physical examination of Mr. Bell, you find no old or recent bruises or other injuries. However, you wonder if he is suffering neglect or financial abuse. What questions could you ask to find out?

CARING

4. *Self-Knowledge*: Think of one patient you have cared for who has something in common with Mr. Bell. Describe the way(s) in which they are alike.

◼ Critical Thinking and Clinical Reasoning

1. Now that you have an understanding of the stages of growth and development, let us return to the three pediatric patients you met in "Meet Your Patients," in Volume 1. All three children are diagnosed with pneumonia. You have introduced yourself to Miguel's and Tamika's caregiver and spoken by phone to Carrie's mother. Each is asking you how this hospitalization will affect their child or grandchild.

   ▪ Tamika, a 3-year-old, lives with her grandparents. Her elderly grandmother is present only during afternoon visiting hours because she must care for her husband, who suffers from numerous health problems. Tamika's grandmother appears unconcerned about her granddaughter's health problems and instead asks questions about her husband's multiple medical diagnoses.
   ▪ Miguel, a 2-month-old, lives with his mother. Since his admission yesterday, his mother has stayed at his bedside and provided most of her son's care. Miguel's mother is 17 years old and is very concerned about her son's condition.
   ▪ Carrie, a 13-year-old, lives with her parents. Both parents are able to visit only during evening visiting hours, when they leave work. Carrie's mother, Elaine, a 45-year-old bank vice president, expresses concern about Carrie's condition and asks whether she will need to be hospitalized long. All of the caregivers seem to lack knowledge of their child's illness and care. You are wondering whether it would be helpful to schedule a group teaching session with the children's caregivers.

   a. Based on Erikson's stages of development, contrast the developmental stages of Miguel, Tamika, and Carrie.

   b. How will nursing care differ for each child?

   c. Analyze each caregiver's developmental stage, and discuss the impact it may have on health teaching.

   d. Would it be a good idea to have the children's caregivers meet for a group teaching session to provide information about pneumonia? Explain.

2. For each of the following concepts, use critical thinking to describe how or why it is important to nursing, patient care, or growth and development. Note these are *not* to be merely definitions.

Ego	Preschooler development
Defense mechanisms	School-age development
Cognitive development	Puberty
Psychosocial development	Adolescent development
Fetal development	Young adult development
Infant development	Middle adult development
Reflexes	Older adult development
Toddler development	

What Are the Main Points in This Chapter?

➤ Growth and development occur across the life span in a predictable pattern.

➤ Developmental theories help nurses identify what to expect behaviorally, cognitively, socially, and morally from patients at various ages.

➤ Fetal growth begins at the time of conception and continues for 10 lunar months until birth.

➤ Critical adaptations at birth include the establishment of respirations and independent circulation, thermoregulation, and the production of urine.

➤ Between birth and 1 year, infants develop a sense of trust when the caregiver provides the child with love, warmth, and food.

➤ The toddler period (12 to 36 months) is the time when the child explores the environment and attempts to become autonomous.

➤ In the preschool period (4 to 5 years) children are able to separate from their parents, communicate needs through language, and control bodily functions.

➤ The school-age child (6 to 12 years) begins to develop relationships outside the home. This leads to increasing confidence and independence.

➤ In the adolescent period (12 to 18 years) children establish their own identities and begin to make decisions that will affect their future.

➤ The young adult (20 to 40 years) leaves home and begins to function as an independent person.

➤ Middle adulthood (40 to 65 years) is a time when people balance aspirations with reality. It is often a time when the needs of children diminish whereas the needs of aging parents increase.

➤ The number of older adults (age 65 and older) has risen significantly because of increasing life expectancy.

➤ Older adulthood is a time of transition. Most health problems experienced by older adults are chronic in nature and often affect the person's ability to live independently.

➤ Growth and developmental differences result in each age group's having specific health problems requiring specific assessment techniques. Data from these assessments are used to plan and provide care and anticipatory guidance that are developmentally appropriate.

➤ Abuse of both children and adults is common. Assess all patients for signs of abuse.

For practice questions for this chapter,

 Go to **NCLEX-Style Chapter Quiz,** on the Student Resource Disk or DavisPlus at http://davisplus.fadavis.com/Wilkinson2

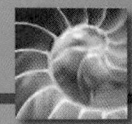

Knowledge Map

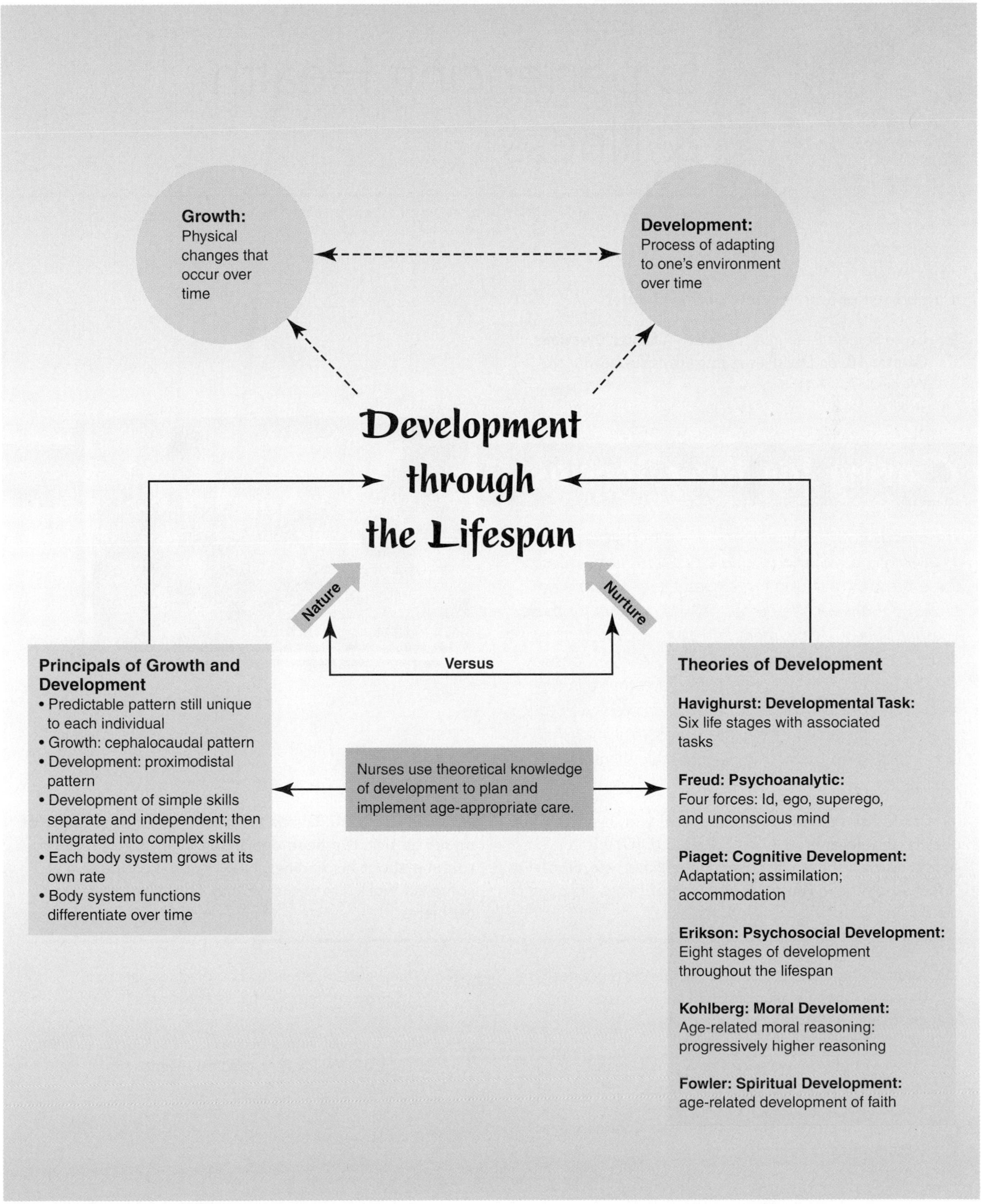

Growth:
Physical changes that occur over time

Development:
Process of adapting to one's environment over time

Development through the Lifespan

Nature

Nurture

Versus

Principals of Growth and Development
- Predictable pattern still unique to each individual
- Growth: cephalocaudal pattern
- Development: proximodistal pattern
- Development of simple skills separate and independent; then integrated into complex skills
- Each body system grows at its own rate
- Body system functions differentiate over time

Nurses use theoretical knowledge of development to plan and implement age-appropriate care.

Theories of Development

Havighurst: Developmental Task:
Six life stages with associated tasks

Freud: Psychoanalytic:
Four forces: Id, ego, superego, and unconscious mind

Piaget: Cognitive Development:
Adaptation; assimilation; accommodation

Erikson: Psychosocial Development:
Eight stages of development throughout the lifespan

Kohlberg: Moral Development:
Age-related moral reasoning: progressively higher reasoning

Fowler: Spiritual Development:
age-related development of faith

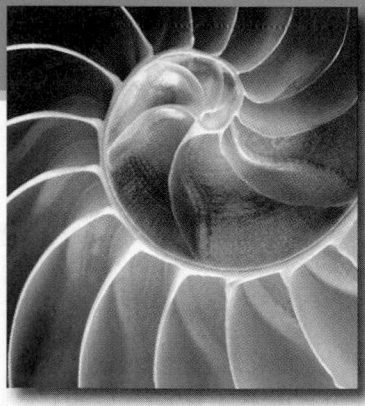

CHAPTER 10

Experiencing Health & Illness

For a podcast of an overview of this chapter,

 Go to Student Resources, **Podcast – Chapter Overviews, Chapter 10,** on DavisPlus at http://davisplus.fadavis.com/ Wilkinson2

Caring for the Garcias

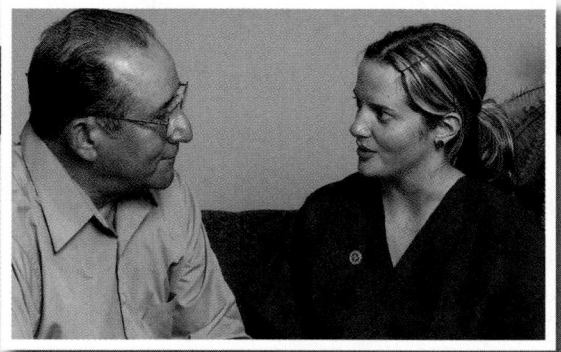

The exercises in this section allow you to practice the kind of thinking you will use as a full-spectrum nurse. Because these are critical-thinking questions, there is usually no single right answer. We do not provide answers for these questions because it is more important for you to think about the questions than to arrive at the "right" answer. These questions are designed to improve your thinking more than to "cover content." Discuss answers with your peers—discussion can stimulate critical thinking. If you have difficulty with any of these questions, consult with your instructor.

Mr. Garcia has recently been diagnosed with hypertension, obesity, and degenerative joint disease (DJD). He is struggling with these diagnoses. He tells his wife, Flordelisa, "I feel so old now. These are the kind of things my parents are dealing with."

At a clinic visit Mr. Garcia tells you, "It's hard to think of myself as sick. I've been depressed ever since Jordan told me about his findings. Now he's asked me to get some lab work. I'm afraid he may find even more problems."

A. Identify the disruptions that Mr. Garcia must deal with based on these diagnoses. Explain your reasons for choosing these disruptions.

B. How would you evaluate Mr. Garcia's health status? To review the concepts of health status,

VOL 1 Go to Chapter 10, **The Health-Illness Continuum and Dunn's Health Grid,** in Volume 1.

C. What kinds of activities could you suggest to Mr. Garcia to improve his health status?

D. What stage of illness behavior is Mr. Garcia exhibiting in regard to his recent medical diagnoses?

Practical **Knowledge**
knowing how

Practical knowledge in this chapter means using the nursing process to apply what you have learned about how people experience health, wellness, and illness.

Procedures

The procedures in this chapter are designed to help you admit, transfer, and discharge patients in such a way that you can begin, at first contact, to establish trust.

Procedure 10-1   Admitting a Patient to a Nursing Unit

➤ For steps to follow in *all* procedures, refer to the Universal Steps for All Procedures found on the inside back cover of Volume 2.

Critical Aspects

- Begin the admission: Introduce yourself, assist the patient into a hospital gown, weigh, assist him into the bed.
- Validate patient identity.
- Obtain a translator, if needed.
- Complete the nursing assessment, including vital signs; validate the admission list of medications.
- Provide information: Room, equipment, routines, Health Insurance Portability and Accountability Act (HIPAA), nurse call system, and advance directives.
- Answer any questions.
- Provide printed information.
- Complete nursing admission paperwork according to agency policy.
- Complete or ensure that admission orders have been completed.
- Inventory the patient's belongings; send home or lock up valuables.
- Finish the admission process.
  - Ensure patient comfort (water, positioning, pain).
  - Make one last safety check: call light, bed position, side rails.
  - Ask: "Is there anything else I can do for you?"

Equipment

- Identifying armband (if this has not been done in the admissions department)
- Patient's chart, including physician's orders and nursing admission record
- Thermometer, blood pressure cuff, and stethoscope
- Scales for height and weight
- Gown
- Admission pack (e.g., bath basin, water pitcher, soap, comb, toothbrush, mouthwash, and facial tissues)
- Nursing care plan or clinical pathway, if one has already been made
- Hospital brochures, Patient Care Partnership, and other forms
- Admission assessment form

Delegation

A registered nurse is responsible for managing medical orders and assessing the patient's need for nursing care in all settings, although this may vary in some specifics according to hospital policy, the law, and regulations. Most other admission activities can be delegated to nursing assistive personnel (NAP) if the patient is stable.

Pre-Procedure Assessments

- Assess for signs of emotional and/or physical distress.
- Assess ability to ambulate and/or move.
- Assess ability to communicate and understand what is occurring.

(continued on next page)

Procedure 10-1 ■ **Admitting a Patient to a Nursing Unit** (continued)

➤ When performing the procedure, always identify your patient according to agency policy and be attentive to standard precautions, hand hygiene, patient safety and privacy, body mechanics, and documentation.

Procedure Steps

1. Ensure placement of patient labels (e.g., on the chart, at the bedside, outside the door).

2. Introduce yourself to the patient and family.
Talking to the patient and family reassures them and provides information about the patient's level of consciousness and awareness, social relationships, and so on.

3. Assist the patient into a hospital gown.
If the patient is able to stand, assist her into a gown before weighing her to obtain the most accurate weight.

4. Measure height and weight while the patient stands on a scale, if possible.
If the patient is able to stand, use a floor scale. If she is unable to stand, transfer her into the bed and measure her weight using a bed scale. Weigh in the same manner each time to ensure accuracy.

5. Assist the patient into the bed.
Get the patient comfortable before continuing the admission to prevent overtiring her.

✚ **6.** Check the patient's identification band to ensure the information, including allergies, is correct. Verify this information with the patient or family.

Questioning the patient about allergies and verifying with the family will ensure that the information is accurate and documented on the wristband and the chart.

7. Measure vital signs.
Measuring the vital signs before completing the rest of the admission ensures that you will be aware of the patient's status. If the vital signs are abnormal, further assess the patient's

condition before continuing. Report your findings to the admitting care provider.

8. Complete the nursing admission assessment, including health history and physical assessment. For inpatients, this must be completed within 24 hours after admission. All patients should be screened on admission for risk for pressure ulcers.
These are needed to identify problems and establish a baseline. The Joint Commission requires that each patient have an admission assessment performed by a registered nurse.

✚ **9.** Check that the list of the patient's current medications (created in the admitting department) is complete and accurate. Usually the patient's own medications are sent home with the family, or they may be sent to pharmacy for storage.

It is important to know what medications the patient has been taking. The pharmacy will identify medicines from home when necessary. When medications are ordered and given during the patient's stay, they are compared to those on the list so any discrepancies can be resolved.

10. Explain equipment, including how to use the call system, and point out the location of personal care items.
These actions ensure that the patient and family will be able to call for assistance if needed and increase the patient's and family's level of comfort and ability to function in the hospital setting.

11. Explain hospital routines, including use of side rails, meal times, and so on. Answer the patient's and family's questions.
Hospitalization takes away control of basic decisions. Knowing the routines and available choices increases patient and family comfort.

12. Verify with the patient that all other admission data on the chart are complete.
Basic data such as name, address, marital status, name of admitting physician, admitting diagnosis, consent to treatment, and so on, will usually be obtained in the admitting office. However, you will need to be sure all the admitting information is complete, and complete it if it is not.

13. Ask the patient if he has an advance directive (e.g., power of attorney or living will). If so, place a copy in the hospital record. If not, explain the purpose of the document and give the patient a form to fill out if he wishes to do so. (See Chapters 15 and 45 if you need more information about advance directives.)
Advance directives enable patients to indicate their preferences about treatments and prolonging life.

14. Advise the patient of his privacy rights under HIPAA. See that he has a written explanation of his privacy rights (see Chapter 45 as needed).

15. Inventory the patient's belongings. Encourage the family to take home valuable items and money. If that is not possible, arrange to have valuables placed in the hospital safe. Most agencies require money in excess of $5.00 to be sent home or to the cashier's office.
Patient belongings, including valuables, are frequently lost during hospitalization. If possible, have the family take them home. Documenting the disposition of everything ensures being able to return the belongings to the patient upon discharge.

16. Complete or ensure that all admission orders have been completed (e.g., laboratory tests, medications, diet and fluid orders).

Unless it is an unscheduled admission, diagnostic tests are usually completed on an outpatient basis before admission to the hospital. However, there may still be some orders that need to be done immediately, while others can be delayed. Make sure the orders are completed in the most appropriate time frame.

17. Ensure patient comfort (e.g., positioning, pain, water at bedside).

18. Make one last safety check (i.e., call light within reach, bed in low position, side rails up as appropriate, equipment functioning properly).

19. Before leaving, ask if there is anything else you can do for the patient and family.

20. Initiate the care plan or clinical pathway.
Identifying the patient's priority problems enables the nurse to develop the most appropriate nursing orders.

What if . . .

■ **The patient may be at risk for falls?**

Perform falls risk assessment as appropriate to the patient, and according to agency policy.

Falls are common in inpatient facilities, especially among older adults. If a patient has falls risk factors, risk reduction measures can be instituted.

■ **The patient has special care needs?**

When the patient has special needs, such as allergies, a "nothing by mouth" order, or an "intake and output" order, post patient care reminders at the head of the bed or at the door to remind other care providers.

■ **The patient needs a more in-depth assessment in some areas?**

Perform special needs assessments as relevant to the care and condition of the patient (social situation, nutrition and hydration status, functional abilities, spiritual and cultural variables). If these are warranted, they must be completed within 24 hours after admission or prior to surgery.

In-depth assessment of these topics is not a part of all admission assessments, but should be done if the patient's condition warrants.

■ **The patient has a learning disability?**

If possible, preadmissions should be arranged for the patient and main caregiver. This allows more time to discuss issues of consent, alleviate anxiety, and set up links with a learning disability specialist or social worker. Whether or not this is possible: Allow more time for the admission process.
   Use short sentences, with one idea at a time.
   Include the caregiver in the admission process, but encourage the patient to participate as much as possible.
   Document the main caregiver and contact numbers.
   Expect the patient to be anxious.
   Include special communication and personal needs in the plan of care.
   Give the patient hospital information with pictures, such as those given to children, if appropriate for her developmental level.

■ **The patient is an older adult?**

Ask all older adults if they have had any falls in the past year. If they report a fall, observe them as they stand up from a chair without using their arms, walk several paces, and return ("get up and go"). If they are steady, no further assessment is required. If there is unsteadiness or if the person reports more than one fall, further assessment is required.

The incidence and severity of fall-related complications rise steadily after age 60. Falls rates in nursing homes and hospitals are almost three times the rate for those living at home.

■ **The patient is a child?**

   Use a friendly approach.

The first priority is to establish a trusting relationship with the child and parents to help relieve fears and anxiety. Children younger than 3 years may fear being separated from parents. Older children usually worry more about what is going to happen to them.

   Explain the visiting and rooming-in policies to the parents.
   Ask about the child's usual routine (e.g., toileting, bedtime rituals, favorite foods).
   Speak to the child directly if she is old enough to understand.
   Direct the family to the bathroom, playroom, television, and snack room, if those are available.
   Encourage the parents to bring toys and other favorite items from home.

It helps the child feel more comfortable in the unfamiliar surroundings.

(continued on next page)

Procedure 10-1 ■ Admitting a Patient to a Nursing Unit (continued)

Documentation

- Document all assessment findings on the admission database provided by the institution. If you need an example, see Nursing Admission Data Form, in Chapter 3.
- Document an admission note and any teaching or other interventions in the nursing notes or flowsheet (according to agency policy).
- Recall that a discharge plan is created on admission. If you need to see a discharge plan, go to Chapter 5, Discharge Planning Form, in this volume.

3/13/11   0345   *Client admitted to room 345 accompanied by wife. He denies pain at this time. Respiratory rate is 24 bpm without retractions or nasal flaring. Pulse 84 bpm, 3+ equal bilaterally. Nursing admission history completed per facility protocol. Encouraged client and family to ask questions. They expressed concern about pending diagnosis and cost of hospitalization. Client was given an overview of the current treatment plan including NPO status. Client correctly stated that NPO means "I may not have anything to eat or drink." Wife stated "I will make sure he does not eat or drink anything." Encouraged client to rest during the next few hours. —*
————————————— Linda Nielsen, RN

Practice Resources

The American Geriatrics Society (2001); U.S. Department of Health and Human Services (2003); The Joint Commission (2008).

Procedure 10-2   Transferring a Patient to Another Unit in the Agency

➤ For steps to follow in *all* procedures, refer to the Universal Steps for All Procedures found on the inside back cover of Volume 2.

Critical Aspects

- Make a final, brief focused assessment.
- Plan ahead the amount of help needed.
- Schedule time of the transfer.
- Make appropriate notifications.
- Gather and label patient medications.
- Gather the patient's belongings, supplies, and treatment equipment.
- Bring the transfer vehicle to the bedside.
- Transfer the patient to the new room.
- Give oral handoff report and make final nursing notes entry.

Equipment

- Medical record or chart
- Care plan
- Patient's medications
- Supplies for any ongoing treatments
- Patient's belongings, clothes, and personal care articles
- Standardized handoff form, if available
- A utility cart, if belongings are numerous
- Wheelchair or transfer cart, if bed is not being moved

Delegation

If the patient's condition allows, you can delegate the physical transfer of the patient and have the nursing assistive personnel (NAP) move the patient's belongings to the other room. However, as the nurse, you are responsible for obtaining and completing the necessary records, making the final assessment, and gathering and checking the medications. You must also give the handoff report to another nurse.

Pre-Procedure Assessment

■ Make a final, brief focused physical assessment.
■ Assess the patient's mobility and ability to assist.

■ Assess for emotional and/or physical distress (administer medications, as needed).
■ Assess the patient's ability to communicate and understand what is occurring.

➤ When performing the procedure, always identify your patient according to agency policy and be attentive to standard precautions, hand hygiene, patient safety and privacy, body mechanics, and documentation.

Procedure Steps

◆ **1.** Obtain the number of personnel needed to make a safe transfer.
For efficiency and patient and staff safety.

2. Gather the patient's medications and label them correctly for the new room.
Ensures availability of medications when the patient arrives at the new unit; helps prevent medication administration errors.

3. Notify the receiving unit of the time to expect the transfer; notify other departments (e.g., dietary, pharmacy, admitting), primary care provider, and family of the transfer.
You need to schedule the transfer with the receiving nurse so he can plan his work and so you can arrange the transfer time to limit the number of interruptions during the handoff. Limiting interruptions minimizes the possibility of failing to communicate or forgetting information. Other departments must have the transfer data so that services such as meals and physical therapy treatments will not be interrupted. The primary care provider and family, of course, need to know where to find the patient.

4. Gather the patient's personal belongings, treatment-related supplies and equipment (e.g., isolation supplies, clean dressings), chart, Kardex, and care plan. Place in a container (e.g., the patient's bath basin) or on a utility cart if necessary.
Having the supplies and equipment "ready to go" makes the transfer more efficient for you and less stressful for the patient.

5. Bring the wheelchair or transfer cart to the bedside and assist the patient to the chair or cart. If using a wheelchair, the patient can hold the pan of supplies; if using a bed or cart, place supplies on the bed.

6. Take the patient to the new room and give the handoff report. Follow agency procedure for handoff reports. However, the method chosen should allow both the giver and receiver of patient information the opportunity for questioning.
  a. If you need to review content of an oral handoff report, see Chapter 16, Clinical Insight 16-1. In general, the report should include name, age, sex, physicians, surgical procedures, medical diagnoses, medications, allergies, laboratory data, special equipment (e.g., oxygen, suction), the patient's current health status, and whether there are advance directives and resuscitation status. Identify the nursing diagnoses and priorities for nursing care.
  b. Consistently use a structured framework or memory aid to guide the handoff process and the oral report.
The objective of a handoff is to provide accurate information about the patient. The information communicated must be accurate in order to ensure patient safety.

◆ c. Be sure to point out to the nurse if patient is taking corticosteroids, anticoagulants, diabetic medications, antibiotics, or narcotic analgesics.

These medications can have serious side effects and need careful monitoring.

What if. . .

■ **The patient has intravenous (IV) lines and other equipment that cannot be turned off?**

It is common to transfer patients with IV lines. Some wheelchairs are equipped with an IV pole; for others, you may need to obtain a rolling pole from the unit supply room. The patient may be able to maneuver the rolling pole. Most beds and transfer carts also have portable IV poles, sometimes stored along the underside. Portable oxygen and suction are also available for patients who must have them even during transfer. Be sure to obtain these, set them up, and check their functioning prior to moving the patient from his bed.

■ **The patient has too many personal belongings for one person to carry?**

If the patient's condition requires two staff members to transfer, one person can manage the utility cart while the other manages the patient. If only one person can make the actual move, load a utility cart and move all the supplies and belongings to the new room before transferring the patient.

■ **The patient is being transferred to the intensive care unit (ICU)?**

If this is an urgent transfer, you may need to notify the receiving nurse and move the patient with his records and medications. Later you can make the other notifications, finish the charting, and move belongings and other supplies. In some ICUs, the family may need to take the patient's personal belongings home.

(continued on next page)

Procedure 10-2 ■ Transferring a Patient to Another Unit in the Agency (continued)

Evaluation

With the receiving nurse, evaluate the patient's response to the move. The receiving nurse will take vital signs and make a preliminary admission assessment.

Documentation

Just before moving, document as much information as you can, including the patient's status at that time. After handoff, document the information reported in handoff, the name and title of the person who received the patient, and your report. Sign the note. Some agencies have a standardized form for the transfer note.

> 3/13/11   1615   Client transferred to room 501 via stretcher with side rails up x2 with assistance x1. Temperature 104.8° F, pulse 100, BP 138/88, and respirations 20 and shallow. Drowsy upon arrival. Responds to verbal stimuli with moaning. Last pain medication administered at 1515. Denies pain when asked. No urine noted since 12:00 pm; will encourage voiding by offering urinal every two hours. #22 IV in RAC and #18 IV in R hand flushed with 3 ml of normal saline and flushes without redness, edema, or induration. Receiving 3 lpm of oxygen during transfer. Placed on 3 lpm in room and will wean oxygen as tolerated. Handoff report given to Linda Hamm, RN. ——
> ———————————— Sarah Fields, RN
>
> X Sarah Fields, RN   Cary Nielsen, LPN

Practice Resources

The Joint Commission (2008); McFetridge, B., Gillespie, M., Goode, D., et al. (2007).

Procedure 10-3   Transferring a Patient to a Long-Term Care Facility

➤ For steps to follow in *all* procedures, refer to the Universal Steps for All Procedures found on the inside back cover of Volume 2.

Critical Aspects

- Plan in advance: notify the patient and family of the impending transfer.
- Prepare the patient's records; copy for the new facility if needed.
- Pack personal items and treatment supplies.
- Coordinate the transfer with the receiving facility and other hospital departments.
- Make the final assessment; document and sign.
- Move the patient to the transportation vehicle.
- Give an oral or telephone report to the receiving nurse; use standardized form if available.
- Notify the long-term care facility if the patient is colonized or infected with methicillin-resistant *Staphylococcus aureus* (MRSA) or other contagious microorganisms.

Equipment

- Medical record or chart
- Care plan
- Patient's medications
- Supplies for any ongoing treatments
- Patient's belongings, clothes, and personal care articles
- Standardized transfer form, if available
- A utility cart, if belongings are numerous
- Wheelchair or transfer cart

Delegation

If the patient's condition allows, you can delegate the physical transfer of the patient and have the NAP move the patient's supplies and belongings. However, as the nurse, you are responsible for obtaining and completing the necessary records, making the final assessment, and gathering and checking the medications. You must also give the handoff report to another nurse.

Pre-Procedure Assessment

- Make a final, brief focused physical assessment.
- Assess the patient's mobility and ability to assist.
- Assess for emotional and/or physical distress (administer medications, as needed).
- Assess the patient's ability to communicate and understand what is occurring.

> When performing the procedure, always identify your patient according to agency policy and be attentive to standard precautions, hand hygiene, patient safety and privacy, body mechanics, and documentation.

Procedure Steps

1. Notify the patient and family well in advance of the upcoming transfer to another facility. Include information about the reasons the patient is being transferred, as well as any alternatives to transfer. You will also need to determine which agency is to arrange transportation for the patient.

Allows them time to adjust emotionally and to make any necessary plans.

2. Prepare the patient's records. You may need to send a copy of the patient's chart to the receiving facility. The original remains with the hospital. You will usually also send a copy of the comprehensive nursing assessment and a detailed nursing care plan, as well as prescriptions and cards for future appointments (e.g., with physicians or social workers).

Ensures continuity of care, thus minimizing patient stress.

3. Gather and pack the patient's personal items and treatment supplies to send to the long-term care facility with the patient.

Having the supplies and equipment "ready to go" makes the transfer more efficient for you.

4. Be certain the medications are labeled correctly.

Ensures availability and correct administration of medications when the patient arrives at the new facility.

5. Coordinate the transfer. Notify the receiving facility of the time to expect the transfer and of any special equipment the patient will need (e.g., IV pole, portable oxygen); notify other hospital departments (e.g., dietary, pharmacy, admitting), primary care provider, and family of the transfer.

You need to schedule the transfer with the receiving agency so they can plan their work and so you can arrange the transfer a time that will limit the number of interruptions during the transfer. Other in-house departments must have the transfer data so that services such as meals and physical therapy treatments will be discontinued. The primary care provider and family, of course, need to know where to find the patient.

6. Just before transfer, make your final quick assessment and sign off your charting (usually there is a preprinted, standardized discharge form for this purpose).

It is important to complete documentation in a timely manner, but it is also important to provide the most recent assessment data to the long-term care facility.

7. When you are notified that transportation has arrived, take the patient off the unit and out of the hospital (or delegate this task). Alternatively, a transporter may come to your unit to get the patient. (Note: some agencies ask you to remove the patient's identification band at time of transfer.)

Keeping the patient on the unit as long as practical helps to minimize his anxiety and fatigue that may occur from a long wait in the hospital lobby.

8. Give an oral report to the nurse at the long-term care facility. You will usually give a telephone report unless a nurse comes to your hospital to accompany the patient. The report should include, as appropriate for the care, treatment, and services provided, the following:

a. The reason the patient is being transferred

b. The patient's physical and psychosocial status

c. A summary of care, treatment, and services provided and progress toward outcomes

d. Referrals, community resources provided to the patient

To ensure continuity of care and provide a baseline for later changes in the patient's health status.

- It is best to consistently use a structured framework or memory aid to guide the handoff process and the oral report.

The objective of a handoff report is to provide accurate information about the patient. The information communicated must be accurate in order to ensure patient safety.

- Notify the long-term care agency if the patient is colonized or infected with MRSA or other contagious microorganisms.

So they can arrange for and communicate any special isolation or care activities to their staff. MRSA is a serious problem for long-term care residents.

(continued on next page)

Procedure 10-3 ■ Transferring a Patient to a Long-Term Care Facility (continued)

◆ ■ Be sure to point out to the nurse if patient is taking corticosteroids, anticoagulants, diabetic medications, antibiotics, or narcotic analgesics. These medications confer particularly high risk of adverse postdischarge drug events, and the long-term-care nurses will need to continue careful monitoring.

What if . . .

■ **The patient has intravenous (IV) lines and other equipment that cannot be turned off?**

It is common to transfer patients with IV lines. Some wheelchairs are equipped with an IV pole; or you may need to hold the IV bag while taking the patient to the transporting vehicle. If so, always hold the bag well above the patient's chest and arm so that blood does not back up in the tubing. Also, you should notify the long-term care facility so they will have the necessary equipment in the transport vehicle. Portable oxygen and suction are also available for patients who must have them. Usually the receiving facility will bring these, but you need to coordinate that in advance.

◆ ■ **When you are ready to transfer the patient, her condition worsens and she becomes unstable?**

Perform interventions to stabilize the patient, call for help if needed, and notify the medical provider. Notify the transporter and the long-term care center of the change and postpone the transfer until further medical assessment is done.

Evaluation

The receiving nurse at the long-term care facility will evaluate the patient's response to the move.

Documentation

Just before the transfer, document your final assessment and complete the agency's discharge summary. You will probably put your final nursing note on a transfer or discharge summary, similar to the ones shown in Assessment Guide & Tools, later in this chapter.

| 3/13/11   1455   Transfer system assessment complete. Temperature 98.6°F, pulse 110, respirations 20 even and unlabored, and blood pressure 110/68. Pulses are 3+ equal bilaterally. Lungs without adventitious sounds. States name, age, date, and location without assistance. Denies pain or discomfort at this time. Wife remains at bedside and will follow ambulance to Shady Grove Long Term Care Facility. Client asks "when will the ambulance arrive to transfer me to Shady Grove?" Explained to client ambulance would be arriving in the next few minutes. Telephone transfer report complete to Chris Queen, LPN. Client requires skilled nursing care. See discharge summary.

    X Sarah Fields, RN   __ L. Nielsen, LPN |

Practice Resources

The Joint Commission (2008); McFetridge, B., Gillespie, M., Goode, D., et al. (2007).

Procedure 10-4 ☐ **Discharging a Patient from the Healthcare Facility**

➤ For steps to follow in *all* procedures, refer to the Universal Steps for All Procedures found on the inside back cover of Volume 2.

Critical Aspects

Notify the patient and family well in advance of the discharge.

A day or two before discharge:

- Arrange for or confirm: transportation and services and equipment needed at home.
- Make referrals.
- Provide teaching about the patient's condition and medications.
- Provide training in use of equipment.
- Ask the caregiver to bring clothing for the patient to wear home.

Day of discharge:

- Make and document final assessments.
- Confirm that the patient has house keys, heat is turned on, and food is available.
- Make final notifications (community agencies, transportation).
- Gather and pack the patient's personal items and treatment supplies.
- Label and give take-home medications to the patient.
- Give the patient prescriptions, instruction sheets, and appointment cards
- Review discharge instructions with the patient.
- Answer questions.
- Document the final nursing note and complete the discharge summary.
- Accompany the patient out of the hospital.
- Notify Admissions of the discharge.
- Ensure records are sent to the medical records department.

Equipment

- Medical record or chart
- Patient's medications
- Supplies for any ongoing treatments
- Patient's belongings, clothes, and personal care articles
- Standardized discharge form, if available, with instructions for patient
- A utility cart, if belongings are numerous
- Wheelchair

Delegation

If the patient's condition allows, you can delegate to the NAP such tasks as packing belongings, helping the patient dress, and taking the patient out of the facility. However, as the nurse, you are responsible for obtaining and completing the necessary records, making the final assessment, gathering and checking the medications, and coordinating care.

Pre-Procedure Assessment

- Make a final, brief focused physical assessment.
- Assess the patient's mobility.
- Assess for emotional and/or physical distress.
- Assess the patient's ability to communicate and understand what is occurring.

➤ When performing the procedure, always identify your patient according to agency policy and be attentive to standard precautions, hand hygiene, patient safety and privacy, body mechanics, and documentation.

Procedure Steps

1. Notify the patient and family as much in advance of the discharge as possible. This is often done early in the hospital stay.
Allows them time to adjust emotionally and to make any necessary plans.

A Day or Two Before Discharge (Steps 2 and 3)

2. Make or confirm necessary arrangements.

a. Arrange for or help the family arrange for services (e.g., home healthcare, physical therapy, intravenous therapy, social worker) that will be needed at home.
Note: To reimburse for home care, insurers require a physician's order for all services, and the patient must meet certain eligibility criteria.

(continued on next page)

Procedure 10-4 ■ Discharging a Patient from the Healthcare Facility (continued)

b. Confirm or arrange for equipment needed in the home (e.g., portable oxygen).

c. Confirm or arrange for transportation.

d. Make necessary referrals (e.g., medical specialists, physical therapists); book appointments, if necessary and if in line with agency policy.

Hospital stays are short, and many patients are still ill enough to require complex treatments and care by family members when they go home.

3. Communicate and provide teaching to the patient and caregivers.

Patients who have a clear understanding of their after-hospital care (e.g., medications, follow-up visits) are 30% less likely to visit the emergency department or be readmitted than patients who lack this information (AHRQ, 2009).

a. Discuss the patient's diagnosis, care needs, and functional abilities with the family/caregiver.

b. Train the patient and caregiver in the use of equipment. Arrange for follow-up evaluation at home to check that equipment is working and being used correctly, and that further training is given if needed.

In the stress of illness and the disruption of transition home, patients may not retain what they are taught in the hospital. Therapies will be ineffective if equipment is used incorrectly, so follow-up is essential to help avoid further illness and hospital readmission.

c. Educate about medication use and side effects.

Medication errors at home are a frequent cause of adverse events and readmissions to the hospital.

d. Ask relatives or the caregiver to bring clothing for the patient to wear home, if needed.

If this was an unplanned admission, the patient may have come in nightwear and a robe.

Day of Discharge (Steps 4 Through 16)

4. Make and document final assessments.

a. Assess that the patient's condition remains as expected.

b. Confirm that the patient has house keys, heating is turned on, and food is available.

c. Follow up on diagnostic and laboratory test results.

5. Bring a wheelchair or other transport device to the bedside.

6. Make final notifications.

a. Contact the family or guardian; confirm transportation.

b. Notify community service agencies and home health nursing of the discharge, as needed.

7. Gather prescriptions, a list of current medications, any other instruction sheets, and appointment cards; give to the patient along with the discharge instructions at discharge. Be certain that either the patient or caregiver can read the instructions.

Inadequate literacy has been shown to be a risk factor for readmission.

8. Gather and pack the patient's personal items and treatment supplies.

Having the supplies and equipment ready to go makes the transfer more efficient for you and less stressful for the patient and family.

✚ **9.** Be certain the patient's medications are labeled correctly; pack them, and record which medications he is taking home.

Ensures availability and correct administration of medications when the patient arrives home. Provides a legal record that the patient left with the medications.

10. Review discharge instructions with patient and caregiver about (and provide a written copy to take home):

a. Medication instructions

b. Symptom management and treatments

c. When and with which care provider for the follow-up appointment(s)

d. How to obtain further care, treatment, and services, as needed

e. How and when to call the physician or primary care provider; including signs of a change in condition

f. Whom to contact in an emergency

g. Diet restrictions

h. Maintenance of hydration

i. Activities of daily living, focusing on safety and mobility

Of course, teaching should occur throughout the hospital stay. However, it is important to reinforce with a last-minute summary and written instructions to take home. With the stress of illness and anticipation of discharge, patients may not retain what they are taught.

11. Address any questions or concerns of the patient and caregiver.

To ensure the ability to transition to home.

12. Give new prescriptions to the patient, as well as reminder cards for outpatient appointments (e.g., with social services, physicians).

Ensures continuity of care, thus minimizing patient stress.

13. Document your final nursing note and complete the discharge summary (the patient often receives a copy of the summary).

It is important to document the patient's condition at the time he leaves the unit. This provides a baseline for comparison if his condition should deteriorate after discharge. The patient needs a copy of (1) his instructions for care at home, which may be called a discharge plan, and (2) his discharge summary, a summary of the progress of his illness and treatment from admission through discharge. Some agencies combine these into one form.

14. When you are notified that transportation has arrived, accompany

the patient off the unit and out of the hospital (or delegate this task).
Keeping the patient on the unit as long as practical helps to minimize the anxiety and fatigue that may occur from a long wait in the hospital lobby while a family member brings a car to the door.

15. Notify the admissions department of the discharge. Depending on agency policy, notify the primary care or admitting physician.
This will stop all scheduled services, such as meals, and notify the housekeeping department that the room needs to be cleaned.

16. Ensure the patient's records are sent to the medical records department.
Whether paper or electronic, the chart is a legal document and remains permanently in storage in the medical records department.

What if. . .

■ ◈ **Near the time of discharge, the patient's condition worsens and he becomes unstable?**
Perform interventions to stabilize the patient, call for help if needed, and notify the provider. Notify the family that discharge will be delayed. Communicate with other hospital departments and community agencies as necessary.

■ **The patient is an older adult?**
  ▪ Allow for more time to dress and leave the hospital.
  ▪ Allow for more time to communicate, teach, and answer questions.
  ▪ Obtain feedback to be certain the caregivers have heard and understood instructions.
  ▪ Consider having a geriatric nurse specialist make follow-up home visits.

Hearing, visual, and mobility deficits become more common with advanced age.

■ ◈ **The patient is taking "high-risk" drugs postdischarge?**
Medications with a high risk of postdischarge adverse events include corticosteroids, anticoagulants, diabetic medications, antibiotics, antianxiety agents, sedatives, and narcotic analgesics.
  ▪ Provide teaching for patient, family, and other caregivers throughout the hospital stay. A day or two before discharge, review teaching with patient and family; evaluate their understanding.
  ▪ On discharge, summarize medication precautions and provide clear written instructions. Be sure the patient and family can read them.

Evaluation

A few weeks after discharge, the facility will contact the patient to evaluate the quality and appropriateness of the discharge process. This may be done by making a home visit, telephoning, or sending a questionnaire. As a nurse, you may or may not be involved in this evaluation. The best evaluation of the multidisciplinary care will be whether the patient must be readmitted to the acute care facility.

Documentation

■ For the medical record, the primary provider will write a discharge progress note that contains the following information:
  Reason for hospitalization
  Significant findings during the stay, including significant changes in status since admission
  Procedures performed; care, treatment, and services provided during the stay
  Status of goals for the stay
  Condition at discharge

■ Agency policy determines the format and content of nursing documentation. This is often a combination of a structured discharge form or checklist and a narrative progress note. Regardless of format, you should document the following information:
  ▪ Your final assessment of the patient's health status
  ▪ Information and teaching provided to the patient and caregivers
  ▪ Referrals, medications
  ▪ How patient left the unit (e.g., in wheelchair) and who accompanied him (e.g., wife, name of staff member)
The Joint Commission recommends standardized formats for documentation (2008, p. 367).
To see examples of discharge summaries, refer to Assessment Guidelines and Tools later in this chapter.

Practice Resources

Agency for Healthcare Research and Quality (2009); Dudas, V. (2001); Greenwald, J., Denham, C., & Jack, B. (2007); The Joint Commission (2008a, 2008b); Naylor, M., Brooten, D., Jones, B., et al. (1994); Phillips, Wright, Kern, et al. (2004); U.S. Department of Health and Human Services (2003); Zwicker, D., & Picariello, G. (2003).

Clinical Insights

Clinical Insight 10-1 ▶ Preparing the Room for a Newly Admitted Patient

Delegation

As a general rule, these tasks can be delegated to NAPs. The nurse is responsible for evaluating and supervising, as well as for setting up special equipment (although the NAP may obtain it from storage).

Clean the Room

Agencies differ; however, it is common for the housekeeping department to clean the room and change the bed linens when a patient is discharged, so you should find the room ready for your preparations. The rest of these guidelines assume that fact.

Prepare the Bed

- Position the bed according to patient status. If the patient is ambulatory, put the bed in the lowest position and lock the wheels. If the patient will arrive on a stretcher, place the bed at stretcher height.
- If necessary, rearrange the furniture to allow easy access to the bed.
- Fold back the top linens to "open" the bed (see the figure).

The patient may need to go to bed immediately, so it should be ready when she arrives.

Prepare Routine Supplies

- Most agencies have an admission pack containing a bath basin, soap, lotion, tissues, water pitcher, and drinking glass. Open it and put it in the room.
- Place a hospital gown on the bed and slippers by the bedside. Patients may choose to wear their own sleep clothing, though.

Prepare Equipment

You will need:

- A stethoscope, thermometer, and blood pressure cuff in the room for taking vital signs
- A scale for measuring and weighing the patient
- Bedpan and urinal if the patient is not ambulatory; possibly a bedside commode
- A clean-catch urine specimen container if laboratory work has not already been done
- Set up and check special equipment (e.g., oxygen, suction, cardiac monitor, pulse oximeter, IV pump).

Prepare the Environment

Turn on the lights, adjust the room temperature. Open or close curtains, as needed.

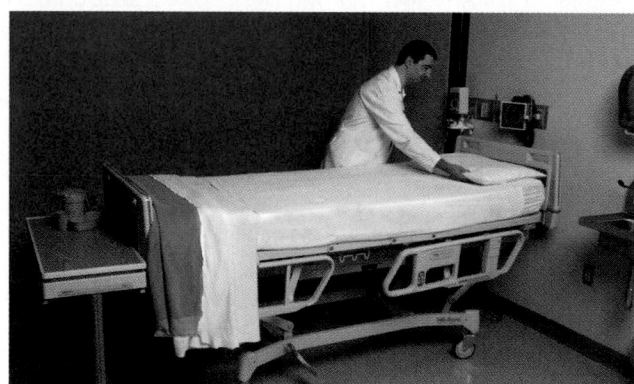

Forms

The forms in this section are copies that are put into the patient's permanent record in paper form. Many agencies have computer-based discharge processes, however.

Fishermen's HOSPITAL

Discharge Assessment/Instructions

Date of Discharge	Time of Discharge	Mode of Discharge ☐ Ambulatory ☐ Wheelchair ☐ Stretcher ☐ Ambulance			Accompanied by:
Belongings sent with patient/family ☐ Yes ☐ No		Personal Medications sent with patient family ☐ Yes ☐ No			
Temp	P	Discharge Destination			Transfer Information Sent
R	BP	☐ Home ☐ AMA ☐ Facility_____ ☐ Home Health			☐ Yes ☐ No

Special Instructions

Patient Assessment and Health Status

	Yes	No		Yes	No		Yes	No
Afebrile	☐	☐	Skin Intact	☐	☐	Hygiene	☐	☐
Able to live independently	☐	☐	Eating Well	☐	☐	Self-Care	☐	☐
Pain Controlled	☐	☐	Adequate Hydration	☐	☐	Assist	☐	☐
Oriented	☐	☐				Total Care	☐	☐
Appropriate Behavior	☐	☐				Adequate Elimination	☐	☐
Functions Independently	☐	☐						

Additional Comments:

Weight monitoring daily   Avoid all tobacco products

Instructions

Diet
☐ No Restrictions

Activity
☐ No Restrictions

Special Equipment/Treatment
☐ No Restrictions

Discharge Medications (Name, Amount, Special Instructions)
☐ No Meds   See Patient Education

Special Instructions/Discharge Summary
Call MD or go to the ER if symptoms worsen

☐ Pt or Caregiver given instructions about and counseled on potential for drug-food interactions

Physician Follow-up Appointment	Outpatient Visit
Referral ☐ None Required	

I have received all personal belongings.
I have received a copy and understand the above Instructions.
I have received a copy of the Patient Education form.

Patient Identification

_____
Signature/Responsible Party

_____
Physician/Nurse Signature   Date

0916065

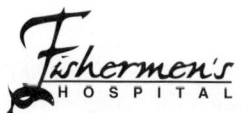

Fishermen's HOSPITAL

3301 Overseas Highway, Marathon, FL 33050 • Ph 305-743-5533 • Fax 305-743-3962

Allergies/Reactions		No known drug allergies ☐		**IN-PATIENT** Circle Y to continue or N to not continue and sign below to authenticate order.		**AT DISCHARGE** Circle Y to continue at same dose or N to not continue or document any changes in dose.		

MEDICATION NAME (Include Herbal, OTC, Vitamins)	**Dose / Route / Freq**	**Reason Taken**	**LAST DOSE DATE/TIME**	**Continue on Admission**		**Continue at home on same dose**		**Continue with the following changes:**
Patient takes no medication ☐								
				Y	N	Y	N	
				Y	N	Y	N	
				Y	N	Y	N	
				Y	N	Y	N	
				Y	N	Y	N	
				Y	N	Y	N	
				Y	N	Y	N	
				Y	N	Y	N	
				Y	N	Y	N	
				Y	N	Y	N	
				Y	N	Y	N	
				Y	N	Y	N	
				Y	N	Y	N	
				Y	N	Y	N	

Source-of-Medication list *(check all used):*
___ Bottles/List
___ Patient/Family
___ Retail pharmacy_____
_____
___ MD office records
___ Previous discharge medical record
___ Medication Administration Record from_____
_____
___ Med Reconciliation Form
Meds:
___ Sent home with_____
___ Removed
    Sent to Pharmacy for approval

New medications prescribed for patient discharge:		
Meds	**Dose / Route / Freq**	**Reason**

ADMITTING NURSE SIGNATURE   DATE

DISCHARGE NURSE SIGNATURE   DATE

Patient Education Form

Page ____ of ____

THINKING CRITICALLY ABOUT EXPERIENCING HEALTH AND ILLNESS

The exercises in the following sections allow you to practice the kind of thinking you will use as a full-spectrum nurse. Because these are critical-thinking questions, there is usually no single right answer. We do not provide answers for these questions because it is more important for you to think about the questions than to arrive at the "right" answer. These questions are designed to improve your thinking more than to "cover content." Discuss answers with your peers—discussion can stimulate critical thinking. If you have difficulty with any of these questions, consult with your instructor.

Applying the Full-Spectrum Nursing Model

PATIENT SITUATION

Recall Evelyn ("Meet Your Patient" in Volume 1). Evelyn is 87 years old and has lived in a nursing home for the last 5 years. She suffers from congestive heart failure (CHF), hypertension, diabetes, macular degeneration resulting in near blindness, a severe hearing deficit, urinary incontinence, and immobility resulting from a hip fracture. Despite these limitations, she keeps current in the lives of all of her family members and friends. At the nursing home, staff members confide in Evelyn and she knows about their children, their romances, and the gossip around the nursing home. Whenever there is an election, she makes sure that she gets to vote. She "reads" every audio book she can get her hands on.

Recently Evelyn was admitted to the hospital in severe CHF. When leaving the nursing home, she told her pastor, "I don't want to die yet. I'm having too much fun!" You notice that the papers from the nursing home do not contain an advance directive, and it was not mentioned in their report to you.

THINKING

1. *Critical Thinking (Considering Alternatives):*

    a. What are some possible reasons that that there is no advance directive?

    b. Which of those seems most likely to you?

    c. How might you finding out about the status of Evelyn's advance directive?

DOING

2. *Nursing Process (Nursing Diagnosis):* On the care plan from the nursing home, there were two nursing diagnoses:

- Urge Urinary Incontinence related to difficulty ambulating to bathroom
- Impaired Skin Integrity related to immobility and incontinence

Which of these can you remove from the care plan for now? Explain your decision.

CARING

3. *Self-Knowledge:* The next day, despite aggressive treatment, Evelyn's condition worsens. She is not responding to verbal stimuli and her oxygen level is decreasing. There is discussion about putting her on a respirator.

    a. What would you be feeling?

    b. If Evelyn has an advance directive that says "no ventilator," how would that change your feelings?

    c. If there is an advance directive that says "do everything possible to keep me alive," how would that change your feelings?

    Note: We are not asking you what you would do; rather, how you would feel.

▓ Critical Thinking and Clinical Reasoning

1. Describe your personal view of health.

2. Identify an individual in your life, personally or professionally, who personifies health. What characteristics do you identify in this individual that represent health? What factors do you think contribute to this individual's health status?

3. Use the nursing process to develop a plan to improve your personal health.

4. What attributes, resources, or life experiences do you have as an individual to offer in your role as a nurse?

5. For each of the following concepts, use critical thinking to describe how or why it is important to nursing, patient care, or experiencing health and illness. Note that these are *not* to be merely definitions.

Health	Hardiness
Wellness	Responses to illness
Illness	Health–illness continuum
Disruptions	

▓ What Are the Main Points in This Chapter?

➤ Health is a complex phenomenon that involves physical, mental, and spiritual aspects. Having good health is an almost universal desire.

➤ Wellness is a way of life oriented toward optimal health and well-being.

➤ Life and wellness require nourishment. Nourishment comes in the form of food, exercise, sleep, relationships, meaningful work, the environment, and memories.

➤ The person with an illness rarely perceives the experience as a medical diagnosis. Instead, illness is usually described in terms of how it makes the person feel, such as pain, sadness, loss, fatigue, or being overwhelmed.

➤ People dealing with life-threatening illness have to figure out how to live and still be dying. Dealing with death is one of the most difficult experiences you will face as a nurse.

➤ One aspect of persevering in illness and life disruption is maintaining as much normalcy as possible. Normalcy helps clients cope with illness.

➤ Nurses deal with people who have been thrust into new life situations, situations they did not ask for and for which they were not prepared.

➤ People who are suffering experience loneliness. Part of aloneness can be related to the actual physical separation, part of it from a sense of the world going on without them, and part of it from a sense of no one really being in their world.

➤ Several factors influence a person's responses to disruptions. These factors include age; family patterns; culture; hardiness; support; access to healthcare resources; the stage and nature of the illness; and the intensity, duration, and multiplicity of the disruption.

➤ Chronic illnesses are a large and growing health care concern, especially among older adults.

➤ The top three risks for functional decline are cognitive impairment, depression, and disease burden.

➤ You can ease patients' disruptions from admission, transfers, and discharge from a healthcare setting by discharge planning, communication, coordination, and teaching.

➤ As a nurse, you will need to cultivate a healing presence. Listening, being attentive, being willing to learn from those in your care, and recognizing and respecting others' ways of coping are behaviors associated with a healing presence.

➤ Most people experience health, illness, and wellness as an ever-changing continuum on which they move.

➤ Communicating genuine care, concern, and sensitivity comes from who you are as a person, not from assuming a professional persona that you "put on" to fulfill a role.

➤ Patients and families may not recognize the strengths and creative abilities that they bring to a situation. Part of the art of nursing is to envision strengths and potential in patients and families who may be too overwhelmed to identify them on their own.

➤ Your healing presence may be the most memorable aspect of nursing care that you have to offer.

For practice questions for this chapter,

 Go to **NCLEX-Style Practice Quiz,** on the Student Resource Disk or DavisPlus at http://davisplus.fadavis.com/Wilkinson2

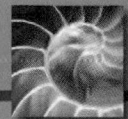 # Knowledge Map

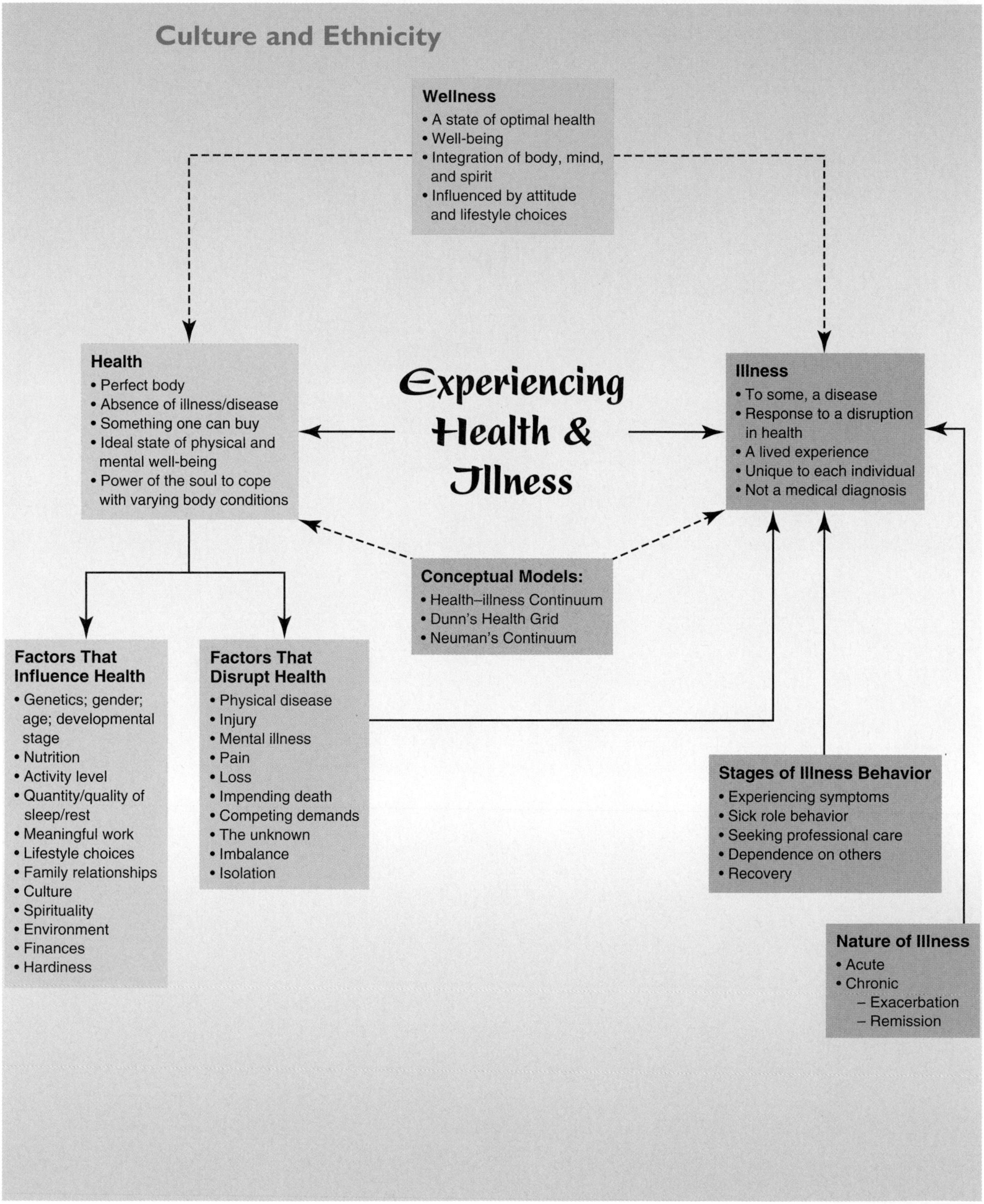

Culture and Ethnicity

Wellness
- A state of optimal health
- Well-being
- Integration of body, mind, and spirit
- Influenced by attitude and lifestyle choices

Experiencing Health & Illness

Health
- Perfect body
- Absence of illness/disease
- Something one can buy
- Ideal state of physical and mental well-being
- Power of the soul to cope with varying body conditions

Illness
- To some, a disease
- Response to a disruption in health
- A lived experience
- Unique to each individual
- Not a medical diagnosis

Conceptual Models:
- Health–illness Continuum
- Dunn's Health Grid
- Neuman's Continuum

Factors That Influence Health
- Genetics; gender; age; developmental stage
- Nutrition
- Activity level
- Quantity/quality of sleep/rest
- Meaningful work
- Lifestyle choices
- Family relationships
- Culture
- Spirituality
- Environment
- Finances
- Hardiness

Factors That Disrupt Health
- Physical disease
- Injury
- Mental illness
- Pain
- Loss
- Impending death
- Competing demands
- The unknown
- Imbalance
- Isolation

Stages of Illness Behavior
- Experiencing symptoms
- Sick role behavior
- Seeking professional care
- Dependence on others
- Recovery

Nature of Illness
- Acute
- Chronic
  - Exacerbation
  - Remission

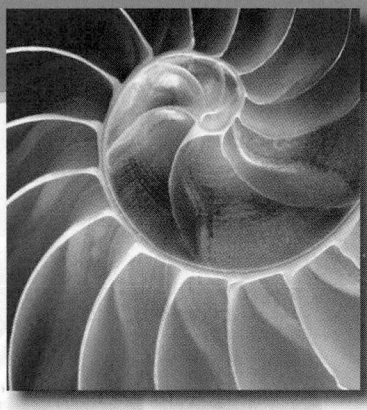

CHAPTER 11

Psychosocial Health & Illness

For a podcast of an overview of this chapter,

 Go to Student Resources, **Podcast – Chapter Overviews, Chapter 11,** on DavisPlus at http://davisplus.fadavis.com/ Wilkinson2

Caring for the Garcias

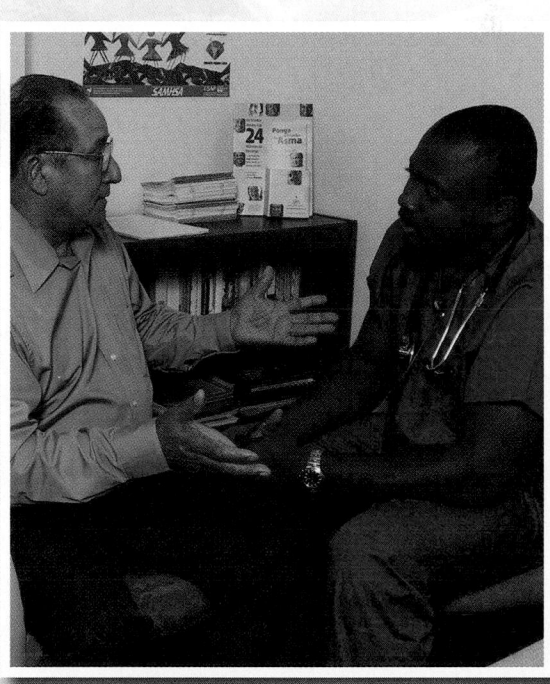

The exercises in the following section allow you to practice the kind of thinking you will use as a full-spectrum nurse. Because these are critical-thinking questions, there is usually no single right answer. We do not provide answers for these questions because it is more important for you to think about the questions than to arrive at the "right" answer. These questions are designed to improve your thinking more than to "cover content." Discuss answers with your peers—discussion can stimulate critical thinking. If you have difficulty with any of these questions, consult with your instructor.

Recall the case of Joseph Garcia. Mr. Garcia has been diagnosed with hypertension, obesity, and degenerative joint disease. At clinic visits he has made the following comments: "Every time I come in here, I get some new diagnosis. I guess it's amazing I'm not dead yet. I thought I had a lot more time left, but I'm not so sure anymore." When you ask him what his main concerns are, he tells you, "Just take a look at me! I'm a mess. Nothing is turning out the way I planned. I might as well just die now. It would save my family a lot of grief."

A. What information do you need in order to respond to Mr. Garcia?

B. How should you respond to Mr. Garcia?

C. What actions should you take?

D. What conclusions can you make about Mr. Garcia's self-concept (body image, role performance, personal identity, and self-esteem? What additional information do you need about his self-concept?

Practical **Knowledge**
knowing how

This section provides guidelines and forms for assessing self-concept, self-esteem, anxiety, and depression. In addition, you will find tables of selected standardized outcomes and interventions to consider when planning care for patients with problems related to self-concept, anxiety, or depression.

Clinical Insights

Clinical Insight 11–1 ▶ **Assessing Self-Concept Problems**

Area of Assessment	Examples of Assessment Questions
Body image	▪ When you look in the mirror, what do you see? ▪ How do you think others see you? ▪ How does your current ability to engage in work and leisure activities compare to how you would like to be?
Role performance	▪ What are your three or four major roles (e.g., daughter, student)? ▪ How successful are you in each of these roles? ▪ How important is it to you to be successful in each of these roles? ▪ What is interfering with your ability to perform any of these roles? What can you do about it?
Personal identity	▪ How did you see yourself before your illness/injury/loss? ▪ How do you see yourself now? ▪ How would you describe yourself to others? ▪ What special abilities do you have? ▪ How do you think others see you?
Self-esteem (also refer to Clinical Insight 11-2)	▪ How do you feel about yourself? ▪ What do you like about yourself? ▪ To what extent do you feel you are in control of your life? ▪ If you could change one thing about yourself, what would it be? ▪ Where would you like to be 5 years from now? ▪ How realistic are your expectations of yourself? ▪ How do you see your illness/injury/loss in relation to yourself?

Clinical Insight 11-2 ▶ Performing a Self-Esteem Inventory

Place a check mark in the column that most closely describes the client's answer to each statement. Each check is worth the number of points listed.

	3 Often or a great deal	2 Some-times	1 Seldom or occasionally	0 Never or not at all
1. I become angry or hurt when criticized.				
2. I am afraid to try new things.				
3. I feel stupid when I make a mistake.				
4. I have difficulty looking people in the eye.				
5. I have difficulty making small talk.				
6. I feel uncomfortable in the presence of strangers.				
7. I am embarrassed when people compliment me.				
8. I am dissatisfied with the way I look.				
9. I am afraid to express my opinions in a group.				
10. I prefer staying home alone rather than participating in group social situations.				
11. I have trouble accepting teasing.				
12. I feel guilty when I say no to people.				
13. I am afraid to make a commitment to a relationship for fear of rejection.				
14. I believe that most people are more competent than I am.				
15. I feel resentment toward people who are attractive and successful.				
16. I have trouble thinking of any positive aspects about my life.				
17. I feel inadequate in the presence of authority figures.				
18. I have trouble making decisions.				
19. I fear the disapproval of others.				
20. I feel tense, stressed out, or "uptight."				

Problems with low self-esteem are indicated by items scored with a 3 or by a total score higher than 46.

Source: Townsend, M. C. (2009). *Psychiatric mental health nursing: Concepts of care* (5th ed.). Philadelphia: F. A. Davis, p. 248.

Clinical Insight 11-3 ▶ Identifying Depressed Patients Who Should Be Referred for Evaluation

One way to identify depression that is more than simple, situational depression is to ask the following two questions. A Yes answer merits a referral.

1. "Over the past 2 weeks, have you felt down, depressed, or hopeless?"
2. "Over the past 2 weeks, have you felt little interest or pleasure in doing things?"

Source: U.S. Preventive Services Task Force. (2002). Screening for depression: Recommendations and rationale. *Annals of Internal Medicine, 1*36(10), 760–764.

Another method is to use the mnemonic SIGECAPS, a concise version of the *DSM-IV-TR* diagnostic criteria. Ask the patient if he has experienced, for 2 or more weeks:

Sleep increase/decrease
Interest in formerly compelling or pleasurable activities diminished
Guilt, low self-esteem
Energy poor
Concentration poor
Appetite increase/decrease
Psychomotor agitation or retardation
Suicidal ideation

Both of the following require referral for evaluation and treatment:

Major depression = depressed mood or interest *plus* 4 SIGECAPS for 2 or more weeks
Mild depression (mood disorder) = depressed mood or interest *plus* 3 SIGECAPS most days for 2 or more years

Source: Brigham and Women's Hospital (2001).

Some people prefer a mnemonic from an older source, IN SAD CAGES, which you would use in essentially the same way. Ask the patient if he has experienced, for 2 or more weeks:

Interest reduced
Negative thoughts
Sleep disturbance
Appetite change
Decreased confidence or self-esteem
Concentration reduced
Affect blunt or flat
Guilt
Energy reduced
Suicidal ideas

The original reference does not include a suggested total that requires referral. However, you can assume that the more symptoms, the more severe the depression. We would suggest the following:

IN (reduced interest and negative thoughts or depressed mood) *plus* 4 of the other **SAD CAGES** requires referral.
Do not try to differentiate mild and major depression with this method.

Adapted from Rund, D. A., & Hutzler, J. C. (1983). *Emergency psychiatry.* St. Louis, MO: C. V. Mosby, p. 144.

Assessment Guidelines and Tools

Anxiety Assessment Guide

Rating Scale: None = 0, Mild = 1, Moderate = 2, Severe = 3, Disabling (Panic) = 4

PHYSIOLOGICAL EFFECTS		PSYCHOLOGICAL EFFECTS	
Shortness of breath (dyspnea)	____	Depersonalization (unreal)	____
Choking sensation	____	Feeling "on edge"	____
Dry mouth	____	Poor concentration	____
Pounding heart, increased heart rate	____	Poor memory	____
Chest pain	____	Depressed mood	____
Increased sweating and clammy	____	Loss of interest	____
Feeling faint, dizzy, unsteady	____	Restlessness	____
Nausea and abdominal upsets	____	Sense of panic	____
Numbness (pins and needles)	____	Worry, anticipation of the worst	____
Hot/cold flashes	____	Irritability	____
Trembling, shaking	____	Nightmares	____
Muscle tension and aches	____	Feeling of fear and foreboding	____
Exaggerated startle response	____	Excessive apprehension	____
Difficulties in falling asleep and staying asleep	____	Feeling lack of control	____

Assessing Overall Scores

0–28	Mild anxiety
29–56	Moderate anxiety
57–84	Severe anxiety
85–112	Disabling anxiety

Creating a total score from this table can help you assess whether overall anxiety is mild, moderate, severe, or disabling. However, individual physiological or psychological symptoms that are rated as severe (3) or disabling (4) may be more important and relevant to your nursing assessment. For example, your patient's overall or total assessment may be 26 (in the mild range, 0–27) but she has rated "Excessive apprehension" as 4 (disabling).

Depression Assessment Guide: Patient Health Questionnaire (PHQ-9)

This is a valid and reliable measure of depression developed in 1999 by Pfizer, Inc. It can be self-administered (Kroenke, Spitzer, & Williams, 2001). It may be useful across cultures (Chen, Huang, Chang, et al., 2006).

Over the past 2 weeks, how often have you been bothered by any of the following problems? (Check or circle your answers.)

	NOT AT ALL	SEVERAL DAYS	MORE THAN HALF THE DAYS	NEARLY EVERY DAY
1. Little interest or pleasure in doing things	0	1	2	2
2. Feeling down, depressed, or hopeless	0	1	2	3
3. Trouble falling or staying asleep, or sleeping too much	0	1	2	3
4. Feeling tired or having little energy	0	1	2	3
5. Poor appetite or overeating	0	1	2	3
6. Feeling bad about yourself—or that you are a failure or have let yourself or your family down	0	1	2	3
7. Trouble concentrating on things, such as reading the newspaper or watching television	0	1	2	3
8. Moving or speaking so slowly that other people could have noticed. Or the opposite—being so fidgety or restless that you have been moving around a lot more than usual	0	1	2	3
9. Thoughts that you would be better off dead or of hurting yourself in some way	0	1	2	3
ADD COLUMNS		[ ] +	[ ] +	[ ]

TOTAL: [   ]

10. If you checked off any problems, how difficult have these problems made it for you to do your work, take care of things at home, or get along with other people?

Not difficult at all   _____

Somewhat difficult   _____

Very difficult   _____

Extremely difficult   _____

(Healthcare professional: For interpretation of TOTAL, please refer to the accompanying score card. *[Note to students: Interpretation requires training. You should report the patient's score to your instructor or your immediate supervising nurse.]*)

Source: Pfizer, Inc. Retrieved from http://www.phqscreeners.com/. Used by permission.

Differentiating Depression and Dementia

This table may help you to identify older adults who should be referred for further evaluation to determine whether symptoms are related to depression or dementia. To screen for depression,

 Go to Chapter 11, **Tables, Boxes, Figures: Geriatric Depression Rating Scale (Short Form),** on the Student Resource Disk or DavisPlus at http://davisplus.fadavis.com/Wilkinson2

To determine whether the patient should be referred to a mental health professional, refer to Clinical Insight 11-3.

CHARACTERISTIC	DEPRESSION	DEMENTIA
Cause/triggers	Loss (e.g., of spouse, of independence); stress	Physiological causes (e.g., Alzheimer's disease, brain infarcts)
Onset	Acute or chronic; can be related to specific events	Chronic, gradual, and insidious
Course	Varies, depending on cause	Progressive, over a long period of time
Alertness	Usually reduced	Usually normal
Memory	Memory loss and forgetfulness	Recent and remote memory impaired; loss of recent memory is first sign; some loss of common knowledge
Thinking	Inability to concentrate	Difficulty with abstraction and word finding, especially nouns; difficulty with calculations; decreased judgment
Response to questions	Often says "I don't know."	Answers inappropriately or with "near misses"
Language	Speaks slowly; slow to respond to verbal stimuli	Disoriented, rambling, incoherent; difficulty using nouns
Sleep	Difficulty falling asleep, early morning awakening, much day sleeping	Sleep fragmented; awakens often during night
Reversibility	Potential	Irreversible, progressive

Source: Adapted from Edwards, N. (2003). Differentiating the three D's: Delirium, dementia, and depression. *MedSurg Nursing.* Retrieved from http://findarticles.com/p/articles/mi_m0FSS/is_6_12/ai_n18616788

Standardized Nursing Language

You can use the tables in this section when planning care for patients with problems of self-concept, anxiety, or depression. The tables provide standardized wording for nursing diagnoses, outcomes, and interventions. You can use the NOC indicators with the outcomes to write goals. Non-NOC outcomes are also suggested. In addition to the broad NIC interventions, the tables also provide specific nursing activities suggested by NIC.

Psychosocial Outcomes: Examples from NOC Taxonomy

From the Psychosocial Health Domain

Abusive Behavior Self-Restraint	Role Performance
Coping	Social Interaction Skills
Child Adaptation to Hospitalization	Social Involvement
Loneliness Severity	Social Support
Psychosocial Adjustment: Life Change	Suicide Self-Restraint

From Other Domains

Family Coping	Family Normalization
Family Functioning	Family Participation in Professional Care
Family Health Status	Family Resiliency

Source: Moorhead, S., Johnson, M., Maas, M. L., & Swanson, E. (Eds.). (2008). *Nursing outcomes classification (NOC)* (4th ed.). St. Louis, MO: C.V. Mosby.

Psychosocial Interventions: Examples from NIC Taxonomy

Behavioral Domain: Care that supports psychosocial functioning and facilitates lifestyle changes

Anger Control Assistance	Decision-Making Support
Anxiety Reduction	Health Education
Behavior Management	Role Enhancement
Conflict Mediation	Socialization Enhancement
Coping Enhancement	Support Group

Family Domain: Care that supports the family

Developmental Enhancement	Family Support
Family Integrity Promotion: Childbearing Family	Family Therapy
Family Involvement Promotion	Normalization Promotion
Family Process Maintenance	Parent Education: Adolescent
Family Mobilization	Parenting Promotion

Source: Bulechek, G. M., Butcher, H. K., & Dochterman, J. M. (Eds.). (2008). *Nursing interventions classification (NIC)* (5th ed.). St. Louis, MO: C.V. Mosby. Used with permission.

Self-Concept Diagnoses: Selected Standardized and Individualized Outcomes

NURSING DIAGNOSIS	NOC OUTCOMES	NOC OUTCOME INDICATORS AND SCALE LETTER*	INDIVIDUALIZED OUTCOMES (NOT NOC)
Chronic Low Self-Esteem	Depression Level	Crying spells mild (n)	Participates and expresses pleasure in activities.
	Quality of Life	Economic status, completely satisfied (s)	Incidence of expressions of worthlessness decreases.
			Reports improved libido.
	Self-Esteem	Verbalizations of self-acceptance often positive (k)	Reports satisfaction with close relationships.
			Makes frequent eye contact.
			Maintains erect posture.
Situational Low Self-Esteem	Adaptation to Physical Disability	Adapts to functional limitations (m).	Accepts help from family members as needed.
	Grief Resolution	Verbalizes acceptance of loss (m).	Verbalizes positive self-description.
	Psychosocial Adjustment: Life Change	Reports feeling useful (m).	Asks for and accepts help from others.
	Self-Esteem	Maintenance of eye contact, often positive (k)	Makes frequent eye contact. Maintains erect posture.
Disturbed Personal Identity	Distorted Thought Self-Control	Refrains from responding to hallucinations or delusions, sometimes demonstrated (m).	Reports when experiencing hallucinations or delusions; describes their content.
			Verbal and nonverbal behaviors are congruent.

Self-Concept Diagnoses: Selected Standardized and Individualized Outcomes—cont'd

NURSING DIAGNOSIS	NOC OUTCOMES	NOC OUTCOME INDICATORS AND SCALE LETTER*	INDIVIDUALIZED OUTCOMES (NOT NOC)
	Identity	Verbalizes clear sense of personal identity, consistently demonstrated (m).	Accurately differentiates self from environment and other people.
	Self-Mutilation Restraint	Refrains from injuring self, consistently demonstrated (m).	Maintains control of urges; does not injure self.
			Reports to nurse when feeling the urge to harm self.
Ineffective Role Performance	Caregiver Lifestyle Disruption	Financial burden to caregiver, moderate (n)	Demonstrates ability to meet role expectations.
			Identifies strategies for role change(s).
	Coping	Identifies effective coping patterns, often demonstrated (m).	Reports comfort with role expectation.
			Verbalizes feeling in control of his life.
	Depression Level	Impaired concentration, none (n)	Identifies and uses effective coping strategies.
	Psychosocial Adjustment: Life Change	Maintains productivity, consistently demonstrated (m).	Demonstrates ability to manage finances.
	Psychomotor Energy	Exhibits ability to accomplish daily tasks, consistently demonstrated (t).	Adapts routine tasks to conserve energy.
	Role Performance	Reported comfort with role expectations, totally adequate (f).	Reports strategies for role changes.
Disturbed Body Image	Body Image	Internal picture of self, often positive (k)	Demonstrates congruence between body reality, body ideal, and body perception.
	Child Development (2 to 17 years)	Balances on one foot, consistently demonstrated (m).	Openly expresses signs of grief over loss of bodily function.
	Grief Resolution	Progresses through stages of grief, consistently demonstrated (m).	Expresses satisfaction with body appearance and function.
	Psychosocial Adjustment: Life Change	(See Situational Low Self-Esteem diagnosis.)	Demonstrates willingness to use strategies to enhance appearance and function.
	Self-Esteem		Verbalizes positive aspects of body.
Risk-Prone Health Behavior	Acceptance: Health Status	Performs self-care tasks, consistently demonstrated (m).	Expresses feelings about illness.
(previously Impaired Adjustment)	Compliance Behavior	Performs treatment regimen as prescribed, often demonstrated (m).	Keeps appointments with healthcare provider.
	Coping	Reports increase in psychological comfort, consistently demonstrated (m).	Follows prescribed regimen for medications and other therapies.
	Grief Resolution	(See Body Image Disturbance diagnosis.)	Maintains usual grooming and hygiene.
	Health-Seeking Behavior	Asks health-related questions when indicated, consistently demonstrated (m).	Requests information about physical condition and measures to maximize health.
	Participation in Health Care Decisions	Seeks reputable information, consistently demonstrated (m).	Participates in making decisions about healthcare.

Continued

Self-Concept Diagnoses: Selected Standardized and Individualized Outcomes—cont'd

NURSING DIAGNOSIS	NOC OUTCOMES	NOC OUTCOME INDICATORS AND SCALE LETTER*	INDIVIDUALIZED OUTCOMES (NOT NOC)
	Psychosocial Adjustment: Life Change	Sets realistic goals, sometimes demonstrated (m).	Identifies barriers to achieving health goals.
	Treatment Behavior: Illness or Injury	Follows recommended treatment regimen, consistently demonstrated (m).	Alters lifestyle to meet treatment requirements.

Sources: Johnson, M., Bulechek, G., Dochterman, J., et al. (2006), *NANDA, NOC, and NIC linkages: Nursing diagnoses, outcomes, and interventions* (2nd ed.). St. Louis, MO: C.V. Mosby; and Moorhead, S., Johnson, M., Maas, M., et al. (Eds.) (2008), *Nursing outcomes classification (NOC)* (4th ed.). St. Louis, MO: C.V. Mosby. Used with permission.

*See NOC Measurement Scales in Chapter 5, Volume 2, for scales to use in describing desired outcomes or goals.

Self-Concept Diagnoses: Selected NIC Interventions and Nursing Activities

NIC INTERVENTION	SELECTED NURSING ACTIVITIES (NIC)
Anticipatory Guidance	Assist the patient to adapt to anticipated role changes.
	Suggest books/literature for the patient to read, as appropriate.
	Schedule visits at strategic developmental/situational points.
Behavior Modification	Determine patient's motivation to change.
	Maintain consistent staff behavior.
	Reinforce constructive decisions concerning health needs.
Body Image Enhancement	Use anticipatory guidance to prepare patient for predictable changes in body image.
	Monitor frequency of statements of self-criticism.
	Assist patient to separate physical appearance from feelings of personal worth, as appropriate.
Coping Enhancement	Use a calm, reassuring approach.
	Assist the patient in developing an objective appraisal of the event.
	Encourage the acceptance of the limitations of others.
Decision-Making Support	Inform patient of alternative views or solutions in a clear and supportive manner.
	Help patient identify the advantages and disadvantages of each alternative.
	Obtain informed consent, when appropriate.
Delusion Management	Establish a trusting, interpersonal relationship with patient.
	Avoid arguing about false beliefs; state doubt matter-of-factly.
	Avoid reinforcing delusional ideas.
Developmental Enhancement	(depends on developmental stage)
Child and Adolescent	Assist each child to become aware he/she is important as an individual.
	Facilitate a sense of responsibility for self and others.
Grief Work Facilitation	Identify the loss.
	Encourage expression of feelings about the loss.
	Instruct in phases of the grieving process, as appropriate.
Hallucination Management	Maintain a safe environment.
	Provide patient with opportunities to discuss hallucinations.
	Provide antipsychotic and antianxiety medications on a routine and PRN (as-needed) basis.
Hope Inspiration	Assist patient or family to identify areas of hope in life.
	Inform the patient about whether the current situation is a temporary state.

Self-Concept Diagnoses: Selected NIC Interventions and Nursing Activities—cont'd

NIC INTERVENTION	SELECTED NURSING ACTIVITIES (NIC)
Mood Management	Assist patient to identify thoughts and feelings underlying the dysfunctional mood.
	Determine whether patient presents a safety risk to self or others.
	Provide opportunity for physical activity (e.g., walking or riding the exercise bike).
Parent Education: Childrearing Family	Facilitate parents' discussion of methods of discipline available, selection, and results obtained.
	Give parents a variety of strategies to use in managing a child's behavior.
Reality Orientation	Inform patient of person, place, and time, as needed.
	Provide a consistent physical environment and daily routine.
	Recommend patient wear personal clothing, assist as needed.
Role Enhancement	Assist patient to identify usual role in family.
	Assist patient to identify role insufficiency.
	Assist patient to identify positive strategies for managing role changes.
Risk Identification	Institute routine risk assessment, using reliable and valid instruments.
	Determine presence and quality of family support.
	Determine financial resources.
Self-Esteem Enhancement	Monitor patient's statements of self worth.
	Convey confidence in patient's ability to handle situation.
	Refrain from teasing.
Values Clarification	Pose reflective, clarifying questions that give the patient something to think about.
	Encourage patient to make a list of what is important and not important in life and the time spent on each.
	Avoid use of cross-examining questions.

Source: Bulechek, G. M., Butcher, H. K., & Dochterman, J. M. (Eds.). (2008). *Nursing interventions classification (NIC)* (5th ed.). St. Louis, MO: C.V. Mosby. Used with permission.

Anxiety-Related Diagnoses: Selected NOC Outcomes and NIC Interventions

CUE CLUSTER	NANDA-I DIAGNOSIS*	NOC OUTCOMES†	SELECTED INDICATORS	NIC INTERVENTIONS AND SPECIFIC ACTIVITIES‡
Susan is pacing the floor and does not make eye contact when she speaks to you. Her hands are shaking. Her BP is 140/88 mm Hg, P is 100 beats/min, and R are 24. She says she is worried.	Anxiety	Anxiety Self-Control **Other Outcomes** Anxiety Level Concentration Coping	(Often demonstrated) ■ Monitors intensity of anxiety. ■ Maintains concentration.	Anxiety Reduction ■ Use a calm, reassuring approach. ■ Explain all procedures, including sensations the patient is likely to experience during the procedure. ■ Help the patient identify situations that precipitate anxiety. **Other Interventions** Anger Control Assistance Anticipatory Guidance Calming Technique Coping Enhancement Emotional Support

Continued

Anxiety-Related Diagnoses: Selected NOC Outcomes and NIC Interventions—cont'd

CUE CLUSTER	NANDA-I DIAGNOSIS*	NOC OUTCOMES†	SELECTED INDICATORS	NIC INTERVENTIONS AND SPECIFIC ACTIVITIES‡
Martin has a terminal illness. He looks very sad. He states that he is worried that his dying will be prolonged and difficult for his family and that he is afraid of dying.	Death Anxiety	Acceptance: Health Status **Other Outcomes** Anxiety Self-Control Comfortable Death Depression Level Dignified Life Closure Fear Self-Control Hope Spiritual Health	(Often demonstrated) ■ Appears peaceful. ■ Reports positive self regard. ■ Clarifies personal values.	Emotional Support ■ Listen to and encourage expressions of feelings and beliefs. ■ Provide support during denial, anger, bargaining, and acceptance phases of grieving. **Other Interventions** Anxiety Reduction Coping Enhancement Decision-Making Support Dying Care Hope Instillation Pain Management Presence Religious Ritual Enhancement Spiritual Support
Ms. Eng says, "I just don't know whether to have this chemotherapy or not. I know I could live a little longer, but the side effects . . ." She has decided twice to do it and each time has changed her mind. She says, "I just can't focus on anything else."	Decisional Conflict	Decision Making **Other Outcomes** Information Processing Participation: Health Care Decisions Personal Autonomy	(Not compromised) ■ Identifies alternatives. ■ Identifies needed resources to support each alternative.	Decision-Making Support ■ Determine whether there are differences between the patient's view of own condition and the views of healthcare providers. ■ Serve as a liaison between the patient and family. ■ Serve as a liaison between patient and other healthcare providers. **Other Interventions** Assertiveness Training Health System Guidance Learning Facilitation Mutual Goal Setting
Bryan is to have his burns débrided today. He is crying. He says, "I wish my mom was here. It hurts so bad when they do that. I'm so scared."	Fear	Fear Self-Control **Other Outcomes** Fear Level Fear Level: Child	(Often demonstrated) ■ Uses relaxation techniques to reduce fear. ■ Maintains concentration. ■ Controls fear response.	Security Enhancement ■ Spend time with the patient. ■ Answer questions about health status in an honest manner. ■ Hold a young child or infant, as appropriate. **Other Interventions** Anxiety Reduction Calming Technique Coping Enhancement Presence

Anxiety-Related Diagnoses: Selected NOC Outcomes and NIC Interventions—cont'd

CUE CLUSTER	NANDA-I DIAGNOSIS*	NOC OUTCOMES†	SELECTED INDICATORS	NIC INTERVENTIONS AND SPECIFIC ACTIVITIES‡
Mr. Paul's blood pressure remains dangerously high, yet he does not make the changes in diet and exercise that are needed, and he often fails to take his pills. "I feel OK. This is a bunch of mumbo jumbo. My folks ate fried foods, and they lived to be over 80."	Ineffective Denial	Health Beliefs: Perceived Threat **Other Outcomes** Acceptance: Health Status Anxiety Self-Control Fear Self-Control Symptom Control	(Strong) ■ Perceived threat to health ■ Perceived vulnerability to progressive health problems ■ Perceived impact on functional status	Self-Awareness Enhancement ■ Assist the patient to identify the values that contribute to self-concept. ■ Assist patient to identify the impact of illness on self-concept. ■ Verbalize the patient's denial of reality, as appropriate. **Other Interventions** Anxiety Reduction Calming Technique Coping Enhancement Counseling Emotional Support Health Education Security Enhancement Self-Awareness Enhancement Self-Modification Assistance Self-Responsibility Facilitation Teaching: Disease Process

*NANDA International. (2009). *Nursing diagnoses: Definitions and classification 2009–2011*. Philadelphia: Author. Used with permission.

†Johnson, M., Bulechek, G., Butcher, H., et al. (2006). *NANDA, NOC, and NIC linkages: Nursing diagnoses, outcomes, and interventions* (2nd ed.). St. Louis, MO: C.V. Mosby; and Moorhead, S., Johnson, M., Maas, M. L., et al. (Eds.). (2008). *Nursing outcomes classification (NOC)* (4th ed.). St. Louis, MO: C.V. Mosby. Used with permission.

‡Johnson, M., Bulechek, G., Butcher, H., et al. (2006). *NANDA, NOC, and NIC linkages: Nursing diagnoses, outcomes, and interventions* (2nd ed.). St. Louis, MO: C.V. Mosby; and Bulechek, G. M., Butcher, H. K., & Dochterman, J. M. (Eds.). (2008). *Nursing interventions classification (NIC)* (5th ed.). St. Louis, MO: C.V. Mosby. Used with permission.

Depression-Related Nursing Diagnoses: Selected NOC Outcomes and NIC Interventions

CUE CLUSTER	NANDA-I DIAGNOSIS*	NOC OUTCOMES†	SELECTED INDICATORS	NIC INTERVENTIONS AND SPECIFIC ACTIVITIES‡
John is dying of AIDS. He sleeps most of the time. During care activities (e.g., bath), he closes his eyes and remains passive. When asked to move or participate, he sighs and says, "I can't." When friends visit, he turns away from them; when they talk to him, he just shrugs. He has quit eating. He says, "It doesn't matter what I do. Nothing can change the way this turns out."	Hopelessness	Hope **Other Outcomes** Depression Level Depression Self-Control Mood Equilibrium Psychomotor Energy Quality of Life Will to Live	(Often demonstrated) Expresses meaning in life. Expresses inner peace. Expresses belief in self. Expresses belief in others. Expresses sense of self-control.	Hope Inspiration ■ Demonstrate hope by recognizing the patient's intrinsic worth and viewing the patient's illness as only one facet of the individual. ■ Help the patient expand spiritual self. ■ Create an environment that facilitates patient practicing religion, as appropriate. ■ Facilitate the patient or family's reliving and savoring past achievements and experiences. ■ Teach the family about the positive aspects of hope (e.g., develop meaningful conversational themes that reflect love and need for the patient). ■ Avoid masking the truth. **Other Interventions** Coping Enhancement Counseling Mood Management Resiliency Promotion Self-Modification Assistance Spiritual Growth Facilitation Values Clarification
Jennifer is 16 and pregnant. She does not follow good health practices. She angrily says, "It's my body, and I don't want this baby. But my parents say abortion is a sin. I should honor my parents, but I hate them. I hate having to depend on them, and I hate being pregnant."	Powerlessness	Health Beliefs: Perceived Control **Other Outcomes** Depression Self-Control Family Participation in Professional Care Health Beliefs Health Beliefs: Perceived Ability to Perform Health Beliefs: Perceived Resources Hope Participation in Health Care Decisions Personal Autonomy	(Strong) Requested involvement in health decisions. Efforts at gathering information. Belief that own actions control health outcomes. Willingness to designate surrogate decision maker.	Self-Responsibility Facilitation ■ Discuss with the patient the extent of responsibility for present health status. ■ Determine whether the patient has adequate knowledge about healthcare condition. ■ Encourage verbalizations of feelings, perceptions, and fears about assuming responsibility. ■ Discuss consequences of not dealing with own responsibilities. ■ Encourage patient to take as much responsibility for own self-care, as possible. ■ Provide positive feedback for accepting additional responsibility and/or behavior change. **Other Interventions** Cognitive Restructuring Decision-Making Support Emotional Support Family Involvement Promotion Financial Resource Assistance Health Education Health System Guidance Hope Inspiration Mood Management Mutual Goal Setting Patient Rights Protection Self-Esteem Enhancement Values Clarification

Selected NOC Outcomes and NIC Interventions—cont'd

CUE CLUSTER	NANDA-I DIAGNOSIS*	NOC OUTCOMES†	SELECTED INDICATORS	NIC INTERVENTIONS AND SPECIFIC ACTIVITIES‡
Tim has attempted suicide twice. He now says, "I will get it right this time. I know where I can get a gun."	Risk for Suicide	Suicide Self-Restraint **Other Outcomes** Mood Equilibrium Will to Live	(Often demonstrated) Obtains assistance as needed. Controls impulses. Refrains from gathering means for suicide. Refrains from giving away possessions. Upholds suicide contract. Expresses feelings.	Suicide Prevention ■ Refer patient to mental healthcare provider . . . for evaluation and treatment. . . . ■ Administer medications to decrease anxiety, agitation, or psychosis and to stabilize mood, as appropriate. ✚ Conduct mouth checks after medication administration to ensure that patient is not "cheeking" the medications for later overdose attempt. ■ Initiate suicide precautions (e.g., ongoing observation and monitoring of the patient, provision of a protective environment) . . . ■ Limit access to windows, unless locked and shatterproof, as appropriate. ■ Monitor patient during use of potential weapons (e.g., razor). ■ Assist patient to identify network of supportive persons and resources (e.g., clergy, family, providers). **Other Interventions** Behavior Management: Self-Harm Hope Inspiration Mood Management Spiritual Support

* NANDA International. (2009). *Nursing diagnoses: Definitions and classification 2009–2011*. Philadelphia: Author. Used with permission.

†Johnson, M., Bulechek, G., Butcher, H., et al. (2006). *NANDA, NOC, and NIC linkages: Nursing diagnoses, outcomes, and interventions* (2nd ed.). St. Louis, MO: C.V. Mosby; and Moorhead, S., Johnson, M., Maas, M., et al. (Eds.). (2008). *Nursing outcomes classification (NOC)* (4th ed.). St. Louis, MO: C.V. Mosby. Used with permission.

‡Johnson, M., Bulechek, G., Butcher, H., et al. (2006). *NANDA, NOC, and NIC linkages: Nursing diagnoses, outcomes, and interventions* (2nd ed.). St. Louis, MO: C.V. Mosby; Bulechek, G. M., Butcher, H. K., & Dochterman, J. M. (Eds.). (2008). *Nursing interventions classification (NIC)* (5th ed.). St. Louis, MO: C.V. Mosby. Used with permission.

THINKING CRITICALLY ABOUT PSYCHOSOCIAL HEALTH & ILLNESS

The exercises in the following sections allow you to practice the kind of thinking you will use as a full-spectrum nurse. Because these are critical-thinking questions, there is usually no single right answer. We do not provide answers for these questions because it is more important for you to think about the questions than to arrive at the "right" answer. These questions are designed to improve your thinking more than to "cover content." Discuss answers with your peers—discussion can stimulate critical thinking. If you have difficulty with any of these questions, consult with your instructor.

Applying the Full-Spectrum Nursing Model

PATIENT SITUATION

Matthew has been admitted to the emergency department with extensive wounds to both forearms, including tendon and vascular damage, from a suicide attempt. Matthew seems very quiet, almost withdrawn, and answers most of your questions in monosyllables.

Matthew reports the following: He is the third child in a family of five. Matthew's middle-class parents are now retired, and his brothers and sisters are scattered across the country in various large cities. Although Matthew claims his schooling years were unremarkable, he reminisces about several occasions when he was bullied and physically beaten by gangs of older adolescents.

Matthew further states that he graduated from Harvard Law School and became vice president of an influential law firm. Despite his apparent success in life, from early childhood he has continued to question his self-worth. Plagued by worries and depression that have increased over the past few years, he says he wrote a note indicating that he now realizes what a failure he is and proceeded to slash both of his forearms with a sharp razor.

Matthew reports that he has not been eating much, feels tired all the time, and has no interest in going outside the house. He says, "I just don't feel like doing anything; I just want to sleep all the time."

THINKING

1. *Theoretical Knowledge*: Using just the information you have in the patient situation, use the SIGECAPS method in Clinical Insight 11-3 to assess Matthew's level of depression. You will need to assume that he is reporting what he has experienced in the last 2 weeks (unless he is obviously referring to the past).

2. *Critical Thinking (Inquiry)*: What items of the SIGECAPS cannot be completed with the information in the Patient Situation? What do you need to ask Matthew to complete them?

DOING

3. *Nursing Process (Interventions)*: Based on your SIGECAPS data, what do you need to do right away (or be certain it was done in the emergency department)?

CARING

4. *Self-Knowledge*: What do you have in common with Matthew that might help you to empathize with him?

5. *Ethical Knowledge*: Try to put aside your own beliefs now, and answer from the perspective of Matthew and one of your nursing colleagues on the unit.

   a. Give one reason to support Matthew's claim that he has a right to commit suicide if his despair is too deep to bear.

   b. Give one reason to support a colleague's claim that he does not have a right to commit suicide, no matter how he feels.

Critical Thinking and Clinical Reasoning

1. Review the scenario about Karli ("Meet Your Patient" from Volume 1):

You are caring for a 16-year-old patient named Karli who is suffering from fractures to both arms and several ribs, as well as extensive first- and second-degree burns to 30% of her body after a motor vehicle accident. Karli was driving her parents' car home from her part-time job when she lost control of the car and crashed into a wall. The car exploded in flames. A passerby quickly reported the accident, and fast action by the emergency response team saved Karli's life.

Karli is suffering from a moderate amount of shock and pain. She alternates among outbursts of anger, self-directed sarcasm, and despondence. She tells you that she cannot understand how the accident happened, that one moment she was adjusting the car radio, and the next moment she awoke in the hospital. Then suddenly she explodes. "It's not fair! I just took my eyes off the road for a second; that's all!" She bursts into tears. Picking at her bandages, she sobs, "No one will ever love me the way I'm going to look. My life is over. I hate myself!" You take her hand. "I used to be pretty," she says, "but now I'll look like a freak! What did I do to deserve this? I know plenty of kids who drive drunk or high all the time. I wasn't doing anything wrong! Why did this happen to me?"

a. Now that you have completed Chapter 11 in Volume 1, make a list of the multiple physical, psychological, and social issues that you would need to consider in developing a comprehensive care plan for Karli.

b. Compare your list with the one you made when you first began reading the chapter. How is it different? Or is it the same?

2. In the "Meet Your Patient" scenario, Karli perceives herself as unlovable "looking this way." Which of the following nursing activities do you think might be helpful in *exploring and changing her perception*? For those you *do not* choose, explain why.

Role Enhancement

- Help the patient distinguish ideal and actual self. Help her describe realistic roles and expectations tailored to specific health changes.
- Compare realistic roles to previous and less functional roles.

Conflict Mediation

- Provide a quiet, private, neutral setting for mediation to take place.
- Maintain your own neutrality in the process; do not "take sides."

Promoting Family Integrity

- Encourage and facilitate communication among family members.
- Encourage family members to care for the patient as much as possible.

Family Mobilization

- Help the family to identify strengths they can use to support the patient.
- Teach family members how to provide home care for the patient.
- Help the family identify community resources and/or support groups.
- Keep the family informed about the patient's progress, with the patient's permission.

Enhancing Socialization

- Explore and reinforce the individual's established relationships.
- Provide opportunities to rehearse relationship-building skills.
- Investigate, assist, and promote any developing relationships with persons of similar interests and goals.
- Provide information and links to community activities that relate to the person's past, current, and future interests.
- Promote access to education in social skills development.

- Encourage the patient to communicate and engage in interpersonal relationship activities by providing ongoing positive feedback.
- Organize small, cohesive group activities.
- Provide or act as a role model where appropriate.

3. Mrs. King is being admitted into the orthopedics unit for a scheduled total knee replacement. Even though she appears to be in good health for a 72-year-old woman, you are concerned about her excessive weight, which can be described as moderate to severe obesity. You are troubled by how the obesity may negatively affect postsurgical recovery, wound healing, and mobility.

   a. What theoretical knowledge will you draw on to plan care to meet her biopsychosocial needs?

   b. What assumptions are you making? What stereotypes do you have that might affect your understanding of Mrs. King's situation?

   c. What do you think might be contributing to Mrs. King's obesity?

   d. What facts do you have to support those ideas?

   e. How could you find out for sure what is contributing to Mrs. King's obesity?

4. Day by day, you notice that your patient is eating less and complaining about constipation and tiredness. You carefully review her nutritional requirements against the food menu, as well as check nursing records for bowel movements. You have exhausted your initial search for obvious reasons why your patient's appetite has changed. After sitting down next to your patient, you cannot help noticing how tired she looks.

   a. What psychosocial problem do you suspect (low self-esteem, depression, anxiety, or disturbed personal identity)?

   b. What data do you have to support your inference in (a)?

   c. Objective data in her chart indicate that the patient has been eating very little and that she has been having bowel movements only every 3 or 4 days—and even then only with a laxative or enema. What other symptom do you need to investigate further?

   d. How could you obtain more information about that symptom?

   e. Think of depressed people you have known or depressed patients you have cared for. What have you found to be difficult about dealing with them?

5. Edna Jackson is 42 years old. She has had a hysterectomy (removal of her uterus). Her surgery was uncomplicated, her overall health is good, and she is expected to make a full and rapid physical recovery.

   Her husband was not present when she was admitted and has not been to see her since the surgery. He did not want her to have the surgery. He told Edna that he doesn't know whether he will want to have sex with her when she is no longer "a whole woman." He has had casual affairs during their marriage, which Edna has tolerated because she feels that difficulty is balanced by the many positive benefits of their relationship, which include a "good sex life."

   Edna has seven brothers and sisters, and she has five children of her own, ages 23, 21, 18, 6, and 4. She comes from a culture and a religion that value children and motherhood. She believes she is a good mother, although she must work full time outside the home.

   Edna is an office manager—respected by her boss and by those who work for her. She has an internal locus of control and evaluates her job performance as "better than most people would do."

   a. Look at the context. What aspects of this situation may negatively impact Mrs. Jackson's recovery?

b. Based on your answers in (a), what nursing diagnoses might be useful in describing the psychosocial aspects of Mrs. Jackson's health? (State both the problem and the etiology.)

c. What strengths does Mrs. Jackson have that may help her to avoid and/or overcome those problems?

6. Matthew has been admitted to the emergency department with extensive wounds to both forearms, including tendon and vascular damage, from an attempted suicide. Matthew seems very quiet, almost withdrawn, and answers most of your questions in monosyllables.

   Matthew reports that he is the third child in a family of five. Matthew's middle-class white parents are now retired, and his brothers and sisters are scattered across the country in various large cities. Although Matthew claims his schooling years were unremarkable, he reminisces about several occasions when he was bullied and physically beaten by gangs of older adolescents.

   Matthew graduated from Harvard Law School and became vice president of an influential law firm. Despite his apparent success in life, he has continued to question his self-worth from early childhood. Plagued by worries and depression that have increased over the past few years Matthew wrote a note indicating that he now realized what a failure he is and proceeded to slash both his forearms with a sharp razor.

   During the nursing assessment, Matthew reports that he has not been eating much, feels tired all the time, and has no interest in getting outside the house. He says, "I just don't feel like doing anything; I just want to sleep all the time."

   a. After Matthew's tendon and vascular repair, Matthew is admitted to your medical–surgical unit. What, broadly speaking, are your first two priorities for Matthew's care?

   b. Which of the following nursing diagnoses would you use, and why? (Consult a NANDA-I handbook, if necessary): Risk for Suicide or Risk for Self-Mutilation

   c. Prioritize the following interventions for Matthew. Rank order them (1 = highest rank, 4 = lowest rank). Explain your thinking.
   Refer to a mental health professional for help with his depression.
   Examine Matthew's belongings and the room for anything he might use to harm himself.
   Encourage Matthew to tell you if he begins having thoughts of suicide.
   Begin establishing a therapeutic relationship and gaining his trust.

   d. Evaluate your self-knowledge. To plan comprehensive care for Matthew, in what areas do you need to increase your theoretical and practical knowledge? How will you do that?

7. For each of the following concepts, use critical thinking to describe how or why it is important to nursing, patient care, or psychosocial health and illness. Note that these are *not* to be merely definitions.

Self-concept	Defense mechanisms
Self-esteem	Depression
Body image	Therapeutic relationships
Biopsychosocial well-being	Hopelessness
Anxiety	

What Are the Main Points in This Chapter?

➤ Health and well-being are influenced by psychological, social, and spiritual development.

➤ Psychosocial theory provides a way to understand people as interactions of psychological and social events.

➤ Self-concept is one's overall view of oneself; it answers the question, "Who do you think you are?"

➤ Self-concept is developed throughout the life span and is influenced by multiple factors. Four dimensions contribute to self-concept: body image, role performance, personal identity, and self-esteem.

➤ Body image is a person's mental image of his physical self.

➤ Role performance consists of the actions a person takes and the behaviors she demonstrates in fulfilling a role, such as the role of a student.

➤ Personal identity is a person's view of himself as a unique human being, different and separate from all others.

➤ Self-esteem evaluations arise from the differences between the ideal and the actual self.

➤ Communication skills are important because psychosocial information is personal and sometimes sensitive.

➤ When you formulate psychosocial diagnoses it is difficult, but important, to determine what is cause and what is effect.

➤ Many of the NOC standardized psychosocial outcomes are found in the domains of Psychosocial Health and Family Health.

➤ Many of the NIC standardized psychosocial interventions are found in the Behavioral and Family domains.

➤ Anxiety is a common emotional response to a (usually unknown) stressor; it results from psychological conflicts, and it is accompanied by physical symptoms (e.g., trembling).

➤ Assessment should identify the presence, level, and cause of anxiety.

➤ Interventions for anxiety should help the patient become aware that he is anxious, identify the source of anxiety, and deal with the symptoms it produces.

➤ Depression is characterized by diminished interest or pleasure in previously enjoyed activities, sadness, emptiness, a flat or hollow feeling (absence of feeling), tearfulness, difficulty concentrating, feelings of worthlessness, and some physical symptoms (e.g., constipation).

➤ Assessment of depression includes a comprehensive history of mood, thoughts, behavior, and physical status.

➤ If you suspect severe depression, you should refer the patient to a mental health specialist; if there is a risk of suicide, referral should be immediate.

➤ In communicating with depressed persons, it is important to not be overly cheerful and to avoid phrases such as "Cheer up."

For practice questions for this chapter,

 Go to **NCLEX-Style Practice Quiz,** on the Student Resource Disk or DavisPlus at http://davisplus.fadavis.com/Wilkinson2

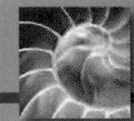

Knowledge Map

Psychosocial Health and Self-Concept

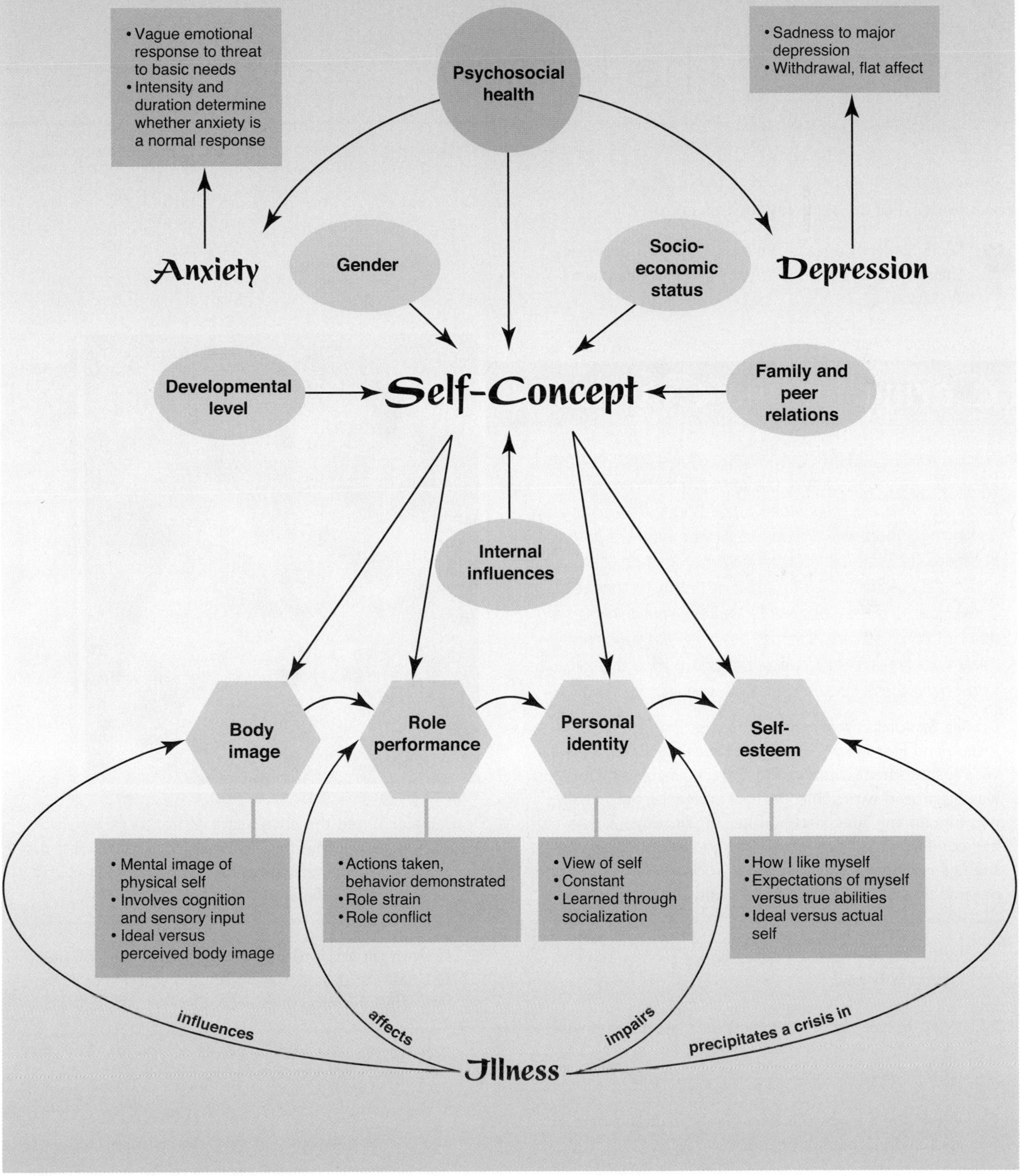

Psychosocial health

- Vague emotional response to threat to basic needs
- Intensity and duration determine whether anxiety is a normal response

Anxiety

- Sadness to major depression
- Withdrawal, flat affect

Depression

Gender

Socio-economic status

Developmental level → **Self-Concept** ← **Family and peer relations**

Internal influences

Body image
- Mental image of physical self
- Involves cognition and sensory input
- Ideal versus perceived body image

Role performance
- Actions taken, behavior demonstrated
- Role strain
- Role conflict

Personal identity
- View of self
- Constant
- Learned through socialization

Self-esteem
- How I like myself
- Expectations of myself versus true abilities
- Ideal versus actual self

influences   *affects*   *impairs*   *precipitates a crisis in*

Illness

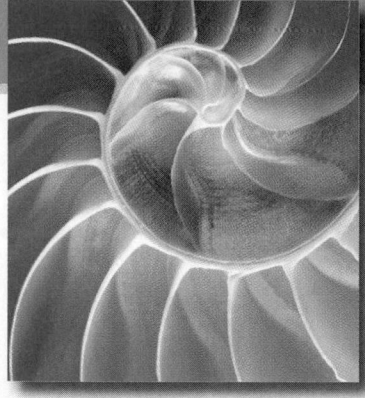
The Family

For a podcast of an overview of this chapter,

 Go to Student Resources, **Podcast – Chapter Overviews, Chapter 12,** on DavisPlus at http://davisplus.fadavis.com/ Wilkinson2

Caring for the Garcias

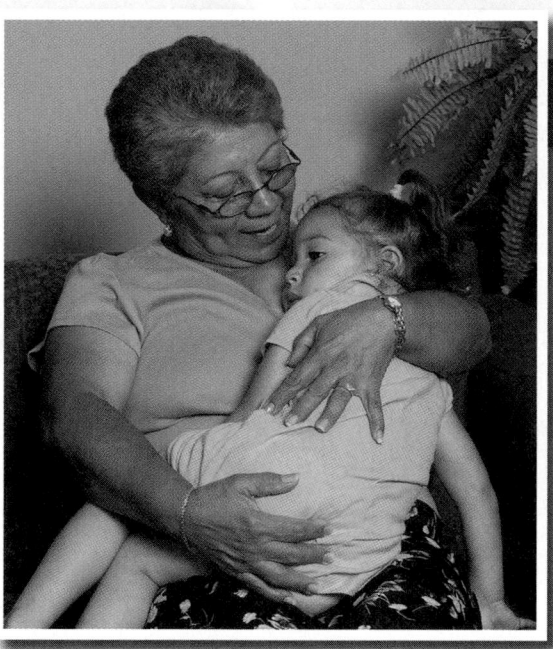

The exercises in the following section allow you to practice the kind of thinking you will use as a full-spectrum nurse. Because these are critical-thinking questions, there is usually no single right answer. We do not provide answers for these questions because it is more important for you to think about the questions than to arrive at the "right" answer. These questions are designed to improve your thinking more than to "cover content." Discuss answers with your peers— discussion can stimulate critical thinking. If you have difficulty with any of these questions, consult with your instructor.

Bettina Sanford, 3 years old, is the first grandchild for Joseph and Flordelisa Garcia. Until recently, Bettina lived with her mother, Corazón, the Garcias' daughter. Corazón was diagnosed with schizophrenia at age 18, but initially was functioning adequately on her medications. However, her condition has been worsening and for the past year she has not been taking her medications. When Corazón became unable to care for herself and Bettina, Joe and

Flordelisa assumed the child's care. Corazón rarely visits Bettina. Joe and Flordelisa convinced Corazón to obtain residential care at a mental health facility. Joe tells you at a clinic visit that he wishes his family were "normal."

A. What do you need to clarify about Joe's statement about his family?

B. What do *you* think Joe means by a "normal" family?

C. How would you respond to Joe's comments?

D. What effect might this new family structure have on Joe's and Flordelisa's health?

E. How might you promote family functioning for the Garcias? What assessments should you make? What interventions should you consider?

F. What personal values or biases do you have that may affect your ability to care for the Garcias?

Practical **Knowledge**
knowing how

Material in this section will help you to assess and plan care for families.

Clinical Insights

Clinical Insight 12-1 ▶ Conducting a Family Assessment

In general, a family assessment should include the following:

Identifying data	Include such information as name, address, phone number, cultural/ethnic background, religious identification, social affliation.
Family composition	For each member of the family, include gender, age, relationship, date and place of birth, occupation, and education.
Family history and developmental stage	This refers to the stages and developmental tasks in the following table, "Family Development."
Environmental data	Include a description of the home, neighborhood, and larger community, as well as the family's social supports and transactions with the community.
Family structure	In addition to identifying the structural type (e.g., traditional nuclear, single-parent, etc.), assess: —Communication patterns: Functional and dysfunctional patterns; the manner in which emotions are expressed, and contextual variables that affect communication —Power and role structures (e.g., How are family decisions made? What are the roles of each member? Have there been changes in these?) —Family values (e.g., What are their values? What are their priorities? How do they compare to the values of their cultural group? Are there value conflicts in the family?)
Family functions	Assess the effectiveness of the family's: —Nurturing (e.g., Are the members close? Are they separate or connected?) —Socialization and child-rearing (e.g., Who is the socializing agent(s) for the children? What are their child-rearing practices? Are needs for play being met?)
Health beliefs, values, and behaviors	How do they define health and illness? What are their dietary, sleep, physical, and drug habits? What are their dental and medical health practices, including physicals, eye exams, immunizations, etc.? Do they have access to health services?
Family stressors and coping	What are their stressors (e.g., financial, family communication or relationships, neighbors, holidays, children's behavior)? What successful coping strategies have they used? What dysfunctional strategies?
Abuse and violence within the family	Because of the prevalence of abuse and because families are likely to be ashamed to discuss it, you should assess every family to see if any abuse or neglect is occurring. For detailed guidelines, go to Procedure 9–1, Assessing for Abuse.

Tables

Family Development		
STAGES	**TASKS**	**CHILDREN'S AGES (IF ANY) (APPROXIMATE)**
Beginning family	▪ Relinquishing the family of origin as the major emotional and economic resource ▪ Gaining a sense of autonomy and independence ▪ Making the relationship/marriage work; investment in spouse as the major emotional resource ▪ Finding a place in the kin network of each partner ▪ Exploring options for career development ▪ Deciding whether to have children	None
Childbearing family	▪ Achieving pregnancy and birth ▪ Adjusting to life changes after birth and to the infant's needs ▪ Determining ways to meet all members' needs ▪ Renegotiating marriage ▪ Increasing contact with extended family	Newborn to 2 years
"No longer newlyweds" (with no children)	▪ Establishing a sense of the permanence of the relationship ▪ Establishing long-term residency ▪ Being involved in the community/promoting the well-being of the community	*Not applicable*
Family with preschool children	▪ Adjusting to increased costs associated with family life ▪ Socializing the preschoolers ▪ Coping with loss of parental energy and privacy	3–5 years
Mature family (with no children)	▪ Renegotiating relationship on basis of more maturity ▪ Adjusting to changing levels of responsibility in work and community ▪ If not done already, achieving financial security	Not applicable
Family with school-age children	▪ Adjusting to the needs and demands of growing children ▪ Promoting joint decision making among parents and children ▪ Encouraging and supporting educational and school-related activities	6–12 years
Family with teenagers and young adults	▪ Maintaining open communication among family members ▪ Reinforcing ethical and moral values ▪ For teens, balancing independence with parental rules	13–20 years
Family launching young adults	▪ Maintaining support to young adults as they leave the security of family ▪ Rediscovering marriage	18–30 years
Postparental family	▪ Preparing for retirement ▪ Adjusting to children's moving into new phases of adulthood, marriage or other relationship, and childbearing and to becoming a grandparent	Adult
Middle-aged couple (with no children)	▪ Accepting that it may be too late to reconsider childbearing or childrearing ▪ Reaching the peak of a career or realizing that the peak may not occur ▪ Planning for retirement	*None*
Aging family (applies to family with no children)	▪ Adjusting to retirement and changes associated with aging ▪ Adjusting to the loss of a spouse and friendships	Adult *(or none)*

Adapted from Friedman, M. M. (2003). *Family nursing: Theory and practice* (5th ed.). Norwalk, CT: Appleton & Lange; Friedman, M. M., Bowden, V. R., & Jones, E. G. (2003). *Family nursing: Research, theory, and practice* (5th ed.). Upper Saddle River, NJ: Prentice Hall; Hanson, S. M. (2005). *Family health care nursing: Theory, practice, and research* (3rd ed.). Philadelphia: F. A. Davis; McGoldrick, M., & Carter, E. (1985). The stages of the family life cycle. In J. Henslin (Ed.), *Marriage and family in a changing society*. New York: Free Press.

Standardized Outcomes and Interventions

NOC Family Health Outcomes		NIC Family Interventions	
CLASS	**OUTCOME LABELS**	**CLASS**	**EXAMPLES OF INTERVENTIONS**
Family Caregiver Status: Outcomes that describe the adaptation and performance of a family member caring for a dependent child or adult	Caregiver Adaptation to Patient Institutionalization	**Childbearing Care:** Interventions to assist in the preparation for childbirth and management of the psychological and physiological changes before, during, and immediately following childbirth	Birthing
	Caregiver Home Care Readiness		Breastfeeding Assistance
	Caregiver Lifestyle Disruption		Childbirth Preparation
	Caregiver–Patient Relationship		Family Integrity Promotion: Childbearing Family
	Caregiver Performance: Direct Care		Family Planning: Contraception
	Caregiver Performance: Indirect Care		Family Planning: Infertility
	Caregiver Stressors		Family Planning: Unplanned Pregnancy
	Caregiving Endurance Potential		Intrapartal Care
Family Member Health Status: Outcomes that describe the physical and emotional health of an individual family member	Abuse Cessation		Labor Induction
	Abuse Protection		Postpartal Care
	Abuse Recovery: Emotional		Prenatal Care
	Abuse Recovery: Financial		Risk Identification: Childbearing Family
	Abuse Recovery: Physical	**Childrearing Care:** Interventions to assist in raising children	Abuse Protection Support: Child
	Abuse Recovery: Sexual		Attachment Promotion
	Caregiver Emotional Health		Developmental Care
	Caregiver Physical Health		Lactation Counseling
	Caregiver Well-Being		Parent Education: Childrearing Family
	Maternal Status: Antepartum		Parenting Promotion
	Maternal Status: Intrapartum		Sibling Support
	Maternal Status: Postpartum		Teaching: Infant Nutrition
	Neglect Recovery		Teaching: Toddler Safety
Family Well-Being: Outcomes that describe the physical, emotional, and social health of a family as a unit	Family Coping	**Life Span Care:** Interventions to facilitate family unit functioning and promote the health and welfare of family members throughout the life span	Caregiver Support
	Family Functioning		Family Integrity Promotion
	Family Health Status		Family Involvement Promotion
	Family Integrity		Family Mobilization
	Family Normalization		Family Process Maintenance
	Family Participation in Professional Care		Family Support
	Family Physical Environment		Family Therapy
Parenting: Outcomes that describe behaviors of parents that promote optimum growth and development	Parenting: Adolescent Physical Safety		Home Maintenance Assistance
	Parenting: Early/Middle Childhood Physical Safety		Respite Care
	Parenting: Infant/Toddler Physical Safety		Risk Identification: Genetic
	Parenting Performance		Role Enhancement
	Parenting: Psychosocial Safety		

Source: Dochterman, J. M., & Bulechek, G. M. (Eds.). (2004). *Nursing interventions classification (NIC)* (4th ed.). St. Louis, MO: C.V. Mosby. Used with permission.

Source: Moorhead, S., Johnson, M., & Maas, M. (Eds.). (2008). *Nursing outcomes classification (NOC)* (4th ed.). St. Louis, MO: C.V. Mosby. Used with permission.

NOC Outcomes and NIC Interventions for Caregiver Role Strain

NOC OUTCOMES	NIC MAJOR INTERVENTIONS
Caregiver Emotional Health	Caregiver Support, Coping Enhancement, Respite Care
Caregiver Lifestyle Disruption	Caregiver Support, Coping Enhancement, Respite Care
Caregiver-Patient Relationship	Coping Enhancement, Presence, Role Enhancement
Caregiver Performance: Direct Care	Anticipatory Guidance, Role Enhancement
Caregiver Performance: Indirect Care	Consultation, Health System Guidance
Caregiver Physical Health	Energy Management, Nutrition Management
Caregiver Well-Being	Caregiver Support, Respite Care, Teaching: Individual

Source: Johnson, M., Bulechek, G., Butcher, H., et al. (2006). *NANDA, NOC, and NIC linkages.* St. Louis, MO: C.V. Mosby. Used with permission.

THINKING CRITICALLY ABOUT THE FAMILY

The exercises in the following sections allow you to practice the kind of thinking you will use as a full-spectrum nurse. Because these are critical-thinking questions, there is usually no single right answer. We do not provide answers for these questions because it is more important for you to think about the questions than to arrive at the "right" answer. These questions are designed to improve your thinking more than to "cover content." Discuss answers with your peers—discussion can stimulate critical thinking. If you have difficulty with any of these questions, consult with your instructor.

Applying the Full-Spectrum Nursing Model

PATIENT SITUATION

Sandra Jackson is the 22-year-old single mother of an 18-month-old child. She has type 1 diabetes mellitus. Sugar control has been brittle at times, primarily during times of stress and illness. Sandra lives with her mother, two younger sisters, and a brother. At times her boyfriend will stay in the home, depending on the status of their relationship. Sandra works part-time at a retail chain, struggling to meet the financial responsibilities of raising a child. She is showing physical signs of depression and distress (e.g., apathy, anorexia, excessive sleeping, and episodes of crying). Sandra says to you during your home visit, "Something is really wrong with me. I can't snap out of this feeling of darkness. Life is too hard for me and is nothing but pain. I can't take it anymore and want it to be over." You believe she needs immediate mental health support.

THINKING

1. *Theoretical Knowledge:*

   a. What facts and principles do you already know about stress and depression?

   b. How does the emotional well-being of one family member affect others living in the home and the family as a whole?

2. *Critical Thinking (Inquiry):*

   a. What are some factors in Sandra's life possibly contributing to her feelings of hopelessness and thoughts of self-harm?

   b. Name at least three nursing diagnoses that would best suit Sandra's health needs.

DOING

3. *Practical Knowledge:* Based on the knowledge you have about stress and depression, How would you explain to the family about how to support Sandra?

4. *Nursing Process (Evaluation).* What measures would you define to determine whether or not your nursing plan of care was effective?

CARING

5. *Self-Knowledge:* How comfortable would you be caring for a patient who is at risk for self injury? What is one problem, not described in the scenario, that could possibly arise?

6. *Ethical Knowledge:* What ethical concerns might you have for a woman with a young child who is at risk for self-injury but yet has no financial resources to cover expenses of mental health care?

Critical Thinking and Clinical Reasoning

1. You are the nurse caring for a 58-year-old woman who was admitted for surgery of the foot. Today is the second day you have cared for the patient. You notice that the family seems quiet and subdued. You ask the client whether something is wrong. She reveals that her 29-year-old niece just lost her job as a TV programming assistant because her employer found out she is HIV positive. Apparently the diagnosis was revealed on her health insurance claim forms when they were processed.

   a. Name two things in this scenario that you, as a nurse, *cannot* change.

   b. Do the client and family have a problem that you *can* help them with? How could you find out?

   c. Imagine you were your client (the aunt). What concerns would you have?

   d. Try to depict this situation by using systems theory. Draw circles for each system involved and show where they interact.

   e. Draw on your self-knowledge. What biases or values do you have that might affect your thinking in this case, either positively or negatively?

2. You are the nurse in the ICU who is caring for a 45-year-old man who was involved in a serious car accident. He suffered severe head trauma and, if he lives, probably will have serious deficits. He was admitted 24 hours ago and has not made significant improvements. The family is aware of his status and likely outcome.

   a. What are some of the concerns this family might have?

   b. Using structural-functional theories, describe how this family might be affected.

   c. How could you help this family?

3. You are the nurse in the emergency department caring for a child who experienced a fall. The 3-year-old child will be OK and is being discharged. As you are reviewing the discharge instructions, the mother reveals that she and the child spent the previous night in a hotel because of violence in the home. She tells you that her husband (the child's stepfather) drinks excessively and at times has become violent, hitting her but not the child. She did not call him when they went to the emergency room, and she is afraid to go home.

   a. What do you think this woman's main concerns might be?

   b. Do you think this is a common or an unusual problem?

   c. What is the developmental stage of this family?

   d. What theoretical knowledge do you need to help this family?

   e. What kinds of help do you think this woman might need if she decides to escape from her husband?

   f. How could you help her at this moment?

4. For each of the following concepts, use critical thinking to describe how or why it is important to nursing, patient care, or the family. Note that these are *not* to be merely definitions.

Family relationships
Blended families
Communication
Systems theory
Structural–functional theory
Family interactional theory
Developmental theory

Family as the unit of care
Family health risk factors
The national economy
Health beliefs
Family coping mechanisms
Unexpected illness

What Are the Main Points in This Chapter?

➤ *Family* is not limited to the traditional definition of husband, wife, and their children; defined more broadly, it is a group of individuals who provide physical, emotional, economic, and/or spiritual support while maintaining involvement in each other's lives.

➤ Families are structured in a variety of ways. Three examples are the traditional nuclear family, dual-earner families, and single-parent families.

➤ Family nursing views the family from three perspectives: as the context for care of an individual, as the unit of care, and as a system.

➤ Wellness of each member is critical to the health of the family unit.

➤ Under general systems theory, the family is viewed as a system in interaction with other systems (e.g., other families, groups, communities, and individuals).

➤ Under structural–functional theories, families are viewed as social systems with a focus on outcomes.

➤ Developmental theories focus on family stages: beginning family, childbearing family, family with preschool children, family with school-age children, family with teenagers and young adults, family

launching young adults, postparental family, and aging family.

➤ Family interactional theory views the family as a unit of interacting personalities with a major emphasis on family roles.

➤ The family teaches health beliefs, values, and behaviors to its individual members.

➤ Assessment of family communication patterns consists of interviewing the family and the individual seeking care, as well as astute observation by the nurse.

➤ How families cope with everyday life situations and hospitalization can influence the effectiveness of care rendered.

➤ Nurses can promote family wellness by addressing both individual and family concerns.

➤ The family can be a source of support or a source of difficulties for the ill person.

For practice questions for this chapter,

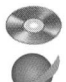 Go to **NCLEX-Style Practice Quiz,** on the Student Resource Disk or DavisPlus at http://davisplus.fadavis.com/Wilkinson2

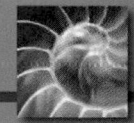

Knowledge Map

Family Health Concepts

Challenges to health
- Poverty
- Disease
- Homelessness
- Violence
- HIV/AIDS
- Developmental changes

Family risk factors
- Adapting to new roles
- Financial needs
- Adolescent's risk-taking behaviors
- Children leaving home
- Illness
- Sandwich generation

Family structures
- Single parent
- Without children
- Extended
- Single individuals
- Gay and lesbian couples
- Families with adopted and foster children

interrelated

occur in response to; and modify

Family coping patterns

affect

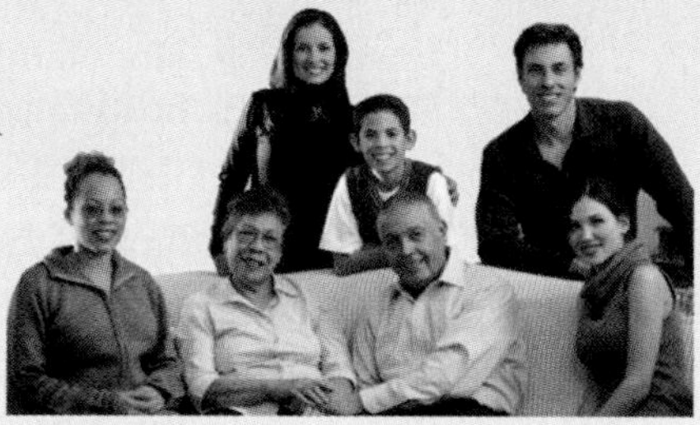

Family communication patterns

influence and reflect

Family Health

guide thinking about

Family theories
- General systems theory
- Structural–functional theories
- Developmental theories
- Family interactional theory

Holistic family nursing

Indicators of family health
- State of family well-being
- Sense of belonging and connectedness
- Shared responsibility
- Trust and respect
- Spending time together, sharing rituals and traditions
- Flexibility
- Commitment: working together to maintain the family
- Spiritual well-being
- Respect for privacy of individual members
- Positive, effective communication
- Ability to compromise and disagree
- Appreciation and affection for each other
- Responding to the needs and interests of all members
- Egalitarian distribution of power
- Health-promoting lifestyle of individual members

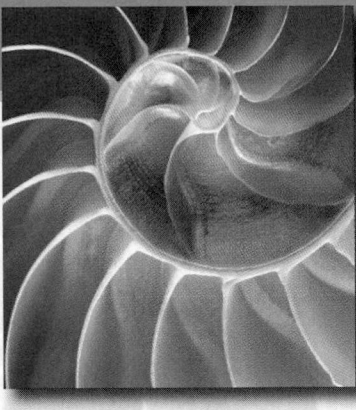
Culture & Ethnicity

For a podcast of an overview of this chapter,

 Go to Student Resources, **Podcast – Chapter Overviews, Chapter 13,** on DavisPlus at http://davisplus.fadavis.com/ Wilkinson2

Caring for the Garcias

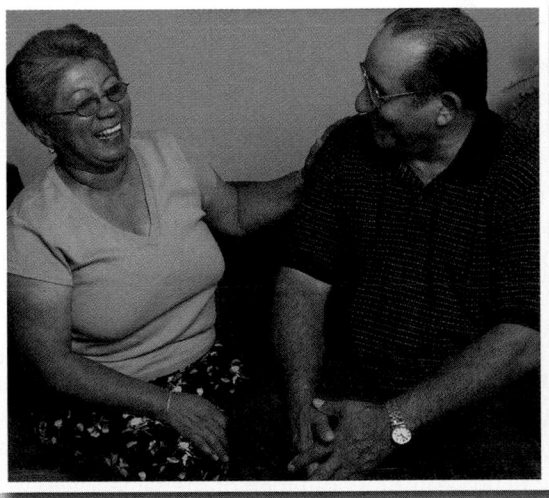

The exercises in this section allow you to practice the kind of thinking you will use as a full-spectrum nurse. Because these are critical-thinking questions, there is usually no single right answer. We do not provide answers for these questions because it is more important for you to think about the questions than to arrive at the "right" answer. These questions are designed to improve your thinking more than to "cover content." Discuss answers with your peers—discussion can stimulate critical thinking. If you have difficulty with any of these questions, consult with your instructor.

Review the initial assessment of Joseph Garcia, found just before Chapter 1 in this volume. Recall that Mrs. Garcia is from Mexico, whereas Mr. Garcia is of Cuban and Irish heritage.

A. How might the Garcias' cultural heritage affect their health beliefs?

B. What factors would you want to consider when performing a cultural assessment of the Garcia family?

Practical **Knowledge**
knowing how

Information in this section may be useful for assessing and communicating with clients of cultures different from your own.

Clinical Insights

Clinical Insight 13-1 ▶ **Assessing for Biological Variations**

People differ genetically and physiologically. Some biological variations create susceptibility to certain diseases and injuries. The following are examples:

Body Build and Structure

- 12% of Native Americans have 25 vertebrae instead of 24, which relates to an increased number of back problems.
- The lower a person's socioeconomic status, the more likely he is to be obese.
- African American and Caucasian men are on average about 3.5 inches taller than Asian American men and 2 inches taller than Mexican American men.

Skin Color

- Darker skin challenges the nurse to be more observant when assessing skin color changes (e.g., when assessing oxygenation or skin rashes). Obtain a baseline skin color by asking a family member or someone who knows the patient well.
- To assess for oxygenation and cyanosis in dark-skinned people, examine the sclera, buccal mucosa, tongue, lips, nail beds, palms of the hands, and soles of the feet.
- To assess for jaundice in Asians, examine the sclera.

Vital Signs

- The average systolic blood pressure of African American men between the ages of 35 and 65 is 5 mm Hg higher than that of European American men of the same age.

Laboratory Tests

- Native Americans, Hispanic Americans, and Japanese Americans, on average, have higher blood glucose levels than Caucasians.
- Bone density is greater in Caucasians than in Chinese, Japanese, and Eskimos.

Susceptibility to Disease

- African Americans have a higher incidence of hypertension and sickle cell anemia.
- Asian Americans have a higher incidence of tuberculosis compared to the white population.

- African Americans, Native Americans, and Mexican Americans are approximately two times as likely to have diabetes mellitus as whites (the prevalence among whites is 7.8%).

Nutritional Variations

- All groups demonstrate food preferences.
- Soy sauce, used in many Asian foods, is high in sodium.
- There is a high incidence of diabetes mellitus in areas where sugar cane is a major crop.

Enzymatic and Genetic Variations and Body Secretions

- Lactose intolerance, caused by a deficiency of the enzyme lactase, is more commonly seen in African Americans, Native Americans, and Asians.

Drug Metabolism

- Native Americans and Asians are more likely to experience facial flushing and palpitations after ingesting alcohol.
- African Americans metabolize alcohol, nicotine, antihypertensives, and beta blockers differently from European Americans; they are more susceptible to side effects of haloperidol and tricyclic antidepressants; and they respond better to diuretic therapy than do Caucasians.
- Asian Americans tend to experience more gastrointestinal side effects from opiates, even though the analgesic effect is less.
- Chinese Americans are more sensitive to the cardiovascular effects of propranolol; they have increased absorption of antipsychotics, antihypertensives, and some narcotics.
- Recall that most drug studies in the past were normed on European Americans, so "variations" refer to differences from those norms.

Practice Resources

Andrews, M. M., & Boyle, J. S. (2007); Purnell, L. D., & Paulanka, B. J. (2008); Spector, R. E. (2004); Suzuki, L. A., & Ponterotto, J. G. (2007).

Clinical Insight 13-2 ▶ Obtaining Minimum Cultural Information

You should obtain at least this much cultural information from every client. For some, you may need a more in-depth assessment.

■ Begin the interview with open-ended questions, such as the following:

  I would like to know more about your family.
  Who will be able to help you when you go home?
  What do you do to help keep yourself well?

Language(s) spoken; proficiency in the language of the host country

Length of time client has been here; where client was raised

Ethnic affiliation and identity

Usual religious practices

Nonverbal communication style

Family roles, primary decision-maker

Social support in the new country

■ When you and the client are comfortable, be sure to ask a question such as, "What concerns you the most about your illness and treatment?" This allows you to focus on the individual rather than just on his culture.

■ You will not need to perform an in-depth cultural assessment on every patient, but you will need to recognize situations in which this is needed. Lipson and Meleis (1985) suggest that the following minimum information is important:

■ What language(s) do you speak?
■ Are you comfortable speaking [English], or would you like to have an interpreter?

■ Where were you raised?
■ How long have you lived here?

■ With what racial and ethnic group(s) do you identify?
■ How closely do you identify with the values of those groups?

■ What religion do you practice, if any?
■ Are there any special rituals or practices you want us to be aware of?

■ You will need to observe the patient and draw on your theoretical knowledge of the patient's cultural group for this information.

■ Who is in your family?
■ What is your role in your family?
■ Who makes most of the decisions?
■ How are decisions made in your family?
■ Whom should I talk to for decisions about your health care?

■ Do you have family and friends here?
■ Whom can you go to when you need help?
■ Where do you work?
■ Will you need any help with your health care expenses?

Practice Resources

Giger, J. N., & Davidhizar, R. (2008); Lipson, J., & Meleis, A. (1985); Spector, R. E. (2004); Suzuki, L. A., & Ponterotto, J. G. (2007).

Clinical Insight 13-3 ▶ Assessing Pain Perception in Selected Cultural Groups

The following are some general cultural beliefs about and responses to pain. Remember that these are only a starting point (archetypes) and that you must never stereotype a person on the basis of culture. Assess each person individually.

Cultural Group	Pain Perception and Responses
African American heritage	Depending on the religion, may believe that pain is inevitable and must be endured; therefore, may tolerate a great deal of pain. Depending on the religion, may seek prayers and the laying on of hands for pain relief. May see pain as a test of faith. May see pain as the only sign of illness or disease, so may not follow medical therapies (e.g., for hypertension) if pain is absent.

(continued on next page)

Clinical Insight 13-3 ▶ **Assessing Pain Perception in Selected Cultural Groups** (continued)

European American heritage, New England subculture	(These are chronic pain responses.) Copes by working and keeping busy. Stoicism; lack of expressiveness and behavioral pain response, including little wincing and groaning. Pain is viewed as a biological abnormality that can be treated and lived with; may be angry with care providers if treatment is ineffective. *Polish American subgroup:* Strong tendency for nonexpressiveness
Arab heritage	View pain as unpleasant and something to be controlled. Expect medical science to be able to relieve their suffering. Express pain openly with family members, less so with health professionals. This may cause the nurse to evaluate pain relief as adequate even though the family may be demanding more medication for the patient.
Chinese heritage	Pain expression is similar to traditional U.S. culture, but description of pain may be different (i.e., described more often as "dull" and "diffuse"). Use external pain relief methods, such as massage, oils, warmth, and relaxation.
Filipino heritage	View pain as a part of living an honorable life or as an opportunity to atone for sins. Commonly tolerate severe pain, with stoic acceptance. May not complain of pain or ask for interventions.
Irish heritage	Value stoic response to pain. Ignore, deny, or minimize pain. Delay seeking treatment.
Italian heritage	Verbalization of pain is common and acceptable, even with chronic pain. Women are especially likely to report and express pain. Expect immediate treatment for pain.
Japanese heritage	It is a virtue, and a matter of family honor, to bear pain without expressing it. There may be taboos against use of narcotics for pain relief. May be more accepting of analgesics if reassured that pain control enhances healing.
Jewish heritage	Verbalization of pain is common and acceptable. Knowing the reason for pain is as important as obtaining relief.
Mexican heritage	View pain as the will of God or a part of life. May view pain as punishment for immoral behavior. May view enduring pain as a sign of strength. May endure pain longer and report it less frequently than other groups, or may express vocally with groaning and crying out. May delay seeking help for pain, hoping it will go away. May interpret pain as a loss of manhood or provider role.
Navajo Indian heritage	View pain as a part of life. Do not express pain openly. May hide the intensity of their pain. May not request pain medication. May prefer herbal medications for pain.
Puerto Rican heritage	Loud and outspoken expression of pain is not an exaggeration, but a socially learned coping mechanism. May experience low self-esteem because of pain. Older or rural people may not be able to interpret pain-rating scales. Most prefer oral or intravenous analgesics to intramuscular or rectal routes. Many use herbal teas, heat, and prayer to manage pain.

Practice Resources

Andrews, M. M., & Boyle, J. S. (2007); Bates (1996); Giger, J. N., & Davidhizar, R. (2008); Purnell, L. D., & Paulanka, B. J. (2008); Spector, R. E. (2004); Todd, K. (1996); Zborowski, M. (1952).

Clinical Insight 13-4 ▶ Performing a Cultural Assessment Using Giger and Davidhizar's Transcultural Assessment Model

Assess information listed in the following categories.

Cultural Uniqueness

- Cultural and ethnic identification
- Place of birth
- Time in country

Communication

- Voice quality
- Pronunciation and enunciation
- Use of silence
- Use of nonverbal communication
- Touch
- Spoken language

Space

- Degree of comfort
- Distance in conversations
- Definition of space
- Body movement

Social Organization

- Normal state of health
- Marital status
- Number of children
- Parents living or deceased
- Friends
- Work
- Leisure

Time

- Orientation to time
- View of time
- Physiochemical reaction to time

Environmental Control

- Locus of control
- Value orientation
- Health and illness beliefs

Biological Variations

- Physical assessment (including body structure, skin color, skin discoloration, hair color and distribution, other visible physical characteristics, weight, height, lab variances)
- Susceptibility to illness
- Nutritional preferences
- Psychological characteristics

Other

In addition to the Giger and Davidhizar categories, obtain information about the following:

- Educational experiences (formal and informal)
- Family patterns of health care
- Family role and function
- Healthcare beliefs and practices (folk and professional)
- Religious practices
- Social networks
- Values orientation

Adapted from Giger, J. N., & Davidhizar, R. E. (2008). *Transcultural nursing: Assessment and intervention* (5th ed.). St. Louis, MO: C. V. Mosby.

Clinical Insight 13-5 ▶ Communicating with Clients Who Speak a Different Language

When possible, use an interpreter or a translator. An **interpreter** is specially trained to provide the meaning behind the words, whereas a **translator** just restates the words from one language to another. An interpreter can serve as a cultural broker by conveying the client's responses to questions, and by providing general information about the client's culture (Munoz & Luckmann, 2004).

When using any type of interpreter, it is important to do the following:

- Have the interpreter spend some time alone with the patient.
- Address your questions to the client, not the interpreter.
- Ask the interpreter to interpret the words used by the healthcare provider as closely as possible, except where literal translation might be offensive or misunderstood. In such cases, an interpreter (as compared to a translator) would provide the meaning of your words in terms acceptable to the client.

- Because of confidentiality issues, avoid asking a family member, especially a child or spouse, to act as an interpreter.
- Avoid using an interpreter who is socially or politically incompatible with the client (e.g., you would not ask an Israeli to interpret for a Palestinian).
- Be aware of gender and age differences. (It usually is preferable to have an interpreter of the same gender as the client.)
- Do not use metaphors ("happy as a clam") or medical jargon.
- Observe nonverbal communication (e.g., body language) when the client is listening and talking to the interpreter.
- Maintain eye contact with both the client and interpreter.
- Speak slowly and distinctly, facing the client; do not speak loudly.
- Ask one question at a time; allow time for interpretation and response from the client before asking another question.

(continued on next page)

Clinical Insight 13-5 ▶ **Communicating with Clients Who Speak a Different Language** (continued)

- Use active rather than passive voice (e.g., say, "The doctor will see you tomorrow." rather than "You will be seen by the doctor tomorrow.")
- Be aware that many clients can understand more English words than they can express.
- Have health education materials translated into the client's language, or have an interpreter audiotape or videotape instructions.

If there is no one available to interpret for you, in addition to the strategies listed above, Munoz and Luckmann (2004) suggest the following:

- Greet the client with respect. Greet the person formally, using Mr., Ms., and so forth, until given permission to do otherwise. People in some groups consider it disrespectful to use a person's first name.
- Identify the client's primary language, and use any words that you are familiar with in her language to show that you are trying to communicate.

- If appropriate, use a third language that both of you speak. For example, some Vietnamese and some Cambodians speak French.
- Speak slowly and clearly, using simple sentences to talk about one question or need at a time.
- Use gestures to help convey meaning.
- Restate in different words, if needed.
- Use pictures or diagrams.
- Be aware that some clients may answer yes even if they don't understand what you have said.

Practice Resources

Munoz, C., & Luckmann, J. (2004); Office of Minority Health & Health Disparities (2001); Purnell, L. D., & Paulanka, B. J. (2008).

THINKING CRITICALLY ABOUT CULTURE & ETHNICITY

The exercises in the following sections allow you to practice the kind of thinking you will use as a full-spectrum nurse. Because these are critical-thinking questions, there is usually no single right answer. We do not provide answers for these questions because it is more important for you to think about the questions than to arrive at the "right" answer. These questions are designed to improve your thinking more than to "cover content." Discuss answers with your peers—discussion can stimulate critical thinking. If you have difficulty with any of these questions, consult with your instructor.

Applying the Full-Spectrum Nursing Model

PATIENT SITUATION

Mrs. Vasquez, a 70-year-old Mexican American woman, has diabetes mellitus and has come to the hospital because of a sore on her lower leg that will not heal. Mrs. Vasquez, a widow, cares for herself at home. She speaks only broken English and has some difficulty understanding your questions. After great effort on your part, you determine that she has missed her last appointment with her diabetes specialist because she has no transportation, so she has just been putting a dressing on the sore. Mrs. Vasquez tells you that she loves to see her grandchildren, who visit often, and that she enjoys cooking and eating Mexican food. She also says that she believes she is sick because she has not pleased God. However, God is a source of comfort and assurance to her. She prays a lot and has rosary beads in her hand.

THINKING

1. *Theoretical Knowledge (Recall of Facts and Principles)*: List six important culture specifics.

2. *Critical Thinking (Application of Knowledge)*: Based on your theoretical knowledge, what are your expectations about communicating with Mrs. Vasquez?

3. *Critical Thinking (Compare and Contrast)*: Compare your expectations to the actual data you have about her ability to communicate.

DOING

4. *Nursing Process (Assessment)*: What are some pertinent cultural data that you should assess for Mrs. Vasquez?

5. *Nursing Process (Analysis/Diagnosis)*: Which nursing diagnosis do you think would be best for planning Mrs. Vasquez's care? (Recall that the etiology should suggest your nursing interventions, and the diagnostic label should suggest the expected patient outcome.) Explain your reasoning.

   - Noncompliance (with clinic appointments) r/t lack of transportation
   - Impaired Skin Integrity r/t self-treatment of ulcer
   - Noncompliance (with clinic appointments) r/t beliefs about God and illness

CARING

6. *Self-Knowledge*: What areas of commonality do you have with Mrs. Vasquez, around which you might form a caring relationship?

7. *Self-Knowledge*: Do you agree with Mrs. Vasquez that illness may be caused by displeasing God?

8. *Ethical Knowledge*: Suppose you do not agree with Mrs. Vasquez that she is ill because she has displeased God. Discuss whether you would explain to her that this is most likely not true and then teach her about the cause of diabetic ulcers.

Critical Thinking and Clinical Reasoning

1. Mrs. Vasquez, a 70-year-old Mexican American woman, has diabetes mellitus and has come to the hospital because of a sore on her lower leg that will not heal. Review the details of Mrs. Vasquez's case in the Full Spectrum Nursing Model "Situation," preceding.

   a. Identify Mrs. Vasquez's cultural data and group it under the following culture specifics:

      Communication

      Space

      Time orientation

      Social organization

      Environmental control

      Biological variations

   b. What does your theoretical knowledge lead you to expect about Mrs. Vasquez's personal space? What, if any, actual patient data do you have about that?

   c. What does your theoretical knowledge lead you to expect about her time orientation, social organization, and environmental control? Compare your expectations to the actual patient data that you have.

   d. What theoretical knowledge do you have regarding biological variations among Hispanic people? How does this compare to the actual data, if any, that you have for Mrs. Vasquez?

   e. You have learned that cultural data can have implications for nursing care. Answer each of the following:

      - What additional information should you assess for in this situation?
      - What biases do you have that affect your thinking in this situation?

2. An Asian woman comes to your clinic for assessment of her blood pressure. In casual conversation, she tells you that her oldest daughter is about to be married. She reveals that her daughter has some type of anemia for which she needs medication. She tells you that she has recently heard terrible stories about sickle-cell anemia and is afraid that this is what her daughter has.

   a. What additional data do you need to collect in order to answer this client's questions?

   b. What are the biological variations that normally affect this cultural group?

   c. What assurances, if any, can you give this client about her daughter?

3. At times we must care for clients who do not speak our language. This poses a challenge to the nurse who strives to provide culturally competent care to all clients. Even with the assistance of interpreters, this can be difficult because of such barriers as differing dialects, street talk, and jargon. Keeping these facts in mind, answer the following questions:

   a. What options do you have when you encounter an individual who cannot speak English?

   b. How do you communicate with such a client if no interpreter is available?

   c. What biases do you have about such a situation? Why?

4. Alma is of European descent; she is white. She is a Roman Catholic and believes abortion is wrong. She believes that it should be illegal to own a gun. She is a nursing student.

   Violetta's parents came to the United States from Europe. They were born in France. Before that, her great-grandparents lived in Africa. Violetta is black. She is Roman Catholic, and she believes that abortion is wrong. She believes that it should be illegal to own a gun. She is a nursing student.

   Darcy is of European descent. She is white. She laughs at the idea of religion, saying "Nobody's 'up there' looking out for me; and when you're dead, you're dead." Darcy is a gang member and carries a gun in her purse or her pocket at all times. She did not finish high school, and by the age of 19 she had had two abortions.

   All of the women live in the United States. Which two women do you think share the most cultural commonalities? Explain your thinking.

5. Helen is 52 years old and African American. She is divorced. Her only child, Tamika, is incarcerated for prostitution and possession of narcotics. Helen is now raising her two grandchildren, Calvin, age 13 years, and Jevetta, age 2. Helen is a nursing assistant at the local hospital. It's hard for her to make ends meet because she has hypertension and diabetes, for which she takes a number of medications, including insulin—that is, when she can afford them. Helen has not applied for medical assistance because she believes she should be able to take care of herself, but she does receive assistance for Jevetta's day-care costs. In addition to her grandchildren, Helen has a large group of friends, many of whom attend her church. She has little time to spend with her friends since she took custody of the children. Jevetta has been admitted to the hospital for asthma. You are Jevetta's student nurse.

   a. Using your data collection skills, identify NANDA-I diagnostic labels that you could apply to Jevetta and to Helen as Jevetta's caregiver.

   b. What resources may be helpful to Helen?

6. Examine the following nursing diagnosis labels. For this set of labels, write an etiology that might be caused by cultural differences. The first one is completed for you as an example.

   - Imbalanced Nutrition: Less than (or More Than) Body Requirements *r/t patient's lack of knowledge about how to adapt his preferred ethnic foods to her prescribed low-fat diet.*
   - Ineffective Health Maintenance
   - Ineffective Role Performance
   - Anxiety
   - Powerlessness
   - Deficient Knowledge

7. For the following set of labels, explain or give an example of how the nurse might misdiagnose or misperceive the data because of cultural differences. The first one is done for you.

   - Decisional Conflict

   The nurse might ask a woman to make some decision about her care. The woman may seem very indecisive and unable to reach a conclusion. The reason may be that the husband is the decision maker in the family. When the husband arrives, the Decisional Conflict ("problem") may disappear.

   - Confusion
   - Effective or Ineffective Breastfeeding
   - Impaired Social Interaction
   - Social Isolation
   - Noncompliance
   - Pain (Acute or Chronic)

8. For each of the following concepts, use critical thinking to describe how or why it is important to nursing, patient care, or cultural competence. Note that these are *not* to be merely definitions.

Culture
Subculture
Ethnicity
Race
Religion
Acculturation
Health and illness belief
Health and illness practice
Phenomena of culture
Ethnocentric
Folk medicine

Cultural competence
Transcultural nursing
Giger and Davidhizar assessment
   model
Biological variations among cultures
Prejudice and racism
Professional (e.g., nursing) subculture
Cultural sensitivity
Cultural awareness
Culture universals
Culture specifics

What Are the Main Points in This Chapter?

➤ The cultural and ethnic composition of North America has changed dramatically over the past several decades, making it essential that nurses understand the healthcare beliefs and practices of diverse populations.

➤ Culture includes shared values, beliefs, norms, and practices that guide a particular group's thinking, decision making, and actions in a patterned way.

➤ Through acculturation, most ethnic and cultural groups modify some of their traditional cultural characteristics, values, beliefs, and practices.

➤ You should be familiar with the common characteristics of different cultural groups in your community.

➤ The U.S. Census Bureau has identified the following racial categories on the 2010 census questionnaire:

White

Black, African American, or Negro

American Indian or Alaska Native

Asian Indian

Chinese

Filipino

Japanese

Korean

Vietnamese

Other Asian

Native Hawaiian

Guamanian or Chamorro

Samoan

Other Pacific Islander (specify, e.g., Tongan)

➤ The two Census Bureau (2010) ethnicity (or "origin") categories are (1) Hispanic, Latino, or Spanish and (2) Not Hispanic, Latino, or Spanish. Subcategories under Hispanic origin are: Mexican, Mexican American, Chicano; Puerto Rican; Cuban; and Another Hispanic, Latino, or Spanish origin.

➤ **Culture universals** (commonalities) are the values, beliefs, and practices that people from *all* cultures share. **Culture specifics** (diversities) are those values, beliefs, and practices that are unique to a culture.

➤ A **cultural archetype**, similar to a model, is an example: something that is recurrent and has its basis in facts. A **cultural stereotype** is a widely held but oversimplified and unsubstantiated belief that all people of a certain racial or ethnic group are alike in certain respects.

➤ Six organizing phenomena of culture that influence health include communication patterns, space, social organization, time, environmental control, and biological variations.

➤ Healthcare providers cannot understand the health beliefs and practices of diverse populations if they view them through the lens of the conventional (Western, U.S.) culture of health care.

➤ A variety of "alternative" healing systems exists. Remedies have been passed down from generation to generation and include the use of herbs, customs, and rituals.

➤ An understanding of cultural concepts, theories, and models can help you develop cultural competence.

➤ Some barriers to culturally competent care include ethnocentrism, stereotyping, prejudice, and racism.

➤ When assessing a client and making nursing diagnoses, you must consider the client's cultural values, beliefs, and practices related to health and healthcare.

➤ Culturally competent care requires a nonjudgmental attitude, self-awareness, sensitivity, respect for differences, theoretical knowledge, and the desire to be culturally competent.

For practice questions for this chapter,

 Go to **NCLEX-Style Chapter Quiz,** on the Student Resource Disk or DavisPlus at http://davisplus.fadavis.com/Wilkinson2

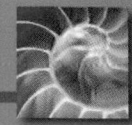

Knowledge Map

Culture and Ethnicity

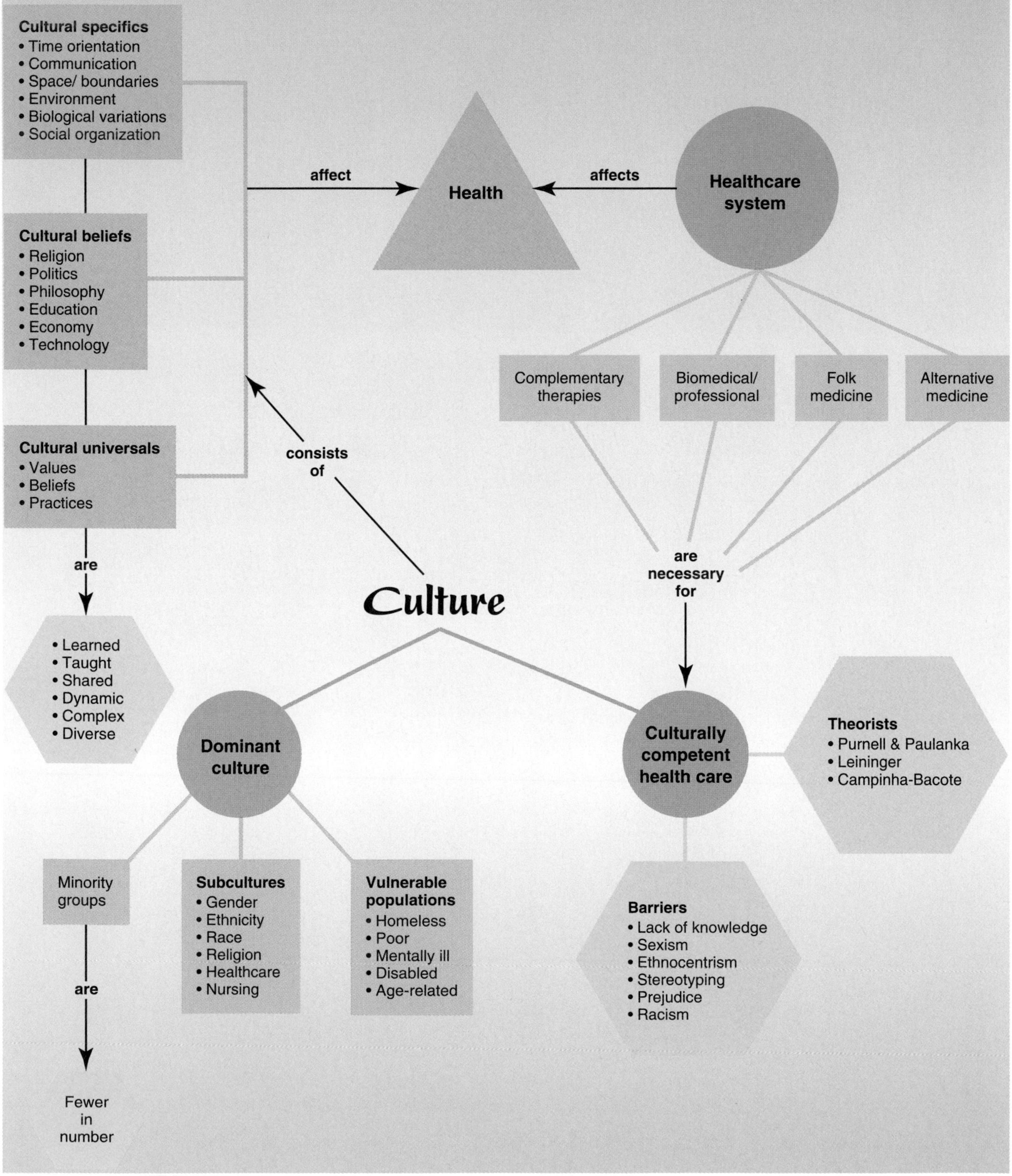

Cultural specifics
- Time orientation
- Communication
- Space/ boundaries
- Environment
- Biological variations
- Social organization

Cultural beliefs
- Religion
- Politics
- Philosophy
- Education
- Economy
- Technology

Cultural universals
- Values
- Beliefs
- Practices

affect → **Health**

Healthcare system *affects* →

Complementary therapies **Biomedical/ professional** **Folk medicine** **Alternative medicine**

consists of

Culture

are
- Learned
- Taught
- Shared
- Dynamic
- Complex
- Diverse

are necessary for

Dominant culture

Culturally competent health care

Theorists
- Purnell & Paulanka
- Leininger
- Campinha-Bacote

Minority groups

Subcultures
- Gender
- Ethnicity
- Race
- Religion
- Healthcare
- Nursing

Vulnerable populations
- Homeless
- Poor
- Mentally ill
- Disabled
- Age-related

Barriers
- Lack of knowledge
- Sexism
- Ethnocentrism
- Stereotyping
- Prejudice
- Racism

are

Fewer in number

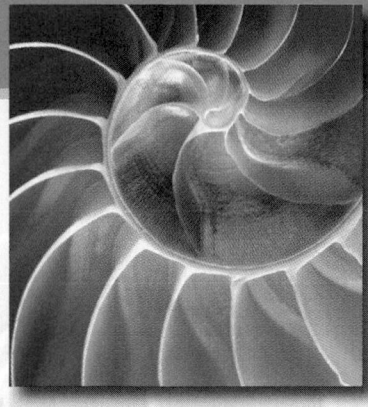

CHAPTER 14

Spirituality

For a podcast of an overview of this chapter,

 Go to Student Resources, **Podcast – Chapter Overviews, Chapter 14,** on DavisPlus at http://davisplus.fadavis.com/ Wilkinson2

Caring for the Garcias

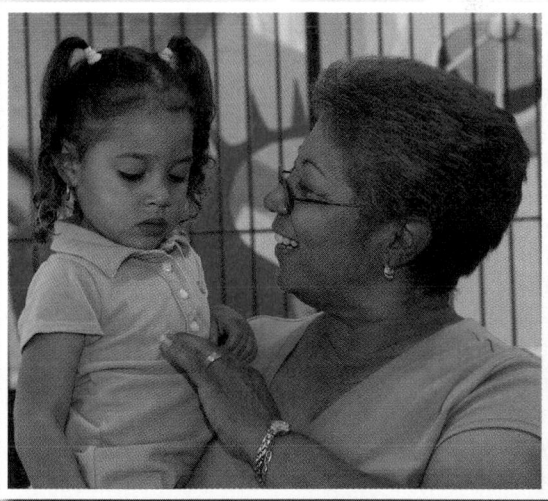

The exercises in the following section allow you to practice the kind of thinking you will use as a full-spectrum nurse. Because these are critical-thinking questions, there is usually no single right answer. We do not provide answers for these questions because it is more important for you to think about the questions than to arrive at the "right" answer. These questions are designed to improve your thinking more than to "cover content." Discuss answers with your peers—discussion can stimulate critical thinking. If you have difficulty with any of these questions, consult with your instructor.

Bettina Sanford is the 3-year-old grandchild of Joseph and Flordelisa Garcia. The Garcias are both practicing Catholics. Bettina's mother, Corazón, is the Garcia's daughter. Corazón feels that Catholicism is "a waste of time" and does not attend church. Bettina has had no formal religious experiences or training.

A. At a clinic visit, Joe asks you what you think about keeping religion away from a child. How would you respond?

B. Joe explains his views on the situation: "If anything were to happen to her, she would go to hell. I think we should take her to Church and get her baptized right away. I don't know how anyone can live like that. She has no connection to God." Do you agree with this statement? Explain your views.

C. Joe asks you to pray for Bettina and her mother. How would you feel about this situation? What would you say to Joe?

Practical **Knowledge**
knowing how

In this section, you will find guidelines for performing spiritual interventions and for performing focused spiritual assessments.

Clinical Insights

Clinical Insight 14-1 ▶ **Using Selected NIC Interventions and Activities to Support Spirituality**

Nursing Diagnoses

Moral Distress
Spiritual Distress
Risk for Spiritual Distress
Readiness for Enhanced
  Spiritual Well-Being

Impaired Religiosity
Risk for Impaired
  Religiosity
Readiness for Enhanced
  Religiosity

Nursing Interventions and Activities

Dying Care

Facilitate obtaining spiritual support for patient and family.
Support the patient and family through stages of grief (see Chapter 15).
Facilitate discussion of funeral arrangements.

Emotional Support

Explore with the patient what has triggered emotions.
Embrace or touch the patient supportively.
Make supportive or empathetic statements.
Encourage the patient to express feelings.

Forgiveness Facilitation

Listen empathetically without moralizing or offering platitudes.
Explore forgiveness as a process.
Assist client to seek out an arbitrator (objective party) to facilitate the process of individual or group concern.
Explore possibilities of making amends and reconciliation with self, others, and/or higher power.

Hope Inspiration

Assist the patient/family to identify areas of hope in life.
Help the patient expand his spiritual self.
Facilitate the patient/family's reliving and savoring past achievements and experiences.
Create an environment that facilitates patient's practicing religion, as appropriate.

Presence

Be physically available as a helper.
Remain physically present without expecting interactional responses.
Offer to remain with the patient during the initial interaction with others in the unit.
Listen to the patient's concerns.
Stay with the patient to promote safety and reduce fear.

Religious Ritual Enhancement

Coordinate or provide healing services, communion, meditation, or prayer in the place of residence or other setting.
Encourage the use of and participation in usual religious rituals or practices that are not detrimental to health.
Assist with modifications of the ritual to meet the needs of the disabled or ill.
Treat the individual with dignity and respect.

Self-Awareness Enhancement

Assist the patient to realize that everyone is unique.
Assist the patient to identify life priorities.
Assist the patient to identify guilty feelings.
Assist the patient to identify his source of motivation.

Self-Esteem Enhancement

Encourage the patient to identify strengths; reinforce strengths that the patient identifies.
Provide experiences that increase the patient's autonomy, as appropriate.
Explore previous achievements of success.
Assist the patient to identify the significance of culture, religion, race, gender, and age on self-esteem.
Monitor the frequency of self-negating verbalizations. [And, replace these thoughts and words with more self-affirming actions.]

Spiritual Growth Facilitation

Encourage conversation that assists the patient in sorting out spiritual concerns.
Assist the patient with identifying barriers and attitudes that hinder growth or self-discovery.
Offer individual and group prayer support, as appropriate.
Encourage participation in devotional services, retreats, and special prayer/study programs.
Assist the patient to explore beliefs as related to healing of body, mind, and spirit.
Refer for pastoral care or primary spiritual caregiver as issues warrant.

Spiritual Support

Be open to the patient's expressions of loneliness and powerlessness.
Encourage chapel service attendance, if desired.
Provide desired spiritual articles, according to individual preferences.

Be available to listen to the individual's feelings.

Listen carefully to the individual's communication, and develop a sense of timing for prayer or spiritual rituals.

Be open to the individual's feelings about illness and death.

Values Clarification

Think through the ethical and legal aspects of free choice, given the particular situation, before beginning the intervention.

Pose reflective, clarifying questions that give the patient something to think about.

Encourage the patient to make a list of what is important and not important in life and the time spent on each.

Encourage the patient to list values that guide behavior in various settings and types of situations.

Avoid use of the [preceding] intervention with persons with serious emotional problems.

Other NIC Spiritual Care Interventions

Active Listening   Crisis Intervention
Anticipatory Guidance   Decision-Making Support

Anxiety Reduction	Emotional Support
Bibliotherapy	Grief Work Facilitation
Coping Enhancement	Guilt Work Facilitation
Counseling	Humor
Meditation Facilitation	Religious Addiction
Mood Management	Prevention
Music Therapy	Religious Ritual Enhancement
Referral	Resiliency Promotion
Role Enhancement	Self-Responsibility Facilitation
Self-Esteem Enhancement	Support Group
Self-Modification	Touch
Assistance	

Sources: Bulechek, G. M., Butcher, H. K., & Dochterman, J. M. (Eds.) (2008). *Nursing interventions classification (NIC)*. St. Louis, MO: C. V. Mosby; National Guideline Clearinghouse (2005). Promoting spirituality in the older adult. Retrieved from http://www.guidelines.gov/summary/summary.aspx?docJ_id=6830&nbr=004197&string=nursing

---

Clinical Insight 14-2 ▶ **Praying with Patients**

Because there is a rich diversity in religious expression, keep the following guidelines in mind when you pray for or with patients:

Ask how the patient prefers to address the divine. Some people prefer the use of parental language in their prayers, for example, *Father God* or *Divine Mother*. Some use the word *Jehovah, Yahweh,* or *Allah.* Hindus may address one or more of multiple gods, each of whom has several names. So don't be afraid to seek direction from the patient in these matters: most people are honored to be able to explain their beliefs and practices to someone who is open to the experience.

Before the prayer begins, ask the patient whether any rituals or religious items are necessary. Muslims may want water to wash the mouth, nostrils, and hands before beginning prayer. Roman Catholics may want to hold their rosary beads while praying, and some Buddhists and Hindus meditate with a set of beads called a mala. Others may have a prayer cloth or other item that needs to be accessible.

Always feel free to pray or not to. Never feel that you are being forced to do or say something that makes you uncomfortable.

Do not be a compulsive "pray-er" or a compulsive avoider of prayer. Always make sure that the patient (and/or family) is comfortable with prayer if he has not yet requested it.

Know that there are appropriate times and places for the offering of prayer. Prayer at the bedside may be most appropriate, although it may make people uncomfortable in a crowded waiting room. Perhaps the statement "I will

be praying for you and your family" might be more appropriate for some patients than actually praying aloud at that moment.

When a patient asks for prayer, consider using this reply: "I would be honored to offer prayer. What would you like me to *especially* address in the prayer?" Knowing what the patient hopes for in prayer gives you an idea of the type of prayer the person is requesting.

When the patient tells you what he wants you to pray for, be sure to focus your prayer around the request. It is always good to summarize the results of previous conversations with the patient and his needs in the course of your prayer. For example, imagine that a patient with cancer who has been treated with chemotherapy now finds his blood counts are coming back to normal levels. The chemotherapy treatment seems successful at this point, but the patient is afraid of a relapse and asks you to pray for the cancer to be cured. There is a lot going on in this situation and it is easy to get lost in the complexity of need. Analyze the situation in terms of what has happened in the past, what is happening now, and what the patient is requesting. This will help you organize your thoughts and then put them into the form of a prayer. Perhaps you would want to take the patient's hand in yours (if appropriate, based on your intuition and the nature of your nurse-patient relationship) and compose a prayer in the following manner: Dear [Lord], I give you thanks that [John] has done so well with his treatments. Please continue to help him be to be strong and open to your healing presence. We pray for his family, doctors, and nurses that all may be a part of [John's] continued healing and

(continued on next page)

Clinical Insight 14-2 ➤ **Praying with Patients** (continued)

sense of comfort. I pray that the treatments that he is receiving, together with the prayers that we are offering, may all be effective in his care and in the treatment of his cancer. Watch over [John], and visit us all at this time with your healing presence. [Amen.]

When a terminally ill patient requests a prayer for a cure, total healing, or a miracle, you may be challenged. Knowing how to offer prayers that are "realistic" allows for the occurrence of miracles and healings of all types while also keeping in perspective the physical realities of the nature of disease and the reality of death.

If composing a prayer is difficult for you, you may want to explore the use of the Psalms in The Hebrew Bible (Old Testament) or some New Testament scriptures, if appropriate for the patient. (See especially Psalms 43, 51, 67, 121). In terms of larger themes, the following sources for patients who profess Christianity may be helpful:

Forgiveness and guilt: Psalm 51, Isaiah 55:7, and Matthew 6:9-15
Comfort: Psalm 23, John 14
Hope: Psalm 42, Romans 15:4
Love and acceptance: Matthew 5:11
Caring: 1 Corinthians 12

For exact quotations of these passages,

 Go to Chapter 14, **Psalms for Prayers,** on the Student Resource Disk or DavisPlus at http://davisplus.fadavis.com/ Wilkinson2

For patients of other religions, ask whether they have examples of their sacred writings from which you might be allowed to read. Perhaps the patient has a favorite prayer or a text from an authoritative source that brings comfort and hope.

It is always good to include in the course of your prayer a request for God's help and direction with the patient's healthcare team, doctors, surgeons, and family members. This expresses the reality that we are all working together for a common good and purpose and that we depend on God and others for our welfare and place in life.

Once the prayer is over, thank the patient for asking you to participate in that way and ask whether you can be of any further assistance.

Assessment Guidelines and Tools

The HOPE Approach to Spiritual Assessment: Examples of Questions

Mnemonic	Examples of Questions
H—Sources of **hope**, meaning, comfort, strength, peace, love and connection	What are your sources of internal support?
	What do you hold on to to get you through difficult times?
	For some people, religious or spiritual beliefs are a source of comfort in dealing with life's ups and downs. Is this true for you?
O—**Organized** religion	Do you belong to a religious or spiritual community? Does it help you?
	How important is this to you?
	What aspects of your religion are helpful to you?
P—**Personal spirituality/Practices**	Do you believe in God? What is your relationship with God?
	Do you have personal spiritual beliefs that are not a part of organized religion? If so, what are they?
	What aspects of your spirituality are most helpful to you (e.g., meditation, prayer, reading scripture, listening to music, nature)?
E—**Effects** on medical care and end-of-life issues	Has your illness affected your relationship with God? Or to do the things that usually help you spiritually?
	Are you concerned about conflicts between your beliefs and your healthcare treatment plan?
	Do you have any dietary restrictions or other practices I should know about in planning your care?
	Would you like to speak to a clinical chaplain (or community spiritual leader)?

Source: Based on Gowry, A., & Hight, E. (2001). Spirituality and medical practice: Using the HOPE questions as a practical tool for spiritual assessment. *American Family Physician, 63,* 36–41.

S-P-I-R-I-T Assessment

- Obtain information from the patient when possible.
- For an emergency admission or if the patient cannot give information, consult the next of kin or a designated power of attorney (DPOA) as soon as possible for information.
- Assess the following key areas.

S—Spiritual/religious belief system

Religion, tradition, sect, or denominational affiliation

Text/writing(s) that provide source of authority and codes for behavior

Name and phone number of supporting or affiliated church, synagogue, temple, or other place of worship

Past experience with a belief system (positive or negative)

Beliefs related to health, illness, healthcare, healthcare providers, Western medicine, adjuvant therapies, herbal or natural healing methods or techniques

Beliefs about suffering, terminal or chronic illness, advanced directives, autopsy, organ donation

Stigmas related to illness, if applicable

P—Personal spirituality

Individual beliefs and practices of affiliation that the patient or family accepts and attempts to follow (may be directly or indirectly related to above assessment areas)

Individual beliefs that may differ or even be contrary to affiliation beliefs

Whether spirituality is a part of personal experience of religion or a separate entity

Level of comfort discussing spirituality

Whether personal spirituality is viewed positively or negatively at the present time

I—Integration within a spiritual community

Name and title of religious or spiritual leader or authority figure(s)

Names and titles of religious groups that may need to be contacted: Stephen Ministry, prayer group leader, prayer chain support person, shaman, medicine man or woman, men's or women's group within denomination

Role of patient or individual in any of above named groups

R—Ritualized practices and restrictions

Activities that patient or family's faith encourages or forbids

Needs for modesty and covering of body parts or appendages

Any special beliefs or needs in relation to drawing blood or to laboratory tests or procedures

Dietary needs and restrictions: food preferences, preparation of foods, and location of food preparation areas

Gender-specific roles and responsibilities of care providers

Prayer needs and restrictions: Who delivers and offers such practices?

Articles or other materials needed for worship, devotion, or prayer (rosaries, prayer beads, prayer books, religious tracts, Bibles, crosses, prayer shawls or cloths)

I—Implications for medical care

Beliefs and practices that healthcare providers should remember while providing care

Specific medications that may not be administered and withheld; implications for pain control

Specific medical procedures or products that may not be administered (abortion, blood products)

Communication patterns and needs for effective care delivery: Who makes decisions? What is the role of parents or guardians when children or other vulnerable populations are the recipients of care? Does the guardian reflect the beliefs of patient, if these are known?

T—Terminal events planning

Wishes for advance directives (cardiopulmonary resuscitation, intubation, ventilator assist, feeding tubes)

Wishes for transplantation or organ donation

Need for religious services (last rites, ministries of healing, baptism, initiation, confession, communion)

Clergy or ministry groups to be contacted and when

Ideas of an afterlife

Treatment of the body at the time of death

Funeral planning

Source: Adapted from Highfield, M. E. F. (2000). Providing spiritual care to patients with cancer. *Clinical Journal of Oncology Nursing,* *4*(3), 115–120.

Sources of Spiritual Data

You can acquire information about a patient's spirituality from a variety of sources other than interviews.

- **Patient's environment.** Observe the patient's environment for hints about her spirituality (e.g., pictures of family and/or pets, the presence of sacred texts or reading materials, articles used in worship [a crucifix, rosary beads, religious medals, statues], or copies of church bulletins/sermon tapes).
- **Patient's questions.** The patient may ask questions that are indicative of spiritual comfort, longing, or distress. For example, the patient may ask if you attend church and if so, whether it provides you with a sense of comfort and meaning.

- **Patient's behaviors, moods, and feelings.** Multiple behaviors/moods/feelings give a clear and certain indication that the patient is struggling with issues that have spiritual overtones. These warrant further assessment and nursing intervention. For example, a patient may ask you if you have ever really felt guilty about something you did as a child.
- **Nonverbal communication.** Body language may indicate hopeful or distressing times. For example, you may observe a patient praying; or when asking about spirituality, you may see the patient rolling his eyes, shaking his head, and demonstrating muscle tension.

THINKING CRITICALLY ABOUT SPIRITUALITY

The exercises in the following sections allow you to practice the kind of thinking you will use as a full-spectrum nurse. Because these are critical-thinking questions, there is usually no single right answer. We do not provide answers for these questions because it is more important for you to think about the questions than to arrive at the "right" answer. These questions are designed to improve your thinking more than to "cover content." Discuss answers with your peers—discussion can stimulate critical thinking. If you have difficulty with any of these questions, consult with your instructor.

Applying the Full-Spectrum Nursing Model

PATIENT SITUATION

Charles Johnson is a 75-year-old African American man with newly diagnosed cancer of the lung. His physicians want to start chemotherapy to try to increase his life span. He is unsure whether he wants to have chemotherapy.

Mr. Johnson was brought up in the Baptist Church but has fallen away from practicing his faith over the years. He has been a heavy drinker all of his adult life and, as a young man, became alienated from churchgoing. He explains: "Church folk are all a bunch of hypocrites, if you ask me. I choose not to be a part of any of that." Nevertheless, he says that he tries to be kind to and tolerant of others. "I've messed up my life, so I figure I don't have any business telling other people how to live. I guess I just figure that how a person lives is between themselves and God."

Mr. Johnson has one surviving relative, a sister, who is concerned about him. His sister is a devout Jehovah's Witness, and she has tried several times to talk to Mr. Johnson about how important Jehovah is in her life. She continually leaves religious pamphlets and materials in his mailbox to encourage him to think about religion again.

Mr. Johnson's wife divorced him 20 years ago because of his drinking behaviors, and he has alienated his two middle-aged children, a son and a daughter. Mr. Johnson has two grandchildren, whom he rarely sees. He lives alone, is retired, and is having some trouble making ends meet financially. He has one avid hobby: he loves to go out in a boat and fish all day with his buddy, Jim. This, he says, is relaxing and gives him peace of mind.

THINKING

1. *Theoretical Knowledge (Recall of Facts and Principles):* Define *forgiveness,* and explain the benefits of forgiving self and others.

2. *Critical Thinking (Application of Knowledge):* Based on your theoretical knowledge about forgiveness, with whom might Mr. Johnson need to reconcile? Why do you think so?

DOING

3. *Practical Knowledge (HOPE Assessment):* Use the HOPE assessment (Clinical Insight 14-1) and enter Mr. Johnson's data. Identify sections for which you need additional data.

CARING

4. *Self-Knowledge:* How is your religious background similar to or different from Mr. Johnson's?

5. *Self-Knowledge:* (a) How would you feel if Mr. Johnson said to you, "Church folk are all a bunch of hypocrites, if you ask me. I choose not to be a part of any of that"? (b) How would you respond?

6. *Ethical Knowledge:* Imagine that Mr. Johnson's sister comes to visit and leaves some religious pamphlets on a chair, where he will not see them before she leaves. What would you do?

Critical Thinking and Clinical Reasoning

1. A 5-year-old boy was admitted to the hospital last night with a fever of 103°F (39.4°C). He was diagnosed with a serious infection that is easily treated with intravenous (IV) antibiotics. However, his parents are Christian Scientists, and they do not want the boy to be given antibiotics. They have called their Christian Science practitioner to visit as soon as possible.

   a. What practical knowledge do you have that will give you some insight into this situation?

   b. What essential piece of knowledge do you need that is *not* given in this scenario?

   c. If the parents do not agree to accepting IV antibiotics for their child, what can you do to (1) ensure that the child receives treatment and (2) support their spiritual needs?

2. A woman is admitted to the emergency department and gives birth to a premature baby boy who is in severe respiratory distress. The woman is a devout Roman Catholic. What interventions could you use to provide holistic spiritual care in such an emergency situation?

3. Interview nurses in the area where you have your clinical experiences. Discuss the interviews with classmates.

   a. Ask them to describe spiritual problems their patients have had.

   b. Ask them to tell you of any spiritual interventions they have used with patients and how effective they believe them to be.

   c. Ask them how comfortable they are in using spiritual interventions, especially prayer.

4. For each of the following concepts, use critical thinking to describe how or why it is important to nursing, patient care, or spirituality. Note that these are *not* to be merely definitions.

   Spirituality and religion

   Nursing research in religion and healthcare

   Major religions and healthcare

   The nurse and spirituality

   Assessment of the spiritual domain of care

   Spiritual care nursing interventions

   Spiritual well-being

What Are the Main Points in This Chapter?

➤ Spirituality is a powerful force in the lives of many patients—a force that has the potential to affect their health and perception of well-being.

➤ Nursing has historical roots in religion and spirituality.

➤ Nurses work with other disciplines to provide spiritual care.

➤ Religion is a sort of "map" that outlines and integrates essential beliefs, values, and codes of conduct into a manner of living.

➤ Spirituality, like a journey, takes place over time and involves the accumulation of life experiences and understandings. It is the attempt to find meaning, value, and purpose in life.

➤ Spiritual development involves struggles with faith, hope, and love.

➤ Religion and spirituality affect health and well-being; and in turn, health and well-being affect a person's religion and spirituality.

➤ Research suggests that religion and spirituality are important to healthcare outcomes; however, it does not explain *how* or *why* this is so.

➤ The more you know about similarities in and differences among the world's major religions, the more you will be able to offer comprehensive, compassionate care to patients.

➤ People, even within the same religion, vary greatly in the degree to which they follow the rituals and practices of their religion.

➤ Self-knowledge helps you to avoid abuses of spiritual care (e.g., imposing your religion on a patient).

➤ Barriers to spiritual care include (1) lack of awareness of spirituality in general and of your own spiritual belief system, (2) differences in spirituality between you (the nurse) and the patient, (3) fear that your spiritual knowledge is insufficient, and (4) fear of where spiritual discussions might lead.

➤ Various ready-made tools are available for performing an in-depth spiritual assessment.

➤ NANDA-I labels describing spiritual needs are Moral Distress, Spiritual Distress, Risk for Spiritual Distress, Readiness for Enhanced Spiritual Well-Being, Impaired Religiosity, Risk for Impaired Religiosity, and Readiness for Enhanced Religiosity. Spiritual Pain is a non-NANDA-I diagnosis that may be useful.

➤ Nursing interventions related to spiritual care require you to be self-aware, fully present, supportive, empathetic, and nonjudgmental and to have a wish to benefit the patient.

➤ When a patient asks you to pray, you must determine whether he wishes you to pray *for* or *with* him, and you should ask what he would like you to *especially* address in the prayer.

➤ A miracle does not necessarily involve the notion of a cure; miracles are more often events that proceed according to natural law but still have a powerful impact on the person's expectations.

➤ Nurses who are open to diversity, who exhibit multiple understandings of religion, and who fashion for themselves different means of spiritual expression are comfortable in the spiritual care domain.

For practice questions for this chapter,

Go to **NCLEX-Style Chapter Quiz,** on the Student Resource Disk or DavisPlus at http://davisplus.fadavis.com/Wilkinson2

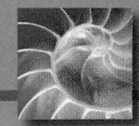

Knowledge Map

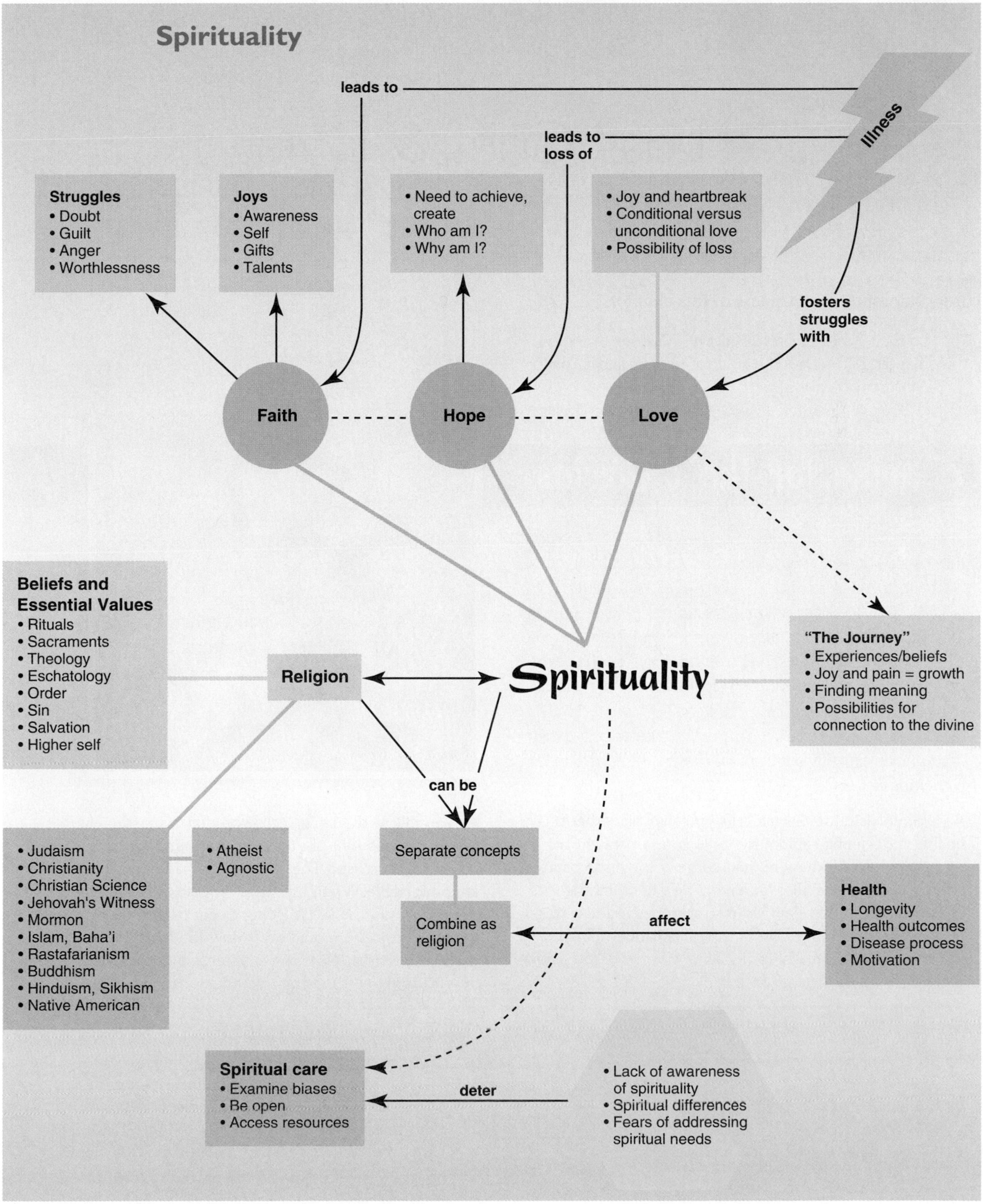

Spirituality

Struggles
- Doubt
- Guilt
- Anger
- Worthlessness

Joys
- Awareness
- Self
- Gifts
- Talents

leads to

- Need to achieve, create
- Who am I?
- Why am I?

leads to loss of

- Joy and heartbreak
- Conditional versus unconditional love
- Possibility of loss

Illness

Faith - - - - - **Hope** - - - - - **Love**

fosters struggles with

Beliefs and Essential Values
- Rituals
- Sacraments
- Theology
- Eschatology
- Order
- Sin
- Salvation
- Higher self

Religion ←→ **Spirituality**

"The Journey"
- Experiences/beliefs
- Joy and pain = growth
- Finding meaning
- Possibilities for connection to the divine

- Judaism
- Christianity
- Christian Science
- Jehovah's Witness
- Mormon
- Islam, Baha'i
- Rastafarianism
- Buddhism
- Hinduism, Sikhism
- Native American

- Atheist
- Agnostic

can be

Separate concepts

Combine as religion

affect

Health
- Longevity
- Health outcomes
- Disease process
- Motivation

Spiritual care
- Examine biases
- Be open
- Access resources

deter

- Lack of awareness of spirituality
- Spiritual differences
- Fears of addressing spiritual needs

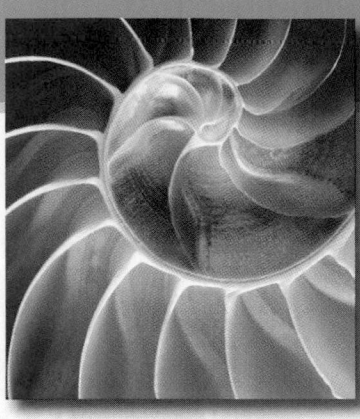

CHAPTER 15

Loss, Grief, & Dying

For a podcast of an overview of this chapter,

 Go to Student Resources, **Podcast – Chapter Overviews, Chapter 15,** on DavisPlus at http://davisplus.fadavis.com/ Wilkinson2

Caring for the Garcias

The exercises in the following section allow you to practice the kind of thinking you will use as a full-spectrum nurse. Because these are critical-thinking questions, there is usually no single right answer. We do not provide answers for these questions because it is more important for you to think about the questions than to arrive at the "right" answer. These questions are designed to improve your thinking more than to "cover content." Discuss answers with your peers—discussion can stimulate critical thinking. If you have difficulty with any of these questions, consult with your instructor.

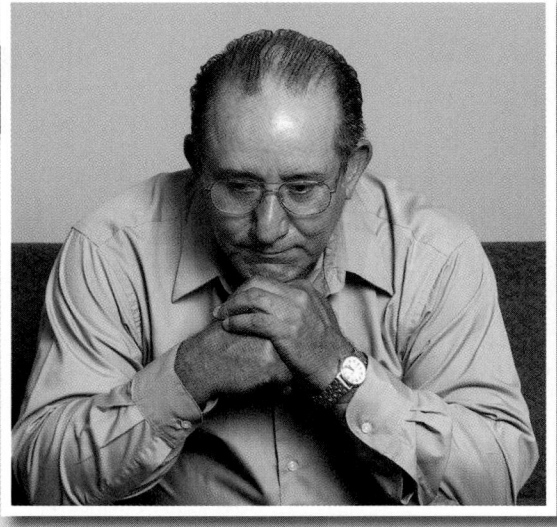

At a clinic visit, Joe Garcia tells you that his father's health is declining rapidly. Joe tells you, "I thought he was doing okay. I knew he had surgery for his prostate, so I thought it was all over. Lately he's been having lots of low back and hip pain. So my mom begged him to go to the doctor, and he told him he has cancer all over." Joe shakes his head and looks away from you. You notice tears in his eyes.

As you talk with him, he tells you that his family has avoided discussions about serious illness and death. "It just never got discussed. The whole idea made my parents uncomfortable. When my father got sick the first time, he refused to discuss it. 'I'm going to get better. Don't even think about it,' he would say." Now Joe feels the need to discuss this situation with his parents but doesn't know how to bring up the topic. He asks for your advice.

A. What would you think and feel when you see Joe's tears and when Joe asks for this advice?

B. What would you advise Joe?

C. What type of grief is Joe experiencing?

D. Examine the factors that affect grief. Apply these factors to Joe's situation. You will need to review the family history included in the introduction to the Garcias (in the front of this book) to fully answer this question. Indicate whether the information for any of the factors to be evaluated is insufficient.

Practical **Knowledge**
knowing how

This section provides guidelines for communicating with people who are grieving, for caring for dying patients and their families, and for providing postmortem care.

Clinical Insights

Clinical Insight 15-1 ▶ Communicating with People Who Are Grieving

Perfect your listening skills.
- Listen for what is *not* said as well as what is said.
- Be alert for nonverbal cues.

Respond to nonverbal cues with appropriate touch and eye contact. A smile, a gentle touch, sitting with a patient, and eye contact all relay a message of genuine care and concern. You may not need to say very much at all.

Encourage and accept expressions of feelings.
- Receiving expressions of intense feelings (e.g., anger and guilt) may be painful for you. It may help to remember that it is therapeutic for people to express their feelings.
- You don't need to change the person's feelings or "make them better." As much as we would like to do this, it is not possible.
- You do need to validate the person's feelings (e.g., "It is normal to feel that way; it is OK").

Reassure the person that it is not "wrong" to feel anger, guilt, relief, or other feelings she may believe to be unacceptable.
- A dying patient might say, "I know it's awful, but I feel so angry with God for giving me this disease." Or a bereaved spouse might admit, "I shouldn't feel this way, but I'm relieved that it's finally over."

- Patients need to hear you say their feelings are not "wrong" or "bad" and that they are going through a normal process.

Increase your self-awareness. Become more conscious of your own attitudes and feelings regarding death and dying. If you are comfortable with your perspective, you will be able to hear patients' expressions of anger, guilt, frustration, fear, and loneliness more comfortably.

Continue to communicate with dying patients even if they are in a coma. Encourage family members to do so as well.
- Talk to the patient. Tell him what is going on around him, what care you are providing, and when you or others enter or are about to leave the room. Research indicates that patients continue to hear even though they cannot respond, sometimes up to the moment of death.
- Avoid discussing the dying person as though he were not present.

(Note: If you need further information about communication techniques, refer to Chapter 18, Volumes 1 and 2.)

Practice Resources
Eisenhandler, S. (2004); Emanuel, L., Ferris, F., von Gunter, C., et al. (2008); The Joint Commission (2008); Kruse, B. (2004); Traylor, E., Hayslip, B., Kaminski, P. L., et al. (2003).

Clinical Insight 15-2 ▶ Helping Families of Dying Patients

View the family as your unit of care.
Family members often rate communication with clinicians as one of their most important needs.

Provide information, support, and a listening ear.
Include specific facts about the patient's condition and prognosis and whom to call about changes in condition.

Communicate medical updates daily.
Information can relieve anxiety and is useful to the family when making decisions.

Encourage family members to help with care if they are able.
This helps meet their need to be useful, promotes family ties, and makes the patient more comfortable. Instruct and supervise as appropriate. If family members are not physically or emotionally able to provide care, accept that.

Encourage family members to ask questions.
They may hesitate to do so for various reasons (e.g., they may not want to interrupt busy care providers).

Listen actively to the patient's and family's concerns.
Make eye content; clarify when you don't understand.
This helps you avoid misinterpreting the family's concerns and needs.

Help the family to understand the goals of care and solve problems when needed.

Follow up with other healthcare team members promptly if the family has questions that are outside your scope of practice.

Arrange for a formal multidisciplinary meeting with the family soon after the patient's admission, if possible. Discussions should cover personal, cultural, and religious

(continued on next page)

Clinical Insight 15-2 ➤ **Helping Families of Dying Patients** (continued)

traditions (e.g., how prayers are to be conducted, how the body is to be handled after death, and so on).

Encourage the family to visit the hospital chapel and to speak with a chaplain or with their own spiritual adviser.

Provide anticipatory guidance regarding the stages of loss and grief, so that they will know what to expect after their loved one dies.

Acknowledge the family's feelings and the loss they are experiencing.
Many times family members begin the grieving process before the loved one dies.

Help the family members explore past coping mechanisms; reinforce successful past coping mechanisms.

Refer for ethics consultation if decision-making may become a problem.

Remind family members and significant others to take care of themselves.
Watching a loved one die is a very difficult experience. A sensitive, caring nurse can make it a little easier.

- Many times they need "permission" to go to eat or to go home and rest.
- If the patient is near death and family and friends do not want to leave the patient's side, make them as comfortable as possible.
- Provide comfortable chairs, coffee, and snacks (according to organizational policy), and be alert for other needs they may have.

Teach the family what to expect with regard to medications, treatments, and signs of approaching death.
If family members know what is normal, they will be less likely to panic or fear the inevitable.

As physical signs of death become apparent, keep the family informed. You may say something like, "Her blood pressure is becoming difficult to hear. That is one of the signs that she is closer to death." Help the family to understand what the patient is experiencing, as this may be very different from what they are seeing.

Reassure families of patients who become withdrawn near the time of death that this does not mean the patient is rejecting them, but only that his body is conserving energy and that he has come to terms with dying and letting go of his connections with life.

When approaching death is apparent, ask family members directly, "Do you want to be present while he is dying?" Tell them what to expect, if they do not know

When an expected death occurs, shift the focus of your care to the family and those who were caregivers.

Practice Resources

Ahrens, T., Yancey, V., & Kollef, M. (2003); Boyle, D. K., Miller, P. A., & Forbes-Thompson, S. A. (2005); Emanuel, L., Ferris, F., von Gunter, C., et al. (2008); Hudson, P. (2006); The Joint Commission (2008); von Gunter, C., Ferris, F., & Emanuel, L. (2000).

Clinical Insight 15-3 ➤ **Caring for the Dying Person: Meeting Physiological Needs**

Active dying usually occurs over a period of 10 to 14 days (although it can take as little as 24 hours). The "final hours" refers to the last 4 to 48 hours of life, in which failure of body systems results in death (Pitorak, 2003). Physiological needs during this time include mobility, oxygenation, safety, nutrition, fluids, elimination, personal hygiene, comfort, and control of pain and symptoms (nausea, vomiting).

Encourage the patient to be as independent as possible, so she will maintain a sense of control.

Provide adequate pain control.
This can be a major issue for patients and caregivers. In fact, dying patients are often more concerned about pain and loss of control than about dying itself. Pain is difficult to assess in semiconscious or unconscious patients. See Chapter 30 if you need more information about pain management.

- Provide education to dispel the myths about pain medication (e.g., addiction, overdose). Effective pain control

medications exist and can be administered by various routes.
- Assure the patient and family that analgesics will not be addictive in this situation.
- Respect the patient's informed decision to refuse pain medications. For example, a patient may prefer to endure pain in order to be awake and alert when his family is at the bedside.
- Follow one of the common pain protocols to ensure that pain is controlled.
- Administer pain medication on a regular schedule instead of waiting until the patient asks (prn), to ensure pain control.
- Teach and perform nonpharmacological pain-relief measures when you judge they may be helpful. These might include meditation, heat/cold therapies, massage, distraction, imagery, deep breathing, and herbal-scented lotions. It may be soothing to play soft music, add "white noise," or turn off the television.

■ Patients who are near death may moan or grunt as they breathe; this does not necessarily indicate pain. Be sure that families understand this. When accompanied by agitation and restlessness, these symptoms may indicate terminal delirium, which may require medications for control.

Monitor the patient's energy level.

Remember that fatigue is a normal part of the dying process. Most dying patients sleep much of the time.

■ Perform hygiene and other care, if the patient tires easily or lacks the energy to care for herself (i.e., activities of daily living).
■ Remove environmental stressors that interfere with sleep (e.g., noise, too much light, a room that is too hot or too cold).
■ Identify psychosocial stressors (e.g., depression, anxiety, fear) that may keep the patient awake (see Clinical Insight 15-4).

Maintain skin integrity.

During the final hours of life, the goal changes from preserving skin integrity to providing comfort. Realize that during this time even excellent care may not prevent skin breakdown.

■ Turn the patient frequently unless contraindicated. Refer to the pain control interventions in the preceding list.
■ Assess for increased diaphoresis and/or incontinence.
■ Maintain adequate nutrition.

If the patient is comatose or unconscious, provide special care for the eyes so they do not become too dry. Many agencies use a form of artificial tears for this purpose.

If the patient is not able to take fluids, wet the lips and mouth frequently with cool water or with a prepared product to prevent dryness and cracking of lips and mucous membranes of the nose, mouth, and eyes.

There is some evidence that glycerin swabs dry the mucous membranes and should not be used.

Provide artificial hydration (unless the patient has an advance directive requesting no artificial hydration) per nasogastric (NG) or IV route.

IV fluids can cause edema, nausea, and even pain in a patient who is actively dying. Dehydration is thought to not cause distress during the last hours, and may even be protective (Emanuel et al., 2008).

Take the vital signs often, unless contraindicated; observe for decreased level of consciousness and pallor.

Assess and provide interventions for constipation, urinary retention, and incontinence.

Constipation may be associated with decreased fluid intake, inactivity, weakness, hypercalcemia, hyperkalemia, and lack of privacy. It can contribute to pain, nausea, vomiting, and anorexia, so intervention is an important comfort measure. Incontinence may occur because of fatigue and loss of sphincter control. It can be distressing to patients and family members.

■ Administer laxatives, stool softeners, and lubricants for constipation.
■ Catheterize the patient if he is unable to void and the bladder becomes distended.
■ Use pads for incontinence, but change them frequently to prevent skin breakdown and, near the end, to promote comfort.
■ Use a rectal tube if diarrhea is severe.

Intervene for "death rattle" if it occurs and if it is distressing to the family.

■ Turn the patient on his side, and elevate the head of the bed.
■ Administer antispasmodic and anticholinergic medications if necessary.

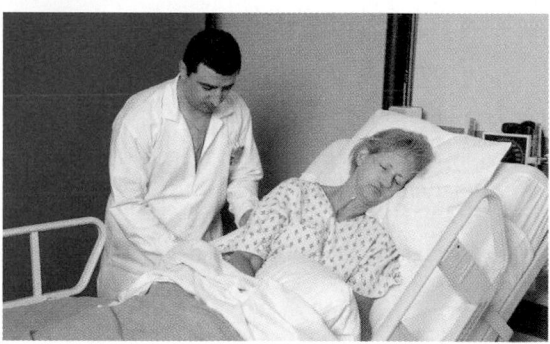

Provide medication for other symptoms, such as nausea and breathlessness.

Continue to speak to the patient as if he can hear.

Do not talk about the patient to others in his presence. The patient is usually able to hear even after he can no longer respond to sounds and other stimuli. Assume the unconscious patient hears everything.

Document changes in vital signs and level of consciousness. Record intake and output, noting changes. Document the times of cardiac arrest and cessation of respirations.

Practice Resources

American Nurses Association (2003); Emanuel, L., Ferris, F., von Gunter, C., et al. (2005); Harvey, J. (2001); The Joint Commission (2008); Qaseem, A., Snow, V., Shekelle, P., et al. (2008).

Clinical Insight 15-4 ▶ Caring for the Dying Person: Meeting Psychological Needs

Patients experience many emotions at end of life, including anger, sadness, depression, fear, relief, loneliness, and grief. At this time, communication and support are most helpful. Discussing concerns and issues is a viable means of coping.

The following interventions are important:

If there is an advance directive or living will, locate the documents. Review the documents to be certain you understand the patent's wishes. If you have not already done so, notify all relevant health professionals of the existence of these documents.

Answer all questions honestly.

Explain all care and treatments even if the patient is unconscious.
He may still be able to hear.

Realize that the patient may feel he is losing control.
- Help the person recognize what he does have control over.
- Include the patient in care decisions as much as he is able.

Attend to social needs.
Relationships are a priority at this time. Some patients may simply need to keep the bonds with family members and friends intact. For other patients, this may be a time to re-establish or mend relationships.

- Notify family members when the patient wishes to see them.
- Allow the patient and family to discuss death at their own pace.
- Offer to contact a chaplain or other spiritual leader if the patient chooses.
- Pray with the patient if he requests it and you are comfortable doing so.

Encourage the patient to express feelings. Be prepared to accept a wide range of feelings, including anger, hopelessness, loneliness, and depression.

Early in the dying process, assess the sources of financial support for the patient and family.
- Finances may be a concern and may place an additional burden on the family.

- The patient may feel he is a burden to care for.

Be aware of sexual needs.
Some people may feel it is not right to have sexual feelings when the person they love is dying. Others may be afraid of harming the patient if they are sexually intimate.

- Provide realistic information about these issues.
- Suggest ways a couple can be close and affectionate at this time
- Be aware that expressions of sexuality may change as a person becomes closer to death.

When the patient is very near death, focus on relieving symptoms (e.g., pain, nausea) and emotional distress.

If the person can communicate, ask about immediate concerns:
- "Are you in pain?" "Are you comfortable?"
- "What are you afraid of now?"
- "What can we do to help you go peacefully?"
- "Who do you want in the room with you right now?"
- If the patient asks whether he is dying, be honest.

If the patient cannot communicate, ask the family what the patient would want. Ask the person most likely to know.

When the patient is very near death, it may be helpful to say something like, "Your family will be fine" rather than, "It is OK for you to go now."
Be aware that some people seem to wait to die until after a significant date (birthday, anniversary, and so on) has passed. Others wait for family to gather, whereas others wait until loved ones leave so they will not upset the family by dying in their presence.

Practice Resources

Duffy, S., Jackson, F., Schim, S., et al. (2006); Emanuel, L., Ferris, F., von Gunter, C., et al. (2008); Hancock, K., Clayton, J., Parker, S., et al. (2007); The Joint Commission (2008); National Guideline Clearinghouse (2005); Pitorak, E. (2003).

Clinical Insight 15-5 ▶ Providing Postmortem Care

Supporting the Family
- **At the moment of death, do not interrupt or intrude on the family.** Wait quietly and observe, or if they would feel more comfortable being alone with the patient, leave the room. Give them as much time as they need. When they move away from the body, or have expressed their last good-byes, then it is time to assess the patient and report the lack of vital signs.
- **Immediately after death, express sympathy to the family.** This is very important. Make a simple statement, such as, "I am sorry for your loss." Avoid statements that interpret the situation for the family, such as, "It's God's

will." Also avoid attempts to mitigate the family member's grief, for example, "It will get better in time," or "You still have your son."
- **If the family wishes to be alone with the body,** straighten the bedcovers and make the patient look as natural as possible.
- **Be accepting of family members' behavior at this time,** no matter how strange it may seem to you. A family might want to take a picture, or the spouse may lie down beside the deceased person.
- **If no family members are present, identify the next of kin** and be sure the family is informed of the patient's death.

- **If family members arrive after the death, offer to take them to the bedside.**
- **If family members wish to be involved in postmortem care,** *encourage them to do so.* This can facilitate their grieving process.
- **Take care to present the patient's body in a way that is appropriate for the family** (i.e., remove any tubes, IV lines, and so on, according to the institution's policy) and have the patient positioned in a way that appears comforting (e.g., bed covers pulled up, hands at the side). Viewing the body is useful to many individuals.
- **Ask whether each family member wishes to spend time alone with the deceased person,** and arrange for them to do so. Never remove the body until the family is ready.
- **Ask, "How can I help?" "What do you need?" "What would you like for me to do?"**
- **Locate personal effects and give them to the family/next of kin.** If you can't remove a ring, wrap it with gauze, tape it in place, and tie the gauze to the wrist to prevent subsequent loss.

Legal Responsibilities

- **Usually the physician must pronounce death;** however, in some areas a coroner or a nurse may also perform this task.
- **The person who pronounces death must sign the death certificate.** In some agencies, the nurse is responsible for checking to see that it has been signed.
- *If the patient is donating organs,* review and make any necessary arrangements.
- *If an autopsy is to be performed,* as a rule, the physician (or other person designated by the institution) is responsible for obtaining signed permission from the next of kin.

Care of the Body

- **Follow agency policies,** *and respect cultural and spiritual preferences.*
- **Wash the body** *if there has been any incontinence or drainage.* Place ABD pads between the buttocks to absorb rectal drainage.

In some cultures, the body is not washed, or family members arrange to have someone special do it; so you should ask the family before performing this task.

- **Dress the body in a clean gown, comb the hair, and straighten the bed linens.**
- **Place the body supine in a natural position.**
  - Place the dentures in the mouth before rigor mortis occurs.
  - Close the eyes and mouth before rigor mortis occurs. Close the eyes by gently pressing on the lids with your fingertips. If they do not stay closed, place a moist compress on the eyelids for a few minutes and then try to close them again.
  - Tie a strip of soft gauze (e.g., Kling) under the chin and around the head if your institution requires it (not all do).

This keeps the mouth set in a natural position in case there is a viewing later. Alternatively, you can place a folded towel under the chin to keep the jaw closed.

- Place a pillow under the head and shoulders.

To prevent blood from settling there and causing discoloration.

- **Be sure that dressings are clean, and unless an autopsy is to be done, remove all tubes and drains.** Be careful when removing tape or dressings. Apply small adhesive bandages to puncture sites.

After death, the skin loses its elasticity and can be torn easily.

- **If the family asks about the coldness** *and color of the body,* explain to them about algor mortis and livor mortis.

Algor mortis occurs when the blood stops circulating. The body temperature drops about 1.8°F per hour until it reaches room temperature. The dependent parts of the body appear bluish and mottled because when the blood stops circulating, the red blood cells break down, releasing hemoglobin. This is called **livor mortis.**

- **After the family has spent time with the body, arrange to have it sent to the morgue,** where either an autopsy will be performed, or, if not, the funeral home in charge of arrangements will arrive to transport the body.
  - Pad the wrists and ankles to prevent bruising; tie them together with gauze.
  - Wrap the body in a shroud or body wrap for transfer to the morgue.
  - If no relatives were present to receive patient belongings, bag them, label the bag, and send with the patient to the morgue.
  - If possible, close doors to adjoining rooms before transport.
- **Make sure there are identification tags, and hazard labels** *if necessary, on the body, on the shroud or body bag, and on the patient's possessions.* Follow agency policy for number and location of tags. They will usually include the patient's name, room and bed numbers, date and time of death, and the physician's name.

Misidentification can create legal problems, for example, if the body is prepared incorrectly for a funeral.

- **Follow institutional policy if the patient has died of a communicable disease.** By law, there are special preparations to perform in such cases.
- **Handle the body with dignity.**
- **Documentation varies among healthcare facilities.** However, you will almost always document the time that you noted absence of heartbeat and respirations, any auxiliary equipment (e.g., mechanical ventilator) still present, the disposition of the patient's possessions (especially money and jewelry), and the date and time the body is transported to the morgue or funeral home.

Practice Resources

College of American Pathologists (2007); Harvey, J. (2001); The Joint Commission (2008).

Forms

DO NOT RESUSCITATE ORDERS
Physician: Complete Part I & II to initiate order. Part III is to be
completed every seven days.

☐ **DNR forms completed on previous admission. Verified by:** _____.
Date of original order: _____.

                                              Signature   **Date**

NOTE: Words that appear in the directions in all capital letters are listed in the DNR definitions.

PART I: ☐ If this patient suffers a cardiac or respiratory arrest, a Cart is not to be called and no resuscitation measures are to be carried out.

PART II: ☐ This order is to be transcribed and instituted immediately. All required documentation is complete.

or

☐ This order is to be transcribed and instituted only after the CONCURRING PHYSICIAN'S statements have been completed.
I have requested Dr. _____ to be the CONCURRING PHYSICIAN.

_____, M.D.   _____, R.N.
   Signature of ATTENDING PHYSICIAN   Signature of Transcribing Nurse

_____   _____   _____   _____
   Date   Time   Date   Time

PART III: Review of DNR ORDER
This is to verify that review and determination of continued appropriateness of the DNR ORDER and the conditions under which it was obtained was done: (to be documented at least every 7 days)

Date	By	Date	By
			Continued on reverse side

PART IV: Wavier to DNR ORDER
I, the undersigned, have previously consented to a DO NOT RESUSCITATE ORDER. During the procedure and until I am returned to my room, I hereby waive my consent to the DO NOT RESUSCITATE ORDER and authorize my ATTENDING PHYSICIAN to write such an order.

_____   _____   _____   _____
Signature of patient or SURROGATE or PROXY   Date   Signature of WITNESS   Date
   (or parent or legal guardian for minor)

☐ DNR ORDER suspended during the peri-operative period, as noted above.

_____, M.D.   _____, R.N.
   Signature of ATTENDING PHYSICIAN   Signature of Transcribing Nurse

_____   _____   _____   _____
   Date   Time   Date   Time

PART V: Revocation of DNR ORDER
I, the undersigned, hereby revoke the DO NOT RESUSCITATE ORDER previously consented to by me.

_____   _____   _____   _____
Signature of patient or SURROGATE or PROXY   Date   Signature of WITNESS   Date
   (or parent or legal guardian for minor)

☐ DNR ORDER revoked.

_____, M.D.   _____, R.N.
   Signature of ATTENDING PHYSICIAN   Signature of Transcribing Nurse

_____   _____   _____   _____
   Date   Time   Date   Time

13610 3/01 side 1 of 2

Assessment Guidelines

You can use these guidelines for assessing dying patients as well as for other types of loss.

Assessing Grief and Loss

1. Assess the patient and significant others for common grief reactions.

PHYSICAL	EMOTIONAL	BEHAVIORS	COGNITION
Loss of appetite	Anger	Forgetfulness	Decreased concentration
Weight loss/gain	Sadness	Withdrawal	Forgetfulness
Fatigue	Guilt	Insomnia or too much sleep	Impaired judgment
Decreased libido	Relief	Dreaming of deceased	Obsessive thoughts of the deceased or lost object
Decrease in immune system	Shock	Verbalizing the loss	
Decreased energy	Numbness	Crying	Preoccupation
Possibly physical symptoms, such as headache or stomach pain	Loneliness	Loss of productivity at work or school	Confusion
	Fear		Questioning spiritual beliefs
	Anxiety		Searching to understand
	Powerlessness		Searching for purpose and meaning
	Helplessness		
	Depression		

2. Assess knowledge base of patient and significant others.
   a. Do the patient and family have the information they need to make informed decisions about healthcare choices? For example, you might ask the following questions:

   - "Tell me what you understand about your illness."
   - "Are there any questions about your illness that you'd like me to answer?"
   - "What are your options for treatment?"
   - "Do you know how to reach your provider if you have questions about your care?"

   b. What and how much do the patient and family want to know?

   Some people wish to have all the details of their condition and care. For others, the details cause anxiety.

3. Assess the history of loss.
   Determine whether the patient or family has sustained recent losses or major changes (e.g., death, moving, divorce, retirement). Ask such questions as:

   - "Have you had any recent changes in your life?"
   - "Tell me about your family."
   - "Are your parents still living?" (as appropriate)
   - "What previous experiences have you had with the loss of someone you loved (or with this condition)?"

4. Assess coping abilities and support systems.
   Some coping assessment questions include the following:

   - "What do you do to help you reduce stress?"
   - "Do you have family/friends you can talk with?"
   - "What would you say is your greatest support when going through difficult times?"
   - "Tell me about a previous loss and what you did to cope with it."
   - "Are you using any community resources to help you get through this? Do you know what they are?"

   The way individuals have coped in the past will affect how they cope with dying or with their current loss. It may also be therapeutic for them to identify their resources and supports.

Continued

Assessing Grief and Loss—cont'd

5. Assess the meaning of the loss or illness.
Be alert for statements such as the following, which may indicate the patient or family is struggling to find meaning:

- "I'm being punished."
- "She doesn't deserve this."
- "Why is this happening to me?"

In trying to "make sense" of their loss or their dying, people try to attach a meaning to their suffering.

6. Differentiate between grief and depressive disorder.
a. Symptoms common to both grief and depressive disorder: sadness, insomnia, poor appetite and weight loss

Feelings of sadness and depression are a normal part of grief, provided the depression does not linger too long.

b. Symptoms that indicate grief, but not depression. An example is a "trigger" event. The person may feel relatively better in certain situations, such as when she is with friends and family. However, triggers, such as the deceased person's birthday, an anniversary, or holidays, cause the feelings to resurface more strongly.

c. Symptoms that indicate depressive disorder:

- The depression is more pervasive. That is, the person rarely gets any relief from the symptoms.
- Feelings of guilt not related to the loved one's death
- Thoughts about own death or of suicide (other than feelings the person would be better off dead now that the loved one is gone)
- Preoccupation with own "worthlessness"
- Sluggishness
- Hesitant and confused speech
- Prolonged and marked difficulty in carrying out activities of daily living
- Hallucinations, other than thinking he hears the voice of or sees the deceased person

Source: Ferszt, G. G., & Leveillee, M. (2006). How do you distinguish between grief and depression? *Nursing2006, 36*(9), 60–61.

7. Perform a physical assessment.
Look for signs of increased stress, such as tension, forgetfulness, distraction, increased or decreased appetite and sleep, weight gain or loss, fatigue, and decreased self-care (e.g., deficient hygiene).

A thorough physical examination adds data to help you determine how well the patient is coping with the loss or illness.

8. Perform a cultural and spiritual assessment.
a. Assess the patient's and family's religious beliefs, any spiritual needs they may have (e.g., forgiveness, hope, meaning, love), and cultural influences that may affect the way they cope.

b. Do not assume that a person adheres closely to the dominant values of his religious or cultural group. Always assess. For example, ask:

- "To what religious and ethnic groups do you belong?"
- "How closely do you identify with those groups?"

See Chapter 13 for details of cultural assessment and Chapter 14 for details of spiritual assessment, if you need them.

9. Perform these specific assessments for dying patients.
For dying patients, in addition to the other assessments in this guideline, you should also assess the following:

a. When the patient and family are ready, encourage them to talk about what the patient might want for burial or cremation or whether there are tasks that the person would like taken care of (e.g., giving away valuables, calling family members).

b. Determine whether the dying person has a living will or advance directives.

c. Discuss with the patient and family the possibility of organ donation if appropriate for the patient's circumstances.

d. Observe for physical changes indicating the approach of death:

1 to 3 months before death: increased sleep, decreased appetite, difficulty digesting food

1 to 2 weeks before death: decreased blood pressure, pulse and respiration changes (decreased or increased), a yellowish pallor to the skin, extreme pallor of extremities, temperature fluctuations, increased perspiration, brief periods of apnea during sleep, rattling breathing sounds, nonproductive cough

Assessing Grief and Loss—cont'd

Days to hours before death: a brief surge of energy and mental clarity, with a desire to eat and talk with family members

- Dehydration, difficulty swallowing, decreasing blood pressure, weak pulse
- Sagging of tongue and soft palate, diminished gag reflex, secretions accumulating in the oropharynx and/or bronchi
- Shallow, rapid, or irregular breathing; Cheyne-Stokes respirations; apnea of 10 to 30 seconds; "death rattle"
- Decreased peripheral circulation, "clammy" skin; extremities cool and mottled; dependent body parts darker than the rest of the body
- Decreased urinary output secondary to decreased kidney function
- Slack facial muscles
- Retained feces; bowel and bladder incontinence
- Blurred vision; eyes open but unseeing
- Restlessness or agitation (check for impacted stool, distended bladder, pain)
- Decreased communication, quiet, withdrawal

Moments before death: Does not respond to touch or sound; cannot be awakened. There may be a short series of long-spaced breaths before breathing stops entirely and the heart stops beating. Auscultate to determine whether apical pulse and respirations are absent.

Standardized Nursing Language

NOC Outcomes and NIC Interventions for Loss and Grieving Diagnoses

NURSING DIAGNOSES	SELECTED NOC OUTCOMES	SELECTED NIC INTERVENTIONS
Grieving ***Defining Characteristics:*** Anger, potential loss of significant object (e.g., job status, body function), denial of potential loss, sorrow, guilt, bargaining, altered eating and sleep patterns, changes in activity level or libido, difficulty taking on new roles	Adaptation to Physical Disability Coping Family Coping Grief Resolution Psychosocial Adjustment: Life Change	Anticipatory Guidance Body Image Enhancement Coping Enhancement Emotional Support Family Integrity Promotion Family Support Grief Work Facilitation Grief Work Facilitation: Perinatal Death

- For Thomas Manning ("Meet Your Patient") in Volume 1, do you see any symptoms of Grieving?

Complicated Grieving ***Defining Characteristics:*** Repetitive use of ineffective coping behaviors, reliving of past experiences with little or no reduction in intensity of grief, prolonged interference with functioning, psychosomatic responses, expressions of grief (e.g., anger, sadness, crying), idealization of lost object or person, labile affect, developmental regression, denial of loss, expression of unresolved issues or guilt	Coping Family Coping Family Resiliency Grief Resolution Psychosocial Adjustment: Life Change Role Performance	Coping Enhancement Family Integrity Promotion Family Support Grief Work Facilitation Grief Work Facilitation: Perinatal Death Resiliency Promotion Role Enhancement Self-Awareness Enhancement

- Notice that most of the outcomes are the same for Grieving and Complicated Grieving.
- How do the interventions differ? Do you understand why? (If not, review the Theoretical Knowledge section of this chapter.)
- Notice that for both diagnoses, many of the defining characteristics include normal grief reactions. But for Grieving, the symptoms occur before the loss. For Complicated Grieving, they continue to occur for a long time after the loss, and/or they are more intense than normal.

Continued

NOC Outcomes and NIC Interventions for Loss and Grieving Diagnoses—cont'd

NURSING DIAGNOSES	SELECTED NOC OUTCOMES	SELECTED NIC INTERVENTIONS
Ineffective Denial *Defining Characteristics:* Does not admit fear of death, makes dismissive comments when speaking of death/loss, minimizes the grief/pain, displaces feelings to body (i.e., somatic and psychosomatic symptoms)	Acceptance: Health Status Anxiety Self-Control Fear Self-Control Health Beliefs: Perceived Threat Symptom Control	Anxiety Reduction Calming Technique Coping Enhancement Counseling Emotional Support Health Education Security Enhancement Self-Awareness Enhancement Self-Modification Assistance Self-Responsibility Facilitation Teaching: Disease Process

■ Does Mr. Manning exhibit any of the defining characteristics for Ineffective Denial?

Hopelessness *Defining Characteristics:* Verbal cues (e.g., "I can't" or "Why go on"), sighing, closing eyes, shrugging, decreased appetite, lack of emotion, increased or decreased sleep, little or no involvement in care, passivity, lack of initiative, seeing no solution or way out	Depression Level Depression Self-Control Hope Mood Equilibrium Psychomotor Energy Quality of Life Will to Live	Counseling Hope Instillation Mood Management Resiliency Promotion Self-Modification Assistance Spiritual Growth Facilitation Values Clarification

■ Does Mr. Manning exhibit any of the defining characteristics for Hopelessness?
■ Which outcome and intervention seem most directly related to Hopelessness?

Powerlessness *Defining Characteristics:* Sees that the situation could be changed but does not think it is within his power to change it; expresses helplessness, anger, frustration over inability to perform previous tasks; does not seek information or participate in care or decisions about care	Depression Self-Control Family Participation in Professional Care Health Beliefs Health Beliefs: Perceived Ability to Perform Perceived Control Perceived Resources Participation in Healthcare Decisions	Cognitive Restructuring Decision-Making Support Family Involvement Promotion Financial Resource Assistance Health Education Mood Management Mutual Goal Setting Self-Esteem Enhancement Self-Responsibility Facilitation Values Clarification

■ Why do you think that Self-Esteem Enhancement is an intervention for Powerlessness but not for Hopelessness?

NOC Outcomes and NIC Interventions for Loss and Grieving Diagnoses—cont'd

NURSING DIAGNOSES	SELECTED NOC OUTCOMES	SELECTED NIC INTERVENTIONS
Caregiver Role Strain *Defining Characteristics:* Fear that loved one may need to be institutionalized; alterations in caregiver's health, ability to give care, or complete caregiving tasks; apprehension about the future	Caregiver Emotional Health Caregiver Lifestyle Disruption Caregiver-Patient Relationship Caregiver Performance: Direct Care Caregiver Performance: Indirect Care Caregiver Physical Health Caregiver Well-Being Parenting Performance Role Performance	Anticipatory Guidance Attachment Promotion Caregiver Support Consultation Coping Enhancement Energy Management Health System Guidance Nutrition Management Respite Care Parenting Promotion Presence Role Enhancement Teaching: Individual

■ Do you know what Respite Care is? If not, look it up on the Internet or in the NIC manual.

Chronic Sorrow *Defining Characteristics:* Periodic, recurrent sadness; feelings of varying intensity that interfere with high-level well being; expresses one or more of the following feelings: anger, being misunderstood, confusion, depression, disappointment, emptiness, fear, frustration, guilt, helplessness, hopelessness, loneliness, low self-esteem, being overwhelmed	Acceptance: Health Status Depression Level Depression Self-Control Grief Resolution Hope Mood Equilibrium Psychosocial Adjustment: Life Change	Coping Enhancement Grief Work Facilitation Grief Work Facilitation: Perinatal Death Hope Instillation Mood Management Spiritual Support
Spiritual Distress *Defining Characteristics:* Nightmares or other sleep disturbances, concern over the meaning of life/death/suffering/existence, gallows humor, questions moral implications of therapeutic regimen, anger at God, desires but unable to participate in usual religious practices	Dignified Life Closure Hope Spiritual Health	Dying Care Emotional Support Hope Instillation Spiritual Growth Facilitation Spiritual Support

Sources: Moorhead, S., Johnson, M., Mass, M., et al. (Eds.). (2008). *Nursing outcomes classification (NOC)* (4th ed.). St. Louis, MO: C.V. Mosby. Used with permission; Bulechek, G., Butcher, H., Dochterman, J. M. (2008). *Nursing interventions classification (NIC)* (5th ed.). St. Louis, MO: C.V. Mosby. Used with permission; Johnson, M., Bulechek, G., Butcher, H., et al. (2006). *Nursing diagnoses, outcomes, and interventions: NANDA, NOC, and NIC linkages* (2nd ed.). St. Louis, MO: C.V. Mosby. Used with permission; NANDA International. (2009). *Nursing diagnoses: Definitions and classification 2009–2011*. Philadelphia: Author. Used with permission.

THINKING CRITICALLY ABOUT LOSS, GRIEF, & DYING

The exercises in the following sections allow you to practice the kind of thinking you will use as a full-spectrum nurse. Because these are critical-thinking questions, there is usually no single right answer. We do not provide answers for these questions because it is more important for you to think about the questions than to arrive at the "right" answer. These questions are designed to improve your thinking more than to "cover content." Discuss answers with your peers—discussion can stimulate critical thinking. If you have difficulty with any of these questions, consult with your instructor.

Applying the Full-Spectrum Nursing Model

PATIENT SITUATION

Marie is 84 years old and has had a right-sided cerebrovascular accident (CVA, or stroke). Doctors say she is unlikely to regain much physical function, if she even awakens from the coma. She was alert and active before her stroke and was able to maintain her independence with the help of a home health aide, who assisted her with ADLs and meal preparation three times a week. Kelly and Dan, her children, have met with the physician, who tells them that Marie's chance of survival is slim. He wants to put a feeding tube into Marie and has asked whether they want Marie to be resuscitated in case of cardiac or respiratory arrest. Kelly wants to do what is best for her mother, but she feels that Marie would not want to be kept alive in the condition she is in. She is also concerned about putting her through uncomfortable procedures if there is no chance of recovery. Her brother, Dan, thinks Marie should have the feeding tube. Kelly asks to speak with you and wants to know the best thing to do for her mother.

THINKING

1. *Theoretical Knowledge (Recall of Facts and Principles)*: If Marie and Dan agree that they do not want Marie to be resuscitated, the physician will complete a DNAR order. What do the letters *DNAR* represent?

2. *Critical Thinking (Problem Solving)*: At this stage of your education, you probably need more information about CVAs and tube feedings. Write a PICO question you could use to search the literature for information about these two topics and how they are related. See Chapter 8 if you need to review PICO questions.

DOING

3. *Practical Knowledge (Nursing Diagnosis)*: Write a possible nursing diagnosis to describe Kelly's situation.

4. *Practical Knowledge (Basic Skills)*: If Marie and Dan agree to tube feedings for Marie, as her nurse, what basic nursing skills will you need to perform? How will you learn to perform these skills, if you do not already know how to do them?

CARING

5. *Ethical Knowledge*: How do you think the situation came to this? What might Kelly, Dan, and Marie have done before the stroke to prevent this confusion and indecision?

6. *Self–Knowledge*: What are your responsibilities in this situation? What could you do to help Kelly and Dan?

Critical Thinking and Clinical Reasoning

1. Jessie McCarthy is a 69-year-old woman who is terminally ill with multiple myeloma. She is currently hospitalized for a week of chemotherapy. Her husband of 49 years is recuperating from recent hip surgery and has difficulty getting around. Her daughter and son-in-law are very close to them, and her granddaughter, 14 years old, has a very special relationship with her "Gammie." The side effects of Mrs. McCarthy's chemotherapy include nausea and headaches. She doesn't like to have people around when she feels this way. Jessie's pastor comes to visit every other day and seems to bring her comfort. Her 50th wedding anniversary will occur when she is in the hospital. She verbalizes fear of "not making it home this time." You are her nurse in a hospital where palliative care is provided. Begin developing a holistic plan of care for Mrs. McCarthy, addressing the main issues noted.

   a. What immediate physical problems does Mrs. McCarthy have? Do not use her medical diagnosis as an answer.

   b. What might you do to meet her physical needs?

   c. What psychological needs does Mrs. McCarthy have: (1) What are her fears? (2) What social and emotional issues is she facing? (3) How might you help meet her needs?

2. You are caring for Jack Wirtz, a 37-year-old man who was admitted to the hospital for a lumbar laminectomy (surgery of his lower spine). As you are doing Jack's preop assessments, he tells you that his 12-year-old son died 6 months ago in an automobile accident in which Jack was the driver. He is a builder and has been out of work since the accident. His wife has gone back to work to help support them. Jack's affect is flat, and he talks in a monotone.

   a. What losses has Jack experienced?

   b. What further assessments need to be made for Jack, and why?

3. A patient requests your participation in a plan for assisted suicide or seeks passive euthanasia. What are your options as a nurse? Use the Internet to get information about this.

   a. List the URLs for the pages you found to be helpful in answering the question. Beside each URL, state the name of the organization, person, or agency to whom the Web site belongs.

   b. For each URL, state what you believe to be the *purpose* of the Web site.

4. Find a partner. Take 5 minutes to describe to her a personal loss you have had (e.g., a person, a pet, an object, an aspect of health). The partner must listen silently and not speak at all during these 5 minutes. When you have finished, answer the following questions:

   a. What did you feel when describing your loss?

   b. Did you feel that the listener was really listening to you?

   c. How did the listener respond to you?

5. Now reverse the process; you become the listener. When you have finished, answer the following questions:

   a. What did you feel while you were listening?

   b. Did the time go quickly or seem long?

   c. What did you learn from this listening experience?

6. John is 17 years old and volunteers at the hospital. He has just moved from another state because of his father's work, so he is a new senior in high school. As you chat with him, he reveals that his mother is getting radiation and chemotherapy treatments for breast cancer and has been very ill. What are some loss issues this young man is facing?

7. Sharon is a 48-year-old woman who is in the hospital for a hysterectomy (removal of her uterus) due to fibroids and heavy bleeding. With teary eyes, she shares with you, her nurse for the evening, that she is feeling "down" and doesn't want any visitors this evening. She says, "I really thought I would feel better after having this surgery done."

a. Why do you think Sharon is teary and feeling "down"?

b. What should you do to begin helping Sharon cope with her loss?

8. You are having lunch with a nursing colleague, who reveals to you that her mother has Alzheimer's disease. Her mother has been placed in a nursing home because she is losing her memory and is not safe at home. Your friend tells you that lately she (the nurse) has been feeling distracted, angry for no reason, and can't seem to shake her feelings of sadness. How would you respond?

a. What might be causing your colleague to feel distracted and angry?

b. How would you respond to her?

9. You are caring for Mr. Bishop, a 57-year-old man who is terminally ill with metastatic bone cancer. He wants to donate his organs for research after his death, but his wife is totally against this.

a. What do you do or say to him to help resolve this issue? Go to the following URL, and download the organ donor brochure for information to use in this situation: http://organdonor.gov/donation/index.htm

b. Now go to the top of the Web page and look at the logo and other information. Who do you think provides and maintains the content for this Web site? What else would give you a clue about the source of the site?

c. Look at the bottom of the Web page. What department of the U.S. government "owns" this page?

10. For each of the following concepts, use critical thinking to describe how or why it is important to nursing, patient care, or loss, grief, and dying. Note that these are *not* to be merely definitions.

Physical loss   Stages of grief
Actual loss   Advanced directives
Complicated grief   Assisted suicide
Disenfranchised grief   Palliative care
Significance of the loss

What Are the Main Points in This Chapter?

➤ How people cope with loss directly affects their healing and well-being.

➤ Loss may be actual or perceived, physical or psychological, external or internal.

➤ Grief is the physical, psychological, and spiritual response to loss.

➤ People do not move neatly from one stage of grief or dying to the next; there is constant movement and overlap between and among them.

➤ The grieving process is affected by the significance and circumstance of the loss, the timeliness of the death, the amount of support for the bereaved, spiritual beliefs, cultural values, the person's developmental stage, and conflicts existing at the time of death.

➤ Patients experience loss of independence, body image, self-esteem, and so on, when they are ill and/or hospitalized. Recognizing these as losses, you can assist the patient with the grieving process, thus promoting physical, emotional, and spiritual healing.

➤ The Uniform Determination of Death Act states that death has occurred when "An individual . . . has sustained either (1) irreversible cessation of circulatory and respiratory functions, or (2) irreversible cessation of all functions of the entire brain, including the brain stem. . . ."

➤ Palliative care means providing comfort care and symptom relief but without further efforts to stop the disease process or prevent death.

➤ Hospice care is a movement and an approach to allow terminally ill persons to face death with dignity and surrounded by the comfort of their home and family.

➤ Healthcare providers are responsible for educating staff and patients about advance directives.

➤ A do not attempt resuscitation (DNAR) order is a specific order to *not* do cardiopulmonary resuscitation.

➤ Nurses should be aware of what is involved with assisted suicide and euthanasia. You should think ahead about what your response might be if a patient wants to discuss these topics. You may find the American Nurses Association (ANA) position statement on assisted suicide and euthanasia helpful.

➤ An autopsy is a medical examination of the body to determine the cause of death.

➤ When a patient is dying or has experienced a loss, you should perform a thorough, holistic assessment.

➤ Most grief is normal, not dysfunctional; you should not diagnose Complicated Grieving for every person who is grieving a loss.

➤ You can facilitate grief work by validating feelings ("It's normal to feel that way") and providing an opportunity and encouragement to talk about the lost person or object.

➤ At the moment of death, do not interrupt or intrude upon the family; give them as much time as they need to say good-bye to their loved one. Express your sympathy.

➤ Active dying usually occurs over a 10- to 14-day period, although it can take as little as 24 hours. During the final 4 to 48 hours, failure of body systems results in death.

➤ When the patient is very near death, focus on relieving physical symptoms and emotional distress. If he can communicate, ask about immediate concerns, such as, "Who do you want in the room right now?"

➤ Care of the body includes making it presentable for the family, carefully placing identification tags, and arranging to have the body sent to the morgue.

➤ The death certificate must be signed by the person who legally pronounced the death (usually a physician).

➤ It is normal for the nurse to feel grief when a patient dies.

For practice questions for this chapter,

 Go to **NCLEX-Style Chapter Quiz,** on the Student Resource Disk or DavisPlus at http://davisplus.fadavis.com/Wilkinson2

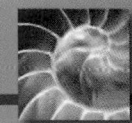

Knowledge Map

Loss, Grief, & Dying

Types of loss
- Actual
- External
- Physical
- Perceived
- Internal
- Psychological

Types of grief
- Complicated
- Uncomplicated
- Disenfranchised
- Anticipatory

- Chronic
- Masked
- Delayed

Factors affecting grief
- Significance of loss
- Support systems
- Existing conflicts
- Circumstances
- Prior losses
- Developmental stage
- Spirituality
- Culture
- Timeliness

Types of loss
- Aspects of self
- Significant relationships
- Environment

Loss

Grief

Theorists
- Engel
- Worden
- Rando
- Bowlby

Legalities
- Organ donation
- Autopsy
- Advanced directives
- Assisted suicide
- Euthanasia

Dying

Self-care for nurses
- Self-knowledge (fears, beliefs)
- Look for support
- Allow own grief

Physiological stages
- Withdrawal
- Systems deterioration
- Cheyne-Stokes breathing
- Mottling
- Organ failure
- Death

Psychological stages (Kübler-Ross)
- Denial
- Anger
- Bargaining
- Depression
- Acceptance

Care
- Mobility
- Oxygenation
- Safety
- Nutrition
- Fluids
- Pain

Palliative care
- Holistic
- Comfort

Hospice care
- "Way" of care
- Dignity
- Quality of life
- Spiritual

Care
- Honesty
- Therapeutic communication
- Spiritual and cultural support

unit **3**

Essential Nursing Interventions

CHAPTER 16

Documenting & Reporting

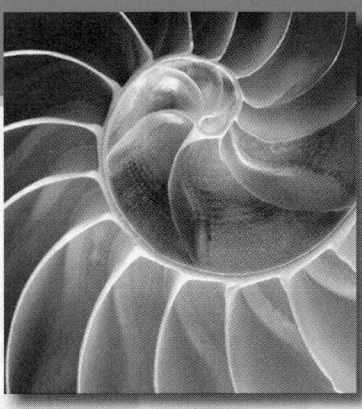

For a podcast of an overview of this chapter,

 Go to Student Resources, **Podcast – Chapter Overviews, Chapter 16,** on DavisPlus at http://davisplus.fadavis.com/Wilkinson2

Caring for the Garcias

The exercises in the following section allow you to practice the kind of thinking you will use as a full-spectrum nurse. Because these are critical-thinking questions, there is usually no single right answer. We do not provide answers for these questions because it is more important for you to think about the questions than to arrive at the "right" answer. These questions are designed to improve your thinking more than to "cover content." Discuss answers with your peers—discussion can stimulate critical thinking. If you have difficulty with any of these questions, consult with your instructor.

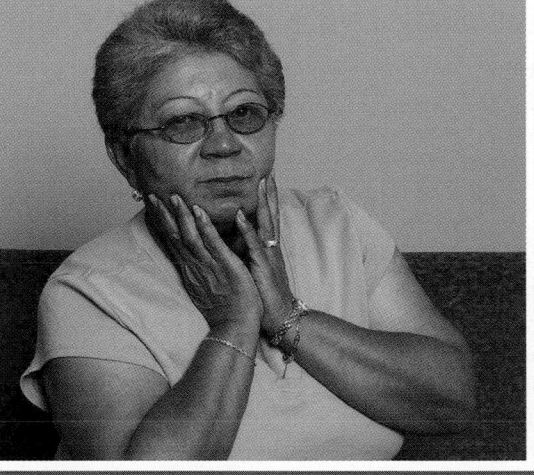

Flordelisa Garcia arrives at the Family Medicine Clinic complaining of pain and drainage from her right eye. She requests an appointment. As part of your clinical experience, you are working as a triage nurse at the clinic. As the triage nurse, you must evaluate the patient's status and determine whether she needs to be seen today. Below is your conversation with Mrs. Garcia.

Mrs. Garcia: I don't have an appointment, but I need to see someone today. My husband is a patient here. I have an appointment in two weeks for a physical, but I've never been here before. I just can't wait two weeks.

You: What seems to be the problem?

Mrs. Garcia: My eye is killing me. My right one. It burns and stings, and there's all this nasty gunk coming out. I think I need some medicine for it.

You: Tell me a little more about this problem. When did this start?

Mrs. Garcia: I woke up yesterday with a painful, itchy eye. I used some saline drops, but the eye seems to be worse. I work at a preschool, and they won't let me work unless I take care of this. I also think I need to be checked for other things. I haven't had an appointment in a long time. I suppose I just need some tests. My husband just

(continued on next page)

Caring for the Garcias (continued)

found out he had high blood pressure, but I don't think I do. I guess I'm not old enough. I'm 50, but my mother got high blood pressure when she was 70.

As she is talking, you notice a large amount of thick, yellow-green drainage in the corner of her right eye and the eye is reddened. She is rubbing this eye vigorously and

dabbing at it with a tissue. The skin is puffy around the eye as well. Her left eye is slightly red, but there is no drainage. Her vital signs are as follows: blood pressure, 132/76 mm Hg; heart rate, 88 beats/min; respirations, 18 breaths/min; and temperature 98.9°F (37.2°C).

Based on your brief assessment, you ask the receptionist to give Mrs. Garcia an urgent appointment.

A. Make two charting entries to describe the above events. First make a brief narrative note.

B. Next, construct a SOAPIER note. Be sure to follow charting guidelines when you prepare your note.

Practical **Knowledge**
knowing how

Clinical Insights

Clinical Insight 16-1 ▶ Giving Oral Reports

1. **For all types of report formats:**
   Remember the acronym CUBAN (Currie, 2002):
   Confidential, **U**ninterrupted, **B**rief, **A**ccurate, **N**amed nurse

2. **Use a Standardized Format.** The following are examples.

   PACE
   Patient/Problem—Include patient's name, room number, diagnosis, reason for admission, and recent procedures. State the present problem. Briefly summarize medical history relevant to the current problem.
   Assessment/Actions—Nursing assessments and interventions directed to the problem.
   Continuing/Changes—Continuing needs and potential changes include:
   ▪ Patient care and treatments that must be monitored on other shifts (e.g., dressing changes)
   ▪ Changes in the patient's condition or the care plan, recent or anticipated (e.g., new orders, changes in discharge date)
   Evaluation—Evaluation of responses to nursing and medical interventions, progress toward goals, and effectiveness of the plan

   SBAR
   Identify yourself, the patient, and the agency.
   Situation—"Here's the situation. . ."
   Background—"The supporting background information is. . ."
   Assessment—"My assessment of the situation is that. . ."
   Recommendation—"I recommend that you. . ."
   For additional information about SBAR, see Clinical Insight 18-3.

3. **Include the following content.**
   In a handoff report:
   ▪ Patient's name, age, and room number
   ▪ Patient's admitting diagnosis—one or several may exist.
   ▪ Patient's relevant past medical history
   ▪ Treatments the patient has received during this admission, such as surgery, line placements, breathing treatments
   ▪ Upcoming diagnostic tests, surgeries, or treatments

   ▪ Patient restrictions, such as diet, bed rest, isolation, activity limits
   ▪ Plan of care, such as IV therapy, pain management, current medications, wound care, and patient or family concerns
   ▪ Significant assessment findings from the previous shifts

   In a transfer report:
   ▪ Your name, facility, and phone number
   ▪ Patient's name, age, gender, and admitting and current diagnoses

- Patient's physician(s), if still following patient
- Procedures or surgeries performed
- Current medications and last date/time each was taken
- Patient status at present as well as progression since admission
- Last set of vital signs, plus any pertinent trends since admission
- Tubes in the patient, such as IVs, catheters, drainage tubes, along with the intake and output of each tube or drain
- Presence of wounds or open areas of the skin plus current interventions for each
- Names and contact numbers for family and significant others
- Special directives, such as code status, preferred intensity of care, or isolation required
- Reason the patient is being transferred

4. When your report is finished:

- Ask the receiving nurse if he has any questions.
- Get the nurse's full name, and then record it plus the transfer date and time in your transfer documentation.

References

Haig, K., Sutton, S., & Whittington, J. (2006). SBAR: A shared mental model for improving communication between clinicians. *Joint Commission Journal of Quality and Patient Safety, 32*(3),167–175.

Kaiser Permanente of Colorado. (unknown). SBAR technique for communication. Institute for Healthcare Improvement. Retrieved August 16, 2008, from http://www.ihi.org/IHI/Topics/PatientSafety/SafetyGeneral/Tools/SBARTechniqueforCommunicationASituationalBriefingModel.htm

Schroeder, S. (2006). Picking up the PACE: A new template for shift report. *Nursing 2006, 36*(10), 22–23.

Clinical Insight 16-2 ▶ Receiving Telephone and Verbal Orders

You should accept verbal and telephone orders only in specific situations when the primary care provider is not able to write or enter the orders personally.

- If possible, have a second nurse listen to the order to verify its accuracy.
- Write or enter the order electronically only if you heard it yourself; no third-party involvement is acceptable.
- Repeat the order even if you believe you have clearly understood it. Spell unfamiliar names to be sure the spelling is correct.
- Pronounce digits of numbers separately. For example, instead of "seventeen," say "one, seven." Mishearing a number can lead to a serious error in medication dosage.
- Make sure the verbal and telephone order makes sense in light of the patient's current status.
- Transcribe the order directly into the chart as quickly as possible. Writing it on a piece of paper, then copying it again onto a paper order sheet introduces an additional chance of error. If entering the order electronically, it's best to have the EHR's order entry area open and begin entering the order as the prescriber is dictating it to you.
- Write the order while the prescriber remains on the telephone or in the building so that you can ask any necessary questions immediately without the need for a return call.
- When writing the order onto a paper order sheet, first document the date and time. Next write the text of the order. Following the text of the order, depending on how

you received the order write "TO" (telephone order) or "VO" (verbal order) followed by the ordering provider's name and then your name. The following is an example of a telephone order:

12/17/11 0815 – Morphine 2 mg IV push ×1 for pain now. ——————————————————
T.O. Dr. Clayton Kent/Sarah Hogan, R.N.

- If entering the order electronically, indicate during order entry that the order was given verbally or over the telephone, the date and time the order was given, and then search for and select the ordering provider's name. Click "sign" or whatever option in your EHR indicates the order is signed and is now active.
- Be sure you have the phone number so that you can reach the provider if future questions arise.
- The physician, physician assistant, or nurse practitioner must countersign all verbal and telephone orders within 24 hours.

References

The Joint Commission (2008a, 2008b). *Hospital Accreditation Program. 2009 chapter. National patient safety goals.* Retrieved July 1, 2008, from http://www.jointcommission.org/NR/rdonlyres/31666E86-E7F4-423E-9BE8-F05BD1CB0AA8/0/09_NPSG_HAP.pdf

The Joint Commission (2008). *2008 hospital accreditation standards*, pp. 116–117. Oakbrook Terrace, IL: The Joint Commission on Accreditation of Healthcare Organizations.

Clinical Insight 16-3 ▶ General Guidelines for Documentation

When to Document

- *After care or assessment.* Chart as soon as possible after you give care or make an observation. Never chart ahead.
- *Beginning of shift.* Begin charting at the beginning of your shift or work time.
- *Chronologically.* On paper, document specific times in chronological order. (Most EHRs automatically insert the current date and time when forms are opened, although those dates and times can be changed if necessary before signing the form.)

- *Avoid "block" charting.* Do not chart in blocks of time, such as "From 1300 to 1500." Each entry between 1300 and 1500 needs to be made individually.
- *Late entries, paper.* Add late entries to the first available line. Record the time and date you are charting, but in the body of the entry clearly designate that this is a late entry.
- *Late entries, EHR.* Open the appropriate form and change the automatically generated current date/time to the date/time your care was actually done; then sign.

What to Document

Your interventions, the patient's responses, and your evaluation of progress toward goals. This is usually done on the Interdisciplinary Plan of Care.

Any significant events or changes in condition. When possible, quote the patient to document his interpretation of the event or change.

Informed consent. If you are asked to obtain informed consent for a procedure, you should document your actions. In most states, your signature (paper or electronic) confirms only that the patient signed the consent. The physician conducting the procedure is legally responsible for discussing the procedure and its risks and benefits. For further discussion on informed consent, see Chapters 44 and 45.

Patient teaching, including medication instruction, instruction about the patient's diagnoses, and discharge teaching. If the patient's physical or cognitive condition prevents teaching, indicate that and explain it in your documentation. Documenting patient teaching can positively affect insurance and other payments to the institution.

Any attempts you have made to contact the primary care provider about the patient's condition or attempts to clarify orders. If you are unable to make contact with the primary care provider, include in your documentation any contact with your charge nurse, nurse manager, supervisor, medical director, and hospital administrator.

Patient leaving the facility against medical advice (AMA). Chart the patient's condition, any explanations of risks and consequences given to the patient, the patient's destination (if known), and your notification of the patient's care providers. Many facilities have specific forms for AMA departures. If possible, use the designated form. If the form is hardcopy paper, have the patient sign the form before leaving.

The patient's refusal of treatment. Quote the exact language the patient used in this situation whenever possible.

Spiritual concerns expressed by the patient and/or family. Document your interventions.

Use of restraints. Most facilities have a separate form that allows you to document the reason for restraint use, the type of restraint, and frequent checks of the patient. The primary care provider must place a signed order for restraints in the chart or in the EHR. Restraint orders must be reordered inside a specific timeframe set by the organization or the restraints are discontinued (see Chapter 21).

"Occurrences" such as falls and medication errors. Chart your findings accurately and objectively, and fill out a separate occurrence form. Do not make reference to the occurrence form anywhere in your charting.

Complete data about medications. When the MAR (medication administration record) is on paper, include the date, time given, medication given, and your initials. If the MAR is electronic, ensure the date, time given, and medication given are accurate, then sign electronically that the administration was accomplished successfully.

PRN, unscheduled, IV infusions, and stat medications may also appear on the paper or electronic MAR. If necessary, include any comments regarding the medication in your narrative charting or insert a comment in your electronic charting. Certain PRN medications require that a follow-up response be documented within a specific period of time after administration. This period of time is set by the organization, usually 15 to 30 minutes after the medication is given.

Any medications that the patient refuses or that are accidentally omitted must be documented on the MAR. If the patient states a reason for refusing the medication, when charting narratively on paper, quote him in your notes. Most electronic MARs include an option to indicate the medication was missed or not given and explain with a selection from a drop-down list such as "Patient refused" or "Patient not available." Some MARs also allow you to explain in a narrative comment why a medication was not given or was missed.

How to Document (General Guidelines)

- **Use accurate, nonjudgmental language.** Avoid labeling patients or members on the care team. Also avoid documenting judgments about decisions made by members of the team.
- **Provide details** about the patient's condition; give examples.
- **Avoid words such as good, average, or normal.** These are vague, subjective terms that do not clearly define the status of the client.
- **Use only the abbreviations authorized by your organization.** See "Abbreviations Commonly Used in Health Care," following Clinical Insight 16-5.
- **Use correct spelling and grammar.** Incorrect spelling may raise questions about what you are attempting to communicate. Incorrect grammar implies carelessness on your part and creates a question of your competence if your chart is reviewed.
- **Date and time all your notes (paper or electronic) accurately.** To avoid confusion between A.M. and P.M., many organizations use a 24-hour clock or military time. The day begins at 0001, which is equivalent to 12:01 A.M., and ends at 2400 (12 midnight). After 12 noon, just add 12 to the P.M. time (e.g., 1:30 P.M. + 12 = 1330 in military time). For an illustration,

 Go to Chapter 16, **Figure 16-5,** in Volume 1.

- **Think about what you say.** Remember that the patient's record is permanent and that the information is confidential.
- **Do not assume that everything you see already documented is correct,** especially if your patient's condition makes the prior documentation illogical or unlikely. Be sure to question this with the appropriate persons, preferably the person who originally made the entry.
- **Chart your own nursing actions.** Never allow anyone to chart for you.
- **Do not document others' actions** as though you had performed them.
- **If you need to document the actions of someone else, be sure to designate that clearly.** For example, if the NAP (nursing assistive personnel) helps the patient ambulate, do not chart "Patient ambulated to bathroom." Instead, chart "J. Scott, NAP, ambulated patient to bathroom." If you are documenting electronically, you can indicate another person performed the action in an added comment, or by searching for and selecting the other care provider in the appropriate field, then signing.
- **Don't chart what someone else said, heard, felt, or smelled** unless the information is critical. If it is, then use quotations and attribute the remarks to the person who made them. For example, "Wife stated, 'My husband told me that he is in a lot of pain, but does not want to bother the nurses.'"

Clinical Insight 16-4 ▶ Guidelines for Documenting in the Paper Health Record

- *Before you begin writing:*
  - Ensure you have the correct form (e.g., I&O sheet, graphic record).
  - Check that the chart and documentation forms are clearly marked with the patient's name and identification number.
- *Write legibly, neatly, in an organized manner.* This enables others to read your entries and use them to make clinical decisions. Sloppy or illegible handwriting creates errors or, at least, leads to poor communication.
- *Keep patient paper records in designated areas to which only healthcare providers have access.*
- *Always use black ink* for handwritten notes (some agencies do permit blue ink). Inks other than black or blue are not legible when a chart is photocopied. DO not use green or red pen. Remember the chart is a legal document.

- *Do not leave blank lines in the narrative notes.* If you need to leave space for clarity, draw a straight line through the area and begin on the next line. Open areas leave an opportunity for later tampering.
- *Draw a line through the incorrect charting and initial it.* Never use a correction fluid, "ink over," or otherwise cover up written notes.
- *Sign all your paper charting entries with your first name, last name, and professional credentials,* such as Judy Long, RN.
- *Don't write in "shorthand" or your own abbreviated symbols.*
- *Use only abbreviations that are approved by your organization.*
- *Recognize good forms.* Paper documentation forms must be efficient, comprehensive, and reasonable, and should prompt nurses to document appropriately.

Clinical Insight 16–5 ▶ Guidelines for Documenting in the Electronic Health Record

To ensure your documentation in the EHR is most efficient and effective, keep the following in mind:

What Skills Do I Need?

- You must have basic computer, mouse, and software skills to document effectively in the EHR. If you are uneasy or more stressed using computers, or unfamiliar with the software it may take you longer to make the transition to documenting in the EHR.
- Help keep patient rooms clutter-free so that you have a place to use a portable computer in the room for direct charting.

What Is Unique About Entering the Data?

- *Before opening charting forms,* ensure that the patient's name, patient identification number, and any other unique health record identifiers are correct.
- *When moving away from the open EHR,* close the screen and temporarily or permanently log off to ensure confidentiality and privacy. Most computer stations will automatically log-off after a specified period of inactivity. This helps keep unauthorized viewers from having access to patient information.
- Some computer screens are equipped with *privacy filters* to protect patient information from the view of non-authorized viewers.
- *If your EHR allows you to save partially completed documentation* before signing it, ensure that you do complete the documentation and sign it as quickly as possible. In most EHR systems, saved documentation is not seen by others until it is signed.
- *Electronic forms and flowsheets are often built in a format similar to a checklist.* This can make it more difficult to capture detailed patient changes and findings.
- *If you make an error* (e.g., if you make entries on the wrong chart or enter and sign the wrong information), *it can be corrected.* The entry can never be completely deleted; however, only the corrected information will be visible to anyone viewing the chart.

What Happens if the Computer Doesn't Work?

- EHR systems can have periodic downtimes due to scheduled maintenance or network or interface problems. Client care does not stop, so you need to know the processes and procedures to follow when the EHR is offline and inaccessible. Follow organization policies regarding the amount of time the EHR needs to be "down" before you begin documenting on paper form.

How Do I Maintain Confidentiality and Data Security?

- *Create a secure password*—not something obvious, such as your birth date, Social Security number, or family members' names. Instead, you might choose a password that is at least six characters long and includes at least one capital letter (if the system is case sensitive), one number, and (if allowed by the system) one symbol. The system you are using will determine the specifications.
- *Change your password at regular intervals* even if your organization does not require it. Some systems will lock you out of the system if your password is not changed as required.
- *Do not share your personal username or password* with anyone. You are responsible for the data recorded and saved using your electronic identity. If someone else enters data or accesses charts under your identity, you will be held responsible for those actions if the patient initiates legal action.
- *Do not leave patient data displayed on the screen where others can see it.*
- *Do not leave the computer unattended after you have logged on.* This allows others access to confidential data, and to document under your name.
- *Do not leave a portable device (e.g., a laptop or PDA) unattended in a public location,* such as on a countertop in the nurses' station. This increases the possibility of theft or unauthorized access to secured patient information.
- *Never access client health records that you have no professional reason to view.* This is a severe breach of client privacy rules. Some states have or are planning harsher penalties for these privacy violations.
- *Become familiar with your organization's policies* regarding network and patient health record information security and confidentiality.

Abbreviations Commonly Used in Healthcare

Abbreviations Commonly Used in Healthcare

ABBREVIATION	MEANING	ABBREVIATION	MEANING
ADL	Activities of daily living	HOH	Hard of hearing
ad lib	As desired, if the patient desires	H&P	History and physical
AKA	Above-knee amputation	hr	Hour
Amb	Ambulation, ambulatory	ht	Height
Amt	Amount	HTN	Hypertension
ASAP	As soon as possible	hyper	Above or high
bid	Twice a day	hypo	Below or low
BM	Bowel movement	ICU	Intensive care unit
BR	Bedrest	I&O	Intake and output
BRP	Bathroom privileges	Isol	Isolation
BSC	Bedside commode	IV	Intravenous
$\bar{c}$	With	IVP	Intravenous push (caution: do not use to mean "IV piggyback")
cal	Calories		
Cath	Catheter	L	Liter
CBC	Complete blood count	lb	Pound
CCU	Critical care unit or coronary care unit	LPN	Licensed practical nurse
c/o	Complaint of	LMP	Last menstrual period
CO_2	Carbon dioxide	LVN	Licensed vocational nurse
CPR	Cardiopulmonary resuscitation	mcg	Microgram
CVA	Cerebrovascular accident (stroke)	MD	Medical doctor
D&C	Dilatation and curretage	med	Medication
DM	Diabetes mellitus	mg	Milligram
dsg or drsg	Dressing	mL	Milliliter
DX or Dx	Diagnosis	MN	Midnight
EBL	Estimated blood loss	NAS	No added salt
EKG/ECG	Electrocardiogram	N/V/D	Nausea, vomiting, diarrhea
ED/ER	Emergency department, emergency room	NKA or NKDA	No known allergies or no known drug allergies
EEG	Electroencephalogram		
EENT	Eyes, ears, nose, throat	NG	Nasogastric
ETOH	Alcohol	NGT	Nasogastric tube
F	Female	noc	At night
FBS	Fasting blood sugar	NPO	Nothing by mouth
Ft	Foot	O_2	Oxygen
Fx	Fracture	OB	Obstetrics
GI	Gastrointestinal	OOB	Out of bed
gtt(s)	Drop(s)	OPD	Outpatient department
GU	Genitourinary	ortho	Orthopedics
GYN	Gynecology	OR	Operating room
HA	Headache	os	Mouth, opening
HMO	Health maintenance organization	OT	Occupational therapy
h/o	History of	oz	Ounce
hob or HOB	Head of bed	pc	After meals

Continued

Abbreviations Commonly Used in Healthcare—cont'd

ABBREVIATION	MEANING
PCA	Patient-controlled analgesia
PO	By mouth
P, p̄	After
PPBS	Postprandial blood sugar
prn	As needed
Pt	Patient
PT	Physical therapy
q	Every
qam	Every morning
qh	Every hour
qid	Four times a day
RN	Registered nurse
R/O	Rule out
RX or Rx	Treatment or prescription
s̄	Without
SCD	Sequential compression device

ABBREVIATION	MEANING
SOB	Short of breath
s̄s̄	One-half
SSE	Soapsuds enema
Stat	Immediately
STI or STD	Sexually transmitted infection or sexually transmitted disease
TB	Tuberculosis
TO	Telephone order
TPR	Temperature, pulse, respirations
tid	Three times a day
VO	Verbal order
VS	Vital signs
WBC	White blood count
w/c	Wheelchair
WNL	Within normal limits
wt	Weight

Caveat: Abbreviations vary among healthcare agencies. Futhermore, they change rather often because of regulating agency guidelines (e.g., The Joint Commission). Therefore, you will need to be familiar with the abbreviations in the agency in which you work.

Charting Forms

Adult admission history electronic screen.

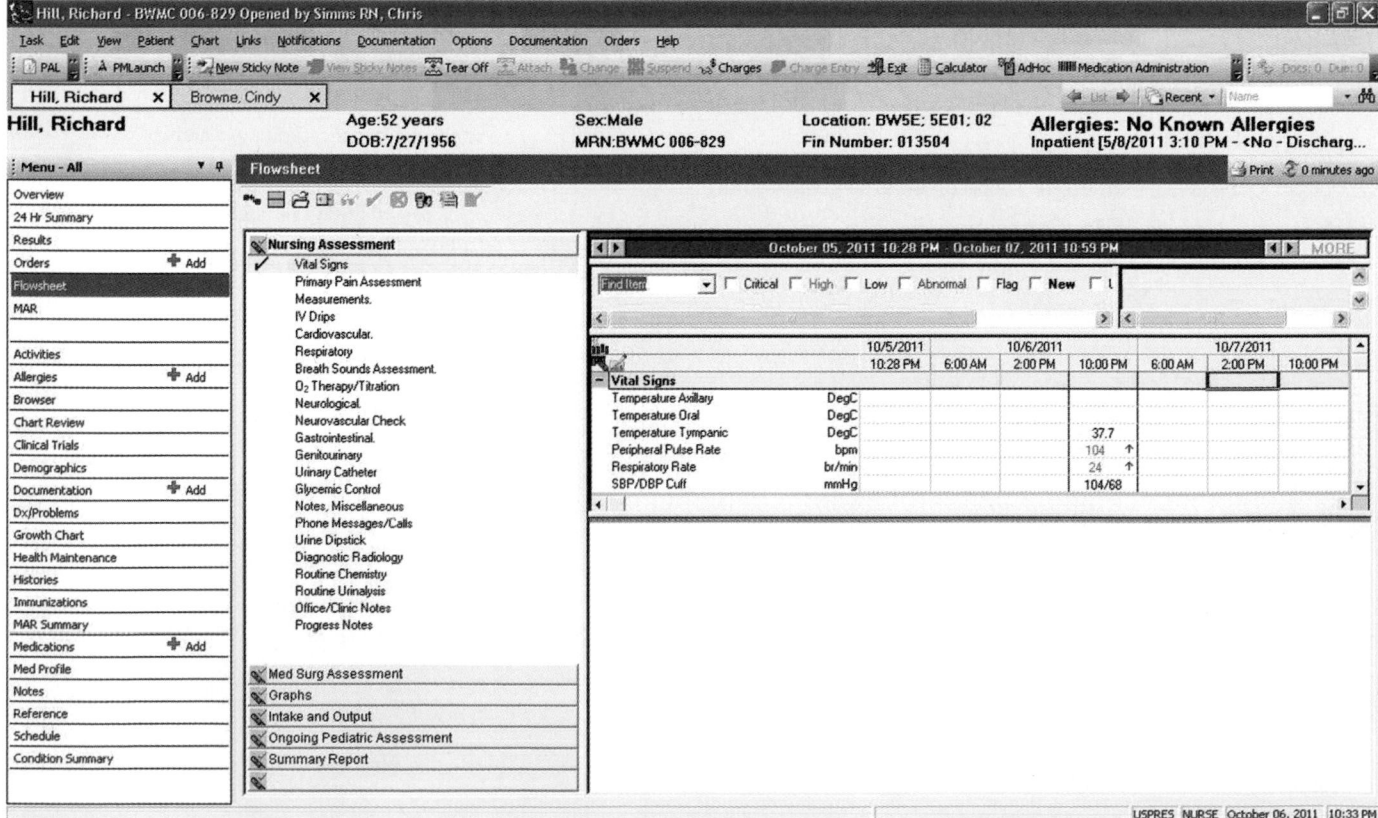

(Courtesy of Cerner Corporation.)

Nurses use intake and output (I&O) records to record data about the patient's fluid status.

INTAKE AND OUTPUT SHEET

DATE	Time	INTAKE						OUTPUT						SIGNATURE OF NURSE
		ORAL	IV	IV MED	BLOOD PRODUCT	OTHER	TOTAL	URINE	EMESIS	STOOL	SUCTION	OTHER	TOTAL	
	6 A.M.-2 P.M.													
	2 P.M.-10 P.M.													
	10 P.M.-6 A.M.													
	TOTAL													
	6 A.M.-2 P.M.													
	2 P.M.-10 P.M.													
	10 P.M.-6 A.M.													
	TOTAL													
	6 A.M.-2 P.M.													
	2 P.M.-10 P.M.													
	10 P.M.-6 A.M.													
	TOTAL													
	6 A.M.-2 P.M.													
	2 P.M.-10 P.M.													
	10 P.M.-6 A.M.													
	TOTAL													
	6 A.M.-2 P.M.													
	2 P.M.-10 P.M.													
	10 P.M.-6 A.M.													
	TOTAL													

A flowsheet used in long-term care.

C.N.A. SIGNATURE	INITIALS

PHYSICAL MOBJ.TRANSF.		SAFETY DEVICE/RESTRAINT	
AMB.	Ambulatory	N	NON-RELEASE
AA	Amb. With Assist	S	SELF-RELEASE BELT
W/C	Wheelchair bound	M	MITTEN
B	Bedfast	W	WRIST
I	Ind. Transfers	GC	GERI-CHAIR/TABLE
A	1 person A with trans	R	RECLINER
D	Dependent transf.	A	ALARM
H	Hoyer Lift transf.	N/A	NONE

MONTH:　　　　**YEAR:**

NIGHT SHIFT	16	17	18	19	20	21	22	23	24	25	26	27	28	29	30	31
Mental Status (Oriented or Confused)																
Quality of Sleep (Slept well or Restless)																
Turn/Reposition(Ind,Assist or Total)																
Safety Device/Restraint (see legend)																
Siderails (Up or Down)																
Behavior(Resists care,Combative or N/A)																
Bladder Function (Inc.,Cont. or Foley)																
Bowel Function (Inc or Continent)																
Bowel Movement (Lrg or Med or Small)																
Certified Nurse Assitant Initials																

DAY SHIFT																
Mental Status (Oriented or Confused)																
Breakfast (percentage eaten)	%	%	%	%	%	%	%	%	%	%	%	%	%	%	%	%
Amt. of assist. (Ind. or Assist or Fed)																
Lunch (percentage eaten)	%	%	%	%	%	%	%	%	%	%	%	%	%	%	%	%
Amt. of assist. (Ind. or Assist or Fed)																
10am Nourishment (% ,Refused or N/A)																
Bathing (Shower, Bedbath or Tub bath)																
Personal Hygiene (Ind., Assist or Total)																
Dressing (Ind or Assist or Total)																
Physical Mobility (see legend)																
Transfer Ability (see legend)																
Toileting (Ind., Assist or Total)																
Safety Device/Restraint (see legend)																
Siderails (Up or Down)																
Turn/Reposition(Ind,Assist or Total)																
Behavior(Resists care,Combative or N/A)																
Bladder Function (Inc. or Cont. or Foley)																
Bowel Function (Inc or Continent)																
Bowel Movement (Lrg or Med or Small)																
Certified Nurse Assistant Initials																

P.M. SHIFT																
Mental Status (Oriented or Confused)																
Dinner (percentage eaten)	%	%	%	%	%	%	%	%	%	%	%	%	%	%	%	%
Amt. of assist. (Ind. or Assist or Fed)																
2pm Nourishment (% or Refused or N/A)																
HS Nourishment (% or Refused or N/A)																
Bathing(Shower or Bedbath or Tub bath)																
Physical Mobility (see legend)																
Transfer Ability (see legend)																
Safety Device/Restraint (see legend)																
Siderails (Up or Down)																
Turn/Reposition(Ind,Assist or Total)																
Behavior(Resists care,Combative or N/A)																
Bladder Function (Inc., Cont. or Foley)																
Bowel Function (Inc or Continent)																
Bowel Movement (Lrg or Med or Small)																
Certified Nurse Assistant Initials																

RT. NAME:	MEDICAL REC. #	RM#	PHYSICIAN

Nursing assessment flowsheets are comprehensive charting documents.

DATE / /										

VS
TIME		
BP		
P R		
TEMPERATURE		

ASSESSMENTS / INTERVENTIONS
ACTIVITY
PAIN LEVEL:
INTERVENTION
RESPONSE
DR. VISIT

LAB

INTAKE
DIET / APPETITE
PO
IV
IV TUBE / SITE CONDITION

OUTPUT
URINE
BM

SAFETY
PERSONAL CARES

RESPIRATORY
☐ HEATED ☐ COOL MIST ☐ CROUP TENT   F102 ✔ LIST
O2   LPM ADJ
O2 SAT   RA O2
INC SPIRO

INITIAL

TIME_____		BREATH			TIME_____		BREATH			TIME_____		BREATH
		LU LL SOUNDS RU RL					LU LL SOUNDS RU RL					LU LL SOUNDS R
PULSE		☐ ☐ CLEAR ☐ ☐			PULSE		☐ ☐ CLEAR ☐ ☐			PULSE		☐ ☐ CLEAR
Before	After	☐ ☐ CRACKLES ☐ ☐			Before	After	☐ ☐ CRACKLES ☐ ☐			Before	After	☐ ☐ CRACKLES
		☐ ☐ RHONCHI ☐ ☐					☐ ☐ RHONCHI ☐ ☐					☐ ☐ RHONCHI
		☐ ☐ WHEEZING ☐ ☐					☐ ☐ WHEEZING ☐ ☐					☐ ☐ WHEEZING
		☐ ☐ DIMINISHED ☐ ☐					☐ ☐ DIMINISHED ☐ ☐					☐ ☐ DIMINISHED
		☐ ☐ ABSENT ☐ ☐					☐ ☐ ABSENT ☐ ☐					☐ ☐ ABSENT

After Treatment Eval | After Treatment Eval | After Treatment Eval
☐ NO CHANGE ☐ IMPROVED ☐ ADVERSE | ☐ NO CHANGE ☐ IMPROVED ☐ ADVERSE | ☐ NO CHANGE ☐ IMPROVED ☐ ADVEF

DRUG		DRUG		DRUG	
☐ P&PD	INITIAL	☐ P&PD	INITIAL	☐ P&PD	INITIAL

PATIENT CARE FLOW SHEET

PUPIL SIZE

1 mm 2 mm 3 mm 4 mm 5 mm 6 mm 7 mm 8 mm

GLASGOW COMA SCALE

Child		Adult	
Eye Opening		**Eye Opening**	
Spontaneous	4	Spontaneous	4
To sounds	3	To speech	3
To painful stimulation	2	To pain	2
None	1	Nil	1
Motor Responses		**Motor Responses**	
Spontaneous Movement	6	Obeys commands	6
Localizes to pain	5	Localizes pain	5
Withdraws	4	Withdrawal	4
Reflex flexion	3	Abnormal flexion	3
Reflex extension (decerebrate)	2	Extensor rigidity	2
None (flaccid)	1	Nil	1
Verbal Responses		**Verbal Responses**	
Appropriate words or social smile; fixes and follows	5	Oriented	5
Cries, but consolable	4	Confused	4
Persistently irritable	3	Inappropriate	3
Restless, agitated	2	Incomprehensible	2
None	1	Nil	1

NEUROVASCULAR RATING SCALE

EXTREMITY: RA, LA, RL, LL CAP REFILL: NOR = <3 SEC * = >3 SEC
COLOR: NOR = NORMAL DU = DUSTY RED = RED PALE = PALE
SENSATION: NOR = INTACT NUMB = NUMBNESS TIN = TINGLING Ø = ABSENT
MOTION: FULL = FULL LTD = LIMITED Ø = NONE PAIN: RATE (0-10)
PULSES: NOR = NORMAL ↓ = DIMINISHED Ø = NOT PALPABLE DOP = DOPPLER

STRENGTH (DESIGNATE EXTREMITY)

5 = NORMAL STRENGTH   2 = LIFTS, FALLS BACK
4 = LIFTS AGAINST RESISTANCE   1 = MUSCLE CONTRACTION, NO MOVEMENT
3 = LIFTS AGAINST GRAVITY   0 = NO MUSCLE CONTRACTION, NO MOVEMENT

ADJUCANTS FOR 02 ADMINISTRATION

NC Nasal Cannula M Mask NRB Non Rebreather
TT Trans Trach ET Endotrachial Tube

Activity	Personal Cares/Safety	Diet
AMB - Ambulating	AM - AM Care	R - Regular
ARMS - Being held	PA - PM/HS Care	S - Soft
BR - Bed rest	CLWR - Call Light Within	NA - Low Sodium
CH - Chair	Reach	LF - Low Fat
L - Lavatory	OR - Oral Care	MS - Mechanical Soft
ROM - Range of motion	SH - Shower	ADA - Diabetic Diet
SLP - Sleeping	SP - Sponge	CL - Clear Liquids
T/P - Turned/Positioned	SK - Skin Care	FL - Full Liquids
↑c̄ - Up with assist	SR↑ - Side rails up	ICE - Ice Chips
↑s̄ - Up without assist	SR↓ - Side rails down	ø - Refused
DA - Dangle	L△ - Linen changed	
CO - Commode	PE - Peri care	
IV Site/Condition	FO - Foley care	**Wound Interventions**
✔ - No redness, swelling,	SN - Snack	DDI - Dressing dry, intact
leakage	BA - Backrub	DRNG - Drainage
DC - Discontinued		D△ - Dressing change
INF - Infiltrated	**Lab Values**	SSG - Serosanguinous
SWL - Swelling	✔ - Physician notified	SWL - Swelling
D△ - Dressing change		O - Odor
T△ - Tubing change		

PAIN ASSESSMENT IN ADULTS

0 NO PAIN 1 2 3 4 5 6 7 8 9 10 WORST PAIN

INIT.	SIGNATURE / TITLE	INIT.	SIGNATURE / TITLE

PATIENT NAME

(Courtesy of Teton Valley Hospital, Driggs, ID.)

THINKING CRITICALLY ABOUT DOCUMENTING AND REPORTING

The exercises in the following sections allow you to practice the kind of thinking you will use as a full-spectrum nurse. Because these are critical-thinking questions, there is usually no single right answer. We do not provide answers for these questions because it is more important for you to think about the questions than to arrive at the "right" answer. These questions are designed to improve your thinking more than to "cover content." Discuss answers with your peers—discussion can stimulate critical thinking. If you have difficulty with any of these questions, consult with your instructor.

Applying the Full-Spectrum Nursing Model

PATIENT SITUATION

Ellen is 85 years old and has sustained a right-sided cerebrovascular accident (CVA, or stroke). Doctors say she is unlikely to regain much physical function, if she even awakens from the coma. Her children, Mary and Dale, have met with the physician, who tells them that Ellen is not likely to survive. The physician wants to insert a feeding tube and has asked whether they want Ellen to be resuscitated in case of cardiac or respiratory arrest. Mary tells you she wants to do what is best for her mother, but she feels that Ellen would not want to be kept alive in the condition she is in. She is also concerned about putting her through uncomfortable procedures if there is no chance of recovery. Her brother, Dale, says, "Mom needs the feeding tube. I can't sit and watch her starve to death. As long as she's alive, there's hope."

THINKING

1. *Theoretical Knowledge (Recall of Facts and Principles)*: You plan to use the Focus Charting® format to document this interaction.

   a. Write the focus for this note.

   b. What does the acronym D-A-R stand for?

2. *Critical Thinking (Contextual Awareness)*:

   a. What aspects of this situation have you experienced or observed before in your role as a caregiver?

   b. How might those past experiences affect your perception in this situation?

DOING

3. *Practical Knowledge (Handoff Report)*: Ellen's last name is Smith; assume her children are also named Smith. Ellen is in room 820. Using the PACE format, what would you say to the oncoming nurse during handoff report? You will be able to address only a small amount of physiological information because the scenario does not provide it.

CARING

4. *Self-Knowledge*: In what way(s) can you identify with any of the people involved?

Critical Thinking and Clinical Reasoning

1. You are caring for a 96-year-old patient, James Wilson. Mr. Wilson has been admitted to the hospital for pneumonia. He is normally alert and oriented to place, time, and person. However, during this admission he has become confused and agitated. He frequently yells at staff and resists care by kicking and hitting. While you are providing morning care, Mr. Wilson becomes very agitated and yells and curses at you. When you attempt to provide oral hygiene, he throws his dentures at you. The dentures break when they hit the floor.

   a. Construct a nurse's note about this situation using the paper charting format you prefer.

   b. You will need to complete an occurrence report regarding the broken dentures. The report asks you to identify actions that you might have taken to prevent this incident. Brainstorm this question with your peers. Identify one or two actions that might have prevented this incident.

2. The physician has written an order on your patient's paper chart that you find illegible. A veteran nurse states that she can read it, and she translates it for you. What factors should you consider before determining how to proceed?

3. For each of the following concepts, use critical thinking to describe how or why it is important to nursing, patient care, or documenting and reporting. Consider both paper and electronic documentation in each. Note that these are *not* to be merely definitions.

Narrative charting

SOAP(IER) charting

Nursing admission form

Medication administration record

Occurrence report

Flowsheets

Charting by exception

Signing documentation forms

Handoff report

Late entry

What Are the Main Points in This Chapter?

➤ The client record is a collection of documents that form a legal record of the client's healthcare experience.

➤ The client record is used by health professionals to communicate about the client's care, to legally document the care delivered to the client and the client's responses to that delivered care, to document care for reimbursement, to educate students, to determine whether care is adequate, as a data source for health research, and as the basis for determining the cost of care.

➤ In source-oriented records, members of each discipline record findings in a separately labeled section.

➤ In problem-oriented records, members of each discipline chart on shared notes, and the record is organized around a problem list.

➤ In electronic health records (EHRs), members of each discipline all chart inside the same EHR. The EHR can be organized as source-oriented, problem-oriented, or a combination of the two.

➤ The EHR can be accessed by many members of the healthcare team at the same time.

➤ In narrative charting, the writer tells the story of what has occurred in a chronological format.

➤ SOAP(IER) is an acronym for Subjective data, Objective data, Assessment, Plan (and Intervention,

Evaluation, and Revision). This format may be used to address a single problem or to document summative notes on a patient.

➤ In Focus Charting®, data is entered in a Data/Action/ Response (DAR) format.

➤ Charting by Exception (CBE) utilizes pre-printed or electronic flowsheets to document most aspects of care. CBE assumes that unless a separate entry is made—an exception—all standards have been met and the patient has responded as expected.

➤ Paper and electronic flowsheets and graphic records are used to record recurring assessments, such as vital signs, intake and output, weight, hygiene, and ADLs.

➤ Paper progress notes are used to document the patient's responses to care. They may be in the form of narrative, SOAP(IER), PIE, or Focus-style notes.

➤ A discharge summary should be completed when the patient is discharged from the organization. A transfer form should be completed when the patient is transferred within the organization.

➤ An occurrence report, or incident report, is a formal record of an unusual occurrence or accident that is not part of the patient's chart.

➤ The most commonly used paper and electronic home health documentation form is OASIS, a federally required form that includes history, assessment, demographics, and information about the client's and caregiver's abilities.

➤ Federal law requires that a resident in long-term care must be evaluated using the Minimum Data Set for Resident Assessment and Care Screening (MDS) within 4 days of admission. The MDS must be updated every 3 months and with any significant change in client condition.

➤ The handoff report is designed to alert the next nurse about the client's status, changes in the client condition, planned activities, tests or procedures, or concerns that require follow-up.

➤ Nurses should not take verbal and telephone orders unless the ordering physician, physician assistant, or nurse practitioner is in a situation where the order can't be written or entered or the patient is in a life-threatening situation.

➤ Telephone orders offer more room for error because of unfamiliar terminology and differences in background noise.

➤ Charting should be accurate and nonjudgmental.

➤ You should document as soon as possible after you make an observation or provide care.

➤ You should never share your electronic username or password with someone else.

➤ Document any significant events or changes in condition, teaching performed, the use of restraints, and patient refusal of treatment or medications.

➤ You are responsible for documenting the care you provided. Never chart the actions of others as though you had performed them.

➤ If you believe a provider's order is inappropriate or unsafe, you are legally and ethically required to question the order.

For practice questions for this chapter,

Go to **NCLEX-Style Chapter Quiz,** on the Student Resource Disk or DavisPlus at http://davisplus.fadavis.com/Wilkinson2

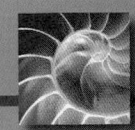

Knowledge Map

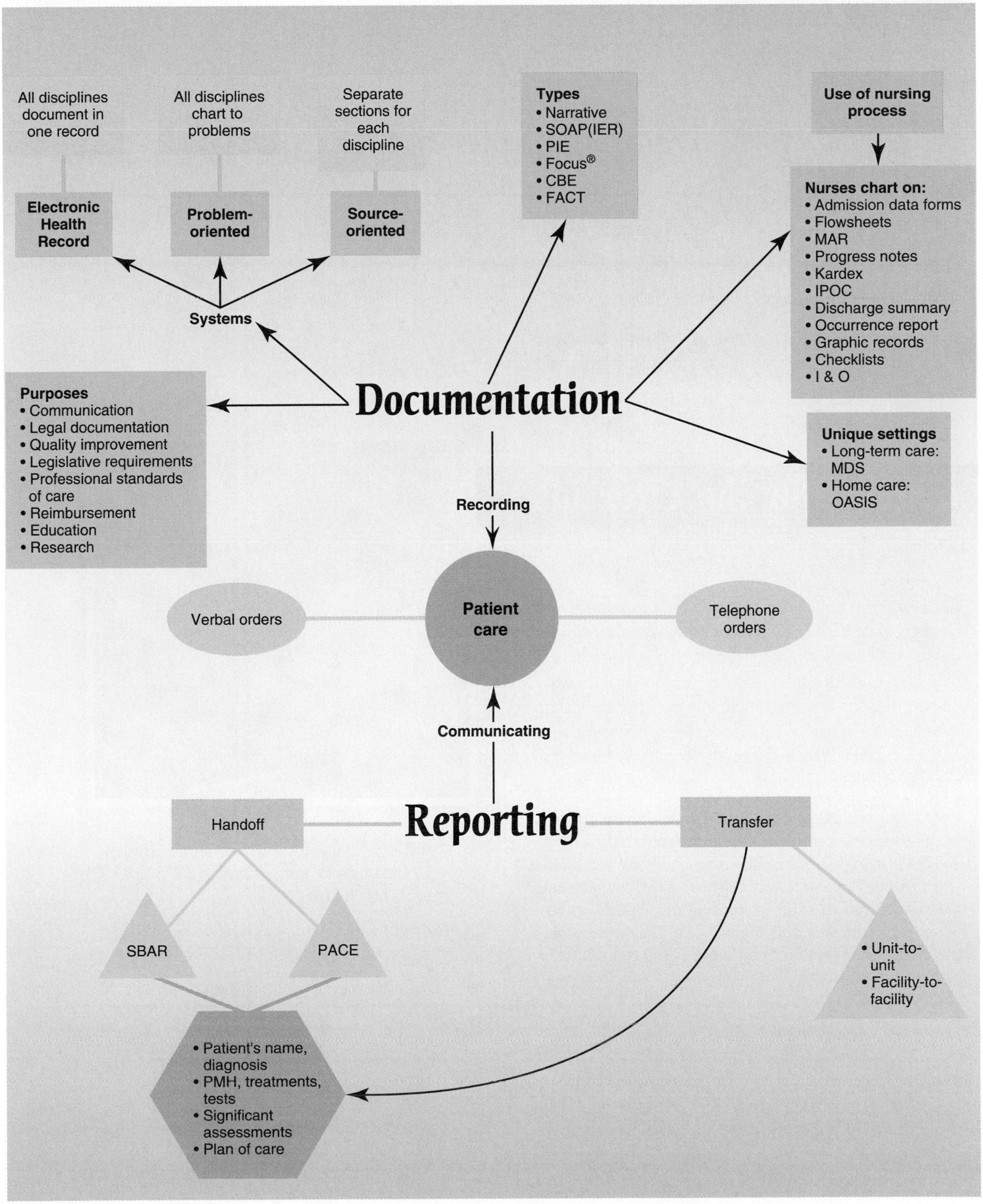

All disciplines document in one record

All disciplines chart to problems

Separate sections for each discipline

Types
• Narrative
• SOAP(IER)
• PIE
• Focus®
• CBE
• FACT

Use of nursing process

Electronic Health Record

Problem-oriented

Source-oriented

Nurses chart on:
• Admission data forms
• Flowsheets
• MAR
• Progress notes
• Kardex
• IPOC
• Discharge summary
• Occurrence report
• Graphic records
• Checklists
• I & O

Systems

Documentation

Purposes
• Communication
• Legal documentation
• Quality improvement
• Legislative requirements
• Professional standards of care
• Reimbursement
• Education
• Research

Unique settings
• Long-term care: MDS
• Home care: OASIS

Recording

Verbal orders

Patient care

Telephone orders

Communicating

Reporting

Handoff

Transfer

SBAR

PACE

• Unit-to-unit
• Facility-to-facility

• Patient's name, diagnosis
• PMH, treatments, tests
• Significant assessments
• Plan of care

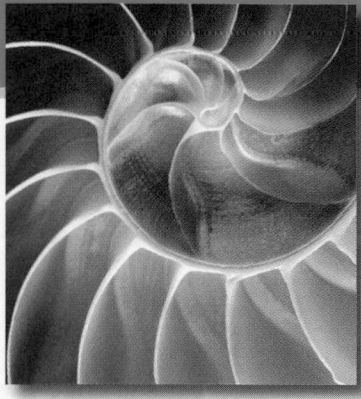

CHAPTER 17

Measuring Vital Signs

For a podcast of an overview of this chapter,

 Go to Student Resources, **Podcast – Chapter Overviews, Chapter 17,** on DavisPlus at http://davisplus.fadavis.com/ Wilkinson2

Caring for the Garcias

The exercises in the following section allow you to practice the kind of thinking you will use as a full-spectrum nurse. Because these are critical-thinking questions, there is usually no single right answer. We do not provide answers for these questions because it is more important for you to think about the questions than to arrive at the "right" answer. These questions are designed to improve your thinking more than to "cover content." Discuss answers with your peers— discussion can stimulate critical thinking. If you have difficulty with any of these questions, consult with your instructor.

Recall that on Joseph Garcia's preliminary visit to the family medicine center, his blood pressure (BP) was 162/94 mm Hg. On subsequent visits, his BP was 168/100 and 174/98. Mr. Garcia was diagnosed with hypertension and prescribed an antihypertension medication, to be taken each morning. This morning Mr. Garcia presents at the clinic for follow-up. The following information is gathered as he checks in for his visit.

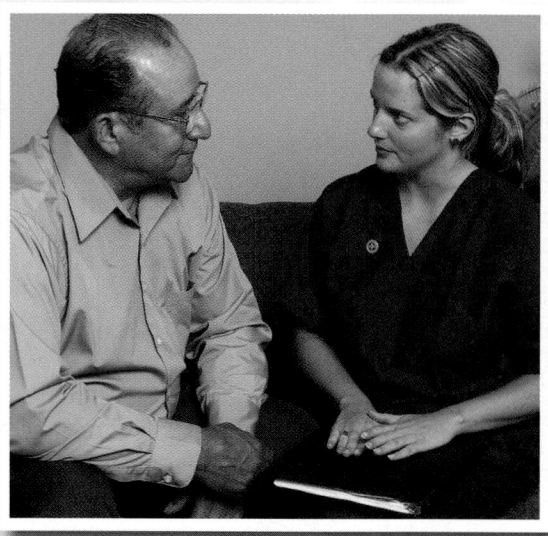

VS: BP, 168/92; pulse, 80 beats/min; respirations, 20 breaths/min; temperature, 98.4°F (36.9°C)
Weight: 231 lb (105 kg)

Review the preliminary data and the preceding information to answer the following questions:

A. What patterns do you see in the data?

B. Do you have enough information to draw any conclusions? If not, what other information should you gather?

C. Identify three alternatives that may explain what is happening with Mr. Garcia's vital signs.

D. How could you determine which of these alternatives provides the best explanation of what is happening?

E. Why is it important to intervene in this situation?

Practical **Knowledge**
knowing how

Use the Procedures, Clinical Insights, and tables in this section when assessing your patients' vital signs.

Procedures

Procedure 17-1 ☐ Assessing Body Temperature

➤ For steps to follow in *all* procedures, refer to the Universal Steps for All Procedures found on the inside back cover of Volume 2.

Critical Aspects

- Clean before and after using, if the thermometer is not disposable.
- Select the appropriate site and thermometer type.
- Turn on, or otherwise ready the thermometer.
- Insert the thermometer in its sheath, or use a thermometer designated only for the patient.
- Insert and leave an electronic thermometer in place until it beeps; for other thermometers use the recommended times.
- Cleanse and store in recharging base (store glass thermometers safely to prevent breakage).
- For an oral temperature, obtain a reading 20 to 30 minutes after the patient consumes hot or cold food or fluids or smokes.
- Hold a rectal thermometer securely in place, and never leave it unattended.

Equipment

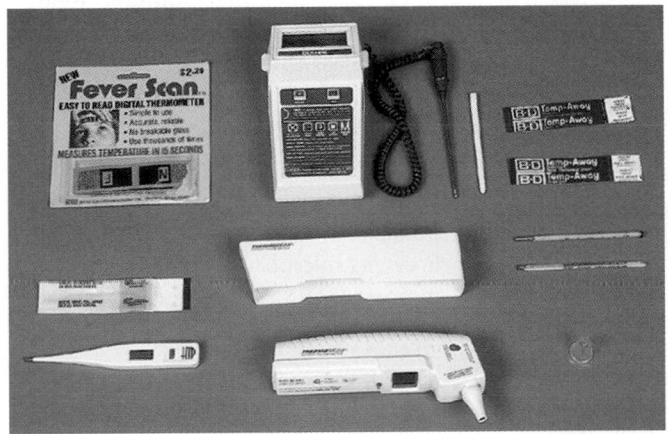

- Thermometer
  An oral thermometer generally has a blue tip.
  A rectal thermometer generally has a red tip.

➕ Glass-and-mercury thermometers should not be used in any healthcare setting, but because many people still use them at home, we include them in this procedure. They should be used with disposable covers, and cleaned and sterilized regularly according to the manufacturer's instructions.

- Thermometer cover, if needed
- Procedure gloves, if taking a rectal temperature or if there is risk of contact with body fluids (e.g., saliva)
- Water-soluble lubricant, if taking a rectal temperature

- Towel, if needed, for taking an axillary temperature (*to dry the axillae*)
- Tissues

Delegation

You can delegate temperature measurement to nursing assistive personnel (NAP) if you conclude that the patient's condition and the NAP's skills allow. Perform the assessments that follow, and inform the NAP of the route and type of thermometer used. Explain any special considerations; for example, tell the NAP to be sure the patient has not had anything to eat or drink in the last 20 to 30 minutes; or inform the NAP if the patient is confused. Ask the NAP to record and report the temperature to you, and to report immediately if the temperature is elevated (e.g., greater than 100°F [37.8°C]).

Pre-Procedure Assessments

- Determine the site that is most appropriate for the patient. Consider patient comfort, safety, and accuracy.
  For example, do not use the oral route for patients who are unable to hold the thermometer properly, for children or others who cannot follow instructions (e.g., unconscious patients), or for patients who use "mouth breathing."

- For an oral temperature: Determine how long it has been since the patient smoked, had anything to eat or drink, or chewed gum.
  Smoking, eating, drinking, and chewing gum can all affect an oral reading. If any of these have occurred, wait 20 to 30 minutes before taking an oral temperature.

(continued on next page)

Procedure 17-1 ■ Assessing Body Temperature (continued)

■ Assess for any contraindications to using the site you have chosen. For example:

Tympanic: Assess for impacted earwax or hearing aid.

Rectal: Check the client record for diarrhea or impacted stool.

Axillary: Check the client record for presence of fever or hypothermia.

Skin: Assess for the presence of conditions that require a very precise, reliable reading (e.g., fever, hypothermia).

Some conditions increase the risk for patient injury; others contribute to inaccurate, unreliable temperature measurement.

■ **What were the previous recordings, if any?**
Noting changes over time is important in all patient assessments.

■ Assess for clinical signs and symptoms of temperature alterations.

■ Procedure 17-1A Taking an Axillary Temperature

➤ When performing the procedure, always identify your patient according to agency policy and be attentive to standard precautions, hand hygiene, patient safety and privacy, body mechanics, and documentation.

Procedure Steps

1. Slide the thermometer into a protective sheath (depending on type of thermometer).
A protective sheath provides a barrier to prevent transmission of organisms.

2. Dry the patient's axilla, as needed.
Moisture from perspiration alters the temperature reading.

3. Position the patient and the thermometer.
   a. Assist the patient to a supine or sitting position.
   b. Place the thermometer tip in the middle of the axilla.
   c. Position the patient's upper arm down, with the lower arm across the chest.
Puts the thermometer in close proximity to the axillary blood vessels,

allowing it to better reflect the core temperature. ▼

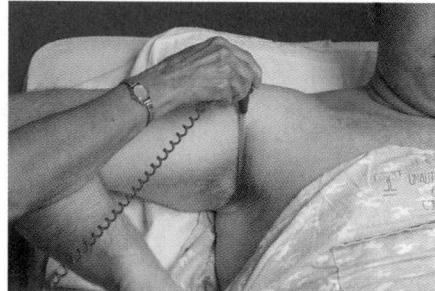

4. Hold the thermometer in place for the recommended time.
   a. Leave an electronic probe in place until it beeps.
   b. Leave a glass thermometer in place for 8 minutes, or according to agency policy (usually 5 minutes for children).

Study findings differ for accuracy of temperature measurements at the axillary site. Follow agency policy.

5. Remove the thermometer.
   a. Discard the thermometer cover.
   b. If there is no cover, wipe the thermometer with a tissue.
Removes any moisture that may have accumulated in 8 minutes' time.

6. Read the temperature.
   a. Electronic thermometer: Read the digital display.
   b. Glass thermometer: Hold at eye level, and rotate it until the markings are clear.

7. Clean and replace the thermometer in the storage base, following agency policy.
Prevents microbial growth on thermometers and recharges the battery.

■ Procedure 17-1B Taking an Oral Temperature

➤ When performing the procedure, always identify your patient according to agency policy and be attentive to standard precautions, hand hygiene, patient safety and privacy, body mechanics, and documentation.

Procedure Steps

1. For a glass thermometer, shake down the liquid if necessary.
   a. Stand in an open area away from tables and other objects.
Prevents thermometer breakage.
   b. Hold the end opposite the bulb between your thumb and

forefinger, and snap your wrist downward.
   c. Shake the thermometer until the reading is less than 96°F (36°C).
The reading must be lower than the anticipated temperature measurement.

2. Slide the thermometer into a protective sheath.

The protective sheath provides a barrier to prevent transmission of microorganisms.

3. Place the thermometer tip under the tongue in the posterior sublingual pocket (right or left of frenulum).
Puts the tip in close proximity to the major blood vessels under the tongue,

allowing the thermometer to reflect the core temperature. ▼

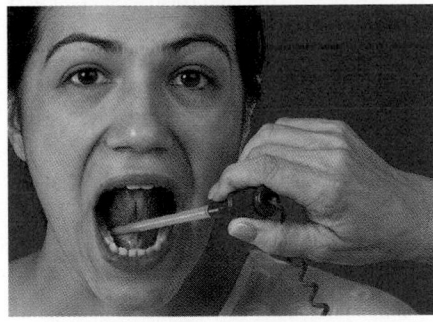

4. Have the patient close his lips around the thermometer, cautioning him not to bite down on it.
Protects the thermometer from exposure to the air, which could alter the reading. Biting may break a glass thermometer, injuring the mouth.

5. Leave the thermometer in place for the recommended time.
  a. Glass thermometer: 5 to 8 minutes
  b. Electronic thermometer: Until it beeps
  c. According to agency policy
Research findings differ on the optimal time for measuring an oral temperature, so follow agency policy.

6. Remove the thermometer; discard the cover. If there is no cover, wipe the thermometer with a tissue.
Wiping removes mucus that can make the markings on a glass thermometer difficult to read.

7. Read the temperature.
  a. Glass thermometer: Position the thermometer at eye level, and

rotate it until the markings are clear. ▼

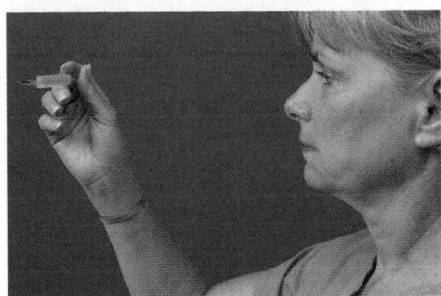

  b. Electronic thermometer: Read the digital display.

8. Clean and replace the thermometer. Follow agency policy.
Prevents microbial growth on thermometers and recharges battery of electronic thermometers.

■ **Procedure 17-1C** **Taking a Rectal Temperature**

➤ When performing the procedure, always identify your patient according to agency policy and be attentive to standard precautions, hand hygiene, patient safety and privacy, body mechanics, and documentation.

➤ *Note:* This procedure primarily describes use of an electronic thermometer.

Procedure Steps

1. Slide the thermometer into a protective sheath.
A protective sheath provides a barrier to prevent transmission of microorganisms.

2. Position an adult patient in Sims' position (on the side with the knees flexed); place a child in the prone position. Drape the patient so that only the anal area is exposed. You can lay a small child face down across your lap or a parent's lap.
Flexing the knees helps relax the muscles to ease insertion and aid in visualization. Draping provides privacy and decreases embarrassment. ➤

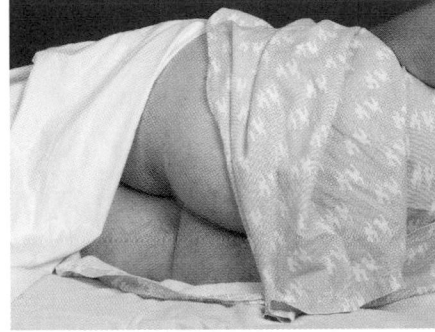

3. Lubricate the tip of the thermometer by squeezing water-soluble lubricant onto a tissue and then applying it to the thermometer.
Prevents injury to the rectal mucosa and eases insertion. Inserting the thermometer into the lubricant container would contaminate contents of the container.

4. Don a procedure glove on your dominant hand, or on both hands if necessary.

5. With your nondominant hand, separate the patient's buttocks to visualize the anus.

6. Gently insert the thermometer approximately:
  Adult: 1 to 1.5 in. (2.5 to 3.7 cm)
  Child: 0.9 in. (2.5 cm)
  Infant: 0.5 in. (1.5 cm)
The thermometer must be placed past the rectal sphincter.

  a. Have the patient take a deep breath. Insert the thermometer as he exhales.
Taking a deep breath helps relax the anal sphincter.

(continued on next page)

Procedure 17–1 ■ **Assessing Body Temperature** (continued)

b. If you feel resistance, do not use force.
Inserting the thermometer too far or forcing against resistance may injure the rectal mucosa. ▼

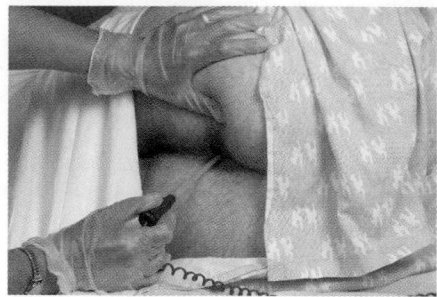

7. Hold the thermometer in place until it beeps. (For a glass thermometer, hold the thermometer 3 to 5 minutes.)
The thermometer must be held in place to prevent inadvertent injury to the patient. An electronic thermometer will beep when a constant temperature is reached. Research differs on the optimal time for measuring a rectal temperature, so follow agency policy.

8. Remove the thermometer, discard the cover, and read the digital display

9. Remove the procedure glove(s) and discard in a biohazards container.

10. Follow agency policy for cleaning and storing thermometers.
Prevents microbial growth on thermometers and recharges electronic thermometer battery.

■ **Procedure 17–1D** **Taking a Temporal Artery Temperature**

➤ When performing the procedure, always identify your patient according to agency policy and be attentive to standard precautions, hand hygiene, patient safety and privacy, body mechanics, and documentation.

Procedure Steps

✚ If the patient has been lying down, do not measure the temperature on the side that was lying on the pillow. Do not measure if a cap or hair has been covering the area over the temporal artery.
These can prevent heat dissipation and produce a falsely high reading.

1. Remove the protective cap from the instrument; clean the lens/probe according to the manufacturer's instructions.

2. Place the probe flat on the center of the forehead, midway between the eyebrow and the hairline. ▼

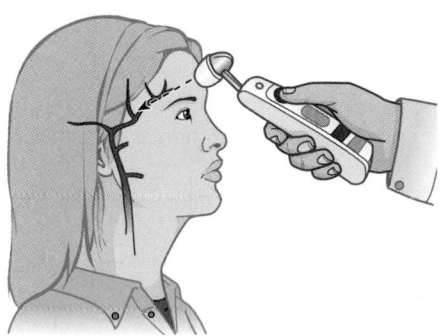

3. Press and hold the button while you stroke the thermometer medially to laterally across the forehead; keep the lens/probe flat and in contact with the skin, and slide in a reasonably straight line until you reach the hairline. ▼

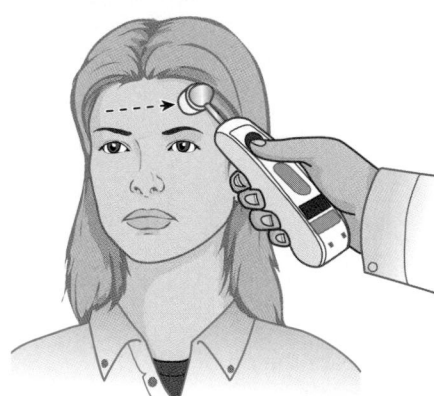

4. Still holding the button, touch the the thermometer lens/probe behind the ear lobe, in the soft depression below the mastoid.

This step is necessary for an accurate reading if there is any moisture at all on the patient's forehead. ▼

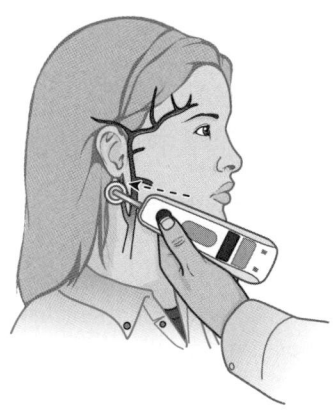

5. Release the button for the temperature reading. ▼

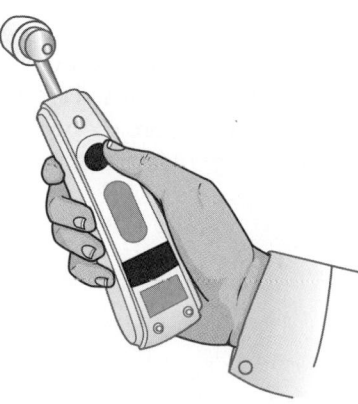

■ Procedure 17–1E   Taking a Tympanic Membrane Temperature

➤ When performing the procedure, always identify your patient according to agency policy and be attentive to standard precautions, hand hygiene, patient safety and privacy, body mechanics, and documentation.

Procedure Steps

1. Make sure the thermometer lens is intact and clean.
Ensures an accurate reading.

2. Place a disposable cover tightly over the lens, making sure the clear film is smooth across the lens.
Ensures an accurate reading.

3. Position the patient's head to one side. If you are right-handed try to use the right ear; if you are left-handed, use the left ear.
This allows you to better visualize the ear canal.

4. Straighten the ear canal, or follow the manufacturer's instructions. As a rule: ▼

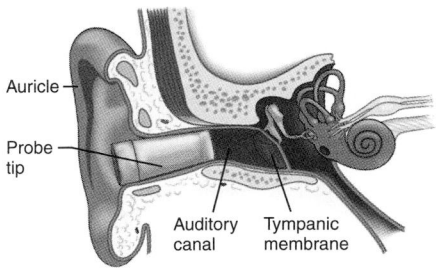

Auricle
Probe tip
Auditory canal   Tympanic membrane

a. For an adult, pull the pinna up and back. ▼

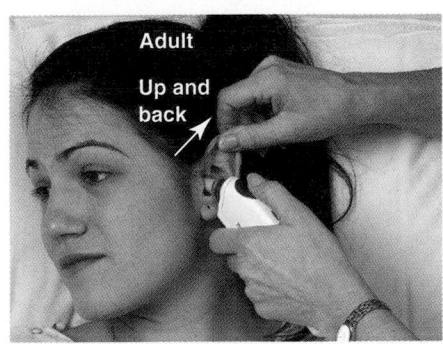

Adult
Up and back

b. For a child, pull the pinna down and back. ▼

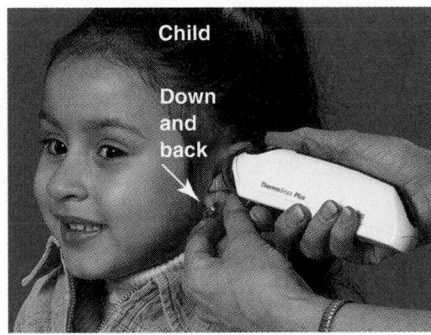

Child
Down and back

Some tympanic thermometers require you to straighten the ear canal; others do not. Some instruct, for adults, to pull the ear up, backward, and slightly away from the head. Some models instruct, for a child, to pull the pinna straight back instead of down and back. The external auditory canal is curved upward in children younger than 3 years of age. In an adult, it is a slightly S-shaped structure.

5. Insert the probe into the ear canal gently and firmly, directing it toward the tympanic membrane and inserting far enough to seal the opening.
Creates a seal to obtain an accurate reading without causing trauma to the ear canal.

6. For some thermometer models, rotate the probe handle toward the jaw. Follow the manufacturer's instructions; not all models require this.
Aims the lens toward the tympanic membrane.

7. Take the measurement.
   a. Press and release the button to obtain the reading.

b. Follow the instructions for the specific tympanic thermometer being used.
Some tympanic thermometers record the reading immediately; for some you must wait for about 3 seconds.

8. When you hear a beep and the display flashes, remove the thermometer. Note the reading in the display window.

9. Repeat the measurement in the other ear.
A study of 132 adults found significant differences in temperature in the left compared with the right ear. In Addition, the left ear tended to register a lower temperature than the right ear at temperatures below 36.7°C (98.1°F) and a higher temperature above 36.7°C (Heusch & McCarthy, 2005).

10. Discard the probe cover (usually you will press an "eject" button to do this), and replace the thermometer in its charging base.
Recharges the battery and protects the instrument.

(continued on next page)

Procedure 17-1 ■ Assessing Body Temperature (continued)

■ Procedure 17-1F Taking a Skin Temperature Using a Chemical Strip Thermometer

➤ When performing the procedure, always identify your patient according to agency policy and be attentive to standard precautions, hand hygiene, patient safety and privacy, body mechanics, and documentation.

Procedure Steps

1. Place the thermometer strip (paper or tape) on the patient's skin, generally on the forehead or abdomen.
The thermometer strip must be in contact with the skin to work properly. ▼

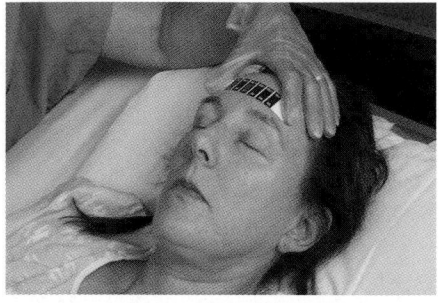

2. Leave the thermometer strip in place 15 to 60 seconds (or as the manufacturer directs).

3. Observe for color changes.
Chemical strips have indicators that change colors to indicate temperature changes.

4. Read the temperature before removing the strip from the patient's skin.
Ensures the most accurate reading. Note that chemical strip thermometers are not very accurate. If the temperature is not within the normal range, retake it with an electronic or other thermometer.

5. Remove and discard the thermometer strip.

What if...

■ **The patient's temperature is not within normal range?**

Identify whether the temperature reading indicates hypothermia, fever, or hyperthermia (e.g., heat stroke).

Perform other assessments to determine the cause or severity of the findings.

Assess for clinical signs to confirm an abnormal temperature reading.

Institute interventions to raise or lower temperature, as appropriate. Provide comfort measures (e.g., change linens if they are wet from diaphoresis).

■ **You are using a glass thermometer?**

Before and after using, shake down the thermometer as needed.

Clean the thermometer before and after using with soap and water or approved solution; rinse.

Use disposable covers, if available.

When reading the thermometer, hold it at eye level and rotate it until the markings are clear and easy to read.

Handle carefully and store in an appropriate container to avoid breakage.

Evaluation

■ Compare to normal range for developmental stage, site used, and client's baseline data.
■ Look for trends to identify potential concerns.

Patient Teaching

■ Inform the patient of the temperature reading.
■ Explain the significance of the temperature reading and any interventions that may be needed.

Home Care

Clients commonly use chemical strip (disposable), glass, or tympanic membrane thermometers at home. Teach the following points:

⬥ Do not use an oral thermometer to take a rectal temperature. Use a specially shaped, more rounded, rectal thermometer *to avoid injury to the rectum.*

⬥ Do not use glass-and-mercury thermometers. If you discover a glass-and-mercury thermometer, urge the client to replace it with a safer instrument. Arrange for an exchange if there is a procedure for this in your agency or community.

Glass-and-mercury thermometers carry the risk of breakage, cuts, and exposure to toxic mercury.

■ Chemical strip thermometers and tympanic thermometers are not very accurate. If you obtain a high or low reading, retake the temperature using a glass or other type of thermometer.
■ Teach the same procedures you have learned for measuring temperature. Observe as the client takes a temperature to ensure correct technique.
■ Clients often use the oral site. Remind them to not drink, eat, or smoke for 30 minutes before taking the temperature.
■ Reinforce the following points about care of reusable thermometers:
  ▪ If you use the same thermometer for more than one person, use disposable covers, if possible; clean the thermometer well between uses.
  ▪ If the person has an infection or communicable illness, soak the thermometer in 70% isopropyl alcohol between uses.
  ▪ Clean the thermometer after each use, even if it is used for only one person. Wash with soap and water, rinse with cold water, dry well, and store in a clean, dry container.

■ If you store a thermometer in alcohol, rinse it with cold water before taking the temperature.

■ Do not use the same thermometer for both oral and rectal temperatures.

Documentation

You will usually record temperature on a graphic flowsheet (see Forms section). In some situations (e.g., a fever), you may need to write a nurse's note. If so, follow these suggestions:

■ Chart the temperature, indicating the route of measurement.

■ Document the temperature according to agency policy.

■ Notify the appropriate person of abnormal findings.

■ Document supporting findings, such as "Skin is hot and dry" and state whether the temperature reading is consistent with the client's condition.

Example

> 9/06/11 1230   Oral temperature 105°F; it has risen steadily since the first elevation at 0630, when it was 100°F. Skin hot and dry. Patient is voiding only small amounts, but states no burning. Urine dark but clear. No chills. I & O begun. Gave Tylenol 650 mg by mouth and notified Dr. Anderson of patient's condition and medication. — Mary Clinton, RN

Practice Resources

Gyi, A. (2007); Heusch, A., & McCarthy, P. (2005); Lockwood, C., Conroy-Hiller, T., & Page, T. (2004); Quatrara, B., Coffman, J., Jenkins, T., et al. (2007); Rabinowitz, R., Cookson, S., Wasserman, S., et al. (1996); Robinson, J., Jou, H., & Spady, D. (2005); Therapeutic Research Center (2007); Vital Signs (1999).

Thinking About the Procedure

 Go to the *Fundamentals of Nursing Skills Videos,* **Temperature: Axillary.**

1. Why did the nurse use the blue thermometer probe instead of the red one?

2. What did the nurse do to ensure that the thermometer probe was in good contact with the axillary skin?

 For suggested responses, go to Chapter 17, **Thinking About the Procedure Suggested Responses,** on the Student Resource Disk or DavisPlus at http://davisplus.fadavis.com/Wilkinson2

Procedure 17-2 | Assessing Peripheral Pulses

➤ For steps to follow in *all* procedures, refer to the Universal Steps for All Procedures found on the inside back cover of Volume 2.

Critical Aspects

■ Make sure the client is resting while you assess the pulse.

■ Count for 15 or 30 seconds if pulse is regular; for 60 seconds if it is irregular.

■ Note pulse rate, rhythm, and quality.

■ Compare pulses bilaterally.

Equipment

■ Watch with a second hand or digital readout

■ Pen, pencil, and flowsheet or personal digital assistant (PDA)

Delegation

You can delegate measurement of pulses to the nursing assistive personnel (NAP) if you conclude that the patient's condition and the NAP's skills allow. For example, if pedal circulation is critical and you suspect it may be difficult to palpate, you should not delegate assessment of the pedal pulse. If you do delegate, perform the following assessments, and tell the NAP which site (e.g., radial, brachial) to use. Inform the NAP of any special considerations (e.g., to note what the patient's activity has been just before taking the pulse). Ask the NAP to record and report the pulse to you and to report immediately if it is outside normal limits (you must specify what is "normal" for each patient).

(continued on next page)

Procedure 17-2 ■ **Assessing Peripheral Pulses** (continued)

Pre-Procedure Assessments

■ Determine why assessment of pulses is indicated. Conditions requiring an assessment of pulses include blood loss, cardiac or respiratory disease, diabetes mellitus, and other conditions that affect oxygenation.

■ Assess factors that may alter the pulse, such as activity and medications. If the client has been active recently, wait 5 to 10 minutes before measuring.
Activity increases the pulse rate; increased intracranial pressure decreases the rate; medications such as digoxin decrease the rate; other medications, such as albuterol, increase the pulse rate.

■ Procedure 17-2A Assessing the Radial Pulse

➤ When performing the procedure, always identify your patient according to agency policy and be attentive to standard precautions, hand hygiene, patient safety and privacy, body mechanics, and documentation.

Procedure Steps

1. With the patient sitting or supine, flex the patient's arm, and place the patient's forearm across his chest.

2. Palpate the radial artery.
The radial site is the most frequently used to calculate the patient's heart rate because it is generally the easiest site to use.

   a. Place the pads of your index or middle fingers (or both) in the groove on the thumb side of the patient's wrist, over the radial artery.
   b. Press lightly but firmly until you are able to feel the radial pulse. Start with light pressure to prevent occluding the pulse, and gradually increase the pressure until you feel the pulse.
The fingertips are the most sensitive parts of the hand to palpate arterial pulsations. Avoid using the thumb, because it has its own pulsation and may interfere with the accuracy of your count. ▼

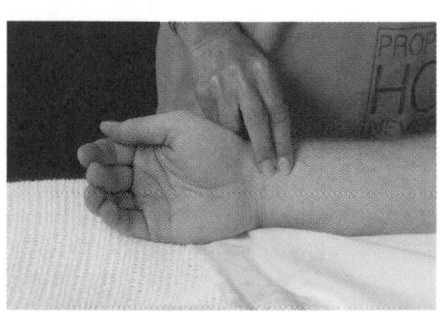

3. Note the rhythm and quality of the pulse. Note whether the thrust of the pulse against your fingertips is bounding, strong, weak, or thready.
The rhythm and quality of the pulse are a reflection of the patient's cardiac output. The strength of the pulse reflects the volume of the blood that is ejected against the arterial wall with each contraction of the heart. An irregular or weak pulse indicates decreased cardiac output. A bounding pulse indicates increased cardiac output.

4. Count the pulse:
   a. Count for 60 seconds the first time you take a patient's pulse. After that, you can count a pulse with a regular rhythm for 15 seconds and multiply by 4, or count for 30 seconds and multiply by 2 to get the beats per minute.
If you do not know the patient well, count for a full minute to be certain to detect any irregularities. Also see Step 4c rationale.

   b. Begin timing with the count of 1—starting with the first beat that you feel.
   c. Count an irregular pulse for a full minute (60 seconds).
Research is conflicting. Some studies indicate that a 60-second count is most accurate; others say that accuracy is not affected by a 30-second, or even a 15-second, count if the

pulse is regular. You must count an irregular pulse for a full minute to be accurate.

5. For an admission assessment or peripheral vascular check, palpate the radial pulses on both wrists simultaneously.
   a. Note any difference in the quality of the pulse between arms. Is the pulse on one side weaker than that on the other?
Palpating simultaneously enables the recognition of small differences in the peripheral circulation.

■ Procedure 17-2B Assessing the Brachial Pulse

➤ When performing the procedure, always identify your patient according to agency policy and be attentive to standard precautions, hand hygiene, patient safety and privacy, body mechanics, and documentation.

Procedure Steps

1. Palpate the brachial artery.
   a. Using firm pressure, press in the inner aspect of the antecubital fossa until you palpate the brachial artery.
   b. If you have difficulty palpating the pulse, ask the patient to pronate the forearm (i.e., turn the palm of the hand downward).

This brings the brachial artery over a bony prominence and makes the pulse easier to feel. ▼

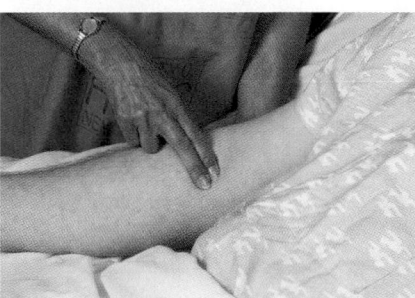

2. Assess pulse rate, rhythm, and quality, and assess bilaterally as for the radial pulse (see Procedure 17-2A). The brachial pulse is used most frequently to assess blood pressure and to identify the presence of a pulse during cardiopulmonary rescuscitation (CPR) in an infant.

■ Procedure 17-2C Assessing the Carotid Pulse

➤ When performing the procedure, always identify your patient according to agency policy and be attentive to standard precautions, hand hygiene, patient safety and privacy, body mechanics, and documentation.

✚ Caution! Do not palpate the carotid pulse except during cardiopulmonary resuscitation in an adult, and in certain situations to assess for circulation to the head. Pressure on the carotid (especially in older adults) can stimulate the vagus nerve, causing the pulse and blood pressure to drop suddenly, and perhaps fainting or circulatory arrest

Procedure Steps

1. Palpate the carotid artery lightly.

a. Place your fingers on the patient's trachea, and slide them to the side into the groove between the trachea and the sternocleidomastoid muscle.
Compressing the carotid arteries can stimulate the carotid bodies and significantly decrease the patient's heart rate and blood pressure.

Compressing the carotid arteries can decrease circulation to the brain. ➤

✚ NEVER compress the carotid artery on both sides of the neck at the same time.

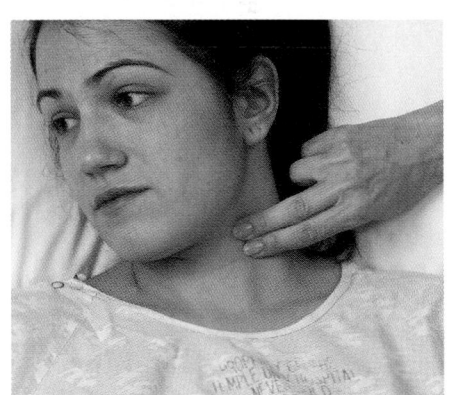

2. Assess the rate, rhythm, and quality, and compare bilaterally as for the radial pulse (see Procedure 17-2A).

■ Procedure 17-2D Assessing the Dorsalis Pedis Pulse

➤ When performing the procedure, always identify your patient according to agency policy and be attentive to standard precautions, hand hygiene, patient safety and privacy, body mechanics, and documentation.

Procedure Steps

1. Palpate the dorsalis pedis pulse.
   a. Run your fingers up the groove between the great and first toes to the top of the foot.
   b. Palpate very lightly.
The dorsalis pedis pulse is easily obliterated, so use very light pressure. The dorsalis pedis pulse is used to access circulation of the foot.

2. Assess pulse rate, rhythm, and quality, and assess bilaterally as

for the radial pulse (see Procedure 17-2A). ▼

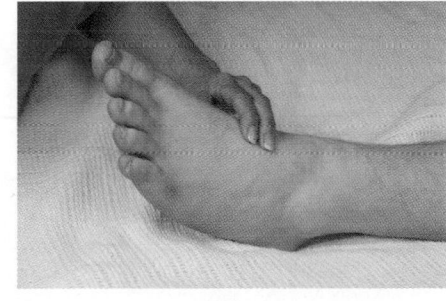

3. If you are unable to palpate the dorsalis pedis pulse, use a Doppler ultrasound device to listen for the pulse.

(continued on next page)

Procedure 17-2 ■ **Assessing Peripheral Pulses** (continued)

■ Procedure 17-2E **Assessing the Femoral Pulse**

➤ When performing the procedure, always identify your patient according to agency policy and be attentive to standard precautions, hand hygiene, patient safety and privacy, body mechanics, and documentation.

Procedure Steps

1. Palpate the femoral pulse by pressing deeply in the groin midway between the anterosuperior iliac spine and the symphysis pubis.
The femoral artery lies very deep and requires significant pressure to palpate. You may need to use both hands to feel the pulse on an adult. ➤

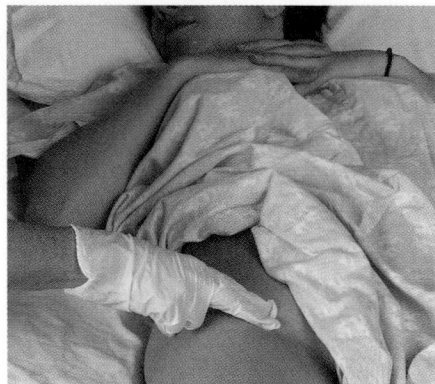

2. Assess pulse rate, rhythm, and quality, and assess bilaterally as for the radial pulse (see Procedure 17-2A). The femoral pulse is used to determine the presence of a pulse during CPR and to assess circulation to the leg.

■ Procedure 17-2F **Assessing the Posterior Tibial Pulse**

➤ When performing the procedure, always identify your patient according to agency policy and be attentive to standard precautions, hand hygiene, patient safety and privacy, body mechanics, and documentation.

Procedure Steps

1. Palpate the posterior tibial pulse by pressing on the inner (medial) side of the ankle below the medial malleolus.
The posterior tibial pulse is usually palpated easily, but it may be deeper in some people. So, press down moderately and then increase pressure until you feel the pulse. It is relatively easy to obliterate. ➤

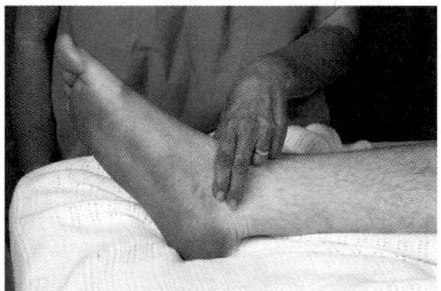

2. Assess pulse rate, rhythm, and quality, and assess bilaterally as for the radial pulse (see Procedure 17-2A). The posterior tibial pulse is used to assess circulation to the lower extremity; it is assessed along with the dorsalis pedis pulse.

■ Procedure 17-2G **Assessing the Popliteal Pulse**

➤ When performing the procedure, always identify your patient according to agency policy and be attentive to standard precautions, hand hygiene, patient safety and privacy, body mechanics, and documentation.

Procedure Steps

1. Palpate the popliteal pulse by pressing behind the knee in the middle of the popliteal fossa.
The popliteal pulse can be difficult to feel. It is used only when specifically indicated because of absence of pedal pulses or for taking a thigh blood pressure. ➤

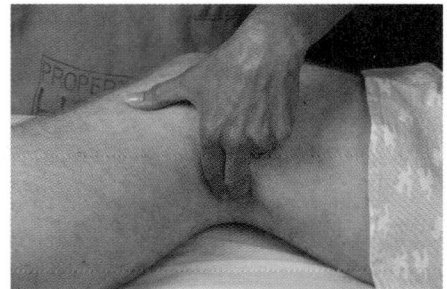

2. Assess pulse rate, rhythm, and quality, and assess bilaterally as for the radial pulse (see Procedure 17-2A). The popliteal pulse is used to assess circulation of the lower leg and auscultate a thigh blood pressure.

■ Procedure 17-2H Assessing the Temporal Pulse

➤ When performing the procedure, always identify your patient according to agency policy and be attentive to standard precautions, hand hygiene, patient safety and privacy, body mechanics, and documentation.

Procedure Steps

1. Palpate the temporal pulse by pressing lightly lateral (outside area) and superior to (above) the eye. ▼

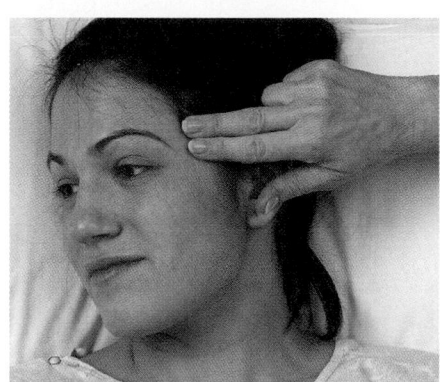

2. Assess pulse rate, rhythm, and quality, and assess bilaterally as for the radial pulse (see Procedure 17-2A). The temporal pulse is easily accessible and is used frequently in infants.

What if...

■ **The patient is an infant or a child younger than age 3 years?**

Auscultate an apical pulse rate. Rates are faster and small arteries more difficult to feel in a child or infant.

If a parent is present, encourage the parent to hold the child to reduce anxiety.

Fear increases the pulse rate.

■ **The patient is an older adult?**

Have the patient at rest for 15 to 20 minutes after activity and before assessing the pulse.

The pulse tends to return to baseline more slowly in older adults.

If the pulse is fast, take repeated measures; if a pattern of fast rate emerges, note this for the primary care provider for further evaluation.

An elevated heart rate is related to increased mortality in older adult women, so it is a simple index of general health status.

■ **The pulse is faint or weak?**

Use a Doppler ultrasound device to detect blood flow.

Lack of pulses indicates inadequate circulation to the lower extremities. If you cannot feel the pulse, you must determine whether the pulse is absent or whether you are having difficulty feeling.

To draw the conclusion that the pulse is "absent," you must use a Doppler.

Apply transmission gel to the end of the probe. Do not use water-soluble lubricant as a substitute for transmission gel.

Place the probe lightly on the skin over the artery you are using.

Turn on the instrument and set the volume control to the lowest setting.

Tilting the probe to a 45° angle to the artery, move the probe slowly in a circular motion to locate the signal (a rhythmic hissing noise). Count for 60 seconds.

Move the probe slowly to avoid distorting the signal.

When you are finished, wipe the gel off the patient's skin. Clean the probe with soapy water or an antiseptic solution. Do not immerse the probe or bump it against anything hard.

Clean the probe to prevent cross-contamination to other patients. Probes are fragile and may malfunction if bumped against a hard surface.

Evaluation

Especially if pedal pulses are decreased, observe for other indications of inadequate circulation, such as cool skin, decreased capillary refill, and bluish or ashen skin tone. You must provide supporting evidence if you chart that pedal pulses are decreased or absent. The complete absence of a pulse requires immediate intervention.

Patient Teaching

■ Teach the patient about the significance of any abnormalities in pulse rate or rhythm.
■ Explain any interventions that may be needed.

Home Care

Assess the skill level of the person who will be assessing the client's peripheral pulses in the home, and provide instruction if necessary.

Documentation

Usually you will document routine vital signs (VS), including pulse, on a flowsheet or graphic. If you record it in a nurse's

note, document the pulse rate, rhythm, quality, and site (e.g., "radial pulse 64 beats/min, regular, and strong bilaterally").

Practice Resources

Best practices (2007); Gyi, A. (2007); Lockwood, C., Conroy-Hiller, T., & Page, T. (2004); Perk, G., Stessman, J., Ginsberg, G., et al. (2003); Trim, J. (2005); Vital Signs (1999).

Thinking About the Procedure

 Go to the *Fundamentals of Nursing Skills Videos,* **Pulse: Carotid.**

1. Why do you think the nurse might be assessing this patient's carotid pulse?

2. What two landmarks does the nurse use to locate the carotid artery?

 For suggested responses, go to Chapter 17, **Thinking About the Procedure Suggested Responses,** on the Student Resource Disk or DavisPlus at http://davisplus.fadavis.com/ Wilkinson2

Procedure 17-3 ☐ Assessing the Apical Pulse

➤ For steps to follow in *all* procedures, refer to the Universal Steps for All Procedures found on the inside back cover of Volume 2.

Critical Aspects

- Position the patient supine or sitting.
- Palpate and place the stethoscope at the 5th intercostal space at the midclavicular line.
- Count for 60 seconds.
- Note pulse rate, rhythm, and quality and the S_1 and S_2 heart sounds.

Equipment

- Watch with a second hand or second readout
- Stethoscope
- Alcohol wipes (to clean stethoscope)

Delegation

You can delegate measurement of the apical pulse to the nursing assistive personnel (NAP) if you conclude that the patient's condition and the NAP's skills allow. First perform the following assessments. Then inform the NAP of any special considerations (e.g., to note what the patient's activity has been just before taking the pulse, or to mark the time exactly so you can compare it to the patient's ECG). Ask the NAP to record and report the pulse to you, and to report immediately if it is outside normal limits (you must specify what is "normal" for each patient).

Pre-Procedure Assessments

- Determine why assessment of the apical pulse is indicated.

Conditions that require assessment of the apical pulse include digitalis therapy, blood loss, cardiac or respiratory disease, or other conditions that affect oxygenation status.

- Assess factors that may alter the pulse, such as activity and medications. If the client has been recently active, wait 10 to 15 minutes before obtaining a measurement.

The apical pulse is generally best heard at the point of maximum impulse (PMI) in the 5th intercostal space at the midclavicular line. The PMI is located over the apex of the heart.

➤ When performing the procedure, always identify your patient according to agency policy and be attentive to standard precautions, hand hygiene, patient safety and privacy, body mechanics, and documentation.

Procedure Steps

1. With the client supine or sitting, expose the left side of the chest, but only as much as necessary.
Prevents distortion of sound from the patient's gown rubbing on the stethoscope, while also protecting the patient's privacy. ▼

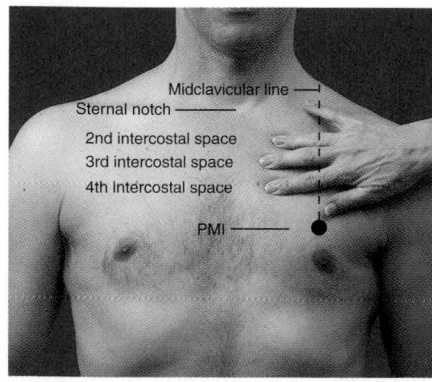

Midclavicular line
Sternal notch
2nd intercostal space
3rd intercostal space
4th Intercostal space
PMI

◆ 2. Wipe the stethoscope with a 70% alcohol or benzalkonium chloride wipe before and after examining the patient.
Cleaning can reduce the bacterial count by up to 100%.

3. Palpate the 5th intercostal space at the midclavicular line for the apical pulse.
The left ventricle of the heart and the point of maximum impulse lie in this area.

a. To locate the 5th intercostal space, slide your finger down from the sternal notch to the angle of Louis (the bump where the manubrium and sternum meet).
b. Slide your finger over to the left sternal border to the 2nd intercostal space.
c. Now place your index or ring finger (depending on which hand you use) in the 2nd intercostal

space, and count down to the 5th intercostal space by placing a finger in each of the spaces.
d. Slide over to the midclavicular line, keeping your finger in the 5th intercostal space.

4. Palpate the apical pulse.
a. The palpated apical pulse is also called the point of maximal impulse (PMI).
b. The pulse area should be about the size of a quarter, without lifts or heaves.
A larger than normal pulsation may indicate ventricular hypertrophy.

5. Warm the stethoscope in your hand for 10 seconds. Then place the diaphragm over the PMI, and listen to the normal S_1 and S_2 heart sounds (lub dub).
A cold stethoscope placed on the skin may startle the patient and increase the heart rate. Heart sounds result

when blood moves through the valves of the heart. The first heart sound is louder at the apical area and should be audible when the pulse is auscultated.

 Go to the sound file, **Heart Sounds,** on the Student Resource Disk or DavisPlus at http://davisplus.fadavis.com/Wilkinson2

6. Count the apical heart rate for 1 full minute.
Ensures accuracy. Because the apical heart rate is needed as an assessment measure for the administration of some medications (e.g., digoxin), accuracy is essential. Some cardiac conditions cause

either slow or irregular rates, both of which must be counted for a full minute to ensure accuracy.

What if . . .

■ **The apical rate is less than 60 beats/min?**
(Note: You may also see "bpm" as an abbreviation for "beats per minute.")
If the patient is on cardiac medications, withhold them and consult with a physician about whether to adjust dosage.

Certain cardiac medications (e.g., digoxin) are given to slow the heart rate; bradycardia may indicate that blood levels are too high.

Assess for chest pain, dizziness, dyspnea. May indicate decreased cardiac output

■ **The apical rate is greater than 100 beats/min?**

Obtain a complete set of vital signs. Assess for pain, anxiety, fever, dehydration, decreased oxygenation, hypotension, and decreased exercise. These factors may increase pulse rate.

Evaluation

■ Are the findings within normal limits?
■ Are there other factors supporting the findings?
■ What are the trends over time?
■ Is the skin pink, warm, and dry?
■ Any cyanosis?

Patient Teaching

■ Teach the patient about the significance of any abnormalities in the pulse rate or rhythm.
■ Explain any interventions that may be necessary.

Home Care

■ Assess the skill level of the person who will be assessing the client's apical pulse in the home, and provide instruction if necessary.

 Teach the home caregiver when to hold medications and/or to call primary care provider (e.g., to hold the digitalis if the rate is <60).

■ Before leaving the home, clean the stethoscope with detergent or disinfectant, when possible; or place it in a plastic bag for transporting to the reprocessing location.

 If the patient has a multidrug-resistant organism infection, reusable equipment such as stethoscopes should remain in the home. If the stethoscope cannot remain in the home, clean and disinfect it before leaving the home, using a low to intermediate level disinfectant. If this is not practical, place the stethoscope in a plastic bag and transport it to another site for cleaning and disinfection.

Documentation

Document the pulse rate, rhythm, and site.

Example:

9/05/11	0900	*Apical pulse regular and*
		strong, rate 64. ——— Janice Jonas, RN

Practice Resources

Best practices (2007); Centers for Disease Control and Prevention (2005); Gyi, A. (2007); Hwu, Y., Coates, V., & Lin, F. (2000); Lockwood, C., Conroy-Hiller, T., & Page, T. (2004); Siegel, J., Rhinehart, E., Jackson, M., et al. (2006); Vital Signs (1999).

Thinking About the Procedure

 Go to the *Fundamentals of Nursing Skills Videos,* **Pulse: Apical.**

1. How does the nurse position the patient in the video?

2. How is this the same as or different from the position described for this procedure in Volume 2?

3. Can you think of any reasons why the nurse in the video may have positioned her client in this manner?

 For suggested responses, go to Chapter 17, **Thinking About the Procedure Suggested Responses,** on the Student Resource Disk or DavisPlus at http://davisplus.fadavis.com/Wilkinson2

Procedure 17-4 ☐ Assessing for an Apical–Radial Pulse Deficit

➤ For steps to follow in *all* procedures, refer to the Universal Steps for All Procedures found on the inside back cover of Volume 2.

Critical Aspects

- Palpate and place the stethoscope over the apex of the heart.
- Palpate the radial pulse.
- Have two nurses carry out the procedure, if possible.
- Count for 60 seconds, simultaneously.
- Compare the pulse rate at both sites; calculate the difference.

Equipment

- Watch or clock with a second hand or second readout
- Procedure gloves, if indicated
- Stethoscope
- Alcohol wipes to clean the stethoscope

Delegation

Instead of delegating measurement of an apical–radial pulse to nursing assistive personnel (NAP), you would most likely ask the NAP to assist you in this procedure because it is best performed by two persons working together.

Pre-Procedure Assessments

- Determine why assessment of pulse deficit is indicated.

Conditions that require assessment of pulse deficit include digitalis therapy, blood loss, cardiac or respiratory disease, and other conditions that affect oxygenation status.

- Assess factors that may alter the pulse, such as activity and medications.

➤ When performing the procedure, always identify your patient according to agency policy and be attentive to standard precautions, hand hygiene, patient safety and privacy, body mechanics, and documentation.

Procedure Steps

✚ **1.** Wipe the stethoscope with a 70% alcohol or benzalkonium chloride wipe before and after examining the patient.

Cleaning can reduce the bacterial count by up to 100% and prevent the transmission of microbes.

2. Expose the left side of the patient's chest, minimizing patient exposure.
Prevents distortion of sound from the patient's gown rubbing on the stethoscope and protects privacy.

3. If two nurses are performing the procedure, place the watch so that the second hand is visible to both nurses.
Using one watch increases accuracy of counts.

4. Nurse I palpates the 5th intercostal space at the midclavicular line for the apical pulse, and firmly holds the diaphragm of the stethoscope in place, using firm pressure.

Aids in hearing high-pitched sounds and ensures good contact between the diaphragm of the stethoscope and the skin. ▼

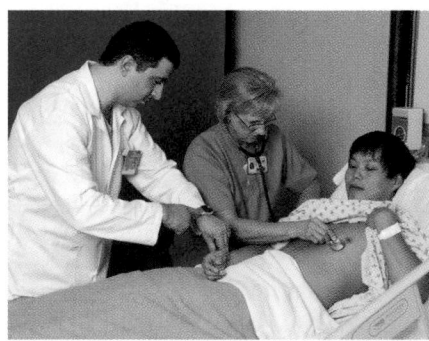

5. Nurse 2 palpates the radial pulse and assesses rate, rhythm, and quality.

6. Nurse 2 says "Start" when ready to begin and "Stop" when finished. Both nurses count the pulse simultaneously for I full minute.
Count simultaneously to ensure accuracy. Counting for I full minute is necessary for an accurate assessment of any discrepancies that may exist between the two sites.

7. To obtain pulse deficit, subtract the radial rate from the apical rate.

Apical Rate – Radial Rate =
Pulse Deficit

Atrial and ventricular dysrhythmias may cause beats that do not perfuse, so although you hear an apical heart beat, you do not feel a peripheral pulse. The pulse deficit is the number of heart beats that do not perfuse.

What if . . .

- **There is not another nurse available to assist?**
- Hold the stethoscope in place with the one hand while palpating the radial pulse with the hand wearing the watch.
Even if you cannot manage to count both rates, you should be able to feel any differences between the apical and radial pulses.

- **There has been an increase in pulse deficit since the last measurement?**

An increase in pulse deficit means that the patient's cardiac output has decreased.

Evaluation

- Identify the presence of an apical-pulse deficit, and compare to previous findings.
- Assess other measures of cardiopulmonary status to identify a decline in the patient's condition
- Look for trends.

The presence of any apical–radial pulse deficit is abnormal.

Patient Teaching

- Teach the patient about the significance of an apical–radial pulse deficit.
- Explain any necessary interventions.

Home Care

- Assess the skill level of the person(s) who will be measuring the client's apical–radial pulse deficit in the home, and provide instruction if necessary.
- Before leaving the home, clean the stethoscope as described in the Home Care section of Procedure 17-3.

Documentation

Document the apical–radial pulse deficit.

Example:

| 9/05/11 | 0900 | Apical-radial pulse deficit |
| | | is 4 beats/minute. ——— Jon Albertson, RN |

Practice Resources

Best practices (2007); Centers for Disease Control and Prevention (2005); Jevon, P., Ewens, B., & Lowe, R. (2000); Gyi, A. (2007); Lockwood, C., Conroy-Hiller, T., & Page, T. (2004); Siegel, J., Rhinehart, E., Jackson, M., et al. (2006); Vital Signs (1999).

Thinking About the Procedure

 Go to the *Fundamentals of Nursing Skills Videos*, **Pulse Deficit: Apical–Radial.**

1. Use the visual (non-narrated) video. How did the nurses show respect for the patient's personhood?

2. What safety measures did they demonstrate?

3. At the end of the procedure, what would you assume they did that was not shown on camera?

 For suggested responses, go to Chapter 17, **Thinking About the Procedure Suggested Responses,** on the Student Resource Disk or DavisPlus at http://davisplus.fadavis.com/ Wilkinson2

Procedure 17-5 ☐ **Assessing Respirations**

➤ For steps to follow in *all* procedures, refer to the Universal Steps for All Procedures found on the inside back cover of Volume 2.

Critical Aspects

- Count unobtrusively (e.g., while palpating the radial pulse).
- Count for 30 seconds if respirations are regular; for 60 seconds if they are irregular.

A 60-second count is recommended for increased accuracy, even for regular respirations.

- Observe the rate, rhythm, and depth of respirations.

Equipment

- A watch with a second hand (or a wall clock)

Delegation

You can delegate the counting of respirations to the nursing assistive personnel (NAP) if you conclude that the patient's condition and the NAP's skills allow. Perform the following assessments, and inform the NAP of any special considerations (e.g., the need to keep the patient in a certain position). Ask the NAP to record and report the respirations to you, and to report immediately if they are not within the normal range for this patient (specify the range).

Pre-Procedure Assessments

- Observe for signs of respiratory distress—breathing faster or slower than normal, gasping breaths, confusion, circumoral (around the month) cyanosis.

Signs of hypoxemia may indicate that the patient is not adequately oxygenated.

- Determine the baseline respiratory rate and character of respirations.
- Assess for factors that may affect the respiratory rate (e.g., pain, activity, fever, respiratory disorders).

(continued on next page)

Procedure 17-5 ■ Assessing Respiration (continued)

➤ When performing the procedure, always identify your patient according to agency policy and be attentive to standard precautions, hand hygiene, patient safety and privacy, body mechanics, and documentation.

Procedure Steps

1. Position the patient.
   a. With the patient in a sitting position (preferably), flex the patient's arm, and place her forearm across her chest.

Aids in counting the patient's pulse rate by making the rise and fall of the chest more discernible and by making the patient less aware that you are measuring the respiratory rate. The patient's awareness might alter the respiratory rate and/or pattern because respirations are partially under voluntary control. ▼

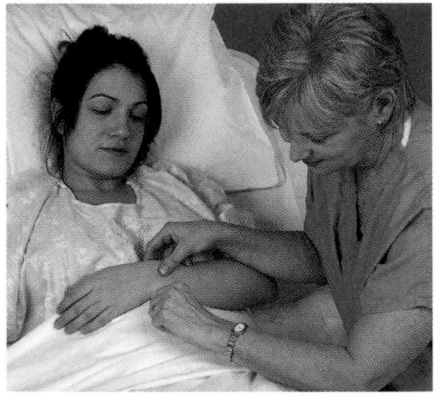

2. Palpate and count the radial pulse; remember that number. Then, keeping your hand on the patient's wrist, count the respirations.
Allows you to count the respirations unobtrusively.

3. Observe the respiratory rate, rhythm, and depth.
   a. Rate: Normal for patient's age, fast (tachypnea), or slow (bradypnea)
   b. Rhythm: Regular or irregular
   c. Depth: Normal, shallow, or deep (e.g., Kussmaul's)
All of these characteristics are necessary to evaluate respiratory status. Different pathologies affect each of these characteristics differently.

4. Count the number of breaths per minute. Begin timing the respirations with a count of 1, not 0, the same as with pulse measurement.
   a. If the respiratory rhythm is regular, count the rate (one inhalation and one exhalation is one respiration) for 30 seconds, and multiply by 2.
   b. If the rhythm is irregular, count the rate for 1 full minute (60 seconds).
Variations in rhythm may cause an inaccurate rate when counted for less than 1 minute.

What if. . .

■ **The patient is an infant?**

Place your hand on the abdomen to assess the respiratory rate. For infants, auscultate breath sounds with a stethoscope.

Infants and young children breathe rapidly and are abdominal breathers, so it is difficult to see each and every rise and fall of the abdomen. Using a stethoscope increases the accuracy of the count, as well as providing information about the breath sounds.

For infants and very young children, count for one full minute.

Infants and young children have irregular respirations. Counting for a full minute provides a more accurate rate for irregular respirations.

■ **The patient is receiving oxygen therapy, or requires careful assessment of respiratory status?**

Apply a pulse oximeter (see Procedure 35-2, Monitoring Pulse Oximetry).

Evidence suggests that pulse oximetry is useful for detecting deterioration of physiological function that might otherwise be missed (e.g., during the perioperatuve period or in seriously ill patients).

Evaluation

■ Compare the respiratory rate and rhythm with previous readings.
■ Note other vital signs, especially temperature.
■ Look for trends, and note whether the respiratory rate and rhythm are changing in conjunction with changes in the other vital signs.
If the patient has an elevated temperature, the respiratory rate will increase. Corresponding elevation in pulse with respiratory rate may indicate hypoxemia. If respirations are not within normal parameters, assess oxygenation with a pulse oximeter.

Patient Teaching

Teach the patient about factors that affect respiratory status, such as smoking and activity.

Home Care

Assess the skill level of the person(s) who will be measuring the client's respiratory rate in the home, and provide instruction as needed.

Documentation

You will document routine VS (including respirations) on a graphic or flowsheet. When a nurse's note is needed, follow these guidelines.
■ Document the respiratory rate and rhythm.
■ Document that respirations are either labored or unlabored; if labored, describe in what way (e.g., intercostal retractions, use of accessory muscles, nasal flaring)

Example:

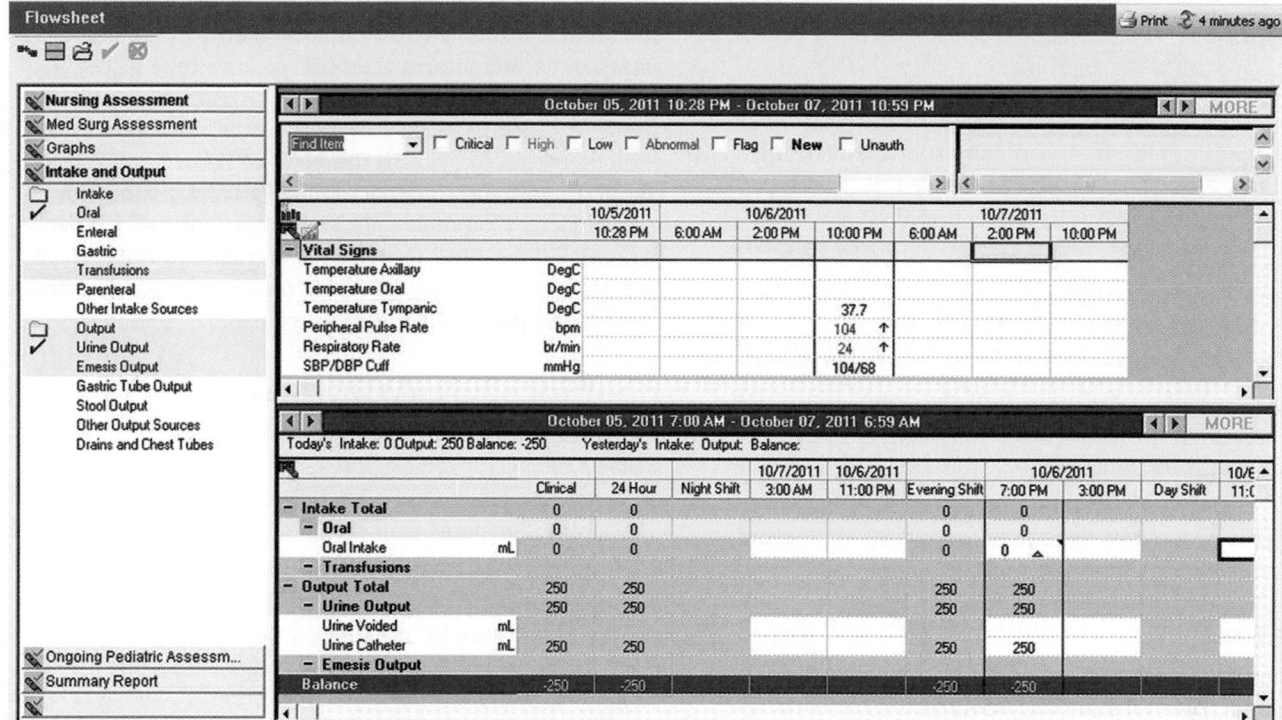

Electronic Flowsheet.

Practice Resources

Centers for Disease Control and Prevention (2005); Gyi, A. (2007); Lockwood, C., Conroy-Hiller, T., & Page, T. (2004); Vital Signs (1999).

Thinking About the Procedure

 Go to the *Fundamentals of Nursing Skills Videos,* **Respirations.**

1. Write an example of a nursing note describing Mr. Johnson's respiratory status. Assume that his rate is 12 breaths/min (it may be difficult to count in the video). What else can you observe?

 For suggested responses, go to Chapter 17, **Thinking About the Procedure Suggested Responses,** on the Student Resource Disk or DavisPlus at http://davisplus.fadavis.com/Wilkinson2

Procedure 17-6 ■ Measuring Blood Pressure

➤ For steps to follow in *all* procedures, refer to the Universal Steps for All Procedures found on the inside back cover of Volume 2.

Critical Aspects

- If possible, place the patient in a sitting position, with the feet on the floor and the legs uncrossed.
- Measure blood pressure (BP) after the patient has been inactive for 5 minutes.
- Support the patient's arm at the level of the heart.
- Use cuff of the appropriate size.
- Wrap the cuff snugly.
- Inflate the cuff while palpating the artery. Inflate to 30 mm Hg above the point at which you can no longer feel the artery pulsating.
- Place the stethoscope on the artery, and release pressure at 2 to 3 mm Hg per second.
- Record systolic/diastolic pressures (first and last sounds heard—e.g., 110/80).
- Wait at least 2 minutes before remeasuring.

(continued on next page)

Procedure 17-6 ■ **Measuring Blood Pressure** (continued)

Equipment

■ Stethoscope

✚ Note: Do not wear a stethoscope around your neck. There is a slight risk that you can entangle it in intravenous and other lines. There is also a risk that a psychotic or delirious patient could use it to harm you. Also, wearing a stethoscope can be a source of cross-contamination.

■ 70% alcohol or benzalkonium chloride wipes.
For cleaning stethoscope before and after use. Clean all parts.

■ Sphygmomanometer with a cuff of the appropriate size. Refer to Clinical Insight 17-2.
Using a cuff that is too small will result in a false-high reading; using a cuff that is too large will result in a false-low reading.

■ NOTE: This procedure describes the use of an aneroid manometer or an electronic measuring device.

Delegation

You can delegate measurement of BP to the nursing assistive personnel (NAP) if you conclude that the patient's condition and the NAP's skills allow. Perform the following assessments, and inform the NAP of the site (e.g., radial, brachial) to use. Inform the NAP of any special considerations (e.g., not to place a BP cuff on the same side as the site of a mastectomy). Ask the NAP to record and report the BP to you, and to report immediately if it is outside normal limits (you must specify what is "normal" for each patient). Tell the NAP that if BP is elevated, to note which arm, the patient's position during measurement, and activity immediately preceding the measurement.

Pre-Procedure Assessments

■ Check for factors or activities that may alter the readings.
Caffeine, smoking, exercise, and stress can all elevate the BP. Be certain the patient has been lying or sitting for at least 5 minutes (30 minutes after strenuous exercise) and is relaxed.

■ Check the previous recording, if any.
Noting changes over time is important with all patient assessments. Because BP changes constantly and because so many factors affect it, you cannot draw conclusions from a single measurement.

➤ When performing the procedure, always identify your patient according to agency policy and be attentive to standard precautions, hand hygiene, patient safety and privacy, body mechanics, and documentation.

➤ *Note:* To improve the accuracy of your readings, also refer to Clinical Insights 17-1 and 17-2.

Procedure Steps

1. Clean the stethoscope before and after the procedure.
Although only a small percentage of microorganisms are pathogenic, cleaning can reduce the bacterial count by 94% to 100%.

2. Position the patient comfortably, ensuring that:
   a. The legs are uncrossed, the back is supported, and the feet are resting on the floor (if the patient is sitting in a chair); or that the patient is supine.
This position allows for the most accurate reading. Crossing the legs may elevate the BP reading.

   b. The measurement arm being is supported at heart level, slightly flexed, with the palm facing upward.
The blood pressure will decrease if the arm is above the heart and increase if the arm is below the heart or not supported.

3. Fully expose the arm, being careful that clothing is not tight. Remove clothing rather than rolling up a sleeve.
Clothing that is tight enough to restrict blood flow will alter the reading.

4. Place the cuff on the upper arm. ▼

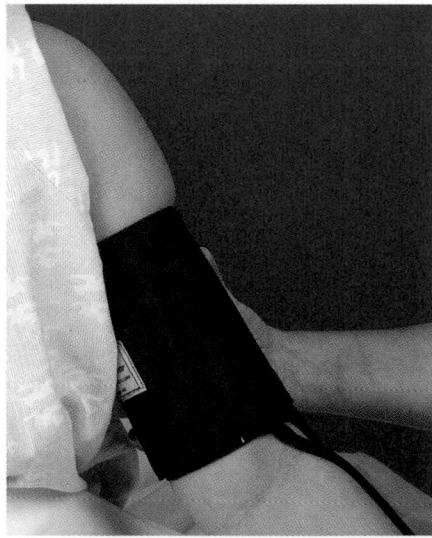

   a. Wrap the cuff snugly.
   b. Ensure that the cuff is totally deflated, and palpate the brachial artery.

   c. Place the bottom edge of the cuff approximately 1 in. (2.5 cm) above the antecubital space.
   d. Place the center of the cuff bladder directly over the brachial artery (the center is often indicated with an arrow on the BP cuff).
The center of the cuff bladder needs to be directly over the brachial artery to obtain an accurate reading. Loose application of the cuff results in overestimation of the pressure.

5. Place the stethoscope ear pieces in your ears, pointing slightly forward.
When the ear pieces point slightly forward, they direct sound into the ear canal, making the sounds more audible.

6. Palpate the brachial artery on the arm with the cuff. (Use the radial artery for this step if you prefer.)
For correct stethoscope placement

7. Inflate the cuff, as follows:
   a. Close the sphygmomanometer valve and inflate the cuff rapidly to about 80 mm Hg.

b. Then palpate the pulse while you continue inflating in 10 mm Hg increments until you no longer feel the pulse.

c. Note the pressure at which the pulse disappears.

d. Go to step 8 or step 8 Variation, as you prefer.

Palpating the artery while inflating the cuff ensures that that the cuff is inflated higher than the systolic BP. If the patient has an auscultatory gap, the systolic pressure can be mistakenly identified as lower than it actually is. Palpation is particularly important if the baseline systolic BP is unknown or if the patient is hypertensive.

8. Continue inflating the cuff to a pressure that is 20 to 30 mm Hg above the level at which the pulse disappeared.

Helps ensure you will not miss an auscultatory gap or a faint first sound.

Step 8 Variation

- Do not continue palpating after the pulse disappears.
- Instead, deflate the cuff rapidly.
- Wait 2 minutes, then place the stethoscope over the brachial artery and inflate the cuff to a pressure that is 20 to 30 mm Hg above the palpated level.
- Continue with steps 9 and 10.

9. Place the stethoscope over the brachial artery as follows: ▼

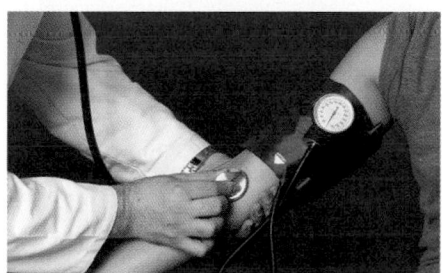

a. Be certain that the stethoscope tubing is not touching anything and that the diaphragm is not tucked under the edge of the cuff.

When the tubing rubs against clothing, for example, it produces artifact sounds that make it difficult to hear the BP sounds. Placing the bell or diaphragm under the cuff can partially occlude the brachial artery, delaying the appearance of the Korotkoff sounds.

b. Using the bell will enable you to hear BP sounds more accurately, especially at diastolic pressures. However, most people use the diaphragm because it is easily placed and because some stethoscopes do not have a bell.

10. Deflate the cuff slowly (2 to 3 mm Hg per second or per beat), listening for the Korotkoff sounds as you deflate. Deflating the cuff more slowly increases patient discomfort and may alter the reading. Deflating the cuff faster may cause errors in hearing the Korotkoff sounds.

a. Note the point on the manometer at which you hear the first sound. This is the systolic BP. (If you are using an electronic BP device, read the digital screen when the numbers appear. Follow the manufacturer's instructions.)

The 1st Korotkoff sound is the systolic pressure.

b. Continue deflating the cuff, and note the level at which the sounds become muffled and disappear. The diastolic pressure is the point at which the sound disappears.

The 5th Korotkoff sound (the disappearance of sound) is the diastolic BP in adults. The 4th Korotkoff sound (the muffling of sounds) is the diastolic BP in children. The AHA recommends recording the first sound, muffling, and last sound in children younger than 13 years, pregnant women, and people with high cardiac output or peripheral vasoconstriction.

11. If you need to repeat the measurement, deflate the cuff completely, and wait 2 minutes before reinflating it. Prevents venous congestion and false high readings.

What if . . .

- **You cannot feel the brachial pulse?**

While supporting the arm at the elbow, have the patient pronate her forearm.

This moves the brachial artery more over a bony prominence, making the pulsation easier to feel.

- **You have difficulty hearing BP sounds for many patients?**

You may need a stethoscope with a built-in amplifier.

- **You are not certain of the systolic reading when you begin to deflate the cuff?**

Do not stop cuff deflation to recheck the systolic reading. Deflate the cuff completely and wait 1 to 3 minutes before taking another measurement.

Stopping deflation and retaking the BP too soon can lead to a muffling of the Korotkoff sounds and inaccurate results.

✚ **You must use a mercury manometer?**

Because mercury is a health hazard, mercury manometers should not be found in healthcare agencies. Use an aneroid manometer or an electronic BP device if one is available. If you must use a mercury manometer, be certain the meniscus of the mercury is at eye level when taking the reading. Take care not to bump equipment against the glass cover over the column of mercury.

- **You are using an automatic blood pressure device?**

Follow the same guidelines as for a manual BP (e.g., cuff size and placement, patient position).

Turn on the machine; be sure the cuff is deflated.

Apply the cuff.

Press the button to start the measurement.

At the tone, read the digital measurement.

- **You do not have a cuff size to fit the upper arm?**

Use the forearm, thigh, or calf. See procedure Variations A, B, and C, respectively.

- **The patient requires contact or isolation precautions?**

Follow agency guidelines for equipment (e.g., stethoscope, BP cuff). Generally the equipment remains in the room with the patient; otherwise it must be disinfected before leaving the room. For information about contact precautions and protective isolation, see Chapter 20 Clinical Insights.

(continued on next page)

Procedure 17-6 ■ Measuring Blood Pressure (continued)

Procedure Variation A. Measuring Blood Pressure in the Forearm

■ Place a properly sized cuff on the forearm, midway between the elbow and the wrist. Auscultate over the radial artery.
■ Note that a forearm reading is not interchangeable with an upper arm reading.

Procedure Variation B. Measuring Blood Pressure in the Thigh

■ Use the thigh or the calf if the cuff will not fit either the upper or lower arm.
NOTE: The thigh systolic measure may be 20 to 30 mm Hg higher than an arm BP reading. The diastolic reading is generally comparable.

■ Place the patient in a prone position. If patient cannot be prone, place supine with knee slightly bent.
■ Choose the correct cuff size. Wrap the cuff snugly around the thigh so that the lower edge of the cuff is approximately 1 in. (2.5 cm) above the popliteal fossa and the center of the cuff bladder is positioned directly over the popliteal artery (often indicated with an arrow on the blood pressure cuff). Palpate and auscultate over the popliteal artery. ▼

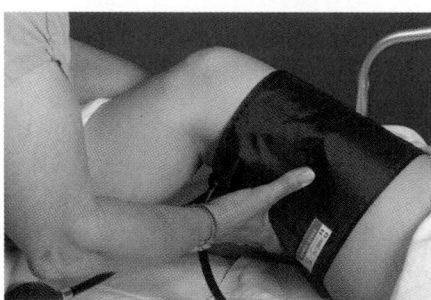

Procedure Variation C. Measuring Blood Pressure in the Calf

■ Use the thigh or the calf if the cuff will not fit either the upper or lower arm.
■ Place the patient supine.
■ Choose the correct size cuff. Wrap the cuff snugly around the calf so that the lower edge of the cuff is approximately 2.5 cm above the malleoli or ankle. Place the stethoscope over either the dorsalis pedis or the posterior tibial artery. Calf BP measurements are not equivalent to upper arm measurements in adults; they tend produce a higher systolic BP.

Evaluation

■ Compare the BP reading with previous readings.
■ Look for trends. Is the BP slowly decreasing (e.g., impending shock) or slowly increasing (e.g., hypervolemia)?
■ Look for a corresponding change in pulse rate, indicating potential hypoxemia.
■ If this is the first BP measurement for the client, check readings in both arms.
A difference of 10 mm Hg or less is normal.
■ Report any significant changes in the BP reading.

Patient Teaching

Teach the patient about:
■ Normal BP values (keep in mind that prehypertension is diagnosed at a lower level when using self-monitored readings).
■ Significance of the BP reading.
■ Further follow-up that may be necessary.

Home Care

■ The American Heart Association (AHA) and other guidelines recommend self-monitoring of BP at home. It is thought that self-measurement of BP provides more reliable data than office BP because of the availability of multiple readings. It is also thought to improve adherence to treatment regimens.
■ If possible, use the same equipment each time to prevent false changes in measurement.
■ Explain the need for frequent recalibration of the home-monitoring device.

■ Assess the skill level of the person(s) who will be measuring the patient's BP in the home, and provide instruction if necessary.
■ Assess whether self-monitoring is causing the client to be anxious.
Some clients do become overly anxious when they know they must monitor their BP, or when they obtain a high reading. Self-monitoring should not be used if it produces too much anxiety; this raises the BP even more.
■ Teach clients not to change their medication dosage without consulting their primary provider when their BP goes up or down.

✚ Before leaving the home, clean the stethoscope and sphygmomanometer with detergent or disinfectant, when possible; or place them in a plastic bag for transporting to the reprocessing location.

✚ If the client has an infection with a multidrug-resistant organism, reusable equipment such as stethoscopes should remain in the home. If the stethoscope and sphygmomanometer cannot remain in the home, clean and disinfect them before leaving the home, using a low to intermediate level disinfectant. If this is not practical, place them in a plastic bag and transport them to another site for cleaning and disinfection.

Documentation

■ You will usually document BP on a flowsheet (such as in Procedure 17-5, Documentation).
■ Document the blood pressure systolic/diastolic readings (e.g., 130/80).

- If you hear the 4th Korotkoff sound or muffling, document systolic/muffling/diastolic (e.g., 130/80/70). If you hear an auscultatory gap, document "systolic/ diastolic with an auscultatory gap from . . ." For example, "170/90 with an auscultatory gap from 170 to 140."
- Follow agency policy regarding the recording of muffled sounds.
- If you chose an alternate site, document the site used and the reason for not using the upper arm.

Practice Resources

American Association of Critical-Care Nurses (2006); American Heart Association (n.d.); British Hypertension Society, Hypertension Influence Team (2006); Centers for Disease Control and Prevention (2005); Gyi, A. (2007); Joint National Committee on Prevention, Detection, Evaluation, and Treatment of High Blood Pressure (2003); Lockwood, C., Conroy-Hiller, T., & Page, T. (2004); Rhinehart, E. (2001); Siegel, J., Rhinehart, E., Jackson, M., et al. (2006); Siegel, J. D., Rhinehart, E., Jackson, M., et al. (2007); Vital Signs (1999).

Thinking About the Procedure

 Go to the *Fundamentals of Nursing Skills Videos*, **Blood Pressure: Manual and Automatic.**

1. At the beginning of the procedure using the manual method (with an aneroid manometer), the nurse places her left hand on the patient's legs for a moment. Why did she do that?

2. What size cuff did the nurse use?

3. When using the automatic device, how many times did the nurse press on the machine? For what reasons?

 For suggested responses, go to Chapter 17, **Thinking About the Procedure Suggested Responses,** on the Student Resource Disk or DavisPlus at http://davisplus.fadavis.com/ Wilkinson2

Clinical Insight 17-1 ▷ Taking an Accurate Blood Pressure

To improve your technique and accuracy of measurement, use the following tips in addition to Procedure 17-6.
- Explain the procedure, particularly on admission or when changing the routine.

Reduces patient anxiety.

- Wait 30 minutes before assessing BP after client has ingested caffeine or smoked.
- Do not assess BP while the client is in pain.
- Apply the cuff over bare skin, if possible. Controversy surrounds this issue, so follow the manufacturer's instructions; advise clients who are home monitoring to apply the cuff over bare skin.
- Instruct the client not to talk during BP measurement. You should not talk either.
- Keep environmental noise and client movement to a minimum.
- Hold the stethoscope lightly but completely against the skin; do not put your thumb on top of the bell or diaphragm. Try not to allow the tubing to brush against your clothing or the bed.

- Do not be influenced by the client's previous BP measurements.
- Use the same limb for each measurement, unless you are comparing arms or averaging readings from both arms.
- For the initial reading, measure the BP in both arms and use the arm with the higher reading for subsequent measurements.
- If you obtain an elevated reading, confirm in the other arm.
- Do not draw conclusions based on one reading. Take two or more readings, at least 2 to 5 minutes apart, and average them. If the readings differ by more than 5 mm Hg, obtain and average additional readings.

Practice Resources

Joint National Committee on Prevention, Detection, Evaluation, and Treatment of High Blood Pressure (2003); Ma, G., Sabin, N., & Dawes, M. (2008); McKay, D. (2008).

Clinical Insight 17-2 ▷ Choosing a Blood Pressure Cuff Size

- The *width* of the bladder should cover approximately two-thirds of the *length* of the upper arm (or other extremity) for an adult, and the entire upper arm for a child.
- Another method for sizing: (1) the cuff width should be 40% of the arm circumference, and (2) the *length* of the bladder should encircle 80% of the arm.
- Perhaps the easiest sizing method is to measure *arm circumference* and follow this guideline from the National Guideline Clearinghouse (2005):

For arm circumference	Cuff should be
22–26 cm (8 ½ × 10 ¼ in.)	"small adult" size: 12 × 22 cm (4 ¾ × 8 ¾ in.)
27–34 cm (10 ½ × 13 ½ in.)	"adult" size: 16 × 30 cm (6 ¼ × 11 ¾ in.)
35–44 cm (13 ¾ × 17 ¼ in.)	"large adult" size: 16 × 36 cm (6 ¼ × 14 ¼ in.)
45–52 cm (17 ¾ × 10 ½ in.)	"adult thigh" size: 16 × 42 cm (6 ¼ × 16 ⅝ in.)

Practice Resources

National Guideline Clearinghouse (2005).

Forms

Graphic Flowsheet

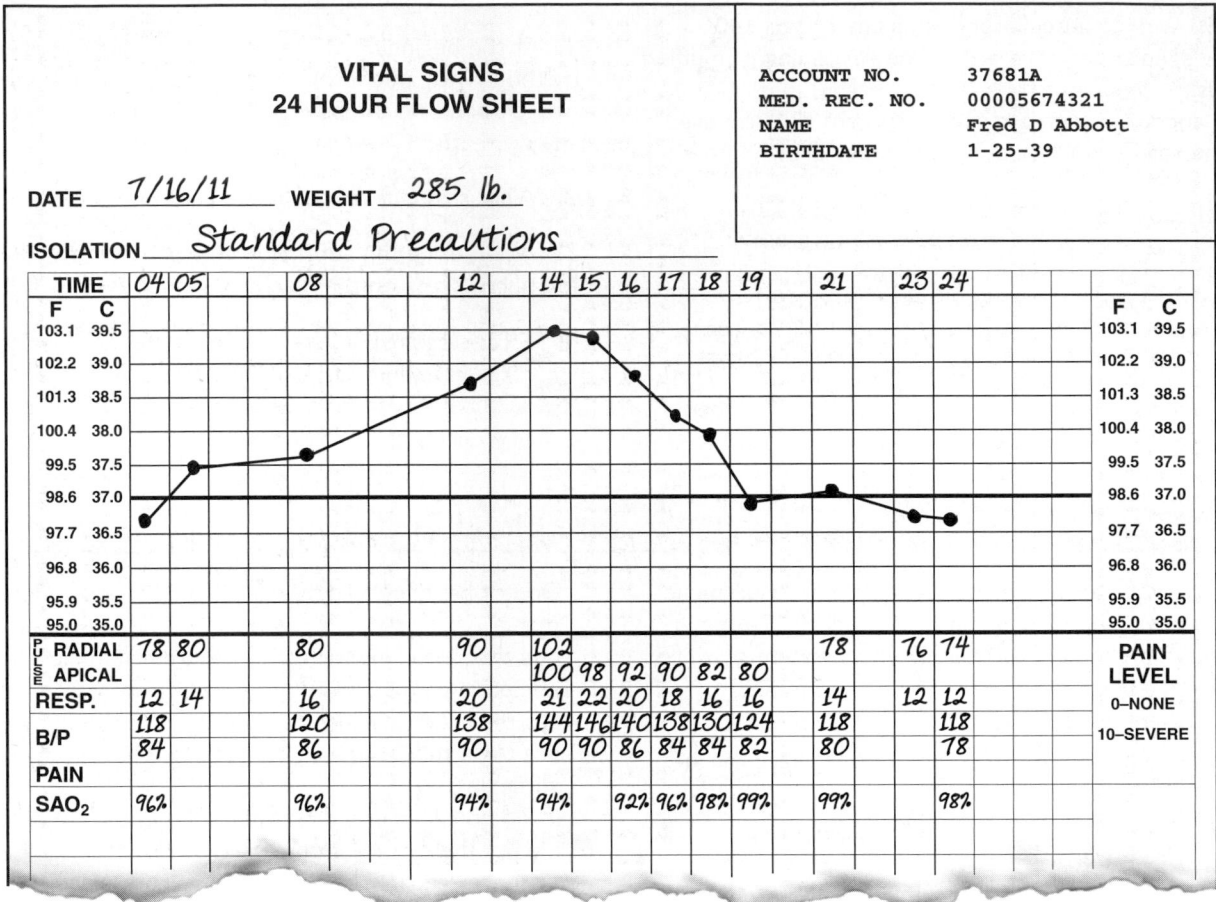

VITAL SIGNS 24 HOUR FLOW SHEET

ACCOUNT NO.	37681A
MED. REC. NO.	00005674321
NAME	Fred D Abbott
BIRTHDATE	1-25-39

DATE __7/16/11__ WEIGHT __285 lb.__

ISOLATION __Standard Precautions__

TIME	04	05		08			12		14	15	16	17	18	19		21		23	24				PAIN LEVEL
PULSE RADIAL	78	80		80			90		102							78		76	74				0–NONE
PULSE APICAL										100	98	92	90	82	80								
RESP.	12	14		16			20		21	22	20	18	16	16		14		12	12				10–SEVERE
B/P	118			120			138		144	146	140	138	130	124		118			118				
	84			86			90		90	90	86	84	84	82		80			78				
PAIN																							
SAO₂	96%			96%			94%		94%		92%	96%	98%	99%		99%			98%				

Temperature graph values (F / C):
103.1 / 39.5
102.2 / 39.0
101.3 / 38.5
100.4 / 38.0
99.5 / 37.5
98.6 / 37.0
97.7 / 36.5
96.8 / 36.0
95.9 / 35.5
95.0 / 35.0

Standardized Language

NOC Outcomes and NIC Interventions Associated with Abnormal Vital Signs		
SELECTED NURSING DIAGNOSES	**SELECTED NOC OUTCOMES**	**SELECTED NIC INTERVENTIONS**
Hyperthermia	**Temperature** Thermoregulation	Fever Treatment
	Thermoregulation: Newborn	Temperature Regulation
	Vital Signs	Vital Signs Monitoring
Hypothermia	Thermoregulation	Hypothermia Treatment
	Thermoregulation: Newborn	Newborn Care
	Vital Signs	Temperature Regulation
		Vital Signs Monitoring
Ineffective Thermoregulation	Thermoregulation	Newborn Care
	Thermoregulation: Newborn	Temperature Regulation
		Temperature Regulation: Intraoperative
Risk for Imbalanced Body Temperature	Thermoregulation	Newborn Care
	Thermoregulation: Newborn	Temperature Regulation
		Temperature Regulation: Intraoperative
		Vital Signs Monitoring

NOC Outcomes and NIC Interventions Associated with Abnormal Vital Signs—cont'd

SELECTED NURSING DIAGNOSES	SELECTED NOC OUTCOMES	SELECTED NIC INTERVENTIONS
Decreased Cardiac Output	**Pulse** Vital Signs	Vital Signs Monitoring
Ineffective Breathing Pattern	**Respirations** Mechanical Ventilation Mechanical Ventilatory Weaning Respiratory Status: Airway Patency Respiratory Status: Ventilation Vital Signs	Airway Management Asthma Management Mechanical Ventilation Respiratory Monitoring Ventilation Assistance Vital Signs Monitoring
Risk for Falls secondary to hypotension	**Blood Pressure** Falls Occurrence	Fall Prevention Risk Identification Self-Care Assistance: Transfer

Sources: NANDA International (2007). *Nursing diagnoses: Definitions and classification 2007-2009*. Philadelphia: Author; Johnson, M., Bulechek, G., Butcher, H., et al. (2006). *Nursing diagnoses, outcomes, and interventions: NANDA, NIC, and NOC linkages* (2nd ed.). St. Louis, MO: C.V. Mosby.

Tables

Centigrade–Fahrenheit Conversion Chart

°CENTIGRADE	°FAHRENHEIT	°CENTIGRADE	°FAHRENHEIT
34.0	93.2	38.8	101.8
34.2	93.6	39.0	102.2
34.4	93.9	39.2	102.5
34.6	94.3	39.4	102.9
34.8	94.6	39.6	103.2
35.0	95.0	39.8	103.6
35.2	95.4	40.0	104.0
35.4	95.7	40.2	104.3
35.6	96.1	40.4	104.7
35.8	96.4	40.6	105.1
36.0	96.8	40.8	105.4
36.2	97.1	41.0	105.8
36.4	97.5	41.2	106.1
36.6	97.8	41.4	106.5
36.8	98.2	41.6	106.8
37.0	98.6	41.8	107.2
37.2	98.9	42.0	107.6
37.4	99.3	42.2	108.0
37.6	99.6	42.4	108.3
37.8	100.0	42.6	108.7
38.0	100.4	42.8	109.0
38.2	100.7	43.0	109.4
38.4	101.1	44.0	111.2
38.6	101.4		

THINKING CRITICALLY ABOUT VITAL SIGNS

The exercises in the following sections allow you to practice the kind of thinking you will use as a full-spectrum nurse. Because these are critical-thinking questions, there is usually no single right answer. We do not provide answers for these questions because it is more important for you to think about the questions than to arrive at the "right" answer. These questions are designed to improve your thinking more than to "cover content." Discuss answers with your peers—discussion can stimulate critical thinking. If you have difficulty with any of these questions, consult with your instructor.

Applying the Full-Spectrum Nursing Model

PATIENT SITUATION

A patient in the critical care unit had a stable pulse and BP for the first few days. He has become more ill and now his pulse and BP are weak and difficult to palpate. His last BP reading was abnormally low, so it must be monitored frequently. He is receiving intravenous fluids in both arms.

THINKING

1. *Critical Thinking (Reflecting and Deciding What to Do)*: Which of the patient's vital signs (TPR and BP) might you be able to delegate to nursing assistive personnel?

DOING

2. *Practical Knowledge*: How would you take the patient's blood pressure? Be specific: (a) What site would you use? (b) What equipment would you use?

3. *Nursing Process (Assessment)*:

   a. Will you need to validate any of the vital signs you obtain? If so, why?

   b. How could you validate those vital signs?

CARING

4. Assume that you are very busy. How would you demonstrate caring to this patient while you are assessing his vital signs (the ones you did not delegate to a NAP)?

Critical Thinking and Clinical Reasoning

1. Recall the clients you encountered at the community health fair (Meet Your Patient, Volume 1). Two-year-old Jason's oral temperature was 102°F (38.9°C); his skin was warm, dry, and flushed. His mother told you that he had been eating poorly and was very irritable. What cues alert you that something is wrong?

2. You have already established (in Volume 1) what, if any, additional information you need to determine the meaning of Jason's temperature elevation.

   a. What theoretical knowledge may account for Jason's temperature?

   b. Are there any actions you should take while meeting with Jason and his mother? If so, what?

   c. What biases do you have that affect your thinking about this situation? (This requires self-knowledge.)

3. Suppose you have the following data: In a long-term-care center, where most patients are older, the average normal oral temperature of the patients is 97.1°F (36.2°C). In a local well-baby nursery, the average skin temperature of the newborns ranges from 97.7° to 98.6°F (36.5°– 37.0°C), but it fluctuates during the first 24 hours after birth. At a walk-in surgery center, the average oral temperature of the healthy clients is 98°F (36.7°C).

   a. What conclusion might you draw about what is causing the differences in average body temperature among these three groups? (*Clue:* First list the average temperatures in order, from highest to lowest.)

   b. What theoretical knowledge did you use to answer that question?

4. Suppose you have the following data about patients' temperatures:

   Patient A, 58 years old: 0600, 97.7°F (36.5°C); 1200, 98.8°F (37.1°C); 2100, 99°F (37.2°C)

   Patient B, 14 years old: 0600, 97.5°F (36.4°C); 1200, 97.9°F (36°C); 2100, 98.4°F (36.9°C)

   Patient C, 80 years old: 0600, 96.4°F (35.8°C); 1200, 96.8°F (37.1°C); 2100, 97.2°F (36.2°C)

   What conclusion can you draw about what is probably affecting the patients' temperatures? (*Clue:* Look at the pattern for each patient. How are the patterns similar?)

5. Organize a small group of classmates. Obtain several different sizes of blood pressure cuffs for each member of the group. Practice checking blood pressures on each other. Vary the size of the cuffs used, and note the variation generated by the change in cuff size. List your findings here (for at least three different people and at least two cuff sizes).

	Cuff Size		
BP Reading	**Large**	**Medium**	**Small**
Person A			
Person B			
Person C			

6. Analyze the following scenario. A 46-year-old man is hospitalized for multiple trauma after a mountain bike accident.

   Vital signs on admission: BP, 138/90; pulse, 108 beats/min; respirations 24 breaths/min; temperature, 37.2°C (98.9°F)

   8 hours later: BP, 162/100; pulse, 122 beats/min; respirations, 26 breaths/min; temperature, 37.9°C (100.2°F)

   He is restless, agitated, and in pain.

   a. What is going on in this situation that may be influencing the VS?

   b. Do you have enough patient information to determine what is happening?

   c. What nursing actions should you consider?

   d. Should you involve others in your discussion of possible actions? If so, who?

   e. What can you delegate in this situation?

   f. Should you report this change in vital signs to the primary care provider? Why or why not?

7. Ms. Alvin is an 80-year-old patient in a long-term care facility. Her blood pressures have been in the range of 120/70 to 130/80 for the past month. When she is newly assigned to your care, you see that according to her chart, she has a history of hypertension. She is taking an antihypertensive medication. You observe that she is very thin, especially her extremities. She weighs only 90 lb (40.8 kg) although she is of average height.

   a. Do you think the charted BPs are probably accurate? Why or why not?

   b. How could you make sure that the recorded BP readings are accurate?

   c. After looking for a small BP cuff, you discover that there is only one size available in the agency: a standard adult size. What should you do?

8. For each of the following concepts, use critical thinking to describe how or why it is important to nursing, patient care, and measuring vital signs. Note that these are not to be merely definitions.

Vital signs	Radial artery
Circadian rhythm	Brachial artery
Metabolism	Apical pulse
Shivering	Diaphragm
Fever	Oxygen saturation and pulse oximetry
Pulse	Blood pressure
Stethoscope	Peripheral resistance

▰ What Are the Main Points in This Chapter?

➤ Vital signs (temperature, pulse, respirations, and blood pressure) are indicators of a person's state of health and functioning of the body systems.

➤ Many factors, such as age, activity, smoking, and gender, cause normal variations in vital signs.

➤ Body temperature is the balance between heat production and heat loss.

➤ Fever is a symptom, but it is also beneficial to the immune response.

➤ A normal pulse rate varies widely according to age, from an average of 120 beats/min for newborns to 80 beats/min for adults.

➤ Assess the pulse for quality, bilateral equality, volume, and rate.

➤ Respiration is the process of supplying the body with oxygen and disposing of carbon dioxide.

➤ Assess respirations for rate, depth, rhythm, and associated clinical signs (e.g., breath sounds, chest movement, cough, pallor, and cyanosis).

➤ Blood pressure is the pressure of the blood as it is forced against arterial walls during cardiac contraction.

➤ Prehypertension is blood pressure ranging between 120 and 139 systolic or between 80 and 89 mm Hg diastolic obtained with two readings taken 6 minutes apart.

➤ Hypertension is persistent elevated BP (> 140 systolic or > 90 mm Hg diastolic) on more than two separate occasions.

➤ Clients can prevent or modify hypertension through certain lifestyle changes (e.g., exercise, weight control, and stress management).

➤ Nurses can delegate the activity of taking vital signs, but the nurse is responsible for evaluating the meaning of the data.

For practice questions for this chapter,

 Go to **NCLEX-Style Chapter Quiz,** on the Student Resource Disk or DavisPlus at http://davisplus.fadavis.com/Wilkinson2

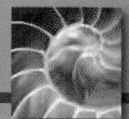

Knowledge Map

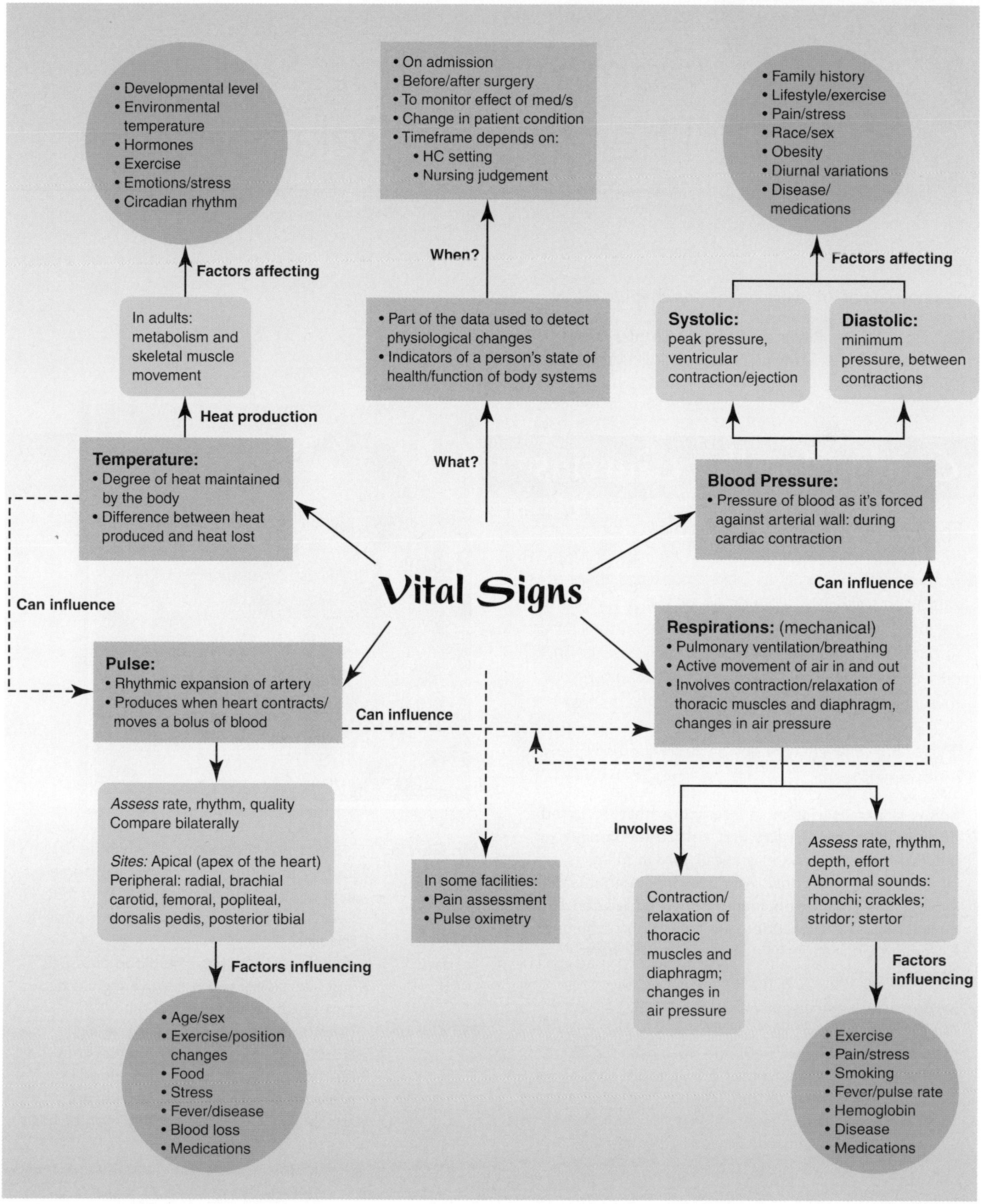

Factors affecting

- Developmental level
- Environmental temperature
- Hormones
- Exercise
- Emotions/stress
- Circadian rhythm

When?

- On admission
- Before/after surgery
- To monitor effect of med/s
- Change in patient condition
- Timeframe depends on:
  - HC setting
  - Nursing judgement

Factors affecting

- Family history
- Lifestyle/exercise
- Pain/stress
- Race/sex
- Obesity
- Diurnal variations
- Disease/ medications

In adults: metabolism and skeletal muscle movement

- Part of the data used to detect physiological changes
- Indicators of a person's state of health/function of body systems

Systolic: peak pressure, ventricular contraction/ejection

Diastolic: minimum pressure, between contractions

Heat production

What?

Temperature:
- Degree of heat maintained by the body
- Difference between heat produced and heat lost

Blood Pressure:
- Pressure of blood as it's forced against arterial wall: during cardiac contraction

Vital Signs

Can influence

Can influence

Pulse:
- Rhythmic expansion of artery
- Produces when heart contracts/ moves a bolus of blood

Can influence

Respirations: (mechanical)
- Pulmonary ventilation/breathing
- Active movement of air in and out
- Involves contraction/relaxation of thoracic muscles and diaphragm, changes in air pressure

Assess rate, rhythm, quality
Compare bilaterally

Sites: Apical (apex of the heart)
Peripheral: radial, brachial carotid, femoral, popliteal, dorsalis pedis, posterior tibial

Involves

In some facilities:
- Pain assessment
- Pulse oximetry

Contraction/ relaxation of thoracic muscles and diaphragm; changes in air pressure

Assess rate, rhythm, depth, effort
Abnormal sounds: rhonchi; crackles; stridor; stertor

Factors influencing

Factors influencing

- Age/sex
- Exercise/position changes
- Food
- Stress
- Fever/disease
- Blood loss
- Medications

Factors influencing

- Exercise
- Pain/stress
- Smoking
- Fever/pulse rate
- Hemoglobin
- Disease
- Medications

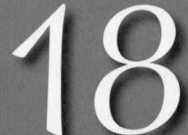

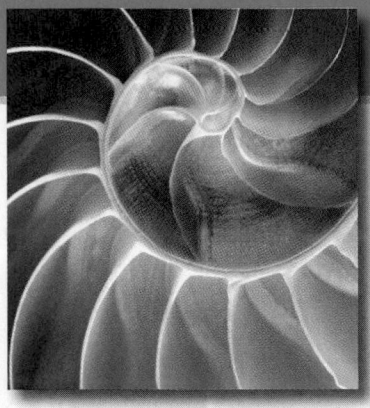

Communicating & Therapeutic Relationships

For a podcast of an overview of this chapter,

 Go to Student Resources, **Podcast – Chapter Overviews,**
Chapter 18, on DavisPlus at http://davisplus.fadavis.com/
Wilkinson2

Caring for the Garcias

*The exercises in the following section allow you to practice
the kind of thinking you will use as a full-spectrum nurse.
Because these are critical-thinking questions, there is
usually no single right answer. We do not provide answers
for these questions because it is more important for you
to think about the questions than to arrive at the "right"
answer. These questions are designed to improve your
thinking more than to "cover content." Discuss answers
with your peers—discussion can stimulate critical thinking.
If you have difficulty with any of these questions, consult
with your instructor.*

Below is a transcript of an interaction that occurred
during Mr. Joseph Garcia's first visit to the family
medical center. As you may recall, Jordan Miller is a
family nurse practitioner who is examining Mr. Garcia.
Analyze the interaction. Identify open-ended and closed
questions and therapeutic communication techniques.
Comment on responses that Jordan might have
improved on.

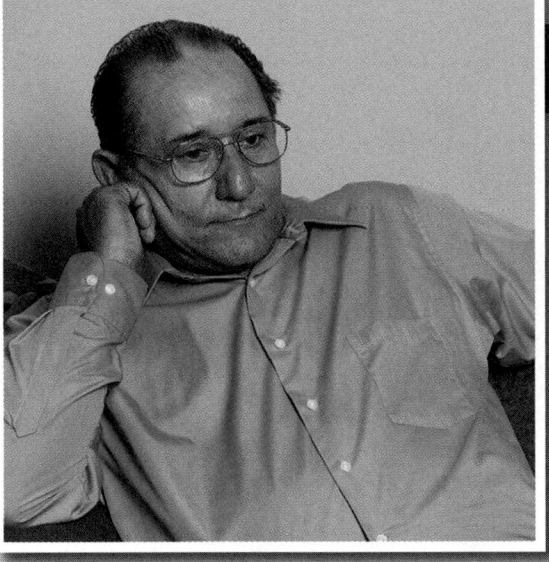

Jordan:	Are your parents still living?
Mr. Garcia:	Yes, they're both alive. My father is 80 years old, and my mother is 76.
Jordan:	I'd like to hear a little more about your family history. Tell me about your father's cancer. How old was he when he was first diagnosed? Has he had treatment?
Mr. Garcia:	He was probably about 60 when he first found out about it. I know he had some kind of surgery and takes medicines, but I don't know the details. He seems all right, though.
Jordan:	Your father also has high blood pressure and heart disease. Please give me a little more history about that.
Mr. Garcia:	My father and mother both have high blood pressure and heart disease. They both take medicines for their blood pressure. My father had a small heart attack about 10 years ago. My mother has

Caring for the Garcias (continued)

Jordan:	never had a heart attack that I know of, but she sometimes has chest pain. Your mother also has diabetes?	**Mrs. Garcia:**	A lot of people in my family have diabetes, too. But so far I'm OK, I think. My family is from Mexico, and I know a
Mr. Garcia:	She's had that for a long time. My parents joke about that. My father is part Cuban and part Irish. A lot of people in his family, especially on the Latin side, have diabetes, but nobody in my mother's family. Yet my mother is the one with the diabetes!	**Jordan:** **Mrs. Garcia:**	lot of diabetics back home. Have you been seen for a health exam lately, Mrs. Garcia? Not in about a year, but I'm going to schedule an appointment here.

Practical Knowledge knowing how

This section provides clinical insights, assessments, outcomes, and interventions for communicating with patients.

Clinical Insights

Clinical Insight 18–1 ▶ Enhancing Communication Through Nonverbal Behaviors

Nonverbal Behaviors	Interpretation
Direct eye contact	Demonstrates interest and attention. The nurse must consider the client's cultural heritage when determining how much eye contact is appropriate.
Concerned facial expression	Lends credibility, if congruent with conversation.
Leaning forward	Shows interest in the conversation.
Personal space	Maintaining a distance of 18 inches to 4 feet allows most clients to feel comfortable during the interaction. Adjust the distance within that range based on the client's preference.
Professional appearance	Gives people an impression of how you may act in your role as a healthcare provider.
Sitting down to talk	Communicates willingness to listen and a sense of not wanting to rush the interaction with the client.
Touch	Conveys caring and concern when used appropriately.

Clinical Insight 18–2 ▶ Assertive Communication

- Maintain eye contact, as culturally appropriate.
- Speak clearly and firmly.
- Project a clear tone of voice.
- Communicate self-confidently.
- Maintain professional composure.
- Communicate in a positive manner.
- Refrain from sarcasm.

- Ensure congruence between verbal and nonverbal messages.
- Guide the direction of the discussion.
- Use "I" statements.
- Focus on the issues.
- Do not invite negative responses.
- Avoid self-effacing statements.

Clinical Insight 18-3 ▶ Communicating with SBAR*

Situation	In 10 seconds, identify yourself and the patient and describe the present situation that prompted you to call. State: your name your unit the patient's name and room number the problem
Background	Give other information pertinent to the situation—not the patient's entire history since admission, but circumstances leading up to the situation (e.g., medications, lab results, current symptoms).
Assessment	State the problem and what you think is causing it. This is an inference rather than traditional data collection.
Recommendation	State what you think will correct the problem, or what you need from the physician.

*If you need other information about SBAR,

 Go to Chapter 16, Volume 1.

Practice Resources

Beyea, S. (2004); Carroll, T. L. (2006); Haig, K. M., Sutton, S., & Whittington, J. (2006); Institute for Healthcare Improvement (2008); Pope, B. B., Rodzen, L., & Spross, G. (2007).

Clinical Insight 18-4 ▶ Communicating with Clients from Another Culture

General Guidelines

- Most important: Be aware of your own cultural beliefs and attitudes.
- Learn about other cultures, especially those in your area.
- Convey empathy and show respect.
- Be certain the communication strategies you usually use are culturally appropriate for the individual.
  Is direct eye contact viewed as aggressive or impolite?
  How much space should you keep between yourself and the patient?
- Use touch cautiously. In some cultures, it is inappropriate to touch certain parts of the body.
- Proceed slowly. Rushing may cause the patient to be more anxious, and is offensive to some.
- Smile and be polite, but not overfriendly or casual. Use the patient's title and last name when introducing yourself.
- Use short words and sentences. Don't give too much information in one sentence.
- Present one idea at a time.
- Provide written teaching materials.

If There Is a Language Barrier

- Written information provided must be appropriate to the population served and the language of the patient (The Joint Commission, 2008, p. 156).
- Use a trained medical interpreter, if possible.
- To review guidelines for communicating with clients who speak a different language, go to Clinical Insight 13-5 in Chapter 13 of this book.
- Some medical dictionaries (e.g., *Taber's Cyclopedic Medical Dictionary*, 2009) have a comprehensive list of English–Spanish phrases.
- The following are some useful Spanish words and phrases.

English	Spanish	English	Spanish
How do you feel?	¿Como se siente?	Cough	Tosa
Good	Bien	Open your mouth	Abra la boca
Bad	Mal	Take a deep breath	Respire profundamente
Have you any difficulty breathing?	¿Tiene dificultad al respirar?	You may eat	Puede comer
Are you thirsty?	¿Tiene sed?	Tea	Té
Have you any pain?	¿Tiene dolor?	Coffee	Café
Show me where	Enséñeme dónde	I will give you something for	Le dare algo para eso
Is it worse now?	¿Está peor ahora?	A pill	Una píldora

Spanish Patient-Education Materials

The following U. S. government sites offer free, reliable patient-education materials. For other online sources:

 Go to Chapter 18, **Resources for Caregivers & Health Professionals,** on the Student Resource Disk or DavisPlus at http://davisplus.fadavis.com/Wilkinson2

■ **http://www.fda.gov/oc/spanish**
Quick Information for Your Health. The Food and Drug Administration (FDA). U.S. Department of Health & Human Services. (Easy to read)

■ **http://www.ahrq.gov/consumer/espanoix.htm**
Spanish Information. Agency for Healthcare Research and Quality (AHRQ), U.S. Department of Health & Human Services. (Topics such as how to prevent medical errors, having surgery, and choosing a health plan)

■ **http://www.cdc.gov/flu/professionals/patiented.htm**
The Flu Gallery: Patient and Provider Education materials. Centers for Disease Control and Prevention. (Information about preventing and treating the flu)

■ **http://www.usa.gov/gobiernousa/Temas/Salud-Nutricion-Seguridad.shtml?toggleTo=en_Health**
Health, Nutrition, and Safety. U.S. General Services Administration, FirstGov.gov site. (Basic health topics, community health services, food safety, and so on.)

■ **http://www.nlm.nih.gov/medlineplus/spanish/healthtopics.html**
Health Topics. MedlinePlus, U.S. National Library of Medicine, National Institutes of Health, Department of Health and Human Services. (Health information sorted by body location and systems, disorders, demographic groups, and so on.)

 Go to Chapter 18, **Resources for Caregivers & Health Professionals,** on the Student Resource Disk or DavisPlus at http://davisplus.fadavis.com/Wilkinson2

Clinical Insight 18-5 ▶ Communicating with Clients Who Have Impaired Speech

Healthcare agencies should address the communication needs of those with vision, speech, hearing, language, and cognitive impairments (The Joint Commission, 2008, p. 156).
■ Nonverbal communication is the key to communication with clients with impaired speech.
■ Ask the client use hand gestures and a picture board, as appropriate.
■ Solicit family assistance in understanding the client's speech.
■ Provide a comfortable environment for the client to practice speaking.

■ Be positive and patient.
■ Although the client may have difficulty speaking, you should continue to speak and explain all procedures.
■ A referral to a speech pathologist may be necessary.

Reference
Adams-Wendling, L., & Pimple, C. (2007, June).

Clinical Insight 18-6 ▶ Communicating with Clients Who Have Impaired Cognition or Consciousness

Clients Who Are Cognitively Impaired

Always try to communicate.	Make every effort to communicate, even if you think that the client cannot understand you.
Don't rush the client.	Provide adequate time to allow the client to communicate. He needs time to respond to your questions or commands.
Use multiple communication modalities.	Provide verbal and written discharge instructions. Review the instructions several times with the client before discharge, and include family members in the teaching.
Provide reminders.	Use memory aids, schedules, and reminder notices to reinforce information.
Orient the client.	Verbally orient to time, person, and place, and provide visual orientation materials, such as a calendar or schedule.
Stimulate memory.	If the client loses his place in the conversation, stimulate memory by repeating his last expressed thought (e.g., "We were talking about your back pain. Tell me more about your back pain").
Use short sentences.	Use short sentences, containing a single thought (e.g., "Are you hungry?"). Avoid complex statements (e.g., "You look hungry. Would you like a sandwich or a milk shake, or can you hold off until dinner?")

(continued on next page)

Clinical Insight 18–6 ▶ **Communicating with Clients Who Have Impaired Cognition or Consciousness** (continued)

Ask "yes/no" questions.	Ask direct questions that require only a "yes" or "no" answer (e.g., "Are you hungry?").
Limit choices.	Limit choices to avoid confusing or frustrating the patient.
Be concrete and specific.	Do not use vague comments to indicate that you are listening. The client may be unable to interpret comments such as, "I see." Instead, repeat the client's words and directly state your response (e.g., "You are cold. I will bring you a blanket").
Avoid slang and jargon.	The client may not understand, and may become anxious.
Use gestures.	Model desired behaviors. You might say "Brush your teeth now" and then pantomime brushing your teeth.
Don't assume.	Bear in mind that the client cannot behave differently and that he may be confused about reality. When the person is talking about superficial, routine matters, he may seem more competent than he is.
For clients with expressive difficulties:	▪ If you are sure of the word the person is trying to say, repeat it. Don't guess, though. ▪ Pay close attention to nonverbal communication. ▪ Assess for and anticipate unmet needs, such as hunger, thirst, and pain. ▪ Respond to the emotion, not the words. ▪ Do not reprimand the patient if she curses or is aggressive.

Patients Who Are Unconscious

▪ Touch and speak to unconscious or sedated patients, and advise them of care you are providing. Although the patient may not be able to respond, she may be able to hear your comments.

▪ Consult with previous caregivers or the family to determine what the patient responds to.

▪ Begin each interaction by identifying yourself and calling the patient by name.

▪ Speak calmly and slowly.

▪ Explain all healthcare procedures.

▪ Provide soothing music and periods of rest.

Practice Resources

Jayasekara, R. (2009); Miller, C. A. (2008); Stern, C. (2006, October).

Assessment Guidelines and Tools

Focused Assessment: Communication

A focused assessment should identify factors that alter a patient's ability to receive, understand, and transmit verbal and nonverbal messages.

Medications	▪ Is the patient taking medications that might interfere with speech, cognition, or level of consciousness?
Language Barriers	▪ What is the patient's primary language? ▪ Does the patient have sufficient command of the dominant language? ▪ Is an interpreter (foreign language or sign language) required? ▪ Can the patient read and write? At what level and in what language?
Cognitive Function	▪ What is the patient's level of consciousness? ▪ Is there short-term or long-term memory loss, or both? ▪ Is intellectual function at, below, or above expectations for age? ▪ Can the patient read simple instructions? ▪ Can the patient follow simple spoken instructions? ▪ Can the patient understand a yes-no choice? ▪ Are there symptoms or a diagnosis of mental illness or dementia? ▪ If the patient is unconscious, are there nonverbal responses that indicate he can hear you (e.g., blinking, moving the head, squeezing your hand)?

Focused Assessment: Communication—cont'd

Hearing	▪ Ask the patient, and observe, whether there are hearing problems.
	▪ Is the patient wearing a hearing aid? If so, is it working properly? Does the patient appear to be reading your lips?
	▪ Is the patient trying to use sign language to communicate?
	▪ Refer to Chapter 19 for tests of hearing (e.g., ticking watch).
Vision	▪ Is the patient wearing glasses or contact lenses?
	▪ Is the patient able to see adequately?
	▪ Refer to Chapter 19 for vision tests.
	▶ Also see **Brief Bedside Assessment,** Skills Videos to Accompany Fundamentals of Nursing.
Aphasia	▪ Is there a history of stroke, or a diagnosis of aphasia?
	▪ Is there receptive aphasia (inability to receive or interpret verbal or nonverbal messages)?
	▪ Is there expressive aphasia (inability to express verbal or nonverbal messages)?
Physiological barriers	Does the patient have conditions that cause difficulty speaking, such as:
	▪ Dyspnea?
	▪ Artificial airway?
	▪ Oral problems, such as poorly fitted dentures?
	▪ Cleft palate or other structural problems?
Communication Style	▪ Is it difficult to understand what the patient says (e.g., slurring words, stuttering, inability to pronounce certain sounds)?
	▪ Does the patient speak readily, or refuse to speak?
	▪ Does the patient speak slowly or rapidly; spontaneously or hesitantly?
	▪ Is the vocabulary adequate for the purpose needed?
	▪ Has the vocabulary changed from the person's normal vocabulary?
Other	▪ Are verbal and nonverbal communication congruent?

Standardized Language

Selected NOC Outcomes and NIC Interventions for Impaired Verbal Communication

NOC OUTCOMES	SELECTED OUTCOME INDICATORS	NIC INTERVENTIONS	SELECTED NIC ACTIVITIES
Communication	Acknowledgment of messages received Exchanges messages accurately with others	Active Listening	▪ Be aware of the tone, tempo, volume, pitch, and inflection of the voice. ▪ Use questions or statements to encourage expression of thoughts, feelings, and concerns.
Communication: Expressive	Use of written language Use of pictures and drawings to communicate	Assertiveness Training	▪ Promote expression of thoughts and feelings, both positive and negative.
Communication: Receptive	Interpretation of spoken language Interpretation of sign language	Communication Enhancement (Hearing Deficit, Speech Deficit, Visual Deficit) Presence Touch	▪ (Hearing) Move close to less affected ear. ▪ (Speech) Give one simple direction at a time, as appropriate. ▪ (Vision) Identify yourself when you enter the patient's space. ▪ Be physically available as a helper. ▪ Give a reassuring hug, as appropriate. ▪ Hold the patient's hand to provide emotional support.

Sources: Bulechek, G., Butcher, H. K., & Dochterman, M. J. (Eds.) (2008). *Nursing interventions classification (NIC)* (5th ed.). St. Louis, MO: C.V. Mosby. Used with permission; Johnson, M., Bulechek, G., Butcher, H., et al. (Eds.). (2001). *Nursing diagnoses, outcomes, and interventions: NANDA, NOC, and NIC linkages* (2nd ed.). St. Louis, MO: C.V. Mosby. Used with permission; Moorhead, S., Johnson, M., Maas, M., et al. (Eds.). (2008). *Nursing outcomes classification (NOC)* (4th ed.). St. Louis, MO: C.V. Mosby. Used with permission; NANDA International. (2007). *Nursing diagnoses: Definitions and classification 2007–2008.* Philadelphia: Author. Used with permission.

THINKING CRITICALLY ABOUT COMMUNICATING AND THERAPEUTIC RELATIONSHIPS

The exercises in the following sections allow you to practice the kind of thinking you will use as a full-spectrum nurse. Because these are critical-thinking questions, there is usually no single right answer. We do not provide answers for these questions because it is more important for you to think about the questions than to arrive at the "right" answer. These questions are designed to improve your thinking more than to "cover content." Discuss answers with your peers—discussion can stimulate critical thinking. If you have difficulty with any of these questions, consult with your instructor.

Applying the Full-Spectrum Nursing Model

Choose *two* of the following communication techniques and plan to consciously use them with your next patient. Use the following thinking, doing, and caring questions to reflect on your interaction.

Active listening	Validating messages
Communicating assertively by making "I" statements.	Sharing observations about body language
	Asking open-ended questions
Restating a message	Using silence
Clarifying messages	Summarizing the conversation

THINKING

1. *Critical Thinking (Contextual Awareness)*: Before you have the conversation, make a note of what is going on in the situation (e.g., values, environment, culture) that might influence the effectiveness of the two techniques you will be using.

DOING

2. *Nursing Process (Assessment)*: Before using the two techniques, assess for factors that might affect the patient's ability to communicate. Make a note of them.

3. *Nursing Process (Implementation)*: As soon as possible after using the techniques, record the conversations. Try to remember the exact words.

4. *Nursing Process (Evaluation)*: Evaluate your ability to use the two techniques you chose.

   a. Did you use them at appropriate time in the conversation: as an appropriate response to something the patient said?

   b. What effect did what you said have on the interaction? How did the patient respond to what you said?

   c. Do you think your communication was therapeutic for the patient?

CARING

5. *Self–Knowledge*:

   a. What were your thoughts and feelings before, during, and after the interaction?

   b. In what way has your comfort level with these two techniques changed?

   c. Describe the type of patient or situation in which you would be the least confident in your ability to communicate therapeutically.

Critical Thinking and Clinical Reasoning

1. Mrs. Washington presents to the clinic complaining of a painful lump in her left breast. She is 40 years old and appears very nervous. She tells you, "I was afraid to come in, but I guess I have to find out what this is."

   a. How might you acknowledge the client's feelings? Give examples.

   b. What might you say to clarify and validate the client's messages?

   c. Write a hypothetical conversation with Mrs. Washington that:

   - Acknowledges her feelings
   - Establishes trust
   - Explores the issue
   - Clarifies and validates the client's messages
   - Uses silence
   - Summarizes the conversation

2. Paramedics bring a 35-year-old man and his 14-year-old son to the emergency department (ED). Both have been involved in a recreational vehicle gas explosion and have suffered burns. The son is placed in one of the trauma rooms adjacent to his father. He has partial and full-thickness burns over his face, neck, chest, arms, and hands, and he is unresponsive. The father has partial-thickness burns on his right hand and forearm. He appears to be in a lot of pain and is screaming for his son in Spanish. He speaks limited English. Thirty minutes later, his wife (and the boy's mother) arrives at the ED. She is crying and asking whether her husband and son will be OK. Her English is fluent.

   a. Identify at least two interventions to help you communicate with the father.

   b. What kind of body language would you expect from the father?

   c. How could you show acceptance of and establish trust with the father?

   d. Identify at least two factors that will influence communication with the son.

   e. Identify at least two communication strategies to use with the son.

   f. Explain or give an example of how to use the following techniques as you communicate with the anxious wife and mother:

   - Establishing trust
   - Using silence
   - Offering nonverbal support

3. For each of the following concepts, use critical thinking to describe how or why it is important to nursing, patient care, or communication. Note that these are *not* to be merely definitions.

Verbal communication	Therapeutic communication
Nonverbal communication	Therapeutic relationship
Intrapersonal communication	Barriers to therapeutic communication
Interpersonal communication	Distance between sender and receiver
Group communication	Communication strategies

What Are the Main Points in This Chapter?

➤ Communication is a dynamic, reciprocal process of sending and receiving messages.

➤ Communication occurs on three levels: intrapersonal, or self-talk; interpersonal (between two or more people); and group communication.

➤ The sender delivers a message to the receiver via verbal and/or nonverbal communication. The receiver provides feedback to the sender.

➤ Verbal communication is the use of spoken and written words.

➤ Nonverbal communication, sometimes called body language, communicates how someone is feeling and gives a more accurate account of an individual's true sentiment.

➤ Physical development, maturity, language skills, intellectual abilities, culture, gender, roles, and relationships influence the communication process

➤ Collaborative professional communication is assertive without being aggressive.

➤ Communication is most successful in a comfortable environment. A favorable environment is quiet, private, free of noxious smells, and at a comfortable temperature.

➤ The distance between individuals engaged in communication is affected by the relationship of the individuals, the nature of the conversation, the setting, and cultural influences.

➤ Relationships affect the choice of vocabulary, tone of voice, use of gestures, and distance associated with the communication.

➤ Therapeutic communication is the use of communication skills that result in a positive effect on client care; it is the foundation of professional nursing practice.

➤ Therapeutic communication occurs in the context of a helping relationship. The helping relationship has four phases: pre-interaction, orientation, working phase, and termination.

➤ Group communication occurs when you are interacting with a family, a community, or a committee. Groups may be focused on a task, self-improvement, coping skills, or work-related issues.

➤ To enhance communication, listen actively, establish trust, be assertive, restate messages, clarify and validate messages, interpret body language, share observations, explore issues, use silence, and summarize the conversation.

➤ Barriers to communication include asking too many questions, asking why, changing the subject inappropriately, failing to listen, failing to probe, expressing approval or disapproval, offering advice, providing false reassurance, stereotyping, and using patronizing language.

➤ Language barriers, sensory perceptual alterations, impaired cognitive skills, and physiological barriers make therapeutic communication challenging, but nursing activities can enhance communication with these clients.

For practice questions for this chapter,

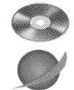

Go to **NCLEX-Style Chapter Quiz,** on the Student Resource Disk or DavisPlus at http://davisplus.fadavis.com/Wilkinson2

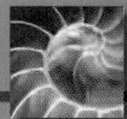# Knowledge Map

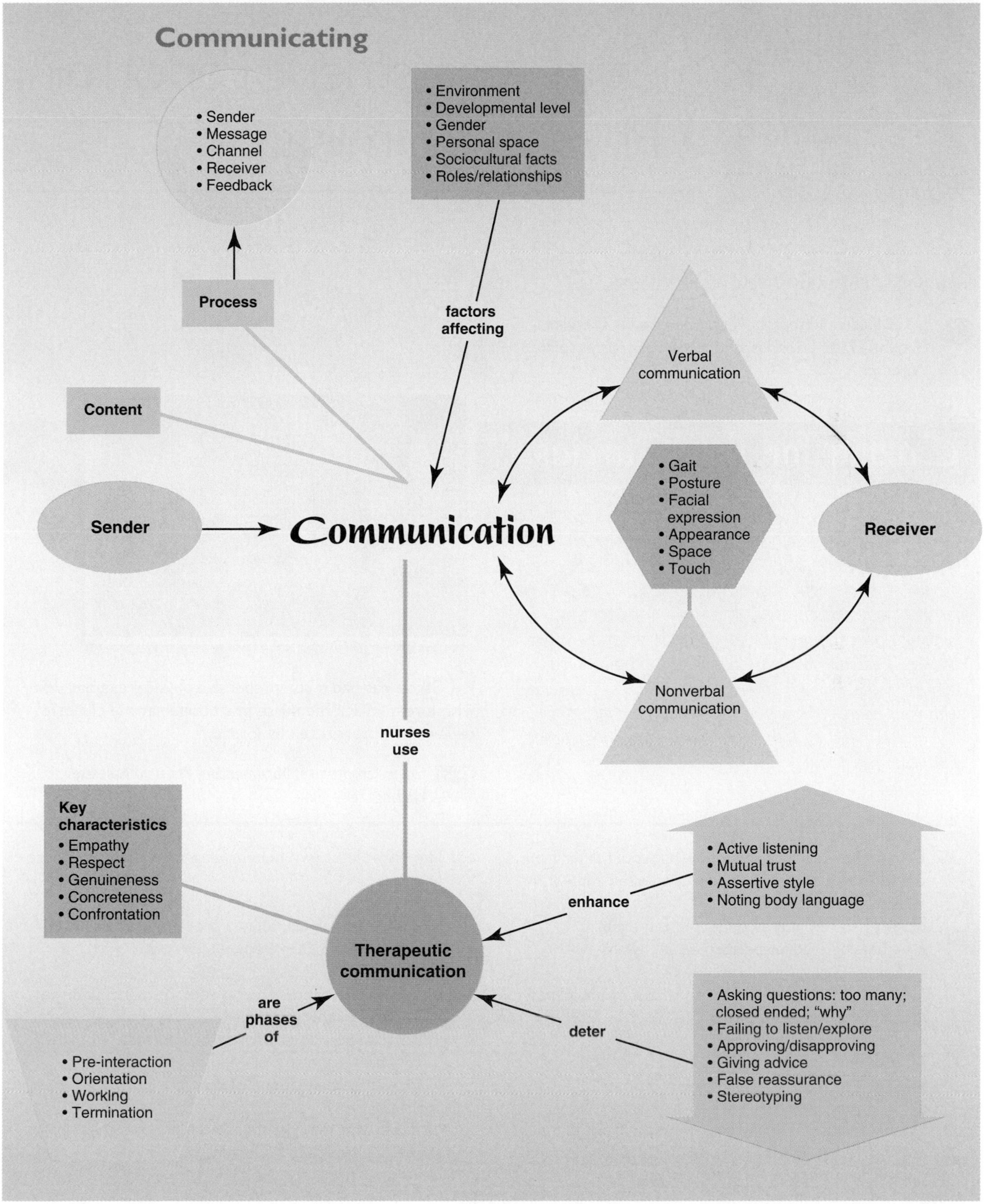

Communicating

- Sender
- Message
- Channel
- Receiver
- Feedback

Process

Content

- Environment
- Developmental level
- Gender
- Personal space
- Sociocultural facts
- Roles/relationships

factors affecting

Sender → **Communication**

Verbal communication

- Gait
- Posture
- Facial expression
- Appearance
- Space
- Touch

Receiver

Nonverbal communication

nurses use

Key characteristics
- Empathy
- Respect
- Genuineness
- Concreteness
- Confrontation

Therapeutic communication

enhance
- Active listening
- Mutual trust
- Assertive style
- Noting body language

are phases of
- Pre-interaction
- Orientation
- Working
- Termination

deter
- Asking questions: too many; closed ended; "why"
- Failing to listen/explore
- Approving/disapproving
- Giving advice
- False reassurance
- Stereotyping

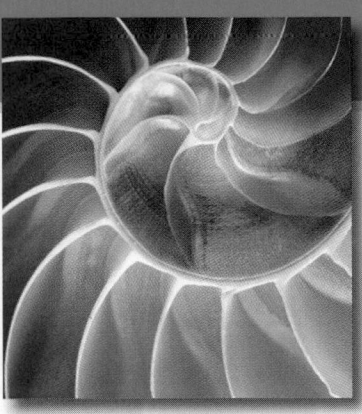

CHAPTER 19

Health Assessment: Performing a Physical Examination

For a podcast of an overview of this chapter,

 Go to Student Resources, **Podcast – Chapter Overviews, Chapter 19,** on DavisPlus at http://davisplus.fadavis.com/ Wilkinson2

Caring for the Garcias

The exercises in the following section allow you to practice the kind of thinking you will use as a full-spectrum nurse. Because these are critical-thinking questions, there is usually no single right answer. We do not provide answers for these questions because it is more important for you to think about the questions than to arrive at the "right" answer. These questions are designed to improve your thinking more than to "cover content." Discuss answers with your peers—discussion can stimulate critical thinking. If you have difficulty with any of these questions, consult with your instructor.

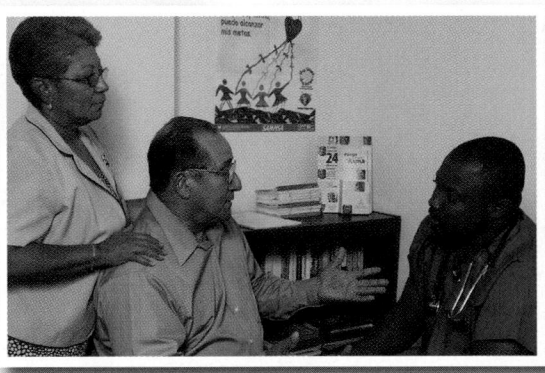

Joe Garcia has had a comprehensive physical examination with Jordan Miller, the nurse practitioner at the clinic. To review the note written by Jordan,

 Go to Chapter 19, **Documenting Physical Assessment Findings,** in Volume 1.

A. Discuss how each of the following would differ from the examination Jordan Miller conducted and what would be expected if:
  - A registered nurse conducted the exam.
  - A nursing student performed the exam.

B. Review Jordan's documentation of the exam. Identify the abnormal findings.

C. Review the laboratory work. Identify the abnormal findings.

D. What conclusions, if any, can you draw from these findings? What actions should you consider based on these conclusions?

E. Identify at least two nursing diagnoses based on these findings.

F. Jordan Miller has identified a problem of Imbalanced Nutrition: More Than Body Requirements for Mr. Garcia.
  - What information do you need to determine the etiology of this problem?
  - Because you do not have that information, write a two-part diagnostic statement describing Mr. Garcia's nutritional status.

G. Now rewrite the nutrition statement as a three-part statement, using "as evidenced by."

Caring for the Garcias (continued)

H. Jordan Miller has identified the diagnosis Acute Pain (knees) for Mr. Garcia. If the pain is caused by a medical condition, osteoarthritis, how would you write a two-part diagnostic statement to describe this health status?

I. How would the examination of Flordelisa Garcia differ from the exam Joe experienced?

J. How would the examination of Bettina Sanford, Joe's 3-year-old granddaughter, differ?

K. If you were responsible for examining Joe Garcia, what aspects of the exam would you find most challenging? Explain why.

Practical **Knowledge**
knowing how

The registered nurse is responsible for patient assessment. As the RN, you should (1) perform the initial assessment to establish a baseline and (2) perform follow-up assessments for any changes. You can instruct nursing assistive personnel (NAPs) to report any changes to you. You can delegate assessment of height, weight, and vital signs to the NAP; however, you should perform the initial admission general survey. You may also want to obtain the first set of vital signs yourself, because they will serve as a baseline.

In this section, you will find all the procedures and assessment guidelines necessary for a complete physical examination (Procedures 19-1 through 19-19). In addition you will find three Clinical Insights to assist you with physical assessment, and an Abnormal Atlas at the end of the chapter. Procedure 19–20 is a brief bedside assessment.

Clinical Insights

Clinical Insight 19–1 ▶ **Performing Percussion**

Direct Percussion

Tap lightly with the pads of the fingers directly on the skin.

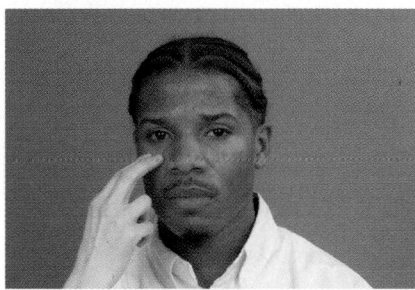

Direct percussion over the sinuses

Indirect Percussion

■ Keep your fingernails short.
■ Strive for a quiet environment: Turn off all entertainment media and music, shut the door, and so on.
This allows you to better perceive the subtle differences in percussion notes.

■ One hand is considered the stationary hand; the other is the striking hand.
■ Hyperextend the middle finger of your stationary hand, and place its distal portion firmly against the client's skin over the area you wish to percuss.
■ Lift the rest of your fingers off the patient's skin.
Prevents dampening the sounds produced.

■ Be sure both of your hands are relaxed to best perform the technique.
Stiff hands will not effectively produce the percussion sounds for assessment.

■ Use the middle finger of your dominant hand as the striking finger **(plexor),** and tap the distal portion of the middle finger of the stationary hand using a quick motion from your wrist.
■ Use enough force to elicit a clear sound.
■ Percuss two times over each location, then move to a new body location and repeat.

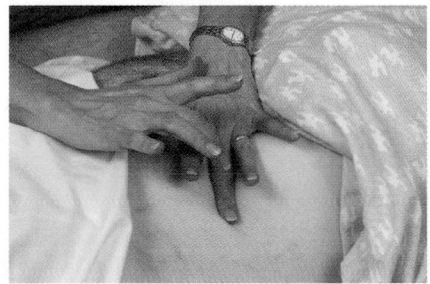

Indirect percussion

Use the terms in the following list to describe the sounds you hear. The terms are based on the components of the sounds produced by percussion:

(continued on next page)

Clinical Insight 19–1 > **Performing Percussion** (continued)

- **Amplitude**—The loudness or softness of a sound
- **Pitch**—The number of vibrations per second; either high or low in nature
- **Quality**—A distinctiveness about the sound produced
- **Duration**—How long the sound lingers

Percussion Notes

SOUND	AMPLITUDE	PITCH	QUALITY	DURATION	EXAMPLE
Resonant	Medium-loud	Low	Hollow	Medium	Normal lung
Hyperresonant	Louder	Lower	Booming	Longer	Hyperinflated lung (as in emphysema)
Dull	Soft	High	Muffled thud	Short	Liver/spleen
Flat	Very soft	High	Absolute dullness	Very short	Thigh or tumor
Tympany	Loud	High	Musical	Longest	Gastric air bubble, intestinal air

To listen to some percussion sounds,

Go to the sound file, **Percussion Notes,** on the Student Resource Disk or DavisPlus at http://davisplus.fadavis.com/Wilkinson2

Clinical Insight 19–2 > **Performing Auscultation**

- Provide a quiet environment to facilitate auscultation.

- Clean your stethoscope with a 70% alcohol or benzalkonium chloride wipe before and after using it to examine a patient. Most stethoscopes are colonized by bacteria, although only a small percentage are pathogenic. Cleaning can reduce the bacterial count by 94% to 100%.

- Use the diaphragm to listen to high-pitched sounds that normally occur in the heart, lungs, and abdomen. Press the diaphragm hard enough to produce an obvious ring on the patient's skin.
- Use the bell to hear low-pitched sounds, such as extra heart sounds (murmurs) or turbulent blood flow (bruits). Apply the bell lightly with just enough pressure to produce an air seal with its full rim.
- Place the earpieces facing forward.
Seals the ear canal and improves detection of sounds.

- Warm the stethoscope before you place it on the client's skin.
- Place the stethoscope directly on the client's skin. Do not listen through clothing.
This can create artifact or reduce the quality of auscultation.

- If body hair prevents good contact with the skin, dampen the hair before you listen.
- Close your eyes as you listen through the stethoscope.
This helps improve your focus.

- Concentrate on one sound at a time. Do not try to evaluate breath and heart sounds at the same time.
Improves the quality of the data.

For examples of heart sounds,

Go to the sound file, **Heart Sounds,** on the Student Resource Disk or DavisPlus at http://davisplus.fadavis.com/Wilkinson2

Practice Resources
Centers for Disease Control and Prevention (2005); Kennedy, K. J., Dreimanis, D. E., Beckingham, W. D., et al. (2003); Rutala, W. A., & Weber, D. J. (2004).

Clinical Insight 19-3 ▶ Assisting with a Speculum Exam

Equipment

- Patient drape
- Nonsterile gloves
- Vaginal speculum (see accompanying figure)

  The speculum may be plastic or metal.

  The size of the speculum depends on the patient's history. Use a small speculum for a woman who has never been sexually active or an older woman who is not sexually active.

  If a culture or a Pap smear is to be obtained, lubricate the speculum with warm water. Otherwise, use a water-soluble lubricant.

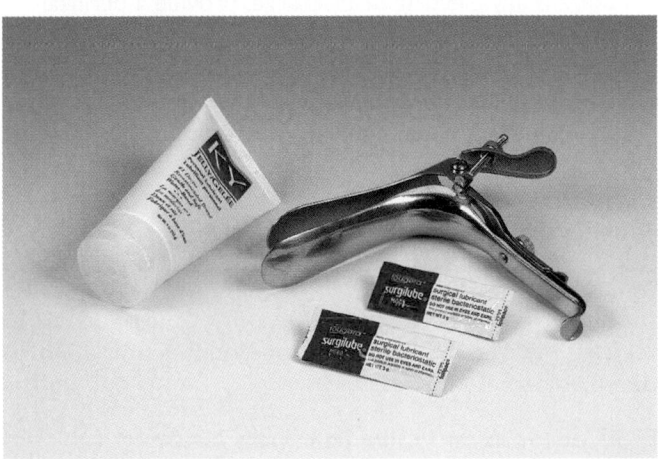

Equipment. A vaginal speculum

- Lubricant
- Pap smear slide, spatula, brush, or specimen broom and container with solution
- Fixative, if the smear technique is used
- Genital culture supplies
- Additional light source

Preparing the Patient

- Explain to the patient that an internal examination of her vagina and pelvic organs will be performed. The examination usually takes only a few minutes, and although it might not be comfortable it should not be painful. Reassure her that you will provide privacy and keep her warm during the procedure.
- Have the woman urinate before the examination if needed.

Emptying the bladder helps the patient to feel more comfortable during the exam.

- Assist the woman to the lithotomy position, and cover her with a drape.

Inserting the Speculum

The speculum is inserted into the vagina to visualize the cervix (see accompanying figure). Once the speculum is

inserted, you may need to adjust the light source for the examiner.

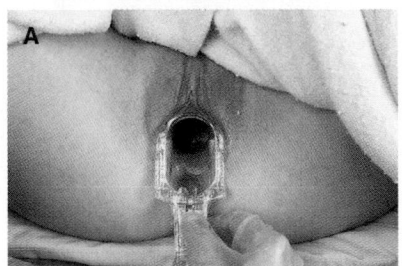

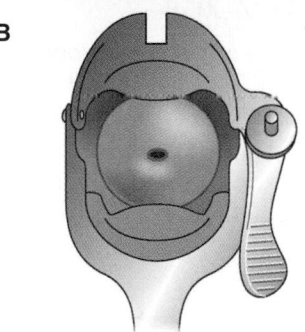

A, A vaginal speculum examination. Placement of the speculum in the vagina. *B*, View through the speculum

Collecting Specimens

If a routine screening for cervical and uterine cancer is being done, a specimen will be collected. Additional cultures or screens may be required if there is unusual discharge or risk of sexually transmitted infection. Genital cultures are endocervical smears.

Pap Smear Procedure

- Most commonly, the examiner inserts a small brush through the cervical os and rotates it to obtain cells from within the cervical canal (endocervical smear). The brush is then rolled onto the slide.

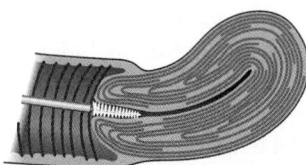

Collecting/broom. Using a specimen broom to obtain endocervical cells

A second specimen may be obtained by lightly scraping the cervix with a wooden spatula to obtain cells from the ecto-cervix (the lowest portion of the cervix that protrudes into the vagina). The spatula is then smeared on the slide. Some examiners use both specimen sources and then apply a

(continued on next page)

Clinical Insight 19-3 ➤ **Assisting with a Speculum Exam** (continued)

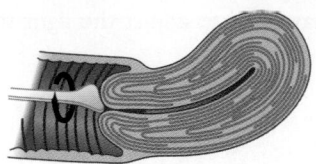

Collecting/spatula. Using a spatula to obtain ectocervical cells

fixative, usually a spray or liquid, on top of the specimen to preserve it for examination. After the samples are obtained, the speculum is removed.

Pap Smear, Alternative Method

▪ The examiner inserts a specimen broom into the cervical os and rotates it. The broom is then inserted into a fixative solution and rotated to disperse cells into the solution. This technique is gaining popularity because it is considered more sensitive for detection of cervical changes. After the samples are obtained, the speculum is removed.

Bimanual Exam

After removing the speculum, the examiner inserts lubricated gloved fingers into the vagina while pressing down on the lower abdomen and suprapubic area. This is known as a **bimanual exam.** It is used to assess the consistency of the cervix; the size of the uterus; and to detect tenderness over the ovaries, fallopian tubes, or with movement of the cervix.

Post-procedure

▪ Assist the woman to a sitting position at the end of the exam.
▪ You may need to assist the woman with perineal care.
▪ If there is any bleeding or discharge, provide a perineal pad.
▪ Document the date and time of the procedure, the name of the examiner, the patient's tolerance of the procedure, and any nursing assessments or interventions performed.

Practice Resources

American College of Obstetricians and Gynecologists (ACOG, 2003).

Procedures

This section presents a comprehensive physical examination you can use for ongoing physical assessments. Procedure 19-20 provides a brief bedside assessment.

When examining each body system be sure to compare findings on both sides of the body. The following procedures are described mainly for adult patients. To review ways in which to adapt your examination to people of different ages,

 Go to Chapter 19, **How Do I Modify Assessment for Different Age Groups,** in Volume 1.

Procedure 19-1   **Performing the General Survey**

> ➤ For steps to follow in *all* procedures, refer to the Universal Steps for All Procedures found on the inside back cover of Volume 2.

Critical Aspects

▪ Observe the patient's apparent age, sex, race, facial expression, body size and type, posture, movements, speech, grooming, dress, hygiene, mental state, and affect.
▪ Identify any signs of distress.
▪ Measure vital signs.
▪ Measure height and weight, and calculate body mass index (BMI).
▪ Consider the client's cultural/ethnic background, gender, and developmental stage.
▪ Review history data that may influence general survey findings, including usual state of health, current health problem, allergies, and unexplained changes in weight.
▪ Perform functional and SPICES assessments for older adults.
▪ Note verbal and nonverbal responses throughout exam.

Equipment

See Equipment Needed for Physical Examination below.

Equipment Needed for Physical Examination

Usual Equipment for Ongoing Assessment

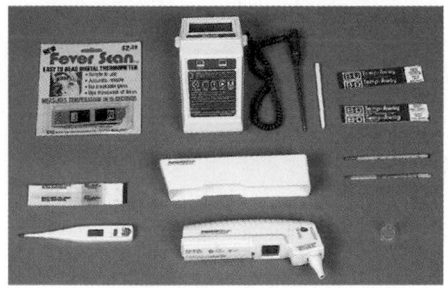

Thermometer (for measuring temperature)

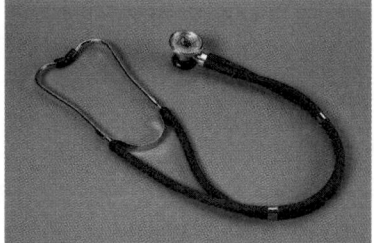

Stethoscope (for measuring blood pressure and listening to heart, lung, and bowel sounds)

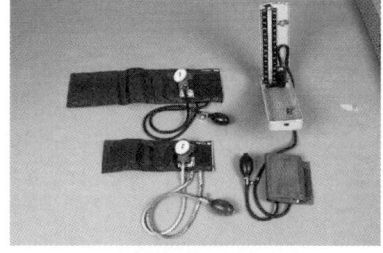

Sphygmomanometer (for measuring blood pressure)

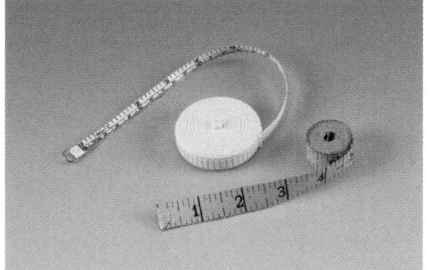

Tape measure (to measure circumference and length)

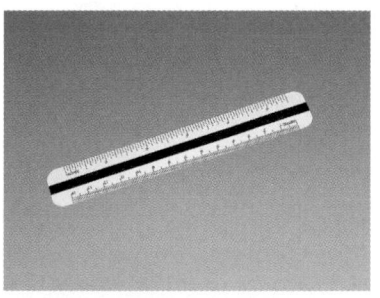

Pocket ruler (to measure size or distance).

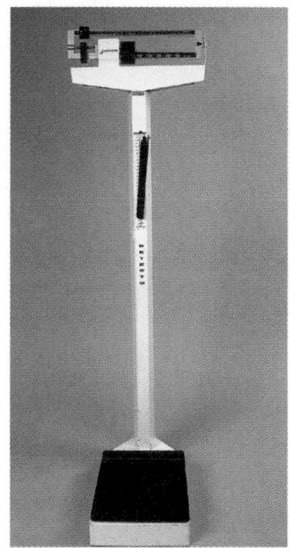

Scale (to measure weight and height)

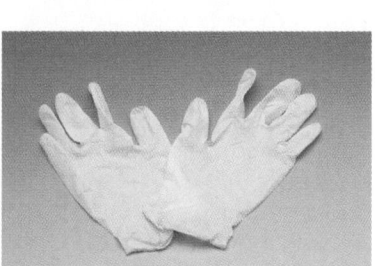

Gloves (to wear if there is any possible exposure to blood or body fluids)

(continued on next page)

Procedure 19-1 ■ **Performing the General Survey** (continued)

Equipment Needed for Physical Examination—cont'd

Additional Equipment for a Comprehensive Assessment

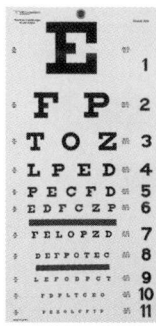

Snellen acuity chart (for screening vision)

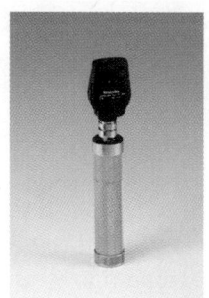

Ophthalmoscope (for inspection of the internal structures of the eye)

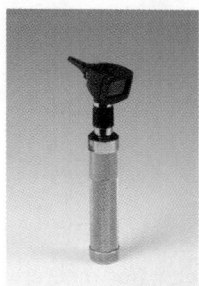

Otoscope (for examining the external auditory canal and tympanic membrane)

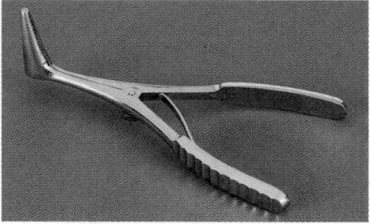

Nasal speculum (for examining the nasal turbinates)

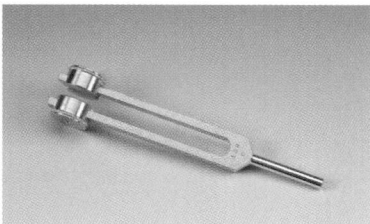

Percussion hammer (for eliciting deep tendon reflexes)

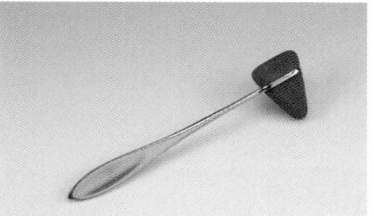

Tuning fork (for auditory screening and assessment of vibratory sensation during the neurological exam)

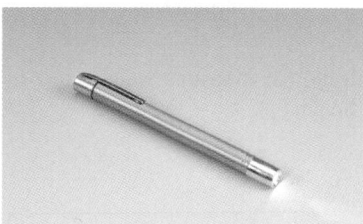

Penlight (for visualizing the eyes and inside of mouth, or highlighting a skin lesion)

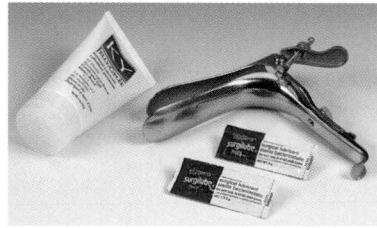

Vaginal speculum and lubricant (for examining the female pelvis; lubricant is also used for rectal exams)

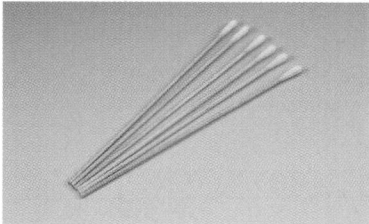

Cotton-tipped applicators (for obtaining specimens)

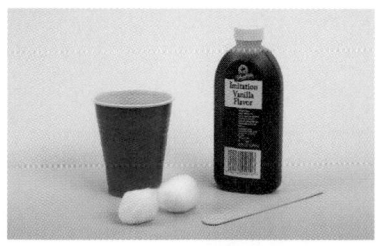

Cotton balls, tongue depressor, strong-smelling substance, a glass of water (for testing various cranical nerves)

Positioning

- Have the client seated as you begin the examination (on an exam table or on the side of the bed).
- If the client is unable to sit, use Fowler's or semi-Fowler's position.

Focused History Questions

- How are you feeling today?
- (If the client is an outpatient) What brings you to the clinic today?
- Are you in any discomfort or pain?
- Have you had any hospitalizations or surgeries?
- What medicines do you take? That means prescribed as well as over-the-counter drugs.
- How much alcohol do you drink per day? Do you smoke cigarettes? If so, how many per day? Do you use drugs for non-medical purposes?
- Do you use any herbal products or natural remedies?
- Do you have any difficulty falling asleep or staying asleep?

This is a common problem for older adults.

Developmental Modifications for Infants and Children

- Encourage the parents to be present for the examination. Position an infant on a padded examination table or held against the parent's chest.

Infants and toddlers usually feel most secure if a parent is present.

- Offer toddlers choices. Involve the parent in the exam. Praise the toddler for cooperation.
- Allow the preschool child to sit in the parent's lap if she wishes. Let the child help with the exam. Give reassurance as you proceed. Compliment the child on her cooperation.

Preschoolers often are fearful of body injury and invasive procedures.

- Support the school-age child's independence. Develop rapport by asking the child about his teacher or favorite school and play activities. Allow the child to undress himself and get up and down from the exam table. Demonstrate your equipment before you use it.
- Adolescents should be examined without parents or siblings present unless they request otherwise. Provide privacy.

Adolescents are self-conscious and introspective.

Developmental Modifications for Older Adults

- Observe the older adult's energy level during the physical examination, and provide rest periods if needed. If the client tires easily, arrange the exam sequence to limit position changes.
- Allow extra time to interview and examine older adults.
- Be aware that stiff muscles and arthritic joints may make it impossible for older adults to assume certain positions.
- Be alert for hearing and vision deficits in older adults, and adapt your interview techniques accordingly (e.g., elicit feedback to be sure the client has heard you correctly).
- Assess the older adult's functional status. You can use the Lawton Instrumental Activities of Daily Living (IADL), found in "Assessment Forms" in Chapter 3 of this volume.
- Work the SPICES assessment into the examination of various body systems: **S**leep disorders, **P**roblems eating or feeding, **I**ncontinence, **C**onfusion, **E**vidence of falls, **S**kin breakdown.

➤ When performing the procedure, always identify your patient according to agency policy and be attentive to standard precautions, hand hygiene, patient safety and privacy, body mechanics, and documentation.

Procedure Steps	Expected Findings
Performing the General Survey	
1. Identify signs of distress (e.g., pain, fear, or anxiety). If signs of distress are present, perform a focused assessment, and address the immediate problem.	The client is in no apparent distress. The client appears relaxed, with no evidence of pain, fear, or anxiety. **Abnormal findings:** Pain, grimacing, breathing problems, skin color changes
2. Observe apparent age, sex, and race. Ask the patient, "What racial or ethnic group do you identify with?" Ask yourself, • Is apparent age consistent with biological age? • Are there cultural or gender-related factors that influence the exam or findings?	Client appears his stated age. Makes eye contact consistent with his cultural norms. Is reasonably comfortable with being examined.

(continued on next page)

Procedure 19-1 ■ **Performing the General Survey** (continued)

3. Note facial characteristics, including facial expression, symmetry of facial features, and the condition and color of the skin. Ask yourself,

- What is the client's face telling me?
- Is the facial expression appropriate to the situation?
- Are facial features symmetrical (palpebral fissure and nasolabial folds)?
- Are there any changes in condition or color of skin?
- Does the client maintain eye contact?

Face is symmetrical; visible skin is intact without excessive wrinkling, discoloration, or deformity.

4. Note body type and posture. Greet the client with a handshake. Be aware that shaking hands is not acceptable in all cultures.

Allows you to assess muscle strength and surface skin characteristics while at the same time conveying that you care.

Ask yourself,

- Is the body build stocky, slender, average, obese, or **cachectic** (very thin, wasted appearance)?
- Are the body parts proportional to the client's overall size?
- Does the client have abnormal fat distribution?
- Does the client assume a specific position for comfort (e.g., sitting versus supine)?

Posture is upright, and body appears proportionate. Grip is strong.

5. Observe gait, and note any abnormal movements. If the client has Impaired Bed Mobility, determine ability to move and amount of assistance needed. Ask yourself,

- Does the client move in a coordinated manner?
- Are there any obvious gait problems?
- Does the client walk with a wide base of support or short stride length?
- Does the client use assistive devices?
- Are there any abnormal or spastic movements?

Movements are coordinated; gait is steady; does not use assistive devices.

Abnormal findings: Unstable or shuffling gait; spastic movements, stiff movements

6. Listen to your client's speech pattern, pace, quality, tone, vocabulary, and sentence structure. Ask yourself,

- Are the responses appropriate?
- Is there any difficulty with speech?
- Does the client's tone of voice match her statements?

Client responds appropriately to questions. Tone of voice matches responses. Speech is clear, evenly paced, and rises and falls based on content.

Abnormal findings: Rapid speech, slow speech, slurred speech

7. Assess mental state and affect.
  a. Determine level of consciousness.
  b. Determine orientation to time, place, and person.
Ask yourself,

- If the client is disoriented, does he reorient easily?
- What is the client's mood? Is it appropriate for the situation?

Many medical conditions and medications can affect mental status. If you note any abnormal findings: during the general survey, be sure to focus on them when you assess mental status during the sensori–neurological examination.

Awake, alert, and oriented to time, place, person, and self. Mood is appropriate for the situation.

Abnormal findings: Confusion and irritability, inability to recall information or provide history, lethargy and somnolence, bizarre responses

8. Observe dress, grooming, and hygiene. Ask yourself,
- Is the client appropriately and neatly dressed?
- Is the client well groomed?
- Are there any unusual odors?

Client is dressed appropriately for the climate. Skin is clean, and clothing is in good repair. No noticeable odor.

Abnormal findings: Poor hygiene, dirty skin or nails, uncombed hair, visible soiling of clothing, mismatched or wrinkled clothing, objectionable odor

9. Measure vital signs: blood pressure, temperature, radial pulse, respiratory rate. If your initial observations and interview indicate that the client is in pain, perform a pain assessment, as well). See Chapter 30.

BP: < 120/80 mm Hg

Temperature: 97.3°–98.6°F (36.3°–37°C) oral

Pulse: 60–100 beats/min, regular, and easily palpated

Respiratory rate: 12–20, regular and even

Abnormal findings: See Chapter 17.

10. Measure height and weight.
   a. For adults: Calculate BMI, or use the accompanying table.

$$\frac{Wt\ (lb) \times 703}{Ht\ (in.)^2} = BMI$$

   b. For children: Plot height and weight on growth chart.

For adults: BMI is 18.5–24.9.

For children: Height and weight are consistent with previous trend on growth chart.

Abnormal findings:

BMI < 18.5 = underweight

BMI 25–29.9 = overweight

BMI ≥ 30 = obese

BMI 30–34.9   Level I Moderate obesity

BMI 35–39.9   Level II Severe obesity

BMI > 40   Level III Morbid obesity

Developmental Modifications

Infants and children
- Weigh infants without clothing; weigh older children in their underwear.
- For infants and children younger than 2 years, position supine to measure height; be sure knees are extended.
- For infants and children youger than age 2, also measure head circumference.

What if . . .

- **There is an apparent language barrier?**

Obtain an interpreter; and refer to Clinical Insight 18-4, in Chapter 18 of this volume.

Use this table to find body mass index, based on height and weight, or use a BMI calculator such as the ones found at, http://www.nhlbisupport.com/bmi/bmicalc.htm and http://www.cdc.gov/nccdphp/dnpa/bmi/adult_BMI/english_bmi_calculator/bmi_calculator.htm ▼

Weight (lb)

Height (ft/in)	120	130	140	150	160	170	180	190	200	210	220	230	240	250	260	270	280	290	300	310	320	330
4'5"	30	33	35	38	40	43	45	48	50	53	55	58	60	63	65	68	70	73	75	78	80	83
4'6"	29	31	34	36	39	41	43	46	48	51	53	56	58	60	63	65	68	70	72	75	77	80
4'7"	28	30	33	35	37	40	42	44	47	49	51	54	56	58	61	63	65	68	70	72	75	77
4'8"	27	29	31	34	36	38	40	43	45	47	49	52	54	56	58	61	63	65	67	70	72	74
4'9"	26	28	30	33	35	37	39	41	43	46	48	50	52	54	56	59	61	63	65	67	69	72
4'10"	25	27	29	31	34	36	38	40	42	44	46	48	50	52	54	57	59	61	63	65	67	69
4'11"	24	26	28	30	32	34	36	38	40	43	45	47	49	51	53	55	57	59	61	63	65	67
5'0"	23	25	27	29	31	33	35	37	39	41	43	45	47	49	51	53	55	57	59	61	63	65
5'1"	23	25	27	28	30	32	34	36	38	40	42	44	45	47	49	51	53	55	57	59	61	62
5'2"	22	24	26	27	29	31	33	35	37	38	40	42	44	46	48	49	51	53	55	57	59	60
5'3"	21	23	25	27	28	30	32	34	35	37	39	41	43	44	46	48	50	51	53	55	57	59
5'4"	21	22	24	26	28	29	31	33	34	36	38	40	41	43	45	46	48	50	51	53	55	57
5'5"	20	22	23	25	27	28	30	32	33	35	37	38	40	42	43	45	47	48	50	52	53	55
5'6"	19	21	23	24	26	27	29	31	32	34	36	37	39	40	42	44	45	47	48	50	52	53
5'7"	19	20	22	24	25	27	28	30	31	33	35	36	38	39	41	42	44	45	47	49	50	52
5'8"	18	20	21	23	24	26	27	29	30	32	34	35	37	38	40	41	43	44	46	47	49	50
5'9"	18	19	21	22	24	25	27	28	30	31	33	34	36	37	38	40	41	43	44	46	47	49
5'10"	17	19	20	22	23	24	26	27	29	30	32	33	35	36	37	39	40	42	43	45	46	47
5'11"	17	18	20	21	22	24	25	27	28	29	31	32	34	35	36	38	39	40	42	43	45	46
6'	16	18	19	20	22	23	24	26	27	29	30	31	33	34	35	37	38	39	41	42	43	45
6'1"	16	17	19	20	21	22	24	25	26	28	29	30	32	33	34	36	37	38	40	41	42	44
6'2"	15	17	18	19	21	22	23	24	26	27	28	30	31	32	33	35	36	37	39	40	41	42
6'3"	15	16	18	19	20	21	22	24	25	26	28	29	30	31	32	34	35	36	38	39	40	41
6'4"	15	16	17	18	20	21	22	23	24	26	27	28	29	30	32	33	34	35	37	38	39	40
6'5"	14	15	17	18	19	20	21	23	24	25	26	27	29	30	31	32	33	34	36	37	38	39
6'6"	14	15	16	17	19	20	21	22	23	24	25	27	28	29	30	31	32	34	35	36	37	38
6'7"	14	15	16	17	18	19	20	21	23	24	25	26	27	28	29	30	32	33	34	35	36	37
6'8"	13	14	15	16	18	19	20	21	22	23	24	25	26	27	29	30	31	32	33	34	35	36
6'9"	13	14	15	16	17	18	19	20	21	23	24	25	26	27	28	29	30	31	32	33	34	35
6'10"	13	14	15	16	17	18	19	20	21	22	23	24	25	26	27	28	29	30	31	32	34	35

Less risk   More risk

Procedure 19-1 ■ **Performing the General Survey** (continued)

Documentation

- Document BP as right or left arm, and note the patient's position: sitting, standing, or lying.
- Document temperature measurement route: oral, rectal, or tympanic membrane.
- For children, document height and weight on a growth chart.

 Go to Chapter 19, **Supplemental Materials: Growth Charts,** on the Student Resource Disk or DavisPlus at http://davisplus.fadavis.com/Wilkinson2

- If you need more information about documenting,

 Go to Chapter 19, **Documenting Physical Assessment Findings,** in Volume 1. Also see Chapter 17 for documenting vital signs on a graphic flowsheet.

Practice Resources

National Guideline Clearinghouse (2006); National Heart Lung and Blood Institute (n.d.).

Procedure 19-2 ☐ **Assessing the Skin**

➤ For steps to follow in *all* procedures, refer to the Universal Steps for All Procedures found on the inside back cover of Volume 2.

Critical Aspects

- Techniques: Inspection, palpation, and olfaction
- Assess both exposed and unexposed areas.
- Inspect skin color; note any unusual odors.
- Inspect and palpate any lesions. Describe their size, shape, color, distribution, texture, surface relationship, and exudate.
- Evaluate the lesions for possible malignancy, remembering the mnemonic ABCDE.
- Use the dorsal aspect of your hand to palpate skin temperature.
- Palpate skin turgor by gently pulling up skin, noting its return when you release it.
- Palpate skin for texture, moisture, and hydration.
- Review history that may influence skin findings.

Equipment

- Nonlatex gloves (if exposure to body fluids is a possibility)
- Flexible transparent ruler—*to measure lesions*
- Penlight—*to provide adequate lighting to unexposed areas*
- Magnifier—*for better visualization of lesions*
- Pen and record form

Focused History Questions

Ask the patient about the history or presence of any:
- Rashes
- History of allergies
- Areas of skin that have changed color
- Skin lesions

- Skin with rough or unusual texture
- Skin that is always warm or cool, regardless of room temperature

Developmental Modifications for Older Adults

- Assess the level of risk for pressure ulcers. For assessment tools (Braden scale, Norton scale), go to Chapter 34 in this volume.

As adults age, the subcutaneous tissue layer thins. The dermal layer loses elasticity as a result of changes in collagen fibers; and the strong bond between the epidermal and dermal layers decreases. These changes make the skin prone to breakdown.

➤ When performing the procedure, always identify your patient according to agency policy and be attentive to standard precautions, hand hygiene, patient safety and privacy, body mechanics, and documentation.

Procedure Steps

1. Inspect skin color, including mucous membranes, tongue, and conjunctiva.
To assess color changes of exposed and unexposed areas. Color changes and odors may indicate underlying disease and should be fully investigated.

Expected Findings

Skin color is uniform, with darker exposed areas. Mucous membranes and conjunctiva are pink and moist. No unusual odors.

a. Provide good lighting.

b. In dark-skinned clients, look for color changes in the conjunctiva or oral mucosa, tongue, lips, nail beds, palms of the hands, and soles of the feet.

Skin color varies widely among individuals by age and ethnicity, but in each individual skin color is fairly uniform over his body. ▼

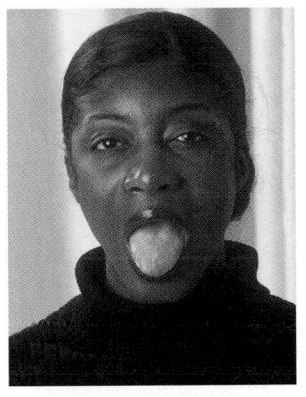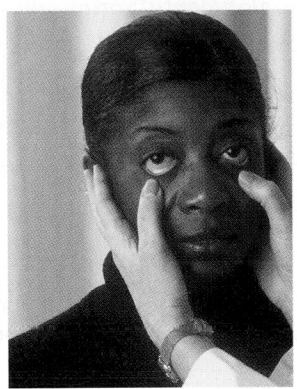

Step 1

c. Note any unusual odors.

d. To assess for cyanosis, be sure to examine the tongue.

Exposure to cold causes the lips to turn blue, but not the tongue. Cyanosis affects the color of the skin, mucous membrane, and tongue.

2. Palpate skin for temperature.

a. Wear procedure gloves and discard after examing any open areas of the skin.

b. Use dorsal aspect of hand or fingers.

c. Compare bilaterally.

The dorsum of the hands and the fingers are most sensitive to temperature variations.

3. Palpate skin for turgor. Test an unexposed area, such as the area below the clavicle, inner thigh, sternum, or forehead, by gently pinching up the skin, noting its return when you release it.

Developmental Modifications

Infants—Check skin turgor on the abdomen.

Older adults—Check skin turgor over the sternum or clavicle.

Developmental Variations

Newborns—May be jaundiced for a few weeks. Blue-black Mongolian spots and pink-red capillary hemangiomas are common and fade with time.

Older adults—May have thin, translucent skin and wrinkles due to loss of elasticity. Fragile skin is not uncommon among lighter skinned, older adults.

Abnormal findings: Pallor, jaundice, cyanosis, erythema, hyperpigmentation, hypopigmentation. If there are abnormal findings, ask the patient (or someone who knows him well) about the baseline skin color. See the Abnormal Atlas: Skin Color Changes at the end of this chapter for examples of color changes.

Skin is warm; temperature is the same bilaterally.

Abnormal findings: Local area(s) that are warmer or cooler than the rest of the skin; generalized temperature increase or decrease. If the skin is excessively warm, assess for fever. Localized warmth with erythema can indicate an infection. Cool skin might be a sign of compromised circulation or dehydration, particularly in the older adult.

Skin returns immediately to its original position.

Developmental Variations

Older adults have decreased skin turgor due to decreased elasticity.

Abnormal findings: Decreased or increased turgor. Tenting (decreased turgor): Skin takes several seconds to return to original position. Decreased turgor or tenting is seen with dehydration or normal aging. It predisposes the patient to skin breakdown.

Increased turgor: Skin tension does not allow the skin to be pinched up. ▼

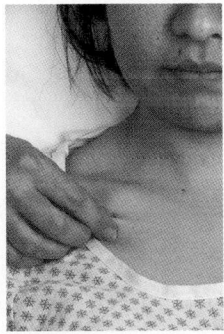

Step 3

(continued on next page)

Procedure 19-2 ■ **Assessing the Skin** (continued)

---

4. Palpate the skin for texture.
Texture varies, depending on the area being assessed and the age of the client.

Skin is smooth and soft. Exposed areas and extensor surfaces (e.g., elbows and knees) are drier and coarser than other areas.

Developmental Variations

Infants and young children—Have smooth skin.

Abnormal findings: Coarse, thick, rough, or dry skin; very smooth, thin, fine-textured, shiny skin

---

5. Palpate skin for moisture/hydration.
  a. Use the dorsum of your hand.

Skin is warm and dry.

Developmental Variations

Older adults—Skin may be dry and flaky because of decreased activity of sebaceous and sweat glands.

Adolescents—May have skin that is oilier than normal.

Abnormal findings: Increased moisture (skin feels damp, visible diaphoresis); decreased moisture (skin feels dry)

---

6. Inspect for edema.
  a. Press firmly with your fingertip for 5 seconds over a bony area, such as the tibia.
  b. Release your finger, and observe the skin for the reaction. Normally there will be no evidence of the pressure once you remove your finger. If pitting edema is present, you will see a depression in the skin.
  c. If edema is present, note the location, degree, and type of swelling. For example, if you observe edema in the lower leg, how far up the leg does it extend?

No edema

Grading System

Trace: Minimal depression with pressure.

+1: 2 mm depression; rapid return of skin to position.

+2: 4 mm depression that disappears in 10–15 seconds.

+3: 6 mm depression that lasts 1–2 minutes. Area appears swollen.

+4: 8 mm depression that persists for 2–3 minutes. Area is grossly edematous.

Abnormal findings: Edema is an abnormal finding.

---

7. Identify any skin lesions.
  a. Inspect and palpate lesions.
  b. When you notice bruises, be alert for signs of abuse (see Chapter 9).
  c. Ask the client: "Do you have any new moles or other lesions? Has there been any change in existing moles/lesions?"
  d. Assess for malignant lesions using ABCDE:

No lesions are present.

Normal variations include moles, freckles, birthmarks, striae (in pregnant women or clients who have lost much weight), and wrinkles.

Developmental Variations

Newborns—**Milia** (tiny collections of sebum, usually on the face) are common.

Adults—**Acrochordons** (skin tags) may be seen around the neck, axillae, skinfolds, or areas where clothing rubs.

A (asymmetry)
B (irregular borders)
C (color variations)
D (diameter: 0.5 cm)
E (elevation) ▼

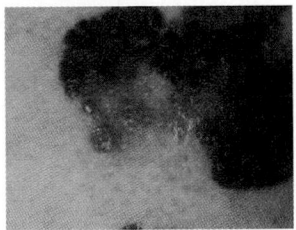

Malignant melanoma

Older adults—Flat beige or brown macules are common on exposed skin areas.

Abnormal findings: See the accompanying Abnormal Atlas: Skin Lesions at the end of this chapter. Also see the table, "Describing Skin Lesions," following this procedure.

Adolescents—Acne is a common abnormal finding among adolescents.

Describing Lesions

When you observe a lesion, evaluate and describe the following:

- **Size.** Measure the length, width, and depth of the lesion.
- **Shape and pattern.** Describe the *shape* of individual lesions. If there are clusters or groups, describe the *pattern*. Is it linear or circular? Are the *borders* distinct, or do they run together? Is the border smooth or irregular?
- **Color.** Describe the color of the lesion, and determine whether there is any variation of color within the lesion.
- **Distribution.** Are the lesions distributed over the entire body? Are they confined to a specific region? What parts of the body are affected?
- **Texture.** The texture (e.g., smooth, rough, scaly) of a lesion helps with classification.
- **Surface relationship.** To assess surface relationship, you will need to palpate the lesion. Is it flat, raised, or depressed? Is it firmly attached to the surrounding skin or mobile?
- **Exudate.** Examine the lesion(s) for signs of drainage. Describe the color, appearance, amount, and odor of drainage, if present.
- **Tenderness, pain, or itching.** Press on the lesion, and determine the patient's reaction. Does touching the lesion cause pain or discomfort?

Patient Teaching

Teach the patient the signs and symptoms of skin cancer, the importance of the skin exam, and preventive measures.

Home Care

- Assess the skill level of the caregiver. Instruct the caregiver in the importance of skin assessment and measures to prevent skin breakdown.
- Be alert for lesions (e.g., burns, bruises) that may signal physical abuse. For more signs of abuse, refer to Procedure 9-1.

Documentation

- If lesions are present, describe the history: onset, duration, associated or aggravating factors (e.g., itching), factors that relieve symptoms, treatments that have been used, and responses to treatment.
- Sketch the location of skin lesions on body diagrams, if available (see example below); or sketch a body if necessary. ▼

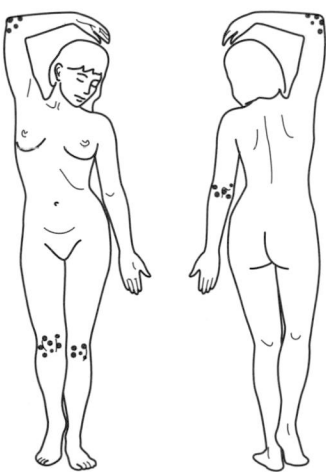

Documentation

If you need more information about documenting,

 VOL 1 Go to Chapter 19, **Documenting Physical Assessment Findings,** in Volume 1.

(continued on next page)

Procedure 19-2 ■ **Assessing the Skin** (continued)

Describing Skin Lesions

TYPES		DESCRIPTION
Primary Lesions		
Macule (nonpalpable, < 1cm) 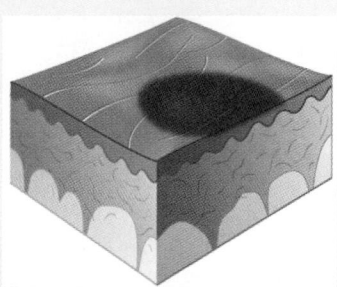	Macule (nonpalpable, < 1 cm) 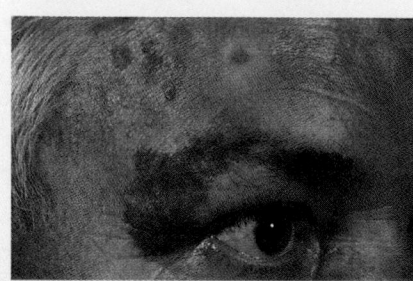	Flat and colored. Examples: freckle, petechiae, birthmark, Mongolian spot
Papule (palpable), < 1 cm; plague, > 1 cm 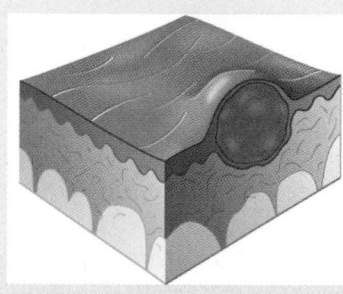	Papules (seborrheic keratosis) 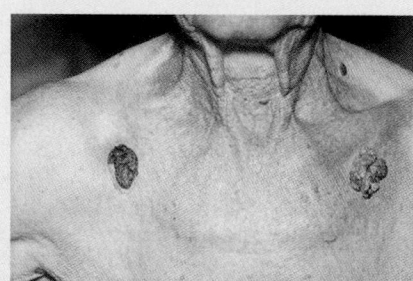	Elevated and raised, but superficial Examples: mole, psoriasis
Vesicle (palpable), < 1 cm; bulla, > 1 cm 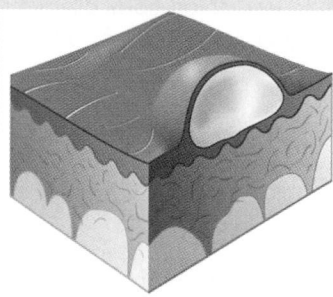	Vesicles (blisters) 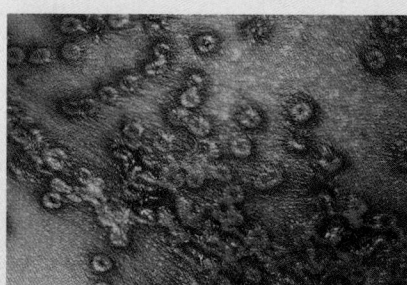 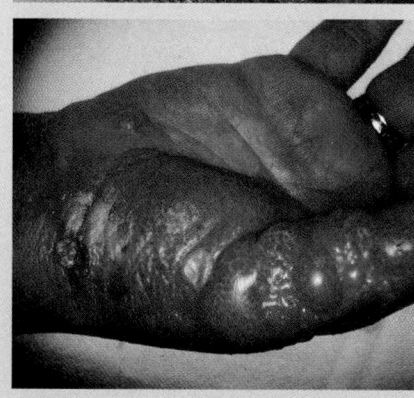	Elevated and filled with serous fluid. Examples: blister, herpes simplex

Describing Skin Lesions—cont'd

TYPES		DESCRIPTION
Cyst (palpable), < 2 cm 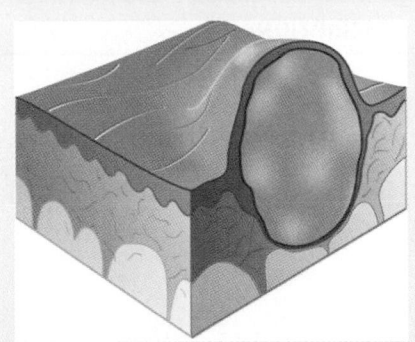	Keratogenous cyst 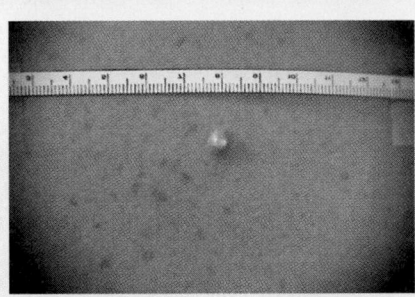	Palpable, fluid-filled, and encapsulated. If not fluid-filled, called a nodule
Pustule (palpable) 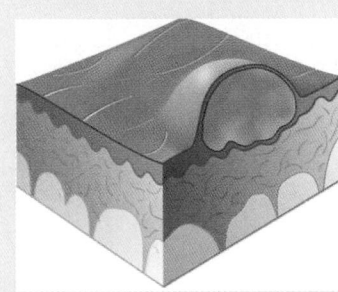	Pustules (acne) 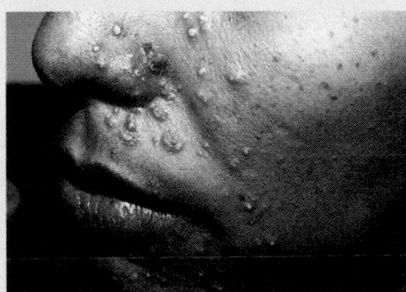	Elevated and filled with pus. Examples: acne, folliculitis, impetigo
	Nodule (palpable) 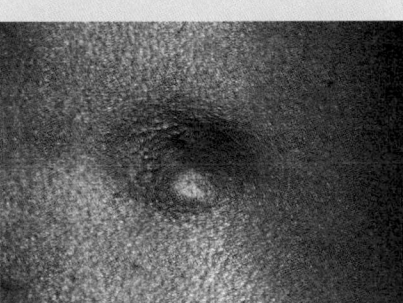	Elevated, solid, and firm, with depth into dermis. Examples: wart, lipoma (fatty cyst)
Wheal 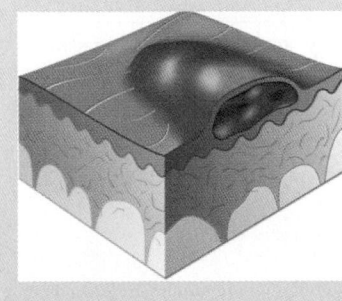	Hive 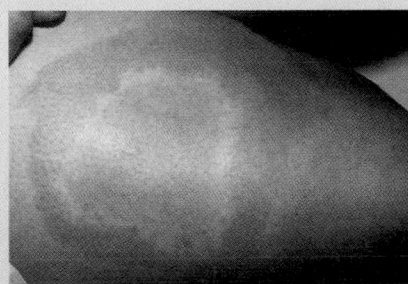	Elevated, superficial, with localized edema. Examples: insect bites, hives

(continued on next page)

Procedure 19-2 ■ **Assessing the Skin** (continued)

Describing Skin Lesions—cont'd

TYPES		DESCRIPTION
Secondary Lesions		
Excoriation 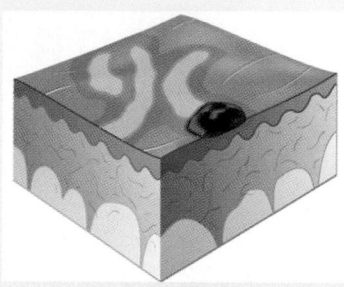	Excoriation from pruritus 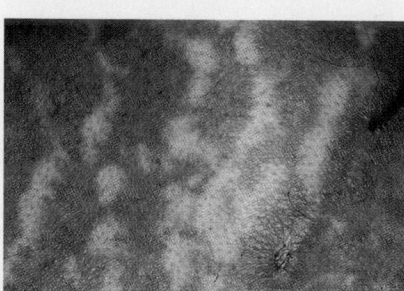	Abrasion or loss of skin that does not extend beyond the superficial epidermis. Examples: scratches, stasis dermatitis, atopic dermatitis
Erosion 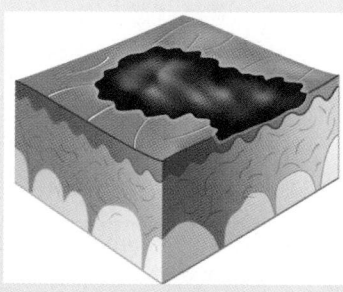	Erosions 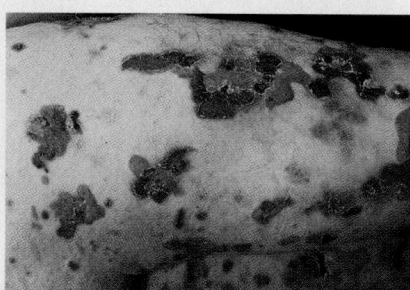	Loss of superficial epidermis, usually secondary to rupture of a blister. Examples: abrasions and impetigo
Fissure 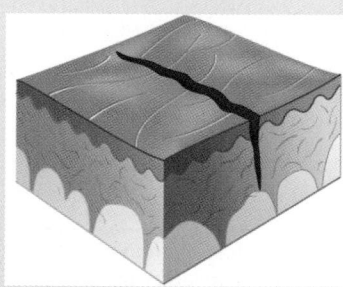	Cheilitis 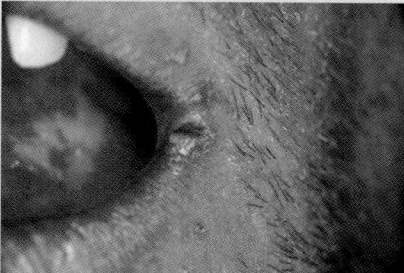	Linear break in the skin ("crack"); may extend to the dermis. Examples: athlete's foot, cheilitis
Ulcer 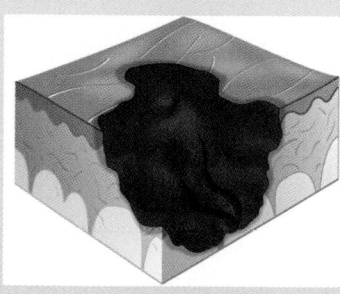	Stasis ulcer 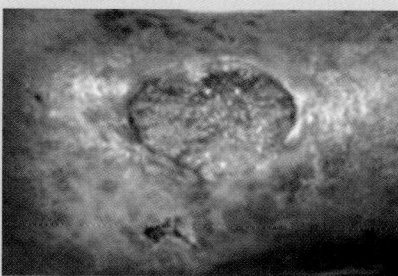	Irregularly shaped with loss of tissue. Graded based on depth and tissue involvement. Examples: pressure ulcers, stasis ulcers

Describing Skin Lesions—cont'd

TYPES		DESCRIPTION
Crust 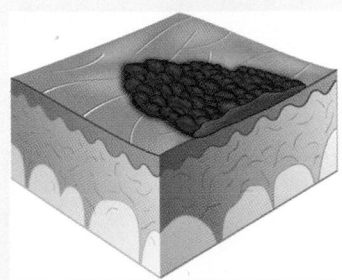	Crust 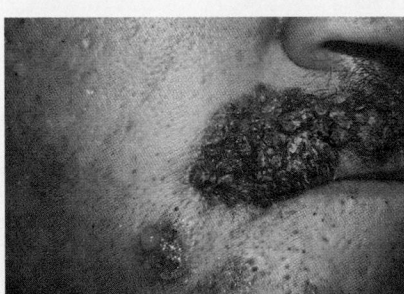	Elevated, rough texture with dried exudate. Examples: impetigo, herpes simplex
Scales 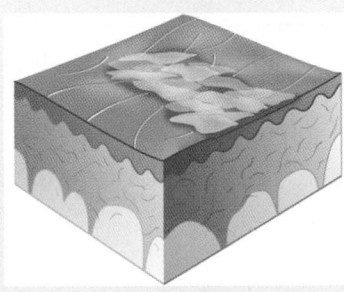	Psoriasis 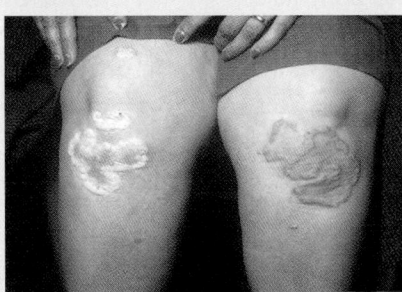	White to tan flaking, dead skin cells; may be adherent or loose. Examples: psoriasis and dandruff
Scar 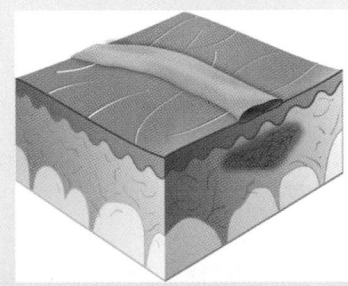		Fibrous tissue at site of injury, trauma, or surgery. Examples: surgical site, trauma site
Keloid 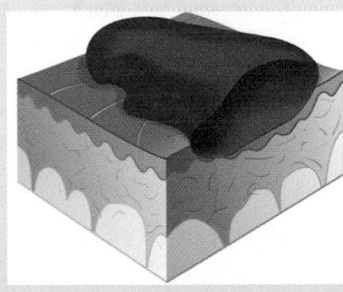	Keloids 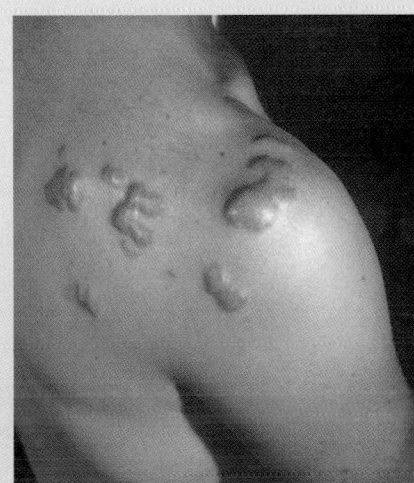	Raised and irregular scar due to excess collagen formation. Examples: surgical scars, ear piercing

Practice Resources
Yifan Xue (2007).

Procedure 19-3 ☐ Assessing the Hair

➤ For steps to follow in *all* procedures, refer to the Universal Steps for All Procedures found on the inside back cover of Volume 2.

Critical Aspects

- Techniques: Inspection and palpation
- Assess scalp hair and body hair.
- Inspect hair for color, quantity, distribution, condition of scalp, and presence of lesions or pediculosis.
- Palpate the texture of the hair.
- Palpate the scalp for mobility and tenderness.

Equipment

- Nonlatex procedure gloves (if exposure to body fluids is a possibility)
- Pen and record form

Focused History Questions

- Have you had any changes in hair texture?
- Have you had any loss of hair?
- Do you use dyes or chemical treatments for curling or straightening?

➤ When performing the procedure, always identify your patient according to agency policy and be attentive to standard precautions, hand hygiene, patient safety and privacy, body mechanics, and documentation.

Procedure Steps

1. Inspect the hair and scalp.
Check the color, quantity, and distribution of the hair and the condition of the scalp. Note the presence of lesions or pediculosis.
Sex, genetics, and age affect hair distribution on the head, legs extremities, pubis, and axillae. With aging, melanocyte function declines and sebaceous gland function decreases.

2. Palpate the texture of the hair.

3. Palpate the scalp for mobility and tenderness.

Expected Findings

The hair is evenly distributed on the scalp, and fine body hair is present over the body. The hair is clean and free of debris or pediculosis.

Developmental Variations

Infants—May have very little scalp hair.

Adolescents—May have oily hair. Puberty marks the onset of pubic hair growth and increased hair growth.

Older adults—Scalp, axillary, leg, and pubic hair may be dry and thin; hair of the ears, nostrils, and eyebrows may become coarse.

Abnormal findings: Generalized hair loss not attributed to genetics or aging; patchy hair loss; **hirsutism** (excess facial or trunk hair). See Abnormal Atlas at the end of this chapter.

Hair texture varies (fine, medium, coarse) depending on genetics and treatments.

Abnormal findings: Very dry, coarse hair; very fine, silky hair

Scalp is smooth, firm, symmetrical, nontender, and without lesions.

Abnormal findings: Tenderness, lesions.

Patient Teaching

If indicated, teach the patient to check for head lice, and provide preventive measures.

Documentation

- If you need more information about documenting,

 Go to Chapter 19, **Documenting Physical Assessment Findings,** in Volume 1. Also see Chapter 17 for documenting vital signs on a graphic flowsheet.

Procedure 19-4 ☐ Assessing the Nails

➤ For steps to follow in *all* procedures, refer to the Universal Steps for All Procedures found on the inside back cover of Volume 2.

Critical Aspects

- Techniques: Inspection and palpation
- Inspect the nails for color, condition, and shape.
- Palpate the texture of the nails.
- Assess capillary refill by pressing on the nail and releasing.
- Assess factors that may alter nail assessment findings (e.g., a cold environment may slow capillary refill).
- Examine nails on both hands and feet.
- You may defer examination of the toenails until you assess peripheral circulation.

Equipment

- Nonlatex gloves (if exposure to body fluids is a possibility)
- Pen and record form

Focused History Questions

- Have you had any recent changes in the way your nails grow or look?
- Have you had any recent trauma to your nails?
- Do you use acrylic nails?
- Do you have any medical problems, such as peripheral vascular disease or diabetes?

➤ When performing the procedure, always identify your patient according to agency policy and be attentive to standard precautions, hand hygiene, patient safety and privacy, body mechanics, and documentation.

Procedure Steps

1. Inspect nails.
   - Check nails for color, condition, texture, and shape.
   - Examine nails on both hands and feet. However, you may defer examination of the toenails until the assessment of peripheral circulation.

For efficiency of the assessment.

Expected Findings

Healthy nail beds are level, firm, and similar to the color of the skin. The shape is convex, with a nail plate angle of about 160°.▼

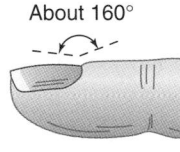

About 160°

Step 1

Developmental Variations

Newborns—Have very thin nails.

Children—May bite their nails. Most children outgrow this habit.

Older adults—Nails grow more slowly, become thicker, and tend to split.

Abnormal findings: Yellow, blue, or black discoloration. White spots may indicate zinc deficiency. Spoon-shaped (concave) nails are associated with iron deficiency. See Abnormal Atlas: Nail Appearance, at the end of this chapter.

(continued on next page)

Procedure 19-4 ■ **Assessing the Nails** (continued)

2. Inspect and palpate for texture.
Grooves or lines in the nails provide information about nutrition and health problems.

Nails are smooth and uniform in texture.

Abnormal findings: Thickened, brittle, or soft nails; nails with deep vertical grooves

3. Assess capillary refill.
Briefly press the tip of the nail with firm, steady pressure; then release and observe for changes in color.
This test assesses circulatory adequacy rather than the nails themselves. However, circulatory insufficiency affects the nails and nailbeds. It is convenient to perform the assessment at this point in the exam.▼

Normal capillary refill is < 2 to *3 seconds.*

Developmental Variations

Older adults—Capillary refill time (CRT) is slower.

Males—CRT faster than in women

Environment—CRT is slower in a cool environment.

Abnormal findings: Delayed capillary refill.

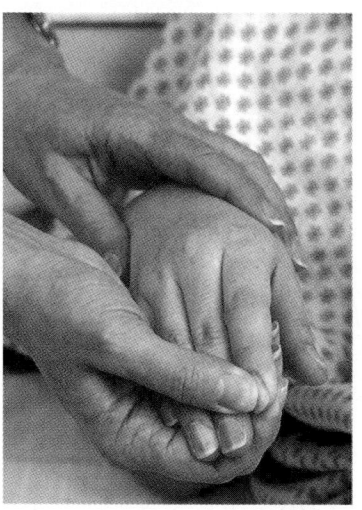

Step 3

Documentation

■ If you need more information about documenting,

 Go to Chapter 19, **Documenting Physical Assessment Findings,** in Volume 1.

Practice Resources
Anderson, B., Kelly, A. M., Kerr, D., et al. (2008).

Procedure 19-5 ☐ **Assessing the Head and Face**

➤ For steps to follow in *all* procedures, refer to the Universal Steps for All Procedures found on the inside back cover of Volume 2.

Critical Aspects

- Techniques: Inspection, palpation, auscultation
- Inspect the head for size, shape, symmetry, and position.
- Inspect the face for expression and symmetry.
- Palpate the head for masses, tenderness, and scalp mobility.
- Palpate the face for symmetry, tenderness, muscle tone, and TMJ function.

Equipment

- Nonlatex gloves (if exposure to body fluids is a possibility)
- Penlight (to transilluminate the sinuses)
- Pen and record form

Positioning

Preferably, the client should be sitting.

Focused History Questions

- Have you had any recent headaches?
- Have you ever had a head injury or loss of consciousness?
- Have you ever had a seizure?
- Do you have jaw or facial pain?

➤ When performing the procedure, always identify your patient according to agency policy and be attentive to standard precautions, hand hygiene, patient safety and privacy, body mechanics, and documentation.

Procedure Steps

1. Inspect the head.
Check for size, shape, symmetry, and position.

Developmental Modifications

- *Newborns and infants*—Assess and transilluminate fontanelles, and measure head circumference.

Expected Findings

There is wide variation in head size and shape, although the shape should be symmetrical and rounded. The head should be erect, midline, and proportional to the body size based on age.

Developmental Variations

Newborns and infants—Cranial bones are not fused at birth, and head shape may reflect normal pressure or trauma during vaginal birth for several weeks. The anterior fontanelle ("soft spot") fuses at about 18 months; the posterior, at about 8 weeks. Infants normally cannot hold their head up until about 6 months of age.

Abnormal findings: Larger or smaller than expected size for age, asymmetry of skull

---

2. Inspect the face.
   a. Note the client's facial expression.
   b. Ask yourself,
- Are the facial features symmetrical?
- Are there any abnormal facial movements?
- Are there any visible lesions of abnormal hair distribution?

Helpful hint: Look for symmetry in the palpebral fissures and the nasolabial folds. ▼

Facial expression is appropriate for the situation. No visible lesions. Facial features and movement are symmetrical.

Abnormal findings: Facial appearance inconsistent with sex, age, or racial/ethnic group; asymmetry of facial features or facial movement ▼

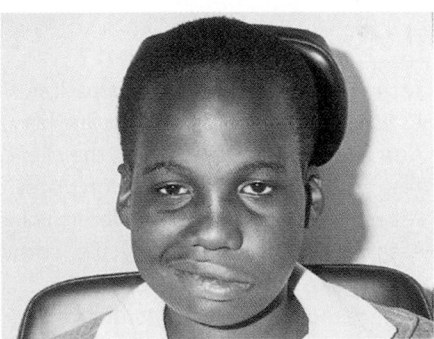

Bell's palsy

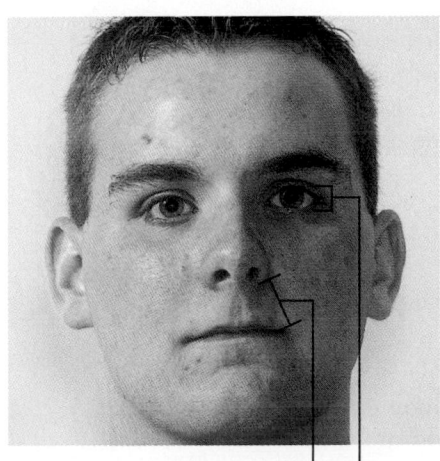

Nasolabial fold

Palpebral fissure

Step 2

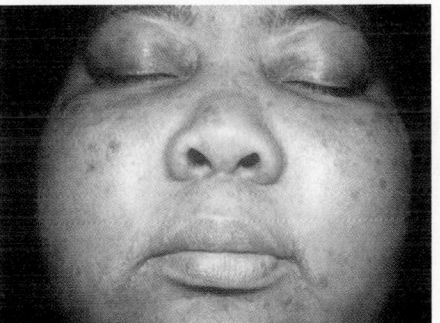

Cushing's syndrome

(continued on next page)

Procedure 19–5 ■ **Assessing the Head and Face** (continued)

3. Palpate the head.
Check for masses, tenderness, and scalp mobility.

Developmental Modifications

■ *Newborns and infants*—Palpate anterior and posterior fontanelles.

The head should be relatively smooth, with no tenderness or lesions.

Abnormal findings: Contour abnormalities (e.g., indentations, "bumps")

---

4. Palpate the face for symmetry, tenderness, muscle tone, and temporomandibular joint function. ▼

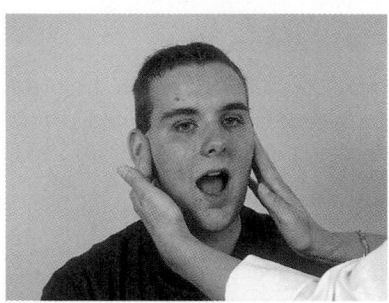

Palpating the TMJ

Smooth, symmetrical movement with no pain, crepitus, or clicking of the jaw

Abnormal findings: Irregular or uneven movement of the jaw; pain or popping with movement

---

Documentation

■ If you need more information about documenting,

 Go to Chapter 19, **Documenting Physical Assessment Findings,** in Volume 1.

Procedure 19-6 ☐ **Assessing the Eyes**

➤ For steps to follow in *all* procedures, refer to the Universal Steps for All Procedures found on the inside back cover of Volume 2.

Critical Aspects

■ Techniques: Inspection and palpation
■ Assess distance vision using a Snellen chart.
■ Test near vision by measuring the client's ability to read newsprint at a distance of 14 inches (35.5 cm).
■ Test color vision by using color plates or the color bars on the Snellen chart.
■ Assess peripheral vision by determining when an object comes into sight.
■ Assess EOMs by examining the corneal light reflex, observing the six cardinal gaze positions, and performing the cover/uncover test.
■ Inspect the external eye structures.
■ Test the corneal reflex with a cotton wisp, if appropriate.
■ Check the pupil reaction for direct and consensual response.
■ Assess accommodation by having the patient focus on an approaching object.
■ Palpate the external eye structures.

Equipment

■ Nonlatex gloves—if exposure to body fluids is a possibility
■ Visual acuity chart with color bars (Snellen)
■ A card—to cover one eye during the acuity exam
■ Penlight
■ Cotton ball and cotton-tipped applicator

■ Ophthalmoscope
■ Pen and form

Position

Preferably, the client should be sitting.

Focused History Questions

- Have you noticed any changes in your vision?
- Do you wear glasses or contact lenses?
- Have you ever had an eye injury?
- Have you ever had an eye infection or stye?
- Do you have problems with excessive tearing or dry eyes?
- Have you ever had eye surgery?
- Have you ever experienced blurred vision?

- Do you have difficulty with nighttime vision?
- Do you ever see halos of light, spots or floaters, or flashes of light?
- Do you have a history of eye problems, such as glaucoma, or medical problems, such as diabetes or hypertension?
- When was your last eye exam?
- Do you use any prescription or over-the-counter eye medications?

➤ When performing the procedure, always identify your patient according to agency policy and be attentive to standard precautions, hand hygiene, patient safety and privacy, body mechanics, and documentation.

Procedure Steps

1. Test distance vision.
   - Depending on patient's age and literacy level, use the Snellen standard eye chart or Snellen E chart (for those who cannot read). Picture charts are available for preschoolers.
   - If the client wears corrective lenses, they should be worn during a test.
     a. Have the patient sit or stand 6 m (20 ft.) from the chart. With a card, cover the eye not being tested; ask the patient to read the smallest line of print that he can distinguish. Consider a line to be read correctly if the client makes no more than two mistakes in that line.
     b. Test the opposite eye.
     c. Test both eyes together.
     d. At the end of each line of the Snellen chart is a fraction—the top line is 20/200. After each test, record the resulting fraction: the number at the end of the smallest line the patient could read with no more than two errors. ▼

Expected Findings

Expect 20/20 vision in the right eye, left eye, and both eyes. The top number of the fraction indicates the distance the person was standing from the chart; the bottom number is the distance from which a person with normal vision would be able to read the chart.

Developmental Variations

Children—Distance vision does not reach 20/20 until around 6 or 7 years of age.

Middle adults—At about middle age, the lens of the eye begins to lose some ability to accommodate to near objects.

Abnormal findings: A smaller fraction (e.g., 20/100) indicates diminished distant vision or myopia. A larger fraction (e.g., 20/15) indicates diminished near vision, called hyperopia.

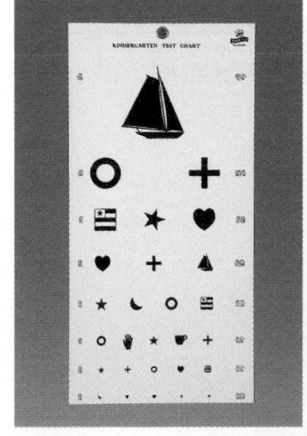

Preliterate chart

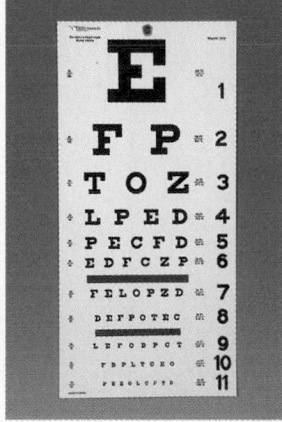

Snellen standard chart

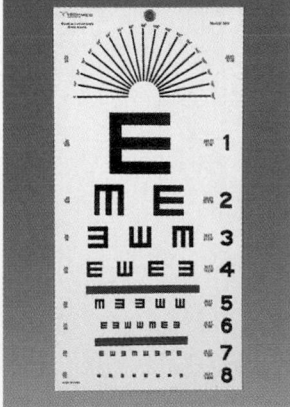

Snellen E chart

2. Test near vision.
Test the client's ability to read newsprint at a distance of 35.5 cm (14 in.) from the eyes. Use print-sized pictures if the patient is unable to read.

The client reads newsprint at a distance of 35.5 cm (14 in.).

Abnormal findings: The need to hold the print at a greater distance indicates hyperopia or presbyopia.

(continued on next page)

Procedure 19-6 ■ **Assessing the Eyes** (continued)

3. Test color vision.
　a. Have the patient differentiate patterns of colors on color cards or identify the color bars on the Snellen eye chart.
　b. Inability to distinguish colors requires a thorough evaluation using the Ishihara cards to determine the scope of the color deficit. ▼

Color vision is intact.

Developmental Variations

Older adults—Experience some decline in color vision, especially in the ability to see purples and pastels.

Abnormal findings: Inability to distinguish colors

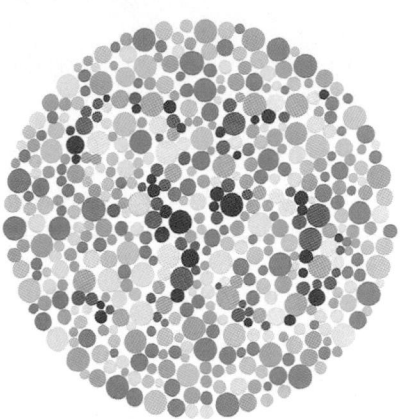

Ishihara card

4. Test peripheral vision.
　a. Seat the client 60–90 cm (2–3 ft.) from you.
　b. Have client cover one eye and fix the gaze straight ahead while you bring an object in from the periphery to the center of the visual fields. Be sure to begin by holding the object well outside the range of normal peripheral vision. Instruct the client to identify when the object becomes visible.
　c. Repeat this in each of the four visual fields, moving clockwise.

Expect no deficits in the visual fields.

Abnormal findings: Loss of peripheral vision. Report gross deficits to an ophthalmologist for further assessment.

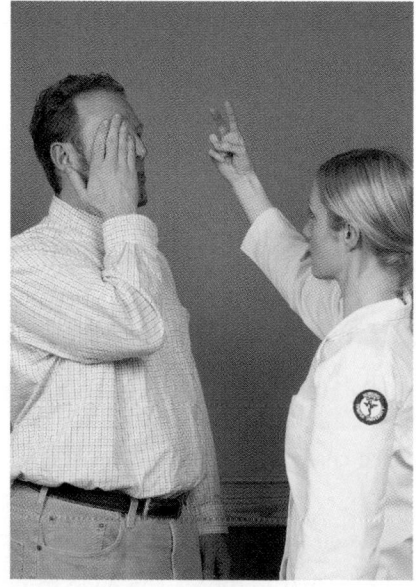

Step 4

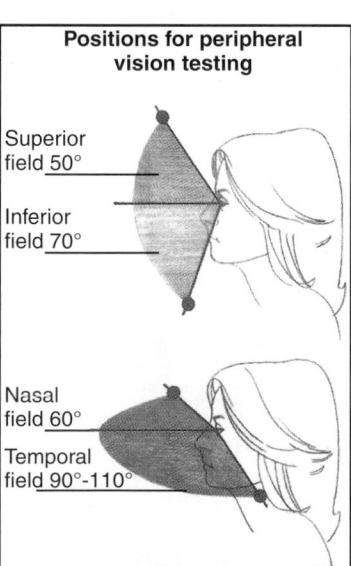

Positions for peripheral vision testing

Superior field 50°
Inferior field 70°

Nasal field 60°
Temporal field 90°-110°

5. Assess extraocular movements.
a. Inspect the eyes for parallel alignment.

b. Test the corneal light reflex by shining a penlight at the bridge of the nose. Note where the light reflects on the cornea of each eye.

c. Test the six cardinal fields of gaze. Stand in front of the patient, and have the patient follow an object through the six cardinal fields without moving his head. ▼

a. The eyes should be in parallel alignment.

b. Corneal light reflex appears at the same position in each eye.

Abnormal findings: An asymmetrical corneal light reflex may indicate weak extraocular muscles or strabismus.

c. The eyes move through all six gaze positions.

Abnormal findings: Inability to move through all gaze positions

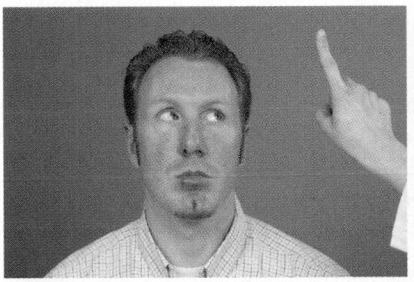

Up left

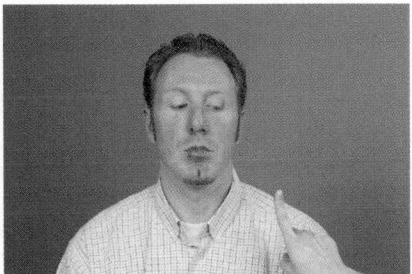

Side left

Down left

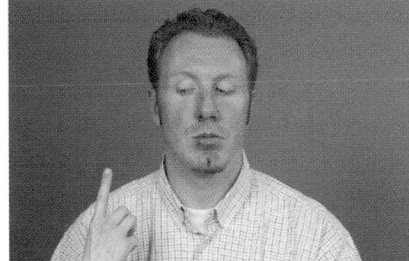

Down right

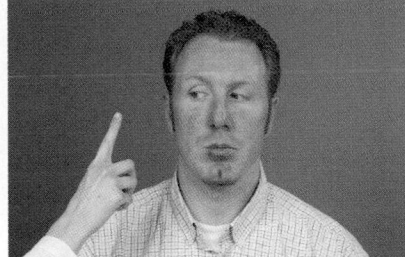

Side right

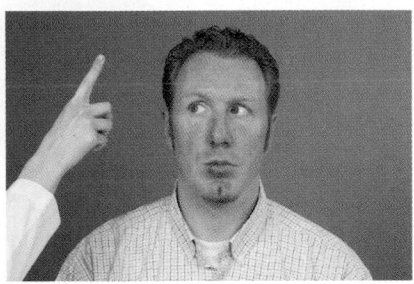

Up right

d. Perform the cover/uncover test. Cover one eye and have the patient gaze at a distant object. Uncover the eye. Repeat on the opposite side.

d. The gaze should be steady when the eye is covered and uncovered.

Abnormal findings: A shift in gaze indicates weak eye muscles.

---

6. Inspect the external structures.
a. General appearance: Check the color and alignment of the eyes.

a. Eyes clear, bright, and in parallel alignment.

Developmental Variations

Older adults—A decrease in periorbital fat may give the eyeballs a sunken appearance.

Abnormal findings: Glazed eyes may indicate a febrile state.

b. Inspect the eyelids. Note the presence of any lesions, edema, or lid lag.

b. No lesions present; lids move freely. Upper eyelid covers half of the upper iris.

Developmental Variations

Older adults—The lower lids may sag; skinfolds are prominent in the upper lids.

Abnormal findings: Asymmetry of lids may result from CN III damage or from a stroke. Lesions may be benign (e.g., a stye) or pathological (e.g., basal cell carcinoma).

(continued on next page)

Procedure 19-6 ■ **Assessing the Eyes** (continued)

c. Inspect the eyelashes. Note symmetry and distribution.

c. Eyelashes are evenly distributed and curve outward. No crustations or infestations are present.

Abnormal findings: Inflammation of the eyelids, which may be caused by infection; inverted eyelashes (entropion); everted eyelashes (ectropion); visible sclera between the iris and upper lid

d. Inspect the lacrimal ducts and glands. Note any edema, excessive tearing, or drainage.

d. No periorbital edema or lesions are present. No drainage

Abnormal findings: Swelling, redness, drainage, or tenderness.

e. Inspect the conjunctivae. Note the color, moisture, and contour of the conjunctivae.

(1) The palpebral conjunctivae cover the lids. To assess, have the patient look up as you place a cotton-tipped applicator on the upper lid, gently grasp the upper lid and lashes, and evert the lid over the cotton-tipped applicator.▼

e. The palpebral conjunctivae are smooth, glistening, and peach in color. Minimal blood vessels are present. The bulbar conjunctivae are clear with few underlying blood vessels and white sclera visible.

Developmental Variations

Older adults—The conjunctivae may be pale or have a slightly yellow tint due to fat deposits.

Abnormal findings: Pallor, dryness, edema; pterygium; subconjunctival hemorrhage

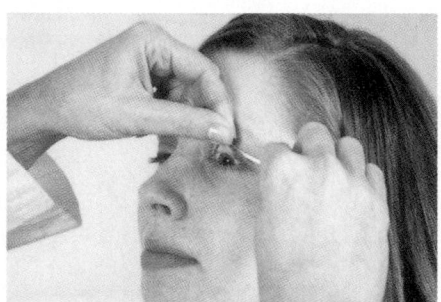

Step 6e(1)

(2) The bulbar conjunctiva covers the eyeball. To assess, pull the lower lid down.▼

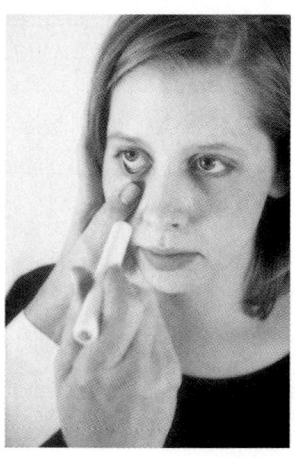

Step 6e(2)

f. Inspect the sclera.
Note the color of the sclera and whether lesions are present.

f. The sclera should be smooth, white, and glistening. Dark-skinned patients may have a yellowish cast to the peripheral sclera or small brown spots more centrally.

Abnormal findings: Yellow (icteric) sclera

g. Inspect the cornea and lens.
As the client looks straight ahead, shine a penlight at an angle to the eye, and move it across the corneal surface. Note the color and whether any lesions are present.

g. The cornea and lens are clear, smooth, and glistening.

Developmental Variations

Older adults—Arcus senilis is a normal variant.

Abnormal findings: Lens opacities (cataracts); roughness or irregularity of the cornea

h. Test the corneal reflex.
Touch the cornea with a wisp of sterile cotton, or use a needleless syringe to shoot a small amount of air over the cornea.

h. Blink reflex is prompt.

Abnormal findings: Failure to blink may result from neurosensory deficits.

◆ NOTE: *This is not routinely performed on conscious patients. A conscious person can blink intentionally, so there is no need. In addition, there is a slight risk of corneal abrasion from cotton.*

i. Inspect the iris and pupils.
Note the color, size, shape, and symmetry.

i. The iris is blue, green, brown, or a combination of these colors; its shape is circular. The pupils are round and of equal size. Unequal pupils (anisocoria) can be a normal variation if the difference is less than 0.5 mm.

Developmental Variations

Older adults—Pigment degeneration may cause the iris to be pale with brownish discolorations.

Abnormal findings: Damage to one eye may cause the iris to be a different color. Absence of part or all of the iris is a congenital problem. Unequal pupils may result from CN III damage, brain herniation, or increased intracranial pressure.

j. Test pupillary reaction.
In a dimly lighted room, have the patient look straight ahead. Bring a penlight in from the side, and shine the light onto one eye. Note the reaction, equality, and speed of response of both eyes. For example, when you shine a light onto the right eye, the right pupil reaction is direct; the left eye is consensual. Repeat the test on the opposite eye. ▼

j. Normal direct and consensual response to light is brisk, with equal constriction of both pupils.

Developmental Variations

Older adults—Pupil reaction may be slower but should be symmetrical.

Abnormal findings: Sluggish or fixed pupils may result from CN II damage or brain injury. Absence of consensual response may result from nerve compression or anoxia.

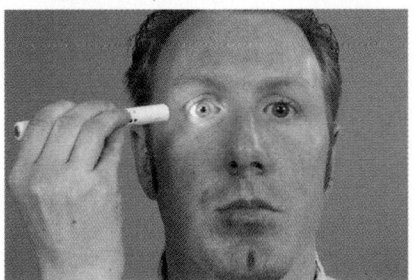

Testing pupillary reaction to light

k. Test pupil accommodation.
Have the patient look straight ahead and focus on an object about 30 cm (12 in.) from his face. Slowly bring the object in toward the patient's eyes. Note pupil size and location.

k. The pupils constrict and the eyes cross as a person attempts to focus on a near object.

Developmental Variations

Older adults—Accommodation may be slow.

Abnormal findings: One or both pupils fail to accommodate, or they accommodate slowly.

l. Inspect the anterior chamber.
Shine a penlight across the eye from the side as the patient looks straight ahead. Observe color, size, shape, and symmetry.

l. The chamber should be clear and symmetrically curved.

Abnormal findings: Blood or pus in the chamber. Also see Abnormal Atlas: Eyes at the end of this chapter.

(continued on next page)

Procedure 19-6 ■ **Assessing the Eyes** (continued)

7. Palpate the external structures.
   a. Gently palpate the globe (eyeball) with your fingertips on the upper lids over the sclera. Note the consistency and any tenderness.
   b. Palpate the lacrimal glands and ducts by palpating below the eyebrow and below the inner canthus of the eye. Note tenderness and excessive tearing or discharge. ▼

The globe is firm and nontender. Lacrimal glands are nonpalpable; no tenderness is present.

Abnormal findings: Firm or tender globe; swelling and tenderness over the lacrimal glands

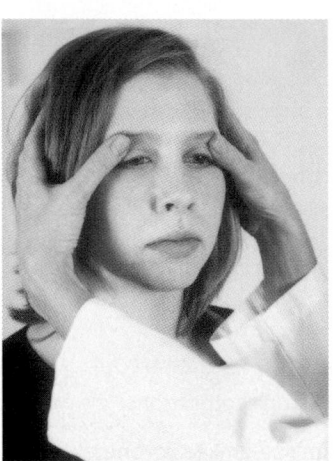

Step 7

8. Assess the internal structures via ophthalmoscopy. This is an advanced physical assessment technique.
   a. Darken the room.
   b. Stand about 1 foot from the patient at a 15° lateral angle.
   c. Dial the lens wheel to zero with your index finger. Hold the ophthalmoscope to your brow.
   d. Have the patient look straight ahead while you shine the light on one pupil and identify the red light reflex. ▼

Expect a positive red light reflex. On internal examination, the optic disk is round with sharp margins. There are no opacities and the cup:disk ratio is 1:2. The disk is yellow with a white cup.

Abnormal findings: Any findings not consistent with the above should be reported promptly.

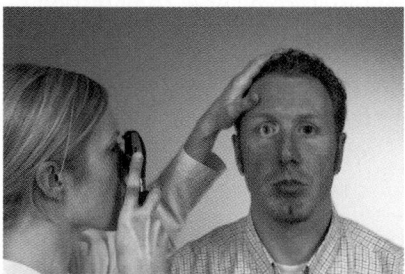

Checking red reflex

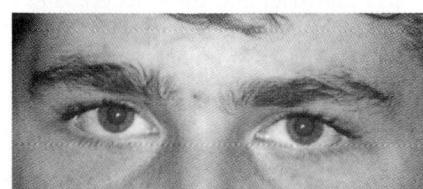

Red reflex over pupil area

e. Once you identify the red light reflex, move in closer to within a few inches of the eye and observe the internal structures of the eye. Adjust the lens wheel to focus as needed. Use your right eye to examine the patient's right eye, and your left eye to examine the patient's left eye. ▼

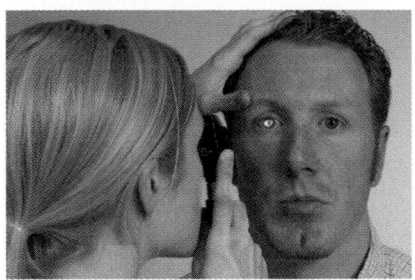

Step 8e: Examining internal structures of the eye

f. Repeat for the opposite eye.

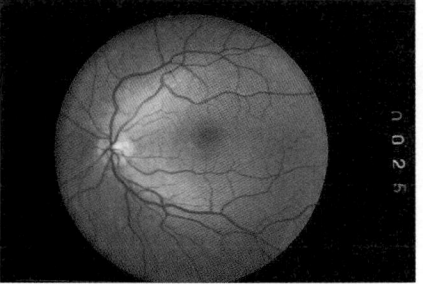

Normal fundus

Patient Teaching

Teach the patient the importance of routine eye examinations.

Documentation

■ If you need more information about documenting,

 Go to Chapter 19, **Documenting Physical Assessment Findings,** in Volume 1.

Procedure 19-7 ■ Assessing the Ears and Hearing

➤ For steps to follow in *all* procedures, refer to the Universal Steps for All Procedures found on the inside back cover of Volume 2.

Critical Aspects

- Techniques: Inspection and palpation
- Inspect the external ear for placement, size, shape, symmetry, and the condition of the skin.
- Palpate the external structures of the ear for skin condition and tenderness.
- Inspect the tympanic membrane and bony landmarks.
- Assess gross hearing with the whisper and watch-tick tests.
- Perform the Weber test to assess hearing loss.
- Perform the Rinne test to identify whether hearing loss is conductive or sensorineural.

Equipment

- Nonlatex gloves (if exposure to body fluids is a possibility)
- Tuning fork
- Watch
- Otoscope with pneumatic tube
- Pen and record form

Position

Have the patient seated, if possible.

Focused History Questions

- Do you have any hearing problems?
- Have you ever had ringing in your ears?
- Have you had any changes in your hearing?
- Do you have any ear drainage? If yes, how much and what color?
- Do you have any ear pain?
- Do you have any balance problems, dizziness, or vertigo?
- Do you have a history of head trauma?
- Are you exposed to noise pollution at work or in your home environment?

(continued on next page)

Procedure 19-7 ■ **Assessing the Ears and Hearing** (continued)

➤ When performing the procedure, always identify your patient according to agency policy and be attentive to standard precautions, hand hygiene, patient safety and privacy, body mechanics, and documentation.

Procedure Steps

1. Inspect the external ear.
   a. Check the placement and angle of attachment of the ear. ▼

Expected Findings

a. The normal angle of attachment is 10°.

Abnormal findings: High or low placement of the ear may be a sign of hearing deficit or genetic problems.

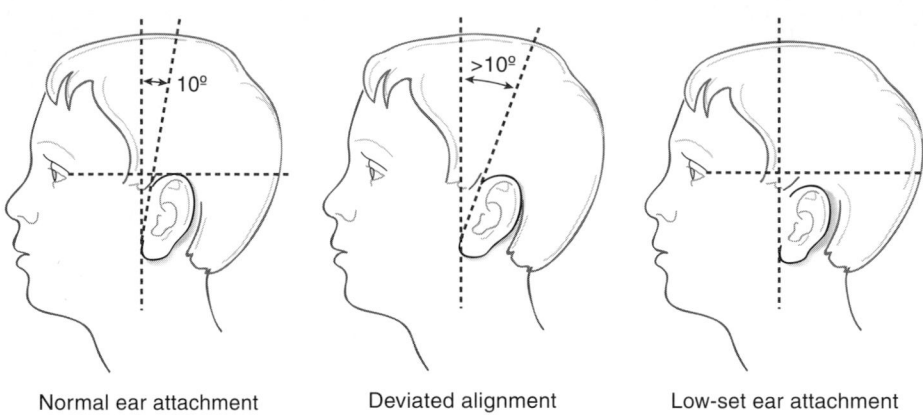

Normal ear attachment   Deviated alignment   Low-set ear attachment

b. Note the shape, size, and symmetry of the ears.

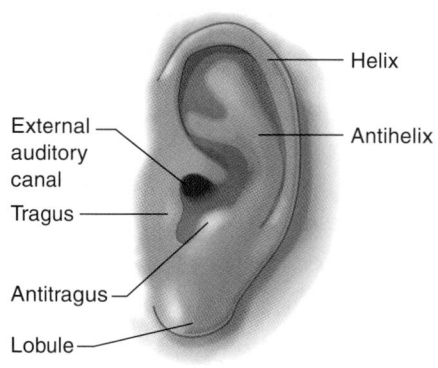

Step 1b

b. The helix, antihelix, antitragus, tragus, and lobule are present. The ears are 4–10 cm in length and symmetrical in size and shape.

Developmental Variations

Older adults—The ear changes shape as the lobe elongates.

Abnormal findings: Absence of any of the landmarks may indicate a hearing deficit. Ears that are < 4 cm long or > 10 cm long may indicate a genetic disorder.

c. Observe the color of the ear.

c. Color is consistent with skin color.

Abnormal findings: Redness may indicate inflammation or infection.

d. Observe the condition of the skin; observe for drainage and visible lesions.

d. Skin is intact with no drainage or lesions. Piercings may be present.

Developmental Variations

Older adults—May have coarse hair on the helix, antihelix, and tragus; skin may be dry.

Abnormal findings: Bloody or purulent drainage; lesions. The ears are a common location for skin cancer.

2. Palpate the external structures of the ear.
  a. Note the consistency of the skin, the presence of lesions, and any signs of tenderness.

Skin is soft, pliable, and nontender. No nodules or lesions are present.

Abnormal findings: Tenderness is often associated with infection.

---

3. Perform an otoscopic exam.
  a. This is an advanced physical assessment technique.
  b. Use a speculum with the largest diameter and shortest length that the ear canal can accommodate. 4 mm is a common size for adults.
  c. Have the patient tilt his head to the side not being examined.
  d. For adults, grasp the pinna and gently pull upward and back. For a child, position the pinna down and back. It positions the ear canal with more direct alignment, allowing for improved visualization.

  e. Insert the speculum no further than halfway into the ear canal. As you advance the speculum, examine the canal for redness, open areas, drainage, foreign objects, and so on. ▼

The ear canal is light in color and patent, with a small amount of yellow cerumen (color may vary). TM is shiny and pearly gray with a cone of reflective light on the nasal aspect that would be 5 o'clock in the left ear and 7 o'clock in the right ear. Bony landmarks are visible. The TM is mobile. No bulging or retraction of the TM. ▼

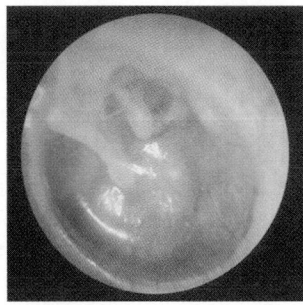

Normal TM left ear

Developmental Variations

Older adults—May have dry ear wax. The TM is translucent, and the light reflex may be diminished.

Abnormal findings: Excessive wax may occlude the canal. TM that is red, with a distorted light reflex, suggests otitis media. A change in the position or shape of the cone of light reflex indicates an imbalance in middle ear pressure. ▼

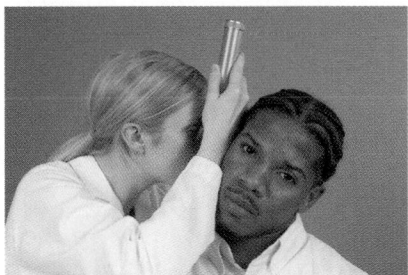

Otoscope insertion with handle up

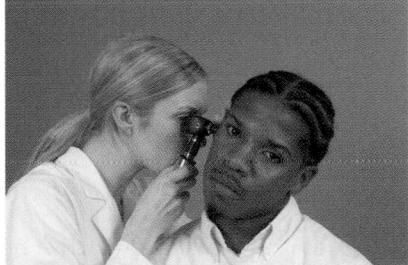

Otoscope insertion with handle down

  f. Look through the magnifying lens.
   (1) Observe the ear canal.
   (2) Observe the tympanic membrane.

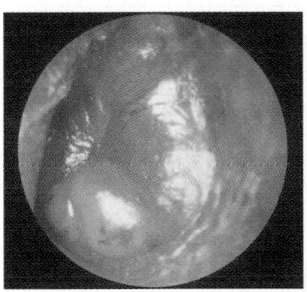

Otitis media

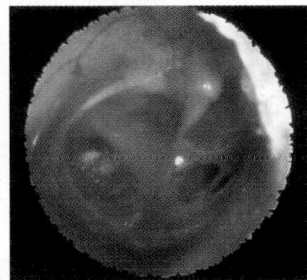

Perforated TM

(continued on next page)

Procedure 19-7 ■ **Assessing the Ears and Hearing** (continued)

g. Test the mobility of the tympanic membrane by using the otoscope's pneumatic tube to gently "puff" air into the external ear canal while observing movement of the cone of light.

NOTE: *The ears are mirror images, with the cone of light at 7 o'clock in the left ear and 5 o'clock in the right ear.*

Developmental Modifications

Children—Many young children fear the otoscopic examination. Demonstrating the procedure on a parent or a doll may relieve their anxiety.

h. Carefully remove the otoscope from the ear canal, being careful not to traumatize the delicate tissue.

---

4. Test gross hearing.
a. Stand 1–2 ft. behind the patient. Have the patient cover one ear as you whisper some words. Repeat on the other side. Have the patient repeat the words she heard.

A test of hearing also indicates cranial nerve XIII is intact.

b. Have the patient occlude one ear. Hold a ticking watch next to the patient's unobstructed ear. Slowly move it away until the patient says she can no longer hear the sound. Repeat for the opposite ear.

Developmental Modifications

Infants—For infants younger than 3 months of age, loudly clap your hands behind the infant and observe whether he startles. After 3 months of age, the infant should turn his head or eyes toward a sound, for example, when the parent stands behind the infant and calls his name.

The patient is able to hear you whisper on both sides. The patient hears the watch at a distance of about 12 to 13 cm (5 in.).

Developmental Variations

Older adults—Often have a generalized loss of hearing. It first occurs in the high-frequency sounds (*f, s, sh,* and *ph*) and then progresses to include all frequencies.

Abnormal findings: Problems with the whisper test indicate low-tone hearing loss. Problems with the watch-tick test indicate a high-pitch deficit.

---

5. Perform the Weber test.
Place a vibrating tuning fork on top of the patient's head. Ask the patient whether the sound is the same in both ears or louder in one ear.

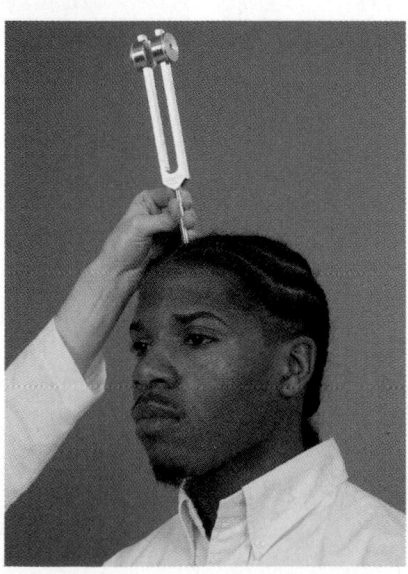

Weber test

The patient hears the sound equally in both ears.

Abnormal findings: Sound is louder in one ear.
■ If there is a conductive hearing loss, the vibration will be louder in the impaired ear. Conductive hearing loss may be caused by external or middle ear problems, such as infection, blockage of the canal by cerumen, or trauma to the TM.
■ If there is a sensorineural hearing loss, the sound will be louder in the unaffected ear. Sensorineural loss may result from inner ear problems or from some medications.
■ Perform the Rinne test to further identify the type of hearing loss.

6. Perform the Rinne test (if the Weber test is positive).
  a. Strike a tuning fork on the table. While it is still vibrating, place it on the patient's mastoid process.
Tests bone conduction of sound.

  b. Measure the elapsed time in seconds that the patient hears the vibration.
  c. Move the tuning fork to 2.5 cm (1 in.) in front of the ear, and measure the elapsed time until the patient can no longer hear the vibration.
Tests air conduction of sound.

  d. Repeat for the opposite ear.▼

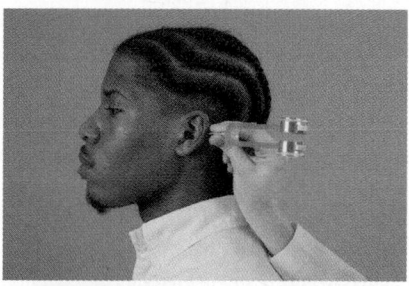

Step 6a

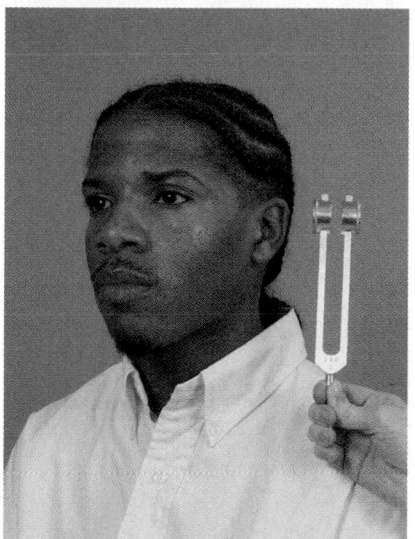

Step 6c

Normally, sound transmission through air (step 6c) is twice as long as transmission through bone (step 6b); that is, AC = 2 × BC.

The ratio of AC to BC is similar in both ears.

Abnormal findings:
- Conductive loss: AC is less than 2 × BC.
- Sensorineural loss: AC is greater than BC but not 2 × longer; or the patient is unable to hear the tuning fork through BC.
- A difference between ears indicates unilateral hearing loss.
- Inability to hear the tuning fork through BC indicates sensorineural hearing loss.

7. Perform the Romberg test.
Have the patient stand with feet together, hands at side, with eyes opened and then with eyes closed. Note the patient's ability to maintain balance.

 Stand nearby in case the client loses his balance.

Tests for balance. Strictly speaking, it does not assess the ears, but the vestibular nerve and other parts of the central nervous system. Therefore, you may prefer to perform the test during the neurological exam.

The patient maintains balance with minimal sway.

Abnormal findings: Positive Romberg (swaying) is seen with vestibular and cerebellar disorders.

Patient Teaching
Teach the patient the importance of routine hearing examinations.

Documentation
- If you need more information about documenting,

 VOL 1 Go to Chapter 19, **Documenting Physical Assessment Findings,** in Volume 1.

Procedure 19–8 ☐ Assessing the Nose and Sinuses

➤ For steps to follow in *all* procedures, refer to the Universal Steps for All Procedures found on the inside back cover of Volume 2.

Critical Aspects

- Techniques: Inspection and palpation
- Insert the speculum about 1 cm, and then open it as much as possible.
- Inspect the external and internal structures of the nose.
- Transilluminate and palpate the sinuses.
- Palpate the external structures of the nose.

Equipment

- Nonlatex procedure gloves (if exposure to body fluids is a possibility)
- Penlight
- Nasal speculum or otoscope with a wide-tipped speculum
- Pen and record form

Position

Have the patient seated, if possible.

Focused History Questions

- Do you have any nasal congestion?
- Do you have a history of nose or sinus problems?
- Do you have problems with seasonal or environmental allergies?
- Do you have a history of sinus headaches?
- Do you experience nose bleeds (*epistaxis*)?
- Have you ever broken your nose?
- Have you had any changes in your sense of smell?
- Do you use any nasal sprays or allergy medications?

➤ When performing the procedure, always identify your patient according to agency policy and be attentive to standard precautions, hand hygiene, patient safety and privacy, body mechanics, and documentation.

Procedure Steps	Expected Findings
1. Position the client for the exam.	
2. Inspect the external nose. Note the position, shape, and size. Observe for discharge and flaring.	The nose is midline and symmetrical. No discharge or flaring **Abnormal findings:** Asymmetry suggests congenital deformity or trauma. Flaring suggests respiratory distress (especially in infants, who cannot breathe through the mouth). Clear drainage suggests allergy; yellow or green drainage suggests upper respiratory infection; bloody drainage may result from trauma, hypertension, or a bleeding disorder.
3. Check for patency of the nasal passages. Ask the patient to close his mouth, hold one naris closed, and breathe through the other naris. Repeat with the opposite naris.	The client breathes freely through both nares.
4. Inspect the internal structures. 　a. Use a nasal speculum or an otoscope with a large speculum (or a penlight with a speculum) to assess the internal structures. 　b. Tilt the patient's head back to facilitate speculum insertion and visualization. 　c. Brace your index finger against the patient's nose as you insert the speculum.	Nasal mucosa is pink and moist. Septum is intact and midline. No lesions **Abnormal findings:** Deviated septum; polyps. Pale boggy mucosa is seen with allergies; bright red mucosa is associated with rhinitis, sinusitis, and cocaine use. Clustered vesicles suggest herpes infection. Erosion of nasal mucosa should signal you to investigate further for other signs or history of crack/cocaine use. Blood in the nasal passage indicates trauma, nose bleeds, or polyps.

d. Insert the speculum about 1 cm into the nares. Use the other hand to position the client's head and to hold the penlight if you do not have a lighted scope. ▼

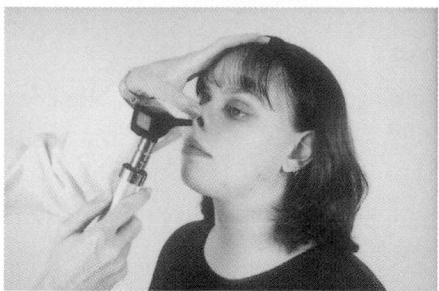

Step 4d

e. Observe the nasal mucosa for color, edema, lesions, erosion or ulceration, blood, and discharge. Inspect the septum for position and intactness.

f. Check for sense of smell using commonly recognized objects, such as a lemon or vanilla. Do not use a noxious odor. You can defer this test until the sensorineurological part of the exam if you choose, but keep the same order for every exam.

Cranial nerve I is intact when the patient shows an ability to detect odor.

Developmental Modifications

Infants and children—You will not need a speculum to examine internal structures. Push the tip of the nose upward with your thumb, and direct a penlight into the nares.

---

5. Transilluminate the frontal and maxillary sinuses.
   a. Darken the room.
   b. Frontal sinuses: Shine a penlight or the otoscope with speculum below the eyebrow on each side. ▼

A red glow is seen above the eyebrow, indicating that the frontal sinus is patent.

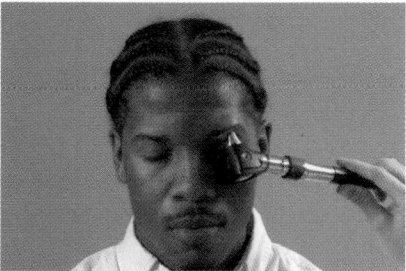

Step 5b

c. Maxillary sinuses: Place the light source below the eyes and above the cheeks. Look for a glow of red light at the roof of the mouth through the client's open mouth. ▼

A red glow may be (but is not always) seen in the roof of the mouth, indicating that the maxillary sinus is patent.

Abnormal findings: Absence of transillumination may result from mucosal thickening or sinusitis.

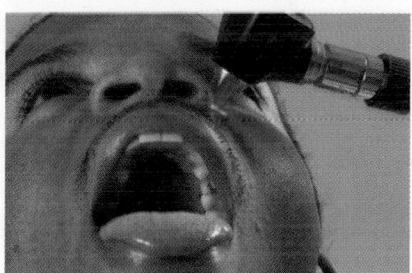

Step 5c

(continued on next page)

Procedure 19-8 ■ **Assessing the Nose and Sinuses** (continued)

6. Palpate the external structures.	No tenderness, lesions, or deformity

7. Palpate the frontal and maxillary sinuses.	No tenderness **Abnormal findings:** Tenderness may indicate infectious or allergic sinusitis.

Documentation
- If you need more information about documenting,

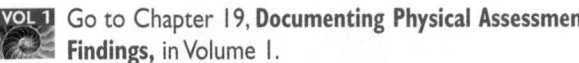 VOL 1 Go to Chapter 19, **Documenting Physical Assessment Findings,** in Volume 1.

Procedure 19-9 ■ Assessing the Mouth and Oropharynx

➤ For steps to follow in *all* procedures, refer to the Universal Steps for All Procedures found on the inside back cover of Volume 2.

Critical Aspects
- Techniques: Inspection and palpation
- Inspect the lips, oral mucosa, gums, teeth, and bite.
- Inspect the hard/soft palate, tonsils, and uvula.
- Inspect the tongue and frenulum; inspect under the tongue.
- Palpate the lips and tongue for tenderness and muscle tone.
- Test the gag reflex by touching the back of the soft palate with a tongue blade.

Equipment
- Nonlatex procedure gloves
- Penlight
- Tongue blade
- Small gauze pad
- Pen and record form

Position
Have the patient seated, if possible.

Focused History Questions
- Do you have any problems with your mouth or teeth?
- When was your last dental exam?
- Do you have any discomfort in your mouth or throat?
- Have you had any recent changes in your mouth or teeth?
- How often do you brush your teeth? Floss?
- Do you smoke or chew tobacco?
- Do you have any sores or irritation in your mouth? If so, when did you first notice this?

➤ When performing the procedure, always identify your patient according to agency policy and be attentive to standard precautions, hand hygiene, patient safety and privacy, body mechanics, and documentation.

Procedure Steps

1. Inspect the mouth externally.
Locate the placement of the lips and their color and condition. Ask the client to purse his lips.

Expected Findings

The lips are midline, symmetrical, moist, and intact with no lesions. Coloring is consistent with ethnic group/race. The client can purse his lips.

Abnormal findings: Asymmetry (may be due to congenital deformity, trauma, paralysis, or surgical alteration); pallor; cyanosis; redness; inability to purse lips (may indicate facial nerve damage); lesions (may be caused by bacteria, viruses, or trauma)

---

2. Note the color and condition of the oral mucosa and gums.
   a. Inspect and palpate the lower lip. Pull the lower lip away from the teeth, and inspect the inner side of the lip. Palpate any lesions for size, mobility, and tenderness.

Oral mucosa is pink, moist, and intact; no lesions. Gingiva is consistent in color with the other mucosae and is intact, with no bleeding. Buccal mucosa is pink and moist, with no lesions. Mucosa is darker in dark-skinned clients.

b. Inspect the buccal mucosa, top to bottom and back to front. ▼

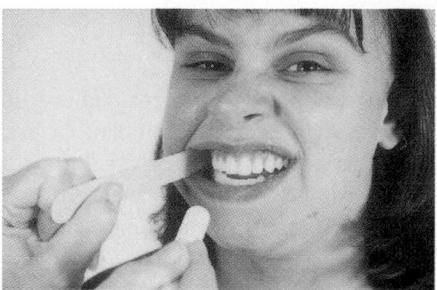

Step 2b

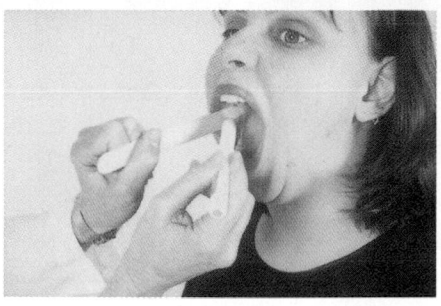

Step 2b

■ Ask the client to open his mouth. Use a tongue depressor to retract the cheek, then shine a penlight onto the mucosa.

■ Using a tongue blade and penlight, inspect the Stensen's duct openings to the parotid glands.

■ Finally, palpate inside each cheek by placing a finger inside and thumb outside. Grasping the cheek between them, move the finger about. Repeat on both sides.
c. As you are inspecting the buccal mucosa, also examine the gums. Check for color, bleeding, edema, retraction, and lesions. Press gum tissue gently with gloved finger or tongue blade to assess firmness.

Developmental Variations

Older adults—Mucosa is drier than in young adults because of decreased salivary gland activity; brownish pigmentation of gums may be seen, especially in dark-skinned people.

Abnormal findings: Receding gums, sponginess, bleeding, inflammatory changes, gingival hyperplasia, ulcerations, or other lesions

Structures of the Mouth and Oropharynx

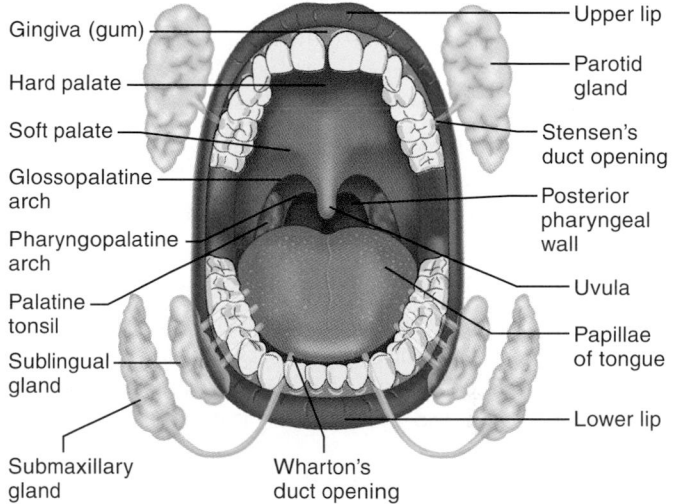

3. Inspect the teeth. You can do this while you are inspecting the oral mucosa and gums, in step 2.
a. Observe the number, color, and condition of the teeth. Note the occlusion ("bite") and any loose teeth.
b. If the client wears dentures, ask her to remove them. Inspect for cracked or worn areas; assess the fit.

Most adults have 28 teeth, or 32 if the wisdom teeth have erupted. Children have 20 teeth. The teeth should be white, in good repair, with no caries and good occlusion. The top front teeth should slightly override the lower ones.

Developmental Variations

Older adults—May have receding gums, so teeth appear longer. Teeth may be chipped, eroded, or stained.

Abnormal findings: Missing or poorly anchored teeth, misalignment, and brown or black enamel (indicative of dental caries or staining, e.g., from taking tetracycline). White spots may indicate excessive fluoride intake.

4. Inspect the tongue and the floor of the mouth.
a. Ask the client to "stick out" his tongue. Examine the upper surface for its color, texture, position, and mobility.
b. Ask the client to roll his tongue upward and move it side to side.

Tongue is moist, and the coloring is consistent with the client's race. Mucosa has no lesions or discoloration. Papillae are intact. Tongue is midline with full mobility. The base of the tongue is smooth with prominent veins. No tenderness; no palpable nodules.

(continued on next page)

Procedure 19-9 ■ **Assessing the Mouth and Oropharynx** (continued)

c. Have the client place the tip of his tongue on the roof of his mouth, as far back as possible. Using the penlight, inspect the underside of the tongue, the frenulum (which fastens the tongue to the floor of the mouth, in the center), and the floor of the mouth.
d. Inspect the two Wharton's duct openings to the submaxillary glands, on either side of the frenulum.
e. Use a tongue blade or gloved finger to move the tongue aside and examine the lateral aspects of the tongue and the floor of the mouth bilaterally. Use caution when placing your finger into the mouth of a noncompliant client.
Ulcers may form on the tongue and on other oral mucosa.

Developmental Variations

Older adults—May have varicosities under the tongue.

Abnormal findings: Red, smooth, or painful tongue; inflamed mucosa or ducts; tongue that is not midline or has restricted mobility; ulcerations of the tongue or the floor of the mouth (e.g., from trauma, viral infection, or cancerous changes); white plaque or black, hairy tongue (fungal infection) ▼

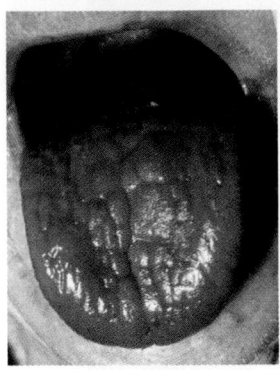 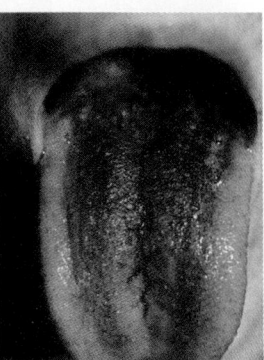

Red, beefy tongue   Black, hairy tongue

---

5. Palpate the tongue and floor of the mouth. Stabilize the tongue by grasping it with a gauze pad. Palpate top, bottom, and sides with your other index finger.

---

6. Inspect the oropharynx (hard/soft palate, tonsils, and uvula). Note the color, shape, texture, and condition.
  a. Have the client tilt his head back and open his mouth as widely as possible. Depress the tongue with a tongue blade, and shine a penlight on the areas to be inspected.
  b. To inspect the uvula, ask the client to say "ah," and watch the uvula as the soft palate rises.
  c. Inspect the oropharynx by depressing one side of the tongue at a time, about halfway back on the tongue.
  d. Note the size and color of the tonsils; note any discharge, redness, swelling, or lesions.
  e. Look and palpate for cleft palate, especially in infants.

Hard and soft palate are pink and smooth. Uvula is midline and rises symmetrically. Tonsils are pink, symmetrical, and without lesions or exudate.

Developmental Variations

Children—Until about age 12, the tonsils may extend beyond the palatine arch.

Abnormal findings: Redness, edema, lesions, plaques, drainage; yellow or greenish streaks on the posterior wall of pharynx (indicate postnasal drainage); tonsils that are red, edematous, or enlarged or have white or pale patches of exudates. Asymmetrical rise of the uvula may indicate a problem with CN IX or X.

---

7. Test the gag reflex by touching the back of the soft palate with a tongue blade.

Positive gag reflex is present.

Developmental Variations

Older adults—May have a slightly slower gag response.

Abnormal findings: Absence of a gag reflex is seen with extreme sedation, head injury, or damage to CN IX and X. Also see Abnormal Atlas: Mouth and Oropharynx, at the end of this chapter. Inability to articulate the specified words indicates CN XII is not intact.

8. Ask the client to repeat the following words: Light, tight, dynamite. Again, you may defer this test to the sensorineurological portion of the exam if you choose.

Patient Teaching

Instruct the patient in the importance of dental care and the need for regular checkups.

Documentation

- If you need more information about documenting,

 Go to Chapter 19, **Documenting Physical Assessment Findings,** in Volume 1.

Procedure 19-10 ___ Assessing the Neck

➤ For steps to follow in *all* procedures, refer to the Universal Steps for All Procedures found on the inside back cover of Volume 2.

Critical Aspects

- Techniques: Inspection and palpation (auscultation as needed)
- Inspect the neck. Note symmetry, range of motion (ROM), and the skin condition.
- Palpate the cervical lymph nodes. Note the size, shape, symmetry, consistency, mobility, tenderness, and temperature of any palpable nodes.
- Palpate the thyroid. If it is enlarged or if there is a mass, auscultate.

Equipment

- Stethoscope
- Pen and record form

Position

- Have the client seated, if possible.
- For infants and children, position supine.

Focused History Questions

- Do you have any difficulty swallowing?
- Do you have any neck pain or stiffness?
- Do you have any neck masses or lumps?
- Do you have any history of thyroid disease?
- Do you have any difficulty swallowing?

➤ When performing the procedure, always identify your patient according to agency policy and be attentive to standard precautions, hand hygiene, patient safety and privacy, body mechanics, and documentation.

Procedure Steps

1. Inspect the neck. Note symmetry, range of motion (ROM), and the condition of the skin.
   a. Inspect the neck in a neutral position.
   b. Inspect the neck when it is hyperextended.
   c. Inspect the neck when the patient swallows water.

Expected Findings

Neck is erect, midline, and symmetrical with full ROM. No masses are present; skin is intact. Larynx and trachea rise with swallowing. Thyroid is not visible.

Abnormal findings: Swollen lymph nodes may be visible. An enlarged thyroid may be visible in the lower half of the neck.

(continued on next page)

Procedure 19-10 ■ Assessing the Neck (continued)

2. Palpate the cervical lymph nodes. Note the size, shape, symmetry, consistency, mobility, tenderness, and temperature of any palpable nodes.

   a. Use light palpation with one or two fingerpads in a circular movement.

   b. Palpate the cervical nodes in the following order:

     (1) *Preauricular*—in front of the ear

     (2) *Posterior auricular*—behind the ear

     (3) *Tonsilar*—at the angle of the jaw

     (4) *Submandibular*—halfway up the lower jaw

     (5) *Submental*—under the tip of the chin

     (6) *Occipital*—at the base of the skull in the occipital area

     (7) *Superficial cervical*—below the tonsilar node over the sternocleidomastoid muscle

     (8) *Deep cervical*—under the sternocleidomastoid muscle

     (9) *Posterior cervical*—in posterior triangle along trapezius muscle

     (10) *Supraclavicular*—above the clavicle

Use the same sequence every time so that the steps will become automatic and you will not omit any area.

Lymph nodes are supple and nontender; no masses are palpable. ▼

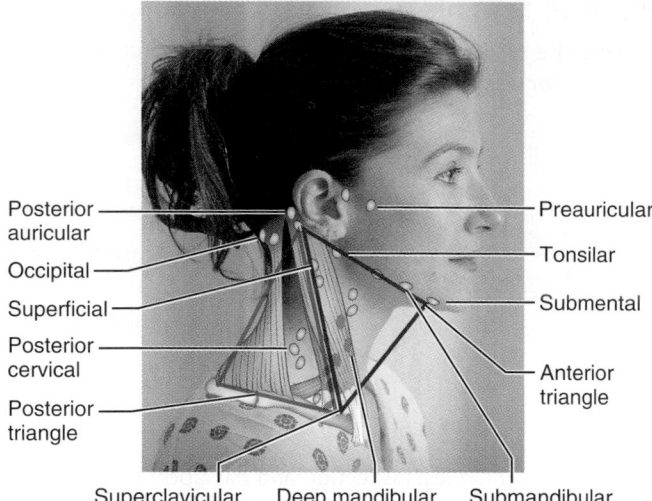

Abnormal findings: Lymphadenopathy (palpable nodes 1 cm or greater). Immobile nodes may indicate malignancy, inflammation, or infection in the area they drain.

---

3. Palpate the thyroid.

To use the posterior approach:

   a. Stand behind the client, and ask her to flex her neck slightly forward and to the left.

   b. Position your thumbs on the nape of the client's neck.

   c. Using the fingers of your left hand, locate the cricoid cartilage, which is located below the thyroid cartilage. Push the trachea slightly to the left with your right hand as you palpate just below the cricoid cartilage and between the trachea and sternocleidomastoid muscle.

   d. Ask your client to swallow (give her small sips of water if necessary), and feel for the thyroid gland as it rises up. ▼

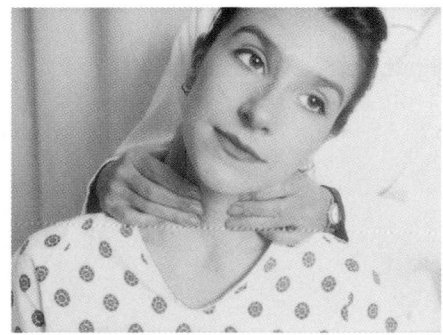

The thyroid is generally nonpalpable. If some tissue is palpable, the consistency is firm and smooth. There is no nodularity, enlargement, or tenderness.

Abnormal findings: An enlarged thyroid may signify a tumor or goiter. A tender thyroid is associated with inflammation. ▼

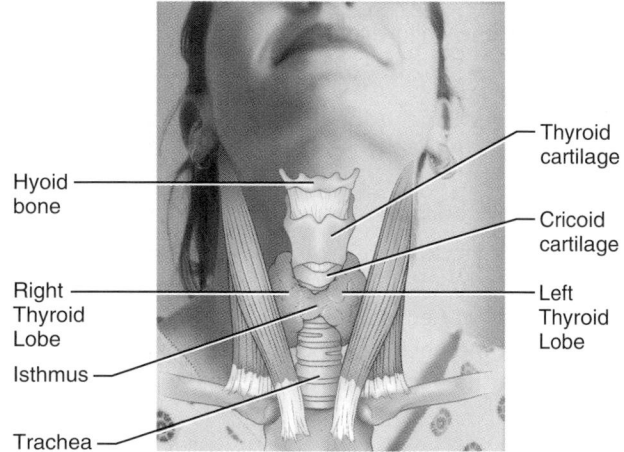

e. Reverse and repeat the same steps to palpate the right thyroid lobe (use the fingers of your left hand to displace the trachea to the right, while using the fingers of your right hand to palpate the thyroid to the right of the trachea).

To use the anterior approach:

f. Stand in front of the client, and ask her to flex her neck slightly forward and in the direction you intend to palpate.

g. Place your hands on the neck, and apply gentle pressure to one side of the trachea while palpating the opposite side of the neck for the thyroid as the client swallows.

h. Reverse and repeat the same steps on the opposite side.

What if. . .

■ **The thyroid gland is enlarged or there is a mass?**

Auscultate the thyroid for bruits using the bell portion of the stethoscope. Ask the client to hold her breath as you auscultate. There should be no bruits.

Patient Teaching

Teach the patient how to perform a "neck check" - self-check the thyroid with a glass of water and a handheld mirror. Tell the patient: "Hold the mirror in your hand and focus on your neck just below the Adam's apple and above your collarbone. Tip your head back, take a drink of water, and swallow. As you swallow look at your neck. Check for any bulges in this area as you swallow." To download Neck Check instructions, and for more information about thyroid health, go to

 http://wwwthyroidawareness.com

Documentation

■ If you need more information about documenting,

 Go to Chapter 19, **Documenting Physical Assessment Findings,** in Volume 1.

Procedure 19-11 ☐ **Assessing the Breasts and Axillae**

➤ For steps to follow in *all* procedures, refer to the Universal Steps for All Procedures found on the inside back cover of Volume 2.

Critical Aspects

- ▪ Techniques: Inspection and palpation
- ▪ Inspect the breasts and axillae for skin condition, size, shape, symmetry, and color.
- ▪ Inspect the nipples for discharge. Culture any discharge, if present.
- ▪ If you notice an open lesion or nipple discharge, wear procedure gloves to palpate the breasts.
- ▪ Palpate the breasts using the vertical strip method, pie wedge method, or concentric circles method.
- ▪ Palpate the nipples, areolae, and lymph nodes.

(continued on next page)

Procedure 19-11 ■ Assessing the Breasts and Axillae (continued)

Equipment

- Nonlatex procedure gloves, if exposure to body fluids is possible
- Glass slide
- Culturette
- Pen and record form

Positioning

The patient must assume several positions during breast examination (see step 1).

Focused History Questions

- Do you have a lump or thickening in your underarm or breasts that persists throughout your menstrual cycle?
- Do you have any breast pain or discharge?
- Have you noticed any changes in the skin on your breasts, nipples, or underarms?
- Have you had any changes in your nipples?
- Have your breasts changed in size, shape, or contour?
- Do you perform breast self-examination (BSE)?
- Are you taking any medications or hormones?
- If you are premenopausal, when was your last period?

> ➤ When performing the procedure, always identify your patient according to agency policy and be attentive to standard precautions, hand hygiene, patient safety and privacy, body mechanics, and documentation.

Procedure Steps

1. Inspect the breasts. Note size, shape, symmetry, and color. Inspect with the client in each of the following positions:

   a. Sitting or standing with arms at her side

   b. Sitting or standing with arms raised slightly but not over her head

   Aids in detecting dimpling or retraction of breast tissue

   c. Seated or standing with her hands pressed on her hips

   Aids in detecting dimpling or retraction of breast tissue

   d. With the client leaning forward

   Helpful when examining large, pendulous breasts

   e. With the client supine with a pillow under the shoulder of the breast being examined

   Helps spread the breast tissue over the chest wall

Expected Findings

The breasts are symmetrical; however, the dominant side may be more developed, resulting in a slightly asymmetrical appearance. Skin color is lighter than exposed areas, and there are no lesions, redness, or edema. Texture is smooth, with no dimpling or retraction. Striae are a normal variation.

Developmental Variations

Newborns—You may see breast enlargement and watery, white discharge from the nipples during the first 2 weeks of life.

Children—Breasts typically begin to develop at about 13 years of age; the breasts may not develop at equal rates.

Pregnancy—Breast size increases; areolae and nipples darken; superficial veins become prominent; stretch marks may be present; colostrum (a thick, yellow precursor to breast milk) can sometimes be expressed as early as the second trimester.

Older adults—Breasts lose firmness and become flaccid and pendulous.

Abnormal findings:

- Asymmetry warrants further investigation.
- Swelling or erythema may be seen in infection (mastitis).
- Peau d'orange (dimpled skin texture) skin changes may be seen with lymphatic obstruction that is present in some forms of breast cancer.
- Puckering, lesions, and retraction may also be seen with breast cancer.
- Gynecomastia (enlargement of breasts in males) may indicate hormone imbalance.

2. Inspect the nipples and areolae. Note color, shape, and symmetry. Observe for any discharge.

The areolae and nipples are darker in color than breast tissue. Nipples are everted and point in the same direction. No discharge is present, except in newborns and during pregnancy and lactation. No lesions or erosion is present.

Abnormal findings:

- Nipple discoloration that is not associated with pregnancy
- Nipples pointing in different directions. Such findings warrant follow-up as a potential sign of an underlying mass.
- Flat or inverted nipples, which are caused by shortening of the mammary ducts. May make breastfeeding difficult.
- Any nipple discharge not associated with newborns, pregnancy, or breastfeeding requires a thorough evaluation
- Cracks and nipple redness, which may occur with breastfeeding

---

3. Inspect the axillae. Note the color, condition of the skin, and hair distribution.

Skin is intact with no lesions or rashes. Presence of hair depends on the age of the client and personal preference. Axillary hair develops with puberty. Some women may choose to shave the hair, whereas others will allow it to grow.

Abnormal findings: Rashes, redness, or unusual pigmentation may indicate infection or allergy to deodorants. Dark-pigmented, velvety skin may be seen with *acanthous nigricans,* a condition associated with obesity and type 2 diabetes mellitus.

---

4. Palpate the breasts, wearing procedure gloves if necessary. Using the fingerpads of your three middle fingers, make small circles with light, medium, and deep pressure. Begin at an imaginary line drawn straight down the side from the underarm; move across the breast to the middle of the sternum. Check the entire breast area, moving down until you feel only ribs and up to the clavicle.

   Follow one of the following three patterns (evidence suggests the vertical strip method is best).

   a. *Vertical strip method:* Start at the sternal edge, and palpate the breast in parallel lines until you reach the midaxillary line. Go up one area and down the adjacent strip (like "mowing the grass").

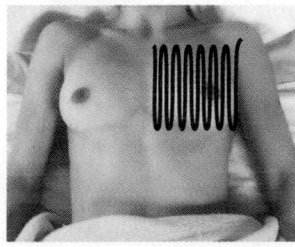

Breasts are soft and nontender with no lesions or masses. Consistency depends on age; premenopausal women have firm and elastic tissue, whereas postmenopausal women have softer tissue that may be stringy or cordlike.

Abnormal findings: Breast lumps or masses may be benign or malignant and require follow-up.

Technique Hints

- Do not remove your fingers from the skin surface once you have begun palpating. Move from area to area by sliding the fingers along the skin.
- Most breast lesions in women are found in the upper outer quadrant.
- Most breast cancer in men occurs in the areola.

(continued on next page)

Procedure 19–11 ■ **Assessing the Breasts and Axillae** (continued)

b. *Pie wedge method:* This method examines the breast in wedges. Move from one wedge to the next. ▼

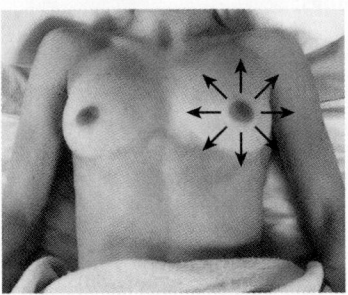

c. *Concentric circles method:* Start at the outermost area of the breast at the 12 o'clock position. Move clockwise in concentric, ever smaller, circles. ▼

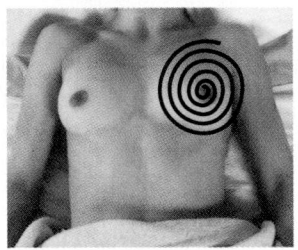

---

5. Palpate the nipples and areolae.
 a. If the woman is supine, place a small pillow or folded towel under the shoulder of the breast you are examining.
 b. Squeeze the nipple gently between your thumb and finger to check for discharge.
 c. Note tissue elasticity and tenderness.

Nipples are elastic and nontender. No discharge is present.

Abnormal findings: Loss of elasticity may indicate underlying malignancy. Bloody, purulent discharge may indicate infection. Other forms of drainage may indicate malignancy. Nipple tenderness is normal when establishing breastfeeding.

---

6. Palpate the axillae and clavicular lymph nodes.
 a. Have the woman sitting with her arms at her sides or supine.
 b. Using your fingerpads, move your fingers in circular fashion.
 - Central nodes: located high in the midaxillary region
 - Anterior pectoral nodes: located on the lower border of the pectoralis major in the anterior axillary fold
 - Lateral brachial nodes: located high in the axilla on the inner aspect of the humerus
 - Posterior subscapular nodes: located high in the axilla on the lateral scapular border
 - Epitrochlear nodes: located above the elbow
 - Infraclavicular nodes: located below the clavicle
 - Supraclavicular nodes: located above the clavicle ➤

Nodes are nonpalpable.

Abnormal findings: Palpable nodes may be seen with infection or malignancy. Enlarged lymph nodes caused by infection are tender.

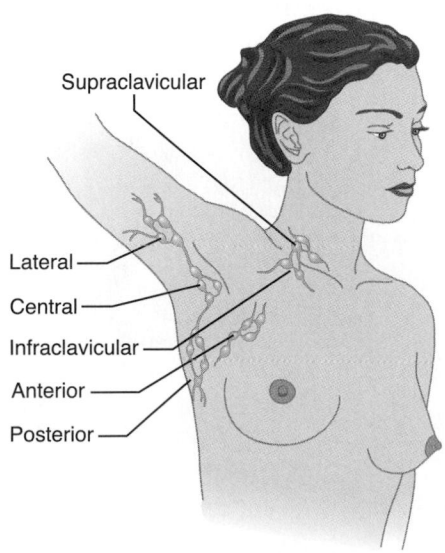

Location of Normal Lymph Nodes

What if. . .

- **There is a nipple discharge?**

If there is nipple discharge in a woman who is not pregnant or breastfeeding, obtain a specimen by placing a glass slide up to the breast to capture a drop of discharge. Transport the slide to the laboratory as soon as possible. If there is ample discharge, obtain a swab of the discharge with a culturette.

Patient Teaching

Instruct the patient in BSE and recommendations for mammograms and clinical breast examinations. The American Cancer Society (2007) recommends that women ages 40 and older have a screening mammogram and a clinical breast examination (CBE) every year (other guidelines recommend every 2 years); and that women ages 20 to 30 have a CBE every 3 years. They consider a monthly BSE to be optional. Stress that BSE does not replace the need for mammograms and CBE. This issue remains controversial. There is evidence that BSE does not decrease the death rate from breast cancer; but there is also evidence that BSE, done correctly, does help women to reduce their individual risk and find cancer at earlier stages, when cure rates are higher (ACOG News Release, 2007).

Documentation

- If you palpate a mass or lump, document its size, shape, symmetry, mobility, tenderness, and skin color changes. To document the location, divide the breast into four quadrants by intersecting vertical and horizontal lines. With the nipple as the center, locate the mass or lump as though the breast were a clock; state the distance in cm from the nipple (e.g., 4 o'clock, 2.5 cm from nipple).
- If you need more information about documenting,

 Go to Chapter 19, **Documenting Physical Assessment Findings,** in Volume 1.

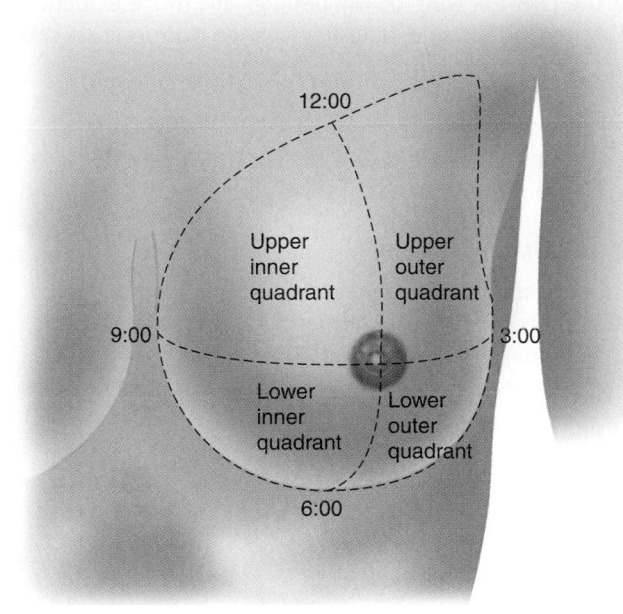

Practice Resources

The American College of Obstetricians and Gynecologists (ACOG, 2007); American Cancer Society (2009); Green, B., & Taplin, S. (2003); Hackshaw, A., & Paul, E. (2003).

Procedure 19-12   ■   **Assessing the Chest and Lungs**

➤ For steps to follow in *all* procedures, refer to the Universal Steps for All Procedures found on the inside back cover of Volume 2.

Critical Aspects

- Techniques: Inspection, palpation, percussion, auscultation
- Assess respirations by counting the rate and observing the rhythm, depth, and symmetry of chest movement.
- Inspect the chest for anteroposterior:lateral ratio, costal angle, spinal deformity, respiratory effort, and skin condition.
- Palpate the trachea.
- Palpate the chest for tenderness, masses, or crepitus.
- Palpate chest excursion.
- Palpate the chest for tactile fremitus.
- Percuss the chest.
- Percuss diaphragmatic excursion.
- Auscultate lung sounds.

(continued on next page)

Procedure 19-12 ■ Assessing the Chest and Lungs (continued)

Equipment

- Stethoscope
- Felt-tipped marker and ruler
- Pen and record form

Position

- Have the client sitting, if possible, and leaning forward for the posterior approach.

If the client is unable to sit up, findings will be distorted.

- If the client is lying down, findings are more evident on the dependent side; help her change positions so that you can assess with each side dependent.

Focused History Questions

- Do you have fatigue or activity intolerance?
- Do you have any current respiratory problems?
- Have you had any recent respiratory problems?
- Do you have a cough?
- Do you have any difficulty breathing?
- What, if anything, causes you to be short of breath?
- Have you had any chest pain?
- Do you have a history of allergies or asthma?
- Do you smoke? If so, how much and for how long?
- If you smoke, have you tried to quit? Would you like to quit?
- Are you exposed to air pollutants at home or at work?

➤ When performing the procedure, always identify your patient according to agency policy and be attentive to standard precautions, hand hygiene, patient safety and privacy, body mechanics, and documentation.

Procedure Steps

1. Count the respiratory rate, and observe the rhythm and depth; observe the symmetry of chest and respiratory movements.
(See Chapter 17 if you need more information about counting respirations.)

Expected Findings

- Respirations are quiet with a regular rhythm and depth.
- Chest movement is symmetrical.
- 12–20 breaths/min for adults. The normal respiratory rate varies by age.

Developmental Variations

Infants and children—A newborn may have a respiratory rate of 40–90. The rate gradually declines as the child matures. Newborns breathe abdominally, so you will see little chest movement.

Older adults—Rate changes very little; however, respirations decrease in depth as muscles become weakened.

Abnormal findings:

- Chest asymmetry may be seen with musculoskeletal disorders of the spine, such as kyphosis or scoliosis.
- Asymmetrical chest movement during breathing is seen in rib fractures, pneumothrax, and atelectasis; affected chest area may not move at all with respiration.
- Sternal and intercostal retractions are seen with hypoxia, respiratory distress, and airway obstruction.
- Respiratory rate may be increased with activity, smoking, fever, pain, or anemia.

2. Inspect the chest.
   a. Inspect the anteroposterior (AP):lateral ratio. To review,

 Go to Chapter 19, in Volume 1.

   a. The normal adult AP:lateral ratio is 1:2.

Developmental Variations

Infants—AP is equal to the lateral diameter

Older adults—Kyphosis and osteoporosis change the size and shape of the chest; weakening thoracic and diaphragm muscles allow the chest to widen and become more barrel-shaped.

Abnormal findings: AP:lateral ratio is increased in COPD (barrel chest).

b. Inspect the costal angle. ▼

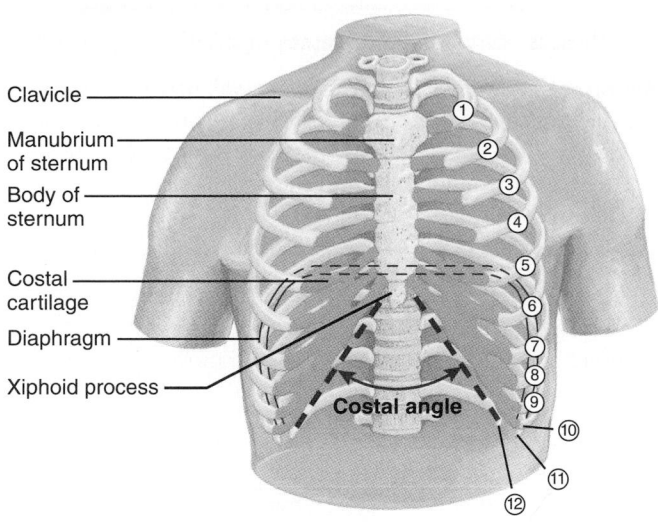

Clavicle

Manubrium of sternum

Body of sternum

Costal cartilage

Diaphragm

Xiphoid process

Costal angle

① ② ③ ④ ⑤ ⑥ ⑦ ⑧ ⑨ ⑩ ⑪ ⑫

c. Identify any spinal deformities.

d. Observe the effort required to breathe.

e. Note the color and condition of skin.

b. The costal angle is < 90°.

Abnormal findings: Costal angle is > 90° in COPD.

c. The spine is straight without lateral curvatures or deformity.

Abnormal findings: Scoliosis is a lateral curvature of the spine. Kyphosis is excessive thoracic curvature. ▼

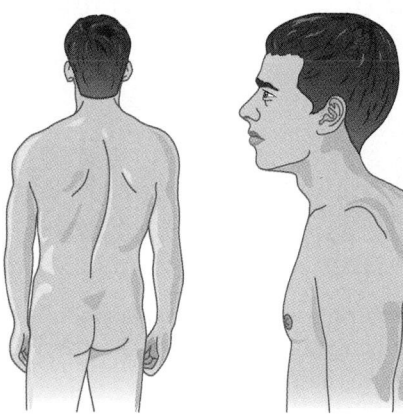

Scoliosis   Kyphosis

d. Respirations appear effortless. There is no retraction or use of accessory muscles.

Abnormal findings: Sternal and intercostal retractions are seen in severe hypoxia or respiratory distress.

e. Skin color and hair distribution are consistent with the client's gender, ethnicity, and exposure to the sun. The skin is intact with no scars.

Abnormal findings: cyanosis of the chest wall (due to extreme hypoxia or cold temperature).

---

3. Palpate the trachea.
Place your fingers and thumb on either side of the trachea and note its position. (In a comprehensive exam, you may have already done this with the neck examination.)

Developmental Modifications

Infants—Neck is short, so it may not be possible to palpate the trachea.

Trachea is in the midline.

Abnormal findings: Tracheal deviation may occur from a mass in the neck (e.g., thyroid enlargement) or from excess pressure in the lungs (e.g., tension pneumothorax).

(continued on next page)

Procedure 19–12 ■ **Assessing the Chest and Lungs** (continued)

---

4. Palpate the chest.
- Observe for tenderness, masses, or **crepitus** (crackling skin due to air in the subcutaneous tissue).
- Palpate the anterior, posterior, and lateral chest by placing your hands on the chest wall.

The chest is nontender. No masses or crepitus is present.

Abnormal findings: Pain in the chest wall may be due to fracture, inflammation, or trauma. Crepitus results from air leaking into the subcutaneous tissue. It is most likely to occur around wounds, central IV line sites, chest tubes, or a tracheostomy.

---

5. Palpate chest excursion (expandability).
a. Place your hands at the base of the client's chest with fingers spread and thumbs about 5 cm (2 in.) apart (at the costal margin anteriorly and at the 8th to 10th rib posteriorly).
b. Press your thumbs toward the client's spine to create a small skinfold between them.
c. Have the client take a deep breath, and feel for chest expansion.
This may be performed on the anterior or posterior portion of the chest, or both. ▼

Chest excursion is symmetrical on the anterior and posterior aspect of the chest (you should feel equal pressure on your hands; thumbs should move apart equal distances).

Abnormal findings: Limited chest excursion may occur with shallow breathing, restrictive clothing, or restrictive airway disease. Asymmetrical excursion may result from airway obstruction, pleural effusion, or pneumothorax.

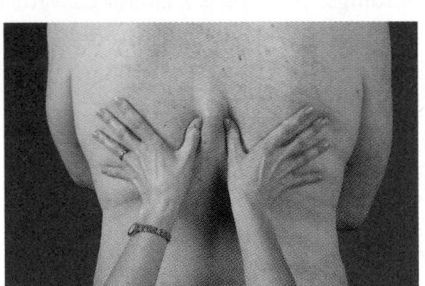

---

6. Follow the same pattern and sequence for palpating fremitus, percussing, and auscultating the chest. See the accompanying diagram. ▼

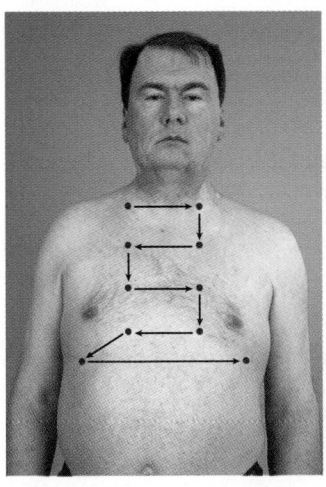 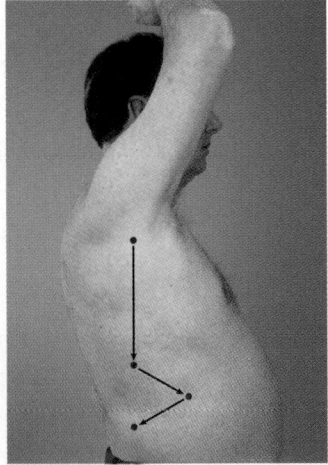 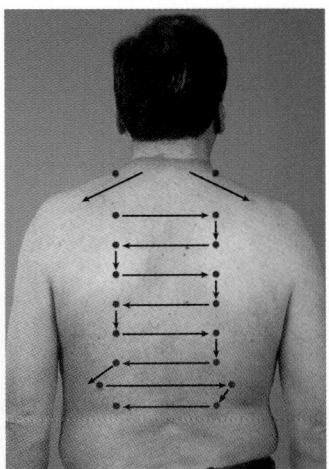

Percussion and auscultation sites

---

7. Palpate the chest for tactile fremitus.
a. Use the palmar surface of your hands, but raise the fingers off the client's chest so that you palpate with the bony metacarpophalangeal joints of your hands.
Bony prominences are best for detecting vibrations.

Tactile fremitus is equal bilaterally on the anterior and posterior chest; it is diminished at midthorax. Fremitus is normally diminished if the chest wall is very thick or the voice very soft.

b. Palpate for vibrations as the client says "99." ▼

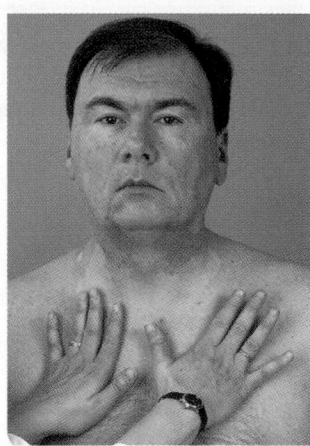

Developmental Modifications

Infants—Place your hand over the chest while the infant is crying.

---

8. Percuss the chest.
  a. Percuss over the intercostal spaces rather than over the ribs.
Percussion over bone produces less resonance.

  b. Use the indirect percussion method on the anterior, posterior, and lateral chest, following the diagram in step 6. Compare the right side to the left side.

---

9. Percuss the posterior chest for diaphragmatic excursion.
  a. Percuss the level of the diaphragm on full expiration. Have the client exhale completely and hold his breath while you percuss (beginning just below the scapula) from resonance over the lung downward toward the diaphragm. The sound will become dull at the diaphragm. Mark the area with a pen.
  b. Percuss the diaphragm level on full inspiration. Have the client take a deep breath and hold it as you percuss again. Mark the location.
  c. Measure the distance between the two marks. ▼

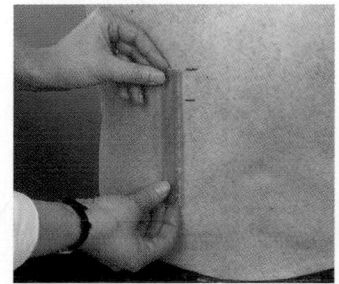

Developmental Variations

Children and thin adults—May have increased fremitus.

Abnormal findings: Increased fremitus occurs with conditions that cause fluid in the lungs (e.g., pulmonary edema). Decreased or absent fremitus occurs when there is decreased air movement or tissue consolidation (e.g., emphysema, asthma).

■ The anterior chest is resonant to the 2nd ICS on the left and to the 4th ICS on the right.
■ The lateral chest is resonant to the 8th ICS.
■ The posterior chest is resonant to T12.

Abnormal findings: Dullness is heard with fluid or masses in the lungs. Hyperresonance is heard with air trapping that occurs with emphysema.

Diaphragmatic excursion (the distance between the two marks) is normally 3–6 cm.

Abnormal findings: Decreased excursion may indicate paralysis, atelectasis, or COPD with overinflated lungs.

(continued on next page)

Procedure 19–12 ■ Assessing the Chest and Lungs (continued)

10. Auscultate the chest.
   a. Follow the pattern in Step 6.
   b. Use the diaphragm of the stethoscope.
   c. Have the client take slow, deep breaths through his mouth as you listen at each site through one full respiratory cycle.
Refer to the tables at the end of this procedure.
To listen to some lung sounds,

 Go to the sound file, **Breath Sounds,** on the Student Resource Disk or DavisPlus at http://davisplus.fadavis.com/Wilkinson2

No abnormal or adventitious sounds are heard. Lung fields are clear to auscultation. *Bronchial* breath sounds are heard over the trachea. *Bronchovesicular* breath sounds are heard over the sternum anteriorly and between the scapulae posteriorly. *Vesicular* breath sounds are heard over most of the lung fields.

Developmental Variations

Infants—Breath sounds are louder than in adults.

Abnormal findings: Crackles or rales, rhonchi, wheezing, stridor, friction rub, grunting

11. Auscultate for abnormal voice sounds if there is evidence of lung congestion. Follow the pattern in Step 6.
   a. Assess for bronchophony by having the client say "1, 2, 3" as you listen over the lung fields.
   b. Assess for egophony by having your client say "eee" as you listen over the lung fields.
   c. Assess for whispered pectoriloquy by having your client whisper "1, 2, 3" as you listen over the lung fields.

No abnormal voice sounds are heard.

Abnormal findings:
   a. **Bronchophony** is present if the words are clearly heard over the lungs.
   b. **Egophony** is present if the sound you hear is "ay."
   c. **Whispered** pectoriloquy is present if you hear, "One, two, three" clearly.

Patient Teaching

Instruct the patient about the dangers of tobacco use, especially smoking; exposure to air pollutants and environmental pollutants, such as radon or asbestos; and the signs and symptoms of lung cancer.

Home Care

■ Instruct clients or caregivers to identify any pollutant within the home that may cause respiratory problems, such as radon, dirty heating/air conditioning systems, or mold.
■ Instruct caregivers or patients with allergies and/or asthma to eliminate potential allergens, such as cigarette smoke, dust, feathers, and pet dander.

Documentation

 Go to Chapter 19, **Documenting Physical Assessment Findings,** in Volume 1.

Normal Lung Sounds			
NORMAL LUNG SOUNDS	**LOCATION**	**DESCRIPTION**	**ILLUSTRATION**
Bronchial or tubular	Heard over the trachea	Blowing, hollow sounds; inspiration is shorter than expiration and lower-pitched.	Inspiration / Expiration
Bronchovesicular	Heard over the 1st and 2nd ICS anteriorly and over the scapula posteriorly	Medium-pitched, medium intensity, blowing sounds; inspiration and expiration are equal length and similar pitch	Inspiration / Expiration
Vesicular	Heard over the lung periphery	Soft, low-pitched sounds; inspiration is longer, louder, and higher-pitched than expiration	Inspiration / Expiration

Abnormal Lung Sounds

ABNORMAL LUNG SOUNDS	CAUSE	CHARACTERISTICS	EXAMPLES
Crackles (sometimes called rales)	Air bubbling through moisture in the alveoli	Bubbling, crackling, popping. Soft, high-pitched, and very brief sounds, usually heard during inspiration	Pneumonia Congestive heart failure (CHF) Bronchitis Emphysema
Rhonchi	Mucus secretions in the large airways	Course, snoring, continuous low-pitched sounds heard during inspiration and expiration. May clear with coughing.	Bronchitis Emphysema Narrowed airways Fibrotic lungs
Wheezes	Narrowing of small airways by spasm, inflammation, mucus, or tumor	High-pitched musical or squeaking sounds heard during inspiration or expiration	Acute asthma Emphysema
Stridor*	Partial upper airway obstruction or tracheal or laryngeal spasm	High-pitched, continuous honking sounds heard throughout the respiratory cycle but most prominent on inspiration	Acute respiratory distress Foreign body in airway Epiglottitis
Friction Rub	Rubbing together of inflamed pleural layers	A high-pitched grating or rubbing sound that may be heard throughout the respiratory cycle. Loudest over lower lateral anterior surface.	Pleuritis
Grunting	Retention of air in the lungs	A high-pitched tubular sound heard on expiration	Emphysema

*Patients with stridor need immediate medical evaluation.

Procedure 19-13 ▢ Assessing the Heart and Vascular System

➤ For steps to follow in *all* procedures, refer to the Universal Steps for All Procedures found on the inside back cover of Volume 2.

Critical Aspects

- Techniques: Inspection, palpation, auscultation
- If possible, work from your patient's right side.
- Inspect the neck for pulsations.
- Measure jugular venous pressure (JVP).
- Inspect the precordium for pulsations.
- Palpate the carotid arteries.
- Palpate the precordium for pulsations, lifts, heaves, or thrills.
- Auscultate the carotid arteries with the bell of the stethoscope.
- Auscultate the jugular veins with the bell of the stethoscope.
- Auscultate the precordium at the apex, left lower sternal border, base left, and base right. Use the bell and then the diaphragm of the stethoscope.
- Palpate the peripheral pulses. Any abnormalities require further evaluation.

(continued on next page)

Procedure 19-13 ■ Assessing the Heart and Vascular System (continued)

Equipment

- Combination stethoscope with bell and diaphragm
- Two rulers
- Pen and record form

✚ Clean stethoscope and rulers before and after using unless they are only used for one patient.

Position

Place the client in three positions: sitting, supine, and left lateral (to facilitate hearing specific sounds).

Focused History Questions

- Have you experienced any fatigue or activity intolerance?
- Do you have a history of high blood pressure or stroke?
- Have you ever passed out or felt light-headed?
- Do you have any problems with your heart or circulation?
- Do you ever experience chest pain? If so, describe the circumstances that triggered the pain.
- What was the pain like? What did you do to relieve it?
- Do you ever experience palpitations or a rapid heart beat?
- Do you ever feel short of breath?
- Do you ever get swelling in your feet?
- What medications are you taking?

➤ When performing the procedure, always identify your patient according to agency policy and be attentive to standard precautions, hand hygiene, patient safety and privacy, body mechanics, and documentation.

Procedure Steps

1. Inspect the neck.
   a. With the patient supine, inspect the carotid and jugular venous system in the neck for pulsations.
   b. Assess jugular flow: Compress the jugular vein below the jaw. The vein collapses, and the jugular wave is more prominent at the supraclavicular area.
   The jugular venous pulse is easily obliterated with gentle pressure. ▼

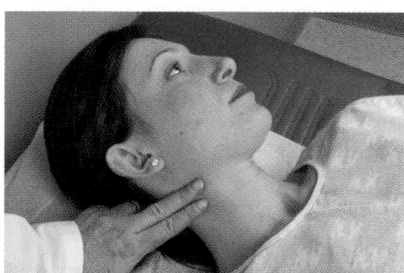

Assessing jugular flow

   c. Assess jugular filling: Compress the jugular above the clavicle. The vein distends and the jugular wave disappears. ▼

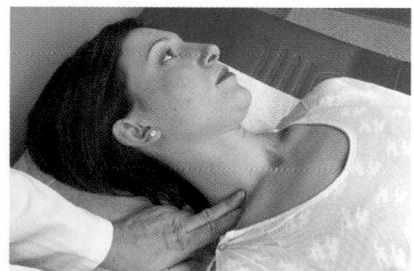

Assessing jugular filling

Expected Findings

Carotid pulsation is easily visible. A slight pulsation in the supraclavicular area or suprasternal notch indicates jugular venous pressure. The pulsation should be easily obliterated when you apply pressure to the area.

Abnormal findings: Significant jugular vein distention suggests right-sided heart failure.

2. Measure jugular venous pressure (JVP).
  a. Elevate the head of the bed to a 45° angle.
  b. Identify the highest point of visible internal jugular filling.
  c. Place a ruler vertically at the sternal angle (where the clavicles meet).
  d. Place another ruler horizontally at the highest point of the venous wave.
  e. Measure the distance in centimeters vertically from the chest wall. ▼

Normal jugular venous pressure is < 3 cm.

Abnormal findings: Elevated JVP (in CHF or constricted flow into the right side of the heart); low JVP (in hypovolemia)

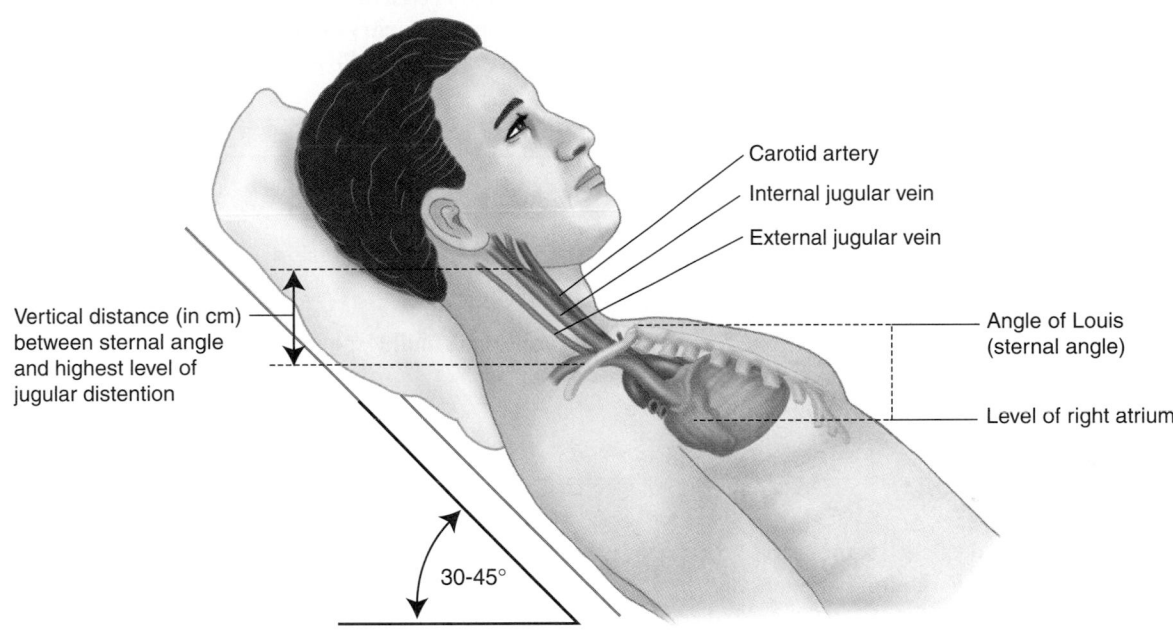

Vertical distance (in cm) between sternal angle and highest level of jugular distention

Carotid artery
Internal jugular vein
External jugular vein
Angle of Louis (sternal angle)
Level of right atrium

30-45°

---

3. Inspect the precordium for pulsations. (Have the patient supine with tangential lighting.)

Visible pulsation at the point of maximal impulse (PMI, the 5th ICS in the midclavicular line)

Developmental Modifications

Children—Look for the PMI more medially and at about the 4th ICS in children younger than age 8.

Developmental Variations

In thin adults and children, a pulsation may also be visible over the base of the heart.

Abnormal findings: A pulsation (a heave or lift) displaced toward the axillary line indicates left ventricular hypertrophy. Pulsations to the right of the sternum may indicate an aortic aneurysm.

---

4. Very gently palpate the carotid arteries.
  a. Palpate each side separately.
Bilateral pressure may impair cerebral blood flow.

  b. Avoid massaging the carotid artery as you palpate.
Increased pressure on the carotid will lead to a drop in the heart rate and blood pressure.

  c. Note the rate, rhythm, amplitude, and symmetry of the pulse.
  d. Note the contour, symmetry, and elasticity of the arteries.
  e. Note any thrills.

- Rhythm is regular with +2 amplitude.
- Contour: There should be a smooth upstroke with less acute descent.
- Symmetry: Pulses are equal bilaterally.
- Elasticity: Carotids are soft and pliable.

Developmental Variations

Pulse rate is age dependent.

Older adults—The carotids may be stiff and cordlike.

Abnormal findings: A thrill indicates turbulent flow.

(continued on next page)

Procedure 19-13 ■ **Assessing the Heart and Vascular System** (continued)

5. Palpate the precordium.
   a. For this part of the examination, have the patient sit up and lean forward. If lying down, have him turn to the left side.
   b. Palpate in all five areas: apex, left lateral sternal border, epigastric area, base left, and base right.
   c. Feel for pulsations, lifts, heaves, and thrills.
Brings the apex of the heart closer to the chest wall.

Helpful hint: Perform cardiac palpation and auscultation from the patient's right side, whenever possible.
This allows you to stretch the stethoscope during auscultation so that you minimize interference and "static."

PMI is palpable at the apex over a 1–2 cm area. Slight pulsation from the abdominal aorta may be felt at the epigastric area. No pulsations, lifts, heaves, or thrills are palpable.

Abnormal findings: A pulsation, lift, or heave may be seen with left ventricular hypertrophy. A ***lift*** is a pulsation that is forceful enough to seem to lift the examiners fingers with palpation. A **heave** is a pulsation that feels rolling under your fingers. A **thrill** indicates turbulent flow and feels like a vibration over the PMI.

---

6. Auscultate the carotids.
   a. Place the bell portion of the stethoscope over the carotid artery to listen for bruits.
Bruits are low-pitched sounds, best heard by the bell portion.

   b. Have the patient hold his breath as you listen.
Breath sounds over the trachea are loud and could interfere with the ability to hear a bruit.

No audible bruit is present.

Developmental Variations

Children—Bruit may be heard because of a high-output state.

Abnormal findings: In adults, a bruit suggests carotid stenosis.

---

7. Auscultate the jugular veins.
   a. Place the bell portion of the stethoscope lightly over the jugular veins to listen for a low-pitched venous hum.
   b. Have the patient hold his breath as you listen.

No venous hum is audible.

Developmental Variations

Children—A venous hum may be heard. This is a benign condition whereby, blood travels to the brain and back down again to the heart, causing the vein walls to vibrate.

---

8. Auscultate the precordium.
To review heart sounds,

 Go to the sound file, **Heart Sounds,** on the Student Resource Disk or DavisPlus at http://davisplus.fadavis.com/ Wilkinson2

  ■ If not already in that position, ask the patient to sit upright and lean forward a bit.
  ■ This will position the heart closer to the chest wall for clearer auscultation.
  ■ Listen for the S_1, S_2, S_3, and S_4 sounds.
  ■ Listen for murmurs.
  ■ Listen with both the bell and the diaphragm at the sites in the following figure:

No extra sounds are heard. No murmurs, clicks, or rubs are present.

Developmental Variations

Infants—You may hear a split S_2 when the child takes a deep breath.

Children—The chest wall is thinner, so heart sounds are louder than in adults.

Older adults—An S_4 sound is considered normal; extra systoles per minute are considered normal.

These sites are located along the pathway the blood takes as it flows through the atria, ventricles, and valves of the heart. ▼

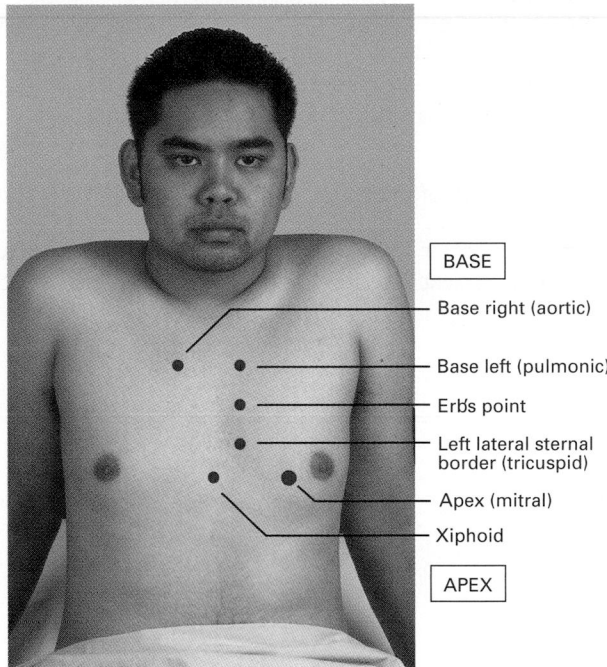

BASE
— Base right (aortic)
— Base left (pulmonic)
— Erb's point
— Left lateral sternal border (tricuspid)
— Apex (mitral)
— Xiphoid
APEX

a. *Base right (aortic valve).* Locate the angle of Louis. (It is the prominence on the sternum, two to three fingerbreadths below the suprasternal notch.) Slide your fingers laterally until you feel the 2nd ICS.

The right 2nd ICS is the best place to auscultate the aortic valve.

b. *Base left (pulmonic valve).* Locate the angle of Louis (the prominence on the sternum, two to three fingerbreadths below the clavicular notch). Slide your fingers laterally until you feel the 2nd ICS.

The left 2nd ICS is the best place to auscultate the pulmonic valve. ▼

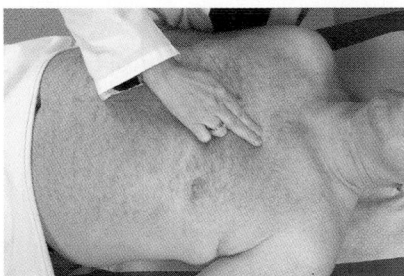

Palpating base left

c. *Apex (mitral valve).* You may be able to locate the apex by observing the pulsation at the PMI. It is at the 5th ICS in the midclavicular line.

a. $S_1 < S_2$

b. $S_1 < S_2$

c. $S_1 > S_2$

Developmental Variations

Children—You will hear S_3 at the apex in about 30% of children.

(continued on next page)

Procedure 19-13 ■ Assessing the Heart and Vascular System (continued)

d. Left lateral sternal border (LLSB) (tricuspid valve).
From the apex, *slide* your finger up to the 4th ICS, then move close to the sternum.

Assessing Murmurs

Auscultating murmurs is an advanced technique that requires practice and experience. However, if you hear a murmur, assess its:

- Location
- Quality
- Frequency (high, medium, or low pitch)
- Intensity (loudness)
- Timing (in relation to S_1 and S_2)
- Duration
- Configuration (constant or crescendo/decrescendo)
- Radiation (can you hear this in other locations?)
- Respiratory variation (does it change with breathing?)

Classifying Murmurs

Grade

$1/6$ Very faint, comes and goes
$2/6$ Quiet, but heard immediately
$3/6$ Moderately loud
$4/6$ Loud, associated with a thrill
$5/6$ Heard with stethoscope half off the chest wall; thrill present
$6/6$ Heard with stethoscope entirely off the chest wall; thrill present

---

9. Inspect the periphery for color, temperature, and edema. (You will probably already have done this when examining the integumentary system.)

---

10. Palpate the peripheral pulses: radial, brachial, femoral, popliteal, dorsalis pedis, and posterior tibial.
   a. Using the distal pads of your second and third fingers, firmly palpate pulses.
   b. Palpate firmly but not so hard that you occlude the artery.
   c. If you have trouble finding a pulse, vary your pressure, feeling carefully at the correct anatomical location.
   d. Assess pulses for rate, rhythm, equality, amplitude, and elasticity.
   e. Describe pulse amplitude on a scale of 0–4:
     0 = absent, not palpable
     1 = weak, barely palpable, easily obliterated by the finger
     2 = normal, obliterated by strong finger pressure
     3 = full, increased, not easily obliterated
     4 = bounding, forceful, obliterated only by strong finger pressure

---

d. $S_1 >$ or $= S_2$. You may hear a split S_1.

Abnormal findings: Extra sounds (S_3 or S_4), murmurs, clicks, or rubs. NOTE: A diastolic murmur or a murmur greater than grade 3/6 is never innocent. Also, *in infants,* a split S_2 sound during normal respirations may indicate an atrial-septal defect.

For a description of murmurs,

 Go to Chapter 19, **Tables, Boxes, Figures: ESG Table 19-1,** on the Student Resource Disk or DavisPlus at http://davisplus.fadavis.com/Wilkinson2

Skin is warm. No edema is present. Color is appropriate for race.

Abnormal findings: Pallor, cyanosis, coolness, shininess, sparse hair growth, and clubbing of the nails (may indicate pulmonary oxygenation problems or impaired central or peripheral circulation)

All pulses are regular, strong, and equal bilaterally. Pulse amplitude is +2.

Developmental Variations

Older adults—Arterial pulses may be difficult to palpate because of decreased arterial perfusion.

Abnormal findings: Weak, absent, or asymmetrical pulses may indicate partial or complete occlusion of the artery. Other signs of arterial occlusion include pain, pallor, cool temperature, paresthesia, or paralysis.

11. Inspect the venous system. If a client has varicosities, assess for valve competence with the manual compression test.
    a. With the client standing, compress the distal portion of the vein.
    b. Still holding the distal portion, compress the proximal portion.

What if. . .

■ **The patient is obese and heart sounds are difficult to hear?**

The larger the body mass over the heart, the more more difficult it is to hear heart sounds clearly. However, it may help to have the patient sit upright and lean forward as you auscultate.

■ **Findings from inspecting and palpating peripheral pulses are abnormal?**

If inspection or palpation findings are abnormal, perform the following more extensive tests.

More Extensive Tests for Abnormal Findings

1. *Perform the capillary refill test* anywhere you note signs of diminished blood flow.
    a. Press the skin with sufficient pressure to produce blanching.
    b. Release the pressure and observe the return of color.

2. *Perform Allen's test* to assess abnormal pulse findings and arterial flow in the hands.
    a. Have the client form a tight fist with one hand.
    b. With her fist still clenched, compress her radial and ulnar arteries.
    c. Ask the client to open her hand; observe for pallor.
    d. Release the ulnar artery and watch for natural color to return.
    e. Then repeat the process, but release the radial artery.

3. *Check the ankle–brachial index (ABI)* to assess circulatory impairment of the feet.
    a. Use a Doppler (hand-held ultrasonic device) to measure blood pressure at the posterior tibialis or dorsalis pedis pulse sites.
    b. Compare that pressure with blood pressure obtained over the brachial artery.
    c. To calculate the ABI, divide the systolic pressure at the ankle by the systolic pressure at the brachial site.

4. *Perform the color change test* to assess arterial circulation in the legs.
    a. While the client is lying supine, elevate the legs to increase venous return.
    b. Have the client quickly move to a sitting position with the feet dangling.

Veins are not distended. Superficial spiderlike veins, especially on the lower extremities, may occur with normal aging.

If the valves are competent, you will not feel backflow. If the valves are incompetent, you will feel a wave pulsation with your lower hand as a result of backflow when you press on the proximal segment of the veins.

Developmental Variations

Older adults—Often have peripheral edema as a result of chronic venous insufficiency.

Abnormal findings: Ropelike, distended, tortuous, or painful veins (**varicosities**)

Color returns in < 3 seconds.

In a healthy individual skin color returns rapidly with each maneuver. Failure to return to normal color indicates impaired flow through the open artery.

Normally pallor resolves in 3–5 seconds.

Normally ankle pressure is higher than brachial pressure. The following is a summary of ABI findings.
    Normal: 1 or greater
    Minimal disease: 0.8–0.95
    Moderate disease: 0.8–0.4
    Severe disease: 0.4–0

Example: If the systolic pressure at the ankle is 75 and at the brachial artery is 100, the ABI is 75/100, or 0.75. This indicates moderate peripheral vascular disease.
    d. Normal color should return to the feet in less than 10 seconds. Pallor with the legs elevated and dependent rubor (reddish-purple color) are signs of arterial insufficiency.

(continued on next page)

Procedure 19–13 ■ **Assessing the Heart and Vascular System** (continued)

Patient Teaching

Instruct the patient in the risk factors of heart disease and stroke and in the signs and symptoms of heart disease.

Documentation

■ If you need more information about documenting,

 Go to Chapter 19, **Documenting Physical Assessment Findings**, in Volume 1.

If you need more information about assessing apical and peripheral pulses and measuring blood pressure,

 Go to the *Fundamentals of Nursing Skills Videos*, **Vital Signs.**

Procedure 19–14   **Assessing the Abdomen**

➤   For steps to follow in *all* procedures, refer to the Universal Steps for All Procedures found on the inside back cover of Volume 2.

Critical Aspects

- Techniques: Inspection, auscultation, percussion, palpation (in that order)
- Have the client void prior to the exam.
- Position the client supine with the knees slightly flexed.
- Inspect the abdomen.
- Auscultate the abdomen for bowel sounds and bruits.
- Use indirect percussion to assess at multiple sites in all four quadrants.
- Using your fist or blunt percussion, percuss the costovertebral angle bilaterally to assess for kidney tenderness.
- Lightly palpate throughout the abdomen by pressing down 1–2 cm in a rotating motion. Identify surface characteristics, tenderness, muscle resistance, and turgor.
- Use deep palpation to palpate organs and masses.

Equipment

- Stethoscope
- Felt-tipped marker
- Tape measure and ruler
- Penlight or examination light
- Pen and record form

✚ Clean stethoscope and other equipment before and after using unless they are only used for one patient

Position

Begin with the client supine, arms at sides, with small pillows under the head and knees.
Relaxes the abdominal muscles.

Focused History Questions

- What types of foods do you typically eat?
- Are there any foods that you cannot eat? If so, why?
- How many cups of coffee, tea, cola, or caffeinated beverages do you drink per day?
- Do you smoke? If so, how much and at what age did you start?
- Do you drink alcohol? If so, how many drinks per day? Per week?

- Do you use any drug for non-medical purposes?
- Do you have any abdominal pain?
- How often do you have a bowel movement (BM)?
- Have you noticed any changes in your BMs?
- Are you having any problems with constipation, diarrhea, or getting to the bathroom in time to use the toilet?
- Have you ever seen blood in your stool or noticed blood when you wipe after a BM?
- Have you ever had black, tarry stools?
- How often do you use antacids, laxatives, enemas, aspirin, or anti-inflammatory medicines such as Anaprox or Motrin?
- What home remedy, herbal, or over-the-counter medicines do you use?
- What prescription medicines do you use?
- Have you ever been immunized for hepatitis?
- Have you ever had a blood transfusion?
- What is your occupation?
- Have you ever been diagnosed with an ulcer, hemorrhoids, hernia, bowel problem, cancer, hepatitis, liver problems, cirrhosis, or appendicitis?
- Have you ever had abdominal surgery? If so, when, what type, and what if any follow-up was done for the problem?

- Do you have any family history of abdominal problems, such as ulcers, gallbladder disease, bowel disease, or cancer?
- Do you ever have trouble with:
  Swallowing?
  Heartburn?
  Nausea?
  Vomiting?
  Diarrhea?
  Bloating?

Excess gas?
Yellowing of the skin?

Developmental Modifications

For older adults, recall that "Problems with eating" is a part of the SPICES assessment. Ask clients, for example:
- Do you have difficulty chewing or swallowing your food?
- How is your appetite?
- Are you able to shop for and prepare your food?

➤ When performing the procedure, always identify your patient according to agency policy and be attentive to standard precautions, hand hygiene, patient safety and privacy, body mechanics, and documentation.

Procedure Steps

1. Have the client void before the exam.
Empties the bladder so that you do not mistake a full bladder for a mass.

2. Position the client supine with the knees slightly flexed.
Relaxes the abdominal muscles.

3. Inspect the abdomen.
   a. Observe the size, symmetry, and contour of the abdomen.
      (1) Stand at the client's side and view across the abdomen.
      (2) If distention is present, use a tape measure to measure girth at the level of the umbilicus.
      (3) Have the client raise his head and check for bulges.
Accentuates hernia, if present.

   b. Observe the condition of skin and skin color. Look for lesions, scars, striae, superficial veins, and hair distribution (if you have not already done this in your examination of the integumentary system).

   c. Note abdominal movements.

Expected Findings

a. Abdomen is flat, slightly rounded, scaphoid (concave), or slightly protuberant; sides are symmetrical. No visible masses or distention are present.

Developmental Variations

Infants and toddlers—Protruberant abdomen is normal.

Abnormal findings: Tumors, cysts, bowel obstruction, or scoliosis may cause asymmetry.

b. Skin color is consistent with ethnicity but is usually lighter in color than exposed areas. No lesions are present. Hair distribution is appropriate for age and gender. Striae, superficial veins, and scars are common variations.

Abnormal findings:
- Skin color changes may be associated with bruising, internal bleeding, or jaundice.
- Striae occur after periods of rapid growth or weight gain. Pink striae are new. Older striae are silver-white in color.
- Dilated veins are associated with liver disease and obstruction of the vena cava.

c. On a thin client, peristalsis and aortic pulsations may be visible. Men tend to use their abdominal muscles for breathing.

Developmental Variations

Infants and children—Peristaltic waves are often visible. Abdominal breathing is common in infants and young children.

Older adults—Abdomen may be more rounded because of decreased muscle tone.

(continued on next page)

Procedure 19-14 ■ **Assessing the Abdomen** (continued)

Abnormal findings:
- Persitaltic waves may be seen if there is intestinal obstruction.
- Abnormal respiratory movements may be seen with respiratory distress.
- Pulsations (in other than a thin client) may indicate an aortic aneurysm.

d. Note the position, contour, and color of the umbilicus. ▼

d. Umbilicus is inverted and in the midline. No discoloration or discharge is present. ▼

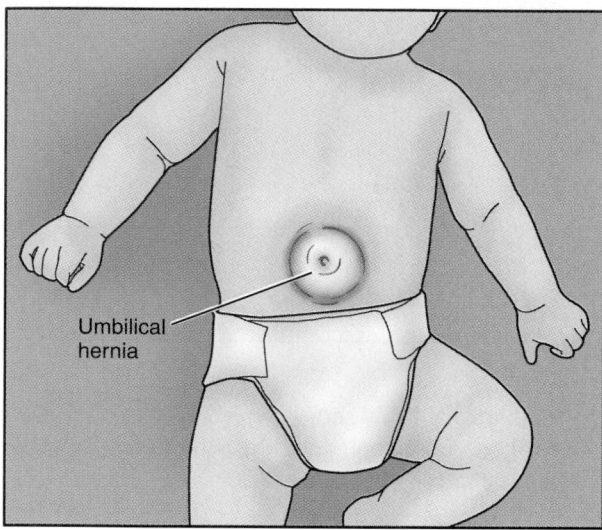

Umbilical hernia

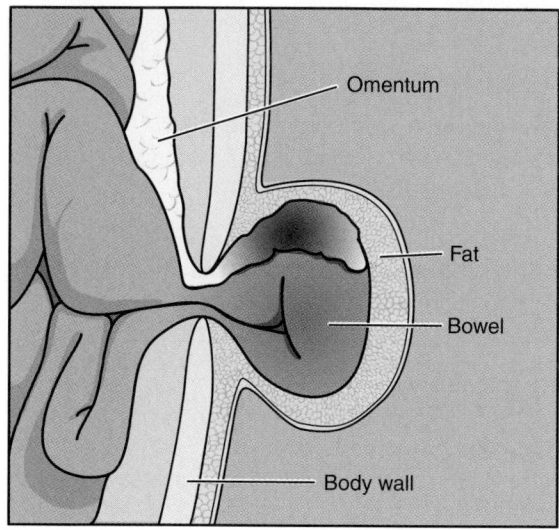

Omentum

Fat

Bowel

Body wall

Abnormal findings: Protrusion of the umbilicus may result from a hernia or underlying mass.

4. Auscultate the abdomen.
   a. Ask the client when he last ate.
Bowel sounds are loudest 5 or 6 hours after the person eats, when the small intestine contents empty through the ileocecal valve into the large intestine. They also increase immediately after eating.

   b. Listen for bowel sounds. To hear a sample of bowel sounds,

 Go to the sound file, **Bowel Sounds,** on the Student Resource Disk or DavisPlus at http://davisplus.fadavis.com/ Wilkinson2

   (1) Using the stethescope diaphragm, listen in several areas in all four quadrants (see the figure).
The diaphragm of the stethoscope is used because bowel sounds are high-pitched.

   (2) If bowel sounds are infrequent or difficult to hear, listen to the right of the umbilicus over the ileocecal valve.

   b. Audible bowel sounds, occuring every 5–15 seconds or 5–30 times per minute in a healthy adult.

Abnormal findings:
- *Hyperperistalsis* (hyperactive bowel sounds): > 2 or 3 sounds per second or > 30 bowel sounds per minute; loud, rushing sounds
- *Hypoperistalsis:* < 5 sounds per minute; faint sounds
- *Absent* bowel sounds: none after listening for 5 minutes

(3) Listen for 5 minutes before concluding that bowel sounds are absent. ▼

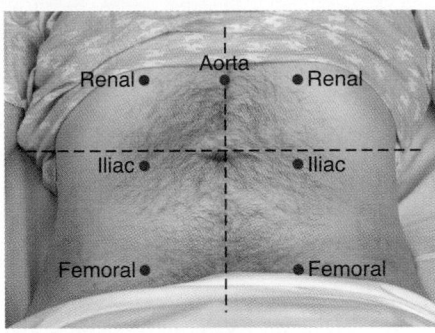

c. Use the stethoscope bell to listen for bruits over the aorta and the renal, femoral, and iliac arteries.

c. No audible bruits are present.

Abnormal findings: A bruit is abnormal and may indicate an aneurysm or altered blood flow.

---

5. Percuss the abdomen. (See Clinical Insight 19-1.)
a. Use indirect percussion to assess at multiple sites in all four quadrants.
b. Estimate organ size by noting the change in sounds as you percuss over the liver, spleen, and bladder. ▼

Tympany, with dullness over organs or fluid, is present. No tenderness

Abnormal findings: Extremely high-pitched tympanic sounds are heard with distention. Extensive dullness indicates organ enlargement or underlying mass.

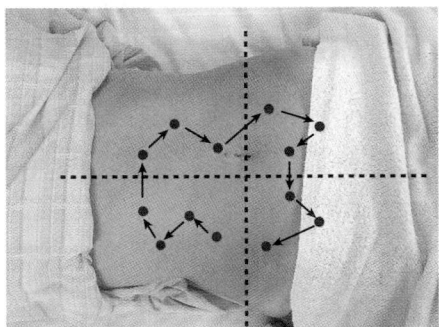

---

6. Using fist or blunt percussion, percuss the costovertebral angle (where the end of the rib cage meets the spine) bilaterally to assess for kidney tenderness. ▼

No costovertebral angle tenderness is present.

Abnormal findings: Pain or tenderness is associated with kidney infection or musculoskeletal problems.

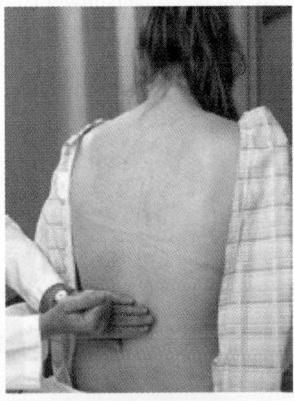

(continued on next page)

Procedure 19–14 ■ **Assessing the Abdomen** (continued)

7. Palpate the abdomen.

   a. Begin with light palpation throughout the abdomen. Identify surface characteristics, tenderness, muscular resistance, and turgor.

     (1) If the client is having pain in one area of the abdomen, palpate that area last.

A guarding response to pain from palpation can interfere with your assessment of the other areas.

     (2) Using your fingertips, press down 1–2 cm in a rotating motion.

     (3) Lift your fingers and move to the next site.

     (4) Palpate the entire abdomen if possible.

     (5) Proceed in an organized fashion through all quadrants, using the same sequence in every examination.

     (6) Observe for grimacing, guarding, or verbal statements of tenderness or pain.

Developmental Modifications

Encourage a child to place her hand lightly over yours as you palpate.

   Caution: Do not palpate the abdomen if the client has a Wilms' tumor, a large diffuse pulsation, or a history of organ transplant

   b. Use deep palpation to palpate organs and masses.

   a. The abdomen is soft and nontender, with no masses. Muscles are easily palpated; no guarding is present.

Abnormal findings: Guarding and rigidity may indicate peritonitis. Tenderness on light palpation indicates the need for further evaluation.

   b. Tenderness may be noted in a normal adult near the xiphoid process and over the cecum and sigmoid colon.

Developmental Variations

Older adults—May have a higher pain threshold, so they may not react to palpation even if there is an abnormality in the abdomen.

Deep Palpation Techniques

DEEP PALPATION: ONE-HANDED TECHNIQUE	**DEEP PALPATION: BIMANUAL TECHNIQUE**

DEEP PALPATION: ONE-HANDED TECHNIQUE

- Using your fingertips, press down 4 to 6 cm in a dipping motion.
- Proceed in an organized fashion through all four quadrants.

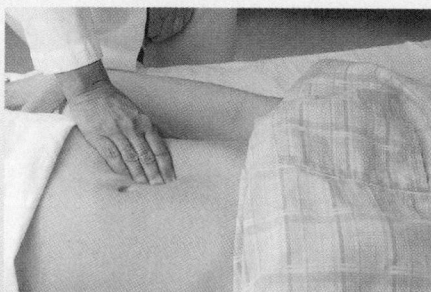

DEEP PALPATION: BIMANUAL TECHNIQUE

- This technique is useful when palpating a large abdomen.
- Place your nondominant hand on your dominant hand.
- Depress your hands 4 to 6 cm (1.5 to 2 in.) in a dipping motion.
- Proceed in an organized fashion through all four quadrants.

What if. . .

- **You palpate a mass? Have the client tighten her abdominal muscles.**

If the mass is in the abdominal wall, it will become easier to palpate. If it is deep in the abdomen, it will be difficult to palpate.

Abnormal findings: A mass indicates the need for further evaluation.

c. **Palpate the liver.**
   (1) Stand at the client's right side.
   (2) Place your right hand at the client's right midclavicular line under the costal margin, parallel to the right costal.
   (3) Place your left hand under the client's back at the lower (11th to 12th) ribs, and press upward. This elevates the liver toward the abdominal wall.
   (4) Ask the client to inhale and deeply exhale while you press in and up, gently but deeply, with your right fingers.

Alternative approach: Hooking technique. Place your hands over the right costal margin, and hook your fingers over the edge. Have the client take a deep breath, and feel for the liver's edge as the liver drops down on inspiration and then rises up over your fingers during expiration. ▼

c. The liver is not normally palpable unless the client is very thin. If it is palpable, the edge should be smooth and nontender.

Developmental Variations

Children—Liver is relatively large and can be palpated 1–2 cm (0.5–1 in.) below the right costal margin.

Abnormal findings: Palpation below the costal margin indicates enlargement.

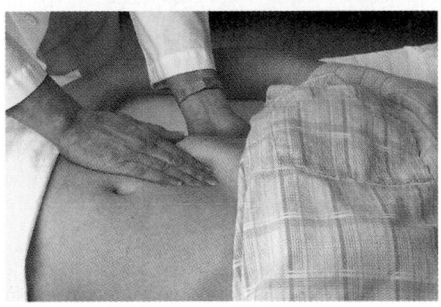

d. **Palpate the Spleen**
   (1) Stand at the client's right side.
   (2) Reach across the client to place your left hand under the costovertebral angle, and pull upward to move the spleen anteriorly.
   (3) Place your right hand under the left anterior costal margin, and have the client take a deep breath.
   (4) During exhalation, press your hands together (inward) to try to palpate the spleen. ▼

d. The spleen is not normally palpable.

Abnormal findings: Splenic enlargement or tenderness may result from infection, enlargement, trauma, or cancer.

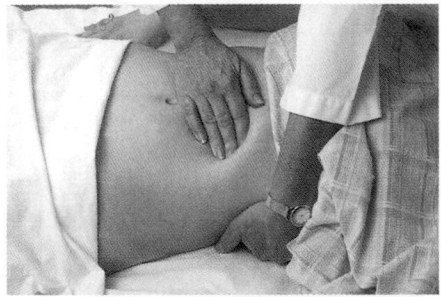

What if . . .

■ **The patient is ticklish or guarding when you palpate the abdomen?**

Distract the person by giving her a task, such as "Count aloud to 10" or "Count backwards from 100." Alternatively, have the client place her hand on her abdomen; place your hand on hers and begin light palpation. When she begins to feel more relaxed, slip your hand underneath hers and continue.

(continued on next page)

Procedure 19-14 ▪ **Assessing the Abdomen** (continued)

▪ **The patient complains of abdominal pain?**

Check for rebound tenderness: Place your hand perpendicular to the abdomen. Press firmly and slowly then release quickly.

If pain increases when you remove your hand, this indicates peritoneal irritation. Rebound tenderness in the right lower quadrant may be a sign of appendicitis.

Patient Teaching

Instruct the patient in the importance of proper diet, the signs and symptoms of colorectal cancer, and the importance of screening colonoscopy.

Documentation

▪ If you need more information about documenting,

 VOL 1 Go to Chapter 19, **Documenting Physical Assessment Findings,** in Volume 1.

Procedure 19-15 ☐ **Assessing the Musculoskeletal System**

➤ For steps to follow in *all* procedures, refer to the Universal Steps for All Procedures found on the inside back cover of Volume 2.

Critical Aspects

- Techniques: Inspection and palpation
- Assess posture, body alignment, and symmetry.
- Assess the spinal curvature.
- Examine the gait by assessing the base of support, stride, and phases of the gait.
- Assess balance through tandem walking, heel-and-toe walking, deep knee bends, hopping, and the Romberg test.
- Assess coordination by testing finger–thumb opposition, rhythmic movements of lower and upper extremities, and rapid alternating movements.
- Test the accuracy of movements by having the client touch his finger to his nose with his eyes closed.
- Measure limb length and circumference. Compare limbs on both sides of the body.
- Inspect muscle symmetry.
- Perform range of motion of all joints.
- Assess muscle strength by having the client perform ROM against resistance.

Equipment

- Tape measure
- Goniometer
- Pen and record form

Developmental Modifications

For older adults, recall that "Problems with falls" is a part of the SPICES assessment. If your facility has a falls assessment tool, perform that focused assessment.

Focused History Questions

- Do you have any difficulty with coordination (e.g., folding clothes, brushing your teeth)?
- Do you now have, or have you ever had, musculoskeletal problems, pain, or disease? If so, what medications or treatments are you using?
- Have you ever injured your bones or joints?
- Do your joints, muscles, or bones limit your activities?
- Do you lose your balance or fall?
- Do you have any occupational hazards that could affect your muscles and joints?

➤ When performing the procedure, always identify your patient according to agency policy and be attentive to standard precautions, hand hygiene, patient safety and privacy, body mechanics, and documentation.

Procedure Steps

1. Assess posture.
   a. Note the body and head position.

   b. Check the alignment and symmetry of the shoulders, scapula, and iliac crests. Inspect from the front, back, and side.

Developmental Modifications

Newborns—Palpate clavicles for fractures that may have occurred at birth. Check for congenital hip dysplasia (dislocation) by examining for asymmetry of the gluteal folds or shortening of the femur.
   c. Assess the spinal curvature by:
      (1) Observing the client's profile while he is standing erect.
      (2) Having the client bend forward at the waist with arms hanging free at the sides. ▼

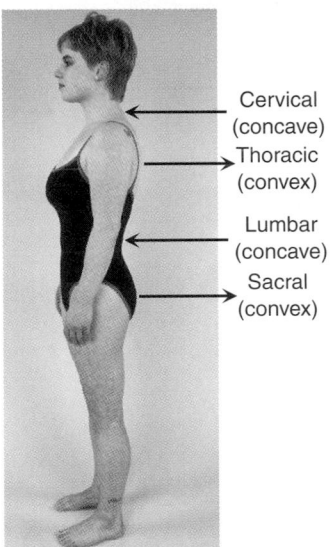 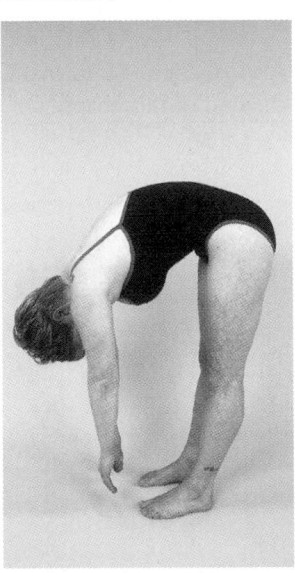

Assessing for normal curves

Cervical (concave)
Thoracic (convex)
Lumbar (concave)
Sacral (convex)

   d. Have the client stand upright with the feet together. Note the position of the knees. ▼

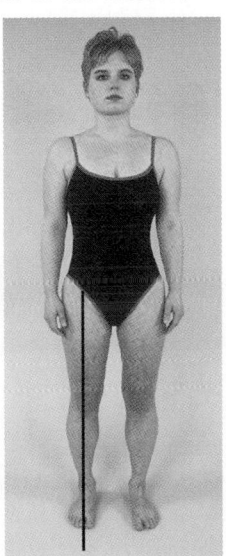

Expected Findings

   a. Posture is erect, with the head in the midline.

   b. The shoulders, scapula, and iliac crests are symmetrical.

   c. Cervical and lumbar curves are concave; thoracic and sacral curves are convex.

Developmental Variations

Children—**Lordosis** (exaggerated lumbar curve) is normal before age 5.

Abnormal findings: Kyphosis, scoliosis, lordosis

Also see **Abnormal Atlas: Musculoskeletal System,** at the end of this chapter.

   d. Patella is in the midline on an imaginary line drawn from the anterior superior iliac crest to the feet.

Developmental Variations

Children—**Genu varum** (bowlegs) is normal for 1 year after a child begins to walk.

(continued on next page)

Procedure 19–15 ■ **Assessing the Musculoskeletal System** (continued)

2. Assess gait by observing the client walking.

Developmental Modifications

Children—Observe them at play.

a. Pay attention to the base of support (distance between the feet) and stride length (distance between each step).

a. Average base of support for an adult is 5–10 cm (2–4 in.). Average stride length is 30–35 cm (12–14 in.); the longer the legs, the longer the stride length.

Abnormal findings: Abnormal gait can be caused by muscle weakness, joint stiffness, pain, deformities, and central nervous system dysfunction. A wide base of support and shortened stride length reflect a balance problem, placing the client at risk for falls.

b. Observe the phases of the gait. ▼

b. Movements are smooth and coordinated, weight is evenly distributed, arms swing in opposition, and toes point forward.

Abnormal findings: Toeing in or out, jerky or shuffling movements, touching the floor first with the toe rather than the heel, arms held out to the side or front.

Also refer to "Abnormal Gaits" on the Abnormal Atlas at the end of this chapter.

Stance phase

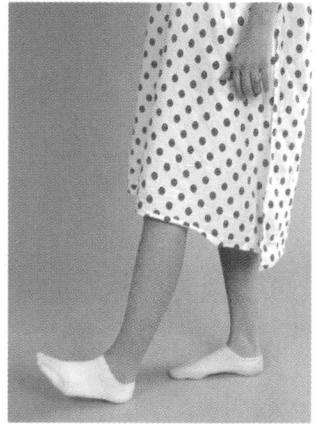

Heel strike

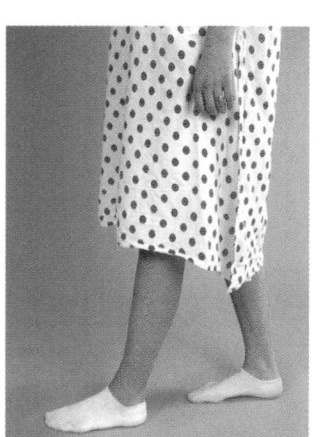

Foot flat

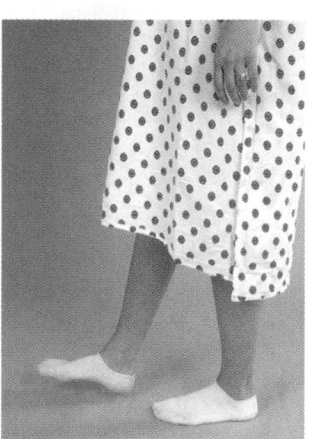

Midstance

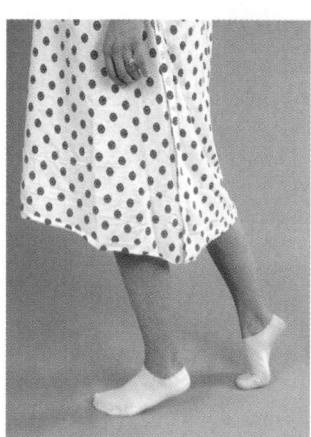

Push-off

Swing phase

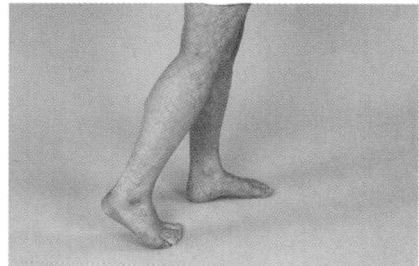

Accelerate

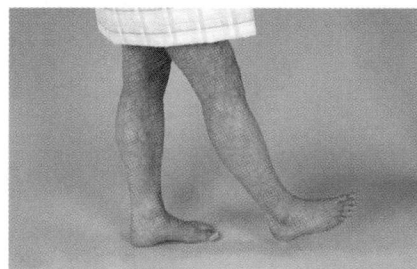

Swing-thru

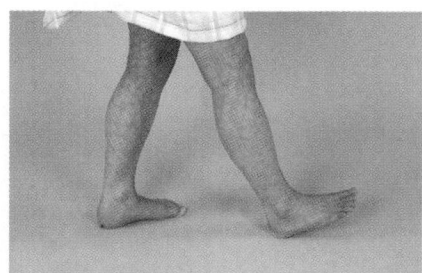

Decelerate

3. Assess balance.

What if . . .

■ **The client was unsteady when walking?**

Do not complete this portion of the exam.

If the client's gait is steady, you may proceed.
  a. Have the client tandem walk heel-to-toe.
  b. Have the client walk alternately on heels and toes.
  c. Ask the client to do a deep knee bend.
  d. Ask the client to hop in place on each foot several times.
  e. Perform the Romberg test (if you did not already do so when examining the ears): Have the client stand with feet together and eyes open. Then have him close his eyes and stand still.

✦ Stand nearby in case the client loses his balance.

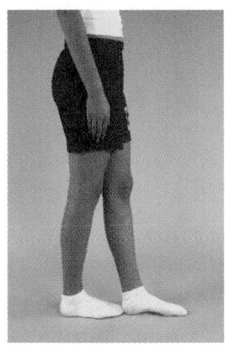 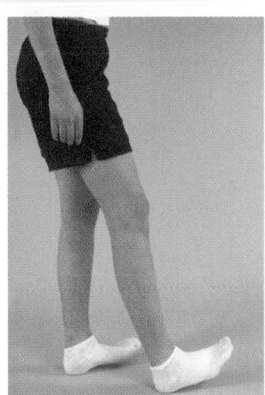 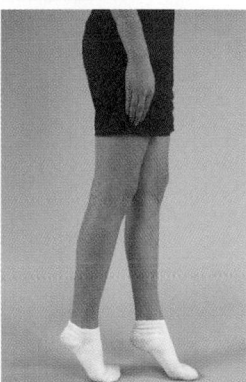

Step 3a. Walking heel-to-toe

Step 3b. Walking on heels

Step 3b. Walking on toes

Developmental Modifications

Infants—Observe sucking, swallowing, and kicking movements.

Children—To assess a child's movement, coordination, range-of-motion, and so on, watch the child at normal play. Cerebellar function cannot be tested on infants and toddlers because of their immature neuromuscular system.

The client is able to perform each of these maneuvers smoothly. The Romberg test (see Procedure 19-7) is negative—the client is able to maintain balance with minimal sway with eyes open and closed.

Developmental Variations

Infants—Should be able to sit alone by age 8 months.

Abnormal findings: Balance problems may indicate a cerebellar disorder, an inner ear problem, or muscle weakness.

---

4. Assess coordination while the client is seated.
  a. Test upper extremity coordination by having the client perform finger–thumb opposition. Test one side and then the other. ▼

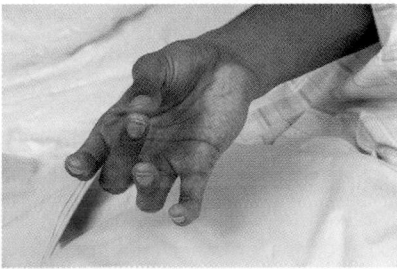

  b. Test rapid alternating movements by having the client alternate between supinating and pronating her hands.
  c. Assess lower extremity coordination by having the client perform rhythmic toe-tapping, one side at a time.
  d. Have the client run the heel of one foot down the shin of the other leg. Repeat on the opposite side.

The client is able to perform these movements smoothly and in a coordinated fashion. The dominant side (usually the right) may be slightly more coordinated.

Developmental Variations

Older adults—Decreased coordination and reaction time may result from slower nerve conduction and loss of muscle tone.

Abnormal findings: Slowness or awkwardness with movement may indicate a cerebellar disorder or muscle weakness.

(continued on next page)

Procedure 19-15 ■ **Assessing the Musculoskeletal System** (continued)

5. Test accuracy of movements. Have the client touch his finger to his nose with his eyes open. Repeat with his eyes closed.

The movement is accurate with eyes open and closed.

Abnormal findings: Inaccurate movements indicate cerebellar dysfunction.

6. Measure the limbs.
  a. Measure arm length from the acromion process to the tip of the middle finger.
  b. *Apparent leg length*—Measure from the umbilicus (a nonfixed point) to the medial malleolus.
  c. *True leg length*—Measure from the anterior superior iliac crest, crossing over the knee to the medial malleolus ▼

a., b., c. The differences in length between the right and left arm and leg are 1 cm or less.

Abnormal findings: Leg length discrepancies may cause back and hip pain and gait problems. A *true leg length* discrepancy results from unequal bone length; an *apparent leg length* discrepancy may result from a pelvic tilt or flexion deformity of the hip.

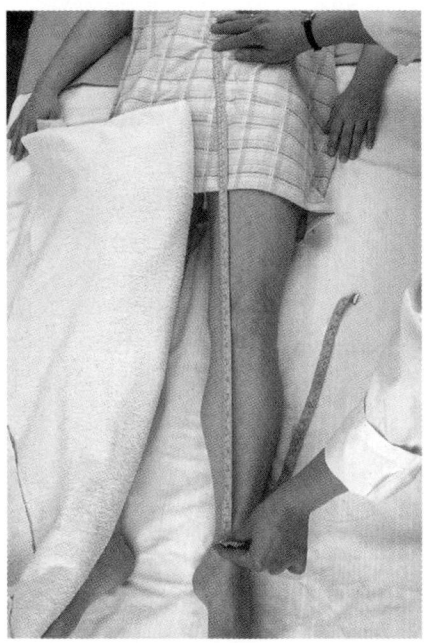   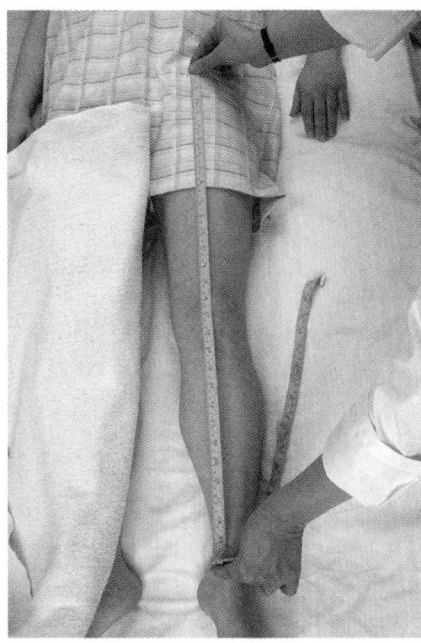

Apparent leg length   True leg length

  d. Measure the circumference of the forearms, upper arms, thighs, and calves.

d. The differences in circumference between the right and left arm and leg are 1 cm or less.

Abnormal findings: Circumference differences >1 cm may reflect atrophy or hypertrophy.

7. Inspect muscles and joints bilaterally for symmetry and shape.

Developmental Modifications

Older adults—Observe for surgical scars indicating joint replacement or joint surgeries.

Size and shape are symmetrical. Muscles and joints are smooth, nontender, and similar in color and temperature to surrounding tissue.

Developmental Variations

Older adults—Muscle mass and tone decrease.

Abnormal findings:
- Hot, red, swollen, stiff, or painful joints may indicate injuries, arthritis, gout, bursitis, or other inflammatory diseases.
- *Heberden's nodes* are hard, painless nodules over the distal interphalangeal joints—usually seen with degenerative joint disease (DJD), but they may be seen with rheumatoid arthritis (RA).
- Severe misalignment and deformity are more often a result of DJD than of RA.
- Crepitus may be heard in DJD.

8. Test active ROM by asking the client to move the following joints through ROM:

a. Temporomandibular joint (TMJ)

b. Neck

c. Thoracic and lumbar spine

d. Shoulder

e. Upper arm and elbow

f. Wrist

g. Hands and fingers

h. Hip

i. Knee

j. Ankles and feet ▼

- *TMJ* —Able to flex, extend, move side to side, protrude, and retract the jaw.
- *Neck*—Flexes, extends, hyperextends, bends laterally, and rotates side to side.
- *Spine*—Able to bend at the waist, stand upright, hyperextend (bend backward), bend laterally, and rotate side to side.
- *Shoulder*—Able to move the arm forward and backward, abduct, adduct, and rotate internally and externally.
- *Upper arm and elbow*—Able to bend, extend, supinate, and pronate the elbow.
- *Wrist*—Flexes, extends, hyperextends, and moves side to side.
- *Hands and fingers*—Able to spread the fingers (abduct), bring them together (adduct), make a fist (flex), extend the hand (extend), bend fingers back (hyperextend), and bring thumb to index finger (palmar adduction).
- *Hip*—Able to extend the leg straight, flex the knee to the chest, abduct and adduct the leg, rotate the hip internally and externally, and hyperextend the leg.
- *Knee*—Able to flex and extend the knee.
- *Ankles and feet*—able to dorsiflex, plantar flex, evert, invert, abduct, and adduct the feet and ankles.

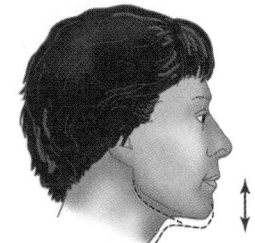

Depression: lowering a body part
Elevation: raising a body part

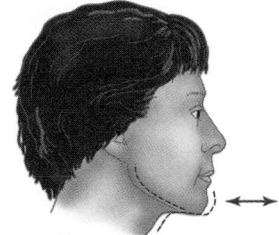

Retraction: moving backward
Protraction: moving forward

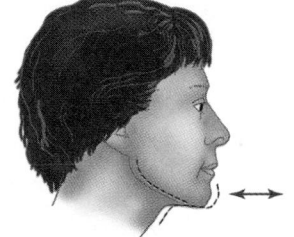

Retraction: moving backward
Protraction: moving forward

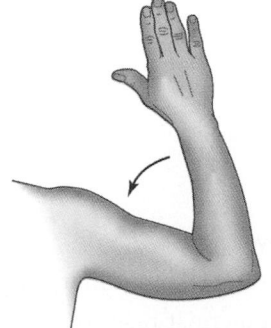

Flexion: bending, decreasing joint angle

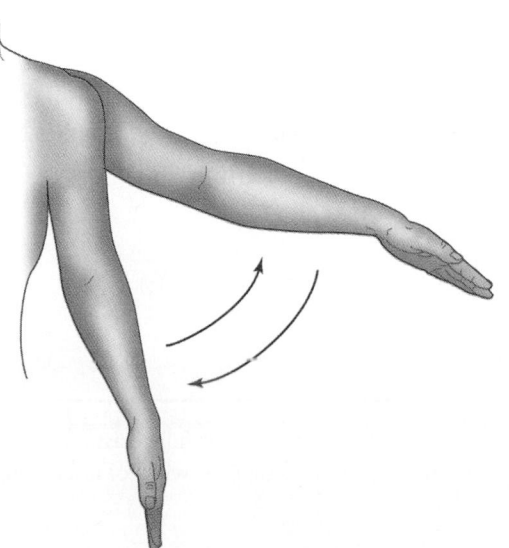

Abduction: moving away from midline
Adduction: moving toward midline

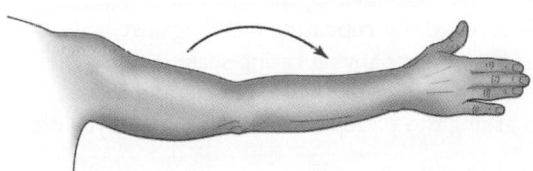

Extension: straightening, increasing joint angle

(continued on next page)

Procedure 19-15 ■ Assessing the Musculoskeletal System (continued)

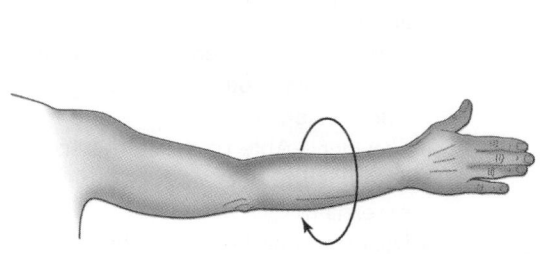

Circumduction: moving in a circular fashion

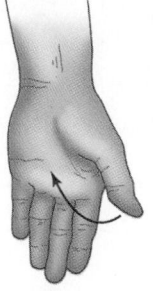

Resposition

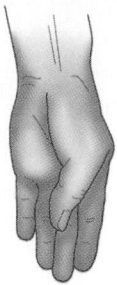

Opposition

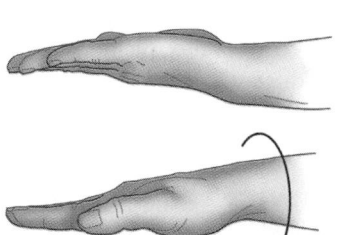

Supination: turning upward

Pronation: turning downward

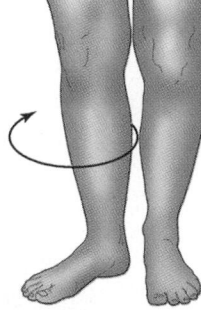

External rotation:
turning away from midline

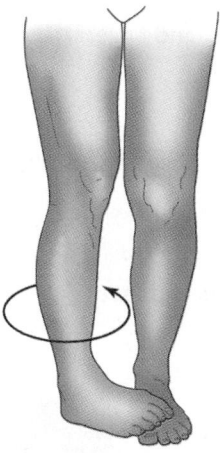

Internal rotation:
turning toward midline

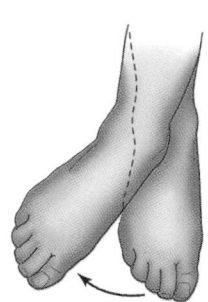

Eversion: turning outward

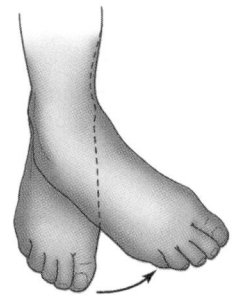

Inversion: turning inward

What if . . .

■ **The client cannot move the limb?**

Put the joint through passive range of motion.

◆ Never force a joint against resistance or if it causes discomfort.

---

9. Test muscle strength by repeating ROM against resistance. Use the accompanying rating scale.
   a. Test hand grip by crossing your middle and index fingers and asking the patient to squeeze. (*Tip: If you are*

Expect active motion against full resistance. There should be no crepitus (clicking) or pain with joint movement.

wearing rings, a strong handgrip on those fingers can be painful.) ▼

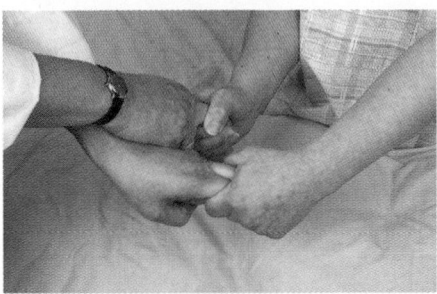

b. Test biceps strength. Place one hand on the client's biceps and have the patient raise the forearm (flex the elbow) as you apply resistance at the wrist.

c. Test triceps strength by having the client straighten the arm at the elbow (extend the elbow) as you apply resistance at the wrist.

d. Test leg strength by having patient raise leg (straighten the knee) against your hand as you apply resistance.

e. Test ankle strength by asking the patient to point the toes downward (plantar flexion) the ankle while you apply resistance to the plantar sufrace of the foot.

f. Test ankle strength by having the client point the toes toward the knee (dorsiflexion) as you apply resistance to the top of the foot.

Muscle Strength Rating Scale		
RATING	**CRITERIA**	**CLASSIFICATION**
5	Active motion against full resistance	Normal
4	Active motion against some resistance	Slight weakness
3	Active motion against gravity	Weakness
2	Passive ROM	Poor ROM
1	Slight flicker of contraction	Severe weakness
0	No muscular contraction	Paralysis

What if. . .

■ **There is limited range of motion in a joint?**

Use a goniometer to measure the limited motion in degrees. Place the goniometer over the joint, matching the angle of the joint.

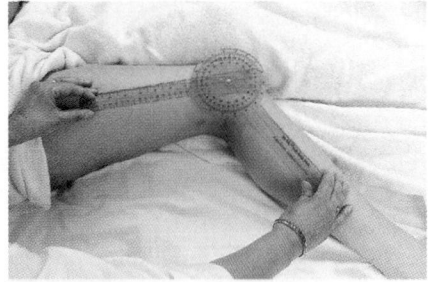

Using a goniometer

Documentation

■ If you need more information about documenting,

 VOL 1 Go to Chapter 19, **Documenting Physical Assessment Findings,** in Volume 1.

Procedure 19-16 Assessing the Sensory–Neurological System

➤ For steps to follow in *all* procedures, refer to the Universal Steps for All Procedures found on the inside back cover of Volume 2.

➤ *NOTE:* This procedure provides guidelines for performing a comprehensive neurological exam. Steps 1–10 assess cognitive status, and the box at the end of the procedure contains questions that are useful for screening cognitive status.

Critical Aspects

- Assess behavior.
- Determine level of arousal.
- Determine level of orientation.
- Assess memory.
- Assess mathematical and calculation skills.
- Assess general knowledge.
- Evaluate thought processes.
- Assess abstract thinking.
- Assess judgment.
- Assess communication ability.
- Test cranial nerves.
- Test superficial sensations.
- Test deep sensations.
- Test discriminatory sensations.
- Test deep tendon reflexes.
- Test superficial reflexes.
- Assess for dementia in institutionalized older adults.

Equipment

- Pen and record form
- Wisp of cotton
- Sharp object, such as a toothpick or sterile needle
- Objects to touch, such as a coin, button, or key
- Something fragrant, such as coffee or rubbing alcohol
- Something to taste, such as sugar, salt, or lemon
- Tongue blade
- Two test tubes
- Reflex hammer
- Ophthalmoscope

Developmental Modifications for Children

- For children younger than age 5 years, use the Denver Developmental Screening Test II to assess neurological and motor function.
- Check the child's ability to understand and follow instructions.

Developmental Modifications for Older Adults

- You may need to perform the sensory–neurologic exam over several sessions. The full exam is lengthy, and older adults fatigue easily. If the client seems to be getting tired, stop the test and finish at a later time.

Focused History Questions

- Do you have any neurological ("nerve") problems?
- Have you ever had head trauma, loss of consciousness, dizziness, headaches, or seizures?
- Do you have memory problems, forgetfulness, or inability to concentrate?
- Have you noticed any changes in your ability to see, smell, taste, hear, feel, or maintain balance?
- Do you have any weakness, numbness, or paralysis?
- Do you have any problems performing activities of daily living (ADLs)?
- Do you have any problems walking?
- Do you have mood problems or depression?
- Do you use alcohol or drugs for non-medical purposes? If so, how much and how often?
- Have you ever been treated for neurological or psychiatric problems?
- Do you have a history of hypertension, diabetes, stroke, or circulation problems?

➤ When performing the procedure, always identify your patient according to agency policy and be attentive to standard precautions, hand hygiene, patient safety and privacy, body mechanics, and documentation.

Procedure Steps

1. Assess behavior. Note the client's facial expression, posture, affect, and grooming.

2. Determine level of arousal (LOA):
  a. Note the client's response to verbal stimuli.
  b. If the client does not respond to verbal stimuli, try tactile stimulation: Gently shake the client's shoulder.
  c. If the client does not respond to tactile stimuli, try painful stimuli: Squeeze the trapezius muscle, rub the sternum, apply pressure on the mandible at the angle of the jaw, or apply pressure over the "moon" of the nail.
The Glasgow Coma Scale and the FOUR Scale at the end of this procedure provide standard references for assessing LOA for a patient with head injury.

3. Determine the level of orientation.

  a. *Orientation to time:* Ask the client to state the year, date, and time of day.

  b. *Orientation to place:* Ask the client to state where he is (i.e., city, state, where he lives).

  c. *Orientation to person:* Ask the names of family members. Ask, "Do you know who I am?" If the client cannot answer these questions, ask him to state his name.
Self-identity remains intact the longest.

4. Assess memory.
  a. *Assess immediate memory* by asking the client to repeat a series of three numbers that you speak slowly (e.g., 1, 5, 8). Gradually increase the length of the series until the client cannot repeat the series correctly. Record the length of the last correct series (e.g., "Successfully repeats a series of 7 numbers correctly.")
  b. Repeat the test, beginning with a series of three numbers, but ask the client to repeat them back to you in reverse order.

Expected Findings

The client is well groomed, with an erect posture, pleasant facial expression, and appropriate affect.

Abnormal findings: Inappropriate behavior may result from neurological or psychological problems, as well as from a variety of medications, alcohol, and street drugs.

The patient is awake and alert and readily responds to verbal stimuli.

Abnormal findings: Lethargy, stupor, or coma may result from trauma, neurological disorder, hypoxia, or chemical substances

✚ A changing level of arousal (along forgetfulness, restlessness, or sudden quietness) is one of the earliest indicators of increased intracranial pressure, which can be life-threatening.

The client is awake, alert (see Step 2), and oriented to time, place, and person (AAO × 3).

  a. Hospitalized patients commonly lose track of date and time of day, but they easily reorient. As a rule, they should at least know the year.

  b. Interpret data carefully. In some situations (e.g., after an automobile accident away from home), the patient may know he is in the hospital but not know which hospital or which city.

  c. Patient should know you are a healthcare worker, but not necessarily your name.

Developmental Variations

Older adults—The stress of an unfamiliar situation can create confusion in an older adult.

Abnormal findings: Disorientation may result from physical or psychological problems. Bizarre responses are usually associated with psychiatric problems.

Immediate, recent, and remote memory are intact. Average series recall is 5–8 numbers in sequence and 4–6 numbers in reverse order.

Developmental Variations

Children—Number of objects recalled is usually fewer than the child's age in years.

Older adults—Loss of immediate and recent memory is common; long-term memory is usually not impaired.

Abnormal findings: Memory problems may be benign or may signal underlying neurological problems. Temporary memory loss may occur after trauma.

(continued on next page)

Procedure 19-16 ■ **Assessing the Sensory–Neurological System** (continued)

c. *Assess recent memory* by naming three items (e.g., "mirror, truck," and "the letter X") and asking the client to recall them later during the exam. Alternatively, you can ask questions such as, "How did you get to the hospital? What did you have for breakfast?" However, you will need to verify the patient's answers.

d. *Assess remote memory* by asking the client his birth date or the date of a major historical event.

Developmental Modifications

Children—Assess memory by using names of toys (e.g., truck, ball, puzzle), names of people in his family, or names of familiar cartoon characters.

---

5. Assess mathematical and calculation skills.

a. Have the client solve a simple mathematical problem, such as 3 + 3.

b. If he is able to solve that problem, present a more complex example, yet simple enough that regardless of math skills the client could still determine the appropriate response, such as, "If you have $3 and you buy an item for $2, how much money will you have left?"

c. To assess both calculation skills and attention span, ask the client to count backwards from 100.

d. A more difficult test is to have the client perform serial threes or serial sevens. Ask him to begin at 100 and keep subtracting 3 (or 7).

Consider the person's language, education, and culture in deciding whether this test is appropriate for him.

Mathematical and calculation ability is appropriate for the patient's age, education level, and language ability. The average adult can solve simple mathematical problems and can complete serial sevens in about 90 seconds with 3 or fewer errors.

Abnormal findings: Inability to calculate at a level appropriate for age and educational level may indicate neurological impairment or developmental delay.

---

6. Assess general knowledge.

You can ask questions directly or work this into the overall interaction with the client.

Ask the client how many days in the week or months in the year.

Vocabulary and general knowledge are intact.

---

7. Evaluate thought processes.

Assess throughout the exam. Notice attention span, logic of speech, ability to stay focused, and appropriateness of responses.

Thought processes are clear, client responds appropriately, and speech is coherent and logical.

Abnormal findings: Alteration in thought processes may be due to physical disorders, such as dementia; psychiatric disorders, such as psychosis; or alcohol and drugs.

---

8. Assess abstract thinking.

Ask the client to interpret a maxim (or saying), such as "A penny saved is a penny earned" or "A rolling stone gathers no moss."

Developmental Modifications

Children—The ability to think abstractly does not develop until the late school-age years or adolescence. To assess a child under the age of 12, ask her to describe things that are like and unlike a named object (e.g., "Tell me something that is like a cup.")

Abstract thinking is intact.

Abnormal findings: Inability to think abstractly is associated with dementia, delirium, mental retardation, and psychoses.

9. Assess judgment.
Ask the client to respond to a hypothetical situation, such as, "If you were walking down the street and saw smoke and flame coming from a house, what would you do?"

Judgment is intact.

Abnormal findings: Impaired judgment may be associated with dementia, psychosis, or substance abuse.

---

10. Assess communication ability.
  a. Listen to the client's speech. Note the rate, flow, choice of vocabulary, and enunciation.

  a. Speech flows easily, and patient enunciates clearly. Vocabulary is consistent with the client's age, education, and language fluency.

Abnormal findings: Problems with flow (e.g., halting speech, stuttering, very rapid speech, slurred words) may be due to language problems, nervousness, anxiety, or neurological problems.

  b. Test spontaneous speech: Show the client a picture, and have him describe it.

  b. Spontaneous speech is intact.

Abnormal findings: Impaired spontaneous speech is associated with cognitive impairment.

  c. Test motor speech by having the client say "Do, re, mi, fa, so, la, ti, do." Assess ability to swallow. Observe for clarity of speech, facial mobility, drooling, and oral hypotonia. Ask the client to repeat a short phrase 2 or 3 times and observe for lack of coordination.
  d. Test automatic speech by having the client recite the days of the week.

  c. Motor speech is intact.

Abnormal findings: Impaired motor speech is associated with problems with CN XII or with coordination of speech muscles.

  d. Automatic speech is intact.

Abnormal findings: Cognitive impairment or memory problems cause difficulty with automatic speech.

  e. Test sound recognition by having the client identify a familiar sound, such as clapping hands.

  e. Sound recognition is intact.

Abnormal findings: Temporal lobe problems may be the cause of impaired sound recognition.

  f. Test auditory–verbal comprehension by asking the client to follow simple directions (e.g., "Point to your nose; rub your left elbow.")

  f. Auditory–verbal comprehension is intact.

Abnormal findings: Temporal lobe problems affect reception. Frontal lobe problems affect expression.

  g. Test visual recognition by pointing to objects and asking the client to identify them.

  g. Visual recognition is intact.

Abnormal findings: Impaired visual recognition indicates parieto–occipital lobe problems.

  h. Test visual–verbal comprehension by having the client read a sentence and explain its meaning.

  h. Visual–verbal comprehension is intact.

Abnormal findings: Impaired visual–verbal comprehension indicates cognitive impairment.

  i. Test writing by having the client write her name and address.
  j. Test ability to copy figures by having the client copy a circle, letter x, square, triangle, and star.

  i. Writing ability is intact.

  j. The client is able to copy figures.

---

11. Test cranial nerve I—olfactory nerve.
Note: You can assess CN I with your examination of the nose and sinuses (see Procedure 19-8).
  a. Before testing, check the patency of the nostrils by gently occluding each nostril and having the client sniff.
  b. Have the client occlude one nostril and hold an aromatic substance (e.g., lemon, coffee, vanilla, alcohol) under the nostril.

The client can identify the substances.

Developmental Variations

Older adults—May have a decreased sense of smell.

Abnormal findings: Anosmia is the loss of the sense of smell. It may be genetic, related to chronic nose or sinus problems, heavy tobacco use, snorting cocaine, or zinc deficiency.

(continued on next page)

Procedure 19–16 ■ **Assessing the Sensory–Neurological System** (continued)

c. Repeat with a different substance under the other nostril. ▼

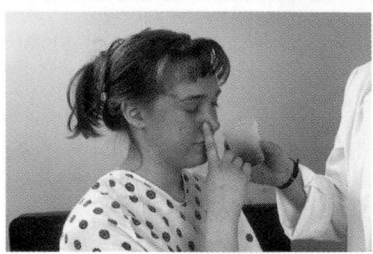

Developmental Modifications

Children—Select a substance that you are certain the child is familiar with (e.g., peanut butter).

---

12.   Test cranial nerve II—optic nerve.
Note: You can assess CN II with your examination of the eyes (see Procedure 19-6).

    a. Test visual acuity by asking the client to identify the smallest print readable on the Snellen chart (use picture chart for small children, Snellen E for school-age children).

    b. Identify visual field by having the client describe the boundaries of the visual field while her eye is in a fixed position.

    c. Perform a fundoscopic exam.

    a. Visual acuity is 20/20 in the right eye, left eye, and both eyes.

Abnormal findings: Many visual deficits are correctable with eyeglasses or contact lenses. They are not necessarily caused by optic nerve damage.

    b. Peripheral vision range is approximately 50° in the superior field, 70° in the inferior field, 60° in the nasal field, and 90–110° in the temporal field.

    c. Disc margins are sharply demarcated. The cup is half the size of the disc or less.

Abnormal findings: CN II deficits may be due to tumor or CVA.

---

13.   Test cranial nerves III, IV, and VI—oculomotor, trochlear, and abducens nerves.
    a. Test EOMs by having the client move the eyes through the six cardinal fields of gaze while holding her head steady. ▼

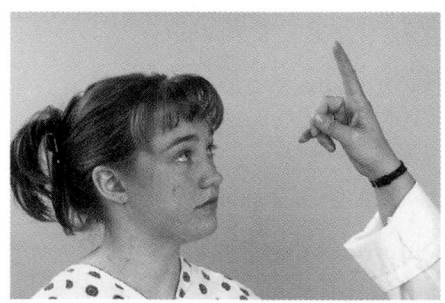

    b. Test pupillary reaction to light and accommodation. See Procedure 19-6 for further details on each of these tests.

Client can move her eyes through the six cardinal fields of gaze. Pupils are equal in size and react to light and accommodation.

Abnormal findings: Changes in intracranial pressure (ICP) may affect EOMs and pupillary reaction.

14. Test cranial nerve V—trigeminal nerve.

    a. Test motor function by having the client move his jaw from side to side, clenching his jaw, and biting down on a tongue blade.

Note: You can assess this function in your examination of the mouth and oropharynx (see Procedure 19-9).

    b. Test sensory function by having the client close her eyes and identify when you are touching her face at the forehead, cheeks, and chin bilaterally—first with your finger and then repeat with a toothpick.

    c. Test the corneal reflex by touching the cornea with a wisp of cotton or puffing air from a syringe over the cornea.

The corneal reflex is not usually tested on a conscious person because the procedure is unpleasant and a corneal abrasion can occur. A conscious person can blink intentionally, so there is no need to stimulate the blink.

Note: You can assess the corneal reflex in your examination of the eyes (see Procedure 19-6).

The client is able to perform all motor functions and can perceive light touch and superficial pain bilaterally; corneal reflex is intact.

Abnormal findings: Inability to perceive light touch and superficial pain may indicate peripheral nerve damage. An absent corneal reflex is an ominous neurological sign.

---

15. Test cranial nerve VII—facial nerve.

    a. Test motor function by having the client make faces, such as smile, frown, or whistle.

Note: You can assess this function in your examination of the head and face (see Procedure 19-5).

    b. Test taste on the anterior portion of the tongue by placing sweet (sugar), salty (salt), or sour (lemon) substance on the tip of the tongue. Do not test taste by using pungent, bitter, or markedly unpleasant flavors.

Note: You can assess this function in your examination of the mouth and oropharynx (see Procedure 19-9).

The client is able to perform all movements and can distinguish sweet, salty, and sour tastes.

Developmental Variations

Older adults—Have decreased taste sensation, especially sweet and salty, due to taste bud atrophy and diminished sense of smell.

Abnormal findings: Asymmetrical movement may be seen with nerve damage from a CVA or Bell's palsy. Impaired taste may be associated with nerve damage, chemotherapy, or radiation to the face or neck.

---

16. Test cranial nerve VIII—acoustic nerve.

Note: You can assess this function in your examination of the ears (see Procedure 19-7).

    a. Perform watch-tick test for hearing by holding a watch close to the client's ear. ▼

Hearing is intact. Romberg test is negative.

Abnormal findings: Hearing loss, loss of balance, or vertigo may result from acoustic nerve damage.

    b. Perform Weber and Rinne tests to assess air and bone conduction.

(continued on next page)

Procedure 19-16 ■ **Assessing the Sensory–Neurological System** (continued)

c. Test balance with the Romberg test, if it has not already been performed.

See Procedures 19-7 and 19-15 for further details on these tests.

Developmental Modifications

Children—Romberg test is appropriate only after age 3.

---

17. Test cranial nerves IX and X—glossopharyngeal and vagus nerves.
   a. Observe ability to talk, swallow, and cough.
   b. Test motor function by asking the client to say "ah" while you depress a tongue blade and observe the soft palate and uvula.
   c. Test sensory function by taking a tongue blade and gently touching the back of the pharynx to induce a gag reflex.
   d. Test taste (sweet, salty, and sour) on the posterior portion of the tongue. Avoid bitter or repulsive tasting substances.

Swallow and cough reflex are intact. Speech is clear. The uvula and soft palate rise symmetrically, and the gag reflex is intact. Taste on the posterior tongue is intact.

Developmental Variations

Older adults—Have decreased taste sensation, especially sweet and salty, due to atrophy of the taste buds and a diminished sense of smell.

Abnormal findings: Damage to CN IX and X impairs swallowing. Damage to CN X changes voice quality.

---

18. Test cranial nerve XI—accessory nerve.
Note: You can assess this motor nerve function with your examination of the musculoskeletal system (see Procedure 19-5).
   a. Place your hands on the client's shoulder, and have the client shrug his shoulders against resistance. ▼

Movement is symmetrical and pain-free. Full ROM of the neck with +5 strength.

Abnormal findings: Asymmetrical movement, pain, or absent movement indicates CN XI disorders.

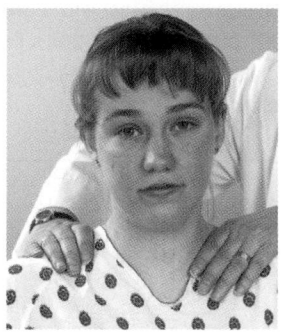

   b. Have the client turn his head from side to side against resistance.

---

19. Test cranial nerve XII—hypoglossal nerve.
   a. Ask the client to say "d, l, n, t."
   b. Have the client protrude the tongue and move it from side to side.

The client can articulate the sounds and move the tongue easily.

Abnormal findings: Tongue paralysis

20. Test superficial sensations. ▼

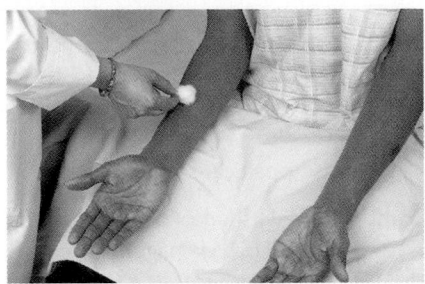

- Begin with the most peripheral part when testing the limbs (e.g., test the foot before the leg).

If the client can feel sensation in the most peripheral part, you can assume the sensory nerve is intact to that point.

- If the client does not perceive the touch in an area, determine the boundaries of the dysfunction by testing at about every inch (2.5 cm). Sketch the area of sensory loss.
- Wait about 2 seconds before moving to each site.

Wait so that you can be sure that the patient is perceiving each stimulus separately.

a. *Light touch:* With the patient's eyes closed, brush a cotton wisp on various areas of the body, comparing sides. Ask the client to say, "Now," when he feels your touch and to point to the spot you are touching.

b. *Pain:* With the patient's eyes closed, use a toothpick (or sterile needle) with dull and sharp ends. Touch various areas of the body (except the face), and have the patient identify whether the sensation is dull or sharp. Alternate the dull and sharp ends as you move from spot to spot. Compare sides of the body.

c. *Temperature sensation:* Test only if the patient's perception of pain is abnormal. Use test tubes filled with hot and cold water. Touch the tube to various areas of the body, comparing sides; have the client say "Hot," "Cold," or "Don't know."

If pain sensation is intact, temperature will be, too, because sensations for pain and temperature are transmitted along the same tracts.

a. Able to identify areas of light touch.

Abnormal findings: Diminished sensation or areas of absent perception

b. The client is able to identify the areas stimulated and the type of sensation.

Abnormal findings:
- **Hyperalgia:** increased pain sensation
- **Analgesia:** no pain sensation
- **Paresthesia:** numbness and tingling

Developmental Variations

Older adults—May have a decreased perception of temperature and deep pain.

---

21. Test deep sensations.

a. *Assess vibratory sensation* by placing a vibrating tuning fork on a metatarsal joint and distal interphalangeal joint. Have the patient identify when she feels the vibration and when it stops. ▼

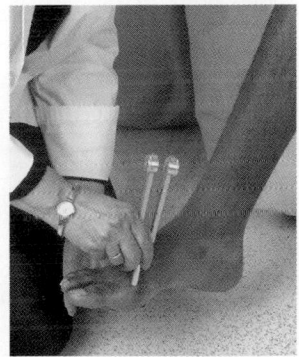

a. Vibratory sense is intact bilaterally in the upper and lower extremities.

Abnormal findings: Diminished or absent vibration sense is seen with peripheral nerve damage from vascular disease, diabetes, alcoholism, or damage to the posterior column of the spinal cord.

(continued on next page)

Procedure 19–16 ■ **Assessing the Sensory–Neurological System** (continued)

b. *Test kinesthetic sensation* (position sense) by holding the client's finger or toe on the sides and moving it up or down. Keeping her eyes closed, have the client identify the direction of the movement. ▼

b. Position sense is intact bilaterally in the upper and lower extremities.

Developmental Variations

Older adults—May lose position sense in the great toes.

Abnormal findings: Diminished or absent position sense indicates nerve or spinal cord damage.

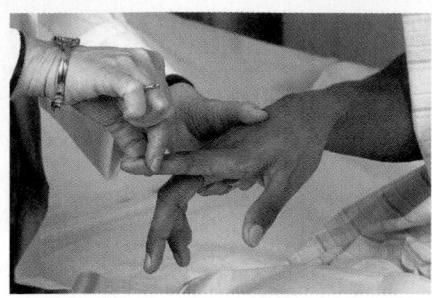

22. **Test discriminatory sensations.**

   a. *Assess stereognosis* by placing a familiar object (e.g., a coin or a button) in the palm of the client's hand and having her identify it.

   b. *Assess graphesthesia* by drawing a number or letter in the palm of your patient's hand and having the patient identify what was drawn.

   c. *Test two-point discrimination* with toothpicks. Have the patient close her eyes. Touch her on the finger with two toothpicks simultaneously. Gradually move the points together, and have the patient say, "One," or "Two," each time you move the toothpicks. Document distance and location at which she can no longer feel two separate points. ▼

   a. Stereognosis is intact bilaterally.

   b. Graphesthesia is intact bilaterally.

   c. Discriminates between two points on fingertips no more than 0.5 cm apart.

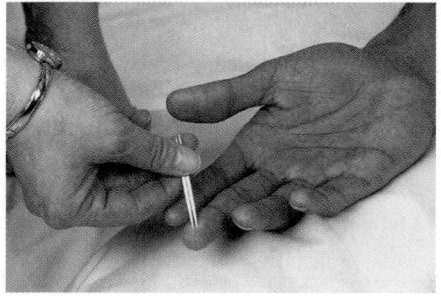

   d. *Test point localization* by having the patient close her eyes while you touch her. Have her point to the area you touched. Repeat on both sides and the upper and lower extremities.

   e. *Test sensory extinction* by simultaneously touching the patient on both sides (e.g., on both hands, both knees, both arms). Have the patient identify where he was touched. ▼

   d. Point localization is intact bilaterally in the upper and lower extremities.

   e. Extinction is intact: Client should feel the sensation on both sides of his body.

Abnormal findings: Abnormalities in any of the discriminatory sensation tests may indicate a lesion or disorder of the sensory cortex or disorder of the posterior column of the spinal cord.

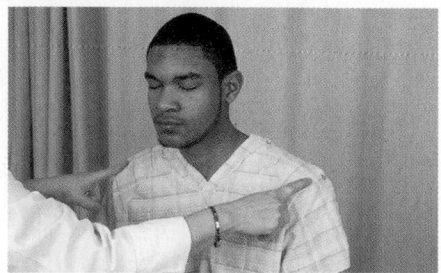

Developmental Modifications

Older adults—May need more time to respond to a stimulus, as reaction time may be slower.

---

23. Test deep tendon reflexes.
(See the accompanying scale to grade responses.)

Deep Tendon Reflex Grading Scale

0   No response detected

+1   Diminished response

+2   Response normal

+3   Response somewhat stronger than normal

+4   Response hyperactive with **clonus** (involuntary contractions that continue after the first contraction is elicited by the hammer)

a. *Biceps reflex* (spinal cord level C5 and C6). Rest the patient's elbow in your nondominant hand, with your thumb over the biceps tendon. Strike the percussion hammer to your thumb. ▼

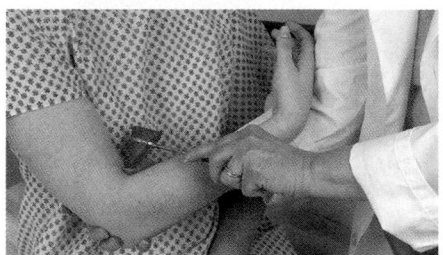

b. *Triceps reflex* (spinal cord level C7 and C8). Abduct the patient's arm at the shoulder, and flex it at the elbow. Support the upper arm with your nondominant hand, letting the forearm hang loosely. Strike the triceps tendon about 2.5–5 cm (1–2 in.) above the olecranon process. ▼

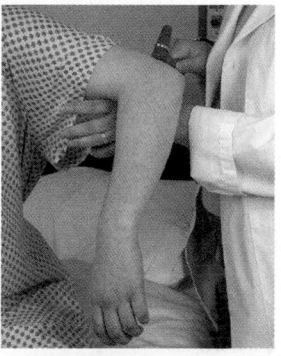

Developmental Variations

Older adults—Reflex responses may not be as strong as in young adults. Reaction time is slower as well.

a. +2 response: You can feel the biceps contract with your thumb; slight flexion of the elbow.

b. +2 response: Contraction of triceps with slight extension at elblow

(continued on next page)

Procedure 19-16 ■ Assessing the Sensory–Neurological System (continued)

c. *Brachioradialis reflex* (spinal cord level C3 and C6). Rest the client's arm on her leg. Strike with the percussion hammer 2.5–5 cm (1–2 in.) above the bony prominence of the wrist on the thumb side.▼

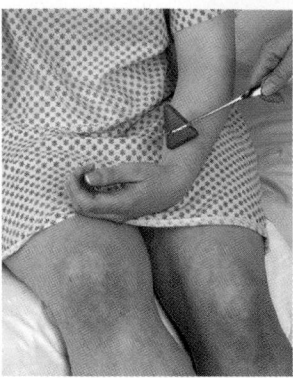

c. +2 response: Flexion at elbow and supination of forearm

d. *Patellar reflex* (spinal cord level L2, L3, and L4). Have the client sit with her legs dangling. Strike the tendon directly below the patella.▼

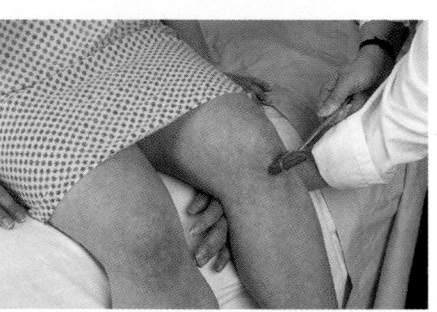

d. +2 response: Contraction of quadriceps with extension of leg

e. *Achilles reflex* (spinal cord level S1, S2). Have the patient lie supine or sit with her legs dangling. Hold the patient's foot slightly dorsiflexed, and strike the Achilles tendon about 5 cm (2 in.) above the heel with the percussion hammer.▼

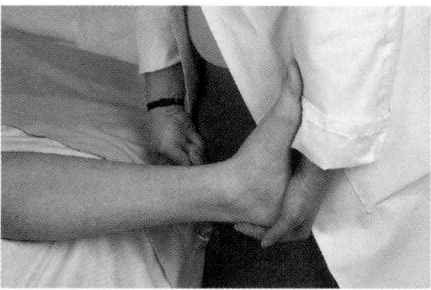

e. +2 response: Plantar flexion of foot.

Developmental Variations

Older adults—May lose this reflex.

Abnormal findings:

■ Absent or diminished responses are seen with degenerative disease, nerve damage, or lower motor neuron disease.

■ Hyperactive reflexes are seen with spinal cord injuries and upper motor neuron disease.

■ Rooting, palmar grasp, and tonic neck reflexes present after 6 months of age.

Developmental Modifications

Newborns—test the following reflexes:

■ **Rooting reflex**—Stroke the cheek; the head should turn to the side you touched.

■ **Palmar grasp**—Place one finger in the baby's hand; his fingers should curl around your finger.

■ **Tonic neck reflex**—Position the baby supine; turn his head to one side. The arm and leg on that side should extend, and those on the other side will flex.

24. Test superficial reflexes.

Plantar reflex (Babinski response): With your thumbnail or pointed object, stroke the sole of the client's foot in an arc from the lateral heel to medially across the ball of the foot. Record a normal response if all the toes curl downward or if there is no response. Record a positive response if there is dorsiflexion of the great toe and fanning of the other toes.▼

Babinski response is negative.

Infants and children—Positive Babinski is normal until age 2 or until the child begins walking.

Abnormal findings: A positive Babinski response is seen with drug or alcohol intoxification or upper motor neuron disease.

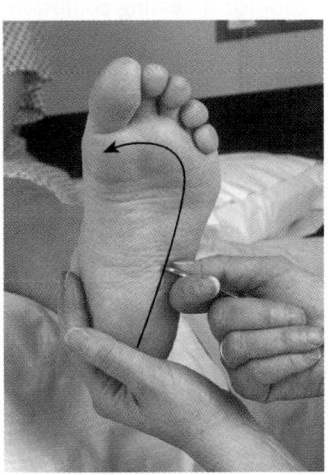

Developmental Modifications

Older adults—This reflex may be difficult to elicit.

25. Mental status screening.

The following questions may be used for a rapid evaluation of cognitive status. You may have already assessed for some aspects of mental status (e.g., orientation to time).

This complete set of questions is included so you can use them for a mental status exam that is not part of a comprehensive assessment. In a comprehensive assessment, do not repeat questions you have already covered in other areas of assessment.

Questions for Evaluating Cognitive Status

QUESTION	FUNCTION ASSESSED
What is today's date?	Orientation to time
What time is it?	Orientation to time
Where are you?	Orientation to place
What is the reason for your visit? (If the patient is hospitalized, modify the question as: Why are you in the hospital?)	Communication, vocabulary, thought processes, recent memory
Ask the patient to count backwards from 100.	Word comprehension, abstract reasoning
Ask the patient to name several objects that you point to. Be sure to use common objects such as a pen, shoe, or window.	Vocabulary, general knowledge, and word comprehension
Write a brief command, such as "Clap your hands," on a slip of paper. Hand the paper to the patient and ask him to follow the instructions.	Reading comprehension
Ask the patient to write the names of his family members, along with their relationship to him.	Writing, thought processes, memory, sound recognition
Ask the patient to name three things that begin with the letter "D."	Auditory comprehension, thought processes
Ask the patient to draw a circle, square, and triangle next to each other on a sheet of paper.	Word comprehension, mathematical and calculation skills, communication (naming)
Difficulty with any of these questions requires further evaluation.	

Procedure 19-16 ■ **Assessing the Sensory–Neurological System** (continued)

What If. . .

■ **The patient is an older adult?**

For a mental-status exam for older adults,

 Go to the link to the Mini-Cog exam in **Chapter 19, Resources for Caregivers & Health Professionals,** on the Student Resource Disk or DavisPlus at http://davisplus. fadavis.com/Wilkinson2

You should also assess older adults for dementia, which is characterized by these four features:
■ Mental status change of sudden onset, or fluctuating course
■ Difficulty focusing attention, distractible
■ Disorganized, illogical thinking

■ Increased or decreased level of consiousness (e.g., hyperalert, lethargic)

Delirium occurs in 15% to 60% of older hospitalized patients. You should assess them frequently to facilitate prompt identification and management of delirium.

For a reliable tool for assessing confusion and dementia in older adults,

 Go to the link for The Confusion Assessment Method Instrument in **Chapter 19, Resources for Caregivers & Health Professionals,** on DavisPlus at http://davisplus.fadavis. com/Wilkinson2

Home Care

Instruct caregivers in home safety if the client has cerebral function deficits or sensory or motor deficits.

Documentation

■ If you need more information about documenting,

 Go to Chapter 19, **Documenting Physical Assessment Findings,** in Volume 1.

Glasgow Coma Scale					
EYE RESPONSE	**SCORE**	**MOTOR RESPONSE**	**SCORE**	**VERBAL RESPONSE**	**SCORE**
Opens spontaneously	4	Obeys verbal commands for movement	6	Oriented and converses	5
Opens to verbal commands	3	Reacts purposefully to localized pain	5	Disoriented but converses	4
Opens to pain	2	Withdraws in response to pain (generalized body response)	4	Uses inappropriate words	3
No response	1	Assumes flexor posture (decorticate posturing—arms flexed to chest, hands clenched and internally rotated) in response to pain. *Indicates problem is at or above the brainstem*	3	Makes incomprehensible sounds	2
				No response	1

Glasgow Coma Scale—cont'd

EYE RESPONSE	SCORE	MOTOR RESPONSE	SCORE	VERBAL RESPONSE	SCORE
		Assumes extensor posture (decerebrate posturing—arms extended, hands clenched and hyperpronated); Indicates problem at the brainstem level	2		
		No response	1		
Totals					

Note: Education is necessary for proper interpretation of this scale.

Sources: Centers for Disease Control and Prevention (CDC). (no date). Glasgow Coma Scale. Last reviewed June 23, 2006. Retrieved from http://www.bt.cdc.gov/masscasualties/gscale.asp (Accessed June 29, 2008); Rauen, C., Chulay, M., Bridges, E., et al. (2008). Seven evidence-based practice habits: Putting some sacred cows out to pasture. *Critical Care Nurse, 28(2),* 98–124; Rowley, G., & Fielding, K. (1991). Reliability and accuracy of the Glasgow Coma Scale with experienced and inexperienced users. *Lancet, 337,* 55–58; Teasdale, G., & Jennett, B. (1974). Assessment of coma and impaired consciousness. *Lancet, 2,* 81–84; Teasdale, G., Kril-Jones, R., & van der Sande, J. (1978). Observer variability in assessing impaired consciousness and coma. *Journal of Neurology, Neurosurgery, and Psychiatry, 41,* 603–610.

Full Outline of UnResponsiveness (FOUR)

Eye Response

4—Eyelids open or opened, tracing, or blinking on command

3—Eyelids open but not tracking

2—Eyelids closed but open to loud voice

1—Eyelids closed but open to pain

0—Eyelids remain closed with pain

Motor Response

4—Thumbs-up, fist, or peace sign

3—Localizing to pain

2—Flexion response to pain

1—Extension response to pain

0—No response to pain or generalized myoclonus status

Brain Stem Reflexes

4—Pupil and corneal reflexes present

3—One pupil wide and fixed

2—Pupil or corneal reflexes absent

1—Pupil and corneal reflexes absent

0—Absent pupil, corneal, and cough reflexes

Respirations

4—Not intubated, regular breathing pattern

3—Not intubated, Cheyne-Stokes breathing pattern

2—Not intubated, irregular breathing

1—Respirations greater than ventilator rate

0—respirations at ventilator rate or apnea

Note: **Education is necessary to use this scale properly.**

Sources:

National Guideline Clearinghouse (2008). Assessing cognitive function. In: *Evidence-based geriatric nursing protocols for best practice.* Agency for Healthcare Research and Quality. Retrieved from http://www.guideline.gov/summary/summary.aspx?view_id=1&doc_id=12266 (Accessed September 1, 2008).

Rauen, C. A., Chulay, M., Bridges, E., et al. (2008). Seven evidence-based practice habits: Putting some sacred cows out to pasture. *Critical Care Nurse, 28(2),* 98–124.

Wijdicks, E. F. M., Bamlet, W. R., Maramattom, B. V., et al. (2005). Further validation of the FOUR Score coma scale by intensive care nurses. *Annals of Neurology, 58(4),* 585–593.

Procedure 19-17 ☐ Assessing the Male Genitourinary System

➤ For steps to follow in *all* procedures, refer to the Universal Steps for All Procedures found on the inside back cover of Volume 2.

Critical Aspects

- Techniques: Inspection and palpation
- Inspect the external genitalia, including color, discharge, and the pattern of hair distribution.
- Palpate for lumps, masses, hernias, or enlarged lymph nodes.

Equipment

- Nonlatex procedure gloves
- Penlight
- Pen and record form

Developmental Modifications for Children

- Obtain the parent's permission to perform this assessment.
- Explain to the child what you are going to do, and expect some resistance or embarrassment.

Children are taught to not let strangers touch their genitals, and many children are modest.

Developmental Modifications for Older Adults

- Assess for incontinence.

Incontinence is one of the elements of the SPICES assessment model for older adults.

Focused History Questions

- Have you noticed any redness, swelling, discharge, or odor in your genital area?
- Have you noticed asymmetry, lumps, or masses in your genitals? If so, describe them, and show me where they are.
- Have you ever been told you have a hernia?
- Have you ever had trauma to your genitals?
- Are you having any problems urinating?
- Are you sexually active? If not, have you ever been?
- Do you have sex with men, women, or both?
- What types of sexual activity do you engage in? Oral, anal, genital?
- Do you have more than one partner? How many partners have you had in the last 6 months?
- Do you use birth control? If so, what type and how often?
- Have you ever been treated for a sexually transmitted infection (STI)? If so, what type?
- Are you concerned about STIs or HIV?
- Do you take any precautions to avoid infections?
- Do you have any concerns about your sexual function?
- Do you have any difficulty achieving or maintaining an erection?
- Have you been taught to examine your testicles?
- How often do you do testicular self-examination?
- Have you had any surgery of your reproductive tract?

➤ When performing the procedure, always identify your patient according to agency policy and be attentive to standard precautions, hand hygiene, patient safety and privacy, body mechanics, and documentation.

Procedure Steps	Expected Findings
1. Instruct the client to empty his bladder and undress to expose the groin area.	
2. Have the patient stand while you sit at eye level to the genitalia; alternatively, the patient can lie supine on the exam table with his legs slightly apart.	
3. Inspect the external genitalia. a. Note the hair distribution pattern and condition of pubic hair. See the table discussing Tanner staging, at the end of this procedure. The appearance of the external genitalia depends on the client's developmental stage.	a. Hair distribution is triangular and appropriate for age. No pediculosis is present. **Abnormal findings:** Sparse or absent hair may result from genetic factors, aging, or local or systemic disease.

b. Inspect the condition of the skin of the penis. Observe for the presence or absence of the foreskin. Note the position of the urethral meatus and any lesions or discharge.

b. Skin is intact with no lesions or discharge. Color is consistent with ethnicity. The urethral meatus is midline. The foreskin may be absent (circumcised); if present, it covers the glans and easily retracts.

Developmental Variations:

Infants—Foreskin is difficult to retract in the uncircumsized male until about age 3 months.

Older adults—Penis and testes decrease in size.

Abnormal findings: Ulcerations or lesions (may be seen with a number of sexually transmitted infections, such as genital warts and genital herpes); **phimosis** (foreskin cannot be retracted and becomes swollen)

c. Observe the condition, size, position, and symmetry of the scrotal skin.

c. The skin should be free of lesions, nodules, swelling, rash, and erythema. The skin is rugated and deeper in color than the rest of the body. Size and shape vary greatly. The left scrotal sac is usually lower than the right.

Abnormal findings: A rash may be caused by **tinea cruris,** a fungal infection often called "jock itch." Swelling may indicate hernia, tumor, or infection.

d. Note the condition of the inguinal areas. Look for swelling or bulges. The best way to do this is to have the client bear down while you palpate the inguinal canal.

d. The inguinal area should be free of swelling or bulges.

Abnormal findings: A bulge may indicate a hernia or enlarged lymph node.

---

4. Palpate the penis.
   a. With a gloved hand, use your thumb and fingers to palpate the shaft of the penis. Note consistency, tenderness, masses, or nodules.
   b. Retract the foreskin if present.

The penis is nontender with no masses or nodules. Pulsations are present on the dorsal side. The foreskin, if present, easily retracts.

Abnormal findings: Inability to palpate a pulse may indicate vascular insufficiency; difficulty retracting the foreskin or problems with its return to position need further evaluation.

---

5. Palpate the scrotum, testes, and epididymis.
   a. Don a procedure glove and use your thumb and fingers to palpate. ▼

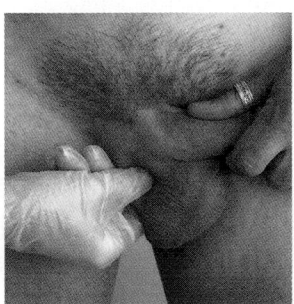

Step 5a

The scrotal skin is rough but without lesions. Each testicular sac contains a testicle and epididymis. The testes are rubbery, round, movable, and smooth. They are sensitive to pressure but nontender. The epididymis is comma shaped. The spermatic cord is smooth and round. There is no swelling or nodules. The left scrotal sac is usually lower than the right.

Abnormal findings:
- A unilateral mass
- Painless intratesticular masses may represent testicular cancer.
- A testicle that is swollen or tender may indicate infection or torsion.

(continued on next page)

Procedure 19-17 ■ Assessing the Male Genitourinary System (continued)

b. Note size, shape, consistency, mobility, masses, nodules, or tenderness. ▼

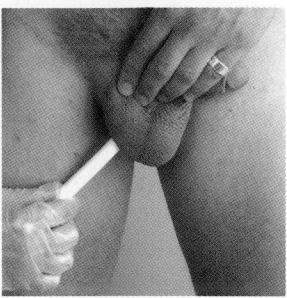

Step 5b

c. Transilluminate any lumps, nodules, or edematous areas by shining a penlight over the area in a darkened room.

6. Palpate the inguinal and femoral area for hernias.
a. Assess for inguinal hernias with a gloved hand. Have the patient hold his penis to one side. Place your index finger in the client's scrotal sac above the testicle, and invaginate the skin. Follow the spermatic cord until you reach a slitlike opening (Hesselbach's triangle). Ask the client to cough or bear down as you feel for bulges.
b. Palpate for femoral hernias by palpating below the femoral artery while having the client cough or bear down. ▼

No bulges or palpable masses are present in the inguinal or femoral area.

Direct hernia: protrusion through the abdominal wall. Indirect hernia: protrusion into the inguinal canal or into the scrotum.

Abnormal findings: A bulge or mass often represents a hernia. Refer to the Abnormal Atlas at the end of this chapter.

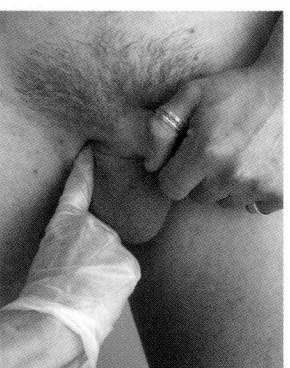

Step 6.

7. Palpate the lymph nodes in the groin area and the vertical chain over the inner aspect of the thigh. ▼

Nodes should be < 1 cm in size and freely mobile.

Abnormal findings: Enlarged or tender lymph nodes may indicate local or systemic disease. Also see Abnormal Atlas: Male Genitourinary System.

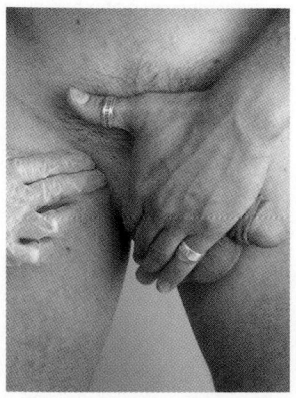 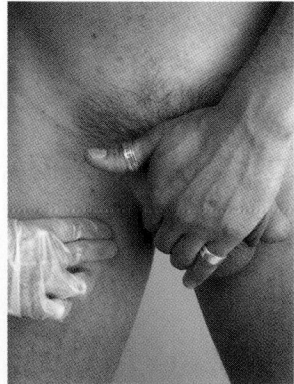

Step 7

Documentation

If you need more information about documenting,

 Go to Chapter 19, **Documenting Physical Assessment Findings,** in Volume 1.

Tanner Staging

STAGE	PUBIC HAIR	PENIS	TESTES AND SCROTUM
Stage 1: Preadolescent	No pubic hair except for fine body hair similar to that on abdomen	Same size and proportions as in childhood	Same size and proportions as in childhood
Stage 2	Sparse growth of long, slightly pigmented, downy hair, straight or only slightly curled, chiefly at base of penis	Slight or no enlargement	Testes larger, scrotum larger, somewhat reddened and altered in texture
Stage 3	Darker, coarser, curlier hair spreading sparsely over pubic symphysis	Larger, especially in length	Further enlarged
Stage 4	Coarse and curly hair, as in adult; area covered greater than in stage 3 but not as great as in adult	Further enlarged in length and breadth, with development of glans	Further enlarged; scrotal skin darkened
Stage 5 Adult	Hair same as adult in quantity and quality, spreading to medial surfaces of thighs but not up over abdomen.	Adult in size and shape.	Adult in size and shape.

Adapted from: Tanner, J. (1962). *Growth at adolescence* (2nd ed.). Oxford: Blackwell Scientific.

Procedure 19-18   Assessing the Female Genitourinary System

➤ For steps to follow in *all* procedures, refer to the Universal Steps for All Procedures found on the inside back cover of Volume 2.

Critical Aspects

- Techniques: Inspection and palpation
- Inspect the external genitalia.
- Palpate lymph nodes and possible hernia sites.

Equipment

- Patient drape
- Additional light source
- Nonlatex procedure gloves (if exposure to body fluids is a possibility)
- Pen and record form

Positioning

Lithotomy position, if possible.

Developmental Modifications for Older Adults

- Assess for incontinence.

Incontinence is one of the elements of the SPICES assessment model for older adults.

- Older women may have arthritis, which, along with muscle weakness, may make it difficult for them to assume the lithotomy position. You may need to use Sims' position and/or provide support for them to maintain a position.

Developmental Modifications for Children

- Obtain parental permission for this examination.
- Explain to the child what you are going to do, and expect some resistance or embarrassment.

Children are taught to not let strangers touch their genitals, and many children are modest.

- Do not perform internal assessment of an adolescent unless the girl is sexually active.

Focused History Questions

- Are you having any problems urinating?
- Have you noticed any redness, swelling, discharge, or odor in your genital area?
- Have you ever been told you have a hernia?
- Have you ever had trauma to your genitals?
- Are you sexually active? If not, have you ever been?
- Do you have sex with men, women, or both?
- What types of sexual activity do you engage in? Oral, anal, or genital?
- How many partners do you currently have?
- How many partners have you had in the last 6 months?
- Do you use birth control? If so, what kind and how often?
- Have you ever been treated for a sexually transmitted infection (STI)? If so, what type?
- Are you concerned about STIs or HIV?
- Do you take any precautions to avoid infection?
- Do you have any concerns about your sexual function?
- Have you had any surgery of your reproductive tract?
- When was your last menstrual period?
- How often are your periods?
- Do you have any problems with your periods, such as cramping, breast pain, or heavy flow?
- How often do you have a gynecologic health exam?
- When was your last Pap smear?
- Have you ever had an abnormal Pap smear? If so, how was it treated?
- How many times have you been pregnant?
- How many children do you have?
- Have you ever had a miscarriage? An abortion?

➤ When performing the procedure, always identify your patient according to agency policy and be attentive to standard precautions, hand hygiene, patient safety and privacy, body mechanics, and documentation.

Procedure Steps

1. Inspect the external genitalia.
   a. Note the hair distribution pattern and the condition of pubic hair. See the table entitled Maturation Status in Females at the end of this procedure.

The appearance of the external genitalia depends on the developmental stage of the client.

Expected Findings

a. Hair distribution in the pubic region is inverse triangular. Some hair may extend onto her abdomen and upper thighs. Hair distribution is appropriate for age. No **pediculosis pubis** (pubic lice).

Abnormal findings: Sparse or absent hair (may result from genetic factors, aging, or local or systemic disease); lice, **nits** (white lice eggs), or flecks of dried blood on the skin.

b. Inspect the condition of the skin of the mons pubis and labia. Observe for color, condition, lesions, and discharge.

b. Skin is intact with no lesions or discharge. Labia majora and minora are symmetrical, with smooth to moderate wrinkling. Skin color is consistent with ethnicity. No ecchymosis, excoriation, nodules, edema, rash, or lesions are present.

Developmental Variations

Older adults—Labia and vulva are atrophied.

Abnormal findings: Ulcerations or lesions may occur with with a number of sexually transmitted infections.

---

2. Inspect the clitoris, urethral meatus, and vaginal introitus.

a. Wearing gloves, use your thumb and index finger to separate the labia and expose the clitoris. Observe the clitoris for size and position. ▼

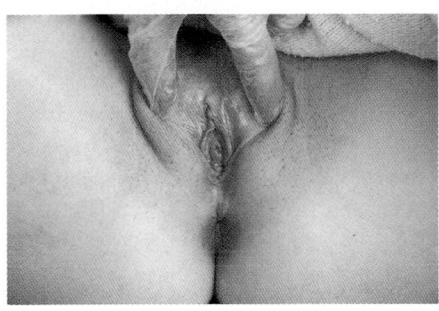

a. The clitoris is about 2 cm long and 0.5 cm in diameter. No redness or lesions are present.

Abnormal findings: Enlargement of the clitoris may result from androgen excess or swelling related to trauma. Absence of the clitoris, along with parts of the labia, is seen with female circumcision.

b. With the labia separated, observe the urethral meatus and vaginal introitus. Observe for color, size, and presence of discharge or lesions.

b. The urethral meatus is slitlike, midline, and free of discharge, lesions, swelling, or erythema. The mucosa of the introitus is pink and moist. Some clear to white discharge may be present and is odor-free.

c. Have the client bear down while you observe the introitus.

c. The introitus is patent, and there is no bulging or discomfort with bearing down.

Abnormal findings: Discharge, redness, or swelling may result from infection. Pale and dry mucosa may result from aging or use of topical steroids. Bulging may indicate prolapse of the uterus, bladder, or rectum.

---

3. Palpate Bartholin's glands, the urethral glands, and Skene's ducts.

a. Lubricate the index and middle fingers of your dominant hand with water-soluble lubricant.

b. To palpate Bartholin's glands, insert your lubricated fingers into the vaginal introitus, and palpate the lower portion of the labia bilaterally between your thumb and fingers. ▼

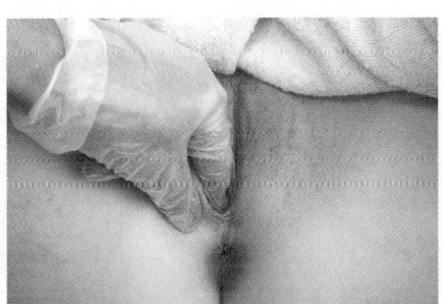

No swelling, masses, or tenderness of the glands is present. There is no urethral discharge. The labia are uniform in texture, and there is no discharge or pain with palpation. The perineum is smooth and firm in **nulliparous** women (women who have had no children), thinner in **parous** women (women who have had children).

Abnormal findings: Pain or discharge from the glands may indicate infection. Fissures or tears in the perineum are painful and require treatment.

(continued on next page)

Procedure 19–18 ■ **Assessing the Female Genitourinary System** (continued)

c. To palpate Skene's ducts, rotate your internal fingers upward, and paplate the labium bilaterally.▼

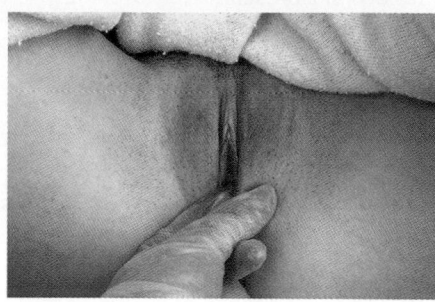

d. To milk the urethra, apply pressure with your index finger on the anterior vaginal wall, and observe for urethral discharge. Culture any discharge you see.

---

4. Assess vaginal muscle tone and pelvic musculature.
a. Insert two gloved fingers into the vagina.
b. Ask the woman to constrict her vaginal muscles and then to bear down as though she were having a bowel movement.

Muscle tone should be strong in women who have never given birth. With increasing **parity** (number of births), pelvic muscle tone diminishes. Diminished tone may also result from injury, age, or medication. No bulges should be noted.

---

5. Palpate the inguinal and femoral area for hernias.

No bulges or palpable masses are present in the inguinal or femoral area.

---

6. Palpate the lymph nodes in the groin area and the vertical chain over the inner aspect of the thigh.

Nodes should be < 1 cm in size and freely mobile.

Abnormal findings: Enlarged or tender lymph nodes may indicate local or systemic disease. Also see Abnormal Atlas: Female Genitourinary System at the end of this chapter.

Documentation

If you need more information about documenting,

 VOL 1 Go to Chapter 19, **Documenting Physical Assessment Findings,** in Volume 1.

Maturation Status in Females		
STAGE OF DEVELOPMENT	**BREASTS**	**PUBIC HAIR**
Stage 1. Prepuberty	Elevation of papilla	No pubic hair except for fine body hair similar to hair on abdomen

Maturation Status in Females—cont'd

STAGE OF DEVELOPMENT	BREASTS	PUBIC HAIR
Stage 2	Breast bud. Elevation of breast and nipple and increased diameter of areola.	Sparse growth of long, slightly pigmented, downy hair, straight or only slightly curled, mostly along labia.
Stage 3	Areola deepens in color and enlarges further. Glandular tissue begins to develop beneath areola.	Hair becomes darker, coarser, and curlier and spreads sparsely over pubic symphysis.
Stage 4	Areola appears as a mound; breast appears as a mound; papilla and areola form a secondary mound.	Pubic hair is coarse and curly as in adults. It covers more area than in stage 3, but does not extend to the medial thighs.
Stage 5. Adult	Mature breast. Areola recesses to general contour of breast; nipple projects forward.	Quality and quantity are consistent with adult pubic hair distribution and spread over medial surfaces of thighs but not over abdomen.

Adapted from: Tanner, J. (1962). Growth at adolescence (2nd ed.). Oxford: Blackwell Scientific.

Procedure 19-19 ☐ Assessing the Anus and Rectum

➤ For steps to follow in *all* procedures, refer to the Universal Steps for All Procedures found on the inside back cover of Volume 2.

Critical Aspects

- Inspect the external anal area, sphincter tone, and stool for occult blood.
- Palpate the anus and rectum for muscle tone and masses.
- For women, assessment of the anus and rectum is usually performed at the end of the internal pelvic exam; for men, it is done after the genitourinary exam.

Equipment

- Water-soluble lubricant
- Hemoccult test
- Nonlatex procedure gloves
- Pen and record form

Developmental Modification for Infants and Children

You will not usually perform a rectal exam on infants and children.

Focused History Questions

- Do you have any pain or discomfort around your anus?
- Do you ever have difficulty passing stool?
- Have you ever noticed blood on your stool or when you wipe?
- Do you have or have you ever been told you have hemorrhoids?
- For men, have you ever had a prostate exam or a prostate-specific antigen (PSA) blood test? If so, what were the results?

➤ When performing the procedure, always identify your patient according to agency policy and be attentive to standard precautions, hand hygiene, patient safety and privacy, and body mechanics.

Procedure Steps

I. Inspect the anus. Note the condition of the skin and the presence of any lesions.

Expected Findings

Anal area is intact, with no inflammation or lesions. Anus is a darker color than surrounding tissue.

Abnormal findings:
- A fissure or tear may be due to trauma, severe constipation, or an abscess.
- External hemorrhoids or skin tags may be visible.

---

2. Palpate the anus and rectum.
   a. For women, change gloves to prevent cross-contamination. Insert a lubricated index finger gently into the rectum. Palpate the rectal wall, noting masses or tenderness.
   b. For males, have the client bend over the exam table or turn on his left side if recumbent. Insert a lubricated index finger gently into the rectum. Palpate the rectal wall, noting, masses or evidence of tenderness. ▼

Good sphincter tone. Rectum is nontender. No palpable masses or hard stool. The stool is brown and negative for occult blood.

Abnormal findings:
- Hard stool in the rectum indicates impaction.
- Positive occult blood indicates bleeding in the GI tract.
- A palpable mass or enlarged prostate gland requires further evaluation.
- Internal hemorrhoids may be present.

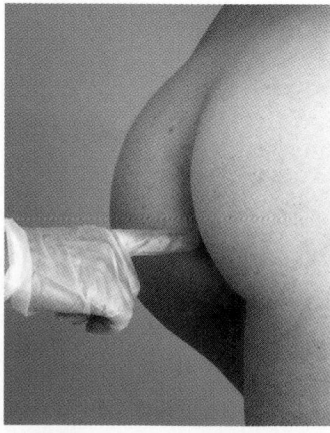
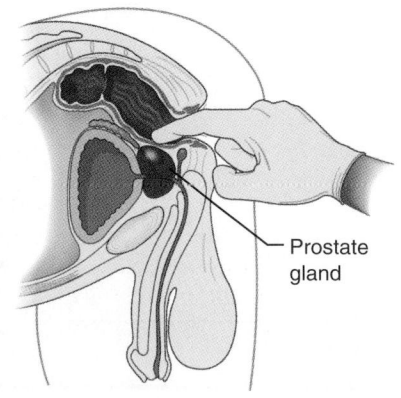

Prostate gland

Step 2b

c. Test any stool on the gloved finger for occult blood. See Procedure 28-1.

Patient Teaching

Instruct the client in the importance of colonoscopy and prostate exam.

Documentation

If you need more information about documenting,

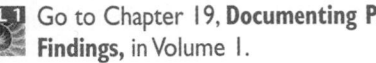 Go to Chapter 19, **Documenting Physical Assessment Findings,** in Volume 1.

Procedure 19-20 ☐ Brief Bedside Assessment

This assessment is not as detailed as in Procedures 19-1 through 19-19. You might perform such an assessment when admitting a patient to a hospital unit. You can also use it for ongoing assessments. For daily patient assessments, you will modify the procedure to fit the patient's health status. You may be able to omit some portions, and you may need to add in-depth, focused assessments of some body systems. The entire assessment should take no more than 15 minutes after you become skilled.

➤ For steps to follow in *all* procedures, refer to the Universal Steps for All Procedures found on the inside back cover of Volume 2.

Critical Aspects

- Modify procedure to fit the patient's health status.
- Observe the environment and the patient's general appearance.
- Measure vital signs, pain status, and pulse oximetry.
- Use a systematic (e.g., head-to-toe) approach.
- Assess the integument.
- Assess the head and neck.
- Assess the back with patient sitting.
- Assess the anterior chest (heart and lungs).
- Assess the abdomen with patient supine.
- Assess urinary status.
- Assess upper extremities, including edema and capillary refill.
- Assess lower extremities, including edema and capillary refill.
- Assess for spinal deformities with patient standing.
- Assess balance, coordination, ROM, and gait.

Equipment

- Thermometer, stethoscope, sphygmomanometer
- Procedure gloves

Focused History Questions

- Ask about any health problems, allergies, or medications.
- Ask your patient how she feels currently and during the previous month and year.
- Ask other questions as you assess each body system.

➤ When performing the procedure, always identify your patient according to agency policy and be attentive to standard precautions, hand hygiene, patient safety and privacy, body mechanics, and documentation.

Procedure Steps

1. Greet the patient and explain what you need to do. Ask the patient her name and confirm by checking her identity band.
Assures that you have the correct patient and also allows you to assess mental status and communication.

2. Observe the environment (e.g., IV lines, oxygen, urinary catheter) and patient's general appearance (including signs of distress).
This allows you to identify any immediate actions you may need to take before performing the assessment.

3. Begin by measuring the vital signs (patient supine or sitting):
   a. temperature, pulse, respirations, blood pressure
   b. pain status
   c. pulse oximetry

4. Now assess each body system
   a. Use a systematic approach such as head-to-toe.
   b. As you assess each system, observe for mobility, range of motion, balance, and coordination.
   c. As you talk with the patient, observe her thought processes and level of consciousness.

Procedure 19-20 ■ **Brief Bedside Assessment** (continued)

5. Assess the integument.
   a. Ask about any hair, nail, or skin changes, including rashes
   b. With each body system, inspect skin color, rashes, and lesions; and palpate for temperature, turgor, and texture. Also inspect the hair and nails in that area (e.g., when assessing the legs and feet).
   c. Assess wounds: appearance, size, drainage, dressings, drains.
   d. Inspect and palpate the hair and scalp

6. Assess the head and neck.
   a. Ask the patient about any problems with the head and neck.
   b. (Reminder: remember to continue assessing mental status and orientation to time, place, and person.)
   c. Inspect the external ears; observe for apparent hearing deficit.
   d. Check the eyes for pupil reaction and cardinal fields of gaze. Ask about and observe for any problems with vision.
   e. Inspect the color of the lips, mucous membranes, and conjunctiva.
   f. Inspect the tongue and oropharynx.
   g. Inspect for hydration, color, and lesions of the mucous membranes.
   h. Lightly palpate the carotid pulse (only if indicated by patient's condition) and listen for carotid bruits.

   ✚ Do not palpate both carotid arteries at the same time. See Procedure 19-13.

7. Assess the back while patient is in the sitting position.
   a. Inspect skin.
   b. Auscultate breath sounds; compare side to side and apex to base.
   c. Assess respiratory rate, rhythm, and effort.
   d. Note cough, secretions, how many pillows used to sleep on, and whether head of bed is elevated for breathing.
   e. Check oxygen order, SaO_2, ability to use incentive spirometer.

8. Assess the anterior chest.
   a. Ask about any respiratory or cardiovascular problems.
   b. Palpate skin turgor, temperature, and PMI.
   c. Auscultate breath sounds.
   d. Auscultate heart sounds. Note rate, rhythm, S_1, S_2, and extra sounds.

9. Assess the abdomen, with the patient supine.
   a. Inspect the size, shape, symmetry, and condition of the abdominal skin.
   b. Observe abdominal movements including respirations, pulsations, and peristalsis.

   c. Auscultate bowel sounds in all four quadrants, and the aorta for bruits.
   d. Palpate all four quadrants for tenderness, guarding, and masses; and inspect for rebound tenderness.
   e. Ask the patient about any weight changes, gastrointestinal (GI) complaints, a change in appetite or diet.
   f. Review the pattern for bowel movements, and when examining a woman, ask of her last menstrual period.

10. Assess urinary status.
    a. Review voiding pattern with the patient (including frequency and dysuria).
    b. If there is an indwelling catheter, observe for patency, kinks in the tubing, and color of urine; monitor intake and output.
    c. Palpate for bladder distention.

11. Assess the upper extremities.
    a. Ask about any problems with the hands and arms, such as weakness, arthritis, change in sensation, temperature or color.
    b. Inspect the condition of the skin and nails.
    c. Palpate skin temperature and bilateral brachial and radial pulses.
    d. Check capillary refill.
    e. Note any stiffness or limited range of motion of the hands and arms.
    f. Test muscle strength by having the patient grip your hands or two fingers.
    g. Note whether the patient has any casts, traction, splints, or slings.
    h. Observe for edema.

12. Assess the lower extremities.
    a. Ask about any problems with the legs, such as weakness, numbness, tingling, arthritis, edema, change in sensation, and temperature or color.
    b. Observe ROM and ability to ambulate or move about in bed.
    c. Inspect the condition of the skin and nails.
    d. Palpate skin temperature and pedal pulses; check capillary refill.
    e. Test for leg strength by asking the patient to raise the leg against your counterpressure. (This is more easily done with the patient sitting.)
    f. Check sensation through light touch, proceeding to pain as needed.
    g. Observe for problems such as paralysis.
    h. Observe for edema.

13. Ask the patient to stand, and inspect for:
    a. Gross spinal deformities.
    b. Balance and coordination of movements.
    c. Range of motion and gait.

14. With the patient seated in bed, legs extended, check for:

    a. Babinski reflex

    b. Homans sign

Documentation

- Document your findings and report any significant changes or findings to the primary care provider. As a student, report your findings to the instructor and the patient's assigned RN for validation and action.

- To print out a form to use as a documentation worksheet when performing a brief physical exam,

 Go to Chapter 19, **ESG Figure 19-2, Documentation Worksheet for Bedside Assessment,** on the Student Resource Disk or DavisPlus at http://davisplus.fadavis.com/Wilkinson2

- If you need more information about documenting,

 Go to Chapter 19, **Documenting Physical Assessment Findings,** in Volume 1.

Thinking About the Procedure

 Go to the *Fundamentals of Nursing Skills Videos,* **Brief Physical Assessment.**

Choose the visual (non-narrated) version from the Main Menu.

1. What equipment did the nurse bring into the room?

2. What position did the nurse use to auscultate the patient's anterior chest? Alternatively, what position could she also have used?

3. Because this was only a brief bedside assessment, what procedure did the nurse omit when palpating the abdomen?

4. Why did the nurse have the patient walk to the wall (near the end of the assessment)?

5. If the nurse had needed to check the patellar reflex, at what point in the exam would this have been most convenient?

 For suggested responses, go to Chapter 19, **Thinking About the Procedure Suggested Responses,** on the Student Resource Disk or DavisPlus at http://davisplus.fadavis.com/Wilkinson2

What Are the Main Points in This Chapter?

➤ A physical examination may be conducted to obtain data about the patient, to further investigate an identified health problem, to monitor a client's health status, or to screen for health problems.

➤ A comprehensive physical assessment includes a complete head-to-toe examination of every body system. Data from a comprehensive physical assessment provide guidance for care and determine the need for further assessment.

➤ A focused physical assessment is performed to obtain data about an actual, potential, or possible problem that has been identified. A focused exam adds to the database created from the comprehensive assessment.

➤ An ongoing assessment is appropriate for periodic reassessment of the client and reflects the dynamic state of the client. This is a less detailed examination than a comprehensive assessment.

➤ Before a physical assessment, you will need to gather equipment, prepare the environment, review the skills you will use, familiarize yourself with the patient situation, review the nursing plan of care, and assist the patient to relax by taking the time to develop a rapport.

➤ *Inspection* is the use of sight to gather data. Inspection begins the moment you meet the client.

➤ *Palpation* is the use of touch to gather data. Use palpation to assess temperature, skin texture, moisture, anatomical landmarks, and abnormalities such as edema, masses, or areas of tenderness.

➤ *Percussion,* tapping on the skin with short strokes from your fingers, produces vibrations that allow you to determine the location, size, and density of underlying structures.

➤ *Ausculation* is the use of hearing to gather data. Direct auscultation is unassisted listening. Indirect auscultation is listening to the sounds produced by the body with the help of a stethoscope.

 Go to Chapter 19, **Resources for Caregivers & Health Professionals,** on the Student Resource Disk or DavisPlus at http://davisplus.fadavis.com/Wilkinson2

For practice questions for this chapter,

 Go to **NCLEX-Style Chapter Quiz,** on the Student Resource Disk or DavisPlus at http://davisplus.fadavis.com/Wilkinson2

Abnormal Atlas

Skin Color Changes

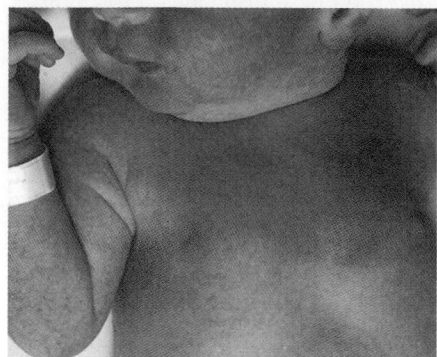

Jaundice

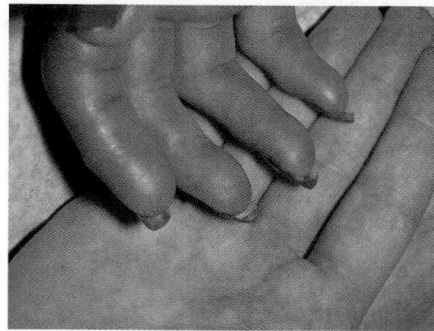

Cyanosis

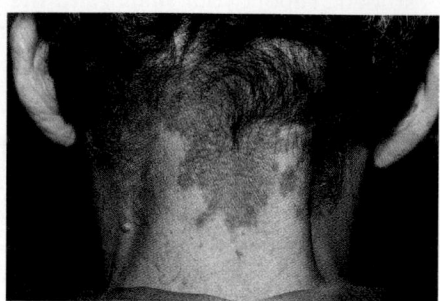

Port-wine stain (nevus flammeus)

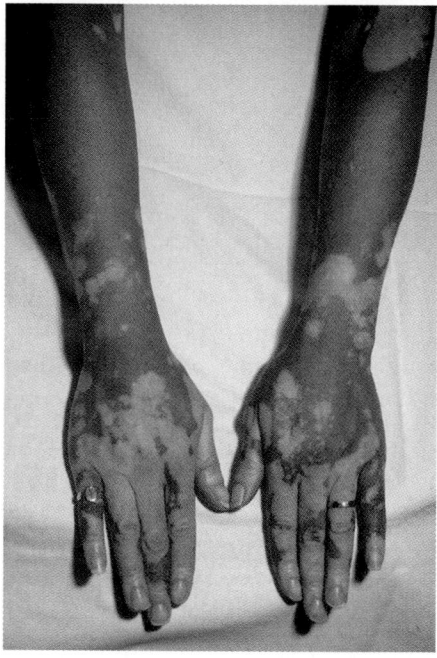

Vitiligo

Skin Lesions

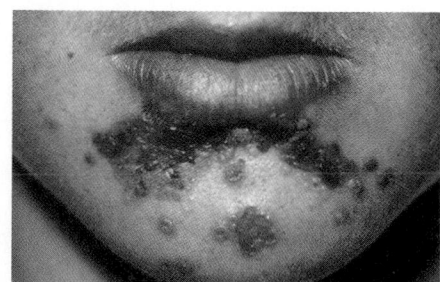

Herpes simplex

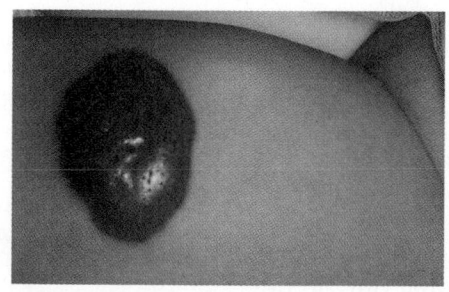

Capillary hemangioma

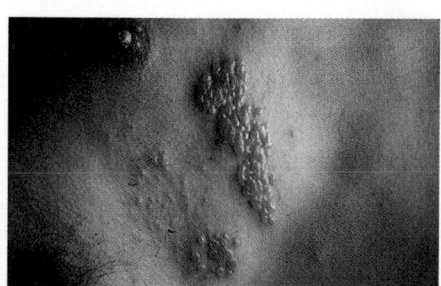

Vescicles (blisters)

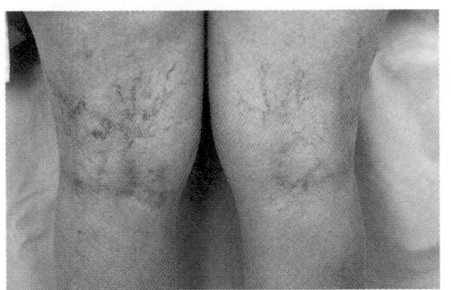

Venous star

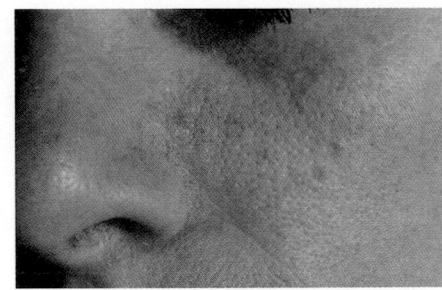

Petechiae

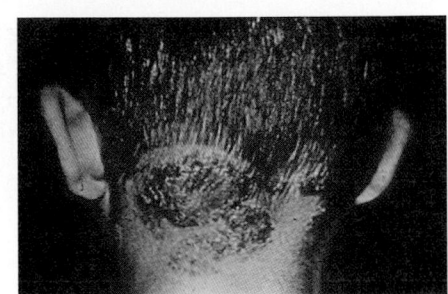

Ringworm

Hair

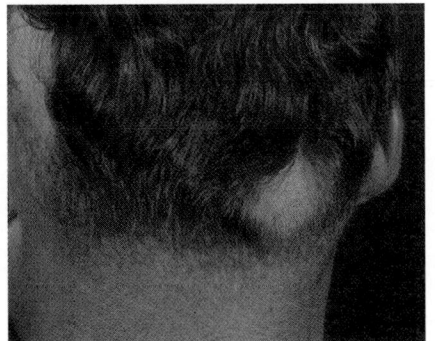

Alopecia areata

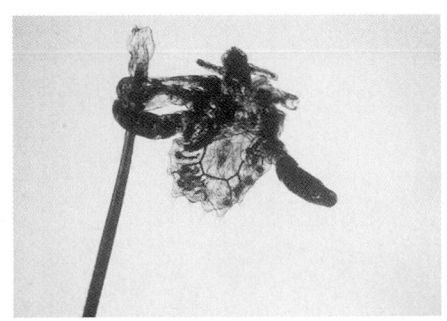

Pediculosis (lice)

Nail Appearance

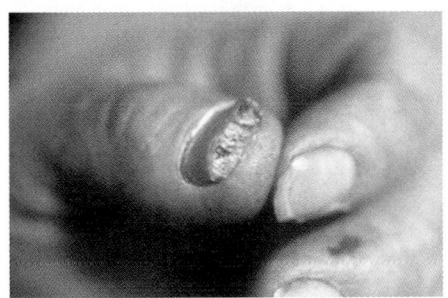

Fungal infection

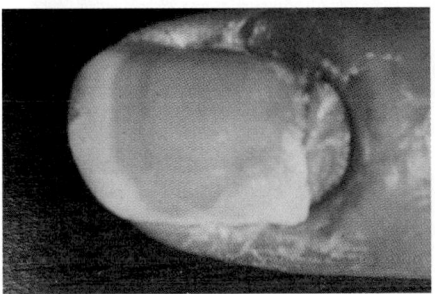

Paronychia

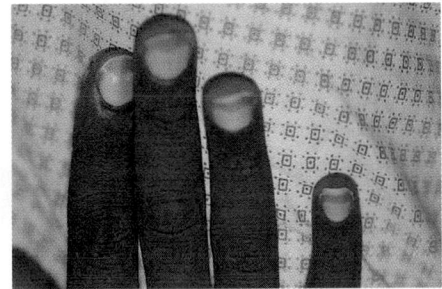

Half-and-half nails

Eyes

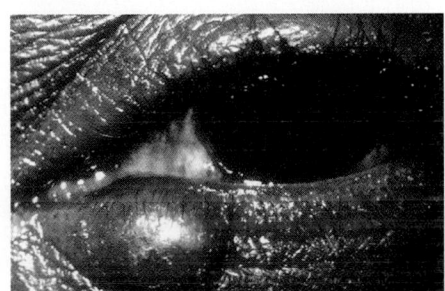

Hordeolum

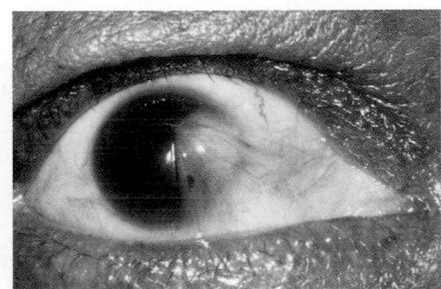

Pterygium

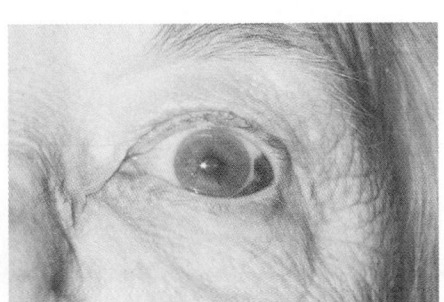

Subconjunctival hemorrhage

Mouth and Oropharynx

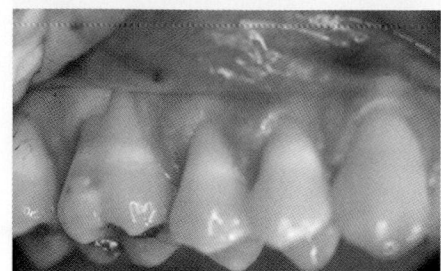

Gingival recession

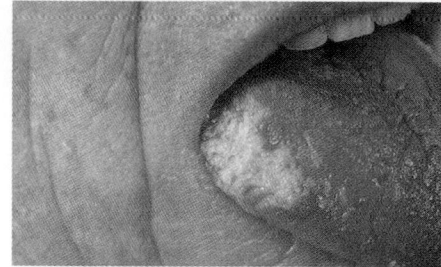

Leukoplakia

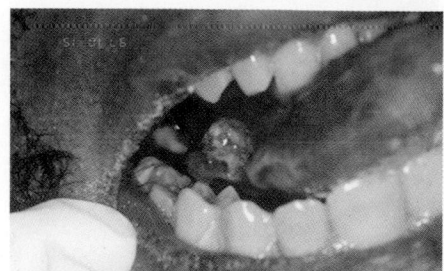

Cancer of the tongue

Musculoskeletal System

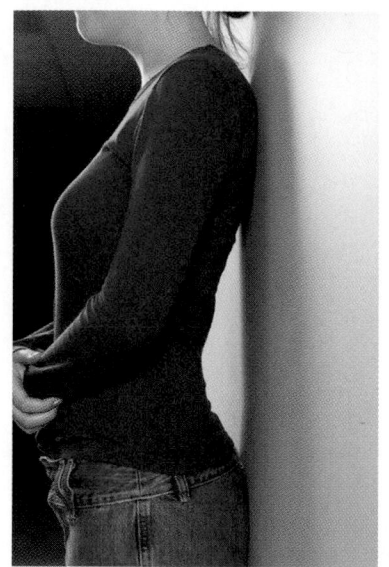

Lordosis

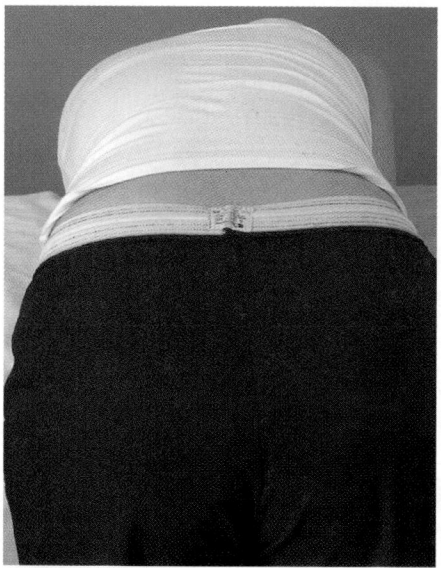

Scoliosis

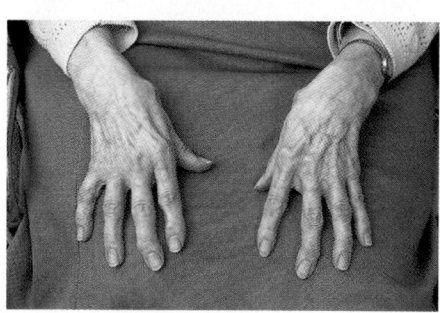

Degenerative joint disease (Heberden's nodes)

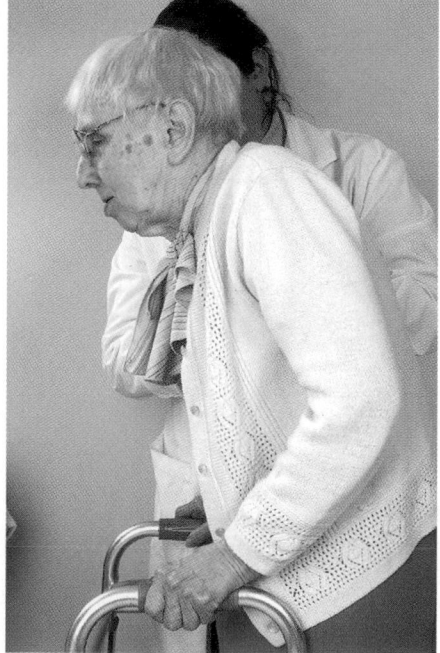

Kyphosis

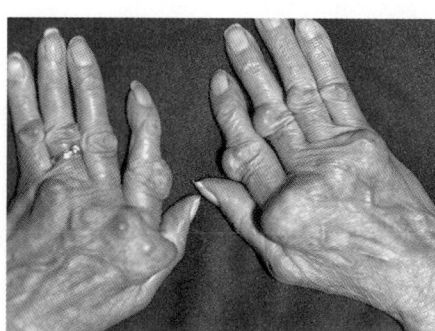

Rheumatoid arthritis

Abnormal gaits

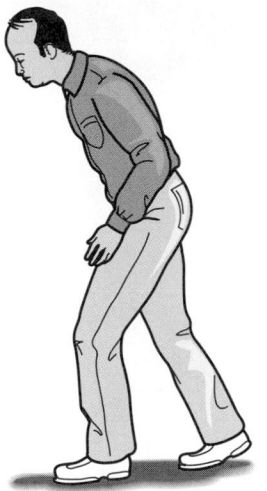

Propulsive gait

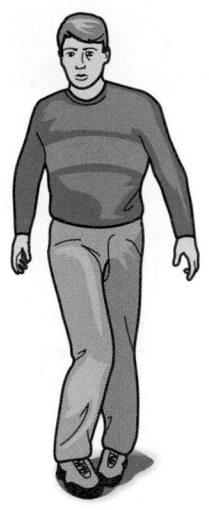

Scissors gait

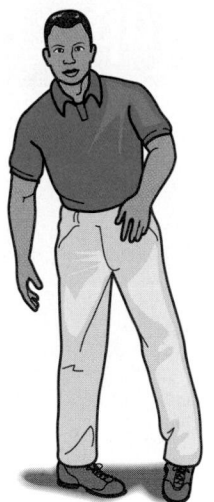

Spastic gait

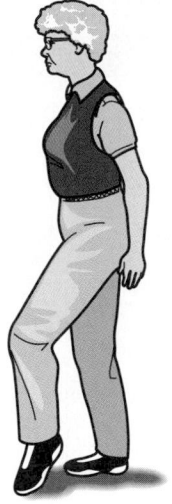

Steppage gait

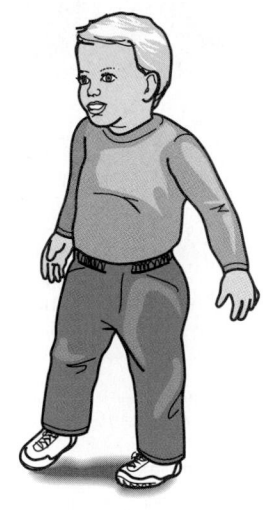

Waddling gait

Male Genitourinary System

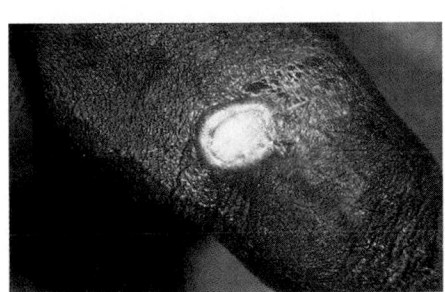

Syphilitic chancre

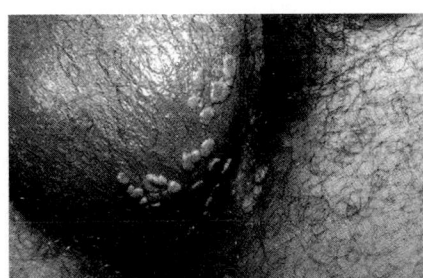

Genital warts

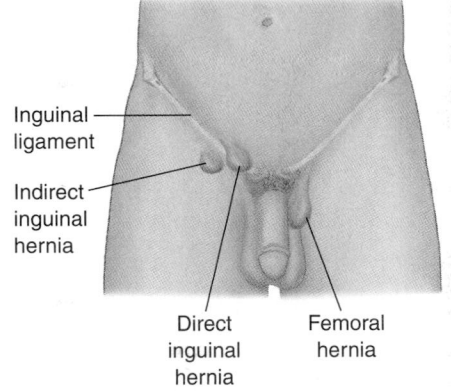

Inguinal ligament

Indirect inguinal hernia

Direct inguinal hernia

Femoral hernia

Locations of direct and indirect hernias

Female Genitourinary System

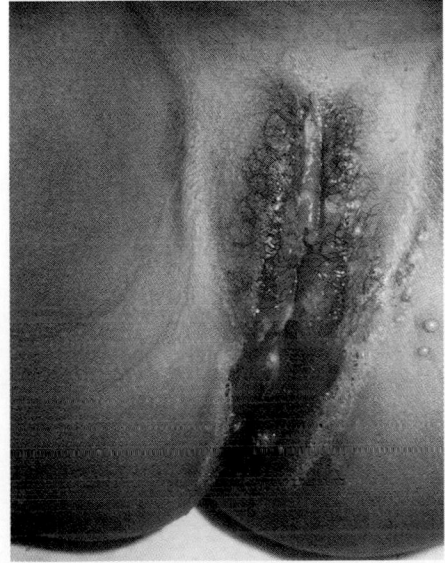

Herpes vulvovaginitis

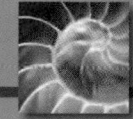

Knowledge Map

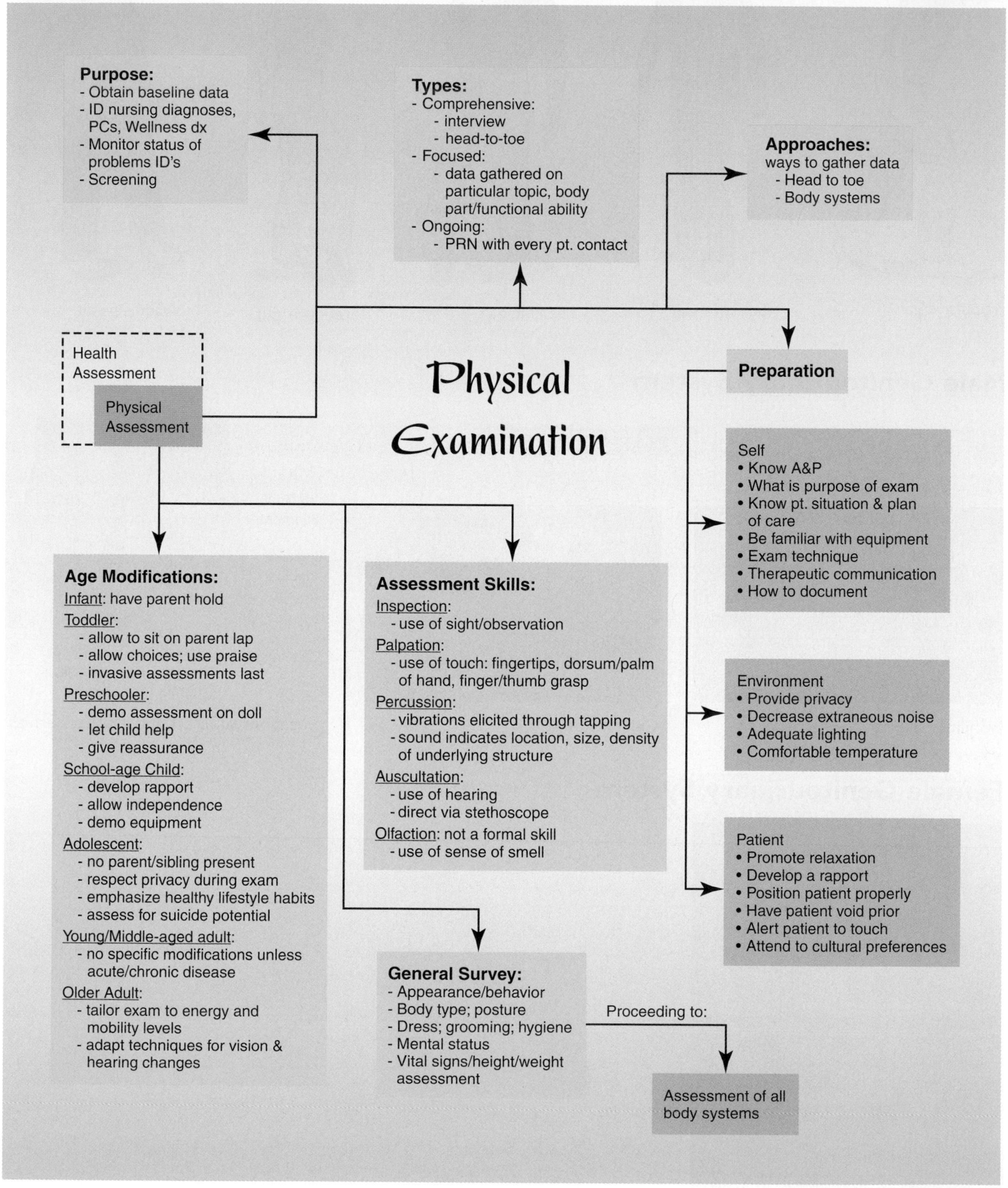

Purpose:
- Obtain baseline data
- ID nursing diagnoses, PCs, Wellness dx
- Monitor status of problems ID's
- Screening

Types:
- Comprehensive:
  - interview
  - head-to-toe
- Focused:
  - data gathered on particular topic, body part/functional ability
- Ongoing:
  - PRN with every pt. contact

Approaches:
ways to gather data
- Head to toe
- Body systems

Health Assessment

Physical Assessment

Physical Examination

Preparation

Self
- Know A&P
- What is purpose of exam
- Know pt. situation & plan of care
- Be familiar with equipment
- Exam technique
- Therapeutic communication
- How to document

Environment
- Provide privacy
- Decrease extraneous noise
- Adequate lighting
- Comfortable temperature

Patient
- Promote relaxation
- Develop a rapport
- Position patient properly
- Have patient void prior
- Alert patient to touch
- Attend to cultural preferences

Age Modifications:
Infant: have parent hold
Toddler:
- allow to sit on parent lap
- allow choices; use praise
- invasive assessments last
Preschooler:
- demo assessment on doll
- let child help
- give reassurance
School-age Child:
- develop rapport
- allow independence
- demo equipment
Adolescent:
- no parent/sibling present
- respect privacy during exam
- emphasize healthy lifestyle habits
- assess for suicide potential
Young/Middle-aged adult:
- no specific modifications unless acute/chronic disease
Older Adult:
- tailor exam to energy and mobility levels
- adapt techniques for vision & hearing changes

Assessment Skills:
Inspection:
- use of sight/observation
Palpation:
- use of touch: fingertips, dorsum/palm of hand, finger/thumb grasp
Percussion:
- vibrations elicited through tapping
- sound indicates location, size, density of underlying structure
Auscultation:
- use of hearing
- direct via stethoscope
Olfaction: not a formal skill
- use of sense of smell

General Survey:
- Appearance/behavior
- Body type; posture
- Dress; grooming; hygiene
- Mental status
- Vital signs/height/weight assessment

Proceeding to:

Assessment of all body systems

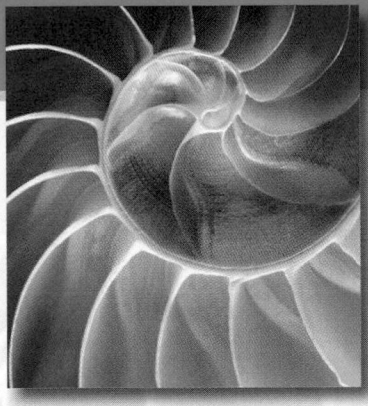

CHAPTER 20

Promoting Asepsis & Preventing Infection

For a podcast of an overview of this chapter,

 Go to Student Resources, **Podcast – Chapter Overviews, Chapter 20,** on DavisPlus at http://davisplus.fadavis.com/ Wilkinson2

Caring for the Garcias

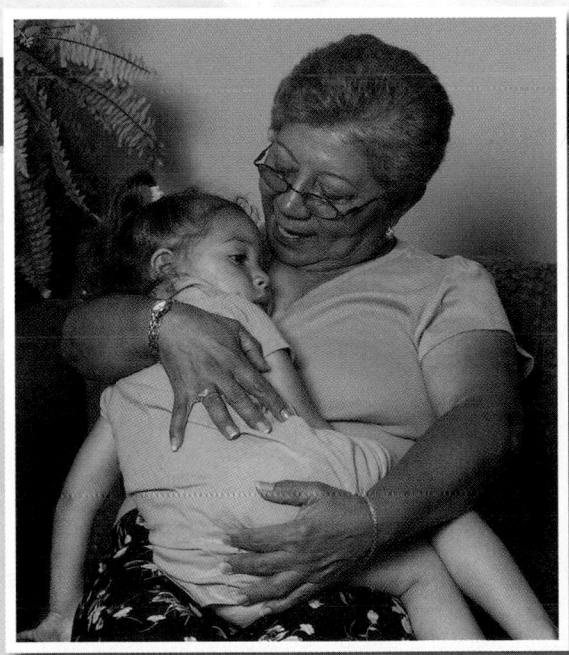

The exercises in the following section allow you to practice the kind of thinking you will use as a full-spectrum nurse. Because these are critical-thinking questions, there is usually no single right answer. We do not provide answers for these questions because it is more important for you to think about the questions than to arrive at the "right" answer. These questions are designed to improve your thinking more than to "cover content." Discuss answers with your peers—discussion can stimulate critical thinking. If you have difficulty with any of these questions, consult with your instructor

Ms. Garcia works as a preschool teacher in her community. Bettina, her grandchild, has been attending the preschool since she came to live with her grandparents. Ms. Garcia tells you at a recent visit to the clinic that Bettina has had "a lot of problems with colds and a runny nose since she started preschool."

A. Based on your theoretical knowledge of asepsis and immunity, what is the most likely explanation for Bettina's symptoms?

B. Do you have enough patient data to make any conclusions? If not, what other information should you gather?

C. Identify three alternatives that may explain what is happening.

D. What strategies could you recommend that Ms. Garcia implement at the preschool to help limit the number of infections? Identify at least two strategies.

Practical **Knowledge**
knowing how

As a nurse, you play a vital role in preventing the transmission of infection. Most infection control measures are independent nursing activities. You do not need a medical prescription for them. You do need theoretical knowledge and scrupulous medical and surgical asepsis technique. The procedures in this section and the clinical insights in the next section provide the guidance you will need to perform this important role.

Procedures

Procedure 20-1   Hand Hygiene

➤ For steps to follow in *all* procedures, refer to the Universal Steps for All Procedures found on the inside back cover of Volume 2. For this procedure, also refer to Clinical Insight 20-1.

Critical Aspects

- Remove your jewelry and watch.
- Wet your hands and wrists under running water.
- Apply 3 to 5 mL of liquid soap (or, typically, 3 to 4 pumps from a dispenser).
- Wash hands for at least 15 seconds, lathering all surfaces of the hands and fingers.
- Clean under your fingernails.
- Rinse and dry your hands thoroughly.
- Turn off the faucet with a dry paper towel.

Equipment

- Liquid soap (antimicrobial)
- Paper towels
- Warm, running water
- Hand moisturizer (optional)

Assessments

- Check your hands for breaks in the skin.
Breaks in the skin provide a route for microbial entry.

- Inspect the condition of your nails.
  —Nails should be no longer than ¼ inch from the fingertips.
  —Do not wear artificial nails or extensions.
  —Nail polish should not be chipped.
  —Preferably, do not use polish.
Research indicates the area under the nails, artificial nails/extensions, and chipped polish act as reservoirs for microorganisms.

Procedure 20-1A Using Soap and Water

➤ When performing the procedure, always identify your patient according to agency policy and be attentive to standard precautions, hand hygiene, patient safety and privacy, body mechanics, and documentation.

Procedure Steps

1. Bare your hands and forearms. Push your sleeves above your wrists, and remove your wristwatch and rings.
Moist clothing facilitates transfer of microorganisms; jewelry harbors bacteria and creates a moist area on the skin, which facilitates bacterial growth.

2. Turn on the water. Adjust the water temperature to warm.
Warm running water opens pores to aid in removing microorganisms without removing excess skin oils. It also reduces chapping.

3. Wet your hands and wrists. Keep your hands below your wrists and forearms.
The hands are considered more contaminated than the wrists and arms, so prevent water from running from your hands onto your wrists and forearms.

   a. Avoid splashing water onto clothing.
   b. Avoid touching the inside of the sink.

Microorganisms travel in moisture. The inside of the sink is considered contaminated. ▼

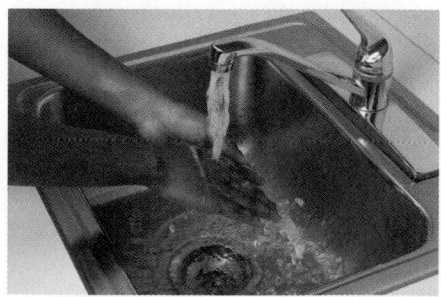

4. Apply 3 to 5 mL of liquid soap, which is typically 3 to 4 pumps using a soap dispenser. Rub the soap over all surfaces of your hands.

Three to 5 mL of liquid soap provides adequate amounts to completely cover the hands for maximum effectiveness to remove transient microorganisms.

5. Vigorously rub your hands together for at least 15 seconds, lathering all surfaces, interlacing fingers, rubbing around each finger and thumb, rubbing the backs and palms of the hands in a circular motion.

Washing for at least 15 seconds is required for mechanical removal of microorganisms and to give antimicrobial products adequate contact with the skin surfaces to be effective. Attention to all areas of the hands is necessary; research indicates areas of the hands most often missed are the thumb, the wrist, and areas between the fingers. ▼

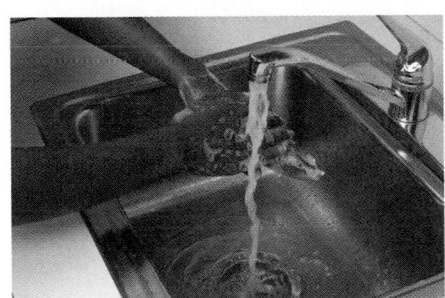

6. Clean under your fingernails, if needed, using a disposable nail cleaner. Areas under the nails harbor high concentrations of microorganisms. Chipped nail polish and artificial nails/extenders support growth of microorganisms, especially gram-negative bacteria.

7. Rinse your hands thoroughly. Keep your hands below your wrists and forearms.

Rinsing hands from wrist to fingertips mechanically washes away debris and microorganisms to flow into the sink and not back up the hand and arm.

8. Dry your hands thoroughly, moving from your fingers up to your forearms and blotting with paper towel.

Move from the area you wish to keep cleanest (hands). Blotting decreases skin irritation.

9. Turn off the faucet with a dry paper towel. Do not handle the paper towel with the opposite hand.

Prevents contamination of hands from the faucet. The paper towel has had contact with the contaminated faucet and may transfer microorganisms to your freshly washed hand. Many pathogens

can live on environmental surfaces, such as faucets and countertops. ▼

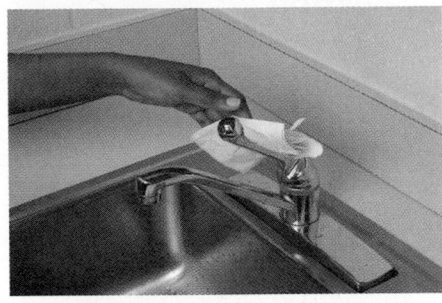

10. Apply a recommended hand moisturizer at least twice daily; use hand care products recommended by infection preventionists.

Hand moisturizer is recommended to prevent skin from drying, which may lead to skin damage and increase the risk for transmission of infection. Petroleum-based products compromise latex gloves, resulting in permeability. Anionic-based moisturizers can neutralize the residual effects of chlorhexidine gluconate and chloroxylenol. In most agencies, you will use the moisturizer recommended by the infection preventionist.

■ Procedure 20-1B Using Alcohol-Based Handrubs

➤ When performing the procedure, always identify your patient according to agency policy and be attentive to standard precautions, hand hygiene, patient safety and privacy, body mechanics, and documentation.

Procedure Steps

1. Use alcohol-based handrubs when hands are not visibly soiled and when certain pathogens are suspected.

Antiseptic solutions are not effective when organic material or dirt from hands is present. Alcohol handrubs cannot remove spores, and therefore should not be used for hand hygiene when Clostridium difficile or Bacillus anthracis is suspected of being present.

2. Bare your hands and forearms. Push your sleeves above your wrists. Remove your jewelry and wristwatch.

3. Apply a sufficient quantity (at least 3 mL) of antiseptic solution to cover the hands and wrists.

All surfaces must be covered with sufficient product to effectively remove microorganisms.

4. Vigorously rub antiseptic solution into for 15 to 30 seconds (or as long as it takes to sing "Happy Birthday" if no clock is available), interlacing fingers, rubbing around each finger and thumb, and rubbing the backs and palms of the hands in a circular motion including under the nails until the solution is completely dry.

Fifteen to 30 seconds is recommended by the Centers for Disease Control and Prevention (CDC) for effective disinfection by alcohol handrubs ▼

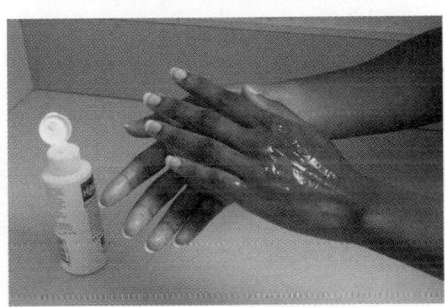

(continued on next page)

Procedure 20-1 ■ Hand Hygiene (continued)

Evaluation

Hands are free of handrub and dry.

Documentation

Hand hygiene is a responsibility of all healthcare providers. It does not require documentation.

Practice Resources

Association of periOperative Registered Nurses (2004); Boyce, J., & Pittet, D. (2002); Larson, E., Girard, R., Pessoa-Silva, L., et al. (2006); Pratt, R., Pellowe, C., Wilson, J., et al. (2007); Siegel, J., Rhinehart, E., Jackson, M., et al. (2007).

Thinking About the Procedure

 Go to the *Fundamentals of Nursing Skills Videos*, **Asepsis: Handwashing.**

1. How does the nurse in the DVD clean her fingernails?

2. Does nurse in the DVD turn off the faucet with a paper towel? What is the reason for what she does?

 For suggested responses, go to Chapter 20, **Thinking About the Procedure Suggested Responses,** on the Student Resource Disk or DavisPlus at http://davisplus.fadavis.com/Wilkinson2

Procedure 20-2 Donning Personal Protective Equipment (PPE)

➤ For steps to follow in *all* procedures, refer to the Universal Steps for All Procedures found on the inside back cover of Volume 2.

Critical Aspects

- Before exposure, don appropriate personal protective equipment according to standard precautions or transmission guidelines.
- Wear an N-95 respirator mask for airborne isolation.
- Wear a surgical mask for droplet isolation.

Equipment

Following CDC recommendations, you will usually use some combination of gloves, gown, mask, and eye protection; depending on the organism and level of precaution. In certain situations, you may need hair covers and shoe covers (e.g., when full barrier precautions are needed).

- Disposable gloves of the proper size
- Disposable isolation gown
- Face mask (or N-95 respirator mask, as indicated)
- Face shield or goggles
- Hair cover
- Shoe covers

➤ When performing the procedure, always identify your patient according to agency policy and be attentive to standard precautions, hand hygiene, patient safety and privacy, body mechanics, and documentation.

Procedure Steps

1. Assess the need for PPE. If you need more information about choosing PPE, refer to Clinical Insights 20-3, 20-4, and 20-5.

   a. **Gloves:** When you may be exposed to any body secretions directly or indirectly

   Gloves provide a barrier against body fluids. All patients are considered potentially infected per Standard Precautions (see Clinical Insight 20-3).

   b. **Gowns:** When your uniform (e.g., scrubs) may become exposed to potentially infective secretions

Examples of such situations include excessive wound drainage, fecal incontinence, or other discharges from the body, or when fluids may be splashed (as in eye irrigation).

   c. **Face mask:** To prevent transmission of pathogens spread through close respiratory (3 ft or less) or mucous membrane contact with respiratory secretions

   Surgical masks provide a barrier to large-particle droplets (> 5 microns in diameter).

   d. **Face shield or eye goggles:** When splashing might occur and

fluids enter your eyes (e.g., blood splashes, respiratory droplets, or wound débridement). To protect the entire facial area, wear a face shield (for maximum protection, it should protect the crown and chin and wrap around the face to the ear).

   Helps prevent pathogens from entering the conjunctiva directly or indirectly.

   e. **N-95 respirator:** When caring for clients infected with airborne organisms (< 5 microns) such as the tuberculosis bacillus.

   This device prevents the airborne transmission of the tuberculosis bacterium. The respirator mask shown is disposable; some are reusable. ▼

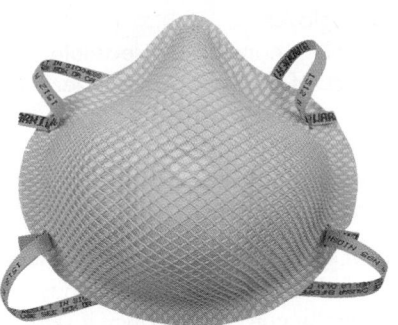

f. **Hair covers:** When there is a potential for spraying or splashing of body fluids

Although this is not in the CDC report (Siegel, Rhinehart, Jackson, et al., 2007), agency policy may advise hair covers in certain situations.

g. **Shoe covers:** When there is a potential for contamination of shoes with body fluids

Although this is not in the CDC report (Siegel, Rhinehart, Jackson, et al., 2007), agency policy may require shoe covers in certain situations. The floor (and anything in contact with it) is considered contaminated. However, certain categories of pathogens require full protective gear, and in those circumstances shoe covers are necessary.

2. Determine the availability of appropriate personal protective equipment.

A patient gown is not a substitute for a disposable isolation gown. Isolation gowns must be made of moisture-repelling materials to prevent contamination of underlying clothing and skin.

3. Don the isolation gown.
While donning PPE, the goal is to not contaminate the PPE.

a. Pick up the gown by the shoulders, allowing the gown to fall open without touching the floor or other surfaces.

Touching the floor or other surfaces will contaminate the gown with environmental pathogens. ▼

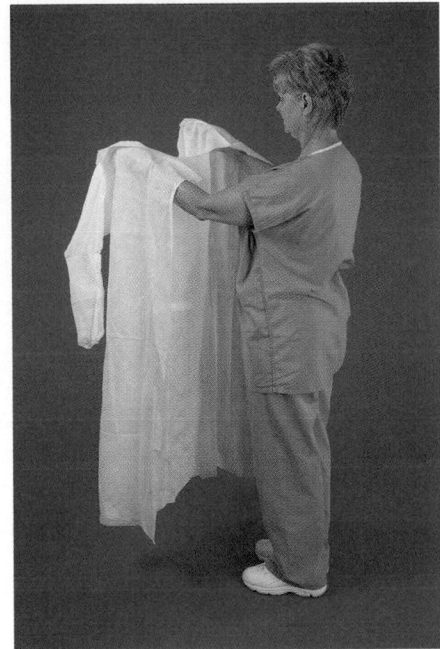

b. Slip your arms into the sleeves. ▼

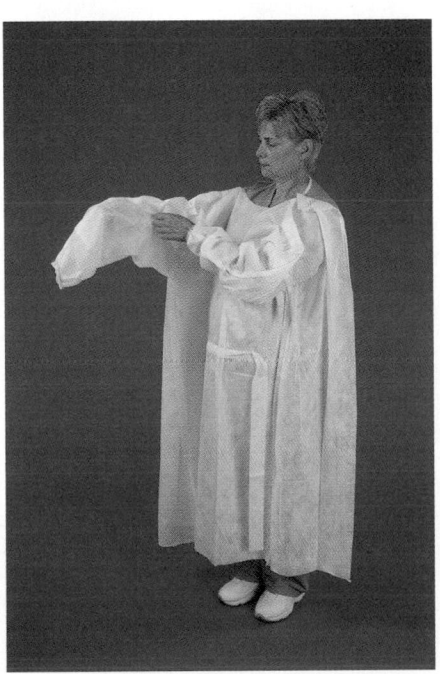

c. Fasten ties at the neck.
d. Position the gown so that it covers the back, and fasten the ties

at the waist. Do not bring ties around to the front of the gown.
The front of the gown is considered contaminated after you enter the patient's room. If the ties are at the front of the gown, they will be contaminated, making it difficult to remove the gown safely.

e. If the gown does not completely cover your clothing in the back, wear two gowns. Put on the first gown so that the opening is in the front, and then place the second gown over the first, so that the opening is in the back.

4. Don the face mask or N-95 respirator.

a. Determine how the mask is secured. Identify the top edge of the mask by locating the thin metal strip (nosepiece) that goes over the bridge of the nose.

Surgical masks may be secured by ties at the back of the head and neck, loops around the ears, or elastic bands.

b. Place the mask over your nose, mouth, and chin. Press the flexible metal strip so that it conforms to the bridge of your nose.

The mask must fit snugly to the face for maximum barrier protection. Correct positioning will also keep your glasses or goggles from fogging. ▼

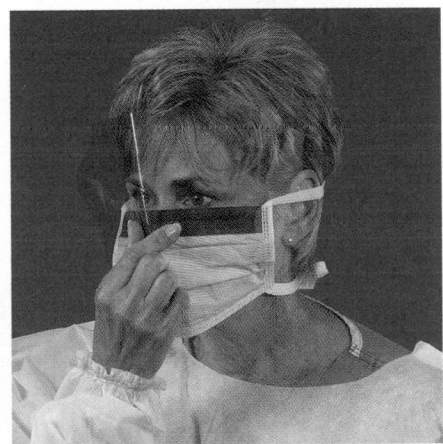

c. Tie the upper ties to the back of your head and the lower ties to the back of your neck or slip the
(continued on next page)

Procedure 20-2 ■ Donning Personal Protective Equipment (PPE) (continued)

loops around your ears or place the elastic bands as with the ties.

d. Place the lower edge of the mask below your chin, and tie the lower ties.

Covering the nose and mouth creates a barrier to prevent droplet pathogens from entering through the nasal and oral mucous membranes or the respiratory system.

5. Don the face shield or goggles.

a. Face shield: Place the shield over your eyes, adjust the metal strip over the bridge of your nose, and tuck the lower edge below your chin. Secure the straps behind your head.

b. Safety glasses or goggles: Set them over the top edge of the mask.

See Step 1c, d, e for rationale.

6. Don hair cover, if indicated. Hair covers can be worn to protect from contamination when you anticipate sprays or airborne exposure.

7. Don shoe covers, if indicated. Wear shoe covers to protect against exposure to airborne organisms or contact with a contaminated environment and as a part of full barrier precautions (e.g., when the patient has hemorrhagic disease or severe acute respiratory syndrome [SARS]).

8. Don gloves.

a. Select nonsterile disposable gloves of the appropriate size. See Clinical Insight 20-3.

The correct size will prevent gloves from falling off or ripping while you are working with the client.

b. If you are wearing a gown, make sure that the glove cuff extends over the cuff of the gown. If skin is visible between the gown and the glove, tape the glove cuff to the gown cuff, covering all visible skin.

To provide complete protection of hands and wrists, no skin should be visible between the glove and gown.

Patient Teaching

Answer questions the patient may have and educate about the need for PPE, his disease process, and the purpose of isolation.

Home Care

- Identify the type of PPE needed, and ensure that the necessary supplies are available.
- Develop a plan with the client and family for using and disposing of personal protective equipment and contaminated items.
- Teach family members to don PPE as needed.
- Obtain referral for a home health agency to provide support.

Documentation

The use of personal protective equipment is generally assumed and does not require documentation.

Practice Resources

Minnesota Department of Health (n.d.); Siegel, J. D., Rhinehart, E., Jackson, M., et al. (2007).

Thinking About the Procedure

 Go to the *Fundamentals of Nursing Skills Videos,* **Asepsis: Personal Protective Equipment, Donning.**

1. When donning PPE, what does the nurse do that indicates that she thinks splashing may occur during her care of the patient?

 For suggested responses, go to Chapter 20, **Thinking About the Procedure Suggested Responses,** on the Student Resource Disk or DavisPlus at http://davisplus.fadavis.com/ Wilkinson2

Procedure 20-3 ■ Removing Personal Protective Equipment (PPE)

➤ For steps to follow in *all* procedures, refer to the Universal Steps for All Procedures found on the inside back cover of Volume 2. For this procedure, also refer to Clinical Insights 20-2 and 20-3 if you need more information.

Critical Aspects

- Remove the PPE at the doorway before leaving the patient's room, or in an anteroom.
- Avoid contaminating self, others, or the environment when removing equipment.
- Always remove gloves first when removing PPE, unless gown ties in front
- Considered contaminated: front areas, sleeves, mask, and gloves of the PPE (as well as head and shoe covers if you are wearing them)
- Considered clean: the inside of the gown, gloves, the ties on the mask, and ties at the back of the gown (as well as the inside of the head and shoe covers if you are wearing them).

➤ When performing the procedure, always identify your patient according to agency policy and be attentive to standard precautions, hand hygiene, patient safety and privacy, body mechanics, and documentation.

Procedure Steps

1. Remove gloves first (unless the gown ties in front; in that case, see "What If...").

Gloves are the most contaminated PPE and must be removed first to avoid contamination of clean areas of the PPE during their removal.

　a. Remove the first glove by grasping the outside cuff of the glove with the opposite gloved hand and pulling downward so that the glove turns inside out. Do not touch the skin of your wrist or hand with your gloved hand.

The outside of both gloves are contaminated. To prevent contamination, touch only the outside (contaminated) surface of first glove to outside (contaminated) surface of second glove. "Dirty touches dirty" and "clean touches clean." ▼

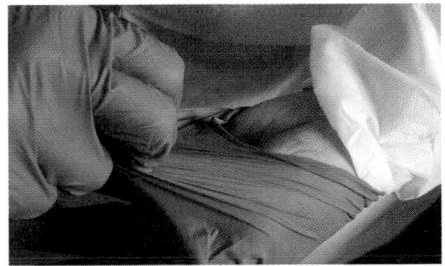

　b. Hold the removed glove in the palm of your gloved hand. Slip two ungloved fingers inside the cuff of the remaining glove. Pull the glove off, inside out, over the glove that hand is holding.

The inside of the gloves are considered "clean" because they have not been in contact with client or contaminated surfaces. Therefore, you can touch the insides with your bare hands. ▼

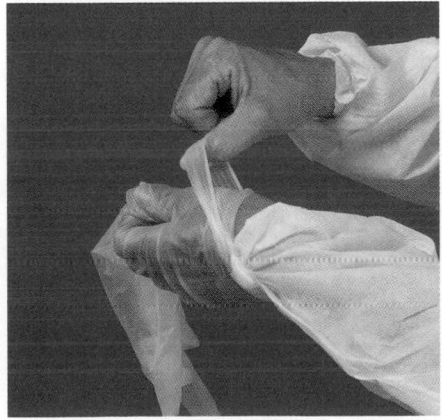

　c. Dispose of the gloves in a designated waste receptacle.

2. Remove the gown:
　a. Release the waist ties and the neck ties of the gown, bending slightly forward to allow the gown to fall forward.

The ties and the inside area of the gown are considered clean areas. Gown front and sleeves are contaminated. Allowing the gown to fall forward exposes the clean area for the hands to grasp more readily.

　b. Slip your hands inside the neck and peel the gown away from the shoulders. Reach inside to pull off the cuff and remove your arm from the sleeve. Repeat the maneuver to remove the second sleeve. Do not touch the front of the gown, even if it is not visibly soiled.

The inside of the gown is clean and will not contaminate your hands. The front of the gown and the sleeves are considered contaminated. ▼

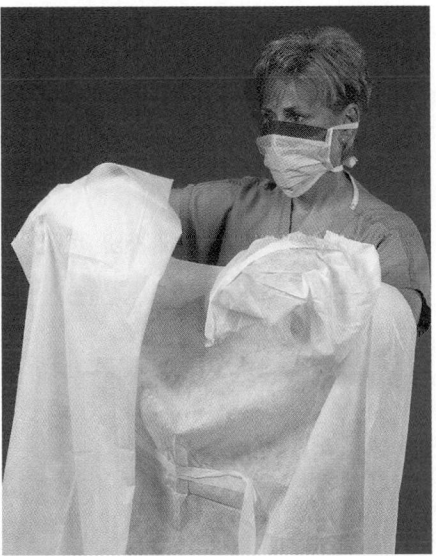

3. Fold the gown so the inside of the gown is to the outside. Holding the gown away from your uniform, roll it up with the contaminated front and sleeves in the center, and place in the designated waste receptacle.

The inside of the gown is considered clean. Folding the gown prevents

contamination of your hands, the clothing, and the environment. ▼

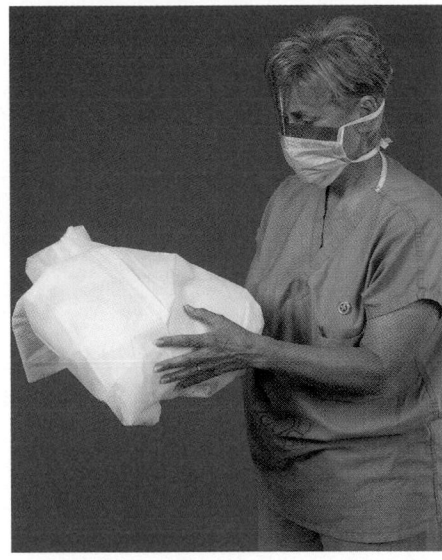

4. Remove goggles (if wearing them). Grasp only the ear pieces (or head band) of the goggles and pull off the face. Place in the receptacle provided for disinfection if the goggles are not disposable.

Earpieces are considered clean. Some goggles are cleaned and reused

5. Remove your mask or face shield (if wearing one). Untie the lower ties first. Untie the upper ties next, being careful not to let go of the ties. Touch only the ties; do not touch the front of the mask. Dispose of the mask by holding on to the ties and placing it in a designated waste receptacle.

Ties are considered clean. The front of the mask is potentially contaminated; do not touch it with your bare hands.

6. Remove your hair covering, if you are wearing one. Slip your bare fingers under the edge of the hair cover, being careful not to touch the outside of it. Lift it up and away from your hair. Touching only the inside of it, place it in a designated waste receptacle.

The inside of the hair covering is considered clean, so you may touch it with your bare hands.

7. Remove shoe covers, if wearing them. Be careful to touch only the insides of the covers.

(continued on next page)

Procedure 20-3 ■ **Removing Personal Protective Equipment (PPE)** (continued)

8. Perform hand hygiene before leaving the room.
Wash your hands after all patient contact even if gloves are worn to prevent contamination.

9. Close the door.
Keeping the door closed contains contaminates and makes signage more visible.

What if . . .

■ **The gown is tied in front?**
This would be an unusual circumstance, but if that occurs, you must untie the front gown ties before removing your gloves; then remove the gloves and untie any back ties (e.g., at the neck). Because the front of the gown (including a front tie) is considered contaminated, once you remove your gloves, you could not use your bare hands to untie a front tie.

■ **You are wearing two gowns (top one tied in back, inner one tied in front)?**
Remove gloves; untie waist ties of outer gown, remove the gown and fold it inside out. Remove the inner gown by untying it in front. Fold inner gown inside out. Take off goggles and face mask or shield.

Patient Teaching
See Procedure 20-2.

Home Care
See Procedure 20-2.

Documentation
The removal of personal protective equipment is generally assumed and does not require documentation.

Practice Resources
Siegel, J., Rhinehart, E., Jackson, M., et al. (2007); U.S. Department of Labor (n.d.a & b).

Thinking About the Procedure

 Go to the *Fundamentals of Nursing Skills Videos*, **Asepsis: Personal Protective Equipment, Removing.**

1. When removing her gloves, how does the nurse protect her hands from contamination?

 For suggested responses, go to Chapter 20, **Thinking About the Procedure Suggested Responses,** on the Student Resource Disk or DavisPlus at http://davisplus.fadavis.com/ Wilkinson2

Procedure 20-4 ■ **Surgical Handwashing: Traditional Method**

➤ For steps to follow in *all* procedures, refer to the Universal Steps for All Procedures found on the inside back cover of Volume 2. For this procedure, also refer to Clinical Insights 20-2, 20-3 and 20-7 if you need more information.

Critical Aspects

- Don surgical shoe covers, cap, and face mask before the scrub.
- Use warm water.
- Perform a prewash, using soap and water.
- Clean under your nails under running water.
- Wet the scrub sponge, and apply a generous amount of antimicrobial soap.
- Using a circular motion, scrub all surfaces of nails, hands, and forearms at least 10 times, or the length of time specified by agency policy.
- Rinse hands and arms by keeping your fingertips higher than your elbow.
- Grasp a sterile towel, and back away from the sterile field.
- Thoroughly dry your hands before donning sterile gloves.

Equipment
- Antimicrobial soap (60% to 95% alcohol, or other FDA-approved for surgical hand asepsis)
- Soft, nonabrasive scrub sponge
- Disposable single-use nail cleaner

- Deep sink with foot or knee controls
- Surgical shoe covers, cap, and face mask
- Sterile gloves of the correct size
- Surgical pack containing a sterile towel

➤ When performing the procedure, always identify your patient according to agency policy and be attentive to standard precautions, hand hygiene, patient safety and privacy, body mechanics, and documentation.

Procedure Steps

1. Determine the agency policy for the duration of the surgical scrub and the type of cleansing agent used.
The type of cleansing agent determines how long to scrub. Typically, an alcohol-based antimicrobial soap requires 2 to 6 minutes.

2. Avoid chipped polish or artificial nails. Trim so nails do not extend beyond fingertips. Remove rings, watches, and bracelets. Preferably, do not wear nail polish.
Rings are a substantial risk factor for harboring moisture and gram-negative bacilli and *S. aureus*; and artificial nails and chipped polish are more likely to carry gram-negative pathogens, including *pseudomonas*, because water collects between the artificial and real nails.

3. Put on surgical shoe covers, cap, and face mask before the surgical scrub.

4. Determine that sterile gloves, gown, and towel are set up for use after the scrub.
To maintain sterility, the sterile towel, gown, and gloves must be ready for use immediately after you scrub. If you need to gather supplies after the scrub, you will need to start the scrub procedure over again.

5. Perform a prewash before the surgical scrub (see Procedure 20-1).
The prewash removes any visible soil, reduces the number of microorganisms on your skin, and allows you to begin the surgical scrub with clean hands.

6. Remove debris from underneath your fingernails using a single-use nail file under running water.

Decreases the number of microorganisms. ▼

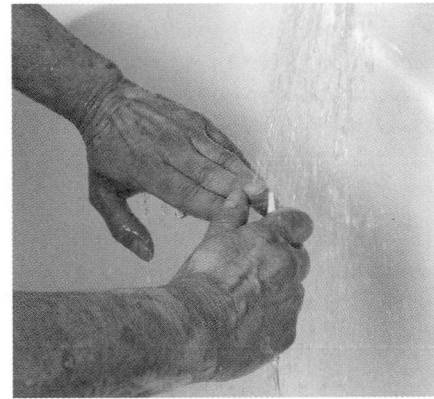

7. To begin the surgical scrub, turn on the water, using the knee or foot controls or motion sensors. Adjust the temperature so that the water is warm.
Hot water removes too many of the skin's protective oils. Knee and foot controls help to prevent contamination of the hands. You cannot touch any unsterile surfaces once you begin the surgical handwash. ▼

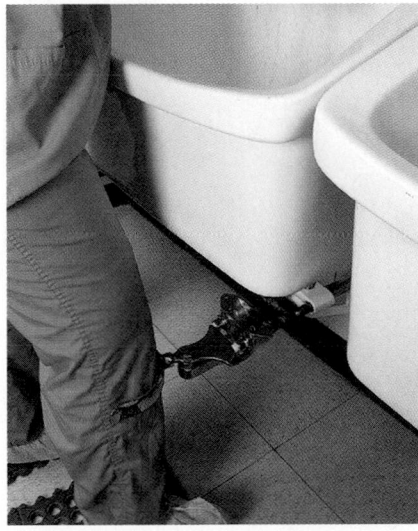

8. Wet your hands and forearms from elbows to fingertips, keeping hands above elbows and away from your body. If using a scrub sponge, wet the sponge.
Prevents water running down from your elbows and forearm over rinsed hands.

9. Apply a liberal amount of antimicrobial soap onto your hands and the sponge; lather well to 2 inches above the elbow. Do not touch the inside of the sink with your fingers, hands, or elbows. Avoid splashing your surgical attire.
Scrub brushes are harsh on the skin. Soft, nonabrasive sponges are recommended instead. Antimicrobial soap reduces the number of microorganisms.

10. Using a circular motion, scrub all the surfaces of one hand and arm. Start at the fingers. Scrub at least 10 strokes each on nail, all four sides of each finger, hands, and arms. When scrubbing the arm, use 10 strokes each for the lower, middle, and upper areas of the forearm. Keep your hands higher than your elbows.
All surfaces of the skin must be scrubbed effectively. ▼

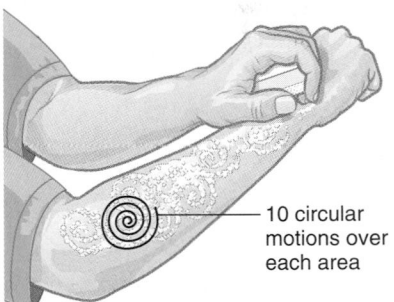

10 circular motions over each area

11. Rinse the brush, and reapply antimicrobial soap. Repeat the scrub on the second hand and arm. Normally the scrub takes at least 2 to 6 minutes.
(continued on next page)

Procedure 20-4 ■ Surgical Handwashing: Traditional Method (continued)

The purpose of the scrub is to decrease the number of microorganisms on the hands. The length of the scrub depends on the time needed for the particular scrub agent to be effective.

12. Rinse your hands and arms, keeping your fingertips higher than your elbows.

Prevents contamination of hands from water running from the upper arm down onto hands. ▼

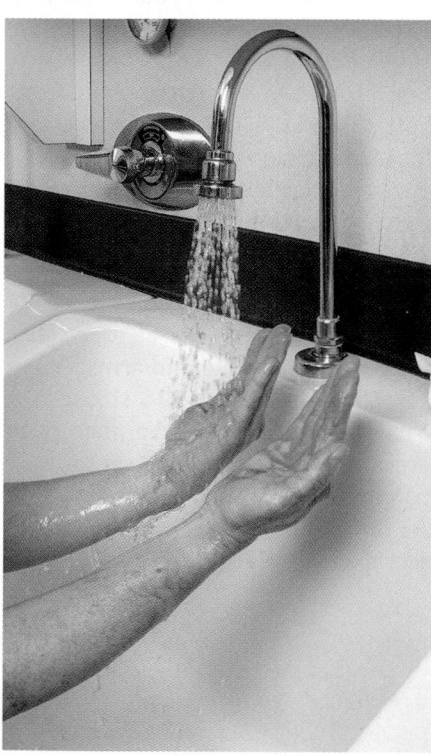

13. Repeat steps 8 through 12 if directed to do so by the soap manufacturer or agency policy.

14. With your arms flexed and your hands held higher than your elbows, move to the area with the sterile towel and gown.

Avoids contamination of hands from water runoff.

15. Grasp the sterile towel, and move away from sterile field.

Moving away keeps the sterile field dry and prevents you from inadvertently brushing against the table, which would contaminate the field. ▼

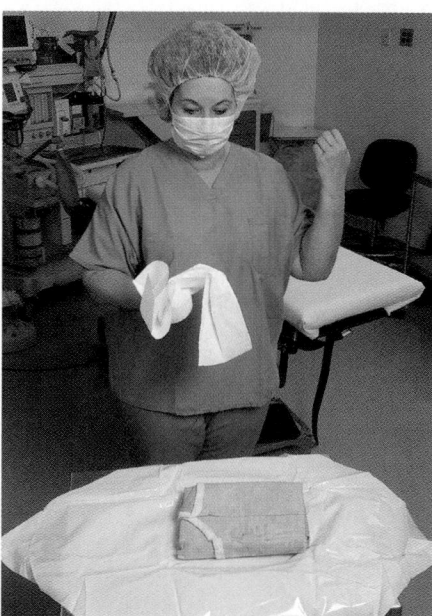

16. Lean forward slightly, and allow the towel to fall open, being careful not to let it touch your clothing.

The towel would be contaminated if it brushed against your uniform.

17. Use one end of the towel to dry one hand and arm. Use the opposite end to dry the other hand and arm. Be certain your skin is thoroughly dry before donning sterile gloves.

Dry skin prevents maceration and allows gloves to go on much more easily. Use a separate section of the towel to prevent rewetting the skin.

What if . . .

■ **The agency uses an alcohol-based surgical hand-scrub product?**

  a. Perform steps 1 through 6. Omit steps 7 through 17.

  b. Using the indicated amount of handrub, rub all surfaces of the hands, including the nails and up the arm to 2 inches above the elbow, according to the manufacturer's recommendations and agency policy.

  Many different products are on the market. Be careful to follow the manufacturer's guidelines for use for maximum effectiveness.

  c. Allow the handrub to dry completely before you don sterile gloves.

Patient Teaching

If the patient is able to observe the procedure, explain the purpose of the surgical scrub and sterility.

Documentation

A surgical hand scrub does not require documentation. Instead, chart the procedure (or surgery) and how the patient tolerated it.

Practice Resources

Association of periOperative Registered Nurses. Recommended Practices Committee (2004); Boyce, J., & Pittet, D. (2002); Siegel, J., Rhinehart, E., Jackson, M., et al. (2007).

Procedure 20-5 ☐ Surgical Handwashing: Brushless System

➤ For steps to follow in *all* procedures, refer to the Universal Steps for All Procedures found on the inside back cover of Volume 2. For this procedure, also refer to Clinical Insights 20-2, 20-3 and 20-7 if you need more information.

Critical Aspects

- Don surgical shoe covers, cap, and face mask before the scrub.
- Use warm water.
- Perform a prewash, using soap and water.
- Clean under your nails under running water.
- Apply a generous amount of antimicrobial soap.
- Using a circular motion, scrub all surfaces of nails, hands, and forearms at least 10 times, or the length of time specified by agency policy.
- Rinse hands and arms by keeping your fingertips higher than your elbow.
- Grasp a sterile towel, and back away from the sterile field.
- Thoroughly dry your hands before donning sterile gloves.

Equipment

- Antimicrobial soap (60% to 95% alcohol, or other FDA-approved for surgical hand asepsis)
- Disposable single-use nail cleaner

- Deep sink with foot or knee controls
- Surgical shoe covers, cap, and face mask
- Sterile gloves of the correct size
- Surgical pack containing a sterile towel

➤ When performing the procedure, always identify your patient according to agency policy and be attentive to standard precautions, hand hygiene, patient safety and privacy, body mechanics, and documentation.

Procedure Steps

1. Determine agency policy for duration of the surgical scrub and the type of cleansing product to be used.
Policies vary from institution to institution, although all should be based on sound principles for infection control designed in accordance with CDC guidelines. The type of cleansing agent determines how long to scrub. Typically, alcohol-based handrub is rubbed onto hands and arms until dry.

2. Before starting the surgical scrub, gather supplies and set up sterile gloves, gown, and towel for use after the scrub.
To maintain sterility of the hands after the scrub, the sterile gloves, gown, and towel must be ready before washing.

3. Observe recommended hygiene.
a. Avoid wearing artificial nails and extenders and chipped polish; nails should not extend beyond the end of the fingers. Preferably, do not wear nail polish.
The Association of Peri-Operative Registered Nurses (AORN) and CDC recommend avoiding these when in direct contact with patients or in high-risk situations, such as the perioperative setting

or among those receiving immunosuppressant therapy. Individuals wearing artificial nails have been shown to harbor more pathogenic organisms in the subungual area than those with natural nails, particularly gram-negative bacilli, especially pseudomonas, and various strains of yeast. Long nails can tear gloves.

b. Remove rings, watches, and bracelets before starting the surgical scrub.
Removing hand jewelry is advised to increase the quality of hand hygiene and reduce the spread of potential pathogens. Risk of infection from microorganisms increases exponentially in relation to the number of rings worn.

4. Don shoe covers, a cap, and a mask. Tuck hair completely under the cap.
Masks filter out possible airborne pathogens carried in the nose or mouth, preventing contamination of sterile areas. Covering the hair reduces the transmission of pathogenic organisms that adhere to the hair shaft or scalp, which is a warm, moist environment for organisms.

5. Perform a prewash before the surgical scrub. Use a pick to remove

dirt and debris from under the nails; discard.
The prewash removes any visible soil, reduces the number of microorganisms on your skin, and allows you to begin the surgical scrub with clean hands. The nail bed harbors dirt and debris in which microorganisms live.

6. Turn on the water, using the knee or foot controls or motion controls. The temperature usually adjusts automatically in a surgical scrub sink. Water temperature that is too hot can cause injury to the skin, making it prone to disruption in the skin integrity. In addition, it can remove the skin's normal flora and natural oil, which has a protectant effect.

7. Wet hands and forearms from the fingertips to elbows, keeping hands above the elbows and away from the body at all times.
Prevents water running down from your elbows and forearm over washed and rinsed hands.

8. Dispense a palmful of antibacterial soap into your dominant hand. Insert the fingertips of your nondominant hand into the soap using a twisting motion to apply the product to the

(continued on next page)

Procedure 20–5 ■ Surgical Handwashing: Brushless System (continued)

fingertips and nails. Then rub the hands together to distribute the soap over the hands. ▼

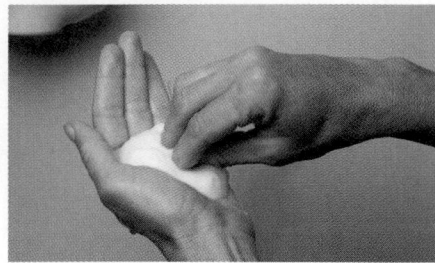

9. Vigorously rub all surfaces of your nondominant hand and fingers, adding water as needed. Be sure to rub each digit on all sides. Do not touch the inside of the sink during the cleansing procedure.

Complete contact and friction are necessary for removal of microorganisms adherent to the skin's surface. The inside of the sink is considered contaminated with microbes and should be avoided. Incidental contact necessitates repeating the cleansing procedure.

10. Rub the hands together and cleanse the back side of the hand and the lower third of your nondominant arm (nearest the wrist).

Although the palmar surface carries more organisms than the back side of the hands and arms, this area, nonetheless, should be cleansed thoroughly to reduce microbial colonization.

11. Rinse using deep basin sink with knee, foot, or motion-operated controls.

Improved adherence to sterile technique commonly results from use of

motion or foot/knee-operated or motion controls for faucets.

12. Repeat the hand cleansing and rinsing process on the dominant hand and forearm.

13. Rinse and dispense soap into hands each time when cleansing a new area. Be sure the soap dispenser is not blocked.

A blocked dispenser can interfere with obtaining the proper amount of product needed for reducing bacterial colonization. Many products are available for the brushless surgical scrub procedure. Adhere to the manufacturer's guidelines for use.

14. Cleanse the remaining two-thirds of the nondominant arm to 2 inches above the elbow. Cover every aspect of the middle and upper third of the forearm.

15. Repeat the wrist-to-elbow scrub on the dominant arm.

16. Rinse each arm thoroughly and independently.

17. Repeat all the scrub steps (8 through 16), stopping before the elbow. The scrub is complete after cleansing every aspect of the hands and forearms for 3 full minutes.

The CDC promotes a 2- to 3-minute scrub time using an antiseptic detergent in order to achieve maximal microbicidal activity while avoiding irritant contact dermatitis associated with use of an abrasive sponge. Reduced time required to perform the surgical scrub often results in increased compliance with the prescribed technique.

18. With the arms flexed and hands held higher than the elbows away from the body, move to the area with the sterile towel and gown.

This position prevents water running down from your elbows and forearm over rinsed hands.

19. Grasp the sterile towel, and move away from the sterile field. Lean forward slightly, and allow the towel to fall open, being careful not to let it touch clothing or gown.

This motion is performed to maintain a dry sterile field and prevent inadvertent brushing against the table and contaminating the field.

20. Use one end of the towel to dry one hand and arm. Dry the other hand and arm with the opposite end of the towel.

Use of a separate section of the towel guards against inadvertently rewetting the skin or contaminating an already clean area.

21. Allow time for the skin to dry thoroughly before donning sterile gloves.

Dry skin prevents maceration and allows the gloves to go on more easily. Moisture left on the skin can be a source of further microbial contamination.

22. Once the brushless scrub is complete, prevent contamination of the hands and forearms when moving from the scrub sink to the sterile table by keeping the hands in front of the body and above the waist. It may be necessary to enter backwards through the door of the surgical suite to prevent contamination of the scrubbed hands.

Documentation

A brushless surgical hand scrub does not require documentation in the patient's medical record. However, you must adherence to the institution's policy for performing the technique.

Patient Teaching

If the patient is able to observe the procedure, explain the purpose of a diligent approach to surgical scrub for promoting a low-risk environment for infection.

Home Care Adaptations

Sinks in the home environment typically do not have knee- or foot-operated controls or motion-sensor on/off devices. Therefore, when scrubbing for a sterile procedure in the home, contact with the faucet handles is performed with barrier objects (e.g., a paper towel) between the clean hands and the environmental surface.

Practice Resources

Association of periOperative Registered Nurses (AORN). Recommended Practices Committee (2004); Centers for Disease Control and Prevention (2002).

Thinking About the Procedure

 Go to the *Fundamentals of Nursing Skills Videos,* **Asepsis: Surgical Hand Washing, Brushless System.**

1. The nurse in the DVD does not dry her hands before she leaves the sink area. Why?

2. How did she dry her hands to keep them surgically clean?

 For suggested responses, go to Chapter 20, **Thinking About the Procedure Suggested Responses,** on the Student Resource Disk or DavisPlus at http://davisplus.fadavis.com/Wilkinson2

Procedure 20-6   Sterile Gown and Gloves (Closed Method)

➤ For steps to follow in *all* procedures, refer to the Universal Steps for All Procedures found on the inside back cover of Volume 2. For this procedure, also refer to Clinical Insights 20-2, 20-3, and 20-7 if you need more information.

Critical Aspects

- Put on shoe covers, hair covers, and mask before the scrub.
- Perform the surgical scrub.
- Grasp the gown at the neckline, and slide your arms into the sleeves without extending your hands through the cuffs.
- Have a co-worker pull the shoulders of the gown up and tie the neck tie.
- Don gloves using the closed method by keeping your hands covered at all times, first with the gown cuffs, and then with the sterile gloves.
- Secure the waist tie on your gown by handing it to a co-worker and turning to receive it.
- Keep your hands within your field of vision at all times.
- Do not turn your back to a sterile field.

Equipment

- Sterile gloves of the right size
- Sterile gown

  (These should be lying on a sterile field. If they are not, you will need to create a sterile field to place them on.)

➤ When performing the procedure, always identify your patient according to agency policy and be attentive to standard precautions, hand hygiene, patient safety and privacy, body mechanics, and documentation.

Procedure Steps

1. Grasp the gown at the neckline. Hold the gown up and allow it to fall open as you step back from the table. Be careful not to allow the gown to come into contact with nonsterile areas while you are lifting it off the table and opening it.

The gown will be contaminated if it touches unsterile objects. ▼

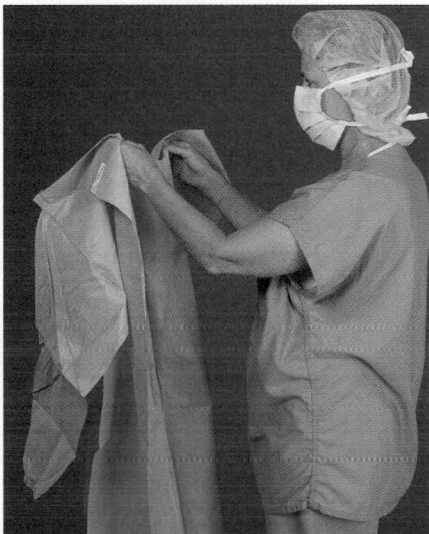

2. Slide both arms into the sleeves, but do not extend your hands through the cuffs. ▼

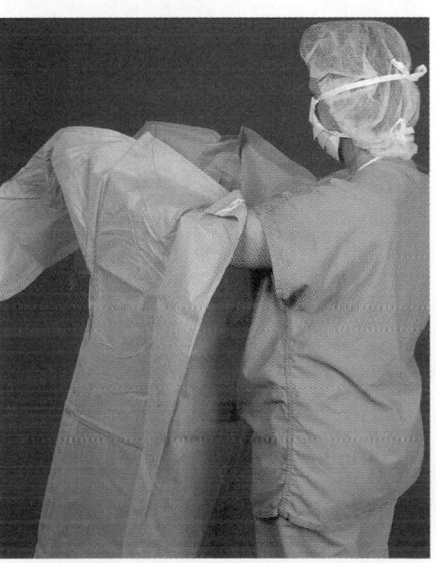

(continued on next page)

Procedure 20-6 ■ Sterile Gown and Gloves (Closed Method) (continued)

3. Keep the sleeves of the gown above waist level.
Hands will contaminate the sleeve edge if allowed to pass through the cuff.

4. Have a co-worker (or the circulating nurse, if you are in the operating room) stand behind you and pull the shoulders of the gown up and tie the neck tie. The co-worker touches only the inside of the gown while pulling it up.
Touching only the inside prevents contamination of the gown with the nurse's hands.

5. Don sterile gloves using the closed method.
   a. Open the sterile glove wrapper, keeping your fingers inside the sleeve of the gown. The outer wrapper has already been discarded.
   b. With your dominant hand, keeping your hands inside the gown sleeves, grasp the cuff of the glove for your dominant hand.
Keeping the hand inside the cuff ensures that you are making contact with the sterile gown; sterile is touching sterile. ▼

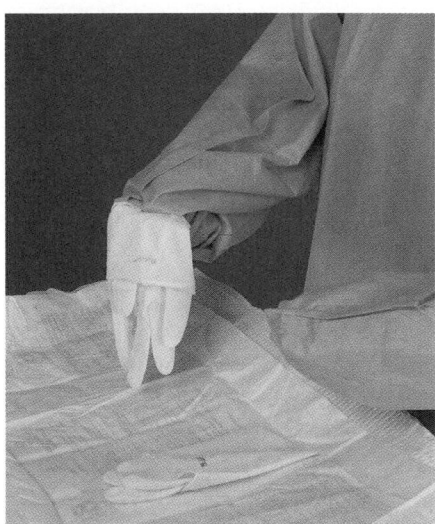

   c. Lay the glove on the dominant hand forearm of the thumb side down with the glove opening pointed toward the fingers and thumb of glove positioned over the thumb of the hand.
   d. With your nondominant hand, grasp the inside glove cuff through the gown, being careful to keep your fingers inside the gown.

Bare fingers would contaminate the sterile glove. ▼

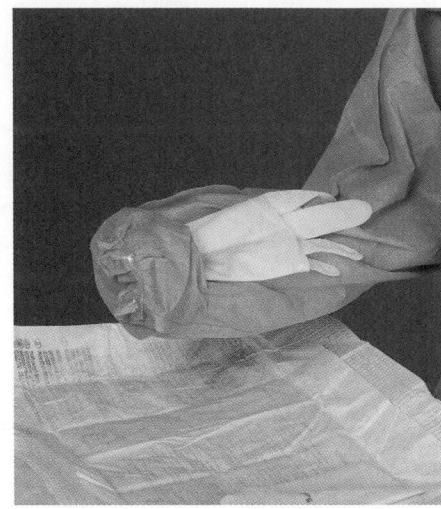

   e. With your dominant hand encased in the gown sleeve, grasp the upper side of the glove cuff and pull it over the cuff of the gown. ▼

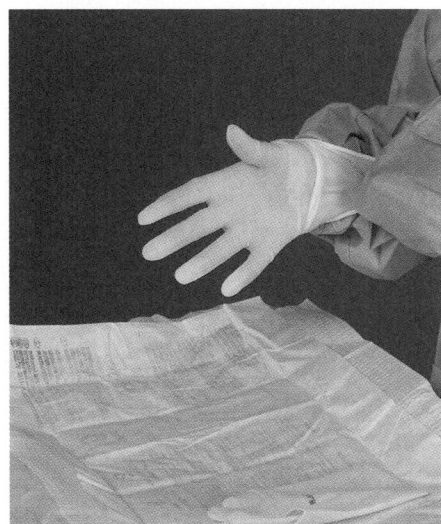

   f. Pull the sleeve of your gown up to assist the cuff over the wrist and move your fingers into the glove.
   g. Place the second glove on the forearm of your dominant hand, thumb side down with the glove opening pointed toward your fingers. Grasp the inside glove cuff with your dominant hand through the gown, being careful to keep fingers inside the gown.
   h. With your nondominant hand, pull the glove cuff over the cuff of the gown.
   i. Grasp the sleeve of your gown and the cuff of the glove, and pull

the glove onto your dominant hand. ▼

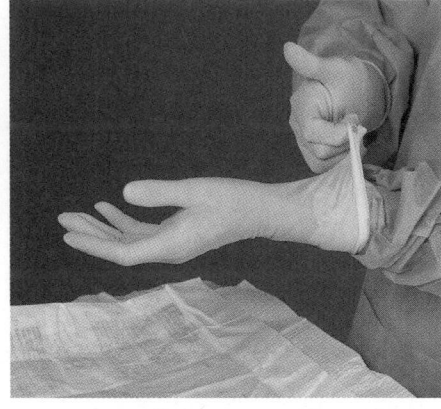

   j. Adjust the fingers in both gloves so the excess glove is pulled over the fingertips.
Maintains sterility of the gown and gloves by maintaining a closed system. The final adjustment of the gloves is done when both gloves are in place, to prevent contaminating the gloves.

6. Grasp the waist tie on the gown, and hand the tie to the circulating nurse or a co-worker who is wearing a hair cover and mask. Your co-worker will grab the tie with sterile forceps. The tie is considered sterile. You will need help pulling it around you. A co-worker can help you. Using sterile forceps keeps the tie sterile.

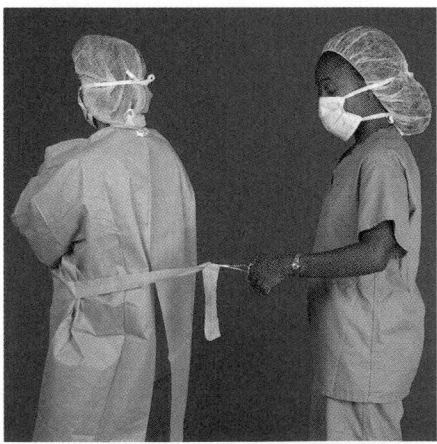

7. Make a three-quarter turn, and receive the tie from your co-worker.
Because only areas within your field of vision are considered sterile, a co-worker must pull the waist tie around you.

8. Secure the waist tie.
Ensures that the gown is secured and will not expose clothing to a sterile field.

Patient Teaching

If the patient is alert during the procedure, explain:

- The need for the sterile procedure
- Why he must not touch the drapes
- Why he must not move or talk once the drapes are in place
- Explain any special precautions during the procedure,

Documentation

- Donning sterile gown and gloves does not require documentation.
- You will need to chart the procedure performed and how the patient tolerated it.
- In the operating room, the circulating nurse charts about the surgery and the patient's response.

What if. . .

- **Your hand inadvertently comes through the cuff opening when putting on the gown?**

Change gowns. The cuff would have been contaminated and would then contaminate your glove.

Practice Resources

The Association of periOperative Registered Nurses (AORN, 2005a, 2005b, 2006); Centers for Disease Control and Prevention (2002).

Thinking About the Procedure

 Go to the *Fundamentals of Nursing Skills Videos,* **Asepsis: Sterile Gown and Gloves, Closed Method.**

1. In the early part of the procedure, a nurse in white is touching the surgical nurse with her hands. Is this an error? Why or why not?

2. After the surgical nurse has gloved, she hands her gown ties to an unsterile co-worker. This person does *not* take the tie with a forceps as the textbook procedure (above) instructs. Why, in this instance, is that acceptable?

 For suggested responses, go to Chapter 20, **Thinking About the Procedure Suggested Responses,** on the Student Resource Disk or DavisPlus at http://davisplus.fadavis.com/Wilkinson2

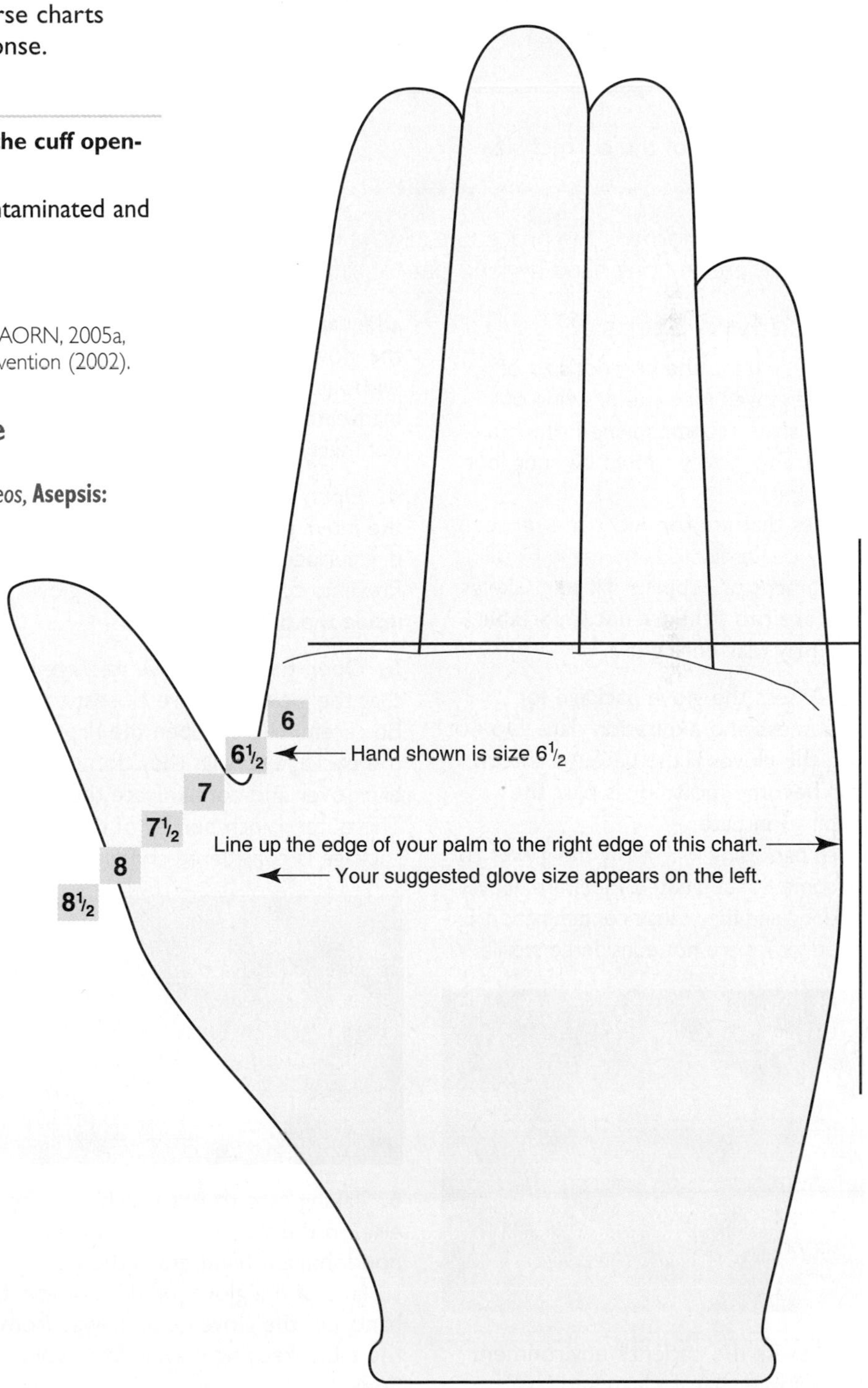

6

6½ ← Hand shown is size 6½

7

7½

8   Line up the edge of your palm to the right edge of this chart. →

8½   ← Your suggested glove size appears on the left.

Sterile glove sizes. This can help you determine the proper size glove you need for your hand.

Procedure 20-7 Sterile Gloves (Open Method)

➤ For steps to follow in *all* procedures, refer to the Universal Steps for All Procedures found on the inside back cover of Volume 2. For this procedure, also refer to Clinical Insights 20-2, 20-3, and 20-7 if you need more information.

Critical Aspects

- Remove all jewelry including rings and watches.
- Place the glove package on a clean, dry surface.
- Open the inner package so that the cuffs are closest to you.
- Apply the glove of your dominant hand first by touching only the inside of the glove (the folded-over cuff) with your nondominant hand.
- Apply the second glove by touching only the outer part of the glove with your already-gloved hand; keep your sterile thumb well away from your bare skin.
- Do not touch the gloves to any unsterile items.

Equipment

- Sterile gloves of the correct size

➤ When performing the procedure, always identify your patient according to agency policy and be attentive to standard precautions, hand hygiene, patient safety and privacy, body mechanics, and documentation.

Procedure Steps

1. Determine the correct size of sterile gloves (see the drawing of glove sizes accompanying Procedure 20-6). The gloves should be snug, but not tight.
Gloves that are too loose are more easily contaminated and make handling equipment or supplies difficult. Gloves that are too tight are uncomfortable and may tear during use.

2. Assess the glove package for intactness and expiration date. Do not use the gloves if the package is torn, has become moist, or is past the expiration date.
Torn packaging may allow the gloves to become contaminated. Moisture allows wicking and may cause contamination. Expired gloves are not considered sterile. ▼

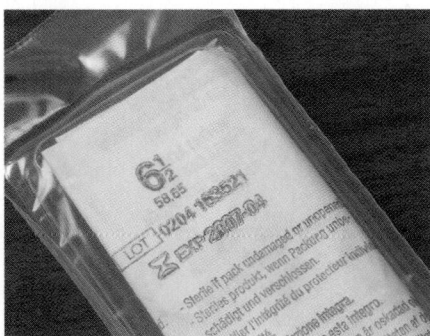

3. Assess the patient's environment for a space that is clean and has

adequate space to allow you to open the glove package. Don the gloves without touching a nonsterile item.
Inadvertently touching a nonsterile item will contaminate the gloves.

4. Open the outer wrapper, and place the inner glove package on a clean, dry surface.
Prevents contamination of the gloves inside the package.

5. Open the inner glove package so that the glove cuffs are closest to you. Be careful to fully open the flaps of the package so that they do not fold back over and contaminate the gloves.
The outer 1 inch border of the glove package is considered contaminated. ▼

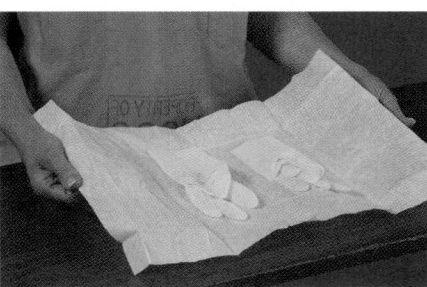

6. Taking care to not touch anything else on the sterile field, with your nondominant hand, grasp the inner surface of the glove for the dominant hand. Lift the glove up and away from the table, keeping it away from your body.

The inside of the glove is not considered sterile because it is in contact with your skin. Lifting the glove up and away from the table prevents you from accidentally touching the table or your clothing while donning the glove and thereby contaminating the glove.

7. Slide your dominant hand into the glove, keeping your hand and fingers above your waist and away from your body.
The area below the waistline is considered contaminated. Keeping gloves away from your body prevents accidental contamination. ▼

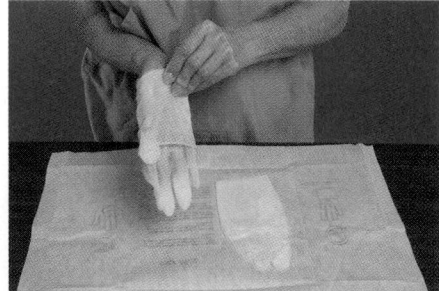

8. Slide your gloved fingers under the cuff of the glove for the nondominant hand, keeping your gloved thumb well away from your ungloved hand. Lift the glove up and away from the table and away from your body.

The outside of the glove is sterile and may be touched with your sterile gloved hand. ▼

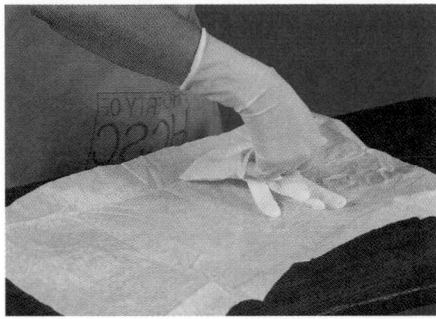

9. With gloved fingers still under the cuff, slide your nondominant hand into

the glove and pull it on, being careful to avoid contact with your gloved hand, especially the thumb. ▼

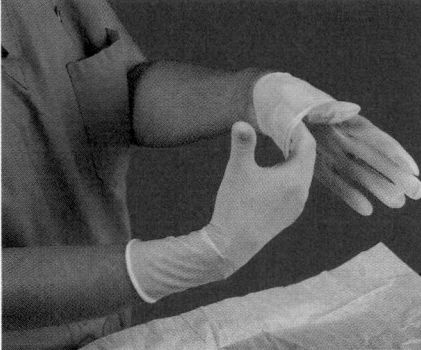

10. Adjust both gloves to fit your fingers. If necessary, pull the fingers of the gloves down so that no excess is at the fingertips.

Adjusting your gloves after both have been donned decreases the risk of contamination and allows for greater dexterity during the procedure.

11. Keep your hands between shoulder and waist level in front of you.

Keeps the gloves within your field of vision to avoid contamination.

Note: To remove soiled gloves after the procedure, refer to Procedure 20-3.

Patient Teaching

Explain the reason sterile gloves are needed for the procedure.

Home Care

- Many home care procedures are clean rather than sterile. The client is in his own environment and not surrounded by other patients, who may serve as hosts for infection.
- You may need to teach caregivers how to apply sterile gloves for some procedures. No modifications are required. Demonstrate the procedure, and have the caregiver do a return demonstration.

Documentation

- No special documentation is needed for sterile gloving.
- Chart the procedure you performed and the patient's response to the procedure.

Practice Resources
Association of periOperative Registered Nurses (AORN, 2005a, 2006).

Thinking About the Procedure

 Go to the *Fundamentals of Nursing Skills Videos,* **Asepsis: Sterile Gloves (Open Method).**

1. At the beginning of the procedure, the nurse opens the outer (clear plastic) glove package and turns the inner (white paper) package out on a table top. Does this break sterile technique? Why or why not?

2. There is no break in sterility, but at one point in the procedure, the nurse almost contaminates a glove. What happened?

 For suggested responses, go to Chapter 20, **Thinking About the Procedure Suggested Responses,** on the Student Resource Disk or DavisPlus at http://davisplus.fadavis.com/Wilkinson2

Procedure 20-8 ■ Sterile Fields

➤ For steps to follow in *all* procedures, refer to the Universal Steps for All Procedures found on the inside back cover of Volume 2. For this procedure, also refer to Clinical Insights 20-2, 20-3, and 20-7 if you need more information.

Critical Aspects

- Prepare the sterile field as close as possible to the time of use.
- Do not cover the sterile field once established.
- Do not turn away from the sterile field.
- Inspect for package integrity, inclusion of sterile indicator, and/or expiration date. Do not use outdated items.
- Clear a space and prepare the patient before setting up the sterile field.
- Establish the sterile field with a sterile drape or sterile package wrapper.
- Add items to the sterile field by gently dropping them onto the sterile field.
- Pour sterile solutions into a sterile bowl or receptacle without touching the bowl or splashing onto the sterile field.
- Don sterile gloves and perform procedure.

(continued on next page)

Procedure 20-8 ■ **Sterile Fields** (continued)

Equipment
■ Package of sterile supplies required for the procedure
■ Sterile gloves of the correct size

■ Procedure 20-8A Setting Up a Sterile Field

➤ When performing the procedure, always identify your patient according to agency policy and be attentive to standard precautions, hand hygiene, patient safety and privacy, body mechanics, and documentation.

Procedure Steps

1. Assess the sterility of all packages and equipment. Check to make sure the packaging is intact and the expiration dates have not passed.
Only sterile items should enter a sterile field. Any compromise in packaging means that the item is assumed not to be sterile.

2. Arrange the environment for performing the sterile procedure.
   a. Clean off the surface you will use to set up the sterile field.
Inadequate space causes inadvertent contamination during sterile procedures.

   b. Position the patient as needed for the procedure.
Allows you to immediately proceed with the planned procedure. Once the sterile field is established, air movement can create contamination of the sterile items.

Procedure Variation
Using Sterile Packaged Equipment

3. Place the sterile package on a clean, dry surface.
Prevents contamination of the sterile item. If a surface is damp, strike-through may occur, making the item unsterile. ▼

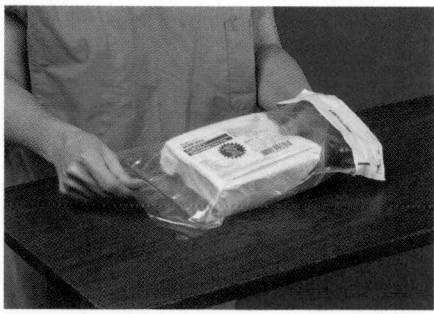

4. Open the flap away from you first to prevent passing an unsterile arm over the sterile items
If you move an unsterile item over a sterile field, the field is no longer considered to be sterile. ▼

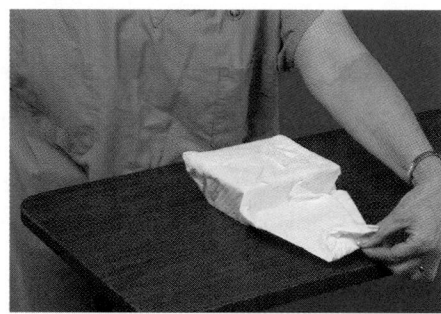

5. Open the side flaps. ▼

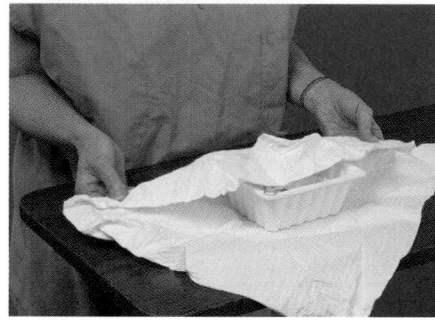

6. Pull the final flap toward you. The wrapper is now the sterile field. The area 1 inch from the edge of the wrapper and 1 inch from the table edge is considered unsterile. Do not readjust the sterile area after the package has been opened.
Only the horizontal surface of the draped area is considered sterile. Any part of the sterile wrapper that falls below the level of the sterile area (e.g., top of the table) is considered

unsterile. If you move the field after opening, the field shifts and places unsterile areas of the wrapper on the surface. ▼

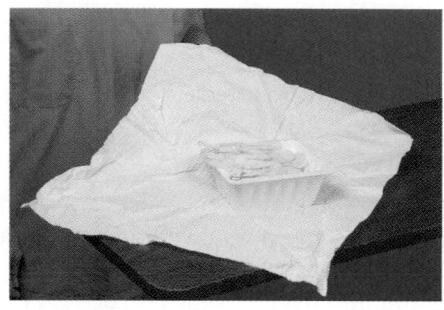

Procedure Variation
Opening a Fabric- or Paper-Wrapped Sterile Package

7. Check and remove the chemical indicator strip.
The indicator tape per manufacturer or institution confirms that the package was sterilized. The pack usually is also dated.

8. Remove the outer wrapper, and place the inner wrapped package on a clean, dry surface.
The outer wrapper is not considered sterile and is discarded.

9. Open the inner wrapper following the same technique described in steps 3 through 6.

Procedure Variation
Using a Sterile Drape
Omit steps 3 through 9.

10. Place the package on a clean, dry surface. Hold the edge of the package flap down toward the table, grasp the top edge of the package, and peel back. The sterile drape is inside the outer wrapper. This maneuver opens the

package without contaminating the sterile drape. ▼

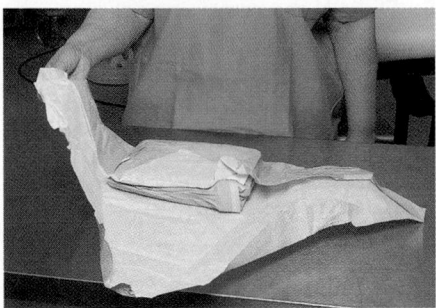

11. Pick up the sterile drape by the corner. Allow the drape to fall open, away from your body and away from unsterile surfaces. Place it on a clean, dry surface by touching only the edge of the drape. Avoid fanning the drape. A 1-inch border around the sterile drape is considered unsterile.

■ **Procedure 20-8B** **Adding Supplies to a Sterile Field**

➤ When performing the procedure, always identify your patient according to agency policy and be attentive to standard precautions, hand hygiene, patient safety and privacy, body mechanics, and documentation.

Procedure Steps

1. Hold the sterile package in your dominant hand. Grasping the corner of the wrapper, peel each corner back with your nondominant hand.
The inside of the wrapper is sterile and will be used as a barrier when placing the sterile item onto a sterile field.

2. Holding the contents several inches above the field, allow the supplies to drop onto the field inside the 1-inch border of the sterile field. Do not let your arms pass over the sterile field.

By holding the package upside down, you ensure that the sterile part of the package is facing the sterile field and that you deposit the item onto the sterile field. ▼

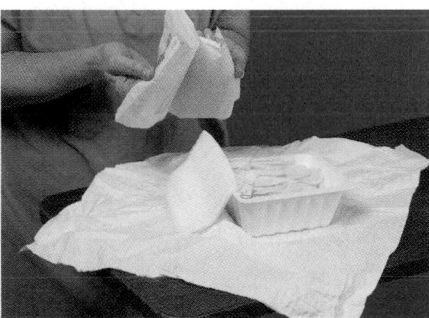

3. Dispose of the wrapper, and continue opening any needed supplies for the procedure.
Once sterile gloves are on, you will not be able to add items without contaminating the gloves.

■ **Procedure 20-8C** **Adding Sterile Solutions to a Sterile Field**

➤ When performing the procedure, always identify your patient according to agency policy and be attentive to standard precautions, hand hygiene, patient safety and privacy, body mechanics, and documentation.

Procedure Steps

1. Use a sterile bowl or receptacle if the sterile field is fabric or at risk for strike-through.
You may add a sterile bowl to the field by unwrapping (as discussed above) and holding the bowl through the sterile wrapper as you place it near the edge of the sterile field. The sterile bowl may also be placed next to the sterile field.
If you place the sterile bowl on the field, place it near the edge so that

you can pour the sterile solution from the back of the sterile field. This prevents you from reaching over and thereby contaminating the field.

2. Check that the sterile solution is correct, and confirm that the expiration date has not passed.
Check the solution as you would a medication. Validate that the solution and concentration are correct and have not expired. ➤

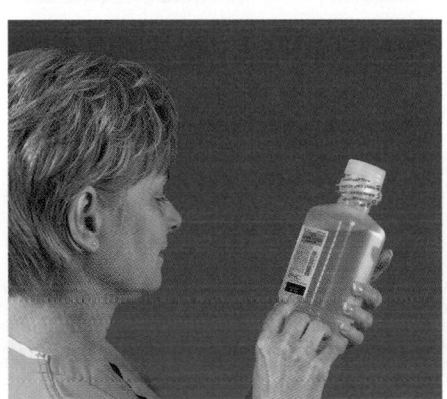

3. Remove the cap off the solution bottle by lifting it directly up and throw it away.

(continued on next page)

Procedure 20-8 ■ Sterile Fields (continued)

The edge of the container is considered contaminated after the contents have been poured and the sterility of the contents cannot be ensured if the cap is replaced.

4. Hold the bottle 4 to 6 inches above the bowl and pour the needed amount of the solution into the bowl. Prevents you from inadvertently touching the sterile bowl with the bottle and thereby, contaminating the bowl. Limited height reduces the risk of splashing, which strikes through and contaminates a cloth or permeable sterile field. A disposable sterile drape

generally has a plastic membrane in the middle to prevent strike-through. ▼

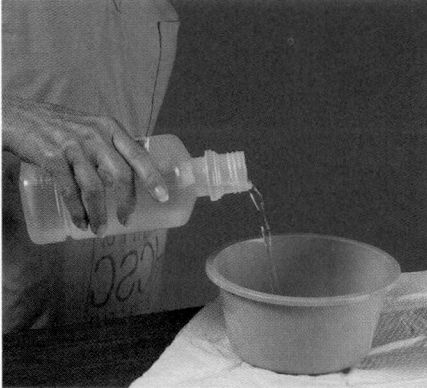

5. Discard the remaining solution. Reusing open containers may cause contamination due to drops contacting the unsterile areas and running back over the container opening.

6. Before donning sterile gloves to perform the procedure, double-check that all supplies have been added to the field. Do not leave the sterile field unattended. Do not turn your back to the sterile field.
If a sterile item is out of your field of vision, it is no longer considered sterile because airborne particles, insects, or liquids could contaminate the field.

Home Care

■ Most sterile procedures in the home are done by visiting nurses.
■ Procedures performed by clients or family members are usually clean rather than sterile.

Documentation

■ You will not document the actual setting up of the sterile field.
■ Document the procedure, your assessment of the patient's tolerance for the procedure, and your assessment of the area being treated by the procedure.

Practice Resources
Association of periOperative Registered Nurses (AORN, 2006).

Thinking About the Procedure

 Go to the *Fundamentals of Nursing Skills Videos*, **Asepsis: Sterile Fields.**

1. When opening the large sterile bowl, what is the first thing the nurse does to ensure sterility?

2. What does the nurse in the DVD do with the cap and the bottle of solution after she pours from it into the sterile bowl? Why does she not set it beside the sterile bowl?

 For suggested responses, go to Chapter 20, **Thinking About the Procedure Suggested Responses,** on the Student Resource Disk or DavisPlus at http://davisplus.fadavis.com/Wilkinson2

Clinical Insights

Clinical Insight 20-1 ▶ Guidelines for Hand Hygiene

Handwashing

When to Wash

■ When hands are visibly dirty or soiled with blood or body fluids
■ When arriving on and leaving the patient care unit
■ Before direct contact with a patient, even if you intend to wear procedure gloves
■ Before donning gloves (either procedure or sterile)
■ After removing gloves
Hand hygiene is required regardless of whether gloves are used or changed.

■ After contact with a patient's intact skin (e.g., when lifting a patient or taking a blood pressure)
■ After contact with body fluids, mucous membranes, nonintact skin, and wound dressings even if hands are not visibly soiled

■ When moving from a contaminated body site to a clean body site during patient care
■ Before and after contact with objects and equipment in the patient's immediate vicinity.
■ Before eating and after using a restroom. Use soap and water.
■ Before and after touching any area on your face and hair

What to Use

■ Use alcohol-based hand rub (at least 60% alcohol) for routine hand hygiene and if hands are not visibly soiled.
■ Use soap and water when hands are dirty or visibly soiled.
■ Use soap and water after using a restroom.
■ Use soap and water if exposure to *Bacillus anthracis* (or other spore-producing bacteria) is suspected or proven.

- Avoid using hot water.
- Use disposable paper towels.

How to Wash

Refer to Procedure 20-1 and

 Go to the *Fundamentals of Nursing Skills Videos,* **Asepsis: Handwashing.**

Fingernails

- Do not wear artificial nails or extenders when caring for patients at high risk (e.g., in intensive care and oncology units). The 2007 epic2 guidelines, in the United Kingdom, recommend that nail polish and artificial nails and extenders not be worn at all. The CDC's position is that although studies provide evidence that wearing artificial nails poses an infection hazard, additional studies are warranted. It is best to not wear nail polish because it chips easily.
- Keep nail tips less than ¼-inch long (CDC). Other researchers suggest nail tip length not more than 2 mm (not past the tips of the fingers).

Longer nails are associated with increased microbial carriage on the hands. The 2007 epic2 guidelines, in the United Kingdom, recommend short nails.

Jewelry

- We recommend that you not wear a watch or rings in the clinical setting, especially rings with stones.

In 2007, the CDC stated that jewelry is still an unresolved issue. They noted that hand contamination with potential pathogens increased when nurses wear rings, but that no studies have related that practice to the transmission of pathogens to patients. However, the 2007 epic2 guidelines, in the United Kingdom advise healthcare workers to remove wrist and hand jewelry.

- If your agency permits you to wear jewelry, clean it thoroughly and often.

Practice Resources

Boyce, J., & Pittet, D. (2002); Pratt, R., Pellowe, C., Wilson, J., et al. (2007); Rupp, M., Fitzgerald, T., Puumala, S., et al. (2008); Siegel, J., Rhinehart, E., Jackson, M., et al. (2007).

Clinical Insight 20-2 ▶ **Providing a Clean Patient Environment**

The following guidelines are used along with standard precautions for all patients. A clean environment includes the surfaces in a patient's room, as well as supplies, equipment, and other objects brought into the room.

Supplies and Equipment

- Do not stock rooms with unnecessary supplies.
- Consider supplies that are brought into a patient's room contaminated. Do not return them to the linen or supply cart; instead, handle them according to agency policy.
- Also consider contaminated any items brought from the patient's home, gifts from visitors, and so forth.
- Mobile computing devices should be cleaned (e.g., pagers, smartphones, point-of-care keyboards, and medication administration devices). However, most hospitals lack infection prevention policies for mobile devices. Be sure to wash your hands after using such a device.

Often, electronic devices cannot be decontaminated without damage; in that case, only hand hygiene can protect you and the patient from these vectors.

- Clean stethoscopes with alcohol before use on a patient. Disposable stethoscopes are commercially available, but not commonly seen in healthcare agencies (some hospitals do have disposable stethoscopes for patients in isolation or on transmission-based precautions).

Stethoscopes are often contaminated with *Staphylococcus aureus* because care providers do not clean them adequately between patients.

- Clean reusable equipment that is soiled with blood or body fluids according to agency policy—typically, autoclaving, ethylene oxide gas, or dry heat.
- Do not reuse equipment for the care of another patient until it has been cleaned and reprocessed appropriately.

- Dispose of single-use equipment that is soiled with blood or body fluids in appropriate biohazard containers.
- Wear gloves when handling equipment that is visibly contaminated. Perform hand hygiene.

Linens

- Carefully handle contaminated linens to prevent skin and mucous membrane exposures, contamination of clothing, and transfer of microorganisms to other patients or the environment.

Linens may harbor microorganisms that may transfer to your clothing, open skin, or mucous membranes, to then be carried to other clients or environment.

Uniforms and Lab Coats

- Do not wear a uniform (e.g., scrubs) or a lab coat for more than one day without laundering.

Care provider clothing is often contaminated as care providers move from patient to patient. The traditional white lab coats are being banned in some hospitals because they are a vehicle for dangerous pathogens. The CDC states that although contaminated clothing has not been implicated directly, the potential exists for it to transfer pathogens to patients.

- If you wash your uniforms at home, they require only washing with warm or hot water and detergent (except in the case of possible exposure to multidrug-resistant organisms, for which you should add bleach).

Spills and Waste

- Empty and clean bedpans, urinals, and emesis basins immediately after use.
- Place soiled dressings, drains, and so forth, in appropriate waterproof bags for disposal. Do not leave such used supplies in an open trash can.

(continued on next page)

Clinical Insight 20-2 ▶ **Providing a Clean Patient Environment** (continued)

■ Bag and remove soiled linens from the room immediately.
■ Wipe up small spills from table tops and floors. Notify the houskeeping or environmental services department for large spills.

Home Care

■ Teach clients and caregivers to keep the home environment clean.
■ To disinfect the home environment, use and teach caregivers to create, a dilute bleach solution. Mix 1 part regular-strength bleach to 50 parts water. The mixture may be stored for a month in an opaque container.

✚ NEVER mix the solution with other household cleaners. Be careful not to splash the bleach because it removes color from fabric and other objects, and keep it out of reach of children.

■ Washing dishware and eating utensils in a dishwasher with hot water and detergents is sufficient decontamination.

■ Healthcare workers in the home are a potential source of pathogens and should use caution to avoid infecting the patient.

Needles and Sharps

✚ Do not recap, bend, break, or hand-manipulate used needles. If recapping is necessary, use a one-handed scoop technique. Place used sharps in puncture-resistant containers.

Practice Resources

Carling, P., Parry, M., & Von Beheren, S. (2008); Centers for Disease Control and Prevention (2008c); Davidson, S., & Malkary, G. (2008); Perry, C., Marshall, R., & Jones, E. (2001); Siegel, J., Rhinehart, E., Jackson, M., et al. (2007).

Clinical Insight 20-3 ▶ **Following CDC Standard Precautions**

Standard precautions (Tier 1) apply to all clients and should be used whenever there is a possibility of coming in contact with blood, body fluids (except sweat), excretions and secretions, mucous membranes, and breaks in the skin.

These precautions are designed to protect you from exposure to potential pathogens, to decrease the likelihood that you will transmit pathogens among patients, and to protect the patient from microorganisms that you may carry.

✚ Assume that every person may be infected or colonized with an organism that could be transmitted to others

TIER 1 COMPONENT	RECOMMENDATIONS
Hand Hygiene	■ Perform hand hygiene after touching blood, body fluids, secretions, excretions, contaminated items; immediately after removing gloves; between patient contacts. Refer to Clinical Insight 20-1 for details.
Respiratory Hygiene/ Cough Etiquette for Patients	■ Instruct symptomatic persons to cover mouth/nose when sneezing/coughing. ■ Provide and use tissues and dispose in a no-touch receptacle. ■ Perform hand hygiene after soiling hands with respiratory secretions or after using a tissue or covering the mouth/nose. ■ Wear a surgical mask if tolerated (some patients may not be able to tolerate the decreased oxygen that is available when breathing room air through a mask), or do not come within 3 feet of another person if possible.
Masks and Eye Protection (for the Nurse)	■ Wear a mask and eye protection or a face shield to protect mucous membranes of the eyes, nose, and mouth during patient care activities that are likely to generate splashes or sprays of blood, body fluids, secretions, and excretions. ■ Barrier protection helps keep microorganisms from accidentally entering your mucous membranes, eyes, nose, or mouth.
Patient Placement	■ Place in a single-patient room if the patient is at increased risk of transmitting or acquiring infection, does not maintain appropriate hygiene, is likely to contaminate the environment, or is at increased risk of developing adverse outcome following infection.
Gowns	■ Wear a clean, nonsterile, nonpermeable gown during procedures and activities when you anticipate contact of clothing or exposed skin with blood or body fluids, secretions, and excretions (e.g., when there is a risk of spray or splash onto clothing). ■ Promptly remove the gown once it is soiled. Avoid contaminating clothing when removing the gown. ■ Wash hands after removing the gown. ■ See Procedure 20-2, Donning and Removing PPE.

TIER I COMPONENT	RECOMMENDATIONS
Needles and Sharps	■ Never recap, bend, or break used needles, or otherwise manipulate them using both hands, or use any other technique that involves directing the point of a needle toward any part of the body. Instead, use either a one-handed "scoop" technique or a mechanical device designed for holding the needle sheath (see Procedure 23-10, Recapping Needles...). ■ Use safety features when available. ■ Place "sharps" (e.g., scalpels, needles, and so on) in puncture-resistant containers for disposal.
Patient Resuscitation	■ Use one-way valve mouthpieces, resuscitation bags, or other ventilation devices as an alternative to mouth-to-mouth resuscitation methods in situations when the need for resuscitation is predictable. To prevent contact between rescuer's and client's mucous membranes and airflow, preventing transmission of microorganisms.
Soiled Patient-Care Equipment, Environment, Textiles & Laundry	■ See Clinical Insight 20-2 for details. ■ Wear gloves if the equipment or laundry is visibly contaminated. ■ Handle equipment, textiles, and laundry in a manner to prevent transfer of microorganisms to others and the environment. ■ Perform hand hygiene. ■ Develop procedures for routine care, cleaning, and disinfection of environmental surfaces, especially frequently touched surfaces in patient-care areas.
Gloves	***When to Wear*** ■ If you have an area of irritation or a break in the skin, wear gloves or apply an occlusive dressing during patient contact. ■ Wear gloves when contact with blood or other potentially infectious materials, mucous membranes, and nonintact skin could occur. ***When to Remove or Change*** ■ Remove gloves immediately after caring for a patient. Avoid touching clean items, environmental surfaces, or another patient. ■ Do not wear the same gloves for care of more than one patient; do not wash gloves and reuse gloves between patient contact. Research shows that washing and reusing gloves between patient contacts results in increased bacterial counts on the hands. ■ Change gloves during patient care if moving from a contaminated body site to a clean. ■ Change gloves between tasks or procedures on the same patient if you have made contact with material that may contain a high concentration of microorganisms. ***Use and Storage*** ■ When preparing for a procedure, first collect equipment and place at the bedside ready for use; then wash your hands and put on gloves just before performing the procedure. Donning gloves ahead of time allows them to become contaminated before the procedure. ■ Do not carry gloves in your pocket. Keep them in their original box and remove them when and where required. ■ Do not store gloves on top of trash containers or on windowsills. ■ Hand washing or disinfection is required regardless of whether gloves are used or changed. Gloves are not completely impermeable to microorganisms; furthermore, they may leak or tear. Hands can be easily contaminated when removing gloves, as well.

COMPARISON OF GLOVE MATERIALS

	Natural Rubber	Synthetic Materials		
Material	Latex	**Nitrile**	**Vinyl**	***Polyethylene (or polythene)
Durability	Flexible, strong, less prone to splitting	Resists tears and punctures	Tear more readily than latex	Prone to splitting; thin, tear easily
Barrier Performance	Greater protection from viruses than vinyl gloves	Comparable to latex	More permeable and provide less protection from bloodborne viruses than other gloves.	Usually loose fitting, so do not protect well from contamination

(continued on the next page)

Clinical Insight 20-3 ➤ **Following CDC Standard Precautions** (continued)

TIER 1 COMPONENT	RECOMMENDATIONS			
Material	**Latex**	**Nitrile**	**Vinyl**	***Polyethylene (or polythene)**
Allergic Reactions	Associated with allergic reactions	Allergic reactions have been reported	Not associated with allergic reactions; good alternative for those with latex sensitivity	Not reported
Fit	Close-fitting; allows for tactile sensitivity and dexterity more than other materials			Loose fitting, less tactile sensitivity and dexterity than other materials
Cost, Compared to Latex	—	More expensive than latex	Comparable to latex	Cheap in comparison to other gloves
Appropriate Uses	▪ When handling infectious materials; use powder-free latex gloves. ▪ Don't use oil-based lotions (they can cause gloves to deteriorate).	When handling infectious materials	Use for activities not likely to involve contact with infectious materials (e.g., food preparation, cleaning)	Use for activities not likely to involve contact with infectious materials (e.g., food preparation, cleaning), but not in healthcare settings.

*Note: Polyethylene gloves are not recommended for use in healthcare settings.

Practice Resources

Best practices: Evidence-based nursing procedures (2nd ed.), (2007); Boyce, J., & Pittet, D. (2002); Occupational Safety & Health Administration, U.S. Department of Labor (n.d.); Pratt, R., Pellowe, C., Wilson, J., et al. (2007); Siegel, J., Rhinehart, E., Jackson, M., et al. (2007); U. S. Department of Labor (n.d.a).

Clinical Insight 20-4 ➤ **Following Transmission-Based Precautions**

Note: Refer to Clinical Insight 20-3 if you need to review standard precautions.

Use transmission-based (Tier 2) precautions when the routes of transmission are not completely interrupted using Standard Precautions alone. Recall from the discussion of the chain of infection, in Volume 1, that pathogens may be transmitted by contact, droplet, or air. Each mode of transmission requires a different approach to prevent infection, and has a different set of precautions. For some diseases, you may need to use more than one of the categories.

For all transmission-based precautions, institute measures to counteract adverse effects of isolation on patients (i.e., anxiety, depression, perceptions of stigma, reduced contact with staff, and increases in preventable adverse events).

Helps to improve acceptance by patients and adherence by staff.

Contact Precautions

Contact precautions are used when direct contact with the patient or the patient's environment can lead to spread of the pathogen. This is the most common form of transmission. Draining wounds, dressings, patient supplies, and secretions are sources of infection. Indirect contact, or contact with fomites, can also transmit pathogens that spread by this method.

Contact precautions include the following:

▪ **Follow all standard precautions.**

Patient Placement and Transport

▪ Place the patient in a private room when available. Otherwise, place in a room with a patient with an active infection caused by the same organism and no other infections.
Ideally, consult with an infection preventionist for patient placement. A private room provides the most effective protection.

▪ When transporting the patient, ensure that infected or colonized areas of the body are contained and covered.
▪ *Ambulatory care*: Place the patient in an exam room or cubicle as soon as possible.

Personal Protective Equipment

▪ Wear clean nonsterile gloves when touching the patient's intact skin. Don gloves on entry to the room.
▪ Wear a clean gown you anticipate your clothing may contact the patient or any contaminated items in the room.
▪ Remove PPE and observe hand hygiene before leaving the room. Take care that your skin and clothing do not contact environmental surfaces on the way out of the room.

Equipment, Supplies, and Environment

▪ Keep contact precaution supplies just outside the patient's room on a cart.

- Double bag all linen and trash (or use a single waterproof bag), and clearly mark them contaminated.
- Use disposable equipment (e.g., blood pressure cuffs) if possible; otherwise, clean and disinfect the equipment per institutional policy before removing them from the room and before use on another patient.
- Ensure that the patient room is cleaned and disinfected at least daily.
- *Home care:* Limit the amount of nondisposable equipment brought into the home. If possible, leave the equipment in the home until discharge from home care.
- *Home care:* If equipment cannot remain in the home, clean and disinfect items before taking them from the home, or place them in a plastic bag for transport to a reprocessing area.

Other

- Follow any additional precautions specific to the microorganism.
- Discontinue contact precautions after signs and symptoms have resolved or according to pathogen-specific recommendations.

Droplet Precautions

Droplet precautions are used when the known or suspected pathogen can be spread via moist, large droplets (e.g., sneezing, coughing, talking). Droplets can spread infection by direct contact with mucous membranes or through indirect contact, for example, suctioning or touching a bedside table that was contaminated with moist droplets and then rubbing your eyes. Droplet precautions include the following:
- **Follow all standard precautions.**
- **Follow all contact precautions.**

Patient Placement and Transport

- If no private room is available and the patient must be placed with patients who have a different infection, ensure that the patients are physically separated by more than 3 feet. Keep the privacy curtain closed.
This minimizes contact between patients. Ideally, consult with an infection preventionist for patient placement. A private room provides the most effective protection.
- Limit transport outside the room to medically necessary purposes; if transport is necessary, the patient should wear a mask. The transporter is not required to mask.

Personal Protective Equipment

- Keep droplet precaution supplies just outside the patient's room on a cart.
- Wear a mask when working within 3 feet of the patient. Don the mask on entry into the room. Whether to wear goggles is an unresolved issue. Follow agency policy.
- Change PPE and perform hand hygiene between contact with patients in the same room, regardless of whether one or both patients are on droplet precautions.

Other

- Instruct patients to observe respiratory hygiene/cough etiquette.

- Discontinue droplet precautions after signs and symptoms have resolved or according to pathogen-specific recommendations.

Airborne Precautions

Airborne precautions are used to control the spread of infections that are transmitted person-to-person on air currents. Airborne infections include tuberculosis, varicella (chickenpox), severe acute respiratory syndrome (SARS), and rubeola (measles). Pathogens that are spread by this method are very small and can be easily transmitted through ventilating systems as well as by any activities that stir the air, such as fanning sheets, shaking out towels, or sweeping the floor. Airborne precautions include the following:
- **Follow all standard precautions.**
- **Follow all contact precautions.**

Patient Placement and Transport

- Place the patient in an airborne infection isolation room (AIIR)—one with negative pressure that discharges and exchanges the air outside or through a high-efficiency particulate air (HEPA) filtration system. Monitor air pressure daily (usually this is via an electronic device with an alarm).
- Keep the room door closed when not required for entry and exit.
To maintain the negative pressure and contain the airborne organisms.

- If such a room is not available, transfer the patient to a facility where one is available.
- In the event of an outbreak involving large numbers of patients who require airborne precautions, consult with infection preventionists for patient placement.
- Limit transport of the patient outside the room to medically necessary purposes; if transport is necessary, cover any infectious skin lesions and have the patient wear a mask. The transporter is not required to mask if the patient is wearing a mask and infectious skin lesions are covered. Notify the receiving department.
So the receiving department can take airborne precautions.

- *Ambulatory care:* Triage and identify patients with suspected airborne precautions upon entry to the agency. Place the patient in an AIIR as soon as possible. If one is not available, place a mask on the patient and place him in an exam room. Do not reuse the room for at least an hour after the patient leaves it.

Personal Protective Equipment

- Keep airborne isolation supplies just outside the patient's room on a cart.
- Don a mask on entering the room. Wear a special, fit-tested, approved mask (e.g., N95 respirator) if the patient is suspected of having pulmonary tuberculosis or smallpox.
- Remove your respirator/mask outside the room after closing the door. If the respirator is not disposable, clean and store according to the manufacturer's instructions.
- When using a respirator mask, check the seal. Hold your hands over the respirator and exhale. If you feel

(continued on next page)

Clinical Insight 20-4 ▶ Following Transmission-Based Precautions (continued)

air around your nose, adjust the nosepiece; if you feel air at the edges, adjust the straps.

■ When the patient has rubeola, chickenpox, or disseminated zoster, CDC makes no recommendation about use of PPE if, based on your history of vaccination or disease, you think you are presumed immune to the disease.

■ If the patient is known to have or is suspected of having measles (rubeola) or varicella (chickenpox), only immune caregivers should provide care. Immune caregivers do not need to wear masks.

Other

■ Discontinue airborne precautions according to pathogen-specific recommendations of the CDC.
■ Tape a waterproof bag to the bedside. *To facilitate proper disposal of tissues*

Practice Resources

American Heart Association (2008); *Best practices: Evidence-based nursing procedures* (2nd ed.) (2007); Pratt, R., Pellowe, C., Wilson, J., et al. (2007); Siegel, J., Rhinehart, E., Jackson, M., et al. (2007); U.S. Department of Labor (n.d.a).

Clinical Insight 20-5 ▶ Preventing Multidrug-Resistant Organism Infections (MDROs)

✚ *Note:* Refer to Clinical Insights 20-1, 20-2, 20-3, and 20-4, which are also followed in preventing the transmission of MDROs. Preventing MDROs requires some measures over and above the other precautions, but does not replace them.

The CDC recommends that hospitals try to reduce infection rates by improving hygiene and standard precautions; and resorting to special measures, such as screening all high-risk patients, only if other methods fail.

■ **Perform meticulous hand hygiene, for *all* patient care.**
■ **Observe standard precautions for *all* patients.** See Clinical Insight 20-2. Standard precautions, including hand hygiene, are absolutely essential in preventing spread of infection. There is some evidence that standard precautions alone may be as effective as isolating MRSA patients in private rooms and wearing PPE (Halcomb, Griffiths, & Fernandez, 2008). However, most studies reporting successful MDRO control used a combination of several control measures.
■ **Observe (or modify) contact precautions** routinely for patients infected or colonized with target MDROs. Usually this continues until the patient has a negative culture for the organism.

The type of organism and extent of disease it causes varies by population and institution. Approaches to prevention and control must be tailored to the needs of individual institutions and populations.

Patient Placement and Transport

■ Assign the patient to a single room, if available. Give highest priority to those having conditions that may lead to transmission of infection (e.g., uncontained secretions or excretions, inability to follow cough hygiene).
■ If no single room is available, place with a patient with the same MDRO.

Personal Protective Equipment

■ Use masks according to standard precautions when performing splash-generating procedures (e.g., wound irrigation). Masks are not recommended for routine care (e.g., upon room entry).
■ Use gloves and gowns according to standard precautions.
■ *Home care and ambulatory care:* Follow standard precautions for PPE.

Equipment, Supplies, and Environment

■ Ensure that patient rooms are cleaned well and often. Disinfect high-touch surfaces (e.g., bed rails, door knobs, bedside commodes) in the room.
■ Dedicate noncritical equipment (e.g., stethoscope, blood pressure cuff) to use on individual patients colonized or infected with MDROs.
■ Follow standard precautions for handling linens and eating utensils.
■ *Home care:* Limit the amount of patient-care equipment brought into the homes of patients infected or colonized with MDROs. See Contact Precautions in Clinical Insight 20-4 to review this.

Other

■ Actively observe for symptoms of infections, such as MRSA. Some institutions require screening cultures at admission, or on admission to certain units (e.g., intensive care).
■ Be aware of and practice preventive measures, such as:
  Use intravenous and urinary catheters only when essential, and with scrupulous sterile technique.
  Special measures to prevent lower respiratory tract infection in intubated patients
  Judiciously select and use antimicrobials.
Note: If MDROs continue to be a problem in spite of diligent infection control measures, your agency might

consider intensifying infection control practices. For example:

- Donning gowns and gloves before or upon entry to the patient's room
- Assigning the same personnel to the care of MDRO patients only
- Stopping new admissions to the unit or facility

- Obtaining environmental cultures
- Screening high-risk patients on admission

Practice Resources

Calfee, D., Salgado, C., Classen, D., et al. (2008); Halcomb, E., Griffiths, R., & Fernandez, R. (2008); Institute for Healthcare Improvement (n.d.a); Institute for Healthcare Improvement (n.d.b); Siegel, J., Rhinehart, E., Jackson, M., et al. (2007).

Clinical Insight 20-6 ▶ Maintaining a "Protective Environment" in Special Situations

The CDC recommends a protective environment (isolation) for a special class of stem cell transplant patients, who are neutropenic (and therefore immunocompromised) secondary to chemotherapy. You may, in some facilities, encounter protective isolation for other types of patients, as well. However, in most instances, standard and transmission-based precautions are adequate protection for those patients. In special situations:

- **Follow standard precautions** meticulously, including hand hygiene before and after patient contact.
- **Follow transmission-based precautions** as indicated by a suspected or proven infection.

Patient Room

- Maintain a protective environment (PE) room.
- Avoid a standing collection of water in the room (e.g., with fresh flowers or humidifiers) to prevent fungi and bacteria typically found in this water.

Personal Protective Equipment

- PPE is not required for care providers or visitors for routine entry into the room, unless approaching the patient.
- If the patient must have diagnostic or other procedures that cannot be performed in the PE room, provide respiratory protection (e.g., an N95 respirator, minimal contact with others).
- Gown, gloves, and mask are used for visitors and care providers according to standard precautions and as indicated for suspected or proven infections for which they are recommended.
- Refer to Clinical Insight 20-2 and Procedure 20-5 to review donning and removing PPE.

Care Providers, Visitors

- Only healthy caregivers should provide care. Do not care for such a patient if you have an upper respiratory infection, for example.

- Healthcare workers caring for patients in protective isolation should not also be providing care for other patients with active infections.
- Restrict visitors who have a cold or contagious illness.

Housekeeping/Environmental Services

- Carpeting in patient rooms or halls traps soil and can wick moisture, creating an environment for growth of microbes.
- Upholstered furniture and furnishings tend to harbor microbes.
- Avoid dusting methods that scatter particles in the air.
- If vacuum cleaning is necessary, use a vacuum cleaner equipped with a HEPA filter.
- Wet-dust horizontal surfaces daily with EPA-registered disinfectant or detergent.

Engineering

- Use of 99.7% efficiency particulate air (HEPA) filters to remove particles for incoming air at a specified flow rate of air
- Well-sealed rooms—no air leaks
- Ventilation as for airborne precautions
- Directed air flow within the room
- Positive room air pressure in relation to the corridor
- Back-up ventilation equipment (e.g., portable fans or filters)
- For patients who require both protected environment and airborne isolation, use an anteroom to control air in and out of the room.

Practice Resources

American Institute of Architects (2006); Siegel, J., Rhinehart, E., Jackson, M., et al. (2007).

Clinical Insight 20-7 ➤ Guidelines for Observing Sterile Technique

For steps in setting up a sterile field and adding supplies and solutions, see Procedure 20-7.
Tip: Sterile touches sterile. Unsterile touches unsterile.

Setting up the Field

■ Close doors and limit foot traffic when setting up a sterile field.
Air currents can carry dust and microorganisms.

■ Prepare a sterile field as close as possible to the time of use.
To minimize the opportunity for contamination via air currents.

■ You may establish a sterile field by using a sterile drape or by using the inner side of a sterile package wrapping. Touch the inside of the wrapper only after you don sterile gloves.

■ When you are placing a sterile drape, protect your gloved hands by cuffing the drape over your hands.

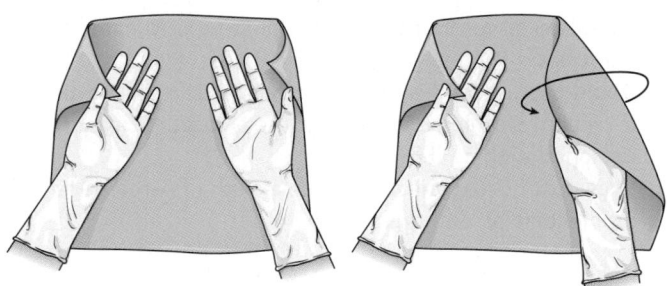

Protecting gloved hands.

What Areas are Considered Sterile?

■ A sterile field is sterile only on the horizontal plane. Consider nonsterile any material that drapes over the horizontal plane.

■ The border of a sterile drape is considered unsterile even if it remains on a horizontal surface. Consider a 1-inch margin around the drape unsterile.
Because it is in contact with contaminated surfaces.

■ If you are wearing sterile attire, only in the front of your body from the chest to the level of the sterile field is considered sterile.

■ Sleeve cuffs are considered unsterile when your hands pass beyond the cuff (they are sterile if you don gloves using the closed method).

Keeping the Field Sterile

■ No one in unsterile garb should come near a sterile field. They should remain at least 1 foot away.

■ Remain at least 1 foot away from nonsterile areas if you are wearing sterile garb.

■ Never turn your back to a sterile field. A sterile field or open sterile items must be kept in constant view.
You are responsible for monitoring and maintaining the sterility. If you cannot see the field, you do not know if it has become contaminated.

■ Keep conversation to a minimum around the sterile field.
To reduce the spread of droplets.

■ Avoid reaching over a sterile field even if you are in sterile garb.

■ Handle sterile equipment only if you are wearing sterile gloves.

■ Limit the amount of time a sterile field remains set up in advance of a procedure.

■ Liquid can act as a wick and contaminate a field. Sterile liquids must be contained in sterile bowls on the field or the sterile drape must be nonpermeable in order to avoid wicking.

Adding Sterile Items

■ Only sterile items can be placed on a sterile field.

■ Before adding items to a sterile field, inspect them immediately for proper packaging, integrity, and inclusion of a sterilization indicator.

■ Never assume an item is sterile. If there is any doubt about its sterility, consider it contaminated.

■ All items applied to a sterile field must be sterilized in an approved manner.

Practice Resources

The Association of periOperative Registered Nurses (AORN, 2006).

Diagnostic Testing

Common Tests for Evaluating the Presence of or Risk for Infection	
TEST	**DESCRIPTION**
White blood cell (WBC) count with differential	A breakdown of the number and types of WBCs; normal WBC count is 5,000–10,000/mm^3.
Blood cultures	A sample of blood placed on culture media and evaluated for growth of pathogens. Normally, should show no growth of infectious microorganisms.
Urine cultures	Urine is normally sterile with no microorganism growth.

Common Tests for Evaluating the Presence of or Risk for Infection—cont'd

TEST	DESCRIPTION
Throat cultures, wound cultures	Presence of microorganisms is normal, but there should be no growth of infectious microorganisms.
Disease titers	Blood tests for specific disease immunity (e.g., to rubella)
Panels to evaluate specific disease exposure	Blood tests to evaluate exposure to specific diseases (e.g., HIV, hepatitis)
Immunoglobulin (IgG, IgM) levels	Blood tests to evaluate humoral immunity status
C-reactive protein (CRP)	A blood test to measure inflammatory change or bacterial infection
Agglutinins, warm or cold	Used to diagnose atypical infections by detecting antigens in the blood
Erythrocyte (red blood cell) sedimentation rate (ESR or sed rate)	A measure of inflammatory changes. Sed rate increases with inflammation. Normally it is @ 15 mm/hr for men and < 20 mm/hr for women.
Iron level	Normally 60–90 grams/100 mg. Lower in chronic infection.

Standardized Language

NOC Outcomes and NIC Interventions for Risk for Infection

NURSING DIAGNOSIS	NOC OUTCOMES*	NIC MAJOR INTERVENTIONS
Risk for Infection: At increased risk for being invaded by pathogenic organisms	Community Risk Control: Communicable Disease	Circulatory Care: Arterial Insufficiency
	Immune Status	Communicable Disease Management
	Immunization Behavior	Health Screening
	Infection Severity	Immunization/Vaccination Management
Risk Factors:	Infection Severity: Newborn	Incision Site Care
Chronic disease	Risk Control: Sexually Transmitted Diseases (STD)	Infection Control
Inadequate acquired immunity		Infection Protection
Inadequate primary defenses (e.g., broken skin)	Wound Healing: Primary Intention	Surveillance: Community
	Wound Healing: Secondary Intention	Teaching: Safe Sex
Inadequate secondary defenses (e.g., low white blood cell count)		Teaching: Sexuality
Increased exposure to pathogens		Wound Care
Immunosuppression		
Invasive procedures		
Insufficient knowledge to avoid exposure to pathogens		
Malnutrition		
Certain medications		
Rupture of amniotic membranes		
Trauma		
Tissue destruction		

*For 5-point scales to use in describing desired outcomes or goals, see Chapter 5, NOC Measurement Scales.

Sources: NANDA International (2009). *Nursing diagnoses: Definitions & classification 2009–2010.* Ames, IA: Wiley-Blackwell; Bulechek, G. M., Butcher, H. K., & Dochterman, J. M. (2008). *Nursing interventions classification (NIC)* (5th ed.). St. Louis, MO: C.V. Mosby; Johnson, M., Bulechek, G. M., Butcher, H. K., et al. (2006). *NANDA, NOC, and NIC linkages* (2nd ed.). St. Louis, MO: C.V. Mosby; Moorhead, S., Johnson, M., Maas, M. L., et al. (2008). *Nursing outcomes classification* (4th ed.). St. Louis, MO: C.V. Mosby. Used with permission.

THINKING CRITICALLY ABOUT PROMOTING ASEPSIS AND PREVENTING INFECTION

The exercises in the following sections allow you to practice the kind of thinking you will use as a full-spectrum nurse. Because these are critical-thinking questions, there is usually no single right answer. We do not provide answers for these questions because it is more important for you to think about the questions than to arrive at the "right" answer. These questions are designed to improve your thinking more than to "cover content." Discuss answers with your peers—discussion can stimulate critical thinking. If you have difficulty with any of these questions, consult with your instructor.

Applying the Full-Spectrum Nursing Model

PATIENT SITUATION

Mr. Long, a frail elderly man, is in the hospital because he has become dehydrated and needs intravenous fluids and other supportive care. The nurse administered intravenous fluids. Mr. Long also has a fairly large decubitus ulcer (bedsore), which was cultured recently and found to be infected with *Staphylococcus aureus*. The nurse wore gloves to treat the ulcer. While doing so, she noticed that the IV was infusing too fast and, without thinking, regulated the IV without removing her soiled gloves. The next nurse to regulate the IV did so with her bare hands, and then, without realizing it, rubbed her neck. Later, the nurse developed a boil on her neck, which was infected with *S. aureus*.

THINKING

1. *Theoretical Knowledge*:

   a. What are the six links in the chain of infection?

   b. Why do you think the *S. aureus* was able to thrive in Mr. Long's decubitus ulcer?

   c. What are the three modes of transmission of microorganisms? Which one is the most frequent mode of transmission?

2. *Critical Thinking (Reflecting)*:

   a. What was the reservoir for the *S. aureus*?

   b. What was the exit from Mr. Long?

   c. What was (were) the fomite(s) for transmission to the nurse?

   d. What was the portal of entry into the nurse?

DOING

3. *Nursing Process (Implementation)*: In addition to wearing gloves, what other PPE (if any) does the nurse need if she is performing decubitus care and changing Mr. Long's bed linens?

CARING

4. *Self-Knowledge and Ethical Knowledge*: Think of one instance in the clinical setting in which you did *not* follow standard precautions? Why do you think that happened?

Critical Thinking and Clinical Reasoning

1. You notice that your clinical instructor is not washing his hands between patients. What should you do?

2. As you are gowning and gloving for your first experience in the operating room, you become nervous and forget the proper procedure for applying sterile surgical garb. How should you handle this situation?

3. What action should you take if you contaminate yourself while gowning and gloving?

4. Refer to Procedure 20-7, the open method for donning sterile gloves. In the photograph at step 7, you can see that the nurse has a sterile glove on her right hand and is touching the glove with her bare left hand. Is the nurse breaking the "sterile-touches-sterile" principle? Explain your thinking.

5. Refer to Procedure 20-6, the closed method of donning a sterile gown and gloves. Examine the very last photograph, in which one nurse is preparing to turn and receive her gown tie from a co-worker. The gowned nurse has already donned sterile gloves, using the closed method. When the gowned nurse turns to receive the tie, what must she take care to not touch? What can she touch?

6. For each of the following concepts, use critical thinking to describe how or why it is important to nursing, patient care, or promoting asepsis and preventing infection. Note that these are *not* to be merely definitions.

Chain of infection	Standard precautions
Pathogens	Transmission-based precautions
Asepsis	Protective isolation
Healthcare-related infections	Sterile
Multiple-drug-resistant organisms (MDROs)	Medical asepsis
Contamination	Surgical asepsis

What Are the Main Points in This Chapter?

➤ Healthcare-related infections (infections that are acquired in healthcare facilities) are a major health problem worldwide.

➤ The chain of infection consists of six links that must all be present for infection to be transmitted from one individual to another: infectious agent, reservoir, portal of exit, mode of transmission, portal of entry, and susceptible host.

➤ Pathogens are strains of bacteria, viruses, fungi, protozoa, helminths, and prions that cause disease.

➤ Drug-resistant and multiple-drug-resistant organisms (MDRO) have mutated to develop resistance to one or more classes of antimicrobial drugs. They are a serious problem because: (1) options for treating MDRO infections are limited; (2) they are associated with increased hospital lengths of stay and hospital charges; and (3) they are associated with serious illness and increased mortality.

➤ Many emerging pathogens are airborne and widely spread by air travel before the carrier shows any symptoms. They have the potential for causing epidemics and pandemics.

➤ Infectious illnesses typically follow five predictable stages: incubation, prodromal stage, illness, decline, and convalescence.

➤ Primary body defenses, such as intact skin and mucous membranes, block entry of pathogens into the body.

➤ Invading microorganisms trigger the body's secondary defenses, which include phagocytosis, the complement cascade, the inflammatory response, and fever.

➤ The humoral immune response results in the production of antibodies that neutralize pathogens or trigger their destruction.

➤ The cell-mediated immune response results in the production of T cells that destroy infected body cells.

➤ Nutrition, hygiene, rest, exercise, stress reduction, and immunization protect the body against infection.

➤ Anything that weakens the body's defenses or increases the person's exposure to pathogens makes the person more susceptible to infection. Such factors include illness, injury, medical treatment, infancy or old age, frequent public contact, and various lifestyle habits.

➤ Medical asepsis requires that objects and surfaces in the healthcare environment be disinfected.

➤ Scrupulous hand washing markedly decreases the transmission of infection and is the most important aspect of medical asepsis.

➤ Standard precautions are used with all clients whenever there is a possibility of coming in contact with blood, body fluids (except sweat), excretions and secretions, mucous membranes, and any break in the skin.

➤ Transmission-based precautions are added to standard precautions when there is concern about transmission of infection via contact, droplets, or air currents.

➤ Isolation precautions are designed to prevent the spread of disease, not to isolate the person who has the disease.

➤ Surgical asepsis is an attempt to prevent the patient from coming in contact with *any* microorganisms.

➤ Sterile technique is required in many patient activities, such as administering an injection, starting an intravenous line, or performing a sterile dressing change.

➤ Exposure to blood, body secretions, or body tissues containing blood or secretions requires immediate action. Minimize the exposure by washing hands or flushing the area thoroughly. Contact the infection preventionist or employee health nurse as soon after the exposure as possible, complete an injury report, and seek medical care.

➤ The task of the infection preventionist is to minimize the number of infections in the healthcare facility.

➤ A key factor in minimizing infectious outbreaks is recognizing unusual disease patterns.

For practice questions for this chapter,

 Go to **NCLEX-Style Chapter Quiz,** on the Student Resource Disk or DavisPlus at http://davisplus.fadavis.com/Wilkinson2

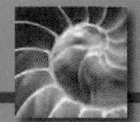

Knowledge Map

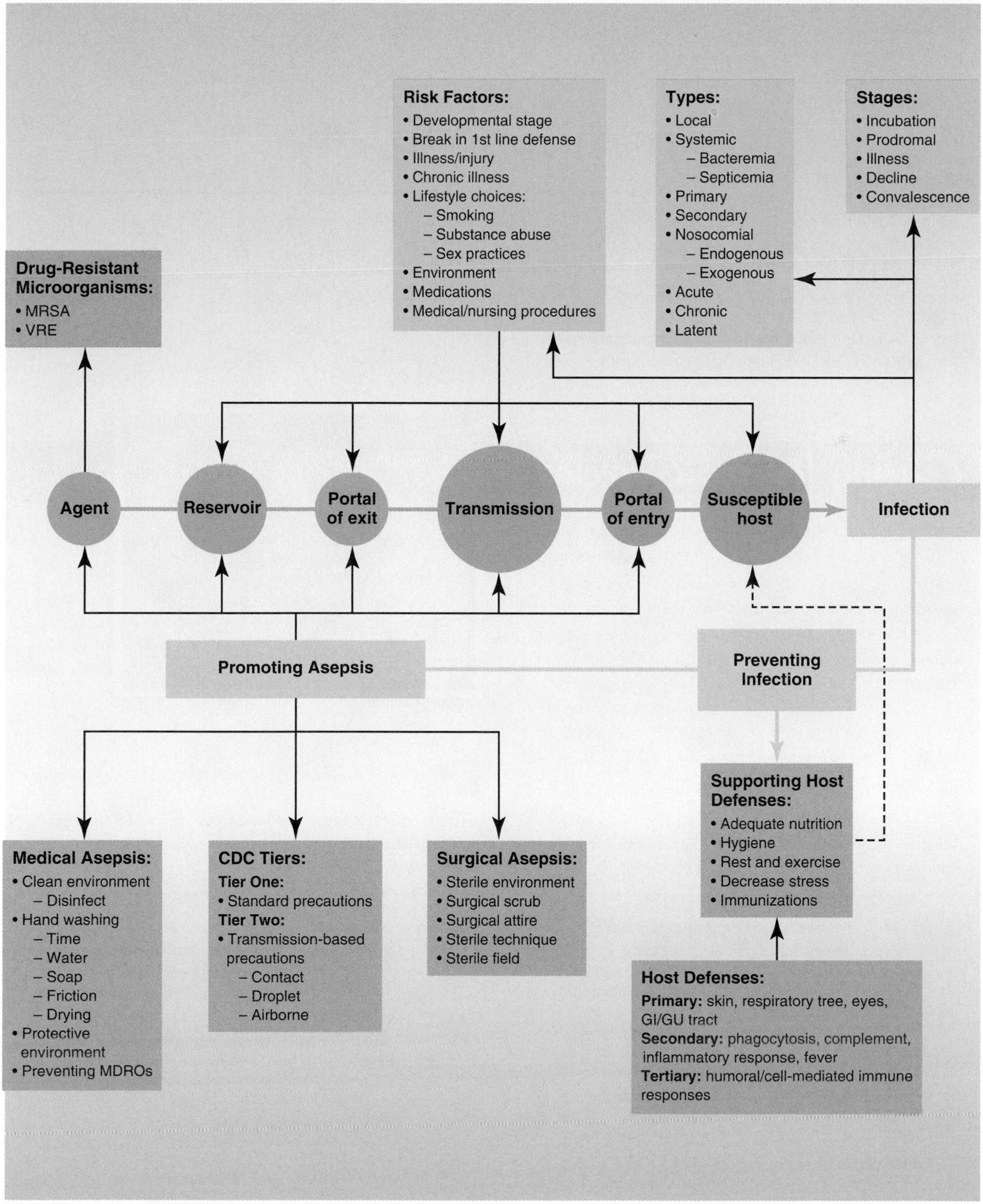

Risk Factors:
- Developmental stage
- Break in 1st line defense
- Illness/injury
- Chronic illness
- Lifestyle choices:
  - Smoking
  - Substance abuse
  - Sex practices
- Environment
- Medications
- Medical/nursing procedures

Types:
- Local
- Systemic
  - Bacteremia
  - Septicemia
- Primary
- Secondary
- Nosocomial
  - Endogenous
  - Exogenous
- Acute
- Chronic
- Latent

Stages:
- Incubation
- Prodromal
- Illness
- Decline
- Convalescence

Drug-Resistant Microorganisms:
- MRSA
- VRE

Agent — **Reservoir** — **Portal of exit** — **Transmission** — **Portal of entry** — **Susceptible host** → **Infection**

Promoting Asepsis

Preventing Infection

Supporting Host Defenses:
- Adequate nutrition
- Hygiene
- Rest and exercise
- Decrease stress
- Immunizations

Medical Asepsis:
- Clean environment
  - Disinfect
- Hand washing
  - Time
  - Water
  - Soap
  - Friction
  - Drying
- Protective environment
- Preventing MDROs

CDC Tiers:
Tier One:
- Standard precautions
Tier Two:
- Transmission-based precautions
  - Contact
  - Droplet
  - Airborne

Surgical Asepsis:
- Sterile environment
- Surgical scrub
- Surgical attire
- Sterile technique
- Sterile field

Host Defenses:
Primary: skin, respiratory tree, eyes, GI/GU tract
Secondary: phagocytosis, complement, inflammatory response, fever
Tertiary: humoral/cell-mediated immune responses

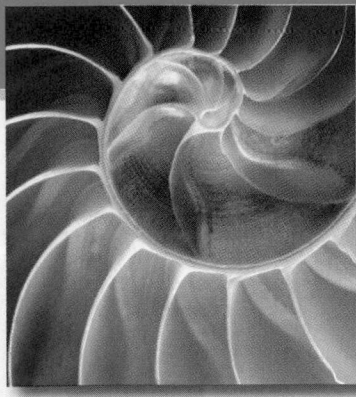

CHAPTER 21

Promoting Safety

For a podcast of an overview of this chapter,

 Go to Student Resources, **Podcast – Chapter Overviews, Chapter 21,** on DavisPlus at http://davisplus.fadavis.com/ Wilkinson2

Caring for the Garcias

The exercises in the following section allow you to practice the kind of thinking you will use as a full-spectrum nurse. Because these are critical-thinking questions, there is usually no single right answer. We do not provide answers for these questions because it is more important for you to think about the questions than to arrive at the "right" answer. These questions are designed to improve your thinking more than to "cover content." Discuss answers with your peers—discussion can stimulate critical thinking. If you have difficulty with any of these questions, consult with your instructor.

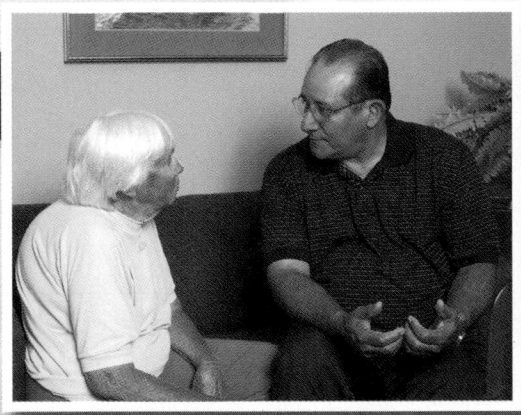

Refer to the database for Joseph Garcia in the front of this volume. Use full-spectrum thinking to identify safety hazards for Mr. Garcia, his 3-year-old grandchild (Bettina Sanford, who lives with him), and his widowed mother, Katherine, who lives alone.

A. Without even using any patient data from the database (except ages), what theoretical knowledge do you have that will help you to identify risks that commonly occur in the developmental stages represented by these three clients?

Mr. Garcia
Mr. Garcia's 3-year-old grandchild, Bettina
Mr. Garcia's widowed mother, Katherine

B. From Mr. Garcia's database, what data can you put together with your theoretical knowledge to identify the most likely safety risks for him? What are those risks?

C. From the risks and possible risks you have identified, for which one do you definitely need more data before deciding whether it increases his risk for

Caring for the Garcias (continued)

accidents? That is, which piece of data is especially vague? What do you need to find out?

D. You know the theoretical (or possible) risks for Mr. Garcia's mother. What data do you need in order to determine her *actual* safety risks?

E. What, if any, data do you have that would help you to identify any *actual* safety risks for Mr. Garcia's grandchild? What, if any, are those risks?

F. What would you want to assess at the preschool to be sure that safety measures exist for preventing falls?

Practical **Knowledge**
knowing why

Nursing interventions to promote safety in the home focus mainly on patient teaching. In hospitals and long-term care facilities, however, you will take a more proactive role in preventing injury to patients. In addition to patient advocacy activities, you will need practical knowledge of measures other than restraints (e.g., bed and chair monitors) you can use to prevent falls. You must also know how to apply and manage restraints safely.

Procedures

Procedure 21-1 ☐ **Using a Bed Monitoring Device**

➤ For steps to follow in *all* procedures, refer to the Universal Steps for All Procedures found on the inside back cover of Volume 2.

Critical Aspects

- Select the correct type of alarm for your patient.
- Explain to the patient and family that a patient monitoring device alerts the staff when the patient tries to get out of the chair or bed.
- Apply or place the device; connect the control unit to the sensor pad.
- Connect the control unit to the nurse call system, if possible.
- Explain that the patient will need to call for assistance when she wants to get up.
- Disconnect or turn off the alarm before assisting the patient out of the bed or chair.
- Reactivate the alarm after assisting the patient back to the bed or chair.
- Understand that bed alarms by themselves do not prevent falls; they are utilized to improve the timeliness of staff response. Patients who are at risk for falls require increased observation and surveillance.

Equipment

Bed or chair exit monitoring device

There are at least four types of staff notification systems that may be utilized to warn caregivers that a patient is leaving a bed or chair: (1) pressure sensitive, (2) posture indicators, (3) motion sensors, and (4) pull-cord and combination alarms.

Delegation

As the nurse, you must determine whether a monitoring device is needed. You must also select the appropriate device and provide ongoing evaluation of its effectiveness. You may delegate to a nursing assistive personnel (NAP) the installation of the device, after verifying the NAP has the necessary knowledge and skill.

Pre-Procedure Assessments

Assess for intrinsic factors that increase the risk for falls:
- Older than age 75
- History of a recent fall or fear of falling
- Bowel and bladder incontinence (particularly urge bladder incontinence)
- Cognitive impairment
- Mood changes, lability
- Dizziness
- Functional impairment
- Medications (especially new medications or changes in regimen)
- Other medical problems (diseases such as dementia, hip fracture, type 2 diabetes, Parkinson's disease, arthritis, and depression)

(continued on next page)

Procedure 21-1 ■ **Using a Bed Monitoring Device** (continued)

Assess for extrinsic environmental factors that increase the risk of falling:

- Use of an assistive device
- Equipment in the room
- Wet or uneven floors
- The use of physical restraints
- Inappropriate footwear
- Poor lighting
- Lack of grab rails and bars in the bathroom

- Furniture and adaptive aids that are in disrepair or unstable (e.g., bed rails, IV poles)
- Clothing that may cause tripping

  Identify factors that increase risk for more severe injury in the case of a fall. These include use of anticoagulants (e.g., Coumadin, Plavix or aspirin) and osteoporosis.

  Check the alarm on the monitoring device to ensure that it is working properly.

> When performing the procedure, always identify your patient according to agency policy and be attentive to standard precautions, hand hygiene, patient safety and privacy, body mechanics, and documentation.

Procedure Steps

1. Apply the device.

Step 1 Variation. Bed or Chair Monitor

Place sensor pads under the patient's buttocks.

The sensor will alarm when the patient attempts to get out of the bed or chair; it alarms when there is no weight on it for more than a few seconds. Many electronic beds have bed exit and patient position monitors for which you must select the desired alarm sensitivity. For example, you may set the system to alarm when the patient exits the bed, when the patient attempts to exit the bed, or even when the patient moves in the bed. ▼

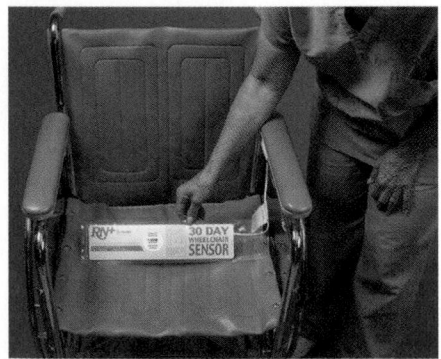

Step 1 Variation. Leg Sensors

Place sensors on the patient's thigh.
The alarm will sound when the leg assumes a near-vertical position. ▼

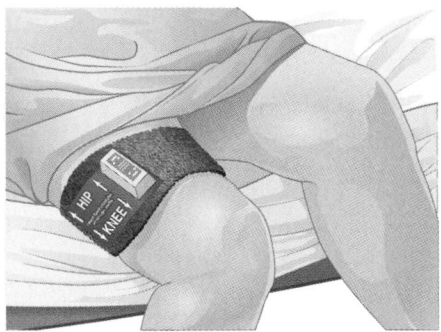

Step 1 Variation. Infrared Beam Detector

Attach next to the bed or on the wall. ▼

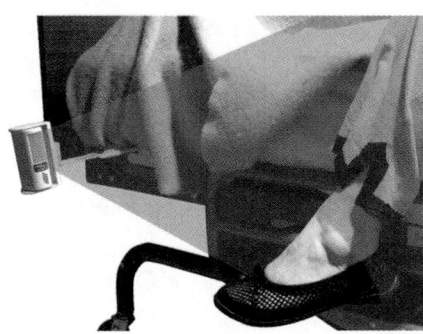

Step 1 Variation. Cord-Activated Sensor

Attach one end of the cord (clip) to the patient's garment. Attach the other end to the control unit. The cord should be long enough to allow moderate movements, but short enough to prevent false alarms. Be sure the cord is free to pull straight out from the monitor and is not blocked by pillows, bedding, or bedrails. The alarm is activated when the patient's movement causes the cord to be detached from the control unit. Some patients will deactivate the alarms, including removing the alarms clipped to their garments. ▼

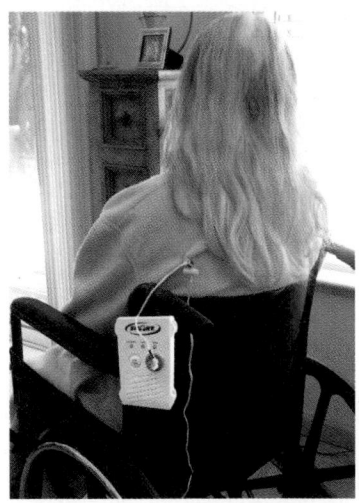

2. Connect the control unit to the sensor pad.

Step 2 Variation. Bed or Chair Monitor

Mount the control unit on the bed or chair.

Step 2 Variation. Leg Sensor

Mount the control unit directly on the leg sensor.

Step 2 Variation. Infrared System

Mount the control unit next to the bed or on the wall.

Step 2 Variation. Cord-Activated System

Mount the control unit next to the bed or on the wall.

3. Connect the control unit to the nurse call system, if possible. Allows for a quicker response; however, not all call systems will accommodate this.

4. Disconnect or turn off the alarm before assisting the patient out of the bed or chair.

Prevents false alarms. Some systems have a standby setting to allow the alarm to be temporarily suspended.

5. Reactivate the alarm after assisting the patient back to the bed or chair.
Helps improve the timeliness of staff response, which may prevent patient falls.

6. Be sure the patient has easy access to the nurse call light.

Evaluation

- Assess the sensitivity of the monitoring device, and adjust as needed to ensure that the alarm is activated if the patient tries to get out of the bed or chair.
- Continue to assess fall risk per agency policy and as indicated by the patient's physical and/or mental status.
- In the event of a fall, perform a post-fall assessment to identify possible causes. Monitor patients closely for 48 hours after a fall.

Patient Teaching

- Explain to the patient and family that a bed or chair exit monitoring device alerts the staff when the patient tries to get out of the chair or bed.
- Explain that the purpose of the device is to help prevent falls using the least restrictive method possible will reassure the patient and family.
- Explain to the patient that she will need to call for assistance when she wants to get up.

Calling for assistance will prevent the alarm from sounding. Summoning for help can prevent the patient from falling.

Documentation

Document the initial sensor placement, including type of sensor used and the location of placement.

- After documenting initial placement, follow agency policy for documenting the use of bed exit monitor. Usually, the minimum documentation for exit monitors is every 8 hours.
- Place the patient on fall risk precautions according to agency policy.
- Document on the fall risk assessment sheet, restraint flowsheet, and nursing notes according to agency policy.

Sample documentation:

8/25/11	1000	*Client becomes easily disoriented while sitting in wheelchair and attempts to rise to a standing position. Safe standing and walking with assistance x1. Reminded to ask for assistance when standing or walking and placed next to nurses station.*
		— *Marsha Klein, RN*
8/25/11	1215	*Continues to be confused and to stand up without assistance. Wheelchair exit alarm placed on wheelchair and monitoring clip attached to back of client's gown. Notified client's daughter, June Kennedy, via telephone. Daughter agreed the exit alarm would help keep her father from falling.*
		— *Marsha Klein, RN*

Practice Resources

Gray-Micelli, D. (2008); FAQs for the 2007 National Patient Safety Goals (updated 2007); The Joint Commission (July 12, 2000); National Guideline Clearinghouse (2005).

Thinking About the Procedure

 Go to the *Fundamentals of Nursing Skills Videos,* **Safety: Bed Monitoring Device.**

1. Where does the nurse attach the bed monitoring device control unit?

2. Where does the nurse put the sensor?

 For suggested responses, go to Chapter 21, **Thinking About the Procedure Suggested Responses,** on the Student Resource Disk or DavisPlus at http://davisplus.fadavis.com/Wilkinson2

Procedure 21-2   Using Restraints

➤ For steps to follow in *all* procedures, refer to the Universal Steps for All Procedures found on the inside back cover of Volume 2.

Caution: This procedure describes Medicare standards, but state and agency policies may be more restrictive.

Critical Aspects

- Follow agency policy, state laws, and professional guidelines.
- Try alternative interventions, such as the following, first:
  - Bed/chair alarms
  - Patient sitters (nonprofessional staff hired to watch the patient)
- Use the least invasive method among the various types of restraints:
  - Verbal restraints
  - Chemical restraints (e.g., antipsychotic or sedative medication)
  - Seclusion (safe containment to de-escalate)
  - Physical restraints (4-point devices, tie-on, Velcro, leather)
- Use restraints only to protect a patient and/or caregiver from injury; not for the convenience of the caregiver or as a punishment.
- Obtain the required consent form.
- Obtain a medical order before restraining, except in an emergency.
- Secure restraints in a way that allows for quick release.
- Ensure that restraints do not impair circulation or tissue integrity.
- Check restraints every 30 minutes.
- A prescriber must reassess and reorder the restraints every 24 hours.
- Release restraints and assess every 2 hours (more often for behavioral restraints).

Equipment

- Restraint of the appropriate size: belt, vest, wrist or ankle, or mitt
- Soft gauze or cotton padding for bony prominences

Delegation

As the nurse, you must determine whether restraints are needed in each specific situation. You must also select the least restrictive type of restraints, evaluate their effectiveness, and continue to assess for complications that may occur. You may delegate to NAP the application and periodic removal of ordered restraints, after verifying that the NAP has the knowledge and skill to do so.

Pre-Procedure Assessments

- Assess the patient's risk for falls, including mobility status and level of awareness.
- Assess for need for restraints: The immediate physical safety of the patient, a staff member, or others is threatened.

If a patient must be temporarily restrained so that a procedure may be performed, this is not considered "restraint."

- Determine that all less restrictive interventions have been tried unsuccessfully.
- Identify the appropriate restraint:
  —The least restrictive possible
  —Does not interfere with care or exacerbate patient's medical condition.
  —Does not pose a safety risk to the patient.
  —Can be changed easily to keep it clean.

➤ When performing the procedure, always identify your patient according to agency policy and be attentive to standard precautions, hand hygiene, patient safety and privacy, body mechanics, and documentation.

Procedure Steps

1. Determine whether dangerous behaviors continue despite attempts to eliminate causal factors using less restrictive interventions.

2. Obtain a physician's prescription for restraint, including type of restraint, indications for use, site of restraint application, and duration. Determine if the restraint is being used for medical–surgical or behavioral reasons.

Federal and state regulations and laws permit healthcare facilities to use restraints only when they are medically needed. Restraints can be used only with a physician's order for a specified and limited time. When you apply restraint in an emergency, obtain the order as the restraint is being applied, or as quickly as possible afterward. When the restraint prescription expires (maximum 24 hours), physician assessment and a new prescription are needed.

3. Notify the family of the change in patient status and the need for restraints. Obtain patient and family consent when clinically feasible. Patients have the right to refuse treatment. Consent may not be necessary if there is an immediate threat to patient safety; however, as a rule, the family must be notified of the use of restraints if the patient has cognitive impairment. Many times family members prefer to sit with the patient as an alternative to restraint.

4. Pad bony prominences and apply the appropriately sized restraint, using appropriate knotting techniques.

✚ a. Use a quick-release knot, such as the half-bow, when tying restraints to the bed frame or wheelchair. Do not tie restraints to the siderails.

A quick-release knot is used to prevent patient injury and for ease of caring for the patient. Tie the knot on an immovable part of the bed to prevent injuring the patient if the siderails or head of bed are lowered. A quick-release knot will not tighten or slip when the patient moves about, but unties quickly when you pull on the loose end. ▼

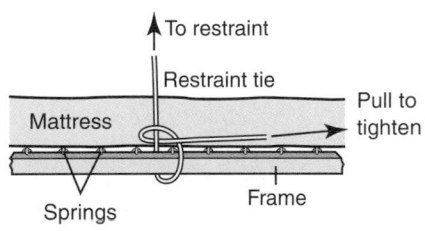
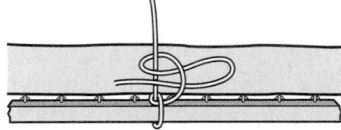
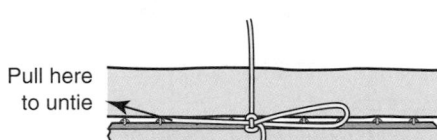

Step 4 Variation. Belt Restraint
a. Place the belt restraint at the patient's waist, removing any wrinkles.
b. Make sure that the belt is snug but does not constrict the patient's waist.
c. Some belts have a key-locked buckle to prevent slipping.

A belt restraint is used mainly to prevent a patient from falling when getting up from a chair or wheelchair and may be used to remind a patient not to get out of bed unassisted. ▼

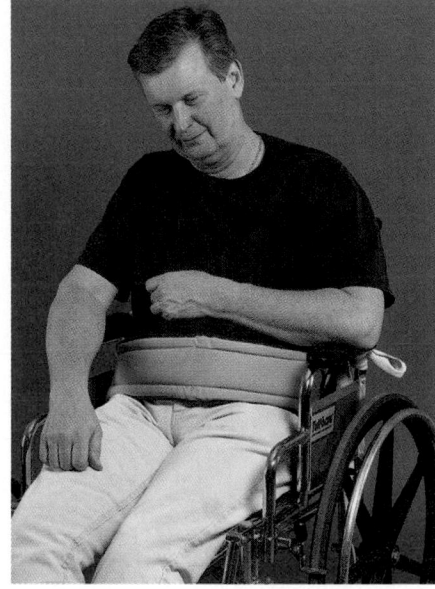

Step 4 Variation. Vest or Jacket Restraint
a. Place the patient in the vest restraint. A zipper-style vest is preferred.

A vest restraint with a rear zipper is less likely to accidentally strangle the patient.

b. Attach the vest straps to the bed or wheelchair.

A vest restraint is used mainly to prevent a patient from falling out of a chair or wheelchair and sometimes to prevent a patient from getting out of bed unassisted. ▼

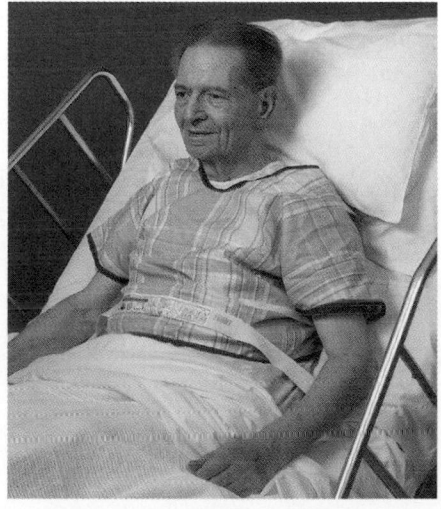

Step 4 Variation. Wrist or Ankle Restraint
a. Apply the padded portion of the wrist or ankle restraint around the patient's wrist or ankle.
b. Make the restraint snug enough to prevent the patient from being able to slip it off, but not tight enough to impair circulation.
c. Attach the restraint strap to the bed frame. Do not attach to bed rails.

A wrist restraint is used mainly to prevent an agitated patient from pulling at tubes, such as IV sites and nasogastric tubes. ▼

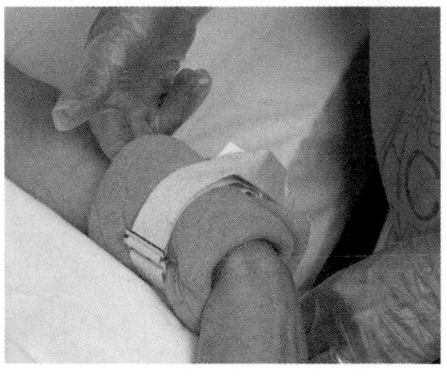

Step 4 Variation. Mitt Restraint
a. Place patient's hand in the mitt restraint, ensuring that fingers are slightly flexed in the mitt.
b. Attach restraint strap to the bed frame if necessary.

A mitt restraint is used mainly to prevent a patient from pulling at tubes, such as IV sites and nasogastric tubes. Mitt restraints limit the use of the fingers, which may be enough to prevent the patient from grasping the tube. If this is the case, mitts that are not tied to the bed frame are the least restrictive restraint. ▼

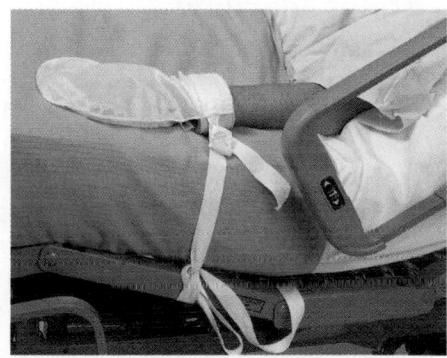

(continued on next page)

Procedure 21-2 ■ Using Restraints (continued)

Step 4 Variation. Enclosed Bed

a. Place patient in the bed and zip all sides. Be sure zippers are completely closed and zipper tabs are positioned in the upper aspects of the net panels out of the patient's reach.

b. Adhere to the manufacturer's minimum height and weight recommendations.

c. Never leave the bed in the high position with the patient unattended.

An enclosed bed is a canopy-like padded bed that is used mainly to keep a patient from wandering or from falling out of bed. The bed has nylon netting on all four sides, with zippered panels that can be opened to provide care. The patient has full freedom of movement and access to all parts of his body. Patients in enclosed beds have a higher risk of becoming entrapped between the bed rails and the mattress, risking suffocation. The dangers are greater for smaller patients and when the bed is left in a high position.

5. Adjust the restraint to maintain good body alignment, comfort, and safety. You should be able to slide two fingers under a wrist or ankle restraint.

The restraint should be snug enough to prevent it from slipping off, but not tight enough to impair circulation.

6. Release restraints and provide skin care, passive and active range of motion, ambulation, toileting, hydration, and nutrition at least every 2 hours. Assess for the continued need for restraint.

Prevents impaired circulation and injury. Medicare- and Medicaid-certified healthcare agencies must ensure that a patient's abilities do not decline unless the decline cannot be avoided because of the patient's medical condition. Patients often lose the ability to bathe, dress, walk, toilet, eat, and communicate when they are regularly restrained. If restraints are necessary, they must be used in a way that does not cause these losses.

7. Place the patient on fall risk precautions according to agency policy.

Patients who are restrained have a higher incidence of falls.

Evaluation

■ Assess the initial restraint placement, circulation, and skin integrity. Observe for pallor, cyanosis, and coolness of extremities when extremities are restrained.

■ Check the restraint every 30 minutes (more often for a behavioral restraint).

■ Reassess the restraint, circulation, the patient's response to the intervention, and the need for continuing the use of the restraint every 2 hours; remove it when it is no longer needed.

Ensures that the restraint is still functioning as intended. Monitoring and reassessment are critical components of caring for patients in physical restraints. Frequency of monitoring is determined by the type of restraint (behavioral vs. medical–surgical). Patients in medical–surgical restraints should be evaluated by an RN at least every 2 hours. Patients in behavioral restraints require more frequent monitoring and in some circumstances require continual observation.

Patient Teaching

■ Explain to the patient and family the need for the restraints.

■ Explain that the restraints will be removed as soon as possible.

Home Care

■ The same guidelines apply to clients in the home.

■ Evaluate caregivers' knowledge and skill in using restraints, and provide teaching as needed (e.g., regarding padding bony prominences and the need to periodically release restraints).

■ If an enclosed bed is used in the home, instruct the caregiver in safe use.

Documentation

Document the following:

■ All nursing interventions that were done to eliminate the need for the restraint (e.g., moving patient closer to the nurses' station, asking a family member to remain with the patient, reorienting the patient)

■ Reasons for placing the restraint (e.g., patient behaviors)

■ The initial restraint placement, location, circulation, and skin integrity

■ The teaching session with the patient and family members

■ Circulation checks, range of motion, and restraint removal per agency protocol

■ Entries on fall risk assessment sheet, restraint flowsheet, and nursing notes according to agency policy

Sample documentation:

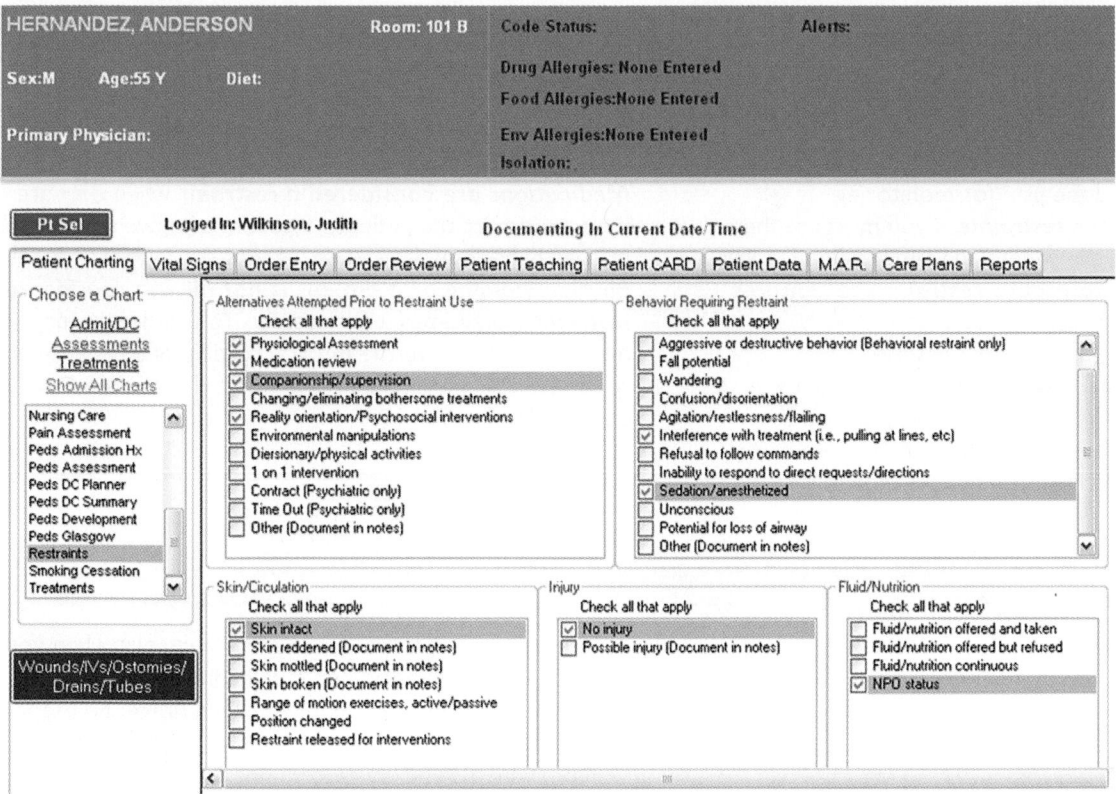

Practice Resources

Centers for Medicare and Medicaid Services, Department of Health and Human Services (2006b); The Joint Commission (2005); National Guideline Clearinghouse (2005); U.S. Food and Drug Administration (2007b).

Thinking About the Procedure

 Go to the *Fundamentals of Nursing Skills Videos,* **Safety: Applying Restraints.**

1. What type of restraint did the nurse use?

2. After putting the restraint on the patient, where did the nurse tie the restraint straps?

 For suggested responses, go to Chapter 21, **Thinking About the Procedure Suggested Responses,** on the Student Resource Disk or DavisPlus at http://davisplus.fadavis.com/Wilkinson2

Clinical Insights

This section includes guidelines for using restraints and for preventing needlestick injuries.

Clinical Insight 21-1 ▶ What You Should Know About Using Restraints

■ **Restraints are a last resort.** The current standard of care is restraint-free. Restraints should be a last-resort intervention.

■ **Individualize care.** Before using restraints, try to understand the message in the patient's behavior. The best way to achieve restraint-free care is to individualize care to avoid the risky behavior.

■ **Try less restrictive interventions** before resorting to restraints. For example, request family involvement as an alternative to restraint. Family members may be able to interpret a patient's gestures or understand what is bothering him. For other suggestions,

 Go to Box 21-6 in Volume 1.

■ **Follow agency policy,** professional guidelines, and state laws for using restraints.

■ **Use restraints only for safety,** to ensure the immediate physical safety of the patient or others.

■ **No standing orders** or "as needed" orders for physical restraint are allowed.

■ **You must obtain a medical prescription** from a physician or other licensed care provider. In an emergency, an RN may initiate a restraint and obtain a prescription either simultaneously or as soon as possible after applying the restraint.

(continued on next page)

Clinical Insight 21-1 ▶ What You Should Know About Using Restraints (continued)

- **Guidelines are more restrictive when restraints are used for behavior management.**
- **You must renew restraint prescriptions every 24 hours** (more often for behavioral restraints).
- **You must modify the plan of care** to reflect the application of restraints and the plan for monitoring.
- **Explain the need for the restraints,** if you must use them.
- **Obtain consent** from the patient and family when feasible.
- **Always use the least restrictive restraint that ensures safety.**
- **Remove the restraint as soon as possible.**
- **Monitor and reassess.** These are critical components of caring for patients in physical restraints. Assess restraints every 30 minutes (more frequently for patients with behavioral restraints, who may need continuous monitoring).

- **Remove restraints for assessment, feeding, toileting, and skin care every 2 hours.** Patients in medical–surgical restraints should be evaluated by an RN at least every 2 hours. Those in behavioral restraints require more frequent monitoring.
- **Medications are considered a restraint** when they are used to restrict the patient's freedom of movement or to manage behaviour.
- **Physical holding of a patient is not always considered restraint.** Sometimes it is necessary to use devices or methods that involve the physical holding of a patient for routine physical examinations or tests. These are not considered restraints.

Clinical Insight 21-2 ▶ Preventing Needlestick Injury

 Use needleless systems (e.g., retractable needles) when possible.
More than 80% of needlestick injuries can be prevented with the use of safe needle devices (ANA, 2002).

- **Before beginning a procedure:**
  —Provide adequate lighting and space to perform the procedure.
  —Place the sharps container near the work area, if it is moveable.
  —Obtain assistance if there is a risk the patient may be uncooperative, combative, or confused.
  —Inform the patient about the procedure and explain the importance of avoiding any sudden movement.
- **During the procedure:**
  —Be sure you can see the sharps container at all times.
  —When handling a sharp, be aware of other persons in the immediate area.
  —Do not hand-pass exposed sharps from one person to another.
  —When using a safety needle, observe for audio or visual cues that the feature has engaged.
- **Handling needles:**
  —Do not shear or break contaminated needles
  —Avoid recapping, bending, or removing contaminated needles and other sharps unless there is no feasible alternative.
  —When you must recap a sterile needle, use a mechanical recapping device or a modified "scoop" technique (see Procedure 23-10).
  —Never carry syringes in your uniform pocket.
- **Sharps containers:**
  —Be sure that puncture-proof needle disposal containers are kept in every room.
  —Place sharps containers at eye level; do not overfill a sharps container.
  —Make sure the container is large enough to hold the entire sharp device.

—Dispose of sharps immediately. For example, when you break an ampule neck, put it immediately in the sharps container. Do not wait until you have drawn up the medication.
—Inspect sharps and waste containers for protruding sharps. If found, notify safety personnel for removal of the hazard.

If your agency does not use needleless systems or protective devices you should do the following:
- Explain the OSHA Bloodborne Pathogens Standard (BPS) to your employer, including the need to provide needleless systems or protective devices for blood products and parenteral medication administration.
- Refer your employer to the OSHA Web site at www.osha.gov/needlesticks/needlefaq.html
- OSHA requires worker involvement in evaluating, selecting, and implementing the use of safer needle products; volunteer to serve on that committee.
- Ask your agency for a copy of their exposure control plan, which is required by the BPS for monitoring compliance with the new law.
- Keep a record of needlestick injuries on your unit and of "near-misses" (e.g., overfilled sharps containers, sharps left on bed or overbed table).
- Submit written concerns to your employer.
- If your employer refuses to purchase safety devices, you may want to file an OSHA complaint (see www.osha.gov/as/opa/worker/complain.html). If you do, refer to Chapter 44, whistleblowing. Complaints can be filed anonymously.

Sources

Adapted from: American Nurses Association (2002); Centers for Disease Control and Prevention (n.d.); National Institute for Occupational Safety and Health (NIOSH) (n.d.); U.S. Department of Labor, Occupational Safety and Health Administration (2001); Wilburn, S. (2004).

Assessment Guidelines and Tools

The "Get Up and Go Test" should be conducted as part of a routine assessment when dealing with older persons. Its purpose is to detect "fallers" and to identify those who need evaluation. The staff should be trained to perform the "Get Up and Go Test" at check-in and query those with gait or balance problems for falls.

Initial Check

All older persons who report a single fall should be observed as they "get up and go":
- Move from a sitting position and stand without using their arms to help them rise and stand.
- Walk several paces, turn, and return to the chair.
- Sit back in the chair without using their arms for support.

Those who have difficulty or demonstrate unsteadiness performing this test require the following follow-up assessment.

Follow-Up Assessment

In the follow-up assessment, ask the person to:
- Sit.
- Stand without using their arms for support.
- Close his eyes for a few seconds, while standing in place.
- Stand with eyes closed, while you push gently on his sternum.
- Walk a short distance and come to a complete stop.
- Turn around and return to the chair.
- Sit in the chair without using his arms for support.

Referring for Comprehensive Evaluation

In any of the following situations, you should refer the patient for a comprehensive fall evaluation. The evaluation should be performed by a practitioner with advanced skills and experience (AHI of Indiana, n.d.; American Academy of Neurology, 2008; Hendrich, 2007; Kenny, Rubenstein, & Martin, et al., 2001).
- The patient is seeking care because of a fall.
- The patient or family reports recurrent falls in the past year.
- The patient's gait or balance are abnormal.

The Timed Up & Go Test for Fall Risk Assessment

Doctors are asked to assess annually all patients who are 65 years or older using the **Timed Up & Go Test.**

Timed Up & Go Test

1. Have the patient in a seated position.
2. Place a visible object 8 feet away from the patient.
3. Ask the patient to get up and walk around the object, and then sit back down.
   - Allow the patient to practice once.

- Then time the patient three times as he performs these steps.
- Scores greater than 8.5 seconds are associated with high fall risk in community-dwelling older adults.

Practice Resources

AHI of Indiana Inc. (n.d.); American Academy of Neurology (2008a, February); American Academy of Neurology (2008b, February); Hendrich, A. (2007); Kenny, R., Rubenstein, L., Martin, F., et al. (2001).

Home Safety Checklist

Home Safety

_____ Are smoke detectors installed in appropriate locations and operating properly?

_____ Is the water heater temperature set at a safe level to avoid scalds?

_____ Do you keep extra fuses on hand?

_____ Do small rugs have nonskid backing?

_____ Do you have a proper stepstool or ladder for in-home use?

_____ Are there covers on electrical outlets where children play?

_____ Are all firearms safely stored and locked according to current regulations?

_____ Are emergency numbers posted at all telephones?

_____ Are all firearms safely stored and locked according to current regulations?

_____ Are emergency numbers posted at all telephones?

Entrances

_____ Is there adequate lighting at entrances?

_____ Are steps well maintained?

_____ Are snow and ice immediately cleared from doorsteps?

_____ Are shoes, boots, umbrellas, and so on neatly stored inside?

_____ Are other tripping hazards (toys, puddles from wet boots, and so on) cleaned away?

Stairways

_____ Are stairways clear of all hazards, such as shoes and toys?

_____ Are there full-length handrails in good repair?

_____ Can stairways be well lighted?

_____ Are treads, risers, and carpeting in good condition?

_____ Are spills and wet surfaces cleaned up immediately?

Continued

Home Safety Checklist—cont'd

Bathrooms

_____ Do you use nonskid mats/surfaces in bathtubs to prevent falls?

_____ Do you have a proper medicine cabinet?

_____ Are expired medications disposed of properly?

_____ Do you keep electrical appliances away from sinks, tubs, and other water receptacles?

_____ Do you use a night-light to illuminate the way to the bathroom at night?

_____ Is a ground fault circuit interrupter (GFCI) installed for bathroom circuits?

Kitchen

_____ Do you clean the stove's exhaust hood and duct frequently?

_____ Are cleaners, disinfectants, and other poisons secured out of reach of children and away from foods?

_____ Do you always use a stepstool for climbing?

_____ Are utensils and knives neatly stored?

_____ Are handles of pots and pans always turned away from stove fronts?

_____ Are cracked or chipped dishes and glassware disposed of immediately?

_____ Are spills wiped up immediately?

_____ Are cupboard contents kept orderly to prevent objects from falling?

_____ Is a fully charged fire extinguisher readily available?

_____ Are matches and lighters kept out of reach of children?

Living Rooms and Bedrooms

_____ Is furniture arranged to avoid bumping the knees and shins?

_____ Are electrical cords kept away from carpets?

_____ Are fireplace screens used effectively?

_____ Are throw rugs avoided to prevent tripping hazards?

_____ Is furniture kept away from windows to prevent young children from falling out?

_____ Are screens and windows secured to prevent young children from falling out?

_____ Have plans been made for a fire escape route from bedrooms?

_____ Are lamps located near beds to prevent tripping in the dark?

_____ Are all chimneys checked for obstructions?

Exterior Building, Cellar, Barn, Garage, Grounds

_____ Are walkways, aisles, and traffic areas clear of obstructions?

_____ Is there adequate lighting in work areas and driveways?

_____ Are stairs in good condition and equipped with handrails?

_____ Are stairs kept clear of objects both on steps and landings?

_____ Are ladders in good condition and inspected regularly?

_____ Are all floors and driveways free of holes, cracks, and other defects?

_____ Are low ceilings and beams marked clearly with signs or fluorescent materials to prevent bumping into them?

_____ Are stored materials properly stacked to prevent them from falling?

_____ Are protrusions, such as nails, removed from walls, railings, and used lumber to prevent contact?

_____ Are spills wiped up immediately?

_____ Is there ample walking space between stored machines and materials?

_____ Are keys removed from stored machines?

_____ Do large doors open smoothly?

_____ Do you keep your tractor and/or other fuel-burning equipment in an outbuilding separate from the barn or other buildings?

_____ Do you avoid storing flammable liquids in garages, barns, or other structures?

_____ Do you keep the garage door down and locked at all times, test the automatic reverse mechanism monthly, and keep remote controls away from children?

_____ Do you always supervise children in the garage, where many hazards exist (e.g., motor oil, insecticides, power tools)?

_____ If you own a pool, is it covered when not in use and/ or enclosed with a fence to prevent access without your knowledge? Is a flotation device or other rescue equipment within immediate reach? Are children always supervised when they are in or near a pool, pond, or other body of water?

_____

Adapted from National Ag Safety Database (NASD, 2003b).

Standardized Language

NANDA-I Diagnoses and NOC Outcomes for Safety Problems

NANDA-I DIAGNOSTIC LABEL	ASSOCIATED NOC OUTCOMES (EXAMPLES)
Contamination	Allergic Response: Localized
	Community Disaster Response
	Gastrointestinal Function
	Kidney Function
	Neurological Status
	Respiratory Status
Risk for Contamination	Community Risk Control: Lead Exposure
	Personal Safety Behavior
	Risk Detection
Hyperthermia	Thermoregulation
Hypothermia	Thermoregulation: Newborn
Impaired Home Maintenance	Family Physical Environment
	Safe Home Environment
Impaired Skin Integrity	Tissue Integrity: Skin & Mucous Membranes
Risk for Impaired Skin Integrity	Wound Healing: Primary Intention
Impaired Tissue Integrity	Wound Healing: Secondary Intention
Ineffective Thermoregulation	Vital Signs
Risk for Imbalanced Body Temperature	Thermoregulation
Ineffective Airway Clearance (choking)	Aspiration Prevention
	Respiratory Status: Airway Patency
	Respiratory Status: Ventilation
Ineffective Protection	Abuse Protection
	Coagulation
	Community Violence Level
	Health Promoting Behavior
	Immunization Behavior
Latex Allergy Response	Allergic Response: Local
Risk for Latex Allergy Response	Allergic Response: Systemic
	Tissue Integrity: Skin & Mucous Membranes
Risk for Aspiration	Aspiration Prevention
	Swallowing Status
Risk for Falls	Balance
	Fall Prevention Behavior
	Falls Occurrence
Risk for Infection	Community Risk Control: Communicable Disease
	Immune Status
	Infection Severity
	Risk Control: Sexually Transmitted Diseases (STDs)
Risk for Injury	Personal Safety Behavior
	Physical Injury Severity
	Risk Control
	Safe Home Environment

Continued

NANDA-I Diagnoses and NOC Outcomes for Safety Problems—cont'd

NANDA-I DIAGNOSTIC LABEL	ASSOCIATED NOC OUTCOMES (EXAMPLES)
Risk for Perioperative Positioning Injury	Circulation Status
	Neurological Status: Spinal Sensory/Motor Function
	Tissue Perfusion: Peripheral
Risk for Poisoning	Safe Home Environment
Risk for Suffocation	Respiratory Status: Ventilation
Risk for Trauma	Personal Safety Behavior
	Physical Injury Severity
	Tissue Integrity: Skin & Mucous Membranes
Risk for Sudden Infant Death Syndrome	Parenting: Infant/Toddler Physical Safety
	Safe Home Environment
Risk for Vascular Trauma	NOC outcomes have not yet been linked to this diagnosis.

Sources: Bulechek, G., Butcher, H., & Dochterman, J. (Eds.). (2008). *Nursing interventions classification (NIC)* (5th ed.). St. Louis, MO: C.V. Mosby; Johnson, M., Bulechek, G., Butcher, H., et al. (2006). *NANDA, NOC, and NIC linkages* (2nd ed.). St. Louis, MO: C.V. Mosby; Moorhead, S., Johnson, M., Maas, M., et al. (Eds.) (2008). *Nursing outcomes classification (NOC)* (4th ed.). St. Louis, MO: C.V. Mosby; NANDA International. (2009). *Nursing diagnoses: Definitions and classification 2009–2011.* Ames, IA: Wiley-Blackwell. Used with permission.

Examples of NIC Interventions Related to Safety

INTERVENTIONS FROM THE SAFETY DOMAIN

Abuse Protection Support (Child, Domestic Partner, Elder, Religious)

Allergy Management

Area Restriction

Aspiration Precautions

Crisis Intervention

Dementia Management

Elopement Precautions

Emergency Care

Environmental Management: Safety

Fall Prevention

Fire-Setting Precautions

First Aid

Infection Control

Latex Precautions

Physical Restraint

Radiation Therapy Management

Sports-Injury Prevention: Youth

Suicide Prevention

Surveillance: Safety

Vehicle Safety Promotion

SAFETY INTERVENTIONS FROM OTHER DOMAINS

Communicable Disease Management

Community Disaster Preparedness

Environmental Management: Community

Environmental Management: Violence Prevention

Environmental Management: Worker Safety

Home Maintenance Assistance

Surveillance: Community

Source: Bulechek, G., Butcher, H., & Dochterman, J. (Eds.). (2008). *Nursing interventions classification (NIC)* (5th ed.). St. Louis, MO: C.V. Mosby. Used with permission.

THINKING CRITICALLY ABOUT PROMOTING SAFETY

The exercises in the following sections allow you to practice the kind of thinking you will use as a full-spectrum nurse. Because these are critical-thinking questions, there is usually no single right answer. We do not provide answers for these questions because it is more important for you to think about the questions than to arrive at the "right" answer. These questions are designed to improve your thinking more than to "cover content." Discuss answers with your peers—discussion can stimulate critical thinking. If you have difficulty with any of these questions, consult with your instructor.

Applying the Full-Spectrum Nursing Model

PATIENT SITUATION

Recall your patient, Alvin Lin, from "Meet Your Patient" in Volume 1. Mr. Lin, a 79-year-old man who was just transferred from a long-term care facility to your medical unit. His admitting diagnosis is dehydration and pneumonia. The report you received stated he had rested well during the night and was alert and oriented. When you enter his room, he is confused and does not know where he is. He is becoming combative and is trying to get out of bed.

THINKING

1. *Theoretical Knowledge*:

   a. What is the pathophysiology of pneumonia?

   b. When the oxygen level of the blood falls, what is the effect on the central nervous system? If you don't know the answer to this question, look it up in a reliable reference.

   c. What are the defining characteristics for the NANDA-I diagnosis, Deficient Fluid Volume?

2. *Critical Thinking (Considering Alternatives)*:

   a. Which the three defining characteristics (in 1c) may increase Mr. Lin's risk for falls? Why?

   b. What else may be increasing his confusion and his risk for falls?

DOING

3. *Practical Knowledge*: Suppose you have tried all the less restrictive restraints, but Mr. Lin still attempts to get out of bed. He has even pulled out his intravenous line. You decide you must apply restraints to keep him safely in bed. You have called the physician, but he has not returned your call. You cannot wait any longer because you have other patients who need you, and yet you must stay with Mr. Lin to keep him from falling. What should you do right now?

4. *Nursing Process (Diagnosis)*: Which nursing diagnosis seems more useful to you in planning care for Mr. Lin?

   Confusion related to disease process

   Risk for Falls related to confusion and possibly r/t weakness

CARING

5. *Self-Knowledge*:

   a. Do you think having a restraint-free facility is a valuable goal, or not? Explain your thinking.

   b. How did you come to believe that?

6. *Ethical Knowledge*: Suppose Mr. Lin is too confused to give consent for restraints, and you cannot reach his family by telephone. How can you justify applying restraints, and what must you do later to follow up?

Critical Thinking and Clinical Reasoning

1. Recall from "Meet Your Patient" in Volume 1 the clients you encountered in the community setting. Teresa was caring for her 2-year-old son and her elderly grandmother. The grandmother has a fear of falling. In Volume 1, we addressed some of the issues related to "child-proofing" the home. You would like to suggest ways for Teresa to make the home safe for her frail grandmother.

    a. Refer to the critical-thinking model and questions on the page facing the inside back cover of Volume 1. What questions in the Inquiry section should you ask before making suggestions to Teresa?

   b. What specific information do you need about the grandmother? About the home?

   c. Once you have the necessary information, what suggestions could you make about home safety measures?

   d. Consider alternatives. What types of assistive devices might be helpful in preventing falls?

   e. Explore the alternatives. For example, are they practical? What do you need to know about this family to determine whether it is practical for them to obtain such devices?

   f. Think now about Teresa. Given the situation, what might create a safety risk for her?

2. Recall Alvin Lin ("Meet Your Patients," in Volume 1), the 79-year-old man you were assigned to care for on your first day on the medical unit. The initial report you received was that he was alert and oriented, but you find that he is now confused and is becoming combative.

   a. What should be your first two priorities in this situation?

   b. What specific patient data do you need to determine what might have caused this change in behavior? How could you get that data?

   c. What alternatives to restraints might you consider?

3. A friend calls to tell you she thinks her 18-month-old daughter swallowed some of her sleeping pills. The child is very sleepy, and your friend is having difficulty arousing her. Your friend has ipecac in her medicine cabinet and wonders whether she should try to get her awake enough to take it.

   a. What is the first thing that you would recommend that the mother do?

   b. What is a major concern with inducing vomiting, given that you must assume from the mother that the child is very drowsy. What could go wrong if the child vomits?

   c. If the mother decides to take the daughter to the hospital instead of taking time to call the poison control center (PCC), what should you remind her to take with her?

4. An older couple has health problems and are taking several medications. The husband has assumed care for himself and his wife, Ethyl, because Ethyl has been exhibiting confusion at times. He says he sometimes becomes overwhelmed with everything he has to do, and he is not sure that he always gives the medicine at the right times.

 a. What information do you need to know to be able help with this situation? About the medications? About resources? How would you obtain the information?

 b. What suggestions can you make to help the husband organize the medications?

5. You are caring for a patient 12 hours after surgery following an abdominal hysterectomy for cancer. She asks you to help her to walk to a chair. You note that she has IV fluids infusing and is receiving narcotics via a patient-controlled analgesia (PCA) pump. She states that she has not been out of bed since surgery and that she has just administered some medication and would like to get up while she has pain relief. You also notice that there is a Foley (indwelling urinary) catheter connected to a bedside drainage.

 a. What environmental factors could be safety hazards when this patient gets out of bed?

 b. What assessments and other interventions would help to ensure safe ambulation despite those obstacles?

6. For each of the following concepts, use critical thinking to describe how or why it is important to nursing, patient care, or promoting safety. Note that these are *not* to be merely definitions.

Environmental hazard	Choking rescue maneuver
Pathogens	Refrigeration
Poisoning	Mosquito control
Scald injuries	Rodent control
Falls	Reduce, reuse, recycle, respond
Teaching firearm safety to children	Back injuries
Pollution	Needlestick injuries
Radiation	Time, distance, and shielding
Restraint	Gang culture
Ambularm	Morse Fall Scale

What Are the Main Points in This Chapter?

➤ Safety is a basic human need.

➤ Unintentional injuries are the fifth leading cause of death in the United States.

➤ Major causes of unintentional deaths in the United States are motor vehicle accidents, poisoning, and falls.

➤ The environment includes the physical and psychosocial factors that contribute to the life and well-being of each person. It may be identified as any setting where the nurse and client interact.

➤ A person's safety is influenced by developmental factors as well as individual factors, such as lifestyle, cognitive awareness, sensoriperceptual status, ability to communicate, mobility status, and sensory losses, particularly hearing and vision losses.

➤ The main safety hazards in the home are poisoning, carbon monoxide poisoning, scalds and burns, fires, falls, firearm injuries, suffocation and drowning, and take-home toxins.

➤ Most fatal home fires occur while people are asleep, and most deaths result from smoke inhalation.

➤ More than half of all falls occur in the home; about 80% involve people older than age 65.

➤ Community hazards include motor vehicle accidents, pathogens, improper sanitation, pollution (air, water, noise, and soil), and electrical storms.

➤ Safety hazards in the healthcare agency include falls, equipment-related accidents, fires and electrical hazards, restraints, mercury exposure, and biological hazards.

➤ When possible, nurses should use alternative interventions instead of restraints.

➤ Medical orders for restraints must be renewed at least every 24 hours.

➤ Workplace hazards to nurses include back injuries, needlestick injuries, radiation injury, and violence.

➤ All inpatients should be assessed for their risk for falls.

➤ Identifying anxiety may allow the nurse to intervene before a patient becomes aggressive.

➤ The Heimlich maneuver differs from the American Red Cross choking rescue maneuver in that the Heimlich does not include back blows.

➤ Nursing interventions for promoting safety in the home focus on client teaching.

➤ Nursing interventions for promoting safety in the healthcare facility focus on assessing for risk and creating a safe environment.

For practice questions for this chapter,

Go to **NCLEX-Style Chapter Quiz,** on the Student Resource Disk or DavisPlus at http://davisplus.fadavis.com/Wilkinson2

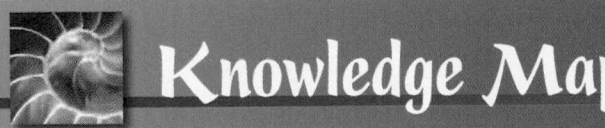

Knowledge Map

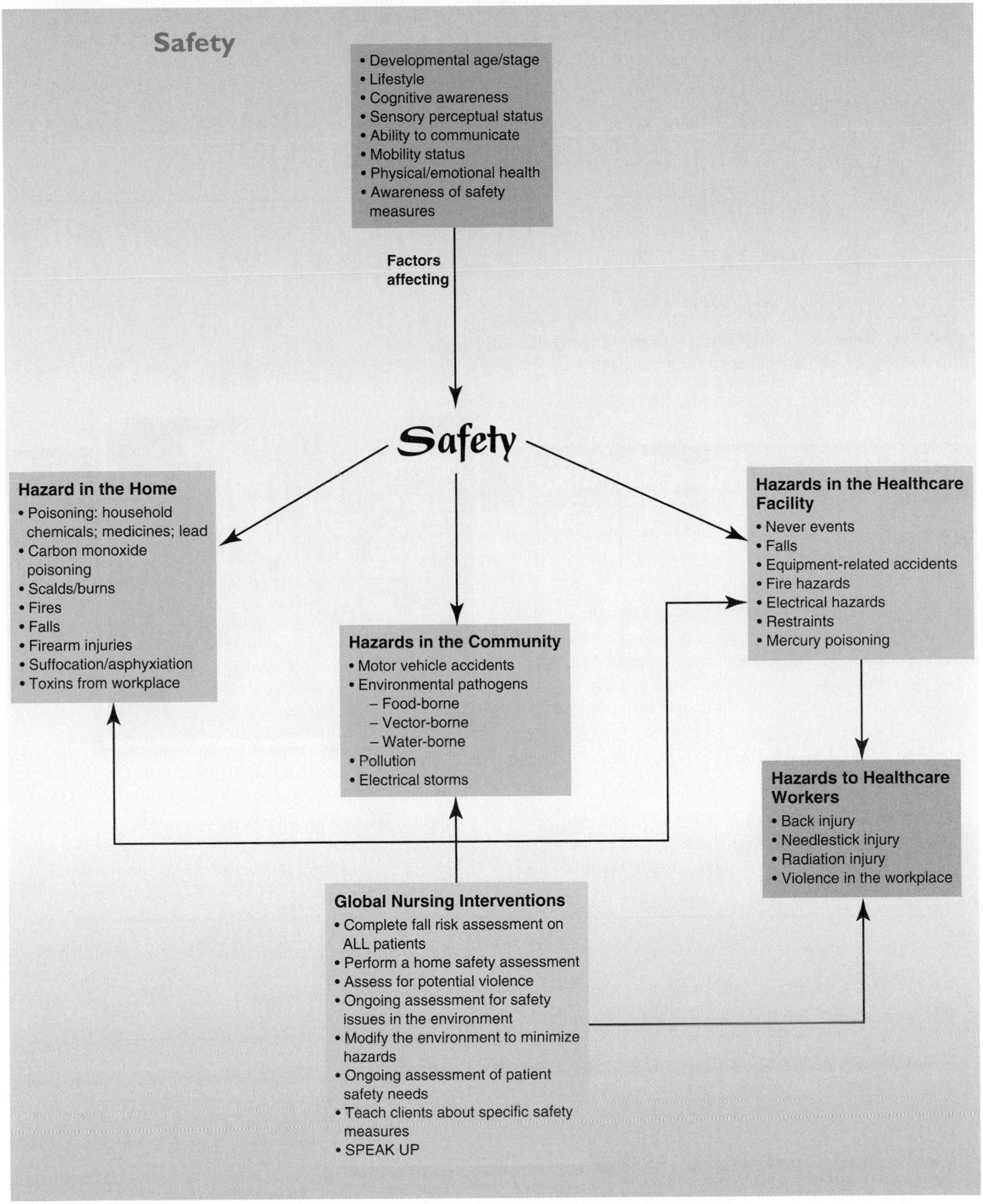

Safety

- Developmental age/stage
- Lifestyle
- Cognitive awareness
- Sensory perceptual status
- Ability to communicate
- Mobility status
- Physical/emotional health
- Awareness of safety measures

Factors affecting

Safety

Hazard in the Home
- Poisoning: household chemicals; medicines; lead
- Carbon monoxide poisoning
- Scalds/burns
- Fires
- Falls
- Firearm injuries
- Suffocation/asphyxiation
- Toxins from workplace

Hazards in the Healthcare Facility
- Never events
- Falls
- Equipment-related accidents
- Fire hazards
- Electrical hazards
- Restraints
- Mercury poisoning

Hazards in the Community
- Motor vehicle accidents
- Environmental pathogens
  – Food-borne
  – Vector-borne
  – Water-borne
- Pollution
- Electrical storms

Hazards to Healthcare Workers
- Back injury
- Needlestick injury
- Radiation injury
- Violence in the workplace

Global Nursing Interventions
- Complete fall risk assessment on ALL patients
- Perform a home safety assessment
- Assess for potential violence
- Ongoing assessment for safety issues in the environment
- Modify the environment to minimize hazards
- Ongoing assessment of patient safety needs
- Teach clients about specific safety measures
- SPEAK UP

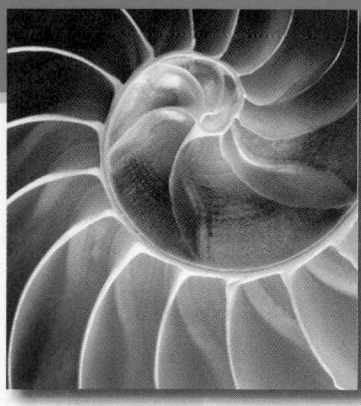

CHAPTER 22

Facilitating Hygiene

For a podcast of an overview of this chapter

 Go to Student Resources, **Podcast – Chapter Overviews, Chapter 22,** on DavisPlus at http://davisplus.fadavis.com/ Wilkinson2

Caring for the Garcias

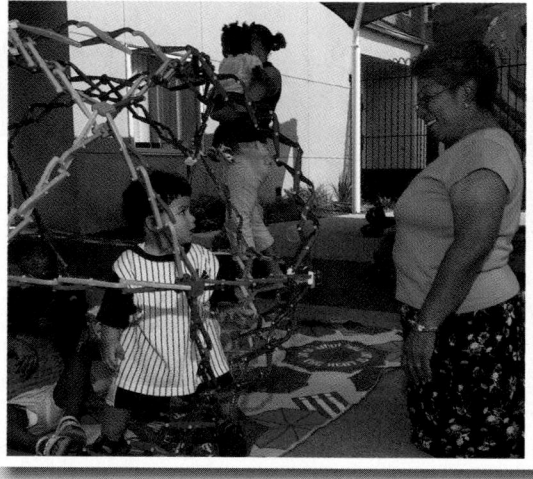

The exercises in the following section allow you to practice the kind of thinking you will use as a full-spectrum nurse. Because these are critical-thinking questions, there is usually no single right answer. We do not provide answers for these questions because it is more important for you to think about the questions than to arrive at the "right" answer. These questions are designed to improve your thinking more than to "cover content." Discuss answers with your peers—discussion can stimulate critical thinking. If you have difficulty with any of these questions, consult with your instructor.

Flordelisa Garcia works as a preschool teacher. She schedules a clinic visit to discuss a variety of concerns. For each of the concerns she mentions, answer the following four questions:

1. What theoretical knowledge do you need?
2. Where could you find it?
3. What, if any, additional patient information do you need?
4. How would you respond to Mrs. Garcia's concerns?

A. Flordelisa tells you that her skin is very dry and irritated.

B. Flordelisa tells you that several of the children at the preschool have recently been diagnosed with head lice. She would like to know how to assess for pediculosis.

C. Flordelisa tells you that her 3-year-old granddaughter, Bettina, frequently refuses to bathe. She asks for advice on how to handle this.

Practical **Knowledge** knowing how

The following procedures and techniques provide the practical knowledge you will need to assist patients with personal cleanliness and grooming. As a nurse you are responsible for providing the necessary assistance and, at the same time, promoting as much self-care as possible. Self-care in activities of daily living (ADLs) promotes increased activity, independence, and self-esteem.

This "Practical Knowledge" section also contains clinical insights for providing hygiene care, a guideline for assessing hygiene needs, and standardized language tables for Self-Care Deficits and nursing diagnoses related to hygiene.

Procedures

Procedure 22-1 ☐ Bathing: Providing a Complete Bed Bath

➤ For steps to follow in *all* procedures, refer to the Universal Steps for All Procedures found on the inside back cover of Volume 2.

Critical Aspects

- Use warm, not hot, water.
- Prevent chilling or tiring the patient.
- Bathe the patient following the principles of "head to toe" and "clean to dirty."
- For extremities, wash and dry from distal to proximal.
- Change the water before cleansing the perineum and whenever the water becomes dirty or cool.
- Perform hand hygiene when moving from a contaminated body part to bathe a clean body part.

Equipment

- Basin for water
- Bath blanket
- Bath towels (2)
- Washcloths
- Soap; or liquid rinse-free soap
- Orangewood stick
- Deodorant, lotion, and/or powder as needed
- Clean patient gown (gown with shoulder snaps or Velcro closures if the patient has an IV line)
- Clean bed linen
- Procedure gloves (for anal and perineal care)
- Bedpan or urinal
- Laundry bag

Delegation

You can delegate this procedure to the NAP if you conclude that the patient's condition and the NAP's skills allow. Perform the following assessments, and inform the NAP of the specific type of bath (e.g., basin, towel, bag bath) and the amount of help the patient needs. Inform the NAP of any special considerations, such as IV lines, drains, and so on. Ask the NAP to report the condition of the patient's skin, level of self-care, and ability to tolerate the procedure.

Pre-Procedure Assessments

Note: Assisting with or supervising the bath provides an excellent opportunity for you to assess the patient's level of consciousness, short- and long-term memory, ability to follow instructions, range of motion, skin condition, activity tolerance, and overall self-care ability.

- Assess the patient's mobility, activity tolerance, type of bath needed, and level of ability to perform bathing self-care.

A patient who has decreased activity tolerance or mobility (e.g., chest pain or shortness of breath with exertion or paralysis) may have limited ability to assist with the bath. Having the patient assist as much as possible increases mobility and sense of control and comfort.

- Check for positioning or activity restrictions (e.g., maintaining hip abduction following a total hip replacement).

Prevents injuring the patient during the procedure.

- Determine the number of people you need to safely bathe and reposition the patient.

Helps prevent injury to the patient or the nurse.

- Assess for personal and cultural issues that may be of concern to the patient regarding the bath.

Bathing may conflict with the patient's sense of privacy or modesty. Cultural norms and individual preferences must be considered.

- Assess for specific patient needs and preferences during a bath, such as special soaps or lotions and extra washcloths or towels.

Advanced age, the presence of skin conditions, or skin breakdown may require special soaps and/or lotions. Incontinence or drainage may require additional washcloths, towels, and precautions. Meeting patient preferences helps prevent depersonalization and promotes patient cooperation with the procedure.

(continued on next page)

Procedure 22-1 ■ **Bathing: Providing a Complete Bed Bath** (continued)

➤ When performing the procedure, always identify your patient according to agency policy and be attentive to standard precautions, hand hygiene, patient safety and privacy, body mechanics, and documentation.

➤ *Note:* You may find that you need to adapt the bathing order and other steps to meet individual needs.

Procedure Steps

1. Provide for patient privacy and comfort.

   a. Close the door or privacy curtains, adjust room temperature, and assist the patient with elimination as needed.

   b. Ask the patient and family if they wish family members to assist with the bath.

Bathing practices differ among cultures and individuals, but are often private. The patient or family may wish to have a family member assist with the bath, or the patient may prefer that they leave the room. Assisting the patient with elimination before beginning the bath helps prevent interruptions during the procedure.

2. Fill the basin with warm water (approximately 105°F, or 41°C). Check the temperature with a thermometer or your hand. If possible, ask the patient to test the water temperature.

Hot water can injure the patient and removes protective skin oils. If the water is too cool, the patient may become chilled. Use water that is comfortable for the patient.

3. Adjust the bed to working height, lower the siderail nearest you, and position the patient supine close to the side of bed you will be working on. ✚ Raise the siderail before you leave that side of the bed.

Prevents you from having to lean over the patient or reach across the

siderail, which can cause back strain or injury. Raising the siderail helps prevent falls. ▼

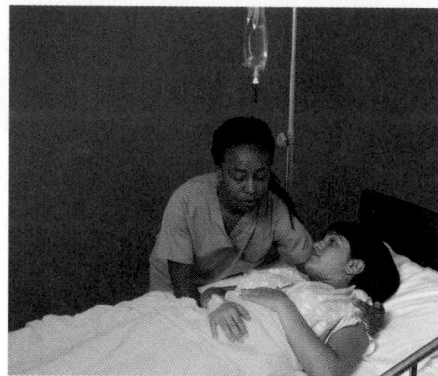

4. Remove the bedspread, and spread the bath blanket over the top sheet; then ask the patient to hold the bath blanket in place while you remove the top sheet.

Protects modesty and prevents chilling. If no bath blanket is available, you can use the top sheet in its place. However, if the sheet becomes wet, it may chill the patient. ▼

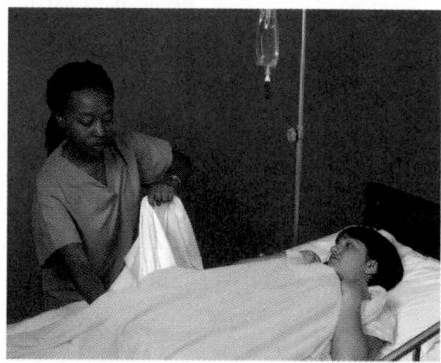

Note: Before proceeding, assist the patient with oral hygiene as needed. See Procedures 22-6 and 22-7, as needed.

5. Remove the patient's gown, keeping the patient covered with the bath blanket. During the bath, expose just the part of the body you are bathing. Maintains the patient's modesty and prevents chilling.

Step 5 Variation. Patient with an IV Line

If the patient has an IV line and is wearing a gown that does not have snap-open sleeves:

■ Remove the gown first from the arm without the IV.

■ Lower the IV container, and pass the gown over the tubing and the container, taking care to keep the container above the level of the patient's arm.

Keeps blood from backing up into the IV line. ▼

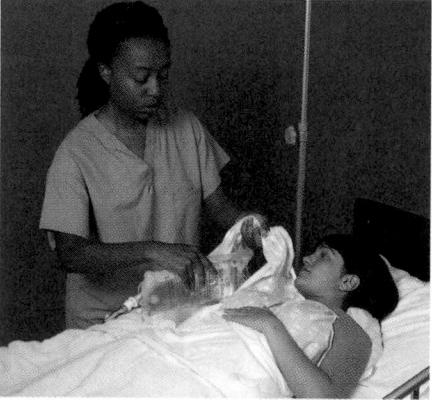

   a. Rehang the container; check the flow rate.

Manipulating the IV equipment may change the flow rate; flow rate must be maintained as prescribed.

✚ b. *Never* disconnect the IV tubing; this breaks the sterile system and provides a portal of entry for pathogens.

   c. After the bath, replace the gown by threading the IV equipment from inside the arm of the gown and onto the affected arm. Then place the unaffected arm through the other arm of the gown.

6. Don procedure gloves if exposure to body fluids is likely or if either you or the patient has any breaks in the skin.

Follows universal precautions; helps prevent transfer of microorganisms.

7. Wash the patient's face, neck, and ears.

  a. Fold the washcloth around the hand to make a mitt, tucking in loose corners.

Keeps loose ends from dragging across the skin. This is uncomfortable because loose ends cool quickly.

  b. Wet the washcloth, wringing out excess water. You may wash the face without soap if the skin is dry or if the patient prefers.

Soap is a drying agent and may be inappropriate to use on the face.

  c. Use a different corner of the washcloth (without soap) to gently wipe each eyelid outward from the inner canthus.

Soap is irritating to the eyes. A major principle is cleaning from "clean to dirty" to prevent contamination of a cleaner area. The inner canthus is considered the cleanest area. Prevents moving debris toward the nasolacrimal duct, which is located near the inner canthus. ▼

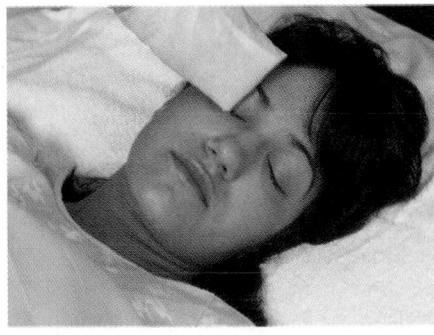

  d. Wash the rest of the patient's face, neck, and ears.

Move sequentially through the bath to make it less tiring for the patient and more efficient for the nurse.

  e. Rinse as needed, and pat face and neck dry.

Some soaps do not require rinsing. Pat the skin dry instead of rubbing to avoid irritation.

8. Wash the patient's arms and chest.

  a. Rinse and wring out the washcloth.

Rinse the washcloth frequently to ensure that it is clean and warm.

  b. Fold the bath blanket off one arm at a time, and place a folded bath towel under the arm. Beginning with the patient's far arm, support the arm, and wash the arm from the hands upward using long strokes.

The folded towel keeps the bottom sheet from getting wet and cold. Long strokes increase circulation in the extremity. Washing from hand upward toward the shoulder increases venous return from the periphery. Lifting the arm provides range of motion to preserve joint mobility.

  c. Continue to support the arm while washing the axilla.

Prevents potential injury to the joints. A sprain, subluxation, or dislocation of the joint can occur when an extremity is not properly supported, especially in older adults.

  d. Rinse as needed, and pat the arms dry.

Rinsing preserves skin integrity by preventing the drying effect of the soap on the skin.

  e. Apply deodorant and/or powder if desired.

Follow patient preferences whenever possible to increase feelings of comfort.

  f. Place the basin of water on the towel. Place the patient's hand in the water. Wash, rinse, and dry. Clean under the nails with an orangewood stick as needed.

Soaking the hand helps with cleaning under the fingernails and promotes comfort.

  g. Repeat the preceding steps 8a–f for the arm nearest you.

  h. Cover the patient's chest with a bath towel, and lower the bath blanket to the patient's waist.

Maintains patient comfort and modesty.

  i. Wash the chest. For women, gently lift each breast to wash the skinfold if needed. Keep the chest

covered between the wash and rinse.

Skinfolds can become reddened and irritated because of skin-to-skin irritation and dampness from perspiration. Skinfolds are also a source of odor. Cover to maintain privacy and warmth.

  j. Rinse and pat the chest dry. Cover with a bath towel.

Rinsing preserves skin integrity by preventing the drying effect of soap on the skin.

9. Wash the abdomen, legs, and feet.
  a. Fold the bath blanket down to the perineal area, and cover the chest with a bath towel.

Maintains patient privacy and warmth.

  b. Wash the abdomen, including the umbilical area; rinse and pat dry. Pay special attention to any skin folds.

Helps promote cleanliness and drying and prevents irritation from soap. Perspiration does not evaporate well from skin folds, nor does bath water, predisposing skinfolds to maceration.

  c. Cover the abdomen and chest with the bath blanket.

Prevents chilling.

  d. Uncover one leg at a time, beginning with the leg farthest from you. Place the bath towel under the leg.

Prevents chilling by keeping the sheet dry under the patient.

  e. Place the basin of water on the towel. Supporting the ankle and heel with your hand, and the leg on your arm, help the patient bend his leg and place his foot in the basin of water to soak.

Support reduces strain on joints. Soaking allows for better cleansing of the foot, especially the toes and nails, and increases patient comfort.

  f. Wash the leg from distal to proximal with long, gentle strokes. Rinse and pat the leg dry.

◆ Do not massage the calves of the legs.

(continued on next page)

Procedure 22-1 ■ **Bathing: Providing a Complete Bed Bath** (continued)

Moving from distal to proximal may help to promote venous return. If a venous thrombus is present, massaging might dislodge the clot and cause an embolus. ▼

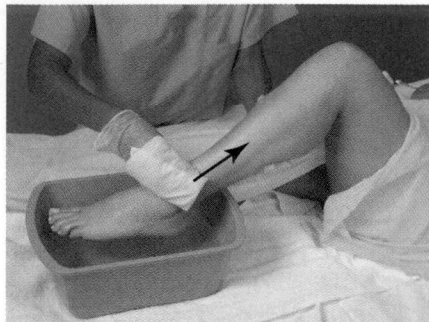

g. Thoroughly wash the foot and toes. Rinse and pat the foot dry; dry well between the toes. Apply lotion as needed.

Maintains healthy skin. Disease processes frequently decrease circulation to the feet and lower legs, increasing the likelihood that minor skin irritations may become more severe. Leaving damp areas between the toes can lead to skin breakdown.

h. Repeat the procedure on the other leg.

10. Wash the back and buttocks.
a. Position the patient on his side with his back facing you, or in the prone position. Make sure the siderail on the far side of the bed, facing the patient, is still up.

Provides for clear visualization of back and access to the area.

b. Exposing only the back and buttocks, place the bath towel under the back and buttocks. Wash the back first and then the buttocks. Rinse and pat dry, paying particular attention to gluteal folds. Observe for redness and skin breakdown in the sacral area.

Maintains the principle of "clean to dirty." The sacral area is a common site of pressure sores. Bath towel keeps

bottom sheet from getting wet and cold. ▼

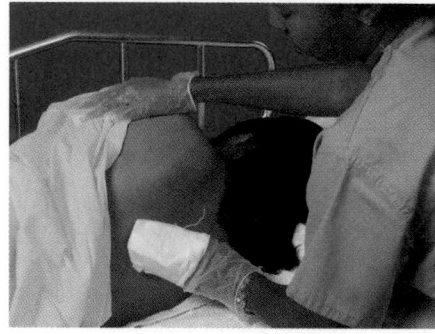

c. Unless contraindicated, give the patient a back rub, applying lotion to the back and buttocks (see Chapter 33, Procedure 33-1: Giving a Back Rub).

Stimulates circulation and maintains the health of the skin. Because the patient is in bed, he is at risk for skin irritation and breakdown from immobility and friction. A back rub may be contraindicated for patients with musculoskeletal injuries or cardiovascular disease.

d. Don procedure gloves if you have not already done so, and wash the rectal area, removing any fecal matter with tissues before washing with the washcloth. Wash from front to back.

Washing the rectal area at this time removes the need for the patient to turn to his side again and helps prevent soiling clean linen when changing the linen in an occupied bed. Fecal matter usually contains microorganisms. Washing from front to back helps prevent transferring bacteria from the rectum to the vagina and urethra. ▼

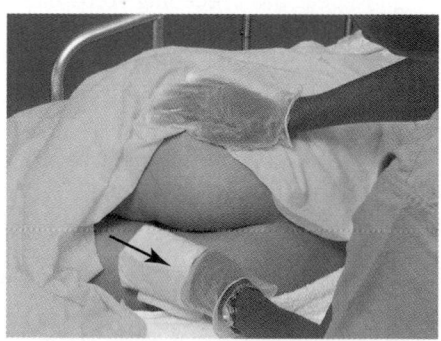

e. Discard the soiled washcloth, and change the bathwater. Wash and wipe out the basin as needed before refilling it. Cover any soiled linen before repositioning the patient.

f. Remove soiled gloves and wash hands or use an alcohol-based hand rub. Don new procedure gloves before providing perineal care.

Prevents transferring microorganisms from anal to genital area—cleansing the gluteal and anal areas contaminates the washcloth, towel, and water. Maintains standard precautions during the bath and prevents soiling of clean linens during bed change and cross contamination to other body sites.

11. Wash the perineal area. See Procedure 22-4: Providing Perineal Care.

12. After providing perineal care, reposition and cover the patient with the bath blanket. Remove soiled gloves and wash hands or use alcohol-based handrub. Help the patient put on a clean gown, and attend to other hygiene needs (e.g., hair grooming).

Prevents contaminating clean linen with soiled gloves. Ensures proper body position and warmth.

13. Change the bed linen as needed, including soiled linen or linen that became damp during the bath. See Procedure 22-14: Making an Occupied Bed.

Ensures patient safety, comfort, and privacy.

What if . . .

■ **You are bathing the patient without assistance, or you are not tall enough to comfortably reach across the patient?**

These situations put you at risk for back strain. Thus, you may want to bathe one side of the body—that is, the right arm, trunk, right leg—and then move to the other side of the bed to bathe the opposite side of the body (instead of the order given in steps 8 and 9). Move the patient close to you before beginning the bath.

- **You are bathing a patient in leg traction?**

You may decide to bathe the arms and trunk first. Then have the patient sit forward so that you can cleanse his back. Then have the patient lift up slightly so that you can wash his buttocks. Finally, wash the lower extremities.

- **You are bathing a patient with dementia?**

Use your knowledge of the person's bathing practices and preferences to determine a time of day and a routine the person will accept. Keep stimulation to a minimum. Turn on some calming music, speak softly and reassuringly, and don't rush. Keep the patient warm. If the patient becomes agitated and you cannot calm him, do not force him to bathe. You may wish to consider a towel bath (Procedure 22-2) for patients with dementia. Also refer to Clinical Insight 22-2.

Many steps in the bathing process may be misinterpreted or stressful for the person with dementia and may present in the appearance of disruptive or agitated behaviors. If forced to bathe, the patient may be upset for hours. Towel baths are effective hygiene measures.

- **Your patient becomes agitated and uncooperative during the bath?**

Speak calmly and softly. Give the patient a few minutes to calm down. Discontinue the bath if the patient remains upset.

- **Your patient is an older adult?**

Consider a bag bath with no-rinse skin cleanser.

These help prevent skin dryness.

a. If you use a tub bath use warm, not hot, water.

Prevents burns (older adults may have decreased sensation in their extremities).

b. Clean the tub well after each use *to prevent infection.*
c. Use antibacterial soap or a mild soap substitute. If you must use soap, it should be unperfumed and rich in moisture. If you use soap, rinse the skin well.
To avoid skin irritation.

d. Pat the skin dry; do not rub.
e. Apply a moisturizer immediately after drying, while there is still moisture in the skin. Wash your hands before applying the moisturizer.
f. Clean the skin immediately after every incident of soiling (e.g., when the patient has a bowel movement).
Prevents maceration and irritation from enzyme activity.

g. Some clinicians recommend bathing older adults every other day instead of daily, and it is generally agreed that they should not bathe more than once a day unless soiling occurs.

Evaluation

- Assess how well the patient tolerated the procedure. Was there any discomfort, shortness of breath, and so on?
- Observe the patient's mobility, both range of motion and ease of movement.
- Note the condition of the patient's skin, including redness and other abnormal findings, especially in skinfolds.
- Ask the patient whether he is comfortable and satisfied.
- If someone other than the nurse performs the procedure, the nurse must still evaluate the care to be certain that it was done and performed satisfactorily.

Patient Teaching

- Discuss the need for activity (e.g., moving about in bed) and the hazards of immobility.
- Discuss usual skin care and how to increase the health of the skin.
- Demonstrate bathing procedure to family or other caregivers.

Home Care

Note: Many of the following apply to older adults and others with self-care deficits.
- Evaluate the home for bathing safety considerations (not limited to bed bath), such as the following:
    Safety bars in the bathroom?
To facilitate transfers and provide support while washing.

A safe water supply for bathing?
Bathing supplies that are available and accessible?
Nonskid mat or abrasive strips for shower or tub?
Helps prevent falls on standing.

Stool for shower; transfer bench or stool for getting into the tub?
Hand-held shower spray?
Facilitates washing and manipulation of bath controls.

Long-handled brush or sponge?
Assists with limitations in ROM.

- Assess the client's ability to help with the bath or to bathe independently.
- Ask how the client usually bathes (e.g., shower, at the sink). Follow the client's preference as much as possible.
- Ask what supplies the client usually uses for the bath, and ask where they are stored. You will need to adapt the procedure depending on the available equipment and supplies.
- Suggest the use of large plastic trash bags or a shower curtain to protect the mattress during a bed bath.
- Instruct caregivers to wear gloves when handling linens that are soiled with blood or other body fluids. Linens should be washed in cold water, separately from other household laundry, and then washed again, using hot water, detergent, and bleach.
Hot water coagulates proteins in the blood and makes it more difficult to remove. Detergent and bleach are used to destroy pathogens.

(continued on next page)

Procedure 22-1 ▪ **Bathing: Providing a Complete Bed Bath** (continued)

Documentation

Chart the type of bath given, how much patient was able to help with the bath, how well the patient tolerated the procedure, the patient's mobility, and any abnormal findings. Hygiene care is charted on checklists and flowsheets in most agencies.

Sample electronic documentation:

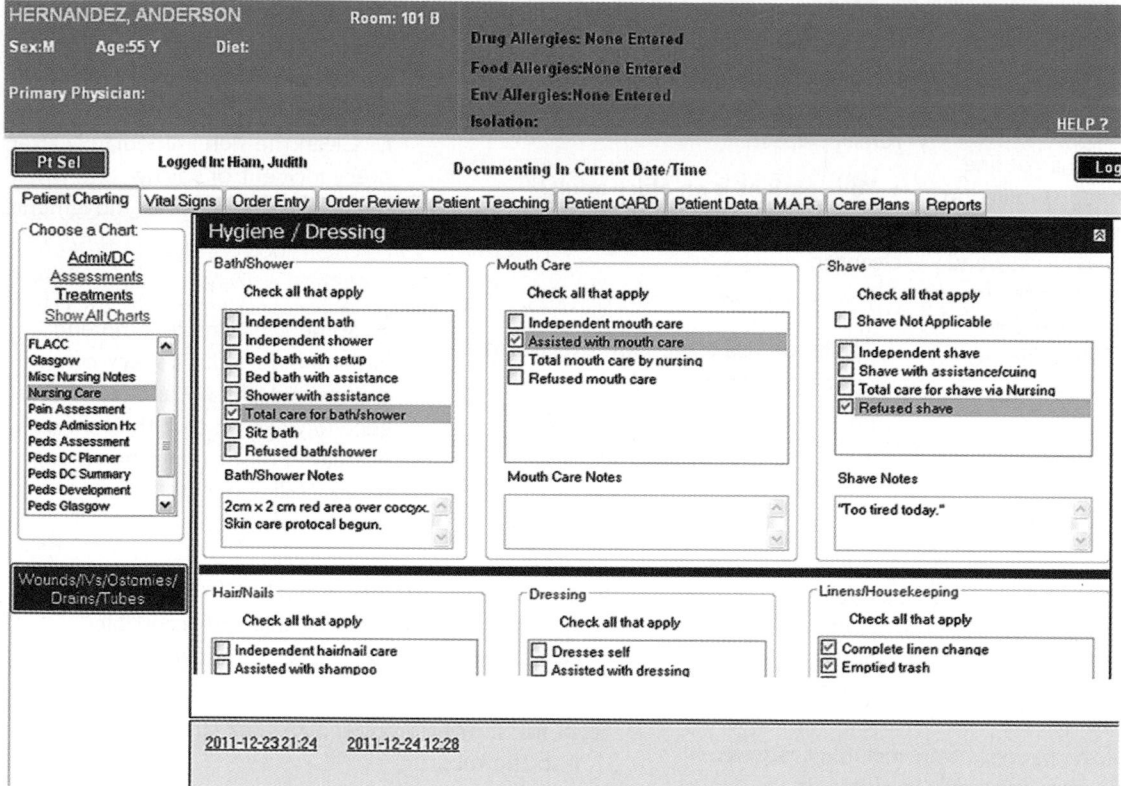

Practice Resources

Downey, L., & Lloyd, H. (2008); Flori, L. (2007); George, M., & Naik, A. (2006); Haas, J., & Larson, E. (2008); O'Flynn, J. (2007); Siegel, J., Rhinehart, E., Jackson, M., et al. (2007); Stern, C. (2007); Thiru-Chelvam, B. (2004).

Thinking About the Procedure

 Go to the *Fundamentals of Nursing Skills Videos*, **Hygiene: Bed Bath, Oral Hygiene, Foot Care, and Back Massage.**

1. After the patient performs oral hygiene, how many basins of water does the nurse fill for the bath? Why?

2. How did the nurse check the temperature of the water?

 For suggested responses, go to Chapter 22, **Thinking About the Procedure Suggested Responses,** on the Student Resource Disk or DavisPlus at http://davisplus.fadavis.com/ Wilkinson2

Procedure 22-2 □ Bathing: Providing a Towel Bath

➤ For steps to follow in *all* procedures, refer to the Universal Steps for All Procedures found on the inside back cover of Volume 2.

➤ *Note:* Because the towel bath is a variation of the bed bath, only the steps differing from a bed bath are listed.

Critical Aspects

- Refer to Procedure 22-1: Bathing: Providing a Complete Bed Bath.
- Check the temperature of the water.
- Begin at the feet and work toward the head (instead of "head to toe" as in Procedure 22-1).

Equipment

- Large plastic bag containing a bath blanket (or a very large towel, about 3 ft × 6 ft), one standard bath towel, and two or three washcloths
- Dry bath blankets (2 or more)
- Dry bath towels
- Pitcher and approximately 2 qt (2000 mL) of warm water (105°F [41°C])
- 30 mL of no-rinse liquid soap or commercial solution of soap, moisturizer, and disinfectant
- Other supplies for a bed bath; see Procedure 22-1.

Delegation

You can delegate this procedure to the NAP if you conclude that the patient's condition and the NAP's skills allow. Perform the following assessments, and inform the NAP of the amount of help the patient needs and any special considerations, such as IV lines, drains, and so on. Ask the NAP to report the condition of the patient's skin, level of self-care, and ability to tolerate the procedure.

Pre-Procedure Assessments

- Assess the patient's mobility and activity tolerance to determine whether she will be able to assist with the bath, whether a bag bath is appropriate, and whether you will need another caregiver to assist.

A patient with decreased activity tolerance or mobility (e.g., because of chest pain or shortness of breath with exertion, or paralysis) may have a limited ability to assist with the bath, making a bag bath the most appropriate choice. For severely compromised patients, having two nurses give the bath will make the procedure much quicker and less demanding on the patient.

➤ When performing the procedure, always identify your patient according to agency policy and be attentive to standard precautions, hand hygiene, patient safety and privacy, body mechanics, and documentation.

Procedure Steps

1. Prepare the bath bag.
   a. Prefold the bath blanket.
   Allows for organized application and ease of handling the blanket.

   ✦ b. Fill a large pitcher with warm water (approximately 105°F [41°C]).
   The amount of water varies depending on the size of the bath blanket and bath towel. Use enough water to saturate them. Hot water can injure the patient and removes more of the skin's protective oils, but if the water is too cool, the patient may become chilled.

   c. Add 30 mL of no-rinse soap or commercial solution to the water according to the manufacturer's instructions.
   Adding a prescribed amount of soap to the water before pouring into the bag prevents excessive sudsing.

   d. Pour the solution into the bag, over the bath blanket and bath towel, to ensure even distribution.

2. If you do not plan to change the linen, work one dry bath blanket under the patient.
   Protects the linen and provides warmth.

3. Spread a dry bath blanket over the patient; remove the patient's clothing, working underneath the blanket.
   Protects privacy and prevents chilling.

4. Replace the dry blanket with the wet blanket:
   a. Take the wet bath blanket or towel out of the bag, squeezing out excess water so that it does not drip.
   b. Push the dry bath blanket down to the patient's waist, and place the wet bath blanket on the patient's chest.

   c. Continue to unfold the wet bath blanket until it covers the patient, pushing the dry bath blanket out of the way as you do so.
   The wet bath blanket will feel warm and relaxing. The dry bath blanket will be used to dry the patient, so you must keep it from becoming damp.

   d. If necessary, place yet another dry blanket on top of the wet one.
   This helps hold in the warmth if the patient is chilling or the room is cool.

5. Bathe the patient, beginning at the feet and working toward the head.
   a. Keeping the patient covered, use the wet bath blanket to wash the legs, abdomen, and chest.
   b. As you work, replace the wet bath blanket with the dry one.

(continued on next page)

Procedure 22-2 ■ Bathing: Providing a Towel Bath (continued)

Keeps the patient from chilling. ▼

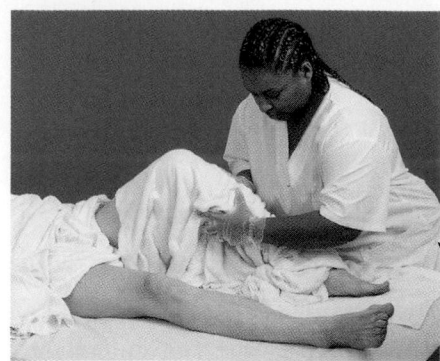

c. Fold the wet bath blanket as each area is bathed, allowing only clean surfaces to contact clean surfaces.

Prevents contamination of the clean side of the wet bath blanket.

d. Use one of the wet washcloths to wash the patient's face, neck, and ears.

Notice that this varies from the order of most baths, which proceed from head to toe. However, this is the most efficient way to accomplish a towel bath. It does not really compromise the clean-to-dirty principle because the legs, abdomen, and chest are usually equally "clean," and you are washing those before the back, buttocks, and perineum. You will use separate, clean cloths to wash the face.

6. Don procedure gloves. Roll the client to one side, unfold the wet bath towel so the clean surface covers the patient, and use the wet bath towel to wash the back and then the buttocks.

7. Change procedure gloves and wash your hands. Wash the perineal area with a washcloth. See Procedure 22-4: Providing Perineal Care.

8. Finish the bath as in Procedure 22-1: Bathing: Providing a Complete Bed Bath. Follow patient preferences whenever possible to increase feelings of comfort.

9. Change linen as needed, including soiled linen or linen that became damp during the bath. You will almost certainly need to change the linen if you have not padded the bottom sheet well before the bath.

Ensures patient safety and comfort. Because the bath is finished rapidly, there is no real need to pad the bottom sheet if you know that you will have time to change the linens after the bath.

What if . . .

■ **Your patient becomes agitated and uncooperative during the bath?**

Speak calmly and softly. Give the patient a few minutes to calm down. Discontinue the bath if the patient remains upset.

See Procedure 22-1: Bathing: Providing a Complete Bed Bath.

Practice Resources

Downey, L., & Lloyd, H. (2008); Flori, L. (2007); The Joanna Briggs Institute (2007).

Procedure 22-3 ■ Bathing: Providing a Packaged Bath

➤ For steps to follow in *all* procedures, refer to the Universal Steps for All Procedures found on the inside back cover of Volume 2.

Critical Aspects

■ Refer to Procedure 22-1, Bathing: Providing a Complete Bed Bath.
■ Check the temperature of the packaged bath after microwaving.

Equipment

■ Packaged disposable washcloths (e.g., Comfort Bath)
■ Lotion
■ Deodorant and/or powder as needed
■ Clean patient gown (gown with shoulder snaps or Velcro closures if the patient has an IV line)
■ Clean linen
■ Procedure gloves
■ Plastic trash bag for used cloths and other disposable soiled items

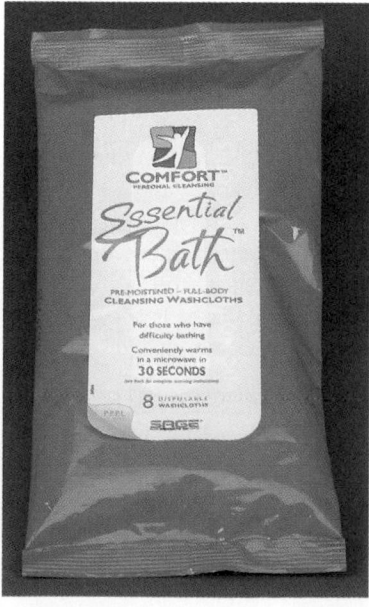

Delegation

You can delegate this procedure to the NAP if you conclude that the patient's condition and the NAP's skills allow. Perform the following assessments, and inform the NAP of the amount of help the patient needs and of any special considerations, such as IV lines, drains, and so on. Ask the NAP to report the condition of the patient's skin, level of self-care, and ability to tolerate the procedure.

Pre-Procedure Assessments

Assessments are the same as in Procedure 22-1, Bathing: Providing a Complete Bed Bath.

➤ When performing the procedure, always identify your patient according to agency policy and be attentive to standard precautions, hand hygiene, patient safety and privacy, body mechanics, and documentation.

Procedure Steps

1. Peel open the label on the commercial bath without completely removing it.

Allows for steam to escape as contents heat without spilling the contents.

2. Warm the solution:

Step 2 Variation. Microwave

◆ Heat the package in the microwave for no longer than 1 minute. The temperature of the contents should be approximately 105°F (41°C). This is controversial. Some references suggest, for safety, using the commercial bag bath at room temperature.

Brings contents to a safe and comfortable temperature.

Step 2 Variation. Warmer Unit

If a warmer unit is used, you do not need step 2 because the bags are always warm.

3. Prepare the patient for the bath as described in Procedure 22-1.

4. Using one washcloth for each body area, wash the patient following the sequence in Procedure 22-1. Or follow the manufacturer's recommended sequence for the number of washcloths in the bag.

5. Allow the areas to air dry; do not rinse.

Prevents the emollient and surfactant skin protectants from being removed.

6. Discard each washcloth after use.

Ensures following the "clean to dirty" principle.

7. Help patient don a clean gown.

What if . . .

■ **A commercial bag bath is not available?**

You can make your own bag bath.
    a. Place eight washcloths in a large self-locking plastic bag.
    b. Mix an emollient or a no-rinse surfactant with warm water, and pour over the washcloths in the bag.
    c. If the water is not warm enough (105°F [41°C]) warm in a microwave oven for 1 to 2 minutes. Check the temperature of the washcloths before using.

Prevents burning the skin.

The washcloths can be prepared ahead of time and kept in a warming unit if one is available. But do not store for longer than 24 hours.

Prevents bacterial growth.

    d. Use each cloth for one of the following areas: face, back, chest, right arm, left arm, right leg, left leg, perineum.
    e. Put used washcloths in the laundry for future use.

For Evaluation, Documentation, and Patient Teaching, see Procedure 22-1: Bathing: Providing a Complete Bed Bath.

Practice Resources

Birch, S., & Coggins, T. (2003); Chu, J. (2004); The Joanna Briggs Institute (2007); Larson, E., Ciliberti T., Chantler, C., et al. (2004).

Procedure 22-4 ■ Providing Perineal Care

➤ For steps to follow in *all* procedures, refer to the Universal Steps for All Procedures found on the inside back cover of Volume 2.

Critical Aspects

- Provide privacy; keep the patient covered as much as possible.
- Place a waterproof underpad to protect the bed linens.
- Use warm water.
- Perform perineal care following the principle of "clean to dirty" (front to back).

Equipment

- Procedure gloves
- Water basin or perineal wash bottle
- Waterproof pad
- Bedpan or portable sitz tub (optional)
- Bath towel
- Washcloth
- Toilet paper
- Cleansing solution or soap
- Perineal ointment or lotion if needed

Delegation

You can delegate perineal care to the NAP if you conclude that the patient's condition and the NAP's skills allow. Perform the following assessments, and inform the NAP of the amount of help the patient needs and any special considerations (e.g., presence of a urinary catheter, vaginal drainage). Ask the NAP to report the condition of the patient's perineum (skin, drainage), level of self-care, and ability to tolerate the procedure.

Pre-Procedure Assessments

- Assess the patient's mobility and activity tolerance. Determine whether the patient will be able to assist with the perineal care. Doing as much self-care as possible increases the patient's sense of independence and maintains modesty.

- Check for positioning or activity restrictions, such as maintaining hip abduction following a total hip replacement.
Prevents injuring the patient during the procedure.

- Assess for psychosocial issues that may be of concern to the patient regarding perineal care.
You must consider cultural norms to ensure that the perineal care is appropriate for the patient. For example, in some cultures a woman would find it completely unacceptable for a male nurse to perform her perineal care (pericare).

- Assess for any specific patient needs for perineal care.
For example, if there are lesions or skin breakdown, you may need to use special soaps and/or lotions. Incontinence or drainage requires assessment and follow-up to prevent Impaired Skin Integrity.

- Assess for the presence of a urinary drainage catheter, perineal surgery, or lesions.
You may need to adapt the procedure to clean around an indwelling urinary catheter or surgical incisions.

➤ When performing the procedure, always identify your patient according to agency policy and be attentive to standard precautions, hand hygiene, patient safety and privacy, body mechanics, and documentation.

Procedure Steps

1. Adjust the room temperature, and assist with elimination as needed.
Assisting the patient with elimination before perineal care helps prevent interruptions during the procedure and allows for thorough perineal care. Adjusting room temperature prevents chilling.

✦ 2. Fill the basin or perineal wash bottle with warm water (approximately 105°F [41°C]).
Hot water can injure the skin, and cool water can cause chilling. Use water that is comfortable for the patient.

3. Wash the perineal area.

a. Position the patient on her back (supine). Place waterproof pads under the patient if they are not already in place. You may wish to place the patient on a bedpan or portable sitz tub, especially if the perineum is grossly soiled.
Placing the patient on a bedpan raises the hips to increase visualization and allows for more thorough cleansing. A bedpan also allows for using additional water when needed.

b. Wear procedure gloves (and other protective wear as needed) when providing perineal care. Wear a procedure gown and

goggles if you are concerned about splashing (e.g., if the patient is confused and may be unable to follow instructions).
Follows standard precautions.

c. Drape the patient to protect privacy.

Step 3c Variation. Female Patient

- Drape the bath blanket so that one point faces the patient's head (drape it in the shape of a diamond).
- Take one of the side points of the diamond, and wrap it around the patient's leg. Anchor the end of the blanket under the patient's foot.

- Repeat on the other leg with other point of the diamond. ▼

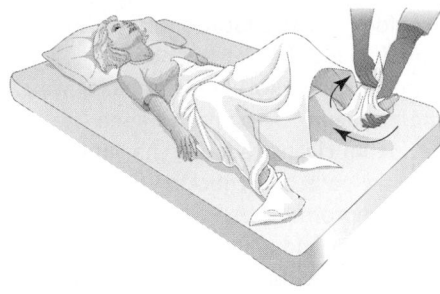

- Fold the center lower point of the diamond up to expose the patient's perineum. ▼

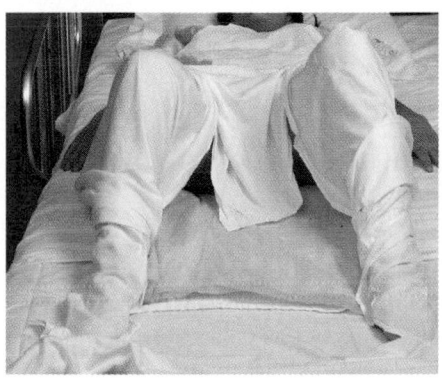

This draping technique covers the patient as much as possible, which helps maintain privacy and prevents chilling during the procedure. The patient can also relax her legs against the bath blanket.

Step 3c Variation. Male Patient

- Place the bath blanket over the patient's chest.
- Fold the bed linens down to expose only the patient's groin.
  d. Remove any fecal material with toilet paper.

Prevents contamination of the perineum with feces, which can lead to bladder or incisional infections. If you are providing perineal care as part of giving a bed bath, you will have cleaned the anal area when the patient was in the lateral position.

  e. Moisten the washcloth with the water in the basin, or spray the perineum with the perineal wash bottle.

Moistens the area or washcloth thoroughly to ensure adequate cleansing.

  f. Wash the perineum.

Step 3f Variation. Female Patient

Wash the perineum from front to back, using a clean portion of the washcloth for each stroke. Cleanse the labial folds and around the urinary catheter, if one is in place.

Prevents contaminating the urethra with fecal material. Any fecal particles that are left can cause skin breakdown due to enzyme activity, and may increase the risk of a urinary tract infection because of the presence of *E. coli* in the feces. ▼

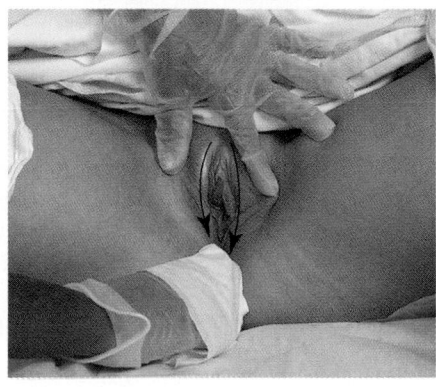

Step 3f Variation. Male Patient

Retract the foreskin, if present, and gently cleanse the head of the penis using a circular motion. Replace the foreskin, and finish washing the shaft of the penis, using firm strokes. Then wash the scrotum, using a clean portion of the washcloth with each stroke. Handle the scrotum with care, because the area is sensitive.

To adequately clean the head of the penis in an uncircumcised male, you must retract the foreskin. After cleaning, replace the foreskin to prevent constriction and edema of the penis. Firm strokes may help to prevent an erection. Using a clean portion of the washcloth for each wipe prevents fecal contamination of the urethra and perineum. ▼

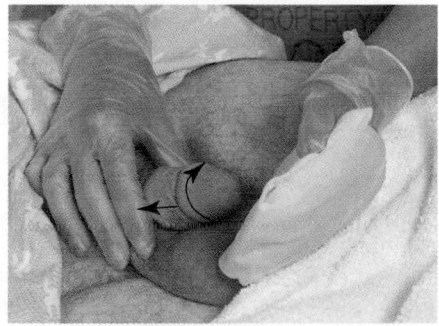

g. In both males and females, cleanse the skinfolds of the groin area thoroughly, and pat dry. Examine the skin creases for redness or excoriation.

Detects and prevents excoriation in skinfold areas, where moisture accumulates.

4. Rinse and pat dry.
Prevents skin injury secondary to maceration. If you are using perineal wash solution, rinsing is not required.

5. If perineal care is being done *not* as part of the bath, also clean the anal area. Ask the patient to turn to the side, and wash, rinse, and dry the buttocks and anal area as needed.
Fecal contamination of the perineum can lead to urinary tract infections and skin irritation. Therefore, the anal area is cleansed last.

6. Apply skin protectants as needed. Powder only if the patient requests it.
If urinary or fecal incontinence is present, skin barriers may be used to prevent urine, feces, or other drainage from contacting the skin. This helps prevent skin breakdown. For female patients, powder is a medium for bacterial growth. In the presence of moisture, it also creates a paste, which irritates the skin.

7. If the patient has an indwelling catheter and if agency policy requires special catheter care, you will usually provide the care at this point. Don clean gloves before providing catheter care, and follow the agency's procedure. For more information about catheter care, see Clinical Insight 27-1, Caring for a Patient with an Indwelling Catheter.

8. Reposition and cover the patient with the bath blanket. Remove soiled gloves, discarding appropriately.
Prevents contaminating clean linen with soiled gloves.

9. Change linen as needed, including soiled linen or linen that became damp during perineal care.
Ensures patient safety, comfort, and privacy.

(continued on next page)

Procedure 22-4 ■ Providing Perineal Care (continued)

What if...

■ **The patient is unable to control bowel and/or bladder?**

Gently cleanse and dry the perineal/perigenital area after each incontinence/soiling and apply a moisture barrier according to agency protocols.

Minimizing contact with irritants such as moisture, urine, and stool can decrease the development of incontinence-associated dermatitis.

Use a spray, no-rinse cleanser and soft wipes.

These aid in preventing irritation from friction, and reducing drying effects on the skin.

Follow agency policy and use skin assessment tools (some geared particularly to perineal skin).

■ Assess for signs of secondary infection in addition to irritation and report as needed.

■ Consider bowel and bladder retraining and scheduling to reduce frequency of incontinence.

■ **The patient is postpartum?**

Provide patient education on perineal care. Include the importance of handwashing before and after cleansing the perineum, measures to keep the perineum clean, frequent changing of sanitary pads, and checking for signs and symptoms of abnormal lochia. If the patient had an episiotomy, laceration, or tear, teaching should also include management of discomfort and signs of wound infection.

Evaluation

■ Assess the patient's responses to the procedure. Was there any discomfort?
■ Observe for difficulty with movement or range of motion during the procedure.
■ Note the condition of the skin, including redness and other abnormal findings.
■ Ask the patient whether she feels comfortable now.

Patient Teaching

■ Discuss adaptations to perineal care. For example, if the area is tender, (1) wash the area with warm water after going to the bathroom, instead of using toilet paper; or (2) use a skin protectant on the area.
■ Review the importance of hand washing after elimination.
■ If appropriate, teach the caregiver how to provide perineal care, including the major concept of cleaning front to back ("clean to dirty"). Stress the importance of wearing gloves and washing hands.
■ Advise women not to douche because it disturbs the balance of normal vaginal flora and can irritate or injure mucosal cells.
■ Explain that scented and deodorant feminine hygiene products are not necessary for cleanliness and may even be harmful. Plain soap and water are the most effective means of odor control.

Home Care

■ Evaluate the ability of the client or caregiver to provide perineal care.
■ If needed, teach the caregiver how to provide perineal care, including the major concept of cleaning front to back ("clean to dirty").
■ Determine the availability of supplies needed for perineal care.
■ You will need to adapt the procedure depending on the available equipment and supplies. Major issues involved in perineal care in the home are the lack of clean water and/or linens. In some instances, you may need to use bottled water or boil water for the

procedure. One option is to use prepackaged moistened towelettes to provide the care (e.g., Comfort Bath towelettes). These products may be heated in a water bath or microwave oven.

Documentation

Usually perineal care is part of routine hygiene care and is charted on a flowsheet. If you need to write a narrative note, chart that perineal care was given, any patient responses to the procedure, and the condition of the perineal area.

Sample documentation:

8/16/11	1430	*Perineal care given. Patient had no c/o discomfort. No redness or discharge noted.* ———— *Nora Noyes, RN*

Practice Resources

Bliss, D., Zehrer, C., Savik, K., et al. (2006); Gray, M., Bliss, D., Doughty, D., et al. (2007); National Collaborating Centre for Primary Care (2006); National Guideline Clearinghouse (2005b); Siegel, J., Rhinehart, E., Jackson, M., et al., Healthcare Infection Control Practices Advisory Committee (2007); Warshaw, E., Nix, D., Kula, J., et al. (2002).

Thinking About the Procedure

 Go to the *Fundamentals of Nursing Skills Videos*, **Perineal Care: Female,** and **Perineal Care: Male.**

1. In the skill, Perineal Care: Female, do you think this patient is incontinent of urine or feces? Why or why not?

2. In the skill, Perineal Care: Male, what did the nurse use to protect the patient's privacy before beginning the procedure?

 For suggested responses, go to Chapter 22, **Thinking About the Procedure Suggested Responses,** on the Student Resource Disk or DavisPlus at http://davisplus.fadavis.com/Wilkinson2

Procedure 22-5 ■ Providing Foot Care

➤ For steps to follow in *all* procedures, refer to the Universal Steps for All Procedures found on the inside back cover of Volume 2.

Critical Aspects

- Inspect the feet thoroughly for skin integrity, circulation, and edema.
- Clean the feet with mild soap; clean the toenails; rinse; and dry well.
- Trim the nails straight across, unless contraindicated. Check institutional policy; many institutions do not allow nurses to trim nails.
- File the nails with an emery board.
- Lightly apply lotion, except between the toes.
- Ensure that footwear or bedding is not irritating to the feet.

Equipment

- Procedure gloves (if there are open lesions)
- Pillow (if procedure is done with the patient in bed)
- Basin for water
- Liquid no-rinse soap
- Bath towel
- Waterproof pad
- Washcloth
- Orangewood stick
- Toenail clippers
- Nail file
- Lotion or prescribed ointment or cream

Delegation

You can delegate foot care to the NAP if you conclude that the patient's condition and the NAP's skills allow. For example, as a rule you should not delegate care if the patient has impaired peripheral circulation or foot ulcers. Perform the following assessments, and inform the NAP of the amount of help the patient needs and any special considerations (e.g., ability to sit in a chair). Ask the NAP to report the condition of the patient's skin and nails, level of self-care, and ability to tolerate the procedure.

Pre-Procedure Assessments

- Assess bilateral dorsalis pedis pulses, skin color, and warmth. Compare right and left feet.

Palpate pulses at the same time bilaterally to determine whether one side is weaker than the other. Decreased circulation to the feet increases the risk for tissue injury and infection. A variety of diseases can cause poor circulation. For example, cardiac or renal disease may cause pedal edema, which impairs circulation to the skin, and diabetes causes vascular changes leading to poor circulation to the lower extremities.

- Thoroughly assess all areas of the feet for skin integrity, edema, condition of toenails, and any abnormalities. Check carefully between the toes.

Decreased circulation in the feet commonly causes such problems as thickened toenails, dry skin, and increased risk of infection. Changes in vision and mobility can increase the

risk for injuries to the feet. Patients with diabetes also may have neuropathy, which prevents them from knowing when they have injured their feet. Identifying abnormalities enables you to provide interventions to help prevent potential problems. ▼

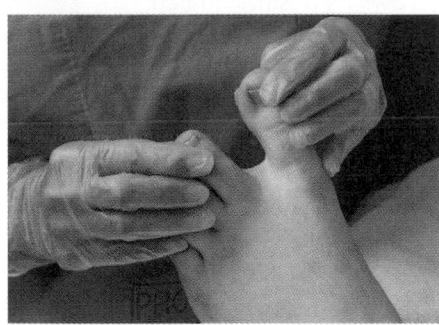

- Check institutional policy to verify whether a nurse is allowed to trim nails. Obtain a primary provider's prescription for trimming the patient's nails, if necessary.

Patients who have diabetes or impaired circulation to the lower extremities require a prescription for trimming their nails. Refer the patient to a podiatrist if the circulation is severely compromised or if edema would make the procedure difficult.

- Assess the patient's usual footwear.

Improperly fitting shoes, especially if they are too tight, are a common cause of foot problems.

- Assess the patient's self-care ability to provide foot care. Evaluate the need for a referral. Determine whether the patient has the necessary vision and mobility to be able provide his own foot care.
- Assess the patient's knowledge about foot care, including usual foot care practices.

Identify potential deficits in understanding of foot care needs that may require additional teaching or referral to a podiatrist, general practice physician, or advanced practice nurse. Many home remedies for foot problems can damage the tissue. For example, corn pads can increase pressure on the tissue, compromising circulation and causing local tissue ischemia. Cutting the sides of the toenails can lead to ingrown toenails.

(continued on next page)

Procedure 22-5 ■ **Providing Foot Care** (continued)

➤ When performing the procedure, always identify your patient according to agency policy and be attentive to standard precautions, hand hygiene, patient safety and privacy, body mechanics, and documentation.

Procedure Steps

1. Wear procedure gloves and other protective wear as needed when providing foot care.
Follows standard precautions. The heel is a common place for skin breakdown, so use gloves if you are unable to see the area without lifting the foot. If the patient has significant drainage to the area, such as a draining wound, you may need to wear a protective gown.

2. Ask the patient to sit in a chair with a waterproof pad or bath towel under the feet, if possible. If the patient is unable to sit in a chair, place him in semi-Fowler's position in bed; place a pillow under his knees.
It is easier to perform the procedure with the patient in a chair. The pillow supports the knee joints and prevents muscle fatigue.

✚ **3.** Fill the basin halfway with warm water (approximately 105° to 110°F [40° to 43°C]).
Hot water can injure the skin. Warm water promotes circulation. Filling the basin halfway prevents spilling when the patient places his foot in the water.

4. Help the patient place one foot in the water, first checking with the patient that the temperature is comfortable.
   a. If the patient is in a chair, place the basin on the floor (on the waterproof pad).
   b. If the patient is in bed, place the basin near the foot of the bed on the waterproof pad; pad the basin with a towel.
The waterproof pad keeps the bed dry. Padding the basin prevents pressure on the back of the leg, which could cause discomfort and interfere with circulation.

5. Allow the foot to soak for 5 to 20 minutes, depending on the patient's tolerance and the condition of his feet.
✚ Soaking is not recommended for patients with diabetes or peripheral vascular disease (PVD).

Soaking softens the skin and helps relax the patient. For patients who have

diabetes or PVD, soaking is not recommended because it may remove natural oils, cause cracking of the skin, and may cause burns even if the water is at the recommended temperature.

6. Clean the foot with mild or no-rinse soap.
Removes loose debris. No-rinse soaps do not dry the skin. ▼

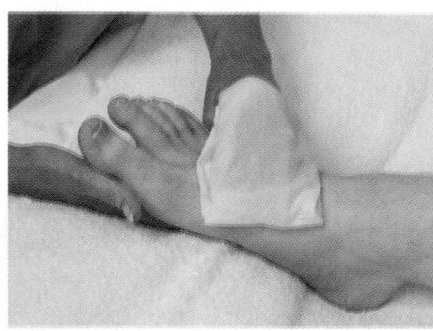

7. Clean under the nails with the orangewood stick while the foot is still in the water.
Water softens the nails and makes cleaning easier.

8. Rinse. Remove the foot from the water, and dry it gently and thoroughly.
Remaining moisture, especially between the toes, can cause maceration and promotes development of fungal infections.

9. Change the water, if necessary.
Ensures proper temperature.

10. Soak the opposite foot while performing steps 11 through 14 for the first (clean) foot.
Saves time.

11. Gently push the cuticles back with the orangewood stick or towel.
Increases cuticle health. Do not damage the cuticle; doing so can increase the risk of infection.

12. Trim the nails straight across with toenail clippers, if not contraindicated by the patient's condition and if permitted by agency policy. Note whether the nail has cut into the skin of the toe being trimmed or the adjacent toes. If the nails are brittle or thick, allow the foot to soak for 10 to 20 minutes before trimming.

Trimming straight across prevents ingrown toenails. Early recognition and treatment of problems will prevent further complications, such as infection. ▼

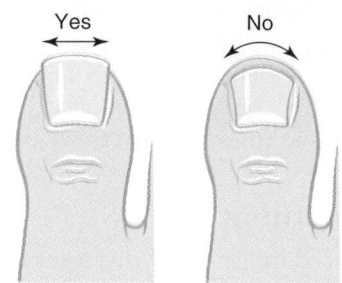

Yes   No

13. File the nails with an emery board.
Smooths the edges to prevent scratching the skin with the toenails.

14. Apply cream, lotion, or foot powder lightly to the feet and toes.
Cream hydrates the skin. Note, however, that excess cream can cause maceration. Foot powder absorbs moisture and functions as a nonirritating deodorant for patients whose feet perspire heavily.

15. Repeat steps 11 through 14 with the second foot.

16. Check the patient's footwear for rough edges that may injure feet.

What if . . .

■ **My patient has Impaired Bed Mobility?**

Apply protective devices (e.g., lamb's wool) as needed.

■ **My patient has an injury, lesions, or pain?**

You may need to use a bed cradle to keep the pressure of the bedding off the patient's feet. Refer to Chapter 34 for other measures to preserve skin integrity.

Protects the feet from further injury from abrasion or pressure.

■ **My patient has diabetes mellitus?**

In addition to controlling blood glucose levels, adhering to a specific foot care plan is essential for people with diabetes. Include the following in your teaching:
■ The importance of inspecting the feet daily

- Ways to protect the feet (e.g., by wearing shoes when out of bed)
- Potential complications involving the feet
- Management of symptoms
- When to seek advice from a healthcare professional
- What to include in the foot care regimen (apply moisturizing lotion

on tops and bottoms of feet but not between toes)—and what not to do (cut corns and calluses, use topical corn removers, or soak the feet)

- Elderly patients with diabetes are especially at risk for development of foot-related complications. Visual changes and loss of flexibility could

make it challenging to bend and visualize the feet. Plastic mirrors may be helpful in this regard.

Early detection and treatment of problems can minimize foot-related complications.

Evaluation

- Observe that feet are clean, smooth, and intact; nails are trimmed and smooth; skin is pink and warm.
- Be sure that foot problems are identified and interventions provided.
- Ask the patient to demonstrate or describe correct foot care.

Patient Teaching

- Reinforce the following as necessary.
  Wash the feet daily with warm water and mild soap.
  Dry the feet well, especially between the toes.
  Inspect the feet daily (using a mirror to check the soles) for cracks, dry skin, cuts, redness, swelling, and change in temperature.
  Keep the toenails trimmed straight across.
  Apply cream lightly to feet daily. Do not apply cream between the toes.
  Report any abnormalities to the healthcare provider: numbness or tingling; decrease in sensation; skin redness, cracks, cuts, swelling; or decrease in skin temperature.
- Discuss the importance of properly fitting footwear and socks.
- Instruct the patient to avoid actions that would decrease circulation to the lower legs (e.g., wearing knee-high stockings, crossing the legs, smoking, sitting in chair without support to the feet).

Home Care

The procedure does not vary in the home. The nurse must:

- Work with the client and care provider to determine the availability of supplies needed for foot care (clean water and so on).
- Identify home care practices, and teach the client and/or caregiver proper foot care techniques. Influencing older adults can be especially difficult if they have usual routines, such as walking barefoot, that put them at risk for injury. For clients with diabetes, the biggest risk to foot health is inadequate regulation of their blood glucose levels.

Documentation

In most agencies you will not document routine foot care (except, perhaps, on a checklist) unless there are problems. If you do document, chart that foot care was given, and chart assessment findings.

Sample documentation:

09/25/11 0900	*Foot care given. 2 cm circular reddened area on right heel. Skin abrasion outer lateral aspect of 5th toe, left foot—bioocclusive dressing applied.*
	— *Ann Hopkins, RN*

Practice Resources

National Collaborating Centre for Primary Care (2004); Plummer, E., & Albert, S. (2008); Siegel, J., Rhinehart, E., Jackson, M., et al. (2007).

Thinking About the Procedure

 Go to the *Fundamentals of Nursing Skills Videos*, **Oral Hygiene, Foot Care, and Back Massage.**

1. The nurse performs foot care near the end of this procedure. Which step was mentioned by the narrator but not demonstrated on the video?
   a. Dry well between the toes.
   b. Trim the nails straight across.
   c. Push the cuticles back with an orangewood stick.
   d. Soak the patient's foot.
   e. Apply lotion to the foot.
   f. File the nails with an emery board.

 For suggested responses, go to Chapter 22, **Thinking About the Procedure Suggested Responses,** on the Student Resource Disk or DavisPlus at http://davisplus.fadavis.com/Wilkinson2

Procedure 22-6 ☐ Brushing and Flossing the Teeth

➤ For steps to follow in *all* procedures, refer to the Universal Steps for All Procedures found on the inside back cover of Volume 2.

Critical Aspects

- Assess the teeth, mucous membranes, and swallowing ability.
- Position the patient to prevent aspiration (sitting or side-lying position).
- Hold the brush at a 45° angle, and brush the patient's teeth (or assist).
- Floss and rinse.
- If the patient is at risk for choking, suction secretions as needed.

Equipment

- Toothbrush or sponge toothettes
- Toothpaste
- Dental floss (two pieces, each about 10 in. long)
- Floss holder (optional)
- Tonsil-tip suction connected to suction source (if aspiration is a concern)
- Emesis basin
- Towel
- Glass of water
- Mouthwash and/or lip moisturizer, if desired
- Procedure gloves; mask and goggles if splashing may occur

Delegation

You can delegate oral hygiene to the NAP if the patient's condition and the NAP's skills allow. Perform the following assessments, and inform the NAP of the specific type of oral care and the amount of help the patient needs. Ask the NAP to report the condition of the patient's mouth, level of self-care, and ability to tolerate the procedure.

Pre-Procedure Assessments

- Assess the patient's ability to assist with oral care.
Having the patient assist whenever possible promotes independence and supports a positive self-image.

- Determine whether the patient has dentures, bridgework, or partial plates.
The presence of these devices determines how you will provide oral care.

- Assess the patient's general oral health, including the presence of the gag reflex and the condition of the teeth, gums, and mucous membranes. If a patient has dentures, examine the mouth with and without the dentures.
To prevent aspiration, you will need a suction set-up if the patient has a hypoactive or absent gag reflex. Any inflammation or lesions in the mouth increase the patient's risk of infection and may make eating difficult or painful, leading to malnutrition. Poorly fitting dentures can cause irritation of the gums.

- Assess the patient's usual oral care, including cultural practices.
Helps determine the type of oral care you will provide and identifies areas of patient teaching needed.

➤ When performing the procedure, always identify your patient according to agency policy and be attentive to standard precautions, hand hygiene, patient safety and privacy, body mechanics, and documentation.

Procedure Steps

1. Position the patient to prevent aspiration: in a high-Fowler's position or in a chair, if possible. Position the patient on her side if the head of bed cannot be elevated.
Prevents aspiration and makes the procedure easier.

2. Set up suction, if needed. Attach suction tubing and tonsil-tip suction; check suction.
Suctioning equipment will be needed if the gag reflex is decreased or absent. Suctioning is done to prevent aspiration of secretions during the procedure.

3. If the patient is able to perform self-care:

    a. Arrange supplies within the patient's reach.

Promotes the patient's ability to do self-care and therefore independence.

    b. Assist the patient with brushing and flossing as needed.
Ensures that the teeth are thoroughly cleaned.

4. For nurse-administered brushing and flossing:

    a. Place the towel across the patient's chest.
Prevents getting the patient's gown or linen wet during the procedure.

    b. Don procedure gloves and other protective garb as needed. Wear gown and goggles if splashing might occur, such as with a confused patient.
Follows standard precautions.

    c. Adjust the bed to working height; lower the siderail nearest you.
Prevents you from having to lean over the patient or reach across the siderail, possibly causing back strain or injury.

    d. Moisten a small, soft toothbrush, and apply a small am ount of toothpaste.
A small toothbrush fits more easily into the mouth and reaches more areas. The soft bristles can be used to brush the tongue and also the gums if the patient is edentulous. Excessive toothpaste does not increase the cleaning, and toothpaste residue has a drying effect on the mucosa. Moistening the toothbrush increases patient comfort because patients frequently have dry mouths.

e. Place, hold, or ask the patient to hold the emesis basis under the chin.

Collects oral secretions and protects clothing and linens.

f. Brush the teeth, holding the bristles at a 45° angle to the gum line.

(1) Using short circular motions, gently brush the inner and outer surfaces of the teeth, from the gum line to the crown of each tooth.

(2) Brush the biting surface of the back teeth by holding the brush bristles straight up and down to the teeth and brushing back and forth.

This is the most effective technique for removing all food particles and plaque from the teeth and gums. Removing debris and subsequent plaque helps to decrease microbial colonization.

(3) If the patient is frail, perform oral suctioning when fluid accumulates in the mouth.

Prevents choking and aspiration.

g. Gently brush the patient's tongue.

Removes coating and accumulated debris that can be a reservoir for bacteria. Brush gently to prevent gagging or vomiting. ▼

Brush teeth, holding bristles at a 45° angle to the gumline. Using short circular motions, gently brush the inner and outer surfaces of the teeth, including the gumline.

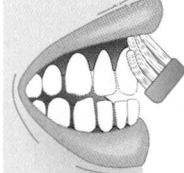

Clean front teeth.

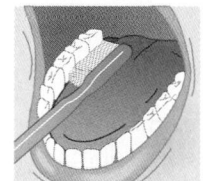

Clean both inner and outer surfaces of the teeth.

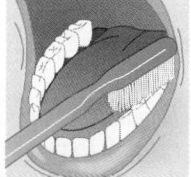

Brush the biting surfaces of the back teeth with the brush bristles straight up and down.

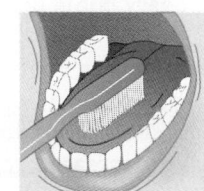

Brush the surface of the tongue.

h. Floss the teeth. Grasp dental floss in both hands, or use a floss holder. ▼

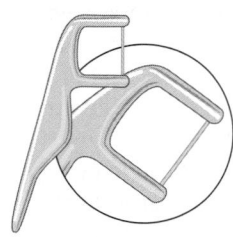

(1) If you are not using a floss holder, wrap one end of the floss around the middle finger of each hand. ▼

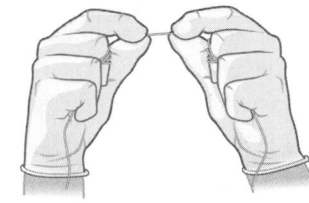

(2) Stretch the floss between your thumbs and index fingers, and move the floss up and down against each tooth. ▼

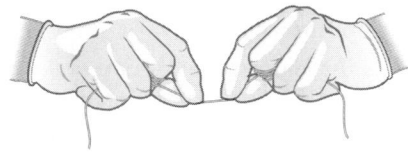

(3) Floss between and around all teeth.

Moving the floss up and down instead of back and forth prevents damaging the gums. ▼

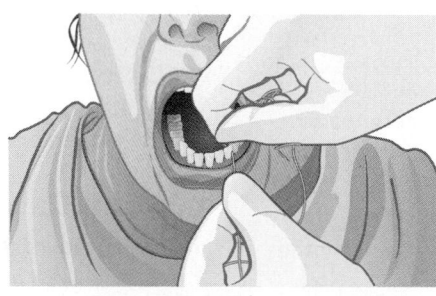

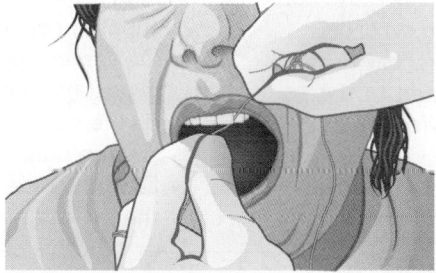

i. Assist the patient in rinsing his mouth, suctioning as needed. Or, ask the patient to rinse vigorously and spit the water into the emesis basin.

Removes food particles from mouth. Suction if the patient has a decreased or absent gag reflex.

5. Offer a mild or dilute mouthwash, and apply lip moisturizer, if desired.

Prevents irritation of the mucous membranes. Apply lip moisturizer for dry lips, for unconscious patients, or those on a ventilator, or per patient preference.

6. Reposition the patient as needed and return the bed to the low position.

Ensures patient comfort and safety.

What if . . .

■ **Your patient has an excessively dry oral cavity?**

You may need to use a saliva substitute.

Aging, adverse medication effects, and illness often lead to decreased salivary production.

■ **Your patient has viscous (thick) mucus?**

Use appropriately diluted sodium bicarbonate to dissolve viscous mucus.

■ ✚ **Your patient has a high risk of gum bleeding (e.g., such as associated with thrombocytopenia), has painful mouth lesions, or toothbrushing is otherwise contraindicated?**

You may use foam or cotton mouth swabs instead of a toothbrush. Do not use glycerin swabs, lemon glycerin swabs, or gauze squares. Use normal saline mouthwash.

Foam swabs are less effective in removing debris and plaque, so it is best to brush when not contraindicated. Lemon glycerin swabs are drying to the mucosa may cause decalcification of tooth enamel. Mouthwashes may be painful.

■ **Your patient has dementia or is uncooperative and agitated for other reasons.**

Use dementia-focused behavior management strategies:

(continued on next page)

Procedure 22-6 ■ **Brushing and Flossing the Teeth** (continued)

Older adults with dementia frequently accumulate greater amounts of plaque and calculus, exhibit a higher incidence of periodontal gingival bleeding, and demonstrate a greater prevalence of denture-related oral mucosal lesions, yet they often resist oral care.

■ Provide oral hygiene at the same time every day, not necessarily at bathing time.
■ Use as many staff members as necessary.
■ Give care in a quiet, distraction-free environment. Keep stimulation to a minimum, turn on some calming music.
■ Speak softly; give directions in short, simple sentences. Give one-step instructions.
■ Use a relaxed, slow approach; be sure your facial expression does not reflect tension.
■ Give reassuring body contact and use gentle touch.

Promotes trust.

■ Provide diversion.

Occupies the patient's hands and prevents "grabbing."

■ ✚ Never place your fingers between the teeth.

■ Try placing a spare toothbrush or a rolled facecloth in the patient's hands while you provide oral care.

Minimizes "grabbing."

■ Use the "hand over hand" technique to gently guide the patient's own hand.
■ Try starting the task (e.g., brushing), then having the resident help finish it.
■ If the procedure is not going well, find another caregiver to come in and attempt the task.
■ Use modified equipment and aids, if available (e.g., mouth props, backward-bent and suction toothbrushes).

■ **Your patient is on a ventilator, is a frail older adult, or has undergone cardiac surgery?**

■ Be certain the teeth are brushed twice a day.
■ In addition to brushing, use moisturizer on lips and oral mucosa every 2 to 4 hours.
■ Apply a 0.12% chlorhexidine gluconate solution twice daily to complement oral care.

■ **Your patient is receiving chemotherapy?**

Stress the importance of good oral hygiene, including brushing the teeth after meals and before going to bed.

Chemotherapy can cause neutropenia (reduced white blood cell count), predisposing the patient to infections. The oral cavity is a common site for infections in patients with neutropenia.

Routine rinses of mouthwashes with chlorhexidine are not recommended. Instead, use a bland rinse of diluted salt and/or sodium bicarbonate. Patients should swish for a minimum of 30 seconds and then expectorate the residue.

Chlorhexidine products have not proved superior to bland rinses in preventing or reducing either chemotherapy/radiation-induced mucositis or yeast colonization. In addition, chlorhexidine products may contain alcohol, may cause discomfort, may alter taste sensations, and may stain teeth. Bland rinses containing one teaspoon of salt or sodium bicarbonate per pint of water reduce the acidity of oral secretions, lessen mucus accumulation, and discourage yeast colonization.

An antifungal agent or a multiagent rinse (sometimes labeled "magic" or "miracle" rinse) may be used, followed by a short NPO period of 30 to 60 minutes. If other mouthwashes or rinses are also being used, allow 30 minutes to pass between their use and the use of an antifungal agent.

✚ *Multiagent rinses typically contain lidocaine. The resulting numbing effect may pose risks for a biting injury or aspiration. These rinses can neutralize antifungal agents.*

Evaluation

■ Inspect the teeth, gums, and mucous membranes to verify that they are free of food particles.
■ Inspect for abnormalities, such as bleeding, that may have been stimulated by the brushing or flossing.
■ Observe for patient discomfort or gagging during the procedure.
■ If the procedure was performed by the NAP, the nurse should still perform an evaluation of the care. This includes a physical assessment of the oral cavity as well as objective and subjective findings related to the patient's tolerance of and satisfaction with the care.

Patient Teaching

■ Discuss the importance of daily oral care.
■ Review any areas of brushing or flossing that the patient has not been performing adequately.

■ Discuss any problems that need further follow-up, such as inflammation, bleeding, dryness, caries, missing teeth, or broken or missing dentures.

Home Care

The procedure does not vary in the home. The issues are that the nurse must:
■ Work with the client and care provider to determine supplies needed for the home.
■ Determine whether suction is needed (e.g., if the client is unconscious or has a decreased gag reflex). Explain to the client and/or caregiver how to obtain a portable suction unit.
■ Demonstrate how to position the client and perform the procedure if the height of the bed is not adjustable or if both sides of the bed are not accessible.

Documentation

Document that oral care was given, the patient's response, any abnormal findings, and nursing interventions. Oral care is usually charted on a flowsheet.

Sample documentation:

12/27/11	0815	*Oral care given. Mucous membranes intact, pink, and dry. No choking or complaints of discomfort. Patient encouraged to increase fluid intake. —— Nancy Botha, RN*

Practice Resources

American Association of Critical-Care Nurses (AACN) (2007); Berry, A. (2007); Chalmers, J. (2005); Coughlan, M., & Healy, C. (2008); Harris D., Eilers J., Harriman, A., et al. (2008); The Joanna Briggs Institute (2004); National Guideline Clearinghouse (2005a); Watando, A., Ebihara, S., Ebihara, T., et al. (2004).

Thinking About the Procedure (Procedures 22-1 through 22-6)

 Go to the *Fundamentals of Nursing Skills Videos*, **Bed Bath, Oral Hygiene, Foot Care, and Back Massage.**

1. How does the nurse protect the patient's gown during oral hygiene?

2. What does the nurse do after the patient uses the mouthwash?

 For suggested responses, go to Chapter 22, **Thinking About the Procedure Suggested Responses,** on the Student Resource Disk or DavisPlus at http://davisplus.fadavis.com/Wilkinson2

Procedure 22-7 ☐ Providing Denture Care

➤ For steps to follow in *all* procedures, refer to the Universal Steps for All Procedures found on the inside back cover of Volume 2.

Critical Aspects

- Refer to Procedure 22-6: Brushing and Flossing the Teeth
- Remove (and replace) the top denture before the lower denture.
- Tilt dentures slightly when removing and replacing.
- Handle dentures carefully, and place the towel in the sink to avoid breaking the dentures if you drop them.
- Use cool water and a stiff-bristled brush.

Equipment

- See Procedure 22-6: Brushing and Flossing the Teeth.
- Denture cup

Delegation

You can delegate denture care to the NAP if the patient's condition and the NAP's skills allow. Perform the following assessments, and inform the NAP of the specific care and the amount of help the patient needs. Ask the NAP to report the condition of the patient's mouth and dentures, level of self-care, and ability to tolerate the procedure.

Pre-Procedure Assessments

See Procedure 22-6: Brushing and Flossing the Teeth.

➤ When performing the procedure, always identify your patient according to agency policy and be attentive to standard precautions, hand hygiene, patient safety and privacy, body mechanics, and documentation.

Procedure Steps

1. Don gloves, and remove dentures (if the client cannot do so).
   a. **Upper denture:** With a gauze pad, grasp the denture with your thumb and forefinger, and move it gently up and down. Tilt the denture slightly to one side to remove it, without stretching the lips. Place the denture in the denture cup.

The gauze gives you a better grip. Breaking the seal on the top dentures can be difficult; movement breaks the suction. Always place dentures in a denture cup as soon

(continued on next page)

Procedure 22-7 ■ **Providing Denture Care** (continued)

as you remove them to prevent accidental breakage. ▼

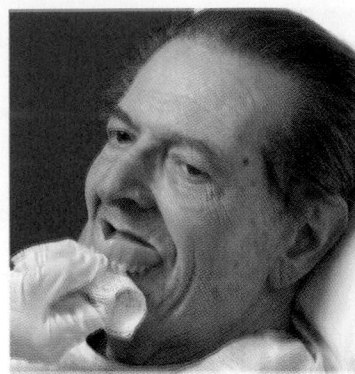

b. **Lower denture:** Use your thumbs to push up gently on the denture at the gum line to release from the lower jaw. Grasp the denture with your thumb and forefinger, and tilt it to remove it from the patient's mouth. Place the denture in the denture cup.

A gauze pad is not usually needed to grasp the lower dentures; however, you can use one if the dentures are difficult to grasp. Pushing up on the dentures breaks the seal. Rotating the dentures is necessary to remove the dentures from the patient's mouth. ▼

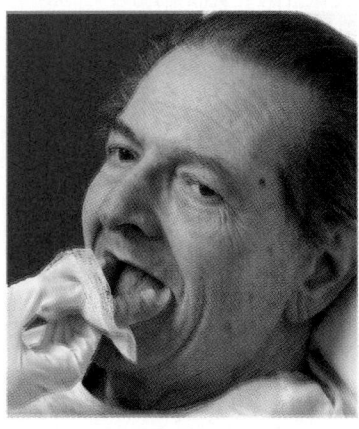

2. Place the towel in the sink, and cleanse the dentures under cool running water.

Heat can damage some dentures. The towel helps prevent the dentures from breaking if they are accidentally dropped. Dentures are expensive and usually not reimbursed by insurance.

a. Apply a small amount of special denture paste to a soft-bristled toothbrush.

Denture paste assists in cleaning. Toothpaste and stiff-bristled brushes may be too abrasive for dentures. However, follow the patient's preference in use of denture cleaner. Some patients prefer to soak their dentures in a cleanser overnight. If dentures have been soaking, rinse them well before placing them in the patient's mouth.

b. Brush all surfaces of each denture.

Loosens all food particles and any old denture adhesive.

c. Rinse thoroughly with cool water.

Removes loosened particles and the cleaning agent. Do not use hot water with dentures, because hot water can react to make the denture material sticky.

Note: You can soak stained dentures in a commercial cleaner, following the manufacturer's instructions. Do not soak the denture overnight if the appliance has metal parts.

Can cause corrosion of the metal parts.

3. Inspect dentures for rough, worn, or sharp edges.

These can irritate the tongue, gums, or mucous membranes of the mouth.

4. Inspect the mouth under the dentures for redness, irritation, lesions, or infection.

If present, refer to a dentist to check the fit of the dentures or to make needed repairs.

5. Apply denture adhesive as needed (ask the patient whether he uses denture adhesive).

Adhesives are needed to "seal" some dentures and prevent slipping and irritation of the gums.

6. Moisten the top denture, if it is dry. Then insert the top denture, at a slight tilt, and press it up against the roof of the mouth.

Moistening the dentures eases insertion. You can tell when you have securely seated the dentures by checking to feel for any slippage or to confirm that the dentures stay in place. Because the top denture is larger, it is removed first and inserted first for ease of insertion.

7. Moisten the bottom denture, if it is dry. Then insert bottom denture, rotating it as you put it in the patient's mouth.

Because it is smaller, the bottom denture is inserted after the top one. ▼

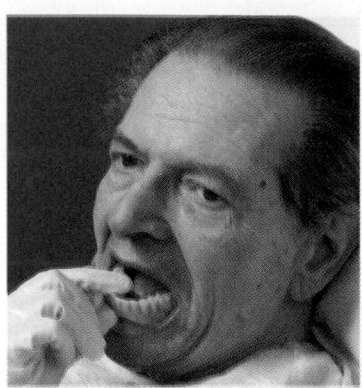

8. Ask the patient whether the dentures are comfortable.

Ensures that the dentures are properly placed.

9. If the patient does not wish to wear the dentures, cover them with water in a clean denture container with a lid. Label the container with the patient's name and the agency identifying number. Place denture container in bedside drawer rather than on top of bedside table for safekeeping.

Drying can cause dentures to warp. Having the denture out of the mouth for several hours a day relieves pressure on the oral tissues, allows saliva to clean the tissues, and helps to minimize gingival irritation.

10. Offer mouthwash.

What if . . .

■ **The patient develops *Candida*-related denture stomatitis?**

Follow agency protocols. Microwave disinfection of complete dentures has been documented as an effective treatment of *Candida*-related denture stomatitis and can reduce the recurrence of infections.

Denture stomatitis ranges in severity. Treatment includes good oral and denture hygiene and administration of antifungal agents. Recurrence of infection after treatment can be due to colonization of Candida *on the dentures.*

Evaluation

- See Procedure 22-6: Brushing and Flossing the Teeth.
- Check to see that dentures are comfortable and fit properly.

For Documentation, Patient Teaching, and Home Care, see Procedure 22-6: Brushing and Flossing the Teeth.

Practice Resources

National Guideline Clearinghouse (2005a); Neppelenbroek, K., Pavarina, A., Spolidorio, D., et al. (2008); Pappas, P., Rex, J., Sobel, J., et al. (2004); Siegel, J., Rhinehart, E., Jackson, M., et al. (2007).

Thinking About the Procedure

 Go to the *Fundamentals of Nursing Skills Videos*, **Oral Hygiene: Denture Care.**

I. In the DVD, how does the NAP protect the dentures from breakage?

2. What did the NAP do to check whether the dentures were securely seated?

 For suggested responses, go to Chapter 22, **Thinking About the Procedure Suggested Responses (Procedure 22-7),** on the Student Resource Disk or DavisPlus at http://davisplus. fadavis.com/Wilkinson2

Procedure 22-8 ☐ Providing Oral Care for an Unconscious Patient

➤ For steps to follow in *all* procedures, refer to the Universal Steps for All Procedures found on the inside back cover of Volume 2.

Critical Aspects

- Assess the condition of the teeth (or dentures), gums, and mucous membranes.
- Assess for the gag reflex.
- Position the patient to prevent aspiration.
- Brush and floss the patient's teeth.
- Suction secretions as needed.

Equipment

- Toothbrush with soft bristles or sponge oral swabs
- Toothpaste
- Denture cup, if the patient has dentures
- 4 in. × 4 in. gauze pad to remove dentures if present
- Tonsil-tip suction connected to suction source (you may use a product that combines the toothbrush or oral swab with the suction device)
- Tongue blade (padded) or bite-block
- Towel
- Waterproof linen protector
- Emesis basin
- Water-soluble lip moisturizer
- Procedure gloves and goggles

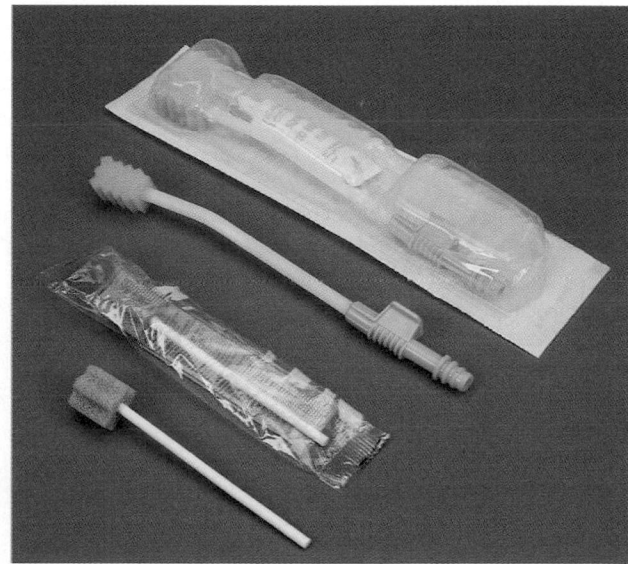

Source: Courtesy of Sage Products, Inc., Cary, IL.

(continued on next page)

Procedure 22-8 ■ **Providing Oral Care for an Unconscious Patient** (continued)

Delegation

As a rule, you probably should not delegate oral hygiene for an unconscious patient to a NAP. However, in some situations it may be acceptable—for example, when the NAP has a great deal of experience caring for unconscious patients and when the NAP's ability to perform oral hygiene safely for them is documented. Perform the following assessments, and inform the NAP of any special considerations for care (e.g., if the patient must have the head of the bed elevated to facilitate breathing). Ask the NAP to report the condition of the patient's mouth and the patient's ability to tolerate the procedure (e.g., ask the NAP to take vital signs before and after the procedure, or to note the oxygen saturation if it is being monitored).

Pre-Procedure Assessments

■ Determine whether the patient has dentures or partial plates.

The presence of these appliances determines how you will provide oral care. You may leave dentures out for an unconscious patient to decrease the risk that the dentures will be damaged or block the airway. However, when possible, keep the dentures in place to help ensure they will fit adequately later. Remove partial plates in an unconscious patient to prevent the plate from causing aspiration or damage to the mouth if it becomes loosened.

■ Assess the patient's gag reflex.

If the patient has an intact gag reflex, the risk of aspiration is lower.

■ Assess the patient's general oral health, including the condition of the teeth and gums, and hydration of the mucous membranes. If the patient has dentures, examine the mouth with and without the dentures.

Unconscious patients tend to breathe through the mouth, so oral mucosa are often dry. Because the oral mucosa act as a barrier against microorganisms, any inflammation or lesions in the mouth increase the risk for infection. The lips, gums, and mucous membranes should be pink, moist, and intact. The teeth should be intact and clean. The condition of the mouth determines what you will use to provide oral care. Assess the fit of dentures and the condition of the skin under the dentures to determine whether the fit is proper and whether any irritation is present.

➤ When performing the procedure, always identify your patient according to agency policy and be attentive to standard precautions, hand hygiene, patient safety and privacy, body mechanics, and documentation.

Procedure Steps

✦ **1.** Position the patient in a side-lying position, with head turned to the side and, if possible, with the head of the bed down.

Secretions will pool in the dependent side of the mouth. This position helps prevent aspiration and facilitates the removal of secretions by gravity.

2. Don procedure gloves and eye goggles.
Follows standard precautions. Eye protection is needed when suctioning because of the risk of splashing.

3. Place a waterproof pad and then a towel under the patient's cheek and chin.
The towel and pad will absorb water and keep the bed linens dry.

4. Set up suction. Attach suction tubing and tonsil-tip suction; check suction.
Suctioning helps ensure that the patient does not aspirate oral secretions during the mouth care procedure.

5. Brush the patient's teeth.
  a. Use a padded tongue blade or bite-block, as needed, to hold the patient's mouth open.
Holding the mouth open provides access for cleaning the oral cavity and keeps the patient from biting the nurse's fingers. ▼

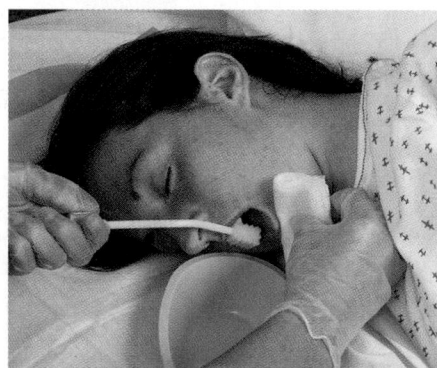

  b. Place an emesis basin under the patient's cheek.
Catches the secretions draining from the patient's mouth.

  c. Moisten the toothbrush, and apply a small amount of toothpaste.

Excessive toothpaste does not increase the cleaning. Brushing the teeth with a soft-bristled brush stimulates the mucosa, which increases the health of the gums.

  d. Brush the teeth, holding the bristles at a 45° angle to the gum line, and using a padded tongue blade or bite-block to hold the patient's mouth open.
  (1) Using short circular motions, gently brush the inner and outer surfaces of the teeth, including the gum line.
  (2) Brush the biting surface of the back teeth by holding the brush bristles straight up and down to the teeth and brushing back and forth.
  (3) Brush the patient's tongue.
This is the most effective technique for removing plaque and debris from the teeth and gums. The tongue can be a reservoir for bacteria. A padded tongue blade or bite block is used to hold the mouth open so you can visualize and reach the different areas of the mouth without injuring the oral mucosa.

✦ e. Perform oral suctioning when fluid accumulates in the mouth.

Removing fluid prevents choking and aspiration.

f. Draw about 10 mL of water or mouthwash (e.g., dilute hydrogen peroxide) into a syringe; eject it gently into the side of the mouth. Allow the fluid to drain out into the basin, or suction as needed.

Rinsing with water or dilute hydrogen peroxide removes any toothpaste residue, which may have a drying effect. Remove all fluid from the mouth to prevent aspiration into the lungs.

6. Provide denture care, if necessary. See Procedure 22-7: Providing Denture Care.

7. Clean the tissues in the oral cavity according to agency policy. Use foam swabs or a moistened gauze square wrapped around a tongue blade. Use a clean swab for each area of the mouth: cheeks, tongue, roof of the mouth, and so on.

Oral tissues may be dry and sticky from mouth breathing. Using separate swabs prevents transfer of microorganisms from one area to another.

8. Remove the basin, dry the patient's face and mouth, and apply water-soluble lip moisturizer.

✦ Use of petroleum-based lip moisturizers (e.g., mineral oil, petroleum jelly) is not recommended because of the possibility of aspiration, which might cause pneumonia. Never use petroleum-based jelly for patients on oxygen therapy; it can cause burns.

9. Remove the waterproof pad and towel; turn off suction equipment; discard gloves and used supplies.

10. Reposition the patient as needed. Maintains good body alignment.

11. Cleanse and store reusable oral hygiene tools in clean containers, separate from other articles of personal hygiene.

Prevents possible contamination from the environment and other personal hygiene tools.

What if . . .

■ **You are providing oral care to a patient receiving mechanical ventilation?**

Provide oral cleansing, including subglottic suctioning, at least every 2 hours and prn. Brush the teeth at least twice a day.

Keeping the oral cavity clean and clear of secretions has been proven to decrease the incidence of ventilator associated pneumonia (VAP). Pooled

oral secretions become rapidly colonized with pathogens that contribute to VAP.

Avoid tap water. Use normal saline or a half strength solution of saline for oral rinses.

Studies show hospital plumbing and tap water are often colonized with microbial organisms.

Apply a 0.12% chlorhexidine gluconate solution twice daily to complement oral care.

■ **It is difficult to floss the patient's teeth, or the patient doesn't tolerate flossing?**

Handheld interdental tools may be used instead of floss. These devices are special small brushes, picks, or sticks.

Toothbrush bristles can't reach between teeth to dislodge food particles and bacteria. Interdental cleaners can be as effective as floss in keeping these areas clean.

■ **Oral tissues are dry and sticky?**

Use appropriately diluted sodium bicarbonate to dissolve viscous mucus.

Evaluation

■ Inspect the teeth, gums, and mucous membranes for cleanliness.
■ Observe the oral mucosa and gums for hydration, inflammation, bleeding, or infection.
■ Observe the patient's overall responses to the procedure (e.g., gagging, coughing, vital signs, skin color).

Patient Teaching

■ Discuss with family members any problems that need further follow-up.
■ Teach oral hygiene measures, as needed.

Home Care

The procedure steps do not vary in the home.
■ Work with the client and caregiver to determine supplies needed for the home.
■ Determine whether suction is needed, and explain to caregivers how to obtain a portable suction unit.

■ Demonstrate how to position the client and perform the procedure if the height of the bed is not adjustable or if both sides of the bed are not accessible.

Documentation

Document that oral care was given, any abnormal findings, and nursing interventions. Typically, though, oral care is documented on a checklist or flowsheet.

Sample documentation:

| 9/16/11 | 0730 | *Oral care given. Mucous membranes pink and moist. White coating on tongue—physician notified. Patient had no coughing during the procedure. Gag reflex is intact. Patient did not aspirate. Respiratory rate 18.* —Susan Hiam, RN |

(continued on next page)

Procedure 22-8 ■ **Providing Oral Care for an Unconscious Patient** (continued)

Thinking About the Procedure

 Go to the *Fundamentals of Nursing Skills Videos*, **Oral Care: Unconscious Patient.**

1. What protective gear does the nurse use?

2. How does the nurse protect the bed linens?

3. Why did the nurse not use the padded tongue blade?

 For suggested responses, go to Chapter 22, **Thinking About the Procedure Suggested Responses,** on the Student Resource Disk or DavisPlus at http://davisplus.fadavis.com/Wilkinson2

Practice Resources
American Association of Critical-Care Nurses (AACN, 2007); American Dental Association (n.d.); Berry, A. (2007); Cason, C., Tyner, T., Saunders, S., et al. (2007); Human, L., & Bell, J. (2007); Slot, D., Dörfer, C., & Van der Weijden, G. (2008).

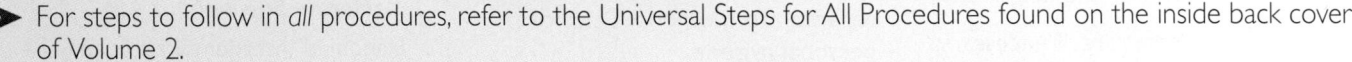

Procedure 22-9 ☐ **Shampooing the Hair**

➤ For steps to follow in *all* procedures, refer to the Universal Steps for All Procedures found on the inside back cover of Volume 2.

Critical Aspects

- Determine the type of procedure needed. Assess the patient's ability to help and the condition of the hair and scalp.
- Identify hair care products needed for the procedure.
- Protect the bed from getting wet.
- Wash the hair with warm water.
- Protect the patient's eyes and ears from soap and water.
- Towel-dry the hair.
- Take care not to burn the patient with the hair dryer, if one is used.

Delegation

You can delegate this procedure to the NAP if you conclude that the patient's condition and the NAP's skills allow. Perform the following assessments, and inform the NAP of the specific type of procedure needed (e.g., in bed, at sink, disposable shampoo equipment) and the amount of help the patient needs. Inform the NAP of any special considerations, such as positions the patient cannot assume or presence of scalp lesions. Ask the NAP to report the condition of the patient's scalp and hair, level of self-care, and ability to tolerate the procedure.

Pre-Procedure Assessments

- Assess for any contraindications to a shampoo. For example, if the patient has scalp sutures, you may need special measures to keep them dry. Or, you might find that a patient has limited head or neck movement. A rinse-free shampoo would be more appropriate in these cases.
- Determine the patient's ability to assist with the procedure.

Promotes independence and provides active range of motion.

- Assess the condition of the patient's hair and scalp.

Dry and brittle hair may indicate hypothyroidism or malnutrition and may require special shampoos or conditioners.

- Note any dryness or irritation of the scalp.
- Determine the need for special hair care products, such as a medicated shampoo.

Dandruff, lice, and dry hair are examples of conditions that require medicated shampoos or conditioners.

- Ask the patient how she normally cares for her hair.

■ Procedure 22-9A **Shampooing the Hair for a Patient on Bedrest**

Equipment

- Shampoo
- Conditioner, optional
- Shampoo tray or commercial system, if available
- Washbasin, plastic pail, small easy to handle plastic container
- Towels (2)
- Washcloth
- Bath blanket
- Waterproof pads or plastic trash bag
- Brush and comb
- Procedure gloves, if indicated by the presence of lesions or infestation
- Hair dryer
- Commercial system, if available
- Follow cultural practices, and identify personal preferences.

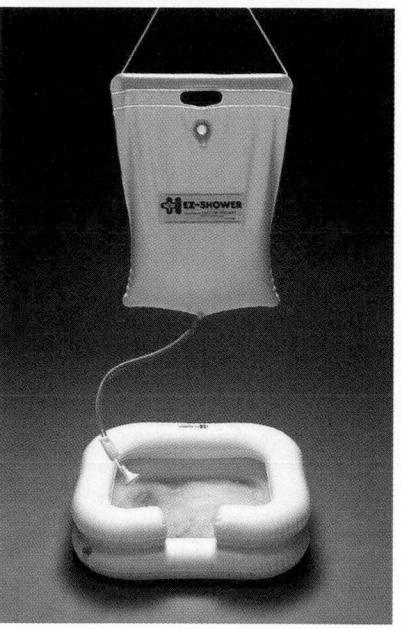

Courtesy of EZAccess, Auburn, WA.

➤ When performing the procedure, always identify your patient according to agency policy and be attentive to standard precautions, hand hygiene, patient safety and privacy, body mechanics, and documentation.

Procedure Steps

1. If lesions or infestation are present, don procedure gloves at this step.
Observes standard precautions.

2. Unless contraindicated (e.g., by a neck condition), lower the head of the bed, take the pillow from under the patient's neck, and place it under her shoulders.
Hyperextends the neck and helps keep water from the eyes.

3. Place the waterproof pad or plastic trash bag under patient's shoulders, and cover with towels. A commercial system will have a drain hose to use.
Protects the bed from getting wet.

4. Collect warm, not hot, water in a container and bring to the bedside.

5. Place the shampoo tray under the patient's shoulders (or head, depending on the type of tray). If you are using a hard plastic tray, pad the neck area with a towel. An inflatable shampoo tray needs minimal padding, but you will need to inflate it before beginning the procedure, either by mouth or with an air pump.

Protects the patient from lying on a hard surface and prevents water from leaking out onto the bed.

6. Ensure that the tray will drain into the washbasin or plastic pail.
Prevents water draining onto the bed or floor.

7. Fold the top linens down to the patient's waist, and cover her upper body with a bath blanket.
Keeps the linen dry; keeps the patient warm.

8. Work your fingers through the patient's hair, or comb the hair to remove tangles prior to washing.
Removing the tangles before washing helps prevent increased tangles while shampooing. Note that very tangled or matted hair may sometimes indicate a lice infestation.

9. Wash the hair.
- Wet the hair, pouring warm water from the pitcher. Do not get water in the person's eyes or ears.
- Next, apply shampoo and lather well, working from the scalp out and from the front to the back of the head.

- Gently lift the patient's head to rub the back of the head.
Cleaning the scalp is the most important part of a shampoo.

10. Rinse thoroughly.
Shampoo is drying if left in the hair. ▼

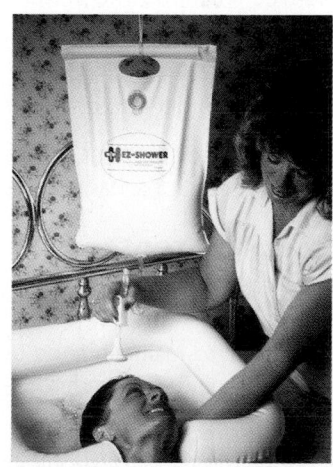

Courtesy of EZAccess, Auburn, WA.

11. If desired, apply conditioner to the hair. Conditioner should be used for patients with hair that tangles easily, such as dry, long, curly, or kinky hair. Rinse if needed. Leave-in conditioner can be used and is recommended for curly hair.

(continued on next page)

Procedure 22-9 ■ **Shampooing the Hair** (continued)

12. Remove the tray, and blot-dry the hair with the towel. Do not use circular motions to dry the hair.
Circular motions will increase tangles.

13. Comb or brush hair to remove tangles, starting at the ends and working toward the scalp.
Prevents excessive pulling on the patient's hair, which may cause breakage.

14. If desired, dry hair with a hair dryer at a medium temperature.
Use a medium temperature to prevent burning the patient.

15. When you are finished, be sure that the patient's clothing and bed linens are dry. Wash the shampoo tray and the brushes and combs.

Procedure Variation
Shampooing the Hair of Black American Clients

16. If the hair is in cornrows or braids, do not take out the braids to wash the hair.

Cornrow braids are left in place during routine hair care.

17. Handle the patient's hair very gently, being careful not to pull on the hair.
Many African Americans have fragile hair that breaks easily. Because it is fragile, apply moisturizer, if needed, to untangle the hair.

18. When shampooing, thread your fingers through the hair from the scalp out to the ends. Do not massage the hair in circular motions.
A circular motion increases tangling.

19. Rinse thoroughly, then apply a conditioner on the hair, if the hair is dry and fragile.
A leave-in conditioner helps minimize tangles and breakage.

20. Comb through the hair.
   a. Do not use a brush or fine-toothed comb on the patient's hair. Use a wide-toothed comb or hair pick.

   b. Part the hair into four sections, and, using a wide-toothed comb or hair pick, begin combing near the ends of the hair, working through each section.
   c. Use additional moisturizer to help soften and ease combing.
Never pull on the hair, because it will break easily.

21. Apply a natural oil to the hair, if desired.
Examples of natural oils are coconut, sweet almond, shea butter, and avocado. There are many commercial products using these oils. Mineral oil and Vaseline tend to clog pores and damage the hair, so use them only if the patient still prefers them after receiving this information.

22. Let the hair air-dry if possible.
Prevents the hair from becoming frizzy. A high temperature, such as from a hair dryer, will also damage the hair.

■ **Procedure 22-9B**   **Shampooing the Hair Using Rinse-Free Shampoo**

Equipment

- Rinse-free shampoo (no water is needed)
- Conditioner, optional
- Bath towel
- Brush or hair pick
- Comb
- Procedure gloves (if scalp lesion or infestation present)

> When performing the procedure, always identify your patient according to agency policy and be attentive to standard precautions, hand hygiene, patient safety and privacy, body mechanics, and documentation.

Procedure Steps

1. If possible, elevate the head of the bed.
Makes it easier to maintain good body mechanics during the procedure.

2. Place a protective pad or bath towel under the patient's shoulders.
Prevents the linen from getting wet from the shampoo.

3. Don procedure gloves if lesions or infestations are present.

4. Work your fingers through the hair, or comb the hair to remove tangles before washing. If the patient has her hair in small braids, do not take out the braids to wash the hair.

5. Apply rinse-free shampoo. Apply enough shampoo to thoroughly wet the hair. One application is usually sufficient to clean the hair.

6. Work the shampoo through the hair, from scalp down to ends.
Helps prevent pulling on and damaging the hair.

7. Dry the hair with a bath towel.
Removes the shampoo. Leaves the hair feeling clean and soft.

■ Procedure 22-9C Shampooing the Hair Using Rinse-Free Shampoo Cap

➤ When performing the procedure, always identify your patient according to agency policy and be attentive to standard precautions, hand hygiene, patient safety and privacy, body mechanics, and documentation.

Procedure Steps

1. Warm the shampoo cap using a water bath or microwave according to package instructions. Be careful to not overheat. Check the temperature before placing on the patient's head to prevent burns.
A commercial no-rinse shampoo cap is a microwavable cap that contains a no-rinse shampoo and conditioner. Different products are available. Be sure to follow the directions on the package.

2. Place the cap on the patient's hair, and gently massage.

The cap contains a no-rinse shampoo and water.

3. Remove the cap, and towel-dry the patient's hair.
Removes the shampoo and excess water.

4. Complete hair care according to the patient's needs (see Procedure 22-9A, Steps 12-14, preceding).

What if. . .

■ **You discover head lice or nits as you begin the shampoo?**

Stop the procedure. Discuss your findings with the patient and offer

reassurance. Leave the patient in a position of comfort and safety. Perform hand hygiene. Report the findings and obtain an order for a prescriptive shampoo.

■ **You do not have a shampoo tray?**

Improvise by using a new bedpan, and reserve it only for washing the hair. Pad it liberally with towels.

Evaluation

■ Observe that the hair is clean, dry, and free of tangles.
■ Observe for patient discomfort or fatigue during the procedure.
■ Ask the patient how the hair and scalp feel.

Patient Teaching

■ Advise patients with coarse hair to wash it less frequently (every 3 to 7 days, depending on dryness). Leave-in conditioners are often recommended for dry, curly, or kinky hair.
■ Discuss potential adaptations in washing hair. Products such as rinse-free shampoos or a shampoo tray can make shampooing easier to accomplish for a bedridden patient.

Home Care

■ In the home care setting, determine how the client usually washes her hair.
■ If the client is confined to bed, work with the caregiver to develop a plan for washing the client's hair that will be effective. For example, if a shampoo tray is not available, you can make one by using a plastic garbage bag and pillows or rolled towels.
■ The newer rinse-free products or the inflatable shampoo tray may be good choices for the client.
■ If the client cannot afford the adaptive equipment needed, refer the caregiver to the local resources, such as senior services.
■ If the client is ambulatory, recommend a shower stool. The stool needs to fit into the shower or bathtub securely, without wobbling, to prevent the client from falling.
■ If the client has only a bathtub, an adaptor for the faucet can be used to attach a hand-held showerhead.

Again, using a shower stool will make the procedure easier.

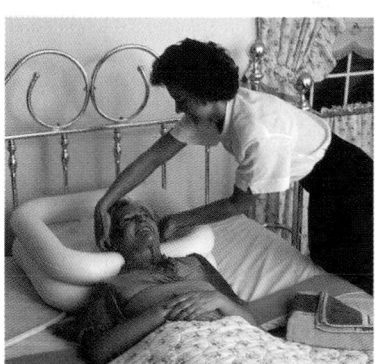

Courtesy of EZAccess, Auburn, WA.

Documentation

Chart that hair was shampooed, the condition of the hair and scalp, and the patient's responses to the procedure.

Sample documentation:

9/16/11   2045   *Hair shampooed. Scalp without signs of irritation. Hair dry. Conditioner applied. No c/o discomfort. Pt states, "My hair feels wonderful now, and my head doesn't itch any more."——Alicia Nelson, RN*

Practice Resources

EZ-Shampoo Instructions for Use (2005); How to shampoo the hair of a person in bed (2008). (Caveat: These are not research articles; they are manufacturers' recommendations.)

(continued on next page)

Procedure 22-9 ■ **Shampooing the Hair** (continued)

Thinking About the Procedure

 Go to the *Fundamentals of Nursing Skills Videos,* **Hygiene: Shampoo Hair in Bed.**

1. This nurse did not have a commercial tray available. What did she use to position the patient for the shampoo, and how did she place it?

2. What did the nurse use as a substitute for a shampoo tray?

3. Specifically, how did the nurse wet the patient's hair?

 For suggested responses, go to Chapter 22, **Thinking About the Procedure Suggested Responses,** on the Student Resource Disk or DavisPlus at http://davisplus.fadavis.com/Wilkinson2

Procedure 22-10 ■ **Providing Beard and Mustache Care**

➤ For steps to follow in *all* procedures, refer to the Universal Steps for All Procedures found on the inside back cover of Volume 2.

Critical Aspects

- Assess the skin for redness, dry areas, or lesions.
- Trim the beard and mustache to the desired length with a comb and scissors or beard trimmer. Follow manufacturer's instructions if using a trimmer or razor.
- Shampoo the beard and mustache.
- Apply conditioner, if desired.
- Towel-dry the beard and mustache, and comb and style as desired.

Equipment

- Scissors or beard trimmer
- Wide-toothed comb
- Mild shampoo
- Basin
- Conditioner for coarse and/or dry hair
- Bath towel
- Procedure gloves (if skin nicks occur, contact with blood may occur)

Delegation

You can delegate beard and mustache care to the NAP if the patient's condition and the NAP's skills allow. Perform the following assessments, and inform the NAP of the specific type of care needed (e.g., in bed, at sink, safety razor, electric razor), and the amount of help the patient needs.

Inform the NAP of any special considerations, such as skin irritation or activity intolerance. Ask the NAP to report the condition of the patient's skin and beard, level of self-care, and ability to tolerate the procedure

Pre-Procedure Assessments

- Ask the patient or family about preferences for beard and mustache care.

Beards and mustaches may have personal and/or cultural meaning. Men in some cultures never cut or trim their beards. Some patients use a comb and scissors to do a slight trim of their beard and/or mustache, whereas others use a beard trimmer for a closer trim.

- Assess the patient's skin and hair condition.

Determine whether the skin has any reddened or dry areas and whether skin treatments are needed.

➤ When performing the procedure, always identify your patient according to agency policy and be attentive to standard precautions, hand hygiene, patient safety and privacy, body mechanics, and documentation.

Procedure Steps

1. Drape the towel around the patient's shoulders.
Protects the patient's clothing from falling pieces of hair and water from shampooing the beard or mustache.

2. Trim the beard and mustache when they are dry.
The beard and mustache are often shorter when dry. If they are cut when wet, they may be shorter than desired after they dry.

Step 2 Variation. Using a Comb and Scissors

a. Comb through the beard, and cut the hair on the outside of the comb. Be conservative; cutting too little is better than cutting too much.

Trimming too much off the beard can be upsetting for the patient, whereas if you cut too little, you can always trim off more.

b. Trim from the front of the ear to the chin on one side, and repeat on the other.
Keeps the beard equal on both sides of the face.

Step 2 Variation. Using a Beard Trimmer

  a. Select the trimming guide to the correct length. Adjust the guide to a longer length rather than a shorter length.

Ensures that you do not cut the beard too short.

  b. Trim from the front of the ear to the chin on one side, and repeat on the other.

3. Trimming the mustache:

  a. Comb the mustache straight down.

Cuts the length equally so that the mustache is just above the upper lip. ▼

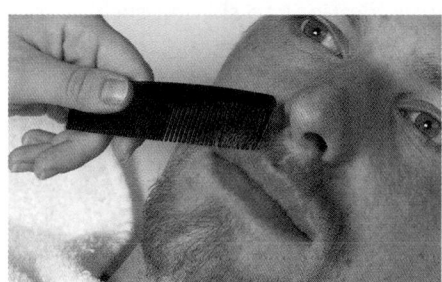

  b. Using either scissors or a beard trimmer, start in the middle, and trim toward one side of the mouth and then toward the other. Do not trim the top of the mustache.

Trimming from the center out toward each side helps you cut both sides equally.

4. Define the beard line by one of the following methods:

  a. Using either the scissors or a beard trimmer, trim the line of the beard so that it is well defined.

Trim very little to ensure that you only define the beard and do not change the length. ▼

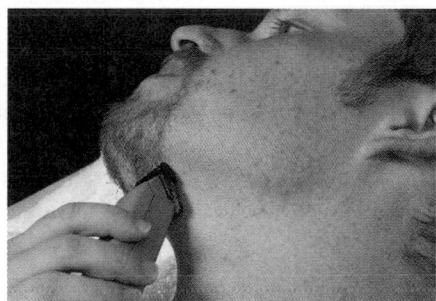

  b. Shave the neck to define the beard line.

This is done particularly for short beards.

5. Apply procedure gloves, if needed, and shampoo the beard and mustache using warm water and a mild shampoo.

The skin under a beard or mustache can be tender, so treat it gently with a mild shampoo. Follow standard precautions, because it is possible to nick the skin and cause bleeding.

6. Rinse well, and pat and wipe the beard and mustache dry with the towel.

Any shampoo left can irritate the skin, as can rubbing motions with the towel.

7. Apply conditioner, if desired.

The hair in many beards and mustaches is coarse.

8. Comb the beard and mustache with a wide-toothed comb or a brush.

Do not use a fine-toothed comb, because it will pull the hair.

Evaluation

- Make sure that the beard and mustache are trimmed to the desired length and are clean.
- Verify that skin problems are identified and treatment initiated.

Home Care

No adaptations are required in the home. The patient's usual supplies are sufficient, as a rule.

Documentation

Chart that beard and mustache were trimmed and shampooed; chart the condition of the skin.

Practice Resources

Procter & Gamble (2008). (Caveat: This is not an evidence-based practice article. It is a manufacturer's recommendation.)

Procedure 22-11 ☐ Shaving a Patient

➤ For steps to follow in *all* procedures, refer to the Universal Steps for All Procedures found on the inside back cover of Volume 2.

Critical Aspects

- Wear procedure gloves.
- Assess the skin for redness or dry areas.
- To soften the beard and moisten the skin:
  - Apply a warm, damp towel to the face.
  - Apply shaving cream or soap.
- To prevent skin irritation:
  - Hold the skin taut, and shave the face and neck.
  - If using a safety razor, hold the blade at a 45° angle to the skin.
  - Shave in the direction of hair growth.
  - Apply after-shave product, if desired.

(continued on next page)

Procedure 22-11 ■ Shaving a Patient (continued)

Equipment

- Safety razor or electric razor
- Shaving cream or soap
- Shaving brush, if desired
- Warm water
- Face towel and bath towel
- After-shave lotion, if desired
- Procedure gloves

Delegation

You can delegate shaving to the NAP if the patient's condition and the NAP's skills allow. Perform the following assessments, and inform the NAP of the specific type of care needed (e.g., safety or electric razor, in bed, or at the sink), and the amount of help the patient needs. Inform the NAP of any special considerations, such as skin irritation or activity intolerance. Ask the NAP to report the condition of the patient's skin, level of self-care, his ability to tolerate the procedure.

Pre-Procedure Assessments

- Determine how much assistance the patient needs.
Aids you in promoting as much independence possible.

- Assess the patient's skin and hair condition for redness, skin lesions, or moles.
Identify skin problems, and determine whether skin treatments are needed or the procedure must be modified. To prevent abrading the skin, do not shave any areas that have skin lesions or moles.

- Assess the patient's usual shaving method, including use of electric razor or safety razor.
When possible, follow the patient's routine. The patient may or may not use shaving cream or shaving soap, shaving brush, and after-shave lotion.

- Check for any contraindications to shaving, such as an increased risk of infection or bleeding (e.g., because of neutropenia, thrombocytopenia, or the administration of anticoagulants, such as warfarin or heparin).

- Assess the direction in which the hair is growing.

➤ When performing the procedure, always identify your patient according to agency policy and be attentive to standard precautions, hand hygiene, patient safety and privacy, body mechanics, and documentation.

Procedure Steps

1. Don gloves.
Skin will bleed if it is nicked or scratched.

2. Place a warm, damp face towel on the patient's face for 1 to 3 minutes.
Opens the pores and softens the beard to prevent pulling. Do not use hot water, because it will dehydrate the skin and can burn sensitive skin.

3. Apply shaving lotion to the face with your fingers or a shaving brush. Lather well for 1 to 2 minutes.
Lathering well helps to further soften the beard. Do not use shaving creams that contain numbing agents, because they close the pores and stiffen the beard.

4. Shave the patient.
a. Pull skin taut with your nondominant hand, and gently pull the razor across the skin. If you are using a safety razor, hold the blade at a 45° angle to the skin.
b. Shave the face and neck in the same direction of hair growth (the direction is not the same for all people). Using short strokes, start shaving at the sideburns, and work down to the chin on each side and then the neck.
c. Last, shave the chin and upper lip.

Usually the hair on the face will grow down toward the chin and on the neck up toward the chin. The hair is generally thickest on the chin and upper lip, so shaving them last allows more time for the shaving cream to soften the hair. Shave in the same direction as the hair is growing to prevent skin irritation. ▼

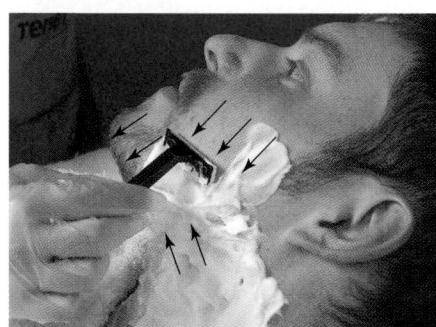

5. Rinse the razor frequently while you are shaving.
Avoids clogging the blade.

6. When you are finished shaving, rinse the patient's face with cool water, and gently pat it dry.
Cool water helps close the pores. Pat dry, do not rub, to prevent irritating the skin.

7. Apply after-shave lotion, if desired.
After-shave lotions that contain alcohol are not recommended, because alcohol

stings and dries out the skin. A moisturizer is recommended.

8. Dispose of the single-use razor in the sharps container.
Prevents cutting injury to others.

Step 8 Variation. Multiuse Razor
Shake the razor to remove excess moisture. Do not bang the razor against objects or dry with a towel. Store the razor in a covered container. Banging or wiping the razor edge will dull the razor and may damage the holding mechanism. A covered container protects others from a cutting injury.

What if . . .

- ✚ **Your patient has a condition that predisposes him to bleeding (e.g., thrombocytopenia) or infection (e.g., neutropenia)?**
Such patients must be shaved carefully using an electric razor, if at all.

A razor scratch or cut causes a break in skin integrity, providing a portal of entry for pathogens. This could be especially serious for a patient whose defenses against infection are compromised. For a patient with a delayed clotting time, a cut could cause excessive blood loss.

Evaluation

- Inspect the patient's face for nicks or cuts.
- Inspect the face for closeness of the shave.
- If the procedure was performed by the NAP, ask the patient about his satisfaction with and tolerance of the care.

Patient Teaching

Teach patients about changes that need to be made in their shaving technique as a result of changes in health status. For example, a patient who has begun taking anticoagulants may need to change from a blade to an electric razor because of an increased risk of bleeding.

Home Care

The procedure does not vary in the home. The nurse must:
- Determine the availability of supplies
- Assess the client's or caregiver's ability to perform the procedure.

Documentation

Chart that the patient was shaved and the condition of the skin. There will probably be a flowsheet or checklist for this information.

Practice Resources

Coughlan, M., & Healy, C. (2008); How to Shave (video, n.d.); 7 Tips for the Best Shave Ever (n.d.). (Caveat: Except for Coughlan & Healy, the preceding are not evidence-based resources. They are information from manufacturers.)

Procedure 22-12 ☐ Removing and Caring for Contact Lenses

> ➤ For steps to follow in *all* procedures, refer to the Universal Steps for All Procedures found on the inside back cover of Volume 2.

Critical Aspects

- Instill one to two drops of wetting solution.
- Gently remove the contact lenses; use your finger pads, not your fingernails.
- Clean and store contact lenses in sterile solution.
- Mark the containers "L" and "R" to identify the correct eye.

Equipment

- Contact lens wetting solution
- Contact lens case
- Contact lens soaking solution
- Contact lens remover (optional)
- Sterile saline (optional)
- Procedure gloves

Delegation

You can delegate this procedure if you conclude that the patient's condition and the NAP's skills permit. For example, if the patient is unconscious, you must determine whether contact lenses are present, and you should not delegate their removal.

Pre-Procedure Assessments

- Determine whether the patient is wearing contact lenses. If the patient is unconscious, examine the eyes for the presence of contact lenses by shining a penlight across the eye. You should be able to see the edge of the lens. Some lenses are larger than others, so examine the surface of the cornea carefully.

- Determine the type of contact lenses in place. Hard lenses are smaller than soft lenses. Each type of contact lens has different care requirements. Hard lenses can be worn for only up to 18 hours. Rigid gas-permeable (RGP) lenses may be worn overnight or for about 7 days, depending on the kind. Soft contacts are used for either short or longer periods.

- Ask the patient whether he is able to remove his contact lenses.

> ➤ When performing the procedure, always identify your patient according to agency policy and be attentive to standard precautions, hand hygiene, patient safety and privacy, body mechanics, and documentation.

> ➤ *Note:* It is difficult to remove a contact lens when wearing procedure gloves. For hard lenses, you can use a suction cup device if one is available. If you must use ungloved hands (e.g., in an emergency situation), it is extremely important to wash your hands thoroughly before and after the procedure. *Do not use your fingernails.*

> ➤ *Note:* Lens cases are marked L and R to indicate left and right lenses. Clean, rinse, and place the lens you remove first into its designated cup before removing the second lens.

(continued on next page)

Procedure 22-12 ■ **Removing and Caring for Contact Lenses** (continued)

Procedure Steps

1. Perform hand hygiene and don gloves.

2. Instill one to two drops of contact lens wetting solution to moisten the lenses.
Moistening the lens aids in removal.

3. Remove the lenses.

Step 3 Variation. Hard or Gas-Permeable Contact Lens

a. ***Alternative 1:*** If the lens is not centered over the cornea, place your finger on the patient's lower eyelid, and apply gentle pressure to move it into position. Place your index finger at the outer corner of the eye, and gently pull sideways toward the ear; position your other hand below the eye to "catch" the lens. Ask the patient to blink. As the skin tightens, the contact will "pop" out.
As the palpebral fissure narrows, the lids catch on the edge of the lens and pop it out.▼

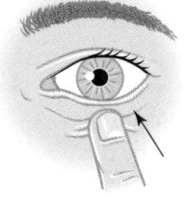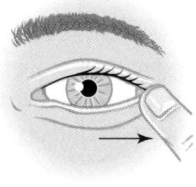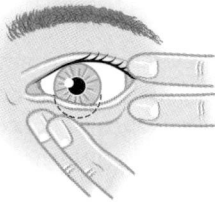

b. ***Alternative 2:*** Use a small suction cup contact lens remover. Gently press the suction cup end of the remover onto the contact lens, and lift straight up off the eye.
c. ***Alternative 3:*** Gently pull the top eyelid up and the lower lid down beyond the top and bottom edges of the lens. Then gently press the lower eyelid up against the bottom of the lens. When the lens is slightly tipped, move the eyelids together. This should cause the lens to slide out.▼

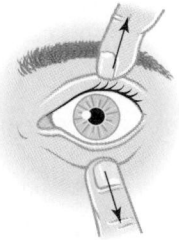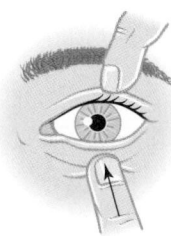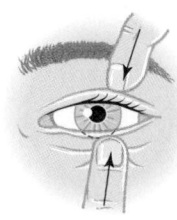

Step 3 Variation. Soft Contact Lens

a. Hold the eye open with your nondominant hand.
Allows you to visualize the contact lens.

b. Gently place the tip of your index finger on the contact lens, and slide it down off the pupil to the white area of the eye.

To prevent potential damage to the eye, do not pinch a lens directly over the pupil.▼

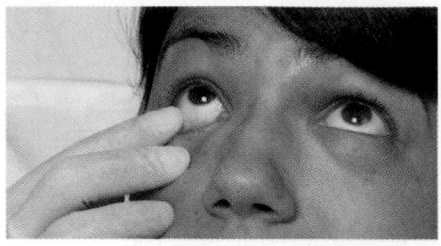

c. Using your thumb and index finger pads, gently pinch the lens, and lift it straight up off the eye. If the edges stick together moisten with a few drops of wetting solution. Rub gently until edges separate.
A soft contact lens is very flexible and pinches easily.▼

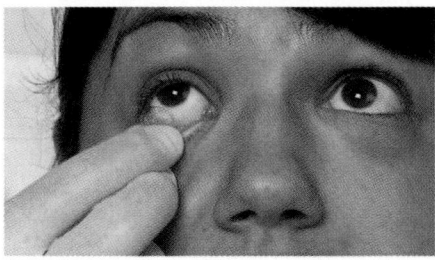

4. Clean the lens according to the instructions on the cleaning solution bottle. If there is no lens cleaner, use sterile saline. Be careful not to tear soft lenses.

5. Rinse the lenses with contact lens solution or sterile saline.
Removes any particles from the lenses.

6. Place the lenses in a contact lens case containing soaking solution or sterile saline (see note above regarding lens cases).
Prevents bacterial growth on the contacts and keeps the lenses from drying out.

Evaluation

Examine the eyes for redness or irritation.

Patient Teaching

- Review with the patient and/or family the importance of keeping the contact lenses clean and moist.
- If hard contact lenses are used, they must be removed at bedtime to prevent hypoxia of the cornea.

Documentation

Chart that contacts were removed, what type of lenses they are, what solution they are stored in, and the condition of patient's eyes.

Practice Resources

Bausch & Lomb (2008, 2009); Holman, C., Roberts, S., & Nicol, M. (2005); Massachusetts Eye and Ear Infirmary (last updated January 5, 2009).

Procedure 22-13 ▪ Making an Unoccupied Bed

➤ For steps to follow in *all* procedures, refer to the Universal Steps for All Procedures found on the inside back cover of Volume 2.

Critical Aspects

- Remove soiled linens without cross-contaminating other items in the room.
- Remake the bed with clean linens.
- Do not "shake" or "fan" linens.
- Work efficiently and safely.
- Ensure that there are no wrinkles in the bottom sheet or drawsheet.

Equipment

- Bottom and top sheets
- Drawsheet
- Pillowcase for each of the pillows
- Linen bag or hamper
- Procedure gloves (if exposure to body fluids is possible)
- Moisture-proof gown (if heavy soiling of linens with body fluids is possible).

Delegation

You can delegate this procedure to the NAP. You are responsible for supervising to ensure that the procedure is performed correctly.

Pre-Procedure Assessments

- Check to see whether the linen (including the mattress pad, blanket, and bedspread) needs to be changed.
- Determine what linens are needed.
- Assess whether the patient is able to be out of bed during the linen change.
- Assess for drainage or incontinence to determine whether personal protective equipment, such as procedure gloves and gown, is needed.

Note: This procedure describes bedmaking by one person. It is more efficient for two people to work together on opposite sides of the bed.

➤ When performing the procedure, always identify your patient according to agency policy and be attentive to standard precautions, hand hygiene, patient safety and privacy, body mechanics, and documentation.

Procedure Steps

1. Assist the patient to a chair. Provide a robe and/or blanket if needed.

Ensures that the patient is comfortable and will be warm enough during the bed change.

2. Prepare the environment: Position the bed flat, raise to appropriate working height, put on the brakes, and lower the siderails. Move the overbed table and other furniture, as needed.

Place the linen bag or hamper conveniently near the bed.

Maintains good body mechanics and prevents back strain during the procedure. Remove obstacles to allow easy access to the bed. Place all items so you can work efficiently, saving time and energy.

3. Don protective gloves and other gear if necessary. Loosen all the bedding.

This observes Standard Precautions and reduces the risk of contaminating your clothing.

4. If the blanket or bedspread is clean, fold it and place it on a clean area (e.g., on the back of a chair). *Do not place on another patient's bed or furniture.*

Reuse the blanket and/or bedspread if it is not soiled. Placing the item on a clean area prevents cross-contamination.

(continued on next page)

Procedure 22-13 ■ **Making an Unoccupied Bed** (continued)

5. Remove the bottom and top sheet, draw sheet, and pillowcases.

a. Do not shake the linens.
Minimizes dispersal of dust, skin cells, and microorganisms into the environment.

b. Holding the items away from your body, place them in a laundry bag or hamper. Place the pillows on a clean area (e.g., on a chair).
Never place linen on the floor, because cross-contamination can occur. Hold dirty linen away from your uniform to prevent contamination. ▼

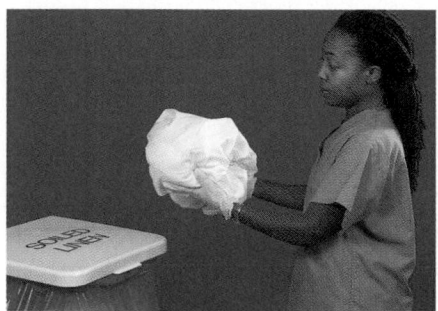

6. From one side of bed:
Placing the linen on one side of the bed uses time and energy efficiently.

Step 6 Variation. Contour-Bottom Sheet

a. Fit the contour-bottom sheet on one side of the bed, and smooth it out over half the mattress.

Step 6 Variation. Flat-Bottom Sheet

b. If you are using a flat-bottom sheet, fold it lengthwise with the center crease in the middle of bed and unfold with the rough side facing down.

c. Position the bottom sheet so that approximately 10 inches hang over at the top and sides. The hem of the bottom sheet should be just even with the bottom edge of mattress.

d. Tuck in the sheet, mitering the sheet at the top corner (see step 11).

When using a flat bottom sheet, having extra sheet at the top helps keep it in place when the head of the bed is raised and lowered. Unfold the sheet rather than shake or fan to reduce dispersing microorganisms into the air. The sheet will not be long enough to tuck in at the bottom.

7. Place the drawsheet with the center fold in the middle of the mattress and unfold. Tuck the side in under the mattress, and smooth out over half of the mattress.
Ensures that all wrinkles are out of the bottom sheet and drawsheet. ▼

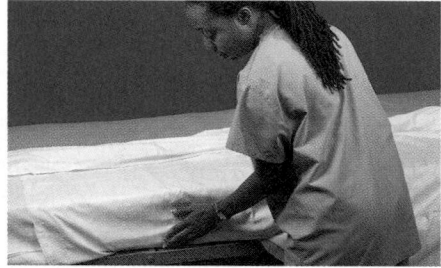

8. Go to the other side of the bed, straighten the linen, and finish tucking in the bottom sheet and drawsheet.

a. Make the drawsheet tight, and smooth any wrinkles in the bottom sheet and drawsheet.

b. If desired, place a waterproof pad on or under the drawsheet.
Pulling the drawsheet tight helps prevent wrinkles from developing under the patient when she moves around in bed. ▼

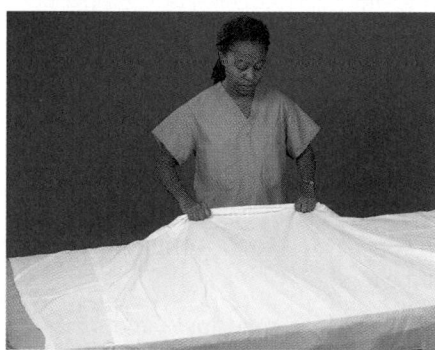

9. Place the top sheet and bedspread along one side of the mattress.
Placing all linen on one side at a time saves steps. Center the top sheet and bedspread, so that when you straighten them from the other side of the bed, they fall equally over each side of the bed. ▼

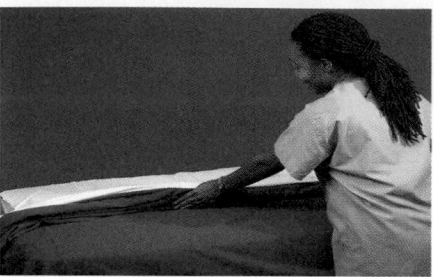

10. At the foot of the bed, make a small pleat in the top sheet and bedspread.
Prevents the top covers from placing pressure on the patient's toes. ▼

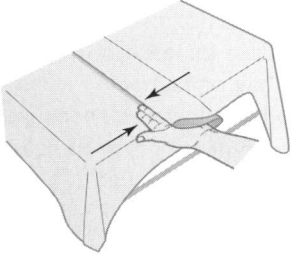

11. Tuck in the top sheet and bedspread at the same time, mitering the corners.

a. Tuck in the sheet and bedspread at the bottom of the mattress. ▼

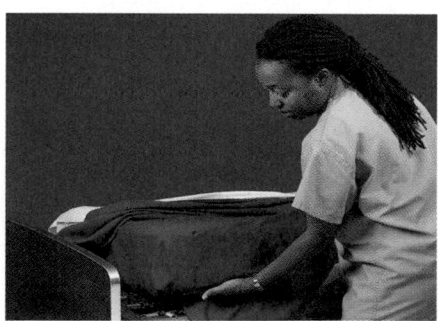

b. Bring the edge of sheet and the bedspread up to make a right angle. ▼

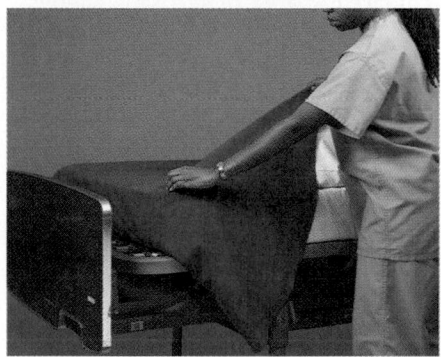

c. Tuck the lower edge of sheet and bedspread under the mattress.
Mitered corners help secure the linen at the foot of the bed. ▼

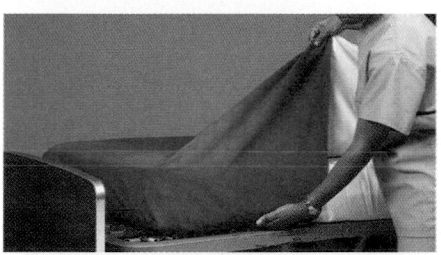

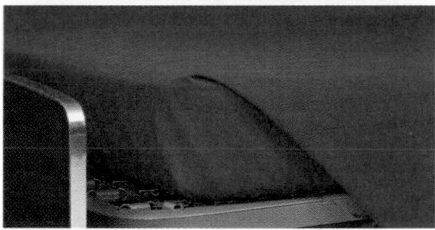

12. Move to the other side of the bed, smooth top linens, and repeat step 11. At the head of the bed, fold the edge of sheet down over the bedspread.
Prevents the bedspread from rubbing against the patient's skin. ▼

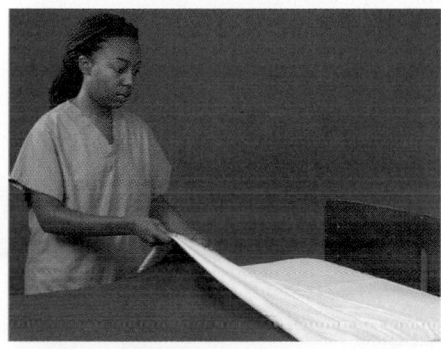

13. Fanfold the top sheet and bedspread back to the foot of the bed.
Makes it easier for the patient to get into bed. ▼

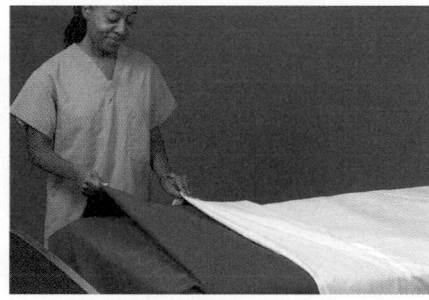

14. Change pillowcases.
a. Turn the pillowcase wrong side out.
b. Grasp the middle of the closed end of the pillowcase.
c. Reaching through the pillowcase, grasp the end of the pillow. ▼

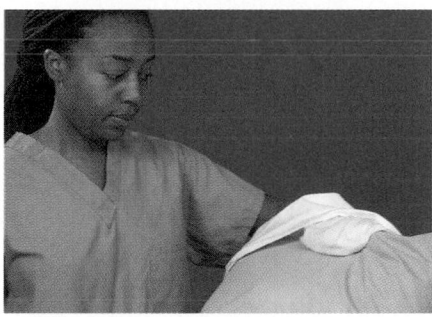

d. Continuing to grasp the end of the pillow, pull the pillowcase down over the pillow.
Do not hold the pillow under your arm or chin to put on pillowcase because contamination can occur. ▼

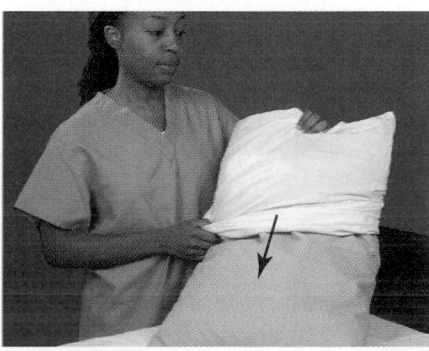

15. Assist the patient back to bed, return the bed to the low position, place the call signal within reach, and place the bedside table and overbed table so that they are accessible to the patient.
Provides for patient comfort and safety.

What if . . .

■ **The linens have been contaminated by body fluids?**

Follow recommended infection control procedures for laundering of linens (e.g., wear procedure gloves, place linen in moisture-proof bags, and so on).

■ **The mattress has become contaminated by body fluids?**

Follow agency policies for cleaning the mattress before putting on clean linens. This often involves notifying another department, such as housekeeping or environmental services, whose members are trained in this procedure.

■ **The patient has a speciality bed or specialty mattress?**

Several products are available with specific criteria to match patients' needs in terms of comfort, prevention or treatment of pressure ulcers, and movement (e.g., specialty beds designed for bariatric patients). Follow the manufacturer's directions (e.g., a recommendation for a specific mattress may be to use only one layer of sheet over the mattress for maximum benefit). If you find the sheets are not large enough to accommodate a specialized mattress, you may need to use two flat sheets to cover it.

(continued on next page)

Procedure 22-13 ■ Making an Unoccupied Bed (continued)

Home Care

The only adaptations at home depend on the type of bed the patient has. If the height of the bed is not adjustable or the bed is not accessible from both sides, the procedure may be more difficult.

Documentation

Linen changes are generally recorded on a checklist, if at all. Additional charting would need to be done only if something abnormal occurred, for example, "The drawsheet had a 20-cm circular area of serosanguineous drainage."

Practice Resources

Bloomfield, J., Pegram, A., & Jones, A. (2008); Schulster, L., & Chinn, R. (2003); Shiomori, T., Miyamoto, H., Makishima, K., et al. (2002); Siegel, J., Rhinehart, E., Jackson, M., et al. (2007).

Procedure 22-14 Making an Occupied Bed

➤ For steps to follow in *all* procedures, refer to the Universal Steps for All Procedures found on the inside back cover of Volume 2.

Critical Aspects

- Maintain patient safety during the procedure.
- Assess the patient's ability to move and the need for assistive equipment and patient-handling devices.
- Position the patient laterally near the far siderail, and roll soiled linens under him.
- Place clean linens on the side nearest you, and then tuck under the soiled linens.
- Roll the patient over the "hump," and position him on his other side, near you.
- Raise the near siderail.
- Move to other side of bed; pull soiled and clean linens through, and complete the linen change as in Procedure 22-13: Making an Unoccupied Bed.
- Place the bed in a low position, raise the siderails, and fasten the call light to the pillow.

Equipment

- Bottom and top sheets
- Drawsheet
- Pillowcase for each of the pillows
- Bath blanket (as needed)
- Linen bag or hamper
- Procedure gloves (if exposure to body fluids is possible)
- Moisture-proof gown (if heavy soiling of linens with body fluids is possible).

Delegation

You can delegate this procedure if you conclude that the patient's condition and the NAP's skills permit. For example, if the patient is very ill, in pain, or requires two people for turning and repositioning, you should assist with or perform the linen change yourself.

Pre-Procedure Assessments

- Determine the patient's ability to assist with the procedure and whether additional help or assistive devices are needed.
- Make other assessments listed in Procedure 22-13: Making an Unoccupied Bed.

➤ When performing the procedure, always identify your patient according to agency policy and be attentive to standard precautions, hand hygiene, patient safety and privacy, body mechanics, and documentation.

➤ *Note:* If linen change is done at the same time as the bed bath, some of these steps will vary.

Procedure Steps

1. Prepare the environment: Move the overbed table and other furniture, as needed, to allow access to the bed. Place the linen bag or hamper conveniently near the bed.

Remove obstacles to allow easy access to the bed. Place all items so you can work efficiently, saving time and energy.

2. Don protective gloves and other gear if necessary.

This observes standard precautions and reduces the risk of contaminating your clothing.

3. Position the bed flat if possible, and raise it to working height. Lower the siderail nearest you.

Maintains good body mechanics and prevents back strain during the procedure. Having the head of the bed flat makes it easier to smooth the bottom sheet. To prevent the patient from falling out of bed, lower the siderails only on the side where you are standing.

4. Disconnect the call device, and remove the patient's personal items from the bed.
Prevents items from getting lost.

5. Check that no tubes (e.g., IV, nasogastric) are entangled in the bed linens.
Prevents dislodging tubes accidentally.

6. If the blanket or bedspread is clean, fold it and place it on a clean area (e.g., the back of a chair); do not place it on another patient's bed or furniture.
Reusing the blanket and/or bedspread if it is not soiled conserves resources.

7. Cover the patient with a bath blanket, if available, or leave the top sheet over the patient.
Covering the patient prevents chilling and preserves modesty.

8. Slide the patient to the side of bed farthest from you, and place him in a side-lying position, facing the siderail. Place a pillow under his head. If needed for support, place a pillow between the patient and the siderail. Placing the patient close to the side rail will allow you to place the clean linen over a larger area, making it easier to roll the patient back onto the clean linen. Patients who cannot maintain the side-lying position should have a pillow placed between their chest and the siderail to prevent them from accidentally rolling into the siderail. ▼

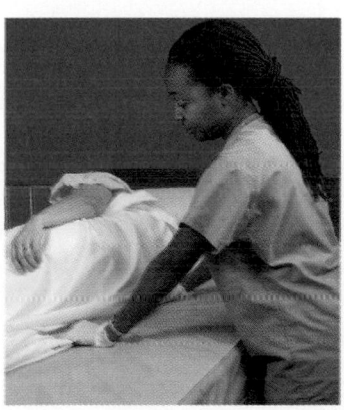

9. Roll or tightly fanfold the soiled linens toward the patient's back. Tuck the roll slightly under the patient. Cover any moist areas with a waterproof pad.
Cover any moist areas to prevent contact with the clean linen or patient.

10. Remove soiled gloves and don clean gloves.

11. Place the clean bottom sheet and drawsheet (or pad) on the near side of the mattress, with the center vertical fold at the center of the bed. Fanfold the half of the clean linen that is to be used on the far side, folding it as close to the patient as possible and tucking it under the dirty linen. Tuck the lower edges of clean linen under the mattress. Smooth out all wrinkles.
Wrinkles under the patient can cause skin irritation. ▼

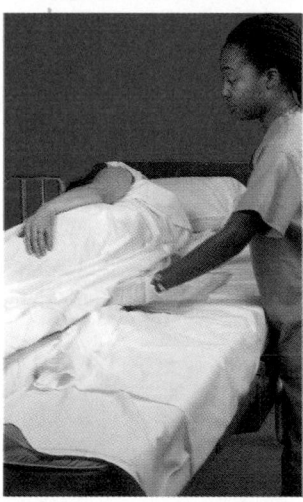

12. Roll the patient over the clean and dirty linen, turning him toward you. Explain to him that he will be rolling over a "lump," and then gently pull the patient toward you so that he rolls onto the clean linen. ▼

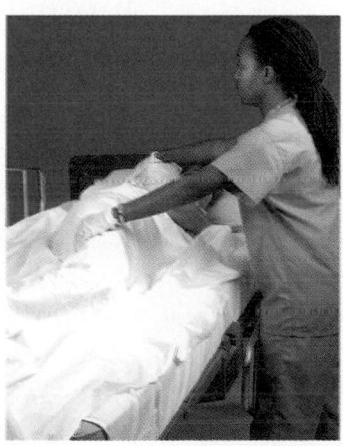

13. Raise the siderail on the clean side of the bed.
Prevents the patient from falling.

14. Move the pillows to the clean side. Position the patient comfortably on his side, near the siderail.
Always ensure patient comfort and safety before going to the other side of the bed.

15. Go to the opposite side of bed, and lower the rail. Pull the soiled linen from under the clean linen, and place it in laundry bag or hamper.
Never place linen on the floor; cross-contamination can occur. ▼

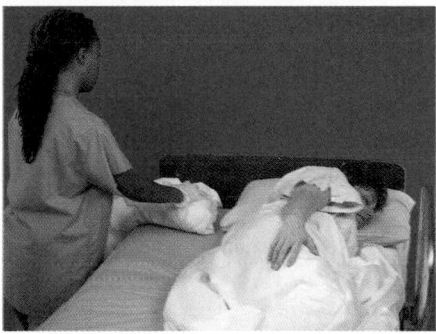

16. Remove soiled gloves and don clean gloves. Pull clean linens through, and tuck them in. Pull taut, starting with the middle section.
Ensures that no wrinkles will be under the patient.

17. Assist the patient to a supine position close to center of the mattress.
Makes it easier to place the top linen. ▼

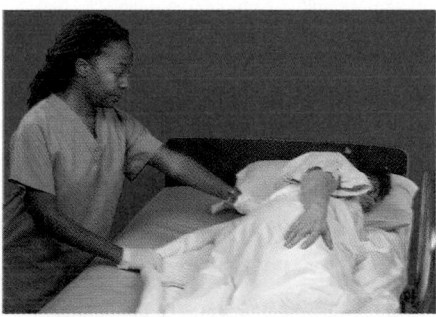

18. Place the top sheet and bedspread along one side of the mattress, and continue making the bed as in Procedure 22-13, steps 9 through 14, *except* remove the bath blanket

(continued on next page)

Procedure 22-14 ■ **Making an Occupied Bed** (continued)

from under the top linens before tucking them in. ▼

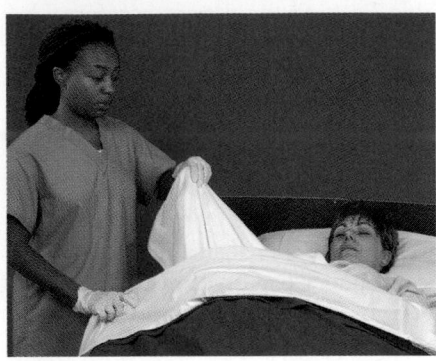

 19. Return the bed to the low position, raise the siderails, and attach the call light within patient's reach. Position the bedside table and overbed table within patient's reach. Ensures patient safety and comfort.

What if . . .

■ **You are making the bed with a patient in leg traction?**

It may be easier to make the bed from top to bottom.

■ Loosen all bed linens and bring the dirty linens from the top of

the bed to hip area. Put the clean bottom sheet on the top corners of the mattress, bring down to hip level and tuck under the dirty linen. Cover any moist areas with a waterproof pad.

■ Ask the patient to grasp the trapeze and raise his buttocks. If the patient is unable to raise his buttocks, use an assistive device per agency policy.

■ Bring the dirty bottom sheet along with the clean bottom sheet toward the foot of the bed. Remove dirty linen and place in the laundry bag.

■ Tuck the clean sheet under the mattress. Cover with the top sheet. To accommodate traction equipment, do not tuck in the top sheet.

■ **You need to move or reposition a patient in bed who is not able to assist or is obese?**

Before making the occupied bed, assess the patient's ability to move.

Use assistive equipment such as friction reducing devices, mechanical

lifts, air powered mattresses and or lateral transfer devices.

These are essential tools in preventing work related injuries. You should limit the need to use your own strength while lifting, turning or repositioning the patient in bed, because the stress placed on the weaker muscles in the arms and shoulders.

Follow agency policies and use of patient moving devices appropriately.

Many healthcare facilities have adopted safe lifting and patient handling policies as a means to protect both the patient and the healthcare worker.

Evaluation

■ Assess how well the patient tolerated the procedure. Was there any discomfort, shortness of breath, and so on?
■ Ask the patient whether he feels comfortable.

Home Care

The only adaptations at home depend on the type of bed the client has. If the height of the bed is not adjustable or the bed is not accessible from both sides, the procedure may be more difficult.

Documentation

Linen changes are usually recorded on a checklist. Additional charting needs to be done only if something abnormal occurred.

Practice Resources

Bloomfield, J., Pegram, A., & Jones, A. (2008); Collins, J., Nelson, A., Sublet, V. (2006); Nelson, A., Lloyd, J., Menzel, N., et al. (2003); Nelson, A., Pragala, G., & Menzel, N. (2003); Siegel, J., Rhinehart, E., Jackson, M., et al. (2007); Trinkoff, A., Brady, B., & Nielsen, K. (2003).

Thinking About the Procedure

 Go to the *Fundamentals of Nursing Skills Videos,* **Linen Change: Occupied Bed.**

1. Where has the nurse placed the clean linen?

2. What did the nurse do to protect the patient's privacy?

For suggested responses, go to Chapter 22, **Thinking About the Procedure Suggested Responses,** on the Student Resource Disk or DavisPlus at http://davisplus.fadavis.com/Wilkinson2

Procedure 22-15 ☐ Caring for Artificial Eyes

➤ For steps to follow in *all* procedures, refer to the Universal Steps for All Procedures found on the inside back cover of Volume 2.

Critical Aspects

- Ask the patient to lie down.
- Remove the artificial eye: Raise the upper eyelid; with the dominant hand, depress the lower lid and apply slight pressure below the eye (or use a small bulb syringe)
- Clean the eye: Clean the eye with saline; store in saline or tap water; label the container.
- Clean the edge of the eye socket with a moistened cotton ball.
- Reinsert the eye: Be sure the prosthesis is wet. Hold it with your dominant hand. Spread the patient's eyelids apart with your nondominant hand, and guide the prosthesis into the eye socket.

Equipment

- Procedure gloves
- Normal saline solution
- Labeled container filled with saline or tap water
- Cotton balls

Delegation

You can delegate this procedure to the NAP if you conclude that the patient's condition and the NAP's skills allow. Perform the following assessments, and inform the NAP of any special considerations. Ask the NAP to report the patient's ability to tolerate the procedure.

Pre-Procedure Assessments

- Assess the patient's activity tolerance and whether you will need another caregiver to assist.

➤ When performing the procedure, always identify your patient according to agency policy and be attentive to standard precautions, hand hygiene, patient safety and privacy, body mechanics, and documentation.

Procedure Steps

1. Wash hands and apply gloves.

2. Position the patient lying down
If you accidentally drop the eye when removing it, it will fall onto the bed instead of the floor.

3. To remove the artificial eye: raise the upper eyelid with your nondominant hand, and depress the lower lid with your dominant hand. Apply slight pressure below the eye to release the suction holding it in place. Catch the eye in the palm of your dominant hand. Alternatively, you can use a small bulb syringe, place it directly on the eye, and squeeze to create suction and

lift the eye straight up from the socket. ▼

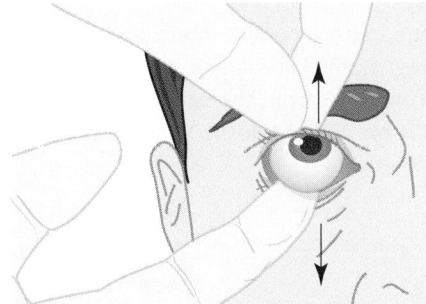

4. Clean the eye with saline, and store it in a labeled container filled with saline or tap water.
✛ Do not use solvents, disinfectants, or alcohol.
These chemicals may irritate the socket or damage the artificial eye.

5. Wipe the edge of the patient's eye socket with a moistened cotton ball, wiping from outer canthus toward the nose.

6. Inspect the socket for redness, swelling, or drainage.
Irritation or infection can occur if debris has entered the socket.

7. To reinsert the eye: remove the prosthetic eye from the container, but do not dry it. Hold the eye between your thumb and the index finger of your dominant hand; with your nondominant hand, pull down on the lower lid while lifting the upper lid and guide the eye into the socket.
The prosthesis will slide into place more easily when it is wet.

Evaluation

- Observe that the eye has been placed correctly in the socket.
- Ask the patient how the eye area feels.
- Observe the eye area for redness or irritation.

Patient Teaching

- Advise the patient to periodically inspect the eye area.
- Review the importance of hand hygiene and proper handling of the eye.
- If the eye wearer experiences dryness or irritation, a lubricant made for ocular prosthetics can be used.

(continued on next page)

Procedure 22-15 ■ **Caring for Artificial Eyes** (continued)

■ If the eye needs to be wiped but not removed, wipe from outer canthus toward the nose.
Wiping outward may dislodge the prosthesis.

■ Encourage the patient to sleep in the prosthesis at night and remove it every 1 to 3 weeks for cleaning (follow prosthesis specialist's advice). Some patients do find that it is necessary to remove and clean the prosthesis every day.
Frequent removal irritates the lining of the socket and increases the amount of discharge produced by the eye socket.

■ The eye should be professionally polished every 6 to 12 months. Symptoms that may indicate the need for a polish are: irritated or itchy lids, increased drainage or discomfort, or changes in the appearance of the artificial eye.

Home Care

■ In the home care setting, determine how the client usually performs eye care.

■ Discuss ways to promote the safety of the artificial eye.

■ Work with the client or caregiver to develop a plan of care for cleaning the eye and care of the area associated with the socket.

Documentation

Chart that the artificial eye was cleansed, the condition of the socket, care given to the area around the socket, and the patient's responses to the procedure.

Practice Resources
Erikson Labs Northwest (2007); Hospital Info (2008); Peters, R. (n.d.).

Procedure 22-16 □ Caring for Hearing Aids

➤ For steps to follow in *all* procedures, refer to the Universal Steps for All Procedures found on the inside back cover of Volume 2.

Critical Aspects

■ Keep hearing aids away from heat and moisture.
■ Clean hearing aids with a damp cloth only.
■ Avoid hairspray and other hair care products.
■ Turn off hearing aids when not in use.
■ Replace dead batteries immediately.
■ Store hearing aids in a case with the battery compartment open.
■ Keep hearing aids and batteries away from children and pets.
■ To clean a hearing aid: Turn it off, remove it from the ear, cleanse the outer ear and the hearing aid, check the battery, reinsert it, turn it on, and check the volume with the patient.

Equipment

■ Face cloth
■ Cotton applicators
■ Dry towel
■ Damp cloth
■ Wax-loop and wax brush, if available
■ Pipe cleaner or toothpick, if wax-loop and wax brush unavailable
■ Procedure gloves (to prevent contact with earwax or ear drainage)

Delegation

You can delegate hearing aid care to the NAP if the patient's condition and the NAP's skills allow. Perform the following assessments, and inform the NAP of the specific type of care needed (e.g., type of hearing aid), and the amount of help the patient needs. Inform the NAP of any special considerations, such as skin irritation or usual volume setting. Ask the NAP to report the condition of the patient's ear, level of self-care, his ability to tolerate the procedure, and his ability to hear in a normal conversation.

Pre-Procedure Assessments

- Determine how much assistance the patient needs.
Aids you in promoting independence as much as possible.

- Determine the type of hearing aid in use. The three common types of hearing aids are (1) postaural hearing aid, (2) in-the-canal hearing aid, and (3) in-the-ear hearing aid.
The cleaning procedure varies according to the type of hearing aid. ▼

- Assess the patient's ear and outer canal for redness, skin lesions, earwax buildup or drainage.
Identify skin problems, and determine whether any symptoms of infection exist. Earwax buildup increases with age and doesn't necessarily indicate a health problem.

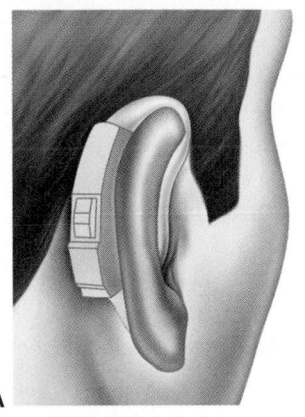 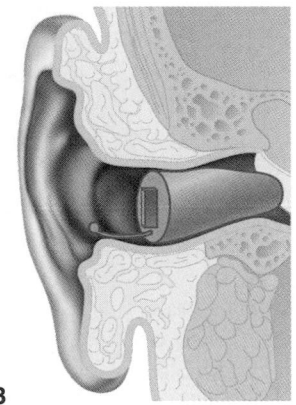 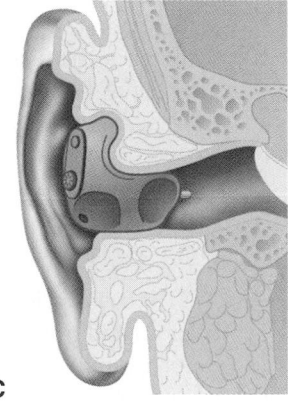

A	B	C
A postaural hearing aid	An in-the-canal hearing aid	An in-the-ear hearing aid

➤ When performing the procedure, always identify your patient according to agency policy and be attentive to standard precautions, hand hygiene, patient safety and privacy, body mechanics, and documentation.

Procedure Steps

1. Don gloves.
The hearing aid may contain earwax buildup or drainage.

2. Place a towel on a nearby table or flat surface.
The towel helps prevent the hearing aid from breaking if it is accidentally dropped. Hearing aids are expensive.

3. To remove the hearing aid:
　a. Turn the hearing aid off by applying slight pressure against the volume control wheel and turning it backward (away from the nose).
Stops the hearing aid from whistling.

　b. Rotate the earmold slightly forward (toward the nose), and gently pull it out. Do not pull on the battery door or the volume wheel.
Pulling on the battery door or the volume wheel may damage the faceplate.

　c. Place the hearing aid on the towel.
The towel will prevent the hearing aid from rolling off the table or banging against the table.

4. Clean the hearing aid.
　a. Wipe all external surfaces with a damp cloth.
　b. Clean the canal portion of the hearing aid using the wax-loop and wax brush, cotton-tipped applicator, pipe cleaner or toothpick. Clean the top portion only. Do not insert anything into the hearing aid itself.
Poking utensils into any part of the hearing aid except for the canal portion may damage the hearing aid.

Step 4b Variation. Detachable Earmold
Disconnect the earmold, and soak it in soapy water. Rinse and dry well, and then reattach it. Do not use alcohol. Never immerse a hearing aid in water, only the earmold.

Detaching an earmold that is glued or fastened by a small metal ring will break the hearing aid. Alcohol will damage the earmold material.

　Check the hearing aid and any tubings for cracks and loose connections. A damaged hearing aid will be less effective and may cause injury to the ear. Early detection of hearing aid damage may allow for repair rather than replacement of the device.

5. Cleanse the outer ear using the corner of a washcloth or a cotton-tipped applicator. Inspect these areas for redness, abrasions, swelling, drainage, or other irregularities.
Poorly fitting or improperly positioned hearing aids may cause trauma to the ear.

6. Insert the hearing aid.
　a. Check that the battery is functioning. Hold the hearing aid in your hand. Close the battery compartment door if open. Turn the power on, turn the volume

(continued on next page)

Procedure 22-16 ■ Caring for Hearing Aids (continued)

high, and listen for a whistling sound.
Whistling indicates proper power level and functioning of the battery.

b. Set the volume control to "Off."
Prevents whistling during insertion and prevents from a sudden, loud noise.

c. Handle the hearing aid by the edges using your thumb and forefinger.
Prevents whistling during insertion.

d. Holding the hearing aid in your dominant hand, use your nondominant hand to gently pull the ear up and back.
Opens the ear canal slightly for an easier insertion and better fit.

e. Insert the canal portion of the hearing aid into the ear. Apply slight pressure and gently rotate the hearing aid back and forth until the canal portion rests flat in the ear.
Allows a better fit and prevents hearing aid from falling out.

Step 6e Variation. Postaural Hearing Aid

Insert the earmold first and then place the earmold over the ear.

Step 6e Variation. In-the-Canal Hearing Aid

Insert with the volume control at the top. The canal should be facing away from your hand.

Step 6e Variation. In-the-Ear Hearing Aid

Insert with the volume control at the bottom.

f. Turn the hearing aid on and adjust the volume by turning the volume control wheel toward the nose. Set the volume control as low as possible.
Normal setting requires a one-third to two-thirds turn of the volume control wheel. A noisier environment requires less volume, or one-fourth turn.

7. Protect the hearing aid from curling irons, hair dryers, hair spray and other hair products.
Heat and moist aerosols will damage the hearing aid.

Procedure Variation
Storing the Hearing Aid

8. Open the battery compartment and place the hearing aid in a closed container labeled with the patient's name.
Saves battery power and allows any moisture to evaporate. Protects the hearing aid from accidental damage or loss.

9. If the hearing aid is to be kept stored and not worn for a week or more, remove the battery completely.
Prevents battery acid from leaking and damaging the hearing aid.

10. Store the hearing aid in a cool, dry place, preferably in the bedside drawer. Keep the hearing aid away from children and pets.
Moisture and heat will damage the hearing aid. Hearing aids and containers are easily lost. A child may choke on the hearing aid. Dogs and cats are attracted to the whistling noise and odor of the hearing aid and sometimes attempt to eat the device.

Procedure Variation
Replacing the Battery

11. Use your finger to swing the battery door open. Never force the door.

12. Peel the tab off the new battery.

13. Hold the battery with the positive (+) side up and slide it into the door, not into the hearing aid itself.

14. Gently close the battery door. Never force the door.

15. Dispose of the old battery in the regular trash.

Guidelines for Care of the Batteries

■ Always dispose of old batteries. Do not throw into a fire.
Minimizes damage from leaking battery acid and prevents mistaking fresh battery from used battery. Heat and fire may cause the battery to explode.

■ Store batteries in a cool, dry place. Do not place zinc-air batteries in the refrigerator.
Heat shortens the life of the battery. Cold batteries warming to room temperature are exposed to condensation and subsequent corrosion.

■ Do not store batteries near coins or other metals.
Contact with other metals can short-circuit the batteries.

■ Do not remove the tab from the battery until the battery is ready for use.
The tab keeps air out of the battery. Once the tab is removed, the battery is activated. Early removal decreases the life of the battery.

■ ◆ Keep batteries away from children, confused adults, and pets.
Minimizes accidental swallowing.

What if . . .

■ **The hearing aid becomes wet?**

Even with considerable care and caution, a hearing aid may become exposed to moisture. In this event, dry the hearing aid as much as possible. Remove the battery and throw it away. Keep the battery door open. Place the hearing aid in its container and allow it to dry overnight. Do not place a new battery in the hearing aid until the next morning.

Moisture will cause the battery to corrode.

■ **The patient wears bilateral hearing aids?**

Be sure to identify which hearing aid is for the left ear and which hearing aid is for the right ear. Most hearing aids have a color marking for easy identification: red = right ear and blue = left ear.

Attempting to force a hearing aid into the wrong ear may cause trauma to the ear.

■ **The patient continues to have hearing difficulties despite hearing aids?**

Hearing aids will not restore full hearing. General tips when communicating with a person with a hearing deficit are listed in Clinical Insight 29-2, Communicating with Clients Who Have Impaired Hearing.

Hearing aids will not block out background noise. A clear, distinct, low-pitched voice helps the client to understand what is being said.

Evaluation

■ Assess how well the patient tolerated the procedure. Was there any discomfort, difficulty with insertion, and so on?
■ Note the condition of the patient's skin, including pain, redness and abnormal discharge.
■ Note the condition of the hearing aid itself.
■ Assess the patient's ability to hear normal speaking voices.
■ Ask the patient whether he feels comfortable and hears satisfactorily.

Patient Teaching

■ Discuss the importance of daily hearing aid care.
■ Review any areas of care that the patient has not been performing adequately.
■ Discuss any problems that need further follow-up, such as earwax build up, faulty or broken hearing aid, or ill-fitting hearing aid.

Home Care

The procedure does not vary in the home. The issues are that the nurse must:
■ Work with the patient and care provider to determine supplies needed for the home.

■ Determine whether further knowledge is required (e.g., if the patient must expose hearing aids to prevailing weather conditions, uses a telephone extensively, must make several adaptations from quiet to noisy environments throughout the day, and so on).
■ Provide a list of available resources (e.g., AARP, National Institutes of Health, Better Hearing Institute).

Documentation

Chart that the patient is wearing a hearing aid, the condition of the ear, and the ability to hear. There will probably be a flowsheet or checklist for this information.

Practice Resources

AARP (2007); Deaf and Hard of Hearing Services Metro (n.d.); Department of Veteran Affairs, (n.d.); National Institute on Deafness and Other Communication Disorders (2007).

Clinical Insights

Clinical Insight 22-1 ▶ Assisting with a Shower or Tub Bath

- Assess the patient's self-care abilities: sensorimotor, musculoskeletal, and cognitive function; activity tolerance; level of knowledge.
- Ensure that the patient has the necessary supplies (e.g., soap, washcloth, towel, clean gown, and so forth).
- Hang a sign on the door to ensure privacy.
- Help wash and dry any areas that the patient cannot reach (e.g., feet, back).
- ◆ Assist the patient to the shower or bathroom as needed.
- Ensure that there is a nonskid surface or mat in the shower or tub.
- For patients who have impaired mobility or activity intolerance, use a shower chair in the shower or tub.
- Be sure that the shower or tub is clean and safe. Most hospitals and long-term care facilities have grab bars and handrails in the bathrooms.
- To avoid burns, verify water temperature for clients with impaired cognition or decreased sensory perception. Water should be 110° to 115°F (43° to 46°C).
- Provide a call device for the patient to obtain help if needed; point out the emergency call device if there is one in the bathroom (usually it is a red button or cord on the wall).

Home Care

- ◆ Encourage clients and families to install hand bars on the sides of the bathtub and on the wall next to the tub. Most hospitals and long-term care facilities have grab bars and handrails in the bathrooms, but these may need to be installed in the home.
- Advise parents never to leave a child alone in the tub or shower and to have a way to unlock the bathroom door from outside the room.
- Advise older adults or those who are ill not to lock the bathroom door while bathing so that help can be summoned if needed (e.g., if they become faint or fall).
- Help families to obtain benches for transferring into the bathtub, or use a plastic chair in the shower.
- Ensure that there is a nonskid surface or mat in the shower or tub.

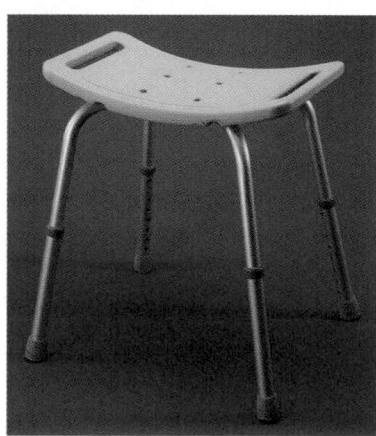

Shower chair

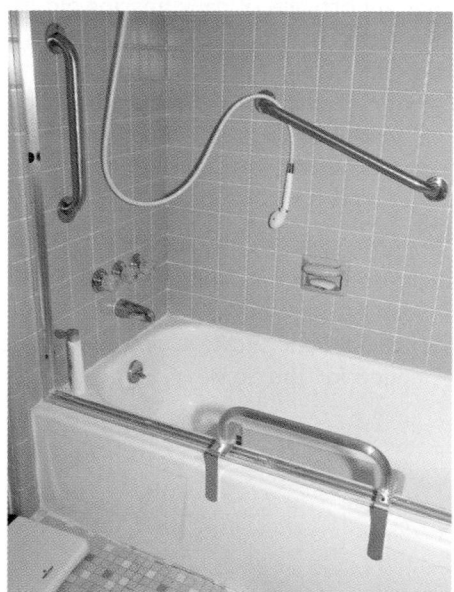

Bathtub with handrail and grab bars

Clinical Insight 22-2 ▶ Bathing a Patient with Dementia

- Focus on the patient, not the task; provide choices.
- Distract with food or by playing relaxing music.
- Use a gentler type of shower head for rinsing.

A strong spray may frighten the patient.

- Avoid sensory overload: Turn down lights, warm the room, play soft music, speak calmly.

People with dementia have trouble processing information. Overloading the senses may trigger aggression.

- Ensure continuity of care.

The patient can build a relationship with the caregiver and reduce fear.

- Encourage the patient to wash her own face if able.

Makes her feel like an active participant, preserves some independence.

- Bathe at a regular time—preferably the same time as when the patient bathed at home.

- Explain the procedure simply, using short sentences.
- Provide privacy.

Patients with dementia do not necessarily lose their modesty and sense of privacy.

- Let the patient know before you touch her or spray her with water.

Sudden actions are often frightening to patients with dementia.

- Do not rush.

The patient will feel the tension and may become agitated.

- Be creative; try bathing one part of the body each day.
- Teach techniques to caregivers at home (e.g., being flexible with time, using a towel bath, etc.)
- Also refer to "What If. . .?" section of Procedure 22-13, Bathing: Providing a Complete Bed Bath.

Assessment Guidelines and Tools

Assessment of Functional Abilities

The Katz Index of Independence in Activities of Daily Living (ADL) is used extensively to assess functional abilities in activities of daily living (bathing/hygiene, dressing/grooming, feeding, toileting). To use the Katz ADL Index,

 Go to Chapter 22, **Tables, Boxes, Figures: ESG Table 22-1,** on the Student Resource Disk or DavisPlus at http://davisplus.fadavis.com/Wilkinson2

 Or go directly to http://www.consultgerirn.org/resources

Assessment Guidelines: Hygiene

Observe Self-Care Abilities

When bathing, dressing, eating, and toileting, which of the following best describes the patient's ability?

- Is completely independent; requires no assistance.
- Requires a device or special equipment (e.g., a walker, a large-handle spoon).
- Requires help, supervision, or teaching from another person.
- Requires help, from another person, as well as a device or special equipment.
- Is totally dependent; does not participate in the activity (e.g., total bed bath).

The Environment

- Is the room temperature comfortable?
- Are the siderails up, when indicated? Is the bed in low position?
- Are bed wheels locked?
- Are bed linens clean and wrinkle free?
- Is the patient's call device within reach?
- Is the overbed table clean and uncluttered?

- Is the walking space uncluttered?
- Are there unpleasant odors?

Skin

Subjective Data

Patients may be sensitive about skin problems or poor hygiene practices, so direct your questions to the patient in a nonjudgmental, respectful manner. General questions to ask include the following:

- How often do you prefer to bathe?
- How do you usually care for your skin?
- What soaps, lotions, or other skin care products do you use?
- Do you have difficulty controlling body odor?
- Have you ever had an allergic skin reaction to food, medications, plants, skin care products, or other materials?
- What problems have you had with your skin in the past?
- What problems are you having with your skin now?
- For each problem identified, ask:

    What symptoms are you having (e.g., any rash or itching)?

    Where is the problem located?

Continued

Assessment Guidelines: Hygiene—cont'd

- How long have you had this problem?
- What have you done to provide relief from the symptoms?
- Do you use any prescription, over-the-counter (OTC), or herbal remedies to treat this problem?
- Have you seen a healthcare provider about this problem?
- Was a diagnosis made? If so, what was it?
- How has this problem affected your life?
- How can I best help you with your skin care?
- Also ask about the presence of diseases or other factors that are known to cause skin problems; for example, decreased mobility, decreased circulation, incontinence, inadequate nutrition, or deficient knowledge.

Objective Data

- Note the skin's overall cleanliness, condition, color, texture, turgor, hydration, and temperature.
- Observe for rashes, lumps, lesions, and cracking.
- Look for drainage from wounds or around tubes.
- Observe for four significant color changes:
  1. **Pallor** in a light-skinned person may appear as pale skin without underlying pink tones. However, in a dark-skinned person, you will need to observe for an ashen gray or yellow color.
  2. **Erythema** is redness of the skin. It is difficult to see in dark-skinned people, so you may discover it by palpating the skin for areas of increased warmth.
  3. **Jaundice,** a yellow discoloration of the skin, is most readily seen in the sclera of the eye.
  4. **Cyanosis,** a bluish coloring of the skin, is caused by decreased peripheral circulation or decreased oxygenation of the blood. In dark-skinned patients, you can most readily see cyanosis by examining the conjunctivae, tongue, buccal mucosa, and palms and soles for a dull, dark color.

Feet

Subjective Data

Ask the patient the following questions or obtain the data from his records:

- What is your normal foot care routine?
- What type of footwear do you usually wear? Observe what the patient is wearing.
- Have you had any foot problems; what treatments have you had for them?
- Do you examine your feet on a regular basis?
- Do you have diabetes mellitus or peripheral vascular disease?

Objective Data

Compare findings for both feet:

- Observe for cleanliness and skin integrity. Note open areas, drainage, or redness.
- Inspect for swelling, inflammation, or infection.
- Palpate for edema.

- Check the skin between the toes for cracks or signs of a fungal infection.
- Notice the color and temperature of the feet; are they the same bilaterally? The color and temperature provide data about circulation and oxygenation. For example, cold, dusky feet may indicate impaired circulation or tissue perfusion secondary to a peripheral vascular disease.
- Check capillary refill. How many seconds does it take for the color to return after you apply pressure?
- Note the presence foot odors, if any.

Nails

Subjective Data

Ask about the patient's usual nail care practices, history of nail problems, and their treatments.

Objective Data

Inspect the nails for the following:

- Shape, contour, and cleanliness
- Presence of broken nails, hangnails, or cracked cuticles
- Hands: Do the fingernails appear neatly manicured, or does the patient bite the nails?
- Feet: Are the toenails trimmed appropriately, straight across?
- Presence of redness or swelling at the nail base or sides

Oral Cavity

Subjective Data

- Usual hygiene practices
- History of periodontal disease or other oral problems
- Financial or insurance problems that limit access to dental care
- Nutritional status and dietary habits (e.g., intake of refined sugars)
- Medications, such as anticonvulsants or diuretics
- Medical treatments, such as radiation therapy, oxygen therapy, and nasogastric tubes
- Other factors known to cause oral problems (smoking, alcohol use, NPO status, dehydration, mouth breathing)
- Self-care deficits (e.g., cognitive impairment, activity intolerance, impaired mobility, depression, lack of knowledge, lack of motivation)

Objective Data

- Observe the lips, which should be pink and moist without lesions.
- Inspect the oral mucosa and gums, which should also be pink, moist, smooth, and free of lesions.
- Healthy gums should have a well-defined margin at each tooth. There should be no visible bleeding.
- Instruct the patient to stick out his tongue and to move it around. It should move freely. The tongue should be symmetrical and pink, with a slightly rough surface.
- Assess the teeth for the presence of any loose, missing, or decaying teeth.

Assessment Guidelines: Hygiene—cont'd

- Examine the hard and soft palates for color, lesions, patches, or petechiae.
- Note any unusual mouth odors or halitosis.

Hair

Subjective Data

- Use of special products or medicated shampoos
- History of hair problems or current conditions needing treatment (e.g., pediculosis)
- History or presence of disease or therapy that affects the hair (e.g., chemotherapy)
- Factors influencing the patient's ability to manage hair and scalp care (e.g., Impaired Mobility)
- Personal or cultural preferences for styling of the hair

Objective Data

- Note the condition, cleanliness, texture, and oiliness of the hair.
- Inspect the scalp for dandruff, pediculosis (head lice), alopecia (hair loss), secretions or lesions.

Eyes

Subjective Data

- If the patient wears glasses, ask when he uses them (e.g., for reading, for driving); and ask how well he sees without them.
- If the patient wears contact lenses, determine:
  - The type of lens (hard, soft, long-wearing, disposable).
  - How often he wears them (daily, occasionally) and for how long at a time. Are they worn during sleep?
  - History of, or present, problems with lens usage (e.g., cleaning, removal).
  - Usual practices for cleaning and storage.
  - History of, or current, problems with the eyes (e.g., redness, tearing, irritation, dryness or "scratchy feeling").

Objective Data

- Inspect the eyes for redness, lesions, swelling, crusting, excessive tearing or discharge.
- Check the color of the conjunctivae.

Standardized Language

Common Etiologies for Self-Care Deficit Diagnoses

Activity Intolerance, Fatigue, decreased strength or endurance (e.g., as in emphysema, pneumonia, heart failure)

Cultural or religious practices and beliefs

Decreased or lack of motivation

Emotional disorders (e.g., anxiety, depression, schizophrenia)

Environmental barriers (e.g., doorway too narrow to accommodate walker, economic status)

Lack of knowledge (e.g., of how to adapt the environment, of adequate hygiene measures)

Limited mobility (e.g., secondary to casts, traction, prescribed bedrest)

Musculoskeletal impairment (e.g., secondary to arthritis, multiple sclerosis)

Neuromuscular impairment (e.g., secondary to spinal cord injury)

Pain and/or discomfort

Perceptual or cognitive impairment (e.g., blindness, Alzheimer's disease)

Personal preferences

Substance abuse

Examples of nursing diagnoses:

   c. Self-Care Deficit (Bathing, Dressing) related to Activity Intolerance secondary to heart failure

   d. Self-Care Deficit (Bathing) related to cognitive and emotional effects of substance abuse

Selected Standardized Outcomes and Interventions for Self-Care Deficit Diagnoses

NANDA-I DIAGNOSIS	NOC OUTCOMES	NIC INTERVENTIONS
Bathing/Hygiene Self-Care Deficit	Ostomy Self-Care	Energy Management
	Self-Care: Activities of Daily Living (ADL)	Eye Care
		Foot Care
	Self-Care: Bathing	Hair Care
	Self-Care: Hygiene	Nail Care
	Self-Care: Oral Hygiene	Oral Health Maintenance
		Ostomy Care
		Bathing
		Ear Care
		Ostomy Care
		Perineal Care
		Self-Care Assistance: Bathing/Hygiene
Dressing/Grooming Self-Care Deficit	Self-Care: Activities of Daily Living (ADLs)	Energy Management
		Environmental Management
	Self-Care: Dressing	Hair Care
		Self-Care Assistance: Dressing/Grooming
Toileting Self-Care Deficit	Knowledge: Ostomy Care	Bathing
	Self-Care: Activities of Daily Living (ADLs)	Bowel Management
		Environmental Management
	Self-Care: Hygiene	Perineal Care
	Self-Care: Toileting	Self-Care Assistance: Toileting
		Urinary Elimination Management

When using NOC outcomes to write goals, rank the patient's abilities by using the NOC scale for self-care indicators: (1) dependent, does not participate, (2) requires assistive person and device, (3) requires assistive person, (4) independent with assistive device, and (5) completely independent. For example:

    Chooses clothing (5)
    Buttons clothing (4)

Sources: NANDA International (2009). *Nursing diagnoses: Definitions & classification 2000–2011*. Philadelphia: Author; Johnson, M., Bulechek, G., Dochterman, J., et al. (2001). *Nursing diagnoses, outcomes, & interventions: NANDA, NOC, and NIC linkages*. St. Louis, MO: C.V. Mosby; Moorhead, S., Johnson, M., Maas, M., et al. (Eds.). (2008). *Nursing outcomes classification (NOC)* (4th ed.). St. Louis, MO: C.V. Mosby; and Bulechek, G., Butcher, H., & Dochterman, J. (2008). *Nursing interventions classification (NIC)*. (5th ed.). St. Louis, MO: C.V. Mosby. Used with permission.

Selected NOC Outcomes and NIC Interventions for Hygiene Problems

NANDA-I DIAGNOSES	NOC OUTCOMES	NIC INTERVENTIONS
Skin		
Impaired Skin Integrity	Immobility Consequences: Physiological	*For Impaired Skin Integrity:*
Risk for Impaired Skin Integrity	Tissue Integrity: Skin and Mucous Membranes	Bathing
	Wound Healing: Primary Intention	Cutaneous Stimulation
	Wound Healing: Secondary Intention	Incision Site Care
		Perineal Care
		Pressure Management
		Pressure Ulcer Care
		Skin Surveillance
		Wound Care
		For Risk for Impaired Skin Integrity, in addition to those above:
		Bed Rest Care
		Circulatory Precautions
		Pressure Ulcer Prevention
		Positioning
Feet		
Impaired Skin (or Tissue) Integrity	Tissue Integrity: Skin and Mucous Membranes	Foot Care
Risk for Impaired Skin Integrity (feet)	Wound Healing: Primary (and Secondary) Intention	Circulatory Care: Arterial Insufficiency
		Circulatory Care: Venous Insufficiency
		Infection Protection
		Self-Care Assistance
		Skin Surveillance
		Teaching: Individual
		Wound Care
Nails		
Risk for Impaired Tissue Integrity	Health-Seeking Behavior	Infection Protection
Risk for Infection	Infection Severity	Nail Care
	Knowledge: Health Behavior	Self-Care Assistance
	Self-Care: Hygiene	Teaching
	Tissue Integrity: Skin and Mucous Membranes	
Mouth		
Risk for Infection	Knowledge: Health Behavior	Oral Health Maintenance
Impaired Dentition	Oral Hygiene	Self-Care Assistance
Impaired Oral Mucous Membrane	Self-Care: Oral Hygiene	Teaching: Individual
Hair		
Impaired Skin Integrity	Tissue Integrity: Skin and Mucous Membranes	Hair Care
Risk for Impaired Skin Integrity		Skin Surveillance
Situational Low Self-Esteem	Self-Esteem	Infection Protection

Continued

Selected NOC Outcomes and NIC Interventions for Hygiene Problems—cont'd

NANDA-I DIAGNOSES	NOC OUTCOMES	NIC INTERVENTIONS
Eyes Disturbed Sensory Perception: Visual	Sensory Function: Vision	Contact Lens Care Eye Care Medication Administration: Eye Prosthesis Care
Ears Disturbed Sensory Perception: Auditory	Sensory Function: Hearing	Ear Care Medication Administration: Ear

Sources: NANDA International (2009). *Nursing diagnoses: Definitions & classification 2000–2011.* Philadelphia: Author; Johnson, M., Bulechek, G., Dochterman, J., et al. (2001). *Nursing diagnoses, outcomes, & interventions: NANDA, NOC, and NIC linkages.* St. Louis, MO: C.V. Mosby; Moorhead, S., Johnson, M., Maas, M., et al. (Eds.). (2008). *Nursing outcomes classification (NOC)* (4th ed.). St. Louis, MO: C.V. Mosby; and Bulechek, G., Butcher, H., & Dochterman, J. (2008). *Nursing interventions classification (NIC).* (5th ed.). St. Louis, MO: C.V. Mosby. Used with permission.

THINKING CRITICALLY ABOUT FACILITATING HYGIENE

The exercises in the following sections allow you to practice the kind of thinking you will use as a full-spectrum nurse. Because these are critical-thinking questions, there is usually no single right answer. We do not provide answers for these questions because it is more important for you to think about the questions than to arrive at the "right" answer. These questions are designed to improve your thinking more than to "cover content." Discuss answers with your peers—discussion can stimulate critical thinking. If you have difficulty with any of these questions, consult with your instructor.

Applying the Full-Spectrum Nursing Model

PATIENT SITUATION

Alice Baker is a frail elderly woman, 93 years old, who lives in a nursing home. She has almost total Self-Care Deficit related to her weakness, painful joints, and dementia. Her mental and physical condition are not likely to improve. Imagine that your charge nurse has instructed you to provide a complete bed bath and other hygiene care for Ms. Baker. When you enter her room with bath supplies and say, "Good morning, Ms. Baker, it's time for your bath," she screams, "Go away from me. I just had a bath. I don't want a bath." You discuss this with the charge nurse, who says, "She has not had a bath, and she needs one today. You will need to do it whether she likes it or not." You tend to agree that Ms. Baker needs a bath because her clothing and linens have food stains, and she smells of urine and perspiration.

THINKING

1. *Theoretical Knowledge*:

   a. What benefits does a bath have for Ms. Baker?

   b. What are the disadvantages of bathing a patient with dementia who is resisting the bath?

2. *Critical Thinking (Considering Alternatives, Deciding What to Do)*:

   a. What do you think Ms. Baker is feeling and experiencing, and how does that help you know what to do?

   b. What are some alternatives to a complete bed bath that would achieve the same purposes?

DOING

3. *Practical Knowledge*: Imagine that you have, indeed, decided that Ms. Baker needs a bath. Which type bath you will give her? What supplies will you need, and where will you find them in the clinical agency you have attended most recently?

CARING

4. *Self-Knowledge*: What is your greatest concern about bathing Ms. Baker; what is the cause of your concern?

Critical Thinking and Clinical Reasoning

1. You are caring for Mrs. Little, a 57-year-old woman who has been experiencing severe arthritic pain. for the past 2 years. She rates her pain at an 8 or 9 on a 10-point pain-rating scale. During your assessment, you notice that Mrs. Little has a moderate body odor, long and untrimmed fingernails and toenails, oily hair, and unshaven legs and axillae. Mrs. Little readily admits that she has neglected her hygiene practices.

a. What is the first hygiene-related nursing diagnosis (problem and etiology) that comes to your mind for Mrs. Little?

b. What data do you have to support a diagnosis of Bathing/Hygiene Self-Care Deficit? What data do you have to support an etiology of "immobility secondary to pain"?

c. With the information in the scenario, how would you rate her Self-Care Deficit: mild, moderate, severe, or total?

d. Anything you could do to help relieve Mrs. Little's pain would facilitate her self-care abilities. However, to plan interventions in which you will assist with her hygiene care, what further patient data do you need?

e. Suppose you assess Mrs. Little further and determine that she has arthritis in multiple joints, including her hands, shoulders, back, knees, and feet. You also determine that she will need a complete bath, either tub or shower, but that she can brush her own teeth if someone provides the necessary supplies. Could you delegate her A.M. hygiene care to an experienced nursing assistive personnel (NAP)? If so, what instructions would you give the NAP?

2. Mr. Thomson is an 87-year-old African American man admitted 2 days ago after being found unconscious in his small apartment. Although Mr. Thomson denies being diabetic, his admission blood sugar was 653 mg/dL. His lower legs are swollen, red, and weeping a clear fluid. His toenails are long, thick, and yellow, and there is a small open sore on the great toe of his left foot. Mr. Thomson's skin is dry and scaly, his hair matted, and he has a strong odor of perspiration and urine. He is uncircumcised. He refuses help with hygiene, saying, "I've taken care of myself for 87 years, and I'll keep doing it. I take my bath once a week on Saturday evening. Now go away!"

a. What theoretical knowledge will you need in order to know what to assess and how to provide his hygiene care?

b. Self-knowledge is important in this case as well. What things in this situation would make caring for Mr. Thomson especially difficult for you? What biases, values, or attitudes might interfere with your ability to give your best care?

3. Your instructor has assigned you to assist the following patients with their hygiene. You must assess the needs of each person, gather information on their bathing habits and preferences, plan nursing measures necessary to meet individual needs, and together with a NAP, provide care.

The first person on your assignment is Mrs. Williams, a 76-year-old Indian American woman who was admitted yesterday after suffering a stroke that paralyzed her right side. Since the stroke, she has been unable to speak clearly and becomes frustrated as she attempts to communicate her needs. Her daughter says Mrs. Williams is a proud, independent, and tidy woman who has been living alone since her husband's death last year. She has been driving her car, cleaning the house, doing her grocery shopping, and maintaining the yard and garden. She wears eyeglasses for reading and driving and has a hearing aid, although she rarely uses it.

The second person on your assignment is Mr. Gold, a 68-year-old man of Orthodox Jewish religion, admitted last week after he experienced a massive heart attack. Although his eyes are open, he is unresponsive to external stimuli. Because of Impaired Swallowing, Mr. Gold is unable to take food or fluid orally; his family has chosen to have a feeding tube placed to ensure adequate nutrition and hydration. His oral mucous membranes and lips are dry and crusty. He is incontinent of urine and stool. Mr. Gold's son, Ira, tells you that throughout his life Mr. Gold adhered to Orthodox Jewish law. The son requests that, in honor of his father, certain aspects of these laws be included in the care plan.

The following questions are about Mrs. Williams.

a. To assess Mrs. Williams' self-care abilities, what important patient data do you still need?

b. What problem has resulted from her stroke that will make it difficult for you to find out about Mrs. Williams' hygiene preferences and practices?

c. From what you know of the patient situation, why do you think Mrs. Williams is becoming frustrated?

d. How do you think you would react if this were to happen to you?

e. How could you provide opportunities for Mrs. Williams to maintain her independence?

The following questions are about Mr. Gold.

a. What additional theoretical knowledge do you need to meet Mr. Gold's religious and cultural needs when providing hygiene care?

b. Where could you obtain such information?

c. If you decide to delegate Mr. Gold's bed bath to a NAP, how could you incorporate his religious and cultural needs into your delegation decisions?

4. For each of the following concepts, use critical thinking to describe how or why it is important to nursing, patient care, or facilitating hygiene. Note that these are *not* to be merely definitions.

Personal hygiene	Patient teaching
Delegation of tasks	Bathing
Cultural differences	Oral care
Skin integrity	Environment and comfort
Life span variables	Hair care
Self-Care Deficits	Nail care
The nursing process	

![icon] What Are the Main Points in This Chapter?

➤ Personal hygiene contributes to physical and psychological well-being by promoting comfort, improving self-image, and decreasing infection and disease.

➤ Although a patient may need assistance with hygiene measures, the goal is to encourage as much independence with these tasks as possible.

➤ Numerous factors influence individual hygiene practices, including personal preferences, cultural/religious/spiritual values and beliefs, economic status, living environment, developmental or knowledge level, and physical and emotional health.

➤ Maintain a respectful, nonjudgmental attitude about cultural and spiritual differences. Avoid the temptation to impose personal values about hygiene practices onto patients.

➤ Consider patients' personal hygiene preferences, and incorporate them into the care plan whenever possible. This reflects caring and promotes maximum participation and independence with ADLs.

➤ Although many hygiene measures can be delegated to NAP, the nurse retains full responsibility for each patient and must instruct the NAP about the patient's limitations and restrictions, amount of assistance necessary, use of any assistive devices, any specific safety precautions to be undertaken, and any other factors influencing the patient's hygiene practices.

➤ The nurse should assess a patient's functional status regularly.

➤ Teaching patients about hygiene is a primary function of the professional nurse.

➤ Intact skin is the body's first line of defense to keep pathogenic microorganisms from entering the body and causing infection.

➤ Bathing removes perspiration and bacteria from the skin surface. It promotes relaxation and comfort, improves circulation, reduces odor, and enhances well-being by increasing self-image. However, it can be stressful for some patients.

➤ You should choose the type of bath to meet the patient's needs (e.g., assist bath, total bed bath, bag bath, and so on).

➤ Bathing is stressful to some patients (e.g., the frail elderly, people with dementia, the morbidly obese). You should focus on the patient's needs for warmth, safety, and comfort, and adapt the bathing procedure to help reduce stress.

➤ Despite common myths, it does not take a lot of water to get a person clean, and not all patients need a complete bath every day.

➤ A complete bath includes perineal care.

➤ Careful assessment of the feet allows for early detection of common foot problems, such as calluses, corns, tinea pedis, ingrown toenail, or foot odor.

➤ Because dirt and debris can collect under the nails and serve as a source of infection, nail care is an important part of hygiene, especially in patients with diabetes mellitus or peripheral neuropathy.

➤ To maintain healthy mucous membranes, teeth, and gums, and to prevent tooth loss and gum disease, regular dental checkups and daily mouth care, including brushing and flossing the teeth, are necessary.

➤ For critically ill and frail elderly patients, as well as those using ventilators, special attention to oral hygiene helps to reduce the risk for pneumonia.

➤ Oral hygiene is challenging for patients with dementia, but it must not be neglected.

➤ The condition of the hair is a measure of an individual's overall health. Shampooing and daily brushing of the hair massages the scalp, stimulates the circulation, and distributes the natural oils.

➤ The eyes normally require very little care; however, when necessary, they may be gently cleansed from the inner to the outer canthus.

➤ Unconscious or critically ill patients who no longer have a blink reflex may need eye care at least every 2 to 4 hours. Keeping the eyes lubricated protects them from corneal abrasions and drying.

➤ Some contact lenses can be worn for only about 12 hours at a time; others may be worn for up to 30 days. Some are disposable; some are not. All types must be cleaned carefully and regularly.

➤ Hearing aids are expensive and should be properly handled and stored. They should not be immersed in water.

➤ When reinserting an artificial (prosthetic) eye, first be certain that it is wet.

➤ Usually no special care is required for the nose. Excess secretions can be removed by gentle blowing with both nostrils open.

➤ Clean, wrinkle-free bed linens help to promote comfort and a sense of well-being.

➤ Room temperature, adequate ventilation, low noise level, and neat and clean surroundings all contribute to a comfortable patient environment.

For practice questions for this chapter,

 Go to **NCLEX-Style Chapter Quiz,** on the Student Resource Disk or DavisPlus at http://davisplus.fadavis.com/Wilkinson2

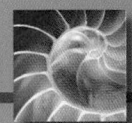

Knowledge Map

Facilitating Hygiene

Factors Affecting Self-Care
- Pain
- Limited mobility
- Sensory alteration
- Impaired cognition
- Emotional dysfunction

Affected by →

Factors Affecting Hygiene
- Preference
- Culture
- Religion
- Economic status
- Developmental level
- Knowledge

Skin Problems:
- Pruritis
- Dryness
- Maceration
- Excoriation
- Abrasions
- Pressure ulcers
- Acne

Perineal Care

Skin Care: Bathing
- Removes bacteria
- Prevents odor
- Friction/warmth dilate surface vessels
- Promotes relaxation
- Enhances well-being
- Type of bath chosen based on nursing judgment

Types of Care
- Early AM
- AM-morning
- PM
- HS
- Bed; shower; tub
- Assist; partial, complete

Hygiene

Hair Care:
- Brushing
- Combing
- Shampoo
- Culturally specific
- Includes shaving

Hair/Scalp Problems
- Dandruff
- Pediculosis
- Alopecia
- Infestation

Foot Care: Focus on Diabetic Patients
- Prevent infection/odor
- Prevent trauma
- Daily inspection
- Wash, rinse, dry
- Water soluble lotion

Foot Problems:
- Corns/calluses
- Tinea pedis
- Ingrown toenail
- Plantar warts
- Odor
- Bunion

Nail Care:
- Daily inspection
- Trim or file
- Remove hangnails
- Clean under nails
- Moisturizing lotion

Oral Hygiene:
- Brushing
- Flossing
- Teaching self-care

Special Considerations:
- Denture care
- Oral care for the unconscious patient: preventing aspiration
- Oral care for the critically ill and frail elderly patient

Oral Problems:
- Halitosis
- Caries/plaque
- Gingivitis
- Pyorrhea
- Stomatitis
- Glossitis
- Cheilosis
- Oral malignancy

Nail Problems:
- Thickened
- Ridged
- Discolored
- Brittle
- Trauma

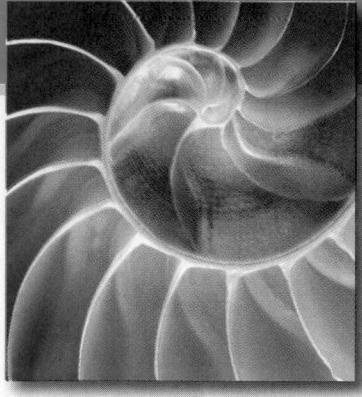
Administering Medication

For a podcast of an overview of this chapter,

 Go to Student Resources, **Podcast – Chapter Overviews, Chapter 23,** on DavisPlus at http://davisplus.fadavis.com/ Wilkinson2

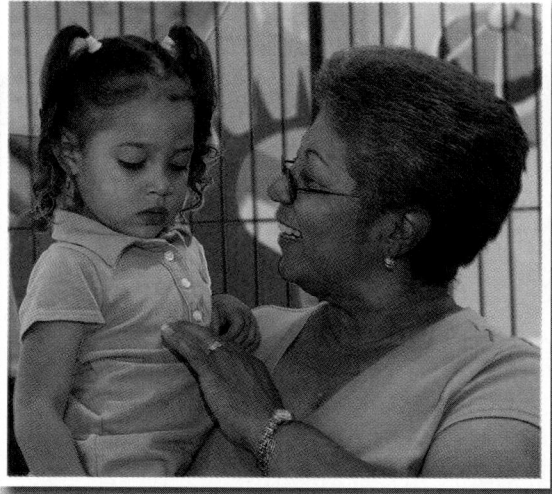

Caring for the Garcias

The exercises in the following section allow you to practice the kind of thinking you will use as a full-spectrum nurse. Because these are critical-thinking questions, there is usually no single right answer. We do not provide answers for these questions because it is more important for you to think about the questions than to arrive at the "right" answer. These questions are designed to improve your thinking more than to "cover content." Discuss answers with your peers— discussion can stimulate critical thinking. If you have difficulty with any of these questions, consult with your instructor.

Bettina Sanford, the 3-year-old granddaughter of Joe and Flordelisa Garcia, has been tired and observed to be sitting down a great deal at preschool. Last week, she developed coughing, wheezing, shortness of breath, nasal congestion, and extreme fatigue. The pediatrician at the Family Medicine Center diagnosed asthma. He prescribed a 5-day tapering course of prednisone, a leukotriene inhibitor (Singulair) 4 mg orally daily at bedtime, and periodic treatments with albuterol through a home nebulizer system.

Joe's mother, Katherine, became very upset when she saw the bottle of prednisone elixir. She was even more upset when she learned that Bettina received an injection of the medicine in the office. She advised Flordelisa not to give Bettina the medicine because, she said, it causes weak bones and stunts growth. Flordelisa has called the clinic asking for advice on how to handle this problem.

A. What theoretical knowledge do you need to answer these concerns?

B. What are some reliable sources where you might find this information?

C. What explanation could you offer to Flordelisa to explain the safety of the prednisone orders? You will need to use a variety of references to answer this question.

D. Flordelisa asks you to explain why Bettina received both a shot and pills. How would you respond?

E. Why is Bettina receiving a leukotriene inhibitor (Singulair) orally and albuterol by nebulizer? Look up the medications, and use your knowledge of different routes of administration.

Practical **Knowledge** **knowing** how

The practical knowledge you will need to administer medications safely and effectively includes procedures and techniques for calculating and measuring dosages and administering medications by a variety of routes. This section also includes information about assessments focused on medications, as well as standardized outcomes and interventions related to medications.

Procedures

Procedures in this section will assist you to prepare, measure, and administer various types of medications, to locate injection sites, and to handle needles safely. Use the following Medication Guidelines for all types and routes.

Medication Guidelines: **Steps to Follow for All Medications (Regardless of Type or Route)**

➤ For steps to follow in *all* procedures, refer to the Universal Steps for All Procedures found on the inside back cover of Volume 2.

➤ **Regardless of the type or route of the medication you are giving, you should always follow the steps below.** For specific routes of administration, refer to the procedures in this chapter.

- Medication administration record (MAR)
- Medication drawer or portable cart with, as needed, keys to the medication drawer
- Procedure gloves, as needed
- Other supplies and equipment needed for the specific procedure (e.g., water, alcohol wipes)

Delegation

As an RN, you can usually delegate administration of medications (except for intravenous medications [IV]) to an LPN/LVN. You cannot delegate this task to nursing assistive personnel (NAP). You can instruct a NAP in the therapeutic effects and side effects of medications and to report any effects observed. Nurse practice acts governing medication administration vary from state to state, and policies vary further among healthcare agencies. For example, in some states, in some situations, LPN/LVNs can administer IV medications. If specially trained NAPs can administer some (e.g., oral or topical) medications in facilities (e.g., in long-term care settings in some states), as the RN you are always responsible for evaluating client responses, which include both therapeutic effects and side effects.

Pre-Procedure Assessments

- Assess your knowledge of the medication (e.g., drug action, purpose, recommended dosage, time of onset and peak action, common side effects, contraindications, drug interactions, and nursing implications).
- Determine whether the prescribed dosage is appropriate for the patient's age and weight.
Dosages are generally decreased for children because of both age and weight. Usually dosing for elderly patients is not based on weight but renal function. Both groups have

less efficient liver and renal function, increasing the length of time a drug stays in the body before being excreted.

- Check for any history of allergies to medications or food. Some medications (e.g., penicillin and cephalosporin) have cross-sensitivity; that is, a patient with a penicillin allergy is at high risk for also being allergic to cephalosporin. Medications can also have cross-sensitivity with certain foods. For more information about how drugs interact with other drugs or with food,

 Go to Chapter 23, **Tables, Boxes, Figures: ESG Table 23-5, Drug–Drug and Food–Drug Interactions,** on the Student Resource Disk or DavisPlus at http://davisplus.fadavis.com/Wilkinson2

- At least on the first administration, assess the patient's knowledge about the medications being given.
The patient will be more likely to take the medication correctly if she understands why she is taking the medication.
- Assess for any factors that would interfere with drug absorption (e.g., diarrhea, inadequate circulation, foods, other medications, etc.).
- Before administering the medication, assess vital signs and check lab studies specific to the medication to determine whether the medication can be safely administered.
- Assess for patient findings that might affect absorption and/or metabolism of the medication, such as impaired liver function, edema, inflammation, or age-related changes.
Medications are metabolized more slowly in a person with decreased liver function.
- Assess for any situations in which administering the medication would not be reasonable, such as oral medications prescribed for a patient who is NPO for surgery or a test, who is vomiting, who has difficulty swallowing, or who is too sedated.

(continued on next page)

Medication Guidelines: ■ **Steps to Follow for All Medications (Regardless of Type or Route)** (continued)

Procedure Steps

1. Check the MAR for the patient's name and identification number, medication, dose, route, time, and drug allergies. The rights of medication administration are: the right patient, right drug, right dose, right route, right time, and right documentation. Initially check the MAR to determine when medications are due **(1st check)**.
Medication prescriptions may change even during your shift; checking the MAR helps ensure that you do not miss medication changes.

2. The prescription should include the patient's name, patient identifier, medication name, dose, route, time, and patient allergies.
This step allows you to clarify any discrepancies before giving the medication.

3. Follow agency policies for medication administration, including the time frame for administration. Most agencies allow medications to be given 30 minutes before or 30 minutes after the time indicated on the MAR. Do not pre-pour medications.
The time of administration is more important for some medications. For example, if an anti-infective agent is given early or late, a therapeutic blood level may not be maintained.

4. Wash your hands.
Hand hygiene minimizes transmission of microorganisms.

5. Access the patient's medication drawer, unlock the medication cart, or log onto the medication dispensing computer.
Depending on the agency, the patient's medications may be in a centralized cart or in a locked drawer in the patient's room. Follow agency policy for obtaining the medication.

6. If administering a narcotic or barbiturate, obtain the narcotic cabinet key and sign out the medication, including the patient's name, drug, dose, and other information per agency policy. Note the drug count when removing a narcotic.

Federal law governs administration of narcotics and barbiturates. All narcotics and barbiturates must be accounted for and witnessed for every shift.

7. Select the ordered medication, and compare medication with the MAR for the first five rights (patient, drug, dose, route, time); check for drug allergies. An inpatient should be wearing an identification band with the drug allergies identified; allergies should be clearly marked in the chart and on the MAR or in the electronic health record (EHR). Question the patient about allergies before giving a newly ordered medication.
This kind of check ensures that the correct drug is being given to the correct patient at the correct time in the correct dose by the correct route.

8. Calculate medication dosage. Double check it. If you are unable to measure the dose exactly, contact the pharmacist.
Verifying dosage will reduce medication errors.

9. Check the expiration date (on the label or on the box) of all medications.
A medication that has expired is no longer guaranteed to be effective.

10. After preparing the medications, do a second check to verify the correct medication, dose, route, and time **(2nd check)**.
Verifies the first five rights of medication administration.

11. Lock the medication cart. Never leave an unlocked medication cart unattended.
Locking the cart guards against pilferage and protects children, older adults with dementia, or anyone wanting to open the cart.

12. Administer the medications.
   a. Take the medication and MAR or hand-held portable device with the electronic health record (EHR) into the patient's room.
You must be able to do the final check in the patient's room and verify that you are administering the correct medication to the correct patient.

   b. Identify the patient using two forms of identification, according to agency policy: checking the identification bracelet, having the patient state her name, comparing the patient to a posted picture of the patient, and checking the patient's date of birth against the MAR.
Agencies may have different means of identifying patients, but you must identify all patients carefully before administering medications. The Joint Commission requires two forms of identification. ▼

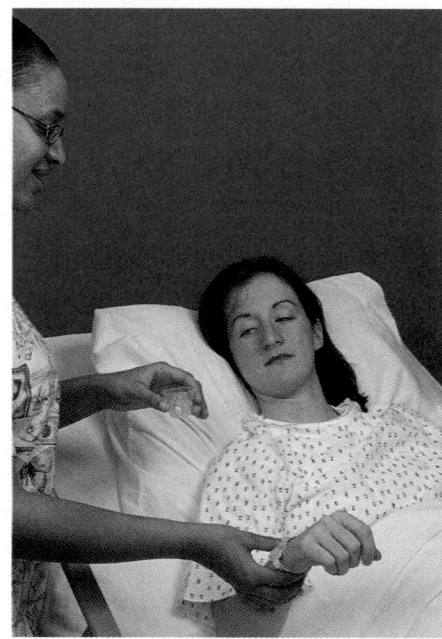

   c. Do a check of the rights of medication for the right patient, right medication, right dose, right route, and right time **(3rd check)**.
Checks for the rights of medication are required for all medications to prevent medication errors. Although an error does not actually occur until the patient has taken a medication, you may be required to file a report for an averted error. Many healthcare facilities are tracking incidents that are near misses. These are errors detected during the checking procedure before drug administration.

   d. Perform any assessments needed, such as checking the pulse or blood pressure.

Some medications can be given only if physical findings or vital signs are within certain parameters. For example, when you administer digoxin you must assess the apical pulse and administer the drug only if the pulse is greater than 60 beats/min; and antihypertensive medications may need to be held if the blood pressure is lower than normal.

e. Explain to the patient that you are there to administer the medication and teach him about the medication.

Patient teaching increases the patient's understanding of and compliance with treatment. Also, the patient may identify potential errors in medication administration. If the patient questions a medication, double-check the medication to be sure you are giving the correct drug and dosage.

f. Administer the medication using appropriate technique (see the procedures for administering medications by the specified route).
g. Remain with the patient until you are sure that she has taken the medication.

If you leave a medication at the bedside, someone else (e.g., another patient or a child) might take it, or the patient might discard it.

h. Document the medication given in the patient's medication record.

If the documentation is not in the patient's record, there is a risk the dose might be given again in error, presuming a missed dose.

What if. . .

- **The patient tells you the pill you are ready to give him is a different color than what he normally takes of a certain prescribed medication?**

Determine why the tablet is different from what the patient is used to taking. Always verify the identity of the drug, especially when it is called into question by the patient who is familiar with the medication he normally takes.

Double checking whenever you are uncertain about a medication you are about to administer helps prevent medication errors; it is possible you have the wrong drug or dosage.

- **The label on the medication shows an expiration date that has passed?**

Do not give the medication. Send it back to the pharmacy for reconstitution or replacement.

Expired medication can lose its potency.

- **The patient refuses to take the prescribed medication?**

Hold the dose and notify the prescriber.

The patient has a right to refuse therapy.

- **You cannot decipher the prescriber's handwritten medication order?**

Hold the dose and notify the prescriber for clarification. Never administer medication if you are not completely sure what is intended.

Handwriting that is hard to read is a common cause of preventable error. Electronic prescribing can help to avoid this.

- **Your patient's medication is not available from the pharmacy at the time the dose is due?**

Do not borrow the medication from another patient's supply. Administer only medication prescribed for that particular patient. Notify the pharmacy of the need to immediately dispense the medication.

This practice increases the risk for medication error because drug dilution or dosage might vary among patients. Or the drug names might be similar sounding, but in fact they are different medications altogether. Also, other patients' medication may then be missing when needed. Incidentatlly, the charges for medication charges might get mixed up.

Evaluation

- Evaluate the therapeutic effects of the medication. For example, check blood pressure after administering an antihypertensive medication, or check pain level after an analgesic.
- Be alert for any adverse reactions, side effects, or allergic reactions. If present, notify the appropriate care provider.

Patient Teaching

- Describe how the drug is prescribed and when the patient should take the medication.
- Discuss the importance of taking the medication as prescribed.
- Explain the need for any laboratory tests for monitoring the medication, such as tests to measure drug level in the blood, if appropriate.
- Explain the purpose, common side effects, and drug interactions of the medications the patient is taking.
- Teach the patient to observe for side effects that signal the need to contact the prescriber.
- Discuss ways to minimize the side effects of a medication, such as avoiding the sun when taking a medication that

causes photosensitivity or rising slowly when taking a medication that causes orthostatic hypotension.
- Discuss potential cultural issues related to taking the medication. An example is the concept of hot and cold conditions and treatments in the Hispanic/Latino culture. If the medication is interpreted as "hot" when the appropriate treatment is "cold," the patient may not take the medication.
- Teach the patient to self-administer medications (e.g., ear drops), as appropriate.

Home Care

- Assess the client's ability to self-administer medications safely.
- Determine the client's financial ability to obtain medications.
- Instruct the client about safe storage of medications.
- Provide instructions for use of each medication.
- Determine whether the client or caregiver has had past problems or present concerns about taking the medications as prescribed.
- If problems have occurred in the past or there are present concerns, discuss possible remedies. For

(continued on next page)

Medication Guidelines: ■ Steps to Follow for All Medications (Regardless of Type or Route) (continued)

example, you might teach the client or caregiver to use a medication storage container with compartments for the times and days of the week, or setting up a system and a schedule that will work for the patient.

Documentation

■ Chart the medication, time, dose, and route given, preadministration assessments, and your signature.
■ Do not document before giving the drug; do not document for anyone else; do not ask another nurse to document a drug you have given. Document only *after* administering the medication.

■ Chart all therapeutic and adverse effects of the medication. Chart your nursing interventions and teaching potential adverse effects.
■ Record the scheduled medications on the MAR. Record PRN medications in the nursing notes and in the MAR, including the reason the medication was given and the patient's response to the medication.
■ If the patient is unable or refuses to take the medication, document on the MAR that the medication was not administered and the reason, and inform the physician.
■ For parenteral medications, chart the site of injection.

Sample EHR documentation:

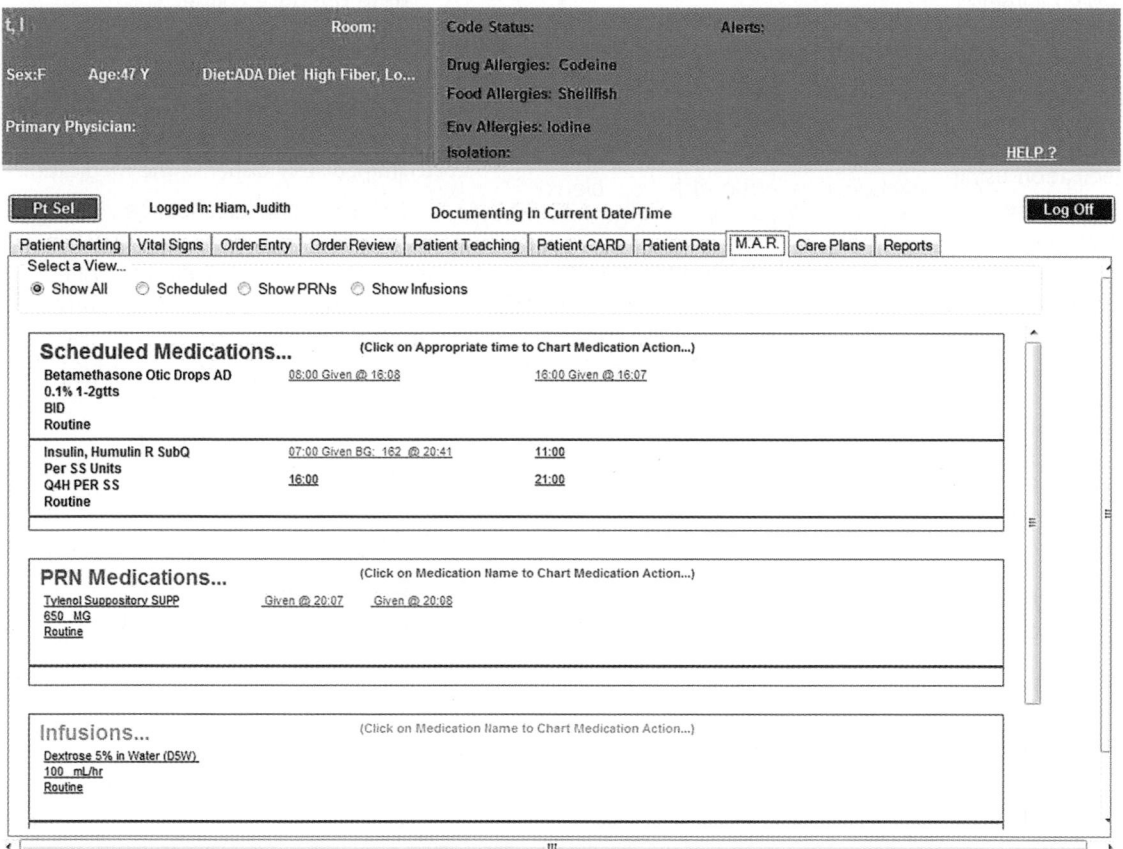

Practice Resources

The Joanna Briggs Institute (2005); The Joint Commission (2006, 2007a, 2007b, 2008); U.S. Food and Drug Administration, Center for Drug Evaluation and Research (2008).

Thinking About the Procedure

 Go to the *Fundamentals of Nursing Skills Videos,* **Medication Guidelines.**

1. Why should the nurse lock the medication dispensing unit after the medication dose is administered?

2. What forms of identification did the nurse check to be sure she is giving the drug to the right patient?

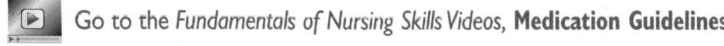 For suggested responses, go to Chapter 23, **Thinking About the Procedure Suggested Responses (Medication Guidelines),** on the Student Resource Disk or DavisPlus at http://davisplus.fadavis.com/Wilkinson2

Procedure 23-1 ☐ Administering Oral Medication

➤ For steps to follow in *all* procedures, refer to the Universal Steps for All Procedures found on the inside back cover of Volume 2. Also refer to Medication Guidelines: Steps to Follow for All Medications (Regardless of Type or Route).

Critical Aspects

- Observe the "three checks" and the "rights of medication": right patient, drug, dose, time, route, and documentation.
- *Tablets and capsules:* Pour the correct number into the medication cup.
- *Liquids:* Hold the plastic medication cup at eye level to measure the dose.
- Assist the patient to a high-Fowler's position, if possible.
- For enterically administered medications, check for correct placement of the nasogastric (NG) or gastric tube (GT).
- Correctly administer the medication.
  Powder: Mix with liquid, and give it to the patient to drink.
  Lozenge: Instruct the patient not to chew or swallow it before dissolving it in his mouth.
  Tablet or capsule: Place the tablet or medication cup in the patient's hand or mouth, and instruct the patient to swallow with sips of liquid.
  Sublingual: Instruct the patient to place the tablet under the tongue and hold it there until it is completely dissolved.
  Buccal: Instruct the patient place the tablet between the cheek and teeth and hold it there until it is completely dissolved.
  Enteral: Make sure the tube is in the proper location before administering medication through it.

Equipment

- Desired liquid for swallowing medications
- Disposable medication cup
- Drinking straw, if needed
- Procedure gloves, if you will need to place a tablet in the patient's mouth
- For enterically administered medications:
  –Water (for diluting and flushing the feeding tube)
  –60-mL catheter-tip syringe
  –Clean gloves
- Stethoscope (*e.g., to check the apical pulse before administering some cardiac medications*)

Delegation

As a rule, you can delegate this skill to an LPN/LVN, depending on the medication, but not to a NAP, except under special policies and situations.

Pre-Procedure Assessments

- Assess the patient's condition to determine whether there are contraindications to oral medications or to the specific medication; for example, the patient's ability to swallow.
Impaired swallowing increases the risk for aspiration.

- Check fluid needs and restrictions. If the patient is NPO (nothing by mouth), check with the prescriber to determine whether the medication should be given by another route or can be given with small sips of water.
A prescriber may decide it is medically necessary to administer oral medication to a patient who is NPO. If there is a fluid restriction, you would need to consider how much fluid you can give with medication. Give additional fluid to a patient with dehydration, and offer only sips for the patient with a fluid restriction.

- For enteral medications, check that the NG tube is in the stomach and is patent.

➤ When performing the procedure, always identify your patient according to agency policy and be attentive to standard precautions, hand hygiene, patient safety and privacy, body mechanics, and documentation.

Procedure Steps

1. Prepare the medication for administration.

Step 1 Variation. For Tablet or Capsule
  a. If you are pouring from a multidose container, do not touch the medication. Pour the tablet into the cap of the bottle, then into the medication cup.
  b. If the medication is unit-dose, do not open the package. Place the entire unit-dose package into the cup.
  c. Many institutions allow combining all tablets or oral caplets scheduled for the same time for the same patient into the same cup. However, even if the agency protocol permits dispensing from a single container, you will need separate cups for medications that require preadministration assessment (e.g., check the apical pulse rate prior to administering digoxin).

(continued on next page)

Procedure 23-1 ■ **Administering Oral Medication** (continued)

When medications are given at the same time, they can be placed in the same cup. If a medication is held because of a preadministration assessment finding, it will be more readily identified when poured into a separate cup.

d. You may break scored tablets with a knife or a pill cutter if necessary.

Only scored tablets may be broken. Breaking an unscored tablet would deliver an imprecise dose.

e. If a patient has difficulty swallowing, check to see whether the pill can be crushed. If so, use a mortar and pestle to grind it. If the pill is in a unit-dose package, grind the pill while it is still inside the package. Mix the ground pill with a small amount of soft food, such as applesauce or pudding.

Some medications, such as capsules, enteric-coated tablets, and sustained-release formulas, cannot be crushed. Crushing such a medication may alter its effectiveness or result in an overdose due to rapid absorption.

Step 1 Variation. For Liquid Medications

f. Check to see whether you must shake the liquid before opening the container.

Some liquids, such as suspensions, will precipitate and need to be shaken to mix the active ingredient with the suspension liquid.

g. Remove the bottle cap, and place it flat side down on the cart or counter.

h. Hold the bottle with the label in the palm of your hand.

Keeping the label on the upward side of the bottle prevents the liquid from dripping down onto the label and obscuring it. ▼

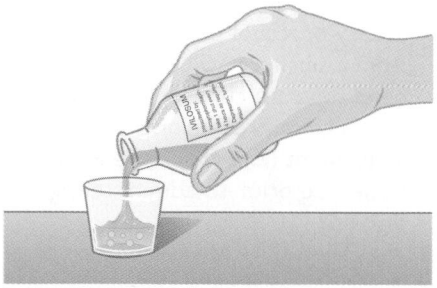

i. Hold or place the plastic medication cup at eye level, and pour the desired amount of medication (or place the cup on a level surface, pour the medication, then hold the cup at eye level to read the amount). Read the dose at the lowest part of the concave surface (meniscus).

Measuring liquids above or below eye level will cause you to read the dose incorrectly and pour too much or too little medication.

j. When you are finished pouring medication, slightly twist the bottle to prevent the medication from dripping down the lip of the bottle. If medication does drip down over the lip, wipe the lip with a tissue or paper towel. Wipe only outside the lip of the bottle.

Wiping the outside of the bottle helps prevent contamination, particularly for thicker solutions, such as elixers or syrups containing sugar.

2. Administer the medication.
   a. Assist the patient to a high-Fowler's position, if possible.

An upright position prevents choking and facilitates swallowing.

b. **Powder:** Mix with liquid at the bedside, and give the mixture to the patient to drink.

Some powders thicken very quickly, so they need to be mixed immediately before administration.

c. **Lozenge:** Instruct the patient not to chew or swallow it whole.

Medication is absorbed through the oral mucosa and is generally inactivated by the acidity in the stomach.

d. **Tablet or capsule:**
   1) If the patient is able to hold the medication in her hand, place the tablet or medication cup in her hand.

Involving the patient in taking the medication encourages independence and is easier for the patient.

2) Give the patient water or other liquid.

Giving the medication with liquid moistens the mouth and helps the patient swallow the pill.

3) If the patient is unable to hold the tablet, place the medication cup up to her lips, and tip the pill into her mouth.

Encourage the patient to do as much as possible. Getting the pill to the back of the mouth will assist in swallowing.

e. **Sublingual medications:** Have the patient place the tablet under the tongue and hold it there until it is completely dissolved.

Sublingual medications are made to be rapidly absorbed through the oral mucosa. The area under the tongue is very vascular, so sublingual medications act very rapidly. Sublingual medications are inactivated by gastric acid if swallowed. ▼

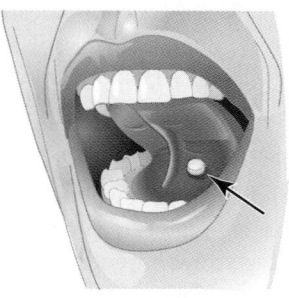

f. **Buccal medications:** Have the patient place the tablet between the cheek and teeth or tongue.

Buccal medications act by being absorbed through the oral mucosa or by being dissolved and swallowed in the saliva. ▼

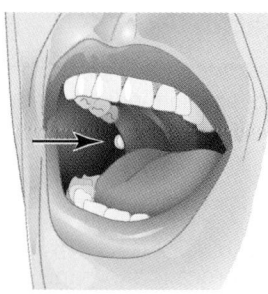

3. Stay with the patient until all medications have been swallowed or dissolved.

Some patients will "chipmunk" the medication in the side of the mouth without swallowing it. Sometimes patient spit it out. Staying at the bedside until the patient swallows oral medication ensures that the patient receives the dose.

■ Procedure 23-1A Administering Medication Through an Enteral Tube

➤ For steps to follow in *all* procedures, refer to the Universal Steps for All Procedures found on the inside back cover of Volume 2. Also refer to Medication Guidelines: Steps to Follow for All Medications (Regardless of Type or Route).

Preparation

■ If the patient is receiving a continuous tube feeding, disconnect it before giving the medications. Leave the tube clamped for a few minutes after administering the medication, according to agency protocol.

■ If the enteral tube is connected to suction, you will usually discontinue the suction for 20 to 30 minutes after administration, and keep the tube clamped, to allow time for the drug to be absorbed.

➤ When performing the procedure, always identify your patient according to agency policy and be attentive to standard precautions, hand hygiene, patient safety and privacy, body mechanics, and documentation.

➤ *Note:* Follow steps 1a through 1j of Procedure 23-1: Administering Oral Medication. Also, follow precautions for administering enteral medications.

Procedure Steps

1. Prepare the medication.
   a. Give the liquid form of medication, if possible. If the solution is hypertonic, be sure to dilute with 10 to 30 mL of sterile water before instilling thorugh a feeding tube.
   Hyperosmolar substances administered too rapidly into the gut can cause bloating, nausea, and osmotic diarrhea.

   b. If pills must be given, verify that the medication can be crushed and given through an enteral tube.
   Some tablets (e.g., sustained-release or enteric-coated tablets) should not be crushed because doing so changes their action.

   c. Crush the tablet and mix it with approximately 20 mL of water or obtain a liquid medication. If you are giving several medications, mix and administer each one separately.
   If you are using a small-bore tube, such as a PEG tube, Keofeed NG feeding tube, or jejunostomy tube, always obtain the liquid form of the medication, because the small-bore tubes clog easily. Ensure that the medication is diluted enough to pass easily through the tube. Instilling drugs one at a time allows you to identify each medication.

2. Don nonsterile procedure gloves.
   Gloving maintains standard precautions.

3. Place patient in a sitting (high-Fowler's) position, if possible.

An upright position reduces the risk for aspiration and choking.

4. For NG tubes, check tube placement (see Chapter 26, Clinical Insight 26-7) by aspirating stomach contents or measuring the pH of the aspirate, if possible. Other, less accurate, methods are injecting air into the feeding tube and auscultating, or asking the patient to speak. ◆ Never rely on only one bedside method for checking tube placement; use a combination of methods.
   NG tubes can become displaced or positioned in the lungs. If medications are given through a misplaced NG tube, the patient may develop aspiration pneumonia.

5. Check for residual volume (see Chapter 26, Procedure 26-3).

6. Flush the tube. Based on the type of tube, use a piston tip or Luer-lock syringe (usually a 30- to 60-mL syringe). Remove the bulb or plunger; attach the barrel to the tube; and pour in 20 to 30 mL of water.
   Flushing ensures patency of the tube and also clears the tube of feeding solution that could clump with medication.

7. Instill the medication by depressing the syringe plunger or using the barrel of the syringe as a funnel and pouring in the medication. A smaller tube or thicker medication will require instilling the medication with a 30 to 60 mL syringe, but when larger

tubes are used, the medication can be poured. ▼

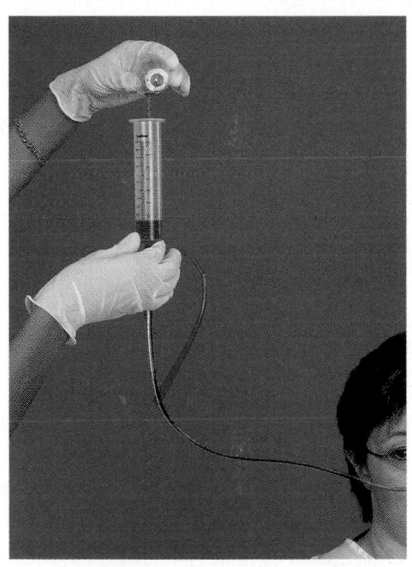

8. Flush the medication through the tube by instilling an additional 20 to 30 mL of water.
   Flushing ensures that all the medication has been administered and prevents the tube from clogging.

9. If there is more than one medication, give each separately, flushing after each.
   Some medications are less effective when given in combination with others, or there may be an additive effect if they have similar actions.

10. Have the patient maintain a sitting position for at least 30 minutes after you administer the medication.
    An upright position minimizes the risk of aspiration.

(continued on next page)

Procedure 23-1 ■ Administering Oral Medication (continued)

What if...

■ **My patient is an older adult who is to receive medication through an enteral tube?**

Check level of consciousness, mentation, or alertness. Check for potential aspiration risk by checking the patient's swallow and gag reflexes.

■ **My patient is a child who is to receive medication through an enteral tube?**

Because of the small size of the feeding tube, only use medications that come in a liquid preparation to prevent occlusion of the tube.

Position an infant in a prone or side-lying position, sitting, or reverse Trendelenburg for 30 minutes to 1 hour following medication administration.

This position facilitates peristalsis and transport of medication through the intestine.

■ **The prescribed medication should be given on an empty stomach?**

If the medication should be taken on an empty stomach, interrupt the feeding 30 minutes before giving the drug. Resume 30 minutes later.

Waiting to give the medication allows time for absorption to occur before the feedings resume.

Evaluation

■ Refer to Medication Guidelines: Steps to Follow for All Medication (Regardless of Type or Route).
■ For medications administered orally:
  –Note whether the patient has difficulty swallowing, gags, or coughs while swallowing oral medication.
  –Evaluate for gastric discomfort.
  –Assess for any signs of drug allergy or intolerance to the medication.
■ For medications administered through a feeding tube, in addition to the preceding assessments, assess that the NG tube is correctly placed and patent before and after administering the medication.

Patient Teaching

■ Refer to Medication Guidelines: Steps to Follow for All Medication (Regardless of Type or Route).
■ Some medications should be given with food; others on an empty stomach. Determine what is prescribed before taking medication.
■ Discuss drug safety measures with the patient, including use of child-safety caps (or using an easy-open cap for an elderly population or with those likely to have difficulty opening containers of this type); keeping the medication in its original container; discarding expired medications; avoiding transferring medication to another container; and carefully reading the label and directions for each medication.
■ Discuss the relationship between food and the medication, if needed. For example, is the medication to be taken with food or not? Does taking medication on an empty stomach contribute to nausea or gastric irritation? Does the medication interact with any foods? For more information about how drugs interact with food,

Go to Chapter 23, **Tables, Boxes, Figures: ESG Table 23-5, Drug–Drug and Food–Drug Interactions,** on the Student Resource Disk or DavisPlus at http://davisplus.fadavis.com/Wilkinson2

For enteral medications:
    Cover the above three topics (for patient teaching about oral medications) plus the following:

■ Discuss the importance of upright positioning for 20 to 30 minutes after taking medication through an enteral tube. This promotes gastric emptying and drug transit from the stomach to the GI tract.
■ Instruct the patient to immediately notify his healthcare provider if he chokes or has difficulty breathing during or shortly after medication is given by enteral tube. The medication should be stopped immediately and emergency care might be necessary.

Home Care

Advise clients who are receiving enteral medication at home to do the following:
■ Notify the healthcare provider if any of the following lasts for more than a day: diarrhea, constipation, nausea, dark urine, bad-smelling urine, or dry mouth.
■ Notify the healthcare provider if the tube becomes clogged or seems to be moving farther out or in.
■ Call the healthcare provider as soon as possible if the feeding tube falls out or you cannot confirm that the end of the tube is in the stomach.
■ To prevent a clogged feeding tube, flush the tube with water each time after giving a medication or feeding.
■ Brush your teeth at least twice daily, if a NG tube remains in place continuously.
■ Clean daily the area where the NG tube goes into the nostrils. Use a cotton-tip applicator moistened with warm water. If your nose becomes sore, you might apply water-soluble lubricant.
■ Change the nasal tape every other day or when it is loose.

Documentation

■ Refer to Medication Guidelines: Steps to Follow for All Medication (Regardless of Type or Route).
■ Often, scheduled medications are recorded only on the MAR.
■ Document the drug, dosage, time, route, and your name as the healthcare provider administering the medication.

- Document any suspected drug reaction, intolerance, or patient response to the medication.
- Be sure to document on the intake and output record the amount of liquid medication and the water used for swallowing medication. Some patients may be fluid restricted, so all intake should be recorded. Be sure to know what is appropriate in your clinical facility.
- For enteral medications: Document patency, residual volume, and placement of tube. Document any difficulty with administering the medications through the feeding tube.
- Be sure to document on the intake and output record the amount of liquid medication and the water used for flushing. Some physicians order a specific amount of water to flush with each medication administration or feeding. Some healthcare facilities use a protocol amount of water to flush gastrostomy tubes. Be sure to know what is appropriate in your clinical facility.

Sample documentation for a PRN oral medication:

> 10/31/12 1800 *Placed client in Fowler's position. Administered Lasix 20 mg. PO tablet with 30 mL water. Patient tolerated medication.* ——— S. Smith, RN

Sample documentation for an enteral medication:

> 8/31/12 1400 *Placed client in Fowler's position. GT placement confirmed with pH of 4.5 using gastric aspirate. Administered 10 mL of liquid medication and flushed with 20 mL of water. Fed 240-mL can of Ensure and flushed GT with 100 mL of water.* ——— S. Smith, RN

What if . . .

- **My patient vomits shortly after taking oral medication?**

Notify the prescriber for instructions regarding giving the dose again or not.

- **My patient is unable to sit upright to take oral medication?**

Assist the patient into a side-lying position and offer a straw to take water with pills or tablets.

- **My patient has difficulty drinking from a cup?**

If the patient has difficulty taking liquids from a cup, use a syringe without a needle to place the medication in his mouth. Place the patient in a side-lying or upright position. Place the syringe between the gum and cheek in the back corner of the mouth, and slowly push the plunger to administer the liquid.

This technique and positioning help prevent aspiration.

- **My patient is on fluid restriction?**

Use the smallest amount of water needed to swallow or dissolve tablets and to flush enteral tubes.

- **My patient is cognitively impaired?**

Request the patient open his mouth to see whether he has swallowed the medication; look under the tongue or side pocket near the inside of the cheek.

Thinking About the Procedure

 Go to the *Fundamentals of Nursing Skills Videos*, **Oral and Sublingual Medications.**

1. How does the nurse in the DVD dispense the tablet from a multidose container and administer to the patient without having to touch it?

 For suggested responses, go to Chapter 23, **Thinking About the Procedure Suggested Responses (Procedure 23-1),** on the Student Resource Disk or DavisPlus at http://davisplus.fadavis.com/Wilkinson2

Procedure 23-2 ■ Administering Ophthalmic Medication

➤ For steps to follow in *all* procedures, refer to the Universal Steps for All Procedures found on the inside back cover of Volume 2. Also refer to the Medication Guidelines: Steps to Follow for All Medications (Regardless of Type or Route).

Critical Aspects

For Instillations

- Use high-Fowler's position, with the head slightly tilted back.
- Work from the inner to outer canthus when cleansing or instilling medication.
- Apply the medication into the conjunctival sac.
- Do not apply the medication to the cornea.
- Do not let the dropper or tube touch the eye.
- For eye drops, press gently against the same side of the nose for 1 to 2 minutes to close the lacrimal ducts. For eye ointment, ask the patient to gently close the eyes for 2 to 3 minutes.

For Irrigations

- Use a low-Fowler's position.
- Check the pH in the conjunctival sac, if indicated.
- Use a Morgan lens or IV tubing to irrigate the eyes.
- For direct-flow irrigation, irrigate from the inner canthus to the outer canthus.
- Irrigate for 20 minutes or until the pH reaches the desired level.

Equipment

- Eye drops or ointment
- Tissue

For irrigation, add:

- Prescribed eye irrigation solution (e.g., 500 to 1000 mL of normal saline or lactated Ringer's solution are commonly used)
- IV tubing or eye irrigation insert, such as the Morgan lens (Follow manufacturer's directions for this specialized equipment.)
- Ocular anesthetic, according to protocol or physician orders
- pH paper
- Basin
- Towel

Delegation

As an RN, you can usually delegate administration of eye instillations to an LPN/LVN. You usually cannot delegate this task to a NAP unless the NAP has special training for a specific, defined situation (e.g., "medication aides" in some long-term-care settings). See Medication Guidelines: Steps to Follow for All Medication (Regardless of Type or Route), at the beginning of the Procedures section.

Pre-Procedure Assessment

- Assess the patient's eyes for redness, discharge, or other signs of irritation.
- Determine whether the eyes need to be cleansed before administration of the medication.

Excess tearing, debris, or excess mucous in the eye could interfere with the effectiveness of the medication.

✚ Check the prescription for where to instill medication (Note: We do not advise using these abbreviations—they have been disallowed by The Joint Commission—but you may still see them written in prescriptions).

OD = right eye
OS = left eye
OU = both eyes

For irrigations, also assess the following:

- Determine the cause of the eye problem—acid, alkaline, or other chemical burn or body fluid splash; or nonembedded foreign body.

Irrigations are generally used to remove chemical or physical irritants, but they may be done following surgery or to treat a severe infection. Normal saline (NS) or lactated Ringer's is the solution generally recommended for high-volume eye irrigations because the pH of 6 to 7.5 is closest to the normal tear pH of 7.1. Volumes of 500 to 1000 mL are generally used.

- Assess the patient's eyes for swelling, redness, drainage, or complaints of pain.

A baseline assessment is useful for determining the need for and effectiveness of irrigation. Sclera should be smooth, white, and glistening.

- Determine the patient's level of discomfort and ability to cooperate with the procedure.

Combative or otherwise uncooperative patients refusing instillation of medication can interfere with the efficiency of the procedure.

- Assess the pain level.

Debris, chemicals, and some liquids in the eye can be extremely painful. The eye may need to be anesthetized before irrigation or a general systemic pain medication given. If the patient cannot hold still for the procedure, he may need to be sedated.

➤ When performing the procedure, always identify your patient according to agency policy and be attentive to standard precautions, hand hygiene, patient safety and privacy, body mechanics, and documentation.

Procedure Steps

1. Assist the patient to a high-Fowler's position, with head slightly tilted back, if possible.
An upright position keeps eye drops in the eye and helps prevent eye drops from draining into lacrimal duct. Do not tilt the head back if the patient has a neck injury or other contraindication.

2. Don procedure gloves.
Gloving complies with standard precautions.

3. Cleanse the edges of eyelid from the inner to outer canthus, if needed.
By following the principle of "clean to dirty," you avoid transferring debris into the nasolacrimal duct.

Procedure Variation
Instilling Eye Drops

(Follow steps 1–3.)

4. Gently rest your dominant hand, with the eyedropper, on the patient's forehead.
Stabilizes the hand in the event the patient moves—prevents accidental injury to the eye.

5. With your nondominant hand, pull the lower lid down to expose the conjunctival sac.
Allows visualization of the area where you will administer the medication.

6. Position the eyedropper about 1.5 to 2.0 cm (½ to ¾ in.) above the patient's eye. Ask the patient to look up, and drop the prescribed number of drops into the conjunctival sac. Do not let the dropper touch the eye.
Keeping the dropping away from the globe of the eye reduces the risk of accidental injury to the eye and avoids contamination of the dropper. Having the patient look up helps to decrease the blink reflex. Instilling the eye drops directly onto the cornea could injure the cornea, so

drops are instilled into the conjunctival sac. ▼

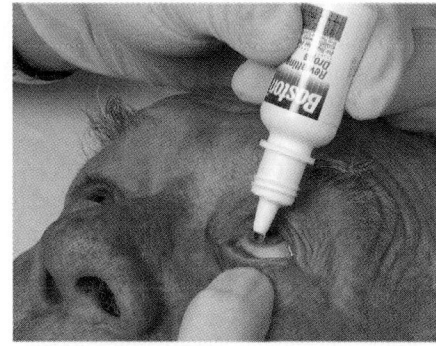

7. Ask the patient to gently close and move his eyes.
Closing the eyes helps to distribute the medication.

8. If the medication has systemic effects, press gently against the same side of the nose for 1 to 2 minutes to close the lacrimal ducts.
This pressure reduces systemic absorption through the lacrimal duct. ▼

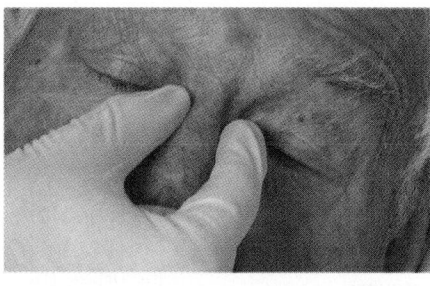

Procedure Variation
Administering Eye Ointment

(Follow steps 1–3).

9. Gently rest your dominant hand, with the eye ointment, on the patient's forehead.
Stabilizing your hand helps to prevent accidental injury to the eye.

10. With your nondominant hand, pull the lower lid down to expose the conjunctival sac.
This position allows visualization of area where you will administer the medication.

11. Ask the patient to look up, and apply a thin strip of ointment—usually

about 2 to 2.5 cm (1 in.)—in the conjunctival sac, and twist your wrist to break off the strip of ointment. Do not let the tube touch the eye.
If the medication ribbon is not broken off, lifting the tube will pull the medication out of the conjunctival sac. ▼

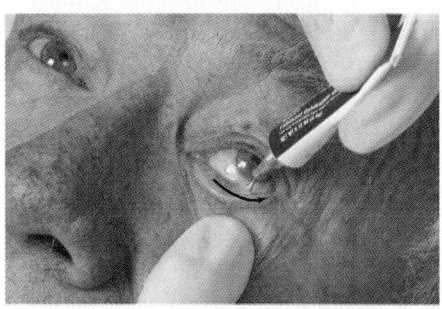

a. Ask the patient to gently close his eyes for 2 to 3 minutes.
Closing the lids helps to distribute the medication.

b. Explain to patient that his vision will be blurred for a short amount of time after administration of ointment.
The viscosity of the ointment can cause blurring.

What if . . .

■ **My patient is a child who won't open his eye for the application?**
Try distracting the child by turning on the television or offering an age-appropriate toy in view.

Distraction and bribery are effective techniques for coaxing a child to cooperate for important matters, such as giving medication.

Ask a family member to help you gain cooperation of the child.

It might be fear or mistrust that is causing him to be unwilling to open his eyes.

■ **My patient wears soft contact lenses?**
Have the patient remove contact lenses before administering the medication and wait at least 15 minutes after instilling eye drops before reinserting the lenses.

(continued on next page)

Procedure 23-2 ■ Administering Ophthalmic Medication (continued)

■ Procedure 23-2A Irrigating the Eyes

➤ When performing the procedure, always identify your patient according to agency policy and be attentive to standard precautions, hand hygiene, patient safety and privacy, body mechanics, and documentation.

Procedure Steps

1. Assist the patient to a low-Fowler's position, with the head tilted toward the affected eye, if possible.
An upright position with the head tilted toward the affected eye helps to drain the irrigating solution from the eye and prevents contamination of the unaffected eye.

2. Place the towel and basin under the patient's cheek to absorb the drainage.
The patient will be more comfortable when he is clean and dry.

3. Check the pH by gently touching the pH paper to secretions in the conjunctival sac.
A litmus test determines the correct irrigating solution and whether the irritant is alkaline or acidic. The normal pH of tears is approximately 7.1.

4. Follow the agency protocol or prescriber's order regarding use of

ocular anesthetic drops.
The ocular anesthetic will be washed out by the irrigation fluid, so it needs to be reinstilled every 2 to 3 minutes, or it can be added to the irrigation solution.

5. Connect the solution and tubing, and prime the tubing.
Priming the tubing prevents blowing air across the cornea, which would be uncomfortable.

6. Irrigate the eye.
   a. Hold the tubing about 2.5 cm (1 in.) from eye.
A safe distance helps prevent accidental trauma to the eye.

   b. Separate the eyelids with your thumb and index finger.
It is easier to irrigate the cornea when the eyelids are separated.

   c. Direct the flow of solution over the eye from the inner canthus to the outer canthus.

The inner canthus is considered clean, primarily because of the open duct in this area. Flowing irrigation solution in this manner follows the principle of "clean to dirty." ▼

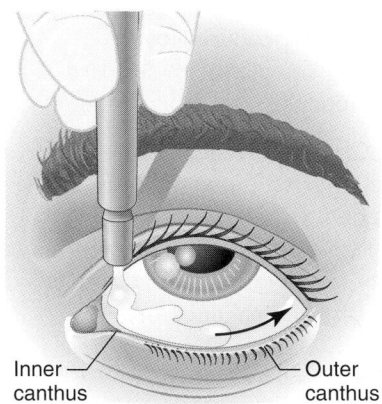

Inner canthus — Outer canthus

7. Recheck pH, and continue to irrigate the eye as needed.
With alkaline or acidic chemical injuries, the pH of the eye needs to be returned to normal as soon as possible to prevent further eye injury.

Evaluation

- Examine the eyes for redness or drainage.
- Observe the patient's ability to follow instructions during the procedure.
- Observe the pain level during the procedure.
- After an irrigation, check for decrease in eye pain.

Patient Teaching

- Discuss with the patient how to prevent contaminating eye drops or ointment.
- Instruct the patient on the best technique for instilling eye drops or ointment.
- If patient needs assistance with instilling drops, discuss use of an eye drop guide.
- Discuss the signs and symptoms with the patient that need to be reported to the physician, including eye pain and increased redness or drainage.

For irrigations:

- Discuss the cause and prevention of eye injuries, including the use of protective goggles.
- Discuss the need for follow-up treatment. If the patient will be instilling eye medications or applying eye patches, ensure that patient is able to use the correct technique.

Home Care

If a splash occurs to the eyes in the home, teach the client to immediately flood his eyes with cool water (as follows):

- Hold your eyelids open and put your head under a faucet or pour water from a clean container.
- Teach the client to roll his eyes as much as possible while running water across your eyes.
- Flood your eyes for at least 20 minutes.
- Get medical help immediately after rinsing your eyes.

Documentation

- For instillations: Chart assessment data before, during, and after instillation. Record on the MAR, as for all medications.
- For irrigations: Chart the condition of the patient's eyes before the irrigation, including the patient's complaints of pain or burning. Document the eye pH, instillation of anesthetic drops, the type and amount of irrigation fluid used, the eye pH following irrigation, and the patient's response. You also need to record other treatment, such as instillation of lubricating and/or antibiotic ointment and application of eye patches.

Sample EHR documentation:

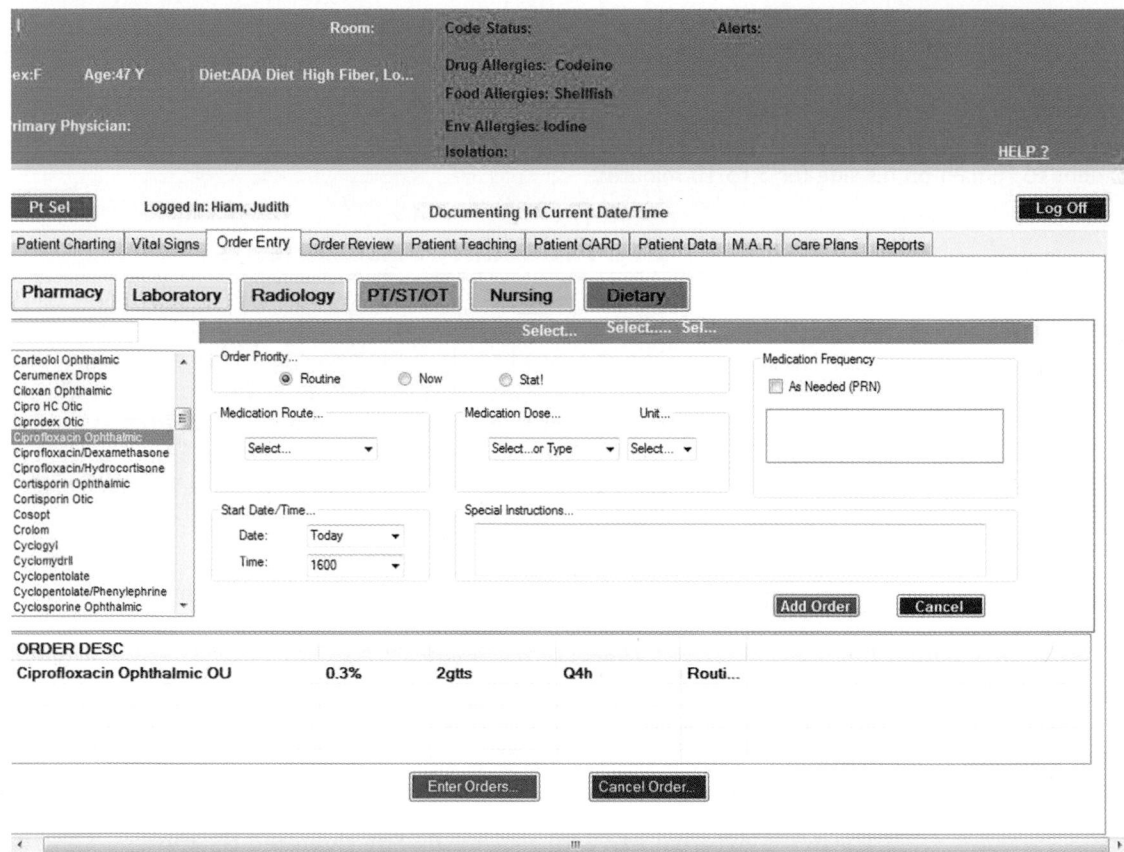

Practice Resource

Michigan Pharmacists' Association (2006).

Thinking About the Procedure

 Go to the *Fundamentals of Nursing Skills Videos*, **Ophthalmic Drops and Ointments.**

1. What does the nurse on the DVD do immediately after instillation of the ophthalmic drops? Why?

2. What hand does the nurse in the DVD use to hold open the eye and expose the conjunctival sac? Why?

 For suggested responses, go to Chapter 23, **Thinking About the Procedure Suggested Responses (Procedure 23-2),** on the Student Resource Disk or DavisPlus at http://davisplus.fadavis.com/Wilkinson2

Procedure 23-3 ☐ Administering Otic Medication

➤ For steps to follow in *all* procedures, refer to the Universal Steps for All Procedures found on the inside back cover of Volume 2. Also refer to the Medication Guidelines: Steps to Follow for All Medications (Regardless of Type or Route).

Critical Aspects

- Warm the solution to be instilled.
- Assist the patient to a side-lying position, with the appropriate ear facing up.
- Straighten the ear canal. For an adult, pull the pinna up and back; for a child 3 years or younger, down and back.
- Instill the ordered number of drops into the ear canal.
- Do not force the solution into the ear or occlude the ear canal with the dropper.
- Instruct the patient to remain on his side for 5 to 10 minutes.

Equipment

- Ear drops
- Dropper with flexible rubber tip
- Cotton-tipped applicators
- Cotton ball

Delegation

As an RN, you can usually delegate administration of otic medications to an LPN/LVN. You usually cannot delegate this task to a NAP unless the NAP has special training for a specific, defined situation (e.g., "medication aides" in some long-term care settings in some states). See the Medication Guidelines at the beginning of the Procedures section.

Pre-Procedure Assessments

- Assess the external ear and canal for erythema, drainage, and cerumen.

You may need to clean the external ear to remove obstructions so that the medication can be distributed throughout the ear canal. Use the otoscope to evaluate the tympanic membrane if the drainage is bloody or the patient complains of pain or decreased hearing acuity. If the tympanic membrane is ruptured, use sterile technique.

- Assess for any ear pain or hearing impairment.
- Establish a baseline that can be used to evaluate the effects of treatment.

➤ When performing the procedure, always identify your patient according to agency policy and be attentive to standard precautions, hand hygiene, patient safety and privacy, body mechanics, and documentation.

Procedure Steps

1. Hold the eardrop bottle in your hand to warm it, or place it in warm water (not hot). Gently shake the bottle before using the drops.
Warm solution is more comfortable than cool. Also, placing cool solutions in the ear can cause dizziness. Gently shaking the bottle disperses the medication throughout the solution.

2. Assist patient to a side-lying position, with the appropriate ear facing up.
This position facilitates administering the drops and prevents drops escaping from the ear.

3. Clean the external ear with a cotton-tipped applicator, if necessary.
Cleaning the ear allows eardrops to reach all areas of the ear canal without trauma. Be careful not to push cerumen further into the ear canal.

4. Fill the dropper with the correct amount of medication.

5. For infants and young children, ask a parent or another caregiver to immobilize the child while you administer the medication.
Mobilization and restraint reduce the risk for injury for the child who struggles during the procedure.

6. Straighten the ear canal.
a. For a child younger than 3 years old, pull the pinna down and back. ▼

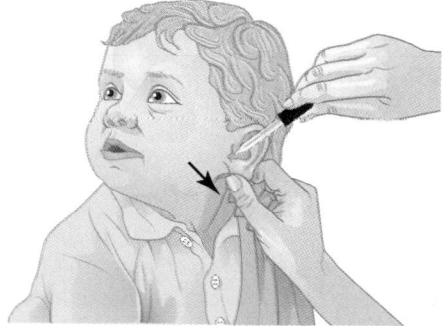

b. For older children and adults, pull the pinna up and back. ▼

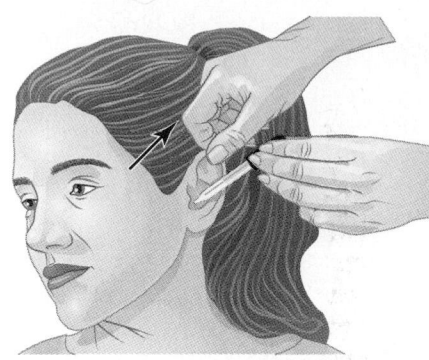

These positions straighten the ear canal for proper channelling of the medication.

7. Instill the ordered number of drops along the side of the ear canal, being careful not to touch the end of the dropper to any part of the ear.
Avoiding contact between the dropper and the ear reduces the risk of contamination of the dropper.

8. Gently tug on the external ear after drops are instilled.
A tug like this facilitates flow of medication into the auditory canal.

9. Instruct the patient to remain on his side for 5 to 10 minutes.
The side-lying position assists in distributing the medication and prevents drops from escaping the ear canal.

10. Place a cotton ball, or a piece of it, loosely at the opening of the auditory canal for 15 minutes.
A cotton ball will absorb excess fluid and keep the medication from rolling out. However, keep in mind that if it is left near an infant it can be a choking hazard if not properly supervised.

What if . . .

- **My patient is a child and rolls over so most of the otic medication rolls back out of the ear?**

Use your best judgment to estimate the amount of the dosage that was lost. Replace it by repeating the procedure for instillation of the medication, except next time position the child securely until you are confident the medication has penetrated the ear canal.

- **There is too much cerumen (ear wax) in the canal to instill otic drops?**

You can use special drops for softening the cerumen and allow for easier removal. Gentle irrigation with warm saline is effective, unless the child has perforation of the tympanic membrane or myringotomy tubes. You should not use a metal syringe (Pomeroy syringe) for the removal of cerumen because (1) this type of syringe is heavy and difficult to control and (2) may be associated with a higher risk of perforations of the tympanic membrane because of the pressure exerted. Oral jet irrigators have been associated with some trauma, including tympanic membrane perforation. You should not attempt to remove impaction by "ear candling," which is the application of hot candle wax.

Evaluation

- Refer to Medication Guidelines: Steps to Follow for All Medication (Regardless of Type or Route).
- Assess for discomfort or pain during the procedure and for relief afterward.
- Evaluate for wax build-up, redness, swelling, or drainage.

Documentation

- Refer to Medication Guidelines: Steps to Follow for All Medication (Regardless of Type or Route).
- Assess the amount, color, character, and odor of drainage, if present.
- Note any swelling or redness in the ear canal.
- Document pain or discomfort and hearing loss.

(continued on next page)

Procedure 23-3 ■ **Administering Otic Medication** (continued)

Sample EHR documentation:

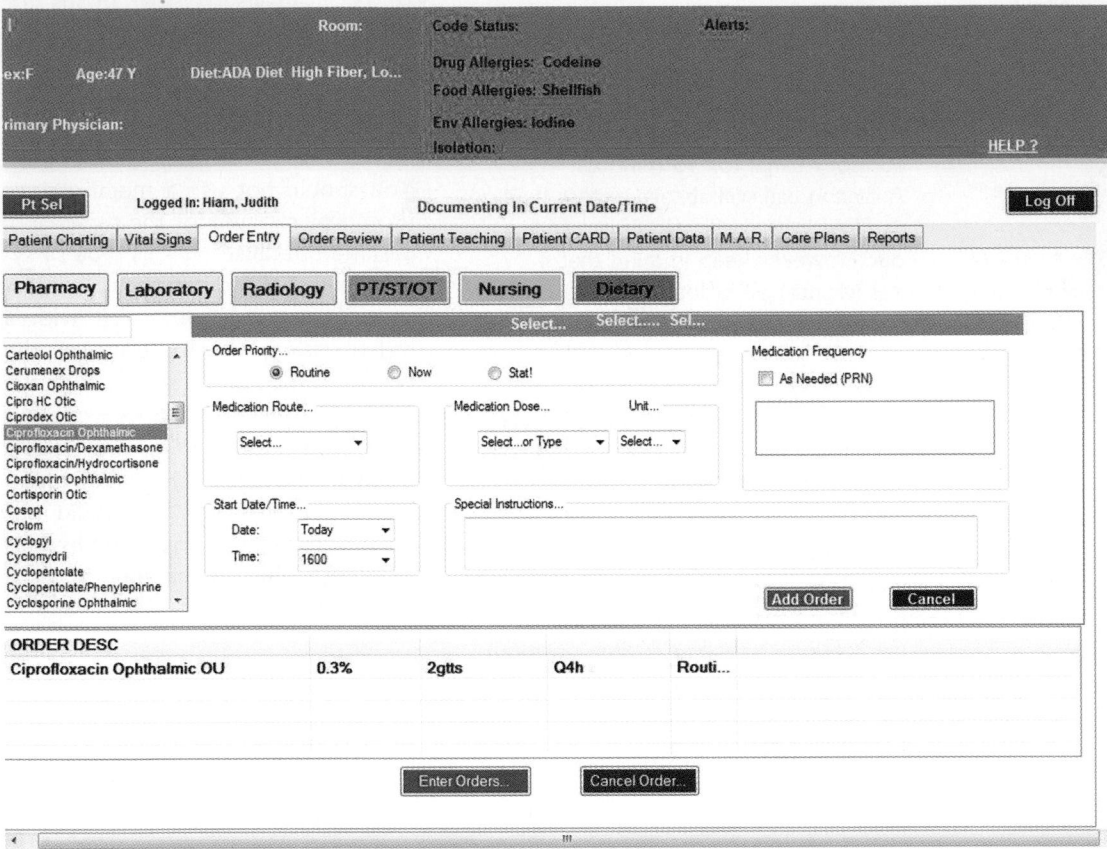

Thinking About the Procedure

 Go to the *Fundamentals of Nursing Skills Videos*, **Medication Administration: Otic Medications.**

1. What risk is there to an infant who receives ear drops and has a cotton ball to absorb residual liquid that can roll out of the ear canal?

2. How does the nurse in the DVD position the ear to instill otic drops?

3. What does the nurse in the DVD do to aid the drops in draining into the ear canal?

For suggested responses, go to Chapter 23, **Thinking About the Procedure Suggested Responses (Procedure 23-3),** on the Student Resource Disk or DavisPlus at http://davisplus.fadavis.com/Wilkinson2

Procedure 23-4 ☐ Administering Nasal Medication

➤ For steps to follow in *all* procedures, refer to the Universal Steps for All Procedures found on the inside back cover of Volume 2. Also refer to the Medication Guidelines: Steps to Follow for All Medications (Regardless of Type or Route).

Critical Aspects

- Determine head position: Consider the indication for the medication and the patient's ability to assume the position.
- Explain to the patient that the medication may cause some burning, tingling, or unusual taste.
- Position the patient with the head down and forward or supine with the head back.
- Place the tip of the sprayer into the right nostril, pointing the tip toward the outside of the nose (toward the outside corner of the right eye). Never point the tip toward the middle of the nose (the septum) or straight up (toward the sinus).
- Have the patient blow his nose, occlude one nostril, and exhale.
- Squirt the spray into the nose while the patient inhales through his other nostril.
- Repeat for the other nostril.

Equipment

- Medication drops, spray, or aerosol
- Tissues

Delegation

As an RN, you can usually delegate administration of nasal instillations to an LPN/LVN. You usually cannot delegate this task to a NAP.

Pre-Procedure Assessments

- Check for nasal obstruction and congestion.

Nasal obstruction or congestion could prevent the medication from reaching the nasal mucosa.

- Assess nasal discharge for color, consistency, and odor.

The appearance of drainage is not always diagnostic of infection, especially for people with chronic sinus problems or polyps.

- Note the color of nasal drainage.

Color can be indicative of the body's response to viral, bacterial, and allergic sources.

- Assess nasal mucous membranes for redness, color, moisture, excoriation, or trauma.

A baseline assessment helps to identifies signs of irritation.

➤ When performing the procedure, always identify your patient according to agency policy and be attentive to standard precautions, hand hygiene, patient safety and privacy, body mechanics, and documentation.

Procedure Steps

1. Explain to the patient the possibility that the medication may cause some burning, tingling, or unusual taste.

The taste of nasal medications can cause patients to become nauseated or vomit after administration. The medication is more likely to cause burning or tingling if the nasal mucosa is inflamed.

2. Don procedure gloves.

Gloving complies with standard precautions.

3. Ask the patient to gently blow his nose.

Removing nasal discharge allows the medication to come into contact with the mucous membranes without traumatizing already inflamed mucosa.

4. Position the patient.
   a. "Head down and forward"— if the patient can comfortably assume this position, ask him to lean forward or kneel on the bed with his head down. Administer the medication, and then ask the patient to tilt his head back to medicate the nasal passages.

Radionuclide studies have demonstrated that using nasal drops or sprays with the patient sitting and leaning the head back causes poor distribution of the medications into the nasal complex and sinuses. ➤

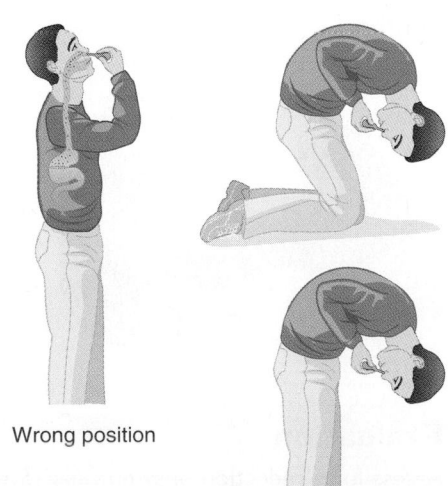

Wrong position

Correct positions

b. To medicate the ethmoid and sphenoid sinuses, assist the patient

(continued on next page)

Procedure 23-4 ▪ **Administering Nasal Medication** (continued)

into a supine position, with his head over the edge of the bed. Support the patient's head. Alternatively, place a towel roll behind the patient's shoulders, and allow the head to drop back. ▼

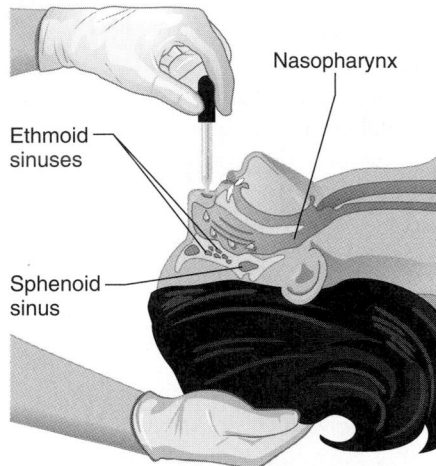

These positions help to prevent straining the neck muscles.

   c. To medicate the frontal and maxillary sinuses, tilt the head toward the affected side.

Titling the head promotes gravity to distribute the medication to the frontal sinuses. ▼

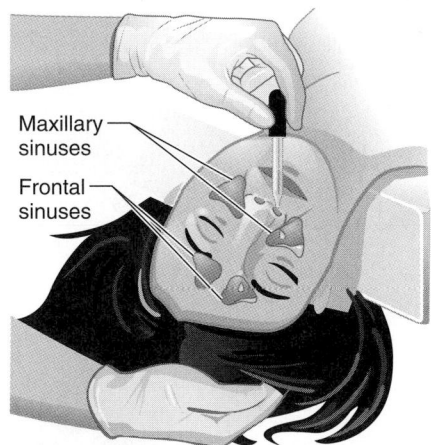

5. Ask the patient to exhale and then close one nostril.

Blocking one nostril provides for deeper inhalation.

6. Administer the spray or drops while the patient breathes through the mouth. If a dropper is used, do not touch the sides of the nostril.

Inhaling through the mouth prevents aspiration of the drops into the trachea and bronchi. Touching the dropper to the nostril will contaminate the dropper.

7. Repeat for the other nostril.

8. If nose drops are used, ask the patient to stay in the same position for 1 to 5 minutes (depending on the manufacturer's guidelines).

Maintaining this position promotes better absorption by using gravity to disperse the medication throughout the nasal passages and sinuses instead of draining out the nose.

9. Instruct the patient to not blow his nose for several minutes.

If the patient blows his nose, he would expel the medication.

What if . . .

▪ **My patient cannot assume the "head down and forward" position in Step 4a?**

Help him to tilt his head upright to administer the drops or spray.

▪ **My patient can taste the medicine after it is administered?**

That means his head was not down enough or he did not inhale long enough. Instruct him to put his head back down and sniff again without the medicine.

▪ **My patient has an excoriated area on the inside septum?**

Assess further, examining other areas of the nasal mucosa. Determine if the patient has a history of substance abuse. Report the findings to the prescriber before administering nasal medication.

▪ **My patient begins to have nosebleeds after using nasal medication?**

First, control the nosebleed. Then hold the medication and notify the prescriber. Assess for other signs of bleeding, bruising, or other petechiae.

Evaluation

Assess for a reduction of symptoms 15 to 20 minutes after administration.

Patient Teaching

▪ Teach the procedure for administering nasal drops or sprays, including proper positioning.

▪ Discuss the correct use of the medication and the adverse effects of overusing nasal decongestants.
▪ Explain the implications of the color of nasal secretions.

Documentation

Chart according to Medication Guidelines: Steps to Follow for All Medication (Regardless of Type or Route). For example, record the administration of the medication on the MAR.

For nasal instillation, document:

- Pre-medication assessment
- Type and amount of solution administered
- Discomfort the patient experienced during the procedure
- Patient's report of response to nasal administrations, such as nasal discharge, obstruction of nasal passage, bleeding, or other complication following the procedure

Sample documentation:

> 10/03/10 1340 *Client complained of nasal stuffiness. Administered mometasone (Nasonex) 2 sprays per nostril as ordered. Client noted nasal tingling following administration of this medication. Client left resting in recliner chair.* —— *H. Peralta, RN*

Thinking About the Procedure

 Go to the *Fundamentals of Nursing Skills Videos*, **Nasal Spray and Drops.**

1. What does the nurse in this DVD use a small towel for?

2. What position is the patient in the DVD in when closing a nostril and inhaling deeply?

 For suggested responses, go to Chapter 23, **Thinking About the Procedure Suggested Responses (Procedure 23-4),** on the Student Resource Disk or DavisPlus at http://davisplus.fadavis.com/Wilkinson2

Practice Resources

American Academy of Family Physicians (2006); Michigan Pharmacists' Association (2006).

Procedure 23-5 | Administering Vaginal Medication

> ➤ For steps to follow in *all* procedures, refer to the Universal Steps for All Procedures found on the inside back cover of Volume 2. Also refer to the Medication Guidelines: Steps to Follow for All Medications (Regardless of Type or Route).

Critical Aspects

- Position the patient in a dorsal recumbent or Sims' position.
- Inspect and cleanse the vaginal area before administering the medication.
- Use a water-soluble lubricant.
- Insert the suppository or applicator along the posterior vaginal wall about 8 cm (3 in.).
- Instruct the patient to maintain the position for 5 to 15 minutes after the medication has been inserted.

For Irrigation (Douche)

- Warm the irrigation solution to approximately 105°F (40.6°C).
- Hang the irrigation solution approximately 30 to 60 cm (1 to 2 ft) above the level of the patient's vagina.
- Position the patient in a dorsal recumbent position on a waterproof pad and bedpan.
- Insert the nozzle approximately 7 to 8 cm (3 in.) into the vagina, and start the flow of irrigation solution.

Equipment

- Medication: foam, jelly, cream, suppository, douche, or irrigating solution
- Applicator (if indicated)

- Washcloth and warm water for perineal care as needed
- Water-soluble lubricant
- Toilet tissue
- Perineal pad
- Bath blanket
- For irrigation: you will also need a waterproof pad, bedpan, vaginal irrigation set (may be disposable; consists of a solution container, nozzle, tubing, and clamp) and IV pole

Delegation

As an RN, you can usually delegate the administration of vaginal medications to an LPN/LVN. You usually cannot delegate this task to a NAP. Nurse practice acts governing

(continued on next page)

Procedure 23-5 ▪ **Administering Vaginal Medication** (continued)

medication administration vary from state to state, and policies vary further among healthcare agencies. However, as the RN you are always responsible for evaluating patient responses, both therapeutic effects and side effects. You can instruct a NAP in the therapeutic effect and side effects of medications and to report any effects observed.

Pre-Procedure Assessments

- Assess for complaints of vaginal burning, pruritus, and pain.

A baseline assessment helps to determine the patient's level of comfort and later the effectiveness of treatment. Infections can cause vaginal burning, itching, and pain.

- Inspect the labia and vaginal orifice for redness and lesions.

This is a good time to assess the perineal area for sign of sexually transmitted infection or other issues requiring healthcare.

- Check for vaginal discharge, including color, amount, consistency, and odor.

➤ When performing the procedure, always identify your patient according to agency policy and be attentive to standard precautions, hand hygiene, patient safety and privacy, body mechanics, and documentation.

Procedure Steps

1. Ask the patient to void before you insert the vaginal medication.
The increased pressure associated with a full bladder could cause discomfort during the instillation of vaginal medications.

2. Position the patient in a dorsal recumbent or Sims' position; drape the patient with a bath blanket so that only the perineum is exposed.
  a. **Dorsal recumbent position**—supine with knees flexed and legs rotated outward.
  b. **Sims' position**—semiprone on the left side with the right hip and knee flexed.
These two positions allow for visualization during administration and promote retention of the medication following administration. Draping respects the patient's modesty.

3. Prepare the medication. Remove the wrapper from the suppository and place the suppository on the wrapper or in a medication cup; or fill the applicator according to the manufacturer's instructions. For irrigation, use a warm solution of approximately 105°F (40.5°C).
Some suppositories come with applicators. Using a warm irrigation solution promotes patient comfort

and prevents injury to the vaginal tissue. ▼

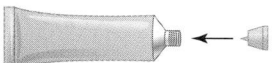

Invert cap and pierce end of medication tube

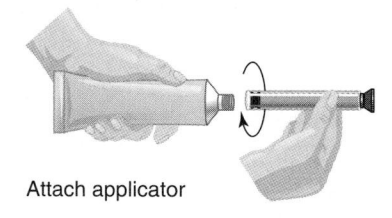

Attach applicator

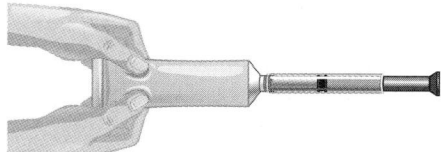

Squeeze medication into applicator

4. Don procedure gloves.
Gloving complies with standard precautions to prevent contaminating your hands and spreading microorganisms.

5. Inspect and clean around vaginal orifice.
Cleaning here prevents the introduction of microorganisms into the vagina during medication administration.

6. Administer the medication.

Step 6 Variation. Suppository
  a. Apply water-soluble lubricant to the rounded end of the suppository and to your gloved index finger on your dominant hand.

Eases insertion and prevents injury to the vaginal tissue.

  b. Separate the labia with your nondominant hand.
Allows visualization of the vaginal orifice.

  c. Insert the suppository as far as possible along the posterior vaginal wall (about 8 cm, or 3 in.) or as far as it will go. If the suppository comes with an applicator, place the suppository in the end of the applicator, insert the applicator into the vagina, and press the plunger.
The posterior vaginal wall is about 2.5 cm (1 in.) longer than the anterior wall. ▼

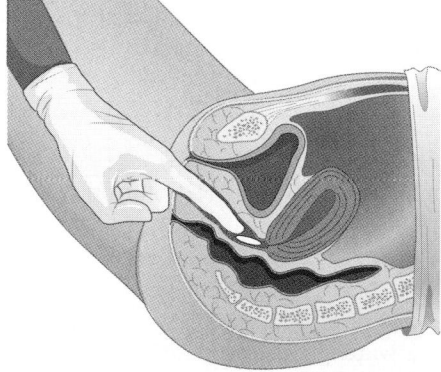

  d. Ask the patient to remain in a supine position for 5 to 15 minutes. You may wish to elevate her hips on a pillow.
Lifting the hips promotes retention and absorption of the medication.

Step 6 Variation. Applicator Insertion of Cream, Foam, or Jelly

  e. Separate the labia with your nondominant hand.

   f. Insert the applicator approximately 8 cm (3 in.) into the vagina along the posterior vaginal wall.

  g. Depress the plunger on the applicator, emptying the medication into the vagina.

  h. Dispose of the applicator, or place it on a paper towel if the applicator is reusable. You will later wash it with soap and water.

  i. Instruct the patient to remain in a supine position for 5 to 15 minutes.

A flat position promotes retention and absorption of the medication.

Step 6 Variation. Irrigation

  j. Hang the irrigation solution approximately 30 to 60 cm (1 to 2 ft) above the level of the patient's vagina.

Hanging the solution high above the site uses gravity to create enough pressure for continuous irrigation without increasing the pressure so much that it causes the patient.

discomfort and possibly damages the vaginal tissue. ▼

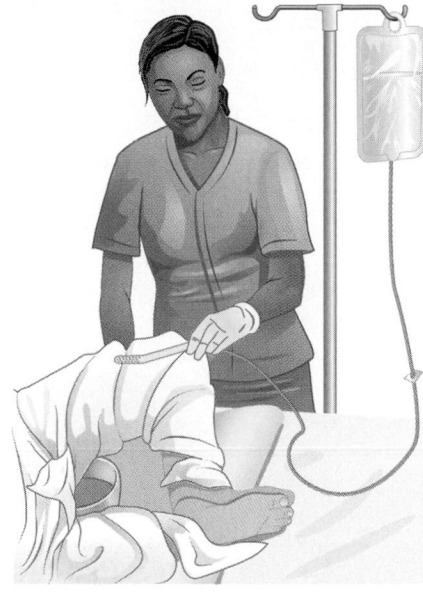

  k. Assist the patient into a dorsal recumbent position, and position a waterproof pad and bedpan under the patient.

The dorsal recumbent position is the easiest for performing a vaginal irrigation. Positioning the patient on the bedpan and using a waterproof pad protects the bedding.

  l. If using a vaginal irrigation set with tubing, open the clamp to allow the solution to completely fill the tubing.

Flushing the tubing prevents introducing air into the vagina, which can cause discomfort.

  m. Lubricate the end of the irrigation nozzle.

Lubrication reduces discomfort and irritation to the vaginal mucosa.

  n. Insert the nozzle approximately 8 cm (3 in.) into the vagina, directing it toward the sacrum.

  o. Start the flow of the irrigation solution, and rotate the nozzle intermittently as solution flows.

The rotation ensures even distribution of the solution throughout the vagina.

  p. After all irrigating solution has been used, remove the nozzle.

  q. Assist the patient to a sitting position on the bedpan.

An upright position promotes removal of all the irrigating solution by gravity.

7. Cleanse the perineum with toilet tissue or with warm water and a washcloth. Dry the perineum.

Drainage could cause skin irritation.

8. Apply a perineal pad if there is excessive drainage.

What if . . .

■ **The labia are reddened?**

Run water over the labia to soothe irritation and cleanse the area.

Evaluation

■ Assess for complaints of vaginal burning, pruritis, or pain.
■ Assess for purulent vaginal discharge.

Patient Teaching

■ Discuss with the patient personal hygiene and pericare.

Documentation

■ For vaginal medications, chart according to Medication Guidelines: Steps to Follow for All Medication (Regardless of Type or Route).
■ For vaginal irrigations, chart assessment; the type and amount of solution administered; discomfort the patient experienced during the procedure; and the patient's report of decreased vaginal pain, itching, and/ or burning following the procedure.

Sample documentation:

08/31/10 1500   *Explained medication and procedure. Client placed in dorsal recumbent position with knees flexed at 90° angle. Vaginal suppository lubricated with water-soluble lubricant and inserted using two fingers. Instructed client to retain suppository as long as possible.*
                                                    — *S. Snider, RN*

Procedure 23-6 ☐ Inserting a Rectal Suppository

➤ For steps to follow in *all* procedures, refer to the Universal Steps for All Procedures found on the inside back cover of Volume 2. Also refer to the Medication Guidelines: Steps to Follow for All Medications (Regardless of Type or Route).

Critical Aspects

- Before inserting the suppository, assess for contraindications, such as rectal surgery, rectal bleeding, or cardiac disease.
- Position the client in Sims' position.
- Lubricate the suppository.
- Insert the suppository past the internal sphincter about ½ to 1 inch in infants and 1 to 3 inches in adults. Never force the suppository during insertion.
- Instruct the patient to stay on his side for 5 to 10 minutes and to retain (not expel) the suppository for about 30 minutes.

Equipment

- Suppository
- Water-soluble lubricant
- Toilet tissue

Delegation

As an RN, you can usually delegate administration of rectal medications to an LPN/LVN. Although in some institutions you can delegate the administration of a glycerine suppository (nonmedicated) to a NAP, you generally cannot delegate administration of rectal medications to a NAP.

Pre-Procedure Assessments

- Determine the presence of contraindications for rectal administration, such as recent rectal surgery, rectal bleeding, or cardiac disease.
- Assess the rectal area for hemorrhoids or irritation.

➤ When performing the procedure, always identify your patient according to agency policy and be attentive to standard precautions, hand hygiene, patient safety and privacy, body mechanics, and documentation.

Procedure Steps

1. Ask whether the patient needs to defecate before the suppository insertion.
Stool in the rectum interferes with insertion of medication against the rectal wall and therefore with retention of the medication.

2. Don procedure gloves.
Gloving prevents exposure to feces and spread of microorganisms; maintains standard precautions.

3. Assist patient to Sims' position—lying on the left side with the right hip and knee flexed—keeping the patient covered as much as possible. Drape the patient.
Sims' position allows visualization of the anus and promotes retention of the medication because the descending colon is on the left side. Sims' position also aids in relaxing the external anal sphincter. Keeping the patient covered prevents chilling and maintains privacy.

4. For an uncooperative patient, such as a confused patient or a young child,

ask someone to help immobilize the patient while you insert the suppository. Help holding the patient allows proper instillation of medication and prevents injury to the rectal mucosa.

5. Prepare the suppository: Remove the wrapper. Using a water-soluble lubricant, lubricate the smooth end of the suppository and the tip of glove on the index finger. If no lubricant is available, apply cool tap water to the rectal opening.
Lubrication eases insertion and prevents friction damage to the rectal mucosa during insertion.

6. Explain that there will be a cool feeling from the lubricant and a feeling of pressure during insertion.
The patient should not experience severe pain with the insertion of a suppository, but will feel the coolness of the lubricant and pressure as the suppository is inserted past the rectal sphincter.

7. Using your nondominant hand, separate the buttocks.
Separation of the buttocks allows you to visualize the anus.

8. Ask the adult patient take deep breaths in and out through the mouth.
Deep breathing relaxes the rectal sphincter. Pushing a suppository through a constricted sphincter produces pain.

9. Insert the suppository:
a. Using the index finger of your dominant hand, gently insert the lubricated smooth end first, or follow the manufacturer's instructions.
Lubrication eases insertion. ▼

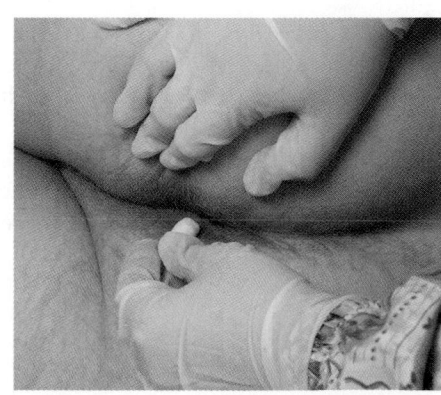

b. Never force the suppository during insertion.
Forcing the insertion of the suppository into a fecal mass would affect absorption. Forcing anything into the rectum may cause rectal irritation.

c. Push the suppository past the internal sphincter and along the rectal wall (½ to 1 in. in infants and 1 to 3 in. in adults).
The suppository must be in contact with the rectal wall for the medication to be absorbed. Inserting the suppository past the internal sphincter promotes retention. For a child, inserting the suppository too far could damage the rectal mucosa. ▼

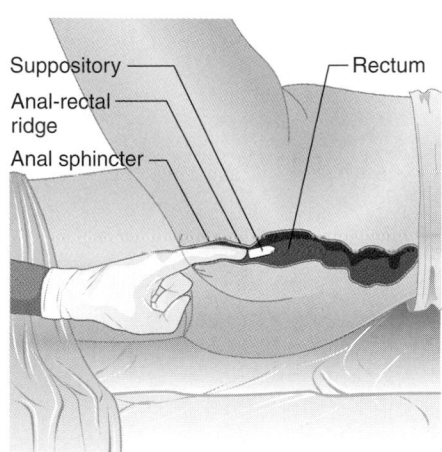

Suppository
Anal-rectal ridge
Anal sphincter
Rectum

10. Ask the patient to try to retain the suppository if he is able. If he has difficulty retaining the suppository, hold his buttocks together for a short time.

11. Wipe the patient's anus with toilet tissue.
Wiping maintains hygiene and comfort.

12. Explain to the patient the need to remain in the side-lying position for 5 to 10 minutes.
Sim's position promotes retention and absorption of the medication. Explanation promotes compliance.

13. Discard used materials into an biohazard receptacle and wash hands thoroughly.

14. Leave the call device within reach and bedpan handy, if the suppository was a laxative.
In case the patient has a sudden urge to defecate or cannot retain the suppository for the recommended time.

What if. . .

- **The prescribed dose is only half of the suppository?**
Cut the suppository lengthwise with a clean, single-edge razor blade.

- **My patient is a child. What is the best way to give a rectal suppository so the child doesn't expel it?**
For pediatric patients, it may be necessary to gently hold the buttocks together for 5 to 10 minutes.

- **My patient is an older adult. Is there anything special I should know?**
Older adults may have difficulty retaining a suppository because of poor sphincter control. You may need to put the bedpan under the patient while you are inserting the suppository.

Evaluation

- Assess for pain or burning during insertion of the medication.
- Determine that the patient retained the suppository for the desired length of time after insertion (reinsertion may be required).
- Assess for rectal pain, if indicated.

Patient Teaching

Explain that suppositories may take up to 30 minutes to be absorbed, depending on the medication.

Documentation

- Refer to Medication Guidelines: Steps to Follow for All Medication (Regardless of Type or Route).
- Chart the condition of anal tissue if abnormalities are present, any complaints of discomfort that are outside of the expected feelings and experience, and the length of time that the suppository was retained.
- Chart responses to medication (e.g., symptom relief, side effects).

(continued on next page)

Procedure 23-6 ■ Inserting a Rectal Suppository (continued)

Sample EHR documentation:

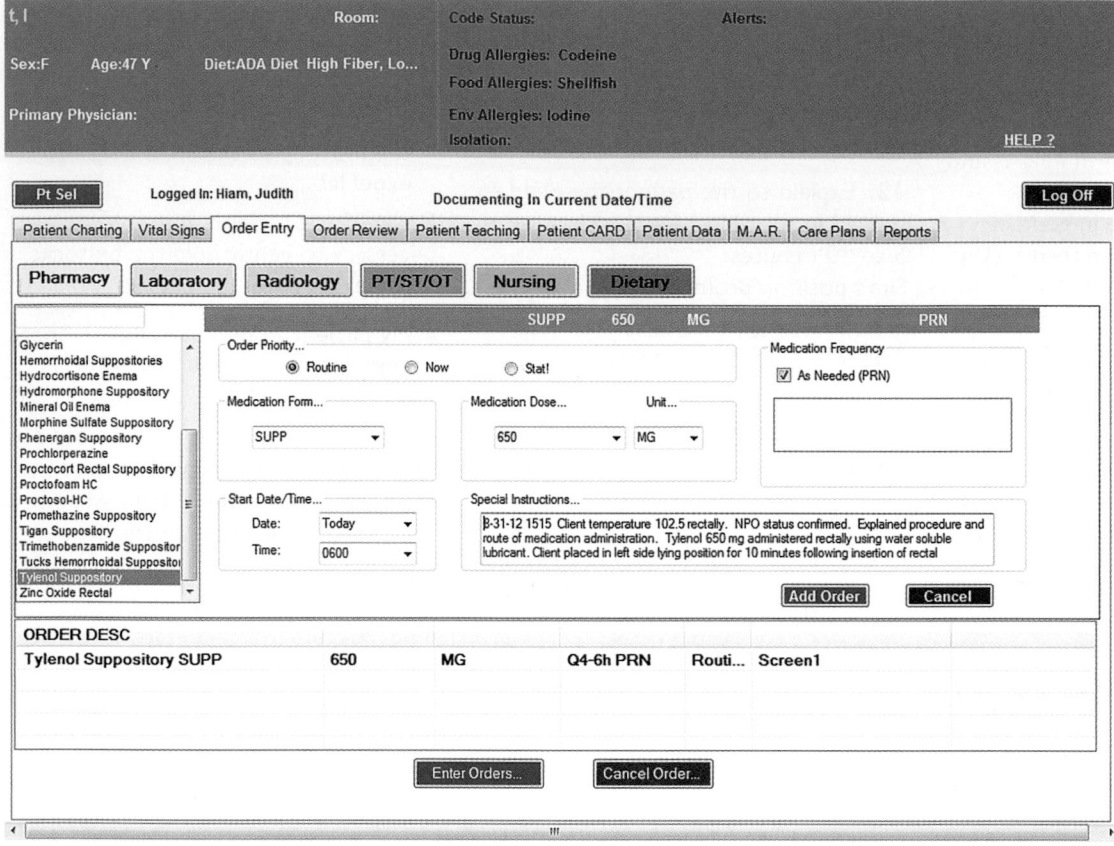

Practice Resources

American Academy of Family Physicians (1992); American Society of Health-System Pharmacists, Inc. (2001); Michigan Pharmacists' Association (2006).

Thinking About the Procedure

 Go to the *Fundamentals of Nursing Skills Videos*, **Rectal Suppositories.**

1. How is the patient in this DVD positioned after insertion of the rectal suppository?

2. Why is he positioned in this manner rather than side lying?

 For suggested responses, go to Chapter 23, **Thinking About the Procedure Suggested Responses (Procedure 23-6),** on the Student Resource Disk or DavisPlus at http://davisplus.fadavis.com/Wilkinson2

Procedure 23-7 Applying Medication to the Skin

➤ For steps to follow in *all* procedures, refer to the Universal Steps for All Procedures found on the inside back cover of Volume 2. Also refer to the Medication Guidelines: Steps to Follow for All Medications (Regardless of Type or Route).

Critical Aspects

- Wear gloves to avoid absorbing the medication through your own skin and to avoid cross-contamination.
- Before applying topical medication, cleanse the skin with soap and water.
- Do not apply medication to skin with open lesions, irritation, or known hypersensitivity.
- Avoid exposure to ultraviolet light/sunlight after applying medication.
- Assess for adverse skin reactions (e.g., hypersensitivity, redness, itching, or local irritation).
- Use gentle technique when applying topical medication to fragile skin, which is typical in older adults. Take care to not over-apply the medication.

Delegation

As an RN, you can usually delegate administration of most topical medications to an LPN/LVN. In many institutions you can delegate the administration of an over-the-counter medication to a NAP. Refer to agency policy regarding administration of topical medication.

Pre-Procedure Assessments

- Assess for skin irritation, open lesions, area of hypersensitivity, or other skin abnormality.
- Determine the presence of contraindications for dermal application; document and report before administering medication.

■ Procedure 23-7A Applying Topical Lotion, Cream, and Ointment

➤ When performing the procedure, always identify your patient according to agency policy and be attentive to standard precautions, hand hygiene, patient safety and privacy, body mechanics, and documentation.

Procedure Steps

1. Don clean gloves.

Gloving complies with universal precautions and protects your skin from the topical medication.

2. Cleanse the skin with soap and water and pat dry before applying to enhance absorption.

Moisture on the skin can interfere with adherence of topical ointment, depending on the product used to suspend the medication.

3. Warm the medication in your gloved hands.

This will be more comfortable for the patient and make the preparation easier to apply.

4. Use gloved hands or an applicator to apply and spread the medication evenly, following the direction of hair growth when coating the area.

Excessive application may irritate the skin. This action will protect you so that you will not absorb the medication through your own skin. ▼

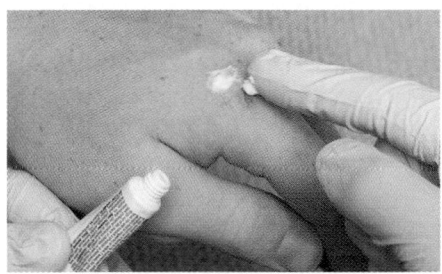

■ Procedure 23-7B Applying Topical Aerosol Spray

➤ When performing the procedure, always identify your patient according to agency policy and be attentive to standard precautions, hand hygiene, patient safety and privacy, body mechanics, and documentation.

Procedure Steps

1. Don clean gloves.

2. Cleanse the skin with soap and water and pat dry before applying to enhance absorption.

3. Shake the container to mix the contents.

Active ingredients might not be evenly distributed throughout the aerosolized suspension and may settle at the bottom of the container.

4. Hold the container at the distance specified on the label (usually 6 to 12 in.), and spray over the prescribed area.

This distance will prevent excess application to a local area.

5. You will need to hold most containers upright when spraying. If you are spraying near the patient's head, cover his face with a towel.

This will prevent him from inhaling the spray.

(continued on next page)

Procedure 23-7 ▪ **Applying Medication to the Skin** (continued)

▪ Procedure 23-7C **Applying Prescribed Powder**

➤ When performing the procedure, always identify your patient according to agency policy and be attentive to standard precautions, hand hygiene, patient safety and privacy, body mechanics, and documentation.

Procedure Steps

1. Don clean gloves.

2. Cleanse the skin with soap and water and pat dry before applying to enhance absorption.

3. Spread apart skinfolds, and apply a very thin layer.
Powder applied to a moist surface creates a pasty solution, which is irritating to skin.

4. Apply the powder to clean, dry skin. Be careful that the patient does not inhale the powder.
Particulate matter, such as powder, can irritate lung tissue and lead to pneumonitis or other inflammatory processes.

▪ Procedure 23-7D **Transdermal Medication**

➤ When performing the procedure, always identify your patient according to agency policy and be attentive to standard precautions, hand hygiene, patient safety and privacy, body mechanics, and documentation.

Procedure Steps

1. Don clean gloves.
Gloving complies with universal precautions and to protect your skin from the topical medication.

2. Remove the previous patch, folding the medicated side to the inside.
This helps to prevent unintentional contact of the medication on a different area of the patient or another's skin.

3. Dispose of the old patch carefully in an appropriate receptacle, keeping it away from children and pets.
Even a used patch has some active medication on it. Proper disposal is important to prevent medication exposure to others.

4. Cleanse the skin of traces of remaining medication. Allow the skin to dry.
A clean, dry surface optimizes the effectiveness of adherence and penetration of the medication via the skin.

5. Remove the patch from its protective covering, and then remove the clear, protective covering without touching the

adhesive or the inside surface that contains the medication. ▼

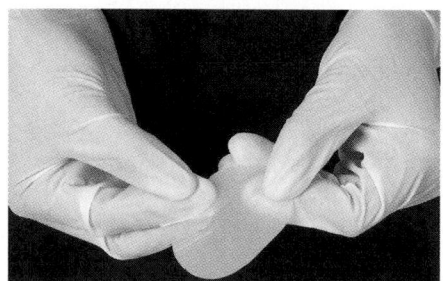

6. Apply the patch to a clean, dry, hairless (or little hair), intact skin area, pressing it down for about 10 seconds with your palm. Be sure the area is free of scars, lesions, and irritation.
A smooth surface maximizes the contact between medication and the skin.

7. Rotate application sites. Common sites are the trunk, lower abdomen, lower back, and buttocks.
Rotating sites prevents irritation to local areas of the skin

8. Avoid areas where lesions are present.
Areas of the skin that are disrupted can become irritated by topical medication.

Other lesions involving thickened layers of skin should be avoided to avoid compromised absorption.

9. Teach the patient to *not* use a heating pad over the area.
Heat can cause some ointments to irritate or even burn the skin.

10. Write the date, the time, and your initials on the new patch.
Complete documentation of the dosage administered can reduce medication errors.

11. Remove gloves and wash your hands again.

12. Observe for local side effects, such as skin irritation, itching, and allergic contact dermatitis.
If an adverse response occurs at the local site, remove the patch, wipe the skin clean, and notify the prescriber.

What if . . .

▪ **The medication is packaged as an ointment form with calibrated paper?**

Wear gloves; apply the ointment in a continuous motion along those marks to measure the required dose. Fold the paper in half to distribute the ointment evenly on the patch.

■ **My patient is a child who does not want the medication to be applied?**

Hold the child securely while medication is applied. Then cover the site with a dressing to keep the child

from disrupting the application of medication.

■ **My patient is an older adult and has fragile skin?**

Avoid areas where penetration of the cream or ointment is likely to be reduced or cause irritation. Be

gentle with application of anything to the skin and diligent with your assessment of the skin response to medication.

Evaluation

■ Assess for rash, excoriation, hives, redness, swelling, or signs of allergy or skin sensitivity to topical medication.
■ Ask the patient if he feels burning, itching, pain, tenderness, or other sensation to skin where medication was applied.
■ Assess for any indication the medication applied is leading to a desired improvement in the patient's condition.

Patient Teaching

■ Explain that topical medication may take up to 30 minutes to be absorbed, depending on the medication.
■ Tell the patient to never ingest or inhale topical medication.
■ Advise the patient to avoid touching his eyes after handling topical medication.
■ Inform the patient to not use more medicine than prescribed or directed.

Over-applying topical medication can sometimes result in an overdose.

Documentation

■ Refer to Medication Guidelines: Steps to Follow for All Medication (Regardless of Type or Route).
■ Record the condition of skin if abnormalities are present and any complaints of discomfort during or after administration.
■ Document responses to medication (e.g., symptom relief, side effects).

Sample documentation:

09/22/12 0835   *Transdermal nitroglycerine patch. 74.6 mg patch applied to upper chest. Pt. instructed to leave patch intact for 12 hours. Patient reported mild, transient headache approximately 45 minutes after application of patch. No evidence of flushing, faintness, or dizziness. Patient denies chest pain.* ———————— M. Finegold, RN

08/01/12 0830   *Fentanyl patch placed on left anterior chest wall below clavicle. Fentanyl patch dated 08/31/08 removed and discarded into narcotic waste bin. Patient stated, "This patch really helps my back feel better."* ———————————— M. Finegold, RN

Thinking About the Procedure

 Go to the *Fundamentals of Nursing Skills Videos,* **Transdermal Medications.**

1. Where does the nurse in the DVD apply the transdermal patch?

2. Why does the nurse apply the medication in this location?

 For suggested responses, go to Chapter 23, **Thinking About the Procedure Suggested Responses (Procedure 23-7),** on the Student Resource Disk or DavisPlus at http://davisplus.fadavis.com/Wilkinson2

Procedure 23-8 ☐ Administering Metered-Dose Inhaler (MDI) Medication

➤ For steps to follow in *all* procedures, refer to the Universal Steps for All Procedures found on the inside back cover of Volume 2. Also refer to the Medication Guidelines: Steps to Follow for All Medications (Regardless of Type or Route).

Critical Aspects

- Identify the number of remaining inhalations in the canister. The "float method" is no longer recommended for determining whether an MDI canister is empty or not.
- Assist the patient to a seated position.
- Shake the inhaler. Remove the mouthpiece cap of the inhaler and insert the mouthpiece into the spacer while holding the canister upright.
- Remove the cap from the spacer.
- Ask the patient to breathe out slowly and completely.
- If the patient is unable to use the MDI independently, time the use of the device with the patient's own respirations.
- Place the spacer mouthpiece into the patient's mouth and ask him to seal his lips around the mouthpiece. Press down on the inhaler canister to discharge one puff of medication into the spacer.
- Ask the patient to slowly inhale and then hold his breath for as long as possible.
- If a second puff is needed, wait at least 1 minute and repeat the previous steps.

Equipment

- Metered dose inhaler
- Spacer
- Tissues

Pre-Procedure Assessments

Assess the patient's respiratory status before administration of medication to establish a baseline that can be used to evaluate the effects of treatment.

Delegation

As an RN, you can usually delegate administration of MDI medications to an LPN/LVN. You usually cannot delegate this task to a NAP unless the NAP has special training for a specific defined situation (e.g., "medication aides" in some long-term care settings in some states). See the Medication Guidelines at the beginning of the Procedures section.

➤ When performing the procedure, always identify your patient according to agency policy and be attentive to standard precautions, hand hygiene, patient safety and privacy, body mechanics, and documentation.

Procedure Steps

1. Identify the amount of medication for inhalation remaining in the canister. Based on the start date and instructions for use, you can determine the number of remaining inhalations. Replace the canister promptly when the canister is nearly empty.
Historically, patients have been instructed to float the canister in water to determine how much medication remains. However, propellants affect the weight of the canister and may lead to false reassurance that there is medication in an empty container. Some MDI medications are used as rescue agents during asthma attacks or periods of dyspnea. It is important to always have medication available for use.

2. Assist the patient to a seated position or high-Fowlers if in bed.
An upright position helps the patient take a deep inhalation when medication administered.

3. Ask the patient to rinse out his mouth and spit the fluid out (not to swallow it).
This helps to prevent transfer of bacteria from the mouth to the inhaler.

4. Shake the inhaler. Remove the mouthpiece cap of the inhaler and insert the mouthpiece into the spacer while holding the canister upright.
A spacer is the most efficient method to deliver inhaled medications. It should be used if the patient has difficulty

coordinating the use of the inhaler, is using a corticosteroid, or if it is prescribed.

Step 4 Variation. No Spacer is Used.
If a spacer is not used, place the canister 1 to 2 inches (2.5 to 5.0 cm) from or directly into the mouth.

5. Remove the cap from the spacer.

6. Ask the patient to breathe out slowly and completely. If a patient is unable to use the MDI independently, time the use of the device with the patient's own respirations.
Deep breathing helps the patient to time the dose with his natural breathing.

7. Place the spacer mouthpiece into the patient's mouth and have him seal his lips around the mouthpiece. Sharply press down on the inhaler canister to discharge one puff of medication into the spacer.
A good seal allows proper delivery of medication. ▼

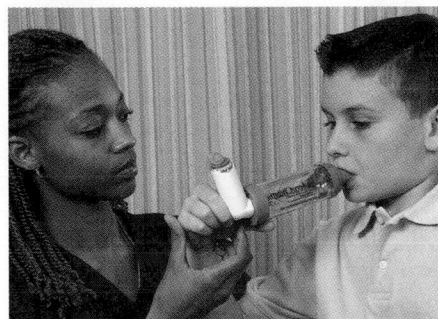

8. Ask the patient to slowly inhale and then hold his breath for as long as possible. Encourage the patient to hold his breath for 10 seconds if possible.
When holding his breath the medication can be delivered deep into the lungs.

9. If a second puff is needed, wait at least 1 minute before repeating steps 6 through 8.
Pausing allows the medication to be absorbed and the canister to recharge.

10. If a corticosteroid inhaler was used, assist the patient to rinse out his mouth with water and spit out the rinse.
Prolonged exposure of this medication to the oral mucosa is irritating and can lead to thrush in some patients.

11. Clear the mouthpiece with a tissue or moist cloth and replace the cap. Periodically rinse the spacer, mouthpiece, and cap with water.
Proper cleaning of the MDI keeps the dispenser from clogging. The following

illustrations summarize the steps for using an MDI. ▼

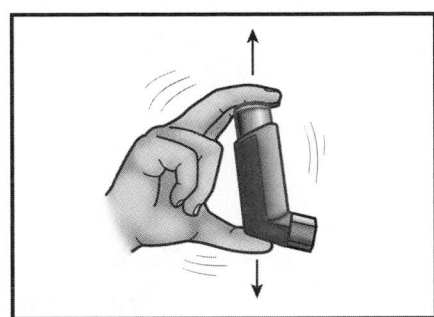

Shake canister.

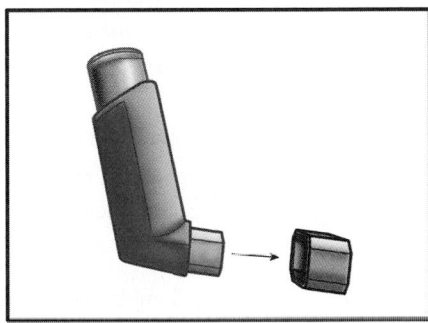

Remove cap. Discharge 2 puffs.

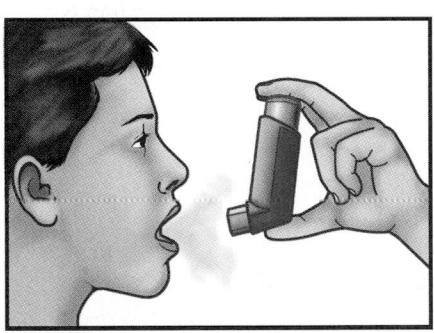

Deep breath out.

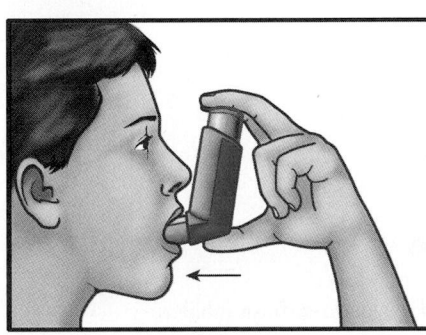

Press top. Inhale med slowly.

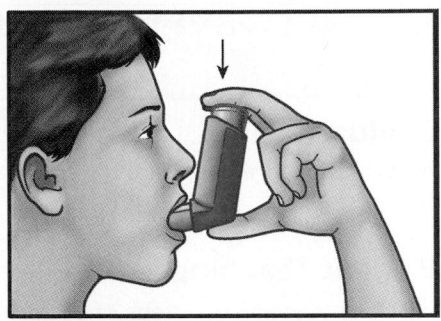

Hold breath. Exhale slowly.

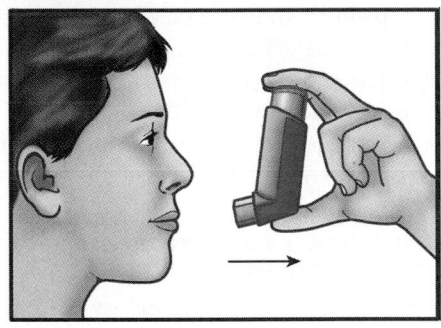

Remove inhaler from mouth.
Wait 1 minute before next puff.

What if . . .

■ **Your client is a small child or frail older adult who is unable to assist with taking medication from the inhaler?**

You may need to time discharge of the medication with the client's inspiration if the patient is unable to administer the medication with his own deep breaths.

■ **Your patient uses an albuterol MDI with chlorofluorocarbon (CFC) as a propellant?**

The FDA made a ruling, effective December 31, 2008, prohibiting use of CFCs in albuterol MDIs. If the patient has an inhaler containing this product, known to be detrimental to the ozone layer, the patient or caregiver can request an alternate prescription.

In addition to the harmful effects of the propellant on the environment, the medication is also likely to be past the expiration date.

(continued on next page)

Procedure 23-8 ■ Administering Metered-Dose Inhaler (MDI) Medication (continued)

Evaluation

Assess for change in respiratory status after medication administration.

Patient Teaching

- Before teaching the steps of the procedure, obtain the appropriate supplies, including the inhaler and tissues.
- Explain to the patient when to use the inhaler and what side effects to anticipate.
- Teach and demonstrate to patients how to correctly use a spacer and MDI.
- Teach patients how to determine if the MDI canister is nearly empty.
- Explain that some inhalers are used in combination with others and must be used in correct order to receive the desired effect.
- Be aware that many patients who have not been taught to use dry powder inhalers do not get any medication into their lungs.
- Errors in using dry powder inhalers increase with age and illness severity. Carefully supervise older adults and very ill patients.

Home Care

General Information to Tell Patients

- Show your healthcare professional how you're using your MDI. If you're having trouble using your MDI, ask for tips or to recommend another device.
- Never puncture or break the canister.
- Do not immerse the MDI in water.
- Keep the MDI somewhere where you can get it quickly when needed, but out of children's reach.
- Store the MDI at room temperature. If it gets cold, warm it by rubbing the canister between his palms. Never use anything else to warm it.

Determining the Number of Remaining Doses

- When you begin using a new MDI, write the start date on the canister.

- The only reliable method for determining the number of doses remaining in a canister is to subtract the number of doses used from the number available. Some devices are equipped with counters. Floating MDIs in water is not accurate for assessing remaining doses and often will clog the valve.

Cleaning the MDI

- Clean your apparatus regularly to avoid drug buildup that might keep the medication from reaching the lungs. Specific maintenance procedures may vary with the manufacturer.
- Remove the metal canister that contains the medication by pulling it out.

Documentation

- Refer to Medication Guidelines: Steps to Follow for All Medications (regardless of Type or Route).
- Document the response to medications.

Sample documentation:

02/02/12   0800   Pt. c/o shortness of breath. RR 26 and labored. Combivent MDI 2 puffs administered with spacer. ————————— ———————————————— S. Smythe, RN
0815   RR 20 regular, even, comfortable. ——————— S. Smythe, RN

Thinking About the Procedure

 Go to the *Fundamentals of Nursing Skills Videos*, **Metered-Dose Inhaler.**

I. What does the nurse in the DVD do after the dose of medication is completely administered by MDI?

 For suggested responses, go to Chapter 23, **Thinking About the Procedure Suggested Responses (Procedure 23-8),** on the Student Resource Disk or DavisPlus at http://davisplus.fadavis.com/Wilkinson2

Practice Resources
Ram, F. S. F., Brocklebank, D. M., White, J., et al. (2002); U.S. Food and Drug Administration, Center for Evaluation and Research (2008); Wieshammer, S., & Dreyhaupt, J. (2008).

Procedure 23-9 □ Preparing, Drawing Up, and Mixing Medication

➤ For steps to follow in *all* procedures, refer to the Universal Steps for All Procedures found on the inside back cover of Volume 2. Also refer to the Medication Guidelines: Steps to Follow for All Medications (Regardless of Type or Route).

Critical Aspects

- Maintain sterile technique.
- Recap the needle or vial access device (VAD) using a needle recapping device or the one-handed method (see Procedure 23-10).
- Change the needle, if indicated.

Drawing Up Medication from Ampules

- Tap the ampule or shake it with a quick snap of the wrist.
- Use an ampule opener or wrap gauze or an unopened alcohol wipe around the neck of the ampule, and snap the ampule away from you.
- Use a filter needle or filter straw.
- Invert or tip the ampule to withdraw all of the medication.
- Dispose of the broken ampule and filter needle in a sharps container.

Drawing Up Medication from Vials

- Clean the rubber top of the vial with an alcohol prep pad or chlorhexidine gluconate (CHG)-alcohol product (for a multidose vial only).
- Draw air into the syringe equal to the amount of medication to be withdrawn.
- Insert the needle or VAD through the rubber top at a 45° to 60° angle, bevel up. Immediately raise to 90 degrees *as* you push to insert the needle.
- Keeping the needle above the fluid line, inject air into the vial and then invert the vial and withdraw the medication.
- Remove bubbles, hold the vial at eye level, and check that the dose is correct before removing the needle.

Mixing Medication in One Syringe

- Make sure the medications are compatible.
- Determine the total volume of all medications to be used.
- Maintain the sterility of the needles and medication.
- Inject air into the second vial, being careful not to let the needle enter the fluid.
- Then inject the air into the other vial; withdraw the dose; expel the air bubbles; and, when the dose is correct, withdraw the needle from the vial.
- Avoid contaminating a multidose vial with a second medication.
- Insert the needle into the second vial.
- Withdraw the second medication very carefully. If there is any excess, you must discard the contents of the syringe and start over.
- When drawing up from a single-dose vial and ampule, draw up from the vial first.
- Do not use prefilled cartridges for intramuscular injections unless they have a safety device; transfer the medication to a syringe with a safety device before administering.
- Always recap a sterile needle using a safety capping device or the one-handed scoop method.

(continued on next page)

Procedure 23-9 ■ **Preparing, Drawing Up, and Mixing Medication** (continued)

Equipment

- Medication vials, ampules, and/or prefilled syringe
- Alcohol prep pad (70% alcohol) or chlorhexidine gluconate (CHG)-alcohol product
- Syringe of the appropriate size for medication volume and viscosity
- Needle of the appropriate size for the site and viscosity to be aspirated through the vial access device (VAD)
- VAD, filter needle, or safety needle.
- Gauze pad or ampule snapper, if you are using ampules

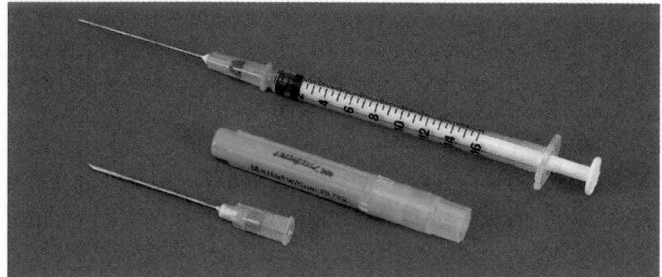

Top: Syringe with a regular needle. Bottom: Filter needle.

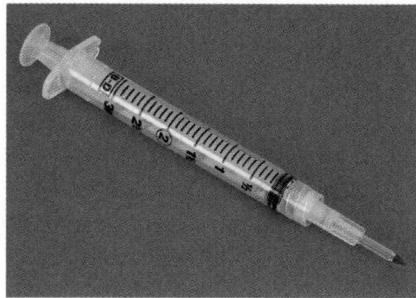

Vial access device.

Delegation

As an RN, you can delegate administration of some parenteral medications to an LPN/LVN. You usually cannot delegate this task to a NAP. Nurse practice acts governing medication administration vary from state to state, and policies vary further among healthcare agencies. Nevertheless, as the RN, you are always responsible for supervising and evaluating delegated care. You can instruct a NAP in the therapeutic effects expected from the medication.

Pre-Procedure Assessments

- Check the ampule or vial for intactness, cloudiness, particles, and color.

A change in color, cloudiness, particles, or cracks indicate the medication is altered or contaminated and should not be used.

- Check the compatibility of the medications.

Some medications are either chemically or physically incompatible and cannot be mixed. Other medications may be compatible for only 20 to 30 minutes, so they must be given promptly after they are mixed. Although physically incompatible medications can frequently be identified by a change in appearance, such as precipitation, no such indication exists for chemically incompatible medications.

- Determine the total volume of medications and whether the total volume is appropriate for the administration site.

Although the reason for mixing medications is to limit the number of injections a patient receives, the total volume of the injections must not be greater than what is appropriate for the site, such as 0.5 to 1 mL for deltoid or 3 to 4 mL for the vastus lateralis or ventrogluteal muscle.

■ *Procedure 23-9A* **Drawing Up Medication from Ampules**

➤ When performing the procedure, always identify your patient according to agency policy and be attentive to standard precautions, hand hygiene, patient safety and privacy, body mechanics, and documentation.

Procedure Steps

1. With your index finger, gently flick or tap the top of the ampule to remove medication trapped in the top of the ampule. An alternate method is to shake the ampule by quickly turning and snapping your wrist, like shaking down a mercury thermometer.
Medication left in the top of the ampule may lead to administering an inadequate dose. All the medication must be in the bottom of the ampule before you open it.

2. Wrap a 2 in. × 2 in. gauze pad (or an unwrapped alcohol wipe) around the neck of the ampule, or slip on an ampule snapper. Snap the top off, breaking it away from you.
Prevents you from accidentally cutting your fingers or spraying glass fragments toward you. Do not use an opened alcohol wipe to break the ampule, because it is not thick enough to prevent injury. ➤

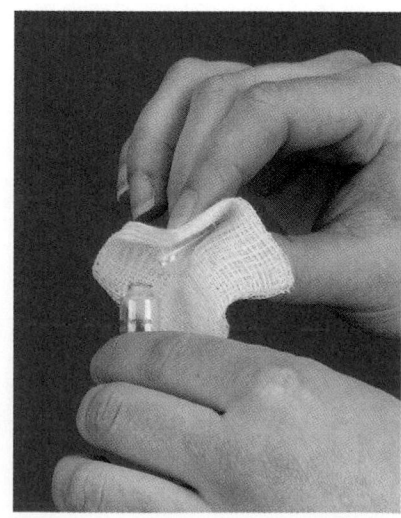

3. Attach a filter needle or filter straw to the syringe. If the syringe has a needle in place, remove both the needle and the cap, and place them on a sterile surface (e.g., a newly unwrapped alcohol pad still in the open wrapper), and attach the filter needle or straw.

The American Society for Health System Pharmacists recommends filtering solutions drawn up from glass ampules to remove glass particles. Opening a glass ampule produces a spray of tiny glass particles. Many of these fractured glass particles can enter the ampule and contaminate the contents. The size of the glass particles increases proportionally with the size of the vial.

4. Withdraw the medication from the ampule by using one of the following techniques. Be careful not to touch the neck of the ampule with the filter straw or needle while withdrawing medication.

Touching the neck of the ampule with the needle or straw increases the risk of contamination.

    a. Invert the ampule, place the needle tip in the liquid, and withdraw the prescribed amount of medication. Be careful not to insert needle through the medication into the air at the top of the inverted ampule.

This method is particularly useful with large ampules. The medication's surface tension will prevent the liquid from leaking from the ampule while the ampule is inverted. However, if you insert the needle too far (into the air

pocket above the medication), the medication will run out. ▼

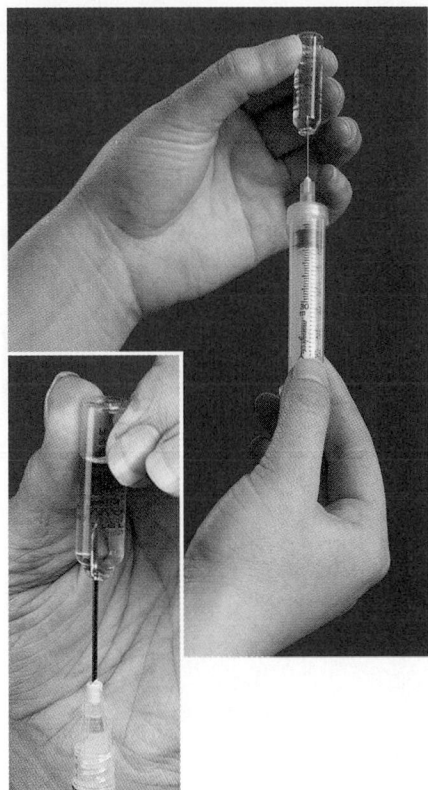

    b. Alternatively, tip the ampule, place a filter needle or straw in the liquid, and withdraw all medication. Reposition the ampule so that the needle or straw tip remains in the liquid.

This method allows for easier stabilization of the ampule while you withdraw the medication, and may help keep you from contaminating the needle on the edge of the vial opening. ▼

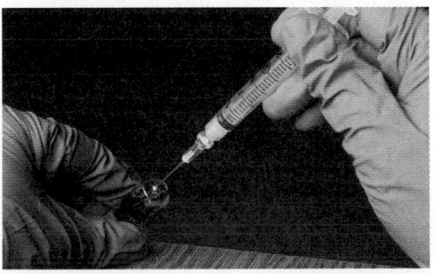

5. Hold the syringe vertically, and draw 0.2 mL of air into the syringe (see Clinical Insight 23-4, Measuring Dosage When Changing Needles).

Draw up and measure the exact medication dose, plus 0.2 mL of air (the syringe plunger should be at 0.2 mL more than the prescribed dose).

6. Remove the filter needle or straw, and reattach the "saved" needle for administering the injection.

7. Eject the 0.2 mL of air, and read the dose. After all of the air is ejected, if you need to eject some medication to make the dose correct, tip the syringe horizontally to eject the medication.

Use a filter needle only to withdraw medication; do not eject medication from it. For injection, use a needle of the correct gauge and length. Pushing the medication out of the syringe with the filter needle in place could cause the filter to break and release the glass fragments. Pulling air into the syringe allows for an exact dose when the medication is injected; the air will clear the needle (after the medication) so that the patient receives all the medication that was drawn up in the syringe. *Note:* This is not the old "air lock" technique; you will eject the air before injecting the medication into the patient.

The syringe must be vertical to eject air; however, if you eject the medication while holding the syringe vertically, the drug will run down the needle and then track through the patient's tissue during the injection.

8. Alternatively, for a medication that is irritating to tissues, you can leave the 0.2 mL of air in the syringe for injection. But be sure to account for the air when you read the dose markings on the syringe.

Parenteral iron is an example of medication that is irritating to the tissue.

9. Dispose of the top and bottom of the ampule and the filter needle in a sharps container.

Disposal into a puncture-proof container prevents accidental needlestick injury.

(continued on next page)

Procedure 23-9 ■ **Preparing, Drawing Up, and Mixing Medication** (continued)

■ Procedure 23-9B **Drawing Up Medications from Vials**

➤ When performing the procedure, always identify your patient according to agency policy and be attentive to standard precautions, hand hygiene, patient safety and privacy, body mechanics, and documentation.

Procedure Steps

1. Mix the solution in the vial, if necessary, by gently rolling the vial between your hands.

Aqueous suspensions will settle to the bottom of the vial, so they need to be mixed. Rolling the vial between your hands will mix the medication without forming air bubbles. Shaking the vial traps air in the medication.

2. Place the vial on a flat work surface and thoroughly scrub the rubber top of the vial with an alcohol prep pad or chlorhexidine gluconate (CHG)-alcohol product.

The alcohol prep pad removes dust, grease, and microorganisms.

3. Uncap the VAD without touching the needle tip or shaft. If you are using a VAD, attach the device to the syringe, and remove the cap.

VADs can be used only with single-use vials, unless the vial is designed for use with access pins, such as a Life-Shield vial.

4. Place the needle or VAD cap on a clean surface, or hold the cap open-side out between two fingers of your nondominant hand.

This method prevents contamination of the cap and the needle during recapping.

5. Draw air into the syringe equal to the amount of medication to be withdrawn from the vial.

Injection of air into the vial makes withdrawing the medication easier. For small unit-dose vials, you may not have to instill air prior to withdrawing the medication, but you will need to maintain backward pressure on the plunger until the needle is completely withdrawn. If you release the plunger, the negative pressure in the vial will pull the medication back into the vial.

6. Maintaining sterile technique, insert the needle or VAD into the vial without coring.

    a. Place the tip of the needle or VAD in the middle of the rubber

top of the vial, with the bevel up at a 45° to 60° angle. ▼

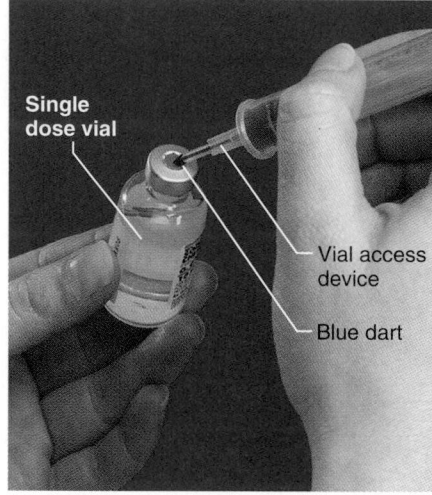

Single dose vial — Vial access device — Blue dart

    b. While pushing the needle or VAD into the rubber top, gradually bring the needle upright to a 90° angle.

This method helps prevent coring, which occurs when a small piece of the rubber top is trapped inside the needle or VAD during insertion. Coring is more likely to occur with large-gauge needles and VADs. ▼

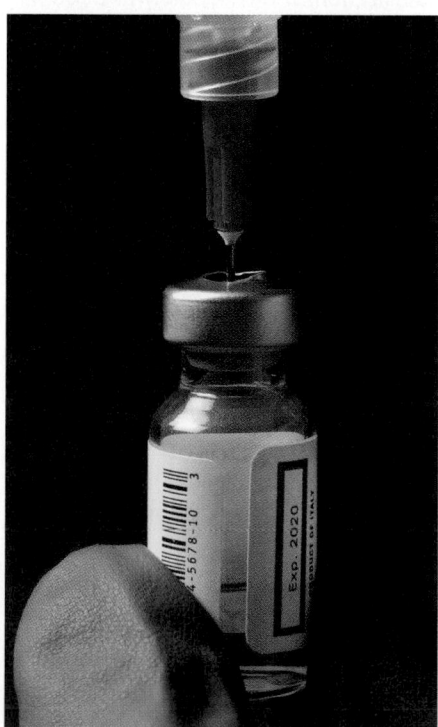

7. With the tip of the VAD above the fluid line, inject the air in the syringe into the air in the vial.

Injecting air into the vial creates positive pressure, making the medication easier to withdraw. Injecting the air into the medication will create air bubbles, which interfere with dosage measurement. ▼

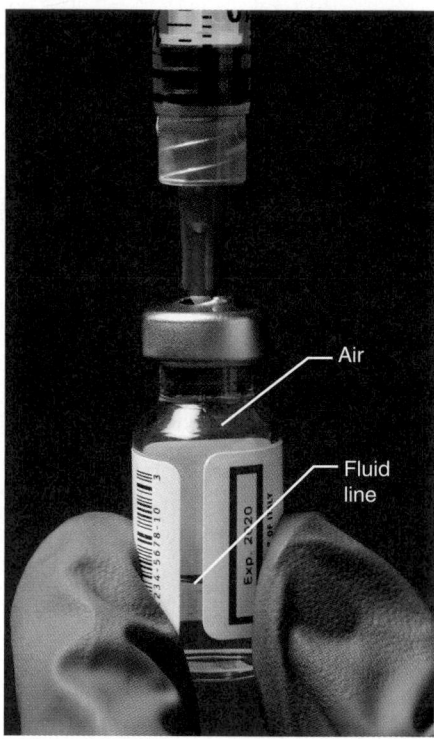

Air — Fluid line

8. Invert the vial, keep the needle or VAD vertical in the medication, and slowly withdraw the medication.

The vial needs to be inverted so that all the medication can be withdrawn. Keeping the needle/VAD in the medication and slowly drawing the medication will help prevent you from drawing excess air into the syringe. ▼

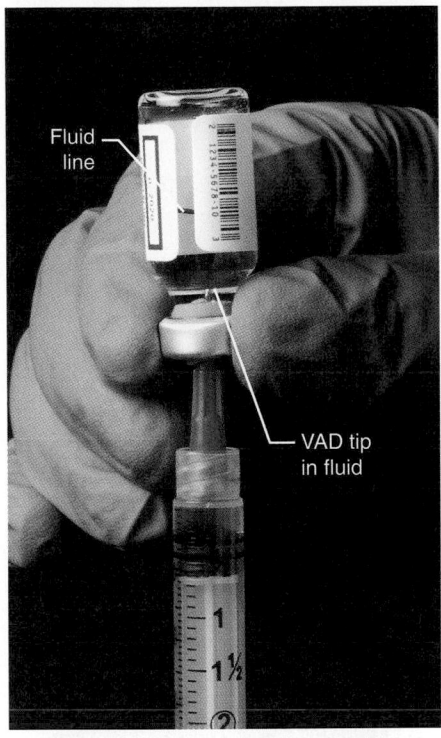

9. Keeping the needle or VAD in the vial, remove any air from the syringe: ▼

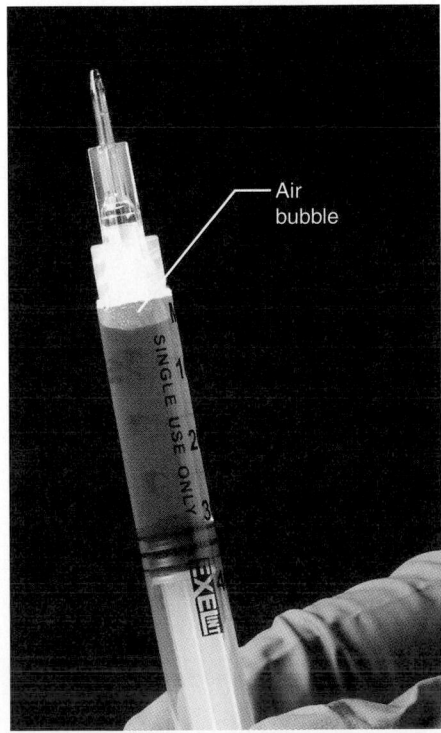

A, **Incorrect**—If syringe is not vertical, air is trapped near the hub.

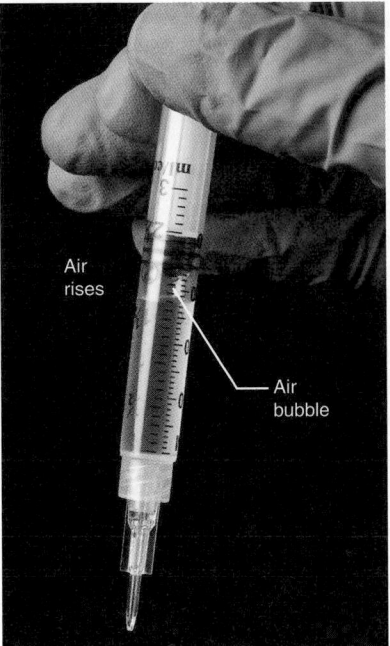

B, **Incorrect**—If tip is down, air is trapped at the plunger.

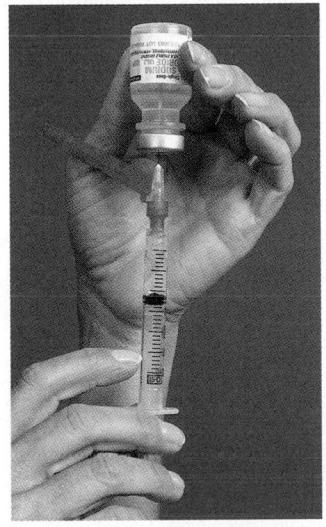

C, **Correct**—Syringe is vertical.

When the VAD is connecting the vial and syringe, a sterile unit is formed. The volume of air in the hub of the syringe and inside the needle/VAD, dead space, will be drawn back into the syringe. Air bubbles alter the dose of medication being administered, so they must be expelled. You can use a pen to tap the syringe if extra force is needed.

a. Carefully stabilize the vial and syringe, and firmly tap the syringe below the air bubbles. When air bubbles are at the hub of the syringe, make sure the syringe is vertical (straight up and down), and push the air back into the vial. Remember that air rises, so if the syringe is tilted, air will be trapped in it.

b. Withdraw additional medication, if necessary, to obtain the correct dose. You can withdraw and eject medication into the vial as many times as needed to expel bubbles from the syringe and obtain the correct dose.

10. When the dose is correct, withdraw the needle or VAD from the vial at a 90° angle. A vertical angle prevents accidental contamination or bending of the needle.

11. Hold the syringe upright at eye level to recheck the medication dose. Reading the syringe at an angle can result in inaccurate measurement.

12. Recap the needle or VAD using a needle recapping device or the one-handed method (see Procedure 23-10). Although recapping a sterile needle does not present a threat of bloodborne pathogen exposure, using a mechanical recapping device or the one-handed method helps develop safe habits.

13. If you are administering an irritating medication or if you used a VAD or filter needle to draw up medication, change the needle before you inject the medication. Before changing the needle, draw back on the syringe plunger to remove all medication from dead space in the old needle (or VAD), remove the old needle, and reattach a new one (see Clinical Insight 23-4). Hold the syringe vertically and expel the air; if it is necessary to expel some medication, hold the syringe horizontally to do so. The difficulty with changing the needles is that you may slightly alter the dose. If you are planning to change the needles, draw slightly more than the ordered dose unless you are combining in one syinge. After changing the needle, remeasure the dose. Holding the syringe horizontally prevents medication from running down the needle and tracking into the patient's skin.

14. Dispose of the vial and filter needle(s) in a sharps container. This prevents sharps injury to healthcare workers or others in the vicinity. Proper disposal also reduces the risk of transmitting infectious organisms.

(continued on next page)

Procedure 23-9 ■ **Preparing, Drawing Up, and Mixing Medication** (continued)

■ Procedure 23-9C **Mixing Medication from Two Vials**

➤ First review Procedure 23-1 (Medication Guidelines: Steps to Follow for All Medications); Procedure 23-9 (Preparing and Drawing Up Medications from Vials); and Procedure 23-10 (Recapping Contaminated Needles).

➤ When performing the procedure, always identify your patient according to agency policy and be attentive to standard precautions, hand hygiene, patient safety and privacy, body mechanics, and documentation.

Procedure Steps

1. Scrub the tops of both vials with an alcohol pad or chlorhexidine gluconate (CHG)-alcohol product. (*Note:* Some experts omit this step for single-dose vials.)
Not all pharmaceutical companies ensure the sterility of the rubber top on vials, even when they are first opened. However, be aware that once your fingers touch the alcohol pad, it is no longer sterile, either; so, you are not sterilizing, but rather are cleaning the vial top.

2. Draw up the same amount of air into the syringe as the total medication doses for both vials (e.g., if the order is for 0.5 mL for vial A and 1 mL for vial B, then draw up 1.5 mL of air). ▼

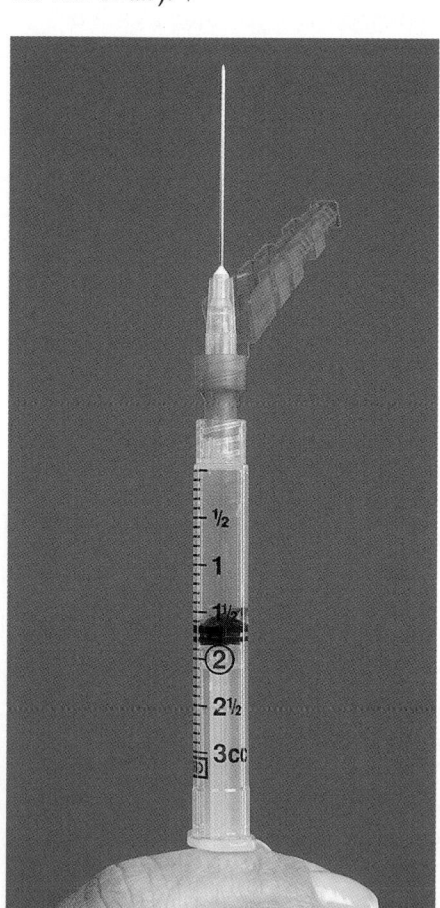

3. Maintaining sterility, insert the needle (or vial access device [VAD]) into the vial in the middle of the rubber top of the vial with the bevel up at a 45° to 60° angle. While pushing the needle (or VAD) into the rubber top, gradually bring the needle upright to a 90° angle.
This method helps prevent coring of the rubber top.

4. Keeping the tip of the safety needle (or VAD) above the medication, inject an amount of air equal to the volume of drug to be withdrawn from the first vial (e.g., 0.5 mL for vial A in step 2); then inject the rest of the air into the second vial (1.0 mL for vial B). Take care to prevent coring. ▼

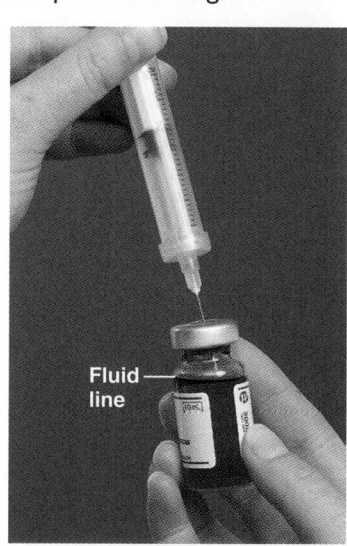

Fluid line

Vial A

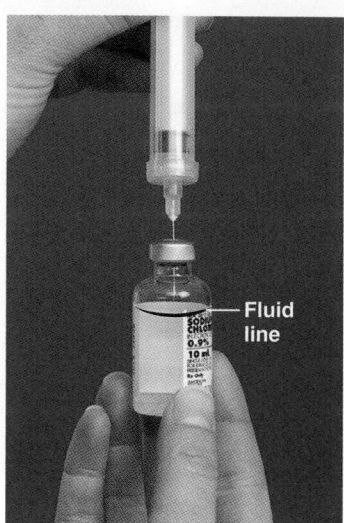

Fluid line

Vial B

Medication is easier to withdraw from a vial with positive pressure. For small unit-dose vials, it may be possible to withdraw the medication without instilling air, but you will need to maintain a slight backward pressure on the plunger until the needle is completely withdrawn. If you release the plunger, the negative pressure in the vial will pull the medication back in. Therefore, it is always safer to instill air.

Steps 3 & 4 Variation. One Multidose Vial and One Single-Dose Vial

Inject air into the single-dose vial first, and change the needle before injecting air into the multidose vial. You must withdraw medication from the multidose vial before withdrawing from the single-dose vial. However, the needle tip should stay above the medication at all times in steps 3 and 4.

This is an extra precaution to prevent contamination of the multidose vial with medication from the single-dose vial.

Steps 3 & 4 Variation. Mixing Two Types of Insulin

If you are mixing two types of insulin at step 3, put air into the regular insulin last (see Clinical Insight 23-5 for mixing two types of insulin).

5. Without removing the needle (or VAD) from the second vial (B), invert the vial and withdraw the ordered amount of medication. Expel any air bubbles, and measure the dose. Remove the VAD from the vial, then pull back on the plunger enough to pull all medication out of the VAD into the syringe (see Clinical Insight 23-4). Read the dose at eye level. Tip the syringe horizontally if you need to eject any medication.

This allows you to withdraw all the medication. Keeping the needle in the medication and slowly withdrawing the medication will help prevent withdrawing excess air into the syringe and prevent bubbles. ▼

6. Insert the needle or VAD into the first vial (A), invert, and withdraw the exact ordered amount of medication, holding syringe vertical. When finished, the plunger should be at the line for the total/combined dose for vials A and B. Be very careful not to withdraw excess medication; keep your index finger or thumb on the flange of the syringe to prevent it being forced back by pressure. If this occurs, you must discard the medication in the syringe and start over. (Using the example in step 2, you would have 1.5 mL of the mixed medications in the syringe.)

Because the medications are mixed, withdrawing extra from the second vial makes the entire mixture incorrect. If you eject excess medication from the syringe, you do not know how much of either medication you have ejected; so, even if you have the correct amount of fluid (e.g., 1.5 mL in our example), you would not know how much of that is medication A and how much of it is medication B.

There is no need to change the needle before step 5 because even if one vial is a multidose vial, you would have withdrawn the medication from it first (in step 4). It will not matter if you track medication into the single-dose vial. ▼

7. Remove the needle or VAD from the vial, and then recap the needle, using a needle capping device or the one-handed scoop method (see Procedure 23-10, Recapping Needles Using One-Handed Technique).

Although recapping a sterile needle does not present a threat of blood-borne pathogen exposure, using a mechanical recapping device or the one-handed method helps develop safe habits. As a rule, we do not recommend using the one-handed scoop for sterile needles; however, this needle will be discarded anyway, so if it is accidentally contaminated with a one-handed scoop, it will not be a major error.

8. Place a new sterile needle on the syringe for the injection.

Obviously, you must replace a VAD with a needle for injection. In addition, if you used a needle, by the time you are finished withdrawing both medications you will have put it through a rubber vial top at least three times. This dulls the needle. A sharp needle causes less trauma to the patient on injection. A new needle also prevents tracking of the medication through the skin and subcutaneous tissues.

9. Hold the needle vertically to expel all air and recheck the dosage (the total for both medications).

The vertical position allows for more accurate accounting of the dose.

10. If you have used a filter needle or VAD, refer to Clinical Insight 23-4, Measuring Dosage When Changing Needles.

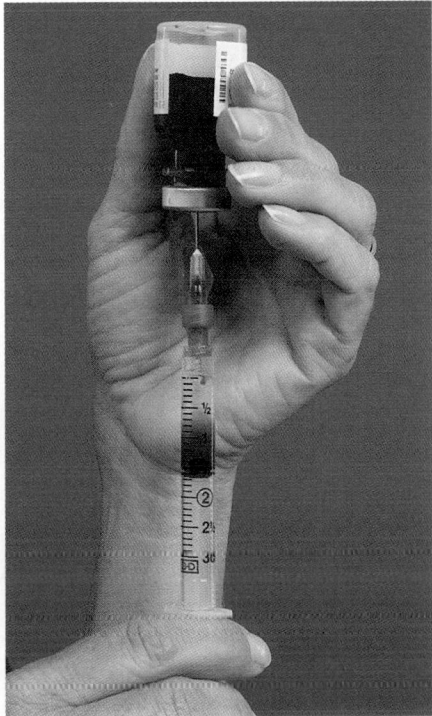

Vial B   **Vial A**

(continued on next page)

Procedure 23-9 ■ **Preparing, Drawing Up, and Mixing Medication** (continued)

■ Procedure 23-9D **Mixing Medication from One Ampule and One Vial**

➤ First review Procedure 23-1 (Medication Guidelines: Steps to Follow for All Medications); Procedure 23-9 (Preparing and Drawing Up Medications from Vials); and Procedure 23-10 (Recapping Contaminated Needles).

➤ When performing the procedure, always identify your patient according to agency policy and be attentive to standard precautions, hand hygiene, patient safety and privacy, body mechanics, and documentation.

Procedure Steps

1. Begin with the vial. Scrub the stopper of a multidose vial using an alcohol wipe or CHG-alcohol combination product. Use povidone iodine only when there is sensitivity to alcohol.
Protects against microbial contamination.

2. Draw up the same volume of air as the dose of medication ordered for the vial.

3. Keeping the tip of the safety needle (or needleless device) above the medication, inject the amount of air equal to the volume of drug to be withdrawn from the vial. The needle should be injecting air-to-air within the vial.
Because you do not need to add air to ampules before drawing up the medication, you should draw from the vial first. In addition, if it is a multidose vial, you would contaminate it with the medicine if you withdrew from the ampule first.

Injecting air into the vial makes withdrawing the medication easier. For small unit-dose vials, it may be possible to withdraw the medication without instilling air, but you will need to maintain a slight backward pressure on the plunger until the needle is completely withdrawn. If you release the plunger, the negative pressure in the vial will pull the medication back into the vial. Therefore, it is safer always to instill air.

4. Invert the vial. Withdraw the prescribed volume (dosage) of medication, keeping the safety needle tip or VAD in the fluid. See Procedure 23-9B.

5. Expel any air bubbles and measure the dose at eye level. Recheck the dosage, and withdraw more or eject the drug as needed.

This prevents air from entering into the needle or VAD.

6. After safely recapping the safety needle, or vial access device (VAD), remove it from the syringe. You may place it on an opened, sterile alcohol pad if you need your hands to open the filter needle packaging.
Keeps the needle sterile, if you are using one; you will reuse it. You would not reuse a VAD from this step on.

7. Attach a filter needle or filter straw to the syringe.
The use of a 5-micrometer (μm) filter minimizes the possibility of withdrawing small glass fragments.

8. Flick or tap the top of the ampule (or snap your wrist) to remove medication from the neck of the ampule.
Flicking the neck of the ampule will help the fluid to drain down into the main part of the ampule, thus, reducing waste.

9. Open the ampule by wrapping the neck with a folded gauze pad or an unopened alcohol wipe or use an ampule snapper. Snap open away from you.
Snapping outward prevents you from accidentally cutting your fingers or spraying glass fragments toward your face. Do not use an opened alcohol wipe to break the ampule, because it is not thick enough to prevent injury.

10. Withdraw the exact ordered amount of medication from the ampule into the syringe (see Procedure 23-9A). Be very careful in drawing up the second medication; if the total amount of the two medications is incorrect, you must discard the syringe contents and start over.

11. Draw 0.2 mL of air into the syringe.

The extra bit of air clears the filter needle (see Clinical Insight 23-4).

12. Confirm the dose is correct by holding the syringe vertically and checking the dose at eye level.
A vertical position ensures the total volume in the syringe equals the ordered amount of both medications plus 0.2 mL of air from the needle.

13. Recap the needle, using a needle capping device or the one-handed technique recommended in Procedure 23-10.
Although recapping a sterile needle does not present a threat of bloodborne pathogen exposure, using a mechanical recapping device or the one-handed method helps develop safe habits. Nevertheless, some scoop techniques pose a significant risk of contaminating the needle, so you must watch carefully that you maintain sterile technique.

14. Remove the filter needle or straw and discard it in a sharps container. Replace with a fresh, safety needle for giving the medication to the patient.
This needle-recapping method prevents accidental needlestick injury. You cannot measure the dose accurately with a filter needle. You should not eject medication through the filter needle because of risk of breaking the filter. See Clinical Insight 23-4, Measuring Dosage When Changing Needles.

15. After placing the administration needle on the syringe eject the 0.2 mL of air and check for the correct dose, if there is excess medication in the syringe, you must discard it and start over.

16. Discard used needles and ampules in a puncture-proof sharps container.

■ **Procedure 23-9E**   **Using a Prefilled Cartridge and Single-Dose Vial—For Intravenous Administration**

➤ *Note:* It is best to not use this technique with multidose vials because there is a risk of contaminating the multidose vial with the cartridge medication.

➤ When performing the procedure, always identify your patient according to agency policy and be attentive to standard precautions, hand hygiene, patient safety and privacy, body mechanics, and documentation.

Procedure Steps

1. Scrub the rubber stopper of the vial thoroughly with an alcohol prep pad or chlorhexidine-gluconate (CHG)-alcohol-based product.

2. Assemble the prefilled cartridge and holder (see Clinical Insight 23-2).

3. Remove the needle cap from the prefilled cartridge, expel the air, and measure the correct dose of medication.
You must confirm that the dose of the first medication is correct before you mix it with the second medication.

4. Holding the cartridge with the needle up, withdraw an amount of air equal to the volume of medication you need from the vial.

5. While continuing to hold the syringe with needle straight up (vertically), insert the needle into the inverted vial, tip of the needle in the air above the medication, and inject the air into the vial. Maintain pressure on the plunger so that air and/or medication does not flow back into the syringe.

Injecting air into the vial makes the medication easier to withdraw. ▼

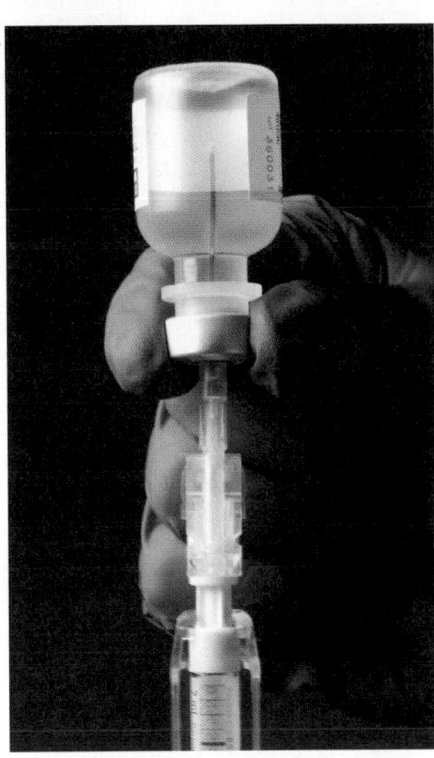

6. While maintaining pressure on the plunger, pull the needle down into the fluid and allow the pressure in the vial to push the medication into the syringe. Withdraw the ordered amount of vial medication, being careful not to withdraw any excess.

7. The pressure will generally push a little less than you need, so carefully withdraw the amount you need for a correct dose – again, do not withdraw any excess.
Withdrawing any excess will result in an altered mixed dose, so you would need to discard the syringe and start over.

8. Recap the needle (use a one-handed method) and if possible, remove the needle from the prefilled syringe and replace with an injection cannula for IV administration. For an IM injection, if the prefilled cartridge does not have a safety needle, you would need to transfer the medication to a new syringe and needle for injection.
VADs and injection cannulas prevent needlestick injury. Unless there is a needle safety device for the prefilled syringe, it is not recommended for IM injections.

What if. . .

■ **You note particulate matter in the ampule or vial?**

Discard the medication and order a new one.

■ **When drawing a second medication from a vial that is to be mixed in one syringe, the medication inadvertently is drawn back into the vial by positive pressure?**

Discard the medication in the syringe and start over.

Documentation

Documentation is per Medication Administration Record.

Thinking About the Procedure

 Go to the *Fundamentals of Nursing Skills Videos,* **Preparing Medications.**

Procedure 23-9A Drawing Up Medications from Ampules.

1. How does the nurse in the DVD safely open the glass ampule? Why does she do it in this manner?

(continued on next page)

Procedure 23-9 ■ Preparing, Drawing Up, and Mixing Medication (continued)

Procedure 23-9B Drawing Up Medications from Vials

1. After injecting medication into a vial, how does the nurse constitute the solution?

2. And why does she do it this way?

Procedure 23-9C Mixing Medication from Two Vials

1. What device does the nurse in the DVD use to extract liquid medication from a vial?

2. After removing the needle from the second vial and pulling back on the plunger enough to pull all medication out of the needle (or access device) into the syringe, how much medication does the nurse in the DVD eject to clear the needle?

3. As a last step after two medications are drawn and mixed in one syringe and the air is expelled, what does the nurse do before administering the dose to the patient?

Procedure 23-9D Mixing Medication from One Ampule and One Vial

1. Why does the nurse insert the needle access device at a 45° angle and then move to 90° angle?

2. How does the nurse in the DVD get rid of air bubbles in the syringe?

 For suggested responses, go to Chapter 23, **Thinking About the Procedure Suggested Responses (Procedures 23-9A, B, C, D),** on the Student Resource Disk or DavisPlus at http://davisplus.fadavis.com/Wilkinson2

Practice Resource
U.S. Food and Drug Administration, Center for Drug Evaluation and Research (2008).

Procedure 23-10   Recapping Needles Using One-Handed Technique

➤ For steps to follow in *all* procedures, refer to the Universal Steps for All Procedures found on the inside back cover of Volume 2. Also refer to Medication Guidelines: Steps to Follow for All Medications (Regardless of Type or Route).

Critical Aspects

Procedure 23-10A: Recapping Contaminated Needles
- Recap a contaminated needle only if you cannot avoid it.
- Do not place either of your hands near the needle cap when recapping the needle or engaging the safety mechanism.
- If you are using a safety needle, engage the safety mechanism to cover the needle.
- Place the needle cap in a mechanical recapping device if one is available.
- If recapping devices are not available and you must recap the needle for your own and/or the patient's safety, use the one-handed scoop technique or one of the methods in Procedures 23-10B.

Procedure 23-10B: Recapping Sterile Needles
- Be sure to keep the needle and cap sterile.
- Do not place your hands near the needle cap when recapping the needle or engaging the safety mechanism.
- Use one of the following methods:
  - Place the needle cap in a medication cup, and recap the needle.
  - Place the cap on a clean surface so that the end of the needle cap protrudes over the edge of the counter or shelf, and scoop with the needle.
  - Use a hard syringe cover: Stand it on end, insert the needle cap into the cover, and then insert the needle.
  - Place the needle cap on a sterile surface, such as on open alcohol prep pad, and use the one-handed scoop technique.

Equipment

- Mechanical recapping device, if available
- Needle cover
- Safety syringe, if available
- Other supplies depending on the method used.

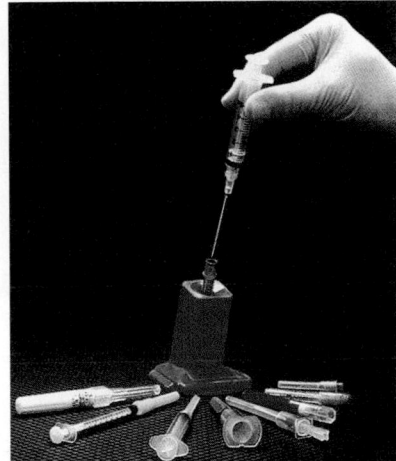

Needle recapping device.

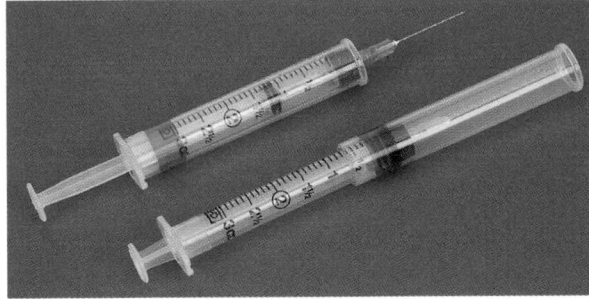

Safety syringe. A, Before injection. B, Cover slides up after injection.

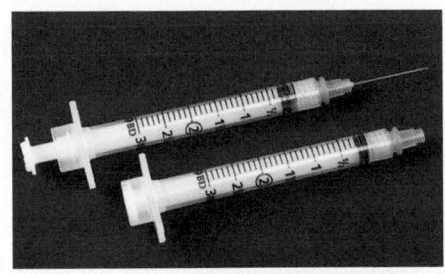

Safety syringe. A, Before injection. B, Needle retracted after injection.

Delegation

Delegation is not usually an issue because recapping needles is done in conjunction with administering parenteral medications, which you will usually not delegate. If you do delegate administration of parenteral medications to an LPN/LVN, you must supervise and evaluate recapping to ensure that the nurse uses proper technique.

Preparation

- Assess the need to recap the needle.

Recap a contaminated needle only if doing so is absolutely unavoidable, according to OSHA standards. As a rule, place a contaminated syringe and needle directly into a puncture-proof sharps container, without capping, bending, or breaking the needle.

- Identify whether the needle is sterile or dirty.

Although a one-handed technique is used to recap both sterile and dirty needles, different considerations exist. When you use the one-handed method for recapping a sterile needle, it is easy to contaminate the needle without realizing it; so, you should modify the technique to help prevent that; the main consideration is to "protect" the needle. The danger in recapping a dirty needle is that you will stick yourself with it, exposing yourself to pathogens. The main consideration is to protect yourself.

- Determine the availability of mechanical recapping device or safety syringe.

Always use a mechanical recapping device or safety syringe, if one is available.

■ Procedure 23-10A Recapping Contaminated Needles

➤ When performing the procedure, always identify your patient according to agency policy and be attentive to standard precautions, hand hygiene, patient safety and privacy, body mechanics, and documentation.

Procedure Steps

1. If you are using a safety needle, engage the safety mechanism to cover the needle. (See Equipment.)
OSHA regulations require the use of safety syringes to prevent needlestick

injuries. You must engage the safety mechanism before placing the needle and syringe into the sharps container.

2. Alternatively, place the needle cap in mechanical recapping device, if one is available. (See Equipment.)

3. If a mechanical recapping device is not available, use the one-handed scoop method to recap the needle.
   a. Place the needle cover on a flat surface.

(continued on next page)

Procedure 23-10 ■ **Recapping Needles Using One-Handed Technique** (continued)

A flat surface keeps the needle cover from rolling during the needle capping procedure. ▼

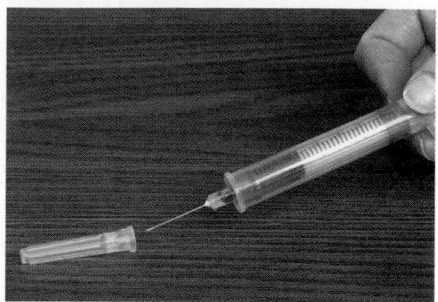

A mechanical recapping device protects against accidental needlestick injury. If it is unavailable, the one-handed method of recapping will prevent accidental injuries when your own or the patient's safety is a concern. ▼

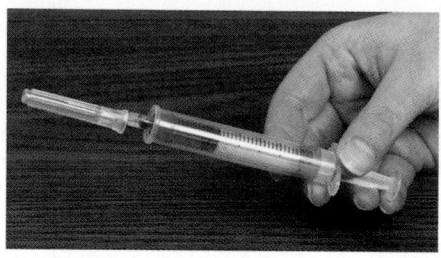

through the needle cap if inserted at an angle. ▼

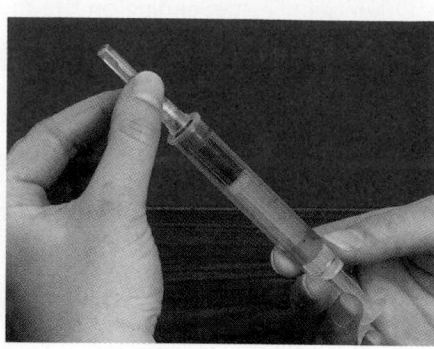

b. Then, holding syringe in your dominant hand, scoop the needle cap onto the needle. Tip the syringe vertically to slip the cover over the needle. Do not hold onto the needle cap with your nondominant hand while scooping.

c. Secure the needle cap by grasping it near the hub.
Prevents an accidental stick if the needle goes through the needle cap. Needles are sharp enough to go

---

■ **Procedure 23-10B** **Recapping Sterile Needles**

➤ When performing the procedure, always identify your patient according to agency policy and be attentive to standard precautions, hand hygiene, patient safety and privacy, body mechanics, and documentation.

Use one of the following techniques to ensure that you do not contaminate a sterile needle.
If you contaminate the needle, microorganisms will be introduced with the injection.

Procedure Steps

1. Place the needle cap in a mechanical recapping device, if one is available.
The device is specially developed to provide safe recapping.

2. Alternative method: Place the cap into a small liquid medication cup with the open end facing up. You can then insert the sterile needle into the cap, keeping your free hand well away from the cup.
This step performs the same function as a mechanical recapping device. The needle and cover need to be taller than the cup you are using, so that the open

end of the cap protrudes above the cup. ▼

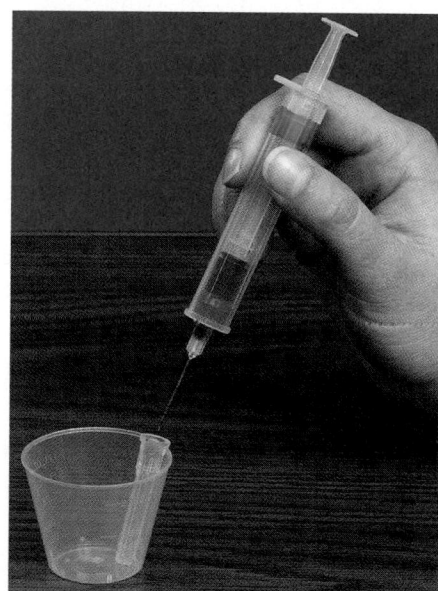

3. Alternative method: Place the cap on a clean surface so that the end of the needle cap protrudes over

the edge of the counter or shelf, and scoop with the needle; keep your free hand well away from the needle and cap as you are recapping.
This method prevents you from inadvertently hitting an unsterile surface with the needle. ▼

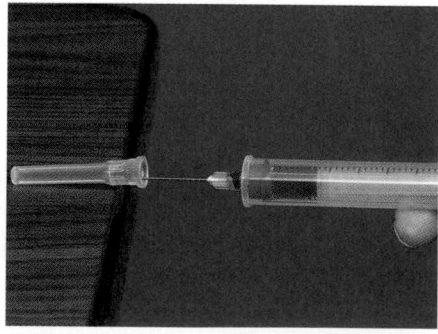

4. Alternative method: If the syringe is packaged in a hard plastic tubular container, stand the container on its large end; invert the needle cap; and place it in the top of the hard container. Insert the needle downward into the cap. ▼

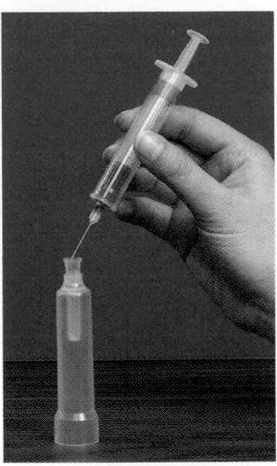

5. Alternative method: Place the needle cap on a sterile surface, such as on open alcohol prep pad, and use the one-handed scoop technique. Be very careful to not touch anything with the needle other than the inside of the needle cap.

The alcohol prep pad provides a sterile barrier. Because you must bring the needle parallel to the flat surface, and because the alcohol pad is so small, it is

easy to contaminate the needle using this method. ▼

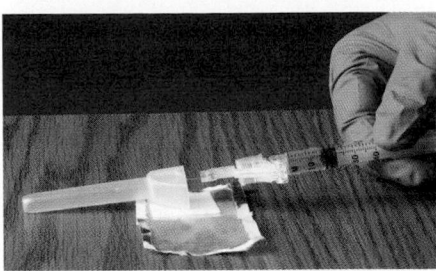

Documentation

No documentation needed for recapping needles.

Practice Resources

U.S. Department of Health and Human Services (DHHS), National Institute for Occupational Safety and Health (NIOSH) (1999, 2000); U.S. Department of Labor, Occupational Safety & Health Administration (OSHA) (2007).

Thinking About the Procedure

 Go to the *Fundamentals of Nursing Skills Videos,* **Recapping Sterile Needles: One-Handed Technique,** and **Recapping Contaminated Needles: One-Handed Technique.**

1. What is the safest method to prevent needlestick injury with a contaminated needle?

2. What are two goals when recapping a sterile needle?

3. If you do not have a safety needle, which method for recapping a sterile needle looks easiest to you?

 For suggested responses, go to Chapter 23, **Thinking About the Procedure Suggested Responses (Procedure 23-10),** on the Student Resource Disk or DavisPlus at http://davisplus.fadavis.com/Wilkinson2

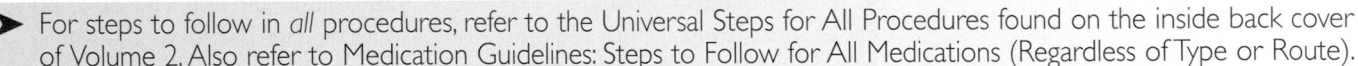

Procedure 23-11   Administering Intradermal Medication

➤ For steps to follow in *all* procedures, refer to the Universal Steps for All Procedures found on the inside back cover of Volume 2. Also refer to Medication Guidelines: Steps to Follow for All Medications (Regardless of Type or Route).

Critical Aspects

- Have appropriate antidotes for certain injections readily available before beginning the procedure.
- Know the location of resuscitation equipment in case of a life-threatening adverse reaction.
- Maintain sterile technique and standard precautions
- Use a 1-mL syringe and a 25- to 28-gauge, ¼ to ⅝-inch needle.
- Be aware that an intradermal dose is small, usually about 0.01 to 0.1 mL.
- Administer the injection on the ventral surface of the forearm, upper back, or upper chest.
- Hold the syringe parallel to the skin at a 5° to 15° angle, with the bevel up.
- Stretch the skin taut to insert the needle.
- Do not aspirate.
- Inject slowly, and create a wheal or bleb.
- Do not massage or bandage the site.

(continued on next page)

Procedure 23-11 ■ **Administering Intradermal Medication** (continued)

Equipment

- Alcohol prep pad or chlorhexidine gluconate (CHG)-alcohol product
- 2 in. × 2 in. gauze pad
- Pen (ink or felt)
- 1-mL syringe (tuberculin) with intradermal needle (25- to 28-gauge, ¼- to ⅝-inch with short bevel)

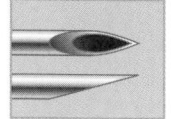 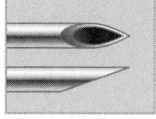 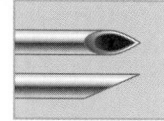

Regular bevel   Intermediate   Short bevel
                 bevel

Delegation

As an RN, you can usually delegate administration of parenteral medications to an LPN/LVN. You usually cannot delegate this task to a NAP.

Pre-Procedure Assessments

- Assess for previous reaction to skin testing.
Some skin tests, such as the tuberculin test, should not be repeated after positive test results.

- Assess for all types of allergies.
Because intradermal injections are also used for allergy testing, a client could have an anaphylactic reaction.

- Assess the skin at intradermal sites for bruising, swelling, tenderness, and other abnormalities.
Do not give intradermal skin tests if skin abnormalities are present. Also avoid giving them in areas where reading the results may be difficult, such as areas of heavy hair growth.

Preparation

- Have appropriate antidotes (usually epinephrine hydrochloride, a bronchodilator, and an antihistamine) readily available before the start of the procedure.
Because many intradermal injections are used for allergy testing, this is an important consideration.

- Know the location of resuscitation equipment (artificial airway, Ambu bag, and code cart)
Allergic reactions can be fatal.

> ➤ When performing the procedure, always identify your patient according to agency policy and be attentive to standard precautions, hand hygiene, patient safety and privacy, body mechanics, and documentation.

Procedure Steps

1. Draw up the medication from the vial (see Procedure 23-9B). The usual dose is 0.01 to 0.1 mL.
Intradermal sites can accommodate only small volumes of medication.

2. Select the site for injection. Usual sites are the ventral surface of the forearm and upper back. The upper chest may also be used. If you need to review site locations,

 Go to Chapter 23, **Figure 23-23**, in Volume 1.

Use areas where subcutaneous fat is less likely to interfere with administration and absorption. The forearm is the standard initial starting point because it has the least amount of subcutaneous tissue. The forearm and upper back usually have little hair, permitting easier visualization to interpret results accurately.

3. Assist the patient to a comfortable position. If you are using the forearm, instruct her to extend and supinate

her arm on a flat surface. If you are using the upper back, ask the patient to lie prone or lean forward over a table or the back of a chair.
This method stabilizes the injection site. The procedure will be more comfortable if the patient is able to relax his muscles. Tension, in general, increases pain perception.

4. Don procedure gloves.
Procedure gloves are not required by OSHA for intradermal injections, but they are recommended by the CDC to prevent accidental exposure to bloodborne pathogens. Remember, gloves cannot prevent needlestick injuries.

5. Cleanse the injection site with an alcohol prep pad or chlorhexidine gluconate (CHG)-alcohol product pad by circling from the center of the site outward. Allow the site to dry before administering the injection.
Cleansing to remove microorganisms, follows the principle of "clean to dirty." Alcohol can interfere with

the test results if a small amount is introduced during the injection; also, if the alcohol has not evaporated, it may cause the skin to sting during the injection.

6. Hold the syringe between the thumb and index finger of your dominant hand.
You must hold the syringe between your thumb and index finger to be able to administer the solution at the correct angle.

7. Hold the client's skin taut by using one of the following methods, with your nondominant hand:
  a. If using the forearm, you may be able to place your hand under the client's arm and pull the skin tight with your thumb and fingers.
  b. Stretch the client's skin between your thumb and index finger.
  c. Pull the client's skin toward the wrist or down with one finger.
A downward motion while stretching the skin eases needle insertion. Holding the skin tight can be difficult because of the low angle of administration.

8. While holding the client's skin taut with your nondominant hand, hold the syringe in your dominant hand with the needle bevel up and parallel to the client's skin at a 5° to 15° angle. Slowly insert the needle. Note that there is some controversy about whether it is better to have the bevel down or bevel up; however, the CDC recommends bevel up.

The low angle of insertion is necessary to place the needle tip in the intradermal layer instead of the subcutaneous tissue. Having the bevel up likely decreases the chance of injecting the medication deeper into the subcutaneous tissue. Patients receiving intradermal injections report bevel up more comfortable. ▼

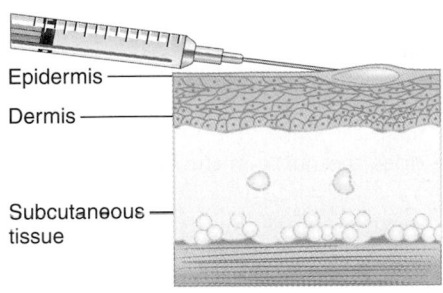

Epidermis
Dermis
Subcutaneous tissue

9. Advance the needle approximately 3 mm (⅛ in.) so that the entire bevel is covered. The bevel should be visible just under the skin.

If the entire bevel is not inserted, the solution will leak out of the tissue. If you can see the bevel under the surface of the skin, you can be sure that the bevel is not in the subcutaneous tissue.

10. Do not aspirate. Hold the syringe stable with your nondominant hand, and release the tightened skin.

This method decreases pressure on the injection site.

11. Slowly inject the solution. You should feel firm resistance. A pale wheal, about 6 to 10 mm (¼ in.) in diameter, will appear over the needle bevel.

The dermis does not have room to absorb the solution, so a wheal forms, stretching the skin. Slow administration gives you time to terminate the injection should a systemic reaction occur. If a bleb (wheal) forms, you have administered the drug properly. The size of the bleb depends on the amount of medication you injected. ▼

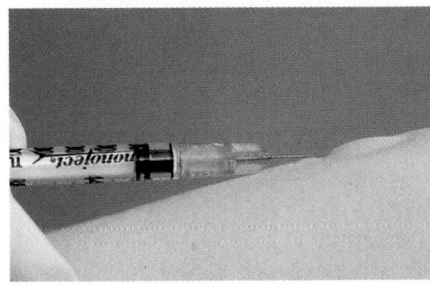

12. Remove the needle, engage the safety needle device, and dispose of the needle in a biohazard, puncture-proof container. If there is no safety device, place the uncapped syringe and needle directly in biohazard, puncture-proof container.

A needle capping device prevents needlestick injuries.

13. Gently blot any blood with a dry gauze pad. Do not rub the skin or cover it with an adhesive bandage.

Rubbing may cause the drug to leak out and alter absorption. An adhesive

bandage can cause irritation and interfere with the skin test.

14. With a pen, draw a 1-inch circle around the bleb/wheal.

Marking the site helps you to identify any change in the size of the wheal at a later time.

What if...

- **My patient has a history of a skin reaction to PPD testing?**

Obtain details about the type and severity of the reaction. If the previous reaction involved ulceration at the site, further Mantoux testing is contraindicated. Report this to the prescriber.

- **My patient is pregnant, is receiving chemotherapy, or has severe eczema?**

Defer tuberculosis skin testing and inform the prescriber.

- **My patient received a live vaccine at the time of tuberculosis skin testing?**

Tuberculosis skin testing should be deferred for one month after live viral vaccines or other major viral infection.

- **My patient has topical anesthetic cream on the skin?**

Use a site where the topical anesthetic cream was not applied or reschedule tuberculosis skin testing for another date.

Evaluation

- Reassess the client 5 and 15 minutes after administration for allergic reactions that may subsequently occur.
- Read the site within 48 to 72 hours of injection, depending on the test.
- Observe that a wheal (about 6 to 8 mm in diameter) forms at the site and that it gradually disappears.
- Observe for minimal bruising that may develop at the site of injection.

Patient Teaching

- Explain when the patient needs to have the intradermal injection read to determine whether the result is positive or negative.
- Explain that mild itching, swelling, or irritation may occur at the injection site and are normal.

If the patient has antigens to the injected solution, a histamine response occurs, causing itching, swelling, or irritation. This response generally subsides within a week.

- Discuss the significance of a positive or negative skin test result.

(continued on next page)

Procedure 23-11 ■ Administering Intradermal Medication (continued)

Explain that some signs of irritation may occur that do not mean a positive test result.

- Instruct the patient not to scratch, apply lotions or creams, cover the site with a bandage, or scrub the site. This might cause irritation and interfere with the test, which may produce false-positive results.

Documentation

- See the information in Medication Guidelines: Steps to Follow for All Medication (Regardless of Type or Route).
- Some medications require documentation of lot numbers (check agency policy).
- Chart when the test is to be read.

Sample documentation:

09/01/11   0800   Explained purpose and procedure for Mantoux skin test. Client stated, "I need a PPD so that I can go to the long term care facility." 0.2 mL of tuberculin purified protein placed in left forearm per physician order. No reaction noted 5 minutes after procedure. Will read test at 0800 on 09/03/11.
—— M. Saleh, RN

Thinking About the Procedure

 Go to the *Fundamentals of Nursing Skills Videos,* **Intradermal Injection: Locating Sites and Administering.**

1. What site does the nurse in the DVD use to inject intradermal medication? And why does she choose that location.

2. For intradermal medication administration, what technique for holding the syringe does the nurse in the DVD use before injection?

3. For intradermal medication administration, what size needle will you typically use?

4. When should you evaluate the site after administering medication intradermally?

 For suggested responses, go to Chapter 23, **Thinking About the Procedure Suggested Responses (Procedure 23-11),** on the Student Resource Disk or DavisPlus at http://davisplus.fadavis.com/Wilkinson2

Practice Resources

Disease Control and Epidemiology, Health and Community Services, Government of Newfoundland and Labrador (2006); Howard, A., Mercer, P., Nataraj, H. C., et al. (1997); National Center for HIV, STD, and TB Prevention, Division of Tuberculosis Elimination (2008).

Procedure 23-12   Administering Subcutaneous Medication

➤ For steps to follow in *all* procedures, refer to the Universal Steps for All Procedures found of the inside back cover of Volume 2. Also refer to Medication Guidelines: Steps to Follow for All Medications (Regardless of Type or Route).

Critical Aspects

- Maintain sterile technique and standard precautions.
- Use a 1-mL syringe and a 25- to 27-gauge needle that is less than 1 inch long (usually ⅜ to ⅝ in.).
- A subcutaneous dose is typically no more than 1 mL.
- Most common injection sites: Use the outer aspect of the upper arms, abdomen, and anterior aspects of the thighs.
- Pinch the skin to inject, as a general rule.
- For an average-weight or thin client, inject at a 45° angle; for an obese client, inject at a 90° angle, as a general rule.
- Aspiration is optional for most medications, but do not aspirate when injecting heparin or insulin.
- Do not massage the site.

Equipment

- Syringe and needle appropriate for volume and site
- Alcohol prep pad or chlorhexidine gluconate (CHG)-alcohol product
- Gauze pad (optional)

Delegation

As an RN, you can usually delegate administration of parenteral medications to an LPN/LVN. You usually cannot delegate this task to a NAP.

Pre-Procedure Assessments

- Check the area for previous injection sites.

Alternating among the arms, thighs, abdomen, and back changes the absorption rate of the medication. Absorption is fastest from the abdomen, then the arms, and lastly the thighs and back. It is recommended that you rotate sites within the same extremity or location, approximately 1 inch from the previous injection. Rotating the site helps prevent the development of lipodystrophy.

- Do focused assessments for the specific medication being administered.
    - *Insulin*—Check capillary blood sugar level, and determine when the patient will be having the next meal; check for signs of hypoglycemia or hyperglycemia.

Insulin must be balanced with food intake to prevent the patient from developing hypoglycemia or hyperglycemia. Different insulins have specific rates of absorption, peak action, and duration. Some insulins, such as Humalog and regular insulin, are rapid acting. Before you administer rapid-acting insulin, the capillary blood sugar must be within the normal range or above, and the patient must be ready to eat. With Humalog, the patient's food tray should be in front of him before you administer the insulin.

- *Heparin*—Check activated partial thromboplastin time (aPTT) and for signs of bleeding, such as bleeding from gums, IV injection sites, and so on.

Heparin is an anticoagulant, so the major side effect is bleeding. Besides overt bleeding, also check for occult blood loss through the urine and stool. The aPTT will not be monitored as frequently with the low-molecular-weight heparins (LMWHs), because bleeding is less likely to occur.

> When performing the procedure, always identify your patient according to agency policy and be attentive to standard precautions, hand hygiene, patient safety and privacy, body mechanics, and documentation.

Procedure Steps

1. Select an appropriate syringe and needle.

   a. For insulin administration, you must use an insulin syringe—typically 0.3, 0.5, or 1.0 mL. Most insulin needles are 28- to 31-gauge. Needle length is often ³⁄₁₆—1 inch. For more information about giving insulin, see Clinical Insight 23-5, Administering Insulin Subcutaneously.

Although both insulin and tuberculin (TB) syringes come in a 1-mL size, they are not interchangeable. Insulin syringes are calibrated in units; they have a permanent (non-removable) needle and a very small amount of dead space.

   b. For other medications, for volumes less than 1 mL, use a tuberculin (TB) syringe with a 25- to 27-gauge, ³⁄₈- to ⁵⁄₈-inch needle.

Because of the small increments on the TB syringe, small doses can be measured more accurately. ▼

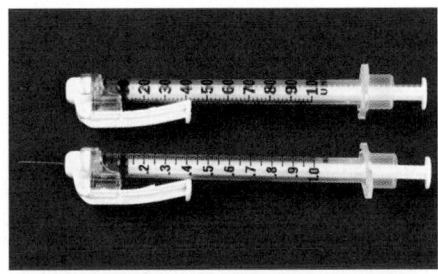

Top: Insulin syringe. Bottom: TB syringe.

   c. For administering a volume of 1 mL, you may use a 3-mL syringe with a 25- to 27-gauge, ³⁄₈- to ⁵⁄₈-inch needle.

Although you can measure 1 mL with a tuberculin (TB) syringe, it will be difficult to handle the syringe because the plunger will be pulled back as far as it can go. It is easy to pull it inadvertently out of the end of the syringe. Some medications are supplied in prefilled syringes. Examples are enoxaparin sodium (Lovenox) and the other low-molecular-weight heparins (LMWHs). These are usually supplied in unit-dose prefilled glass syringes.

2. Draw up the medication. See Procedure 23-9.

3. Select an injection site with adequate subcutaneous tissue. If you need to review site locations,

 Go to Chapter 23, **Figure 23-24,** in Volume 1.

Helps you avoid accidentally injecting into the muscle.

   a. The usual sites are the outer aspect of the upper arms, abdomen (at least 2 inches away from the umbilicus), anterior aspects of the thighs, and high on the buttocks near waist level.

These areas usually have good circulation and are easily accessible. The buttocks are more convenient when someone is giving the injection other than the patient.

The anterolateral and posterolateral abdomen ("love handles") sites are the only subcutaneous site used for administering heparin or low-molecular-weight heparins (LMWHs). For more information about giving heparin, see Clinical Insight 23-6, Administering Anticoagulant Medication Subcutaneously.

The subcutaneous tissue 2 inches away from the umbilicus poses less risk of

(continued on next page)

Procedure 23-12 ■ **Administering Subcutaneous Medication** (continued)

bleeding when an anticoagulant is administered.

b. Check the site for inflammation, bruising, lumps, or other abnormalities.

Avoid areas with skin abnormalities, which may alter the absorption rates or increase patient discomfort during the injection.

4. Position the patient so that the injection site is accessible and the patient is able to relax the appropriate area.

5. Don procedure gloves.

Procedure gloves are required to prevent exposure to bloodborne pathogens. You may prefer to don gloves before step 5; however, you can also do so after step 6 while waiting for the alcohol to dry.

6. Cleanse the injection site with an alcohol prep pad or chlorhexidine gluconate (CHG)-alcohol product by circling from the center of the site outward. Allow the site to dry before administering the injection.

7. Remove the needle cap.

The needle cap is more difficult to remove when using a one-handed technique.

8. With your nondominant hand, pinch the tissue at the injection site,

and determine the angle at which to inject the needle. Insert the needle using a 90° angle. If the adipose tissue pinches 2 inches or more (client is obese), use a longer needle and spread the skin taut instead of pinching. Grasping and lifting the tissue prevents you from accidentally injecting into the muscle. Also, the subcutaneous injection must be given in the fatty tissue and not into intradermal layer. Traditionally, injections had been using a 45° angle to ensure medication is deposited into the subcutaneous layer. ▼

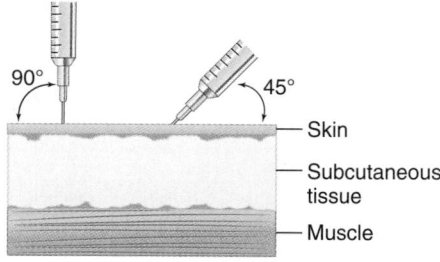

9. Holding the syringe between thumb and index finger of your dominant hand like a pencil or dart, insert the needle at the appropriate angle into the skinfold.

Quickly inserting the needle through the skin minimizes discomfort.

10. Using the thumb or index finger of your dominant hand, press the plunger slowly to inject the medication.

Alternatively, after inserting the needle, you can continue to hold the barrel with your dominant hand and use your nondominant hand to depress the plunger.

Slow administration allows the medication to disperse and decreases discomfort. Subcutaneous injections do not need to be aspirated beforehand, because accidental entry into a blood vessel is rare.

11. Remove the needle smoothly along the line of insertion.

This action prevents pulling against the skin and tissue and thus minimizes discomfort.

12. Gently wipe the site with gauze if needed. Do not massage the site unless directed otherwise.

Occasionally there will be blood at the site after the needle is removed. You might have nicked a surface blood vessel when you injected, and blood is following the needle track out to the surface. Massaging or rubbing the site will alter the rate of absorption of the medication.

13. Engage the needle safety device, and dispose of the needle in biohazard container. If there is no safety device, place the uncapped syringe and needle directly into a biohazard, puncture-proof container.

A sharps container prevents needlestick injuries.

Evaluation

■ Observe for minimal bruising that may develop at the site of injection.
■ Reassess the patient for anticipated response and adverse reaction to medication.
  ■ For insulin, observe for signs that patient's blood sugar level has returned to normal and for signs of hypoglycemia.
  ■ For heparin, observe that patient has no signs of bleeding.
  ■ For other medications, observe for side effects.

Patient Teaching

■ Discuss possible lifestyle adaptations that the patient may need to undertake while receiving the medication, such as diet and exercise recommendations for managing diabetes mellitus.

Home Care

■ Discuss with the client or caregiver the options for insulin administration to determine the most appropriate choice for the person administering the injections.

Many options are available, including specially designed syringes that are easier to handle and read, pen injectors, and prefilled syringes.

■ In the home environment the client might not routinely use an alcohol wipe to cleanse the site. This is acceptable as long as the skin is clean.

In the home environment there is less risk for superinfection with resistant strain organisms, and other hospital-acquired infections.

■ Do not encourage reusing needles and syringes. However, if the client or caregiver believes they need to reuse syringes and needles in the home, teach them

how to safely do so. Teach them the guidelines in Clinical Insight 23-1, Reusing Needles and Syringes.
Determine whether reusing syringes is appropriate for the patient. Contraindications include inadequate hygiene, immunocompromised status, and difficulty handling equipment to prevent contamination of the needle. The very small insulin needles (30-gauge) bend very easily and are not recommended for reuse.

■ Discuss safety concerns regarding subcutaneous medication administration in the home, such as how to dispose of biohazardous wastes correctly and where to obtain a puncture-proof biohazard container.

The patient or caregiver may use a large plastic bottle or a coffee can. Local regulations regarding disposal must be followed.

■ Discuss with the patient the need to rotate sites. For insulin, explain to the patient that alternating among arms, thighs, and abdomen causes different absorption rates. The recommendation is to give the injections due at the same time of the day in the same body location about 1 inch from the previous injection site.

Repeatedly giving the medication in the same site can cause abnormalities in the tissue and alter absorption rates.

■ If the patient is receiving heparin or low molecular weight heparins (LMWHs), discuss the need to avoid nonsteroidal anti-inflammatory medications, such as acetylsalicylic acid (aspirin) and ibuprofen (Motrin, Advil).

These drugs increase the risk of bleeding.

■ For patients receiving heparin or LMWHs, discuss home safety and the need to avoid falls.

The patient is at risk for bleeding and needs to follow safety guidelines to prevent injury.

Documentation

■ Chart according to Medication Guidelines: Steps to Follow for All Medication (Regardless of Type or Route).
■ Some agencies have a specific code for documenting subcutaneous injections, which allows exact site documentation on an outline of the body.
■ In the nursing notes, document any related patient assessment findings, such as capillary blood sugar, signs of hypoglycemia or hyperglycemia, bruising, and so on.
■ Document in the nursing notes as well as MAR any medication that was given PRN.

Sample EHR documentation:

(continued on next page)

Procedure 23-12 ■ Administering Subcutaneous Medication (continued)

Practice Resources
Chan, H. (2001); Cocoman, A., & Barron, C. (2008); Zaybak, A., & Khorshid, L. (2008).

Thinking About the Procedure

 Go to the *Fundamentals of Nursing Skills Videos*, **Subcutaneous Injection: Locating Sites** and **Subcutaneous Injection: Administering.**

1. What are the most common sites for subcutaneous injection? Which site does the nurse demonstrate the procedure?

2. For subcutaneous medication administration, what size needle does the nurse in the DVD say you will typically use, excepting insulin?

 For suggested responses, go to Chapter 23, **Thinking About the Procedure Suggested Responses (Procedure 23-12),** on the Student Resource Disk or DavisPlus at http://davisplus.fadavis.com/Wilkinson2

Procedure 23-13 ☐ Locating Intramuscular Injection Sites

➤ For steps to follow in *all* procedures, refer to the Universal Steps for All Procedures found on the inside back cover of Volume 2. Also refer to Medication Guidelines: Steps to Follow for All Medications (Regardless of Type or Route).

Critical Aspects

- Always palpate the landmarks and the muscle mass to ensure correct placement.

Procedure 23-13A: Locating the Ventrogluteal Site
- On adults, a triangle formed between your fingers when you place your palm on the head of the trochanter, index finger on the anterior superior iliac spine, and middle finger on the iliac crest. This is the preferred site for adults and children older than 7 months.

Procedure 23-13B: Locating the Deltoid Site
- The injection site is an inverted triangle on the upper arm. The base is two to three fingerbreadths below the acromion process, and the tip is even with the top of the axilla. This is a good site in healthy adults for small volume injection, especially when other sites aren't easily accessible because of drains or dressings.

Procedure 23-13C: Locating the Vastus Lateralis Site
- Midlateral thigh: On adults, one handbreadth below the head of the trochanter and one handbreadth above the knee. The site is the middle third of this area lateral to midline of the leg. This is the preferred site for infants who are not walking.

Procedure 23-13D: Locating the Rectus Femoris Site
- Middle third of the anterior thigh. Use this site only if no others are accessible. It is more painful than other sites.

Delegation

As an RN, you can usually delegate administration of parenteral medications (including locating injection sites) to an LPN/LVN. You usually cannot delegate this task to a NAP. If you delegate the skill, you are responsible for evaluating the LPN/LVN's ability to locate injection sites correctly.

Assessment

Always palpate the landmarks and the muscle mass to ensure correct placement of the needle. Because patients body shapes differ, the site locations will vary slightly.

■ Procedure 23-13A Locating the Ventrogluteal Site

➤ When performing the procedure, always identify your patient according to agency policy and be attentive to standard precautions, hand hygiene, patient safety and privacy, body mechanics, and documentation.

Procedure Steps

1. Ask the patient to assume a side-lying position with the legs straight, if possible.
This position makes the site easier to locate.

2. Locate the greater trochanter, anterior superior iliac spine, and the iliac crest.

3. Place the palm of your hand on the greater trochanter, your index finger on the anterior superior iliac spine, and your middle finger pointing toward the iliac crest. (Use your right hand on the patient's left hip; use your left hand on the patient's right hip.) Note that if your hands are very large or very small, the location of the "triangle" will be higher or lower on the hip. Be sure you locate it well in the muscle mass. ➤

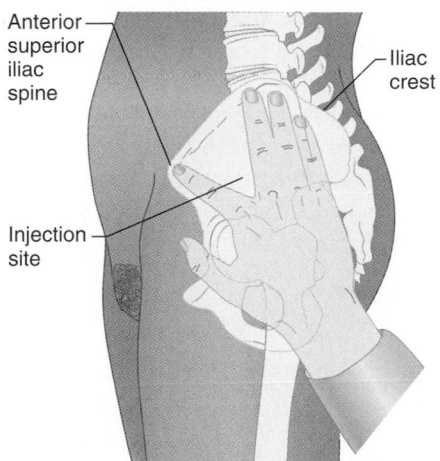

Anterior superior iliac spine

Iliac crest

Injection site

4. The middle of the triangle between your middle and index fingers is the injection site.
This is a safe site for IM administration because it is not in close proximity to any major blood vessels or nerves. The landmarks are easy to find. This large muscle can take volumes up to 5 mL in

the average adult. It is safe for patients of all ages and the preferred site for adults and children older than 7 to 12 months (there is some disagreement over the age; always palpate to assess adequacy of muscle mass, regardless of age). ▼

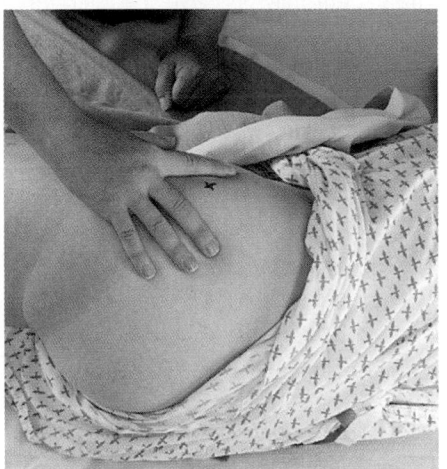

■ Procedure 23-13B Locating the Deltoid Site

➤ When performing the procedure, always identify your patient according to agency policy and be attentive to standard precautions, hand hygiene, patient safety and privacy, body mechanics, and documentation.

Procedure Steps

1. Completely expose the patient's upper arm. Remove the garment; do not roll up the sleeve.
Incomplete exposure of site and landmarks creates a risk of injecting into other than muscle tissue. This is a small site, and it is easy to make an error in location.

2. Locate the lower edge of the acromion process (knobby part of shoulder), and go two to three fingerbreadths down (3 to 5 cm). ▼

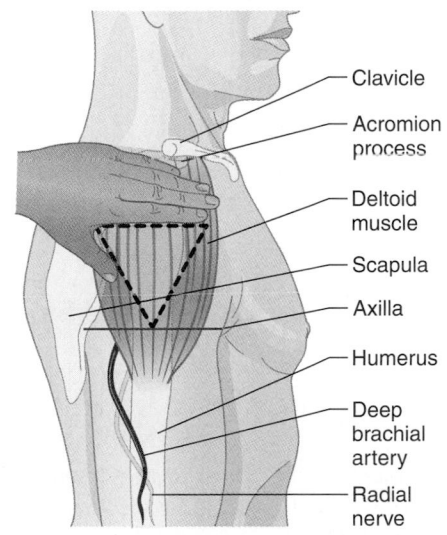

Clavicle

Acromion process

Deltoid muscle

Scapula

Axilla

Humerus

Deep brachial artery

Radial nerve

3. Draw an imaginary line from the anterior axillary crease to the posterior axillary cease.

4. The deltoid site is the resulting inverted triangle.

5. An alternative approach is to place four fingerbreadths across the deltoid muscle, with your top finger on the acromion process. The injection goes three fingerbreadths below the process in the midline of the upper arm.
Locates the appropriate site while avoiding the radial nerve and deep brachial artery. Because it is a fairly small muscle, only 0.5 to 1 mL of medication can be administered.

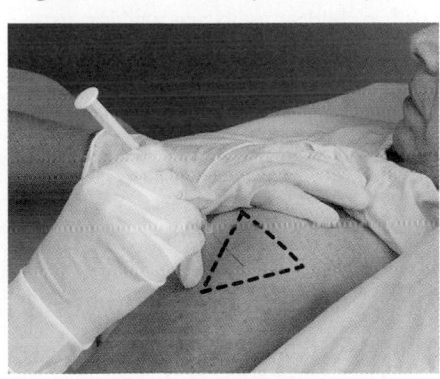

(continued on next page)

Procedure 23-13 ■ **Locating Intramuscular Injection Sites** (continued)

■ *Procedure 23-13C* **Locating the Vastus Lateralis Site**

➤ When performing the procedure, always identify your patient according to agency policy and be attentive to standard precautions, hand hygiene, patient safety and privacy, body mechanics, and documentation.

Procedure Steps

1. Position the patient lying supine or sitting.
The patient may perceive the injection as less painful if supine because he cannot see the needle enter his leg. For some people this provokes anxiety and intensifies pain.

2. Locate the greater trochanter and the lateral femoral condyle.

3. Place your hands on the thigh, with one hand against the greater trochanter, and the other edge of hand against the lateral femoral condyle.

4. Visualize a rectangle between your hands across the anterolateral thigh. The index fingers of your hands form the smaller ends of the rectangle. The long sides of the rectangle are formed by (1) drawing an imaginary line down the center of the anterior thigh and (2) drawing another line along the side of the leg, halfway between the bed and the front of the thigh. This box marks the middle third of the anterolateral thigh, which is the injection site.
The rectus femoris lies on the top (or anterior) portion of the thigh and partially covers the edge of the vastus lateralis. Therefore, do not inject too near the midline of the anterior thigh.

Because it is not near any major blood vessels or nerves, the vastus lateralis site is safe for patients of all ages and recommended site for children younger than 7 months. ▼

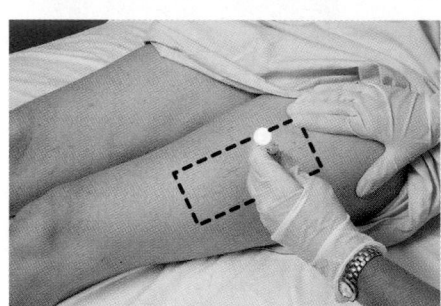

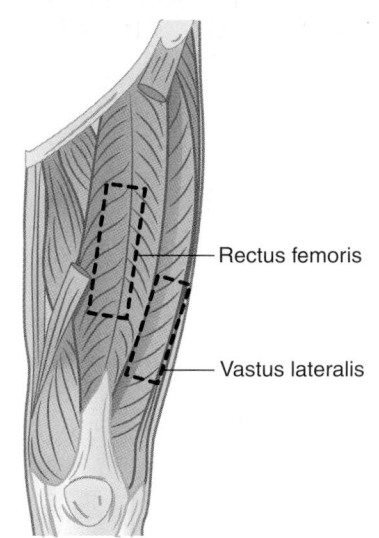

Rectus femoris

Vastus lateralis

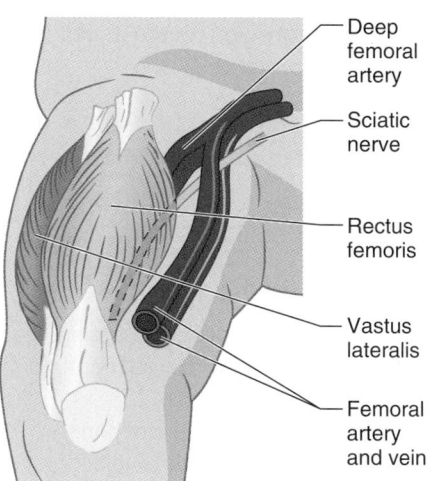

Deep femoral artery

Sciatic nerve

Rectus femoris

Vastus lateralis

Femoral artery and vein

■ *Procedure 23-13D* **Locating the Rectus Femoris Site**

➤ When performing the procedure, always identify your patient according to agency policy and be attentive to standard precautions, hand hygiene, patient safety and privacy, body mechanics, and documentation.

✛ Use this site only if no other sites are accessible and no other medication routes are feasible.

  a. Divide the top of the thigh from the groin to the knee into thirds, and identify the middle third.
  b. Visualize a rectangle in the middle of the anterior surface of the thigh. This is the location of the

injection site. Refer to the drawing of the adult thigh in Procedure 23-13C.

What if. . .

■ **My patient is a child. What is the best site to give an IM injection?**

Because an infant's muscles are not fully developed, site selection is limited.

(1) For children who are walking, use the ventrogluteal site.
(2) For children who are not yet walking: Do not use the ventrogluteal site. Use the vastus lateralis until the gluteal muscles develop further.

Thinking About the Procedure

 Go to the *Fundamentals of Nursing Skills Videos*, **Intramuscular Injections: Locating Sites.**

1. What does the nurse in the DVD say is the best way to ensure correct hand placement when giving IM injections?

2. Which two sites should be avoided for intramuscular injection?

 For suggested responses, go to Chapter 23, **Thinking About the Procedure Suggested Responses (Procedure 23-13),** on the Student Resource Disk or DavisPlus at http://davisplus.fadavis.com/Wilkinson2

Procedure 23-14 ■ Administering an Intramuscular Injection

➤ For steps to follow in *all* procedures, refer to the Universal Steps for All Procedures found on the inside back cover of Volume 2. Also refer to Medication Guidelines: Steps to Follow for All Medications (Regardless of Type or Route).

Critical Aspects

- Maintain sterile technique and standard precautions.
- Use a 1- to 5-mL syringe and a 21- to 25-gauge, 1- to 3-inch needle (longer needle if the patient is obese).
- The usual volume per injection is no more than 3 mL per injection.
- Select an appropriate injection site, and identify the site using anatomical landmarks:
  - The ventrogluteal site is preferred except in special circumstances (e.g., for many adult immunizations).
  - The deltoid site is acceptable for doses of 1 mL or less.
- Aspirate the needle before injecting. If blood appears, withdraw the needle, discard the syringe, and start over.
- Inject at a 90° angle.
- Z-track technique:

  Deliver   **D**isplace
  All   **A**spirate
  Injections   **I**nject (wait 5 to 10 seconds)
  With   **W**ithdraw
  Responsibility   **R**elease

Equipment

- Syringe and needle appropriate for volume and site
- Alcohol prep pad or chlorhexidine gluconate (CHG)-alcohol product
- Gauze pad or adhesive bandage
- Medication
- Procedure gloves
- Biohazard (sharps) container
- Small piece of gauze or cotton ball
- Small adhesive bandage

Delegation

As an RN, you can usually delegate administration of parenteral medications to an LPN/LVN. You cannot delegate this task to a NAP.

Pre-Procedure Assessments

- Identify the site of the previous injection.
- Assess the site for adequate muscle mass, bruises, edema, tenderness, redness, or other abnormalities.

Muscle mass must be large enough to absorb the amount of medication prescribed. Abnormalities at the site increase patient discomfort and alter the absorption rate of the medication.

- Assess for factors that might affect absorption of the medication, such as decreased intramuscular blood flow, as found in shock or muscle atrophy.

Decreased peripheral circulation or muscle atrophy decreases the absorption of the medication.

■ Procedure 23-14A Intramuscular Injection: Traditional Method

➤ When performing the procedure, always identify your patient according to agency policy and be attentive to standard precautions, hand hygiene, patient safety and privacy, body mechanics, and documentation.

Procedure Steps

1. Select the appropriate syringe and needle.

a. The usual syringe size is 1 to 3 mL, depending on volume of medication to be given. For doses

less than 1 mL, you can use a tuberculin syringe with an intramuscular needle.

(continued on next page)

Procedure 23-14 ■ **Administering an Intramuscular Injection** (continued)

b. The needle size is usually 21- to 25-gauge, 1½ inch in length for adults (or 1 in. for deltoid site) but a longer needle (3 in.) might be necessary to penetrate the muscle if the patient is obese.

For IM administration, the needle gauge must be appropriate for the viscosity of the medication, and the needle must be long enough to deliver the medication into the muscle.

c. Some medications are supplied in prefilled syringes, which are used for administration.

2. Draw up the medication (see Procedures 23-9A and 23-9B) or obtain prescribed unit dose and verify medication. If the volume for injection is more than 3 to 5 milliliters, divide the dose for separate injections.

3. Don procedure gloves.

Procedure gloves are required by OSHA to prevent exposure to bloodborne pathogens. You may prefer to don gloves at step 6, while waiting for the antiseptic to dry.

4. Using appropriate landmarks, identify the injection site (see Procedure 23-13).

If the client is to receive more than one injection, rotate sites.

Volumes of 1 to 5 mL may be given, depending on the muscle size (for adults, 0.5 to 1 mL in the deltoid and up to 5 mL in the vastus lateralis site). If the volume for injection is more than 3 to 5 mL, then divide the dose for a separate injection. Rotating sites reduces discomfort and tissue trauma.

5. Position the patient so that the injection site is well exposed and the patient is able to relax the appropriate muscles. Be sure the lighting is adequate. When the patient's muscles are relaxed (and not tense), it is easier to perform the injection and it helps to decrease patient discomfort.

a. *Deltoid site:* Position the patient with the arm relaxed at the side or resting on a firm surface, and completely expose the upper arm.

b. *Ventrogluteal site:* Position the patient on the opposite side, with the upper hip and knee slightly flexed.

This position may cause the trochanter to become more prominent, making it easier to locate the site.

c. *Vastus lateralis:* Position the patient supine or sitting, if the patient prefers.

d. *Rectus femoris:* Position patient supine. Because this site often causes more discomfort than others, use it only if all other sites are inaccessible and no other route is feasible.

✚ e. *Dorsogluteal:* Do not use this site because the sciatic nerve and major blood vessels are located near this site.

You must be able to fully visualize and safely access the site. A relaxed muscle decreases patient discomfort while you administer the injection.

6. Vigorously scrub the injection site with a CHG-based antiseptic or an alcohol prep pad. Place the alcohol wipe on the patient's skin outside the injection site, with a corner pointing to the site. Allow the site to dry before administering the injection.

Cleanse to remove microorganisms; follow the principle of "clean to dirty." Leaving the alcohol prep pad on the skin with a corner pointing to the injection site helps identify the location for the injection. If the alcohol has not evaporated, it may cause the skin to sting during injection.

7. Remove the needle cap.

8. With your nondominant hand, spread the skin taut between your thumb and index finger.

It is quicker, easier, and less painful to insert a needle through the skin that is taut.

9. After telling the patient what you are going to do and that he'll feel a prick as you insert the needle, hold the syringe between thumb and fingers of your dominant hand like a pencil or dart and insert the needle at a 90° angle to the skin surface. Insert fully.

Quickly inserting the needle through the skin minimizes discomfort. A 90° angle is needed for the needle to penetrate through the subcutaneous and adipose tissue to the muscle.

10. Stabilize the syringe with your nondominant hand.

This prevents the needle from moving around in the tissue, thereby causing discomfort and possible tissue trauma.

11. Aspirate by pulling back on the plunger and waiting for 5 to 10 seconds. If you obtain a blood return, remove the needle, discard the syringe, and prepare the medication again. If there is no blood return, continue with step 12.

Aspirating blood indicates that the needle is in a blood vessel. Injecting would result in administering the medication intravenously instead of intramuscularly. If the needle is in a small vessel, it may take a few seconds for the blood to appear in the syringe. There are variations in practice regarding technique for pulling back the plunger to aspirate for blood. Be sure to check with your instructor or the institution's protocol for the recommended method.

12. Using the thumb or index finger of your dominant hand, press the plunger slowly to inject the medication (5 to 10 seconds/mL).

Slow administration allows the medication to disperse and decreases discomfort.

13. Remove the needle smoothly along the line of insertion and retracting needle carefully.

Removing the needle in this way prevents pulling against the skin and tissue and minimizes discomfort.

14. Engage the safety needle device, and dispose of the entire syringe in a biohazard container. If there is no safety device, place the uncapped syringe and needle directly into a biohazard puncture-proof container.

The biohazard sharps container prevents needlestick injuries.

15. Gently blot the site with a gauze pad, and apply an adhesive bandage as needed.

Apply pressure to stop the bleeding but do not massage or rub the site after IM injection. This can cause medication to disperse into the subcutaneous tissue where the needle was injected, which might be irritating to the tissue.

16. Watch for an adverse reaction at the site for 10 to 30 minutes after the injection.

■ Procedure 23-14B Intramuscular Injection: Z-Track Method

➤ When performing the procedure, always identify your patient according to agency policy and be attentive to standard precautions, hand hygiene, patient safety and privacy, body mechanics, and documentation.

Procedure Steps

1–7. Follow Procedure 23-14A, traditional method, preceding.

8. With the side of your nondominant hand, displace the skin away from the injection site, about 2.5 to 3.5 cm (1 to 1.5 in.).
This displaces the skin and subcutaneous tissue over the muscle, so that when it is released after the injection, the medication is sealed in the muscle. ▼

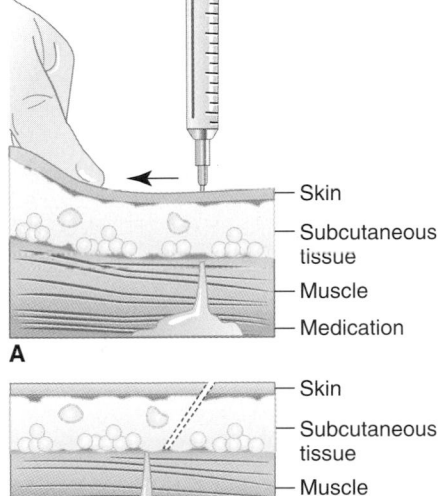

A

B

9. Holding the syringe between the thumb and fingers of your dominant hand like a pencil or dart, insert the needle at a 90° angle to the skin surface. Insert fully.
Quickly inserting the needle through the skin minimizes discomfort. A 90° angle is needed for the needle to penetrate through the subcutaneous and adipose tissue to the muscle.

10. Stabilize the syringe with the thumb and forefinger of your nondominant hand. Keep displacing the skin with your other three fingers.
Stabilizing the needle reduces discomfort and possible tissue injury. You must keep the skin retracted to create a seal after the medication is injected and the skin released.

11. Aspirate by pulling back slightly on the plunger for 5 to 10 seconds. If

you obtain a blood return, remove the needle, discard the syringe, and prepare the medication again.
Aspirating blood indicates that the needle has penetrated a vein. Continuing could result in administering the medication intravenously instead of intramuscularly. ▼

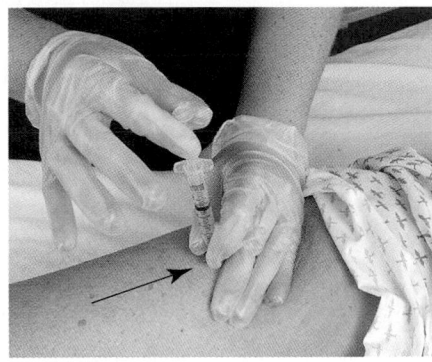

12. Using the thumb or index finger of your dominant hand, press the plunger slowly to inject the medication (5 to 10 seconds per mL).
Slow administration allows the medication to disperse and decreases discomfort.

13. Wait for 10 seconds, then withdraw the needle smoothly along the line of insertion; then immediately release the skin.
Waiting before removing the needle leaves a zig-zag needle track that traps the medication in the muscle, preventing it from leaking up into the subcutaneous tissue.

14. Engage the safety needle device, and dispose of it in a biohazard container. If there is no safety device, place the uncapped syringe and needle directly in a biohazard puncture-proof container.

15. Hold a cotton ball with light pressure over the injection site. Do not massage the site. Apply an adhesive bandage if necessary.
Light pressure will stop superficial bleeding at the injection site. Massaging and rubbing can force medication into the subcutaneous tissues.

What if . . .

■ **My patient is unable to cooperate during the procedure?**
Ask another healthcare provider or family member to help keep the patient from moving during the injection or to help position the patient.

■ **I obtain a blood return when aspirating?**
Stop aspirating. Immediately remove the needle and syringe and discard into a "sharps" container. Obtain new medication and begin the procedure again.

■ **My patient is a child; is there anything different about giving an IM injection?**

▪ Adapt the procedure to decrease pain: Apply Topical anesthetic cream (e.g., EMLA) of a topical cooling spray if time permits. If not, distract the child with conversation, or give him something to do, such as squeeze a hand. Or apply a cold compress over the site.

▪ Adapt the way you spread the skin to inject: In infants and small children, grasp the muscle with your thumb and index finger; in obese children, spread the skin and then grasp the muscle.

▪ Adapt the medication volume: Inject no more than 1 mL in a single injection, 0.5 mL in a small infant

▪ Be aware of the controversy about needle size: The CDC (2007) recommends 1- and 1¼-inch needles for children 1 year old or younger. Follow agency procedures.

■ **My patient is an older adult?**

1. Many adults have decreased muscle mass, so use a shorter needle; spread the skin and grasp the muscle to localize and stabilize the site for injection.

2. Older adults tend to bleed from the site after injection because of reduced tissue elasticity. Apply a small pressure bandage if needed.

(continued on next page)

Labels for figure (left illustration):
— Skin
— Subcutaneous tissue
— Muscle
— Medication

— Skin
— Subcutaneous tissue
— Muscle
— Medication

Procedure 23-14 ■ **Administering an Intramuscular Injection** (continued)

Evaluation
- Observe for minimal bruising or oozing that may occur at the site of injection.
- Observe for local reactions at site (e.g., pain, swelling, redness).

Patient Teaching
- Refer to Medication Guidelines: Steps to Follow for All Medications (Regardless of Type or Route).

Home Care
- Discuss safety concerns with administering medication intramuscularly in the home, such as correct disposal of biohazardous wastes and where they can obtain a puncture-proof biohazard container.

The caregiver or patient can use a large plastic bottle. The local regulations must be followed for disposal.

- Discuss with the client the need to rotate sites.

Repeatedly giving the medication in the same site can cause abnormalities in the tissue and alter absorption rates.

Documentation
- Refer to Medication Guidelines: Steps to Follow for All Medications (Regardless of Type or Route).

- Document related assessment findings, such as pain level or presence of nausea.
- Unless the medication is PRN, you will typically document it only on the MAR.

Sample documentation for PRN medication:

08/31/10 1600 *Client reports nausea following walking 150 feet with assistive device. Phenergan 25 mg administered PO. See MAR.*
08/31/10 1700 *Client reports "I don't feel like I'm going to vomit anymore."* ————— *M.Santos, RN*

Practice Resources
Floyd, S., & Meyer, A. (2007); Kroger, A.T., Atkinson, W. L., Marcuse, E. K., et al.; Advisory Committee on Immunization Practices (ACIP) Centers for Disease Control and Prevention (2006); Nicholl, L. H., & Hesby, A. (2002); Nisbet, A. C. (2006); Wynaden, D., Landsborough, I., McGowan, S., et al. (2006).

Thinking About the Procedure

 Go to the *Fundamentals of Nursing Skills Videos*, **Intramuscular Injection: Traditional** and **Z-Track.**

1. How does the nurse in the DVD mark the site for injection after locating it using landmarks? Do you see any problem with this method?

2. Does the nurse in the DVD pinch the skin or spread it taut when giving an IM injection using the traditional method?

3. In what instance would you use the Z-track method for administering IM medication?

4. Which IM site does the nurse in the DVD use to inject medication using the Z-track technique?

5. What hand does the nurse use to inject IM Z-track medication? And what hand does she use to stabilize the syringe?

 For suggested responses, go to Chapter 23, **Thinking About the Procedure Suggested Responses (Procedures 23-14A and B)**, **Intramuscular Injection**, on the Student Resource Disk or DavisPlus at http://davisplus.fadavis.com/Wilkinson2

Procedure 23-15 ■ **Adding Medications to Intravenous Fluid**

➤ For steps to follow in *all* procedures, refer to the Universal Steps for All Procedures found on the inside back cover of Volume 2. Also refer to Medication Guidelines: Steps to Follow for All Medications (Regardless of Type or Route).

Critical Aspects
- Check the compatibility of the IV solution and medication.
- Refer to agency policy regarding maximum number of meds that can be added to one IV solution.
- Assess the patency of the IV site.
- Maintain the sterility of IV fluids and medication admixture.
- Affix the medication label to the bag, with the name and dose of medication, date and time administered, and your name or initials.

Equipment

- Prescribed IV solution
- Syringe for measuring medication
- Needleless access device or safety needle (if a VAD is not available)
- Antimicrobial swab
- Label with medication, dose, date, time, and your initials

Delegation

As an RN, you should usually not delegate adding medications to IV fluids to LPN/LVNs. Nurse practice acts governing IV medication administration vary from state to state, and policies can further vary among healthcare agencies regarding which additives may be added by LPN/LVNs. Even if you delegate the skill, as the RN you are always responsible for evaluating the patient's responses, both therapeutic effects and adverse effects.

Pre-Procedure Assessments

- Assess the patency of the IV site.
- Assess the appearance of the IV site.
- Check the medication insert or PDR for appropriate time or rate for infusion and for preparation.

■ Procedure 23-15A   Adding Medication to a New IV Bag or Bottle

> When performing the procedure, always identify your patient according to agency policy and be attentive to standard precautions, hand hygiene, patient safety and privacy, body mechanics, and documentation.

Procedure Steps

1. Determine whether the medication(s) are compatible with the IV solution and with each other.
Not all medications or other additives can be mixed with the glucose or saline normally found in the primary IV bag. Multiple additives increase the possibility of incompatibility.

2. Calculate or verify the amount of medication to be instilled into the IV solution, and the rate of administration.
Verifying the dose and the rate of infusion prevents medication errors.

3. Remove any protective covers, and inspect the bag or bottle for leaks, tears, or cracks. Inspect the fluid for clarity, color, and presence of any particulate matter. Check the expiration date.
Double-checking the IV solution reduces the risk of infusing contaminated or expired solutions.

4. Using the appropriate technique, draw up the prescribed medication (see Procedures 23-9A and 23-9B, as needed). Alternatively, insert a VAD transfer device into the medication vial. Medications can come in vials, ampules, or bags.

5. Scrub all surfaces of the IV additive port with an alcohol or chlorhexidine gluconate [CHG]-alcohol combination product.
Diligent scrubbing with antimicrobial products reduces the transmission of microorganisms and helps maintain the sterility of the solution.

6. Remove the cap from the syringe, insert the needle or the needleless access device into the injection port, and inject the medication into the bag, maintaining aseptic technique. ▼

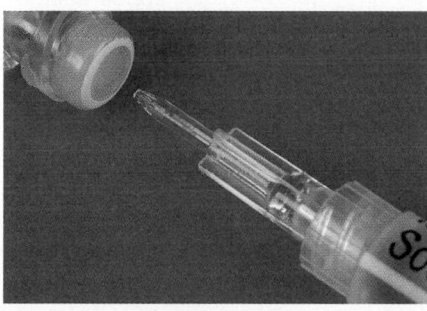

7. Mix the IV solution and medication by gently turning the bag from end to end.
Turning the bag ensures even distribution of the medication or additive into the solution.

8. Place a label on the bag so that it can be read when the bag is hung; include the medication name, dose, route, and your name. Be sure the label does not cover the solution label or volume marks.
A label informs you of additives to IV solutions. ▼

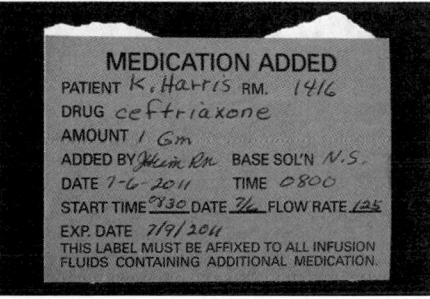

MEDICATION ADDED
PATIENT K. Harris RM. 1416
DRUG ceftriaxone
AMOUNT 1 Gm
ADDED BY JKim RN BASE SOL'N N.S.
DATE 7-6-2011   TIME 0800
START TIME 0830 DATE 7/6 FLOW RATE 125
EXP. DATE 7/9/2011
THIS LABEL MUST BE AFFIXED TO ALL INFUSION FLUIDS CONTAINING ADDITIONAL MEDICATION.

9. Dispose of used equipment, syringe, or VAD appropriately.

■ Procedure 23-15B Adding Medication to a Running IV

> When performing the procedure, always identify your patient according to agency policy and be attentive to standard precautions, hand hygiene, patient safety and privacy, body mechanics, and documentation.

Procedure Steps

1. Determine the compatibility of the medication being added to the existing solution.
Not all medications and solutions are compatible.

2. Note the volume in the existing IV bag and the amount needed for dilution of medication.
Adequate solution is needed to dilute the medication.

3. Clamp the running IV line.
Clamping prevents medication from directly infusing into the patient.

(continued on next page)

Procedure 23-15 ■ Adding Medications to Intravenous Fluid (continued)

4. Scrub all surfaces of the IV additive port with the antimicrobial swab (alcohol or chlorhexidine gluconate [CHG]-alcohol combination product).
Vigorous scrubbing decreases the transmission of microorganisms and maintains the sterility of the solution.

5. Remove the cap from the syringe, insert the safety needle or the VAD into the injection port, and inject the medication into the bag, maintaining aseptic technique. ▼

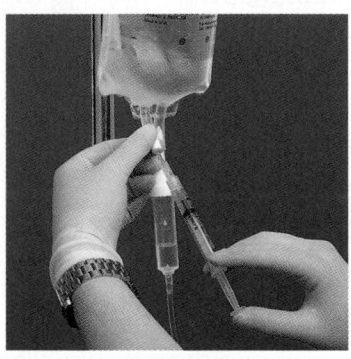

6. Mix the IV solution and medication by gently turning the bag from end to end. Keep the bag above the level of the patient's IV insertion site and do not invert the drip chamber.
Turing the IV bag ensures even distribution of the medication or additive into the solution. The height of the bag keeps blood from backing up in the IV tubing.

7. Place the label on the bag so that it can be read when the bag is hung. Be sure the label does not cover the solution label or volume marks.
A label provides information regarding additives to IV solutions.

8. Unclamp the IV line, and run the IV at the prescribed rate.

9. Dispose of used equipment, syringe, needle or VAD appropriately.

What if. . .

■ **The IV fluid infiltrates into a peripheral site?**

Discontinue the infusion. Restart the peripheral IV, making sure you have good blood return and the line flushes easily. Some IVs are positional. This means the flow may be partially obstructed when the cannula in the vein lodges against the vein wall. In this case, the rate the IV fluid to be delivered is likely to be compromised.

If the tissue at the site of infiltration appears to be swollen and tender, you might apply a cool compress to the site. If the infusion contained irritating substances, such as calcium, dopamine, or various chemotherapy agents, you might need to inject antidote medication into the intradermal layer. Call the prescriber for an order, if this is necessary.

Evaluation

■ Check the IV line at least once every hour to ensure that the ordered or calculated rate is maintained.
■ Assess the patient for complaints of pain at the infusion site.

Patient Teaching

■ Discuss reasons the medication is being given intravenously.
■ Let the patient know whether it is a continuous or intermittent infusion.
■ Explain the need to report immediately any reactions to the medication, such as breathing problems, rashes, or pain at the IV insertion site.

Documentation

■ Document information according to Medication Guidelines: Steps to Follow for All Procedures (Regardless of Type or Route).
■ If you added medication to an existing IV setup, document related patient assessment findings, such as appearance of IV site and complaints of pain or discomfort during administration.
■ Findings are usually documented on an IV flow record rather than in the nursing notes. Chart a nursing note only if there is something outside of the expected findings (e.g., if the IV has infiltrated).

Practice Resources
Infusion Nurses Society (2006a, 2006b).

Procedure 23-16 ■ Administering IV Push Medication

➤ For steps to follow in *all* procedures, refer to the Universal Steps for All Procedures found on the inside back cover of Volume 2. Also refer to Medication Guidelines: Steps to Follow for All Medications (Regardless of Type or Route).

Critical Aspects

■ Determine the type and amount of dilution needed for the medication.
■ Determine the amount of time needed to administer medication.
■ Ensure the patency of the line before administration.
■ Flush the line before and after administering the medication.
■ Maintain sterility.

Equipment

- Syringe appropriate for medication volume and the type of line (e.g., peripheral IV, PICC, etc.)
- If you are administering through an intermittent device:
  - Two 5- to 10-mL syringes, or one 10-mL syringe with 2 to 10 mL of normal saline for flushing the line

Although either is acceptable, separate syringes pose less risk of contamination.

  - Depending on site and facility policy, one 5- to 10-mL syringe containing 2 to 5 mL of heparin flush (or saline) solution

Agency procedures differ: Some use saline to flush; others use heparin.

- Alcohol prep pad, or CHG-alcohol combination product and gauze pad
- Procedure gloves

Delegation

As an RN, you may, in some situations, be able to delegate administration of parenteral medications to an LPN/LVN. However, this is not a common practice.

Pre-Procedure Assessments

- Check the compatibility of the medication with the existing IV solution, if it is infusing.

Medications can be physically or chemically incompatible with the IV solution. Physical incompatibility will often be obvious because precipitation may occur. Chemical incompatibility is not obvious and may result in the medication's having a weaker or a stronger effect than anticipated.

- Assess the patency of the IV line.

If the line is occluded, you will not be able to instill the medication.

- Check the site for redness, swelling, tenderness, and other signs of infiltration or phlebitis.

Some medications are irritating and may be toxic to the tissue. If the IV line is infiltrated, the medication may leak into the tissue and cause injury. IV medications can also irritate the veins and cause phlebitis. Do not infuse a medication into a compromised site.

■ Procedure 23-16A Administering IV Push Through an Infusing Primary IV Line

➤ When performing the procedure, always identify your patient according to agency policy and be attentive to standard precautions, hand hygiene, patient safety and privacy, body mechanics, and documentation.

Procedure Steps

1. Determine how fast the medication may be administered and whether the medication needs to be diluted for administration. Also, check to be sure the medication is compatible with the solution infusing.

IV push medications are frequently injected over 1 minute. Some medications must be administered over a longer time period, and some require diluting before administration. Giving an IV push medication too fast and/or undiluted can result in local or systemic adverse reactions.

2. Prepare the medication from a vial or ampule or obtain the prescribed unit dose and verify medication with the order (refer to Procedure 23-9A and Procedure 23-9B). Dilute as needed. Temporarily pause the infusion

pump to administer the medication.

3. Don procedure gloves. Thoroughly scrub all surfaces of the injection port closest to the patient with the alcohol prep pad or CHG-alcohol combination product. Use povidone-iodine solution (Betadine) only if the patient is sensitive to the other products.

Follow agency policy. Some facilities require nurses to cleanse the port for 1 minute when accessing venous access devices. Using the port closest to the patient minimizes the distance the medication must travel and gets it into the patient's circulation faster. You must use an injection port, which is self-sealing. If you puncture the plastic IV tubing, it will leak.

4. Insert the medication syringe into the injection port. If a needleless

system is not available, use a syringe with a safety needle.

Using a needleless system prevents needlestick injuries.

5. Pinch or clamp the IV tubing between the IV bag and the port. Occluding the tubing upline of the port prevents the medication from being injected back toward the IV bag. ▼

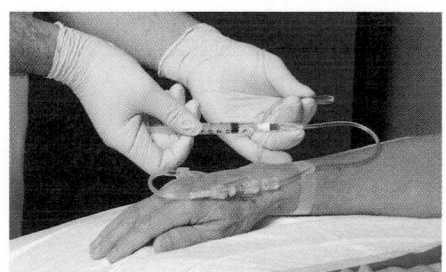

(continued on next page)

Procedure 23-16 ■ Administering IV Push Medication (continued)

6. Gently aspirate by slowly pulling back on the plunger to check for a blood return.
(1) A blood return is one indication that the IV catheter is in the vein. An IV site may still be patent if no blood is returned, and an infiltrated IV line may have a blood return. Use the blood return as one indication of patency (Phillips, 2010). (2) Injecting an IV medication into an IV site that is not patent administers the medication into the local tissue at the IV site. Some medications will cause tissue irritation and even necrosis if infused into the subcutaneous tissue. In addition, the patient would not receive

the immediate therapeutic benefit from the drug

7. If blood is returned, administer a small increment of the medication while observing for reactions to the medication.
Slow injection allows you to observe adverse reactions to the medication before all the medication has been injected. Administering IV push medications carries the highest potential risk to the patient because immediate, life-threatening reactions can occur.

8. Administer another increment of the medication (you may pinch the tubing while injecting medication and

release it when not injecting; this is optional).

9. Repeat steps 7 and 8 until the medication has been administered over the correct amount of time. Medications require different administration times. Follow agency guidelines, physician orders, and pharmaceutical information regarding whether the medication needs to be diluted and the rate of administration.

10. If you clamped the IV tubing during the infusion, open it now and reset it resume at the correct infusion rate.

■ **Procedure 23-16B** **Administering IV Push Through an Intermittent Device (IV Lock) When No Extension Tubing Is Attached to the Venous Access Device**

➤ When performing the procedure, always identify your patient according to agency policy and be attentive to standard precautions, hand hygiene, patient safety and privacy, body mechanics, and documentation.

Procedure Steps

1. Check compatibility of the medication with the existing intravenous solution, if one is infusing. Determine how fast the medication may be administered and whether the medication needs to be diluted for administration.
IV push medications are frequently injected over 1 minute. Some medications must be administered over a longer time period, and some medications must be diluted before administration. Giving an IV push medication too fast and/or undiluted can result in an adverse local or systemic reaction..

2. Prepare the medication from a vial or ampule. Dilute as needed. Refer to Procedures 23-9A and 23-9B.

3. Select the appropriate size of syringe for flush solution.
Smaller syringes exert more pressure against the wall of the IV catheter than do larger syringes. Check with the IV catheter company for specific recommendations, and follow agency policy.

4. Don procedure gloves. Thoroughly scrub all surfaces of the injection port

closest to the patient with an alcohol prep pad or CHG-alcohol combination product. Use povidone-iodine solution (Betadine) only when the patient cannot tolerate an alcohol-based disinfectant.
Follow agency policy. Some facilities require nurses to scrub all surfaces of the port with an alcohol-based antimicrobial product for 1 minute when accessing venous access devices. Using the port closest to the patient minimizes the amount of medication in the IV line.

5. Insert the flush syringe into the injection port.
Flushing the line allows you to check for patency before injecting the medication.

6. Gently aspirate by pulling back on the plunger to check for a blood return.
A blood return is an indication that the IV catheter is in the vein. An IV site may still be patent if no blood is returned, and an infiltrated IV may have a blood return. Use the blood return as one indication of patency.

7. Administer a flush solution to clear the line if blood return is obtained. Use a forward pushing

motion on the syringe, with a slow, steady injection technique. If blood is not returned, see "What If..." at the end of Procedure 23-16.
(1) Rapid flushing causes a jet effect that can cause the catheter tip to migrate to other venous locations; this should be avoided. (2) Injecting an IV medication into an IV site that is not patent administers the medication into the local tissue at the IV site. Some medications will cause tissue irritation and even necrosis if infused into the subcutaneous tissue.

8. Continuing to hold the injection port; remove the flush syringe; scrub the port with the alcohol prep pad or CHG-alcohol based product. Use povidone-iodine only when the patient is sensitive to alcohol-based disinfectants; and attach the medication syringe.
Cleansing the port reduces the risk of introducing microorganisms into the bloodstream.

9. Administer the medication in small increments over the correct time interval.
For example, if 1 mL of the medication is to be given over 1 minute,

inject approximately 0.25 mL every 15 seconds. ▼

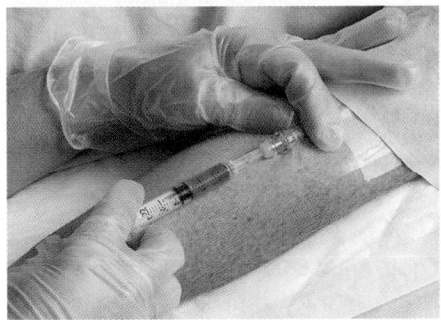

10. Continuing to hold the injection port, remove medication syringe, and scrub all surfaces of the port with

alcohol prep pad or CHG-alcohol-based product. Attach the flush syringe. Vigorous scrubbing reduces the chance of contamination of the port.

11. Administer the flush solution.
Flushing ensures that all the medication has been administered and prevents occlusion of the IV catheter.

12. Use positive-pressure technique when removing the syringe by placing your thumb or index finger to avoid movement of the plunger. Follow equipment guidelines; you may not always need to do this.
This technique prevents blood backflow into the IV catheter, which

might cause an occlusion. Follow equipment guidelines because some injection ports maintain positive pressure by removing the syringe and then closing the clamp. ▼

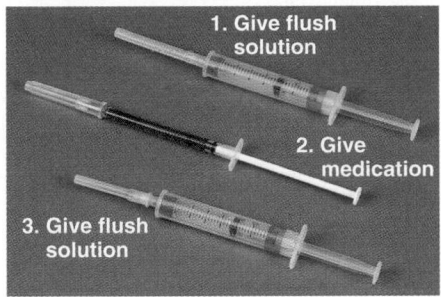

1. Give flush solution
2. Give medication
3. Give flush solution

■ **Procedure 23-16C** **Administering IV Push Through an Intermittent Device with IV Extension Tubing**

➤ When performing the procedure, always identify your patient according to agency policy and be attentive to standard precautions, hand hygiene, patient safety and privacy, body mechanics, and documentation.

Procedure Steps

1. Check the compatibility of the medication with the existing intravenous solution, if one is infusing. Determine how fast the medication may be administered and whether the medication needs to be diluted for administration.
IV push medications are frequently injected over 1 minute. Some medications must be administered over a longer time period, and some medications require diluting prior to administration. Giving an IV push medication too fast and/or undiluted can result in a local or systemic adverse reactions.

2. Prepare the medication from a vial or ampule. Dilute as needed. Refer to Procedures 23-9A and 23-9B.
Some medications must be diluted to prevent adverse reactions during administration.

3. Determine the volume of any extension tubing attached to the access port.
The volume of extension sets can be greater than the IV push medication being given. If not accounted for, all the medication may be injected into the patient's bloodstream at once when the second flush solution is given.

4. Don procedure gloves.

5. Scrub all surfaces of the injection port with an antiseptic wipe.

6. Administer the flush after gently pulling back on the plunger to check for a blood return. If blood is not returned, assess patency by administering a small amount of the flush solution and monitoring for ease of administration, swelling at the IV site, or patient complaint of discomfort at the site.

7. Again scrub the port. Attach the medication syringe and inject a volume of medication equal to the volume of the extension set at the same rate as the flush solution.

This clears the line of saline solution and fills it with medication; it also flushes the IV catheter with saline as the medication pushes the saline through the catheter. When using a 5-mL syringe for peripheral lines and a 10-mL syringe for central lines, administer the flush solution briskly. When you use a smaller syringe, use a slower rate to prevent excess pressure damaging the vein or shearing of the IV cannula. ▼

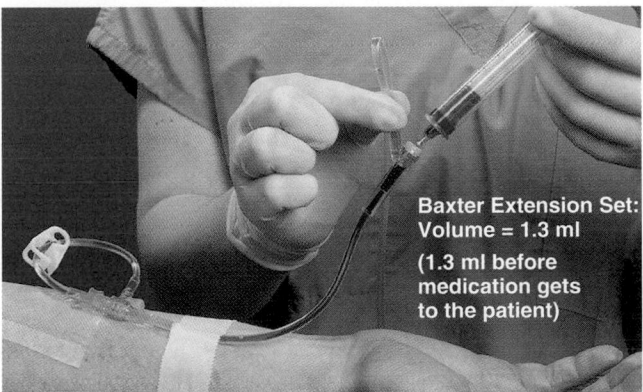

Baxter Extension Set: Volume = 1.3 ml
(1.3 ml before medication gets to the patient)

8. Using a slow, steady injection technique, administer the remainder of the medication over the prescribed time interval for the specific medication. Never force the flush solution into the venous access device if you feel resistance. If you feel any resistance when flushing the line, look
(continued on next page)

Procedure 23-16 ■ Administering IV Push Medication (continued)

for a closed clamp on the catheter or tubing. Or you may check to see if an inline filter is clogged. Do not proceed with the medication infusion until you are sure the catheter is still correctly positioned and that the fluid pathway is unobstructed.

Rapid flushing can create a jet effect that can cause the catheter tip to migrate to an unintended venous location.

9. Continuing to hold the injection connector, remove the medication syringe, vigorously scrub all surfaces of the injection connector for at least 15 seconds and attach the flush syringe. The only time the catheter hub should be opened is when the needleless connector or primary continuous IV set must be changed usually at 96 hour intervals.

10. Administer the same amount of flush solution at the same rate as the medication, using a slow, steady injection technique. Then administer the remainder of the flush solution. For example, if the extension tubing has a volume of 1.3 mL, give the first 1.3 mL of the flush solution at the same rate as the medication.
(1) At this step, the extension tubing contains all the medication. Administering the flush solution all at once pushes the medication too fast (it will enter the vein

all at once). (2) Once you have cleared the medication from the extension tubing and all the medication is already in the vein, then the rate no longer matters as far as the medication is concerned.

11. Use a slow steady injection pressure technique when removing the syringe. Continue to administer the flush solution while withdrawing the syringe cannula from the injection port. Follow equipment instructions regarding the method and order of removing the syringe, closing the clamp, maintaining positive pressure.

12. Discard the flushing syringe from the needleless connector into a safety disposal container.

What if . . .

■ **No blood is returned when I aspirate?**

■ Do not give IV push medication until you can verify the patency of the IV site. If the patency of the IV site is questionable, restart the IV at another site.

■ Further assess the patency of the IV line by administering a small amount of the saline flush and monitoring for ease of administration, swelling at the IV site, or patient complaint of discomfort at the site.

■ Another technique to determine patency is to lower the IV bag below the level of the IV site—a blood return should occur

■ If the IV catheter is a small gauge, a blood return may not always be aspirated.

■ **The IV infusing a dextrose solution infiltrates into the surrounding tissue of a peripheral catheter?**

Immediately stop the running fluid and remove the catheter. Initially apply a cool, moist compress to the site and later use heat to promote comfort.

If the IV line is infiltrated, it can cause tissue injury, inflammation, and edema. Medications and even IV fluids leaking into tissues can be irritating or even lead to tissue necrosis and sloughing.

■ Some medications, such as vasopressors (e.g., dopamine), might need intradermal injection of an antidote, such as phentolamine (Regitine), to reverse the effects of extravasation.

■ If the IV fluid contains dextrose at > 10% concentration, calcium salts, potassium salts, sodium bicarbonate, blood, and parenteral nutrition, then contact the primary care provider, who will likely prescribe injection of hyaluronidase (Amphadase) into the surrounding tissue.

Evaluation

■ Assess the patient for complaints of pain or discomfort at the site.

Patient Teaching

■ Discuss why the medication is being administered intravenously.
■ Explain the need to report immediately any reaction to the medication.

Home Care

■ Discuss with the client and/or caregiver how to care for the IV site, including flushing. Many IV push

medications need to be administered by a nurse. However, cost-cutting efforts have led to short hospital stays, and some clients are now being taught to give their own IV antibiotics at home.
■ Explain how to identify problems with the IV site, such as infiltration and phlebitis.
■ Determine whether the client has adequate facilities for storing the medication, such as refrigeration if needed.
■ Discuss safety issues, such as keeping medications and needles and syringes secure and away from children and pets.

Documentation

Besides charting according to Medication Guidelines: Steps to Follow for All Medications (Regardless of Type or Route), document related patient assessment findings, such as the appearance of the IV site and patient complaints of pain or discomfort during IV administration. You will usually document on an IV flow record and/or MAR rather than in the nursing notes. Chart a nursing note only if there is a problem (e.g., if the patient experiences pain when you administer the medication).

Practice Resources
Infusion Nurses Society (2006a, 2006b); Phillips, D. (2010).

Thinking About the Procedure

 Go to the *Fundamentals of Nursing Skills Videos*, **IV Push Through a Primary Line** and **IV Push Through an IV Lock.**

1. When administering an IV push through a primary IV line, what is the technique the nurse in the DVD uses to ensure the line is patent and the medication doesn't cause an immediate adverse effect?

2. When administering medication by IV push through an intermittent device (IV lock), the nurse in the DVD aspirates blood back into the extension tubing to check for IV patency. How does she clear the tubing of the blood and why?

 For suggested responses, go to Chapter 23, **Thinking About the Procedure Suggested Responses (Procedures 23-16A and B),** on the Student Resource Disk or DavisPlus at http://davisplus.fadavis.com/Wilkinson2

Procedure 23-17 — Administering Medications by Intermittent Infusion

➤ For steps to follow in *all* procedures, refer to the Universal Steps for All Procedures found on the inside back cover of Volume 2. Also refer to Medication Guidelines: Steps to Follow for All Medications (Regardless of Type or Route). For step-by-step instructions in using volume-control devices (pumps), see Procedure 36–9.

Critical Aspects

- Ensure the compatibility of the IV solution and medication, in both the primary and secondary (tandem and piggyback) systems.
- Assess the IV site and the patency of the line.
- Calculate the amount of medication to add to the solution.
- Use the correct amount and type of diluent solution.
- Use the correct rate of administration.
- Determine the correct primary line port in which to infuse the medication.
- Affix the correct label to the secondary bag, identifying the infusate, patient name, start date and hour, discard date and hour, and your initials.

Equipment

- Correct size syringe for measuring medication
- Needleless access cannula or safety needle
- Volume-control IV set (e.g., Buretrol, Volutrol, Soluset) or small bag of diluted medication with piggyback or tandem tubing
- Primary IV solution and tubing (unless one is already infusing)
- Antimicrobial swabs
- Labels for the IV tubing and medication administration system

Delegation

Nurse practice acts governing IV medication administration vary from state to state, and policies can further vary among healthcare agencies, regarding which medications or methods of administration the LPN/LVN/LVN may perform. You should not delegate this procedure to a NAP.

Pre-Procedure Assessments

- Check the compatibility of the medication with the IV solution.

Medications can be physically or chemically incompatible with the IV solution. Physical incompatibility will be obvious if precipitation occurs. Chemical incompatibility is not obvious and may result in the medication's having a weaker or a stronger effect than anticipated.

- Assess the patency of the IV line.

If the line is occluded, or if the fluid has infiltrated, the medication will not infuse.

- Check the site for redness, swelling, tenderness, and other signs of infiltration or phlebitis.

Some medications are irritating to the tissue. If the IV fluid has infiltrated, medication would leak into the tissue and cause injury. IV medications can also irritate the veins and cause phlebitis. Do not infuse a medication into a compromised site.

(continued on next page)

Procedure 23-17 ■ Administering Medications by Intermittent Infusion (continued)

- Determine the amount of IV solution needed to administer the specific medication.

Most medications specify (on the order or on the label) specific dilution to prevent potential harm to the patient.

- Determine the time period over which the solution needs to be infused.

Infusing a medication too slowly may result in an inadequate blood level to achieve therapeutic levels, and infusing a medication too rapidly can cause harm.

- Perform assessments that will provide a basis for evaluating the drug's effectiveness, such as checking blood pressure after administering an antihypertensive agent.

■ Procedure 23-17A Using a Volume-Control Administration Set

➤ For step-by-step instructions in using volume-control devices (pumps), see Procedure 36-9. If you have not already done so, affix a label to the secondary bag indicating the name and amount of medication, date and time given, and your name or initials.

➤ When performing the procedure, always identify your patient according to agency policy and be attentive to standard precautions, hand hygiene, patient safety and privacy, body mechanics, and documentation.

Procedure Steps

1. Prepare the volume-control set tubing if they are not already closed.
   a. Close both the upper and lower clamps on the tubing.

Clamping prevents air bubbles from forming in the tubing.

   b. Open the clamp of the air vent on the volume-control chamber.

Venting allows air to escape, which lets the IV solution enter the chamber.

   c. Maintaining sterile procedure, attach administration spike of the volume-control set to the primary IV bag.
   d. Fill the volume-control chamber with the desired amount of IV solution by opening the clamp between the IV bag and the volume-control chamber. When the correct amount of solution is in the chamber, close the clamp.

The drip chamber provides solution for priming the tubing and diluting the IV medication.

   e. Prime the rest of the tubing by opening the clamp below the chamber and running the IV fluid until all the air has been expelled.

Priming clears the IV tubing of air.

   f. Recheck the amount of fluid in the volume control chamber, and, if needed, add more fluid to the desired amount.

Priming the tubing alters the volume in the chamber. You must fill to the desired amount.

2. With an alcohol or chlorhexidine gluconate-alcohol swab, vigorously scrub all surfaces of the injection port closest to the patient.

Vigorous cleansing is necessary to remove microorganisms and particles from the IV port, which could potentially enter the patient's bloodstream.

3. Connect the end of the volume-control IV line to the patient's IV site. Attach it directly to the IV catheter, to the extension tubing, or to the injection port closest to patient.

4. Scrub the injection port on the volume-control chamber, attach the medication syringe (preferably with a blunt, needleless device), and inject the medication into the solution in the chamber.

5. Gently rotate the chamber to mix the medication in the IV solution.

Rotating the IV bag distributes the medication within the IV solution.

6. Open the lower clamp, and start the infusion at the correct flow rate.

Unclamping allows the infusion of the medication. A correct flow rate infuses the medication over the correct amount of time and prevents a toxic reaction to it.

7. Label the volume-control chamber with the date, time, medication and doses added, and your initials, according to agency policy.

8. When the medication has finished infusing, add a small amount of the primary IV fluid to the chamber, and flush the tubing. For the flush volume, use two times the volume in the dead space of the tubing; check the tubing package for the amount.

Flushing the line ensures all the medication is given to the patient and does not adhere to the tubing. ▼

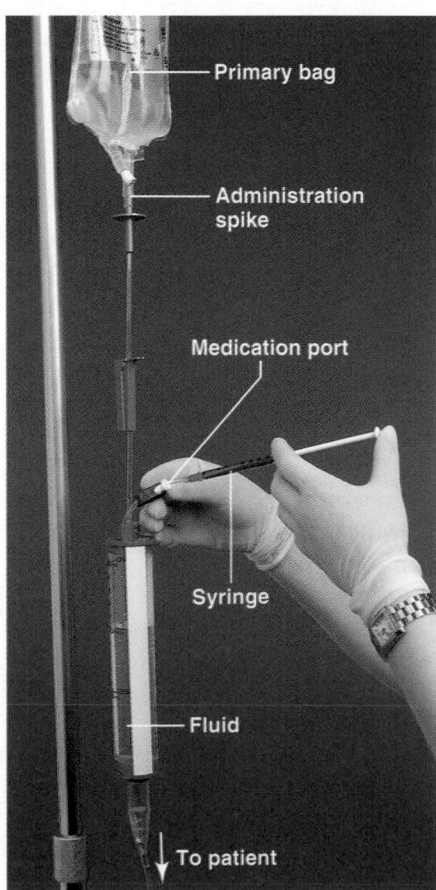

- Primary bag
- Administration spike
- Medication port
- Syringe
- Fluid
- To patient

Thinking About the Procedure

 Go to the *Fundamentals of Nursing Skills Videos,* **Administration Sets: Volume-Control.**

1. When using a volume-control administration set to infuse medication, what does the nurse do to ensure the patient has received the entire medication dose?

 For suggested responses, go to Chapter 23, **Thinking About the Procedure Suggested Responses (Procedure 23-17A),** on the Student Resource Disk or DavisPlus at http://davisplus.fadavis.com/Wilkinson2

■ Procedure 23-17B Using a Piggyback Administration Set

➤ For step-by-step instructions in using intermittent infusion devices (pumps), see Procedure 36–3. If you have not already done so, affix a label to the secondary bag indicating the name and amount of medication, date and time given, and your name or initials.

➤ When performing the procedure, always identify your patient according to agency policy and be attentive to standard precautions, hand hygiene, patient safety and privacy, body mechanics, and documentation.

Procedure Steps

1. Draw up the medication, and inject it into the piggyback solution (see Procedure 23-15). This step is not necessary if the medication comes premixed from the pharmacy, which is frequently the case.

2. Be sure you have the correct tubing. Attach the piggyback tubing to the medication bag. Do not touch the spike.
Tubing connects the piggyback to the primary line. Prevents contamination of tubing and solution. Piggyback tubing is short. Tandem tubing is long.

3. Be sure the slide clamp is closed. Squeeze the drip chamber, filling it one-third to one-half full.
Clamping prevents excess air coming into the line when you are priming the tubing.

4. Open the clamp and prime the tubing, holding the end of the tubing lower than the bag of fluid. Do not let more than one drop of fluid escape from the end of the tubing. Close the clamp.

Step 4 Variation. "Backflushing" the Piggyback Line

a. As an alternative, you can clamp the piggyback tubing, scrub all surfaces of the primary "Y" port, and attach the piggyback setup with the needleless system.

b. Open the clamp on the piggyback tubing, and lower the bag below the primary to prime the piggyback line.
c. Once the line is primed, clamp the piggyback tubing.
Priming removes air from the tubing and maintains sterility of the system. Medications are diluted in small amounts of fluid (usually 50 to 100 mL), so you should take care not to waste any medication. The backflush method ensures you will not lose any of the medication.

5. Label the bag with the date, the medication, the dosage, and your initials. Label the tubing with the time, the date, and your initials.
Tubing used for intermittent infusions can be used for 48 to 72 hours, depending on facility policy; labeling allows the nurse to know when it must be changed.

6. Hang the piggyback container on the IV pole. Lower the primary IV container to hang below the level of the piggyback IV.
Gravity causes the higher bag (the piggyback IV setup) to flow instead of the primary IV setup. When the piggyback IV solution has infused, the primary IV line will resume infusing.

7. Open the clamp of the piggyback line, and regulate the drip rate with the roller clamp on the primary line.

Regulate to the prescribed infusion rate for the medication. ▼

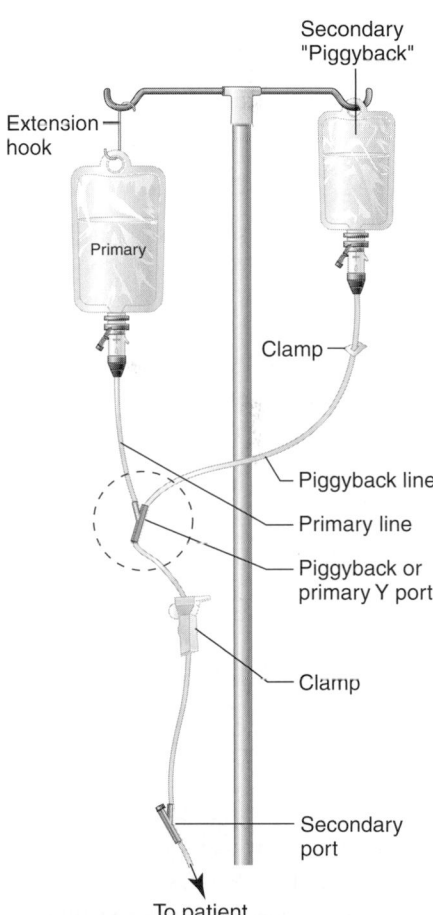

Because the piggyback is the only bag running, the primary roller clamp regulates the speed of the piggyback bag.

(continued on next page)

Procedure 23-17 ■ **Administering Medications by Intermittent Infusion** (continued)

---

8. At the end of the infusion, clamp the piggyback tubing, and move the primary tubing back to its original height. Use the roller clamp to reset the primary bag to its correct infusion rate.

This ensures that the primary fluids flow at their ordered rate rather than flowing at the rate the piggyback medication was flowing—which would probably be either faster or slower than the prescribed primary fluid rate.

Thinking About the Procedure

 Go to the *Fundamentals of Nursing Skills Videos*, **Administration Sets: Piggyback.**

1. In the DVD, which bag was hung in a higher position? Why?

2. How is the primary bag in the DVD hung below the level of the piggyback bag?

 For suggested responses, go to Chapter 23, **Thinking About the Procedure Suggested Responses (Procedure 23-17B),** on the Student Resource Disk or DavisPlus at http://davisplus.fadavis.com/Wilkinson2

■ Procedure 23-17C Using a Tandem Administration Set

➤ For step-by-step instructions in using intermittent infusion devices (pumps), see Procedure 36-3. If you have not already done so, affix a label to the secondary bag indicating the name and amount of medication, date and time given, and your name or initials.

➤ When performing the procedure, always identify your patient according to agency policy and be attentive to standard precautions, hand hygiene, patient safety and privacy, body mechanics, and documentation.

Procedure Steps

1. Draw up the medication, and inject it into the tandem solution (see Procedure 23-15A). This step is not necessary if the medication comes premixed from the pharmacy, which is frequently the case.

2. Be sure you have the correct tubing. After closing the clamp on the tubing, attach the tandem tubing to the (medication) bag. Do not touch the spike.
Tubing connects the tandem set to the primary line. Prevents contamination of tubing and solution. Tubing for the tandem set is longer so the bag can be hung for gravity infusion, if a pump is not in use.

3. Squeeze the drip chamber, filling it one-third to one-half full.
Fluid in the drip chamber prevents excess air in line when priming tubing.

4. Open the clamp and prime the tubing, holding the end of the tubing lower than the bag of fluid. Do not let more than one drop of fluid escape from the end of the tubing. Close the clamp.

Step 4 Variation. "Backflushing" the Tandem Line

a. As an alternative, you can clamp the tandem tubing, scrub the tandem port (the one nearest the patient), and attach the tandem tubing with the needleless system.
b. Open the clamp on the tandem tubing, and lower the bag below the primary line to prime the tandem line.
c. Once the line is primed, clamp the tubing.
Priming removes air from the tubing and maintains sterility of the system. Medications are diluted in small amounts of fluid (usually 50 to 100 mL), so you should take care not to waste any medication. The backflush method ensures that you will not lose any of the medication while clearing the line of air.

5. Label the bag with the date, the medication, the dosage, and your initials. Label the tubing with the time, the date, and your initials.
Tubing used for intermittent infusions can be used for 48 to 72 hours, depending on facility policy; allows the nurse to know when it must be changed.

6. Hang the tandem bag at the same height as the primary bag. ▼

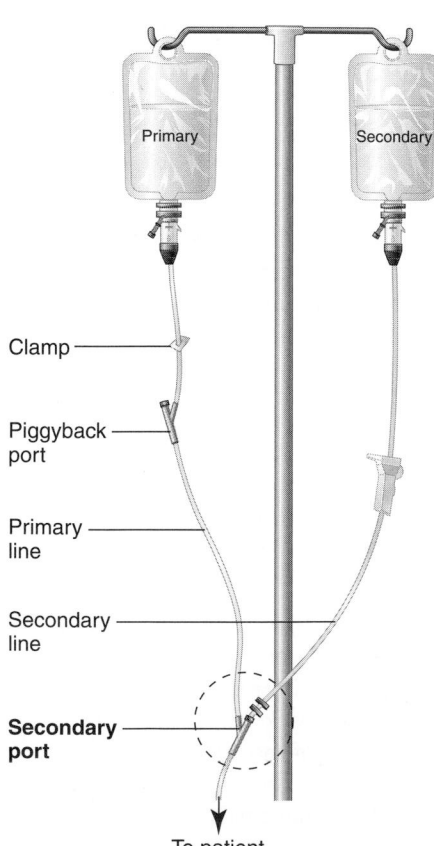

To patient

7. Scrub all surfaces of the lower port of the primary line with an antimicrobial swab, and connect the tandem tubing to this port with needleless system. (If you back-flushed in step 4, the tubing will already be connected.)
Scrubbing prevents contamination.

8. When you are using a tandem set, both the tandem and primary sets run simultaneously. Unclamp the tandem tubing, and regulate the tandem rate at its prescribed infusion rate—the tandem line has its own roller clamp.

You also need to verify the primary set flow rate.
Verifying the medication dosage ensures that the medication is administered at a rate that will provide desired therapeutic effects and reduce possibility of adverse reactions. Infusing the tandem set may change the rate of infusion of the primary set.

9. At the end of the infusion, clamp the tandem tubing. The primary bag should continue to flow at its prescribed rate.

10. Dispose of used supplies safely and according to agency procedures.

What if. . .

- **The medication is not compatible with the primary infusion?**
- Stop and disconnect the primary infusion. Hang a compatible flush solution in its place.
- Connect the tandem (medication) tubing to the flush solution tubing, and hang the tandem bag.

Evaluation

- Assess for patient complaints of pain or discomfort at the site.
- Intermittent infusions are generally infused over 15 to 60 minutes; therefore, you need to assess the patient as soon as the medication begins infusing and every 15 to 20 minutes until it is absorbed.

Patient Teaching

- Discuss why the medication is being administered intravenously.
- Explain the need to report immediately any reaction to the medication.

Home Care

- Discuss with the client and/or caregiver how to care for the IV site. Only a nurse should add medications to the IV.
- Explain how to identify problems with the IV site, such as infiltration and phlebitis.
- Assess whether the client has adequate facilities for storing the medication, such as refrigeration if needed.
- Discuss safety issues, such as keeping medications, needles, and syringes secure and away from children and pets.

Documentation

- Chart information according to Medication Guidelines: Steps to Follow for All Medications (Regardless of Type or Route).
- Document related patient assessment findings, such as the appearance of the IV site and patient complaints of pain or discomfort during the administration.

Practice Resource
Infusion Nurses Society (2006a).

Thinking About the Procedure

 Go to the *Fundamentals of Nursing Skills Videos,* **Administration Sets: Tandem.**

1. When priming the tubing of a tandem administration set, where does the nurse in this DVD do with the solution flushed through the line? Why?

 For suggested responses, go to Chapter 23, **Thinking About the Procedure Suggested Responses (Procedure 23-17C)**, on the Student Resource Disk or DavisPlus at http://davisplus.fadavis.com/Wilkinson2

Procedure 23-18   Administering Medication Through a Central Venous Access Device

➤ For steps to follow in *all* procedures, refer to the Universal Steps for All Procedures found on the inside back cover of Volume 2. Also refer to Medication Guidelines: Steps to Follow for All Medications (Regardless of Type or Route).

Critical Aspects

- First verify the medication can be administered safely through a central site.
- Scrub all surfaces of the catheter connector, with an alcohol or CHG-alcohol combination product every time you enter the line.
- Flush the line before and after administering medication. Use saline, heparinized flush solution, or solution from the infusing IV line.
- Clamp the line between the IV infusion set and the medication port. Open the clamp after medication is administered.
- After administration, monitor and report suspected CVAD dislodgement, line-related infection, or other complications.

Equipment

- Syringe appropriate for medication volume
- Needleless device or safety syringe with a filter needle for drawing up the medication (you would also need a sterile needle for injection).
- Two syringes for the flush solution
- Saline or heparin flush solution, as prescribed
- Alcohol prep pad or CHG-alcohol combination product and gauze pad
- Procedure gloves

Pre-Procedure Assessment

- Carefully palpate the area around the insertion site through the dressing. If the patient has tenderness, assess further for other signs of infection. Check the surrounding catheter insertion site for redness, swelling, warmth, or drainage.
This can indicate catheter-related infection.

- For all types of CVADs, assess the patient's external chest wall for engorged veins at the surface of the skin. Also check for difficulty moving the neck or jaw, headache, or ear pain.
This can indicate vein thrombosis.

- Conduct a comprehensive pain assessment, looking for unusual pain or discomfort.
Chest discomfort could be associated with the catheter's position in the vein, especially if the line is not in an optimal position.

➤ When performing the procedure, always identify your patient according to agency policy and be attentive to standard precautions, hand hygiene, patient safety and privacy, body mechanics, and documentation.

Procedure Steps

1. Prepare the medication.
   a. Check compatibility of the medication with the existing IV solution, if one is infusing.
   b. Verify the medication can safely be administered through a central site. Double check the infusion rate as well.
Some medication might be incompatible with infusion solution or additives. Because dosage may be different for medications given centrally versus peripherally, and because the medication enters the heart almost instantly, any error is potentially life threatening.

   c. Draw up the medication using a needleless device or needle with a filter. Then change to a sterile needle or needleless device for administering the medication.
Filter needles prevent small particles from entering into the line.

   d. Recap needles throughout, using a needle capping device or approved one-handed technique that has a low risk of contaminating the sterile needle (see Procedure 23-10A: Recapping Sterile Needles).
Recapping prevents needlestick injury, and performed correctly, maintains the sterility of the needle.

   e. Dilute medication, if needed. Fill the medication syringe to the exact volume to be infused; expel excess volume.

   f. Label the syringe with the contents, including medication name, dilution, time to be administered, route, name of person constituting the medication.
Excess volume of medication in the syringe is a risk for inadvertent overdosing.

2. Flush the line.
   a. Obtain heparinized or saline solution for flushing the CVAD, following the institution's protocol or as prescribed.
The usual concentration for heparin is 10 to 100 units/mL of solution for adults. The recommended volume of flush varies by institution. Most facilities recommend 3 to 5 mL of solution to

flush the catheter, although some are flushed with 10 mL to flush the line. Some medication might be incompatible with infusion solution or additives. Because dosage may be different for medications given centrally versus peripherally, and because the medication enters the heart almost instantly, any error is potentially life threatening.

◆ Using heparin flush in venous access devices is becoming more controversial because of the potential for heparin-induced thrombocytopenia. Be sure to follow the prescriber's order and the policy of your institution.

b. Before flushing the CVAD, examine the syringe for bubbles. Remove them by flicking the syringe. Eject the bubbles, but be sure you have enough flush solution remaining in the syringe.
This allows the bubbles to rise to the top. Remove bubbles from the syringe before giving medication through the CVAD port to avoid injecting air into the patient's vein.

c. With clean procedure gloves, using pressure and friction, vigorously scrub all surfaces of the CVAD connectors as well as the leur locking threads, or the Luer lock, including the extension "tail," with an alcohol wipe, CHG-alcohol combination product, or other antimicrobial product for at least 15 seconds. Then let it dry for 15 seconds. Do not touch this connector after cleansing.
Antimicrobial swabs reduce the risk of line-related infection by decreasing colonization of the port and tubing.

d. Insert the flush syringe at a vertical angle into the port using a needleless system or safety syringe.
A 90° angle reduces stress on the access port, which may cause shearing or mechanical trauma to the material.

e. Open the clamp between the syringe and the patient.
The clamp between the access port and the tubing that goes to the patient needs to be patent for medication to be injected through the CVAD.

f. Check for blood return by pulling syringe plunger back.
Aspiration of blood ensures catheter placement is in the vein (in most cases).

g. Inject saline or heparinized flush solution into the line, per agency protocol or provider's orders. Some catheter types (e.g., Groshong) do not require heparin in the flush solution. Close the clamp.
Saline or heparin flush is used, depending on the type of CVAD, institutional protocol, and manufacturer recommendations. If blood is likely to draw back into the line, then heparin might be used in the flush solution in order to reduce the risk of clot formation. Saline is generally indicated when simple clearing of the line is needed. Most often heparin is used for implanted CVAD to reduce the risk of occlusion from a clot forming on the device. Different catheters require different volume of flush solutions. Some are more prone to clot formation, depending on whether they are open or closed system devices. The initial flush maintains patency of the line and removes any heparin left if the catheter was used previously.

◆ Never force the flush solution into the venous access device if you feel resistance because you risk rupturing the catheter. Look for a closed clamp on the catheter or tubing. Check to see if an inline filter is clogged.

If using a needleless connector, do one of the following:

Step 2g Variation. Negative Fluid Displacement Devices
Use a positive-pressure technique:
(1) For a blunt cannula with split septum, or mechanical valve, withdraw the cannula before the syringe is completely empty, keeping your thumb on the syringe plunger.
(2) For a mechanical valve device with negative displacement, maintain pressure on the syringe plunger, close the clamp on the IV line between the needleless connector and the patient; and then disconnect the syringe.

Step 2g Variation. Positive Fluid Displacement Devices
Do not use a positive-pressure technique. Wait a short time to allow fluid displacement to occur. Disconnect the syringe; then close the clamp.
The positive-pressure technique would keep the internal mechanism from functioning properly.

Step 2g Variation. Neutral Fluid Displacement Devices
Any flushing technique can be used. The clamping and disconnecting sequence does not matter.
The clamping sequence is directly dependent upon the needleless connector being used and is critical for the final locking solution.

h. After removing the flush syringe from the port, discard it into a safety disposal container.

3. Administer medication through the CVAD.
a. Scrub all surfaces of the needleless connector and extension with an alcohol swab or CHG-alcohol combination product for at least 15 seconds. Allow the port to dry for 15 more seconds.
Antimicrobial swabs reduce the risk of line-related infection by decreasing colonization of the port and tubing.

b. Close the clamp to the infusion if a primary IV is running.
The med could travel back up the line rather than infuse into the patient if the clamp is open.

c. Inject medication into the port, according to the medication order (infusion time).
Some medication is infused bolus; other medication is given over a period of time.

4. After scrubbing all surfaces of the port again with an alcohol pad or other CHG-alcohol product, administer the second syringe of flush solution.
The flush prevents incompatible medication or fluid from mixing at later administrations and ensures that all of the medication clears the catheter and enters the bloodstream.

(continued on next page)

Procedure 23-18 ■ Administering Medication Through a Central Venous Access Device (continued)

5. Clamp the tubing between the syringe and the CVAD port, making sure the tubing is open between the IV fluid and the patient, if there is a running IV.

What if . . .

■ **My patient is a child; how should I secure the line?**

Dress infants and younger children in a one-piece undershirt that fastens between the legs and tape the line to the shirt, leaving a little bit of slack to allow for movement.

■ **The line does not flush easily?**

■ Make sure all clamps are unclamped.
■ Check to see if the central line is kinked or twisted.
■ After straightening lines, attempt to flush the central line again. If the flush solution cannot be injected easily from the syringe into the CVAD, do not force the flush.

Too much flush pressure may dislodge a clot that has formed in the central line.

■ Check to see if an inline filter is clogged.
■ Assess the insertion site to see if the stabilization device or dressing may be causing the occlusion.
■ Try to reposition the patient to lying down and turn to one side.
■ You might also or have the patient lift his arms above his head and then attempt to flush the central line.
■ If it is still difficult to flush after repositioning, notify the physician.

■ **The central line inadvertently comes out?**

Hold firm, constant pressure on the site to control bleeding. Have a colleague notify the physician immediately.

■ **The central line is cracked or leaking?**

Close the clamp between the break or leakage in the line and the patient's line insertion site. Wrap an alcohol wipe and gauze around the broken part of the line. Immediately change the tubing.

■ **The clamp on the line is broken?**

Change the tubing.

A clamp that works properly is essential for patient safety.

■ **The central line gets caught on or pulled by the patient's clothing?**

Loop the tubing over the dressing and secure with tape.

■ **The patient is short of breath or complains of chest pain?**

Notify the physician immediately.

These symptoms could be a sign of fluid overload or other complications, such as a dislodged clot or embolism.

■ **The patient feels pain in the neck or ear on the side where an implantable CVAD is located. Or the patient hears swishing noises or has palpitations?**

Notify the physician immediately.

In this case, the implanted device might be dislodged. Placement must be confirmed by x-ray.

Patient Evaluation

■ Monitor for signs of catheter complications (e.g., shortness of breath, chest pain, and palpitations).
■ Monitor for signs of catheter dislodgement (e.g., neck swelling or pain, bleeding at the site or within the line, palpitations, or gurgling noise).
■ Assess for signs of catheter-related infection (e.g., fever, increased WBC count, redness, warmth at the site).
■ Observe for leaking or blood back-up at the injection ports, tubing connections, and the site.
■ Observe for bleeding at the CVAD site.
■ Assess for sign of allergic response or adverse effects to medication.

Patient Teaching

■ Teach patients, families, and caregivers that the overall goal is to maintain a patent CVAD that is free of infection, occlusion, or dislodgement.
■ Avoid obtaining blood pressure readings in the arm where a percutaneously inserted central catheter (PICC) line is inserted.
■ If a PICC line is in place, do not immerse the arm in water. The patient may shower if the site is covered by an occlusive dressing.

■ No activity restrictions are needed for patients with a CVAD.
■ Teach signs of catheter complications including line-related infection, thrombosis, and accidental dislodgement.
■ Teach signs of catheter dislodgement include pain or swelling in the neck or area near the ear of the affected side of the CVAD. Gurgling sounds might also indicate a problem with the placement of the CVAD.

Home Care

■ The goals of home care for clients receiving medication through a CVAD are medication safety and maintaining an infection-free line.
■ Candidates for home IV therapy through a CVAD are those who:
  ■ Have a family member or other caregiver who can competently provide or assist with care of the line.
  ■ Have telephone access—either via land line or cell phone.
  ■ Have access to reliable transportation in case of a line-related emergency.

- Ideally, caregivers should be able to read instructions for home care.
- Procedures in the home environment are similar to the hospital setting, except clean technique is used instead of sterile.
- Home health supplies may be different than the ones used in the hospital.
- After discharge, follow-up care in the home environment is important to ensure safety.

Documentation

- Document any sign of allergic response to or adverse effects of medication.
- Note any signs of catheter complications.
- Note any signs of catheter dislodgement.
- Document signs of catheter-related infection.
- Record the date and time tubing and port cap are changed.
- Document all medications infused through the CVAD.

Thinking About the Procedure

 Go to the *Fundamentals of Nursing Skills Videos,* **Administering Medication Through a Central Venous Access Device.**

1. What one essential action must the nurse do before administering medication through a CVAD?

 For suggested responses, go to Chapter 23, **Thinking About the Procedure Suggested Responses (Procedure 23-18),** on the Student Resource Disk or DavisPlus at http://davisplus.fadavis.com/Wilkinson2

Practice Resources

Infusion Nurses Society (2006a, 2006b); National Guideline Clearinghouse, Central Venous Access Device Guideline Panel (2006).

Clinical Insights

This section suggests techniques for reconstituting, mixing, measuring, and administering various medications, including insulin and heparin.

Clinical Insight 23-1 ▶ **Reusing Needles and Syringes: Home Care**

Many people (e.g., those who have diabetes) must give themselves repeated injections, perhaps several each day. Supplies for home use are expensive. Insurance may or may not cover the cost, or the person may not have insurance. Therefore, although health professionals and manufacturers recommend that disposable syringes and needles be used only once, some people find it practical to reuse needles and syringes. If they do, you can help them to do it more safely.

Assess for the following:
- Assess whether the patient is capable of safely recapping a syringe. This requires adequate vision, manual dexterity, and no obvious tremor.
- Assess for contraindications to needle reuse. Patients with poor personal hygiene, an acute illness, open wounds on the hands, or decreased resistance to infection should not reuse a syringe or needle.

Teach your patient the following:
- Consult your healthcare provider before beginning this practice.
- Recap the needle immediately after use if you plan to use it again.
- To recap a needle, hold the syringe in one hand, rest that arm or hand on a solid surface, and with the other, replace the cap with a straight motion of the thumb.

Advise the patient *not* to guide both the needle and cap to meet in midair, because this frequently results in needlestick injury.
- Discard needles when they become dull. Usually they cannot be used more than 10 times.
- Examine the needle carefully before reusing it. The new 30- and 31-gauge needles can easily be bent at the tip to form a hook, which can lacerate tissue or break off within the skin. Never reuse a needle that is deformed in any way.
- When a needle hurts too much, it means that the silicone coating is wearing off and it's time to discard it.
- Do not reuse a needle if it has come in contact with anything other than the injection site.
- Do not use alcohol to cleanse the needle. Alcohol may remove the silicone coating that makes for less painful skin puncture. It is best to not clean the needle after use; just carefully recap it.
- The syringe and needle may be stored at room temperature. The potential benefits or risks of refrigerating the syringe are unknown.
- Be aware that reusing needles and syringes increases the risk of infection, although most insulin preparations have bacteriostatic additives that inhibit growth of bacteria commonly found on the skin.

(continued on next page)

Clinical Insight 23-1 ▶ Reusing Needles and Syringes: Home Care (continued)

- Inspect injection sites for redness or swelling. If these signs are present, do not reuse a needle; consult your healthcare provider.
- Never share syringes or needles with another person. This poses a risk of acquiring a bloodborne viral infection (e.g., hepatitis).
- Dispose of needles safely. Do not bend or break a needle;

doing so increases the chance of injury. Use a coffee can or other puncture-proof container with a lid to dispose of needles (see Chapter 21 if you need to review).
- Do not mix insulin types if you reuse needles and syringes. Use one syringe for each insulin type. That means more injections, but certain insulins cannot be mixed without reducing their effectiveness.

Clinical Insight 23-2 ▶ **Using Prefilled Unit-Dose Systems**

Prefilled systems are most limited to some office practices and self-administration. They are used infrequently in healthcare facilities, because the manipulation required to remove the cartridge from the holder creates a needlestick risk for nurses. Because you may encounter these systems in some clinical sites, we include the technique.

1. Check each medication cartridge and dose carefully, because all of the cartridges look alike.
2. No medication preparation is necessary.
3. Insert the cartridge into the holder.
4. Swing or twist the plunger into place, depending on the type of syringe you use. Lock it securely at the needle end.
5. Attach the plunger, if necessary. (The system may come with plunger attached.)

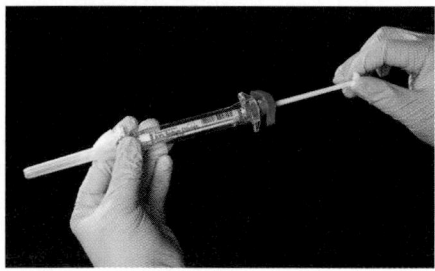

6. Expel air and excess medication.
7. Don gloves.
8. Administer the medication.
9. Dispose of the empty cartridge. Some types are available for reuse.

What if . . .

- **The needle gauge or length is not correct for the patient?**

You can transfer the medication into a regular syringe, maintaining sterile technique. There are two ways you can do it.

Cartridge without removable needle:

1. Pull back on the plunger of the regular syringe and keep a capped, sterile needle ready.

2. Insert the cartridge needle through the open tip of the regular syringe.

3. Eject the medication into the regular syringe.

4. Replace the capped needle onto the regular syringe.

5. Eject the air and check for the correct dosage.

Cartridge with removable needle:

The needle and cap can be removed from some prefilled cartridges, allowing the cartridge to be used as a vial. This allows you to draw the medications into a different syringe. Do not inject air into a cartridge, because the excess pressure may eject the movable bottom.

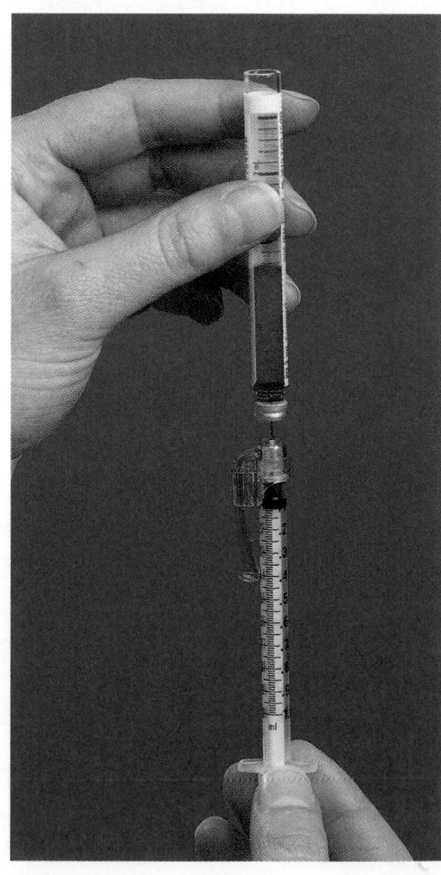

Clinical Insight 23-3 ▶ Reconstituting Medication

1. Remove the caps of both the medication and diluent vials.
2. If a multidose vial is used, scrub the tops of both vials with alcohol wipe or other antiseptic.
To clean the cap of dust and reduce the number of microorganisms.
3. Use a VAD, or if agency policy allows, attach a filter needle to the syringe.
To prevent withdrawing glass and rubber particles, which have been found in medications withdrawn from vials and ampules.
4. Draw up the diluent into the syringe:
   a. Draw air into the syringe in a volume equal to the amount of diluent you will be withdrawing.
   b. Insert the safety needle (or VAD) carefully through the center of the rubber cap, and, keeping the bevel of the needle (or cannula) above the diluent, inject the air.
The air prevents negative pressure inside the vial when you withdraw the diluent, allowing you to withdraw the diluent easily. Keeping bevel above diluent helps prevent bubbles.
   c. Withdraw the diluent in the specified amount.
5. Insert the VAD carefully through the center of the rubber cap, and inject the diluent into the medication vial.

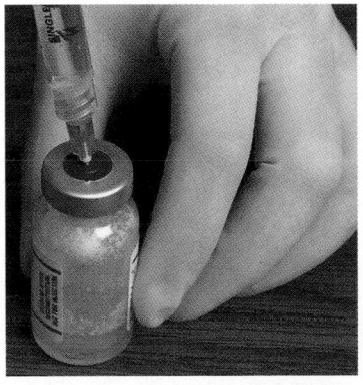

6. Mix the medication, taking care not to create bubbles (e.g., roll, do not shake, the vial). If medication does not mix easily, remove the needle or cannula from the vial, and place the syringe and needle on a sterile field (e.g., the wrapper the syringe came in) while you mix more. Alternatively, recap the sterile needle (see Procedure 23-10A).

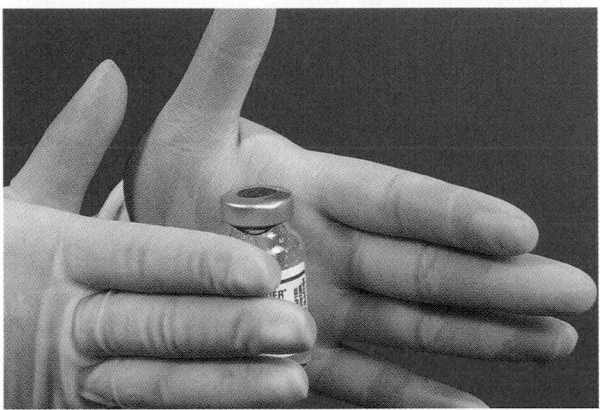

7. Reinsert filter needle or VAD if it was removed), and withdraw the reconstituted medication into the syringe.
8. Remove the filter needle or the cannula from the syringe, and replace it with a sterile needle before measuring the medication.
This ensures that the dose is correct and minimizes discomfort. It also prevents tracking of medication through the tissues; filter needles are usually larger than you will need for an injection. In addition, you should not eject fluid through a filter needle.
9. Hold the syringe vertically, and carefully eject all air from the syringe, but do not eject the medication. Read the dosage.
10. If necessary, hold the syringe horizontally to eject unneeded medication from the syringe to reach the prescribed dose.

Clinical Insight 23-4 ▶ Measuring Dosage When Changing Needles

Note: These are not the old "air lock" techniques.
You should always use a filter needle to withdraw medications, if one is available. However, to give the injection, you must use a needle of the correct gauge and length. You must also eject air to measure the medication; however, pushing medication out of the syringe with the filter needle in place could cause the filter to break and release glass (and other) fragments. In the following method, pulling air into the syringe allows for exact dosage when the medication is injected; when ejected, the air will clear the needle so that the patient receives all the medication that is in the syringe.

For a Nonfilter Needle

When drawing medication from a multidose vial, you may sometimes need to use 2 regular needles. Alternately, you may use a needleless reconstitution device that is designed with a dispensing spike instead of a needle on one end, and a Luer-lock port on the other end that attaches to the syringe. You will use one needle (or needless reconstitution device) for drawing up the medication; and the other for injecting the medication into the patient.

1. To draw medication out of a vial, inject air into the air pocket within the vial. Then withdraw the correct

(continued on next page)

Clinical Insight 23-4 ➤ **Measuring Dosage When Changing Needles** (continued)

amount of medication from the vial using the first needle. Be sure to keep the tip of the needle in the fluid in order to avoid aspirating air bubbles into the syringe.

2. After drawing up the medication dose, tap on the barrel of the syringe to remove air bubbles, if necessary. Then eject the air out of the syringe (keeping the syringe vertical) while retaining the correct amount of medication in the syringe. Check the volume closely at eye level.

3. Remove the first needle and discard it into a needle-safe container. Put on a fresh needle for injection.

4. Pull back on the plunger, and draw an extra 0.2 mL of air to account for the air within the needle.

5. Check the medication dosage. Your plunger should be 0.2 mL more than the ordered dose.

6. When you inject the patient, she will receive the correct dose; the air will drive the medication from the needle into the patient's tissues. This is important when giving irritating medications, such as iron.

This is an air lock.

For a Filter Needle

Use one filter needle (or filter cannula) and one regular needle.

1. With the filter needle (or cannula), withdraw the exact amount of medication. Eject air bubbles (keeping the syringe vertical) as needed to obtain correct dose.

2. Pull back on the plunger to withdraw all the medication from the filter needle (or filter cannula) into the syringe. Depending on the size of the access cannula, this may be as much as 0.2 mL. It will now appear that you have more than the ordered dose in the syringe (but you do not; the air is taking up some of the space).

3. Change to the needle you are going to use for injection.

4. Hold the syringe vertically, and eject air until you see a drop of medication at the tip of the needle ("drop to the top").

5. Measure the medication. It should be at the correct syringe marking. If it is not, then tip the syringe horizontally, and eject the medication until the dose is correct.

6. When you inject the patient, she will receive the correct dose even though some medication will remain in the needle.

7. If you are giving an irritating medication (e.g., iron) draw 0.2 mL of air into the syringe before giving the injection.

This is an air lock.

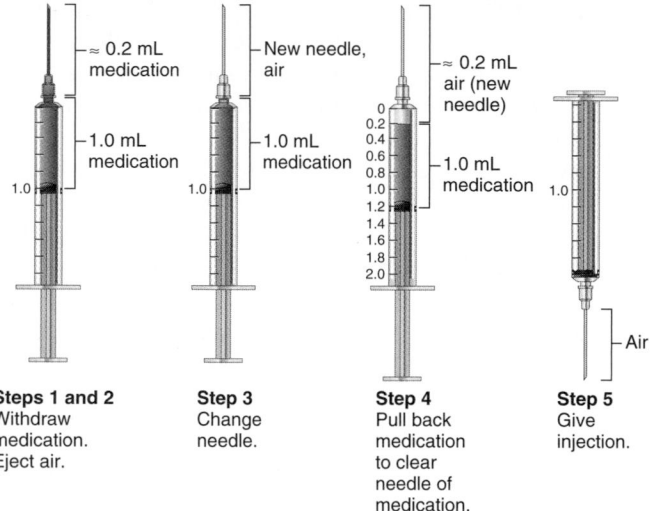

Nonfilter needles.

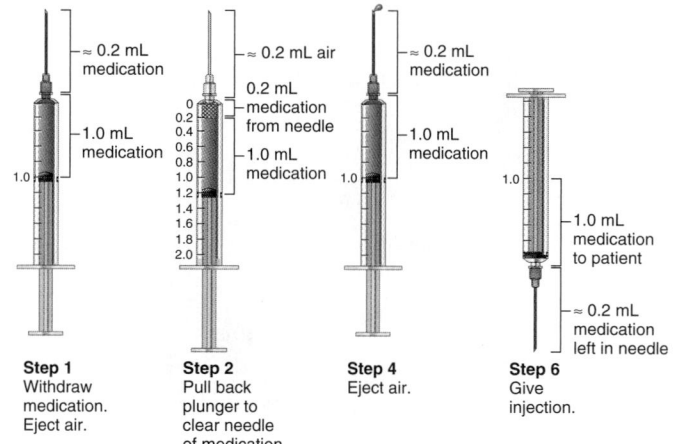

Filter needles.

Clinical Insight 23-5 ▶ Mixing Two Kinds of Insulin in One Syringe

What You Should Know

Various combinations of rapid-acting, intermediate-acting, and long-acting insulin may be prescribed. Some can be mixed; some cannot.

- Lente insulins (Lente and Lantus) can be mixed with each other, but not with neutral protamine hagedorn (NPH).
- Although they are compatible, do not mix Lente with regular insulin except for patients who are already controlled on this mixture. Lente will bind with regular insulin, delaying the onset of action.
- A general rule is "clear before cloudy." Regular insulin is clear; all other types are cloudy. Therefore, you would draw up regular insulin into the syringe before Lente or NPH (neutral protamine Hagedorn) insulin, which are modified. If you draw up a modified type first, the needle may transfer it into the unmodified (regular) vial.

What You Should Do

Follow these steps when drawing up insulin from two vials into one syringe. The procedure assumes you are mixing regular (unmodified) insulin with a modified (e.g., NPH) insulin.

1. Maintain sterile technique throughout.
2. Before preparation, rotate the insulin vials between the palms of your hands for at least 1 minute, and invert them to ensure an adequate concentration. Do not shake the vials because this can create bubbles, which take up space and make it difficult to measure the dose precisely.
3. Scrub vial stoppers with alcohol or other antiseptic (they are usually multidose vials).
4. Using an insulin syringe and needle, inject an amount of sfrom the vial of modified insulin (cloudy vial). Do not allow the needle tip to touch the insulin.
5. Using the same syringe, inject the appropriate amount of air into the vial of regular insulin (clear vial).
6. Do not withdraw the needle; withdraw the correct dose of regular insulin.
7. Remove the syringe from the regular insulin. Eject air, and remove all air bubbles to measure the correct dose.

8. Calculate the total amount on the syringe that the combined types of insulin should measure.
9. Return to the (first) vial of modified insulin (cloudy), and draw the correct dose into the syringe. (For example, if you have 5 units of regular insulin in the syringe and you need 10 units of NPH, the plunger should be at the 15-unit mark when you have drawn up the NPH.)
10. Recall that you have already added air to this vial in a previous step. Draw up the medication slowly and exactly to the total dose, being very careful not to create bubbles and to withdraw only the amount needed. You cannot return any excess to the vial because it is now a mixture of two medications.
11. Administer the insulin mixture within 5 minutes after preparation. Even NPH insulin will bind with regular insulin and delay the onset of its action.

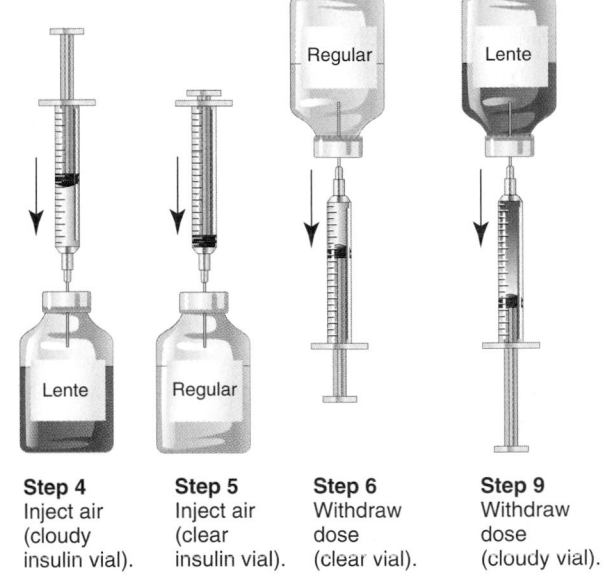

Step 4
Inject air
(cloudy
insulin vial).

Step 5
Inject air
(clear
insulin vial).

Step 6
Withdraw
dose
(clear vial).

Step 9
Withdraw
dose
(cloudy vial).

Total dose is mixture of clear and cloudy insulins.

Clinical Insight 23-6 ▶ Administering Anticoagulant Medication Subcutaneously

Because of the anticoagulant properties of heparin and enoxaparin (Lovenox), you will need to adapt your technique for subcutaneous injections in the following ways:

- To avoid the loss of drug when using prefilled syringes, do not expel the air bubble from the syringe before the injection.
- Enoxaparin-prefilled syringes and graduated prefilled syringes are available with a system that shields the needle after injection.
- Use a ³⁄₈-inch, 25- or 26-gauge needle.
- After drawing up the correct dose, add 0.2 mL of air to the syringe to ensure that all of the medication is injected

into the subcutaneous tissue and is not tracked into the superficial tissue.

- With your nondominant hand, pinch or spread the skin and insert the needle at a 90° angle, using your dominant hand. If the patient has very little subcutaneous tissue, use a ⁵⁄₈″ needle and insert it at a 45° angle. Introduce the whole length of the needle into a skinfold held between the thumb and forefinger; hold the skinfold throughout the injection.
- Alternate administration among sites on the abdomen. Give the injection subcutaneously deep on the abdomen, at least 2 inches away from the umbilicus.

(continued on next page)

Clinical Insight 23-6 ▶ Administering Anticoagulant Medication Subcutaneously (continued)

- Do not aspirate before injecting, because doing so can traumatize tissue and cause bruising.
- Do not massage the site after injecting, because doing so can cause bleeding and bruising. It may also cause the heparin to be absorbed more rapidly than desired.
- Keep a record of the sites used. Most agencies have a chart of the body on which to record the sites injected.

Several mix-ups between heparin and insulin have been reported. To help avoid this (in addition to observing the "3 checks and 6 rights"): (1) Do not store heparin and insulin vials beside each other, (2) have another RN check your preparation before administering IV heparin or insulin, (3) think critically (for example, ask yourself if giving heparin—or insulin—makes sense given the patient's diagnosis) (Cohen, 2007).

Clinical Insight 23-7 ▶ Guidelines for Avoiding Medication Errors

To prevent making a medication error, you should develop a set routine for administering medications. Learn from your mistakes and the mistakes of others. Many errors occur as a result of interruption or distraction. It is best not to stop what you are doing when preparing or giving medication. You might even wear a bright yellow sash to alert people not to disturb you when preparing or giving medication. To administer medications safely, always practice the "three checks" and "rights of medication" of medication administration, and incorporate the following actions into your practice:

1. Right Drug

The following are ways to ensure that you give the correct drug:

Think Critically.

- Review orders often to see whether there have been changes in the medication dosage, route, and so forth—especially after days off, after working a different shift, and after a break.
- If you must take a verbal order, always repeat it back to the prescriber to be sure you have heard correctly. Spell the medication name. Many medication names sound the same when you hear but are actually very different drugs (e.g., Isordil, Isuprel).
- Ask yourself if the medication order is suitable for the patient's condition. If not, question the prescriber.
- Participate in daily patient rounds so you will be better informed about your patient's plan of care and why the medications are ordered.
- Be familiar with the drugs you administer. If you don't know, look it up.

Be aware of the pitfalls in abbreviations, units of measurement, and handwriting.

- Double-check all prescriptions transcribed by hand to the MAR, especially when decimal points are involved.
- Do not attempt to decipher illegible handwriting. The chance of misinterpretation is great, so when in doubt, ask the prescriber to clarify.
- Be alert for names that look very similar (e.g., Keflex and Keflin). It may be impossible to differentiate them when they are hand-written.
- Do not administer a drug ordered by a nickname. Always be sure it is written out in full.
- Clarify abbreviations that may be confusing.

- Do not confuse measurements. It is easy to misread "mg" instead of "mL." There is a significant difference between 1 mg and 1 mL of IV morphine, for example.
- Write out "international units" instead of abbreviating IU. IU can be confused with IV.

Perform the "three checks" of the label against the MAR.

- Read the label before and after you prepare the medication, and again at the bedside to verify that you selected the correct product name and strength.
- Select the prescribed medication from the patient's drug drawer (unless it is a stock drug). Do not "borrow" from another patient's drawer.
- Do not substitute one medication for another.
- Avoid selecting medications based on size and color because many medications are the same size, shape, and color as others.
- Be alert for similar-looking labels. If you are accustomed to withdrawing oxytocin (given IV to stimulate uterine contractions) from a small vial with a green label, you might be surprised to find that the small, green-label vial in your hand is actually hydroxyzine (Vistaril), which would harm the patient if given IV.
- If a label is hard to read or comes off the container, return the container to the pharmacy. Never give a medication from such a container.
- Do not transfer medications from one pharmacy container to another.
- Physically separate the highly concentrated heparin sodium (10,000 units/mL in 1-mL vials) from the more diluted 1 mL vials for flushing heparin locks. There is a risk for fatal hemorrhage if the highly concentrated heparin solution is mistakenly used to flush an IV line. FDA-approved labeling now includes new color and design in order to distinguish various heparin concentrations in the vials.
- Be extremely careful when administering heparin to infants and children.

2. Right Dose

The right dose is the dose prescribed for the particular patient.
- Perform the "three checks" of the dose.
- Question prescriptions for multiple tablets or vials as a single dose; most doses are one or two tablets or one single-dose vial.

- Question abrupt and excessive increases in dosage; most dosages increase gradually.
- Question prescriptions that are not consistent with the standard (protocol) dosage range for the patient's age, weight, and condition. Those who prescribe, dispense, and administer drugs use standardized protocols to describe medications suitable for certain conditions, including customary doses and dilutions.
- Ask another nurse to check your calculations when you must calculate a dosage.
- Know when to use a zero.
  - Always write a zero before a decimal point. It is easy to mistake .15 for 115 if the decimal point is written large or the 1 is written small (e.g., write "Lanoxin 0.125 mg," not "Lanoxin .125 mg").
  - Never write a zero and a decimal point after a whole number. The decimal point may be mistaken for a 1 (e.g., write "5 mg," not "5.0 mg").
  - How you prepare medications can affect the dose.
- *Breaking tablets:* When you must break a tablet, use a knife or a cutting device. If the tablet does not break evenly, you should discard it. Keep in mind, discarded medication must be accounted for, particularly controlled substances.
- Crushing tablets: When crushing a tablet to mix with liquid or food, clean the crushing device completely before and after using it to remove any pieces of a previously crushed drug.
- Use smart infusion pumps to help ensure correct dosing. Enter various drug protocols into the pump; the protocols are linked to a drug library with predefined dosing limits. If you attempt to program outside that parameter, the pump halts or triggers an alarm.
- Examine the standards of care and practice in your institution to see if they comply with the intent of The Joint Commission's 2008 National Patient Safety Goal 3e related to safe dosing with anticoagulation therapy.

3. Right Time

Check the order for the time to give the drug, and document the exact time of administration on the MAR.

- If the drug is not charted, never assume the patient received the drug as scheduled. If you assume the drug has been given, the patient may not receive an essential medication. If you assume the drug has not been given, and give it, the patient may receive an overdose.
- If a dose has been delayed (e.g., because of a diagnostic test), check with the prescriber to clarify when the next dose should be administered. Medications are designed to be given at specific times to maintain constant therapeutic blood levels.
- Give scheduled medications within a "window" of one-half hour before and one-half hour after the scheduled time, as a rule.

- Time oral medications with meals. Give drugs that are irritating to the stomach (e.g., potassium, aspirin) with food; give drugs that absorb better on an empty stomach (e.g., tetracycline, iron supplement) before meals.
- Determine whether your patient is scheduled for any diagnostic procedures, surgery, or blood tests that require him to remain NPO. If so, you may need to hold oral or enteral medications, or have them changed to another route.

4. Right Route

Drug absorption is affected by the route of administration.

- Perform the "three checks" for the route.
- Be sure the drug is in proper form for the route ordered, especially with time-released drugs. For example, cephalexin (Keflex), an antibiotic, comes in capsules, suspensions for oral use, and injectable forms for intramuscular and IV administration. By contrast, the antibiotic penicillin G procaine (Crysticillin) is prepared for IM injection and is *not* to be given intravenously.
- If the order does not specify a route, do not assume. Always clarify with the prescriber.
- Right route also includes right site. If an IM injection is ordered, for example, be sure the site is appropriate for the age of the patient (child, adult, elderly) and the medical condition. For example, if an extremity is traumatized, burned, or with compromised circulation, you would not administer the injection on that side.
- Draw up oral liquids into an oral syringe to avoid inadvertent IV administration.

5. Right Patient

- Perform the "three checks" of the medication label and the MAR for the patient's name and room number.
- Just before giving the medication, always double-check the patient's identification (ID) bracelet to ensure that you have the correct patient. The Joint Commission (2007) recommends using two methods of patient identification; so, also ask the patient to state his name. It is best to say, "Please tell me your name." Never skip this step.
- Do not leave medications at the patient's bedside. If you must leave the room before administering the drug, take it with you.
- Be alert for patients with the same last names. It is common to have two patients with same or similar last names (e.g., Williamson, Wilkinson, Wilson, Wilkerson). Look for and place special alerts on charts and MARs to call attention to similar names.
- Computerized prescriber order entry (CPOE) and bar code medication administration provides a nearly full-proof system for identifying the right patient and transfers data electronically. However, you must ensure order entry is made in the correct patient record.

(continued on next page)

Clinical Insight 23-7 ➤ **Guidelines for Avoiding Medication Errors** (continued)

6. Right Documentation

Most nurses consider documentation the sixth right.

■ After administering a medication, document it immediately on the patient's MAR. Do not wait to chart all medications at the end of a shift, for example.

■ Never document a drug before you give it.

■ Never document a medication given by someone else; do not ask someone else to document medications you administer.

■ As for all charting, write legibly in ink, preferably black but many agencies permit blue ink.

■ If for some reason you do not administer an ordered medication, document that information on the MAR and write a nursing note explaining the reason it was not given.

■ You are responsible for documenting the patient's responses to all medications, including therapeutic effects, side effects, and unexpected or adverse reactions.

Clinical Insight 23-8 ➤ **Taking Action After a Medication Error**

■ First check the patient. Take his vital signs, and perform assessments related to the medication that was given.

■ If you are unfamiliar with the side effects of the medication, consult a drug reference source.

■ Verify that you have made a medication error, and identify the type of error.

■ Notify the nurse in charge for guidance if this is your first error.

■ Notify the prescriber and follow her orders for intervention.

■ Document on the chart that the medication was given, but do not indicate that it was given in error. This alerts anyone reviewing the chart that an error was made.

■ Complete an incident report according to the facility's policies. Ask for assistance if you are unfamiliar with the format or requirement of this form. It is important that the information you provide is factual and accurate.

■ Do not document in the patient's chart that an incident report was filed. This alerts anyone reviewing the chart that an error was made and makes the incident report available for legal review in the event of a lawsuit.

■ When you are calmer and can think clearly, critically review the error. Identify the influences that led to your making the error. Were you rushed? Did you check the prescription? Did you follow the rights of medication? Whatever the reason, use this situation as a learning experience to improve your practice.

Medication-Related and Other Abbreviations

Because abbreviations can be easily misread, it is better to write words in full, especially when you are working with medications. However, you might still see the following abbreviations, so you should be familiar with them. Be sure you are familiar with the list of abbreviations approved for use in your particular agency. Abbreviations should be used cautiously and avoided when possible.

Institute for Safe Medication Practices (ISMP) List of Error-Prone Abbreviations, Symbols, and Dose Designations			
ABBREVIATIONS	**INTENDED MEANING**	**MISINTERPRETATION**	**CORRECTION**
μg	Microgram	Mistaken as "mg"	Use "mcg."
AD, AS, AU	Right ear, left ear, each ear	Mistaken as OD, OS, OU (right eye, left eye, each eye)	Use "right ear," "left ear," or "each ear."
OD, OS, OU	Right eye, left eye, each eye	Mistaken as AD, AS, AU (right ear, left ear, each ear)	Use "right eye," "left eye," or "each eye."
BT	Bedtime	Mistaken as "BID" (twice daily)	Use "bedtime."
cc	Cubic centimeters	Mistaken as "u" (units)	Use "mL."
D/C	Discharge or discontinue	Premature discontinuation of medications if D/C (intended to mean: "discharge") has been misinterpreted as "discontinued" when followed by a list of discharge medications	Use "discharge" and "discontinue."
ij	Injection	Mistaken as "IV" or "intrajugular"	Use "injection."

Institute for Safe Medication Practices (ISMP) List of Error-Prone Abbreviations, Symbols, and Dose Designations—cont'd

ABBREVIATIONS	INTENDED MEANING	MISINTERPRETATION	CORRECTION
IN	Intranasal	Mistaken as "IM" or "IV"	Use "intranasal" or "NAS."
HS	Half-strength	Mistaken as bedtime	Use "half-strength."
hs	At bedtime, hours of sleep	Mistaken as half-strength	Use "bedtime."
IU	International units	Mistaken as IV (intravenous) or 10 (ten)	Use "International units."
o.d. or OD	Once daily	Mistaken as "right eye" (OD-oculus dexter), leading to oral liquid medications administered in the eye	Use "daily."
OJ	Orange juice	Mistaken as OD or OS (right or left eye); drugs meant to be diluted in orange juice may be given in the eye	Use "orange juice."
Per os	By mouth, orally	The "os" can be mistaken as "left eye" (OS-oculus sinister)	Use "PO," "by mouth," or "orally."
q.d. or QD	Every day	Mistaken as q.i.d., especially if the period after the "q" or the tail of the "q" is misunderstood as an "i"	Use "daily."
qhs	Nightly at bedtime	Mistaken as "qhr" or every hour	Use "nightly."
qn	Nightly or at bedtime	Mistaken as "qh" (every hour)	Use "nightly" or "at bedtime."
q.o.d. or QOD	Every other day	Mistaken as "q.d." (daily) or "q.i.d." (four times daily) if the "o" is poorly written	Use "every other day."
qld	Daily	Mistaken as q.i.d. (four times daily)	Use "daily."
q6PM, etc.	Every evening at 6 PM	Mistaken as every 6 hours	Use "6 PM nightly" or "6 PM daily."
SC, SQ, sub q	Subcutaneous	SC mistaken as SL (sublingual); SQ mistaken as "5 every"; the "q" in "sub q" has been mistaken as "every (e.g., a heparin dose ordered sub q 2 hours before hours before surgery) surgery" misunderstood as every 2	
ss	Sliding scale (insulin)	Mistaken as "55"	Spell out "sliding scale"; use "one-half."
SSRI, SSI	Sliding scale regular insulin	Mistaken as selective-serotonin reuptake inhibitor; mistaken as Strong Solution of Iodine (Lugol's)	Spell out "sliding scale (insulin)."
i/d	One daily	Mistaken as "tid"	Use "1 daily."
TIW or tiw	3 times a week	Mistaken as "3 times a day" or "twice in a week"	Use "3 times weekly."
U or u	Unit	Mistaken as the number 0 or 4, causing a 10-fold overdose or greater (e.g., 4U seen as "40" or 4u seen as "44"); mistaken as "cc," so dose given in volume instead of units (e.g., 4u seen as 4cc)	Use "unit."

Continued

Institute for Safe Medication Practices (ISMP) List of Error-Prone Abbreviations, Symbols, and Dose Designations—cont'd

DOSE DESIGNATIONS OR OTHER INFORMATION	INTENDED MEANING	MISINTERPRETATION	CORRECTION
Trailing zero after decimal point (e.g., 1.0 mg)	1 mg	Mistaken as 10 mg if the decimal point is not seen expressed in whole numbers	Do not use trailing zeros for doses.
No leading zero before a decimal dose (e.g., .5 mg)	0.5 mg	Mistaken as 5 mg if the decimal point is not seen	Use zero before a decimal point when the dose is less than a whole unit.
Drug name and drug dose run together (e.g., Inderal 40 mg)	Inderal 40 mg	Mistaken as Inderal 140 mg	Place adequate space between the drug name, dose, and unit of measurement.
Numeric dose and unit of measurement run together (e.g., 10 mg)	10 mg	The "m" can be mistaken for a zero, leading to a 10-fold dosing error	Place adequate space between the drug name, dose, and unit of measurement.
Abbreviations, such as mg. or mL. with a period following the abbreviation	mg or mL	The period is unnecessary and could be mistaken as the number 1 if written poorly.	Use mg, mL, etc. without a period.
Large doses without properly placed commas (e.g., 100000 units or 1000000 units)	100,000 or 1,000,000 units	100000 has been mistaken for 10,000 or 1,000,000; 1,000,000 has been mistaken for 100,000.	Use commas for dosing units at or above 1,000 or use such words as 100 "thousand" or 1 "million" to improve readability.

DRUG NAME ABBREVIATIONS	INTENDED MEANING	MISINTERPRETATION	CORRECTION
NOTE: PHARMACIES DO NOT ACCEPT ORDERS FOR ABBREVIATED MEDICATIONS			
ARA A	vidarabine	Mistaken as cytarabine (ARA C)	Use the complete drug name.
AZR	zidovudine (Retrovir)	Mistaken as azathioprine or aztreonam	Use the complete drug name.
CPZ	prochloperazine (Compazine)	Mistaken as chlorpromazine	Use complete drug name.
DPT	Demerol-Phenergan-Thorazine	Mistaken as diphtheria-pertussis-tetanus	Use complete drug name.
DTO	Diluted tincture of opium, or deodorized tincture of opium (Paregoric)	Mistaken as tincture of opium	Use complete drug name.
HCl	hydrochloric acid or hydrochloride	Mistaken as potassium chloride (The "H" is misinterpreted as "K.")	Use complete drug name unless expressed as a salt of a drug.
HCT	hydrocortisone	Mistaken as hydrochlorothiazide	Use complete drug name.
HCTZ	hydrochlorothiazide	Mistaken as hydrocortisone (seen as HCT 250 mg)	Use complete drug name.
$MgSO_4$	magnesium sulfate	Mistaken as morphine sulfate	Use complete drug name.
MS, MSO_4	morphine sulfate	Mistaken as magnesium sulfate	Use complete drug name.
MTX	methotrexate	Mistaken as mitoxantrone	Use complete drug name.
PCA	procainamide	Mistaken as patient-controlled analgesia	Use complete drug name.
PTU	propylthioracil	Mistaken as mercaptopurine	Use complete drug name.

Institute for Safe Medication Practices (ISMP) List of Error-Prone Abbreviations, Symbols, and Dose Designations—cont'd

DRUG NAME ABBREVIATIONS	INTENDED MEANING	MISINTERPRETATION	CORRECTION
T3	Tylenol with codeine No. 3	Mistaken as liothyronine	Use complete drug name.
TAC	trimcinolone	Mistaken as tetracaine, adrenaline, cocaine	Use complete drug name.
TNK	TNKase	Mistaken as "TPA"	Use complete drug name.
ZnSO$_4$	zinc sulfate	Mistaken as morphine sulfate	Use complete drug name.

STEMMED DRUG NAMES	INTENDED MEANING	MISINTERPRETATION	CORRECTION
"nitro drip"	nitroglycerine infusion	Mistaken as sodium nitroprusside infusion	Use complete drug name.
"Norflox"	norfloxacin	Mistaken as Norflex	Use complete drug name.
"IV Vanc"	intravenous vancomycin	Mistaken as Invanz	Use complete drug name.

SYMBOLS	INTENDED MEANING	MISINTERPRETATION	CORRECTION
ʒ	dram	Symbol for dram mistaken as "3"	Use the metric system.
♏	Minim	Mistaken as "mL"	Use the metric system.
×3d	for 3 days	Mistaken as "3 doses"	Use "for 3 days."
< and >	greater than and less than	Mistaken as opposite of intended; mistakenly using incorrect symbols	Use "greater than" or "less than."
/ (slash mark)	separates two doses or indicates "per"	Mistaken as the number 1 (e.g., "25 units/10 units" misread as "25 units and 110" units	Use "per" rather than a slash mark to separate doses.
@	at	Mistaken as "2"	Use "at."
&	and	Mistaken as "2"	Use "and."
+	plus or and	Mistaken as "4"	Use "and" or "plus."
°	hour	mistaken as zero (e.g., q2° seen as q 20)	Use "hr", "h", or "hour."

Source: Institute for Safe Medication Practices. (2004). *IMSP List of Error-Prone Abbreviations, Symbols, and Dose Designations.* Retrieved from www.ismp.org/PDF/ErrorProne.pdf

Common Medication-Related Abbreviations

ABBREVIATION	EXPLANATION	EXAMPLE OF ADMINISTRATION TIME
ac	before meals	0700, 1100, 1700 hours
ad lib	as desired	
AM	Morning	
bid	twice a day	0900, 2100 hours
c̄	with	
fl oz	fluid ounce	
g, gm, or GM	gram	
gtt	drop	
h, hr	hour	
IM	intramuscular	
IV	intravenous	
IVPB	intravenous piggyback	
Kg or kg	kilogram	
KVO	keep vein open	
L or l	liter	
mEq	milliequivalent	
mL or ml	milliliter	
OTC	over-the-counter	
oz	ounce	
pc	after meals	0900, 1300, 1900 hours
PM	evening	
po or PO	by mouth	
PRN	as needed	
qh, qr (q1h, q1hr)	every hour	
q2h, q2hr	every 2 hours	0800, 1000, 1200 hours, etc.
q3h, q3hr	every 3 hours	0900, 1200, 1500 hours, etc.
q4h, q4hr	every 4 hours	0200, 0600, 1000, 1400, 1800, 2200 hours
q6h, q6hr	every 6 hours	0600, 1200, 1800 hours, 2400.
qid or QID	four times a day	1000, 1400, 1800, 2200
qs	sufficient quantity	
s̄	without	
Stat or STAT	at once	
sup or supp	suppository	
susp	suspension	
tab	tablet	
Tbsp	tablespoon	
Tid or TID	three times a day	1000, 1400, 1800 hours
T or tsp	teaspoon	

Standardized Language

Standardized Diagnoses, Outcomes, and Interventions Related to Medication Administration

NURSING DIAGNOSIS	NOC OUTCOMES	NIC INTERVENTIONS
Deficient Knowledge r/t lack of motivation to learn and/or decreased energy available for learning	Knowledge: Medication Knowledge: Treatment Regimen	Teaching: Individual Teaching: Prescribed Medication Teaching: Psychomotor Skill
Noncompliance with medication schedule r/t (e.g., lack of confidence in its effectiveness, forgetfulness, denial of illness, cost of medications, visual impairment)	Adherence Behavior Compliance Behavior Motivation Treatment Behavior: Illness or Injury	Culture Brokerage Discharge Planning Health System Guidance Patient Contracting Self-Modification Assistance Teaching: Prescribed Medication Telephone Consultation Values Clarification
Ineffective Therapeutic Regimen Management r/t polypharmacy, deficient knowledge, confusion, sensory deficits, self-treatment	Adherence Behavior Compliance Behavior Knowledge: Treatment Regimen Participation in Health Care Decisions Treatment Behavior: Illness or Injury	Behavior Modification Decision-Making Support Health System Guidance Mutual Goal Setting Patient Contracting Self-Modification Assistance Self-Responsibility Facilitation Teaching: Procedure/Treatment
Risk for Poisoning r/t polypharmacy, confusion, impaired memory	Knowledge: Medication Medication Response Risk Control: Drug Use Risk Detection Self-Care: Non-Parenteral Medication Self-Care: Parenteral Medication	Environmental Management Safety Health Education Medication Management Surveillance: Safety
Anxiety r/t learning to self-administer insulin (or other parenteral drugs)	Anxiety Self-Control Coping Impulse Self-Control	Anxiety Reduction Teaching: Prescribed Medication
Risk for Aspiration r/t decreased level of consciousness, impaired swallowing	Aspiration Prevention Respiratory Status: Airway Patency Self-Care: Non-Parenteral Medication Swallowing Status	Airway Management Aspiration Precautions Positioning Respiratory Monitoring Surveillance Swallowing Therapy Vomiting Management
Risk for Injury r/t adverse and/or toxic effects of medications	Risk Control	Health Education Risk Identification
Constipation r/t narcotic usage	Bowel Elimination Hydration	Constipation/Impaction Management Medication Management Nutrition Management

Continued

Standardized Diagnoses, Outcomes, and Interventions Related to Medication Administration—cont'd		
NURSING DIAGNOSIS	**NOC OUTCOMES**	**NIC INTERVENTIONS**
Impaired Comfort: pruritus r/t allergic reaction to medication	Comfort Level	Pruritis Management
Bowel Incontinence (or Diarrhea) r/t side effect of antibiotic therapy	Bowel Continence Bowel Elimination	Bowel Incontinence Care Bowel Management Diarrhea Management Perineal Care
NOC Measurement Scales		

Sources: Johnson, M., Bulechek, G., Butcher, H., et al. (2006). *NANDA, NOC, and NIC linkages* (2nd ed.). St. Louis, MO: Mosby; Moorhead, S., Johnson, M., Maas, M., et al. (Eds.). (2008). *Nursing outcomes classification (NOC)* (4th ed.). St. Louis, MO: C.V. Mosby; Bulechek, G. M., Butcher, H. K., & Dochterman, J. M. (Eds.). (2008). *Nursing interventions classification (NIC)* (5th ed.). St. Louis, MO: C.V. Mosby; NANDA International (2009). *Nursing diagnoses: Definitions and classification 2009–2011,* Oxford, UK: Wiley-Blackwell. Used with permission.

Measuring and Calculating Dosage

Medications are not always available in the exact dosage the patient needs. Therefore, you must be proficient in calculating drug dosages to be sure your patients receive the correct amount of medication.

Drugs in solid form (e.g., pills, powders) are measured by weight (e.g., milligrams, grains). Drugs used for irrigation, infusion, and injection are liquids (usually solutions), measured by volume, generally milliliters. When measuring and calculating, you can think of solutions as a quantity of "solid" drug dissolved in a quantity of "liquid" diluent. The diluent merely carries the medication. When you see a vial marked "50 mg/mL," for example, you will know this means that in each milliliter of diluent there are 50 mg (in weight) of the solid, active, medication. Your task is to determine how many milliliters of liquid you need to give the patient the number of milligrams of active drug ordered.

A solution can be either a solid dissolved in a fluid or a given volume of one liquid dissolved in a given volume of another liquid. Solution concentrations may be expressed as a proportion. A 1/100 solution is a solution of 1 gram of solid dissolved in 100 mL of fluid, or 1 mL of fluid mixed with 100 mL of another fluid.

Medication Measurement Systems

Medications are usually ordered and measured using the metric system; however, there are still a few medications that use the apothecary and household systems, so you need to learn how to work with all three systems.

Metric System

The metric system is the preferred system. The basic metric units of measurement are the **meter** (the unit for linear measurement), the **liter** (for capacity or volume), and the **gram** (for weight). A meter is a little longer than a yard, a liter a little larger than a quart, and a gram a little more than the weight of a steel paper clip. The metric system promotes accuracy by allowing for calculation of small drug dosages. A disadvantage of this system in the United States is its limited use among people outside of healthcare. The following are the metric units you will use in preparing medications.

Weights
1 mg (milligram)	=	1000 mcg or (micrograms)
1 gm (gram)	=	1000 mg (milligrams)
1 kg (kilogram)	=	1000 g or gm (grams)

Volume
1000 mL (milliliters)	=	1 L (Liter)
1000 (cubic centimeters)	=	1 L (Liter)

The following are examples of medication orders using the metric system:

Milk of Magnesia 30 mL orally daily at bedtime
Ancef 1 gm IV q8hr

Apothecary System

The British apothecary system of measurement has been in use in the United States since Colonial times. Only a few medications (e.g., aspirin) are measured using this system because it is less precise. Prescribers usually write apothecary measurements using Roman numerals, but you may also see them in Arabic numerals. The system uses fractions (e.g., gr 1/4) instead of decimals (e.g., 0.25 gr). Keep in mind the apothecary abbreviations are prone to misinterpretation and error because they are used infrequently. The following are the units used in preparing medications:

Volume
1 minim (m)	=	1 drop (gtt)
1 fluid dram (dr)	=	60 minims
1 fluid ounce (oz)	=	8 fluid drams

Weight

1 dram (dr)	=	27.34 grains (gr)
1 grain	=	60 milligrams (mg)

The following are Roman numerals you will use most often:

M	=	1000	x	=	10
D	=	500	v	=	5
C	=	100	i	=	1
L	=	50	ii	=	2

The following are examples of medication orders using the apothecary system:

Aspirin grains V orally q4hr PRN for fever greater than 101°F

Chloramphenicol otic 2 gtts in each ear 3 × daily

Many institutions are no longer using the apothecary system of measurement. If a prescription contains this unit of measurement, verify the intended dose with the prescriber and pharmacist.

Household Measurements

Because most people are familiar with the household system, it is easier to teach a patient about home medications using this system. However, nurses use it only occasionally because dosages measured in this system are usually only approximate. The following are household units of measurement with metric conversion:

Volume

1 tsp (t)	=	5 mL		
1 tablespoon (tbsp or T)	=	3 teaspoons (tsp)	=	15 mL
6 tsp or 2 T	=	1 ounce (oz)	=	30 mL
16 T or 8 oz	=	1 cup (c)	=	240 mL
16 T or 8 oz	=	1 glass	=	240 mL
2 C	=	1 pint (pt)	=	480 mL
2 pt	=	1 quart (qt)	=	946.4 mL
4 qt	=	1 gallon (gal)		

Weight

1 oz	=		=	28.35 gm
16 oz	=	1 pound (lb)	=	0.45 kg

Length

12 inches (in.)	=	1 foot (ft)	=	30.5 cm
3 feet (ft)	=	1 yard (yd)	=	91.4 cm

The following is an example of a medication order using the household system:

Amoxicillin 250 mg per 5 mL. Give 1 tsp PO tid

Special Measurements: Units and mEq

Insulin, a drug used by diabetics to assist in the control of blood sugar, is measured in **units,** with 100 international units (U100) being the standard strength preparation. In this strength, 1 mL of the fluid medication contains 100 units of insulin. Heparin (an anticoagulant) and penicillin are also ordered in units.

Be aware that not all units are the same. You must always read the container label to know the number of units per milliliter.

The following are medication orders using units:

NPH insulin 14 units subcutaneous q morning
Heparin 4000 units subcutaneous 2 × per day

Milliequivalents (mEq) indicate the strength of the ion concentration in a drug. A milliequivalent is the number of grams of a solid contained in one milliliter of a solution. Electrolytes, such as potassium chloride (KCl), are measured in mEq. The following are medication orders using mEq:

KCl 20 mEq orally 2 × daily
D_5W 1000 mL with KCl 40 mEq q8hr

Note that units and mEq *cannot* be directly converted to the apothecary, metric, or household systems.

Calculating Dosages

You should be able to calculate accurately using several different methods and formulas. Inaccurate calculations result in incorrect dosages and could harm the patient. One easy formula to remember is the following:

$$\frac{\text{Dose on hand}}{\text{Quantity (or volume) on hand}} = \frac{\text{Desired dose}}{\text{Quantity (or volume) desired}} \quad \text{or} \quad \frac{\text{DH}}{\text{QH}} = \frac{\text{DD}}{\text{X}}$$

Remember:

You must pay attention to *both* the milligrams (weight of the drug) marked on the medication container *and* the milliliters (amount of liquid in which the medication is dissolved). For example, suppose you have a prefilled syringe containing 50 mg of meperidine (Demerol) in 1 mL volume, but you wish to administer only 25 mg to the patient. How much of the liquid (how many mL) would you give?

$$\frac{\text{DH}}{\text{QH}} = \frac{\text{DD}}{\text{X}} \quad \text{or} \quad \frac{50 \text{ mg}}{1 \text{ mL}} = \frac{25 \text{ mg}}{\text{X}}$$

Therefore (recalling your algebra),

$$50X = 25 \text{ mL,}$$
$$\text{so } X = 25 \text{ divided by } 50,$$
$$\text{so } X = 0.5 \text{ mL}$$

Here is an alternative formula you can use for calculating dosages:

$$\frac{\text{Dose desired (DD)}}{\text{Dose on hand (DH)}} \times \text{quantity on hand (QH)} = \text{desired quantity}$$

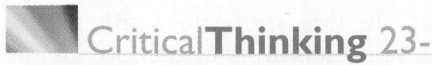

CriticalThinking 23-1

Mr. Pearson ("Meet Your Patients") has been ordered nifedipine (Procardia XL) 60 mg orally daily. You have available Procardia XL (extended-release nifedipine) 30-mg tablets. Calculate the number of tablets you will need for one dose. How many tablets per day?

Conversions Within One System

When a drug prescription is written in the same system as the preparation you have on hand, you can easily make conversions. For example, in the metric system, if you want to convert grams to milligrams, you simply multiply by 1000 (because 1 g = 1000 mg). So, if you have 2.5 grams,

$$2.5 \text{ gm} \times 1000 = 2500 \text{ mg}$$

To change milligrams to grams, *divide* by 1000—move the decimal three places to the left. For example, if you wanted to know, in grams, the equivalent of 250 mg:

You know that 1000 mg = 1 g
By dividing: 250 mg ÷ 1000 mg = 0.25 g

Or by moving the decimal point three places to the left: 250.0 mg = 0.250 g

Use exactly the same procedures to convert liters (L) and milliliters (mL). For example, if you wanted to know how many milliliters are the equivalent of 0.25 L:

You know that 1 L = 1000 mL
By multiplying: 0.25 L × 1000 = 250 mL

By moving the decimal point three places to the right, 0.250 L = 250 mL (Notice that you must add a zero to *have* three places to the right.)

Within the apothecary system or the household system, use the equivalents and follow a similar process of multiplying and dividing (of course, you cannot just move the decimal in these systems). For example, suppose you have a dr ii (2 dram) tablet and you need to know how many grains you have (apothecary system). You know that 2 dram = 27.3 gr, so multiply:

$$2 \text{ dr} \times 55 \text{ gr} = 110 \text{ gr}$$

In the household system, suppose you have 4 tbsp of a liquid and you need to know what part of a cup that represents. You know that 1 cup = 16 tablespoons, so substitute the equivalent and divide:

16 tbsp = 1 cup

So,

4 tbsp = 16 ÷ 4 = 1/4 cup

KnowledgeCheck 23-1

Lanoxin 0.25 mg orally daily is prescribed for a patient with congestive heart failure. The label on the package you have reads

"Lanoxin 0.125 mg." How many tablets will you give? Use the "dose on hand (DOH)" formula.

Go to Chapter 23, **Knowledge Check Response Sheet and Answers,** on the Student Resource Disk or DavisPlus at http://davisplus.fadavis.com/Wilkinson2

Conversions Between Systems

You will sometimes need to make conversions from one measurement system to another. For example, you may need to convert pounds to kilograms because many medications are ordered as milligrams per kilograms (e.g., "Give 2 mg per kg of body weight").

The following are the basic methods for converting between systems.

- **Metric and Apothecary—Weights**
  Grams and grains
  (Memorize: 1 g = 15 gr)
  To convert grams to grains—*multiply* the grams by 15
  To convert grains to grams—*divide* the grains by 15
  Grains and milligrams
  (Memorize: 1 gr = 60 mg)
  To convert grams to milligrams—*multiply* the grains by 60
  To convert milligrams to grains—*divide* the milligrams by 60
- **Metric and Apothecary and Household—Liquid Volume**
  Liters and ounces
  (Memorize: 1 L = 34.4 oz)
  To convert liters and quarts to ounces—*multiply* the liters by 33.4
  To convert ounces to liters and quarts—*divide* the ounces by 34.4
  Ounces and milliliters
  (Memorize: 1 oz = 30 mL)
  To convert ounces to milliliters—*multiply* the ounces by 30
  To convert milliliters to ounces—*divide* the milliliters by 30
  Milliliters and drops
  (Memorize: 1 mL = 15 drops or 15 minims)
  To convert milliliters to minims or drops—*multiply* milliliters by 15
  To convert minims and drops to milliliters—*divide* the minims or drops by 15

KnowledgeCheck 23-2

Work the following conversions:
- How many drops in 4 mL?
- How many mL in 2 oz?
- Convert 16 oz to liters.
- You have 3 g. How many grains is this?
- You have 10 mg. How many grains is this?

Go to Chapter 23, **Knowledge Check Response Sheet and Answers,** on the Student Resource Disk or DavisPlus at http://davisplus.fadavis.com/Wilkinson2

How Should I Calculate Dosage for a Child?

You must be very careful when calculating medication dosages for children and infants. Most drug references list normal pediatric ranges, which can serve as additional verification.

You should rarely need to calculate a child's dosage on the basis of an adult dose, because medication orders should specify the exact dosage for the individual child. However, you can use either the Body Surface Area Formula by using the nomogram for Children or Clark's Rule for Children to verify the safety of pediatric orders. To find a child's BSA using the nomogram, you must know the child's height and weight.

 To use the nomogram, go to Chapter 23, **Tables, Boxes, Figures: ESG Figure 23-2: Nomogram,** on the Student Resource Disk or DavisPlus at http://davisplus.fadavis.com/Wilkinson2

Orders for pediatric dosages are usually either calculated by the prescriber or stated in terms of "milligrams per kilogram of body weight." For example, you might have an order for "Erythromycin 30 mg/kg of body weight." You know that 1 kg equals 2.2 lb. If the child weighs 44 lb, then to convert to kilograms you divide 44 by 2.2; the child thus weighs 20 kg. So, 30 mg/kg would be 30 mg × 20, or 600 mg (the dosage for a 20-kg child).

For Clark's Rule, you would apply a formula using the child's weight in pounds. If you want to use Clark's Rule,

 Go to Chapter 23, **Tables, Boxes, Figures: ESG Box 23-2,** on the Student Resource Disk or DavisPlus at http://davisplus.fadavis.com/Wilkinson2

For a Web-based dose calculator,

 Go to Manuel's Web site at http://www.manuelsweb.com/nrs_calculators.htm

The Student Resource Disk contains several practice problems for calculating adult and child dosages.

 Go to Chapter 23, **Practice Dosage Problems,** on the Student Resource Disk or DavisPlus at http://davisplus.fadavis.com/Wilkinson2

If you cannot work the practice problems easily, you should obtain a dosage calculation book and practice the various formulas until you are proficient with conversion.

THINKING CRITICALLY ABOUT ADMINISTERING MEDICATIONS

The exercises in the following section allow you to practice the kind of thinking you will use as a full-spectrum nurse. Because these are critical-thinking questions, there is usually no single right answer. We do not provide answers for these questions because it is more important for you to think about the questions than to arrive at the "right" answer. These questions are designed to improve your thinking more than to "cover content." Discuss answers with your peers—discussion can stimulate critical thinking. If you have difficulty with any of these questions, consult with your instructor.

Applying the Full-Spectrum Nursing Model

PATIENT SITUATION

Leonard LeMonte is a 57-year-old, African American man who has come to his primary care provider because of persistent headaches that increase in intensity as it gets later in the day. His overall health has been good, although he is approximately 50 to 60 pounds overweight. Past medical history is significant for borderline primary hyptertension and non-insulin-dependent diabetes, type 2 (diet controlled). Leonard tells you he works in a high-stress envrionment. He shares great concern with you that he fears losing his job and not being able to pay his bills and meet other financial commitments for his family. Mr. LeMonte tells you he has little time for hobbies or recreational outlets because he works so many hours.

THINKING

1. *Theoretical Knowledge (Facts and Principles):* You see in the chart that the prescriber has been ordering metformin (Glucophage), 1000 mg daily, to treat Mr. LeMonte's diabetes. By what route is this medication given?

2. *Critical Thinking (Inquiry):* If you did not know the answer to the first question, specifically how did you get that information? State your source.

DOING

3. *Nursing Process (Assessment):* To evaluate Mr. LeMonte's responses to his diabetes medication, what questions do you need to ask him?

4. *Practical Knowledge (Skills):* Mr. LeMonte tells you that he forgot to take his Glucophage this morning and also at lunchtime. What should you do?

CARING

5. *Self-Knowledge:* In what areas do you feel compassion for Mr. LeMonte, on which you might build a caring relationship?

6. *Self-Knowledge:* What do you identify as your strength in dealing with Mr. LeMonte's healthcare needs?

7. *Ethical Knowledge:* Mr. LeMonte tells you that he frequently skips doses of his Glucophage because he can't afford the expense. He asks you not to tell his wife about this because he doesn't want her to worry? What will you do?

Critical Thinking and Clinical Reasoning

1. Your patient is ordered Humulin R insulin 30 units subcutaneously. You have available in a multidose vial Humulin R insulin; the label reads "100 units per mL."

   a. What equipment and supplies do you need to give this medication? Be specific.

   b. What practical knowledge (psychomotor skills) will you need?

c. With regard to the psychomotor skills, what are the two aspects that require the most careful attention? Explain your thinking.

d. What will you do to ensure that you have the correct dosage?

e. What specific technique steps will you take to decrease the risk for infection?

f. Suppose that after drawing the insulin into the syringe, you see that instead of the 30 units ordered, you have only 20 units in the syringe. What will you do?

2. The physician orders heparin 4000 units subcutaneous q12hr for Mr. Dale. You have on hand heparin 10,000 units/mL. How many milliliters should you draw up?

VOL 1 Recall the patients from **Chapter 23, Meet Your Patients,** in Volume 1. Exercises 3 through 6, and 8 following refer to those patients. They are listed here for your convenience.

- Margaret Marks is an 82-year-old woman who has a fractured hip and experiences periods of confusion throughout the day. She has returned home. She tries to be compliant with her medications but has limited income and many times is unable to purchase all of her medication.
- Cary Pearson is a 70-year-old man with feeding and swallowing difficulties. He uses a gastrostomy tube to receive his medications. He lives in an assisted living facility, where a personal aide assists him with his care and medications.
- Cyndi Early is a 32-year-old woman with diabetes who is scheduled for surgery at 1000 today. Cyndi was admitted to the hospital for right upper quadrant abdominal pain associated with nausea and vomiting. She is scheduled today for a cholecystectomy (removal of the gallbladder).
- James Bigler is a 44-year-old man who has had a repair of a compound fracture of the right arm and is receiving IV fluids and medications, including narcotics and antibiotics.
- Rebecca Jones is an 84-year-old woman with compression fractures of the vertebrae resulting from a fall. She has returned to an assisted living facility. Rebecca has hearing and vision problems; she does not always see her medications clearly and frequently takes them according to color and tablet size rather than reading the label.

3. It is 0800, and you have begun organizing your medication pass for this shift by verifying the MAR entries against the physician's orders. You notice that Mr. Bigler has been ordered Toradol 30 mg IM q6hr. His last dose was supposed to have been given at 0600, and there is no documentation that the medication was administered.

a. What should you do?

b. Should you assume the night shift nurse gave the medication but forgot to document that she had given it, and give the 0600 dose late? Why or why not?

c. When should the next dose be given?

d. If the night nurse did *not* give the medication as ordered, what type of medication error did she make? What are some of the things that could have caused this error?

e. Assuming that the nurse *did* give the medication as ordered at 0600, what error did the night nurse make? Which of the "rights of medication" was violated?

4. You receive the laboratory results for Cary Pearson's potassium level and find it to be 3.1 mEq/L. You notify the physician and receive a verbal order to add 20 milliequivalents of KCl to the running IV of D$_5$ ½NS (5% dextrose in half-strength normal saline [0.45% saline]) to infuse at 125 mL/hr. The running IV is in a new 1000 mL bag that is still almost full.

a. Write the order as you would write it on the order sheet.

b. What information must you put on the additive label for this bag?

c. Suppose the situation were slightly different. There is only 100 mL of IV fluid left in Mr. Pearson's IV bag when you call the physician. The physician says to you, "Add 10 mEq to the IV, and infuse it at 125 mL/hr" Would you ask for clarification of this order? Why or why not?

d. Change the situation again. You have taken the order in this way: "Add 20 mEq of KCl to 1000 mL of D_5 ½NS and run at 125 mL/hr." You are preparing this medication and find that Mr. Pearson currently has 500 mL remaining in his IV. Should you add the KCl to this infusing IV or wait until you hang a new 1000-mL bag? If you do add it, how much KCl will you add? What is your rationale for your decision?

e. You begin preparing the infusion with the 20 mEq of KCl to be added and find you have available only a vial containing KCl 40 mEq in a 10-mL vial. How many milliliters of KCl will you add to the bag of fluids?

5. Dr. Xi has ordered heparin 8000 units subcutaneous q12hr for Mrs. Marks.

a. You have vials of heparin containing 10,000 units/mL. How many mL of heparin will you administer?

b. To prevent tissue trauma and hematoma, and to help ensure adequate absorption, what precautions should you take while administering heparin?

c. What syringe and needle will you select for administration, and why?

6. You are checking Mrs. Early's chart and find that the physician has ordered a medication the patient lists as an allergy. What steps should you take?

7. A patient has been taking warfarin sodium (Coumadin) 3 mg daily for the past 3 years. She has tolerated the medication well, but recently she has noticed more bleeding tendencies, such as nosebleeds and hematuria (blood in the urine). You assess the patient and find that she has gross hematuria today and numerous bruises over her body. To answer the following questions, what theoretical knowledge do you need, and where can you find it? (Note: After you get the information you need, answer the following questions.)

a. What could be causing these bleeding episodes?

b. What laboratory test is indicated in this situation, and what do you expect the result to be?

c. What actions should you take in this situation?

8. James Bigler ("Meet Your Patients") has had a postoperative repair of a compound fracture of the right arm and is receiving IV fluids and medications, including opioid analgesics and antibiotics. Coincidentally, he has for some time now had a herniated intervertebral disk, and he has begun to have severe muscle spasms. He was given his first dose of an oral muscle relaxant, cyclobenzaprine (Flexeril) 10 mg at midnight. At 0800 he received another dose. At 0900 he received an IV antibiotic, and, while awake, he has been self-administering his opioid analgesic by IV pump about every 4 hours in a low dose. Consider these facts:

- The most common side effect of Flexeril is drowsiness. It has a half-life of 24 to 72 hours.
- Common side effects of opioids are drowsiness, decreased respiratory rate and depth, decreased blood pressure, and constipation (if taken long term).

■ Aside from allergies, the most common adverse effect of Mr. Bigler's antibiotic is diarrhea.

Mr. Bigler's muscle relaxant (Flexeril) is to be given every 8 hours. When you enter his room to give it again at 1600, you find that he is extremely sleepy. He will awaken when you shake him or speak to him, but he falls right back to sleep, and he is slurring his words. These are new symptoms for him.

a. Is there anything obvious about his medical diagnosis that might be producing these symptoms. If so, what?

b. Which of his medications could cause these symptoms, and why?

c. What would you do? Would you give the 1600 dose of cyclobenzaprine (Flexeril)?

9. Mrs. Jones lives alone and until a few months ago was able to take care of herself. When her eyesight began to deteriorate, she experienced difficulty self-administering her medications.

a. Discuss the assessment required to determine whether she is at risk for ineffective management of her medication regimen.

b. Mrs. Jones has an order for lorazepam (Ativan) 1 mg orally. Is this prescription complete? If not, what is missing? What actions should you take?

c. Mrs. Jones has an order for digoxin (Lanoxin) 1.25 mg orally each A.M. You have available Lanoxin 0.25 mg, and you calculate that the dose to be given would be 5 tablets. You check a drug guide and find that the usual dose is 0.125 mg to 0.25 mg orally daily. What actions should you take?

10. Calculate dosages for the following medications that you will be administering during your medication pass today. Are there any orders you would question? If so, why?

a. Cephalexin (Keflex) 500 mg IV q6hr. You have on hand Keflex 1 gm in 1 mL of solution.

b. Furosemide (Lasix) 280 mg orally daily. You have 40-mg tablets of Lasix available.

c. Meperidine (Demerol) 10 mg intramuscularly, to a child. You have Demerol 25 mg/mL available in a prefilled syringe. In addition to calculating the dosage, describe the equipment you would use to administer the Demerol to a child.

d. Morphine gr ¼. You have morphine labeled 10 mg/mL. How many milliliters of morphine will you give?

11. Describe the procedure for giving meperidine (Demerol) 50 mg and hydroxyzine (Vistaril) 50 mg intramuscularly using the same syringe. The Demerol is in a prefilled 2.5-mL injectable cartridge containing 50 mg of Demerol in 1 mL of fluid. The Vistaril is in a single-dose vial containing 50 mg of Vistaril in 1 mL of fluid.

12. You have an order to give injectable phenytoin (Dilantin) and furosemide (Lasix). You would like to give them in the same syringe. What theoretical and practical knowledge do you need to decide whether you can do this?

13. For each of the following patient problems, (1) state what you think might be the cause and (2) state one thing you might have done to prevent the problem.

a. When you give Mrs. King an intramuscular injection in her ventrogluteal muscle, she complains of pain.

b. Several weeks after receiving an intramuscular injection in the dorsogluteal site, Mr. Aguilar begins having pain in his left lower back and hip; the pain proceeds down his leg. He is beginning to limp when he walks.

c. Several days after receiving a subcutaneous injection, Patti Deal's upper arm is red, hot, painful, and swollen. There is pus oozing from the injection site.

d. Immediately after an intramuscular injection, a patient starts showing severe, unexpected symptoms.

14. For each of the following concepts, use critical thinking to describe how or why it is important to nursing, patient care, or administering medications. Note that these are *not* to be merely definitions.

Pharmacology
Drug classification systems (e.g., according to use or chemical traits)
The *United States Pharmacopoeia (USP)* and the *National Formulary* (US), the *British Pharmacopoeia*, and the *Canadian Formulary*
Drug excretion
Therapeutic levels

Side effects and adverse reactions
The apothecary system
Household measurements
Units and milliequivalents
Standing orders
"Rights of medication" administration
Ventrogluteal site for intramuscular injection
Medication errors

What Are the Main Points in This Chapter?

➤ Drugs are classified according to their use, body systems, and chemical or pharmacological traits. Learning the classifications helps you to remember the characteristics of individual drugs.

➤ The form (preparation) of a drug affects its speed of onset, intensity of action, and route of administration.

➤ In the United States, the Food and Drug Administration (FDA) regulates the manufacturing, sale, and effectiveness of all medications. Various state and federal agencies and legislation also regulate the administration of medications.

➤ Controlled substances must be stored, handled, disposed of, and administered according to regulations established by the U.S. Drug Enforcement Agency (DEA).

➤ In general, IV medications are absorbed most rapidly, followed by intramuscular, subcutaneous, buccal, and oral medications.

➤ Metabolism is the chemical inactivation of a drug into a form that the body can excrete; drug metabolism takes place mainly in the liver.

➤ The primary route of drug excretion is from the kidneys; other routes are the liver, gastrointestinal tract, lungs, and exocrine glands.

➤ The therapeutic level of a drug is the concentration in the blood serum that produces the desired effect without toxicity.

➤ Medication effects can be primary (therapeutic and intended) or secondary (nontherapeutic and unintended). Secondary effects include side effects, adverse reactions, toxic reactions, allergic reactions, and idiosyncratic reactions.

➤ The metric system is preferred for medications; however, for a few medications, the apothecary and household systems are still used.

➤ You are legally responsible for the medications you administer. You must question orders you believe to be incorrect.

➤ To help prevent medication errors, observe the "three checks" (before and after pouring or drawing up a medication, and at the bedside) and "rights of medication" (right drug, right dose, right time, right route, and right patient, as well as right documentation immediately after giving the medication).

➤ If you make a medication error, it is absolutely necessary that you immediately assess the patient's vital signs and physical status; report findings to the primary care provider; and notify the nurse manager of your unit.

➤ The oral route is the one most commonly used; it is convenient and safe.

➤ Buccal and sublingual medications are held in the mouth so that they will be absorbed through the mucous membrane.

➤ For patients who cannot swallow or who have feeding tubes, you can give oral medications through enteric (e.g., NG and gastrostomy) tubes; the medications are given one at a time; the tube must be flushed before and after each medication.

➤ Topical medications may have local and systemic effects; transdermal patches are applied for their systemic effect.

➤ Nebulization is the production of a fine spray, fog, powder, or mist from a liquid drug.

➤ Parenteral medications require the use of sterile technique to prevent infection. *veins or layersgin*

➤ Needle length and gauge are chosen based on the type of medication, the route of administration, and the amount of adipose and muscle tissue the patient has.

➤ Needleless systems and safety syringes reduce the likelihood of needlestick injury.

➤ Always dispose of needles in special "sharps" containers. If you must recap a needle, use a one-handed technique.

➤ The ventrogluteal site is the preferred intramuscular injection site for adults. Other sites are the vastus lateralis and the deltoid. Use the rectus femoris site only if no other sites are available, and never in infants and children. Do not use the dorsogluteal site.

➤ Experts agree the anterolateral thigh (vastus lateralis) is preferred for infants who are not walking. For older infants, there is some controversy about when to begin using the ventrogluteal site. Some say it is the preferred site after the gluteal muscles increases in mass; others continue to recommend the anterolateral thigh throughout childhood. The deltoid can be used for older children if you are certain that the muscle mass is adequate.

➤ Medications may be given intravenously by adding the medication to a large-volume (primary infusion), by the IV push technique, or by intermittent (piggyback and tandem setup) infusion.

➤ You should report medication errors immediately after they occur; a risk management process for monitoring causative factors should be in place.

➤ The most common reasons for a patient to have a central venous access device (CVAD) are:

- To give long-term IV therapy
- To provide total parenteral nutrition when the patient cannot eat normally
- To have blood drawn without the trauma and complications of repeated venipuncture
- When peripheral IV placement is difficult

For practice questions for this chapter,

Go to **NCLEX-Style Practice Quiz,** on the Student Resource Disk or DavisPlus at http://davisplus.fadavis.com/Wilkinson2

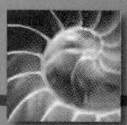 **Knowledge Map**

Drug Names:
- Chemical name
- Generic (official) name
- Brand name (trade)

Drug Classifications:
- By their use
- By body systems
- By pharmacological traits

Efficacy influenced by:
- Pharmacokinetics
    - absorption
    - distribution
    - metabolism
    - excretion
- Pharmacodynamics
    - interaction with target cells
    - how biological response occurs

Factors Contributing to Drug Safety:
- Reliable drug info
    - USP; national formulary; PDR; drug reference books
- State/Federal Regulation
    - Nurse Practice Act
    - U.S. drug laws
    - Regulation of controlled substances
- Improved storage/ distribution systems

DRUGS
- Prescription
- Non-prescription (OTC)

Medication Administration

Medication Orders

Administration Safeguards

Routes of Administration

Error Prevention

Types:
- Standard written
- Verbal
- Telephone
- Standing
- One-time

Correct components:
- Patient name
- Date/time
- Drug name
- Dose and frequency
- Route
- Signature of prescriber

Preparing: Three Checks →
- Label against MAR prior to pouring
- Label against MAR AFTER preparing med at the bedside

Administration: Six Rights →
- Drug
- Dose = accurate calculations
- Time → know "window"
- Route
- The Joint Commission two patient identifiers
- Documentation

Non-Parenteral:
- Oral
    - buccal
    - sublingual
- Topical
    - cream/ointment
    - transdermal
- Ophthalmic
- Otic
- Nasal
- Vaginal/rectal
- Inhaled

Parenteral:
- Intradermal
- Subcutaneous
- Intramuscular
- Intravenous

- 3 checks/6 rights
- Check calculations w/second person
- Watch look-alike, sound-alike drugs
- Check decimals; use correctly
- Question multiple vials/tabs if single dose
- Question abrupt increase in doses

Nursing Skills:
- Appropriate needle/syringe
- Withdrawal from amp/vial
- Correct site
- Correct administration technique

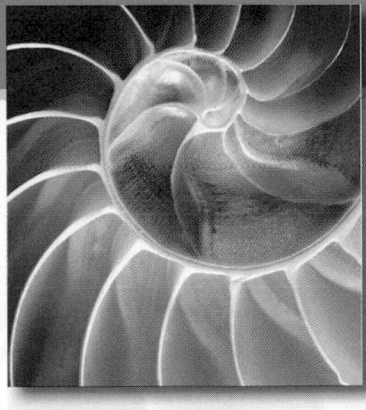

CHAPTER 24

Teaching Clients

For a podcast of an overview of this chapter,

 Go to Student Resources, **Podcast – Chapter Overviews, Chapter 24,** on DavisPlus at http://davisplus.fadavis.com/ Wilkinson2

Caring for the Garcias

The exercises in the following section allow you to practice the kind of thinking you will use as a full-spectrum nurse. Because these are critical-thinking questions, there is usually no single right answer. We do not provide answers for these questions because it is more important for you to think about the questions than to arrive at the "right" answer. These questions are designed to improve your thinking more than to "cover content." Discuss answers with your peers— discussion can stimulate critical thinking. If you have difficulty with any of these questions, consult with your instructor.

Joe Garcia has medical diagnoses including hypertension, type 2 diabetes mellitus, obesity, osteoarthritis. There is a positive history of tobacco abuse. Based on the information you know about Joe and his family, consider the following questions.

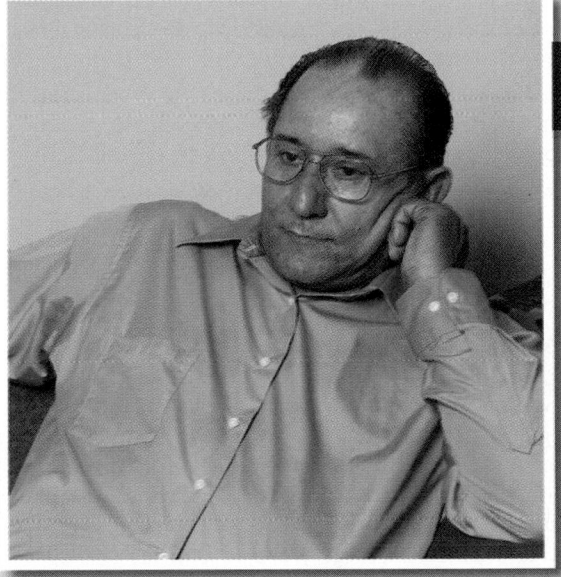

A. What kinds of information does Joe probably need?

B. What would be the best approach to teach Joe about his healthcare conditions?

C. You have been asked to teach Joe about weight loss. What theoretical knowledge must you have, and where can you obtain it?

D. What patient information do you need to know before planning your teaching?

E. Joe tells you that he feels overwhelmed with his recent diagnoses. He does not believe he can begin a weight loss program or attend any teaching sessions. How might you handle this concern?

F. Joe has been prescribed the following medicines:

Lisinopril 20 mg PO daily
Hydrochlorothiazide 25 mg PO daily
Metformin 500 mg PO bid

Devise one or more teaching sessions focused on these medications. You will need to use your pharmacology reference books to devise this plan. As you plan your teaching, recall that Joe is overwhelmed by his recent diagnoses.

Practical **Knowledge**
knowing how

Assessment Guidelines and Tools

Learning Assessment Guidelines

Pre-assessment

Before assessing the learner, think about the following:

- *Time constraints.* How much information do you need to present? How much time do you have to do it?

- *Available resources.* What equipment and supplies do you have to work with? Do you have audiovisual equipment? A chalkboard? A copy machine? Books?

Assessing the Learner

You can assess the learner in several ways: through informal conversations, structured interviews, focus groups, questionnaires, tests, observations, and information obtained from the client's chart. You will pick up many cues in your initial comprehensive assessment of the client. A teaching/learning assessment should include the following:

- *Intended audience.* Who are you teaching? What is the person's age, occupation, developmental level, and cultural affiliation? Will you be teaching a person or a group?

- *Learning needs.* The client's need for information is based on actual or anticipated healthcare or developmental needs. What is the client's medical (or other) problem? What behavioral changes are needed? What self-care knowledge and skills does the client need?

- *Client's knowledge level.* Determine what the client already knows so that you can reinforce correct information, correct misinformation, and adapt the teaching plan to the client's learning needs. Ask questions such as: "What do you think caused your health problem? What are your concerns about it? How has the problem affected your usual activities? What are your concerns about treatment (tests, surgery, and so on)?"

- *Health beliefs and practices.* Teaching will not be effective unless it falls into the range of beliefs and practices that are acceptable to the client. People are unlikely to incorporate changes that do not fit into their value system. Ask the client to give a general description of her health. Ask: "What do you usually do to stay healthy? What problems do you think you are at risk for? What lifestyle changes would you be willing to make in order to improve your health?"

- *Physical readiness.* The client must have adequate concentration, manual dexterity skills, and minimal pain to be able to listen and learn.

- *Emotional readiness.* Find out if the client is experiencing anxiety or emotional distress that will interfere with the learning process. Also ask the client whether she would like a family member or friend to be present during the learning.

- *Ability to learn.* What are the learner's cognitive and psychomotor developmental level and ability? How does the client learn best (e.g., by memorization or recall, or by problem solving or applying information)? How well does the client recall previously presented material?

- *Health literacy level.* Does the patient have the ability to understand basic health information and services needed to make appropriate health care decisions? Is the information the healthcare provider offers in the patient's primary language? Is the health teaching provided in a format the patient can understand? Is medical jargon or unnecessary technical information used? Can the person read and write?

  Adults who have low health literacy may react to learning situations by withdrawal, avoidance, or repeated noncompliance. They may claim that they were too tired, were too busy, or just didn't feel like reading. They may also ask you to read to them with the excuse that their eyes are tired, they are not interested, or they have no energy. They may fail to ask questions or ask for clarification.

- *Neurosensory factors.* What is the client's ability to feel, see, hear, and grasp? Does the client have a medical condition that causes neurosensory compromise?

- *Learning styles.* Ask the person: "How do you prefer to learn new things? For example, do you prefer to read about them, talk about them, watch a video, be shown how to do it, listen to the teacher, or use a computer? Do you like to read? Where do you get information about your health—from books, magazines, your family, your healthcare provider? Do you learn best alone or with other people?"

Standardized Language

NOC Outcomes for Health Knowledge

Health Knowledge outcomes are those that describe a client's understanding in applying information to promote, maintain, and restore health. They are as follows:

Knowledge: Arthritis Management

Knowledge: Asthma Management

Knowledge: Body Mechanics

Knowledge: Breastfeeding

Knowledge: Cancer Management

Knowledge: Cancer Threat Reduction

Knowledge: Cardiac Disease Management

Knowledge: Child Physical Safety

Knowledge: Conception Prevention

Knowledge: Congestive Heart Failure Management

Knowledge: Depression Management

Knowledge: Diabetes Management

Knowledge: Diet

Knowledge: Disease Process

Knowledge: Energy Conservation

Knowledge: Fall Prevention

Knowledge: Fertility Promotion

Knowledge: Health Behavior

Knowledge: Health Promotion

Knowledge: Health Resources

Knowledge: Illness Care

Knowledge: Infant Care

Knowledge: Infection Management

Knowledge: Labor and Delivery

Knowledge: Medication

Knowledge: Multiple Sclerosis Management

Knowledge: Ostomy Care

Knowledge: Pain Management

Knowledge: Parenting

Knowledge: Personal Safety

Knowledge: Postpartum Maternal Health

Knowledge: Preconception Maternal Health

Knowledge: Pregnancy

Knowledge: Pregnancy & Postpartum Sexual Functioning

Knowledge: Prescribed Activity

Knowledge: Preterm Infant Care

Knowledge: Sexual Functioning

Knowledge: Substance Use Control

Knowledge: Treatment Procedure

Knowledge: Treatment Regimen

Knowledge: Weight Management

Source: Moorhead, S., Johnson, M., Maas, M., et al. (Eds.). (2008). *Nursing outcomes classification (NOC)* (4th ed.). St. Louis, MO: C.V. Mosby, p. 115. Used with permission.

NIC Interventions for Patient Education

The following are interventions to assist another to build on his own strengths, to adapt to a change in function, or to achieve a higher level of function.

Chemotherapy Management

Family Planning: Contraception

Health Education

Learning Facilitation

Learning Readiness Enhancement

Parent Education: Adolescent

Parent Education: Childrearing Family

Parent Education: Infant

Preparatory Sensory Information

Teaching: Disease Process

Teaching: Foot Care

Teaching: Group

Teaching: Individual

Teaching: Infant Nutrition*

Teaching: Infant Safety*

Teaching: Infant Stimulation*

Teaching: Preoperative

Teaching: Prescribed Activity/Exercise

Teaching: Prescribed Diet

Teaching: Prescribed Medication

Teaching: Procedure/Treatment

Teaching: Psychomotor Skill

Teaching: Safe Sex

Teaching: Sexuality

Teaching: Toddler Nutrition*

Teaching: Toddler Safety*

Teaching: Toilet Training

*Note: NIC provides activities appropriate to specific age groups (e.g., 0–3, 4–6, 7–9, 10–12 months for infants and 13–18, 19–24, 25–36 months for toddlers).

Source: Bulechek, G., Butcher, H., & Dochterman, J. M. (2008). *Nursing intervention classification (NIC)* (5th ed.). St. Louis, MO: C.V. Mosby, p. 121. Used with permission.

THINKING CRITICALLY ABOUT TEACHING CLIENTS

The exercises in the following sections allow you to practice the kind of thinking you will use as a full-spectrum nurse. Because these are critical-thinking questions, there is usually no single right answer. We do not provide answers for these questions because it is more important for you to think about the questions than to arrive at the "right" answer. These questions are designed to improve your thinking more than to "cover content." Discuss answers with your peers—discussion can stimulate critical thinking. If you have difficulty with any of these questions, consult with your instructor.

Applying the Full-Spectrum Nursing Model

PATIENT SITUATION

Katrina Peplowsi is a 22-year-old college student from the Ukraine who is transported to the emergency department of a local hospital after passing out in her dorm room. Katrina had been sick with a viral illness and she had a fever for 5 days with nausea, vomiting, and diarrhea. She had been drinking large amounts of Gatorade because of her insatiable thirst, thought to be related to the fever and vomiting. Before the illness, Katrina's friends and family had been commenting about her remarkable weight loss since she started school 2 months earlier in spite of her increased appetite. On arrival to the emergency department, Katrina's blood sugar is 585 mg/dL. She is diagnosed with diabetes mellitus, type 1. After stabilization of her blood sugar with fluid therapy and insulin infusion, Katrina regains consciousness. Although Katrina speaks some English, her proficiency is somewhat limited.

THINKING

1. *Theoretical Knowledge (Recall of Facts and Principles):* As your patient is newly diagnosed with diabetes mellitus, type 1, there are many areas in which Katrina will need healthcare education. List at least six important topics that are relevant to her care.

2. *Critical Thinking: (Application of Knowledge):* What considerations do you make as you are devising a teaching plan for Katrina?

3. *Critical Thinking: (Synthesis of Knowledge):* What would factors would you consider important for customizing her teaching plan, considering the extent of her ability to communicate?

DOING

4. *Nursing Process (Assessment):* What are some pertinent personal factors that you should assess for Ms. Peplowski when devising a teaching plan that is best suited to her learning needs?

5. *Nursing Process (Planning):* When setting up a teaching plan involving other members of the healthcare team, how would you plan to optimize Katrina's motivation to learn how to best manage her diabetes after discharge?

CARING

6. *Self-Knowledge:* What areas of commonality do you have with Katrina, around which you might form a caring relationship?

7. *Ethical Knowledge:* Suppose Katrina refuses to receive information from you about diabetes mellitus. She states she is not interested in knowing how to give herself insulin because she doesn't want to give herself injections at home. How should you best respond to Katrina's requests?

■ Critical Thinking and Clinical Reasoning

1. For the following NOC standardized outcomes (Moorhead, Johnson, & Maas, 2008), try to figure out which NANDA-I diagnoses might be linked to each outcome. Consult the NANDA-I handbook as necessary.

Knowledge: Breastfeeding
Knowledge: Child Physical Safety
Knowledge: Diabetes Management
Knowledge: Diet
Knowledge: Disease Process

Knowledge: Energy Conservation
Knowledge: Health Behavior
Knowledge: Illness Care
Knowledge: Infant Care
Knowledge: Infection Management

2. Recall that Heather ("Meet Your Patient" in Volume 1) is a 20-year-old mother of a 4-year-old preschooler. They have come to a family practice clinic for a well-child check-up. You notice that the child speaks in one- or two-word phrases. Heather is impatient with her and repeatedly tells her to "stop using that baby talk." Your nursing instructor tells you that you need to assess for teaching needs and provide anticipatory guidance to the mother regarding safety, nutrition, and normal preschooler growth and development.

   a. Heather says, "I don't know what I'm doing wrong. All her little friends are taller and talking more. She was even small when she was born, so I suppose it's my fault." How do you assess Heather's learning needs without reinforcing her feelings of self-blame?

   b. Your assessment shows that although the child is below the 5th percentile for height and weight, she has grown appropriately since her last clinic visit. What teaching could you provide that might help address her mother's learning needs related to childhood growth and development?

   c. In addition to information on growth and development, your anticipatory guidance should include safety measures and nutrition for a 4-year-old. How can you evaluate whether your teaching has been effective and further promote Heather's retention of all of this new information?

3. As a student, you have learned about discharge planning. Your instructor tells you that you need to begin teaching for discharge as soon as the client is admitted. You hear the nurses complaining that they just don't have time for any teaching. So where do you begin? You will need to use the teaching process for your assigned client.

   Your client is a 9-year-old girl who is being admitted to the outpatient procedures unit for testing because of chronic recurrent urinary tract infections. She receives daily an antibiotic, methylphenidate (Ritalin) for attention-deficit disorder, and an asthma inhaler for sports activities. She is accompanied by her mother and father, a younger sister, and her big, pink teddy bear. She is scheduled for x-ray studies and blood work. Depending on the results of her tests, she may require surgery or dilatation of her ureters. The parents appear very anxious and tell you that their daughter is "a little slow and needs a lot of repetition." You have an hour to prepare her for the procedures and testing.

   a. Assessment

      (1) What information do you already have that will be significant for your teaching plan?

      (2) What other information will you need to gather?

   b. Diagnosis

      (1) What possible diagnoses are involved in this situation? Consider a diagnosis for your client and another one for at least one of her family members.

   c. Planning

      (1) What information will you present first?

      (2) What teaching techniques would you use for this situation?

(3) Who would you include in the teaching?

(4) Where would you complete the teaching?

d. Goals and interventions

(1) Write an appropriate goal for your client (the child). Remember to make the goal client-centered, timed, and realistic. You have only an hour to complete this teaching.

(2) What content and methods would you include in your teaching plan?

(3) How can you incorporate a stuffed teddy bear in your teaching?

e. Evaluation

(1) How would you determine whether your teaching was effective?

(2) What further teaching do you need to continue to prepare your client for discharge?

4. For each of the following situations, determine which teaching techniques would be most effective.

a. A group of adolescents with diabetes need to plan for their prom. The after-prom party lasts until 6:00 AM and will interfere with their usual schedule for insulin administration. You need to help them decide how to manage this problem. They are all busy with after-school activities and attend three different schools.

b. An 80-year-old man has experienced a cerebrovascular accident (CVA) (stroke) with right-sided weakness. He will need mobility training and assessment of his home situation for safety hazards. Currently he lives alone.

c. A new mother must learn how to feed her infant, who has a cleft palate. She is in considerable pain after an emergency caesarean section and unexpected blood loss.

5. You are assigned to a client with a diagnosis that you are unfamiliar with. You are expected to prepare a teaching session for this client and family as well as for your classmates. How should you prepare for this assignment?

6. Give an example of teaching content you might need to present to a 58-year-old patient who has been diagnosed with hypertension. What chapters in this text (Volume 1) might be useful if you need theoretical knowledge about hypertension to answer this question? Where would you look to verify where this information is located?

7. Do you think it is appropriate for a nurse to offer personal experiences in the teaching process? Explain your thinking.

8. A client refuses to make eye contact during a teaching session. This makes it difficult for you to determine whether she is actually paying attention to what you are saying. How can you assess whether she is focused on the teaching session?

9. For each of the following concepts, use critical thinking to describe how or why it is important to nursing, patient care, or teaching clients. Note that these are *not* to be merely definitions.

Role of teaching in nursing practice
Principles of teaching and learning
Factors that affect the learning process
Factors that affect the teaching process
Timing

Choice of techniques
Relevance
Learning styles
Amount of information to be presented

What Are the Main Points in This Chapter?

➤ Teaching is an essential component of professional nursing.

➤ Nurses do formal and informal teaching for individuals and groups.

➤ To be effective, teaching requires cooperation between the learner and the teacher.

➤ Learning is a change in behavior, knowledge, skills, or attitudes that occurs as a result of exposure to environmental stimuli.

➤ Bloom and Krathwohl (1956) identified three domains of learning: cognitive, psychomotor, and affective.

➤ Teaching includes motivating the learner.

➤ Teaching is interactive and requires communication.

➤ Readiness means that the learner is both motivated and able to learn at a specific time.

➤ Other factors that affect learning include emotions, timing, active involvement, feedback, repetition, environment, amount and complexity of the content, communication, developmental stage, culture, and literacy.

➤ Common barriers to teaching in the hospital setting include failure to see teaching as a priority and lack of time, preparation, space, privacy, and third-party reimbursement for teaching.

➤ Barriers to learning include illness, physical discomfort, anxiety, low health literacy, environmental distraction, overwhelming amount of behavioral change needed, lack of positive reinforcement, and feelings of discouragement.

➤ The teaching process is similar to the nursing process.

➤ The nursing diagnosis Deficient Knowledge may be the primary problem or the etiology of other problems; this diagnosis is often used incorrectly.

➤ A teaching plan is similar to a nursing care plan, except that (1) interventions are actually teaching strategies and (2) the plan includes the content of the teaching, the sequencing of the content, and the materials to be used.

➤ Demonstration and return demonstration are the most effective strategies for teaching psychomotor skills.

➤ A certain amount of forgetting is normal. You can aid learner retention by using strategies that require learner participation and by providing printed materials to use at a later time.

➤ It is important to document specifically what teaching you did as well as your evaluation of the learning that occurred.

For practice questions for this chapter,

 Go to **NCLEX-Style Chapter Quiz,** on the Student Resource Disk or DavisPlus at http://davisplus.fadavis.com/Wilkinson2

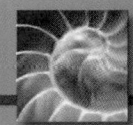

Knowledge Map

Teaching and Learning

Standards
- ANA
- The Joint Commission
- Patient Care Partnership
- Pew Commission

Informal

independent nursing action

Formal

Teaching
Interactive process/activity intended to meet outcomes

using

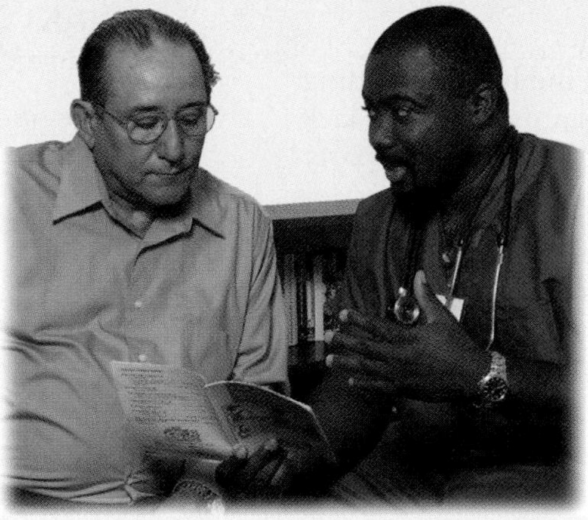

Teaching strategies
- Lecture
- Group/individual discussion
- Demo/return demo
- Multimedia
- Pamphlets, instruction sheets
- Simulation
- Role-playing
- Independent instruction
- Use of Internet
- Gaming

Use a combination of strategies to affect all three domains

Cognitive domain
Storage and recall

Psychomotor domain
Physical skill

Affective domain
Change in attitude, feeling, or belief

Learning
Change in behavior, knowledge, skill, or attitude

Factors affecting learning
- Motivation
- Readiness
- Environment
- Timing/scheduling
- Use of feedback, repetition
- Content and how it is communicated
- Developmental stage
- Culture
- Literacy

Is learning successful?

Evaluate using
- Written tests
- Oral interview/questionnaires
- Return demonstration
- Analysis of client report

How Nurses Support Physiological Functioning

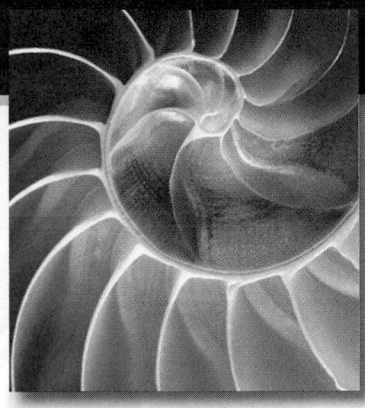

CHAPTER 25

Stress & Adaptation

For a podcast of an overview of this chapter,

 Go to Student Resources, **Podcast – Chapter Overviews, Chapter 25,** on DavisPlus at http://davisplus.fadavis.com/ Wilkinson2

Caring for the Garcias

The exercises in the following section allow you to practice the kind of thinking you will use as a full-spectrum nurse. Because these are critical-thinking questions, there is usually no single right answer. We do not provide answers for these questions because it is more important for you to think about the questions than to arrive at the "right" answer. These questions are designed to improve your thinking more than to "cover content." Discuss answers with your peers— discussion can stimulate critical thinking. If you have difficulty with any of these questions, consult with your instructor.

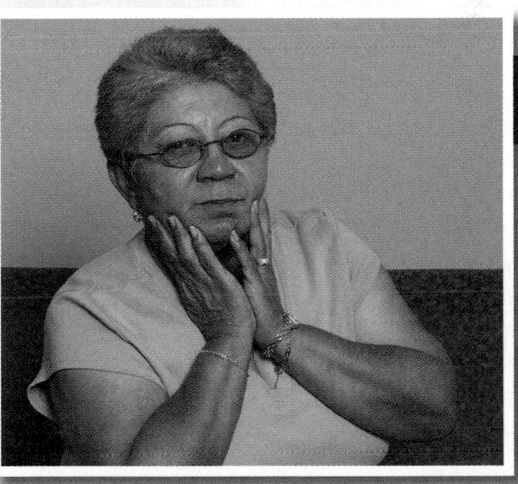

After having a comprehensive physical exam at the family health center, Flordelisa Garcia has been scheduled to have a mammogram and screening laboratory work. When she arrives at the clinic for her mammogram, she tells you she is very nervous. "I have a good friend who just found out she has breast cancer. She's very depressed now. Do I really have to do this test?"

A. What kind of stress is Flordelisa experiencing?

B. Three days later, the radiologist contacts Flordelisa requesting that she return to the family health center for additional films of the upper outer quadrant of the right breast. "There are some calcifications I want to check out," explains the radiologist.
- What factors might affect Flordelisa's adaptation to this stress?
- Evaluate what you know about Flordelisa's perception of her stress, her overall health status, her support

system, and her coping methods. What more do you need to know about these topics to fully answer this question?

C. Later, Flordelisa calls the office frantically explaining that she is very upset about this recent event. She says, "Not knowing is killing me. I'm so nervous I can't stand it. I can't sleep. I can't eat." She asks how she can handle the stress until she comes in for the additional tests next week. What strategies would you recommend to help Flordelisa deal with the stress?

Practical **Knowledge**
knowing how

Clinical Insights

Clinical Insight 25-1 ▶ Dealing with Angry Patients

■ **Be aware of how you are responding to angry patients.** Are you relieving your own stress, or are you relieving the client's stress? If you respond angrily to relieve your own stress, you may provoke further anger in the patient and even escalate the situation to the point of violence.

■ **Keep reminding yourself not to take anger personally;** remind family members of this as well.

■ **Recognize anger and anxiety are normal feelings** when facing adversity, such as a life-threatening or debilitating illness. Do not discount feelings by saying something like, "Please, don't be so angry," or "You shouldn't talk like that." Or, "Everything will be OK. Don't worry."

■ **Encourage the client and family to express feelings** verbally and appropriately.

■ **Listen instead of defending.** If the patient yells, "Everything about this place stinks," don't respond with something like, "This hospital is highly rated by The Joint Commission," or, "We really are all trying to do the best we can for you." Instead, say something to encourage the person to express his feelings or give you more information: "You seem really angry; what's going on?" or "Maybe I can help. Tell me a little more about what stinks."

■ **Do not take responsibility for the patient's anger.** It is not your fault, so don't apologize (unless you really *do* have something to apologize for). In the preceding example, for instance, it is not your fault that "the place stinks" or that the patient feels that way. So do *not* say, "I'm sorry we haven't been meeting your expectations."

■ **Remain calm;** this reassures the patient.

■ **Help the patient identify what is causing the anger** and try to meet those needs.

 ■ **Be alert to your own and to the patient's safety needs.**

■ If the person seems violent, do not allow him to get between you and the door.

■ Be sure you know how to call for help from staff or security personnel if you think you or someone else is in danger.

■ Do not wear a stethoscope around your neck, dangling jewelry, or anything a patient might use to hurt you.

■ Do not go into a room alone with an angry patient who seems to have a potential for violence.

■ Remain at least an arm's length away from an angry and potentially violent patient.

■ Do not turn your back on an angry patient.

■ **If you believe the patient's anger may escalate to violence,** your priority is your own safety and the safety of others in the area.

In addition to the above, if you want more information,

VOL 1 Go to Chapter 21, **Box 21-8,** in Volume 1.

Also refer to the NIC intervention, Anger Control Assistance (Bulechek, Butcher, & Dochterman, 2008, pp. 134–135).

Clinical Insight 25-2 ▶ Crisis Intervention Guidelines

For nurses who are at an entry level of practice, the goals of crisis intervention include the following (Brammer, 2003; Neeb, 2006):

1. Assess the situation.
   What is the nature of the patient's condition and the severity of the crisis?

2. Ensure safety.
   ■ Call for help if you or the patient is in physical danger.
   ■ Do not leave the patient unless you think you are in imminent danger.
   ■ First ensure your own safety; then provide for the patient's safety.

3. Defuse the situation.
   ■ Keep in mind that a person in crisis may not be in control of his actions.
   ■ Try to calm the person verbally.

■ Attempt physical restraint only as a last resort and only when there is enough help to do it safely for both the staff and the patient.

4. Decrease the person's anxiety.
   ■ Reassure the person that he is in a safe place and that you are concerned and want to help.
   ■ Explain gently but firmly that you need his help and cooperation.
   ■ Help the person to vent feelings of fear, guilt, and anger.
   ■ Use physical contact very cautiously. The person in turmoil may interpret touch as aggression or a sexual approach.

5. Determine the problem.
   ■ Find out what the patient believes to be the cause of the crisis.

■ Remain calm, and do not pressure the patient to give reasons. Any tension on your part will create further panic in the patient.

6. Decide on the type of help needed.
   ■ You may be able to calm the person enough for him to understand what just happened, or you may not. Evaluate your ability to calm the patient based on your assessment of his coping skills and resources.
   ■ Put in place the help needed to restore the person to a minimal level of functioning. This may require long-term treatment. In that case, make the referrals.

7. Return the person to his precrisis level of functioning. This may involve crisis counseling and/or home crisis visits.
   ■ The goal of crisis counseling is to provide immediate relief, solve the most urgent problems, and give long-term counseling if needed. Crisis centers often rely on telephone counseling ("hotlines").
   ■ If telephone counseling is not adequate or if observations of the home environment are needed, home visits may be necessary.

Assessment Guidelines and Tools

The Holmes–Rahe Social Readjustment Scale

This is a way to check your stress level, measured in "life change units." Of course it is not possible to score the exact "amount" of stress. However, this will give you a general idea of your stress level and should provide some insight about the sources of your stress. The following are based on the number of life change units over a 1- to 2-year period:

Over 300 points (major amount of change): 80% chance of major illness
200–299 (Moderate amount of change): 50% chance of major illness
150–199 (Mild amount of change): 33% chance of major illness
0–149 (Insignificant amount of change): Minimal chance of major illness

Of course, your personality and your ability to cope also determine the likelihood of your becoming ill.

LIFE EVENT	LIFE CHANGE UNITS
Death of spouse	100
Divorce	73
Marital separation	65
Imprisonment	63
Death of a close family member	63
Personal injury or illness	53
Marriage	50
Dismissal from work	47
Marital reconciliation	45
Retirement	45
Change in health of family member	44
Pregnancy	40
Sexual difficulties	39
Gain of new family member	39
Business readjustment	39
Change in financial state	38
Change in number of arguments with spouse	35
Major mortgage	32
Foreclosure of mortgage or loan	30
Change in responsibilities at work	29
Son or daughter leaving home	29
Trouble with in-laws	29
Outstanding personal achievement	28
Spouse begins or stops work	26
Begin or end school	26

Continued

The Holmes–Rahe Social Readjustment Scale—cont'd

LIFE EVENT	LIFE CHANGE UNITS
Change in living conditions	25
Revision of personal habits	24
Trouble with boss	23
Change in work hours or conditions	20
Change in residence	20
Change in schools	20
Change in recreation	19
Change in church activities	19
Change in social activities	18
Minor mortgage or loan	17
Change in sleeping habits	16
Change in number of family reunions	15
Change in eating habits	15
Vacation	13
Christmas	12
Minor violation of the law	11

Source: Reprinted from Holmes, T., & Rahe, R. (1967). Social readjustment rating scale. *Journal of Psychosomatic Research, 11*(2), 213–218. Reprinted with permission from Elsevier.

Assessing for Stress: Questions to Ask

1. **Assess stressors and risk factors.** Ask the client to complete a stress inventory, such as the preceding Holmes-Rahe Social Readjustment Scale. Then ask the client the following questions:

   - What is causing the most stress in your life?

   - On a scale of 1 to 10 (where 1 is "not much" and 10 is "extreme"), rate the stress you are experiencing in each of these areas: work or school, finances, community responsibilities, your health, health of a family member, family relationships, family responsibilities, relationships with friends.

   - How long have you been dealing with the stressful situation(s)?

   - Can you track the accumulation of stress in your life?

   - How long have you been under this stress?

   - Note the client's developmental stage, and determine whether he is functioning as expected for this stage. Review the expanded version of Chapter 9 if you need help to identify developmental milestones. To help you assess for stressors that can be predicted to occur in each stage, you might ask questions such as:

     What challenges do you face as a result of your life and your age?

     Have you had recent life changes?

     Do you anticipate any life changes?

To review developmental stage changes,

Go to **Chapter 9, Expanded Discussion,** on the Student Resource Disk or DavisPlus at http://davisplus.fadavis.com/ Wilkinson2, and

Go to Chapter 25, **Box 25-1: Stressors Throughout the Life Span,** in Volume 1.

2. **Assess coping methods and adaptation.**

   - What coping strategies have you used previously? What was successful, and what was not successful?

   - Tell me about previous experiences you have had with stressful situations in your life.

   - What do you usually do to handle stressful situations? (If the client needs prompting, you can ask, "Do you cry, get angry, avoid people, talk to family or friends, do physical exercise, pray? Some people laugh or joke, others meditate, others try to control everything, others just work hard and look for a solution. What is your usual response?")

   - How well do these methods usually work for you?

   - What have you been doing to cope with the present situation?

   - How well is that working?

   - During the interview, you should also observe for the use of psychological defense mechanisms.

Assessing for Stress: Questions to Ask—cont'd

To review psychological defense mechanisms,

 Go to Chapter 25, **Table 25-1: Psychological Defense Mechanisms,** in Volume 1.

- If the patient has not exhibited any defense mechanisms, you could ask about the common ones. For example, "Do you ever cope with a situation by denying it exists or just by trying to put it out of your mind?"
- Also ask the client about physiological changes and diseases caused by ongoing stress. Check the client's records for a history of somatoform disorders. Ask the client:

    What physical illnesses do you have? How long have you had them?

    What, if any, physical changes have you noticed?

    Do you have other physical conditions, for example, hypertension, cardiac disease, diabetes, arthritis, joint pains, cancer?

To review findings that might indicate maladaption to stress,

 Go to Chapter 25, **Stress-Induced Organic Responses,** in Volume 1.

3. Assess physiological responses to stress.

The following are examples of questions you should ask:

- What do you do to stay healthy?
- Tell me about your health habits.
- How often do you have a checkup?
- What are your health concerns?

4. Assess emotional and behavioral responses to stress.

Emotional Responses

Observe for:

- Anger
- Anxiety
- Depression
- Fear
- Feelings of inadequacy
- Low self-esteem
- Irritability
- Lack of motivation
- Lethargy

Behavioral Responses

Observe for:

- Crying, emotional outbursts
- Dependence
- Poor job performance
- Substance use and abuse
- Sleeplessness (or sleeping too much)
- Change in eating habits (e.g., loss of appetite, overeating)
- Decrease in quality of job performance
- Preoccupation (i.e., daydreaming)
- Illnesses
- Increased absenteeism from work or school
- Increased number of accidents
- Avoiding social situations or relationships
- Rebellion, acting out

Examples of Assessment Questions

- Do you smoke?
- How much alcohol do you drink every day?
- What do you eat? What is your typical eating pattern?
- How much fluid do you drink daily?
- How many hours do you sleep at night? Do you feel rested when you wake up?
- Do you often wake up very early in the morning and have difficulty getting back to sleep?
- What prescribed medications, vitamins, over-the-counter medications, or herbs do you take?
- What regular physical activity or exercise do you engage in?
- How much time do you spend at work versus at leisure and play?
- Do you constantly take work home with you? Or think about work almost all the time?
- How do you relax?
- Have you given up activities and relationships you previously enjoyed because you "don't have enough time" or are too tired?
- How do you express anger?
- Do you try to be perfect?
- Would you describe yourself as having the stress-filled lifestyle of a type A personality?
- How often do you find yourself feeling hopeless? Sad?

5. Assess cognitive responses to stress.

Observe for the following responses when you assess other functional areas:

- Difficulty concentrating
- Poor judgment
- Decrease in accuracy (e.g., in counting money)
- Forgetfulness
- Decreased problem-solving ability
- Decreased attention to detail
- Difficulty learning
- Narrowing of focus
- Preoccupation, daydreaming

6. Assess support systems.

Ask the following questions:

- Tell me about your home. Describe your living environment. (Make a home visit if possible, or contact the case manager or social worker to arrange a home evaluation.)
- Who are the persons that provide the most support for you? In what ways do they support you?
- What support is available from family, friends, significant others, community agencies, and clergy that you may not have required until now?
- Do you have or do you seek spiritual support?
- How has your stress affected the family?
- What are your financial resources? What are your financial obligations?

Standardized Language

NANDA-I Nursing Diagnoses Associated with Stress

Physical

Constipation

Deficient Fluid Volume

Delayed Growth and
Development

Diarrhea

Disturbed Energy Field

Disturbed Sleep Pattern

Fatigue

Imbalanced Nutrition (can be
More Than or Less Than
Body Requirements)

Nausea

Pain (e.g., backache)

Risk for Injury

Sleep Deprivation

Behavioral

Decisional Conflict

Impaired Home Maintenance

Impaired Verbal
Communication

Ineffective Coping

Ineffective Health
Maintenance

Ineffective Self-Health
Management

Ineffective Therapeutic
Regimen Management

Risk-Prone Health Behavior

Self-Neglect

Cognitive

Acute Confusion

Disturbed Thought Processes

Impaired Memory

Emotional

Anxiety

Defensive Coping

Disturbed Body Image

Disturbed Personal Identity

Fear

Grieving, Complicated

Ineffective Coping

Ineffective Denial

Low Self-Esteem (Chronic or
Situational)

**Interpersonal
Relationships**

Caregiver Role Strain

Compromised or Disabled
Family Coping

Dysfunctional Family
Processes

Impaired Parenting

Impaired Social Interaction

Ineffective Community
Coping

Interrupted Family Processes

Post-Trauma Syndrome

Relocation Stress Syndrome

Risk for Compromised
Resilience

Risk for Other-Directed
Violence

Risk for Self-Directed
Violence

Risk for Suicide

Social Isolation

Stress Overload

Spiritual Domain

Hopelessness

Spiritual Distress

Impaired Religiosity

Adapted from NANDA International (2009). *Nursing diagnoses: Definitions and classification 2009–2011*. Oxford: Wiley-Blackwell. Used with permission.

Standardized Outcomes and Interventions for Stress-Related Nursing Diagnoses

Examples of NOC Outcomes		**NIC Interventions Listed Under "Stress" in the NIC Index**	
Anxiety Level	Family Resiliency	Anxiety Reduction	Counseling
Caregiver Stressors	Nutritional Status	Art Therapy	Dementia Management
Coping	Psychosocial Adjustment: Life Change	Caregiver Support	Emotional Support
Decision-Making		Case Management	Relocation Stress Reduction
Family Coping	Rest	Cognitive Restructuring	Resiliency Promotion
	Sleep	Coping Enhancement	Sleep Enhancement

Adapted from: Moorhead, S., Johnson, M., Maas, M., et al. (Eds.). (2008). *Nursing outcomes classification (NOC)* (4th ed.). St. Louis, MO: C.V. Mosby; Bulechek, G., Butcher, H., & Bulechek, G. (Eds.). (2008). *Nursing interventions classification (NIC)* (5th ed.). St. Louis, MO: C.V. Mosby. Used with permission.

THINKING CRITICALLY ABOUT STRESS AND ADAPTATION

The exercises in the following sections allow you to practice the kind of thinking you will use as a full-spectrum nurse. Because these are critical-thinking questions, there is usually no single right answer. We do not provide answers for these questions because it is more important for you to think about the questions than to arrive at the "right" answer. These questions are designed to improve your thinking more than to "cover content." Discuss answers with your peers—discussion can stimulate critical thinking. If you have difficulty with any of these questions, consult with your instructor.

Applying the Full-Spectrum Nursing Model

PATIENT SITUATION

Mrs. Williams is a 76-year-old Indian American woman who was admitted yesterday after suffering a stroke that paralyzed her right side. She has had diabetes and high blood pressure for many years. Since the stroke, she has been unable to speak clearly and becomes frustrated as she attempts to communicate her needs. Her daughter says Mrs. Williams is a proud, independent, and tidy woman who has been living alone since her husband's death last year. Until her stroke, she had been driving her car, cleaning the house, doing her grocery shopping, and maintaining the yard and garden. She wears eyeglasses for reading and driving and has a hearing aid, although she rarely uses it.

THINKING

1. *Theoretical Knowledge*:

   a. What stroke risk factors probably functioned as stressors for Mrs. Williams? (*Hint*: Look up stroke risk factors in a medical–surgical nursing or pathophysiology text, or online.)

   b. What are common stressors for patients who must be hospitalized?

2. *Critical Thinking (Contextual Awareness)*:

   a. Now that Mrs. Williams is in the hospital, what new stressors might she have?

DOING

3. *Practical Knowledge*: What might you advise Mrs. Williams' daughter to do to help her mother adapt more comfortably to the stressors in the hospital?

4. *Nursing Process (Diagnosis)*: Based on just the data in the scenario, write one actual nursing diagnosis for Mrs. Williams. Do not use potential diagnoses. Remember, the defining characteristics must be present in the scenario. State the data you would need in order to make the diagnosis more descriptive.

CARING

5. *Self-Knowledge*: Imagine yourself in Mrs. Williams' situation.

   a. What is the one thing that would cause you the most stress? Why would that be the most stressful thing?

   b. What is the single most important thing you would want your nurse to do for you?

Critical Thinking and Clinical Reasoning

1. (From "Meet Your Patient" in Volume 1.) Gloria and her husband, John, live in a residential community from which John commutes to work in a nearby city. Gloria runs an accounting business from their home. They have two teenage boys, who are active in sports, church activities, Boy Scouts, and the school band. The boys need transportation to activities. Gloria and John teach Sunday school and are Boy Scout leaders. Gloria's mother needs knee

replacement surgery and so cannot take care of Gloria's father, who is in the early stage of Alzheimer's disease. In addition to her own home responsibilities, Gloria must go to her parents to prepare meals and to provide care for her parents during the day. Gloria's sister comes at 8:00 P.M. to sleep in the parents' home during the night.

a. What resources may be available to help Gloria?

b. What stress-reducing techniques can you suggest to help Gloria?

c. What may reduce John's stress?

d. On a scale of 1 to 10 (1 being low and 10 being high), what number will you give to Gloria's stress level?

2. Look again at Gloria and John's situation. Using the following defense mechanisms, create a possible scenario for each. That is, what might Gloria (or John) say and/or do if they use the defense mechanism in this situation? If you need to review ego defense mechanisms,

 Go to **Table 25-1,** in Volume 1.

a. **Avoidance**—unconsciously staying away from events or situations that might open feelings of aggression or anxiety.

b. **Conversion**—changing emotional conflict into physical symptoms that have no physical basis.

c. **Denial**—transforming reality by refusing to acknowledge thoughts, feeling, desires, or impulses. This is unconscious; the person is *not* consciously lying.

d. **Displacement**—"kicking the dog." Transferring emotions, ideas, or wishes from one original object or situation to a substitute inappropriate person or object that is perceived to be less powerful or threatening.

e. **Reaction formation**—similar to compensation, except the person develops the exact opposite trait. The person is aware of her feelings but acts in ways opposite to what she is really feeling.

3. Mary is a nursing student. She works part time to maintain health insurance coverage for herself and her children and to earn tuition money for school. She has to do her studying after the children are in bed, so she gets little sleep herself. Her grades are low and do not reflect Mary's true knowledge level. Nursing faculty suggest that Mary seek counseling for exam anxiety and test-taking strategies. Mary realizes she may fail out of nursing school without this counseling, but she does not know how she will fit weekly sessions into her already full schedule.

a. List Mary's stressors.

b. Self-knowledge:

  ■ What life experiences do you have that may help you to understand Mary's situation?
  ■ How could these same life experiences interfere with your empathy for and understanding of Mary?
  ■ How much of Mary's story can you identify with as being part of your own experience now?

c. Which type of intervention do you think would be most helpful to Mary: (1) helping her to change her perception of her stressors, or (2) the health promotion activities discussed in Volume 1? Explain your reasoning.

d. Before deciding specifically how to help Mary, what data do you still need?

e. Based on the information you have, what do you think Mary's two most important goals are?

f. If you discover that Mary's most important goals actually are to (1) provide for her children and (2) succeed in nursing school, how might you use this information to help her?

4. *Self-knowledge*: In Volume 1, you listed your stressors. Let's assess further.

a. What are your two (or three) *most* important goals? List them in order of importance.

b. What support do you have that can help you to achieve each of these goals?

5. *Self-Knowledge and Theoretical Knowledge*: Use the "Script for Visualization" to lead a partner through a visualization exercise; then reverse roles, and have your partner lead you through it. To see the script,

 Go to Chapter 25, **Tables, Boxes, Figures: ESG Box 25-2,** on the Student Resource Disk or DavisPlus at http://davisplus.fadavis.com/Wilkinson2

a. Before beginning, what were your thoughts and feelings about the exercise?

b. After doing the visualization exercise, how did you feel? Did you feel more relaxed?

c. How do you think your attitudes and perceptions prior to the exercise affected how you felt *after* the exercise?

6. For each of the following concepts, use critical thinking to describe how or why it is important to nursing, patient care, or stress and adaptation. Note that these are *not* to be merely definitions.

Stress   Inflammatory response
Developmental stressors   Somatoform disorders
Coping strategies   Relaxation techniques for stress reduction
Ego defense mechanisms

▮ What Are the Main Points in This Chapter?

➤ Stress is a disturbance in normal homeostasis caused by internal or external stimuli called stressors.

➤ Adaptive coping techniques are those that offer healthy choices to the person and reduce the negative effects of stress.

➤ Approaches to coping include altering the stressor, adapting to the stressor, and avoiding the stressor.

➤ Whether the outcome of stress is positive (adaptation) or negative (disease) depends on the balance between the strength and duration of the stressors and the effectiveness of the person's coping methods.

➤ The three stages of Selye's general adaptation syndrome (GAS) are alarm, resistance, and exhaustion. Each stage in the GAS produces different physical or psychological responses.

➤ In the alarm stage of the GAS, responses are produced primarily by adrenal hormones, epinephrine, mineralocorticoids, and the sympathetic nervous system.

➤ The exhaustion stage can lead to stress-induced illness, burnout, or death.

➤ The two most common responses of the local adaptation syndrome (LAS) are the reflex pain response and the inflammatory response.

➤ Examples of psychological responses are anxiety, fear, anger, and ego defense mechanisms.

➤ Ego defense mechanisms are unconscious mental mechanisms that help to decrease the inner tension associated with stressors; when overused, they are maladaptive.

➤ Unsuccessful adaptation can lead to crisis, organic disease (e.g., stomach ulcers), somatoform disorders (e.g., hypochondriasis), and psychological disorders (e.g., mental illness).

➤ Crisis exists when (1) an event in a person's life drastically changes his or her routine and is perceived as a threat to self, and (2) the person's usual coping methods are ineffective, resulting in high anxiety and reduced ability to function.

➤ Burnout occurs when nurses or other professionals cannot cope effectively with the demands of the workplace.

➤ You should assess for data about the patient's stressors, risk factors, coping and adaptation, support systems, and psychosocial and physiological responses to stress.

➤ Interventions for stress must be individualized to the patient. They include (1) health promotion activities for preventing and improving the ability to cope with stressors; (2) managing anxiety, fear, and anger; (3) stress management techniques that focus on discharging tension or producing relaxation; (4) techniques to alter perception (i.e., cognitive restructuring and positive self-talk); (5) identifying and using support systems; (6) reducing the stress of hospitalization; (7) providing spiritual support; (8) crisis intervention; (9) stress management in the workplace; and (10) making referrals.

For practice questions for this chapter,

 Go to **NCLEX-Style Chapter Quiz,** on the Student Resource Disk or DavisPlus at http://davisplus.fadavis.com/Wilkinson2

To practice documentation for a patient experiencing stress,

 Go to **Practice Documentation,** on the Student Resource Disk or DavisPlus at http://davisplus.fadavis.com/Wilkinson2

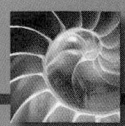

Knowledge Map

Stress & Adaptation

Coping strategies
• Alter stressor
• Adapt to stressor
• Avoid stressor

Types of stress
• Distress
• Eustress
• Internal
• External
• Developmental
• Situational
• Physiological
• Psychological

Stress

Influencing factors
• Overall health
• Support system
• Perception of stressor
• Age
• Life experience
• Developmental
  level

Potential outcome

increases

Adaptation

Responses

When it fails

Disease

Physiological responses
• Selye's GAS: autonomic nervous system
  and endocrine system; alarm, resistance,
  recovery/exhaustion
• Local adaptation: reflex pain and
  inflammatory response

Psychological disorders
• Crisis
• Burnout
• Post-traumatic stress
  disorder

Spiritual responses
• Prayer
• Meditation
• Religious affiliation

Somatoform
• Hypochondriasis
• Somatization
• Pain disorders
• Malingering

Psychological responses
• Anxiety
• Fear
• Ego defense mechanisms
• Anger
• Depression

Organic responses
• Heart disease
• Diabetes
• Irritable bowel syndrome
• Ulcers
• Autoimmune disorders

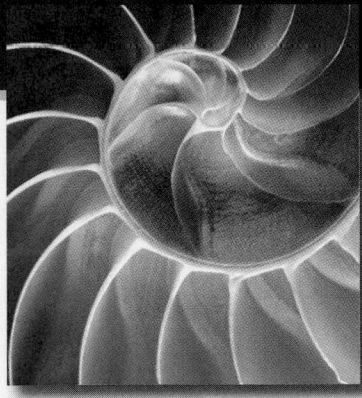

CHAPTER 26

Nutrition

For a podcast of an overview of this chapter,

 Go to Student Resources, **Podcast – Chapter Overviews, Chapter 26,** on DavisPlus at http://davisplus.fadavis.com/ Wilkinson2

Caring for the Garcias

The exercises in the following section allow you to practice the kind of thinking you will use as a full-spectrum nurse. Because these are critical-thinking questions, there is usually no single right answer. We do not provide answers for these questions because it is more important for you to think about the questions than to arrive at the "right" answer. These questions are designed to improve your thinking more than to "cover content." Discuss answers with your peers—discussion can stimulate critical thinking. If you have difficulty with any of these questions, consult with your instructor.

Joseph Garcia has been diagnosed with hypertension, type 2 diabetes mellitus, obesity, osteoarthritis, and tobacco abuse.

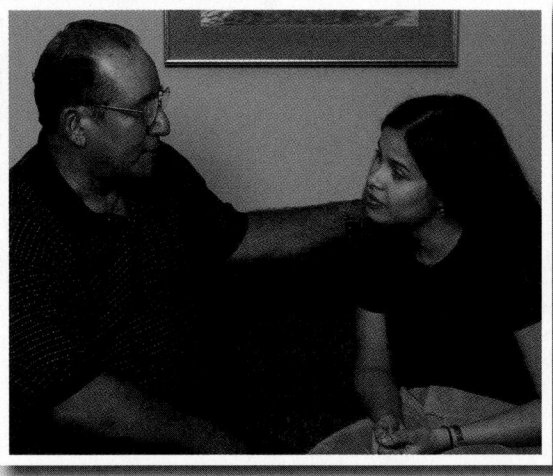

Jordan Miller has advised an 1800-kcal diabetic diet with no added salt and a brisk daily 30-minute walk. Mr. Garcia discusses these challenges with his daughter, Carmen.

A. Why might Jordan have selected this diet plan? Discuss the rationale for each component (i.e., 1800 kcal, diabetic diet, no added salt).

B. Mr. Garcia's diet is complex. He tells you he is overwhelmed by the many changes asked of him. How might Jordan streamline his instructions about Mr. Garcia's diet?

C. Mr. Garcia asks what is the best way for him to monitor his weight loss progress at home and how Jordan Miller will monitor his progress. How would you respond?

D. Identify teaching tools that might help Joe understand his diet.

Practical **Knowledge**
knowing how

To support patient nutrition, you will need to master techniques for assessing nutritional status, feeding patients, administering supplemental feedings, and working with nasogastric and nasoenteric tubes.

Procedures

Procedure 26-1 ☐ Checking Fingerstick (Capillary) Blood Glucose Levels

➤ For steps to follow in *all* procedures, refer to the Universal Steps for All Procedures found on the inside back cover of Volume 2.

Critical Aspects

- Ask the patient to wash his hands with warm soap and water. Dry well with a clean towel.
- Don procedure gloves
- Cleanse the patient's finger with an alcohol prep pad if agency policy requires.
- Prepare the lancet and meter and obtain a clean test strip that is recommended for the meter.
- Stick the side of the fingertip.
- Wipe off the first drop of blood; then place the second drop on the test strip.
- At the indicated time, read the glucose level on the digital display. (Follow the manufacturer's instructions.)

Equipment

- Blood glucose meter
- Test strip
- Sterile lancet (and injector, if available)
- Alcohol (or other antiseptic) pad, if required by policy
- 2 in. × 2 in. gauze pad or cotton ball
- Procedure gloves

✦ Glucometers should be assigned to individual patients. If this is not possible, you must clean and disinfect the device between patients. Injectors, too, should be assigned to individual patients; if possible, use single-use lancets that permanently retract upon puncture. Keep trays or carts with these supplies outside patient rooms. Do not carry supplies in your pocket. If there are unused supplies after the procedure, leave them in the room; do not use them for another patient.
These measures help prevent needlestick injury and transmission of blood-borne pathogens (CDC, 2005).

Delegation

You can delegate this procedure to a licensed practical nurse (LPN) or nursing assistive personnel (NAP) who have been adequately trained in performing the skill if the patient's condition allows. Assess the patient first; if the patient's condition is critical, do not delegate the procedure. Most patients perform this procedure independently at home.

Pre-Procedure Assessments

- **Assess the patient's comprehension of the procedure.** Understanding reduces anxiety and promotes cooperation.

- **Assess potential puncture sites for bruising, inflammation, open lesions, poor circulation, or edema.** Avoid such sites because of risk for infection and inaccurate results.

- **Check for factors such as anticoagulant therapy, bleeding disorders, or low platelet count.** These place the patient at risk for bleeding after skin puncture.

➤ When performing the procedure, always identify your patient according to agency policy and be attentive to standard precautions, hand hygiene, patient safety and privacy, body mechanics, and documentation.

➤ *Note:* The steps of this procedure will vary, depending on the type of glucose meter used.

Procedure Steps

I. Verify the medical prescription for frequency and timing of testing.
A prescription is necessary for testing. Timing and frequency of testing are crucial for accurate insulin dosing.

2. Ask the patient to wash her hands with soap and warm water, if able and to dry completely using a clean towel.
Reduces the risk for infection and dilates capillaries at the puncture site.

Also ensures that the testing site is free of any sugar residue.

3. Turn on the blood glucose meter. Calibrate it according to the manufacturer's instructions.

(continued on next page)

Procedure 26-1 ■ Checking Fingerstick (Capillary) Blood Glucose Levels (continued)

Calibration readies the meter for testing.

4. Check the expiration date on the container of reagent strips. If the strips are expired, replace them. Check that the strip is the correct type for the monitor.
Expired strips may alter test results. Different brands of monitors use different kinds of reagent strips.

5. Don procedure gloves.
Gloving protects against exposure to blood.

6. Remove the reagent strip from the container and place it into the blood glucose meter. Then tightly seal the container.
A tight seal protects reagent strips from exposure to air and light.

7. Select and clean a fingerstick site with an alcohol (or other antiseptic) pad, according to facility policy. Let it dry thoroughly.
Helps protect the patient from infection by removing some surface microorganisms. Allowing the alcohol to dry thoroughly will decrease pain of the skin puncture. Using alcohol is controversial, however, because it may interfere with the reagent on the strip, giving a false low reading; and it dries the skin. Follow agency policy and consult practice guidelines periodically.

8. Use a different site each time you check the glucose.
Adult and child: the lateral aspect of a finger (palmar surface, distal phalanx)
Infant: heel or great toe

The lateral aspect of the finger contains fewer nerve endings than the central fingertip, so it hurts less. Capillaries in infants are too small to obtain an adequate blood sample.

9. Position the finger in a dependent position, and massage from the base toward the tip of the finger.
A dependent position promotes blood flow to the site via gravity and pressure, ensuring an adequate specimen. The massaging action increases blood flow to the tip of the finger, which may prevent the need for repuncture.

10. Prick the finger (or other site) with the lancet:

Step 10 Variation. Exposed-Blade Disposable Lancet
  a. Remove the cover from the lancet, if there is a cover.
  b. Place the back of the patient's hand on the table, or otherwise secure the finger (e.g., hold the finger and hand firmly).
  c. Use a darting motion to puncture the site, at a 90° angle to the skin.

Step 10 Variation. Semi-automatic Injector
  d. Engage the sterile injector and remove the cover.
  e. Place the disposable lancet firmly in the end of the injector.
  f. Place the back of the patient's hand on the table, or otherwise secure the finger (e.g., hold the finger and hand firmly).
  g. Position the end of the injector firmly against the skin, perpendicular (at a 90° angle) to the chosen puncture site.
  h. Push the release switch, allowing the needle to pierce the skin.

Proper positioning and stabilization of the site ensure that the lancet pierces to the correct depth. This prevents patient injury and allows for adequate blood sampling. Patients

tend to pull away as you perform the puncture. ▼

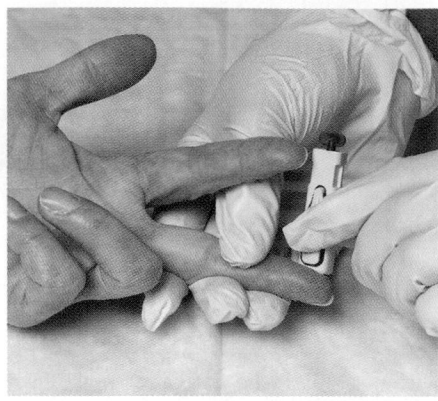

11. Lightly squeeze the patient's finger above the puncture site until a drop of blood has collected.
Squeezing promotes a better blood sample for testing without causing injury to the puncture site.

12. Wipe away the first drop with clean gauze and squeeze again to form another droplet.
The first drop of blood contains more serous fluid and can alter test results.

13. Place the reagent strip test patch close to the drop of blood. Allow contact between the drop of blood and the test strip. Do not "smear" the blood over the reagent strip.
This ensures adequate blood sample for testing. ▼

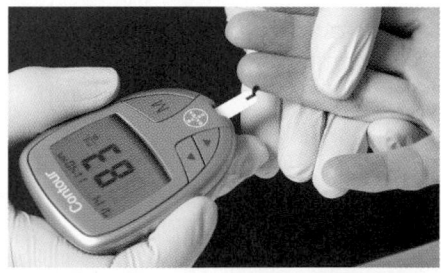

14. Insert the strip into the meter, if it is not already inserted (follow the manufacturer's instructions); allow the blood sample to remain in contact with the test strip for the amount of time specified by the manufacturer. For some meters you insert the test strip before pricking the finger; with others you put the blood on the reagent strip and then insert the strip into the meter. The blood sample must be on the reagent strip for the specified amount of time to ensure accurate test results.

15. Using a gauze pad, gently apply pressure to the puncture site. Pressure stops the bleeding by promoting coagulation.

16. After the meter signals, read the blood glucose level indicated on the digital display. ▼

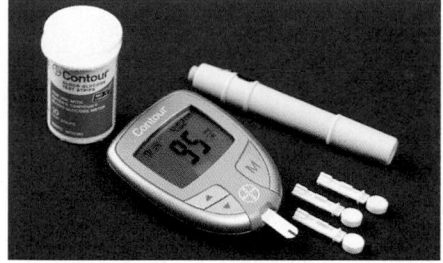

17. Turn off the meter, and dispose of the reagent strip, gauze pad,

alcohol pad, and lancet in the proper containers (e.g., a sharps container for the lancet). Proper disposal prevents sharps injury and the spread of infection via blood-borne pathogens.

18. Remove the procedure gloves, and dispose of them in the proper container. Perform hand hygiene. Hand hygiene and gloving reduce the transmission of microbes.

What if. . .

■ **The patient has poor circulation or is a child or older adult?**

Place a heel warmer or warm cloth on the site for about 10 minutes before obtaining the blood sample. Alternatively, position the patient's hand below the waist for 1 minute.

Capillaries in infants are very small; older adults may have poor peripheral circulation. The warmth may dilate the capillaries, helping you obtain an adequate amount of blood; the dangling of extremities allows blood to pool in the extremity, making it easier for you to obtain the quantity of blood needed.

■ **The patient is taking an anticoagulant such as warfarin sodium (Coumadin)?**

After the procedure, hold pressure for 2 minutes and then apply a pressure bandage if needed. Recheck the site after 5 minutes to make sure bleeding has stopped.

■ **The monitor shows an extremely unusual result or an error message?**

Repeat the process using a different finger or site.

■ **The patient uses a noninvasive method to measure blood glucose?**

A new tool called a continuous blood glucose monitor is now available. It is worn like a wristwatch. Using an electrical current, it pulls fluid from the skin to give a blood glucose reading. It will take readings automatically every 20 minutes for up to 12 hours. Advise the patient to shave his arm if it is very hairy, or the reading may not be accurate. The patient should wear the device for a 3-hour warmup before taking a reading, and should not bathe or swim during that time. This does *not* replace the patient's fingerstick method. Its purpose is to track trends in the blood glucose.

Evaluation

■ Assess the puncture site for bleeding or bruising.
■ Evaluate the patient's understanding of the procedure and the test results.
■ Promptly notify the physician of abnormal test results, or administer insulin based on test results, if prescribed.

Patient Teaching

■ Explain the procedure, test results, and treatment to the patient.
Informing the patient allows the patient to participate in his plan of care, and typically increases adherence to the therapeutic regimen.

■ If the patient will be performing fingerstick blood glucose testing at home, teach the patient how to perform the procedure. Ask the patient to perform a return demonstration.
■ Discuss the importance of maintaining glycemic control.
■ Teach the patient to do the following:
  ■ Read the manufacturer's instructions carefully and call their toll-free number if he has any questions.
  ■ Always use the test strips that are recommended for the meter.

■ Take your meter to your health provider's office so she can make sure you are measuring your blood sugar correctly.
■ Perform quality control checks (read the instructions) to make sure the meter is measuring accurately.
■ Clean the meter according to the manufacturer's directions. Some meters will give you an electronic alert telling you when to clean them.

Home Care

■ Assess the client's ability to perform fingerstick blood glucose monitoring independently.
A change in the patient's condition may not allow the patient to perform testing. Certain conditions, such as arthritis and limited vision, may limit dexterity.

■ Advise the patient about purchasing home glucose monitoring equipment.
■ Explain how to dispose of lancets in a labeled, puncture-proof container, such as an empty bleach container.
■ Instruct caregivers to wear gloves when obtaining a blood sample for glucose monitoring.
■ At home, patients do not need to cleanse their fingers with an alcohol wipe before puncturing it. However,

(continued on next page)

Procedure 26-1 ■ **Checking Fingerstick (Capillary) Blood Glucose Levels** (continued)

they should wash their hands with soap and water and dry well.

Documentation

■ Record the fingerstick blood glucose result in the progress notes or special flowsheet, including the date and time the test was performed.

■ Note whether the physician was notified and record any treatment given.
■ Document patient teaching.
■ If the fingerstick is performed in response to patient symptoms, you may need to write a narrative note.

Sample documentation:

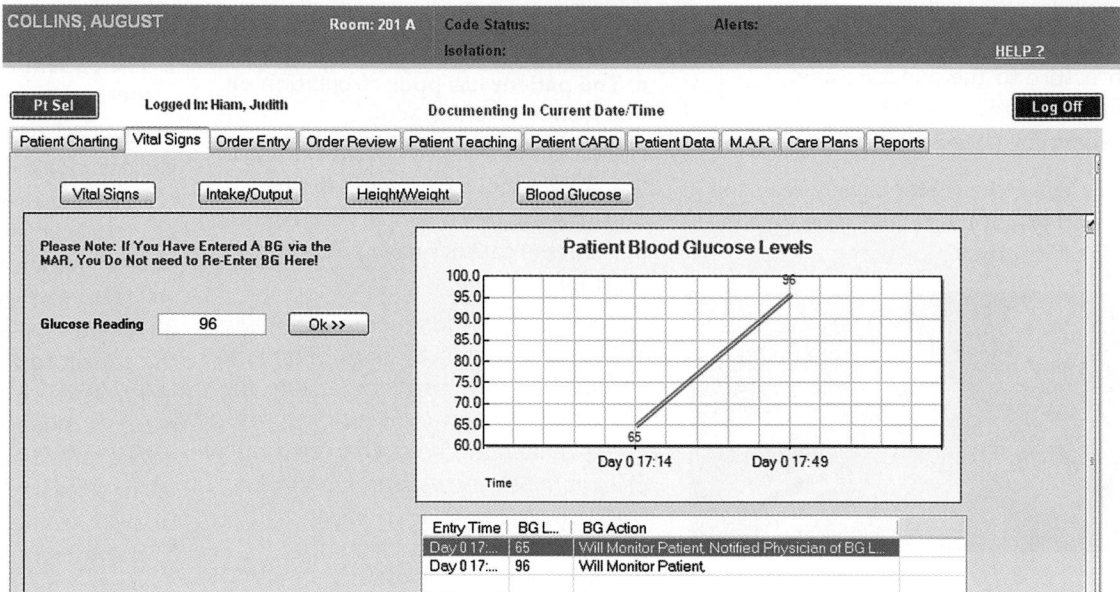

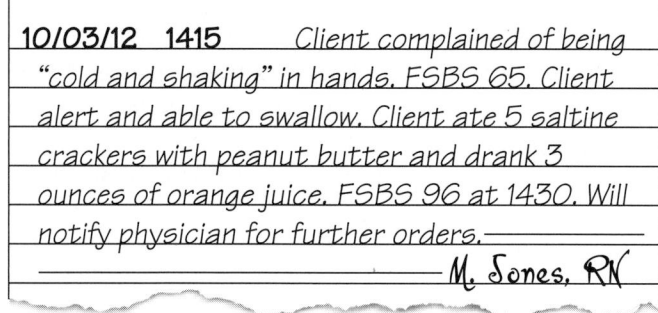

Practice Resources

American Diabetes Association (n.d.); Centers for Disease Control and Prevention (2005); GlaxoSmithKline (last updated 2008); U.S. Food and Drug Administration (2007b).

Thinking About the Procedure

 Go to the *Fundamentals of Nursing Skills Videos,* **Nutrition: Checking Fingerstick (Capillary) Blood Glucose Levels.**

1. When did the nurse don procedure gloves?

2. What is the latest point in the procedure at which the nurse could have donned her gloves?

 For suggested responses, go to Chapter 26, **Thinking About the Procedure Suggested Responses (Procedure 26-1),** on the Student Resource Disk or DavisPlus at http://davisplus.fadavis.com/Wilkinson2

Procedure 26-2 ■ Inserting Nasogastric and Nasoenteric Tubes

➤ For steps to follow in *all* procedures, refer to the Universal Steps for All Procedures found on the inside back cover of Volume 2.

Critical Aspects

- Place the patient in a sitting or high-Fowler's position.
- Measure the length of the tube:
  Nasogastric (NG) tubes: Measure from tip of the nose to earlobe and from earlobe to xiphoid process.
  Nasoenteric (NE) tubes: Add 8 to 10 cm (3 to 4 in.) to the NG measurement, as directed.
- Lubricate the tube with water-soluble lubricant.
- Ask the patient hyperextend the neck and breathe through the mouth.
- Insert the tube gently through the nostril, advance the tube as the patient swallows.
- Instruct the patient to tilt the head forward, drink water, and swallow.
- Withdraw the tube immediately if respiratory distress occurs during or immediately after insertion.
- Confirm tube placement initially by radiograph. Always reconfirm tube placement with a combination of bedside methods before giving feedings or medicine.
- Secure the tube to the nose and to the patient's gown.

To watch an animated demonstration of inserting a nasogastric tube,

 Go to **Animations: Inserting a Nasogastric Tube,** on DavisPlus at http://davisplus.fadavis.com/Wilkinson2

Equipment

- Nasogastric tube (commonly 16 or 18 Fr for adults, but sometimes smaller) or nasoenteric (small bowel) tube (8 Fr, 10 Fr, or 12 Fr)
- Stylet or guidewire (for small-bore tubes), according to agency policy
- Procedure gloves
- Linen-saver pad or towel
- Water-soluble lubricant
- 50- to 60-mL catheter-tip syringe or bulb syringe for Salem sump tubes; 30-mL Luer-lock syringe for small-bore feeding tubes
- Hypoallergenic tape (about 2.5 cm [1 in.] wide) or tube fixation device
- Indelible marker
- Skin adhesive
- Stethoscope
- Emesis basin
- Basin with warm water (for plastic tube) or ice (for rubber tube). Most tubes are plastic.
- Glass of water with a straw
- Penlight
- Tongue blade
- pH test strip
- Tissues
- Safety pin
- Gauze square or small plastic bag
- Rubber band
- Suction equipment (if tube is being connected to suction)

Delegation

This procedure should not be delegated because it requires knowledge of anatomy and physiology and the ability to adapt the procedure based on patient responses. You can, however, delegate associated oral hygiene needs.

Pre-Procedure Assessment

- Verify the medical prescription for type of tube to be placed and whether it is to be attached to suction or drainage.
- Verify the patient's need for NG or NE intubation (e.g., surgery involving the gastrointestinal (GI) tract, impaired swallowing, or decreased level of consciousness).

NG or NE intubation decreases the risk for aspiration in these patients. In many institutions, only specially trained nurses are allowed to place small-bowel feeding tubes.

- Assess each naris for patency, deviated septum, and skin breakdown. Ask the patient to close each nostril alternately and breathe. Select the nostril with the greatest air flow. Ask the patient to blow her nose, if not contraindicated.

A septal defect or facial fracture may cause obstruction, placing the patient at risk for nasal membrane trauma if insertion is attempted through the affected naris.

- Check medical history for anticoagulant therapy, coagulopathy, nasal trauma, nasal surgery, epistaxis, or deviated septum.

Patient history may place the patient at risk for injury during NG or NE insertion. Contraindications to NG insertion by a nurse include maxillo-facial disorders, surgery, or trauma; esophageal tumors or surgery; laryngectomy; skull fracture; unstable high cervical spinal injuries; and esophageal varices (although these patients may have tubes placed by a medical professional via endoscope or fluoroscope).

(continued on next page)

Procedure 26-2 ■ **Inserting Nasogastric and Nasoenteric Tubes** (continued)

■ Assess the level of consciousness and ability to follow instructions.

■ Assess for a gag reflex, using a tongue blade.

Absence of gag reflex places the patient at risk for aspiration.

➤ When performing the procedure, always identify your patient according to agency policy and be attentive to standard precautions, hand hygiene, patient safety and privacy, body mechanics, and documentation.

Procedure Steps

1. Prepare the tube.

Step 1 Variation. Plastic Tube
Wrap the tube around your index finger and then unwrap it and proceed or place in a basin of warm water for 10 minutes and proceed.

Step 1 Variation. Rubber Tube
Place in a basin of ice for 10 minutes.

Step 1 Variation. Small-Bore Tube
Insert a stylet or guide-wire and secure into position, according to agency policy. (Small-bore tubes may come with the guidewire in them. If so, flush the tube with tap water to lubricate the wire for easy removal. Leave the wire in place until the tube is positioned and its placement has been checked on x-ray film. Once the guidewire is removed, do not reinsert it.) Agency policy determines which nurses are authorized to place small-bore tubes.
Warm water softens a plastic tube, and ice stiffens the rubber tube to make it easier to insert. (Most tubes are polyurethane or silicone-based.) Wrapping a plastic tube around your index finger helps the tube flex into a curve and aid in insertion. A guidewire facilitates passage of small-bore tube but can cause trauma if not secured in a proper position.

2. Assist the patient into a high-Fowler's position with pillow behind the head and shoulders. Raise the bed to a comfortable working level.
This position facilitates tube insertion and prevents aspiration should the patient vomit during tube insertion. Gravity facilitates passage of the tube. Raising the bed reduces strain on the nurse's back.

3. Measure the tube for placement.

Step 3 Variation. Nasogastric Tube
Measure the length of the tube to be inserted by measuring from the tip of the nose to the earlobe, and from the earlobe to the xiphoid process. Mark the length with tape or indelible ink.
This measurement indicates the distance the tube must be inserted to reach the stomach. ▼

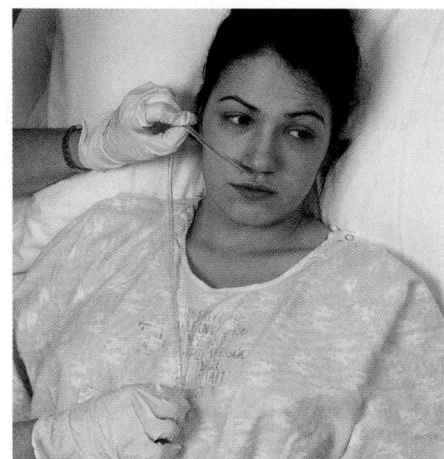

Step 3 Variation. Nasoenteric Tube
Add 8 to 10 cm (3 to 4 in.) to the NG tube measurement, as directed, and mark the tube.

4. Stand on the patient's right side if you are right-handed and on the left side if left-handed. Drape a linen saver pad over the patient's chest, and hand her an emesis basin and facial tissues.
Draping protects the patient's gown from becoming soiled during tube insertion.

5. Prepare the fixation device. Cut a 10-cm (4-in.) piece of hypoallergenic tape if securing tube with tape; split the bottom end lengthwise 2.5 cm (2 in.). If using a commercial feeding tube attachment device, have it ready at this time.
To secure the tube after insertion.

6. Arrange a signal by which the patient can communicate if she wants to stop (e.g., raising her hand).
Relieves anxiety by giving the patient some control over the procedure.

7. Don procedure gloves if you have not already done so.
Reduces the spread of microorganisms.

8. Wrap 10 to 15 cm (5 to 6 in.) of the end of the tube tightly around your index finger, then release.
Forms the tube into a curve that helps it conform more easily to the shape of the nasopharynx.

9. Lubricate the distal 10 cm (4 in.) of the tube with a water-soluble jelly.
Lubrication eases the passage of the tube and prevents injury to the nasal mucosa. Water-soluble lubricant will dissolve if it is aspirated, whereas oil-based lubricants do not dissolve in the respiratory tract and would cause inflammation and blockage of airways if they enter the lungs. Some nurses prefer water as a lubricant because aqueous jelly dries and can block nasal passages, which is irritating to the patient. Some tubes have a surface lubricant and require only that you dip them in room-temperature water.

10. If the patient is awake, alert, and able to swallow, hand her a glass of water with a straw.
Instructing the client to swallow water during insertion eases passage.

11. Instruct the patient to hold her head straight up and extend her neck back against the pillow (slightly hyperextended).
   a. Grasp the end of the tube above the lubricant with the curved end pointing downward.
   b. Carefully insert the tube along the floor of the nasal passage, on

the lateral side, aiming toward the ear.

c. You will feel slight resistance when the tube reaches the nasopharynx; use gentle pressure, but do not force the tube to advance. The patient's eyes may tear; if so, provide tissues.

d. Continue insertion of the tube until just past the nasopharynx by gently rotating the tube toward the client's opposite naris.

Hyperextending the neck straightens the curve where the nasal passage meets the pharynx (nasopharyngeal junction). Gentle insertion prevents trauma to the nasal mucosa. Forcing against resistance can traumatize the mucosa. Tears are normal. ▼

This maneuver closes the trachea and opens the esophagus. ▼

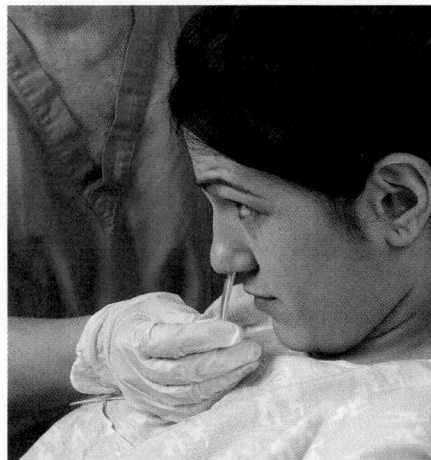

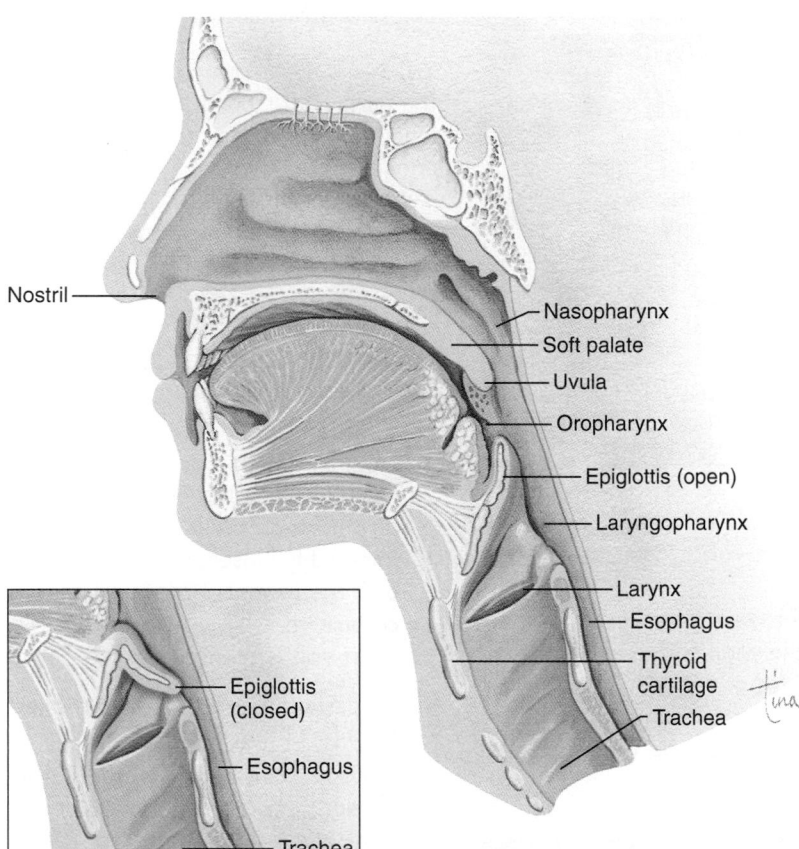

Nostril

- Nasopharynx
- Soft palate
- Uvula
- Oropharynx
- Epiglottis (open)
- Laryngopharynx
- Larynx
- Esophagus
- Thyroid cartilage
- Trachea

- Epiglottis (closed)
- Esophagus
- Trachea

12. Stop for a moment to allow the patient to relax, and perhaps use tissues. Explain that the next step requires her to swallow.

Stopping to relax can give the patient a feeling of control. Also, the rest can reduce gagging.

13. Instruct the patient to flex her head toward the chest, take a small sip of water, and swallow.

14. Rotate the tube 180°.

Rotation helps to redirect the tube so that it will not enter the patient's mouth.

15. Direct the patient to sip and swallow the water as you slowly advance the tube. (If the patient is not allowed water, instruct her to dry swallow or suck air through the straw.) Advance the tube 5 to 10 cm (2 to 4 in.) with each swallow until the tube is advanced the desired distance. Moving the tube with each swallow uses normal peristaltic movement to help advance the tube into the stomach. Swallowing closes the epiglottis so that the tube cannot advance into the trachea.

16. Continue advancing the tube to the desired distance.

♦ **17.** Temporarily secure the tube with one piece of tape. Then verify tube placement (see Clinical Insight 26-7). Never rely on a single bedside method. You can use a combination of the following methods to verify placement at the bedside; however, radiographic verification is the only reliable method and should be done before medications or fluids are given through the tube (Rauen, Chulay, Bridges, et al., 2008).

If you do not secure the tube, at least temporarily, it may move out of position—especially if you are waiting for placement to be confirmed by x-ray film.

a. **Inspect the posterior pharynx for presence of coiled tube.**

Visualization confirms that the tube has gone beyond the oropharynx.

b. **Aspirate gently to withdraw stomach contents and measure aspirate pH.** Aspirate gently over a period of up to 5 minutes, if necessary, to obtain gastric fluid.

The pH of stomach contents is normally 1 to 5.5; however, many situations commonly alter the pH of gastric contents, so the usefulness of this method is limited. pH testing is helpful only if the fluid is acidic; if it is alkaline, the gastric contents may have been altered (e.g., by enteral feedings or antacids and other medications), or

(continued on next page)

Procedure 26-2 ■ **Inserting Nasogastric and Nasoenteric Tubes** (continued)

the tube may be in the lung. This procedure does not reliably confirm gastric placement and should be used in combination with other methods.

   c. **Take note of the amount, color, and consistency of the aspirate.** Gastric aspirates are often white or greenish and may be curdled. Intestinal aspirates will be smaller in quantity, yellowish due to the presence of bile, and not curdled.

   d. **Inject air into the NG tube.** Use this only to confirm other methods; do not use as the primary method of verification because it is the least reliable method.

If the tube is in the stomach, injecting 5 to 30 mL of air with the syringe should produce a gurgling sound audible by listening with a stethoscope over the stomach. However, because the lungs and stomach are so close together, a tube inadvertently placed in the respiratory tract or esophagus can transmit a sound similar to that of air in the stomach.

   e. **Ask the patient to speak.** If she can do so, the tube is probably in the stomach. Use this only to confirm other methods; it is not reliable enough to use as the primary method of verification.

18. If the tube is not in the stomach, advance it another 2.5 to 5 cm (2 to 4 inches) and repeat steps 17a through 17e.

19. After you confirm proper placement, clamp the end of the tube or connect it to the drainage bag, feeding, or suction machine.

20. Secure the tube using one of the following methods.

Step 20 Variation. Securing the Tube with 1-inch (2.5 cm) Tape

   a. Apply skin adhesive to the patient's nose, and allow it to dry.
A skin adhesive helps the tape to adhere and protects skin from breakdown.

   b. Use the 5 cm (2 in.) piece of hypoallergenic tape, split lengthwise for 2.5 cm (1 in.) at one end.

A split tape can be wrapped around the tube in opposite directions to hold the tube in place more securely.

   c. Apply the intact end of tape to the patient's nose.

   d. Wrap the split strips around the tube where it exits the nose.

Step 20 Variation. Securing the Tube with ½-inch Tape

   e. Use half-inch (1.3 cm) tape, 4 inches (10 cm) long. Apply one end of tape to the patient's nose and wrap the other end downward around the tube and then back up to secure on the opposite side of the nose (see photo). ▼

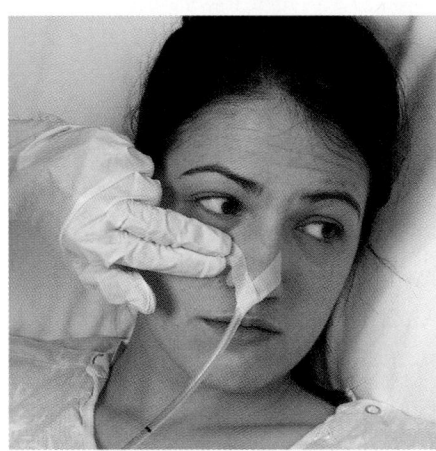

Step 20 Variation. Securing the Tube with a Tube Fixation Device

   f. Peel the backing off the pad and place the wide end of the pad over the bridge of the nose.

   g. Position the connector around the NG or NE tube where it exits the nose. ▼

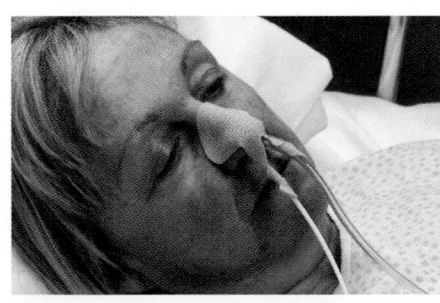

21. Curve and tape the tube to the patient's cheek (not necessary with some commercial tube fixation devices).

Securing the tube to the cheek reduces the tension on the naris.

22. Fasten the tube to the patient's gown: Tie a slipknot around the tube with a rubber band. Loop a rubber band in a slip knot near the connection. (Alternatively, wrap a short piece of tape around the tube to form a tab.) Then fasten the rubber band or the tab to the gown with a safety pin (or tape).
Reduces discomfort produced by the weight of the tube and prevents movement that may cause dislocation of the tube and irritation of the nose.

23. Elevate the head of the bed 30° unless contraindicated.

24. Mark the tube where it enters the naris with tape, or measure the length from the naris to the connector.
A marked tube allows you to easily notice whether tube placement has changed.

What if . . .

■ **The patient is confused, combative, or comatose?**

   a. If the patient is comatose, place him into a semi-Fowler's position. Have a co-worker use a pillow to help position the patient's head forward for insertion.

   b. If the patient is confused and combative, ask a co-worker to assist you with insertion.

■ **The patient gags, coughs, or chokes (at steps 11 and 15)?**

   a. Stop advancing the tube. Ask the patient to take deep breaths and drink a few sips of water.
Helps suppress the gag reflex.

   b. Instruct the patient to breathe easily and take some sips of water.

   c. If coughing continues, pull the tube back slightly.

   d. If gagging continues, use a tongue blade and penlight to check the tube position in the back of the throat.
The tube may be coiled in the back of the throat.

e. Continue to advance the tube to the desired distance.

⬥ f. However, if the tube is coiled in the back of the throat, the patient coughs excessively during insertion, the tube does not advance with each swallow, or the patient develops respiratory distress (e.g., gasping, coughing, or cyanosis), withdraw the tube completely and allow the patient to rest before reinserting.

The tube may be in the patient's trachea.

■ **You are unable to obtain an aspirate (at step 17b) when confirming tube placement?**

a. Use a 50-mL syringe and aspirate very slowly over at least 5 minutes.

b. Flush the tube with air, then aspirate.

c. Turn the patient to the left side, wait 20 minutes, then aspirate again.

■ **The prescription states the tube needs to be in the jejunum?**

a. To advance the tube into the jejunum after the tube has been placed in the stomach, position the patient on the right side.

Positioning on the right side allows gravity to assist tube passage through the pyloric sphincter.

b. Advance the tube 5 to 7.5 cm (2 to 3 in.) hourly, over several hours (up to 24 hours) until radiographic study confirms placement.

Weighted tubes will advance by gravity and peristalsis if a loop of the designated length is made at the entrance to the naris. After reading the initial x-ray, the radiologist or primary physician can provide the measurement needed to advance the tube to the desired position. Note that specially trained nurses usually place these tubes at the bedside.

■ **The procedure is anticipated to cause pain or discomfort?**

Commercial hurricane spray or viscous lidocaine are sometimes used to aid in patient comfort. Some practitioners use them for all NG insertions.

a. You may insert 2% viscous lidocaine into the nasal passage with a syringe before tube placement.

b. Alternatively, you can apply an anesthetic spray to the nasal and oropharyngeal mucosa.

■ **The patient is a child?**

a. Children usually require a smaller diameter tube.

b. Encourage parents to comfort infants and children and participate in their care.

c. You may need to apply restraints during insertion.

To prevent dislodging of the tube.

d. Monitor more frequently for complications.

Small children are not able to communicate problems with the tube.

Evaluation

■ Assess how well the patient tolerated the procedure (e.g., discomfort, gagging, coughing?)

■ Note the color, consistency, and pH of NG or NE aspirate.

■ Ask the patient whether she feels comfortable.

■ Assess respiratory status.

Patient Teaching

■ Explain that the sensation of the tube should decrease with time.

■ Explain the importance of immediately reporting tension on the tube or displacement of the tape or fixation device.

■ Discuss the need for frequent mouth care while the tube is in place.

Home Care

■ Assess the client or caregiver's ability to maintain an NG or NE tube at home.

■ Assess the home environment to determine the client's risk for infection.

■ Instruct the client or caregiver about aspirating stomach contents and measuring pH.

■ Teach the client or caregiver how to verify tube placement.

■ Explain to the client or caregiver how to properly secure the NG or NE tube.

■ Reinforce the need for frequent mouth care.

Documentation

Chart the date and time of insertion, size and type of the NG or NE tube and insertion site (which naris), length of tube from tip of the nose to the end of the tube, tolerance of the procedure, any abnormal findings, and methods for confirming NG or NE tube placement. Document description of gastric contents and respiratory status. NG or NE tube insertion is documented in the progress notes and flow sheets in most agencies.

(continued on next page)

Procedure 26-2 ■ **Inserting Nasogastric and Nasoenteric Tubes** (continued)

Sample EHR documentation:

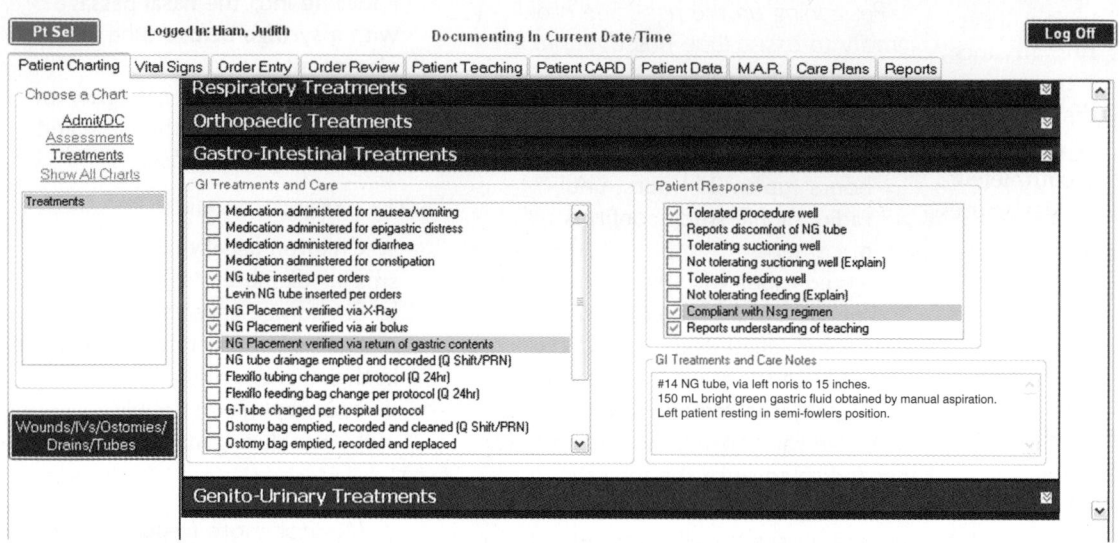

Practice Resources

American Association of Critical-Care Nurses (2005); Cullen, L., Taylor, D., Taylor, S., et al. (2004); Rauen, C., Chulay, M., Bridges, E., et al. (2008); Shlamovitz, G. Z., & Shah, N. R. (2008); Wiegand, D., & Carlson, K. (Eds.) (2005); Wolfe, T., Fosnocht, D., & Linscott, M. (2000).

Thinking About the Procedure

   Go to the *Fundamentals of Nursing Skills Videos,* **Nutrition: Nasogastric Tubes: Inserting and Checking Placement.**

1. What were the patient's responses as the tube advanced down into her throat?

2. What did the nurse do?

3. Why do you think the nurse continued to advance the tube instead of completely withdrawing the tube and starting the procedure all over?

   For suggested responses, go to Chapter 26, **Thinking About the Procedure Suggested Responses (Procedure 26-2),** on the Student Resource Disk or DavisPlus at http://davisplus.fadavis.com/Wilkinson2

Procedure 26-3 ▢ Administering Feedings Through Gastric and Enteric Tubes

➤ For steps to follow in *all* procedures, refer to the Universal Steps for All Procedures found on the inside back cover of Volume 2.

Critical Aspects

- Check the medical prescription for the type of formula, rate, route, and frequency of feeding.
- Check the chart to make sure a confirmation x-ray of tube placement was performed.
- Confirm tube placement at the bedside before administering the feeding.
- Elevate the head of the bed at least 30° to 45° while administering the feedings and for an hour after administration.
- Check residual volume before feeding for intermittent feedings.
  For continuous feeding: Check gastric residual volume at least once every shift. If the residual is 10% greater than the formula flow rate for 1 hour (or alternatively, a total of 150 mL), hold the feeding for 1 hour and recheck. Notify the physician if the residual is still not within normal limits.
  For gastrostomy and percutaneous endoscopic gastrostomy (PEG) tubes and gastrostomy buttons (G-buttons): Check residual volume every 4 hours.
  For jejunostomy tubes: Residual volumes are not checked.
- Flush tubing with 30 mL of water before and after feeding (every 4 hours for continuous feedings), and before and after medication administration. Some closed continuous feeding systems run sterile water tandem with the tube feeding; you can program the pump to deliver flushes according to the feeding protocol.
- Change the tube feeding administration set and other supplies a minimum of every 24 hours.
- Continuous feedings should be infused by pump.

Equipment

- Prescribed feeding formula at room temperature
- Filtered water or prescribed diluent, if ordered
- Tube feeding administration set and bag
- 60-mL Luer-lock or catheter-tip syringe (two needed for syringe feeding)
- Connector to connect administration set to the feeding tube
- Stethoscope
- Enteral feeding infusion pump (if used). Recommended for all continuous feedings.
- IV pole
- Linen-saver pad
- Graduated container
- pH strip
- *For gastrostomy and jejunostomy tubes:* a small precut gauze dressing

Delegation

You can delegate the procedure to the NAP or LPN if the patient's condition is stable and the NAP's skills allow. You must verify peristalsis, tube placement, and feeding tube patency before the feeding is started. Remind the NAP to position the patient upright and to report patient discomfort and any difficulty with the infusion.

Pre-Procedure Assessment

- Check the chart to determine that tube placement has been confirmed by radiography.

This is the only reliable method for confirming placement (Rauen, Chulay, Bridges, et al., 2008).

- Check the length of the exposed tube: (1) Compare the length from the naris to the connector recorded after x-ray confirmation of placement; or (2) Observe the mark that was made on it where it entered the nostril after insertion.

These methods confirm that the tube has not become displaced since radiography. If there is significant change in length, tube position must again be confirmed by radiography.

- Assess fluid status by checking breath sounds, mucous membranes, skin turgor, edema, and intake and output.

These signs indicate fluid volume excess or insufficiency.

- Obtain baseline weight and laboratory studies.

Weight change is a sensitive measure reflecting fluid and nutritional status.

- Monitor vital signs before and after feedings.

Vital signs may vary from baseline due to pain, impaction, or dehydration.

- Auscultate for bowel sounds before each feeding or every 4 to 8 hours for continuous feedings. Also check for distention, nausea, vomiting, and diarrhea.

These symptoms may indicate intolerance of tube feedings. If GI motility is impaired, feedings accumulate in the stomach along with gastric secretions, predisposing the patient to reflux and aspiration. Some medications (e.g., opioids) also slow gastric emptying.

(continued on next page)

Procedure 26-3 ■ **Administering Feedings Through Gastric and Enteric Tubes** (continued)

■ Assess frequency of bowel movements.
Diarrhea may indicate intolerance of the formula, excessive feeding, or gastrointestinal disease.

■ Check patient history for food allergies.
Helps prevent allergic reaction to ingredients in the feeding formula.

■ *For gastrostomy and jejunostomy tubes:* Assess the exit site at every shift. Report redness or drainage to the physician.
Leaking of gastric or intestinal contents may cause skin breakdown.

➤ When performing the procedure, always identify your patient according to agency policy and be attentive to standard precautions, hand hygiene, patient safety and privacy, body mechanics, and documentation.

Procedure Steps

1. Check the medical prescription for the type of feeding, rate of infusion, and frequency of feeding.
A medical prescription is required for enteral feedings. Rate and frequency of feeding are crucial for providing adequate nutrition.

2. Check the expiration date of the tube feeding formula.
Expired formula should be discarded.

3. Prepare the formula.
   a. Shake the feeding formula well.

Step 3 Variation. Intermittent Feedings
   b. Warm the formula to room temperature.
Because the formula goes directly into the stomach and is not warmed by the mouth and esophagus, cold formula may cause abdominal cramping and increase the risk for diarrhea.

Step 3 Variation. Continuous Feedings
   c. Keep continuous-feeding formulas cool, but not cold (don't use ice).
Heat can coagulate some feedings (e.g., those containing egg). Cold feedings may cause vasoconstriction and cramps. Commercially prepared formulas are stored at room temperature.

4. Prepare the equipment for administration.

Step 4 Variation. Open System with Feeding Bag
   a. Fill a disposable tube feeding bag with a 4- to 6-hour supply of feeding formula and prime the tubing.
Limit hang-time to help prevent bacterial growth and prevent air from entering the GI tract.

   b. Label the feeding bag with the date, time, formula type, and rate.
Labeling identifies the formula and helps avoid administering formula past the expiration date.

   c. Hang the disposable tube-feeding bag on an IV pole.

Step 4 Variation. Open System with Syringe
   d. Remove the plunger.

Step 4 Variation. Closed System with Prefilled Bottle with Drip Chamber
   e. Attach the administration set to the prefilled bottle of feeding formula, and prime the tubing.
   f. Hang the prefilled bottle on an IV pole. A prefilled container can safely hang for 24 to 36 hours (some agencies allow for 48 hours).
Closed systems decrease the risk of contamination and prevents air from entering the GI tract.

5. Elevate the head of the bed at least 30° to 45° unless contraindicated.
A position in which the stomach is higher than the gut reduces the risk for aspiration of gastric contents, a serious risk factor for pneumonia. It also promotes digestion.

6. Place a linen-saver pad under the connection end of the feeding tube. Don procedure gloves. Remove the cap from the end of the feeding tube or disconnect it from the suction equipment.
Draping prevents soiling of the patient's bed linens and gown. Clamping the tube prevents air from entering the stomach or gastric contents from leaking out.

✛➤ **7.** Before the first feeding, tube placement must be verified by radiography. For the first feeding after radiography, you can confirm tube placement by checking the chart for x-ray confirmation and reconfirming at the bedside, using a combination of methods: measuring pH of aspirate, asking the patient to speak, observing for unexpected changes in residual volume, observing whether the external length of the catheter has changed, and using the "whoosh" test. (See Clinical Insight 26-7 for complete instructions.)
Only the x-ray method is reliable for verifying that the tube is in the correct position, so use the other methods in combination to confirm each other.

8. For subsequent feedings, aspirate and measure gastric residual volume. Also use other confirmatory methods, such as pH paper, asking the patient to speak, and so on (see step 7, preceding).
   a. Connect the syringe to the proximal end of the feeding tube, slowly draw back on syringe to aspirate contents.
   b. Measure the volume of aspirated contents using a syringe (if volume is more than 60 mL, use a graduated container).
   c. Reinstill aspirate unless the volume is more than the formula

flow rate for 1 hour (or more than 150 mL, or if patient is nauseated). If the residual is too high, see "What if. . .?"

Allows you to aspirate gastric contents, helps assess gastric emptying, and verifies tube placement. Reinstilling aspirate prevents fluid and electrolyte imbalance. Refer to Clinical Insight 26-7 for more rationale.

Step 8 Variation. Jejunostomy Tube

a. Do not measure residual volume.

Residual volumes evaluate gastric emptying. The feeding is directly into the small intestine (the jejunum), which isn't normally a reservoir; therefore, no residual volume is present in the jejunum. In addition, feedings via small bowel feeding tubes should be administered as a continuous infusion via pump.

b. After initial confirmation by x-ray, check placement using pH indicator strips and measuring length of tube from the naris to the connector.

A pH of 7 to 8 is a normal value for the small bowel.

9. Irrigate the feeding tube with 30 mL of tap water.

Irrigation maintains tube patency.

Procedure Variation A
Infusion Pump

10. To begin the feeding, hang the bag on the infusion pump and prime the tubing with supplement (if not already done in step 4).

You can use a pump with a prefilled bag or bottle or an open system with a feeding bag.

11. Thread the bag tubing through the infusion pump according to the manufacturer's instructions. Pinch off the end of the feeding tube.

Pinching the end prevents air from entering the feeding tube. ▼

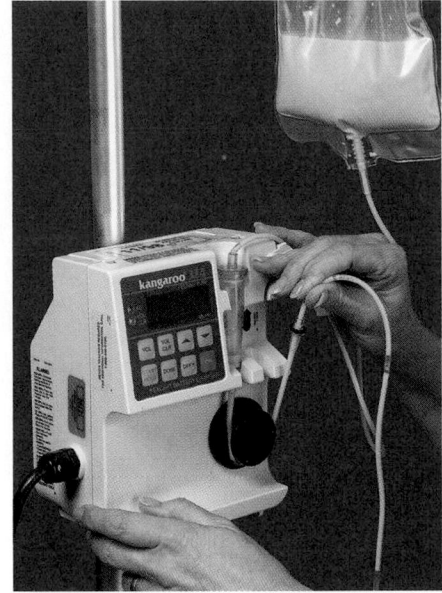

12. If needed, attach a connector to the proximal (open) end of the feeding tube. Connect the distal end of the bag tubing to the connector or directly to the NG or NE tube.

✛ Trace the tubing from the bag back to the patient before starting the feeding.

This ensures that you have not inadvertently hooked the feeding bag to the intravenous line.

13. Turn on the infusion pump. Set the correct infusion rate and volume to be infused.

14. Unclamp the tube and begin the infusion.

An infusion pump delivers continuous tube feeding at the prescribed rate and volume.

Procedure Variation B
Open-System Syringe

15. To begin feeding, clamp or pinch off the end of the feeding tube

Prevents air from entering the feeding tube.

16. Attach the syringe to the proximal end of the feeding tube.

17. Fill the syringe with the prescribed amount of formula.

18. Unclamp the feeding tube, and elevate the syringe. Do not elevate the syringe more than 18 inches above the insertion site. Allow the feeding to flow slowly.

Gravity allows the formula to flow through the feeding tube. Rate of flow is determined by the height of the syringe. Feeding slowly prevents sudden stomach distention, which can lead to diarrhea, cramping, nausea, and vomiting. ▼

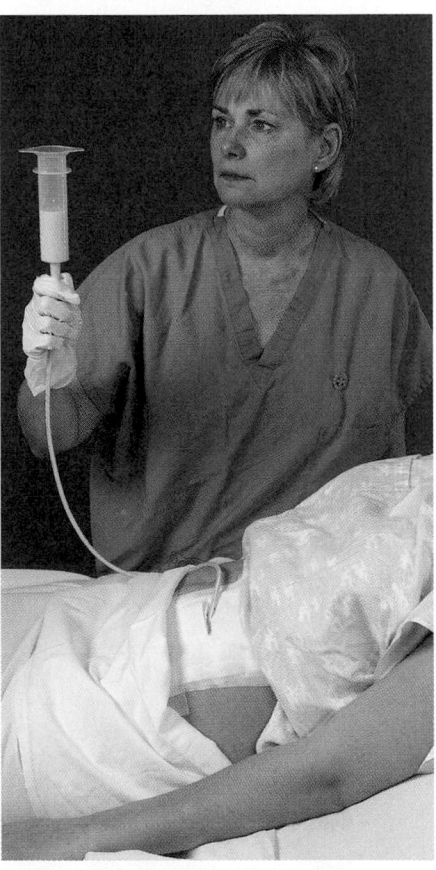

19. When the syringe is nearly empty, refill the syringe until the prescribed amount of feeding has been administered.

If the tubing runs dry, air may enter the stomach and cause discomfort associated with gas.

(continued on next page)

Procedure 26-3 ■ Administering Feedings Through Gastric and Enteric Tubes (continued)

Procedure Variation C Closed System with Prefilled Bottle with Drip Chamber

20. Pinch off or clamp the end of the feeding tube.

Prevents air from entering the feeding tube.

21. Attach administration tubing to the bottle and prime the tubing, using sterile technique.

22. Connect the distal end of the administration tubing to the feeding tube. If needed, first attach a connector to the proximal (open) end of the feeding tube. Trace the tube from the bag back to the patient.

23. Begin the infusion.

Step 23 Variation. Infusion Pump

a. Turn on the infusion pump. Set it the correct infusion rate and volume to be infused. ▼

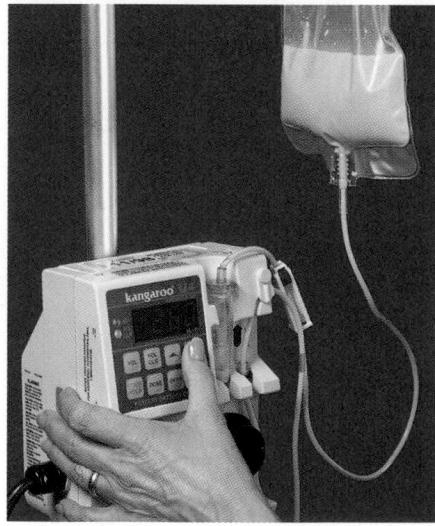

Step 23 Variation. Gravity Drip

b. If your institution uses gravity to infuse prefilled bottles, adjust the drip rate by opening the roller clamp and regulating the flow rate manually.

Ensures administration at the prescribed rate.

24. When the feeding is infused, stop the flow, flush the tube, and disconnect the feeding, as in the following variations:

Pinching or clamping the tubing prevents air from entering the feeding tube, and fluid and gas from leaking out. Instilling water helps maintain feeding tube patency and provides the patient with free water to maintain fluid and electrolyte balance.

Step 24 Variation. Infusion Pump

a. Turn off the pump before pinching, then pinch off the proximal end of the feeding tube.
b. Flush feeding tube with the prescribed amount of water (typically 50 to 100 mL).

Step 24 Variation. Open-System Syringe

c. Disconnect the syringe from the feeding tube.
d. Flush the feeding tube with 50 mL of tap water.

Step 24 Variation. Closed System with Prefilled Bottle with Drip Chamber

e. Turn off pump or turn roller clamp off.
f. Disconnect the feeding tube from the administration tubing.
g. Flush the feeding tube with the prescribed amount of water.

Step 24 Variation. Continuous Feeding

h. If administering a continuous feeding, flush the tube with the prescribed amount of water (typically 50 to 100 mL) every 4 to 6 hours.

25. Cap the proximal end of the feeding tube.

Prevents spillage of gastric contents and stops air from entering the stomach.

26. Keep the head of the bed elevated at least 30° to 45° for 1 hour after administering the tube feeding.

Elevation reduces the risk for aspiration of gastric contents.

27. Provide or assist with regular oral hygiene and encourage frequent gargling.

Oral care reduces oropharyngeal discomfort from the tube.

What if . . .

■ **When checking for residual, the volume is more than the formula flow rate for 1 hour or more than 150 mL?**

Hold the feeding for 1 hour, then recheck the residual. Notify the medical provider if the residual is still elevated. You will likely reinstill the residual very slowly, over a period of time, as the patient tolerates.

High residual volumes indicate delayed gastric emptying.

■ **When checking for residual, none is obtained?**

Use a large syringe and inflate 20 mL of air into the tube; this may move the tube away from the gastric wall or clear the tube of any residual formula, medication, or water.

■ **When irrigating the feeding tube (at step 9), resistance is met? Or when instilling the feeding, the fluid does not flow?**

Do not force the solution. Do not use any fluid other than water for flushing. Check for kinks in tubing and that the pump is working correctly. Turn the client onto his left side. Remove any enteral feeding solution remaining in the tube. Try instilling 5 mL of warm water into the tube and clamping the tube for 5 minutes. Then apply gentle negative pressure to the tube with a syringe. Try flushing with a smaller (e.g., 10 or 20 mL) syringe. If these measures fail, the tube may need to be removed and a new one inserted; contact the primary care provider. (Note: There are other methods, such as the alkalinized enzyme method; they require a medical prescription.)

Do not force the solution because this may damage the tube. However, you can use a smaller syringe to exert slightly more pressure.

■ **The patient has a cuffed tracheostomy tube?**

Inflate the cuff before administering the feeding, and keep the cuff inflated at for least 15 minutes afterward.

Cuffing helps to prevent aspiration.

■ **During the feeding, the patient vomits or complains of nausea or feeling too full?**

Stop the feeding and assess the patient's condition. Flush the tube, wait an hour, then measure gastric contents and restart the feeding at a slower rate. You may need to obtain a medical order to decrease the volume of the feedings.

■ **The patient has a jejunostomy tube?**

Do not instill air into the tube or check for residual before feeding.

The tube is in the jejunum rather than the stomach, and the jejunum isn't normally a reservoir; therefore, no residual volume is present in the jejunum. Gastrostomy and jejunostomy tubes are often placed through the upper abdominal wall; these tubes, of course, cannot inadvertently migrate into the airway. Injecting air into the tube is not necessary and

introduces air into the GI tract, causing the patient discomfort from gas.

Clean the insertion site daily with soap and water. You may apply a small, precut gauze dressing to the site.

Helps prevent bacterial growth; prevents infection.

Be aware that the delivery rate will likely be slower for jejunostomy tubes because of the loss of the stomach as a reservoir.

Evaluation

■ Evaluate the patient's tolerance to the tube feeding; did the patient have any abdominal discomfort, nausea, vomiting, or diarrhea?
■ Auscultate bowel sounds and vital signs every 4 hours.
■ Check gastric residual volume every 4 hours.
■ Monitor intake and output every 8 hours.
■ Weigh patient at least 3 times per week.
■ Assess the exit site for signs of skin breakdown.
■ Assess frequency of bowel movements.
■ Check laboratory values to evaluate nutritional status.

Patient Teaching

■ Demonstrate the procedure to the patient and caregiver if the patient will be continuing tube feedings at home.
■ Explain the importance of flushing the feeding tube with tap water every 4 hours while the patient is awake to maintain tube patency and fluid and electrolyte balance.
■ Discuss the importance of remaining upright for at least 1 hour after the feeding.

Home Care

■ Provide written instructions.
■ Be sure the client has a 7-day supply of enteral feedings.
■ Identify with the client the person who will be responsible for care of the enteral tube and administration of feedings at home.

■ Explain to the client and caregiver how to measure the prescribed amount of tube feeding formula and water for flushes by using household measuring equipment.
■ Explain the importance of washing reusable equipment thoroughly with soap and water to prevent the spread of infection.
■ Discuss how and where to purchase and store the formula.
■ If home feedings are to be delivered by pump:
  ■ Facilitate a home care visit to provide training for the feeding pump.
  ■ Arrange for delivery of the feeding pump before discharge (or refer to the appropriate professional for this).
  ■ Ensure that the client has a 7-day supply of disposable feeding sets and 50-mL syringes upon discharge.

Documentation

■ Chart the type of tube feeding, rate and volume of infusion, amount of gastric residual volume (if any), and tolerance of procedure.
■ Tube feeding intake is documented on the intake and output portion of the flowsheet in most agencies.
■ Record all flushes as intake. Subtract any liquids that you aspirate and do not reinstill (e.g., when gastric residual is too high).

(continued on next page)

Procedure 26-3 ■ **Administering Feedings Through Gastric and Enteric Tubes** (continued)

Sample EHR documentation:

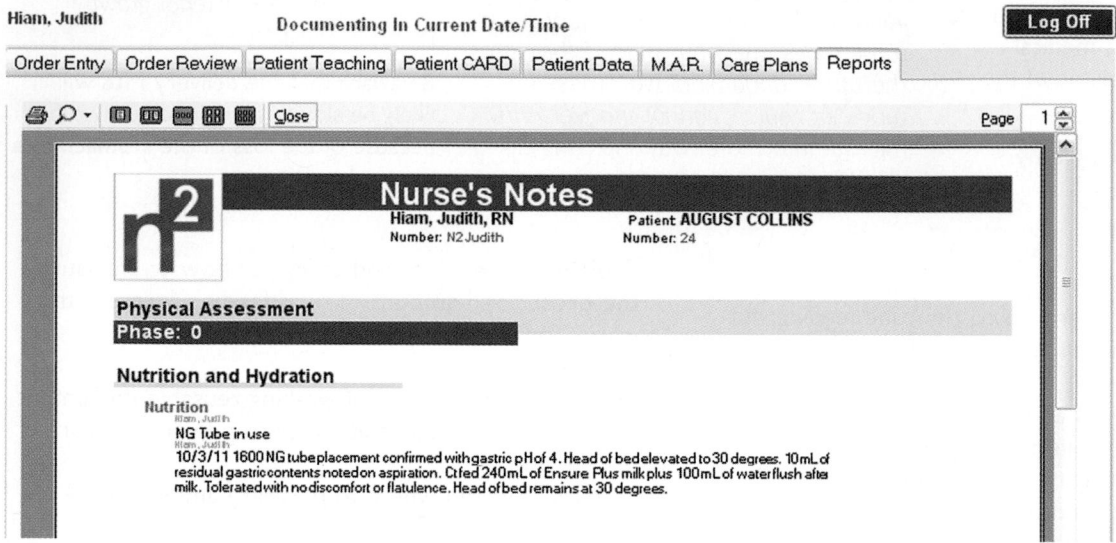

Practice Resources

American Association of Critical-Care Nurses (2005); American Society for Parenteral and Enteral Nutrition (A.S.P.E.N.) (2009a); Griffiths, R., Thompson, D., Chau, J., et al. (2006); Metheny, N. (2006); National Guideline Clearinghouse (NGC) (n.d.), Complete Summary...; Rauen, C., Chulay, M., Bridges, E., et al. (2008).

Thinking About the Procedure

 Go to the *Fundamentals of Nursing Skills Videos,* **Nutrition: Tube Feeding.**

1. What type of feeding system did the nurse use?

2. What did the nurse do next after turning on the pump and setting the rate?

 For suggested responses, go to Chapter 26, **Thinking About the Procedure Suggested Responses (Procedure 26-3),** on the Student Resource Disk or DavisPlus at http://davisplus.fadavis.com/Wilkinson2

Procedure 26-4 ☐ **Removing a Nasogastric or Nasoenteric Tube**

➤ For steps to follow in *all* procedures, refer to the Universal Steps for All Procedures found on the inside back cover of Volume 2.

Critical Aspects

- Verify the primary provider's order for removal of NG or NE tube.
- Assist the patient to a sitting or high-Fowler's position.
- Clear the tube of secretions by injecting 10 mL of air through the main lumen.
- Ask the patient to hold his breath, and gently, but quickly, withdraw the tube.
- Discard the equipment.
- Provide or assist with care of the nose and mouth.

Equipment

- Linen-saver pad
- 60-mL Luer-lock or catheter-tip syringe
- Procedure gloves
- Stethoscope
- Disposable plastic bag
- Emesis basin
- Gauze square

Delegation

This procedure should not be delegated to the LPN or NAP.

Pre-Procedure Assessments

- Auscultate the abdomen for the presence of bowel sounds.

Bowel sounds confirm peristalsis, which indicates bowel function is present.

- Assess the patient's ability to consume an oral diet.

Confirms readiness for discontinuing the NG or NE tube.

- Determine how long it has been since the patient's last enteral feeding.

Wait at least 30 minutes after a feeding to remove the NG tube.

➤ When performing the procedure, always identify your patient according to agency policy and be attentive to standard precautions, hand hygiene, patient safety and privacy, body mechanics, and documentation.

Procedure Steps

1. Check the patient's health record to confirm removal of the tube. For feeding tubes, make sure tube feeding has been stopped at least 30 minutes before removal.

2. Assist the patient to a sitting or high-Fowler's position.
Proper body alignment facilitates tube removal.

3. Place the plastic bag and emesis basin on the bed or within reach. Hand the patient facial tissue. Explain that the procedure may cause some gagging or nasal discomfort, but it will be brief.
Patients often need to blow their nose after this procedure.

4. Drape a linen-saver pad or towel across the patient's chest, and don procedure gloves.
Draping protects the gown and linens from soiling. Maintains universal precautions.

5. If you have not already done so, wash your hands and put on gloves.

6. If the NG tube is connected to suction, turn off suction and disconnect the tube.

7. Stand on the patient's right side if you are right-handed and left side if left-handed.

8. Attach the syringe to the proximal end of the NG or NE tube and flush the tube with 10 mL of water, normal saline, or air.
Flushing clears the tube of feeding formula or gastric secretions that could cause irritation or be aspirated during tube removal.

9. Unpin the tube from the patient's gown, and then untape the tube from the patient's nose. Use an adhesive-remover pad to help loosen the tape as necessary.

10. Clamp or pinch the end of the tube in your hand. Hold gauze up to the patient's nose and be ready to grab the tube with the towel in the opposite hand upon removal.
This prevents gastric fluids from leaking out the end of the tube onto the nurse or patient.

11. Ask the patient to take a deep breath and hold it.
Breath holding closes the epiglottis to prevent aspiration.

12. Quickly, steadily, and smoothly withdraw the tube and place it in the plastic bag.
Rapid removal in one steady motion prevents tissue trauma. The plastic bag acts as a barrier to gastric fluids until the tube can be placed in the trash. Seeing and smelling the tube may cause the patient to become nauseated.

13. If the patient cannot do so, clean her nares and provide mouth care. Remove the tape residue from her nose with adhesive remover.
Promotes patient comfort and prevents infection.

14. If the NG tube was connected to suction, measure the drainage and note the character of the content. Dispose of the tube and drainage equipment according to facility policy.
For patients receiving enteral feedings or gastric suction, record their intake and output. Proper equipment disposal prevents the spread of infection.

15. Remove and dispose of gloves in the nearest receptacle.

Evaluation

- Assess the nares for signs of skin breakdown or bleeding.
- Monitor the patient for signs of GI dysfunction, such as food intolerance, nausea, vomiting, and abdominal distention. Auscultate for bowel sounds.
GI dysfunction could necessitate reinsertion of the tube.
- Monitor intake and output every 8 hours.
- Weigh the patient regularly.
- Check laboratory values to evaluate nutritional status.

Patient Teaching

- Instruct the patient or caregiver on how to remove the feeding tube.
- Explain the importance of reporting nausea, vomiting, food intolerance, or abdominal distention to the physician.
- Explain the importance of and procedure for drinking fluids, if not contraindicated.

(continued on next page)

Procedure 26-4 ▪ **Removing a Nasogastric or Nasoenteric Tube** (continued)

Home Care

- The procedure does not require special adaptation for home care, except that you might want to place the tube in a plastic zippered storage bag before discarding it in the trash receptacle.

Documentation

- Chart the date and time of removal as well as the patient's tolerance of the procedure.
- Document the amount of drainage if the tube was connected to suction.
- Note any complications following NG or NE tube removal, such as food intolerance, nausea, vomiting, and abdominal distention.

Sample documentation:

10/03/11   1430   Explained to client and wife NG tube was to be removed and procedure for removing NG tube. Client stated "I am ready to get this thing out." Untaped NG tube from gown and client's nose. Removed NG tube while asking client to hold his breath. Client tolerated procedure without vomiting, gagging, or bradycardia. Provided mouth care and facial cleansing.————————A. Hiam, RNC

10/03/11   1645   Taking clear liquids since 1430 with no nausea, vomiting, or abdominal distention. Bowel sounds faint, but audible in all 4 quadrants.————————A. Hiam, RNC

Practice Resources

Collins, J.W., Nelson, A., & Sublet, V. (2006); *Best practices* (2007).

Thinking About the Procedure

 Go to the *Fundamentals of Nursing Skills Videos,* **Nutrition, Nasogastric Tubes: Removing.**

1. What was the patient's position for this procedure?

2. What did the nurse use to clear the NG tube before removing it?

3. How did the nurse keep the NG tube out of the patient's sight after removing it?

 For suggested responses, go to Chapter 26, **Thinking About the Procedure Suggested Responses (Procedure 26–4),** on the Student Resource Disk or DavisPlus at http://davisplus.fadavis.com/Wilkinson2

Procedure 26-5 ☐ Administering Parenteral Nutrition

➤ For steps to follow in *all* procedures, refer to the Universal Steps for All Procedures found on the inside back cover of Volume 2.

Critical Aspects

- Perform pre-procedure assessments: Check the patient record (e.g., to confirm CVC tip placement), check blood glucose, and assess patency of the line.
- Perform hand hygiene and don procedure gloves.
- Position the patient supine.
- Examine the parenteral (PN) solution for leaks, cloudiness, and particles. If the solution contains lipids, also look for a brown layer, oil droplets, or oil on the surface. Have a co-worker verify.
- Identify the patient, using two identifiers; have identification verified by a second staff member.
- Compare the bag to the patient's ID band and with the original prescription.
- Observe meticulous sterile technique in the appropriate steps of the procedure. During all steps, observe careful aseptic (clean) technique. Or follow agency policy.
- Use a filter.
- Attach the new administration set to the new bag.
- Prime the tubing (either now or after placing in the pump).
- Place the tubing in the infusion pump; set the rate.
- Clamp the catheter and the old administration set.
- Remove gloves, perform hand hygiene, and don clean (or sterile) gloves.
- Observe meticulous sterile technique in the appropriate steps of the procedure. During all steps, observe careful aseptic (clean) technique.
- Scrub all surfaces of the needleless connector and the Luer-locking threads for 15 seconds with an antiseptic pad.
- Determine patency of the IV line.
- Trace the tubing back to the patient, attach the new infusion tubing to the designated PN lumen (usually the largest one), and secure the Luer-lock connection. Have the patient perform the Valsalva maneuver when connecting the tubing for the new infusion.
- Start the infusion.
- Label the tubing.

Equipment

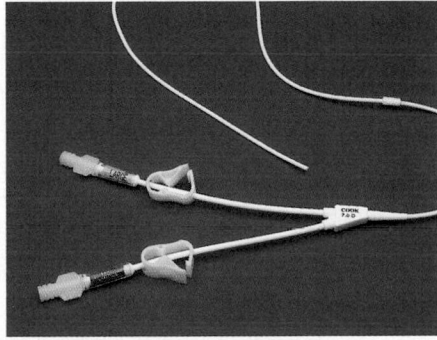

A two-lumen CVC. Note clamps, threaded lumen ends, and color-coded lumens to aid in identification of correct line for PN.

- Parenteral nutrition solution
  - Keep the PN solution refrigerated until 60 minutes before use; do not give cold. Do not hasten warming by placing in a microwave oven or hot water bath.
  Cold solution can cause pain, hypothermia, and venous spasm. Nutrients in PN solution are stable only for this short period of time. Nutrients could precipitate, causing catheter blockage or emboli.

  - Some pharmacies deliver the solution before infusion. Be sure the PN has not been mixed more than

24 hours beforehand. However, in home care you may find that solutions are mixed and delivered weekly.

- Procedure gloves
- Sterile gloves
  (*Note:* If the central line has an injection cap and if IV tubing is connected onto the cap via Luer lock, some agencies do not require gloves.)
- Intravenous administration set, extension set if indicated (free of plasticizers, such as DEHP, when fat emulsion is to be infused)
- 0.22-micron filter (1.2-micron filter if solution contains albumin or lipids)
A 0.22-micron filter will remove most particulates and microorganisms that might have been introduced during mixing, but it is too fine for larger-molecule lipids to infuse properly.

- Time tape
Even though the PN is delivered by infusion pump, there have been numerous recalls of infusion pumps because of malfunction. This simple tape provides valuable information quickly and is an additional safety measure.

- 70% alcohol pads or chlorhexidine gluconate (CHG)-based pads (e.g., 2% CHG in 70% isopropyl alcohol)
- Infusion pump
- 10-mL syringe and saline

(continued on next page)

Procedure 26–5 ■ **Administering Parenteral Nutrition** (continued)

To check for catheter patency

- Blood glucose testing monitor
- Intake and output record
- Transparent dressing or sterile gauze and tape (if dressing is to be changed)
- Catheter stabilization device (e.g., StatLock)

These are recommended for all catheters and must be changed with each dressing change.

- If the dressing is to be changed, you also need a transparent dressing or sterile gauze, tape, and a mask.

Delegation

Do not delegate this skill to the LPN or NAP because administration of parenteral nutrition requires advanced assessment and critical-thinking skills. The LPN or NAP can assist by monitoring vital signs and verifying patient identity with you. Instruct them about complications associated with PN and ask them to inform you of any signs or symptoms or change in the patient's condition.

Pre-Procedure Assessments

- Assess nutrition status and nutritional needs (e.g., daily weights, I&O, lab results). Patients requiring PN have

complex nutritional needs, and actual nutritional status is assessed by a nurse or dietician specializing in nutritional support.

- Check the prescriber's orders for type and concentration of additives in each container and for rate of infusion. (Standardized order forms are recommended by the American Society for Parenteral and Enteral Nutrition.)
- Check the patient's record to confirm that proper central venous catheter (CVC) tip placement has been established before the initial PN administration.
- Check agency policy.

A few may require tubing and filter change with every bottle or bag. The CDC recommends changing the PN set every 72 hours and a fat emulsion set at least every 24 hours.

- Check the blood glucose level.
- Assess for apparent patency of the IV site.

If PN is being administered continuously by pump and the infusion is running and there is no leakage from the insertion, you can begin the first few steps of the procedure. *Actual* patency is checked at step 14.

➤ When performing the procedure, always identify your patient according to agency policy and be attentive to standard precautions, hand hygiene, patient safety and privacy, body mechanics, and documentation.

Procedure Steps

1. Gather equipment and place at the bedside.
Promotes efficient use of time.

✚ **2.** Identify the patient, using two identifiers, according to agency policy. Some institutions require, as an extra precaution, that two people identify the patient.
Multiple patient identifiers helps to avoid "wrong-patient" errors. PN solutions are mixed to meet individual needs.

3. Explain to the patient the procedure and the rationale for it.
Respects the patient's right to be informed.

4. Perform hand hygiene and don procedure gloves.
Reduces transmission of infectious microorganisms.

5. Position the patient supine in bed.

6. Obtain and examine the PN container. Check for leaks, cloudiness,

or floating particles. Do not use if any of these are present. Some agencies require that two people examine the solution.

Step 6 Variation. Solutions Containing Lipids (3-in-1 Admixture)

✚ Do not administer the admixture if it has a brown layer, oil droplets, or oil on the surface. This indicates that the emulsion has "broken," and the large lipid droplets can cause fat emboli if administered. Also note that this solution requires a 1.2-micron filter.
To reduce the risk of adverse events such as fat emboli.

7. Compare the bag to the patient's identification band; check for correct bag number, expiration date, and additives and their concentration. Compare with the original prescription. Have a co-worker verify with you.

Ensures that the correct solution is administered. Check the expiration date to ensure that the solution will be discarded after that date and time. PN solutions are carefully calculated and prepared using the latest recommendations for sterile compounding of solutions. Therefore, no medications should be added to the bag by the nurse either before it is hung or while it is infusing.

8. Connect the IV tubing to the PN solution; prime the tubing. Note that priming may be done manually now or later (on the pump after the tubing is loaded into the pump), depending on the design of the pump.

✚ Be sure to identify the correct port and IV line. Trace the PN tubing from the bag to the patient.

Priming tubing removes air bubbles and prevents air from entering the patient's bloodstream, possibly causing air embolism. If there is PN already infusing, the old tubing must be removed from the pump and the rate regulated manually for the short period it takes to prime the new administration set.

Step 8 Variation. IV Tubing Without an Inline Filter

If the IV tubing does not have an inline filter, attach the filter and the extension tubing before priming. Attach the filter as close to the catheter site as possible.

9. Place the IV tubing in the infusion pump. (Prime the tubing if not done in step 8.) Set the pump to the prescribed rate.

> ⬙ Administration via pump (preferably volumetric) helps prevent complications associated with too-rapid infusion. PN solutions must be administered by infusion pump with reliable, audible alarms. Catheter tip placement must be confirmed before initial PN administration.

10. Identify the correct IV catheter and lumen for the PN. This is usually a PICC line or a centrally inserted venous line designated solely for PN. PN is administered via a central venous catheter (e.g., subclavian catheter, internal jugular, or PICC) whose tip is positioned in the superior vena cava/right atrial juncture. Most guidelines state that a specific intravenous line be reserved for parenteral nutrition and not used for any other purpose. If a single-lumen catheter is used, it is used only for PN. If a multilumen catheter is used, one lumen will be dedicated for the PN, and blood and other fluids should not be given through that lumen.

11. Clamp the catheter and the old PN administration set, if still connected, before disconnecting the tubing.
  a. A clamp should be present on the central line catheters with valves built into the catheter itself.
  b. As an additional safety measure, instruct the patient to perform the Valsalva maneuver just as you change the tubing (step 14).
  c. If Valsalva is contraindicated for a patient, instruct the patient to exhale at a specific time when the lumen is open.

The central line for the PN should already be clamped if no PN is running. If a previous bag is running, always clamp the PN line near the patient before disconnecting. Clamping prevents air from entering the catheter when you open the connection. The Valsalva maneuver increases intrathoracic pressure and creates positive pressure in the central vessels, also helping prevent air embolism.

12. Remove and discard gloves. Perform hand hygiene.
In steps 1 through 11, you were observing universal precautions. From this step forward, the emphasis is on preventing the introduction of microorganisms into the catheter lumen or the catheter insertion site.

13. Don clean gloves (or sterile gloves, if your agency policy requires them). Disconnect the old administration set. Using an alcohol-chlorhexidine pad or a 70% alcohol pad, thoroughly cleanse all surfaces of the central line injection cap and extension leg (in a needleless system) or the Luer-lock, including threads. Because PN solutions are a good medium for growth of pathogens, and because the IV line enters the central circulation, the risk for sepsis is relatively high.

14. Determine patency of the line. Use a 10-mL syringe to aspirate for blood, looking for a brisk return; then flush with saline. If the PN is running continuously on a pump, there are no occlusion alarms, and the dressing is dry and intact, these are also signs—but not proof—of patency.
When PN is running continuously on a pump, the pump creates a constant fluid flow through the lumen to help keep it patent. There is some controversy about this step. Some experts prefer to aspirate for blood only for the first bag of a continuous infusion, and thereafter to flush without aspirating. As always, follow agency policy.

15. Attach the infusion tubing to the designated PN port and then turn the Luer lock to secure the connection. "Luer-slip" connections should not be used. Do not use tape. Trace the tubing from the patient back to the PN container to be certain you are using the correct lumen.
Securing the connection with a Luer-lock connection prevents separation of the connection and decreases the risk for sepsis or embolism. Tape, even sterile tape, has been found to be a medium for bacterial colonization.

Step 15 Variation. Previous Infusion is Still Connected

Be sure the access line and the line to the "old" infusion bag are clamped (step 11). Quickly disconnect from the central line, thoroughly cleanse the port, and connect the new infusion.

16. Trace the tubing from the bag back to the patient. Then start the infusion. Check again to make sure the catheter-tubing connection is secure. Infuse at the rate prescribed (depending on the patient's tolerance, PN is usually started at a rate of 40 to 50 mL/hr and then advanced 25 mL/hr every 6 hours).
PN solutions may contain as much as 70% dextrose. A gradual rate increase allows the patient's pancreatic beta cells time to increase their insulin output to handle the increased glucose load. For lower concentrations of dextrose, you can usually run the same rate for the complete 24-hour volume.

17. Label the tubing with the date and time of change (if it is new tubing or if you have changed the tubing).
Labeling allows other nurses to know when tubing is due to be changed and a new solution must be hung.

18. Remove and discard gloves. Perform hand hygiene.

What if . . .

■ ⬙ **When you flush the catheter (at step 14), you meet resistance?**
Examine the insertion site for leaking fluid or inflammation. Aspirate and try again to flush *gently*. Never forcibly flush against resistance. Reposition the patient and ask him to cough. Roll the patient's shoulder or raise the arm on the same side the catheter is on. If these measures fail, notify the primary care provider.

Occlusion may be caused by a clot; drug precipitation; or catheter migration, kinking, or compression. Forceful flushing may discharge a clot into circulation. Other measures to clear a catheter require a medical order.

(continued on next page)

Procedure 26-5 ■ Administering Parenteral Nutrition (continued)

■ ◆ **The rate falls behind or the pump gives occlusion alarms?**

First check to be sure the pump is turned on, the bag is not empty, and all clamps are fully open. Change the filter if it is clogged. Perform the steps in the preceding item. If those measures do not work, change the pump and send it to biomedical engineering to be checked. Do not attempt to catch up by increasing the rate.

A slow rate may indicate a clogged filter or injection cap, a kinked catheter, or a malfunctioning pump. A clogged filter must be changed; you cannot run the PN without a filter.

■ **The 24-hour total deviates from the prescribed infusion rate by 10% or more?**

Notify the primary provider or nutrition support team.

■ **A PN solution must be discontinued abruptly for any reason?**

Notify the primary provider or nutrition support team. Another solution of 5% or 10% dextrose may be started.

The dextrose solution is started to prevent rebound hypoglycemia. Note that if it is a catheter complication that requires this discontinuation, 10%

dextrose is the highest concentration that can be infused through a peripheral vein because infiltrated hyperosmolar fluid causes tissue injury.

■ **The patient no longer needs parenteral nutrition?**

You may need to decrease the rate gradually, perhaps over 48 hours, before discontinuing the infusion completely. Be sure the patient either receives enteral nutrition or consumes food during the next few hours after stopping PN.

To prevent rebound hypoglycemia.

Evaluation

These are post-procedure evaluations. For ongoing monitoring, see Clinical Insight 26-10.

- Assess vital signs, I&O, and weight.
- Observe that the solution is infusing at the prescribed rate.
- Assess patient's tolerance to the infusion (e.g., observe for pulmonary edema; check lab results).
- Observe for skin rashes, flushing, color changes, or other signs of allergic reactions; notify the primary provider. *Note:* These are not common.
- Monitor blood glucose and do not increase the infusion rate until glycemic control is established.

Patient Teaching

- Inform the patient and family of the purpose and duration of the nutritional support.
- Teach them to recognize and report to the nurse symptoms of complications associated with PN.
- Teach the patient that the dressing must remain occlusive, and to notify nurse if it comes loose or gets wet.
- Teach the patient the importance of measures to prevent blood infections.

Home Care

- The home environment must provide dry storage space for supplies, a refrigerator for storing admixtures, a clean low-traffic area for procedure preparation, and electronic outlets for any electronic equipment.
- Teach safe disposal of supplies.
- Provide verbal and written instructions of the procedures; demonstrate and ask for a return demonstration. Role play "what would you do if. . ." situations with the patient.
- Clients at home often administer their daily 24-hour total over 12 to 16 hours during the night. This allows

them to disconnect from the infusion in the morning, flush the central line, and be free to pursue their usual activities during the day.

- Instruct about solution hang time and management of the access device.

Depending on the anticipated length of therapy, patients may be sent home with a permanent venous access device.

- Provide 24-hour phone numbers for the primary care provider and home care agency.
- Home PN is less expensive than treatment in the hospital, and in many cases is associated with a lower risk of infection.
- Home nutritional support is usually under the direction of specialized nutrition support teams.

Documentation

- A special form may be used for documenting PN administration.
- Bag number, date and time hung, volume, type of fluid, rate of delivery, additives
- Date and time of dressing or tubing change (if performed)
- Patient's tolerance of procedure
- Pre- and post-administration assessment data, including complications and response to therapy
- Results of fingerstick blood glucose checks
- If insulin is required, type, amount, and route/site administered
- Weight
- I&O

Practice Resources

American Society for Parenteral and Enteral Nutrition (A.S.P.E.N.) Board of Directors (2009a); A.S.P.E.N. Board of Directors and Task Force on Parenteral Nutrition Standardization (2007); Infusion Nurses Society (2006a, 2006b); National Guideline Clearinghouse (2005b, 2006, 2008a, 2008b); Task Force for the Revision of Safe Practices for Parenteral Nutrition (2004).

Procedure 26-6 ░ Administering Lipids

➤ For steps to follow in *all* procedures, refer to the Universal Steps for All Procedures found on the inside back cover of Volume 2.

➤ *Note:* If administering through a central line, refer to Procedure 26-5 for precautions associated with central lines.

➤ *Note:* This procedure is for administering fat emulsions. If you are administering an admixture with the parenteral nutrition solution, use Procedure 26-5.

Critical Aspects

- Lipids require a special administration set.
- Position the patient supine.
- Be certain lipids are not cold.
- Examine bottle for a layer of froth or separation into fat globules or layers.
- Complete the infusion within 20 hours.
- Use new tubing for each bottle of lipids.
- If infusing simultaneously with PN, use a separate port below the PN filter.
- Take vital signs before infusing, then every 10 minutes for 30 minutes, and observe for side effects.
- Begin the infusion slowly. If no reactions occur after 30 minutes, adjust to the prescribed rate.

Equipment

- Intravenous lipid solution (not refrigerated)
- Special tubing (infusion set) for lipids

Must be without plasticizers (DEHP). Set should be labeled to that effect.

- Needleless cannula (if using a split septum needleless connector that requires it)
- 70% isopropyl alcohol pads or chlorhexidine gluconate
- Procedure gloves
- Time tape
- Infusion pump
- Intake and output record
- If a filter is a used, it must be a 1.2-micron filter

Lipid particles are large and will clog a smaller size.

Delegation

Do not delegate this skill to the LPN or NAP because administration of lipids requires advanced assessment and critical-thinking skills. The LPN or NAP can assist by monitoring vital signs and verifying patient identity with you.

Instruct them about complications associated with lipids and ask them to inform you of any signs or symptoms or change in the patient's condition.

Pre-Procedure Assessments

- Assess for rash; eczema; dry, scaly skin; poor wound healing; and sparse hair.

These are signs of essential fatty acid deficits.

- Check the history for anemia; coagulation disorders; and abnormal liver, pancreatic, or respiratory function.

These factors predispose to fat emboli. Your role as a staff nurse is to be certain the PN prescriber is aware of these factors; they do not necessarily contraindicate giving the PN.

- Check peripheral IV site for erythema, infiltration, and patency. Check the central venous access site for erythema or other signs of infection.
- Take baseline vital signs just before infusing the lipids.

An immediate reaction can occur upon starting the infusion. Note that not all guidelines require this action.

➤ When performing the procedure, always identify your patient according to agency policy and be attentive to standard precautions, hand hygiene, patient safety and privacy, body mechanics, and documentation.

Procedure Steps

1. Review the prescriber's orders, identify the patient, and explain the purpose of the procedure.
Verifying helps to prevent dosage and wrong-patient errors. Explaining respects the patient's right to be informed and encourages cooperation.

2. Gather equipment and place at bedside. Adjust lighting as needed.

Organization promotes efficient use of time.

3. Perform hand hygiene and don procedure gloves.
Hand hygiene and gloving reduces transmission of infectious microorganisms.

4. Position the patient supine in bed.

5. Be certain lipids are not cold.
Cold infusion can cause discomfort.

6. Examine the bottle for a layer of froth or for separation into fat globules or layers.
Do not use the lipids if these occur.

7. Label the bottle with the patient's name, room number, date, time, rate, and start and stop times. Label the tubing with date and time. *Note:* When lipids are infused with parenteral nutrition, the lipid infusion must be completed within 12 hours.

(continued on next page)

Procedure 26-6 ■ **Administering Lipids** (continued)

Labeling ensures accurate identification.

8. Compare the lipids bottle to the patient's wrist band (bag number, expiration date); compare to the original prescription. Have a colleague verify.

9. Determine patency of the IV line (see Procedure 26-5).

10. Cleanse the stopper on the IV bottle with an antiseptic swab; allow to dry.

11. Connect the special DEHP-free lipids-infusion tubing to the bottle, twisting the spike as you insert it. *Note:* You must use new tubing for each bottle.

Twisting the spike helps ensure that particles from the stopper do not fall into the bottle. New tubing reduces the growth of microorganisms (the feeding provides a medium for fungal growth).

12. Place the primed tubing in the pump and attach the tubing to the IV catheter lumen.

✚ Identify the correct IV line and port for the infusion. Trace the tubing from the bag back to the patient.

a. Thoroughly scrub the catheter injection port or hub and the Luer-lock threads with an antiseptic wipe.
b. If you are infusing lipids simultaneously with PN, attach the primed lipid tubing to the injection port/hub closest to the patient, below the tubing filter, or through a Y-connection at the catheter hub.
c. Turn the Luer-lock to secure the connection.

✚ d. *Note:* If a previous infusion has been running, clamp the catheter lumen and the old administration set tubing before disconnecting and changing the tubing.

Lipids are compatible with PN and you can piggyback them into the same tubing. However, the lipids must be below the filter because their large particles will not go through a PN filter.

13. Begin the infusion. Ideally, infuse slowly at first: 1.0 mL/min for adults and 0.1 mL/min for children (or as prescribed by the physician). Check again to be sure the catheter-tubing connection is secure.

Slow infusion allows time to assess if the patient will have an adverse reaction to the lipids. Nausea, vomiting, and elevated temperature have been reported when lipids are infused quickly.

14. Take the vital signs now, then every 10 minutes for 30 minutes. Observe for side effects (e.g., chills, fever, flushing, dyspnea, nausea, vomiting, headache, back pain).

15. If no reactions occur, adjust to the prescribed infusion rate and continue monitoring according to your agency's protocol.

16. Remove gloves and perform hand hygiene.

17. When the infusion is finished, discard the bottle and IV administration set.

Formula contains sugars that are a medium for growth of pathogens.

What if . . .

■ **The entire bottle of lipids is not used?**

Discard partially used bottles.

Prevents contamination.

Evaluation

■ If ordered, monitor serum lipids 4 hours after discontinuing the infusion.
■ Monitor the IV site for infection, inflammation, and infiltration.
■ Monitor for symptoms of fat emboli.
■ Monitor the IV line for patency.
■ Monitor for allergic reactions (nausea, vomiting, headache, chest pain, back pain, fever).
■ Monitor for lipid intolerance (triglyceride levels, liver function tests, hepatosplenomegaly, decreased coagulation, cyanosis, dyspnea).

Patient Teaching

■ Inform the patient and family of the purpose and duration of the nutritional support.
■ Teach the patient to recognize and report symptoms of complications associated with lipids infusion.

Home Care

■ The home environment must provide dry storage space for supplies, a refrigerator for storing solutions, a clean low-traffic area for procedure preparation, and electronic outlets for any electronic equipment.
■ Teach safe disposal of supplies.
■ Provide verbal and written instructions for the procedures; demonstrate and ask for a return demonstration.
■ Instruct about solution hang time and management of the access device.
■ Provide 24-hour phone numbers for the primary care provider and home care agency.

Documentation

■ A special form may be used for documenting lipids and PN administration.

- Bottle number, date and time hung, volume, type of fluid, and rate of delivery
- Status of dressing, and date and time of dressing or tubing change (if performed)
- Patient's tolerance of the procedure and any problems encountered
- Pre- and post-administration assessment data and blood tests, if any
- Condition of the IV site

- Weight
- I&O

Practice Resources

American Society for Parenteral and Enteral Nutrition (A.S.P.E.N.) Board of Directors (2009a); A.S.P.E.N. Board of Directors and Task Force on Parenteral Nutrition Standardization (2007); Infusion Nurses Society (2006a, 2006b); National Guideline Clearinghouse (2005b, 2006, 2008a, 2008b); Task Force for the Revision of Safe Practices for Parenteral Nutrition (2004).

Clinical Insights

Clinical Insight 26-1 ▶ Serving Sizes for Daily Food Choices

FOOD GROUP	WHAT COUNTS AS A SERVING	RECOMMENDATIONS FOR IMPROVING THE DIET†	MAJOR NUTRIENTS PROVIDED
Fats, oils, sweets *27 g. Use sparingly.	No serving sizes are given. Amounts consumed should be determined by individual energy needs, and these foods should not replace any from other groups	Use canola, peanut, and olive oil instead of margarine and butter.	Essential fatty acids
Milk, yogurt, and cheese 3 cups/day*	1 cup (8 oz) milk or yogurt 1½ oz natural cheese (6 stacked dice) 2 oz processed cheese (8 stacked dice) 2 cups cottage cheese 1 cup custard/pudding	■ Use nonfat or low-fat dairy products.	Protein, calcium, riboflavin, potassium, zinc, iron, fats
Meat, poultry, fish, dry beans, eggs, nuts 5.5 oz/day*	2–3 oz cooked meat, poultry or fish (3 oz is the size of a deck of cards.) ¼ cup cooked dry beans (e.g., navy beans, lima beans) 1 Tbsp peanut butter ¼ cup tofu 1 egg ½ oz nuts (size of ½ a golf ball)	■ Eat lean meat; cut off fat before cooking. ■ Use soy products as meat substitutes. ■ Eat two servings of fatty fish (salmon, tuna, herring, swordfish) per week	Protein, niacin, iron, vitamin B₆, zinc, thiamin, vitamin B₁₂ (only in animal foods)
Vegetable group 2.5 cups/day* (5 servings)	½ cup chopped raw or cooked vegetables (e.g., broccoli, green beans, potatoes, squash, carrots) (looks like the size of a fist) 1 cup raw leafy vegetables (e.g., turnip greens, cabbage, lettuce, broccoli) (4 lettuce leaves) ¾ cup vegetable juice (small Styrofoam cup)	■ Include one serving of a green leafy vegetable daily. ■ Eat one good source of vitamin A daily (green or orange vegetables such as carrots, sweet potatoes, spinach, broccoli, or red cabbage).	Vitamin A, vitamin C, folate, magnesium, fiber
Fruit group 2 cups/day* (4 servings)	½ cup dried fruit (the size of an egg) ½ cup chopped, cooked or canned fruit (looks like half of a fist) ¾ cup fruit juice (small Styrofoam cup) 1 medium apple, banana, orange ½ grapefruit ½ banana ½ cup berries ¼ cup dried fruit 1 melon wedge	■ Eat fresh fruit; avoid fruit with added sugar. ■ Choose one or two sources of vitamin C daily (oranges, grapefruit, cantaloupe, strawberries, or citrus fruit juice).	Vitamin C, potassium (bananas, apricots), fiber

(continued on next page)

Clinical Insight 26-1 ▶ **Serving Sizes for Daily Food Choices** (continued)

FOOD GROUP	WHAT COUNTS AS A SERVING	RECOMMENDATIONS FOR IMPROVING THE DIET†	MAJOR NUTRIENTS PROVIDED
Breads, cereals, rice, and pasta 6 oz/day* (3 servings whole grains & 3 other)	1 slice of bread ½ hamburger bun or English muffin 1 small roll, biscuit, or muffin 5 to 6 small crackers 1 cup of ready-to-eat cereal ½ cup cooked cereal, rice, or pasta (looks like an ice cream scoop)	■ Use whole-grain breads and pasta. ■ Eat oatmeal or bran cereal each day. ■ Eat at least ½ cup of dried beans, peas, or lentils daily.	Starch, thiamin, riboflavin (if enriched), iron, niacin, folate, magnesium, fiber (especially in whole grains)

*For a 2000-calorie diet, these amounts are recommended in MyPyramid.

†Suggestions in this column are not from the MyPyramid food guide. They offer information for choosing the most nutritious foods within a group.

Sources: Adapted from Shaw, Fulton, Davis, et al. (n.d.); U.S. Department of Agriculture (2005); and United States Department of Health and Human Services and U.S. Department of Agriculture (2005).

Clinical Insight 26-2 ▶ **Skinfold Measurement**

■ Take measurements directly on the skin, not through clothing.
■ Take each reading as soon as the jaws of the caliper come into contact with the skin and the reading has stabilized.
■ In each site, take three readings in quick succession, and average the results to the nearest 0.1 mm.
■ Add the averages of all skinfold sites to arrive at a total skinfold measurement.
■ To determine the percentage body fat, compare the final calculated measurent with the values in the appropriate body fat and skinfolds table for the age and gender of the patient.

Measuring Triceps Skinfold

■ Locate the midpoint on the posterior side of the dominant upper arm.
■ With the client's arm hanging loosely at the side, palpate the measurement site at the midpoint to become familiar with distinguishing muscle from adipose soft tissue.
■ From 1 cm above the midpoint, grasp a vertical pinch of skin and only the subcutaneous fat layer between the thumb and index finger. Gently pull the skinfold away from the underlying muscle.
■ Place the skinfold caliper at the midpoint, and slowly release the jaw of the caliper while maintaining a grasp of the skinfold (see the figure).

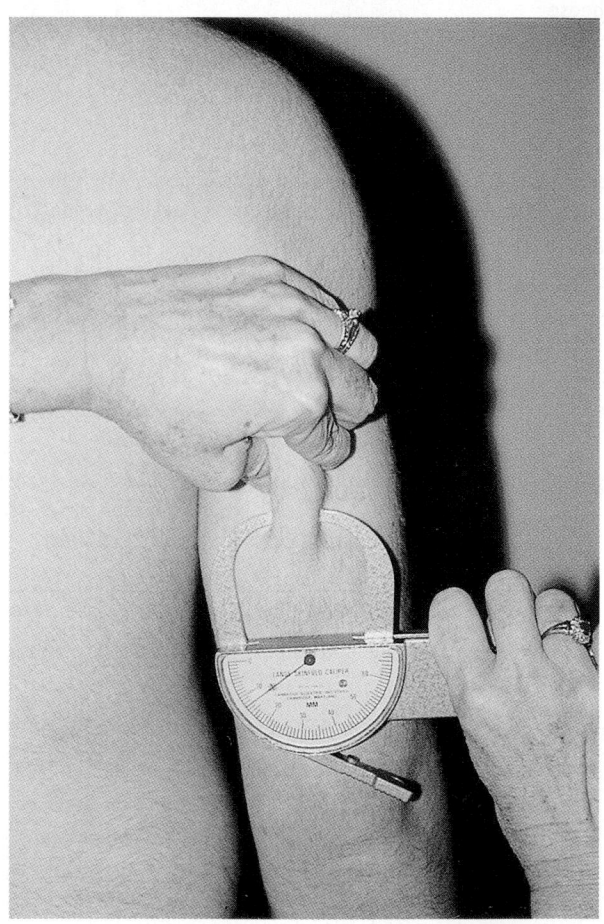

Triceps skinfold

Measuring Subscapular Skinfold

■ Follow the same procedure, except measure on the back, just under the shoulder blade. Grasp below the tip of the inferior angle of the scapula 45° to vertical.

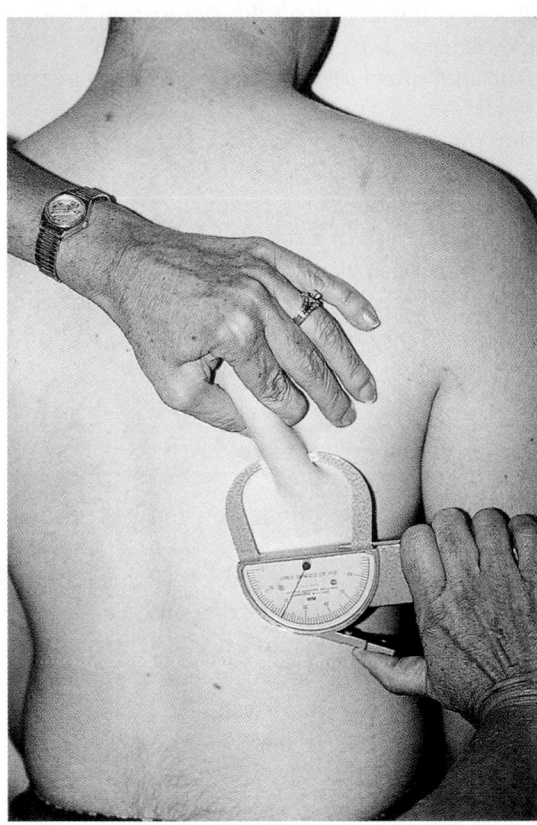

Subscapular skinfold

Measuring Biceps Skinfold

■ Follow the same procedure, except measure the muscle belly of the biceps. With the patient's arm hanging loosely at the side, grasp the skin and subcutaneous fat layer on the front of the upper arm, over the biceps, about level with the nipple.

Measuring Suprailiac Skinfold

■ Follow the same procedure, except measure approximately 1 inch above the hipbone, above the iliac crest in the mid-axillary line.

Calculating Body Mass Index

Calculate the BMI using this formula:
BMI = weight in kilograms ÷ (height in meters)²

Clinical Insight 26-3 ▶ Measuring Circumferences to Evaluate Body Composition

Measuring Mid-Upper Arm Circumference

■ Keeping the client's dominant arm parallel to the body, bend the elbow 90°.
■ Using a tape measure, measure the distance between the **acromion** (the bony protrusion of the back of the upper shoulder) and the **olecranon process** (tip of the elbow).
■ Mark the midpoint between these two landmarks.
■ Ask the client to relax the arm, so that it hangs loose and parallel to the body.
■ Position the tape around the upper arm at the marked midpoint. Make sure the tape is snug but not so tight as to indent or pinch the skin.
■ Record the circumference to the nearest 0.1 cm.

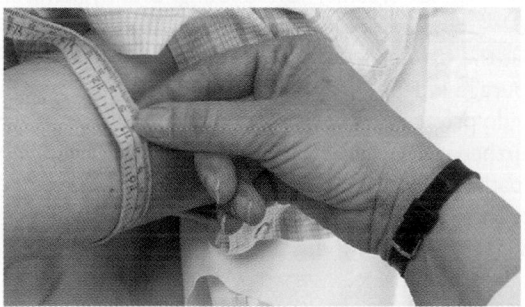

Calculating Waist-to-Hip Ratio (WHR)

■ Use a tape measure to measure the circumference of the waist (at the umbilicus with stomach muscles relaxed).
■ Use a tape measure to measure the circumference of the hips at their widest point.
■ Calculate the waist-to-hip ratio using the following formula:
waist circumference (in.)÷ hip circumference (in.)
Example: Robert's waist measurement is 32 inches, and his hip measurement is 34 inches. His WHR is 32 ÷ 34 = 0.94.
(Obesity = greater than 1.0 in men and greater than 0.8 in women)

Clinical Insight 26-4 ▶ Interventions for Patients with Impaired Swallowing

Nutritional support for patients with Impaired Swallowing includes the following activities from the NIC intervention Swallowing Therapy (Bulechek, Butcher, & Dochterman, 2008, pp. 707–708):

- Provide/use assistive devices, as appropriate.
- Avoid use of drinking straws.
- Assist the patient to position head in forward flexion in preparation for swallowing (chin tuck).
- Assist patient to place food at the back of the mouth and on the unaffected side.
- Monitor the patient's tongue movements while she is eating.
- Check mouth for pocketing of food after eating.
- Monitor body weight.

- Monitor body hydration (e.g., intake, output, skin turgor, mucous membranes).

In addition, you must also take Aspiration Precautions (Bulechek, Butcher, & Dochterman, 2008, p. 145):

- Monitor level of consciousness, cough reflex, gag reflex, and swallowing ability.
- Position the patient upright 90° or as far as possible.
- Keep suction setup available.
- Feed in small amounts.
- Avoid liquids or use of a thickening agent.
- Cut food into small pieces.
- Keep head of bed elevated for 30 to 45 minutes after feeding [your text recommends 1 hour].

Clinical Insight 26-5 ▶ Interventions for Patients Who Have Nausea

- Determine the cause of the nausea (e.g., anxiety; pain; constipation; cough; dehydration; electrolyte disorders; treatments, such as surgery, radiotherapy, or chemotherapy; disease processes, such as peptic ulcer or pancreatitis).
- Keep tissues and water to rinse the mouth at the bedside.
- Maintain a calm environment.
- Provide cool, fresh air.
- Instruct the patient to wear loose clothing.
- Avoid wearing strong perfumes.
- Immediately remove any food that the patient cannot or will not eat. The sight and smell of food can induce nausea.
- Provide or assist with frequent oral hygiene.
- Ask the patient to sit in an upright position for 30 to 45 minutes after eating, unless contraindicated.
- Provide small, frequent meals; avoid greasy, warm, spicy, or aromatic foods. In some cases cold food is better tolerated. Allow the patient to eat what she finds appetizing and tolerates well.
- Provide cool (not cold or iced) cola to drink.
- Have the patient suck on an ice cube, sorbet, or a piece of frozen fruit (pineapple, kiwi, or apple).

- Recommend a dietary consultation if nausea and vomiting persist.
- For malnourished patients, consult a dietitian. Consider dietary supplements; however, these are often poorly tolerated and may sometimes cause even more nausea.
- Assess for dehydration; you may need to administer parenteral fluid and electrolytes.
- Certain psychological techniques may be effective when the nausea is related to anxiety, stress, or anticipation of nausea. The following may be helpful: distraction, relaxation techniques, guided imagery, systematic desensitization, self-hypnosis, biofeedback, and music therapy.
- Administer antiemetics as ordered or per protocol.

Reference

Adapted from Editorial Board Palliative Care (2006, Jan. 12). Practice guidelines: Nausea and vomiting. Utrecht, The Netherlands: Association of Comprehensive Cancer Centres (ACCC). Guideline summary: Nausea and vomiting. In: National Guideline Clearinghouse (NGC) website. Rockville, MD. Retrieved February 14, 2009, from http://www.ngc.gov/summary/summary. aspx?doc_id=11793&nbr=006067&string=nausea+and+vomiting

Clinical Insight 26-6 ▶ Assisting Patients with Meals

General Guidelines

- Recommend having one staff person for every two or three patients who need assistance, allowing about 20 to 30 minutes to feed a patient. Prolonged meal times do not promote appetite; nor does hurrying.
- Feeding assistants should be supervised by an RN or LPN.
- Do not interrupt meals with medications.
- Encourage family members to share mealtimes.
- If the patient's condition allows, encourage him to get out of bed for meals.
- Encourage residents in long-term care settings to eat meals in the dining room instead of in the bedroom.

Preparation

- Assess for rituals used before meals (blessings of food, and so on).
- Provide an opportunity for toileting, oral hygiene, and hand washing before meals.
- Assist the patient to eat and drink only as necessary; encourage independence.
- Provide privacy during meals if the patient is embarrassed; to further maintain dignity, use a napkin, not a bib, over the patient's clothes.
- Check for proper fit of dentures.
- Provide music during the meal if the patient wishes.

■ Demonstrate the use of assistive devices and alternative methods for eating and drinking.

Assisting the Patient

■ If the patient must eat in bed, place the head of the bed at the highest tolerable level, and adjust the overbed table to be in easy reach.
■ If the patient can feed himself, prepare the food on the tray for him (e.g., open food containers, cut the meat, peel an orange, open the milk and butter containers, mash food if needed).
■ If the client is visually impaired, identify the locations of the meal on the tray based on a clock face (e.g., "The coffee is at 1 o'clock above the plate on the right").

Feeding the Patient

■ Feed the patient if she is unable to feed herself.
　■ Sit down while feeding the patient; do not rush.
　■ Position yourself so you can make eye contact.
　■ Be sure to provide adequate time for her to chew and swallow.
　■ If possible, ask her what food she would like next.
　■ Serve one food at a time; serve small amounts.
　■ Serve finger foods (e.g., fruit, bread) to promote independence.
　■ Cue older adults whenever possible with words or gestures.
　■ Have casual conversation with the patient while feeding her to make mealtime more pleasant and relaxed.

After the Meal

■ Help the patient to wash hands or use the rest room after the meal.
■ Record the amount of food and fluid the patient consumed.
■ Document feeding behaviors.
■ Document changes in nutritional status.
■ Document staffing and staff education, and availability of a supportive interdisciplinsary team.

Assisting Older Adults with Dementia

As do all people, older adults with dementia differ in their abilities to eat and communicate. The following are general tips, but you should tailor interventions to each person's specific abilities to achieve the best results. In addition to many of the preceding interventions, try some of the following measures.

■ Assess the patient's self-feeding abilities.
■ Assess the patient's cognitive limitations and communication abilities.
■ Assess for and treat pain.
■ Minimize distractions: Turn off the TV; discourage people from entering the room.
■ Help the patient to a comfortable chair if possible.
■ Assist with oral hygiene and hand hygiene.
■ Remove any unnecessary eating utensils; serve only one food at a time.
■ Remove items that should not be eaten (e.g., packets of salt or pepper), and hot items that could be spilled.
■ Cue the patient verbally to help with self-feeding (e.g., "take a bite," "chew," "swallow").
■ Pantomime eating motions so the patient can imitate them.
■ Place your hand over the patient's to begin and guide self-feeding (hand-over-hand).
■ When assisting, sit at eye level and interact socially with the patient.
■ Involve family members if they have assisted with feeding at home.
■ Train and supervise NAPs in interacting with and feeding patients with dementia.
■ Do not assist too soon – give the patient time to eat independently.
■ Do not feed too fast. Feed at a rate that is safe and comfortable for the patient.

References

Amella, E. (2007). Eating and feeding issues in older adults with dementia: Part II: Interventions. *Try This: Best Practices in Nursing Care for Hospitalized Older Adults With Dementia, D11.2.* The John A. Hartford Institute for Geriatric Nursing and the Alzheimer's Association. Retrieved February 18, 2009, from www.hartfordign.org.

Ebersole, P., Hess, P., Touhy, T., et al. (2005). *Gerontological nursing & healthy aging* (2nd ed.). Philadelphia: Elsevier.

National Guideline Clearinghouse (2001). [Reviewed 2006]. Brief summary: Altered nutritional status. In: National Guideline Clearinghouse (NGC) website. Rockville, MD; Retrieved February 21, 2009, from http://www.guidelines.gov/summary/summary.aspx?doc_id=3304&nbr=002530&string=enteral+AND+feedings

---

Clinical Insight 26-7 ▶ **Checking Feeding Tube Placement**

◆ Because none of the following methods is foolproof, always use a combination. Auscultate as you are injecting air before aspiration; aspirate fluid; check the pH, and so on. Tube placement should be verified by x-ray before the initial feeding is given.

Aspirate and Inspect Stomach Contents

■ Don procedure gloves. This is a clean, not sterile, technique.

■ Just before feeding, draw up 10 to 30 mL of air in a 30- to 60-mL syringe, insert the syringe in the distal end of the feeding tube, and inject air.
To flush out formula, medications, and other substances. This also helps keep a small-bore tube from collapsing when you aspirate.

■ With the same syringe, aspirate the air and 20 to 30 mL of stomach or intestinal contents. Use slow, gentle suction—over 3 to 5 minutes if necessary.

(continued on next page)

Clinical Insight 26-7 ▶ Checking Feeding Tube Placement (continued)

It can take a long time to obtain enough fluid, especially from a small-bore tube.

- ■ If you could not aspirate any fluid, inject another 20 mL of air and use a smaller syringe to aspirate again.

Using a small (< 10 mL) syringe for very small tubes creates less negative pressure and makes it less likely the tube will collapse.

- ■ If you still do not aspirate fluid, repeat the procedure with this variation: Insert air with the large syringe; insert the small syringe into the end the tubing, and leave it for 15 minutes before aspirating.

To allow fluid to accumulate before aspirating.

- ■ If you are still unsuccessful, reposition the patient and try again after 20 minutes.

Repositioning may move the tube into a place where fluid has pooled.

- ■ Inspect the aspirate. Gastric contents are normally greenish brown and liquid.

Intestinal contents are usually yellow-green because of the influence of bile.

- ■ If the patient is receiving enteral feedings, gastric contents should be curdled and white or a greenish color; intestinal contents will be a more yellow (bile) color with no curdling.
- ■ The colors of gastric and pulmonary secretions are altered by a variety of conditions, so this is not a very reliable method.

Measure the pH of the Aspirate

- ■ Follow the preceding procedure for aspirating stomach contents.
- ■ Measure the pH of the aspirated fluid by using nitrazine paper. See the accompanying figure.

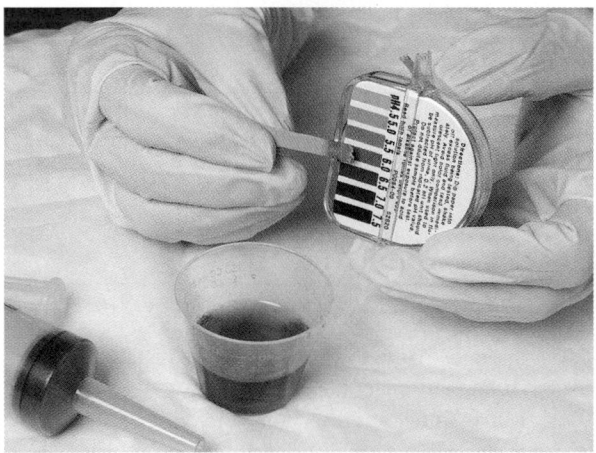

- ■ The lower the pH, the more likely that the tube is in the stomach. However, keep the following variables in mind:
  - ■ If the client is receiving medications to control stomach acidity (e.g., antacids, H$_2$ blockers, or

proton pump inhibitors), the gastric pH may be as high as 6.

- ■ Intestinal contents usually have a pH of 6 or greater.
- ■ The pH of respiratory secretions is 7 or higher; however, respiratory secretions may occasionally have a pH as low as 6.
- ■ If blood is present, either from epistaxis or from gastric bleeding, the pH of the gastric aspirate will not be helpful, because it will rise to resemble the pH of blood (7.35).
- ■ pH testing is useful only if the fluid you aspirate is acidic, indicating gastric placement.

Because of the action of hydrochloric acid in the stomach, gastric contents measure a pH of 1 to 5.5. If the fluid is alkaline, it might be because the gastric contents are alkaline or because the tip of tube is in the small intestine or the lung. Because such situations occur frequently, even this method should be used in combination with other verification methods (Clarke, 2007; Guedon, 2000; May, 2007; Schmieding, Waldman, & Desaulles, 1997).

Inject Air into the Feeding Tube

Although some professionals still inject air into the feeding tube, this method is the least accurate of the bedside methods. Never rely on this method (or any other bedside method) alone.

Because the lungs and stomach lie close together, the sounds created by sending air through the tube can easily be transmitted to nearby areas of the body, causing you to err in determining tube placement.

- ■ Draw 5 to 30 mL of air into a syringe; place the tip of the syringe in the end of the feeding tube.
- ■ Place a stethoscope over the stomach.
- ■ Listen with stethoscope as you inject the air through the tube.

Air injected into the stomach produces a gurgling or whooshing sound in the left upper quadrant. If the tube is in the lungs, you will hear no gurgling.

Other Bedside Methods

The following require repeated assessments over time to be useful for confirming other methods of tube placement.

- ■ ***Observe for respiratory distress***. Note cyanosis or difficulty breathing, coughing, choking.
  - ■ The presence of these symptoms is a good indicator that the tube is in the respiratory tract; but keep in mind that the tube could instead be in the stomach and the symptoms caused by something else.
  - ■ Absence of symptoms does not necessarily indicate correct placement in the stomach.

The tube might be in the airway and not be causing any respiratory symptoms.

- *Measure the residual volume of the aspirate.* Observe for unexpected changes in volume. Gastric volumes will generally be larger than intestinal or esophageal volumes. (Also see Procedure 26-3 and Clinical Insight 26-8 regarding residual volumes.)
- *Measure and observe the length of the tube that extends from the body.* When the tube is inserted, it should be marked with indelible marker where it exits the body (e.g., the naris), and the external length recorded. Compare the external length with previous measure-

ments and with the mark made on the tube when it was inserted. If tube placement does not change, the external length should remain the same.

If the tube is not well secured, it may migrate either up or down, so a consistent measurement of the external tube may help verify tube placement (Peter & Gill, 2009).

- *Assess whether the patient can speak.* Keep in mind that some clients can speak even when the tube is in a lung (Rombeau and Rolandelli, 1997).

Clinical Insight 26-8 ▶ Monitoring Patients Receiving Enteral Nutrition

For patients receiving enteral nutrition, monitor the following:

- *Position of the feeding tube.* Periodically check the placement of the tube. As a rule, check on each shift or at each intermittent feeding. For double-lumen tubes, keep the air vent above the level of the patient's stomach so it will not act as a siphon and leak stomach contents.
- *NG or NE tube insertion site.* An NG or NE tube is secured by adhesive to the nose. Regularly check the skin, gently cleanse the area (with soap and water, as for normal washing; avoid harsh skin cleansers), and retape the tube as needed. Report tissue breakdown, epistaxis (nosebleed), or sinusitis.

They may signal a need for insertion of a percutaneous endoscopy gastrostomy (PEG) tube.

- *Gastrostomy tube, PEG/PEJ insertion site.* Inspect the insertion site for erythema or drainage, which are signs of infection. Clean it daily with soap and water.
- *Fluid balance.* Measure all intake and output.
- *Weight.* To assess the adequacy of the feeding, regularly weigh patients receiving enteral nutrition. There is usually a medical prescription for frequency of weighing. Frequent weight checks allow adjustment of the feeding orders to achieve the desired goal.
- *Tube feeding residual volume.* To assess residual volume, aspirate the feeding tube to determine the amount of feeding remaining in the stomach.

If you are able to aspirate a quantity equal to or greater than the formula flow rate for 1 hour (or alternatively, a total of 150 mL), the patient may be receiving too much fluid or may have delayed gastric emptying. However, you

should not automatically stop the feeding; if you obtain a single sample of an increased residual volume, recheck it in 1 hour. See Clinical Insight 26-7.

- *Frequency of bowel movements.* Bowel movements should occur regularly.
  - Constipation is usually due to inadequate water or fiber. Some commercial feedings contain fiber. To alleviate constipation, you may add free water and perhaps fiber to the formula.
  - Diarrhea may indicate intolerance of the formula, excessive feeding, or gastrointestinal disease.
- *Bowel sounds.* Check before each feeding, or every 4 to 8 hours for continuous feedings. Peristalsis must be present.
- *Abdominal distention.* Measure abdominal girth daily, at the umbilicus.
- *Serum electrolyte levels.* Monitor regularly (per protocol or precription).
- *Urine for sugar and acetone.* This is sometimes done as a bedside screen for hyperglycemia. However, treatment is based on blood sugar levels.
- *Skin turgor, hematocrit, and urine specific gravity.* These are indicators of dehydration and overhydration. Dehydration may occur, for example, if the patient is not consuming enough water, dehydration may occur.
- *Serum blood urea nitrogen (BUN) and sodium levels.* This is especially important for high-protein formulas. Insufficient fluid intake combined with high protein intake may overload the kidneys so that nitrogenous wastes are not excreted adequately.

Clinical Insight 26-9 ▶ Preventing Infection in Patients Receiving Enteral Feedings

Enteral feeding solutions provide an ideal medium for bacterial growth. Contamination of the feeding can have serious consequences for a patient.

- Check dates on feeding solutions and supplies. Do not use any that are outdated.
- Use sterile equipment and supplies; once you have opened them, handle them as little as possible.
- Disposable feeding equipment is meant for one-time use. Do not wash and reuse.

- Use meticulous hand hygiene; wear nonsterile gloves.
- Replace feeding equipment after 24 hours.
- Store opened feeding solutions in the refrigerator in covered and labeled containers. Allow to return to room temperature before giving it to the patient. Discard after 24 hours.
- Keep unopened solutions at room temperature.

(continued on next page)

Clinical Insight 26-9 ➤ **Preventing Infection in Patients Receiving Enteral Feedings** (continued)

- Follow agency policy regarding how long a solution may be left hanging. Usually:
  - Sterile feedings may be hung for up to 24 hours (or unit policy).
  - Nonsterile feedings (i.e., reconstituted powder feedings) may hang for up to 4 hours (or unit policy).
  - Label the feeding containers with the patient's name and the date and time hung; document the time in the patient record.
- Use sterile water for (1) patients who are immunocompromised, (2) patients receiving jejunal feeds, or (3) initially following a gastrostomy insertion.

- Never allow a feeding to hang below the height of the patient's stomach.
- Do not transfer sterile feedings into a second container.
- Replace the feeding tubes according to the manufacturer's recommendations (or agency policy if that is sooner).

Reference

Nunwa, A. (2005). Adult enteral nutrition guidelines. Harrow, Middlesex, England. The Burdett Institute of Gastrointestinal Nursing. St. Mark's Hospital.

Clinical Insight 26-10 ➤ **Monitoring and Other Interventions for Patients Receiving Parenteral Nutrition**

Monitoring

For patients receiving PN, you will need to monitor the following:
- **Catheter insertion site**
  - Assess catheter insertion site for swelling, redness, drainage, or tenderness.
    Signs of infection (and/or phlebitis in PICC lines). The hypertonic PN creates a risk for phlebitis.
  - Observe for swelling in the extremity on the same side of catheter insertion.
    This is a sign of infiltration or phlebitis.
  - Observe for catheter retraction from the vein; observe the length of the catheter from the insertion site to the hub at insertion and periodically.
- **Supplies and equipment**
  - Monitor tubing connections to see that they are secure.
  - Monitor to see that the dressing is secure and dry.
  - Check the rate and amount infused at least hourly.
To ensure the line is patent, the PN is flowing freely, and the pump is functioning properly.
- **Weight.** Regularly weigh the patient (according to medical order or agency policy, but commonly daily or 3 times per week).
(1) Frequent weight checks allow for assessing the adequacy of the formula and make adjustments as needed to achieve the desired goal. (2) Because of the hypertonicity of the solutions, fluid overload can occur. Rapid weight increase is an indicator.
- **Glucose.** Check blood glucose every 4 to 6 hours until stable, and then at least daily.
The high proportion of glucose in the formulas can cause hyperglycemia, the most common complication of PN. You may need to administer regular insulin according to a sliding scale (or the pharmacist may add it directly to

the PN solution). The risk for hyperglycemia is less with 3:1 PN solutions.
- **Diuresis and dehydration.** These can occur if hypertonic dextrose is infused too rapidly.
- **Intake and output.**
To evaluate nutrient intake, fluid balance, and renal function.
- **Lab values.** Patients receiving PN require regular lab studies (the following are examples and not a comprehensive list). The frequency of the studies depends on the patient's condition.
  - Electrolytes, blood sugar, albumin, BUN, and creatinine
    These values are used for formula adjustment and to evaluate electrolyte balance and glucose metabolism.
  - Albumin, transferrin, transthyretin (prealbumin), or retinol-binding protein
    May be used to assess visceral protein status.
  - 24-hour urine for urine urea nitrogen (weekly)
    To assess for nitrogen balance.
  - Complete blood count (CBC) and differential.
    To monitor changes in immune function.
  - Liver function studies
  - Serum zinc
  - Plasma urea
  - Plasma and urine osmolality
  - Blood gases
- **Symptoms of complications:**
  - *Electrolyte imbalances.* Symptoms depend on the electrolytes affected. Monitor lab values.
  - *Sepsis:* Temperature greater than 100°F (37.8°C) orally, rapid pulse from baseline, chills, hypothermia, edema or erythema of skin, exudate from catheter insertion site, malaise, leukocytosis (increased white blood cell count), altered level of consciousness.

- *Air embolus*: Cyanosis, tachypnea, hypotension, heart murmur
- *Catheter dislodgement or thrombosis*: Swelling of arm or neck, pain, difficulty flushing catheter, difficulty infusing PN
- ***Nutritional status***:
  - Calculate the daily calorie intake.
  - Perform nutritional assessment at 2-week intervals.
  - Possibly measure arm circumference and triceps skinfold thickness.
  - Most agencies have specialized nutrition teams who will monitor these parameters.

Maintenance

- Change the dressing over the catheter every 24 hours or according to agency policy; or when it becomes wet, soiled, or nonocclusive. Use sterile technique.
- Secure connections with Luer-lock connectors; do not use tape.
- Change the filter every 24 hours.

- Do not hang PN bottles for more than 12 hours (some guidelines and agency policies specify 24 hours).

PN solutions are prepared in batches under strict aseptic conditions. Its high nutrient concentration makes PN an excellent feeding alternative; however, it also makes the solution ideal for bacterial growth.

- Use sterile aseptic technique when changing the dressing for a central line, as well as when changing the solution and tubing.
- Do not use the PN infusion line for administering any other medicines or solutions.

To decrease the risk of contamination and infection.

- Infuse PN by pump with a reliable, audible alarm.

To protect against "free flow."

- If an infusion falls behind schedule, do not increase the rate in an attempt to catch up. This can cause osmotic diuresis and dehydration.
- When PN is discontinued, it may be done gradually (perhaps over as many as 48 hours). To prevent a sudden drop in blood sugar.

Assessment: Screening for Nutritional Problems

Clients who have risk factors for nutritional problems should be evaluated using one of the methods in this section: Subjective Global Assessment, Nutrition Screening Initiative (NSI), Nutrition Screening for Older Adults with Dementia, and Mini-Nutritional Assessment.

Subjective Global Assessment

Using the subjective global assessment (SGA) method, an experienced clinician examines the general medical history and physical examination to evaluate a client's nutritional status. There are six components pertinent to nutritional status:

1. *Weight history*—over previous 6 months
2. *Dietary history*—including a comparison of usual, recommended, and current intake, as well as changes in eating patterns over the last weeks or months
3. *Gastrointestinal symptoms history*—anorexia, nausea, vomiting, and diarrhea
4. *Energy level*—including activity level and functional abilities
5. *Existing disease*—evaluation of the metabolic demands of any disease states along with acute stressors that may alter those demands

6. *Physical examination data*—regarding loss of fat stores, muscle wasting, and the presence of edema and ascites

As a clinician, you would analyze these components to rate the client's nutritional status as normal, mild, moderate, or severe. The effectiveness of this method depends largely on the experience of the clinician (Barone, Milosavljevic, & Gazibarich, 2003; Detsky, McLaughlin, Baker, et al., 1987). For a link to view this tool online and use with patients,

 Go to Chapter 26, **Resources for Caregivers and Health Professionals, Subjective Global Assessment,** on the Student Resource Disk or DavisPlus at http://davisplus. fadavis.com/Wilkinson2

Nutrition Screening Initiative (NSI), for Older Adults: Indications of Impaired Nutritional Status

Recognizing the importance of nutrition in our aging population, the American Academy of Family Physicians, the American Dietetic Association, and the National Council on Aging developed the Nutrition Screening Initiative (NSI) (1995). The NSI includes (1) a self-administered checklist to evaluate risk, (2) the Level I Screening Tool designed for health professionals, and (3) a Level II Screening Tool for use in healthcare facilities.

The NSI addresses nutritional concerns associated with chronic diseases that older adults frequently experience. The NSI requires collection and evaluation of data in four areas: clinical, dietary, body composition, and biochemical. In addition, it identifies indicators of impaired nutritional status (following).

MAJOR INDICATORS	MINOR INDICATORS	SYMPTOMS	PHYSICAL SIGNS	LAB VALUES
■ Significant weight loss over time ■ Significant high or low weight for height ■ Significant change in functional status ■ Significant and inappropriate food intake ■ Significant reduction in midarm circumference ■ Significant decrease in skinfold ■ Osteoporosis or osteomalacia ■ Folate or vitamin B deficiency	■ Concurrent syndromes ■ Alcoholism ■ Cognitive impairment ■ Chronic renal insufficiency ■ Multiple concurrent medications ■ Malabsorption syndromes	■ Anorexia, nausea, or dysphagia ■ Early satiety ■ Changed bowel habits ■ Fatigue or apathy ■ Memory loss	■ Poor oral or dental status ■ Dehydration ■ Poorly healing wounds ■ Loss of subcutaneous fat or muscle mass ■ Fluid retention	■ Reduced levels of serum albumin, transferrin, or prealbumin ■ Folate deficiency ■ Iron deficiency ■ Zinc deficiency ■ Reduced levels of ascorbic acid

To learn more about the NSI and for tools to use for nutritional screening of older adults,

Go to Chapter 26, **Tables, Boxes, Figures: ESG Table 26-2, Nutrition Screening Initiative (for older adults),** on the Student Resource Disk or DavisPlus at http://davisplus.fadavis.com/Wilkinson2

Mini Nutritional Assessment

The Mini Nutritional Assessment (MNA®) is a quick and easy method of identifying individuals with nutritional risk or with malnutrition. (See the accompanying figure.) This tool was developed primarily for use with older clients. It consists of two parts. The first part screens for nutritional risk. The second part is completed only if the individual is identified to be at risk. The final score, which tallies the scores of both parts, is the Malnutrition Indicator Score. Indications of malnutrition require multidisciplinary follow-up.

NESTLÉ NUTRITION SERVICES

Nestlé

Mini Nutritional Assessment
MNA®

Last name: _____ First name: _____ Sex: _____ Date: _____

Age: _____ Weight, kg: _____ Height, cm: _____ I.D. Number: _____

Complete the screen by filling in the boxes with the appropriate numbers.
Add the numbers for the screen. If score is 11 or less, continue with the assessment to gain a Malnutrition Indicator Score.

Screening

A Has food intake declined over the past 3 months due to loss of appetite, digestive problems, chewing or swallowing difficulties?
0 = severe loss of appetite
1 = moderate loss of appetite
2 = no loss of appetite

B Weight loss during the last 3 months
0 = weight loss greater than 3 kg (6.6 lbs)
1 = does not know
2 = weight loss between 1 and 3 kg (2.2 and 6.6 lbs)
3 = no weight loss

C Mobility
0 = bed or chair bound
1 = able to get out of bed/chair but does not go out
2 = goes out

D Has suffered psychological stress or acute disease in the past 3 months
0 = yes   2 = no

E Neuropsychological problems
0 = severe dementia or depression
1 = mild dementia
2 = no psychological problems

F Body Mass Index (BMI) (weight in kg) / (height in m)^2
0 = BMI less than 19
1 = BMI 19 to less than 21
2 = BMI 21 to less than 23
3 = BMI 23 or greater

Screening score (subtotal max. 14 points)
12 points or greater   Normal – not at risk – no need to complete assessment
11 points or below   Possible malnutrition – continue assessment

Assessment

G Lives independently (not in a nursing home or hospital)
0 = no   1 = yes

H Takes more than 3 prescription drugs per day
0 = yes   1 = no

I Pressure sores or skin ulcers
0 = yes   1 = no

J How many full meals does the patient eat daily?
0 = 1 meal
1 = 2 meals
2 = 3 meals

K Selected consumption markers for protein intake
• At least one serving of dairy products (milk, cheese, yogurt) per day?   yes ☐   no ☐
• Two or more servings of legumes or eggs per week?   yes ☐   no ☐
• Meat, fish or poultry every day   yes ☐   no ☐
0.0 = if 0 or 1 yes
0.5 = if 2 yes
1.0 = if 3 yes

L Consumes two or more servings of fruits or vegetables per day?
0 = no   1 = yes

M How much fluid (water, juice, coffee, tea, milk...) is consumed per day?
0.0 = less than 3 cups
0.5 = 3 to 5 cups
1.0 = more than 5 cups

N Mode of feeding
0 = unable to eat without assistance
1 = self-fed with some difficulty
2 = self-fed without any problem

O Self view of nutritional status
0 = views self as being malnourished
1 = is uncertain of nutritional state
2 = views self as having no nutritional problem

P In comparison with other people of the same age, how does the patient consider his/her health status?
0.0 = not as good
0.5 = does not know
1.0 = as good
2.0 = better

Q Mid-arm circumference (MAC) in cm
0.0 = MAC less than 21
0.5 = MAC 21 to 22
1.0 = MAC 22 or greater

R Calf circumference (CC) in cm
0 = CC less than 31   1 = CC 31 or greater

Assessment (max. 16 points)

Screening score

Total Assessment (max. 30 points)

Malnutrition Indicator Score
17 to 23.5 points   at risk of malnutrition
Less than 17 points   malnourished

Ref.: Guigoz Y, Vellas B and Garry P J. 1994. Mini Nutritional Assessment: A practical assessment tool for grading the nutritional state of elderly patients. *Facts and Research in Gerontology.* Supplement #2:15-59.
Rubenstein LZ, Harker J, Guigoz Y and Vellas B. Comprehensive Geriatric Assessment (CGA) and the MNA: An Overview of CGA, Nutritional Assessment, and Development of a Shortened Version of the MNA. In: "Mini Nutritional Assessment (MNA): Research and Practice in the Elderly". Vellas B, Garry PJ and Guigoz Y, editors. Nestlé Nutrition Workshop Series. Clinical & Performance Programme, vol. 1. Karger, Bâle, in press.

© Nestlé, 1994, Revision 1998. N67200 12/99 10M

References: Guigoz, 2006; Rubenstein, Harker, Salva, et al., 2001; Vellas, Villars, Abellan, et al., 2006.
Literature related to the MNA® is regularly updated at www.mna-elderly.com

Nutrition Screening for Older Adults with Dementia

For a tool to use in assessing nutritional status for patients with dementia,

 Go to **Try This, Issue D11.1: Eating and Feeding Issues in Older Adults with Dementia: Part I: Assessment,** at http://www.hartfordign.org/Resources/Try_This_Series/

Focused Nutritional Assessment

If you identify nutritional problems or risks using the screening tools, you should perform a more in-depth nutritional assessment, such as the following.

Focused Nutritional Assessment

Nutritional History

Item	Components
Demographic data	Name, date, age, sex, date of birth, address, occupation, workplace
Chief complaint	Client's subjective statement of health problem, including onset and duration
Present illness and current health	Detailed data about chief complaint as it relates to nutrition status
	Recent diet changes and reasons
	Recent weight loss or gain and over what period of time
	Usual body weight: 20% above or below desirable weight?
	Change in appetite
	Unusual stress/trauma (surgery, job, family)
	Medications, prescriptions
	Alcohol, nicotine, caffeine consumption
Health history	Previous illnesses, trauma, major dental problems, or issues that could interfere with ability to shop, prepare food, chew, or swallow
	Allergies (i.e., environmental, foods, drugs)
	Eating disorders
	Chronic disease or surgery that affects gastrointestinal tract
	Substance abuse
	Nutritional programs
	Depression
Family health history	Genetic/familial disorders that could affect nutritional status: cardiovascular or gastrointestinal disorders, Crohn's disease, diabetes, cancer, sickle cell anemia, allergies, celiac disease, other food intolerances, obesity
Dietary history	Current food intake pattern using one of the following methods: 24-hour–7-day recall, as appropriate; food frequency questionnaire; food record; and comparison to dietary guidelines and DRIs
	Special dietary considerations, restrictions
	Fad diets
	Vitamin and mineral supplements
	Commercial dietary supplements
	Nonconventional dietary supplements
	Food preferences, dislikes
	Dietary influences from ethnic, cultural, or religious practices
	Counseling needs (based on food knowledge)
Medication history	Recent use of steroids, immunosuppressants, chemotherapy, anticonvulsants, or oral contraceptives
Socioeconomic factors	Adequate food storage, refrigeration, food preparation, payments:
	Supplemental Security Income (SSI), food stamps, WIC
	Who shops for, prepares, and cooks food?

Focused Nutritional Assessment—cont'd

| Personal factors | Stress/coping mechanisms, self-concept, social supports |
| | Daily activity level and exercise regimen |

Nutrition-Focused Physical Examination

Correlate the following physical examination findings with the dietary history, screening methods, anthropometric measurements, and laboratory results.

I. The General Survey

Assess vital signs, height, weight, and overall impressions.

- *Overall appearance.* Does the client look ill? Does he appear adequately nourished? You will want to investigate any hunches as you move through the physical exam.
- *Temperature.* An increase in temperature raises the client's metabolic rate and need for fluid, is a sign of infection, and may decrease the client's appetite.
- *Blood pressure (BP) and heart rate* are affected by fluid status. An elevated BP may be related to fluid volume excess; a low BP may be a sign of dehydration. Heart rate usually increases when fluid volume is low.
- *Height and weight.* Calculate the body mass index (BMI) on the basis of these measures:

BMI = weight in kilograms ÷ (height in meters)²

Classification of Body Mass Index Values

Classification	BMI (kg/m²)	Risk of Comorbidities
Underweight*	<18.5	Low
Normal weight	18.5–24.9	Average
Pre-obese	25.0–29.9	Mildly increased
Class I obesity	30.0–34.9	Moderate
Class II obesity	35.0–39.9	Severe
Class III obesity	≥40.0	Very severe

*Note: In adults in long-term care settings or with serious illness, nutritional support should be implemented for those with a BMI less than 21. In this population a BMI of less than 21 is associated with increased mortality (National Guideline Clearinghouse, 2005).

II. Integumentary System

- *Skin turgor* is an indicator of fluid status. Poor skin turgor may result from dehydration. Swelling may result from overhydration.
- *Skin integrity* reflects overall nutritional status. Poor wound healing may suggest inadequate intake of protein, vitamin C, or zinc. Patients with uncontrolled diabetes often experience slow-healing wounds, especially in the feet and legs.
- *Areas of warmth or erythema.* These are signs of inflammation or infection.
- *Other nutrition-related skin changes* include red, swollen skin lesions (due to niacin deficiency); excessive bleeding seen as petechiae or ecchymoses (due to vitamin K or C deficiency); and xerosis (dry skin).
- *Abnormal nail findings* include spoon-shaped, brittle nails (due to iron deficiency); dull nails with transverse ridge (due to protein deficiency); pale, poor blanching, or mottled nails (due to vitamin A or C deficiency); bruising or bleeding beneath nails (due to protein or caloric deficiency); and splinter hemorrhages (due to vitamin C deficiency).
- *Hair* will grow slowly, thin, or break easily if protein is deficient.

III. The Head and Neck

The condition of the mouth, teeth, and gums has a major effect on a client's choice of food, ability to chew, and ability to swallow.

- *Facial paralysis or drooping* of one side of the face may be a result of stroke, injury, or nerve irritation, which also affects the ability to chew and swallow (dysphagia).
- *Enlarged thyroid gland.* Look for swelling of the thyroid, which may be related to hypothyroid or hyperthyroid states. Both disorders affect metabolic rate and energy requirements.
- *Eyes.* Nutritional deficits may cause the eyes to be red and dry and the conjunctiva pale.
- *Lips and tongue.* The lips may be chapped, red, or swollen. The tongue may be bright red, purple, or swollen or may have longitudinal furrows.
- *Teeth and gums.* Look for cavities, mottled or missing teeth, and for spongy, bleeding, or receding gums.
- *Lymph nodes.* Palpate for enlarged or tender lymph nodes under the chin and along the neck. Nodes that are swollen can signal infection, such as a sore throat.

Continued

Focused Nutritional Assessment—cont'd

IV. Cardiovascular System

You will have gained initial information about the cardiovascular system by taking the vital signs. As you follow up and listen to the heart and check pulses, you should explore any abnormal vital signs.

- *Bounding pulses* are associated with fluid overload, fever, and hypertension.
- *Weak, thready pulse* may indicate dehydration, shock, or hypotension.
- *Edema in the extremities* may be a sign of fluid overload, inadequate protein stores, or electrolyte imbalance.

V. Abdominal Exam

- A *scaphoid or concave abdomen* indicates loss of subcutaneous fat, possibly caused by malnutrition.
- A *round or protuberant abdomen* points to obesity due to excess caloric and/or high fat intake.
- A *generalized enlarged abdomen* may signify **ascites** (fluid in the abdominal cavity) due to liver malfunction. Ascites results from three mechanisms: abnormal movement of protein and water into the abdomen; sodium and fluid retention; and decreased albumin production in the liver.
- *Hyperactive bowel sounds* are heard with gastrointestinal infection, laxative use, and malabsorption disorders.
- *Hypoactive bowel sounds* suggest sluggish motility in the GI tract.

VI. Musculoskeletal System

- *Thin extremities with excess skinfolds* may indicate muscle atrophy and fat loss related to malnutrition, especially protein and calories. This may also occur as a result of prolonged bed rest and inadequate food intake. Skinfold measurement is also useful in assessing muscle and fat stores.
- Look for any obvious *swelling, deformities, or limitation in range of motion* of the joints.
- *Kyphosis* of the spine may indicate osteoporosis and possible insufficient calcium intake.
- *Joint pain* on palpation or with movement is a sign of arthritis or gout. Arthritis may affect ability to shop for groceries, prepare food to eat, and use utensils for eating and drinking. Gout is often induced by diets high in **purines** (food substances that break down into uric acid), obesity, and excess alcohol intake.

VII. Neurological System

The neurological examination will give you insight into the client's ability to perform independent tasks.

- Look for *altered level of consciousness or signs of behavioral disturbances and dementia* through general conversation and appropriateness of answers to specific questions.
- Assess *coordination and reflexes*.
- Assess for *cognitive deficits or severe psychiatric disorders*. A client with cognitive deficits or severe psychiatric disorders may have difficulty preparing food or judging appropriate nutrient choices.
- Assess for *motor or sensory deficits*. Clients with motor or sensory deficits may be unable to purchase, prepare, or eat a variety of foods.
- *Confusion, weakness, diminished reflexes, paresthesia, and sensory loss* may be cues to vitamin B deficiencies.
- *Tetany or severe and generalized muscle spasm* may indicate calcium or magnesium deficits.

VIII. What Are the Signs of Severe Malnutrition?

Malnutrition is a condition of impaired development or function caused by a long-term deficiency, excess, or imbalance in energy and/or nutrient intake.

- Symptoms of undernutrition due to insufficient food include reduced physical activity, weight loss, and reduced height.
- Children, older adults, and people with chronic illnesses such as cancer, HIV infection, and chronic obstructive pulmonary disease (COPD) are most likely to experience malnutrition.
- To assess for malnutrition in children, compare weight, height, and head circumference to the standards (norms) for the child's age.
- Other indicators in children include the presence of iron-deficiency anemia.
- In adolescents, look for a delay of stages of sexual maturation.

Diagnostic Testing

Tests Reflecting Nutritional Status: Norms

Note: Norms are for adults (ages 19 to 65) unless otherwise noted.

■ Blood glucose	70 mg/dL to 100 mg/dL. Capillary blood sugar is frequently assessed at the bedside with a simple fingerstick. Serum blood glucose levels are assessed by drawing a venous blood sample. The level is measured in the laboratory.
	The American Diabetes Association (2006) recommends for diabetic patients a preprandial plasma glucose level of 70 to 130 mg/dL.
■ Serum albumin	3.4–4.8 g/dL
■ Prealbumin	12–42 mg/dL (age 6 years–adult)
■ Globulin	2.3–3.4 g/dL
■ Blood urea nitrogen (BUN)	5–18 mg/dL (children)
	8–21 mg/dL (age 14 – adult);10–31 mg/dL (adult older than 90)
■ Creatinine	0.5–1 mg/dL (female)
	0.6–1.2 mg/dL (male)
■ Hemoglobin	13.2–17.3 g/dL (male)
	11.7–15.5 g/dL (female)
	12.6–17.4 g/dL (male, older adult)
	11.7–16.1 g/dL (female, older adult)

Standardized Language

NOC Outcomes and NIC Interventions Related to Nutrition

NOC OUTCOMES	NIC INTERVENTIONS
The following outcomes are directly linked to nutritional diagnoses:	**The following interventions are directly linked to nutrition problems:**
Appetite	Behavior Modification
Knowledge: Diet	Eating Disorders Management
Nutritional Status	Electrolyte Management
Nutritional Status: Biochemical Measures	Electrolyte Monitoring
Nutritional Status: Food and Fluid Intake	Fluid/Electrolyte Management
Nutritional Status: Nutrient Intake	Fluid Monitoring
Self-Care: Eating	Nutrition Management
Weight: Body Mass	Nutrition Therapy
Weight Control	Nutritional Counseling
	Nutritional Monitoring
	Nutritional Therapy
	Self-Care Assistance: Feeding
	Teaching: Individual
	Teaching: Prescribed Diet
	Weight Gain Assistance
	Weight Reduction Assistance

Continued

NOC Outcomes and NIC Interventions Related to Nutrition—cont'd

The following interventions are also found in the class, Nutrition Support. They address specific etiologies of nutrition problems.

Diet Staging

Enteral Tube Feeding

Feeding

Gastrointestinal Intubation

Swallowing Therapy

Total Parenteral Nutrition (PN) Administration

Tube Care: Gastrointestinal

Weight Gain Assistance

Weight Management

Sources: Bulechek, G., Butcher, H., & Dochterman, J. (Eds.). (2008). *Nursing interventions classification (NIC)* (5th ed.). St. Louis, MO: C.V. Mosby; Johnson, M., Bulechek, G., Butcher, H., et al. (2006). *NANDA, NOC, and NIC linkages.* (2nd ed.). St. Louis, MO: C.V. Mosby; Moorhead, S., Johnson, M., & Maas, M., et al. (Eds.). (2008). *Nursing outcomes classification (NOC)* (4th ed.). St. Louis, MO: C.V. Mosby. Used with permission.

NOC Outcomes and NIC Interventions for Adult Failure to Thrive, Overweight/Obesity and Underweight/Malnutrition

FOR ADULT FAILURE TO THRIVE

Nursing Diagnosis	Adult Failure to Thrive
NOC Outcomes	Appetite
	Cognition
	Nutritional Status
	Nutritional Status: Food and Fluid Intake
	Physical Aging
	Self-Care: Activities of Daily Living (ADLs)
	Will to Live
NIC Interventions	■ Cognitive Stimulation
	■ Environmental Management
	■ Fluid Monitoring
	■ Home Maintenance Assistance
	■ Hope Instillation
	■ Nutrition Management
	■ Nutrition Therapy
	■ Nutritional Monitoring
	■ Risk Identification

FOR OVERWEIGHT/OBESITY

Nursing Diagnoses	Imbalanced Nutrition: More Than Body Requirements
	Risk for Imbalanced Nutrition: More Than Body Requirements
NOC Outcomes	Nutritional Status
	Nutritional Status: Food and Fluid Intake
	Nutritional Status: Nutrient Intake
	Weight Control

NOC Outcomes and NIC Interventions for Adult Failure to Thrive, Overweight/Obesity and Underweight/Malnutrition—cont'd

FOR OVERWEIGHT/OBESITY

NIC Interventions	▪ Behavior Modification—to promote change in eating and exercising behaviors
	▪ Nutritional Counseling—to provide information based on identified knowledge deficits regarding nutrition
	▪ Nutrition Management—to balance metabolic needs with nutrient intake
	▪ Nutritional Monitoring—to analyze patient data to facilitate weight loss and prevent malnourishment
	▪ Weight Management—to balance caloric intake and energy expenditure
	▪ Weight Reduction Assistance—to balance caloric intake and energy expenditure

FOR UNDERWEIGHT/MALNUTRITION

Nursing Diagnoses	Imbalanced Nutrition: Less Than Body Requirements
	Risk for Imbalanced Nutrition: Less Than Body Requirements
NOC Outcomes	Appetite
	Breastfeeding Establishment: Infant
	Nutritional Status
	Nutritional Status: Biochemical Measures
	Nutritional Status: Food & Fluid Intake
	Nutritional Status: Nutrient Intake
	Self-Care: Eating
	Weight: Body Mass
NIC Interventions	▪ Breastfeeding Assistance and Lactation Counseling—are used when breastfeeding difficulties are the etiology of an infant's undernutrition.
	▪ Eating Disorders Management—if anorexia nervosa or bulimia nervosa is present
	▪ Enteral Tube Feeding, Gastrointestinal Intubation, Total Parenteral Nutrition (TPN) Administration, and Tube Care: Gastrointestinal—are used when the patient cannot tolerate oral feedings
	▪ Fluid Monitoring, Fluid/Electrolyte Management, Electrolyte Management, and Electrolyte Monitoring—are used when intake is severely limited and deficits are suspected, when enteral or parenteral feedings are used, or when there is diarrhea or vomiting (e.g., self-induced vomiting in bulimia)
	▪ Nutrition Management—to balance metabolic needs with nutrient intake
	▪ Nutrition Therapy—for the treatment of nutritional imbalance
	▪ Nutritional Counseling—to provide information based on identified knowledge deficits regarding nutrition
	▪ Nutritional Monitoring—to evaluate the effectiveness of the counseling and nutritional therapy
	▪ Self-Care Assistance: Feeding—used when inability to feed self is the etiology of undernutrition
	▪ Swallowing Therapy—to treat dysphagia or difficulty swallowing
	▪ Weight Gain Assistance—used when the focus is to help the client gain weight
	▪ Weight Management—used to maintain a balance in caloric intake and energy expenditure

Sources: Bulechek, G., Butcher, H., & Dochterman, J. (Eds.). (2008). *Nursing interventions classification (NIC)* (5th ed.). St. Louis, MO: C.V. Mosby; Johnson, M., Bulechek, G., Butcher, H., et al. (2006). *NANDA, NOC, and NIC linkages.* (2nd ed.). St. Louis, MO: C.V. Mosby; Moorhead, S., Johnson, M., & Maas, M., et al. (Eds.). (2008). *Nursing outcomes classification (NOC)* (4th ed.). St. Louis, MO: C.V. Mosby; NANDA International (2009). *Nursing diagnoses definitions and classification 2009–2011.* Ames, IA: Wiley-Blackwell. Used with permission.

THINKING CRITICALLY ABOUT NUTRITION

The exercises in the following sections allow you to practice the kind of thinking you will use as a full-spectrum nurse. Because these are critical-thinking questions, there is usually no single right answer. We do not provide answers for these questions because it is more important for you to think about the questions than to arrive at the "right" answer. These questions are designed to improve your thinking more than to "cover content." Discuss answers with your peers—discussion can stimulate critical thinking. If you have difficulty with any of these questions, consult with your instructor.

Applying the Full-Spectrum Nursing Model

PATIENT SITUATION

Mrs. O is a 75-year-old retired schoolteacher who suffered a stroke 8 months ago. Since leaving the hospital, she has been living in a nursing home. Mrs. O has residual weakness on the right side—her dominant side—and has not mastered the use of tableware with her left hand. On admission to the nursing home 7 months ago, she weighed 150 pounds. Today she weighs only 125 pounds. Mrs. O refuses to go to the dining room for meals. The NAPs report that she eats a few bites of most foods, but never eats more than half of anything.

THINKING

1. *Theoretical Knowledge*:

   a. Based on Mrs. O's gender, age, and activity level, make a rough estimate of the number of kcal/day she needs.

   b. What are two other, more precise, ways you could determine Mrs. O's ideal body weight?

2. *Critical Thinking (Considering Alternatives)*: What are some possible explanations for why Mrs. O is not eating all her food?

DOING

3. *Practical Knowledge*:

   a. Suppose you have decided to use the general ideal weight guide to determine Mrs. O's ideal weight. What, specifically, would you need to do? You do not need to actually calculate; just list the action steps.

   b. Suppose you have decided to determine Mrs. O's body mass index (BMI). What equipment would you need?

   c. What is the formula for calculating BMI from the height and weight?

4. *Nursing Process (Diagnosis)*: Write a nursing diagnosis for Mrs. O. Use just the data provided in the situation. Assume her BMI is 20.

CARING

5. *Self-Knowledge*: What would you be feeling if you were in Mrs. O's situation?

6. *Ethical Knowledge*: What are one or two things you would do to help Mrs. O feel cared for and cared about?

Critical Thinking and Clinical Reasoning

1. Recall the employees interviewed in the "Meet Your Patient" scenario in Volume 1. In addition, you now have two more patients, Wakenda Pierre and Luceno Jarin. Their information is provided below.

   - Isaac Schwartz, a 50-year-old accountant, works long hours. He describes a sedentary lifestyle, no tobacco use, infrequent alcohol use, no medical problems, and a nutritional history of skipping meals and daily consumption of restaurant food. You measure his height as 69 inches and weight, 245 lb.
   - Sujing Lee, a 29-year-old project manager, regularly works 65 hours per week. Sujing is 30 weeks pregnant. She does not smoke or drink and has never been hospitalized or had surgery. She has gained a total of 25 pounds so far this pregnancy. Her diet consists mainly of traditional Chinese food. She eats three meals a day and always brings lunch from home. Lately she has felt "tired all the time." At the screening, she weighs 126 lb and measures 63 inches tall.
   - Wakenda Pierre is a 38-year-old administrative assistant. She exercises at the gym 4 to 5 days per week, smokes an occasional cigarette, has two to three drinks every night before dinner, struggles with keeping her blood pressure under control, and eats fast food for breakfast and lunch every day. She is 72 inches tall and weighs 165 lb.
   - Luceno Jarin is a 65-year-old business executive. He tells you he was diagnosed with type 2 diabetes mellitus 5 years ago. He is struggling to follow his prescribed diet. He drinks alcohol sporadically and walks briskly 30 minutes every day of the week. He is 67 inches tall and weighs 205 pounds.

   a. Determine each client's BMI. Based on these results, what conclusions can you make about their weight status?

   b. What are the likely causes of each person's weight status?

   c. What additional workup would be recommended for each individual?

   d. What indications would lead you to believe that each client has adopted a healthier lifestyle?

2. The following are three clients admitted to the medical–surgical unit of your local hospital. On their admission, the primary nurse collected the following information.

	Client 1	Client 2	Client 3
Weight	175 lb	100 lb	250 lb
Height	70 inches	59 inches	65 inches
Gender/Age	Male/40 years old	Female/18 years old	Male/65 years old
Usual Daily Caloric Intake	2500 kcal	1000 kcal	2500 kcal
Usual Activity Level	Moderate	High	Light
Serum Albumin	Normal	Low	Normal
Serum Glucose	Normal	Low	High

   a. Identify which client(s) is/are at risk for nutritional imbalance.

   b. Which client is at risk for developing malnutrition?

   c. What additional information would support this conclusion?

   d. What nursing interventions would you initiate at this time?

3. After 3 days, you examine how well each of these clients is doing using the same parameters as admission day.

	Client 1	Client 2	Client 3
Weight	170 lb	103 lb	250 lb
Current Daily Caloric Intake	2500 kcal	1500 kcal	1500 kcal
Intake (mL)	2000	2000	1000
Output (mL)	1800	1900	500
Current Activity Level	Up as tolerated	Up as tolerated	Bed rest
Serum Albumin	Normal	Low	Normal
Serum Glucose	Normal	Low	High

a. In comparison with the admission data, there are some changes. Which client's health status is a priority now, and why?

b. What is the most likely cause(s) of this concern?

c. Which nursing interventions should be initiated for this client while hospitalized? Focus on nutritional needs.

d. Identify appropriate education that should begin during hospitalization for this client.

4. For each of the following concepts, use critical thinking to describe how or why it is important to nursing, patient care, or nutrition. Note that these are *not* to be merely definitions.

Energy balance
Basal metabolic rate
Body mass index
Nutrients
Weight management
Nutritional history

Body weight standards
Enteral feedings
Parenteral nutrition
Special diets
Nutritional screening

What Are the Main Points in This Chapter?

➤ Reliable guidelines for designing a nutritious diet include the Dietary Reference Intakes (DRIs), Food Guide Pyramids, the USDA Dietary Guidelines, Canada's Food Guide for Healthy Eating, and the Nutrition Facts panel found on packaged foods in the United States.

➤ MyPyramid is a food guide that illustrates healthful dietary choices. It stresses six concepts for healthy eating: activity, moderation, personalization, proportionality, variety, and gradual improvement.

➤ Energy nutrients are carbohydrates, proteins, and fats (lipids). Other important nutrients are water and the micronutrients: fat-soluble vitamins, water-soluble vitamins, and minerals.

➤ Carbohydrates include simple sugars called monosaccharides and disaccharides and complex carbohydrates called polysaccharides.

➤ Glucose, a monosaccharide, is the primary source of energy for the brain, as well as for the body during moderate-to-intense physical activity.

➤ Proteins are made up of amino acids and are required for cell and tissue growth, maintenance, and repair. They also act as buffers in acid–base balance. Proteins are an energy source.

➤ Lipids, including fats and oils, are classified as glycerides, sterols, and phospholipids. They are essential components of cells, fuel the body at rest and during light activity, aid in absorption of fat-soluble vitamins, and promote a sense of satiety when eaten. Low-density lipoproteins (LDLs) are the "bad" cholesterol. High-density lipoproteins (HDLs) are the "good" cholesterol.

➤ Saturated fats and *trans*-fats are less healthful lipid choices than mono- and polyunsaturated fats.

Saturated fats and *trans*-fats raise LDL cholesterol levels in the blood.

➤ The essential fatty acids omega-6 and omega-3 help protect against heart disease when they replace *trans*-fats in the diet. They are found mainly in vegetable oils, nuts, seeds, and fatty fish.

➤ Nutrients must be consumed at least at a minimal level in order to meet the body's physiological needs. This level is called Dietary Reference Intake (DRI).

➤ The fat-soluble vitamins are A, D, E, and K. Water-soluble vitamins are C and the B-complex vitamins.

➤ Minerals (e.g., calcium, iron, magnesium) are important for transmitting nerve impulses, regulating fluid balance, strengthening bones, and producing energy.

➤ The basal metabolic rate (BMR) is a measure of the energy required by resting tissue to maintain basic function.

➤ Factors influencing a client's nutritional status include developmental stage, pregnancy and lactation, education, lifestyle choices, vegetarianism, dieting for weight loss, culture, religion, disease processes, functional limitations, economic factors, and modified or special diets.

➤ Many people must follow a modified diet to assist in managing their illness. In addition, all inpatients must have a diet prescribed by their primary care provider.

➤ When examining an individual's nutritional balance, it is important to screen for nutritional problems. When risk factors are present, thoroughly assess nutritional history, physical findings, anthropometric measurements, imaging techniques, and biochemical values.

➤ A food record is the most accurate method of obtaining data about a client's actual food intake.

➤ The body mass index (BMI), skinfold measurements, and body part circumferences are estimates of body composition.

➤ Laboratory or biochemical indicators of nutritional status include blood glucose and serum protein levels or indices such as albumin, urea, and hemoglobin.

➤ Vitamin and mineral supplementation may be appropriate for some people, but they do not replace the need for a balanced diet.

➤ Government programs provide some assistance for clients who cannot afford to buy food.

➤ Nutritional requirements of older adults are similar to those for all adults, with a slight reduction in the need for calories, and the more likely need for nutrient supplementation. Nutritional problems are also similar, but the incidence is higher among older adults.

➤ Nurses can help support nutrition for patients who have Self-Care Deficits or Impaired Swallowing by assisting patients with meals and providing swallowing therapy.

➤ Nutritional imbalance can range from either inadequate or excessive amounts of a single nutrient relative to overall caloric intake.

➤ Overweight and obesity are a major problem in the United States, both in children and adults.

➤ Interventions for underweight/undernutrition include measures to improve the patient's appetite, assisting with meals, and providing enteral and parenteral nutrition.

➤ Nasogastric tubes are inserted to lavage the stomach; collect a specimen of the stomach contents, or prevent nausea, vomiting, and gastric distention. They are also placed to facilitate enteral feeding.

➤ The most accurate way to check enteral tube placement is by radiographic (x-ray) verification; but this is too expensive and time consuming for ongoing bedside use.

➤ To check enteral tube placement at the bedside, you should use a combination of techniques: aspirate stomach contents to observe color and measure the pH (normally 1 to 5.5 for stomach contents); the "whoosh test"; serial observations for respiratory distress, residual volume, length of tube extending outside the body; and capnometry. Do not rely on a single technique.

➤ Potential complications associated with enteral feedings include aspiration, infection, diarrhea, and electrolyte imbalance.

➤ You must follow meticulous sterile technique when administering parenteral nutrition because the solution is delivered into a large central vein; if infection occurs, sepsis is almost immediate.

For practice questions for this chapter,

 Go to **NCLEX-Style Chapter Quiz,** on the Student Resource Disk or DavisPlus at http://davisplus.fadavis.com/Wilkinson2

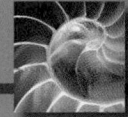

Knowledge Map

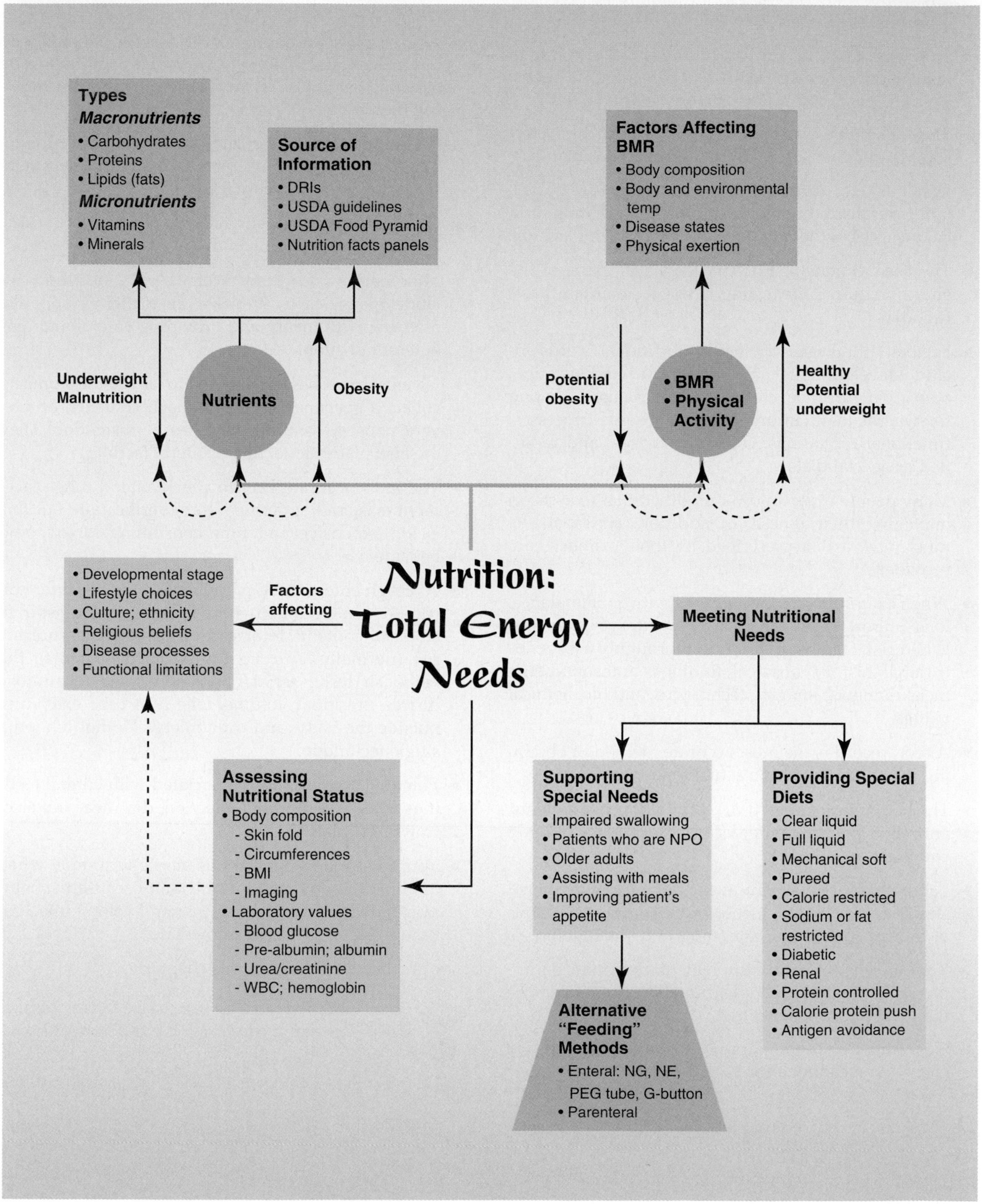

Types
Macronutrients
- Carbohydrates
- Proteins
- Lipids (fats)

Micronutrients
- Vitamins
- Minerals

Source of Information
- DRIs
- USDA guidelines
- USDA Food Pyramid
- Nutrition facts panels

Factors Affecting BMR
- Body composition
- Body and environmental temp
- Disease states
- Physical exertion

Underweight Malnutrition

Nutrients

Obesity

Potential obesity

- **BMR**
- **Physical Activity**

Healthy Potential underweight

- Developmental stage
- Lifestyle choices
- Culture; ethnicity
- Religious beliefs
- Disease processes
- Functional limitations

Factors affecting

Nutrition: Total Energy Needs

Meeting Nutritional Needs

Assessing Nutritional Status
- Body composition
  - Skin fold
  - Circumferences
  - BMI
  - Imaging
- Laboratory values
  - Blood glucose
  - Pre-albumin; albumin
  - Urea/creatinine
  - WBC; hemoglobin

Supporting Special Needs
- Impaired swallowing
- Patients who are NPO
- Older adults
- Assisting with meals
- Improving patient's appetite

Providing Special Diets
- Clear liquid
- Full liquid
- Mechanical soft
- Pureed
- Calorie restricted
- Sodium or fat restricted
- Diabetic
- Renal
- Protein controlled
- Calorie protein push
- Antigen avoidance

Alternative "Feeding" Methods
- Enteral: NG, NE, PEG tube, G-button
- Parenteral

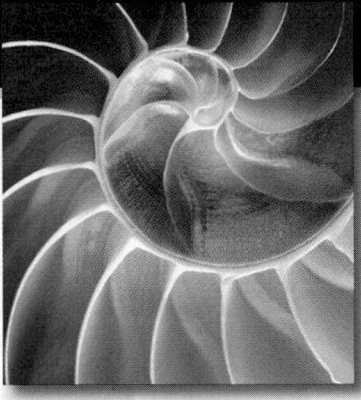

CHAPTER 27

Urinary Elimination

For a podcast of an overview of this chapter,

 Go to Student Resources, **Podcast – Chapter Overviews, Chapter 27,** on DavisPlus at http://davisplus.fadavis.com/Wilkinson2

Caring for the Garcias

The exercises in the following section allow you to practice the kind of thinking you will use as a full-spectrum nurse. Because these are critical-thinking questions, there is usually no single right answer. We do not provide answers for these questions because it is more important for you to think about the questions than to arrive at the "right" answer. These questions are designed to improve your thinking more than to "cover content." Discuss answers with your peers—discussion can stimulate critical thinking. If you have difficulty with any of these questions, consult with your instructor.

At a recent visit to the Family Health Center, Joe and Flordelisa Garcia confide that Joe's mother, Katherine, has had several "accidents." She has denied the problem but Flordelisa tells you that she helped her mother-in-law with laundry recently and many of the clothes smell of urine. They ask you how to approach Katherine about this problem.

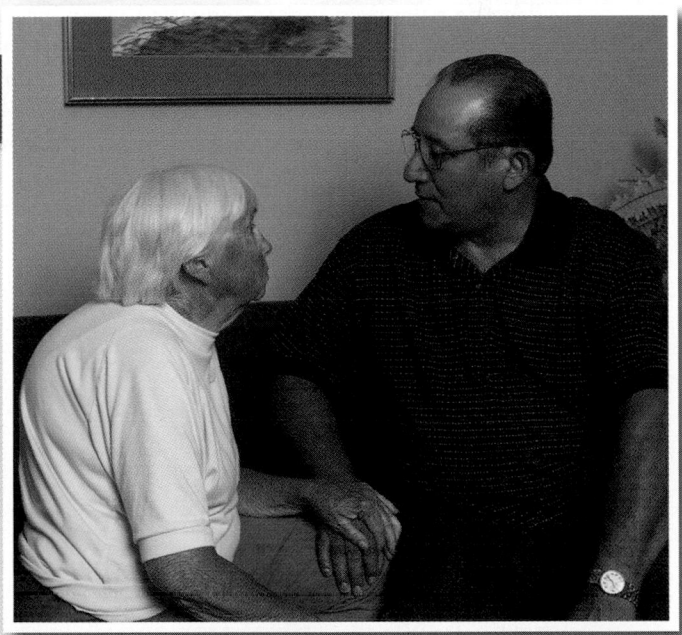

A. How would you respond?

B. What suggestions, if any, could you make to the Garcias about treatment for Katherine?

C. Flordelisa says that she has been told that surgery is the best form of treatment. She asks you whether this is true. How would you answer her question?

Practical **Knowledge**
knowing how

This section provides procedures and clinical insights you will need to support your patients' urinary function. You will also find assessment guidelines, information about diagnostic tests of urinary function, and standardized nursing language tables.

Procedures

Procedure 27-1	**Measuring Urine**

> ➤ For steps to follow in *all* procedures, refer to the Universal Steps for All Procedures found on the inside back cover of Volume 2.

Critical Aspects

- Don clean procedure gloves.
- Record the amount of urine on the input and output (I&O) flowsheets.

Procedure 27-1A: Measuring Urine Output from a Bedpan or Urinal

- Place the bedpan or urinal in the proper position and encourage your patient to begin voiding. Instruct the patient to press the call light button when finished or remain close by.
- Pour the urine from the bedpan or urinal into a graduated measuring device for easy measurement. Place on a flat even surface and read the amount at eye level.

Procedure 27-1B: Measuring Urine from an Indwelling Catheter

- Open the drainage spout and allow urine to drain into the measuring device, being careful to avoid touching the spout to the inside of the container.
- Pour the urine from the bedpan or urinal into a graduated measuring device for easy measurement. Place on a flat even surface and read the amount at eye level to accurately determine how much urine was voided.

Equipment

- Bedpan or urinal
- Clean procedure gloves
- Graduated container
- Toilet paper, as indicated
- Washcloth or towel
- Mild soap and water for patient's hands

Delegation

The procedure may be delegated to nursing assistive personnel (NAPs), but you must be sure that that they know how to perform the procedure correctly, including proper cleansing of the bedpan/urinal and the graduated container according to the facility's policies. Complete the following assessments and instruct the NAP to report any abnormalities seen in the urine (e.g., blood, foul odor, mucus). In addition, the NAP should report any complaints of dysuria by the patient.

Pre-Procedure Assessments

- **Cognitive status**

To determine whether the patient can be instructed to complete this procedure on her own and/or whether she can follow directions.

- **Mobility status**

To determine whether the patient can be permitted to get out of the bed to use the toilet.

- **Urinary status**

To determine the patient's ability to control bladder function.

■ Procedure 27-1A Measuring Urine Output from a Bedpan or Urinal

➤ When performing the procedure, always identify your patient according to agency policy and be attentive to standard precautions, hand hygiene, patient safety and privacy, body mechanics, and documentation.

Procedure Steps

1. Wash your hands and don clean procedure gloves.
Hand hygiene and gloving prevents transmission of bacteria.

2. Place a bedpan or urinal in the appropriate position.
See Procedure 28-2 for placing a patient on the bedpan.

3. Remove the bedpan or urinal, being careful not to spill the urine. Reposition the patient and transport the urine to the bathroom.

4. While still wearing procedure gloves, pour the urine into a graduated cylinder or calibrated measuring container.
   a. Be sure that the measuring device is labeled with the correct patient information (in many institutions, labels are preprinted or barcoded).
   b. Do not use a measuring device for more than one patient.

5. Place the measuring device on a flat surface (e.g., shelf, table), and read the amount at eye level.
When looking at fluid level from an angle, the meniscus may appear falsely low or high.

6. Observe the urine for color, clarity, and odor.

7. Discard the urine in the toilet. If a specimen is required, transfer at least 30 mL of urine to the designated container.

8. Clean the measuring container and store in the patient's bathroom.

9. Remove gloves. Wash your hands.

10. Record the time and amount on the I&O record.

■ Procedure 27-1B Measuring Urine from an Indwelling Catheter

➤ When performing the procedure, always identify your patient according to agency policy and be attentive to standard precautions, hand hygiene, patient safety and privacy, body mechanics, and documentation.

Procedure Steps

1. While wearing clean gloves, place the drainage spout for the collection bag inside a calibrated measuring container. Avoid touching the spout to the inside of the container.
Prevents transmission of bacteria.

2. Unclamp the drainage spout, and direct the flow of urine into the measuring device, still keeping the spout away from the sides of the container.
Prevents transmission of bacteria when unclamping the drainage spout. ▼

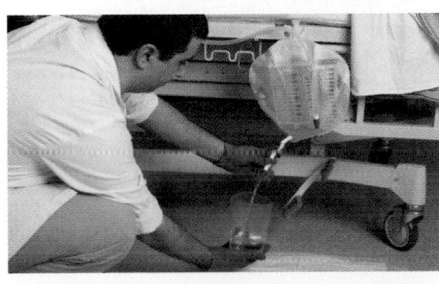

3. Reclamp the spout when the collection bag is empty.

4. Wipe the drainage spout with an alcohol pad, and replace the spout into the slot on the collection bag.
A clean spout reduces transmission of bacteria when the nurse touches it.

5. Measure urine output from the indwelling catheter at the end of each shift unless otherwise ordered. ▼

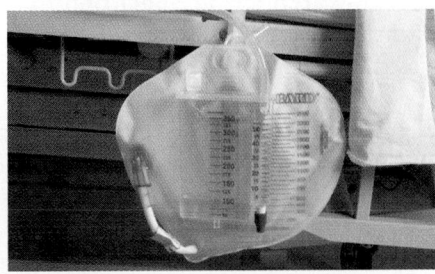

6. Discard the urine in the toilet.

7. Remove gloves and wash your hands.

What if. . .

■ **The provider's orders hourly monitoring of the patient's urine output?**

You will need to obtain a special collection bag with a small measuring chamber; document urine output on the I&O record every hour.

(continued on next page)

Procedure 27-1 ■ **Measuring Urine** (continued)

Evaluation

- Note any unusual characteristics of the urine (e.g., color, odor, presence of sediment or mucus).
- Note any difficulties with urination (e.g., pain, dribbling, difficulty beginning urination).
- Continue to assess that drainage from the indwelling catheter is not obstructed and that the drainage bag is below the level of the bladder.
- Assess for bladder distention.

Bladder distention indicates poor bladder emptying. Note: Some facilities have a bladder-scanning device that will allow you to determine whether there is residual urine.

Home Care

- Teach the client and/or the primary caregiver how to collect and measure the urine.
- Instruct the client and/or primary caregiver to document the urine intake and output on the I&O record.

Documentation

- Document urine volume and the record the time and date the specimen collected, per agency policy.

You may chart specimen collection in the patient's health record (nurse's notes) or a patient graphic flow sheet, depending on the agency.

- Document the characteristics of the urine: color, odor, particulate matter, blood, clarity, or other qualities.

- Document any difficulty with voiding, including pain or burning with urination, frequency, or difficulty starting the urine flow.

Sample documentation:

12/15/12	1330	Pt. voided 40 mL of cloudy, tea-colored urine with a foul odor and no particles or blood noted in urinal. Pt. denies difficulty urinating, pain, and burning.————————————————— B. Tran, RN
12/15/12	1400	Unclamped urine drainage bag and emptied 200 mL of dark brown, cloudy, urine with strong ammonia smell into graduated cylinder. Urine without particles or blood. Drainage bag clamped, cleansed drainage clamp, and replaced drain into slot.————————————————— B. Tran, RN

Practice Resources

Siegel, J. D., Rhinehart, E., Jackson, M., et al. & the Healthcare Infection Control Practices Advisory Committee of the Centers for Disease Control and Prevention (2007).

Procedure 27-2 ▢ **Obtaining a Urine Specimen for Testing**

➤ For steps to follow in *all* procedures, refer to the Universal Steps for All Procedures found on the inside back cover of Volume 2.

Critical Aspects

- Don clean procedure gloves.

Procedure 27-2A: Collecting a Clean-Catch Urine Specimen

- Wash the perineum or the end of the penis first with soap and water if soiled; otherwise, use an antiseptic towelette. (For women, wash from front to back; for men, use a circular motion from urethra outward.)
- Ask the patient to begin voiding. After the stream begins, collect a 30- to 60-mL specimen.
- Maintain sterility: Do not touch the inside of the container or the container lid.
- Pour the urine into a specimen container that is labeled with the patient's name, the date, and the time of collection.
- Place a lid on the container and transport it to the lab in a timely manner.
- Follow agency policy on additional packaging. (Many facilities require packaging the container in a specimen handling bag.)

Procedure 27-2B: Obtaining a Sterile Urine Specimen from a Catheter

- Empty the drainage tube of urine.
- Don clean gloves, and swab the specimen port with an antiseptic swab.
- Insert the needleless access device with a 20- or 30-mL syringe into the specimen port, and aspirate to withdraw the amount of urine you need.
- Transfer the specimen into a sterile specimen container.

- Maintain sterility: Do not touch the needleless access device, the inside of the container or the container lid.
- Transport the specimen to the lab as soon as possible.
- Label the specimen container with the correct patient identification, date and time of collection, and transport it to the lab.

Procedure 27-2C: Collecting a 24-Hour Urine Specimen
- Ask the patient to void. Record the time. Discard this first voiding.
- Collect all urine voided during the next 24 hours.
- Apply a label, identifying the patient's name, date, and time the test ended on the storage container. Transport the specimen to the lab after the collection is complete. Otherwise, place urine in a refrigerator designated for specimen storage.

Equipment

Collecting a Clean-Catch Urine Specimen

- Prepackaged collection kit
- If no kit is available:
  - Sterile specimen container
  - Antiseptic solution
  - Sterile cotton balls or 2 in. × 2 in. gauze pads
- Washcloth or towel
- Mild soap and water
- Two pairs of clean procedure gloves
- Patient identification labels
- Bedpan or bedside commode for an immobile patient

Obtaining a Sterile Urine Specimen from a Catheter

- Clean gloves
- Antiseptic swab
- Sterile specimen container with a lid
- Patient identification label
- Sterile syringe with a sterile 21- to 25-gauge needleless access device (a 5- to 10-mL syringe is usually sufficient)

Collecting a 24-Hour Urine Specimen

Note: Some tests require using a double-storage container. Be sure to find out if you need a double-storage container, preservative, or if there are special instruction for collection of the sample.

- Basin and ice, possibly. Check with the laboratory to determine whether the specimen needs to be kept in a basin of ice during the 24-hour collection.
- Large collection container.

Delegation

This procedure may be delegated to the NAP but you must be sure they know how to perform the procedure correctly, including proper cleansing and maintaining sterility of the container. You must complete the following assessments and instruct the NAP to report any abnormalities seen in the urine (e.g., blood, foul odor, mucus). In addition, the NAP should report any complaints of dysuria by the patient and bring the specimen to you for inspection.

Pre-Procedure Assessment

- Cognitive status
Knowing whether the patient can follow directions or not, helps you to determine whether the patient can be instructed to complete this procedure on her own.

- Mobility status
Knowing whether the patient can get out of bed or not, helps you to determine where the specimen will be collected (e.g., bed, commode, bedpan).

- Urinary status
Patients with impaired ability to control urinary flow may not be able to collect a specimen in this manner.

■ Procedure 27-2A Collecting a Clean-Catch Urine Specimen

➤ When performing the procedure, always identify your patient according to agency policy and be attentive to standard precautions, hand hygiene, patient safety and privacy, body mechanics, and documentation.

Procedure Steps

1. Don procedure gloves.

2. Open the prepackaged kit (if available), and remove the contents.

3. Cleanse, or instruct the patient to cleanse, around the urinary meatus. Allow the area to dry.
Cleansing prevents contamination of the specimen with surface bacteria.

Step 3 Variation for Women
  a. Wash the perineal area with warm water and mild soap, if soiled.
Cleansing the perineum will help healthcare providers to determine whether bacteria found in the specimen could be assumed to have come from the bladder and urethra rather than the perineal skin.

b. Open the antiseptic towelette provided in the prepackaged kit. If there is no kit, pour the antiseptic solution over the cotton balls.
  To cleanse the perineum, wipe down one side of the meatus using one pad and discard it. Then wipe the other side with a second pad. Wipe down the center over

(continued on next page)

Procedure 27-2 ■ **Obtaining a Urine Specimen for Testing** (continued)

the urinary meatus with the third pad; then discard it.

Clean the perineal area at least twice. Use each towelette or cotton ball only once.
Following the "clean-to-dirty" principle decreases the likelihood of contamination of the specimen with feces. Antiseptic helps reduce the number of bacteria. ▼

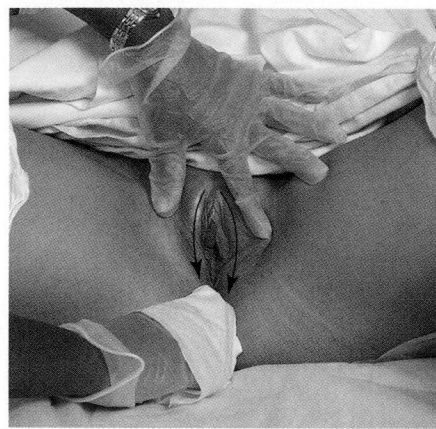

Step 3 Variation for Men

c. If the penis is uncircumcised, retract the foreskin back from the end of the penis.
Retracting the foreskin allows for better access when cleansing the area around the meatus.

d. Use the towelette provided in the prepackaged kit or pour antiseptic solution over cotton balls. You might also use 2 in. × 2 in. gauze pad soaked with povidone-iodine to cleanse the periurethral area.

✚ Before using an iodine-based solution, be sure to check the patient's health history for allergy to iodine.

e. With one hand, grasp the penis gently. With the other hand,

cleanse the meatus in a circular motion from the meatus outward, and cleanse for a few inches down the shaft of the penis. Cleanse around the meatus at least twice, using each towelette or cotton ball only once. Use each time with a fresh 2 in. × 2 in. gauze pad, towelette, or cotton ball.
Cleansing the site helps in this manner prevent contaminating the specimen with bacteria.

4. Remove gloves. Wash your hands, and don the second pair of clean procedure gloves.
Gloving prevents transmission of bacteria.

5. Open the sterile specimen container, being careful not to touch the inside of the lid or container.

6. Holding the container near the meatus, instruct the patient to begin voiding.

Step 6 Variation for Men

a. Keep the foreskin retracted during voiding, if uncircumcised. For a male patient who is unable to assist, it will be necessary to hold the penis.

Step 6 Variation for Women

b. Separate and hold the labia apart, or have the patient do so.
Clearing the distal urethra of bacteria keeps bacteria from contaminating the urine specimen.

7. Allow a small stream of urine to pass; and then without stopping the urine stream, place the specimen container into the stream, collecting approximately 30 to 60 mL.

Midstream urine collection prevents specimen contamination.

8. Remove the container from the stream, and allow the patient to finish emptying the bladder. *Note:* For men, if the penis is uncircumcised, replace the foreskin over the glans when the procedure is finished.

9. Carefully replace the container lid, touching only the outside of the cap and container. Avoid touching the rim of the cup to the genital area. Do not get toilet paper, feces, pubic hair, menstrual blood, or anything else in the urine sample.
These measures maintain sterility of specimen and prevent cross-contamination of others with urine.

10. Label the container with the correct patient information (in many institutions, labels are preprinted or bar-coded). Place the container in a facility-specific carrier (usually a plastic bag) for transport to the lab.

11. Remove your gloves and wash your hands. If the specimen has been obtained from a patient on a bedpan, leave your gloves on until you have removed, emptied, and stored the bed-pan properly.

12. Assist the patient back to bed, or remove the bedpan or urinal, if applicable. (See Procedure 28-2 for removing a bedpan.)

13. Transport the specimen to the lab in a timely manner.
Delayed testing can cause inaccurate results (e.g., casts in the urine will break up if urine is allowed to sit for an extended period of time).

■ *Procedure 27-2B* **Obtaining a Sterile Urine Specimen from a Catheter**

➤ When performing the procedure, always identify your patient according to agency policy and be attentive to standard precautions, hand hygiene, patient safety and privacy, body mechanics, and documentation.

Procedure Steps

1. Empty the drainage tube of urine.

2. Clamp the drainage tube below the level of the specimen port for 15 to

30 minutes to allow a fresh sample to collect. If the client's urine is flowing briskly, you may not need to clamp the catheter.

3. Don clean gloves, and swab the specimen port with an antiseptic swab.

4. Insert the needleless access device with a 20- or 30-mL syringe into the specimen port, and aspirate to withdraw the amount of urine you need. ▼

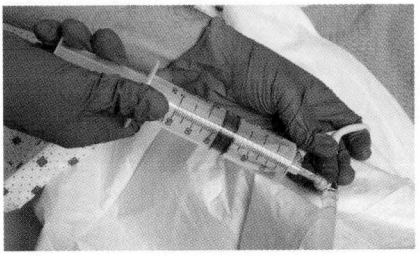

5. Once you have the sample, transfer the specimen into a sterile specimen container.

6. Discard the needleless access device and syringe in a safe container. To avoid accidental needlestick injury.

7. Tightly cap the specimen container. To avoid an incomplete 24-hour urine sampling.

8. Remove the clamp from the catheter.

✦ Be sure to unclamp the tubing of the urinary collection bag after you obtain the sample. Urine backflow can cause bladder distention and lead to stasis-induced urinary tract infection.

9. Label and package the specimen with the correct patient identification according to agency policy. To avoid a wrong-patient error.

10. Transport the specimen to the lab. If immediate transport is not possible, refrigerate the sample.

✦ Never disconnect the catheter from the drainage tube to obtain a sample. Interrupting the system creates a portal of entry for pathogens, thereby increasing the risk of contamination.

■ **Procedure 27-2C** **Collecting a 24-Hour Urine Specimen**

➤ When performing the procedure, always identify your patient according to agency policy and be attentive to standard precautions, hand hygiene, patient safety and privacy, body mechanics, and documentation.

Procedure Steps

1. Use a large collection container (usually supplied by the lab), and collect all urine voided in the 24-hour period. If you need to use more than one container during the 24-hour period, use one container at a time. When it is full, collect your urine in the next container. Occasionally you will be asked to collect each voiding in a separate container.

2. To begin collection, have the client void, and record the time. Discard this first voiding. This marks the beginning of urine collection period.

3. Collect all urine voided during the next 24 hours (e.g., if the first voiding was at 9:00 A.M. on Monday, collect all urine voided until 9:00 A.M. on Tuesday).

4. Inform the client and all staff about the collection. Communication can help to prevent accidental discarding of urine.

5. Post signs in prominent locations, such as the client's bathroom or entry door, to remind staff of the ongoing collection.

It is essential that none of the urine voided during the 24-hour period is accidentally discarded.

6. Apply a label on the specimen, with the patient's name, date, and time the test ended on your storage container.

What if. . .

■ **A urine culture is ordered on the specimen?**

Be sure to list current antibiotic therapy on the laboratory request form.

This information is important to determine sensitivity of the microorganisms.

■ **A clean-catch urine sample is needed for an immobile patient?**

For the patient using a bedpan, raise the head of the bed to a semi-Fowler's position.

Facilitates correct direction of urine flow down into the specimen container you are holding. In addition, this is the anatomical position for voiding.

■ **The catheter drainage tube is made of rubber and has no sampling port?**

In that case, you can obtain the specimen directly from the rubber catheter. Be sure to properly cleanse the tubing with an antiseptic pad before

inserting a needle at a 45° angle. Withdraw the specimen. Put the sterile specimen into a sterile container; label it with the correct patient identification. Send it to the lab or put it on ice until it is transported.

✦ Never insert a needle into the shaft of the catheter because this can puncture the lumen and cause damage to the balloon holding the catheter in place.

Catheters made of materials other than rubber. will leak after you take the needle out.

■ **You need to collect a urine sample from an infant?**

1. Remove the paper covering adhesive patches on the back side of the specimen bag before applying it to the clean and dry perineal area. Start at the narrow area between the anus and vaginal or penile area. Press the adhesive sides firmly against the skin while avoiding wrinkles in the skin against the patch.

(continued on next page)

Procedure 27-2 ■ **Obtaining a Urine Specimen for Testing** (continued)

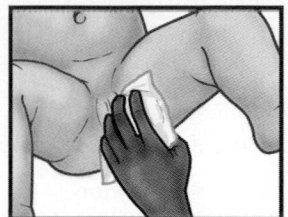 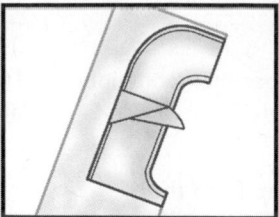 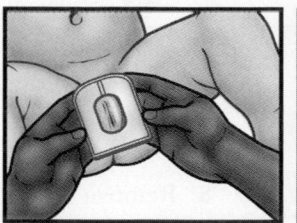 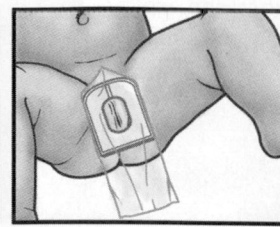

2. It is easier to apply the lower portion of the bag first. The area must also be dry in order for the adhesive to stick to the skin. Since infants urinate frequently, it is best to work quickly to catch the specimen.

3. After the specimen bag is adhering to skin, put a diaper on the infant/

child. Remember to check the collection bag every 15 to 30 minutes to see if there is a specimen. If the infant has not urinated in 2 to 3 hours, discard the bag, re-cleanse the area, and apply a new bag.

It is possible there was a leak in the seal between the skin and the adhe-

sive sides of the specimen collection bag.

4. Once a specimen is obtained in the bag, remove it gently and pour the urine into a sterile specimen cup. Label it with the patient identifying information. ▼

Evaluation

- Note any unusual characteristics of the urine (e.g., color, odor, clarity, crystals, blood, mucus).
- Note any difficulties with urination (e.g., pain, burning, dribbling, difficulty beginning).

Patient Teaching

- For clean-catch and 24-hour urine specimens, teach the patient the steps of the procedure, focusing on how to maintain sterility of the specimen.
- Tell the patient to refrigerate a urine specimen for up to 24 hours until it can be transported to the lab. Instruct the patient to place the specimen in a plastic bag, separate it from food items, and label it appropriately.
- Explain that prepackaged antiseptic wipes cannot be flushed down the toilet.
- For clean-catch and 24-hour urine specimens, instruct a menstruating woman that perineal cleansing is especially important. The woman may use a tampon to prevent leakage during specimen collection. Instruct her to notify the lab that she is menstruating.

Documentation

- Document urine volume in the patient record, per agency protocol, the time and date that the specimen was collected.

Some facilities use the Kardex to indicate the urine collection is either needed, in progress, or completed. Other facilities have nurses chart specimen collection in the nursing notes or electronic health records.

- Document the characteristics of the urine: color, odor, particulate matter, blood, clarity, or other qualities.
- Document any difficulty with voiding, including pain or burning with urination, frequency, or difficulty starting the urine flow.

Sample documentation:

12/10/12   0800   *Order noted for clean-catch urine specimen. Explained to client the procedure for cleaning and obtaining urine specimen. Client stated "I must clean my bottom from front to back using the toilette in here. Then begin to void and stop voiding. Then void directly into this container." Assisted client to bedside commode. 100 mL of clear yellow urine without foul odor, blood, or particles collected. Pt. denies difficulty voiding, pain, and burning. Urine container labeled per protocol and sent to laboratory.* ————————— L. Schaaf, RN

12/10/12   1000   *Order noted for sterile urine specimen. Foley catheter clamped for 15 minutes. Port on Foley cleansed with antiseptic agent. 30 mL of pink tinged urine without foul odor or sediment removed. Specimen labeled per protocol and sent to laboratory.* ————— L. Schaaf, RN

12/10/12   1200   *Order noted for 24-hour urine collection. Explained procedure to client. Client stated, "I will call you when I void. This first void will be flushed and the test will begin. During the test, I will void in the white hat that is in the commode. Then every time that I void, I will call you to empty the urine into the big container. The big container for the urine must be kept cold with ice."* ——— L. Schaaf, RN

Practice Resources
National Institutes of Health, Warren Grant Magnuson Clinical Center (2009); Saint Jude's Children's Research Hospital (2004).

Procedure 27-3 ☐ Testing Urine at the Bedside

➤ For steps to follow in *all* procedures, refer to the Universal Steps for All Procedures found on the inside back cover of Volume 2.

Critical Aspects

- Follow the manufacturer's directions carefully regarding the amount of urine needed.

Procedure 27-3A: Dipstick Testing of Urine
- Read the kit label to be certain that you are using the correct reagent and that the kit has not passed the expiration date.
- To ensure accuracy, the reagent strip should be read at the exact time indicated on the label. You will need adequate lighting to evaluate the results.
- Dipstick testing is considered a preliminary test for screening.

Procedure 27-3B: Measuring Specific Gravity of Urine (Refractometer)
- Before use, be sure the equipment is calibrated to 1.000 according to the manufacturer's instructions.
- Use fresh urine; if you cannot perform the test within 1 hour, refrigerate the specimen.
- Place a drop of urine on the glass plate and close the flap.
- Hold the refractometer up to the light when looking through the eyepiece.
- Read the specific gravity by looking for the point where the contrast line between the dark and light fields crosses the scale.
- Clean the instrument when finished.

Equipment

Dipstick Testing

- Procedure gloves
- Dipstick testing kit

Refractometer Testing

- Refractometer
- Procedure gloves
- Distilled water
- Dropper
- Small urine sample

Delegation

You may delegate bedside urine testing to the NAP if you know that he has the knowledge and skill to perform the procedure. Ask the NAP to report the test results to you and to save the urine sample in case you should need to repeat the test.

Pre-Procedure Assessment

- **Mobility status**
Knowing whether the patient can get out of bed or not, helps you to determine where the specimen will be collected (e.g., toilet, bedside commode, bedpan).

- **Urinary status**
Knowing whether the patient has an indwelling urinary catheter or not, helps you to determine how the specimen will be collected.

■ Procedure 27-3A Dipstick Testing of Urine

➤ When performing the procedure, always identify your patient according to agency policy and be attentive to standard precautions, hand hygiene, patient safety and privacy, body mechanics, and documentation.

Procedure Steps

1. Read the instructions on the diagnostic kit and obtain the reagent and a test strip.

2. Wash your hands and don clean procedure gloves.
Hand hygiene and gloving prevents the transmission of bacteria.

3. Have the patient void into the collection container or obtain urine from the indwelling urinary catheter.

See Procedure 27-1A and B for measuring urine.

4. Obtain a test strip from the kit and dip into the urine, and begin timing. Follow the manufacturer's directions regarding the time needed for the reagent to develop.

5. At the specified time, compare the results to the color chart. You will need good lighting to evaluate the results. ➤

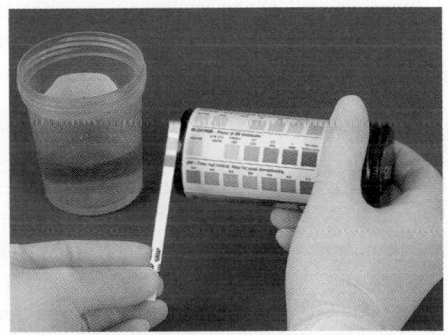

6. Document the test results.

(continued on next page)

Procedure 27-3 ■ Testing Urine at the Bedside (continued)

■ Procedure 27-3B   Measuring Specific Gravity of Urine

➤ When performing the procedure, always identify your patient according to agency policy and be attentive to standard precautions, hand hygiene, patient safety and privacy, body mechanics, and documentation.

Procedure Steps

1. Clean the equipment lens with distilled water and dry with dry lens paper or a soft, nonabrasive cloth.
To ensure accurate results.

2. Before use, confirm the refractometer calibration by testing with distilled water and commercial urinalysis controls (follow the manufacturer's instructions).
When calibrated the refractometer should read 1.000.

3. Wash your hands and don clean procedure gloves.
Hand hygiene and gloving prevent the transmission of bacteria.

4. Use fresh urine; if you cannot perform the test within 1 hour, refrigerate the specimen. Wearing procedure gloves, use the dropper to place one or two drops of urine on the prism surface (at the notched bottom of the cover).

5. Hold the refractometer horizontally, and turn toward the light. Rotate the eyepiece until the scale is in focus.

6. Read the scale at the point where the dividing line between bright and dark fields crosses the scale.
The scale reads from 1.000 to 1.035 in increments of 0.001.

7. Record the results.

8. When you are finished, dry the refractometer, and add a drop of distilled water to cleanse the prism. Dry the equipment with lens paper.

What if . . .

■ **The diagnostic kit for dipstick testing is outdated?**

Contact the pharmacy and/or work with the patient's caregiver to obtain a valid kit.

Evaluation

■ Characteristics of urine output (e.g., volume of output, color, clots, mucus).
■ Abnormally concentrated or dilute urine

Patient Teaching

■ Explain test procedures to the patient and the patient's caregiver and family members as indicated.
Telling the patient what to expect helps to reduce anxiety.

Home Care

■ Teach the client or caregiver the steps of the procedure.
■ Tell the client or caregiver the urine must be tested within an hour or refrigerate the specimen to test later.
■ Instruct the client or caregiver that the specimen should be tested as ordered by the healthcare provider.
■ Teach the client or caregiver to record results on the flow sheet per agency protocol.

Documentation

■ Document urine volume in the patient record, per agency protocol, and the time and date that the specimen was collected.
Some use the Kardex or a procedure checklist to indicate the urine collection is either needed, in progress, or completed. Other facilities have nurses chart specimen collection in the nursing notes.

■ Document the urine specific gravity and pH and note the presence of hemoglobin, glucose, ketones, protein, white blood cells, bilirubin, casts, crystal, and nitrites.
■ Chart other characteristics of the urine: color, odor, clarity, particulate matter, gross blood, mucus shreds, or other qualities.
■ Document any difficulty with voiding, including pain or burning with urination, frequency, or difficulty starting the urine flow.

Sample documentation:

12/10/12   1600   Patient voided in bedside commode. Urine is yellow with sediment. Urine has no odor, blood, or mucus. Urine dipstick completed. No hemoglobin, glucose, ketones, protein, WBC, bilirubin, casts, or crystal nitrates noted on urine dipstick test. Urine dipstick notes +3 RBC, pH 6.5, and specific gravity 1.015. —————— L. Schaaf, RN

Practice Resources

Point of care (2003); Stuempfle, K. J., & Drury, D. G. (2003).

Procedure 27-4 ☐ Inserting a Urinary Catheter

➤ For steps to follow in *all* procedures, refer to the Universal Steps for All Procedures found on the inside back cover of Volume 2.

Critical Aspects

- Allow adequate time for these procedures: Experienced nurses need at least 15 minutes. You will need more time if problems arise—and even more time if you are a novice.
- Take an extra pair of sterile gloves and an extra sterile catheter into the room.
- Be sure to have good lighting.
- Work on the right side of the bed if you are right-handed; and on the left side if you are left-handed.
- Drape the patient for privacy.
- Perform perineal care before the procedure.
- Don sterile gloves and maintain sterile technique while manipulating the supplies in the kit and performing the procedure.
- For indwelling catheterization, pretesting the balloon by inflating it before insertion is not necessary, especially with silicone catheters, because the practice can cause the balloon to form cuffs. Cuffing can cause harm to the patient's urethra.
- Lubricate the catheter tip before insertion.
- Insert the catheter 5 to 7.5 cm (2 to 3 in.) for women, 17 to 22.5 cm (7 to 9 in.) for men, until urine flows—use the smallest size catheter possible.
- Once you have touched the patient's perineum with your nondominant hand, do not remove that hand from the patient.
- Drain the bladder; collect needed samples; measure urine; and connect the drainage bag as needed or remove the catheter if the catheterization is intermittent.

Equipment

Intermittent Urinary Catheter (Straight Catheter)

- Washcloth and towel
- Soap and water
- Procedure gloves, at least two pairs
- Catheter insertion kit containing:
  - Sterile gloves
  - Urinary catheter
  - Antiseptic cleansing agent
  - Forceps
  - Cotton balls
  - Sterile waterproof drapes
  - Sterile lubricant
  - Urine receptacle
  - Specimen container

- Extra pair of sterile gloves and extra sterile catheter
Obtaining extra supplies prevents the need to leave the bedside to obtain additional supplies should the gloves or catheter become contaminated.

- Bath blanket
- Procedure lamp or flashlight
- 2% lidocaine (Xylocaine) gel (according to agency policy and patient need)

Indwelling Urinary Catheter

An indwelling catheter is designed to remain in the urinary bladder. Therefore, in addition to the supplies contained in a straight-catheter kit, an indwelling catheter kit will include the following:

- A double-lumen or triple-lumen catheter with a balloon tip for inflation instead of a single-lumen rubber catheter
- A syringe prefilled with sterile water (to inflate the catheter balloon)
- Urine collection bag with drainage tubing attached; often the tubing is also attached to the catheter
- Tube holder, tape, or leg strap (to secure the catheter)

Straight catheter kit

(continued on next page)

Procedure 27-4 ■ **Inserting a Urinary Catheter** (continued)

- Safety pin and elastic band (if needed to secure the tubing to the bed; you can usually use the clamp on the drainage tubing)

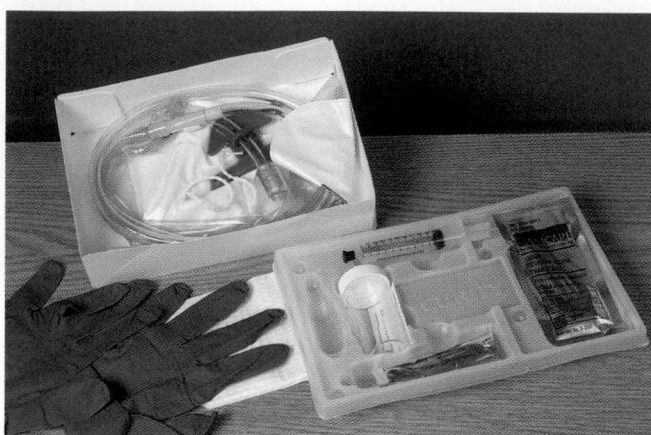

Indwelling catheter kit

Delegation

In some institutions, NAPs undergo special training to learn this skill. In such instances, you may delegate this task to the NAP. However, you must complete the following assessments and instruct the NAP when to stop the procedure and what abnormal findings to report. Otherwise, you should not delegate catheter insertion to a NAP. If you do delegate to an NAP, you must from time to time supervise to ensure that the procedure is being performed correctly.

Pre-Procedure Assessments

- Assess the patient's cognitive level.
To determine whether the patient will be able to follow instructions.

- Assess for the presence of conditions that may impair the patient's ability to assume the necessary position.
To determine whether you will need assistance to help the patient maintain the correct position for catheter insertion.

- Assess the presence and degree of bladder distension.
To establish a baseline against which to evaluate future data.

- Determine time of last voiding or last catheterization.
- Assess the general body size of the patient and size of the urinary meatus.
To determine whether you need to choose a different size catheter.

✚ Determine whether the patient has an allergy to iodine (if that is the antiseptic solution in the kit). Use a different solution if the patient is allergic to Betadine.
- Determine whether the patient is allergic to latex. Many catheters are made of latex.

- Note signs and symptoms of bladder infection (e.g., elevated temperature, urinary frequency, dysuria).
- Note conditions (e.g., enlarged prostate in men) that may make it difficult to pass the catheter.
- Assess the need for additional lighting.
It is sometimes difficult to visualize a woman's urinary meatus. Supplemental, direct lighting helps.

■ Procedure 27-4A **Inserting an Intermittent Urinary Catheter (Straight Catheter)**

➤ When performing the procedure, always identify your patient according to agency policy and be attentive to standard precautions, hand hygiene, patient safety and privacy, body mechanics, and documentation.

➤ Note: The following steps are described for a **female** patient. For steps with an asterisk (*), if your patient is a male, refer to the "Variations for Males" list, immediately following the procedure steps.

Procedure Steps

*1. Place the patient supine, in a position to allow you to see the urinary meatus:
   a. Flex the patient's knees, and place her feet flat on the bed (dorsal recumbent position).
   b. Instruct the patient to relax her thighs and allow them to rotate externally. Obtain help if the patient is confused, unable to cooperate or follow directions, or unable to hold her legs in a correct position.

The urinary meatus is sometimes difficult to visualize on women because it may resemble skinfolds or other anatomical landmarks in the area.

2. If you are right-handed, stand and work at the patient's right side; if you are left-handed, stand and work on the patient's left side.

*3. Drape the patient. Fold the blanket in a diamond shape, wrapping the corners around the patient's legs and folding the upper corner down

over the perineum. (To review draping, see Procedure 22-4.) ▼

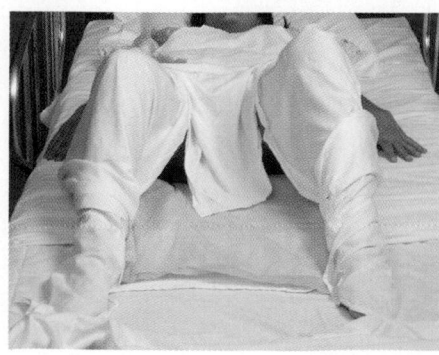

*4. Don clean procedure gloves. Lift the corner of the privacy drape to expose the perineum; wash the perineal area with soap and water; dry. At the same time, visualize and locate the urinary meatus.

Cleansing the perineum before inserting the catheter will reduce the number of skin bacteria, thereby helping to prevent transmission of microorganisms into the bladder. Locating the meatus during this step, when the patient is a woman, will help prevent delays at subsequent steps when it is important to maintain sterile technique.

5. Remove and discard gloves. Wash your hands.

To prevent the transmission of microbes.

6. Organize your work area.
   a. Arrange the bedside table or overbed table within your reach.
   b. Open the sterile catheter kit according to directions, and place it on the bedside table.
   c. Position a biohazard bag or other trash receptacle so that you will not have to reach across the sterile field (between the patient's legs) to dispose of soiled cotton balls and so forth. For example, you may have a trash can on the floor beside the bed, or a trash bag on the bed near, but not between, the patient's feet.

Carrying contaminated objects above a sterile field can contaminate the field. The outer wrapping of the catheter kit may be used for collecting discarded waste.

   d. Position the procedure light positioned at the perineum.

To allow better visualization of the site.

*7. Apply sterile underpad and drape. (Note: This step assumes the waterproof drape is packed as the top item in the kit. If your kit is different, see the What if... section.)

These drapes provide sterile work surfaces and help prevent contaminating your gloves and sterile supplies.

   *a. Place the sterile underpad: Remove the underpad from the kit carefully, allowing it to fall open as you remove it. Do not touch other kit items. Place it flat on the bed,

shiny side down, and tuck the top edge under the buttocks, taking care to touch only the corners of the drape.
   b. Lift the corner of the privacy drape to expose the perineum.
   c. Remove the sterile glove package, and don sterile gloves (see Procedure 20-7). Note: Once you have donned the sterile gloves, you may touch items inside the catheter kit, arranging the supplies as needed.
   *d. Place the fenestrated drape: This has a hole in the center. Pick up the drape, allowing it to unfold as you remove it, without touching any other objects from the kit. For women, place the drape over the perineum with the hole over the labia. ▼

The fenestrated drape provides a sterile barrier to protect you from contaminating your sterile gloves.

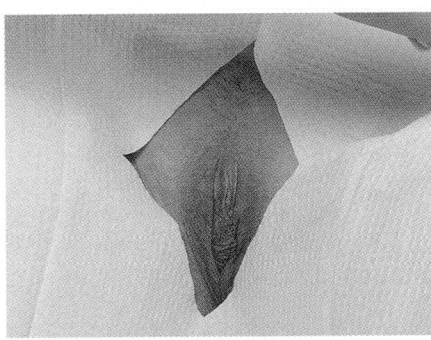

*8. Organize kit supplies on the sterile field, and prepare the supplies in the kit.
   a. Pour antiseptic solution over the cotton balls.
   Note: Some kits contain a packet of sterile antiseptic swabs. Open the end of the packet where you feel the "stick," leaving the swab covered by the packet.

⬥ Before using antiseptic containing povidone iodine (Betadine), verify the patient does not have an iodine allergy.

   b. Lay the forceps near the cotton balls.
   c. Open the specimen container if you need to collect a specimen.
   d. Remove any unneeded supplies, such as the urine specimen container, from the urine collection basin.

   e. Remove the plastic covering (if there is one) from the catheter.
   f. Open the packet or uncap the syringe filled with sterile lubricant.
   *g. Squeeze sterile lubricant into the kit tray; roll the catheter slowly in the lubricant. Lubricate the first 2.5 to 5 cm (1 to 2 in.) of the catheter. Leave the catheter tip in sterile lubricant or on the sterile field until ready to use.

Lubrication allows for ease of insertion of the catheter. Prevents trauma to the mucosa.

   *h. Touching only the box or sterile side of the wrapping, place the sterile catheter kit down onto the sterile field between the woman's legs or bedside.

This approach allows you to reach supplies during catheter insertion. It also extends the sterile field created by the sterile underpad.

*9. Cleanse the urinary meatus.
   a. Place your nondominant hand above the labia, and with your thumb and forefinger spread the patient's labia, pulling up (or anteriorly) at the same time, to expose the urinary meatus. Hold this position throughout the procedure—firm pressure is necessary. If the labia slip back over the urinary meatus, it is considered contaminated, and you will need to change gloves and repeat the cleansing procedure.

When a woman is supine, gravity may cause tissues above the meatus to fall downward and obscure the meatus from sight. Once placed on the patient's perineal area, your hand is considered contaminated.

   b. With your dominant hand, pick up a moistened cotton ball with the forceps and cleanse the perineal area, taking care not to contaminate your sterile glove.

   —Use one stroke and a new cotton ball for each area.
   —Wipe from front to back (clitoris to anus).
   —Wipe in this order: far labium majora, near labium majora, inside far labium, inside near labium, and directly down the center over the urinary meatus. If the kit has only
(continued on next page)

Procedure 27-4 ■ Inserting a Urinary Catheter (continued)

three cotton balls, cleanse only the inside far labium minora, inside near labium minora, and down the center of the urethral meatus.
—Discard the used cotton balls as you use them. Be careful not to move them across the open and sterile kit.

Because the urethra is close to the anus in female patients, thorough cleansing of the perineum is very important to reduce contamination of the catheter and prevent bacteria from being introduced into the urethra. Following the "clean-to-dirty" principle prevents recontamination of the cleansed area.▼

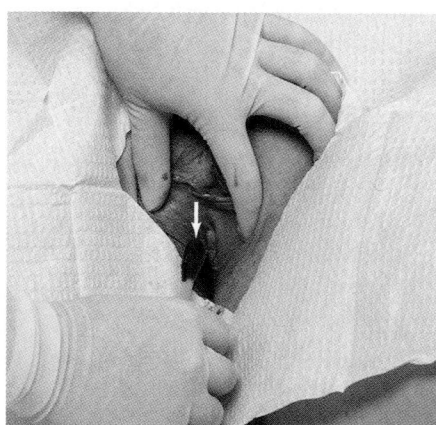

10. Prepare the urine receptacle. Place it 10 cm (4 in.) from the meatus (for women); between the patient's thighs (for men).
The end of the catheter will need to reach into the container to catch the draining urine.

*11. Insert the catheter.▼

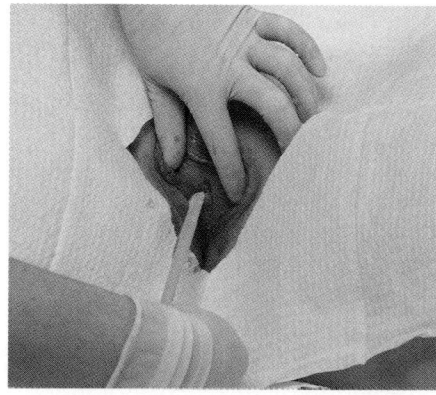

a. Ask the woman to bear down as though she is trying to void.

Grasp the catheter with your dominant hand, no more than 3 to 5 cm (1½ to 2 in.) from the distal end holding it in a coil in your palm. Slowly insert the end of the catheter into the meatus. Ask the patient take slow, deep breaths until the initial discomfort has passed.
Bearing down helps relax the external sphincter and makes insertion easier and more comfortable. Holding the catheter close to the distal end will help to keep the tip stable and prevent it from being inserted into the vaginal opening.

b. Continue inserting the catheter gently until urine flows, for a distance of 5 to 7.5 cm (2 to 3 in.). After you see urine, insert the catheter another 2.5 to 5 cm (1 to 2 in.).

✚ You may feel slight resistance as the catheter goes through the sphincters. Twist the catheter slightly or apply gentle pressure, but do not force the catheter while inserting it. You might need to remove it and cautiously attempt the insertion action again using a new catheter.

Deep breathing helps to relax the sphincters. Forcing may damage mucosa. Insert the catheter more deeply after urine flow to be sure the catheter is well into the bladder so that the bladder can empty completely. The catheter might not advance while inserted when it is misplaced in the vagina or if there is a stricture within the urethra or sphincter spasm.

c. If the catheter touches the labia or unsterile linens, or if you inadvertently place it in the vagina, it is contaminated; you must insert a new, sterile catheter. Leave the contaminated catheter in the vagina while you are inserting the new one into the meatus.
Leaving the catheter in the incorrect location helps to serve as a visual landmark and helps you to avoid making the same mistake again.

12. Manage the catheter and or/urine collection device.

a. Continue to hold the catheter securely with your nondominant hand while the urine drains from the bladder.
Hold the catheter like this prevents the catheter from being expelled by bladder or urethral contractions.

b. If you are to collect a urine specimen, use your dominant hand to take the specimen container and put it into the flow of urine until you obtain the correct amount of urine. Cap the container, maintaining sterile technique. See Procedure 27-2B.

c. When the flow of urine has ceased and the bladder has been emptied, pinch the catheter and slowly withdraw it from the meatus. Discard the catheter in an appropriate receptacle.
Withdrawing slowly promotes adequate urinary drainage, preventing urinary stasis. Pinching prevents urine from dribbling out of the end of the catheter.

d. Remove the urine-filled receptacle, and set it aside outside the patient care area to be emptied when the procedure is finished.
Moving the urine collection receptacle keeps it from spilling onto the bed.

13. Cleanse the patient's perineal area as needed; dry.
This removes residual antiseptic solution from the area, an especially important step if you used povidone-iodine (Betadine). Betadine left on intact healthy skin can cause irritation.

14. Remove and discard disposable supplies (e.g., drapes).

15. Remove your gloves and wash your hands.
Hand hygiene and gloving prevent transmission of bacteria.

16. Return the patient to a position of comfort.

Procedure Variations for Men (Straight Catheter)

Procedure
Step (above)   Nursing Action

1. Position the patient. Position the patient supine, legs straight and slightly apart.

3. Drape the patient. Cover the patient's upper body with a blanket; fold bed sheets down to expose the penis.

4. Wash the perineum. Wash the penis and perineal area with soap and water; dry. If you are using 2% lidocaine (Xylocaine) gel, use a syringe (no needle) to insert it into the urethra now.

7a. Place the sterile underpad. Drop the sterile underpad across the thighs.

7d. Place the fenestrated drape. Place the fenestrated drape with the center hole over the penis. Lift the penis up and through the opening when cleansing the meatus.

8g. Lubricate the catheter. Do not lubricate the catheter if you have already inserted a lubricant (lidocaine-based product) directly into the urethra. Otherwise, you will instill lubricant into the urethra at step 11.

8h. Place the catheter kit on the sterile field. Touching only the box or sterile side of the wrapping, place the sterile catheter kit down onto the sterile field at the bedside or on top of the thighs. You may, as an alternative, set up the sterile field between his legs.

9a. Expose the urinary meatus. With your nondominant hand, reach through the opening in the fenestrated drape and grasp the penis, taking care not to contaminate the surrounding drape. If the penis is uncircumcised, retract the foreskin to fully expose the meatus. If the foreskin accidentally falls over meatus and does not remain retracted or if you drop the penis during cleansing, you must change gloves and repeat the cleansing procedure.

9b. Cleanse the urinary meatus. Continuing to hold the penis with your nondominant hand, hold the forceps in your dominant hand and pick up a cotton ball. Starting at the meatus, cleanse the glans in a series of circular motions and partially down the shaft of the penis. Repeat with at least one more cotton ball.

11a. Grasp the penis and the catheter. Using your nondominant hand, hold the penis gently but firmly at a 90° angle to the body, exerting gentle traction. To gain firm control of the catheter, grasp the catheter 1½ to 2 inches from the proximal end, with the remainder coiled in the palm of the hand.
Holding the penis upright and supporting the shaft with the fingers straightens the urethra, easing insertion of the catheter. Grasping the catheter close to the distal end of the catheter allows for control and helps to avoid inadvertent contamination.

11b. Insert the lubricant. If you have not inserted lidocaine gel into the urethra, make sure the kit contains a prefilled syringe of lubricant rather than a packet of lubricant. Gently insert the tip of the prefilled syringe into the urethra and instill the lubricant.

Step 11b Variation. Lubricant in a Packet
If the kit contains only a single packet of lubricant and if no other kits are available, then lubricate 12.5 to 17.5 cm (5 to 7 in.) of the catheter. This is not the technique of choice, however.

11d. Insert the catheter. Ask patient to bear down as though trying to void; slowly insert the end of the catheter into the meatus. Have the patient take slow, deep breaths until the initial discomfort has passed. Helps relax the external sphincter and makes insertion easier and more comfortable.

◆ If you feel resistance, withdraw the catheter. Do not force against resistance.

Continue inserting the catheter to about 17.5 to 22.5 cm (7 to 9 in.) or until urine flows, then lower the penis.

When bladder is drained, replace the foreskin.

(continued on next page)

Procedure 27-4 ■ **Inserting a Urinary Catheter** (continued)

■ Procedure 27-4B **Inserting an Indwelling Urinary Catheter**

➤ When performing the procedure, always identify your patient according to agency policy and be attentive to standard precautions, hand hygiene, patient safety and privacy, body mechanics, and documentation.

➤ Note: The following steps are described for a **male** patient. For steps with an asterisk (*), if your patient is a female, refer to the "Variations for Females" table, immediately following the procedure steps.

Procedure Steps

*1. Place the patient supine with legs straight and slightly apart. If the patient is confused, unable to follow directions, or unable to hold his legs in correct position, obtain help with the procedure.
This position allows easy access.

2. If you are right-handed, stand and work at the patient's right side; if you are left-handed, stand and work on the patient's left side.

*3. Drape the patient. Cover the patient's upper body with a blanket; fold the bedsheets down to expose the penis.
Covering the patient preserves modesty and a enhances a feeling of security, while ensuring that you can expose the urinary meatus easily.

*4. Don clean procedure gloves. Wash the penis and perineal area with soap and water; dry.
Cleansing the area of skin bacteria reduces the risk of transmitting microbes into the bladder.

5. If you are using 2% Xylocaine gel, use a syringe (no needle) to insert it into the urethra now.
This is frequently used for men to provide local anesthesia. You will need to wait at least 5 minutes for the gel to take effect before inserting the catheter.

6. Remove and discard gloves. Wash your hands.
To protect the transmission of microbes.

7. Organize your work area:
   a. Arrange the bedside table or overbed table within your reach.
   b. Open the sterile catheter kit according to the directions, and place it on the bedside table.

c. Position a plastic bag or other trash receptacle so that you will not have to reach across the sterile field to dispose of soiled cotton balls and so forth. For example, you may have a trash can on the floor beside the bed, but not where you could trip on it or a trash bag on the bed near, but not between, the patient's feet.
Carrying contaminated objects above a sterile field can contaminate the field. The outer wrapping of the catheter kit may be used for collecting discarded waste.

*8. Place the waterproof underpad and sterile drape(s). (Note: This step assumes the waterproof drape is packed as the top item in the kit. If your kit is different, see the What if... section.)
These drapes provide sterile work surfaces and help prevent contaminating your gloves and sterile supplies.

   *a. Remove the underpad from the kit carefully, allowing it to fall open as you remove it. Do not touch other kit items. Drop the underpad across the patient's thighs, touching only the corners.
   b. Remove the sterile glove package and don sterile gloves (see Procedure 20-7).
   Note: Once you have donned the sterile gloves, you may touch any items inside the catheter kit, arranging the supplies as needed.
   *c. Place the fenestrated drape: This has a hole in the center. Pick up the drape, allowing it to unfold as you remove it, without touching any other objects. Place the drape with the center hole over the penis.

The drapes serves as a barrier to protect your gloves during the procedure.

*9. Organize the kit supplies on the sterile field, and prepare the supplies in the kit.
   a. Pour antiseptic solution, such as Betadine, over the cotton balls.

✚ Before using povidone iodine for cleansing, verify the patient does not have an allergy to iodine.

   Note: Some kits contain a packet of sterile antiseptic swabs. Open the end of the packet where you can feel the "stick," leaving the swabs covered by the remainder of the packet.
   b. Lay the forceps near the cotton balls.
   c. Open the specimen container, if you are to collect a specimen.
   d. Remove any unneeded supplies, such as the specimen container, from the kit. Remove the packaging from the catheter, if it is covered.
   *e. Do not lubricate the catheter if you have already inserted a lubricant (Xylocaine gel) directly into the urethra. If you did not do that, be certain that the lubricant in the kit is packaged in a syringe rather than a packet.
   *f. Touching only the box or sterile side of the wrapping, place the sterile catheter kit down onto the sterile field on top of the man's thighs. You may, as an alternative, set up the sterile field between his legs.
Placement of supplies in this manner allows you to reach supplies during catheter insertion.

   g. If the bedside bag is preconnected to the catheter itself, leave the bag on or near the sterile field until after the catheter is inserted.

10. Cleanse the urinary meatus. Discard the used cotton balls as you use them, taking care not to move them across the open and sterile kit. Disposing of the used cotton balls reduced the risk for contaminating the sterile field. ▼

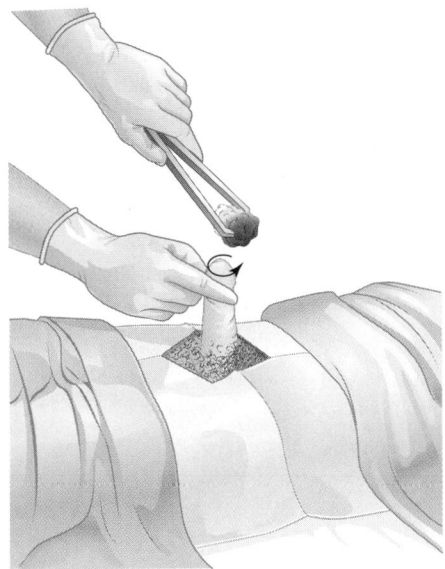

*a. With your nondominant hand, reach through the opening in the fenestrated drape and grasp the penis. Be careful not to contaminate the surrounding drape. If the penis is uncircumcised, retract the foreskin to fully expose the meatus. If the foreskin accidentally falls over the meatus or if you drop the penis during cleansing, you must change gloves and repeat the cleansing procedure.
Retracting the foreskin allows for full cleansing of the area.

*b. Continuing to hold the penis with your nondominant hand, hold the forceps in your dominant hand and pick up a cotton ball. Starting at the meatus, cleanse the glans in a series of circular motions from the inside to the outside and partially down the shaft of the penis. Repeat with at least one more cotton ball. Discard the cotton balls or swabs as they are used. Do not move them across the open sterile kit and field.

Following the "clean-to-dirty" principle prevents recontamination of the cleansed area.

c. Continue to grasp the penis with your nondominant hand. This glove is no longer sterile.

11. Instill lubricant (if not done previously).

Step 11 Variation. Lubricant Packaged in a Syringe
Before beginning the procedure, you should have made sure that the catheter kit contains a prefilled syringe of lubricant rather than a packet of lubricant. Gently insert the tip of the prefilled syringe into the urethra and instill the lubricant (unless you have already inserted Xylocaine gel).

Step 11 Variation. Lubricant Packaged in a Packet
If the kit contains only a single packet of lubricant and if no other kits are available, then lubricate 12.5 to 17.5 cm (5 to 7 in.) of the catheter. This is not the technique of choice, however.

*12. Insert the catheter. ▼

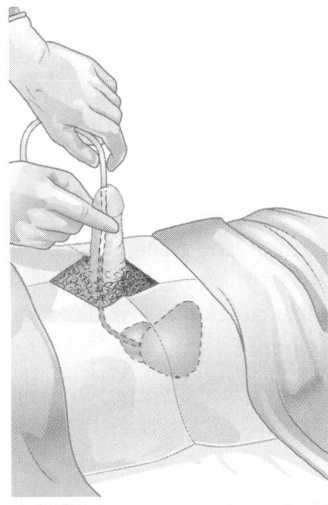

a. With your dominant hand, stabilize the catheter before inserting it by holding the catheter approximately 7.5 cm (3 in.) from the proximal end. Keep the rest of the catheter coiled in the palm of your hand or make sure the distal end of the catheter is connected to the drainage bag.
Coiling the catheter in your hand keeps you from contaminating the catheter.

When you preconnect the drainage bag before you in insert the catheter, you keep the urine from draining onto the bed. Frequently the catheter and drainage bag are connected by the manufacturer.

b. With your nondominant hand, hold the penis gently but firmly at a 90° angle to the body, exerting gentle traction.
Supporting the shaft with the fingers straightens the urethra, easing insertion of the catheter.

c. Ask the patient to bear down as though trying to void; slowly insert the end of the catheter into the meatus. Ask the patient to take slow deep breaths until the initial discomfort has passed.
These are strategies to help the patient to relax the external sphincter and make insertion easier and more comfortable.

d. Continue inserting the catheter to about 17 to 22.5 cm (7 to 9 in.) or until urine flows. You will feel slight resistance at the level of the external sphincter. Continue to advance to the bifurcation (Y connector).

✛ You will commonly feel resistance at the prostatic sphincter. Hold the catheter firmly against the sphincter until the sphincter relaxes. Then advance it, but do not force it.

e. Lower the penis and replace the foreskin.
This prevents compromised circulation and painful swelling.

13. Manage the catheter.
a. Continue to hold the catheter securely with your nondominant hand to stabilize the catheter's position in the urethra. Use your other hand to pick up the saline-filled syringe and inflate the catheter balloon.
By holding the catheter until the balloon is inflated, there is less of a chance of the catheter being expelled by the bladder or urethral contractions. The inflated balloon prevents the

(continued on next page)

Procedure 27-4 ■ **Inserting a Urinary Catheter** (continued)

catheter from slipping out of the bladder. ▼

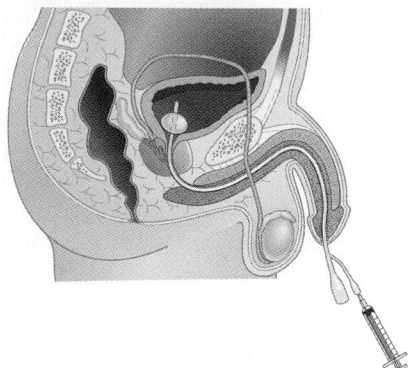

A Catheter placement, male

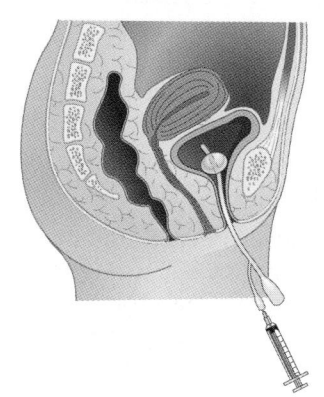

B Catheter placement, female

✚ b. If the patient complains of pain on inflation of the balloon, withdraw the water from the balloon, and reposition the catheter by advancing it 2.5 cm (1 in.).

Pain usually indicates that the balloon was in the urethra instead of in the bladder.

14. Connect the drainage bag to the end of the catheter if it is not already preconnected. Hang the drainage bag on the side of the bed, below the level of the bladder.

Hanging the drainage bag below the bladder promotes adequate urinary drainage by gravity, preventing urinary stasis.

***15.** Using hypoallergenic, medical tape or a catheter strap, secure the catheter to the thigh or the abdomen. Securing the catheter prevents urethral irritation related to tugging or pulling of the catheter.

16. Cleanse the patient's perineal area as needed; dry. Cover the patient with a gown.

Removes residual antiseptic solution from the area, an especially important step if you used povidone-iodine (Betadine), which is not commonly used for this procedure. Betadine left on intact healthy skin can cause irritation.

17. Return the patient to a comfortable position.

18. Remove your gloves and discard them with supplies into biohazard receptacle. Wash your hands.

Gloving and hand hygiene reduce the transmission of bacteria.

Procedure Variations for Women

Procedure Step (above)	Nursing Action
1. Position the patient.	Flex the patient's knees, and place her feet flat on the bed (dorsal recumbent position). Instruct the patient to relax her thighs and allow them to rotate externally. *Note:* If the patient is confused, unable to follow directions, or unable to hold her legs in the correct position, obtain help.
3. Drape the patient.	Fold the blanket in a diamond shape, wrapping the corners around the patient's legs and folding the upper corner down over the perineum (see Procedure 27-4A).
4. Wash the perineal area.	Don clean procedure gloves. Lift the corner of the privacy drape to expose the perineum; wash the perineal area with soap and water; dry. At the same time, visualize and locate the urinary meatus (for women).
8a. Place the underpad and sterile drape.	(This step assumes the sterile underpad is packed as top item in the kit. If it is not, see the What if...? section.) Remove the sterile underpad from the kit carefully before donning sterile gloves. Do not touch other kit items. Allow the umderpad to fall open as you remove it from the kit. Place it flat on the bed shiny side down, and tuck the top edge under the buttocks, taking care to touch only the corners of the drape. Lift the corner of the privacy drape to expose the perineum.
8c. Place the fenestrated drape.	Don sterile gloves. Pick up the drape, allowing it to unfold as you remove it, without touching any other objects. For women, place the drape over the perineum with the hole over the labia.

9e. Lubricate the catheter.	Squeeze sterile lubricant into the kit tray; roll the catheter slowly in the lubricant. Lubricate the first 2.5 to 5 cm (1 to 2 in.) of the catheter. Leave the catheter tip in sterile lubricant or on the sterile field until ready to use.
9f. Move the catheter kit to the bed.	Touching only the box or sterile side of the wrapping, place the sterile catheter kit down onto the sterile field between the woman's legs.
10a. Spread the labia.	Place your nondominant hand above the labia, and with your thumb and forefinger spread the patient's labia, pulling up (or anteriorly) at the same time, to expose the urinary meatus. Hold this position throughout the procedure—firm pressure is necessary. If the labia slip back over the urinary meatus, it is considered contaminated, and you will need to repeat the cleansing procedure. *When a woman is supine, gravity may cause tissues above the meatus to fall downward and obscure the meatus from sight. Once placed on the patient's perineal area, your hand is considered contaminated.*
10c. Cleanse the perineal area.	With your dominant hand, pick up a wet cotton ball with the forceps and cleanse the perineal area, taking care not to contaminate your sterile glove. 1) Use one stroke and a new cotton ball for each area. 2) Wipe from front to back (clitoris to anus). 3) Wipe in this order: far labium majora, near labium majora, inside far labium, inside near labium, and directly down the center over the urinary meatus. 4) If the kit has only three cotton balls, cleanse only the inside far labium minora, inside near labium minora, and down the center of the urethral meatus. *Because the urethra is close to the anus in female patients, thorough cleaning of the perineum is very important to reduce contamination of the catheter and prevent it from it from being introduced into the urethra.*
12. Insert the catheter.	a. Ask the woman to bear down as though she is trying to void. Grasp the catheter no more than 4 or 5 cm (1½ or 2 in.) from the distal end. Slowly insert the end of the catheter into the meatus. Ask the patient to take slow, deep breaths until the initial discomfort has passed. *Bearing down and deep breathing helps relax the external sphincter and makes insertion easier and more comfortable. Holding the catheter close to the distal end will help to keep the tip stable and prevent it from being inserted into the vaginal opening.* b. Continue inserting the catheter gently until urine flows, for a distance of 5 to 7.5 cm (2 to 3 in.). After you see urine, insert the catheter another 2.5 to 5 cm (1 to 2 in.). c. If the catheter touches the labia or unsterile linens, or if you inadvertently place it in the vagina, it is contaminated; you must insert a new, sterile catheter. Leave the contaminated catheter in the vagina while you are inserting the new one into the meatus. *Leaving the catheter in the incorrect location serves as a visual landmark and helps you to avoid making the same mistake again.*
15. Secure the catheter.	Using a tape or catheter strap, secure the catheter to the thigh.

What if . . .

- **The sterile gloves are packed as the top item in the catheter kit?**
- Don sterile gloves: Remove the sterile glove package and don sterile gloves (see Procedure 20-7). *Note:* Once you have donned the sterile gloves, you may touch any item inside the catheter kit, arranging the supplies as needed.
- Place the sterile underpad: Grasp the edges of the sterile drape. Fold the entire edge down 2.5 to 5 cm (1 to 2 in.) and toward you, making

a "cuff" to protect your gloves. Take care not to touch unsterile objects with your gloves or the drape.
- *For women:* Carefully slide the drape under the patient's buttocks without contaminating your gloves. Ask the patient to raise her hips slightly if she can.
- *For men:* Drop the sterile underpad across thighs. ➤

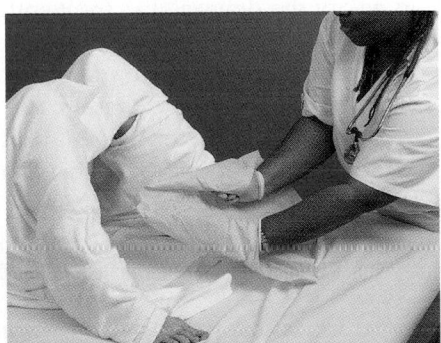

- Place the fenestrated drape: Pick up the drape, allowing it to unfold as you remove it, without touching any objects. Protect sterility as you

(continued on next page)

Procedure 27-4 ■ **Inserting a Urinary Catheter** (continued)

did with the underpad (preceding step).
- *For women*: Place the fenestrated drape over the perineum so that the hole is over the labia.
- *For men*: Place the fenestrated drape so that the center hole is over the penis. You will pull the penis up and through the opening when cleansing the meatus.

■ **A woman is unable to maintain a dorsal recumbent position?**

Use Sims' position (side-lying with the upper leg flexed at the hip). Cover the rectal area.

Prevents contamination from the rectal area to the urethra.

■ **The patient is having a menstrual period?**

Note on the lab form that the patient is having a menstrual period before sending a specimen for diagnostic testing.

Blood in the urine from a menstrual period might lead to misinterpretation of the result.

Evaluation

■ Note any difficulty with catheter insertion.
This can indicate structural problems, especially in an older male patient with an enlarged prostate gland.

■ Note the characteristics of the urine obtained (e.g., amount, color, odor, presence of sediment or mucus).
■ Assess for absence of bladder distention.
Palpating the bladder helps you to determine if it has been emptied. Note: Some facilities have a bladder-scanning device that will allow you to determine whether residual urine remains.

■ For indwelling catheters, continue to assess that drainage is not obstructed and that the drainage bag is below the level of the bladder

Home Care

Indwelling Catheter

For inserting indwelling catheters in the home, teach clients:
■ When to change the catheter
Clients who are at higher risk for catheter blockage may need to change catheters more frequently than the usual 4-week period.

■ How to prevent catheter blockage (e.g., increase fluid intake, use bladder irrigation)
Fluids increase the urine volume, helping to reduce the deposit of sediment or other particles in the tubing.

■ To empty the drainage bag frequently and to keep the bag below the level of the bladder
■ How to prevent urinary tract infections (e.g., use new silver/hydrogel-coated catheters, use clean technique when inserting catheter, prevent blockage of urine outflow, avoid carbonated beverages)
■ To take a shower rather than a bath, to decrease the risk for UTIs
■ How to prevent discomfort at the urethra
■ Use of a leg bag
■ To eat foods that help acidify the urine: meat, eggs, cheese, prunes, cranberries, and whole grains

Documentation

■ Document the time and date of the procedure.
■ Document the size of catheter used.

■ Record the amount of urine obtained on the I&O portion of the graphics sheet. Record the color of urine, odor, presence of mucus, blood, and so on, in the nursing notes.
■ Record the patient's subjective statements.
■ Document if you collected a specimen, and note the time it was sent to the lab.
For an indwelling catheter: In addition, some facilities require that you record the amount of saline used to inflate the balloon.

Sample documentation:

12/28/12   0800   *Order noted for insertion of indwelling catheter. Explained procedure and reason for Foley catheter to client and client verbalized an understanding of the procedure and need for the catheter. Placed client in dorsal recumbent position with blankets to keep client warm. Perineal care completed. 14 Fr Foley catheter inserted using sterile technique per protocol. Foley draining dark yellow urine with sediment and foul odor. No mucus or blood noted in urine. Bladder is not distended. Client returned to semi-Fowler's position and no needs were noted at this time. Taught client to call nurse if there is any discomfort associated with urinary catheter. Call light placed in client's dominant hand.——— L. Chin, RN*
12/28/12   2000   *Client attempted to void in bedpan without success. Bladder palpated right below umbilicus. Order for intermittent urinary catheterization noted. Explained procedure to client. Client stated, "They had to do this last night too." Perineal care complete. Inserted 10 Fr straight catheter using sterile technique. 600 mL of clear, yellow urine without foul odor drained immediately. Client voiced relief and bladder no longer palpable. Catheter removed and perineal care complete. Client resting quietly in supine position.——— L. Chin, RN*

Practice Resources
Grabe, M., Bishop, M. C., Bjerklund-Johansen, T. E., et al. (2008); Lo, E., Nicolle, L., Classen, D., et al. (2008).

Thinking About the Procedure

 Go to the *Fundamentals of Nursing Skills Videos,* **Urinary Elimination: Intermittent Catheterization (Male).**

1. When preparing equipment for inserting a straight catheter, what additional item might you bring with you? Why would this be a good idea?

2. What does the nurse in the DVD do to help relax the patient before starting the procedure?

 Also go to the *Fundamentals of Nursing Skills Videos,* **Urinary Elimination: Indwelling Catheterization (Female): Inserting.**

1. How does the nurse in the DVD position the patient when inserting a urinary catheter?

2. Is it necessary for the patient to be shaved before inserting the urinary catheter?

3. The nurse in the DVD uses which hand to spread the urinary meatus?

4. What does the nurse in the DVD do to make sure the catheter is secure?

 For suggested responses, go to Chapter 27, **Thinking About the Procedure Suggested Responses (Procedure 27-4),** on the Student Resource Disk or DavisPlus at http://davisplus.fadavis.com/Wilkinson2

Procedure 27-5 — Applying an External (Condom) Catheter

> ➤ For steps to follow in *all* procedures, refer to the Universal Steps for All Procedures found on the inside back cover of Volume 2.

Critical Aspects

- Clean and dry the penis before catheter application.
- When applying the condom, stabilize the penis with your nondominant hand.
- Leave a gap of 2.5 to 5 cm (1 to 2 in.) between the condom and the tip of the penis to prevent skin irritation.
- Use only the tape supplied in the application kit to secure the catheter.
- For condom catheters that contain adhesive material on the inside of the condom, grasp the penis and gently compress the condom onto the shaft and roll the condom on.
- Be certain that the tubing from the end of the catheter to the drainage bag is free from kinks.

Equipment

- Condom catheter
- Two pairs of clean procedure gloves
- Washcloth and towel
- Basin of soap and water
- Bath blanket
- Urine collection bag (e.g., bedside drainage bag or leg bag)
- Disposable tape measure
- Skin prep (per agency policy)
- Scissors
- Commercial leg strap

Delegation

You may delegate the application of a condom catheter to the NAP once you have assessed the NAP's skill level and completed the following assessments. Instruct the NAP to report any alterations in the skin integrity along the shaft of the penis.

Pre-Procedure Assessments

- Assess the patient's cognitive status.

Knowing whether the patient can follow directions helps you to determine how to approach the procedure and also to know if the patient may be prone to pulling on the catheter.

- Assess pattern of voiding (e.g., degree and time of incontinence).

Knowing how often and how much the patient voids, helps you to determine when the condom catheter should be applied.

- Assess the skin along the shaft of the penis, the glans, and the meatus (for swelling or excoriation).

The condom catheter cannot be used on excoriated, irritated skin or over areas of impaired skin integrity.

(continued on next page)

Procedure 27-5 ■ **Applying an External (Condom) Catheter** (continued)

■ Note whether and how much the penis is retracted towards the body.

There is an increased risk of nonadherence and leakage of urine in a patient with a retracted penis.

■ Assess for the presence of neuropathy.

Patients with neuropathies that affect sensation in the penis may not feel skin irritation from the condom catheter and will need to be assessed more frequently.

➤   When performing the procedure, always identify your patient according to agency policy and be attentive to standard precautions, hand hygiene, patient safety and privacy, body mechanics, and documentation.

Procedure Steps

1. Don procedure gloves and determine appropriate size of the external catheter by measuring the circumference of the penis using a disposable paper tape. Obtain a correctly sized catheter.

A catheter that is too small impairs circulation. A catheter that is too large allows leakage of urine.

2. Wash your hands and don clean procedure gloves.

Hand hygiene and gloving prevents the transmission of bacteria.

3. Organize supplies and prepare the leg bag or bedside drainage bag for attachment to the condom catheter by removing it from the packaging and placing the end of the connecting tubing near the perineal area.

4. Place the patient supine. If the patient has difficulty breathing, raise the head of the bed to 30°.

5. Fold down the bedcovers to expose the penis, and drape the patient using the bath blanket.

Covering the patient reduces patient embarrassment.

6. Gently cleanse the penis with soap and water. Rinse and dry it thoroughly. If the patient is uncircumcised, retract the foreskin, cleanse the glans, and replace the foreskin. Excess hair along the shaft of the penis may be carefully clipped off with the scissors.

Cleansing the penis not only helps to prevent infection but it also help the condom catheter to adhere better to the shaft.

7. Wash your hands and change procedure gloves.

8. Apply skin prep (if used by your agency), and allow it to dry. *Note:*

Some external condom catheters require the placement of the special adhesive strip onto the penis before the application of the condom. Read the manufacturer's directions.

9. Hold the penis in your nondominant hand. With your dominant hand, place the condom catheter at the end of the penis, and slowly unroll it along the shaft toward the patient's body. Leave 2.5 to 5 cm (1 to 2 in.) between the end of the penis and the drainage tube on the catheter.

Careful unrolling in this manner helps to prevent irritation of the glans due to rubbing and allows for expansion of the penis if an erection were to occur. ▼

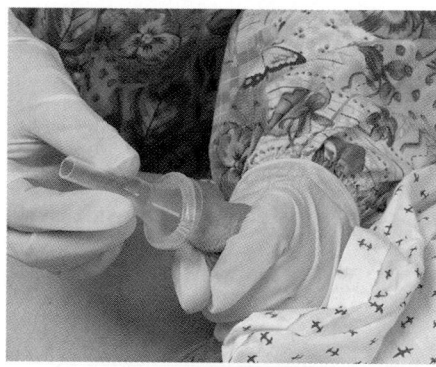

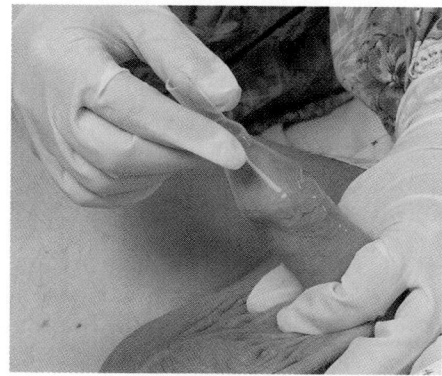

10. Secure the condom catheter in place on the penis.

 a. Ensure that the condom is not twisted.

Twisting can obstruct urine flow.

 b. Do not use regular bandage or surgical dressing tape to hold an external condom catheter in place.

Regular surgical dressing does not expand and could lead to decreased blood flow to the penis.

Step 10 Variation. Catheter with Internal Adhesive

 c. Gently grasp the penis and compress so that the entire shaft comes in contact with the condom.

Step 10 Variation. Catheter with External Adhesive Strip

 d. Wrap the strip around the outside of the condom in a spiral direction, taking care not to overlap the ends.

Avoiding overlapping prevents constriction of blood flow to the penis.

11. Assess the proximal end of the condom catheter. If a large portion of the condom is still rolled above the adhesive strip, you may need to clip the roll (McConnell, 2001).

Clipping the roll prevents constriction of blood flow.

12. Attach the tube end of the condom catheter to a drainage system (e.g., a leg bag). Make sure there are no kinks in the tubing.

Kinks impede the flow of urine. Urine that does not drain away from the meatus can cause irritation and skin breakdown and possibly cause the condom catheter to fall off.

13. Secure the drainage tubing to the patient's thigh using tape or a commercial leg strap (follow facility protocol).

Tape or a leg strap controls movement of the tubing and accidental pulling on the condom catheter. ▼

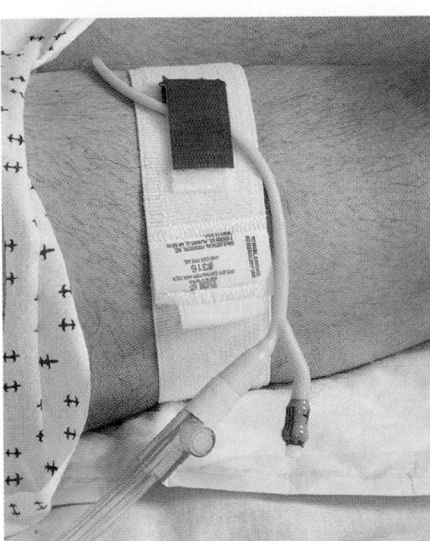

14. Cover the patient and return him to a comfortable position. Raise the siderails and lower the bed.

15. Remove your gloves and wash your hands.

16. Change the condom daily or more often if needed.
This helps to prevent urinary tract infection.

What if...

■ **The urine flow becomes obstructed?**
Check the catheter and collecting tube for kinking; readjust if needed. If that does not solve the problem, irrigate the tubing (see Procedure 27-7). Replace the catheter and tubing, if necessary.

Evaluation

Within 30 minutes of condom application, assess for:
■ Urine flow (should not be obstructed)
■ Swelling or discoloration of the penis
Swelling or discoloration might indicate that the condom is too tight.

Monitor:
■ Penis for circulatory changes
■ Position and patency of the drainage tubing
■ Characteristics of the urine (e.g., amount, color, odor, bleeding)
■ Patient comfort
■ Leakage of urine

Home Care

■ Clients and caregivers should wash their hands before and after any manipulation of the penis or apparatus.
■ Daily bag decontamination with a diluted (1:10) bleach solution has been found effective in reducing bacteria.
■ Teach the client and caregiver to recognize the signs and symptoms of skin irritation and excoriation, as well as the symptoms of urinary tract infection.
■ Teach the client/caregiver to notify the care provider and discontinue use of the condom catheter if skin

irritation or swelling occurs; if the urine becomes thick and cloudy, pink or red; if the urine has mucus in it; or if no urine has drained from the catheter in 6 to 8 hours.
■ Change the external condom catheter every 24 hours. Use paper tape to secure the condom catheter to the inner thigh if you do not have a commercial leg strap.
■ Keep the collecting bag below the level of the bladder.
■ Empty the urine collection device.
■ Regularly empty the collection bag before it becomes completely full.
■ Never allow the draining spigot to come in contact with the nonsterile collecting container.
■ Disinfect the catheter–tubing junction before disconnecting them (if they must be disconnected).
■ Avoid disconnecting the catheter and drainage tube unless the catheter must be irrigated.

Documentation

■ Document the date and time of application of the external catheter in the nursing notes.
■ Note any unusual findings in your assessment of the skin on the penis.
■ Document characteristics of urine (e.g., color, odor, consistency, blood).

(continued on next page)

Procedure 27-5 ■ Applying an External (Condom) Catheter (continued)

Sample EHR documentation:

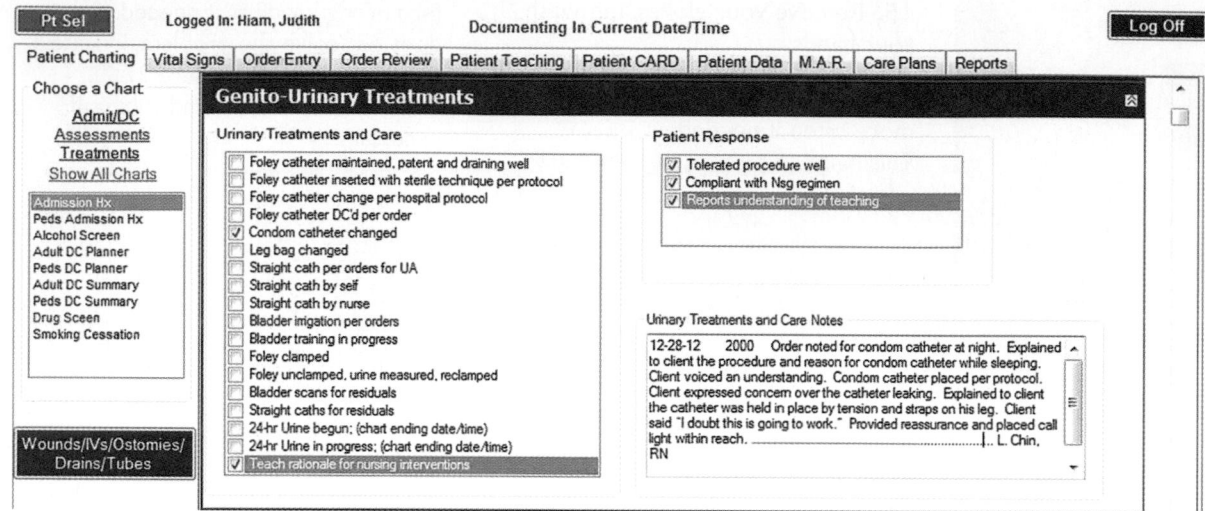

Practice Resources

Madigan, E., & Neff, D. (2003); Wong, E. S. (1981, updated 2005).

Thinking About the Procedure

 Go to the *Fundamentals of Nursing Skills Videos,* **Urinary Elimination: Catheter: External Condom.**

1. What does the nurse do in the DVD before applying the condom catheter?

2. What type of adhesive for the condom catheter did the nurse use for the patient in the DVD?

 For suggested responses, go to Chapter 27, **Thinking About the Procedure Suggested Responses (Procedure 27-5),** on the Student Resource Disk or DavisPlus at http://davisplus.fadavis.com/Wilkinson2

Procedure 27-6 ■ Removing an Indwelling Catheter

➤ For steps to follow in *all* procedures, refer to the Universal Steps for All Procedures found on the inside back cover of Volume 2.

Critical Aspects

- Use clean technique. Wash hands before and after removing the catheter. Wear clean procedure gloves.
- Be sure to remove the tape securing the catheter to the patient.
- Obtain a sterile specimen if needed.
- Deflate the balloon completely by aspirating the fluid.
- Check the balloon size on the valve port to verify that all fluid has been removed.
- If you cannot aspirate all the fluid, do not pull on the catheter. Report to the charge nurse or the primary care provider before continuing.
- Observe the first few voidings after the catheter is removed.

Equipment

- Syringe (5 to 30 mL, depending on balloon size)
- Towel or drape (and a towel as a receptacle for the catheter, such as an emesis basin)
- Hygiene supplies (washcloth, warm water, towel)

Delegation

In some institutions, unlicensed NAPs undergo special training to learn this skill. In such instances, you may delegate this task to the NAP. However, you must complete the following assessments and instruct the NAP about what abnormal findings to report.

Pre-Procedure Assessment

■ Assess the patient's cognitive level.
Knowing whether the patient can follow directions or not, helps you to determine how to approach the procedure and also to know if the patient may be prone to pulling on the catheter or your hands when you are removing the catheter.

■ Assess for the presence of conditions that may impair the patient's ability to assume the necessary position.

Knowing if there are physical limitations helps you to determine whether you will need assistance to help the patient maintain the correct position for catheter insertion.

■ Assess the condition of bladder (e.g., distention), perineum, and meatus (e.g., color, swelling, crusting, drainage, lesion).
This information helps you to establish a baseline for later assessment.

➤ When performing the procedure, always identify your patient according to agency policy and be attentive to standard precautions, hand hygiene, patient safety and privacy, body mechanics, and documentation.

Procedure Steps

1. Wash hands before and after removing the catheter.
For mechanical removal of microorganisms.

2. Wear clean gloves during the removal.
Gloving prevents transmission of bacteria.

3. Explain that this procedure is nearly always pain-free.

4. Instruct the patient to assume a supine position.

5. Place the catheter receptacle near the patient (e.g., on the bed).

6. Place a towel or waterproof drape between the patient's legs and up by the urethral meatus.
These methods preserve modesty and a feeling of security and prevent soiling of the bed.

7. Obtain a sterile specimen (see Procedure 27-2B), if needed. Some agencies require a culture and sensitivity test of the urine when an indwelling catheter is removed.

8. Remove the tape or device securing the catheter to the patient.

9. Deflate the balloon completely by inserting a syringe into the balloon valve and aspirating the fluid. Verify that the total fluid volume has been removed by checking the balloon size written on the valve port.
If water remains in the balloon, it will traumatize the urethra.

10. Ask the patient to relax and take a few deep breaths as you slowly withdraw the catheter from the urethra.
Deep breathing helps the patient to relax the sphincters.

11. Wrap the catheter in the towel or drape.

12. Use warm water and a washcloth to cleanse the perineal area. A mild soap may also be used. Be sure to rinse well if you use soap.
Cleansing the perineum prevents transmission of bacteria.

13. Measure the urine and then empty it in the toilet; discard the catheter, drainage tube, and collection bag in the biohazard waste.

14. Explain to the patient the need to monitor the first few voidings after catheter removal. If the patient toilets independently, place a receptacle in the toilet or beside commode; ask him to notify the nurse when he voids and to save the urine.

15. Remove and discard gloves; wash your hands.

16. Record the date and time of the procedure; the volume, color, and clarity of the urine; and your patient teaching.

17. Return the patient to a position of comfort.

What if. . .

■ **You cannot aspirate all the fluid from the balloon?**

Do not pull on the catheter. Report to the charge nurse or the primary care provider before continuing the procedure.

Pulling on the catheter could cause injury to the urethra.

Evaluation

■ Observe for signs and symptoms of infection.
Signs of UTI include urinary WBCs and pyuria. Signs of fever, bacteriuria and abnormal blood values do not predict catheter-associated UTIs (Madigan & Neff, 2003). Such infection in otherwise healthy patients is often asymptomatic and is likely to resolve spontaneously with the removal of the catheter. Occasionally, infection persists and leads to such complications as prostatitis, epididymitis, cystitis, pyelonephritis, and gram-negative bacteremia, particularly in high risk patients (Wong, 2005).

■ Observe the condition of the meatus.
■ After removing the catheter, monitor the next few voidings. Place a collection container in the commode if the patient is ambulatory.
■ Assess the characteristics of the urine at the time the catheter is removed. Then note the time of the first voiding and the amount voided, and observe the urine for color, amount, odor, and presence of blood.
■ Compare voidings over the next 8 to 10 hours to the patient's intake.
■ Monitor for bladder distention.

(continued on next page)

Procedure 27-6 ■ Removing an Indwelling Catheter (continued)

Patient Teaching

- Explain to the patient that you need to monitor the first few voidings after catheter removal to ensure that he does not have difficulty re-establishing bladder control.
- Teach the patient to notify you when he voids and to save the urine (if the patient toilets independently)

Home Care

For clients who will have catheters at home, teach the family the steps for removing the catheter:

- To remove the catheter, deflate the balloon completely by inserting a syringe into the balloon valve and aspirating the fluid. Verify that the total fluid volume has been removed by checking the balloon size written on the valve port.
- Notify a healthcare provider if the client is unable to urinate within 8 hours after catheter removal, or if his abdomen becomes distended and painful.
- Recognize signs and symptoms of urinary tract infection

Not everyone with a urinary tract infection develops recognizable signs and symptoms, but most people have some. Signs and symptoms of a urinary tract infection develop rapidly and can include a strong, persistent urge to urinate; a burning sensation when urinating; passing frequent, small amounts of urine; blood in the urine (hematuria); cloudy, strong-smelling urine; or bacteria in the urine.

- Increase fluid intake if not contraindicated by other health conditions.

The client should never remove a catheter unless trained by a healthcare provider. Remove the catheter only when prescribed by the provider.

Documentation

Document the following:

- Date and time the catheter was removed
- Amount of urine (on the I&O portion of the graphics sheet)
- Characteristics of urine (e.g., color, odor, cloudiness, turbidity, or blood)
- The time the specimen was sent to the lab
- The amount of fluid removed from balloon, client response to removal of the indwelling urinary catheter, urine in drainage bag, and notification of first void
- Any unusual findings in your assessment of the perineum
- How the patient tolerated the procedure
- Patient teaching

Sample EHR documentation:

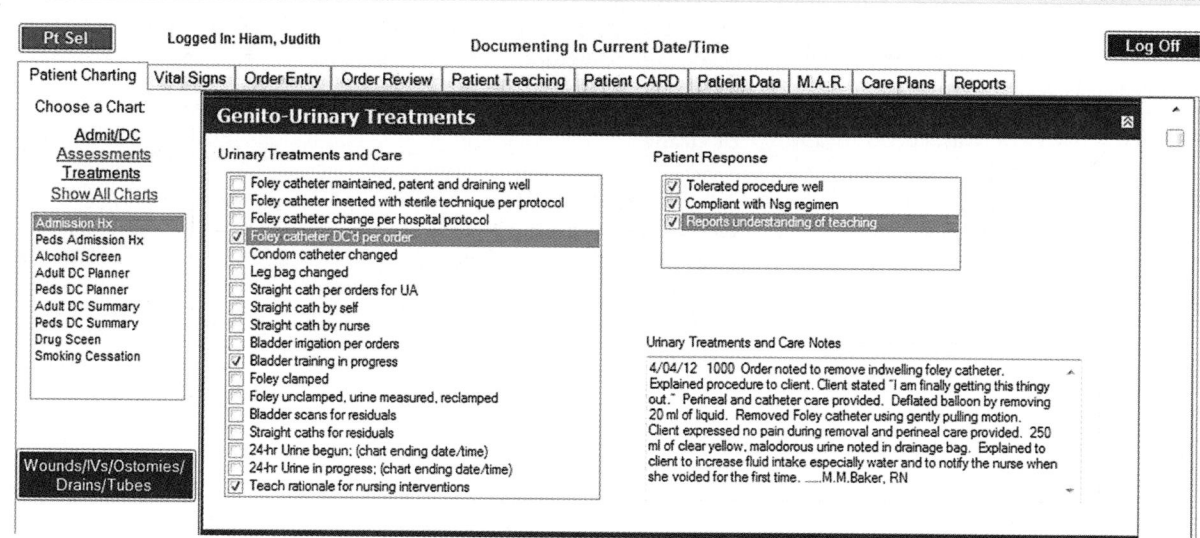

Practice Resources

Griffith, R., & Fernandez, R. (2007, republished 2009, January); Madigan, E., & Neff, D. (2003); Moore, K. N., Fader, M., & Getliffe, K. (2007); Publisher (2008); Wong, E. S., & Hooton, T. M. (1981, updated 2005, April 1).

Thinking About the Procedure

Go to the *Fundamentals of Nursing Skills Videos*, **Urinary Elimination: Indwelling Catheterization: Removing.**

1. What does the nurse do in the DVD that you would not do in real life with a patient?

2. Before removal, would the nurse tell the patient that removing the catheter is painful or pain-free?

3. Where did the nurse dispose of the catheter after removal?

For suggested responses, go to Chapter 27, **Thinking About the Procedure Suggested Responses (Procedure 27-6),** on the Student Resource Disk or DavisPlus at http://davisplus.fadavis.com/Wilkinson2

Procedure 27-7 □ **Irrigating the Bladder or Catheter**

➤ For steps to follow in *all* procedures, refer to the Universal Steps for All Procedures found on the inside back cover of Volume 2.

Critical Aspects

Intermittent Irrigation
- Establish a sterile field under the specimen removal port or the irrigation port on a three-way catheter.
- Because of the risk of infection, never disconnect the drainage tubing from the catheter.
- Use a sterile irrigation solution, warmed to room temperature.
- Instill the irrigation solution slowly.
- Repeat the process as necessary.

Continuous Irrigation
- Drape the patient, exposing only the irrigation port of the catheter.
- Using aseptic technique, attach the connecting tubing to the irrigation solution container.
- Prime the tubing.
- Don clean procedure gloves.
- Pinch the irrigation port of the catheter and connect the irrigation tubing to the port.
- Regulate the flow of the irrigant.
- Monitor urine output.

Equipment

Intermittent Irrigation Through a Three-Way Catheter

- Bag of sterile irrigation solution
- Connecting tubing (to connect the bag to the irrigation port)
- IV pole
- Antiseptic swabs
- Bath blanket

Intermittent Irrigation via the Specimen Port Using a Syringe

- Sterile container
- Sterile 60-mL syringe with large-gauge needleless access device
- Two pairs of clean procedure gloves

Continuous Bladder Irrigation

- Three-way (or triple-lumen) indwelling catheter in place
- Sterile irrigation solution at room temperature
- Connecting tubing
- Antiseptic swabs
- IV pole
- Bath blanket
- Measuring container
- Pair of clean procedure gloves

Delegation

Irrigation of an indwelling catheter requires nursing assessment and clinical decision-making. Because of the high potential for urinary tract infection, you should not delegate this procedure to the NAP. Bladder/catheter irrigation may be delegated with supervision to qualified LPNs who are trained in the procedure.

Pre-Procedure Assessment

- Note the characteristics of the urine (e.g., amount, color, odor, presence of clots or mucus).
  Assess for the presence and degree of bladder distension.

This information helps you to establish a baseline for assessment.

- Note patient complaints of discomfort.
- Assess the patient's cognitive status.

Knowing whether the patient can follow directions or cooperate for the procedure, helps you determine whether she can remain still during the procedure and the likelihood of the sterile field being disrupted.

- Check the chart for the amount and type of sterile solution to use.
- Determine whether the irrigant is to remain in the bladder for any length of time.

(continued on next page)

Procedure 27-7 ■ Irrigating the Bladder or Catheter (continued)

■ Procedure 27-7A Intermittent Bladder or Catheter Irrigation

➤ When performing the procedure, always identify your patient according to agency policy and be attentive to standard precautions, hand hygiene, patient safety and privacy, body mechanics, and documentation.

➤ Note: This is the procedure for the closed methods of irrigation. The "open" method is no longer recommended. Because of the risk for infection, you should never disconnect the drainage tubing from the catheter.

Procedure Steps

Procedure Variation
Three-Way (Triple-Lumen) Indwelling Catheter

1. Before starting bladder irrigation, prepare the connection tubing and irrigation solution warmed to room temperature.
   a. Close the clamp on the connection tubing.
   b. Spike the tubing into the appropriate portal on the irrigation solution bag, using aseptic technique.
   c. Invert the solution and hang it on an IV pole.
   d. Remove the protective cap from the distal end of the connection tubing. Hold the end of the tubing over the sink or trash receptacle. Open the roller clamp, and allow the solution to fill the tubing. Be sure to keep the end sterile.
   e. Reclamp the roller on the tubing to stop the flow of irrigation solution.
   f. Recap the tubing.

2. Wash your hands and don procedure gloves.
To reduce the transmission of microbes.

3. Position the patient supine.

4. Drape the patient so only the connection port on the indwelling catheter is visible.
Protects patient privacy.

5. Before beginning the flow of irrigation solution, empty any urine that is in the drainage bag, and wash your hands. Then document the volume on the I&O record.
Starting the procedure with an empty draining bag gives you a baseline for

correct calculation of true urine output during irrigation.

6. Cleanse the catheter port with antiseptic solution.

7. Connect the irrigation tubing to the catheter port.

8. Slowly open the roller clamp on the irrigation tubing to the desired flow rate.
Slow instillation prevents patient discomfort.

9. Instill or irrigate with the prescribed amount of irrigant. If the irrigant is to remain in the bladder for a certain time period, clamp the drainage tubing for that time.

10. When the correct amount of irrigant has been used and/or the goals of the irrigation have been met, close the roller clamp on the irrigation tubing, leaving the tubing connected to the catheter for use during the next irrigation.
You can assess whether the goals of irrigation have been met by inspecting the color of the urine and assessing for presence of clots, mucus, or blood. Clamping the drainage tubing prevents immediate outflow.

11. Remove gloves, wash your hands, and return the patient to a position of comfort.

Procedure Variation
Two-Way Indwelling Catheter

12. Don clean procedure gloves. Empty any urine currently found in the bedside drainage bag.
Emptying the bag will ensure accurate output results.

13. Wash your hands and then apply clean gloves.

Gloving prevents the transmission of microorganisms.

14. Drape the patient so that only the specimen removal port on the drainage tubing is exposed. Place a sterile waterproof drape beneath the exposed port.
Draping ensures patient privacy and prevents soiling of the bed linens.

15. Open the sterile irrigation supplies. Pour approximately 100 mL of the irrigating solution, warmed to room temperature, into the sterile container, using aseptic technique.
Warm solution is more comfortable to the patient.

16. Scrub all surfaces of the specimen removal port with antiseptic swab.
Cleanings the port reduces the risk of transmission of pathogens into the bladder.

17. Draw up irrigation solution into the syringe. Connect the syringe to the specimen port. For catheter irrigation, use a total of 30 to 40 mL; for bladder irrigation the amount is usually 100 to 200 mL.

18. Clamp or pinch the drainage tubing distal to the specimen port.
Clamping prevents irrigant from going down into the drainage bag instead of into the catheter and/or bladder.

19. Inject the solution into the port. Hold the specimen port slightly above the level of the bladder. If you meet resistance, have the patient turn slightly, and attempt a second time. If resistance continues, stop the procedure and notify the primary care provider.

Holding the port above the level of the bladder enhances gravitational flow of irrigant into the bladder. ▼

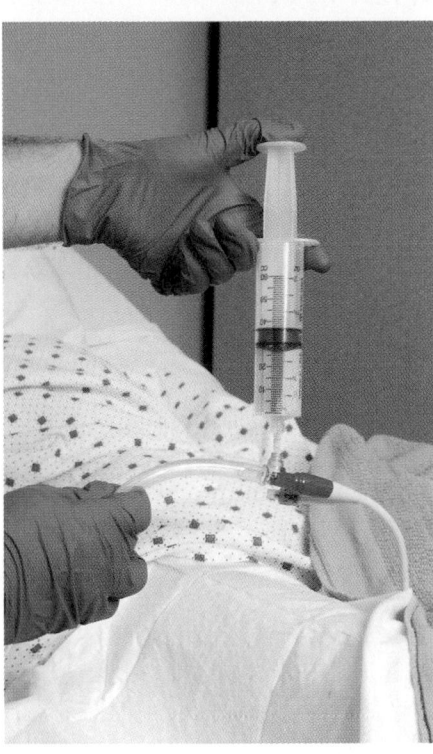

20. When the irrigant has been injected, remove syringe. Refill the syringe if necessary.

21. Unclamp or release the drainage tubing, and allow the irrigant and urine to flow into the bedside drainage bag by gravity. (If the solution is to remain in the bladder for a prescribed time, leave the tubing clamped for that time period.)

22. Repeat the procedure as necessary until the prescribed amount has been instilled or until the goal of the irrigation is met (e.g., removal of clots and mucus, free flowing of urine).

23. Remove gloves, wash your hands, and return the patient to a position of comfort.

■ **Procedure 27-7B Continuous Bladder Irrigation**

➤ When performing the procedure, always identify your patient according to agency policy and be attentive to standard precautions, hand hygiene, patient safety and privacy, body mechanics, and documentation.

Procedure Steps

1. If one is not already present, insert a three-way (triple-lumen) indwelling catheter.
A triple-lumen catheter provides an access for the irrigation solution without disrupting the sterile drainage unit.

2. Prepare the irrigation fluid and tubing:
a. Roll the clamp on the connecting tubing to the "closed" position.
Clamping the tubing prevents air from filling the tubing.

b. Spike the tubing into the portal on the irrigation solution container, using aseptic technique.
This prevents the introduction of microorganisms into the solution.

c. Invert the container, and hang it on the IV pole.

The elevated bag allows the solution to flow by gravity.

d. Remove the protective cap from the distal end of the connecting tubing. Hold the end of the tubing over a sink or other receptacle. Open the roll clamp slowly, and allow the solution to fill the tubing completely. Recap the tubing.
Priming the tubing flushes air from tubing, preventing bladder distension.

3. Perform hand hygiene and don clean procedure gloves.
These two actions prevent the spread of microorganisms.

4. Place the patient supine and drape the patient so that only the connection port on the indwelling catheter is visible.
Draping prevents exposure of the genital area and protects patient privacy.

5. Place a waterproof barrier drape under the irrigation port. However, if the irrigation kit comes with a sterile drape, use that. Pinching the tubing and using aseptic technique, connect the end of the irrigation infusion tubing to the side port of the catheter.

6. Before beginning the flow of irrigation solution, empty any urine that may be in the bedside drainage bag, and document the volume on the I&O record.
Starting the procedure with an empty bag gives you a baseline for correct calculation of true urine output during irrigation.

7. Remove your gloves and wash your hands.
Gloving and handwashing prevents the transmission of microorganisms.

(continued on next page)

Procedure 27-7 ■ **Irrigating the Bladder or Catheter** (continued)

8. Cover the patient, and return him to a position of comfort.

9. Open the roll clamp on the tubing, and regulate the flow of the irrigation solution to meet the desired outcome for the irrigation.

The goal of continuous bladder irrigation for patients who have had a trans-urethral resection of the prostate is to keep the urine light pink to clear. ▼

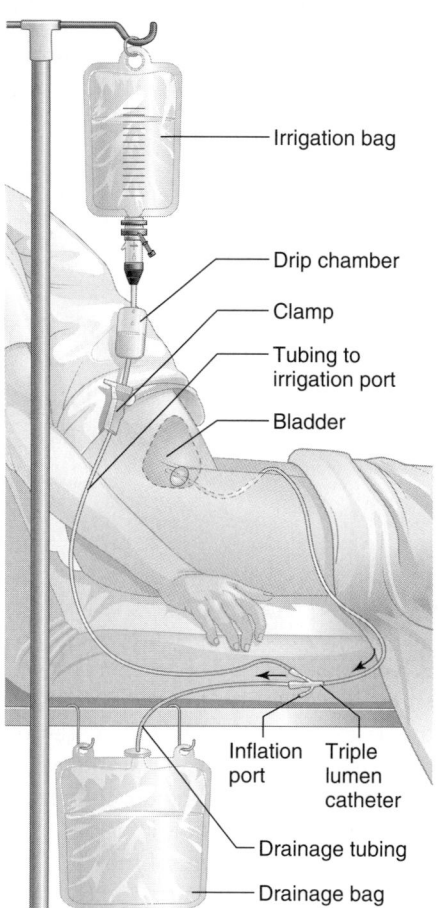

Irrigation bag

Drip chamber

Clamp

Tubing to irrigation port

Bladder

Inflation port

Triple lumen catheter

Drainage tubing

Drainage bag

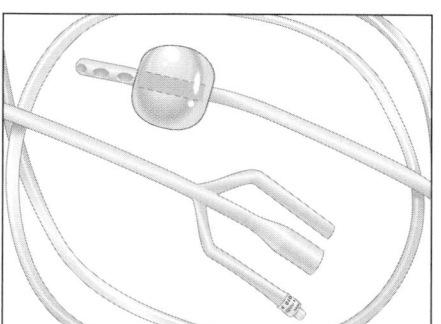

10. Monitor the flow rate for 1 to 2 minutes to ensure accuracy.

Infusing irrigation fluid for a minute or two prevents rapid introduction of solution into the bladder, which would cause patient discomfort.

What if . . .

- **The draining irrigant solution and/or urine looks like it has red blood cells in it?**

Stop the irrigation and report to the primary care provider.

Signs of increased red cells in urine may indicate bladder irritation and possible trauma to the inner mucosal lining of the bladder.

- **If you meet resistance when irrigating?**

Ask the patient to turn slightly, and attempt a second time. If resistance continues, stop the procedure and notify the primary care provider.

Evaluation

- Note the flow rate of irrigant and/or inability to instill irrigant into the catheter.
- Note the characteristics of urine output (e.g., presence of output, color, amount, clots, mucus).
- Note patient report of discomfort (e.g., pain, spasms).
- Assess for development of bladder distention accompanied by lack of urine outflow.

Home Care

For clients who will have continuous bladder irrigation at home, you will need to teach the family the necessary steps of the procedure. Also teach them to:
- Empty the urine collection device before beginning the procedure.
- Utilize strict aseptic technique when irrigating the bladder or catheter.
- Irrigate the catheter using the closed method, which carries the least risk for introducing bacteria into the bladder.

- Identify signs and symptoms of urinary retention and urinary tract infection.
- Wash their hands before and after any manipulation of the catheter site or apparatus.
- Be certain to maintain unobstructed flow.
- Not disconnect the catheter and drainage tube.
- For the syringe method, the client will need access to syringes and needleless access devices and a process to dispose of them properly.

Documentation

- Document the date and time of procedure, the type of irrigant, and the total volume infused.
- Document the characteristics of the urine (e.g., color, odor, clarity, sediment, presence of clots or mucus).
- Record evidence of catheter patency (e.g., flow of urine, absence of distension).

Sample EHR documentation:

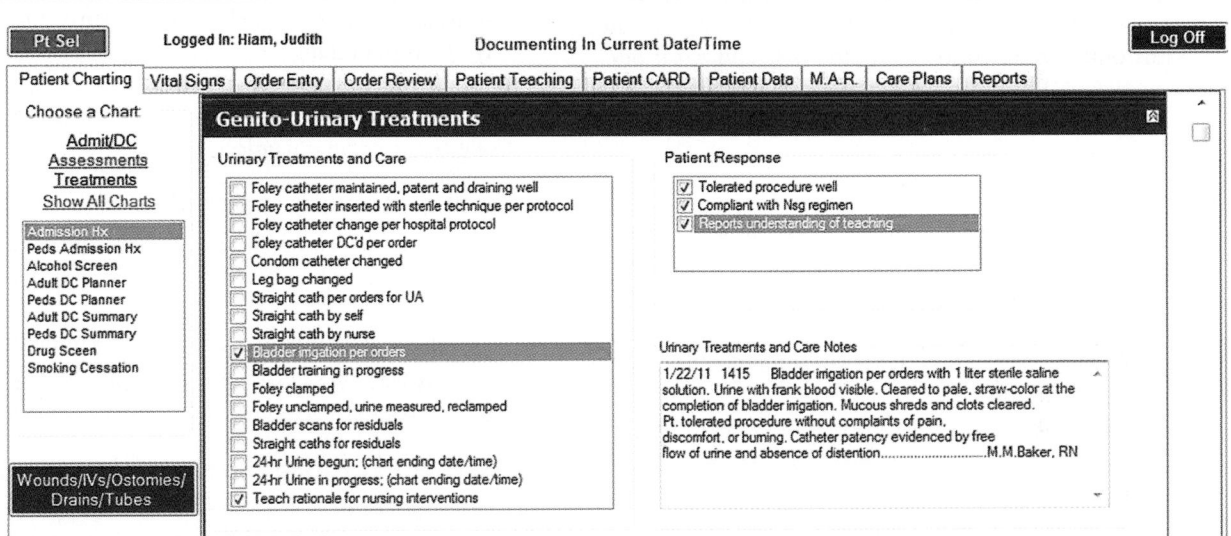

Practice Resources

Jahn, P., Preuss, M., Kernig, A., et al. (2007); Sinclair, L., Cross S., Hagen S., et al. (2006, amended 2009); Wong, E. S., & Hooton, T. M. (1981, last modified 2005).

Thinking About the Procedure

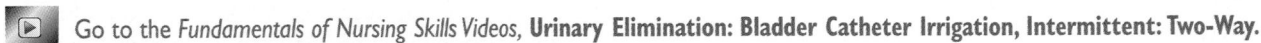

Go to the *Fundamentals of Nursing Skills Videos,* **Urinary Elimination: Bladder Catheter Irrigation, Intermittent: Two-Way.**

1. What does the nurse do after draining the urine out of the drainage collection bag?

2. What size syringe does the nurse in the DVD use to draw up the irrigation solution?

3. What do you notice different about the urine before and after the bladder irrigation procedure?

Go to the *Fundamentals of Nursing Skills Videos,* **Urinary Elimination: Bladder Catheter Irrigation, Intermittent: Three-Way.**

1. What does the nurse do with the clamp if the irrigation solution is not to remain in the bladder?

For suggested responses, go to Chapter 27, **Thinking About the Procedure Suggested Responses (Procedure 27-7),** on the Student Resource Disk or DavisPlus at http://davisplus.fadavis.com/Wilkinson2

Clinical Insights

An indwelling catheter is connected to a drainage tube and collection bag, which constitute a closed system.

Goal 1: Prevent urinary tract infection.

▪ Do not disconnect the tubing or open the drainage system (e.g., to obtain specimens or measure the urine).
A closed system minimizes the chance for pathogens to enter the system and infect the urinary tract.

▪ Regularly check connections between the catheter and drainage tubing and the drainage tube and collection bag.
Loose connections cause leaks and serve as entry points for pathogens.

▪ If the system becomes disconnected, wipe the ends of both tubes with antiseptic (e.g., alcohol or chlorhexadine-gluconate-alcohol combination product) before reconnecting them.

▪ If the catheter becomes soiled from drainage or feces, cleanse it with mild soap and water by cleaning from the meatus outward. Rinse the catheter well, and pat it dry.
This removes the medium for growth of microorganisms.

▪ Empty the collection bag at least every 8 hours and more frequently if urine output is high.
This prevents stagnation of urine.

▪ When emptying the collection bag, avoid touching the spout to any surfaces. If the spout is accidentally contaminated, cleanse it with an antiseptic (e.g., alcohol or chlorhexadine-gluconate-alcohol combination product).

▪ Keep collection bag below the level of the bladder. Never place the bag on the bed.
This prevents backflow of stale urine into the bladder.

▪ Assist the patient to take a shower regularly if his condition permits.

▪ Encourage patients with recurrent UTIs to drink cranberry juice.
Although the evidence of effectiveness is scant, the hippuric acid in cranberry juice prevents bacteria from adhering to the walls of the bladder for some strains resistant to certain antibiotics.

▪ Teach the patient to report signs of UTI (e.g., burning at the meatus); observe for cloudy, strong-smelling urine, chills, or fever.

▪ Change the indwelling catheter only when necessary. Some agencies have a policy specifying that catheters be changed at specified intervals (e.g., weekly). However, this is not advisable because the more often a catheter is changed, the more likely an infection will develop. Change the catheter when any of the following occurs:
  ▪ Sediment collects in the tubing or the catheter.
  ▪ The urine does not drain well.
  ▪ The sandy particles that build up inside the drainage tubing cannot be freed by rolling the tubing between your hands.

Goal 2: Maintain free flow of urine.

Maintaining free flow of urine prevents backflow of urine into the bladder, which can cause bladder distention and injury. Stasis of urine also provides a medium for growth of microorganisms. Note that some of the interventions in this section are the same as those for preventing infection (goal 1).

▪ Make sure the tubing and bag remain below the level of the bladder to prevent backflow.
Urine drains by gravity in this system.

▪ If the collecting bag must be higher than the bladder at any time, you must clamp the catheter.
Clamping prevents backflow of stagnant urine into the bladder.

▪ Frequently inspect the tubing to ensure that urine flows freely in the tubing.
Any kinks, coils, or compression of the catheter or tubing may impede flow and cause backup into the bladder.

▪ If urine is not flowing, check to be sure the patient is not lying on the tubing.

▪ Do not allow the collection bag to lie on the floor.
This decreases the effect of gravity. It also increases the likelihood of contamination.

Goal 3: Prevent transmission of infection.

When providing catheter care, observe universal precautions:
▪ Wear gloves when handling the catheter or drainage system.
Gloving prevents possible exposure to body fluids.

▪ Always wash your hands before and after providing care to any patient, including one with an indwelling catheter.

Goal 4: Promote normal urine production.

Adequate urine production flushes pathogens out of the bladder, provides natural irrigation of the tubing, and prevents stasis of urine.

▪ Unless contraindicated by other health problems, encourage oral intake of at least 8 to 10 glasses (approximately 3000 mL) of fluid per day. For patients who are unable to take oral liquid, provide an equivalent amount of parenteral or enteral fluids.

▪ Monitor intake and output at least every 8 hours. More frequent monitoring may be required if the patient is experiencing fluid and electrolyte problems.

▪ For accurate determination of output, empty the urine into an accurately calibrated container.
Although the urine collection bag has volume markings, they are only approximate.

▪ Observe the urine output for color and characteristics. Report evidence of blood, sediment, or infection to the primary care provider.

▪ Encourage the patient to be active and out of bed as much as possible.

Goal 5: Maintain skin and mucosal integrity.

Perineal skin and mucosa can be irritated by feces and by movement or encrustation of the catheter.

■ Secure the tubing by taping it to the thigh or applying a Velcro band to the thigh through which the tubing is secured. For men, if the catheter will remain in place for an extended period, secure the tubing to the abdomen to prevent damage to the penile–scrotal juncture.

Failure to secure the tubing may cause significant injury to the bladder neck and urethra. Although the inflated balloon helps maintain the catheter in the bladder, you will need to secure the tubing to the leg to prevent traction on the bladder.

■ Routine hygiene care normally provides adequate cleanliness. Cleanse the area around the meatus with mild soap and water daily, after each bowel movement, and more often if there is drainage or excessive sweating. Be sure to rinse well and pat dry.

Rising helps to avoid irritating the skin with soap residue.

■ Avoid using powders or lotions in the perineal area.

Topical products can be irritating to the skin.

■ Monitor the urethral meatus and upper drainage tube.

Encrustation, as evidenced by sandy particles at the meatus, is irritating to the mucosa and signals a need to change the catheter.

Clinical Insight 27-2 ▶ Caring for Patients with Urinary Incontinence

Most urinary incontinence (UI) is managed with skin care and behavioral interventions, but medications and other collaborative treatments are sometimes used.

Perineal Skin Care

■ Provide dry clothing and bedding as soon as possible after incontinence occurs.

■ Wash the perineum with soap and warm water after each episode and rinse and dry well.

Washing removes urine from the skin.

■ Use a skin moisturizer.

■ Use petroleum-based ointment on dry skin.

This can be an effective moisture barrier.

■ Antifungal creams (e.g., nystatin [Mycostatin]) may be prescribed for fungus growth.

Normal urine is acidic. When it remains in contact with the skin, it becomes alkaline, causing encrustations to collect on the skin. The skin then becomes macerated and excoriated.

Lifestyle Modification

Make the following recommendations to clients:

■ Increase daily oral fluids (to 8 to 10 glasses, or 3000 mL), as tolerated.

High fluid intake is good for flushing of the bladder.

■ Limit daily caffeine intake to less than 100 mg. This is about one cup of coffee or two 12 oz. cans of cola.

Caffeine is a diuretic and a bladder stimulant.

■ Try limiting the intake of alcohol, artificial sweeteners, spicy foods, and citrus fruits.

These are thought to irritate the bladder.

■ Lose weight (for persons with a BMI > 30). Studies have shown this to be more effective for women than for men.

■ Stop smoking.

Smoking has been linked to stress UI and urge UI among women, and to urge UI in men.

■ Take prescribed diuretics early in the morning.

Diuretics taken at night can cause nocturia and lead to interrupted sleep.

■ Avoid constipation. (See Chapter 28 for interventions to promote normal bowel elimination.)

Fecal impaction and chronic constipation, especially in older adults, are associated with increased risk of UI.

■ Be aware that high-impact exercise (e.g., running, jumping rope) is associated with increased stress UI.

Bladder Training

The goal of bladder training is to enable the patient to hold increasingly greater volumes of urine in the bladder and to increase the interval between voidings. This involves patient teaching, scheduled voiding, and self-monitoring using a voiding diary.

■ Teach the mechanisms of urination.

■ Teach distraction and relaxation strategies to help inhibit the urge to void. For example:

  ■ Instruct the patient to perform serial subtractions or become involved in an activity that requires concentration (e.g., a crossword puzzle) when she feels the urge to void.

  ■ Alternatively the patient might perform several rapid pelvic floor muscle contractions to quiet the sensations from the bladder.

  ■ Other techniques include deep breathing and guided imagery.

■ **Scheduled voiding** is a form of bladder training involving timed voiding and habit retraining. The patient must be mentally and physically capable of self-toileting.

  ■ Assist the patient to the toilet, commode, or bedpan on a timed schedule. Initially this may be every 2 hours or even more often.

  ■ As a pattern develops and the person gains greater control, the length of time between voiding may be increased.

  ■ Scheduled voiding is usually combined with other techniques, including lifestyle adjustments and pelvic muscle exercises.

■ Ask the patient to keep a daily record of her adherence to the schedule and of the number of incontinence episodes.

(continued on next page)

Clinical Insight 27-2 ▶ **Caring for Patients with Urinary Incontinence** (continued)

■ If the patient can adhere to the schedule without frequent changes due to urgency, the voiding interval can be increased by 15 to 30 minutes each week.

Kegel Exercises

Pelvic floor muscle exercises (PFMEs) strengthen perineal muscles and help to prevent and treat stress, urge, and mixed UI. Kegel exercises are the most commonly used.

Teach patients the following routine to strengthen pelvic floor muscles:

■ Imagine that you are urinating and wish to stop the flow; also tighten your rectum as though you are trying to keep from passing gas. The muscles you contract to interrupt flow are the pelvic floor muscles. (*Note:* Caution the patient against doing Kegel exercises while actually urinating because this may cause backflow of urine.)

■ You should feel your rectum tighten. Women may also feel the vagina tighten. Your abdomen should not tighten—check by placing your hand lightly on your abdomen. Do not contract the thigh and gluteal muscles.

■ Hold each contraction for 5 to 10 seconds and then rest for 5 to 10 seconds. Some people may be able to hold for only 3 seconds at first. Count, "one-and-two-and-three . . ." Keep contraction and relaxation times equal. That is, if you hold a contraction for 5 seconds, rest 5 seconds before the next contraction.

■ A recommended daily exercise routine is to perform 40 to 60 PFMEs divided into two to four sets of 15 exercises each time. Do one set sitting, one standing, and one lying down. Do not do all 40 to 60 exercises at one time; spread them out through the day.

■ One way to remember to perform your exercises it to associate them with an activity. For example, do Kegels at every stoplight or stop sign when you are in the car. Or, do some Kegels every time you go to the bathroom—but not while you are urinating.

Devices

■ **Vaginal weight training** is another form of PFME. The woman inserts a small cone-shaped weight in the vagina for two 15-minute periods per day. The woman must contract the pelvic floor muscles to keep the weight in her vagina. Some women prefer this form of PFME because it helps them identify the correct muscles for contraction. However, this method has not been shown to produce better outcomes than Kegel exercises.

■ A **pessary** is a removable device inserted into the vagina. It is designed to relieve pressure of the pelvic organs on the urethra, which reduces the urge to urinate. When used long term, monitor for vaginal infection and ulceration.

■ An **intravaginal support device** is particularly helpful for women experiencing exercise-related stress incontinence.

■ **Self-intermittent catheterization** can be used to drain the bladder and prevent leakage of urine, especially for those with overflow incontinence.

Medications

■ **Anticholinergics** inhibit involuntary contractions of the bladder, increase capacity of the bladder, and delay the urge to void for people with urge incontinence. Oxybutynin chloride comes in an oral form (Ditropan) or a transdermal patch (Oxytrol) to relax bladder smooth muscle. Transdermal medication is used to treat urge incontinence caused by overactive bladder. The patch relieves symptoms up to 4 days.

■ **Antidepressants** (dulxetine or imipramine) can reduce stress incontinence by causing bladder muscles to relax. Some drugs work by stimulating the nerve that controls the urethral sphincter.

■ **Antispasmotics** help to relax the bladder and prevent urge incontinence. Propantheline bromide (Pro-Banthine) is prescribed to stop bladder muscle contractions (overactive bladder). The typical dosage is 7.5 to 30 mg taken without food three to five times per day.

■ **Muscarinic receptor antagonists** (tolterodine tartrate) block nerve receptors in the smooth muscle of the bladder. These medications control bladder contraction and reduce urinary frequency for people suffering from overactive bladder and urge incontinence.

■ **Estrogen** is used to improve the blood flow and thickness to urethral tissues. Estrogen is not FDA-approved for treatment of stress incontinence, although may be prescribed for other reasons.

■ **Botulinum toxin** injections control spasms of overactive bladder by relaxing the muscles. It is currently not FDA-approved for incontinence, although a therapeutic benefit has been shown.

Surgical Options

■ **Sling procedures**. Placing a urethral sling treats incontinence by lifting the urethra back to a normal position and relieving pressure.

■ **Augmentation of the bladder**. This procedure is reserved for those who do not benefit from other bladder therapies, medication, or self-catheterization. Segments of the bladder are surgically enlarged to improve the bladder capacity. A segment of the bowel is wrapped around the bladder neck to improve the muscle-squeezing action of the bladder.

■ **Injection of bulking agents**. Collagen is injected alongside of the urethra. Effectiveness often lasts a period of years with few complications.

Complementary Alternative Methods

■ **Acupuncture.** In a review comparing 232 published research studies, acupuncture was shown to be the sole complementary and alternative medicine treatment, among reflexology and hypnosis, with early evidence of benefit for incontinence.

■ **Biofeedback** is sometimes used as an adjunct to PFME. Small electrodes are attached to the skin on the

perineum. The electrodes detect a pelvic floor contraction and provide feedback to the patient about the strength of the contraction and the accuracy of the movement.
- **Sacral nerve stimulator.** This electronic device is used for patients who do not respond to behavioral treatment or medication for urge incontinence. The lead wire is placed near the sacral nerve and acts like a bladder pacemaker for better urinary control.

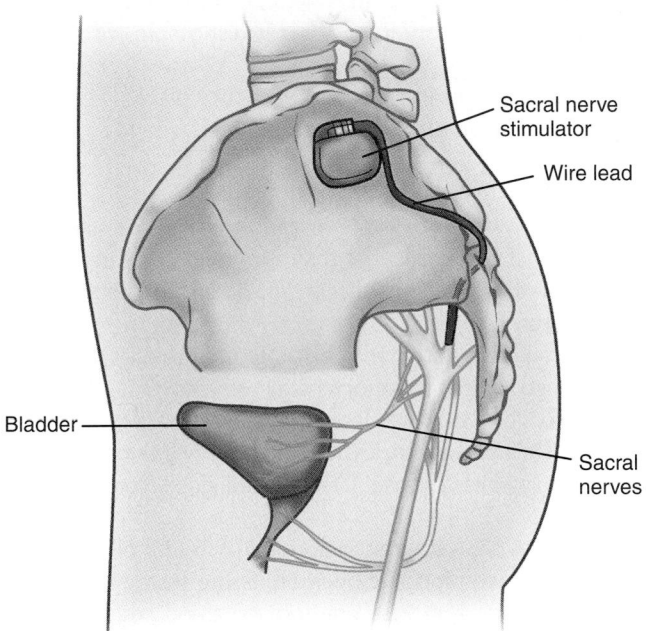

Supportive Interventions

Supportive interventions focus on helping the patient reach the toilet and perform toileting self-care.
- Provide a bedside commode, raised toilet seat, bedpan, urinal, or other aids to make it easier to urinate independently.
- Advise and assist the patient with gait and strength training to improve the person's ability to reach the toilet in time.
- When continence cannot be achieved, provide absorbent products with waterproof coverings. Meticulous skin care must be given when these are used. Under no circumstances should you refer to these as "diapers," as this is disrespectful of the patient's dignity.
- Men with urinary incontinence can use a drip collector, which is a small pocket of padding worn over the penis and held in place with underwear.
- Reassure the patient that urinary incontinence is not inevitable or shameful. It is treatable, and, if not, manageable with medication and/or various devices and behavioral approaches.

References

Hartmann, K. E., McPheeters, M. L., Biller, D. H., et al. (2009, August). Treatment of overactive bladder in women. Evidence Report/Technology Assessment No. 187 (Prepared by the Vanderbilt Evidence-based Practice Center under Contract No. 290-2007-10065-I.) AHRQ Publication No. 09-E017. Rockville, MD: Agency for Healthcare Research and Quality. Retrieved on December 7, 2009, from http://www.ahrq.gov/CLINIC/tp/bladdertp.htm

Lewis, L. (2003). Managing incontinence at home. *American Journal of Nursing*, 3(suppl.), 41.

Clinical Insight 27-3 ➤ Caring for Patients with Urinary Diversions

The overall goals are for the patient to become comfortable with his changed body and to assume self-care.
- Perform a thorough assessment. A healthy stoma ranges in color from deep pink to brick red, regardless of skin color, and is shiny and moist at all times. A pale, dusky, or black stoma often indicates inadequate blood supply; immediately document and report such findings to the surgeon.
- Assess the skin surrounding the stoma for signs of irritation, such as redness, tenderness, and skin breakdown.

When the normally acid urine remains in contact with the skin, it becomes alkaline. Encrustations collect on the skin, and the skin becomes macerated and excoriated. Skin breakdown may lead to infection, pain, and leakage.

- A moisture-proof skin barrier is usually placed around the stoma.

Moisture on the skin can lead to irritation and maceration.

- Be available to discuss the patient's reaction to the stoma.
- Be careful your nonverbal facial expressions do not convey disgust or disapproval when working with the patient and the stoma.
- Closely assess the skin surrounding the stoma.
- Be certain that the collection device fits snugly against the skin.
- Monitor the amount and type of drainage from the stoma.
- Empty the device frequently during the day; connect it to a larger collection bag during the night when the patient is sleeping.
- Provide ample time to explain stoma care and use of ostomy appliances.

For most patients this is a life-long task; therefore patient teaching is essential.

- Barrier creams may be prescribed for irritated skin; if fungal infection develops, nystatin may be prescribed.

Clinical Insight 27-4 ▶ Teaching Your Client About Clean, Intermittent Self-Catheterization

You will need to teach self-catheterization to clients who have compromised ability to spontaneously empty their bladders. In the home setting this is a clean procedure rather than a sterile one. It is referred to as clean, intermittent self-catheterization (CISC). The goals of intermittent self-catheterization are to (1) completely empty the bladder and (2) prevent urinary tract infections.

▪ In teaching the steps of the procedure, consider the client's physical ability to manipulate the catheter and reach the urethra and manipulate the equipment (e.g., range of motion, fine motor skills, degree of sensation).

▪ Encourage the client to drink 8 to 10 eight-ounce glasses of fluid without caffeine each day to ensure a quantity of urine adequate to flush the bladder.

▪ Teach the client to report the signs and symptoms of urinary tract infection: burning, frequency, urgency, dull abdominal ache, fever, or malaise; or urine contains sediment or becomes cloudy, or burning on urination or a fever occurs). Older adults may experience confusion before the other signs and symptoms occur.

▪ Advise the client to contact a healthcare provider if there is bleeding, pain, or difficulty inserting the catheter.

▪ Some CISC catheters can be reused; some are disposable.

▪ Catheterize as often as needed—perhaps every 2 to 3 hours at first.

▪ Discard a reusable catheter when it becomes difficult to clean or difficult to insert. A CISC catheter may be reused for 2 to 4 weeks.

▪ Soak the catheter in a white vinegar solution once a week to control odor and remove encrustation or mucus deposits.

Procedure for Men

1. Try to void before catheterization. If you are unable to void or if the amount is less than 3 ounces (or the amount specified by your healthcare provider), then insert the catheter.
2. Assemble the catheter, lubricant, and drainage receptacle.
3. Thoroughly wash your hands with soap and water; cleanse the penis and the urethral opening.
4. Lubricate the catheter to 6 inches (15 cm).
5. Stand over the toilet or assume a comfortable position (e.g., sitting on the toilet).
6. Hold the penis perpendicular (at a right angle) to your body.
7. Gently insert and advance the catheter.
8. When you meet resistance, at the level of the prostate, take deep breaths to try to relax, and advance the catheter.

9. When urine flow starts, advance the catheter 1 inch (2.5 cm) more; return the penis to its natural position; hold the catheter in place until the urine flow stops and bladder is empty.
10. Withdraw the catheter slowly in small increments to be sure the entire bladder empties.
11. Wash the catheter with soap and water, if it is reusable. Rinse and dry it well. If it is disposable, discard it immediately.
12. Store catheters in a clean, dry, secure place.
13. Record the amount of urine obtained.

Procedure for Women

1. Try to void before catheterization. If you are unable to void or if amount is less than 3 ounces (or the amount specified by your healthcare provider), then insert catheter.
2. Assemble the catheter, lubricant, and drainage receptacle; a good light is important for women.
3. Thoroughly wash hands with soap and water; cleanse your labia and urethra with soap and water or with a moist towelette; rinse. Cleanse and rinse from front to back.
4. Lubricate the catheter to about 1 inch (2.5 cm).
5. Assume a comfortable position. Some women perform CISC standing up with one foot on the toilet.
6. Use a hand mirror to locate the urethral opening, which is between the clitoris and the vagina.
7. Spread your vaginal lips (labia) with the second and fourth fingers; use the middle finger to feel for the urethral opening.
8. Gently insert the catheter into the opening, guiding it upward toward your umbilicus (belly button). This is usually 2 or 3 (5 to 8 cm) inches past the urethral opening.
9. When urine flows, advance the catheter another 1 inch (2.5 cm); hold it in place until the urine stops and your bladder is empty.
10. Withdraw the catheter slowly, in small increments, to be sure the entire bladder empties.
11. If the catheter is reusable, wash it with soap and water; rinse and dry it well. If it is disposable, discard it immediately.
12. Store catheters in a clean, dry, secure place.
13. Record the amount of urine obtained.

Reference

Gilbert, S. M. (2008, May 22). Medical encyclopedia: clean intermittent self-catheterization. Review provided by VeriMed Healthcare Network. Retrieved from http://www.nlm.nih.gov/medlineplus/ency/article/003972.htm.

Assessment Guidelines and Tools

Urinary Elimination History Questions

Usual Urination Pattern

- How often do you urinate?
- Do you get up in the middle of the night to urinate?
- Do you have difficulty getting to the bathroom in time to urinate?
- Do you ever leak urine when you cough, laugh, or exercise?
- Do you ever leak urine on the way to the bathroom?
- Do you need to use pads or tissue in your underwear to catch urine?
- Do you have any difficulty starting to void?

Appearance of Urine

- How would you describe your urine?
- Have you noticed unusual odor with urination?

Changes in Urination Habits or Urine Appearance

- Have you experienced any changes in your voiding pattern recently?
- Have you experienced any changes in the appearance or odor of your urine?

History of Urination Problems

- What has been your experience with urination problems?
- Have you experienced any problems with urinary tract infections or kidney and bladder problems?
- Have you ever lost control of your urination?

- Have you ever had urinary tract surgery or diagnostic procedures?

Use of Urination Aids

- What aids, if any, do you use to help you urinate?
- What is your usual fluid intake over the course of a day?
- What medications are you taking? Have they had any effect on your urination pattern?

Lifestyle Questions

- Where is your bathroom located? Can you get to it easily?
- Can you manage your clothing when you go to the bathroom?
- How much fluid do you drink each day?
- How many caffeinated beverages do you drink?
- Do you smoke?
- Are you bothered with constipation?
- Do you do high-impact exercise (e.g., jogging)?

Presence of Urinary Diversions

- Have you ever had surgery of your urinary tract?
- If so, what and when?

For Infants and Young Children

- Has the child been toilet-trained?
- What elimination routines have been established?

Guidelines for Physical Assessment for Urinary Elimination

Physical assessment for urinary elimination includes examination of the kidneys, bladder, urethra, and skin surrounding the genitals, as appropriate. For a complete discussion of physical examination of the genitourinary system, see Chapter 19, Procedures 19-17 and 19-18, in this volume.

The Kidneys

Technique	Rationale
The **costovertebral (CV) angle** is formed by the junction of the 12th rib and the spine on both sides of the back. Place one palm flat on the CV angle and lightly strike it with the closed fist of the other hand (see the accompanying figure).	You cannot usually palpate the kidneys. Instead, examine them by assessing for costovertebral angle tenderness (CVAT). If kidney inflammation is present, percussion of this angle produces pain.

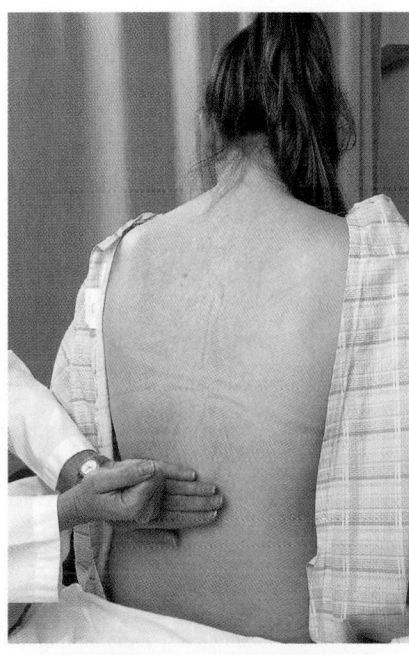

Continued

Guidelines for Physical Assessment for Urinary Elimination—cont'd

The Bladder

Inspect, palpate, and percuss the lower abdomen. Correlate your findings with data about the client's fluid intake and voiding.

▪ Inspect the lower abdomen.	An empty bladder, or one with limited urine, is small and sits below the symphysis pubis. In contrast, a distended bladder rises above the symphysis pubis. If it is very distended, you may be able to see a rounded swelling above the symphysis pubis.
▪ Lightly palpate the lower abdomen to define the bladder margin. Observe the patient's response to palpation, noting signs of tenderness or discomfort.	An empty bladder, or one with limited urine, will not be palpable.
▪ Percuss the area.	A distended bladder produces a dull sound as opposed to the normal tympanic sound of intestinal air.

The Urethra

▪ Inspect the urethral orifice. Look for erythema, discharge, swelling, or odor.	These are all signs of infection, trauma, or inflammation.

The Perineal Area

▪ Frequently inspect skin color, condition, texture, turgor, and presence of urine or stool.	Clients who have urine leakage or a urinary catheter are at risk for perineal skin problems. Ammonia in the urine may result in skin excoriation, skin breakdown, and subsequent infection. If both urine and stool are present on the skin, the likelihood of skin breakdown increases.

Diagnostic Testing

Urinalysis

Characteristic	Expected Findings	Variations
Color	A freshly voided sample is pale yellow to deep amber.	Urine becomes lighter in color and may even be clear if fluid intake is high or urine output is excessive. Urine becomes dark in color as it becomes more concentrated with decreased fluid intake or excessive fluid loss. Color is also affected by diet and medications.
pH	5.0–9.0, with an average of 6.0	Indicates kidneys' ability to help maintain balanced hydrogen ion concentration in the blood. The pH increases (more alkaline) if the client eats dairy products or citrus fruits or has a vegetarian diet. The pH decreases (more acidic) if the client eats a high-protein diet or consumes cranberry juice.
Specific gravity	1.001–1.035	This is a reflection of the kidney's ability to concentrate urine. Specific gravity rises with limited fluid intake or dehydration. It may also rise with kidney disease. Specific gravity decreases as fluid intake increases.
Clarity	A freshly voided sample should be translucent. If the urine sits for a period of time, it will become cloudy.	Cloudiness in a freshly voided sample indicates the presence of other constituents in the urine. These may include bacteria, RBCs, WBCs, sperm, prostatic fluid, or vaginal discharge.
Odor	Fresh urine is aromatic.	Certain foods, such as garlic, onions, and asparagus, may give urine a distinctive odor. Bacteria will give urine an ammonia-like odor. A sweet syrup odor may indicate a congenital metabolic disorder.

Diagnostic Testing

Diagnostic Testing

Protein	< 20 mg/dL	Proteinuria is the most common indicator of renal disease. Protein is increased in diabetic nephrophty, glomerulonephritis, nephrosis, and toxemia of pregnancy. May be increased in benign proteinuria secondary to stress or physical exercise.
Glucose	Negative	Glucose is found in the urine with elevated blood sugars and diabetes.
Ketones	Negative	Presence of ketones indicates impaired carbohydrate metabolism. Ketones may be detected with diabetes, fever, fasting, high-protein diets, starvation, vomiting, postanesthesia period.
Hemoglobin	Negative on dipstick If RBCs are assessed via microscopic exam: < 5 per high-power field	Hemoglobin may be detected with infection of the urinary tract, disease of the bladder, glomerulonephritis, pyelonephritis, trauma, nephrolithiasis, hemolytic reactions, or trauma. It also may be present in samples from women who are currently menstruating.
Bilirubin	Negative	Increased bilirubin occurs with liver disease.
Urobilinogen	Up to 1 mg/dL	Increased is found in cirrhosis, heart failure, liver disease, infectious mononucleosis, malaria, and pernicious anemia.
Nitrite	Negative	Nitrite is used to test for bacteriuria. Increased in the presence of nitrite-forming bacteria.
Leukocyte esterase	Negative If WBCs are assessed via microscopic exam: < 5 per high-power field	Leukocytes are increased in bacterial infection, calculus formation, fungal or parasitic infection, glomerulonephritis, interstitial nephritis, or tumor.
Renal cells	None seen	Renal cells come from the lining of the collecting ducts. Their presence indicates damage to the tubular network.
Transitional cells	None seen	Transitional cells line the renal pelvis, ureter, bladder, and proximal urethra. Their presence is seen with infection, trauma, and malignancy.
Squamous cells	Rare	Typically insignificant: Squamous cells line the vagina and distal portion of the urethra.
Casts	Rare hyaline; otherwise negative	Large numbers of hyaline casts are seen in renal disease, hypertension, with diuretic use, and fever. Granular casts are seen in renal disease, viral infection, or lead intoxication.
Crystals	Absent in freshly voided sample	Crystals in the urine may indicate an old sample, stone formation in the urinary tract, gout, high dietary intake of oxalates, liver disease, or side effect of chemotherapy.
Bacteria, yeast, parasites	None seen	Microbes in the urine indicate an infection of the urinary tract.

Source: Adapted from Van Leeuwen, A., Kranpitz, T., & Smith, L. (2006). *Davis's comprehensive handbook of laboratory and diagnostic tests with nursing implications* (2nd ed.). Philadelphia: F. A. Davis.

Diagnostic Testing

Blood Studies: BUN and Creatinine

Normal Ranges		**Levels may be increased in:**	**Levels may be decreased in:**
Blood urea nitrogen (BUN)	8–20 mg/dL	➤ Renal failure	➤ Inadequate protein intake
Creatinine	0.5–1.1 mg/dL	➤ Impaired renal perfusion	➤ Malabsorption syndromes
		➤ Kidney infection or inflammation	➤ Liver disease
		➤ Kidney obstruction	
		➤ Dehydration	
		➤ Excessive protein intake	
		➤ Use of total parenteral nutrition (TPN)	

Source: Adapted from Van Leeuwen, A., Kranpitz, R., & Smith, L. (2006). *Davis's comprehensive handbook of laboratory and diagnostic tests with nursing implications* (2nd ed.). Philadelphia: F. A. Davis.

Studies of the Urinary System

Direct Visualization Studies

Cystoscopy—Direct visualization of the urethra, bladder, and ureteral orifices by insertion of a scope. May be used to obtain biopsies and treat pathology of visualized areas.

Preparation

➤ Instruct the patient the procedure is performed under anesthesia.

➤ Ensure that a signed consent form is on the chart.

➤ Restrict food and fluids for 8 hours if the patient is receiving general anesthesia. For local anesthesia, allow only clear liquids for 8 hours before the procedure.

Post-Procedure Care

➤ Monitor vital signs and intake and output (I&O).

➤ Observe the characteristics of urine after the procedure.

➤ Encourage increased fluid intake.

➤ Report suprapubic or flank pain, chills, or difficulty urinating.

Cystometry—Urodynamic testing of bladder function; measures bladder pressure and volume.

Preparation

➤ Ensure a signed consent form is on the chart.

➤ Explain that patient cooperation with positioning and activity is crucial during the test.

➤ There are no food or fluid restrictions before the test.

Post-Procedure Care

➤ Monitor vital signs and I&O.

➤ Encourage increased fluid intake.

➤ Report suprapubic or flank pain, chills, or difficulty urinating.

Indirect Visualization Studies

Intravenous pyelogram (IVP)—Uses radiopaque contrast medium to visualize the kidneys, ureters, bladder, and renal pelvis. Evaluates renal function by analyzing flow of contrast over time.

Retrograde pyelogram—Uses radiopaque contrast medium to visualize the renal collecting system. Contrast media is injected via a ureteral catheter inserted through a cystoscope.

Preparation

➤ Obtain history of allergies. This test is contraindicated for patients with allergies to shellfish or iodinated dye.

➤ Ensure baseline BUN and creatinine results are available. This test is contraindicated for patients who are in renal failure.

➤ Ensure that a signed consent form is on the chart.

➤ NPO 8 hours before the procedure.

➤ Some patients may require a laxative the evening before the surgery to clear the GI tract and improve visualization.

Post-Procedure Care

➤ Encourage increased fluid intake.

➤ Monitor vital signs and I&O.

➤ Observe for reactions to the contrast media: rash, nausea, hives.

➤ For a retrograde pyelogram, ureteral catheters may be in place. They will require separate monitoring of I&O for each side.

Ultrasound—Uses sound waves to produce an image of the organs

Preparation

➤ Ensure a signed consent form is on the chart.

➤ Fluid restrictions may be applied based on the organ to be scanned.

Post-Procedure Care

➤ No special care is required.

Computerized tomography—Using contrast media, examines body sections from different angles using a narrow x-ray beam to produce a three-dimensional picture of the area of the body being scanned.

Preparation

➤ Obtain history of allergies. This test is contraindicated for patients with allergies to shellfish or iodinated dye.

➤ Ensure a signed consent form is on the chart.

➤ NPO 8 hours before the procedure.

➤ Remove all metal objects from the patient's body (e.g., eyeglasses, rings, safety pins).

Post-Procedure Care

➤ Monitor vital signs and I&O.

➤ Observe for reactions to the contrast media: rash, nausea, hives.

Renal biopsy—Removal of a piece of kidney tissue for microscopic evaluation.

Preparation

➤ Ensure baseline coagulation studies and hemoglobin results are available.

➤ Ensure a signed consent form is on the chart.

➤ NPO 8 hours before the procedure.

➤ Instruct the patient that sedation and/or pain medication may be given.

Post-Procedure Care

➤ Monitor vital signs and I&O.

➤ Have patient rest in bed on affected side for at least 30 minutes with a pillow or sandbag under the site to prevent bleeding.

➤ The patient should be on bedrest for 24 hours.

➤ Monitor biopsy site for bleeding.

➤ Monitor urine for presence of blood.

Source: Van Leeuwen, A., Kranpitz, R., & Smith, L. (2006). *Davis's comprehensive handbook of laboratory and diagnostic tests with nursing implications* (2nd ed.). Philadelphia: F. A. Davis.

Standardized Language

Interventions When Altered Urination Is the Problem

Biofeedback

Bladder Irrigation

Environmental Management

Fluid Management

Fluid Monitoring

Medication Administration

Medication Management

Pelvic Muscle Exercise

Pessary Management

Prompted Voiding

Self-Care Assistance: Toileting

Urinary Incontinence Care:
  Enuresis

Specimen Management

Teaching: Individual
  Tube-Care: Urinary

Urinary Bladder Training

Urinary Catheterization

Urinary Catheterization:
  Intermittent

Urinary Elimination
  Management

Urinary Habit Training

Urinary Incontinence Care

Urinary Retention Care

Weight Management

Interventions When Altered Urination Is the Etiology of Other Problems

Fluid Management

Infection Protection

Ostomy Care

Perineal Care

Self-Esteem Enhancement

Skin Care: Topical Treatments

Skin Surveillance

Source: Bulechek, G., Butcher, H., & Dochterman, J. (2008). *Nursing interventions classification (NIC)* (5th ed.). St. Louis, MO: C.V. Mosby. Used with permission.

THINKING CRITICALLY ABOUT URINARY ELIMINATION

The exercises in the following section allow you to practice the kind of thinking you will use as a full-spectrum nurse. Because these are critical-thinking activities, there is usually no single right answer. We do not provide answers for these questions because it is more important for you to think about the questions than to arrive at the "right" answer. These questions are designed to improve your thinking more than to "cover content." Discuss answers with your peers—discussion can stimulate critical thinking. If you have difficulty with any of the questions, consult with your instructor.

Applying the Full-Spectrum Nursing Model

PATIENT SITUATION

You are providing care to an older-adult woman, Mrs. Patel, who has a number of health concerns, including diabetes and obesity. Mrs. Patel seeks healthcare because she is experiencing burning with urination, frequency, and urgency. You explain to her these are signs of a urinary tract infection. You discover while taking your nursing history that she also has difficulty with urinary continence. When asking her about toileting habits, she tells you she often doesn't "make it to the bathroom" even while at home. This has been going on for about 3 years now. She has trouble getting up and walking upstairs to the bathroom because of a foot ulcer that doesn't seem to be healing well. Mrs. Patel's affect is flat with little expression. During your time with her, she seems to have little interest in talking about her health concerns. When you ask her about what she does to get out or socialize, she admits to being hesitant to go far because she is afraid of wetting without knowing it and carrying an odor that would be embarrassing to her.

THINKING

1. *Theoretical Knowledge (Recall of Facts and Principles):*

a. What kind(s) of incontinence is this patient likely to have?

b. What are this patient's risk factors for incontinence?

2. *Critical Thinking (Contextual Awareness):*

a. What aspects of this situation have you experienced or observed before in your role as a caregiver?

b. How might those past experiences affect your perception in this situation?

DOING

3. *Practical Knowledge (Patient Teaching):*

a. How could you encourage this woman to seek healthcare for managing her urinary incontinence?

b. What might you ask your patient to do in order to get a better idea of her bladder history and toileting habits?

c. By looking at Mrs. Patel's bladder diary, you see a pattern suggestive of urinary incontinence. What other behavioral strategies might you suggest to improve her ability to have control of her bladder?

CARING

4. *Self-Knowledge:*

a. Have you ever personally experienced urinary urgency when you had trouble getting to the bathroom in time? Reflect on this experience and examine how you might feel if you were incontinent much of the time.

b. In what way(s) can you show compassion for the patient who has urinary incontinence?

Critical Thinking and Clinical Reasoning

1. You receive a report from the NAP that a patient with no history of urinary elimination problems has had 150 mL of oral liquids in 6 hours and has voided 100 mL of clear, dark amber urine. His vital signs at the start of the shift were as follows: blood pressure, 108/76 mm Hg; pulse, 72 beats/min; respirations, 18 breaths/min; temperature, 98.6°F (37.0°C). The most recent check revealed blood pressure, 112/80 mm Hg; pulse, 88 beats/min; respirations, 22 breaths/min; and temperature, 100.4°F (38.0°C).

   a. What conclusion might you draw about what has caused these symptoms?

   b. What actions should you take?

2. As you make patient rounds, you discover a collection bag for an indwelling catheter placed on the bed above the level of the patient's bladder.

   a. What should you do first? What assessments should you make?

   b. What teaching would be important in this situation?

3. Nursing assistive personnel (NAP) complain that Mr. Jones, a patient with dementia, keeps urinating in his trash can and in the hallway.

   a. What special measures could be taken to assist Mr. Jones in finding the bathroom?

   b. What data could be helpful in developing a plan for Mr. Jones?

4. For each of the following concepts, use critical thinking to describe how or why it is important to nursing, patient care, or urinary elimination. Note that these are *not* to be merely definitions.

Blood pressure	Hydration
Kidney tubules	Specific gravity
Developmental stage	Urinary incontinence
Privacy	

What Are the Main Points in This Chapter?

➤ The urinary system consists of two kidneys, two ureters, the urinary bladder, and the urethra.

➤ The kidneys filter nitrogen and other metabolic wastes, toxins, excess ions, and water from the bloodstream and excrete them as urine.

➤ The bladder has a normal average storage capacity of 500 mL (1 pint), but it may distend, when needed, to a capacity twice that amount.

➤ Voiding occurs when contraction of the detrusor muscle pushes stored urine through the relaxed internal urethral sphincter into the urethra.

➤ The kidneys produce urine at a rate of approximately 60 mL per hour, or 1500 mL per day. Most people urinate about five to six times per day.

➤ Voiding and control of urination require normal functioning of the bladder and the urethra, as well as an intact brain, spinal cord, and nerves supplying the bladder and urethra.

➤ As an adult ages, the number of functional nephrons gradually decreases, along with the ability to dilute and concentrate urine. The potential volume of the bladder also decreases as the bladder wall loses elasticity; thus, older adults need to urinate more frequently.

➤ Substances that contain caffeine act as diuretics and increase urine production.

➤ A diet high in salt causes water retention and decreases urine production.

➤ Medications with anticholinergic effects inhibit the free flow of urine and may contribute to urinary retention.

➤ An adequately hydrated adult produces clear yellow urine. Concentrated urine is darker in color, but dilute urine can appear colorless.

➤ A clean-catch urine specimen is preferred for many diagnostic tests. To collect this specimen, the client must cleanse the genitalia before voiding and collect the sample in midstream.

➤ Sterile urine specimens may be obtained by inserting a catheter into the bladder or withdrawing a sample from an indwelling catheter.

➤ 24-hour urine collection requires collection of all urine voided in the time period. The start time of the 24-hour collection begins when the first-voided urine is discarded.

➤ A routine urinalysis is one of the most commonly ordered laboratory tests. It is used as an overall screening test as well as an aid to diagnose renal, hepatic, and other diseases.

➤ Normal urine is free of bacteria, viruses, and fungi. Urinary tract infections are often caused by the introduction of *Escherichia coli (E. coli)*, which normally live in the colon, into the urethra and bladder.

➤ Urinary retention is an inability to empty the bladder. It may be due to obstruction, nerve problems, infection, surgery, medications, or anxiety.

➤ Urinary catheterization is the introduction of pliable tube (catheter) into the bladder to allow drainage of urine.

➤ Urinary incontinence (UI) is a lack of voluntary control over urination. Nurses can independently perform the primary interventions to manage UI.

➤ A urinary diversion, or urostomy, is a surgically created opening for elimination of urine.

➤ A patient with a urinary diversion requires physical and psychological care. The goal is to have the patient become comfortable with his changed body and assume self-care.

For practice questions for this chapter,

 Go to **NCLEX-Style Chapter Quiz,** on the Student Resource Disk or DavisPlus at http://davisplus.fadavis.com/Wilkinson2

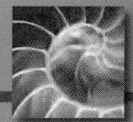 # Knowledge Map

Urinary Elimination

Structures:
Kidneys – filter; regulate
Nephrons – urine formation
Ureters – urine transport
Bladder – urine storage
Urethra – urine transport
Sphincters – flow control

Urination

Factors Affecting:
- Developmental stage: infants, elders
- Personal; sociocultural; environmental
  - time; privacy; loss of dignity
- Nutrition; hydration
- Activity
- Medications
- Surgery/ anesthesia

Pathological Conditions Affecting Urination:
- UTI
- Calculi
- BPH
- Cardiovascular & metabolic diseases
- Neurogenic bladder
- Impairments: mobility, communication, cognition

Assessing Urine:
• Intake and output
• Urine studies
  - analysis
  - specific gravity
  - dipstick
• Specimens from:
  - fresh-voided
  - clean catch
  - sterile specimen
  - 24-hour collection

Promoting Normal Urination:
• Provide privacy
• Position properly
• Establish toileting routines
• Provide adequate fluids/ nutrition
• Assist with voiding

Urinary catheterization
- Straight catheter
- Indwelling catheter
- Suprapubic catheter

- Skin care
- Lifestyle changes
- Bladder training
- Scheduled voiding
  Kegels
- Biofeedback
- Anti-incontinent devices

Common Urinary Problems:
• Urinary tract infections
  - urethritis; cystitis; pyelonephritis

• Urinary retention

• Urinary incontinence:
  - urge
  - stress
  - overflow
  - functional
  - transient
  - reflex
  - enuresis

• Urinary diversions
  - cutaneous ureterostomy
  - ileal conduit
  - Kock pouch (continent urostomy)

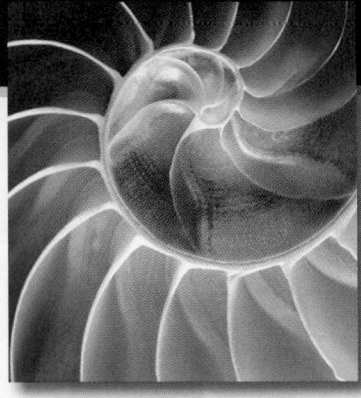

CHAPTER 28

Bowel Elimination

For a podcast of an overview of this chapter,

 Go to Student Resources, **Podcast – Chapter Overviews, Chapter 28,** on DavisPlus at http://davisplus.fadavis.com/ Wilkinson2

Caring for the Garcias

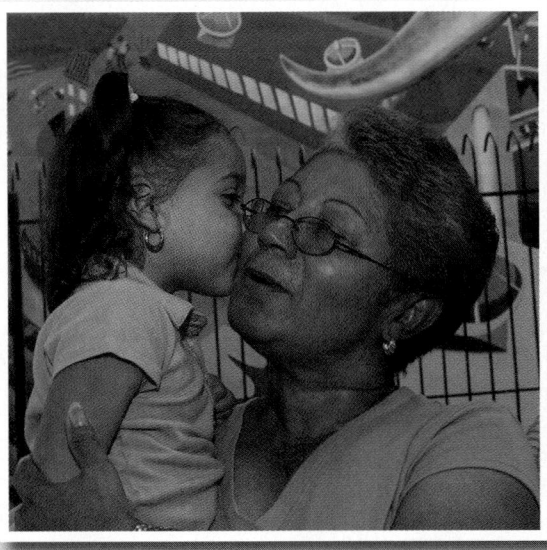

The exercises in the following section allow you to practice the kind of thinking you will use as a full-spectrum nurse. Because these are critical-thinking questions, there is usually no single right answer. We do not provide answers for these questions because it is more important for you to think about the questions than to arrive at the "right" answer. These questions are designed to improve your thinking more than to "cover content." Discuss answers with your peers—discussion can stimulate critical thinking. If you have difficulty with any of these questions, consult with your instructor.

Flordelisa Garcia arrives at the family health center for a scheduled appointment, accompanied by her granddaughter, Bettina. Recently, Flordelisa has been constipated and has had several episodes of bleeding with bowel movements (BMs). She has read that a change in bowel habits is a sign of colon cancer and is worried about that. She brought her granddaughter along because she is also having bowel problems. Bettina's bowel habits are erratic. At times she has a soft BM daily. However, she has also had bouts of constipation and diarrhea. Flordelisa would like advice on her granddaughter's elimination status. As a critical thinker, you will begin by obtaining accurate, credible information.

A. What history questions would be appropriate to ask Flordelisa regarding her bowel concerns? What data do you need? How can you get it? Are the data accurate? What information is important; what is not? Write some specific questions, just as you would ask them in an interview.

Caring for the Garcias (continued)

B. What physical assessments would you conduct for Flordelisa to add to, and possibly to validate, your subjective data?

C. Now you must consider the context. What factors must you consider when gathering a history on Bettina?

D. The family nurse practitioner (FNP) examines Flordelisa and determines that she has external hemorrhoids that have been bleeding because of recent straining at stool. The FNP orders rectal suppositories to decrease the swelling of the hemorrhoids and asks you to teach Flordelisa about

necessary lifestyle changes. What additional information will you need to gather to provide this teaching? Recall that you have already obtained a significant amount of information from the history questions. Again, think about context: Whatever the content of your teaching, Flordelisa will be using that information to care for herself and her granddaughter in her home.

E. The FNP examines Bettina and tells you that the examination is normal. Use your theoretical knowledge of bowel elimination and Bettina's developmental stage to think of possible reasons for her erratic bowel pattern.

Practical **Knowledge**
knowing how

To help you promote normal bowel elimination and support patients who have bowel elimination problems, this section provides practical knowledge of procedures and clinical insights for identifying problems and providing interventions. You will also find in this section assessment guidelines for assisting patients who are having diagnostic studies of the gastrointestinal system and a list of NANDA-I diagnoses, NOC outcomes, and NIC interventions associated with bowel elimination.

Procedures

The procedures in this chapter will help you provide care to patients who have problems with bowel elimination.

Procedure 28-1 Testing Stool for Occult Blood

➤ For steps to follow in *all* procedures, refer to the Universal Steps for All Procedures found on the inside back cover of Volume 2.

➤ *Note:* According to colorectal screening guidelines, all persons age 50 or older should be screened every 1 to 2 years for occult (hidden) blood in the stool. The 2008 National Guideline Clearinghouse (NGC) and the 2007 American Cancer Society recommendations are for annual screening after age 50. High-risk groups require initial screening at a younger age, and should perhaps undergo genetic testing.

Critical Aspects

- Patients should avoid foods that may alter the accuracy of the test for 3 days before collecting a stool specimen.
- Review the patient's medications. If the patient is taking salicylates, nonsteroidal anti-inflammatory drugs (NSAIDs), iron, anticoagulants, and colchicines, consult with the physician.
- Take care that the sample is not contaminated by urine or menstrual blood.
- Test two small stool samples from separate areas of the large sample.
- Following the manufacturer's directions, place the correct number and size of drops of developer solution into the "windows" of the opposite side on the Hemoccult slide.
- Record a positive result if the slide windows turn blue.

(continued on next page)

Procedure 28-1 ■ **Testing Stool for Occult Blood** (continued)

Equipment

- Clean gloves
- Tongue blade or other wooden applicator
- Clean, dry collection container to place in the commode, or a clean, dry bedpan
- Facility-specific fecal occult blood test (FOBT) slide or test paper
- Developing solution

Delegation

You can delegate the collection and testing of a stool sample for occult blood to the unlicensed assistive personnel (NAP) if the NAP has the necessary skills and the patient's condition is stable. Inform the NAP of any special considerations (e.g., the need to assist the patient with ambulation or the need for a bedpan). Instruct the NAP to inform you if there is visible blood in the stool and to show you the FOBT slide for evaluation of results when the test is complete.

Pre-Procedure Assessment

- **Assess the patient's mobility status.**
Determines the patient's ability to participate in stool collection, the need for a bedpan or commode, and so forth.

- **Assess the patient's dietary history for the past 24 to 48 hours.**

Some foods, such as red meat, chicken, fish, horseradish, turnips, or raw vegetables, may lead to a false-positive reading. Vitamin C in excess of 250 mg per day can produce a false-negative result.

- **Assess medication history.**
If the patient is taking medications, such as salicylates, NSAIDs, iron, oxidizing drugs, reserpine, corticosteroids, anticoagulants, colchicines, and high doses of vitamin C, consult with a physician. These medications may cause a false-positive reading. If possible, they will be discontinued for 7 days before the test. If the patient must have them, then the results must be interpreted taking them into consideration.

- **Assess for the presence of hemorrhoids.**
Bleeding hemorrhoids will cause a positive hemetest. Hemoccult is intended to detect blood in the intestines, which is not always visible when passed through the stool from higher up in the intestine.

- **If the patient is female, ask whether she is menstruating.**
Menstrual blood may cause a false-positive result for intestinal bleeding.

- **Check the expiration date on the developing solution for the FOBT test slide.**
- **Assess the patient's or family's understanding of the need for the stool test.**
Provides a baseline for health teaching.

➤ When performing the procedure, always identify your patient according to agency policy and be attentive to standard precautions, hand hygiene, patient safety and privacy, body mechanics, and documentation.

Procedure Steps

1. Determine whether the test will be done by the nurse at the point of care (e.g., in the home or at the bedside) or by lab personnel.
Because of the regulatory and billing practices in some settings, this test may be completed by lab personnel.

2. Ask the patient to void before collecting the stool specimen.
Helps prevent contaminating the stool with urine.

3. Don procedure gloves and place a clean, dry container for the stool specimen into the toilet or bedside commode in such a manner that any urine falls into the toilet and the fecal specimen falls into the container. Obtain a clean, dry bedpan for a patient who is immobile.

Using a sample of stool that comes in contact with either urine or water may produce an inaccurate test result.

4. Instruct the patient to defecate into the container, or place the patient on the bedpan. Do not contaminate the specimen with toilet tissue.

5. Once the specimen has been obtained, wash your hands, and don clean procedure gloves.
Prevent the spread of intestinal bacteria.

6. Gather the necessary testing supplies. Be sure you understand the directions for the testing kit you are using.
This procedure gives instructions for using the FOBT slide method.

7. Explain the purpose of the test. Explain to the patient that serial specimens may be needed.
Testing serial specimens decreases the chances of a false-negative finding.

8. Open the specimen side of the FOBT slide. With a tongue depressor or other applicator, collect a small sample of stool and spread it thinly onto one "window" of the FOBT slide.

9. With a different applicator or the opposite end of the tongue blade, collect a second small sample of stool from a different location in the large sample. Spread the second sample thinly onto the second "window" of the slide.

Reduces the possibility of a false-negative result. ▼

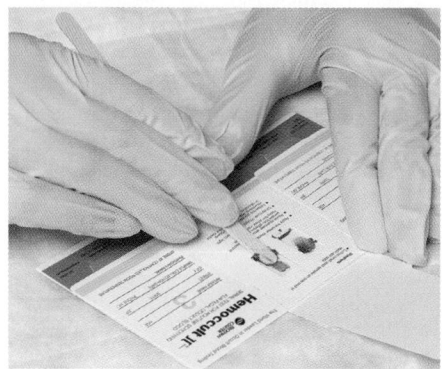

10. Wrap the tongue depressor in tissue and a paper towel; place it in a waste receptacle. Do not flush it. *Prevents transfer of microorganisms. Flushing would likely clog the plumbing.*

11. Close the FOBT slide. *Prevents the transfer of microorganisms from the specimen smears on the slide.*

12. If the test is to be done by laboratory personnel, transfer the specimen to a clean dry container, being careful not to contaminate the outside of the container with feces. Label the specimen in the presence of the patient according to agency policy, and place it into the proper receptacle for transportation to the lab.

13. If you are to perform the test, turn the slide over, and open the opposite side of the FOBT slide. Place one or two drops of developing solution onto each

"window." Follow the directions on the package regarding the number of drops of the developing solution. *Ensures an accurate reading.* ▼

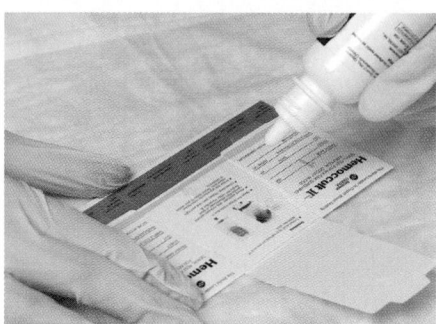

Evaluation

- Observe the color of the paper inside the FOBT slide windows for 30 to 60 seconds.
- If the paper turns blue, consider the test for occult blood to be positive.

Patient Teaching

- Inform the patient of the reasons for performing the test.
- Explain the possible implications of a positive occult blood test, if one is obtained.

Home Care

- Determine the client's level of cognition and manual dexterity to assess his ability to follow instructions and physically perform the test.
- Explain necessary dietary and medication restrictions (see the "Pre-Procedure Assessment" section of this procedure).
- Instruct the client to collect the specimen in a clean, dry container. If an appropriate container is not available, the client may use the toilet.
- If defecating in the toilet, the client should flush it immediately prior to obtaining the sample. If commercial toilet bowl cleaners are in use, remove them from the tank, and flush twice. Then lay rice paper (from the kit) directly on the water; it is okay to get it wet. When using the probe to take the stool sample, take the sample from any area of stool that is above the water line.

- Protect the slide from heat, light, and household chemicals.
- Home collection slides come in a kit, connected together as a set of three. Instruct the client not to tear them apart.
- Emphasize to the client that each sample should be from separate bowel movements on separate days.
- After all three specimens have been collected over the course of at least 3 days, store the slide in a paper envelope to air-dry.
- The client must place the slides in the special mailing pouch that comes with the slides, if they are to be sent back to the lab. The slides should be returned to the care provider or lab no later than 14 days after the first sample was collected.

For additional instructions,

 Go to the **Hemoccult Web site** at www.hemoccultfobt.com

Documentation

- Document the date and time of the specimen collection, both in the patient record and on the specimen container or FOBT kit.
- Note the appearance of the stool (e.g., color, odor) and the presence of blood, mucus, or other abnormal constituents.
- Note any rectal bleeding or discomfort during and after defecation.
- Document the test results on the appropriate agency form.
- Notify the appropriate care provider of the results.

(continued on next page)

Procedure 28-1 ■ Testing Stool for Occult Blood (continued)

Sample documentation:

06/14/12   0915   *Specimen taken from 2 separate sections of yellowish brown soft stool containing mucus. No rectal bleeding or discomfort with defecation. Specimen sent to lab; test results pending.* — S. Hoeszle, RN

Practice Resources

The American Cancer Society (2008); Foran, M., Petersen, J., & Llewandrowski, K. (2006); Gomella L., & Haist, S. (n.d.); Institute for Clinical Systems Improvement (ICSI) (2008); The Joint Commission (2008); Kaiser Permanente Care Management Institute (2006); Siegal, J., Rhinehart, E., Jackson, M., et al. (2007); Sinawer, S., Fletcher, R., Rex, D., et al. (2003).

Procedure 28-2 ■ Placing and Removing a Bedpan

➤ For steps to follow in *all* procedures, refer to the Universal Steps for All Procedures found on the inside back cover of Volume 2.

Critical Aspects

- Determine whether the patient will need to use a regular bedpan or a fracture pan.
- Don clean procedure gloves.
- Help the patient to achieve a position on the bedpan that will be most helpful in facilitating urinary or bowel elimination. Place the patient in a semi-Fowler's position whenever possible. Modify the position based on the patient's condition.
- Provide toilet tissue, clean washcloths, and towels for the patient to perform personal hygiene when elimination is complete. Assist if the patient cannot perform these tasks independently.

Equipment

- Bedpan
- Two pairs of clean gloves
- Toilet tissue
- Two washcloths, towel, and basin
- Waterproof pad
- Bedpan cover

Delegation

You may delegate the placement and removal of a bedpan to the NAP after ensuring that the NAP has the necessary skills and that the patient's condition is stable. Complete the following assessments, and inform the NAP of any special considerations (e.g., medical or surgical conditions that will necessitate the use of a fracture pan, extra care with turning or required positioning based on medical condition).

Pre-Procedure Assessments

- Assess the patient's level of consciousness, ability to follow directions, and mobility status.

Helps determine whether one or two persons are needed to complete the procedure.

- Determine the patient's comfort level—note the presence of rectal or abdominal pain, hemorrhoids, or perianal irritation.

Pain can cause difficulty with positioning and bearing down during defecation. Any unexplained pain should be evaluated by the primary care provider.

- Assess the physical size of the patient and whether the patient can sit up or lie flat when using a bedpan.

Determines the type of bedpan to use and whether you need additional personnel to assist.

- Identify factors that will necessitate the use of a fracture pan. (Examples include a fractured pelvis; total hip replacement; lower back surgery; presence of casts, splints, or braces on lower limbs; or an obese patient who cannot be placed on a regular bedpan.)
- Auscultate bowel sounds, and palpate for distention if necessary.

The colon when full with fecal matter is a rounded, firm mass. A smooth, round mass above the symphysis pubis is a distended bladder.

- Review the patient's chart to determine the need to obtain a stool specimen.

Promotes efficiency by allowing you to obtain a specimen container before placing the patient on the bedpan.

■ Procedure 28-2A Placing a Bedpan

➤ When performing the procedure, always identify your patient according to agency policy and be attentive to standard precautions, hand hygiene, patient safety and privacy, body mechanics, and documentation.

Procedure Steps

1. Obtain the necessary supplies, and take them to the patient's room. Leave clean washcloths, towel, and basin with warm water at the bedside for use during bedpan removal.
The patient will need to wash her hands after using the bedpan.

2. If the bedpan is metal, place it under warm, running water for a few seconds. Then dry it, making sure bedpan is not too hot.
A metal bedpan is very cold. Running it under warm water allows the patient to be more comfortable and helps relax the anal sphincter. Most bedpans now are made of disposable plastic.

3. Raise the siderail on the opposite side from where you are working.
Prevents patient from falling out of bed and gives the patient something to hold onto while moving around in bed.

4. Raise the bed to a comfortable height.
Allows you to use good body mechanics and prevents muscle strain.

5. Prepare the patient by folding down the covers to a point that will allow for placement of the bedpan.

6. Wash your hands and don clean procedure gloves.
Prevents the spread of microorganisms via contact with urine or feces.

7. Observe for the presence of dressings, drains, intravenous fluids, and traction.
These appliances may hinder the patient from assisting with the procedure and may create the need for assistance from another caregiver.

Procedure Variation
For the Patient Able to Move/ Turn Independently in Bed

8. Position the patient.

Step 8 Variation. Supine Position
a. Lower the head of the bed, placing the patient in a supine position.

b. Ask the patient to lift her hips. The patient may need to raise her knees to a flexed position, place her feet flat on the bed, and push up. You can also assist the patient to raise her hips by sliding a hand under the small of her back.

Step 8 Variation. Semi-Fowler's Position
c. Place the bed in a semi-Fowler's position.
d. Ask the patient to raise her hips by pushing up on raised siderails or by using an overhead trapeze.

9. Place the bedpan.

Step 9 Variation. Regular Bedpan
a. Place the bedpan under the patient's buttocks so that the wide, rounded end is toward the back. Do not push the pan under the patient's buttocks.

Step 9 Variation. Fracture Pan
b. When using a fracture pan, place the wide, rounded end toward the front.

10. Instruct or assist the patient to lower her hips onto the bedpan. Move to step 16.

Procedure Variation
For the Patient Unable to Move/ Turn Independently

11. Ask for help from another healthcare worker if the patient's condition warrants.

12. With the patient in the supine position, lower the head of the bed.

13. Assist the patient to the side-lying position. Use a turn sheet, if necessary.

14. Place the bedpan.

Step 14 Variation. Regular Bedpan
a. Place the bedpan under the patient's buttocks so that the wide, rounded end is toward the back.

Do not push the pan under the patient's buttocks. ▼

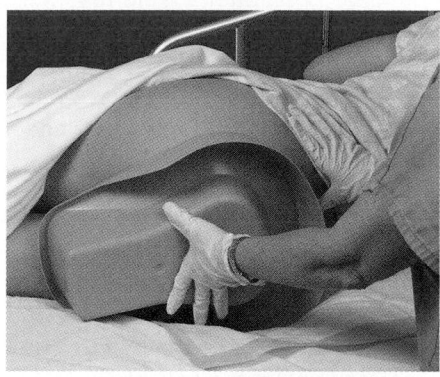

Step 14 Variation. Fracture Pan
b. When using a fracture pan, place the wide, rounded end toward the front. ▼

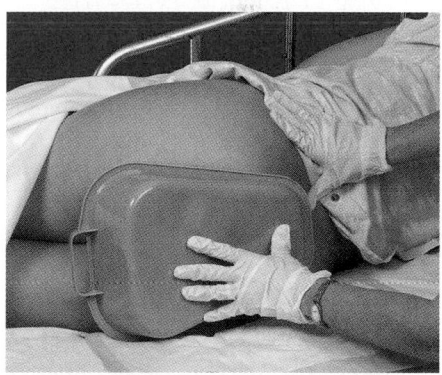

15. Holding the bedpan in place, slowly roll the patient back and onto the bedpan.

16. Replace the covers; raise the head of the bed to a position of comfort for the patient. Place a rolled towel, blanket, or small pillow under the sacrum (lumbar curve of the back). Place the call light and toilet tissue within the patient's reach. Make certain that the bed is returned to its lowest position and that the upper siderails are raised.
Provides privacy, comfort, and safety.

17. Remove your gloves and wash your hands.
Prevents the transmission of intestinal bacteria.

(continued on next page)

Procedure 28-2 ■ **Placing and Removing a Bedpan** (continued)

■ *Procedure 28-2B* **Removing a Bedpan**

➤ When performing the procedure, always identify your patient according to agency policy and be attentive to standard precautions, hand hygiene, patient safety and privacy, body mechanics, and documentation.

Procedure Steps

1. Don clean procedure gloves. Wet the washcloths with warm water and place them near the work area.

2. If the patient is immobile, lower the head of the patient's bed. Pull down the covers only as far as needed to remove the bedpan.
Lowering the head of the bed is necessary only if the patient is immobile.

3. Offer the patient toilet paper. Assist patients who are unable to complete this task independently.

4. Ask the patient to raise her hips. Stabilize and remove the bedpan. If the patient is unable to raise her hips, stabilize the bedpan and assist her to the side-lying position.

Stabilizing the bedpan prevents spillage of urine.

5. Cleanse the buttocks with a warm, wet washcloth. Dry with a towel.
Provides comfort and hygiene and decreases the risk of skin irritation and breakdown.

6. Replace covers, and position the patient for comfort. Offer the patient the second washcloth moistened with warm water to cleanse her hands.
Encourages independence with personal hygiene and decreases transmission of bacteria.

7. Empty the bedpan into the patient's toilet. Measure the output if measuring I&O is part of the treatment plan. Clean the bedpan, following facility-specific guidelines.

If there is no toilet in the patient's room, cover the bedpan and carry it to the nearest toilet or soiled utility room for emptying.

8. Remove the soiled gloves and wash your hands.
Prevents transmission of infectious microorganisms.

What if . . .

■ **Your patient is an older adult?**
Offer a bedpan at set intervals, perhaps in conjunction with a turning schedule. For elderly clients with limited mobility you may wish to keep the bedpan readily available.

To minimize episodes of incontinence and/or falls. Trying to get out of bed to use the toilet is a common cause of falls.

Evaluation

■ Assess the amount and characteristics of any urine and/or stool.
■ Observe the skin on the perineum and buttocks for redness and breakdown.

Home Care

Teach the patient's family the steps of this procedure.

Documentation

■ Document the amount of urine voided if intake and output are being recorded.
■ Note the presence of any unusual characteristics of either stool or urine, and include in the nursing notes. If there are no unusual characteristics, document the passage of stool or urine in the graphic records.

Practice Resources

Ayello, E., & Sibbald, R. (2008); Balas, M., Casey, C., & Happ, M. (2008); Gray-Micelli, D. (2008); Siegel, J., Rhinehart, E., Jackson, M., et al. and the Healthcare Infection Control Practices Advisory Committee (2007).

Thinking About the Procedure

 Go to the *Fundamentals of Nursing Skills Videos*, **Bowel Elimination: Bed Pan.**

1. What kind of bed pan did the nurse use: regular bed pan or fracture pan?

2. Describe the method the nurse used to move the patient so she could place the bed pan.

 For suggested responses, go to Chapter 28, **Thinking About the Procedure Suggested Responses (Procedure 28-2),** on the Student Resource Disk or DavisPlus at http://davisplus.fadavis.com/Wilkinson2

Procedure 28-3 ▪ Administering an Enema

➤ For steps to follow in *all* procedures, refer to the Universal Steps for All Procedures found on the inside back cover of Volume 2.

Critical Aspects

- Generously lubricate and insert the rectal tube gently.
- Instill warm solution at a slow rate.
- For best results:
  - Be sure patient is properly positioned
  - Instruct her to retain the solution for 3 to 15 minutes, depending on the type of enema.
  - Assist the patient in a sitting or squatting position to promote defecation.
- Before leaving the bedside, implement fall prevention measures that are appropriate for your patient.
- Use nursing judgment to modify the procedure based on the patient's mobility and ability to follow your instructions.

Equipment

- Enema administration container, correct enema solution, or prepackaged enema—depends on the type of enema ordered.
  - Enema kit: This may be a grouping of supplies that includes a small plastic bucket or a 1-liter plastic bag with attached tubing, disposable toweling, lubricant, and castile soap.
  - Prepackaged enema solution: If a prepackaged enema (e.g., Fleets) is ordered, you may need to obtain the preparation from the pharmacy or central supply department.
- Washcloths, towels, disposable towelettes and/or toilet tissue
- Bath blanket
- Waterproof pad
- Bedpan with cover or bedside commode, if needed
- Water-soluble lubricant
- Clean procedure gloves
- IV pole

Delegation

You may delegate this procedure to the NAP if the patient is stable. Complete the following assessments, and instruct the NAP about conditions under which the procedure should be stopped (e.g., severe abdominal pain occurs, bleeding is seen, or the patient is unable to retain the solution). Instruct the NAP to report the results of the enema and show you any stool that appears to be abnormal (e.g., containing blood or pus).

Pre-Procedure Assessments

- Assess for history of bowel disorders (e.g., diverticulitis, ulcerative colitis, recent bowel

surgery, abdominal pain, abdominal distention, hemorrhoids).
Some disorders put the patient at risk for complications, such as mucosal irritation or perforation. Abdominal pain along with hypoactive bowel sounds and distention could indicate a bowel obstruction.

- Inspect the abdomen for the presence of distention.
Establishes baseline for effectiveness of the enema.

- Review the patient's chart for the presence of increased intracranial pressure, glaucoma, or recent rectal or prostate surgery.
These conditions contraindicate an enema.

- Review lab results, paying particular attention to BUN, creatinine, and electrolytes.
Hypertonic and hypotonic enemas have been linked to fluid and electrolyte changes. Phosphate enemas (Fleets) have been associated with hyperphosphatemia and hypocalcemia.

- Note the date and time of the patient's last bowel movement, recent bowel movement pattern, and bowel sounds.
Establishes baseline for evaluating bowel function.

- Assess the patient's cognitive level and mobility status.
Determines the patient's ability to follow instructions and the need for placing him on a bedpan for the enema.

- Assess the patient's degree of rectal sphincter control.
Will determine whether you need to administer the enema with the patient on the bedpan. Influences the amount of solution to instill.

- Assess for the presence of a fecal impaction.
May necessitate the need to obtain a prescription for a different type of enema.

(continued on next page)

Procedure 28-3 ■ Administering an Enema (continued)

■ Procedure 28-3A   Administering a Cleansing Enema

➤ When performing the procedure, always identify your patient according to agency policy and be attentive to standard precautions, hand hygiene, patient safety and privacy, body mechanics, and documentation.

Procedure Steps

1. Place the bedpan nearby or the commode near the bed.
So you can reach the bedpan during the procedure; or so the patient can easily get to the commode.

2. Open the enema supplies or kit. Attach the tubing to the enema pail, if you are using a pail.
The 1-liter enema bag comes with preconnected tubing.   .

3. Close the clamp on the tubing, and fill the container with 500 to 1000 mL of warm solution. The water temperature should be lukewarm—105° to 110° F (40° to 43° C).
✚ Check the temperature with a bath thermometer. Never warm the enema solution in a microwave oven.

   a. For infants: Use 50 to 150 mL of solution.
   b. For toddlers: Use 250 to 350 mL of solution.
   c. For school-age children, use 300 to 500 mL of solution.
Cold solution causes intestinal cramping. Very hot solution can damage the intestinal mucosa. Use the correct amount of solution to decrease the necessity of repeating the procedure.

4. Add castile soap (or the soap solution used by your facility) to the fluid at this time if a soapsuds enema has been prescribed.
Soap causes mucosal irritation, which stimulates peristalsis and defecation.

5. Hang the container on the IV pole. Holding the end of the tubing over a sink or waste can, open the clamp and slowly allow the tubing to prime (fill) with solution. Reclamp the tubing when the tubing is filled.
Expresses air from the tubing. Air introduced into the bowel may cause intestinal distention and discomfort.

6. Don clean procedure gloves.
Prevents the transmission of intestinal bacteria.

7. Position the patient: Ask the patient to turn, or assist the patient to turn, to a left side-lying position with the right knee flexed.
Allows the enema solution to fill the rectum and lower intestine following the natural flow of gravity.

   a. If the patient has shortness of breath associated with a respiratory condition, elevate the head of the bed very slightly. Avoid the semi-Fowler's position.
The semi-Fowler's position increases the likelihood that gravity will cause the solution to leak out.

   ✚ b. Do not administer the enema with the patient on the toilet.
The curved rectal tubing can scrape the rectal wall.

   c. If the patient has poor sphincter control, position him on the bedpan in a comfortable dorsal recumbent position.
He will not be able to retain all of the enema solution.

8. Place the waterproof pad under the patient's buttocks or hips.
Prevents soiling of bed linens.

9. Drape the patient with the bath blanket, exposing only the buttocks and rectum. See Procedure 22-4 to review the procedure for draping.
Promotes patient privacy.

10. Depending on the patient's mobility status, place the bedpan flat on the bed, directly beneath the rectum, up against the patient's buttocks.

11. Lubricate the tip of the enema tubing generously.
Allows for ease of insertion and decreases patient discomfort.

12. If necessary, lift the superior buttock to expose the anus. Slowly and gently insert the tip of the tubing approximately 7 to 10 cm (3 to 4 in.) into the rectum. Have the patient take slow, deep breaths as you complete this step. If the tube does not pass with ease, do not force it. Allow a small amount of fluid to infuse and then try again, inserting the tube slowly.
Helps the patient to relax, provides additional lubrication, and decreases reflex tightening of the anal sphincter. ▼

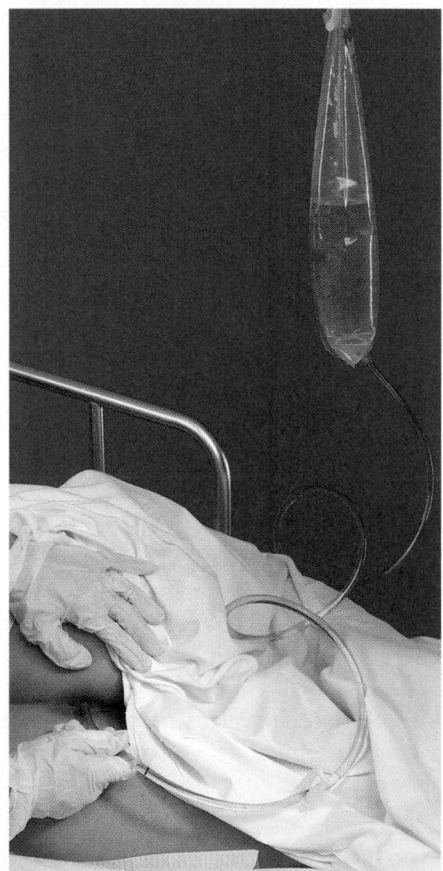

13. Remove the container from the IV pole, and hold it at the level of the patient's hips. Unclamp to begin instilling the solution.
Lowering the container slows the force of the instillation, decreasing pressure,

cramping, discomfort, and reflex expulsion of the solution.

14. Slowly raise the level of the container, so that it is 30 to 45 cm (12 to 18 in.) above the level of the hips. Adjust the pole and re-hang the container. Continue a slow, steady instillation of the enema solution.
The height of the container determines the speed of the flow. A slow, steady rate of infusion decreases cramping and increases the patient's ability to retain the solution.

15. Continuously monitor the patient for pain or discomfort. Assess his ability to retain the solution. If the patient has difficulty with retention, lower the level of the container, stop the flow for 15 to 30 seconds, and then resume the procedure.

✚ If the patient feels pain or you meet with resistance at any time during the procedure, stop and consult with the primary care provider.
Allows the patient to rest and adjust to the sensation of rectal fullness, increasing the patient's ability to retain the solution. Prevents injury.

16. When the correct amount of solution has been instilled, clamp the tubing, and slowly remove it from the rectum. If there is stool on the tubing, wrap the end of the tubing in a washcloth or toilet tissue until it can be rinsed or disposed of.
Prevents transmission of pathogens.

17. Clean the patient's rectal area, recover the patient, and instruct him to hold the enema solution for approximately 5 to 15 minutes. Place the call light within reach.
Retention of the enema solution will distend the bowel and increase the stimulus to defecate. Leaving the solution in the bowel too long may result in fluid and electrolyte complications. Retaining hypertonic solutions may result in dehydration related to large amounts of fluids moving from the capillary bed into the bowel. Excessive retention of hypotonic solutions may cause fluid overload.

18. Dispose of the enema supplies or, if they are reusable, clean and store them in an appropriate location in the patient's room.
Maintains a pleasant environment and helps prevent transfer of pathogens.

19. Remove your gloves and wash your hands.
Prevents transmission of intestinal pathogens.

20. Depending on the patient's mobility status, assist him onto the bedpan, to the bedside commode, or to the toilet when he feels compelled to defecate. Wash your hands and use clean procedure gloves as necessary.

21. After the patient has defecated, inspect the stool for color, consistency, and quantity.

■ **Procedure 28-3B** **Administering a Prepackaged Enema**

➤ When performing the procedure, always identify your patient according to agency policy and be attentive to standard precautions, hand hygiene, patient safety and privacy, body mechanics, and documentation.

Procedure Steps

1. Open the prepackaged enema. Remove the plastic cap from the container. The tip of the prepackaged enema container comes prelubricated. However, you may need to add extra lubricant.
Extra lubricant decreases discomfort and eases insertion of the tube into the rectum.

2. Follow steps 6 through 12 of Procedure 28-3A (regarding gloving, positioning, draping, and inserting the enema tip).

3. Tilt the container slightly and slowly roll and squeeze the container until all of the solution is instilled.

Ensures that the container empties completely and that an adequate amount of solution is instilled. ▼

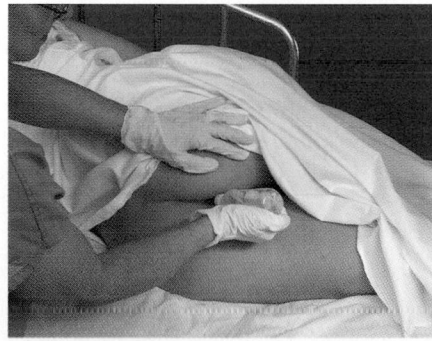

4. Withdraw the container tip from the rectum. Wipe the area with a wash-cloth or toilet tissue.
Prevents transmission of pathogens.

5. Re-cover the patient, and instruct him to hold the enema solution for approximately 5 to 10 minutes. Place the call light within reach.
Retention of the enema solution will distend the bowel and increase the stimulus to defecate. Retaining the solution for longer than the prescribed time has been associated with dehydration and electrolyte imbalances.

6. Dispose of the empty container.
Maintains a pleasant environment.

7. Follow steps 18 through 20 of Procedure 28-3A (regarding equipment disposal, assisting the patient, and observations of stool).

(continued on next page)

Procedure 28-3 ■ **Administering an Enema** (continued)

■ *Procedure 28-3C* **Administering an Oil-Retention Enema**

➤ When performing the procedure, always identify your patient according to agency policy and be attentive to standard precautions, hand hygiene, patient safety and privacy, body mechanics, and documentation.

➤ *Note:* An oil-retention enema may be administered to help a client pass hard stool; it also may be administered before digital removal of stool; or it may be given at least 1 hour before a cleansing enema. See Procedure 28-4 for digital removal of stool.

Procedure Steps

1. Obtain a commercial oil-retention enema kit; these kits include a small rectal tube. If a commercial kit is not available, use a small tube and about 90 to 120 mL of the prescribed solution.
A small tube allows for slower infusion, which minimizes cramping and thereby promotes retention.

◆ 2. Warm the oil to body temperature by running warm tap water over the container. Test a drop on your arm.
If the oil is too cold, it will cause cramping and expulsion of the oil. If it is too warm, it may injure the patient.

3. Follow steps 6 through 12 of Procedure 28-3A (regarding gloving, positioning, draping, and inserting the enema tip).

4. Instill the oil into the rectum.
The oil will soften stool and lubricate the rectum for easier passage of stool.

5. Withdraw the container tip from the rectum. Wipe the area with a washcloth or toilet tissue.

6. Instruct the patient to retain the oil for at least 30 minutes.

7. Follow steps 18 through 20 of Procedure 28-3A (regarding equipment disposal, assisting the patient, and observations of stool).

■ *Procedure 28-3D* **Administering a Return-Flow Enema**

➤ When performing the procedure, always identify your patient according to agency policy and be attentive to standard precautions, hand hygiene, patient safety and privacy, body mechanics, and documentation.

➤ *Note:* A return-flow enema, also known as a Harris flush, may be ordered to help a patient expel flatus and relieve abdominal distention.

Procedure Steps

1. Obtain a rectal tube and solution container (e.g., bag or pail).

2. Prepare 100 to 200 mL (for adults) of tap water or saline.

3. Follow steps 6 through 12 of Procedure 28-3A (regarding gloving, positioning, draping, and inserting the enema tip).

4. Instill all the solution into the patient's rectum.

5. Lower the tube and container below the level of the rectum, and allow the solution to flow back into the container.

6. Repeat this process several times, or until the distention is relieved.

7. Follow steps 18 through 20 of Procedure 28-3A (regarding equipment disposal, assisting the patient, and observations of stool).

What if. . .

■ **The solution for a return-flow enema becomes thick with fecal matter?**
Discard it and begin again with new solution.

Evaluation

■ Observe the amount, color, and consistency of the stool.
■ Evaluate the patient's tolerance of the procedure (e.g., amount of cramping, discomfort).
■ Determine whether the prescriber's orders require subsequent enema administration.
■ Some bowel exams require repeated enemas or enemas administered until the returns are "clear." For the latter, you will need to examine the return and determine whether stool particles are still present. "Clear" does not mean absence of color, but rather absence of stool particles and transparency of the liquid.

Patient Teaching

■ Teach the patient that dependence on enemas to achieve a regular bowel elimination pattern can disrupt the normal process that stimulates defecation.

- Teach dietary and lifestyle changes that promote regular elimination (e.g., increased fluid intake, diet high in fiber, increased exercise).

Home Care

- Show the patient the box for a prepackaged enema, and instruct him that he may purchase this type of enema at a local grocery or pharmacy.
- Assess the patient's ability to administer his own enema. If you determine that he will be unable to do so, encourage him to seek assistance and instruct the caregiver in the task.
- Teach the patient or caregiver proper handwashing. Encourage them to purchase nonsterile procedure gloves.

Patients and caregivers may not be aware of the serious infections that can be caused by gram-negative intestinal bacteria.

- If the patient will be attempting to self-administer a cleansing enema, help him determine how and where to hang the container so that it is at the proper height.
- If a soapsuds enema is to be administered in the home setting, teach the patient which household soaps may be substituted for castile soap.

Some soaps used in the home for cleaning purposes may be too harsh and irritating to the intestinal mucosa.

Documentation

- Document on the nursing notes the type of enema given and, if applicable, the amount of the solution instilled.
- For prepackaged enemas, some facilities require documentation (of the time given and the nurse's initials) on the medication administration record (MAR).
- Document the patient's tolerance of the procedure.
- Document the characteristics and amount of the stool.
- If the prescription is to administer enemas until the returns are clear, document the color of the return solution and the amount of stool seen.

Sample documentation:

06/04/11 0825   Fleets enema administered (see MAR). Patient had no cramping; retained enema for 5 minutes. Passed moderate amount of solid, formed, brown stool with no mucus, but with a streak of bright red blood on the surface. ———————— R. Kline, RN

Thinking About the Procedure

 Go to the *Fundamentals of Nursing Skills Videos,* **Bowel Elimination: Cleansing Enema.**

1. What did the nurse use to drape the patient and protect his privacy?

2. Where was the bag of enema solution when the fluid first began flowing?

 For suggested responses, go to Chapter 28, **Thinking About the Procedure Suggested Responses (Procedure 28-3),** on the Student Resource Disk or DavisPlus at http://davisplus.fadavis.com/Wilkinson2

Procedure 28-4 ☐ Removing Stool Digitally

➤ For steps to follow in *all* procedures, refer to the Universal Steps for All Procedures found on the inside back cover of Volume 2.

Critical Aspects

- Be aware that this procedure is both painful and embarrassing to your patient.
- Trim and file your fingernails so they do not extend over the ends of your fingertips.
- Obtain baseline vital signs, and determine whether the patient has a history of cardiac problems or other contraindications.
- Determine whether the procedure will be accompanied by suppository insertion or enema administration.
- Use only one or two fingers, and remove stool in small pieces.
- Allow the patient periods of rest, and monitor for signs of vagal nerve stimulation.
- Teach the patient lifestyle changes necessary to prevent stool retention.

(continued on next page)

Procedure 28-4 ■ **Removing Stool Digitally** (continued)

Equipment

- Two pairs of clean procedure gloves
- Water-soluble lubricant (containing lidocaine, if agency policy permits)
- Bedpan and cover
- Washcloth, soap, and towel or toilet tissue (or moistened towelettes)
- Basin of warm water
- Bath blanket
- Waterproof pad

Delegation

This procedure should not be delegated to a NAP. Ongoing assessment of the patient by the professional nurse is required when stool is manually removed from the rectum. The nurse must monitor the patient for complications, such as bleeding and vagal nerve stimulation. Nursing judgment is necessary in determining the need to halt the procedure.

Pre-Procedure Assessments

- Assess the patient's baseline vital signs and history of heart disease. Be sure to monitor the patient's pulse before and during the procedure.

Digital removal of stool can stimulate the vagus nerve, causing bradycardia. Patients who have a history of heart disease or dysrhythmia are at greater risk.

- Assess the patient's white blood cell (WBC) count.

If the patient has a compromised immune status, evidenced by a low WBC count, you should discuss this procedure with the primary care provider to evaluate the risks and benefits of the procedure.

- Assess the patient's cognitive level and mobility status.

Determines the patient's ability to follow directions and turn in bed.

- Determine the time of the patient's last bowel movement.

Infrequent defecation increases the chance that hard stool may form in the rectum.

- Assess the patient for history of fecal impaction.

Can be a recurrent problem for immobile, disabled, or institutionalized patients.

- Assess stool consistency.

Patients who are immobilized may become incontinent of watery stool. They may be able to pass small sections of hard stool or small quantities of watery stool. The latter, which may be intermittent or continuous, is a symptom of high colon impaction.

- Assess the patient's ability to defecate: Does the patient have the desire but is unable to have a BM?

Large amounts of stool can cause distention in the rectum.

- Determine whether the patient experiences pain on defecation.

Pain can exacerbate the problem because the patient tends to suppress defecation.

- Assess the patient's pattern of bowel movements, diet, exercise, mobility status, and medications (e.g., iron supplements or narcotic analgesics).

You should determine whether any of these factors contribute to the problem and then add this information to the nursing care plan to help prevent recurrence.

- Assess bowel sounds and any abdominal distention.

There can be peristalsis without gastrointestinal patency, which creates distention. Abdominal distention can aggravate constipation.

Guidelines

- Prevention of fecal impaction is the best treatment, but if impaction has occurred, the stool must be removed. The procedure is both painful and embarrassing to your patient.
- Some practitioners may prescribe an oil-retention enema before the procedure to soften and moisten the stool, making removal easier.
- Also, many advise that you follow digital removal of stool with either an oil-retention and/or tap water enemas. Enema(s) given after the procedure ensure the evacuation of stool that may not have been reached by digital removal.
- Trim and file your fingernails if they extend past the end of your fingertips.

➤ When performing the procedure, always identify your patient according to agency policy and be attentive to standard precautions, hand hygiene, patient safety and privacy, body mechanics, and documentation.

Procedure Steps

1. Determine whether lubricant containing lidocaine is to be used, and obtain the correct lubricant.
May decrease rectal discomfort for the patient.

2. Drape the patient with the bath blanket. Go to Procedure 22-4 to review the procedure for draping. Assist him to turn on his left side, with his right knee flexed toward his head. Place the waterproof pad halfway beneath his left hip.
Provides privacy and exposes the anus for visualization. The pad protects the bed from being soiled.

3. Don clean procedure gloves. Some sources recommend double-gloving.
Prevents the transmission of intestinal bacteria.

4. Expose the buttocks. Place a clean, dry bedpan on the waterproof pad next to the buttocks in line with the rectum.

The bedpan serves as a receptacle for stool that is removed.

5. Wet a washcloth, or have toilet tissue or moist towelettes ready to cleanse the rectal area when you complete the procedure.

6. Generously lubricate either the gloved forefinger and/or middle finger on your dominant hand.

Helps prevent discomfort, pain, and mucosal injury.

7. Slowly slide one lubricated finger into the rectum. Observe for perianal irritation.

The patient may need skin care to reduce pain during additional bowel evacuation. ▼

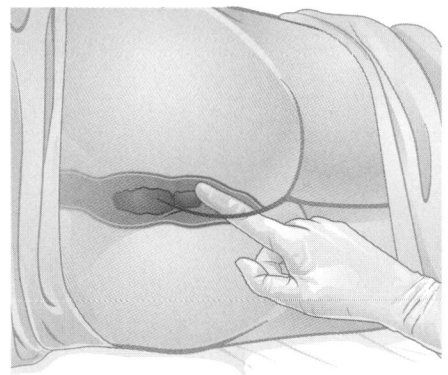

8. Gently rotate your finger around the mass and/or into the mass.

Assists in determining the amount and texture of the fecal bulk.

9. Begin to break the stool into smaller pieces. At this point, you may insert a second finger and gently "slice" apart the stool, using a scissoring motion. Remove pieces of stool via the rectum as they become separated, and place them in the bedpan. ▼

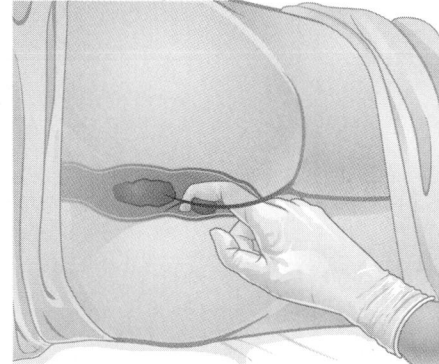

10. As you proceed, instruct the patient to take slow, deep breaths.

Helps the patient to relax his anal sphincter.

11. Continue to manipulate and remove pieces of stool, allowing the patient to rest at intervals. Reapply lubricant (containing lidocaine, if permitted) each time you reinsert your fingers.

Rest periods allow for assessment of and attention to the patient's comfort level and tolerance for the procedure.

12. Assess the patient's heart rate at regular intervals.

Stimulation of the vagus nerve may cause bradycardia and poses a risk for dysrhythmias in susceptible patients.

Stop the procedure if the patient's heart rate falls or the rhythm changes from your initial assessment.

Caution: Some resources suggest that this procedure should be done in small steps (no more than 4 finger insertions in one session), giving a series of suppositories in between stool removal episodes.

Prevents patient fatigue and pain. Reduces the risk of injury to the rectal tissue and vagal stimulation.

13. When removal of stool is complete, cover the bedpan and set it aside. Use a washcloth and/or toilet tissue to cleanse the rectal area.

Provides personal hygiene and decreases transmission of pathogens.

14. Assist the patient to return to a position of comfort. Note the color, amount, and consistency of the stool, and dispose of it properly.

15. Remove your gloves and wash your hands.

Prevents transmission of intestinal pathogens.

What if . . .

■ **The patient is an infant?**

When treating infants with fecal impactions, avoid enemas and mineral oils. Glycerin suppositories may be used to soften the stool before removal.

Evaluation

■ Determine whether evacuation of the retained stool was complete. Perform a rectal exam to assess for presence of stool.
■ Reassess vital signs, and compare the results to the initial assessment. Continue to monitor for 1 hour for bradycardia.
■ Assess bowel sounds.
■ Palpate the abdomen for nontenderness and softness.
■ Ask the patient whether he feels relief from rectal pressure or abdominal discomfort.

Patient Teaching

Retained stool is most often the result of poor dietary habits, lack of fluid intake, lack of exercise, inattentiveness to the urge to defecate, and laxative abuse. Focus patient teaching on lifestyle changes that will facilitate a regular bowel elimination pattern (e.g., high-fiber foods, drinking at least eight glasses of water per day).

Home Care

Home care should focus on preventing constipation that would require the digital removal of stool. Teach clients

(continued on next page)

Procedure 28-4 ■ **Removing Stool Digitally** (continued)

about high-fiber foods, adequate water intake, and the importance of exercise. Digital removal of stool may be necessary for some clients as part of a bowel program (e.g., patients who are paraplegic or quadriplegic). You can teach this procedure to the care provider in the home.

Documentation

- Document the bowel movement on the graphic record.
- Document the procedure and the patient's tolerance for the procedure in the nursing notes.
- Document the patient's pulse rate on the vital signs record.
- Document any unusual characteristics of the stool (e.g., black or green color, blood, or mucus).

Sample documentation:

07/11/12   6:15 P.M.   *Impacted stool removed digitally. No perianal irritation noted. Removed moderate amount (approximately 6 oz [170g]) dry, hard, gray-colored stool. Pulse 78 before removal; 84 after. Encouraging 8 oz fluids every hour.* ———————— *C. Bryan, RNC*

Practice Resources

Creason, N., & Sparks, D. (2000); National Guideline Clearinghouse (NGC), Brief guideline summary: Evaluation and treatment of constipation... (n.d.); Siegal, J., Rhinehart, E., Jackson, M., et al. (2007).

Procedure 28-5   **Inserting a Rectal Tube**

➤ For steps to follow in *all* procedures, refer to the Universal Steps for All Procedures found on the inside back cover of Volume 2.

Critical Aspects

- A rectal tube may be used to facilitate the passage of gas for clients experiencing intestinal distention.
- Position the patient on his left side.
- Lubricate the tip of the tube; insert 10 to 12.5 cm (4 to 5 inches).
- Attach the collecting device to the end of the tube.
- Leave the tube in place for 15 to 20 minutes.
- Assist the patient to move about in bed; the knee–chest position is ideal if tolerated.

Equipment

- 22- to 34-French rectal tube for adults. Choose the size according to the size of the client. For children or petite adults, a smaller size tube (12- to 18-Fr) may be required.
- Water-soluble lubricant
- Procedure gloves
- Toilet paper
- Skin care items (e.g., soap, skin cleanser, water, wipes)
- Collecting device (waterproof pad, graduated cylinder partially filled with water, a urine collection bag nicked at the top to vent)
- Paper tape
- Stool specimen container if needed

Pre-Procedure Assessments

- Obtain baseline vital signs.
- Auscultate bowel sounds; percuss for tympany.
- Observe and palpate the degree of abdominal distention.
- Assess discomfort caused by flatulence.
- Ask whether the patient is passing any flatus.
- Assess the condition of perianal tissues.
- Assess the history of cardiac disease.

Insertion of a rectal tube can stimulate the vagus nerve, causing bradycardia.

➤ When performing the procedure, always identify your patient according to agency policy and be attentive to standard precautions, hand hygiene, patient safety and privacy, body mechanics, and documentation.

Procedure Steps

1. Wear procedure gloves.
Follows standard precautions.

2. Ask the patient to lift his hips or roll from side to side to place a waterproof pad.
Protects against soiling of linens.

3. Attach a collecting device to the end of the rectal tube: Tape a plastic bag or urine collection bag around the distal end of the rectal tube and vent the upper side of the bag; or insert the tube into the specimen container; or place the end of the tube in a graduated container partially filled with water.

Collects small pieces of stool expelled with flatus. Venting the plastic bag prevents overinflation and bursting the bag. An advantage of using water in the container is that gas generates bubbles, and you will be able to assess the effectiveness of the rectal tube based on the amount of bubbling in the container.

4. Place patient in left side-lying position. Drape for privacy.

Allows the tube to follow the normal curve of the rectum and sigmoid colon when inserted.

5. Lubricate the tip of the rectal tube.

Prevents trauma to the rectal mucosa.

6. Separate the buttocks and ask the patient to take a deep breath. Gently insert the tube into the rectum.
Adults: 10 to 12.5 cm (4 to 5 in.)
Children: 5 to 10 cm (2 to 4 in.).

Deep breaths relax the anal sphincter and ease tube insertion.

7. For adults, tape the tube in place; for children, hold it manually.

8. Leave the rectal tube in place for 15 to 20 minutes. If distention persists, you may reinsert the tube every 2 to 3 hours.

Leaving the tube in place for more than 20 minutes may cause pressure necrosis of the mucosa; prolonged stimulation of the anal sphincter may result in loss of the neuromuscular response.

9. Assist the patient to move about in bed to promote gas expulsion. A knee–chest position is ideal.

Because gas is lighter than fluid or solid, the position promotes passage of flatus. Unfortunately, many patients cannot tolerate this position.

10. Remove the tube, wipe the patient's buttocks with tissue, and assist to clean the rectal area as needed.

Prevents transmission of microorganisms from feces; promotes patient comfort and skin integrity.

11. Dispose of used equipment; or clean it if it is to be reused. Follow agency procedures for cleaning.

Evaluation

- Evaluate the patient's response to the procedure (e.g., vital signs, fatigue).
- Assess abdominal distention and abdominal comfort.

Patient Teaching

- Teach the patient that chewing gum, sucking on hard candy, using a straw, smoking, and drinking carbonated beverages increase air swallowing and abdominal distention.

- Teach factors that promote normal elimination (e.g., exercise, increased fluid intake, adequate dietary fiber).

Documentation

Record the following:
- Date and time tube inserted
- Size of tube and characteristics of feces collected
- Abdominal distention before and after the procedure
- Pulse and respiratory rates before and after the procedure
- Tolerance of procedure and any complications
- Patient and family teaching

Procedure 28-6 ☐ **Changing an Ostomy Appliance**

➤ For steps to follow in *all* procedures, refer to the Universal Steps for All Procedures found on the inside back cover of Volume 2. Also see Clinical Insight 28-3: Guidelines for Ostomy Care.

➤ *Note:* Some pouches come with the wafer attached, some without. These instructions assume that the wafer is attached.

Critical Aspects

- Change the pouch every 3 to 5 days, as a general rule.
- Empty the old pouch before removing it, if possible.
- Remove the wafer or pouch, pulling down from the top with one hand while holding counter-tension with the other.
- Assess the stoma and the peristomal skin area (e.g., for discoloration, swelling, redness, irritation, excoriation, bleeding).
- Use a measuring guide to determine the size of the stoma.
- Trace the size of the opening onto the back of the wafer, and cut the wafer opening about 2 to 3 mm (¹⁄₁₆ to ⅛ in.) larger.
- Apply the new wafer with gentle pressure.

 Also go to **Animations: Colostomy,** on DavisPlus at http://davisplus.fadavis.com/Wilkinson2

Procedure 28-6 ■ **Changing an Ostomy Appliance** (continued)

Equipment

- Ostomy pouch
  - One-piece pouch with the wafer attached, or a two-piece system with a separate wafer and pouch
  - Clamp for pouches with an opening at the bottom (a new clamp is not used each time; usually one clamp is packaged with each box of pouches)
- Skin care items per agency protocol or recommended by the enterostomal therapist (e.g., pH balanced skin cleanser, skin prep, skin barrier wipe, adhesive remover, adhesive paste, and stoma paste if needed to fill and smooth skin surface)
- Stoma measuring guide (or precut template)
- Scissors
- Pen or pencil
- Two pairs of clean procedure gloves
- Washcloth, towel, basin with warm water
- Toilet tissue
- 4 in. × 4 in. gauze pad
- Bedpan or container for effluent
- Plastic bag (for disposal of used pouch)
- Plastic bag for disposal of other contaminated articles
- Waterproof pad
- Ostomy deodorant
- Hypoallergenic paper tape (optional) or ostomy belt
- Bath blanket

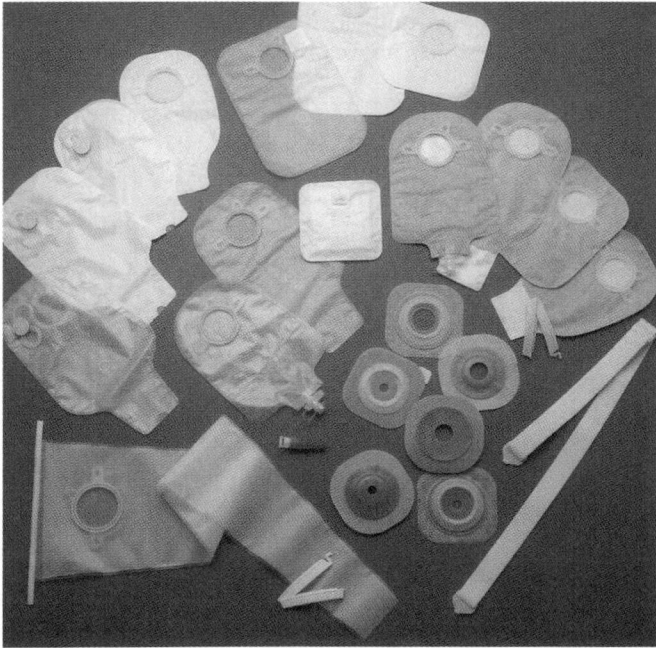

Delegation

During the immediate postoperative period, the professional nurse must assess the newly created stoma and peristomal skin area and use clinical judgment when changing a pouch. You may delegate to a NAP if it is a preexisting, stable stoma and if you are sure the NAP is qualified to perform the task. If you do delegate this task, instruct the NAP to report any changes or unusual findings (e.g., changes in stoma color, swelling, peristomal redness, excoriation, deviations from expected amount) and color and consistency of drainage from the stoma.

Pre-Procedure Assessments

- Assess the type of stoma (e.g., ileostomy, colostomy, urostomy), number of stomas, and location on the abdomen (e.g., is the stoma near structures that will impact care?).

Determines the type of pouch or system to use.

- Assess stoma color, shape, size, and/or length of protrusion or retraction; stoma construction (end, loop, double barrel); direction of stoma lumen; and discharge. Does the stoma lie flat or does it protrude?

The stoma should be moist and red or pink. Alterations in stoma color (purple, black, or blue) may indicate poor circulation and possible necrosis and should be reported to the primary provider.

- Assess peristomal skin for redness, rash, irritation, or excoriation. Observe the existing skin barrier and pouch for leakage and length of time in place. You may have to remove the pouch to observe the stoma fully, depending on the type of pouch (i.e., if the pouch is opaque). Notify the provider or an ostomy specialist immediately if you note peristomal skin abnormalities.
- Determine the changing schedule for the pouch.
- Measure the stoma with each pouching system. Follow the manufacturer's directions and measuring guide for the size of ostomy pouch and the patient's stoma size.

Determines the correct size of equipment needed.

- Observe abdominal shape and incision, if present.

Abdominal shape determines the proper placement of the pouch. Because of stomal and abdominal characteristics, some patients may need convexity in their ostomy pouching system to avoid leakage.

- Assess the patient's willingness to look at the stoma, touch the appliance, and discuss or participate in the task.

May indicate a readiness or desire to learn.

- Assess the patient's condition and self-care ability. Consider vision, dexterity or mobility, and cognitive ability.

Helps determine best type of appliance to use.

- Auscultate for bowel sounds.

Determines the presence of peristalsis.

- Observe for effluent from the stoma, and document your findings.

Change the skin barrier pouch at times of lower effluent output. Avoid changing after meals, when the gastrocolic reflux increases chance of fecal effluent output. Mucous secretion is normal.

- Assess whether a new clamp will be needed or the one on the pouch can be used again.

➤ When performing the procedure, always identify your patient according to agency policy and be attentive to standard precautions, hand hygiene, patient safety and privacy, body mechanics, and documentation.

Procedure Steps

1. Wash your hands and don clean procedure gloves.

Prevents transmission of pathogens.

2. Fold down the bed covers to expose the ostomy site. Place a clean towel across the patient's abdomen under the existing pouch.

Helps prevent spilling effluent onto the patient.

3. Position the patient so that no skinfolds occur along the line of the stoma.

Ensures an adequate seal between the wafer and the skin, preventing leakage.

4. If the present ostomy pouch is drainable, empty it into the bedpan.

Pouches should be drained when they are one-third to one-half full because the weight of the contents may dislodge the skin seal; ostomy drainage is irritating to the skin. The pouch also collects flatus, which needs to be expelled because it can disrupt the skin seal.

   a. To calculate the amount of output in milliliters for an ostomy with a liquid effluent (e.g., ileostomy or urostomy), use a graduated measuring container.

   b. For pouches that you open by unrolling them at the bottom, you must remove a clamp to empty the pouch. Save this clamp for reuse. *Note:* Some pouches cannot be drained.

5. Using a silicone-based (hexamethyldisiloxane) adhesive remover, remove the appliance by applying the adhesive remover with one hand as you press the skin away from the wafer barrier with your other hand. Avoid pulling the appliance straight off. Begin at the top and work downward.

Silicone-based adhesive removers are preferred over alcohol- or oil-based products. Pulling the appliance from the skin tends to strip the loosely bound epidermal skin layers, making the skin more susceptible to moisture loss and irritation from effluent. Silicone-based products reduce the bind strength, whereas alcohol dissolves the adhesives; thus alcohol may cause dryness and irritation. It also causes pain if the skin is not intact. If you use an oil-based solvent, the new pouch will not adhere to the oily skin. ▼

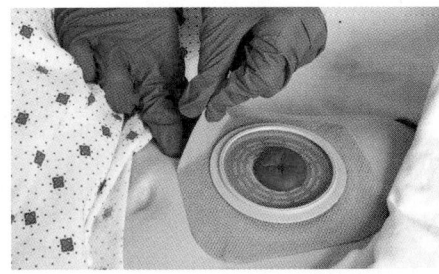

6. Place the old pouch and wafer in the plastic bag for disposal. If you were unable to drain the pouch, dispose of it according to agency protocol.

Prevents transmission of infections caused by fecal bacteria.

7. Inspect the stoma and peristomal skin area (see "Assessment," preceding).

8. Cleanse the stoma and surrounding skin using warm water. Allow the area to dry. You may use a skin cleansing agent with a pH of 5.5 that is designed to both cleanse and moisturize the skin.

Removes old adhesive and any effluent that has leaked. Helps prevent skin irritation and/or breakdown and maintain skin moisture. Select cleansing agents that protect the stratum corneum lipids and proteins.

9. Measure the size of the stoma. You can accomplish this in several ways.

   a. Place a standard stoma measuring guide over the stoma.

   b. Reuse a previously cut template.

   c. Measure the stoma from side to side (approximating the circumference).

The stoma may need to be remeasured frequently during the initial postoperative period because the size of the stoma may change as edema subsides. ▼

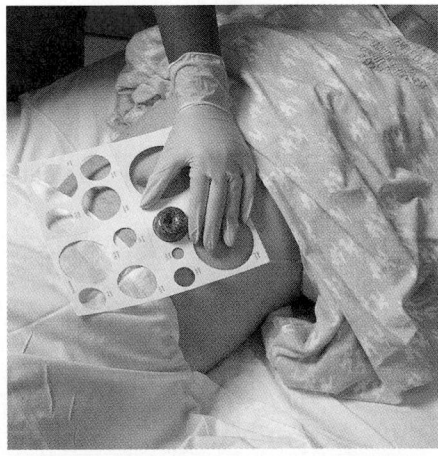

10. Place a clean 4 in. × 4 in. gauze pad over the stoma.

Gauze will absorb any leaking effluent, keeping the skin clean and dry during application of the new pouch.

(continued on next page)

Procedure 28-6 ■ **Changing an Ostomy Appliance** (continued)

11. Remove your gloves and wash your hands.

Decreases the spread of intestinal bacteria.

12. Trace the size of the opening obtained in step 9 onto the paper on the back of the new wafer. Cut the opening. The opening in the wafer should be approximately $1/16$ to $1/8$ inch (1.5 to 3 mm) larger than the circumference of the stoma.

Allows for skin movement with activity and prevents impaired circulation to the stoma.

13. Peel the paper off the wafer. Some resources suggest first holding the wafer between the palms of your hand to warm the adhesive ring.

Enhances the integrity of the seal by making the ring more "sticky" so that it will bond better with the skin.

Note: Some ostomy wafers come with an outer ring of tape attached. Do not remove the backing on this tape until the wafer is securely positioned (see step 16).

14. Don clean procedure gloves.

15. At this time, you may apply ostomy skin care products per your clinical judgment, hospital protocol, or following the recommendations of the enterostomal therapist (e.g., wipe around stoma with skin prep, apply skin barrier powder or paste, or apply extra adhesive paste).

These products prevent or treat excoriated skin and/or ensure a tight seal between the wafer and the skin.

16. Remove the gauze. Center the wafer opening around the stoma, and gently press it down. Press your hand firmly against the newly applied wafer and hold for 30 to 60 seconds

Heat from the hand activates the adhesive ring, making it adhere better thus promoting optimal wear time. Some sources also suggest taping down the edges of the wafer.

Step 16 Variation. One-Piece Pouch

  a. Make sure the bag is pointed toward the patient's feet.

Step 16 Variation. Two-Piece System

  b. Place the wafer on first. When the seal is complete, attach the bag following manufacturer's instructions.

Step 16 Variation. Open-Ended Pouch

  c. Fold the end of the pouch over the clamp, and close the clamp, listening for a "click" to ensure that it is secure.

17. Remove your gloves and wash your hands.

18. Return the patient to a comfortable position. Dispose of the used ostomy pouch following your facility's policy for biohazardous waste.

What if . . .

■ **At step 8, you notice that the stoma is bleeding?**

Slight bleeding of the stoma is normal; report excessive bleeding to the primary care provider.

Evaluation

Make the following observations:

■ Characteristics of stoma: color, size, presence of edema, and shape
■ Presence of blisters, redness, or excoriation on peristomal skin
■ Amount and characteristics of effluent: color, odor, consistency
■ Whether the patient expressed a desire to participate in the task
■ Whether the patient demonstrated nonverbal cues that she is ready to learn about the task (e.g., looking at the stoma)

Patient Teaching

Patient teaching is aimed at preparing the patient to complete this skill at home. She will need to be instructed in how to complete all the steps of the procedure.

Home Care

■ Help the client establish a routine for changing the stoma wafer/pouch. In general, experts recommend changing it twice weekly, or as determined by the physician or ostomy specialist.
■ Advise the client to change the pouch immediately if it begins to leak. The average wear-time in the United States is 4.5 days for a colostomy and 5 days for an ileostomy or urostomy (Richbourg, Fellows, & Arroyave, 2008).
■ The client can complete the removal of her pouch and cleansing of the peristomal skin in the shower.
■ The client may need to stand in front of a mirror or sit to change her ostomy appliance if she is unable to view the stoma easily.
■ Teach the client that slight bleeding is normal when the stoma is washed.
■ The client should not use soaps and lotions containing oils. They decrease the adhesiveness of the wafer.
■ The appliance and wafer cannot be flushed down the toilet.
■ Teach the client to report changes in the color or size of the stoma and/or the presence of peristomal irritation or skin breakdown to the primary care provider.

- Provide information about community support groups, such as Ostomates.
- Provide contact information for ostomy supply vendors.

Documentation

Document the following:
- Your assessment of the stoma and peristomal skin area
- Patient's tolerance of the procedure
- Type of appliance used, including the manufacturer and part number
- Use of any special ostomy skin care products
- Amount of liquid effluent on the I&O portion of the graphics record
- Patient teaching and the degree to which the patient participated in the procedure

Sample EHR documentation:

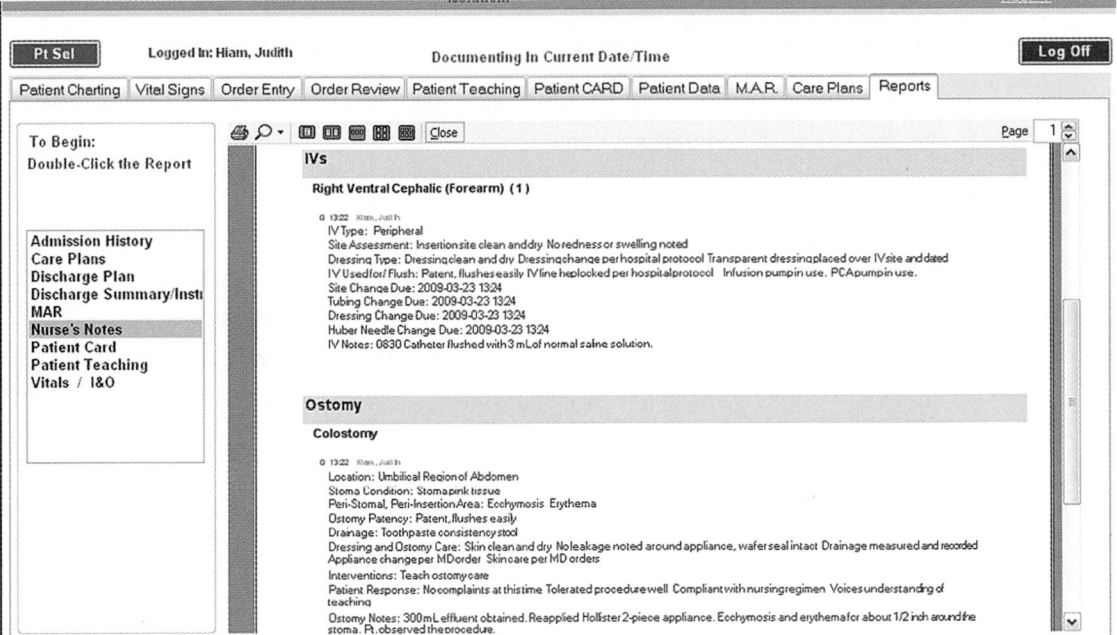

Practice Resources

Black, P. (2008); Burch, J., & Sica, J. (2008); Cronin, E. (2008); Karadag, A., Mentex, B., & Ayaz, S. (2005); Kent, M. (2008); Pulen, R. (2006); Richbourg, L., Fellows, J., & Arroyave, W. (2008); Siegal, J., Rhinehart, E., Jackson, M., et al. (2007).

Thinking About the Procedure

 Go to the *Fundamentals of Nursing Skills Videos,* **Bowel Elimination: Colostomy Appliance, Changing.**

1. What did the nurse do to protect the patient's privacy?

2. How did the nurse determine the size of the opening in the new appliance?

3. When applying the new appliance, which direction did the nurse point the drainage end of the pouch: toward the patient's head, left side, right side, feet?

 For suggested responses, go to Chapter 28, **Thinking About the Procedure Suggested Responses (Procedure 28-6),** on the Student Resource Disk or DavisPlus at http://davisplus.fadavis.com/Wilkinson2

Procedure 28-7 ▪ Irrigating a Colostomy

➤ For steps to follow in *all* procedures, refer to the Universal Steps for All Procedures found on the inside back cover of Volume 2. Also see Clinical Insight 28-3: Guidelines for Ostomy Care.

Critical Aspects

- Consult with the ostomy nurse and/or physician to see if colostomy irrigation is appropriate for your patient.
- Determine the patient's normal bowel pattern before surgery.
- Prime the tubing before irrigation, using 500 to 1000 mL, preferably 1000 mL, of warm tap water.
- Position the patient in front of or on the toilet or bedside commode. If the patient is immobile, place her in left side-lying (Sims') position, and use a bedpan.
- Prepare the new appliance before removing the existing one.
- Examine the stoma and periostomal skin.
- Lubricate the cone at the end of the tubing and insert it gently.
- Allow approximately 30 minutes for evacuation.
- Remove the sleeve, and rinse, dry, and store it.

Equipment

- Irrigation equipment
  - One-piece system with a fluid container connected to tubing with cone or two-piece system with a container separate from tubing with cone
  - Irrigation sleeve; a sleeve without adhesive backing requires a belt to hold it in place
  - Clamp for a sleeve with an opening at the top
  - Prescribed irrigating solution (usually 500 to 1000 mL warm tap water, 100° to 105°F (37.8° to 40.6°C)
- IV pole or other equipment to hang the irrigation container
- Chair
- Water-soluble lubricant
- Silicone-based adhesive remover
- Skin cleansers and barriers as recommended by your agency
- Toilet tissue
- Washcloth, towel
- Waterproof pad
- Two pairs of clean procedure gloves
- Toilet facilities that include a flushable toilet and a hook or some other device to hold the irrigation container; or bedpan or bedside commode (for patients with impaired mobility)
- New ostomy appliance and skin barrier or stoma cap cover
- Ostomy deodorant (optional)
- Plastic bag for disposal of the used pouch

Delegation

The initial irrigation of a newly created colostomy requires nursing judgment and clinical decision making. Initially, this procedure should not be delegated to the NAP, although in some situations it may be delegated to an LPN, depending on agency policy.

Pre-Procedure Assessments

- Evaluate the defecation pattern (or absence) nature of stool, placement of stoma, abdominal distention, and nutritional pattern.

Findings may indicate the need to irrigate to stimulate elimination function; consistency of stool varies along the length of the GI tract.

- Assess the type of ostomy.

Many patients with left-end colostomies may be safely irrigated as a method of continence management. However, do not irrigate an ileostomy.

- Assess the patient's usual bowel pattern.

The purpose for irrigating a colostomy is to promote a regular pattern for bowel elimination.

- Assess for abdominal distention.

Report distention to the primary care provider, as it may indicate excess gas or inflammation.

- Assess hydration status.

The colon may absorb some of the irrigation fluid if the patient is very dehydrated.

- Assess cognitive level and mobility status.

Determines the necessity for a bedpan or bedside commode. Also determines whether patient teaching will be effective.

- Assess the patient's ability to maintain a sitting position.
- Assess the characteristics of the stoma (see Clinical Insight 28-3).

➤ When performing the procedure, always identify your patient according to agency policy and be attentive to standard precautions, hand hygiene, patient safety and privacy, body mechanics, and documentation.

Procedure Steps

1. Place the IV pole near the location of the procedure (e.g., in the bathroom, next to the bedside commode, or next to the bed).
Allows you to work efficiently.

2. If possible, assist the patient to the bathroom or commode. Ask the patient if she prefers to sit directly on the toilet or on a chair in front of it. If the patient must remain in bed, elevate the head of the bed.
Patients with impaired mobility can sit directly on or in front of the bedside commode, or they may remain in bed in the side-lying position.

3. Prepare the irrigation container.
a. For two-piece systems, connect the tubing to the container. Clamp the tubing. Fill the container with 500 to 1000 mL of warm tap water.
Water that is too cold will cause cramping, nausea, and discomfort. Water that is too hot will damage the intestinal mucosa. Note: Some ostomy resources suggest that using 1000 mL of water will promote a more effective irrigation of the entire colon and decrease the necessity to irrigate more than once a day.

b. Prime the tubing. Unclamp the tubing to allow it to fill.
Removes air from the tubing, preventing gas pains.

4. Hang the solution container on the IV pole. Adjust the IV pole so that it reaches the height of the patient's shoulder (approximately 45 cm [18 in.], above the stoma).
The height of the container regulates the force of the flow.

5. Wash your hands and don clean procedure gloves.
Prevents the transmission of pathogens.

6. Remove the existing colostomy appliance (if the patient is wearing one) following the steps in Procedure 28-6.

Inspect the stoma and surrounding skin area.
Use of ostomy skin care preparations may be needed when you replace the pouch.

7. Dispose of the used colostomy appliance properly. Empty the contents into the bedpan or toilet, and discard the pouch in a moisture-proof (e.g., plastic) bag.
Prevents transmission of intestinal bacteria.

8. Apply the colostomy irrigation sleeve, following the manufacturer's directions.

Step 8 Variation. Sleeve with Adhesive Backing
a. Apply according to the steps described in Procedure 28-6.

Step 8 Variation. Sleeve Without an Adhesive Backing
b. Place the belt around the patient's waist, and attach the ends to the pouch flange on either side.

Step 8 Variation. Patient Sitting on a Toilet or Bedside Commode
c. The end of the sleeve should hang down past the patient's pubic area, but not down into the water. Place a waterproof pad under the sleeve over the patient's thighs.
Prevents leakage and spilling of irrigation fluid and effluent.

Step 8 Variation. Patient in Bed
d. The end of the sleeve should go into the bedpan.

9. Generously lubricate the cone at the end of the irrigation tubing with water-soluble lubricant.
Prevents irritation and damage to the stoma and intestinal lumen.

10. Open the top of the irrigation sleeve; insert the cone gently into the colostomy stoma, and hold it solidly in place.

Gentle insertion prevents damage to the mucosa. ▼

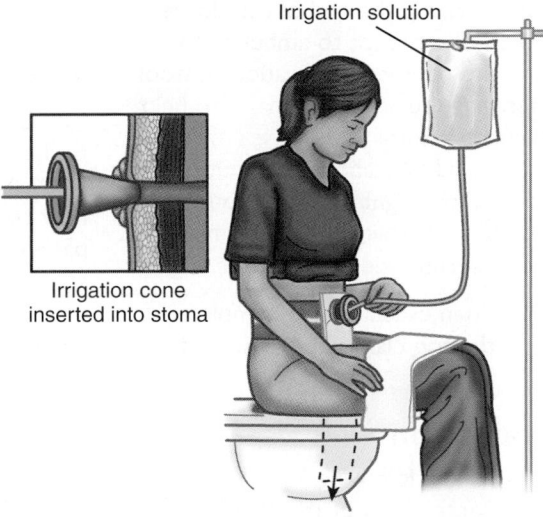

Irrigation solution

Irrigation cone inserted into stoma

11. Open the clamp on the tubing, and slowly begin the flow of water. The fluid should flow for about 10 to 15 minutes or as the patient can tolerate.
Proceeding slowly allows the patient to adjust to the distention of the bowel.

12. If the patient complains of discomfort, stop the flow for 15 to 30 seconds, and ask the patient take deep breaths.
Allows the patient to rest and adjust to the pressure of solution. Cramping may indicate that the bowel is ready to empty, the water is too cold, the flow is too fast, or the tube contains air.

13. When the correct amount of solution has instilled, clamp the tubing, and remove the cone from the stoma.

14. Wrap the end of the cone in tissue or paper towel until you can clean or dispose of it properly.
Prevents transmission of intestinal bacteria.

15. Close the top of the irrigation sleeve with a clamp.
Prevents spillage of irrigation fluid and feces.

(continued on next page)

Procedure 28-7 ■ **Irrigating a Colostomy** (continued)

16. Ask the patient remain sitting until most of the irrigation fluid and bowel contents have evacuated. Alternatively, you can clamp the end of the sleeve and ask the patient to ambulate to stimulate compete evacuation of stool. Massaging the abdomen may also help stimulate return.

This should take about 30 minutes on average. You might wait for about an hour to be certain all the fecal material has been returned.

17. When evacuation is complete, open the top clamp, and rinse and remove the irrigation sleeve. Set it aside.

The irrigation sleeve is reusable, but it should be rinsed promptly to make thorough cleansing easier in the following steps.

18. Cleanse the stoma and peristomal skin area with a warm washcloth. Prep the skin and apply a new colostomy appliance, if the patient is wearing one, following the steps in Procedure 28-6. Otherwise, cover the stoma with a small gauze bandage.

19. Clean the irrigation sleeve with mild soap and water. Allow it to dry. Place the irrigation supplies in the proper place (e.g., in a plastic container or plastic bag).

The irrigation sleeve is reusable, but it must be cleaned well to avoid odors and transmission of pathogens.

20. Remove your gloves and wash your hands.

Prevents healthcare-associated infections.

21. Assist the patient back to a position of comfort.

Evaluation

Observe the following:

- Characteristics of the stool: color, amount, consistency
- Signs of bleeding from stoma or bowel
- Presence or absence of abdominal distention
- Patient's tolerance of procedure (e.g., cramps, fatigue)
- Patient's ability to participate in the irrigation

Patient Teaching

- Teach the patient the purpose for the procedure.
- Explain that using sufficient fluid will decrease the need for multiple irrigations during the day.
- Teach the steps of the irrigation procedure to prepare the patient to complete the task at home.
- Explain that it takes approximately 6 to 8 weeks to achieve bowel regulation with irrigations.

Home Care

- Help the client determine where this procedure will be completed in the home setting.
- Make sure the client has resources for purchasing the supplies for the irrigation. Provide contact information.
- Help the client locate a place to hang the irrigation container. There may be a hook on the bathroom wall, for instance.
- If the irrigating solution does not flow well, the client should:
  - Check the tubing for kinks.
  - Change the position of the cone.
  - Put the container at a slightly higher level.

- Explain and demonstrate how to care for the irrigation supplies (e.g., how to rinse and clean the sleeve and/or belt, if used).

Documentation

Document:

- Your assessment of the stoma and peristomal area
- The amount of irrigation solution used
- The date and time that you performed the irrigation
- Characteristics of the stool returned in the irrigation fluid
- Patient teaching

Sample documentation:

06/14/11   8:30 A.M.   Ostomy irrigated with 750 mL warm tap water. Small amount of loosely formed, flaky stool returned in the fluid, with some undigested food apparent. No blood; very small amount of mucus. Stoma pink, peristomal area without redness. Explained procedure steps to patient as it was performed. Patient stated he will do some of the steps tomorrow. ——— C. Hiam, RNC

Practice Resources

Black, P. (2008); Burch, J., & Sica, J. (2008); Cronin, E. (2008); Karadag, A., Mentex, B., & Ayaz, S. (2005); Kent, D. (2008); Richbourg, L., Fellows, J., & Arroyave, W. (2007); Siegal, J., Rhinehart, E., Jackson, M., et al. (2007).

Procedure 28-8 ▢ Placing Fecal Drainage Devices

➤ For steps to follow in *all* procedures, refer to the Universal Steps for All Procedures found on the inside back cover of Volume 2.

Critical Aspects

Procedure 28-8A: External Device
- Select the fecal management system appropriate for the patient.
- Obtain assistance as needed.
- Place the patient side-lying.
- Cleanse and dry perineal area; clip hair as needed.
- Spread the buttocks and apply the device; avoid gaps and creases.
- Hang drainage bag lower than the patient.

Procedure 28-8B: Indwelling Device
- Select the fecal management system appropriate for the patient.
- Obtain assistance as needed.
- Place the patient left side-lying.
- Remove any indwelling device.
- Cleanse and dry perineal area; clip hair as needed.
- Prepare the device according to instructions (e.g., remove residual air from the balloon).
- Lubricate the balloon generously with water-soluble lubricant.
- Spread buttocks and gently insert the balloon end of the catheter.
- Inflate the device with water or saline.
- Remove the syringe from the inflation port; gently tug the catheter.
- Position the tubing, avoiding kinks; position the collection bag lower than patient.

Equipment

External Fecal Collection Device

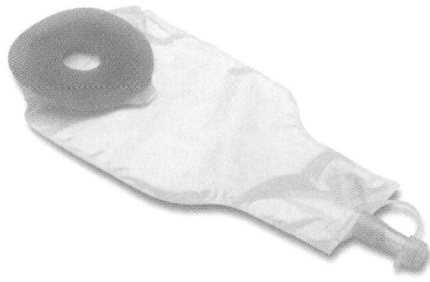

External fecal collection device

- pH-balanced soap and water or recommended skin cleanser
- Skin protection wipes (e.g., peristomal wipes to protect skin and improve adherence)
- Self-adhesive fecal containment device
- Procedure gloves
- Linen-saver pad
- Scissors

Internal Fecal Collection System

- Fecal device kit: Contains soft silicone catheter tube assembly, a syringe, and a collection bag.
- Water-soluble lubricant
- Approximately 100 mL container of tap water or saline. (Follow the manufacturer's directions for amount and type of solution.)

- 500 mL of lukewarm irrigant (water or saline)
- 60-mL Luer-tip syringe and a catheter tip syringe (if not contained in the kit)
- Protective skin-care dressing (e.g., Stomahesive®, DuoDerm®)
- Tape
- Procedure gloves, mask, and goggles
- pH-balanced soap and water or recommended skin cleanser
- Scissors
- Linen-saver pad

Delegation

Application of an external fecal collection system may be delegated to the NAP. Insertion of a internal fecal collection device is usually performed by a professional nurse, but may be delegated to an LPN depending on agency policy.

Pre-Procedure Assessments

- Assess the patient's bowel patterns.

Fecal diversion is indicated when the patient is incontinent of liquid or semi-liquid stools (flowing).

- Assess for allergies to silicone. If the patient is sensitive or allergic to any of the materials in the device, it cannot be used.
- Inspect perirectal skin.

External devices should not be used in patients with impaired skin integrity.

(continued on next page)

Procedure 28-8 ■ Placing Fecal Drainage Devices (continued)

For Indwelling Devices, in Addition:

■ Assess whether the patient has had a recent bowel movement.

Patients who have not had a bowel movement for two or more days should be considered as having firm stool and will likely be given a bowel prep or enema before insertion of the indwelling device.

■ Check for the presence of any indwelling anal or rectal device (e.g., thermometer for continuous temperature monitoring).

The treatment plan may need to be changed. If suppositories or enemas are a part of the current treatment plan, collaborate with the physician as these medication delivery mechanisms will need to be changed.

✦ ■ Identify factors that increase your patient's risk for bleeding, including medications (anticoagulant and/

or antiplatelet therapy) and lab results (PT, PTT, platelets).

Patients with an increased risk of bleeding should be monitored carefully.

✦ ■ Check the chart for contraindications to an indwelling fecal management system (e.g., proctitis, lacerations, rectal surgery in the past year, large or painful hemorrhoids).

If your patient has a history of any of these problems, contact the primary care provider immediately. You may elect to use an external device, but an internal fecal catheter is contraindicated.

✦ ■ Internal fecal catheters should not be used for children.

■ Procedure 28-8A Applying an External Fecal Collection System

➤ When performing the procedure, always identify your patient according to agency policy and be attentive to standard precautions, hand hygiene, patient safety and privacy, body mechanics, and documentation.

Procedure Steps

1. Recruit another nurse or nursing assistant to help you. Assist the patient to a side-lying position and drape to expose the buttocks.

For successful application (without leakage) it is best to have one caregiver position the patient and a second person apply the device.

2. Don procedure gloves.
Observes standard precautions.

3. Cleanse the perineal area and dry well. If perianal hair is present, trim it away.

To obtain a leakproof seal, the device should be attached to clean, dry skin.

4. Spread the buttocks apart to expose the rectum. Apply the fecal bag, being careful to place the opening in the bag over the anus and to avoid gaps and creases.

Careful application helps to obtain a leakproof seal.

5. Release the buttocks. Connect the fecal incontinence pouch to a drainage bag. Hang drainage bag below patient.

To collect and promote gravity drainage of fecal material.

■ Procedure 28-8B Inserting an Indwelling Fecal Drainage Device

➤ When performing the procedure, always identify your patient according to agency policy and be attentive to standard precautions, hand hygiene, patient safety and privacy, body mechanics, and documentation.

➤ Note: Because devices differ markedly, it is best to follow the manufacturer's instructions for placing the device. The following are generic instructions.

➤ Note: Also see Clinical Insight 28-2: Caring for a Patient with an Indwelling Fecal Drainage Device.

Procedure Steps

1. Ensure that a primary care provider has performed a digital rectal exam.

To assess for the presence of contraindications and to check sphincter tone. When sphincter tone is compromised, the patient may not be able to retain the device.

2. Don procedure gloves, mask, and goggles.

To protect from splatters when irrigating or disconnecting the device. Usually the devices are used for incontinence of loose, if not liquid, stool.

3. Position the patient in the left side-lying position.

Allows access to the rectum.

4. Remove any indwelling device.

The presence of a foreign body between the inflated balloon and rectum may damage rectal mucosa and a seal cannot be maintained.

5. Depending on the type of device, verify proper inflation and deflation of the intralumenal balloon. Attach the syringe, inflate with the recommended amount of air, deflate, and remove the syringe.

6. Again depending on the device, fill the retention cuff with 35 to 40 mL of water; disconnect syringe and check for leaks. After verifying function, slowly and completely aspirate all fluid from cuff and balloon and disconnect the syringe.

7. Connect the indwelling tube to the collection bag. Clamp and hang the bag lower than the level of the patient.

8. Some systems have an "introducer," which you must inflate with about 25 mL of air through a connector on the tube. Disconnect the syringe. ▼

9. Insert your lubricated, gloved index finger into the balloon cuff finger pocket (located above the position indicator line) and coat the balloon generously with lubricant.

This allows for digital guidance during insertion.

10. Gently insert the balloon end of the catheter through the anal sphincter until the balloon is beyond the anus and well inside the rectal vault.

This helps prevent accidental expulsion of the device.

11. Inflate the retention cuff with water or saline per the manufacturers guidelines. Do not overfill. If the catheter will not accept the recommended amount of fluid, see "What if..." at the end of this procedure. ▼

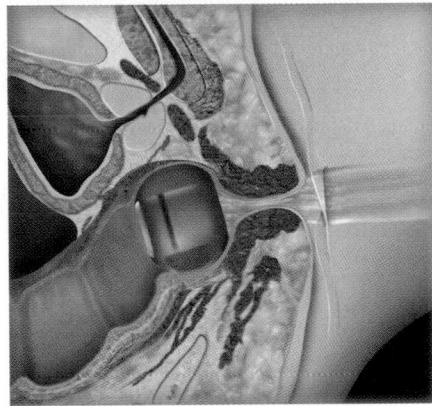

Indwelling fecal drainage device inserted in rectum, with retention cuff inflated. (Courtesy of Hollister Incorporated, Libertyville, IL.)

12. Remove the syringe from the inflation port and put gentle traction on the catheter.

To determine whether the balloon is securely in the rectum and appropriately positioned against the rectal floor.

13. If you inflated an intralumenal balloon or introducer in Step 8, you must now completely aspirate the air from it.

✚ Do not leave an air-inflated intralumenal balloon inflated in an unattended patient.

An inflated balloon can cause tissue necrosis after a period of time.

14. If the device has anchoring straps, apply protective skin care dressing and tape one strap to each of the patient's buttocks.

Prevents internal migration of the tube and occlusion by twisting of the tube.

15. Position the tubing along the patient's leg, avoiding kinks and obstruction and position the collection bag lower than the patient.

Promotes flow of stool from the rectum to the collection bag.

What if...

- **When irrigating, the catheter will not accept the recommended amount of fluid?**

Deflate the balloon and reposition the catheter.

The catheter is probably not positioned correctly. Do not use more than the recommended amount of fluid, as this would result in excessive pressure on the rectal vault and may cause mucosal or sphincter damage.

- **Rectal bleeding occurs with an internal fecal management device?**

Discontinue the device and notify the physician.

Bleeding may indicate pressure necrosis from the device.

Connector to drainage bag

Connector cap

Port to inflate intralumenal balloon (for air)

Sheet clip

Irrigation connector

Retention cuff connector (to fill with water)

Retention cuff

Anchor straps

An indwelling fecal drainage device. (Courtesy of Hollister Inc., Libertyville, IL.)

(continued on next page)

Procedure 28-8 ■ **Placing Fecal Drainage Devices** (continued)

Evaluation

- Confirm catheter/bowel lumen patency by irrigating the bowel according to manufacturer's instructions and physician order. Regular irrigation is required to facilitate evacuation through most devices.

Stool needs to be of loose consistency to pass through the indwelling tube.

- Assess how well the patient tolerated the procedure.
- Note the color, consistency, and odor of stool.
- Monitor the amount of stool in the collection bag. When the collection bag is approximately two-thirds full, change it.
- Monitor for abdominal distention and pain.
- Regularly assess that connections are secure and that the device is not leaking.

In addition, for indwelling devices monitor:
- Length of time the device is in place

Not intended for use longer than 29 days.

- Rectal bleeding

May indicate tissue necrosis, bowel perforation, or fistula formation; device must be removed.

Documentation

- Date, time, and type of collection device used
- Your assessment of the perineal skin
- Patient's tolerance of the procedure
- Characteristics and amount of stool in the collection bag (output)
- Patient/family teaching

Sample EHR documentation:

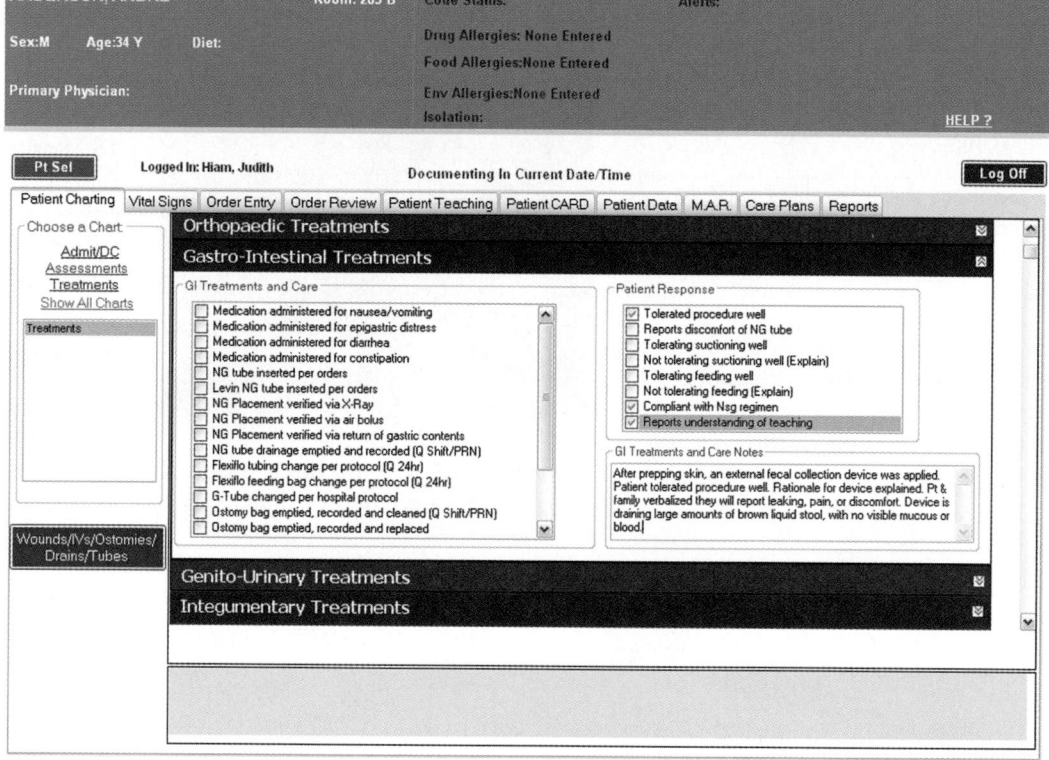

Practice Resources

Benoit R., & Watts, C. (2007); Keshava, A., Renwick, A., Stewart, P., et al. (2007); Siegal, J., Rhinehart, E., Jackson, M., et al. (2007); Wishin, J., Gallagher, T., & McCann, E. (2008); Wound, Ostomy and Continence Nurses Society (2003).

Clinical Insights

Clinical Insight 28-1 ▶ Testing for Pinworms

Pinworms (an intestinal parasite) live in the cecum and migrate to the anal area to deposit eggs during the night; they go back into the rectum during the day. Pinworm infestation is frequently seen in children. The test may need to be repeated on several consecutive days.

- While the child is sleeping, spread the buttocks, and examine the anus to see whether any pinworms are visible to the naked eye. You will need a flashlight to visualize the site.

- Test in the morning, as soon as the person awakens and before he gets out of bed to use the bathroom or bathe. Press clear (not frosted) cellophane tape against the anal opening. Remove it immediately and place it on a slide. Eggs will be visible.
- Alternatively, or in addition, insert a cotton-tipped swab gently into the rectum for not more than 2.5 cm (1 in.). Smear the specimen on a slide to inspect for parasites and eggs.

Clinical Insight 28-2 ▶ Caring for a Patient with an Indwelling Fecal Drainage Device

A catheter is present in the rectum and is connected to a drainage tube and collection bag.

Nursing Goal 1: Prevent injury to rectal sphincter and/or rectal mucosa.

- Do not add air or fluid to the balloon port of the catheter.
- Check the catheter frequently for kinks or obstructions.
- Monitor for signs of complications and notify the healthcare provider immediately if patient experiences:
  - Rectal pain
  - Rectal bleeding
  - Abdominal distention and or/pain.
- Monitor stool for change in consistency (solid or soft-formed stool cannot pass through the catheter and will cause an obstruction).
- How to discontinue the catheter:
  1. Attach a 60-mL syringe to the balloon inflation port and deflate the retention balloon by pulling back on the plunger.
  2. Grasp the catheter as close to the patient as possible and slowly slide it out of the anus.
  3. Dispose of the device accordance to the agency policy for disposal of medical waste.

Nursing Goal 2: Maintain free flow of liquid stool.

- Monitor the patient for changes in stool consistency. If the stool is no longer liquid and flowing, the device must be discontinued.
- Make sure the tubing and bag remain below the level of the patient.
- Irrigate the tube as often as necessary to maintain patency:
  1. Fill a 60-mL syringe with room-temperature tap water.
  2. Attach it to the irrigation port of the catheter and flush by depressing the plunger.

✚ Be sure you are using the irrigation port, NOT the balloon inflation port.

  3. Be sure to subtract the irrigation fluid from the stool volume to maintain an accurate record of intake and output.
- Change the collection bag when it is three-fourths full.
  1. Remove the collection bag from the tubing. Snap the cap onto the used bag and dispose of according to agency policy for medical waste.
  2. Snap new collection bag securely onto the device.

Nursing Goal 3: Prevent transmission of pathogens to others.

- Follow the agency protocol for hand hygiene. Always wear clean procedure gloves when handling the fecal management device.
- Monitor stool cultures and implement isolation protocols as indicated. If a stool sample is ordered, you may obtain it from the collection bag:
  1. If the collection bag is more than 24 hours old, place a new collection bag before obtaining sample.
  2. Cut the collection bag at the bottom and transfer stool to an appropriate container for transport to the lab.
  3. Apply a new collection bag to the connector at the end of the catheter.

Nursing Goal 4: Maintain perineal skin integrity or prevent wounds from being contaminated by stool.

- Monitor insertion site for leakage and signs of infection.
- If perineal wounds are present, keep clean and dry; notify the primary provider if signs of infection are present.
- Perform perineal care according to agency policy

Clinical Insight 28-3 ▶ Guidelines for Ostomy Care

Assess stoma appearance.

- The stoma should be moist and red or pink. Alterations in stoma color (purple, black, or blue) may indicate poor circulation and possible necrosis and should be reported to the healthcare provider.
- Protruding or retracted stomas will need special adjustments in wafer measurement and placement. It is normal for a new stoma to have yellow or blood-tinged mucus or dried blood on it.

Preserve peristomal skin.

- Preserving peristomal skin is critical because skin excoriation may cause an ineffective seal between the wafer and the skin and leakage of effluent. This in turn causes more skin and tissue damage. Leakage may indicate the need for a different type of pouch system or sealant.

Change the pouch as scheduled.

- Pouches are usually changed every 3 to 5 days, preferably before leakage occurs. Frequency also depends on the type of stoma, the equipment used (e.g., one- or two-piece pouch), the effluent, the patient's preference, and the climate (i.e., pouches are changed more frequently during the summer).
- To decrease skin irritation, avoid changing the entire system. In a one-piece or two-piece pouching system, change the skin barrier only every 3 to 7 days, never daily.

Assess the patient's self-care ability.

- Patients with poor vision may need to use magnification mirrors and yellow-tinted sunglasses to help reduce glare and improve contrast when they perform stoma care.

- Patients with immobility or spinal cord injury may need equipment that has a longer pouch that the patient can easily empty independently when sitting.
- Impaired dexterity or vision may warrant the use of a one-piece system or precut pouch and skin barrier, whereas a two-piece system may be better for patients who need to keep the skin barrier in place for several days and change just the pouch.
- Patients who are blind can be taught to change their own equipment.

Plan when to change the pouch.

- Change the skin barrier pouch at times of lower effluent output.
- Avoid changing after meals, when the gastrocolic reflux increases chance of fecal effluent output. Mucous secretion is normal.

Determine whether the ostomy should be irrigated.

- Consult a peristomal nurse or the primary care provider to determine whether an ostomy should be irrigated.
- Many patients with left-end colostomies may be safely irrigated as a method of continence management. An ileostomy, however, drains liquid containing high concentrations of sodium, chloride, potassium, magnesium, and bicarbonate.

✚ Ileostomies should never be irrigated, except in cases of food blockage near the stomal outlet. Only a qualified person, such as an enterostomal therapy nurse, may perform a gentle lavage. For lavage, normal saline is preferred because excessive lavage could lead to a serious fluid and electrolyte imbalance.

Assessment Guidelines and Tools

Focused Assessment: Bowel Elimination

Nursing History

Ask questions such as the following:

1. **Normal bowel pattern**
   - How often do you have a bowel movement (BM)?
   - What time of day do you usually have a BM?
   - Do you follow any routines to help you have a BM?

2. **Appearance of stool**
   - How would you describe your stool?
   - What color is your stool?
   - How would you describe the texture of your stool—hard, soft, or watery?
   - What shape is the stool?
   - Have you noticed unusual odor with your stool?

3. **Changes in bowel habits or stool appearance**
   - Have you had any changes in your bowel pattern recently?

- Have you noticed any changes in the appearance, texture, or odor of your stool?

4. **For clients with a bowel diversion,** you will also gather data on the client's usual care of the stoma, use of appliances, and adjustment to the ostomy.

5. **History of elimination problems**
   - What has been your experience with bowel elimination problems?
   - Have you had any problems with constipation, diarrhea, or severe bloating or gas?
   - Have you ever lost control of your bowels?
   - Have you ever had bowel surgery or diagnostic procedures of the digestive tract?

6. **Use of bowel elimination aids,** including diet, exercise, medications, and remedies
   - What aids, if any, do you use to help you have a BM?
   - What foods help you maintain your bowel pattern?

Focused Assessment: Bowel Elimination—cont'd

- What foods do you avoid? What effect do these foods have on you?
- What is your usual fluid intake over the course of a day?
- What is your usual exercise pattern?
- What medications are you taking? Have they had any effect on your bowel elimination pattern?
- What is your current stress level? What effect does stress have on your bowel elimination pattern?

Physical Assessment

Examine the abdomen, rectum, and anus.

- Recall that in abdominal assessment, the order of the exam is inspection, auscultation, percussion, and palpation.
- Observe the size, shape, and contour of the abdomen, and listen to bowel sounds.
- Percuss and palpate the abdomen for tenderness, presence of air or solid, and presence of masses.

- Inspect the anus for signs of hemorrhoids.
- Depending upon the policies of your institution as well as your skill with assessment, you might also palpate the anus and rectum for the presence of stool or masses. When listening to bowel sounds, note the presence and timing of the sounds and the presence of any bruits.

Normal bowel sounds are high-pitched, with approximately 5 to 15 gurgles every minute.

Hyperactive bowel sounds are very high-pitched and more frequent than normal. They may occur with small-bowel obstruction and inflammatory disorders.

Hypoactive bowel sounds are low-pitched, infrequent, and quiet. A decrease in bowel sounds indicates decreased peristalsis.

- If, after listening for 3 to 5 minutes, you hear no bowel sounds, you can describe them as *absent*.

For a complete discussion of physical examination of the abdomen, rectum, and anus, see Procedures 19-14 and 19-19.

Diagnostic Testing

Direct Visualization Studies of the Gastrointestinal Tract

➤ Because all of the following studies are invasive procedures, you should ensure that the patient has signed an informed consent.

➤ All of the procedures require some degree of advance preparation, such as fasting. Check agency policy, because preparation may vary.

➤ Preparing the patient includes telling him what he will experience and feel during the procedure.

➤ When the patient is sedated (e.g., with midazolam or diazepam), a emergency medical cart ("crash cart") must be in the room during the procedure, and the patient monitored with pulse oximetry.

➤ All of the procedures require teaching for aftercare.

➤ For all tests, explain that rectal bleeding is normal for a few days if polyps were removed or a biopsy was taken.

For nursing responsibilities before, during, and after each test,

 Go to Chapter 28, **Tables, Boxes, Figures: ESG Box 28-1: Direct Visualization Studies of the Gastrointestinal Tract,** on the Student Resource Disk or DavisPlus at http://davisplus.fadavis.com/Wilkinson2

Esophagogastroduodenoscopy (EGD)

Provides direct visualization of the upper GI system. A *fiberoptic endoscope*, a long flexible tube with a light and lens, is introduced through the mouth and advanced for visualization of the esophagus, stomach, and duodenum. The physician may also perform tissue biopsies or coagulate bleeding sites through the endoscope.

Sigmoidoscopy

Allows visualization of the anal canal, rectum, and sigmoid colon. A rigid metal scope or a flexible fiberoptic scope may be used. The patient is usually not sedated. During the exam, the physician may perform a biopsy, remove polyps (small growths), or coagulate sources of bleeding in the area. A sigmoidoscopy is recommended as a screen for colon cancer for middle and older adults. Subsequent screening depends on the findings of the sigmoidoscopy as well as patient and family history; however, it is commonly done every 5 years.

Fiberoptic Colonoscopy

Provides direct visualization of the rectum, colon, entire large intestine, and distal small bowel. A flexible scope is inserted through the rectum and advanced to the cecum. Colonoscopy is useful in detecting lower GI disease. Many patients and healthcare providers choose a colonoscopy for cancer screening instead of a sigmoidoscopy, because colonoscopy provides greater visualization of the colon. This is the preferred test for clients with suspected problems above the level of the sigmoid colon. It may be done in a clinic or physician's office.

Source: The American Cancer Society (2008). *Detailed guide: Colon and rectum cancer: revised 04/21/2008.* Retrieved from http://www.cancer.org/docroot/CRI/content/CRI_2_4_7x_CRC_Colorectal_Cancer_PDF.asp; Van Leeuwen, A., Kranpitz, T., & Smith, L. (2006). *Davis's comprehensive handbook of laboratory and diagnostic tests with nursing implications* (2nd ed.). Philadelphia: F. A. Davis.

Diagnostic Testing *(side tab)*

Diagnostic Testing

Indirect Visualization Studies of the Gastrointestinal Tract

For nursing responsibilities before, during, and after each test,

 Go to Chapter 28, **Tables, Boxes, Figures: ESG Box 28-2: Indirect Visualization Studies of the Gastrointestinal Tract,** on the Student Resource Disk or DavisPlus at http://davisplus.fadavis.com/Wilkinson2

Abdominal Flat Plate

An anterior to posterior (AP) x-ray view of the abdomen is used to detect gallstones, fecal impaction, and distended bowel. This test requires no preparation and no special post-test care.

Barium Enema (BE)

A barium enema is a radiological examination of the rectum, colon, and distal small bowel. A rectal tube is inserted into the rectum or an existing ostomy. Barium (a contrast medium) is instilled. The patient must retain the barium through several position changes while air is instilled and radiographs are obtained. The test is especially useful for visualizing polyps, diverticula, and tumors. In addition, it may be used to reduce certain obstructions. As a rule, patients are not sedated. The test is invasive, so a signed informed consent is necessary.

Ultrasonography (Ultrasound)

Ultrasonography detects tissue abnormalities such as masses, cysts, edema, or stones. An ultrasound probe, called a transducer, is moved over the skin surface of the abdomen. The probe emits a sound wave that abdominal tissue and organs reflect back based on their density. The sound waves may be transformed into images visible on a computer screen.

Computed Tomography (CT) Scan

Computed tomography (CT) examines body sections from different angles using a narrow x-ray beam. It produces a three-dimensional picture of the area of the body being scanned. This test is useful in diagnosis of many abdominal disorders. A CT scan may be enhanced by injecting contrast dye that allows for improved visualization of circulatory function. The patient needs to lie very still during the procedure.

Magnetic Resonance Imaging (MRI)

Magnetic resonance imaging (MRI) produces cross-sectional images of the body. MRI utilizes a strong magnetic field and radio waves. This type of diagnostic test does not use ionizing radiation, so it is free of the hazards of x-rays. MRIs are very sensitive and may be used to detect edema, hemorrhage, blood flow, infarcts, tumors, and infections in organ structures. When used, the contrast medium is noniodinated, and it is administered intravenously to enhance contrast between normal and abnormal tissues. The patient must lie still in a narrow tube, sometimes for up to an hour.

Source: Van Leeuwen, A., Kranpitz, T., & Smith, L. (2006). *Davis's comprehensive handbook of laboratory and diagnostic tests with nursing implications* (2nd ed.). Philadelphia: F. A. Davis.

Standardized Language

Nursing Diagnoses Associated with Bowel Elimination

LABEL, DEFINITION, DISCUSSION	DEFINING CHARACTERISTICS/RISK FACTORS	ETIOLOGIES/RELATED FACTORS
Bowel Incontinence. Change in normal bowel habits characterized by involuntary passage of stool	*Subjective*: Urgency, inability to recognize the urge to defecate or inability to feel rectal fullness *Objective*: Constant dribbling of soft stool, red perianal skin, fecal odor, fecal staining of clothing or bedding, and inability to delay defecation	High abdominal or intestinal pressure, chronic diarrhea, colorectal lesions, dietary habits, medications, decline in muscle tone, immobility (inability to get to the bathroom), inaccessibility of bathroom facilities, impaction, stress, Toileting Self-Care Deficit, impaired cognition, laxative abuse, loss of rectal sphincter control, and motor nerve damage

Nursing Diagnoses Associated with Bowel Elimination—cont'd

LABEL, DEFINITION, DISCUSSION	DEFINING CHARACTERISTICS/RISK FACTORS	ETIOLOGIES/RELATED FACTORS
Constipation. Because frequency of bowel elimination varies, constipation is usually defined as a decrease in the frequency of bowel movements resulting in the passage of hard, dry stool. Stools become dry and hard when peristalsis slows and too much water is reabsorbed from the fecal mass. Unrelieved constipation may eventually result in a **fecal impaction,** in which dry, hard stools lodged in the rectum cannot be passed.	*Subjective:* Abdominal pain, a feeling of rectal fullness, straining or pain with defecation, and some rectal bleeding. The person may report needing to perform manual maneuvers to pass stool (e.g., pressing on the anus or pressing on the posterior vaginal wall).	Abdominal muscle weakness, ignoring the urge to defecate, insufficient physical activity, depression, emotional stress, medications, changes in eating patterns, and insufficient fiber or fluid intake. Habitual laxative use may also cause constipation as the colon becomes responsive only to the stimulating effect of the laxative.
Risk for Constipation. At risk for a decrease in normal frequency of defecation accompanied by difficult or incomplete passage of stool and/or hard dry stool.	*Risk factors:* Abdominal muscle weakness, habitually ignoring the urge to defecate, insufficient intake of fluid and fiber, dehydration, and certain medications (e.g., opioids, anticholinergics, calcium channel blockers), surgery. Constipation is more common among women than men, and increases with age. It is associated with depression, lower socioeconomic status, and lower education levels.	Not applicable
Perceived Constipation is an appropriate diagnosis for a client who makes a self-diagnosis of constipation and uses laxatives, suppositories, or enemas to ensure a daily bowel movement.	*Subjective:* Expectation of a daily bowel movement, or at the same time every day; overuse of laxatives, enemas, or suppositories	Cultural and family health beliefs and impaired thought processes
Diarrhea is the passage of loose, unformed or watery stools. Persistent diarrhea threatens fluid and electrolyte balance, especially in young children and older adults.	*Subjective:* Abdominal pain, cramping, and urgency *Objective:* At least three loose, liquid stools per day; and hyperactive bowel sounds. The patient may also experience bloating, fever, and blood in the stools, depending on the cause of the diarrhea.	Anxiety, high stress levels, radiation, toxins, travel, tube feedings, medication side effects, alcohol abuse, contaminants, laxative abuse, infections, inflammation, irritation, malabsorption, parasite. The most common cause is GI infection; however, diarrhea may occur with a chronic disease, such as celiac disease or irritable bowel syndrome.
Dysfunctional Gastrointestinal Motility is the increased, decreased, ineffective, or absence of peristaltic activity within the GI system. If you use this label, you need to specify whether the GI motility is increased, decreased, and so on (e.g., Dysfunctional GI Motility: Increased).	Because the diagnosis is defined so broadly, defining characteristics include symptoms of both diarrhea and constipation, as well as nausea, regurgitation, vomiting, increased gastric residual, bile-colored gastric residual, and accelerated gastric emptying.	Aging, anxiety, tube feedings, food intolerance (e.g., lactose intolerance), immobility, contaminates (e.g., in food), malnutrition, medications, anesthesia, surgery prematurity, sedentary lifestyle
Risk for Dysfunctional Gastrointestinal Motility is the risk for increased, decreased, ineffective, or lack of peristaltic activity within the GI system.	*Risk Factors:* Abdominal surgery, aging, anxiety, change in food or eater, decreased GI circulation, diabetes mellitus, food intolerance, gastroesophageal reflux disease (GERD), immobility, infection, medications, prematurity, sedentary lifestyle, stress, or unsanitary food preparation	Not applicable

Continued

Nursing Diagnoses Associated with Bowel Elimination—cont'd

LABEL, DEFINITION, DISCUSSION	DEFINING CHARACTERISTICS/RISK FACTORS	ETIOLOGIES/RELATED FACTORS
Toileting Self-Care Deficit is impaired ability to perform or complete own toileting activities. Strictly speaking, this is not a bowel problem. Bowel function may be normal, but the person simply cannot manage toileting.	Use this diagnosis for patients who cannot manipulate their clothing for toileting, carry out proper toilet hygiene, flush the toilet, get to the toilet or commode, or sit on or rise from the toilet or commode.	Cognitive impairment, decreased motivation, environmental barriers, fatigue, impaired mobility, musculoskeletal or neuromuscular impairment, pain, perceptual impairment, severe anxiety, developmental disability, lack of motivation, weakness

Selected Standardized Outcomes and Interventions for Bowel Elimination Diagnoses

NURSING DIAGNOSIS	NOC OUTCOMES AND SCALE*	NOC OUTCOME INDICATORS	NIC INTERVENTIONS AND ACTIVITIES
Bowel Incontinence	Bowel Continence (m and t)	Recognizes urge to defecate. Maintains control of stool passage. Responds to urge in timely manner.	***Bowel Incontinence Care*** Determine . . . cause of fecal incontinence. Keep bed and clothing clean. Place on incontinent pads as needed.
	Bowel Elimination (a and n)	Control of bowel movements Elimination pattern Diarrhea Mucus in stool	***Bowel Management*** Teach patient/family members to record color, volume, frequency, and consistency of stools ***Bowel Training*** Initiate an uninterrupted, consistent time for defecation.
	Tissue Integrity: Skin and Mucous Membranes (a and n)	Skin integrity Erythema Skin lesions	Teach patient/family the principles of bowel training.
Constipation	Bowel Elimination (a and n)	Stool soft and formed Ease of stool passage Pain with passage of stool Passage of stool without aids	***Bowel Management*** Monitor BMs, including frequency, consistency, shape, volume, and color, as appropriate. Instruct the patient on foods high in fiber, as appropriate. Insert rectal suppository, as needed.
	Hydration (a and n)	Skin turgor Moist mucous membranes Fluid intake Dark urine	***Constipation/Impaction Management*** Monitor for . . . impaction Institute a toileting schedule as appropriate. Teach patient/family on the relationship of diet, exercise, and fluid intake to constipation/impaction.

Selected Standardized Outcomes and Interventions for Bowel Elimination Diagnoses—cont'd

NURSING DIAGNOSIS	NOC OUTCOMES AND SCALE*	NOC OUTCOME INDICATORS	NIC INTERVENTIONS AND ACTIVITIES
	Symptom Control (m)	Uses symptom relief measures	**Fluid Management**
		Reports symptoms controlled.	Monitor hydration status (e.g., moist mucous membranes . . .).
			Promote oral intake (e.g., . . . offer fluids between meals).
Constipation, Perceived	Health Beliefs (l)	Perceived importance of taking action	**Teaching: Individual**
			Determine patient's learning needs.
		Perceived threat from inaction	Determine . . . ability to learn specific information (i.e., developmental level, pain, fatigue, emotional state . . .).
		Perceived benefits of action	Reinforce behavior as appropriate
	Bowel Elimination (a and n)	Abuse of elimination aids	**Values Clarification**
		Passage of stool without aids	Encourage the patient to list values that guide behavior in various settings and types of situations.
		Elimination pattern	Encourage consideration of the issues and consequences of behavior.
Diarrhea	Bowel Elimination (a and n)	Elimination pattern	**Bowel Management**
		Fat in stool	Monitor BMs, including frequency, consistency, shape, volume, and color, as appropriate.
		Blood in stool	**Diarrhea Management**
		Mucus in stool	
		Diarrhea	Evaluate medication profile for gastrointestinal side effects.
	Electrolyte and Acid–Base Balance (b and n)	Apical heart rate and rhythm	Encourage frequent, small feedings, adding bulk gradually.
		Respiratory rate, rhythm	Suggest trial elimination of foods containing lactose.
		Serum Na⁺, K⁺, Ca²⁺ (etc.)	
		Impaired cognition	Instruct the patient to notify the staff of each episode of diarrhea.
		Muscle strength	
	Fluid Balance (a and n)	24-hour intake and output balance	Monitor the skin in the perianal area for irritation and ulceration. Measure diarrhea/bowel output.
		Skin turgor	**Fluid/Electrolyte Management**
		Moist mucous membranes	Monitor for abnormal serum electrolyte levels, as available.
	Symptom Severity (n)	Symptom intensity	Consult the physician if signs and symptoms of fluid and/or electrolyte imbalance persist or worsen.
		Impaired life enjoyment	

Continued

Selected Standardized Outcomes and Interventions for Bowel Elimination Diagnoses—cont'd

NURSING DIAGNOSIS	NOC OUTCOMES AND SCALE*	NOC OUTCOME INDICATORS	NIC INTERVENTIONS AND ACTIVITIES
Dysfunctional Gastrointestinal Motility†	Bowel Elimination (a and n)	Bowel sounds	**Bowel Management**
		Elimination pattern	Monitor bowel sounds
	Gastrointestinal Function (a and n)	Abdominal distention	Monitor bowel movements. Note preexisting bowel problems, bowel routine, and use of laxatives.
		Increase in visible peristalsis	
			Evaluate medication profile for GI side effects.
		Regurgitation	Monitor for signs and symptoms of diarrhea, constipation, and impaction.
		Frequency of stools	
		Gastric aspirates: amount of residuals	**Nausea Management**
	Nausea & Vomiting Severity	Frequency of nausea	Perform complete assessment of nausea...
		Frequency of vomiting	Identify factors (e.g., medication...) that may cause... nausea
		Fecal odor of emesis	Instruct in high-carbohydrate and low-fat food...
		Excessive secretion of saliva	**Vomiting Management**
			Measure or estimate emesis volume
			Use oral hygiene to clean mouth and nose
			Control environmental factors that may evoke vomiting (e.g., ... smells...)
Toileting Self-Care Deficit	Refer to Chapter 22.		

Sources: Bulechek, G., Butcher, H., & Dochterman, J. (Eds.). (2008). *Nursing interventions classification (NIC)* (5th ed.). St. Louis, MO: C.V. Mosby; Moorhead, S., Johnson, M., Maas, M., et al. (Eds.). (2008). *Nursing outcomes classification (NOC)* (4th ed.). St. Louis, MO: C.V. Mosby; NANDA International. (2009). *NANDA nursing diagnoses: Definitions and classification 2009–2011.* Ames, IA: Wiley-Blackwell. Used with permission.

*For a list of NOC measurement scales, see Chapter 5, Volume 2.

†This is a new nursing diagnosis. NOC outcomes have not yet been linked to it; these are only suggestions.

THINKING CRITICALLY ABOUT BOWEL ELIMINATION

The exercises in the following sections allow you to practice the kind of thinking you will use as a full-spectrum nurse. Because these are critical-thinking questions, there is usually no single right answer. We do not provide answers for these questions because it is more important for you to think about the questions than to arrive at the "right" answer. These questions are designed to improve your thinking more than to "cover content." Discuss answers with your peers—discussion can stimulate critical thinking. If you have difficulty with any of these questions, consult with your instructor.

Applying the Full-Spectrum Nursing Model

PATIENT SITUATION

Lucy Franklin is a frail elderly woman, a long-time resident in a long-term care facility. She can no longer communicate and lies however the NAPs place her in bed, seldom moving. She is very thin, does not eat or drink, and is being fed entirely through a gastrostomy tube. She is incontinent of both stool and urine, and has recently started having copious diarrhea, probably from the tube feedings, but that has not been established definitely. The skin on Lucy's back, buttocks, and perineum is still intact, but it is quite red now. The healthcare team is considering various measures for controlling the diarrhea, but until that can be achieved, nurses want to protect her skin integrity.

THINKING

1. *Theoretical Knowledge*:

   a. Other than tube feedings, what else could be causing Lucy's diarrhea?

   b. In addition to Impaired Skin Integrity, what are some other risks associated with diarrhea?

   c. Why is fecal incontinence, especially with diarrhea, a risk factor for Impaired Skin Integrity?

2. *Critical Thinking*:

   a. *(Contextual Awareness)*: What other factors in Lucy's situation do you think might make her even more vulnerable to Impaired Skin Integrity? If you do not yet have the theoretical knowledge you need, draw on your own experiences—and think carefully about everything you know about Lucy.

   b. *(Considering Alternatives)*: A fecal incontinence pouch is being discussed as an intervention to preserve Lucy's skin integrity. Do you think it should be an external system or an internal system? Why?

DOING

3. *Practical Knowledge*:

   It has been decided that an external fecal collection system will be used. Describe the steps you will take to apply this system after you have made the necessary assessments.

4. *Nursing Process (Assessments)*:

   What ongoing assessments will you need to make after the fecal collection system is applied?

CARING

5. *Self-Knowledge*:

   How comfortable would you be applying Lucy's fecal collection system? What aspects of the situation make you most uncomfortable?

Critical Thinking and Clinical Reasoning

1. Your neighbor is aware that you are a nursing student and calls you for advice. She has a 12-year-old daughter with diarrhea. "Everything runs through her," states the mother. There are also two other children in the house, ages 6 years and 18 months. Both have had watery stools this morning. Your neighbor explains that her husband has an ileostomy and has been hospitalized since yesterday. Your neighbor has no symptoms but is very worried. She asks, "Do we all need to go to the hospital?"

   a. Consider alternatives. What are the most likely explanations for the diarrhea?

   b. Based on your theoretical knowledge, how would you explain why her husband was hospitalized, while the rest of the family members, who have the same symptoms, remain at home?

   c. After reassuring her, what advice should you offer your neighbor about self-care for her and the children's elimination problem?

2. Consider the following patients:

   ■ A 54-year-old man diagnosed with colon cancer who now has a new sigmoid colostomy
   ■ A 21-year-old woman with Crohn's disease (an inflammatory bowel disorder) who has just had an ileostomy
   ■ A 36-year-old trauma victim who has a new double-barreled transverse colostomy

   a. How are these patients similar?

   b. In regard to their surgery, what nursing care priorities do these patients share?

   c. How do the major concerns for these patients differ? (Consider the context. How are their surgical and self-care situations different?)

3. For each of the following concepts, use critical thinking to describe how or why it is important to nursing, patient care, or bowel elimination. Note that these are *not* to be merely definitions.

   Digestion (in the mouth, esophagus,   Location of a bowel diversion
      stomach, and small intestine)   Bowel sounds
   Large intestine (colon)   Providing privacy
   Rectum and anus   Diarrhea
   Fluid intake

What Are the Main Points in This Chapter?

➤ Bowel elimination is a normal process by which waste products are eliminated from the body.

➤ Feces is a mixture of insoluble fiber and other indigestible material, bacteria, and water.

➤ During defecation, the internal and external anal sphincters relax; the rectum contracts; and peristalsis increases in the sigmoid colon, propelling feces through the anus.

➤ The frequency of BMs varies. As long as stools are passed without excessive urgency, with minimal effort and no straining, and without the use of laxatives, bowel function is regarded as normal.

➤ The bowel pattern set in childhood normally continues into adulthood. Adequate fiber, fluid, and exercise are required to maintain this pattern.

➤ Factors affecting bowel function include developmental stage, personal and sociocultural factors, nutrition, hydration, activity level, stress, anesthesia, medications, pregnancy, surgery and other procedures, and pathological conditions.

➤ To promote regular defecation, provide privacy for the patient and allow time to use the toilet.

➤ Constipation is a decrease in frequency of BMs and the passage of dry, hard stool that requires more effort to pass.

➤ Bulking agents are the preferred medication for treating constipation.

➤ Habitual use of laxatives, with the exception of bulking agents, may cause reliance on medication for bowel elimination.

➤ Fecal impaction is detected by digital examination of the rectum. To treat a fecal impaction, enemas or digital removal of stool is required.

➤ An enema is the introduction of solution into the rectum to soften feces, distend the colon, and stimulate peristalsis and evacuation of feces.

➤ Flatulence can be managed by avoiding foods that trigger this response and maintaining regular bowel movements.

➤ Diarrhea is the passage of frequent, watery stools.

➤ Monitor patients with diarrhea for intake and output, body weight, and vital signs to assess for fluid losses; provide hygiene measures to protect the skin.

➤ Bowel incontinence may be managed by providing assistance to the bathroom at regular intervals and at the times BMs are most likely to occur, and by beginning a bowel training program.

➤ External or internal fecal collection devices can be used to protect perianal skin or to collect large stool samples. They minimize odor, allow for accurate measurement of output, and improve patient comfort.

➤ A bowel diversion is a surgically created opening for elimination of digestive waste products.

➤ The effluent of an ostomy ranges from liquid to solid, depending on the part of the bowel that is being diverted.

➤ A healthy stoma ranges in color from deep pink to brick red and is shiny and moist at all times.

➤ A moisture-proof skin barrier is usually placed around a stoma to protect surrounding skin.

➤ A client with a bowel diversion must adapt to the stoma for elimination and learn to care for the stoma.

For practice questions for this chapter,

Go to **NCLEX-Style Chapter Quiz,** on the Student Resource Disk or DavisPlus at http://davisplus.fadavis.com/Wilkinson2

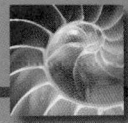

Knowledge Map

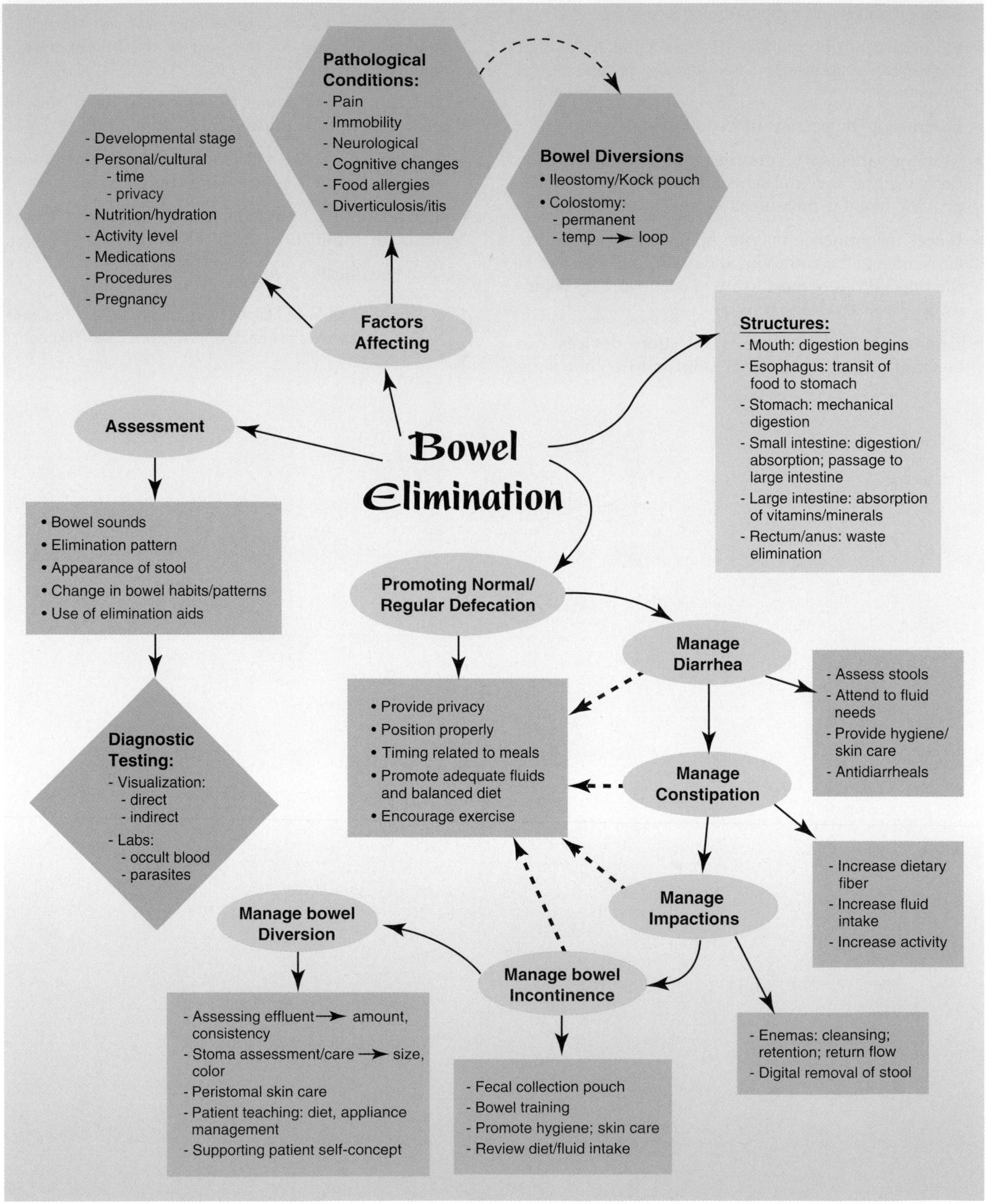

Factors Affecting

- Developmental stage
- Personal/cultural
   - time
   - privacy
- Nutrition/hydration
- Activity level
- Medications
- Procedures
- Pregnancy

Pathological Conditions:

- Pain
- Immobility
- Neurological
- Cognitive changes
- Food allergies
- Diverticulosis/itis

Bowel Diversions

- Ileostomy/Kock pouch
- Colostomy:
   - permanent
   - temp → loop

Structures:

- Mouth: digestion begins
- Esophagus: transit of food to stomach
- Stomach: mechanical digestion
- Small intestine: digestion/ absorption; passage to large intestine
- Large intestine: absorption of vitamins/minerals
- Rectum/anus: waste elimination

Bowel Elimination

Assessment

- Bowel sounds
- Elimination pattern
- Appearance of stool
- Change in bowel habits/patterns
- Use of elimination aids

Diagnostic Testing:

- Visualization:
   - direct
   - indirect
- Labs:
   - occult blood
   - parasites

Promoting Normal/ Regular Defecation

- Provide privacy
- Position properly
- Timing related to meals
- Promote adequate fluids and balanced diet
- Encourage exercise

Manage Diarrhea

- Assess stools
- Attend to fluid needs
- Provide hygiene/ skin care
- Antidiarrheals

Manage Constipation

- Increase dietary fiber
- Increase fluid intake
- Increase activity

Manage Impactions

- Enemas: cleansing; retention; return flow
- Digital removal of stool

Manage bowel Diversion

- Assessing effluent → amount, consistency
- Stoma assessment/care → size, color
- Peristomal skin care
- Patient teaching: diet, appliance management
- Supporting patient self-concept

Manage bowel Incontinence

- Fecal collection pouch
- Bowel training
- Promote hygiene; skin care
- Review diet/fluid intake

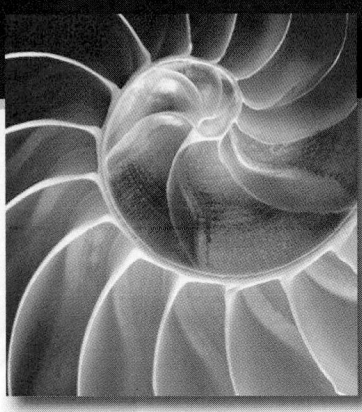

Sensory Perception

For a podcast of an overview of this chapter,

 Go to Student Resources, **Podcast – Chapter Overviews,
Chapter 29,** on DavisPlus at http://davisplus.fadavis.com/
Wilkinson2

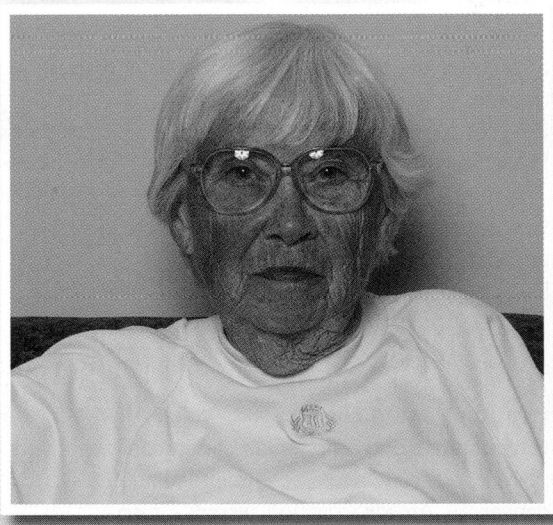

Caring for the Garcias

*The exercises in the following section allow you to practice
the kind of thinking you will use as a full-spectrum nurse.
Because these are critical-thinking questions, there is usually
no single right answer. We do not provide answers for these
questions because it is more important for you to think
about the questions than to arrive at the "right" answer.
These questions are designed to improve your thinking more
than to "cover content." Discuss answers with your peers—
discussion can stimulate critical thinking. If you have difficulty
with any of these questions, consult with your instructor.*

Katherine Garcia, Joe Garcia's mother, has been
experiencing blurred vision. At a recent ophthalmology
appointment, she was told she has bilateral cataracts that
will require surgical removal. She reports to the primary
care clinic today, accompanied by her son, Joe. Katherine
tells you, "I don't know what happened. I was pulling into a
parking space at the grocery store, and the next thing you

know, I hear this loud boom. I don't know how I did it, but
I hit the car next to me. I just didn't see it."

Joe is very concerned and questions whether his mother
should be allowed to drive. Katherine is visibly upset. "I
don't want to hurt anyone, but I don't want to lose all my
freedom." Joe insisted on this appointment to discuss his
concerns.

A. What data will you need to gather from Katherine
and Joe?

B. What assessments will you need to perform?

C. How will cataract surgery most likely affect Katherine?
You will need to learn about the surgery and recovery

to answer this question. Use a textbook, or, for a list
of helpful Web sites you can access,

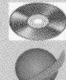 Go to Chapter 29, **Resources for Caregivers and
Healthcare Professionals,** on the Student Resource Disk
or DavisPlus at http://davisplus.fadavis.com/Wilkinson2

D. What information would you offer to Katherine and Joe?

Practical **Knowledge**
knowing how

To provide support for patients with sensorineural alterations, you will need practical knowledge about assessing and diagnosing sensorineural functions. Nursing interventions involve caring for patients who have vision and hearing deficits. This section includes a procedure for otic irrigations, which may be used to correct hearing loss resulting from a cerumen-blocked ear canal. Some procedures to support sensory function, such as instilling medications and irrigating the eye, are presented in the procedures in Chapter 23 of this volume. For other interventions,

 Go to **Chapter 23: Administering Medications,** and **Chapter 29: Sensory Perception,** in Volume 1.

In this section you will also find techniques for communicating with patients who have visual or hearing deficits, assessment guidelines, and standardized language tables.

Procedures

Procedure 29-1 ▪ **Performing Otic Irrigation**

➤ For steps to follow in *all* procedures, refer to the Universal Steps for All Procedures found on the inside back cover of Volume 2.

Critical Aspects

- Warm the irrigating solution to body temperature.
- Assist the patient into a sitting or lying position, with the head tilted away from the affected ear.
- Straighten the ear canal by pulling up and back on the pinna. For a young child, pull down and back to straighten the canal.
- Instruct the patient to notify you if he experiences any pain or dizziness during the irrigation.
- Place the tip of the nozzle (or syringe) into the entrance of the ear canal, and direct the stream of irrigating solution gently along the top of the ear canal toward the back of the client's head.
- Continue irrigating until the canal is clean.
- Perform an otoscopic examination.
- Place a cotton ball loosely in the outer ear.

Equipment

- An ear irrigation system, such as the Welch Allyn ear wash system or an electronic jet ear irrigator.

Using a metal syringe is no longer recommended and is considered dangerous. An ear irrigation system is also preferred over an Asepto or bulb syringe because of the better ability to control pressure and remove cerumen (Harkin, 2008).

- Asepto syringe, or rubber bulb syringe (if an ear irrigation system is not available)
- Irrigating solution (usually water, but may be an antiseptic solution), warmed to 98.6°F (37°C).
- Bath towel and moisture-resistant towel
- A headlight if one is available
- Emesis basin
- Otoscope
- Cotton balls
- Procedure gloves

Delegation

You must assess the client before performing this procedure and evaluate client responses during and after the procedure. The procedure requires knowledge of

anatomy and physiology, use of an otoscope, and, sometimes, use of sterile technique. Therefore, you should not delegate otic irrigation to nursing assistive personnel (NAP).

Assessment

- **Determine whether there are contraindications for ear irrigation.**

Contraindications include ruptured tympanic membrane, present or recent middle ear infection, prior surgery on the ear, cleft palate, or acute inflammation of the ear canal.

- ◆ Assess the external ear for drainage.

Do not irrigate the ears if drainage is present. Drainage from the ear may be a sign of rupture of the tympanic membrane.

- Assess the external ear for cerumen.

Impacted cerumen is the most common reason for performing an ear irrigation.

- ◆ Assess the external ear canal for redness, swelling, or foreign objects; visualize the tympanic membrane. If a foreign object is present, attempt to remove it before irrigation.

Establishes the baseline. If you irrigate with a foreign object in the ear, it may cause the object to swell and become more difficult to remove. Also, if you cannot visualize the tympanic membrane, it may be perforated; if so, otic irrigation is contraindicated.

■ Assess for pain or hearing loss.
Establishes the baseline. Cerumen blockage in the ear canal may result in a conductive hearing loss.

➤ When performing the procedure, always identify your patient according to agency policy and be attentive to standard precautions, hand hygiene, patient safety and privacy, body mechanics, and documentation.

Procedure Steps

1. Warm the irrigating solution to body temperature (98.6°F [37°C]), and fill the reservoir of the irrigator.
Placing cool solutions in the ear can cause dizziness.

2. Assemble the irrigator if necessary, and place a clean disposable tip on it.

3. Assist the client into a sitting or lying position, with the head tilted slightly toward the affected ear. Explain what you are going to do.
Positioning facilitates administering the solution and allows fluid to run along the roof of the ear canal. Knowing what to expect may decrease patient anxiety and improve his ability to cooperate during the procedure.

4. Don gloves; put on the headlight.
The gloves are needed because of the risk of exposure to body fluids. The headlight facilitates direct vision.

5. Drape the client with a plastic drape, and place a towel on the client's shoulder on the side being irrigated. Ask the client to hold an emesis basin under his ear to collect the irrigating fluid that drains out of the ear.
Note: An emesis basin is not necessary if a comprehensive ear wash system is used.
Drape and towel protect the client's clothing.

6. Set the irrigator pressure to the minimum level. Let it run for 20 to 30 seconds to prime the tubing or nozzle before irrigation. (If you must use an Asepto or rubber bulb syringe, fill the syringe with about 50 mL of the irrigating solution, and expel any remaining air.)

7. Straighten the ear canal.
  a. For a child younger than 3 years old, pull the pinna down and back.
  b. For older children and adults, pull the pinna upward and outward.
Straightens the ear canal so that the solution can flow through the length of the canal.

8. Instruct the client to notify you if he experiences any pain or dizziness during the irrigation. Explain to the client that he may feel warmth, fullness, or pressure when the fluid reaches the tympanic membrane.
Pain or dizziness may indicate a contraindication to the procedure.

9. Place the tip of the nozzle (or syringe) about 1 cm (½ in.) above the entrance of the ear canal, and direct the stream of irrigating solution gently along the top of the ear canal toward the back of the client's head.
  a. Do not occlude the ear canal with the nozzle.
  b. Instill the solution slowly.
  c. Allow the solution to flow out as it is instilled.
  d. Repeat these steps for 5 minutes or until you can see cerumen in the return solution.

✚ Directing the flow directly onto the tympanic membrane could injure the membrane. Strong pressure can cause discomfort and may even damage the tympanic membrane. ▼

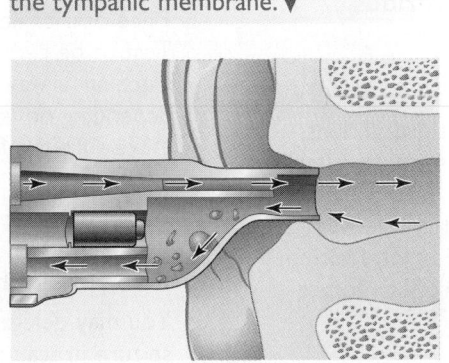

10. Inspect the ear with an otoscope to evaluate cerumen removal. See Procedure 19-7 if you need to review otoscopic examination.
Allows visualization of the canal.

11. Continue irrigating until the examination indicates the canal is cleaned of cerumen and debris.
The irrigating solution will soften the cerumen, easing removal. Blocking the canal prevents the outward flow of the solution.

12. Place a cotton ball loosely in the ear canal, and ask the client to lie on the side of the affected ear.
The cotton ball will absorb excess fluid that drains by gravity.

13. Clean and disinfect the irrigator, according to the manufacturer's instructions or agency protocols. Dispose of the disposable tips.

What if . . .

■ **The cerumen is very hard or you have difficulty removing it?**

The irrigating solution will help soften it, so you may attempt again after 15 minutes.

■ **The patient is an infant or young child?**

Ask another caregiver to immobilize the child during the irrigation.

(continued on next page)

Procedure 29-1 ■ **Performing Otic Irrigation** (continued)

Evaluation

■ Observe the quantity and quality of ear cerumen you removed.
■ Observe the appearance of the ear canal.
■ Assess for complaints of pain or dizziness.
■ Assess for improvement in hearing acuity.
■ Reassess for drainage on the cotton ball.

Patient Teaching

■ Avoid use of cotton-tipped swabs.

They simply push cerumen deeper into the ear.

■ Keep the ear dry for a few days. Use cotton balls coated with petroleum jelly when bathing.

Exposure to a wet environment, such as a swimming pool, may increase the risk of bacterial or fungal infection. Petroleum jelly serves as a barrier to keep water from entering the ear.

■ Clean ears daily with washcloth, soap, and water. If earwax is a problem, over-the-counter preparations (oils) can be used to prevent wax buildup.

■ ✚ Notify the primary care provider if you experience ear pain, vertigo, or "ringing in the ears."

Ear irrigation is an invasive procedure and may result in otitis media, trauma to the external meatus, vertigo, tinnitus, and perforation of the tympanic membrane, although this is not common.

Home Care

■ Provide the caregiver with instructions on ear care as stated above.
■ Teach parents that it is best to avoid irrigation in young children unless absolutely necessary. Oil- or water-based ear drops may be used to treat a wax problem in a child, applying the oil when the child is asleep.

Documentation

■ Document the ear solution used, the quantity, character, and odor of cerumen or drainage.
■ Chart the condition of the ear canal and tympanic membrane after the irrigation.

Sample documentation:

10/18/12   1400   Pt. c/o bilateral decreased hearing acuity. External ear canals occluded with dried cerumen. Irrigated with warm water using electronic jet ear irrigation system. Large amount of dry, brown cerumen removed with irrigation. External canals and tympanic membrane intact to otoscopic inspection after irrigation.————————N. Ephrain, RN

Practice Resources

Burtin, M., & Doree, C. (2009); Harkin, H. (2008).

Clinical Insights

Clinical Insight 29-1 ▶ Seizure Precautions

✚ Institute seizure precautions for patients with a new diagnosis of a seizure disorder or any seizure activity within the past 12 months; frequent seizure activity; history of head trauma (including surgery) within the past 3 years; withdrawal of antiseizure medication or adjustment of the medication regimen.

The goal of seizure precautions is to protect the patient from injury and prevent serious complications.

Before a Seizure Event

■ Explain to the patient the reasons for the precautions.
■ If the patient has frequent or prolonged seizures, establish IV access.

To provide a route to administer medications (e.g., diazepam [Valium]) in the event of a seizure. For intermittent episodes, you can use rectal diazepam (Diastat), lorazepam (Ativan), or midazolam (Versed).

■ Obtain a bed with full-length siderails.

■ Cover the headboard, footboard, and siderails with commercial pads or bath blankets. Tape the blankets in place.

Padding protects the patient's limbs and head from injury if he has a seizure.

■ Keep the rails raised and the bed in low position.

To prevent falls and minimize injuries.

■ Place oral or nasal suction equipment at the bedside. Test to be certain it is working.
■ Place an airway at the bedside or tape to the wall, depending on your agency protocol.
■ Make sure the family knows how to use a call bell.

To summon help in the event of a seizure.

■ Assign the patient to a room in close proximity to the nurses' station.

To allow closer monitoring.

■ You may delegate to the NAP the tasks of setting up seizure precautions.

When a Seizure Occurs

- If you are present when the patient reports having an aura, help him into bed, lower the head, and raise the siderails. Or if in another location, help him to the floor and put something soft under his head.
To keep the head from being injured by hitting the floor.

- Provide privacy.
- Stay with the patient.
- You may insert an oral airway.
To keep the tongue from blocking the airway.

- Don't put anything into the patient's mouth and don't force the airway in place.
This might break the teeth or cause other injury.

- Don't try to hold the jaw open or put your hands in the mouth.
You may be bitten.

- Turn the patient on his side.
This allows secretions to drain and the tongue to fall forward, keeping the airway patent.

- Loosen restrictive clothing.
- Move hard or sharp objects out of the way.
- Do not try to restrain the patient or control his movements.
This might cause muscle and joint injury.

- If the seizure is prolonged or hypoxemia is present, administer oxygen as prescribed.
To avoid hypoxia during the event.

- Usually little nursing action is required beyond preventing physical injury and maintaining a patent airway. The exception is with status epilepticus, in which the patient has repeated seizures without regaining consciousness. In that event, notify a physician immediately.
- Observe the characteristics of the seizure: how it started, location and duration of motor activity type of movements (e.g., stiffening, jerking, twitching, loss of muscle tone), crying out, visual and auditory symptoms, tachycardia, pupil dilation, change in level of consciousness). Note the first symptom and how the seizure progressed.

To help identify the area of the brain involved.

- You cannot delegate care of a patient who is having a seizure. Nursing assessments and interventions are required. You can ask the NAP to obtain help.
- Administer diazepam (Valium) as prescribed if the seizure is prolonged, typically > 6 minutes.

After the Seizure

- Turn the patient on his side and apply suction, if needed.
To allow secretions to drain and maintain a patent airway.

- Reorient and reassure the patient, and make him comfortable. If the patient was incontinent, change bedding and clothing.
- Examine for injuries.
- Keep the room quiet and the lighting dim.
- Stay with the patient, as he may be sleepy or confused.
- Do not give any food or drink until the patient is fully conscious and alert.
- Monitor vital signs and mental status every 15 to 30 minutes for 2 hours. You can delegate this activity to a NAP.
- Observe post-seizure behavior: Evaluate muscle strength, ability to speak, memory, and orientation.
- Pad the siderails, if not already done.
- Ask the patient whether he experienced an aura and what activities preceded the seizure. The type of aura helps locate the area in the brain where the seizure originated.
- Document what happened and your post-procedure assessment.

Lifestyle Management

Sleep deprivation lowers the threshold for seizure activity. The patient should have sufficient rest and a healthy diet. Advise the patient to visit his primary care provider regularly and avoid excess alcohol and any drugs that may interact with seizure medications.

References

American Association of Neuroscience Nurses (2007). *Care of the patient with seizures*. Glenview, IL: Author. Retrieved April 24, 2009, from http://www.aann.org/pubs/cpg/seizures.pdf

Wiegand, L. (2005). *AACN procedure manual for critical care*. Philadelphia: W. B. Saunders.

Clinical Insight 29-2 ▶ Communicating with Visually Impaired Clients

The Joint Commission (2008) requires that institutions address the communication needs of patients with impaired vision.

- Introduce yourself when you enter the room.
- Call the client by her name so that she can be certain you are addressing her.
- When you enter a room with a client who is visually impaired, describe the room, room layout, and activities that are occurring.
- Explain unfamiliar sounds, such as the paging system and monitor and pump alarms.
- If the client has limited vision, be sure to position yourself in the client's field of vision.

- Speak to the visually impaired person before you touch her so that she is prepared for your touch.
- Do not speak loudly unless the client has a hearing impairment.
- Let the client know when you are leaving the room.
- Use the words "see" and "look" as you would with a sighted person.
- Avoid expressions, such as "over there" or "right here." Guide the client to the location or place her hand on the object.

Clinical Insight 29-3 ▶ Communicating with Hearing-Impaired Clients

Healthcare agencies should address the communication needs of those with vision, speech, hearing, language, and cognitive impairments (The Joint Commission, 2008, p. 156).

Assess the patient's method of receiving speech.

- If the patient wears a hearing aid, check to see that it is turned on.
- If not, does the patient read lips or use sign language? Remember that only about ⅓ of spoken words can be understood by speech reading.
- If possible, arrange a hearing evaluation for the client and construction of any required hearing aids.

Position yourself and minimize noise.

- Don't chew gum or eat while talking. Many clients use lip reading to help them interpret your speech.
- Make sure you are clearly visible to the client before you start speaking. Use touch to get the client's attention.
- Face the client directly; keep your hands away from your mouth.
- If the hearing deficit is predominantly in one ear, move closer to the less affected ear.
- Minimize environmental noise (e.g., turn off the TV).

Send the message.

- Speak slowly and articulate clearly, in a natural way. Don't shout. Shouting distorts your words.
- Don't drop your voice at the end of a sentence.
- Use simple, plain language, but longer phrases (e.g., "Would you like for me to get you a drink of water?" instead of "Do you want a drink?")
- Use gestures to provide visual cues (e.g., act out what you want the patient to do).
- Use paper, pencil, or computer communication when necessary. Consider literacy skills.

Interpret the client's responses.

- Observe the client's verbal responses, facial expressions, and body language for clues to understanding. An inappropriate response indicates misunderstanding.
- Be aware the person may nod agreement or say "yes" even when she does not understand what is being said.
- Confirm that the client understood you by asking her to repeat what you said, especially if you are giving specific information, such as a time or place. Many numbers and words sound alike (e.g., "fifteen" and "fifty"; or "Prozac" and "Prograf").
- If the person does not understand what you've said, rephrase your statement. Don't repeat the same words.

For older adults: Use a low-pitched voice. The ability to hear high-pitched tones is lost first with aging.

Assessment Guidelines and Tools

As a nurse, you should always consider your client's sensory–perceptual status. Sensory deficits and excess or inadequate stimulation have a significant influence on quality of life and may be especially troublesome for institutionalized clients.

Screening Hearing in Older Adults

To find a useful tool to screen hearing in older adults,

 Go to http://www.hartfordign.org/Resources/Try_This_Series/

Using this tool, a patient scores 1 point for each of the following: older than 70 years, male, did not attend 12th grade, and cannot hear and understand (without seeing the face) what a person whispers from across the room. Two points are given for ever seeing a doctor because of trouble hearing and being unable to hear and understand (without seeing the face) a person talking in a normal voice from across the room. A total of 3 points indicates the need for further evaluation.

Nursing History: Sensory Perceptual Status

Usual Sensory Function	Ask questions such as the following: ■ How would you rate your vision? ■ How would you evaluate your ability to see objects up close or at a distance? ■ Do you have any difficulty hearing conversations or listening to the radio or television? ■ Have you experienced any difficulty locating sounds? ■ Do you experience ringing or buzzing in your ears? ■ Do you enjoy the taste of food? ■ Do you notice any difficulty with your ability to smell? ■ Are you experiencing any pain or discomfort? ■ Do you have any areas of numbness or tingling on your body? ■ Do you have any difficulty with sensing hot or cold? ■ Describe your level of coordination. ■ What medications are you taking? Have they had any effect on your vision, hearing, sense of taste, smell, touch, or balance? ■ What is your current stress level? ■ What is your usual activity level? ■ What is your preferred activity level?
Risk Factors for Impaired Sensory Function	Assess: ■ Developmental level (e.g., older adults) ■ Health status (usual and current state of health, current health concerns (e.g., Ménière's disease), history of hospitalizations and surgeries) ■ Medications (i.e., look up side effects to determine what, if any, effect the medications have on sensory function) ■ Stress (current and usual stress level, major sources of stressors, usual coping mechanisms) ■ Lifestyle (normal activity, noise, interaction levels, hobbies, and usual lifestyle)
History of Sensory Problems	■ Have you experienced any problems with blurred vision, double vision, sensitivity to light, blind spots, objects moving in front of your eyes, or eye pain? ■ Have you ever felt unable to follow a conversation because of difficulty hearing? ■ Have you ever had problems with your ability to taste or smell? ■ Have you ever had areas of numbness or tingling? ■ Has anyone in your family ever been diagnosed with a stroke or circulation problem? ■ Have you ever had episodes of confusion or disorientation?
Use of Sensory Aids, Including Diet, Exercise, Medications, and Remedies	■ Does the client wear glasses or contact lenses at any time? If so, determine the following: When was the client's last eye exam? Are the glasses clean and in good repair? Are the glasses within easy reach? Are contact lenses in good condition? Is the client able to care for them? ■ Does the client wear a hearing aid? If so, determine the following: Can the client hear adequately with the hearing aid in place? Are the batteries working? Is the hearing aid clean? How much help does the client need to place the aid in his ear? ■ Does the client use a cane or walker? If so: Has the cane or walker been properly fitted to the client? How often does the client use the device when walking? ■ What factors determine when the device will be used?

Continued

Nursing History: Sensory Perceptual Status—cont'd

Assess Mental Status	■ Assess behavior, appearance, response to stimuli, speech, memory, and judgment. If you need more specific instructions, see Procedure 19-16, steps 1–10 and Questions for Evaluating Cognitive Status, at the end of the procedure.
	■ *For older adults,* a tool called the Mini-Cog is especially useful (Borson, Scanlan, Brush, et al., 2000). It consists of 3 memory questions and instructions to draw a clock face. To use this tool,
	Go to http://consultgerirn.org/uploads/File/trythis/try_this_3.pdf
	■ Assess level of orientation: Have the client tell you his name, the date, and his current location. If he can answer these questions correctly, describe him as "awake, alert, and oriented to person, place, and time" (AA&Ox3).
	■ Assess level of consciousness:
	Alert — Is the patient awake and aware of the environment and himself, speaking clearly, making eye contact?
	Confused — Are actions and speech inappropriate?
	Lethargic — Is speech slow or sluggish? Are mental processes and movements sluggish?
	Obtunded — This is a low level of awareness and response to environment. Document it if it occurs.
	Stuporous — This occurs when the patient can be aroused by vigorous stimulation but seems confused during periods of arousal.
	Comatose — In this state, there is no spontaneous movement, no verbalization, and only nonpurposeful movement with stimulation. (Huntley, 2008)
	■ Also see Chapter 19, Procedure 19-16, Assessing the Sensory-Neurological System, Glasgow Coma Scale and Full Outline of UnResponsiveness Scale.
Assess Support Network for Clients with Sensory Deficit	■ Are there support persons to help the client by assuming chores he can no longer perform?
	■ Are there people who provide comfort to ease the client's distress about sensory losses?
	■ Who can provide sensory stimulation?
	■ Who can help reorient and calm the client?
	■ Does the client need help with transportation in order to maintain social contact?

Bedside Assessment of Sensory Function

SENSE	ASSESSMENT PROCESS
Vision	Use the Snellen chart, or have the client read a newspaper.
	Observe for squinting.
Hearing	Perform the whisper test.
	Inspect the ear canals for hardened cerumen.
	Observe client conversations. Are there frequent requests for repeating information or misunderstandings?
	How loud is the client's radio or television?
Smell	Ask the client to close his eyes and identify common smells (e.g., coffee, vanilla, cloves, tobacco).
Taste	Ask the client to close his eyes and identify common tastes (e.g., salt, lemon, and sugar). Give water between tastes.
Tactile	With his eyes closed, touch the client with a wisp of cotton. Have him identify when you have touched him. Repeat this process with a sharp object, such as a needle.
	With his eyes closed, ask the client to identify where you are touching his body.
Kinesthesia	Have the client perform the Romberg test. See Procedure 19–7.
	Have the client perform alternating rapid motions, such as tapping heels or clapping.
	Observe the client's gait and movement.

Standardized Language

Selected NOC Outcomes and NIC Interventions for Sensory Perceptual Nursing Diagnoses

NANDA-I NURSING DIAGNOSES

Disturbed Sensory Perception (specify): Visual, Auditory, Kinesthetic, Gustatory, Tactile, Olfactory. A change in the amount or patterning of incoming stimuli accompanied by a diminished, exaggerated, distorted, or impaired response to such stimuli. Use this diagnosis when there is excessive or insufficient environmental stimuli or when the patient has altered sensory reception, transmission, and/or integration; biochemical or electrolyte imbalances; or psychological stress.

Acute Confusion. The abrupt onset of a cluster of global, transient changes and disturbances in attention, cognition, psychomotor activity, level of consciousness, and/or sleep/wake cycle. This diagnosis may be used for clients experiencing delirium, severe pain, sleep deprivation, dementia, or intoxication associated with alcohol or drug use.

Chronic Confusion. Irreversible, long-standing, and/or progressive deterioration of intellect and personality characterized by decreased ability to interpret environmental stimuli and decreased capacity for intellectual thought processes. It is manifested by disturbances of memory, orientation, and behavior. This diagnosis may be used for clients with Alzheimer's disease, Korsakoff's psychosis, multi-infarct dementia, cerebrovascular accident, and head injury.

Impaired Environmental Interpretation Syndrome. A consistent lack of orientation to person, place, time, or circumstances over more than 3 to 6 months, necessitating a protective environment. This diagnosis includes, but is broader than, Chronic Confusion. It also includes Impaired Memory and inability to reason and concentrate. It often accompanies depression, Huntington's disease, and dementia.

Impaired Memory. The inability to remember or recall bits of information or behavioral skills. Impaired memory may be attributed to pathophysiological or situational causes; it may be either temporary or permanent. Impaired memory may be seen with fluid and electrolyte imbalance, excessive environmental disturbances, certain medications, or age-related changes.

Risk for Peripheral Neurovascular Dysfunction. Can be used when the patient is at risk for disruption in circulation, sensation, or motion of an extremity. Risk factors include trauma, orthopedic surgery, vascular obstruction, burns, immobilization, and mechanical compression (e.g., from a tourniquet, cast, or restraint).

Unilateral Neglect. A lack of awareness and attention to one side of the body. It is manifested by consistent inattention to stimuli on the affected side and may be caused by neurological illness or trauma, one-sided blindness, and effects of other disturbed perceptual abilities.

NANDA-I DIAGNOSES	NOC OUTCOMES	NIC INTERVENTIONS
Disturbed Sensory Perception (specify):		
Visual	Sensory Function: Vision	Communication Enhancement: Visual Deficit
	Vision Compensation Behavior	Environmental Management
		Fall Prevention
Auditory	Communication: Receptive	Communication Enhancement: Hearing Deficit
	Hearing Compensation Behavior	Ear Care
	Sensory Function: Hearing	Environmental Management
Kinesthetic	Balance	Body Mechanics Promotion
	Body Positioning: Self-Initiated	Exercise Promotion: Strength Training
	Coordinated Movement	Exercise Therapy: Balance
	Sensory Function: Proprioception	Environmental Management
Gustatory and Olfactory	Appetite	Environmental Management
	Nutritional Status: Food & Fluid	Feeding
	Intake	Nausea Management
	Sensory Function: Taste & Smell	Nutrition Management

Continued

NANDA-I DIAGNOSES	NOC OUTCOMES	NIC INTERVENTIONS
Tactile	Sensory Function: Cutaneous	Environmental Management: Safety
		Lower Extremity Monitoring
		Peripheral Sensation Management
Acute Confusion	Cognitive Orientation	Cognitive Stimulation
	Distorted Thought Self-Control	Delirium Management
	Information Processing	Delusion Management
	Neurological Status: Consciousness	Environmental Management
		Reality Orientation
Chronic Confusion	Cognition	Anxiety Reduction
	Cognitive Orientation	Cognitive Stimulation
	Concentration	Decision-Making Support
	Decision-Making	Dementia Management
	Information Processing	Environmental Management
	Memory	Memory Training
	Neurological Status: Consciousness	Reality Orientation
Impaired Environmental Interpretation Syndrome	Cognitive Orientation	Dementia Management
	Concentration	Dementia Management: Bathing
	Fall Prevention Behavior	Reality Orientation
	Memory	
	Neurological Status: Consciousness	
Impaired Memory	Cognition	Memory Training
	Memory	Neurologic Monitoring
	Neurological Status	Surveillance: Safety
Risk for Peripheral Vascular Dysfunction	Body Positioning: Self-Initiated	Exercise Therapy: Joint Mobility
	Neurological Status: Cranial Sensory/ Motor Function	Lower Extremity Monitoring
	Neurological Status: Spinal Sensory/ Motor Function	Neurologic Monitoring
		Peripheral Sensation Management
	Adaptation to Physical Disability	Unilateral Neglect Management
	Body Positioning: Self-Initiated	Environmental Management: Safety
	Coordinated Movement	Positioning
		Touch

Sources: Bulechek, G., Butcher, H., & Dochterman, J. (2008). *Nursing interventions classification (NIC).* (5th ed.). St. Louis, MO: C. V. Mosby; Johnson, M., Bulechek, G., Butcher, H., et al. (2006). *NANDA, NOC, and NIC linkages.* St. Louis, MO: C. V. Mosby; Moorhead, S., Johnson, M., Maas, M., et al. (2008). *Nursing outcomes classification (NOC)* (4th ed.). St. Louis, MO: C. V. Mosby; NANDA International. (2009). *Nursing diagnoses: Definitions and classification 2009-2011.* Ames, IA: Wiley-Blackwell. Used with permission.

THINKING CRITICALLY ABOUT SENSORY PERCEPTION

The exercises in the following sections allow you to practice the kind of thinking you will use as a full-spectrum nurse. Because these are critical-thinking questions, there is usually no single right answer. We do not provide answers for these questions because it is more important for you to think about the questions than to arrive at the "right" answer. These questions are designed to improve your thinking more than to "cover content." Discuss answers with your peers—discussion can stimulate critical thinking. If you have difficulty with any of these questions, consult with your instructor.

Applying the Full-Spectrum Nursing Model

PATIENT SITUATION

Clint Gossage is an 85-year-old man who lives at home alone. His wife moved to a nursing home a year ago. Although Mr. Gossage has many self-care deficits, he is still able to live at home, with regular visits from a home health nurse and community services to help with some meals and bathing. When you visit him, you notice that he shouts when talking to you, looks at you intently when you speak, and constantly asks you to repeat what you say. You examine his external ear canal and note that there is some hardened cerumen in the canal. He is not wearing a hearing aid. The patient record reveals tympanic membrane scarring and a diagnosis of conductive hearing loss.

THINKING

1. *Theoretical Knowledge*: Describe the pathophysiology of conductive hearing loss.

2. *Critical Thinking (Considering Alternatives)*: Based on your knowledge of conductive hearing loss and your assessment of Mr. Gossage, what is the first follow-up question you would ask him about his hearing?

DOING

3. *Practical Knowledge*: At a subsequent visit, you discover that Mr. Gossage has impacted cerumen in his left ear. After obtaining a medical order, you prepare to perform an otic irrigation.

   a. To what temperature will you warm the solution?

   b. What position would you use for Mr. Gossage?

   c. Describe how you would place the tip of the syringe (or ear wash system) for irrigating.

   d. After the ear is cleared of cerumen and you have finished irrigating, what should you do next? And what position will you have Mr. Gossage assume when you do it?

4. *Nursing Process (Diagnosis)*:

   a. Write a nursing diagnosis that focuses on Mr. Gossage's safety and that relates to hearing.

   b. Based on your nursing diagnosis, what safety measures would you recommend for Mr. Gossage's home? (Do not address the hearing aid issue here.)

CARING

5. *Ethical Knowledge*: Now think back to the first visit with Mr. Gossage. What are some reasons that he might not have been wearing a hearing aid? Consider physical changes associated with aging.

▨ Critical Thinking and Clinical Reasoning

1. Review the following client scenarios.

   ■ Client A is 84 years old. She is a retired school teacher who loves to read, work in her garden, and volunteer at the local children's hospital. She has developed macular degeneration and is progressively losing her sight.

   ■ Client B is 55 years old. He is a former guitar player in a heavy-metal band. He now works in music production. He has significant hearing loss related to chronic exposure to loud music. Most recently he has developed tinnitus, which has exacerbated his hearing loss.

   ■ Client C is 31 years old. He is a chef at a local four-star restaurant. He suffered a head injury in a motor vehicle accident and has lost his sense of smell.

   ■ Client D is 26 years old. She is a licensed architect working for a firm in the downtown area. She has been taking birth control pills for 5 years. Recently she has been under a great deal of stress. She began drinking lots of coffee, smoking cigarettes, and working long hours. She was admitted to the hospital with right-sided weakness and slurred speech. She is being evaluated for a cerebrovascular accident.

   ■ Client E is 15 years old. He has cerebral palsy. As a result, he has a "scissor walk" and dysarthric speech. He has recently had a series of falls due to increasing problems with balance.

   a. For each client, write a nursing diagnosis to reflect his or her sensory perception problem. Write one other nursing diagnosis that might result from the sensory perception problem. Explain your thinking.

   b. Each of the clients is experiencing a sensory deficit. What interventions would be most appropriate to address each client's concerns?

   c. Which client(s) is/are most likely to have difficulty adapting to the sensory deficit? How would you determine how each client is adapting?

   d. Which client, if any, is most likely to be experiencing sensory overload?

2. Examine the clinical unit that you are visiting for your current clinical rotation. What unit factors contribute to the development of sensory overload?

3. What factors in the clinical unit contribute to the development of sensory deprivation?

4. For each of the following concepts, use critical thinking to describe how or why it is important to nursing, patient care, or sensory perception. Note that these are *not* to be merely definitions.

   Sensory stimulation   Sensory deficits
   Sensory overload   Sensory aids
   Sensory deprivation

▨ What Are the Main Points in This Chapter?

➤ The purpose of sensation is to allow the body to respond to changing situations and maintain homeostasis.

➤ A sensory experience involves four components: stimulus, reception, perception, and an arousal mechanism.

➤ Reception is the process of receiving stimuli from nerve endings in the skin and body.

➤ Perception is the ability to interpret the impulses transmitted from the receptors and give meaning to the stimuli.

➤ Humans respond to sensations when they are alert and receptive to stimulation. The response to a stimulus is based on intensity, contrast, adaptation, previous experience, illness, or injury.

➤ Sensory deprivation is caused by a deficiency of meaningful stimuli.

➤ Sensory deprivation can be due to environmental conditions or to interference with the reception or perception of stimuli.

➤ Sensory overload develops when either environmental or internal stimuli—or a combination of both—exceed a level that the client's sensory system can effectively process. It can also occur in clients with neurological or psychiatric disorders who are unable to adapt to continuing, nonmeaningful stimuli.

➤ Impaired vision and hearing are the sensory deficits most commonly encountered in nursing practice.

➤ The client with impaired vision, hearing, tactile sensation, olfactory sensation, or kinesthesia is at risk for injury.

➤ Visual and hearing changes may diminish the ability to communicate and may hamper social interaction.

➤ Developmental issues, culture, health status, medications, stress level, and individual preferences affect sensory perception.

➤ To assess sensory perceptual function, assess factors affecting sensory perception, mental status, recent changes in sensory stimulation, use of sensory aids, the client's environment, and the support network.

➤ Nursing strategies to address impaired sensory perception include activities to promote sensory function, prevent and treat sensory overload and deprivation, assist clients with sensory deficits, and communicate with clients with altered mental status.

For practice questions for this chapter,

Go to **NCLEX-Style Chapter Quiz,** on the Student Resource Disk or DavisPlus at http://davisplus.fadavis.com/Wilkinson2

To practice documentation for a patient experiencing probable sensory overload,

Go to **Practice Documentation,** on the Student Resource Disk or DavisPlus at http://davisplus.fadavis.com/Wilkinson2

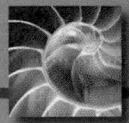

Knowledge Map

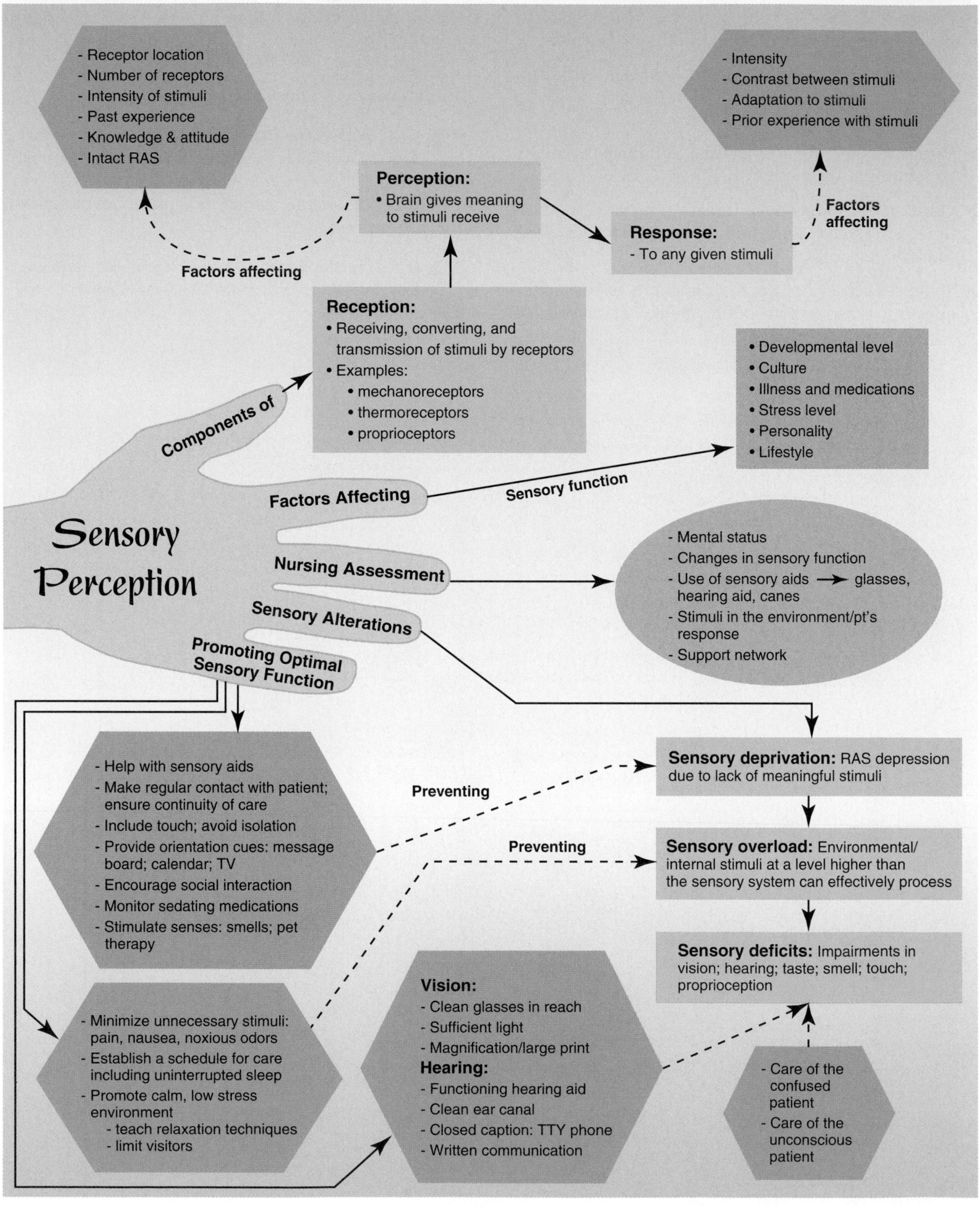

- Receptor location
- Number of receptors
- Intensity of stimuli
- Past experience
- Knowledge & attitude
- Intact RAS

- Intensity
- Contrast between stimuli
- Adaptation to stimuli
- Prior experience with stimuli

Perception:
- Brain gives meaning to stimuli receive

Factors affecting

Response:
- To any given stimuli

Factors affecting

Reception:
- Receiving, converting, and transmission of stimuli by receptors
- Examples:
  - mechanoreceptors
  - thermoreceptors
  - proprioceptors

Components of

- Developmental level
- Culture
- Illness and medications
- Stress level
- Personality
- Lifestyle

Sensory Perception

Factors Affecting   **Sensory function**

Nursing Assessment

Sensory Alterations

- Mental status
- Changes in sensory function
- Use of sensory aids → glasses, hearing aid, canes
- Stimuli in the environment/pt's response
- Support network

Promoting Optimal Sensory Function

- Help with sensory aids
- Make regular contact with patient; ensure continuity of care
- Include touch; avoid isolation
- Provide orientation cues: message board; calendar; TV
- Encourage social interaction
- Monitor sedating medications
- Stimulate senses: smells; pet therapy

Preventing

Sensory deprivation: RAS depression due to lack of meaningful stimuli

Preventing

Sensory overload: Environmental/internal stimuli at a level higher than the sensory system can effectively process

Sensory deficits: Impairments in vision; hearing; taste; smell; touch; proprioception

- Minimize unnecessary stimuli: pain, nausea, noxious odors
- Establish a schedule for care including uninterrupted sleep
- Promote calm, low stress environment
    - teach relaxation techniques
    - limit visitors

Vision:
- Clean glasses in reach
- Sufficient light
- Magnification/large print

Hearing:
- Functioning hearing aid
- Clean ear canal
- Closed caption: TTY phone
- Written communication

- Care of the confused patient
- Care of the unconscious patient

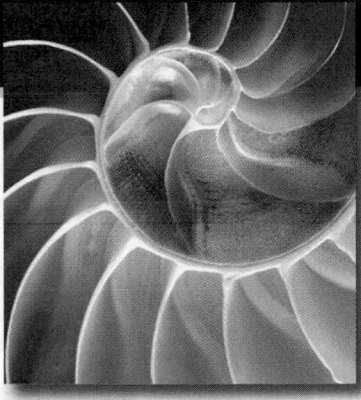

CHAPTER 30

Pain Management

For a podcast of an overview of this chapter,

 Go to Student Resources, **Podcast – Chapter Overviews, Chapter 30,** on DavisPlus at http://davisplus.fadavis.com/Wilkinson2

Caring for the Garcias

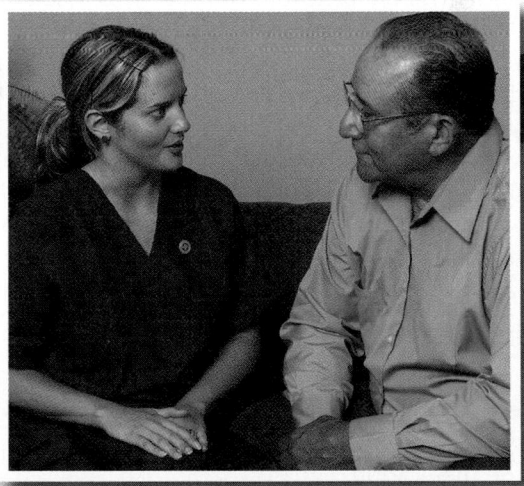

The exercises in the following section allow you to practice the kind of thinking you will use as a full-spectrum nurse. Because these are critical-thinking questions, there is usually no single right answer. We do not provide answers for these questions because it is more important for you to think about the questions than to arrive at the "right" answer. These questions are designed to improve your thinking more than to "cover content." Discuss answers with your peers—discussion can stimulate critical thinking. If you have difficulty with any of these questions, consult with your instructor.

Review the introduction to the Garcias at the front of this volume. Joseph Garcia has bilateral knee pain secondary to osteoarthritis. To develop a pain management plan, what patient data do you need to know?

A. How will you get the data you need? What sources should you use?

B. What types of nursing knowledge (theoretical, practical, ethical, or self-knowledge) are needed to develop a pain management plan?

Practical **Knowledge**
knowing how

When caring for patients with pain, you will need to be skilled in medication administration, including use of patient-controlled analgesia (PCA) pumps and caring for patients who have an epidural catheter.

Procedures

Procedure 30–1 □ Setting up and Managing Patient-Controlled Analgesia by Pump

➤ For steps to follow in *all* procedures, refer to the Universal Steps for All Procedures found on the inside back cover of Volume 2.

Critical Aspects

- Determine the patient's baseline vital signs, cognitive status, physical mobility, and pain level.
- Review the prescriber's order for PCA, including the initial bolus (loading) dose, the basal rate, the demand dose, the lockout interval between each dose, and the 1-hour or 4-hour lockout dose limit.
- Verify PCA with two nurses before initiation, upon discontinuation, at change of shift, and when wasting the remainder.
- Determine if the patient has an allergy to medication.
- Insert the medication cartridge/syringe into the pump, prime the connecting tubing, and lock the pump.
- Set the pump for the loading dose (if prescribed), basal rate, demand dose, lockout interval, and the 1-hour or 4-hour lockout dose limit.
- Connect the tubing into the patient's maintenance IV line.
- Start infusing the medication (loading, then basal, dose).
- Place the button that controls dosing within reach of the patient.
- Change tubing per facility protocol.

Equipment

- PCA pump (infuser and central unit)
- Manufacturer's instructions for the pump
- Cartridge, syringe, or other type of sealed unit containing the medication
- Connecting tubing (to connect the PCA device to the patient's IV line)
- Maintenance IV supplies (if patient does not already have an IV line)
- IV pole
- Antiseptic swab
- Flowsheet
- 1 pair of clean procedure gloves (if venipuncture is necessary)

Delegation

PCA is a system by which a narcotic medication is delivered intravenously to the patient. This procedure is outside the scope of practice of nursing assistive personnel (NAP) and should never be delegated. Furthermore, the NAP should not administer a dose for the patient, even if he asks her to do so. You can inform the NAP of expected side effects and ask her to report her observations to you.

Pre-Procedure Assessment

- Assess physical conditions that can affect respirations.
Respiratory diseases (e.g., chronic obstructive pulmonary disease (COPD) and asthma) and conditions, such as head injury and sleep apnea, increase the risk for respiratory depression with opioid use.

- Assess the level of consciousness and cognitive level.
Determines whether the patient will be able to follow directions for self-dosing.

- Review lab values reflecting liver and kidney function, such as blood urea nitrogen [BUN], creatinine, liver enzymes).
Narcotic analgesics are typically metabolized through the liver or kidneys.

- Assess the baseline respiratory rate, pulse, blood pressure, and oxygen saturation.
A change in vital signs (e.g., hypotension, respiratory rate below 12) may indicate adverse responses to narcotic administration.

- Be aware of the patient's age and weight.
Age is a factor when you are verifying the dose. Older patients and very young children are at increased risk for respiratory suppression, so require lower doses.

- Assess the patient's baseline pain level using a standardized pain assessment tool or numeric scale ranging from 0 to 10.
- Assess the patient's manual dexterity.

Patients with impaired fine-motor control or upper extremity injury may not be able to operate the self-dosing mechanism.

- Review medications currently in use.

The risk of respiratory suppression increases when a PCA pump is used in conjunction with other CNS depressants, such as diazepam (Valium).

Determine the presence and/or involvement of the family. Identify any family anxiety over the patient's degree of pain. Reinforce that only the patient should use the PCA button.

Only the patient should administer the medication. "PCA by proxy" (someone other than the patient pushing the dosing button) is a major factor contributing to adverse patient outcomes (Hagle, Lehr, Brubakken, et al., 2004).

> When performing the procedure, always identify your patient according to agency policy and be attentive to standard precautions, hand hygiene, patient safety and privacy, body mechanics, and documentation.

Procedure Steps

1. Don clean procedure gloves, and initiate IV therapy if the patient does not currently have an IV solution infusing. Refer to Procedure 36-1 as needed.

2. Obtain the medication prescribed and double check it with original order. You may need to remove air from the vial by pushing the injector into the vial. Connect the PCA tubing to the vial (or cartridge).

Some vials may not be completely filled with medication. Ejecting the air makes it faster to prime the connecting tubing.

3. Double-check your dose calculation with another nurse before starting the infusion or wasting medication.

To prevent medication errors in dosing.

   a. One-time "bolus" (or *loading*) dose, which you administer after setting up the pump
   b. Basal rate (the amount of medication to be delivered automatically by the pump over 1 hour)
   c. "On-demand" dose (the amount of drug to be delivered with each push of the button)
   d. The "lock-out" interval (the number of minutes allowed between each administration of an on-demand dose [e.g., q10 min]). Even if the patient pushes the button more frequently, the PCA pump will not administer a dose until the preset time between doses has been met.
   e. The 1-hour or 4-hour lock-out dosage limit (the maximum dose allowed in that time frame). For

example, if the patient has a 4 mg on-demand dose with a 10-minute lockout interval, the patient can receive a maximum of six 4-mg doses per hour for a total of 24 mg/hr and a maximum dose of 96 mg in 4 hours.

Note: PCA prescriptions are usually written in milligrams; however, pump settings may be in milliliters. In such cases, you must verify the concentration (milligrams per milliliter) to set the pump correctly.

4. Prime the tubing; then clamp the tubing above the connector.

Priming prevents air from entering the pump and causing malfunction. Clamping prevents accidental bolus of medication to the patient.

5. Insert the cartridge or vial injector into the pump, and lock the pump. Follow the manufacturer's instruction manual (e.g., some pumps can be set only if the door is closed and locked).

Depending on the pump, it may be a syringe, a cartridge, or other sealed container that can be "locked" into the pump. Locking the pump prevents unauthorized access to the narcotic and dosing features.

6. Turn the pump on, and set the parameters according to the prescriptions and your calculations. The settings may include:
   a. One-time bolus dose
   b. Basal rate
   c. On-demand
   d. The lock-out interval
   e. The 1-hour or 4-hour lock-out dosage limit

7. Scrub the port on the IV tubing closest to the patient, using alcohol or

chlorhexadine alcohol-based product and connect the PCA pump tubing.

Removes gross contamination and discourages growth of pathogens.

8. Open the clamp and administer the bolus (loading) dose if prescribed. Remain with the patient as the dose is delivered. To administer a loading dose, set the pump lockout time to 0 minutes. Set the volume to be delivered as the bolus volume you calculated (e.g., if 10 mg = 0.2 mL, set the volume to 0.2 mL); press the button that controls the loading dose.

A loading dose is usually larger than the basal and on-demand doses because pain is likely to be more severe before the pump is initiated. Remaining with the patient allows you to observe for adverse effects.

9. Close the pump door, and lock the machine with the key.

10. Check for flashing lights or alarms that may indicate the need to correct settings.

11. If you clamped the tubing, be sure to release tubing clamps; press the start button to begin the basal infusion.

12. Ensure that the battery life is sufficient or that the pump in plugged into an appropriate electrical outlet. When possible, plug the pump into an electrical outlet.

To avoid battery failure.

13. Put the control button for on-demand doses within the patient's reach. Be sure the PCA cord is placed away from the call bell.

(continued on next page)

Procedure 30-1 ■ Setting up and Managing Patient-Controlled Analgesia by Pump (continued)

To avoid error in self dosing with PCA. ▼

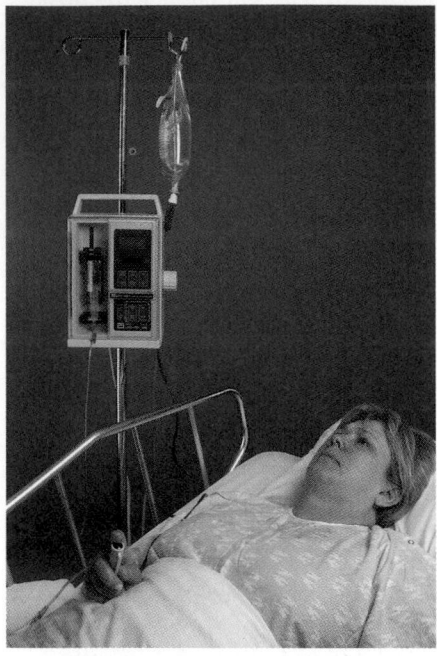

What if. . .

■ **The patient could not verbally communicate pain status?**

Use an alternate standardized pain tool, such as the FACES pain scale or a behavioral measure to determine pain level.

Pain assessment in patients who are noncommunicative may include behavioral or physiological indicators to assess and monitor the effectiveness of pain medication.

■ **The infusion infiltrates?**

Discontinue the IV and establish another IV site. Follow facility policy for application of cold or warm compresses to the infiltrated area. Assess pain level. You may need to contact the prescriber for a bolus dose if the IV has been interrupted for an extended period or the patient has insufficient pain relief.

Evaluation

■ Monitor the patient's pain level, sedation level, and respiratory rate at least every hour for the first 24 hours or according to facility policy after initiating PCA.

Promotes the early detection of respiratory depression, oversedation, or inadequate pain control.

■ Perform routine assessment of number and frequency of doses and pump settings per facility protocol.
■ Check the IV site for redness, infiltration, or phlebitis.
■ Check the IV tubing for patency (e.g., for kinks) to be sure the medication is infusing.

Patient Teaching

Patients who are candidates for use of PCA should be trained before surgery rather than in the immediate postoperative period, when the effects of anesthesia impair learning. Reinforce or teach the patient and family the following:

■ Safe and correct use of the PCA pump
■ The benefits of PCA for controlling pain
■ The pump will deliver only the amount of medication prescribed. Pushing the button too many times will not result in overdosing.
■ The patient cannot accidentally roll over on the button and unintentionally give additional medication.
■ If pain is not being relieved, the patient should tell the nurse so adjustments can be made to the PCA.
■ The pump will alarm when nearly empty, alerting nurses to change the syringe.

■ The PCA button is to relieve pain—not to help the patient sleep.
■ Signs and symptoms of allergic reaction and which ones to report.
■ How to rate pain using a standard pain scale
■ Why family members should not give "doses by proxy"
■ The patient is the only one who can push the pain dosing button.

Documentation

You will usually document PCA initiation on a specialized flowsheet. Items charted include:

■ Time the infusion was begun, including the drug, the loading dose, the basal dose, and lockout and hourly limit
■ Patient's baseline pain level and evaluation of subsequent pain level performed at intervals determined by facility policy
■ Baseline respiratory rate, pulse, blood pressure, and oxygen saturation; routine evaluation of subsequent vital signs performed at intervals determined by facility policy
■ Sedation level
■ Continuous monitoring of vital signs, level of consciousness, and pain status, as well as the number and frequency of doses
■ Unusual occurrences (e.g., oversedation, IV infiltration) in the nursing notes

Sample EHR documentation:

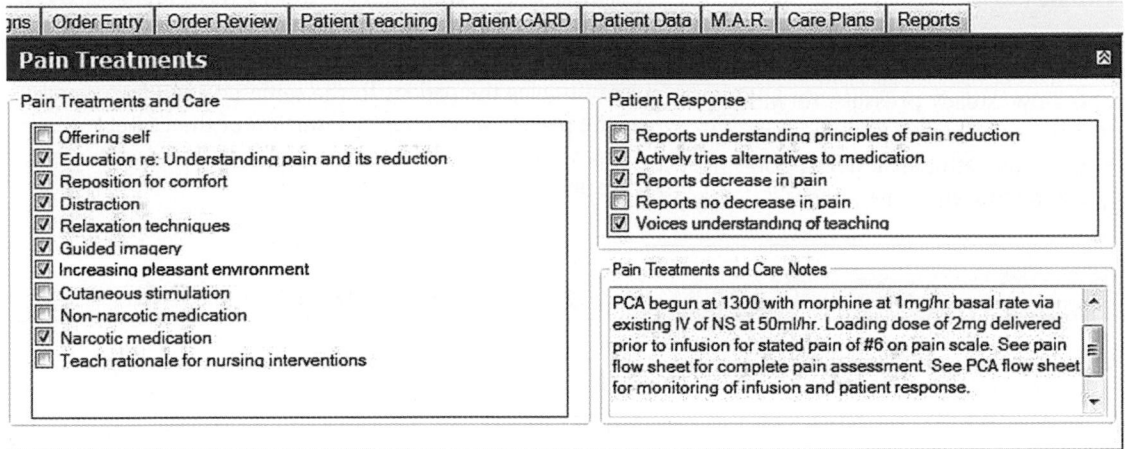

Thinking About the Procedure

 Go to the *Fundamentals of Nursing Skills Videos,* **Patient-Controlled Analgesia.**

1. Why does the nurse close the door of the pump before priming the IV tubing?

2. What vital step does the nurse do before connecting IV tubing to the patient's IV line?

 For suggested responses, go to Chapter 30, **Thinking About the Procedure Suggested Responses (Procedure 30-1),** on the Student Resource Disk or DavisPlus at http://davisplus.fadavis.com/Wilkinson2

Practice Resources

Cohen, M. R., Weber, R. J., & Moss, J. (2006); National Guideline Clearinghouse (NGC) (2009).

Clinical Insights

Clinical Insight 30–1 ▶ Caring for the Patient with an Epidural Catheter

✚ Intraspinal analgesia is contraindicated in patients who received anticoagulant therapy or who have spinal defects, local or systemic infections, or increased intracranial pressure.

Monitoring

- Monitor for respiratory depression (every hour for the first 24 hours, then every 4 hours if the patient is stable).
- Monitor the site for leaking or drainage.
- Check connections for leaks. This can be fixed by carefully retightening connections. If the filter is cracked, replace with a new one using sterile technique.
- Assess for urine retention. Keep careful intake and output (I&O) records.
Urinary retention is one side effect of epidural opioids.
- Observe for signs of headache in the patient as a result of dural puncture. Treatment consists of bed rest, analgesics, and liberal hydration. Caffeine is also helpful and may be

administered IV. If unresolved after 72 hours, patient might receive an epidural blood patch.
- Watch the site for leakage or drainage.
- Observe for signs of catheter migration: nausea, a decrease in blood pressure, and a loss of motor function without a recognizable cause.

Prevention

- Mark all epidural lines *clearly,* for patient safety.
This line must not be confused with an arterial or venous catheter.
- Ensure the tape on the tubing connected to the patient is secure.
To prevent catheter migration.
- Use strict aseptic technique when changing tubing, including mask and sterile gloves for access and maintenance procedures.
Prevents infection.

(continued on next page)

Clinical Insight 30-1 ▶ **Caring for the Patient with an Epidural Catheter** (continued)

Discontinuing the Catheter

▪ If you are specially trained to remove an epidural catheter, first loosen the tape securing the catheter. While wearing clean gloves, apply slow, steady pressure to withdraw the catheter. Inspect the catheter on removal. You must be able to see the tip of the catheter. If not, a portion of the catheter may still be lodged in the patient's

epidural space. Notify the anesthesia team immediately of this finding.

▪ If the catheter cannot be withdrawn with minimal force, try repositioning the patient to the same position for removal as the patient was in during insertion of the catheter.

▪ Cleanse the insertion site, and cover with a dry sterile dressing.

Clinical Insight 30-2 ▶ **Guidelines for Assessing for Nonverbal Signs of Pain**

When assessing for nonverbal signs of pain, keep the following guidelines in mind:

▪ **Facial expression, posture, and body position are reliable indicators of the intensity of pain.** Basic and common facial expressions that signal pain are lowering the brow, wincing, clenching jaws, and closing eyelids (Institute for Clinical Systems Improvement, 2008). Guarding a painful site or maintaining a tense position are signs of pain.

▪ **Changes in vital signs generally last only a short time.** The body seeks equilibrium; thus, after more than an hour, the vital signs typically return to what they were previously even though the patient may still be in pain. Continuous, severe pain may elevate the vital signs again from time to time, but they rarely remain elevated. Normal vital signs do *not* mean that the patient is free of pain.

▪ **Patients may be in pain even if they don't "act like" they are.** Too often, nurses expect patients to "act like" they are in pain. Unfortunately it has been well documented that healthcare professionals fail to assess pain and tend to underrate the pain the patient is experiencing (American Geriatric Society, Panel on Persisten Pain in Older Persons, 2002; McCaffery & Pasero, 1999). They expect to see frowning, crying, or scowling. Patients who use laughter, distraction, or even sleep to cope with their pain

are often undertreated. To assess pain accurately, you must ask your patients and then believe them.

▪ **Use an interpreter if the patient speaks a different language.** Ask the interpreter to explain to the patient that it is important to manage pain and that you will be using a pain scale regularly to assess the patient's pain. Have the interpreter write out the explanation and directions for the pain scale so that you can refer to these when you assess your patient. With written directions, patients can simply point to a face or numeric line to tell you about their pain when no one is present to translate.

▪ **Some patients feel that they are being "bad" or "weak" if they express pain.** Such patients may withdraw or become stoic. It is important that you establish a trusting relationship with them. Convey your concern, and acknowledge that they are experiencing pain. If the patient trusts you, she will feel free to verbalize thoughts and feelings.

▪ **Remember to assess for depression** (see Chapter 11 if you need to review). Depression is often overlooked in the patient in pain. If depression is not treated aggressively, efforts to manage the pain may not be successful. Avoid the misconception, however, that pain is the cause of the depression and that controlling the pain will eliminate the depression. This is rarely the case.

Assessment Guidelines and Tools

Taking a Pain History

Taking a pain history is the most effective way to perform an assessment. Each agency has a different assessment form for this history, but the questions typically will include the following:

Do you have pain now?

When did the pain begin?

Where is the pain located?

How do you rate your pain? (Use a pain scale.)

How would you describe your pain? Sharp? Dull? Achy? Burning?

How often do you have pain? Is it constant or intermittent?

Is there a rhythm or pattern to your pain?

What makes the pain better?

What makes it worse?

How many days this past week has pain interfered in your ability to do what you would like to do?

Does pain interfere with your ability to take care of yourself?

Does pain wake you up at night?

Does pain interrupt your concentration and reduce your ability to think clearly?

Have you experienced this type of pain in the past?

Do you have any other associated symptoms (such as nausea and vomiting) when you are experiencing pain?

Taking a Pain History—cont'd

Does pain prevent you from participating in pleasurable activities, hobbies, and socializing with friends?

Have you used any medications to treat the pain? If so, were they effective? How often do you need to take pain relievers?

What, if any, alternative treatments have you used for pain?

What past experiences or cultural factors, if any, influence the pain?

Observing for Nonverbal Indicators of Pain

Physiological (Involuntary) Responses
Sympathetic Responses (Acute Pain)

Increased systolic blood pressure

Increased heart rate and force of contraction

Increased respiratory rate

Dilated blood vessels to the brain, increased alertness

Dilated pupils

Rapid speech

Parasympathetic Responses (Deep or Prolonged Pain)

Decreased systolic blood pressure, possible syncope

Decreased pulse rate

Changeable breathing patterns

Withdrawal

Constricted pupils

Slow, monotonous speech

Behavioral Responses (Voluntary)

Withdrawing from painful stimuli

Moaning

Facial grimacing

Crying

Agitation

Guarding the painful area

Psychological (Affective) Responses

Anxiety

Depression

Anger

Fear

Exhaustion

Hopelessness

Irritability

Using Pain Scales

The most commonly used pain scales are the visual analog scale (VAS), the numerical rating scale (NRS), the simple descriptor scale (SDS), and the Wong-Baker FACES rating scale.

The Visual Analog Scale

The Visual Analog Scale (VAS) is a 10-cm horizontal line in which "No pain" is written on the left side and "Worst pain imaginable" is written on the right. Patients point to a location on the line that reflects their current pain. Although this rating system is simple and quick, some patients have problems with the abstract nature of the scale.

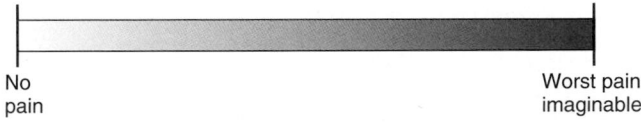

No pain

Worst pain imaginable

The Numerical Rating Scale

The Numerical Rating Scale (NRS) is a line numbered from 0 to 10. Zero indicates no pain at all, whereas a 10 indicates the worst possible pain. Patients choose a number from 0 to 10 to denote their level of pain. To use this scale, the patient must be

able to count to 10. A scale of 0 to 5 may be more helpful for cognitively impaired patients.

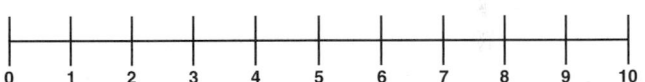

The Simple Descriptor Scale

The Simple Descriptor Scale (SDS) is a list of adjectives that describe different levels of pain intensity. The simplest version of this scale uses the words *mild, moderate,* and *severe.* An SDS with many words is not recommended; it is time-consuming to describe and may not be understood by many patients.

The Wong-Baker FACES Pain Rating Scale

The FACES scale uses simple illustrations of faces to depict various levels of pain. It requires no numerical or reading skill. Initially developed for use with children older than the age of 3, the scale has proven to be extremely useful for adults with communication and cognitive impairments as well.

Continued

Taking a Pain History—cont'd

Wong-Baker FACES Pain Rating Scale

  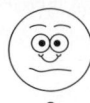 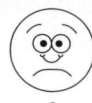  

0	1	2	3	4	5
No hurt	Hurts little bit	Hurts little more	Hurts even more	Hurts whole lot	Hurts worst

Explain to the person that each face is for a person who feels happy because he has no pain (hurt) or sad because he has some or a lot of pain. Face 0 is very happy because he doesn't hurt at all. Face 2 hurts a little more. Face 3 hurts even more. Face 4 hurts a whole lot. Face 5 hurts as much as you can imagine, although you do not have to be crying to feel this bad. Ask the person to chose the face that best describes how he is feeling. Rating scale is recommended for persons age 3 and older.

From Hockenberry MJ, Wilson D: (2009). *Wong's Essentials of Pediatric Nursing* (8th ed.). St. Louis, MO: Mosby. Used with permission. Copyright Mosby.

Revised Faces Pain Scales

We commonly ask patients to rate their pain on a scale of 0 to 10. However, the Wong-Baker FACES scale uses a 0 to 5 scale. To see a revised faces scale adapted to a 10-point scoring system, see Spragud, Piira, & Baeyer (2003). Children's self-report of pain intensity, *American Journal of Nursing, 103*(12), 62–64; or

 Go to the **Pediatric Pain Sourcebook Web site** at www. painsourcebook.ca

To see FACES scales using photos of children of various ethnicities,

 Go to the **OUCHER! Web site** at www.oucher.org

Sedation Rating Scale

1 = Awake and alert

2 = Slightly drowsy, easily aroused

3 = Frequently drowsy, arousable by voice

4 = Arousable by shaking

5 = Somnolent, not arousable

If the score on the sedation scale is 4, or higher, stimulate the patient and notify the physician. Before administering another dose, consider lowering the opioid dose, and investigate other potential causes of sedation.

If the respiratory rate is less than 8 to 10 breaths per minute, respirations are shallow, or the patient is unresponsive to stimulation, attempt to stimulate the patient, notify the physician, and consider administering naloxone (Narcan).

Adapted from *Pocket guide to pain management.* (2004). Distributed by Tufts-New England Medical Center Pain Clinic. Used with permission.

Standardized Language

NANDA-I Diagnoses, NOC Outcomes, and NIC Interventions Associated with Pain

Pain as the Etiology of Other NANDA-I Diagnoses (Examples)

- *Self-Care Deficit (Bathing/Dressing/Grooming)* related to pain in hands secondary to arthritis
- *Sleep Deprivation* related to chronic back pain of more than a year's duration
- *Impaired Walking* related to hip pain secondary to joint deterioration
- *Ineffective Airway Clearance* related to ineffective cough secondary to postsurgical incisional pain
- *Ineffective Coping* related to overwhelming nature of painful uterine contractions during labor as manifested by crying, moaning, thrashing about in bed
- *Impaired Home Maintenance* (difficulty cleaning, shopping, and so forth) related to unremitting pain (headache)
- *Ineffective Sexuality Pattern* related to pain in joints

NOC Outcomes and NIC Interventions for Pain Diagnoses

NANDA-I DIAGNOSIS	NOC OUTCOMES	NIC INTERVENTIONS
Acute Pain	Comfort Status: Physical	Analgesic Administration
	Pain Control	Sedation Management
	Pain: Disruptive Effects	Medication Management
	Pain Level	Pain Management
		Patient-Controlled Analgesia (PCA) Assistance
Chronic Pain	Comfort Status: Physical	Behavior Modification
	Pain Control	Cognitive Restructuring
	Depression Level	Patient Contracting
	Depression Self-Control	Pain Management
	Pain: Adverse Psychological Response	Coping Enhancement
	Pain: Disruptive Effects	Mood Management
	Pain Level	

Sources: Johnson, M., Bulechek, G., Butcher, H., et al. (2006). *NANDA, NOC, and NIC linkages* (2nd ed.). St. Louis, MO: C. V. Mosby; Moorhead, S., Johnson, M., Maas, M., et al. (Eds.). (2008). *Nursing outcomes classification (NOC)* (4th ed.). St. Louis, MO: C. V. Mosby; Bulechek, G. M., Butcher, H. K., & Dochterman, J. M. (Eds.). (2008). *Nursing interventions classification (NIC)* (5th ed.). St. Louis, MO: C. V. Mosby; NANDA International (2009). *Nursing diagnoses: Definitions and classification 2009–2011*, Oxford: Wiley-Blackwell. Used with permission.

THINKING CRITICALLY ABOUT PAIN MANAGEMENT

The exercises in the following sections allow you to practice the kind of thinking you will use as a full-spectrum nurse. Because these are critical-thinking questions, there is usually no single right answer. We do not provide answers for these questions because it is more important for you to think about the questions than to arrive at the "right" answer. These questions are designed to improve your thinking more than to "cover content." Discuss answers with your peers—discussion can stimulate critical thinking. If you have difficulty with any of these questions, consult with your instructor.

Applying the Full-Spectrum Nursing Model

PATIENT SITUATION

Dieter Schmidt is a 48-year-old with a 2-year history of cervical spine injury that began after a motor vehicle accident. Three years before the accident, Dieter fell through a roof to the cement basement when inspecting a building under construction. Presenting symptoms were neck pain when turning his head, bicep weakness, and pain down the arm with tingling into the fingertips. He is unable to sit for extended periods or walk distances. Initially he received treatment with medication, TENS to the site, physical therapy, and cervical fusion. Despite trying all treatments available to him, including surgery, Dieter continues to suffer chronic pain and fatigue. After prolonged suffering with no relief, Mr. Schmidt develops a cynical attitude toward healthcare. He begins missing more and more scheduled appointments for physical therapy. He describes stress he feels from the economic downturn impacting his land development business and fears bankruptcy. As a result, he has given up previous hobbies and most social activities. His relationships with his family and friends are increasingly strained as the pain persists over time.

THINKING

1. *Theoretical Knowledge*:

What is the mechanism that explains how pain is transmitted in the spine?

2. *Critical Thinking (Considering Alternatives, Deciding What to Do)*:

a. When planning care for Dieter, what approach would you take in helping him to set goals for his rehabilitation?

b. Why do you think Dieter displays a negative attitude and reduced compliance toward rehabilitative therapies?

DOING

3. *Practical Knowledge*:

a. (*Nursing Process: Assessment*): What questions would you ask Dieter to assess the impact of pain on his daily living and quality of life?

b. (*Nursing Process: Interventions*): In addition to drug therapy, what other measures might you teach your patient to do to control his pain and increase his comfort?

CARING

4. *Self-Knowledge*:

Have you ever experienced chronic pain, such as back pain, fibromyalgia, arthritis, migraines, sports injuries, or other types? If so, how has it affected your daily life? Has your pain impacted your relationships? Has it interfered with your job or recreational activities? In what other ways would you say chronic pain has reduced the quality of your life?

Critical Thinking and Clinical Reasoning

1. Mrs. J is a 29-year-old woman with terminal metastatic breast cancer. She knows she is dying. She has a devoted husband and two children, ages 2 and 4. Her husband has been taking care of her at home, but she is currently hospitalized for intractable pain. She does not want to be heavily sedated because she wants to spend as much time with her family as she can. She has no pain management plan.

    a. What is it about the patient's situation that may intensify her pain?

    b. Would you suggest using alternative therapies? Why or why not?

2. Mr. L is a 39-year-old construction worker who fell from a roof at a construction site 8 months ago and is still having back pain from the accident. To manage pain, he is prescribed an oral opioid every 4 hours on a prn basis. He is still out of work and has great difficulty walking, so that he spends most of the day in a recliner watching TV and drinking beer. Mr. L also sleeps most nights in the recliner. He states that the alcohol is the only thing that helps his pain. How would you alter his pain management plan to get better relief? What is your rationale for these changes?

3. How might you encourage a facility to enact a pain assessment strategy of pain as the fifth vital sign if this is not their current policy?

4. If you were delegating vital signs to nursing assistive personnel (NAP), what instructions would you give?

5. For each of the following concepts, use critical thinking to describe how or why it is important to nursing, patient care, or pain management. Note that these are *not* to be merely definitions.

Nociceptive pain	Opioid pain medications
Neuropathic pain	Adjuvant therapies
Unrelieved pain	Pain as the fifth vital sign
Fear of addiction	Pain scales
Nonpharmacological pain management	Pain flowsheets
Nonopioid pain medications	

What Are the Main Points in This Chapter?

➤ Pain is whatever the person says it is and exists whenever the person says it does.

➤ Pain has a protective function, warning us of potential or actual tissue damage and prompting us to take action.

➤ Pain can be classified by its origin, cause, duration, and quality.

➤ Pain begins when mechanical, thermal, or chemical stimuli activate nociceptors, which send pain impulses to the spinal cord.

➤ Fast-pain impulses are carried on large-diameter A-delta fibers, whereas slow-pain impulses are carried on thinner C fibers.

➤ Perception of pain occurs in the frontal cortex of the brain.

➤ Pain can be modulated by the endogenous analgesic system or by the gate-control mechanism.

➤ Some of the factors that influence pain are emotional factors, lifespan variations, past pain experiences, sociocultural factors, inability to communicate, and cognitive impairment.

➤ Serious physiological as well as psychological problems can result from unrelieved pain.

➤ Nonpharmacological pain relief measures include cutaneous stimulation, immobilization, and cognitive–behavioral intervention.

➤ Pharmacological measures include nonopioid analgesics, opioid analgesics, and adjuvant analgesics.

➤ Local and regional anesthesia, nerve blocks, and ablation therapy can relieve short- and long-term pain.

➤ Surgical interruption of pain conduction pathways is an option for intractable pain. Options depend on the type and location of pain.

➤ Opioid addiction among individuals being treated for pain is rare.

➤ Pain should be considered the fifth vital sign and assessed when the patient is admitted to a healthcare facility, with each vital signs check, before and after an intervention, and when the patient complains of pain.

➤ The patient's self-report is the most reliable indicator of pain, especially for those suffering chronic pain.

➤ Misconceptions about pain can interfere in pain management.

➤ Older adults are at risk for under-treatment of pain.

➤ Planning for the patient's pain management program includes discovering the patient's own goals, educating the patient and family, and developing a nursing plan of care.

➤ It is important to assess continually the effectiveness of pain management strategies.

For practice questions for this chapter,

 Go to **NCLEX-Style Chapter Quiz,** on the Student Resource Disk or DavisPlus at http://davisplus.fadavis.com/Wilkinson2

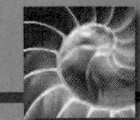

Knowledge Map

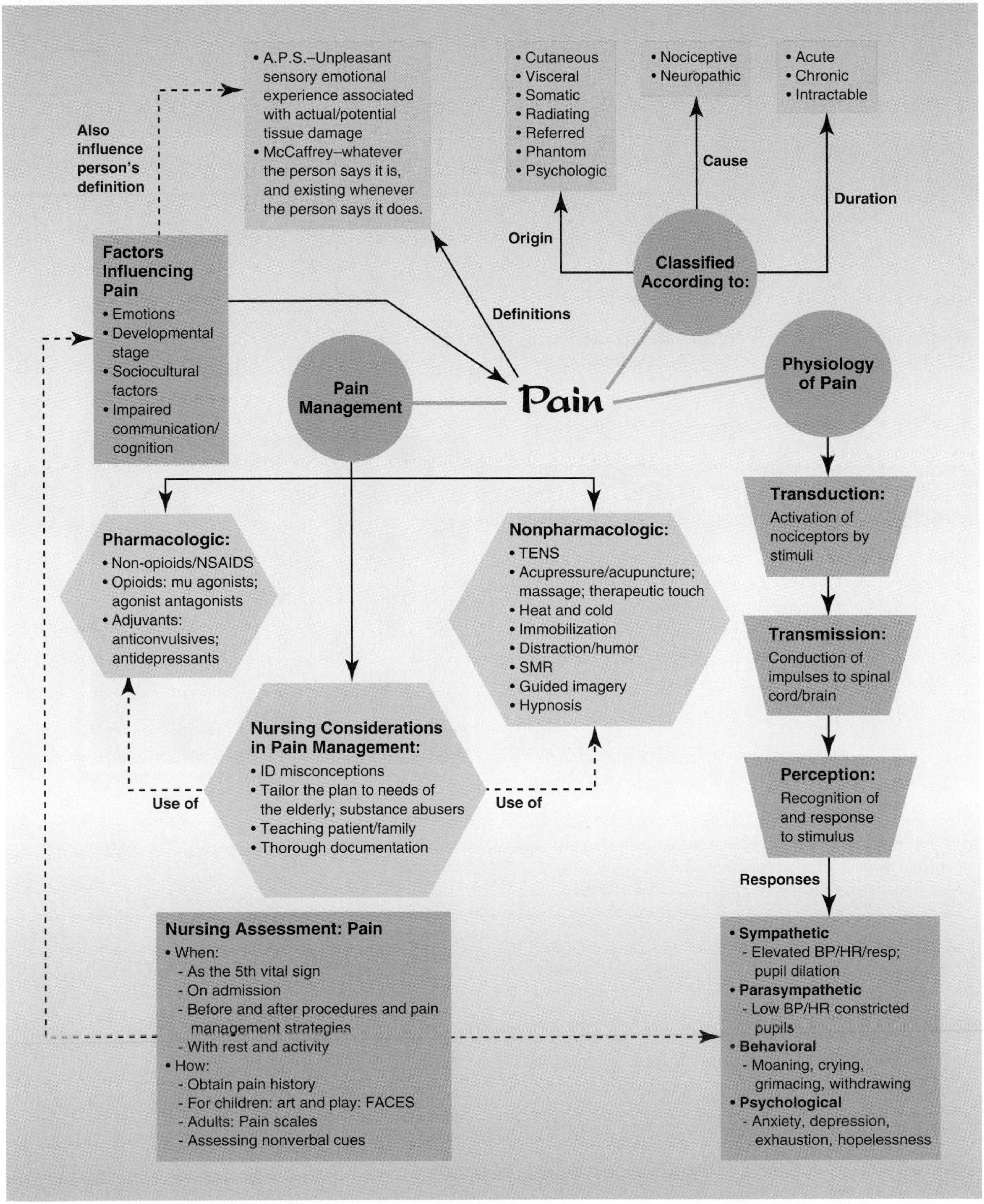

Factors Influencing Pain
- Emotions
- Developmental stage
- Sociocultural factors
- Impaired communication/cognition

Also influence person's definition

- A.P.S.–Unpleasant sensory emotional experience associated with actual/potential tissue damage
- McCaffrey–whatever the person says it is, and existing whenever the person says it does.

- Cutaneous
- Visceral
- Somatic
- Radiating
- Referred
- Phantom
- Psychologic

- Nociceptive
- Neuropathic

- Acute
- Chronic
- Intractable

Cause

Duration

Origin

Classified According to:

Definitions

Pain Management

Pain

Physiology of Pain

Pharmacologic:
- Non-opioids/NSAIDS
- Opioids: mu agonists; agonist antagonists
- Adjuvants: anticonvulsives; antidepressants

Nonpharmacologic:
- TENS
- Acupressure/acupuncture; massage; therapeutic touch
- Heat and cold
- Immobilization
- Distraction/humor
- SMR
- Guided imagery
- Hypnosis

Transduction:
Activation of nociceptors by stimuli

Transmission:
Conduction of impulses to spinal cord/brain

Nursing Considerations in Pain Management:
- ID misconceptions
- Tailor the plan to needs of the elderly; substance abusers
- Teaching patient/family
- Thorough documentation

Use of

Use of

Perception:
Recognition of and response to stimulus

Responses

Nursing Assessment: Pain
- When:
  - As the 5th vital sign
  - On admission
  - Before and after procedures and pain management strategies
  - With rest and activity
- How:
  - Obtain pain history
  - For children: art and play: FACES
  - Adults: Pain scales
  - Assessing nonverbal cues

- **Sympathetic**
  - Elevated BP/HR/resp; pupil dilation
- **Parasympathetic**
  - Low BP/HR constricted pupils
- **Behavioral**
  - Moaning, crying, grimacing, withdrawing
- **Psychological**
  - Anxiety, depression, exhaustion, hopelessness

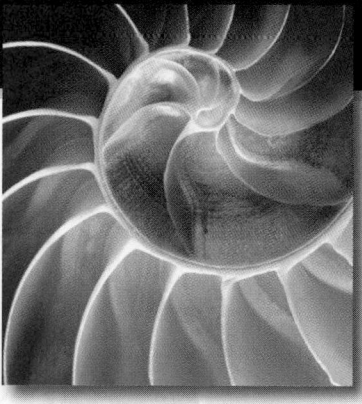

CHAPTER 31

Activity & Exercise

For a podcast of an overview of this chapter,

 Go to Student Resources, **Podcast – Chapter Overviews, Chapter 31,** on DavisPlus at http://davisplus.fadavis.com/ Wilkinson2

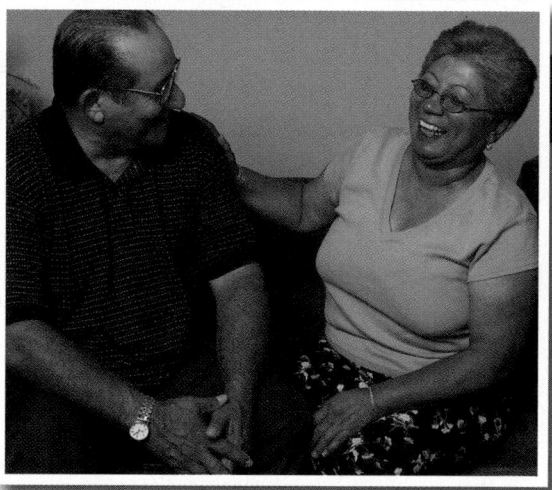

Caring for the Garcias

The exercises in the following section allow you to practice the kind of thinking you will use as a full-spectrum nurse. Because these are critical-thinking questions, there is usually no single right answer. We do not provide answers for these questions because it is more important for you to think about the questions than to arrive at the "right" answer. These questions are designed to improve your thinking more than to "cover content." Discuss answers with your peers—discussion can stimulate critical thinking. If you have difficulty with any of these questions, consult with your instructor.

As you may recall, Joe Garcia has been advised to diet and exercise as part of the treatment plan for hypertension, type 2 diabetes mellitus, obesity, and osteoarthritis.

Jordan Miller's exam has revealed no other cardiovascular problems.

A. Design an exercise program for Joe. Describe the program in detail. Recall that Joe has been relatively sedentary.

B. Compare the type of program you would recommend for Joe with the type of program appropriate for his granddaughter, Bettina.

C. What type of exercise program would be most appropriate for Katherine Garcia, Joe's mother? What additional information do you need to know to answer this question?

Practical **Knowledge**
knowing how

In the next sections you will learn about procedures and techniques for positioning, moving, turning, transferring, and ambulating patients safely. Although the American Nurses Association (ANA, 2005) recommends that you use assistive equipment for all patient lifting and transferring, you may encounter situations in which equipment is not available or you do not have time to get it. In such situations, using good body mechanics may help you decrease the risk of injury to you and the patient.

Procedures

Procedure 31-1 □ Moving and Turning Patients in Bed

➤ For steps to follow in *all* procedures, refer to the Universal Steps for All Procedures found on the inside back cover of Volume 2.

Critical Aspects

Procedure 31-1A: Moving a Patient Up in Bed
- Use a friction-reducing device to move the patient if the patient can assist with movement. Use a full body sling if the patient cannot assist.
- Remove the pillow. Have the patient flex her neck, fold her arms across her chest, and place her feet flat on bed.
- Position a nurse on either side of the patient.
- Use a wide base of support.
- Have the patient, on the count of 3, push off with his heels as you shift your weight forward.

Procedure 31-1B: Turning a Patient in Bed
- Use a friction-reducing device and drawsheet to move the patient. Position at least one nurse on each side of the bed.
- Place the patient's near leg and arm (e.g., the left arm and leg when turning to the right) across his body, and abduct and externally rotate the far shoulder.
- Each nurse places one arm at the level of the patient's shoulders and the other at the level of the patient's hips. Each nurse shifts her weight as both simultaneously roll the patient in the intended direction.

Procedure 31-1C: Logrolling a Patient
- Move the patient as a unit to the opposite side of the bed; raise the siderail on that side.
- Move to the side of the bed that the patient will be turning toward; lower the siderail.
- Each staff member evenly distributes his arms across the patient's length. One nurse is responsible for moving the head and neck as a unit.
- Shift your weight backward as you roll the patient toward you.

Equipment
- Nonlatex gloves, if you may be exposed to body fluids
- Friction-reducing device, such as a transfer roller sheet or scoot sheet
- Pull or lift (draw) sheet
- Pillows, as needed

Delegation
You may ask nursing assistive personnel (NAP) to assist with moving a patient up in bed, turning a patient, or log-rolling a patient after ensuring that the NAP has the necessary skills and that the patient's condition is stable. Complete the assessment, and inform the NAP of any special considerations when moving the patient.

Pre-Procedure Assessment
- Assess the patient's level of comfort.
If the patient is uncomfortable, you may need to administer an analgesic before moving.

- Assess the patient's level of consciousness, ability to follow directions, and ability to assist with the move.
- Assess for any restrictions in movement or position by asking the patient and checking the provider's orders.
- Assess the physical size of the patient and the assistive devices available.
- Review the patient's medical diagnoses. Identify problems that may affect positioning (e.g., respiratory or cardiac problems, pain).

(continued on next page)

Procedure 31-1 ■ **Moving and Turning Patients in Bed** (continued)

■ Observe for the presence of equipment such as IV setups, pumps, or casts and know what must be moved with the patient.

The preceding assessments all help determine how many assistants and equipment you need, the patient's ability to assist in the procedure, and how to proceed with the move safely.

■ Procedure 31-1A **Moving a Patient Up in Bed**

➤ When performing the procedure, always identify your patient according to agency policy and be attentive to standard precautions, hand hygiene, patient safety and privacy, body mechanics, and documentation.

➤ *Note:* This procedure employs the use of a transfer roller sheet. This device is inexpensive and readily available. Scoot sheets further reduce the risk of back and musculoskeletal injury; however, their availability varies. However, having a second person to help move a patient up in bed is the safest approach for staff and patients. Also follow the guidelines in Clinical Insight 31-1.

Procedure Steps

■ Medicate the patient for pain, if needed, before moving the patient in bed.

1. Lock the bed wheels. Lower the head of the bed, and place the patient in a supine position. Position one nurse on each side of the bed. Lower the siderails on the "working" side of the bed. Raise the height of the bed to waist level.
Lowering the siderails and raising the bed allows you to move the patient while maintaining good body mechanics and working with gravity.

2. Ensure that a friction-reducing device, such as a transfer roller sheet, is in place under the drawsheet. If it is not in place, turn the patient from side to side to place the device under the drawsheet. You can improvise this device by placing a clean, unused plastic bag or plastic film under the drawsheet.
A transfer roller sheet facilitates movement by reducing friction. This also helps to reduce back injury to the nurse.

3. Remove the pillow from under the patient's head. Place it at the head of the bed.
A pillow prevents patient from hitting his head on the head board.

4. Instruct the patient to fold his arms across his chest. If an overhead

trapeze is in place, ask the patient to hold the trapeze with both hands if able. Have the patient bend his knees with feet flat on the bed. ▼

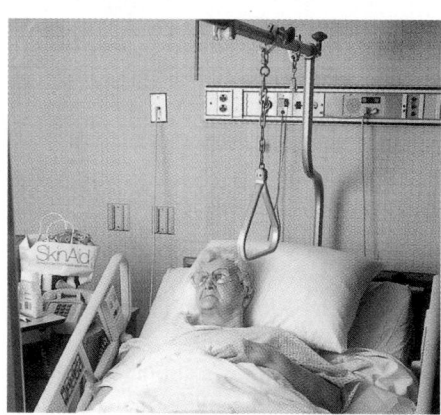

This position facilitates patient's assistance with move.

5. Instruct the patient to flex his neck.
Flexion protects the the neck with movement.

6. With a nurse positioned on either side of the patient, grasp and roll the drawsheet close to the patient.

7. Instruct the patient, on the count of 3, to lift his trunk and push off with his heels toward the head of the bed.

8. Position your feet with a wide base of support. Point your feet toward the direction of the move. Flex your knees and hips.

Allows you to maintain proper body mechanics and prevents injury while moving the patient. ▼

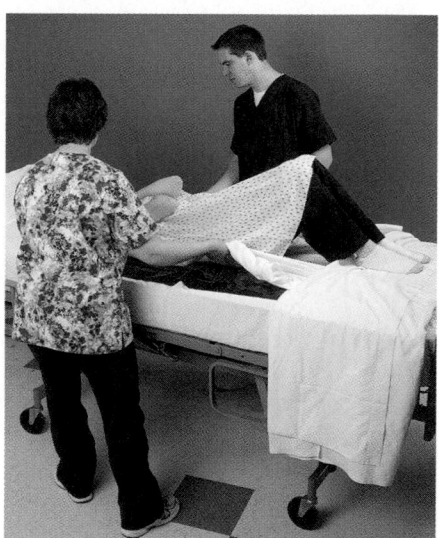

9. Place your weight on your foot nearest to the foot of the bed. Count to 3, and shift your weight forward toward the head of the bed.
Shifting your weight allows you to use your momentum to move the patient, which helps protect your back from injury.

10. Repeat until the patient is positioned near the head of the bed. If you used a plastic bag or film to reduce friction, remove it now.
Plastic is water impermeable, so it allows moisture to pool under the patient. This creates a risk for Impaired Skin Integrity.

11. Straighten the drawsheet, and tuck it in tightly at the sides of the bed.
A wrinkle-free sheet prevents uneven pressure, discomfort, and skin irritation.

12. Place a pillow under the patient's head, and assist him to a comfortable position.
A pillow provides comfort and good body alignment.

13. Place the bed in low position, and raise the siderail.
Helps prevent falls.

14. Place the call light in a position where the patient can easily reach it.
Allows patient to call for help, if needed.

Procedure Variation
Use of an Approved Mechanical Lifting Device

15. Lock the bed wheels. Lower the head of the bed, and place the patient in a supine position. Position at least one nurse on each side of the bed. Lower the siderails. Raise the height of the bed to waist level.

16. Using the drawsheet, turn the patient to one side of the bed. Position the midline of the full body sling at the patient's back. Tightly roll the remaining half of the sling, and tuck the fabric under the drawsheet. ▼

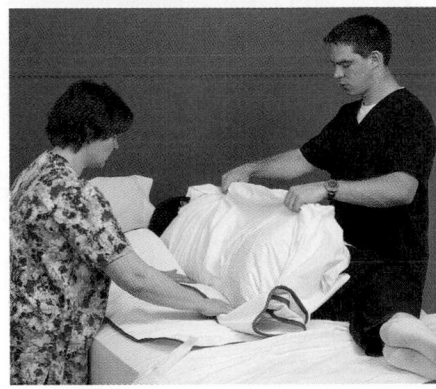

17. With a second nurse positioned on either side of the patient, use the drawsheet to turn the patient to the opposite side of the bed. Unroll the full body sling, and reposition the patient supine.

18. Attach the sling to the overbed lifting device or mechanical lift.

19. Engage the lift to raise the patient off the bed. Advance the lift toward the head of the bed until the patient is at the desired level. ▼

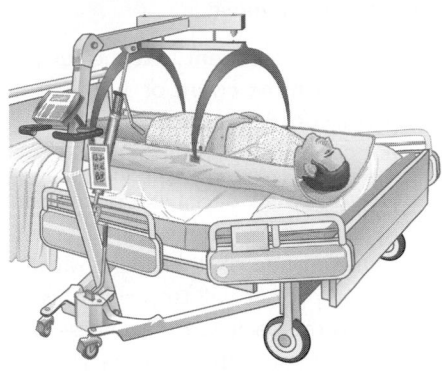

20. Lower the lift, and turn the patient to the desired position. You may leave the sling in place for future movement, or you may remove it by turning the patient from side to side.

Note: If a full body sling is not available, use a friction-reducing device, such as a transfer roller sheet, and at least three staff members.

■ Procedure 31-1B Turning a Patient in Bed

➤ When performing the procedure, always identify your patient according to agency policy and be attentive to standard precautions, hand hygiene, patient safety and privacy, body mechanics, and documentation.

➤ *Note:* This procedure describes the use of a transfer roller sheet. This device is inexpensive and readily available.

Procedure Steps

1. Lock the bed wheels. Lower the head of the bed, and place the patient in a supine position. Position one nurse on each side of the bed. Lower the siderails. Raise the height of the bed to waist level.
Lowering the siderails and raising the bed allow you to move the patient while maintaining good body mechanics and working with gravity to prevent injury.

2. Remove the pillow from under the patient's head and place it at the head of the bed. Roll the patient side to side and place a friction-reducing device under the drawsheet. You can improvise this device by placing a large, clean plastic bag or plastic film under the drawsheet. Move the patient to the side of the bed you are

turning him away from by rolling up the drawsheet close to the patient's body and pulling it. Align the patient's legs and head with the trunk.
This allows you to position the patient in the center of the bed after turning. ▼

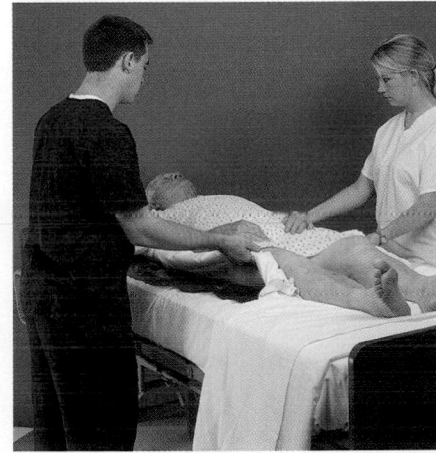

3. Place the patient's near leg and foot across the far leg (e.g., when turning the patient to his right, place his left leg over his right leg).

4. Place the patient's near arm (e.g., left when turning right) across his chest. Abduct and externally rotate the other arm and shoulder.
Positioning the patient's legs and his near arm facilitates turning. Abducting and rotating the other arm prevents it from being caught under the patient during the turn.

5. Each nurse positions her feet with a wide base of support with one foot forward of the other. Bend from the hips, and place one hand on the drawsheet at the level of the patient's hip and the other at the level of the shoulder.

(continued on next page)

Procedure 31-1 ■ **Moving and Turning Patients in Bed** (continued)

A wide base of support allows you to maintain good body mechanics while performing the move.

6. Instruct the patient that the turn will occur on the count of 3.
Counting coordinates and facilitates patient cooperation with the move.

7. On the count of 3, flex your knees and hips and shift your weight. The nurse positioned on the side toward which the patient will turn shifts his weight to the back foot. The nurse on the opposite side shifts her weight forward.

Provides the best leverage to turn the patient. ▼

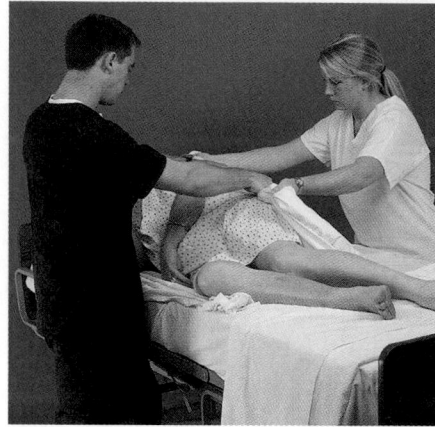

8. If a plastic film is used, remove it after you turn the patient.

9. Position the dependent shoulder forward. Place pillows behind the

patients back and between legs to maintain the patient in the lateral position. Replace the pillow under the patient's head.
Positioning ensures that patient is not putting excess pressure on the inferior shoulder. Pillows help maintain good body alignment.

VOL 1 Go to Chapter 31, **Table 31-2: Positioning a Bed-Bound Patient,** in Volume 1.

10. Place the bed in low position, and raise the siderail.
Helps ensure patient safety.

11. Place the call light in a position where the patient can easily reach it.
Allows patient to call for help, if needed.

■ *Procedure 31-1C* **Logrolling a Patient**

➤ When performing the procedure, always identify your patient according to agency policy and be attentive to standard precautions, hand hygiene, patient safety and privacy, body mechanics, and documentation.

Procedure Steps

1. Lock the bed. Lower the head of the bed with the patient supine. Lower the siderail on the side where you are standing, but keep the opposite rail in the up position. Raise the height of the bed to waist level.
Lowering the siderail and raising the bed allows you to move the patient while maintaining good body mechanics and working with gravity to prevent back injury.

2. You should already have a drawsheet with an underlying friction-reducing device, such as a transfer roller sheet, to move the patient to the side of the bed on which you are standing. (You can improvise this device by placing a clean, unused plastic bag or plastic film under the drawsheet.) Position one staff member at the patient's head and shoulders; she is responsible for moving the head and neck as a unit. Position the other person at the

patient's hips. If you need three staff members, position one at the shoulders, one at the waist, and the third at thigh level. One staff member must maintain the patient's head and neck in alignment. The other members assist with moving the rest of the body in alignment. ▼

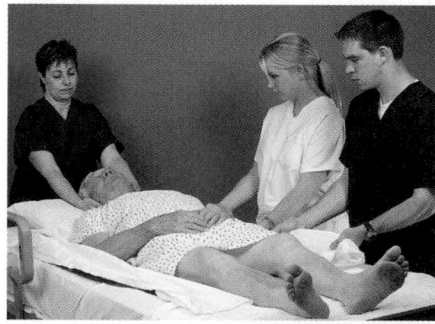

3. Each nurse should position her feet with a wide base of support with one foot slightly more forward than the other.
Facilitates proper body mechanics and minimizes risk of injury to staff members.

4. Use the drawsheet or transfer sheet to move the patient to the side of the bed on which the nurses are standing. The move must be smooth so that the patient's head and hips are kept in alignment. Position the patient's head with a pillow.
A transfer sheet maintains straight alignment of the spine.

5. Instruct the patient to fold his arms across his chest.

6. Place a pillow between the patient's knees.
A pillow prevents internal rotation of the hip and spine with movement. Maintains straight alignment of the spine.

7. Raise the siderail, and move to opposite side of the bed.
Siderails keep the patient from falling out of bed.

8. Lower the siderail on the "new" side of the bed, and face the patient. All nurses should position their feet with a wide base of support, with one foot forward of the other. Place your weight on the forward foot. Bend from the hips, and position your hands evenly along the length of the drawsheet.

Provides the best leverage to turn the patient while maintaining spine alignment.▼

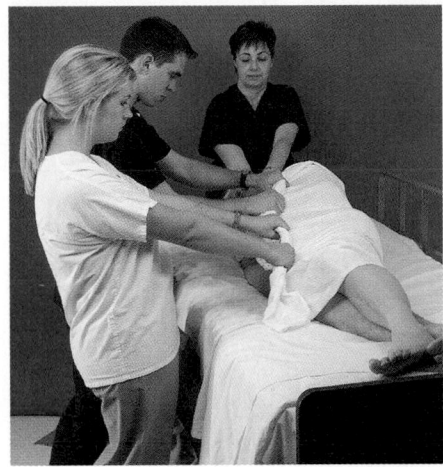

9. All nurses flex their knees and hips and shift their weight to the back foot on the count of 3. Be sure to support the head as the patient is rolled to his side.

Allows you to maintain straight alignment and body mechanics while performing the move.

10. Place pillows to maintain the patient in the lateral position.

 Go to Chapter 31, **Table 31-2: Positioning a Bed-Bound Patient,** in Volume 1.

A pillow provides support and maintains proper alignment.

11. Place the bed in low position, and raise the siderail.

12. Place the call light in a position where the patient can easily reach it. *Allows patient to call for help, if needed.*

What if . . .

■ **Your facility has instituted a no-lift policy and you have to pull the patient up in bed?**

Use assistive equipment, such as friction-reducing devices, mechanical lifts, air-powered mattresses, and/or lateral transfer devices to help prevent work-related injuries.

■ **Your patient is obese or unable to assist (totally dependent) and you need to lift him?**

Minimize manual lifting in all cases and eliminate it where feasible. Therefore, follow facility recommendations/

protocols and use approved devices. You should be familiar with the lift devices in your facility.

■ **The patient has had a total hip replacement and you have to turn or log roll your patient?**

Maintain the affected leg in abduction, by using a pillow or abduction wedge between the legs.

To ensure the hip will not become dislocated during turning.

■ **The patient has a cast or is in traction and you have to turn or log roll your patient?**

Designate a third person to assist in the turning by guiding the affected extremity.

■ **The patient has an external fixation device and you have to turn or log roll your patient?**

Secure the device in place to keep it from moving when lifting or moving the limb as needed.

By holding onto the device to secure it and keep it from moving, there is less movement of the healing bone, and therefore less trauma and pain.

Evaluation

■ Assess the patient's comfort level after the position change.
■ Assess body position and alignment after position change.
■ Assess skin for pressure areas.

Patient Teaching

■ Explain to the patient the importance of maintaining spine alignment.
■ Explain to the patient the importance of frequent position changes.
■ Instruct the patient to ask the nurse when she needs to be turned sooner than scheduled.
■ Teach the patient how she can assist with moving and turning.

Home Care

■ Instruct the family member or caregiver in the techniques for moving, turning, or logrolling the client.
■ Discuss the shearing effects on the skin from sliding down in bed (see Chapter 34).
■ Provide instruction on importance of changing position and maintaining proper body alignment.

Documentation

Repositioning and turning patients are considered routine aspects of care and are not usually charted every time they are done. However, document in the nursing notes any problems with positioning the patient or any areas of skin breakdown. You might also chart turning as an intervention when charting to a specific problem. For example, if the patient has Impaired Skin Integrity, you might describe the skin and chart, "Position changed hourly." Some facilities have flowsheets on which you indicate by a checkmark each time a patient is repositioned.

(continued on next page)

Procedure 31-1 ■ Moving and Turning Patients in Bed (continued)

Sample documentation:

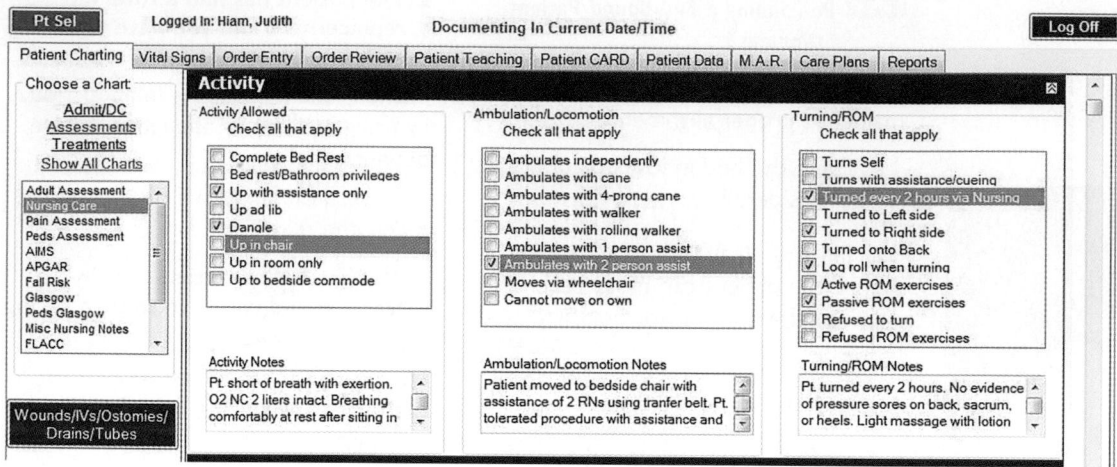

Practice Resources

Collins, J. W., Nelson, A., & Sublet, V. (2006); Nelson, A. & Baptiste, A. S. (2004).

Thinking About the Procedure

 Go to the *Fundamentals of Nursing Skills Videos*, **Moving a Patient Up in Bed; Moving a Patient Up in Bed: Mechanical Lift; Logrolling.**

Turning a Patient in Bed

1. When the nurse positions the patient to prepare for turning in bed, where does she place the arms when turning to the left? How does she position the legs?

Moving a Patient Up in Bed; Moving a Patient Up in Bed: Mechanical Lift

1. When does the nurse first lower the siderails when moving a patient up in bed?

2. In what instance is the mechanical assist used to move a patient up in bed?

Logrolling

1. What might the nurses do to improve the positioning of the patient during and after logrolling?

 For suggested responses, go to Chapter 31, **Thinking About the Procedure Suggested Responses (Procedure 31-1C),** on the Student Resource Disk or DavisPlus at http://davisplus.fadavis.com/Wilkinson2

Procedure 31-2 Transferring Patients

➤ For steps to follow in *all* procedures, refer to the Universal Steps for All Procedures found on the inside back cover of Volume 2.

Critical Aspects

Procedure 31-2A: Transferring a Patient from Bed to Stretcher

- Move the patient to the side of the bed where the stretcher will be placed.
- Position the stretcher next to the bed, and lock it in place.
- Keep the destination device (i.e., bed to stretcher or vice versa) situated a little lower than the surface the patient is on to reduce the workload of the transfer.
- Using the drawsheet, roll the patient away from the stretcher.

- Place the transfer board against the patient's back halfway between the bed and stretcher. Position a friction-reducing device over the transfer board. Turn the patient to his back and onto the transfer board with the drawsheet.
- On a count of 3, use the drawsheet to slide the patient across the transfer board onto the stretcher.

Procedure 31-2B: Dangling a Patient at the Side of the Bed

- Place the patient in a supine position, and raise the head of the bed to 90°.
- Apply a gait transfer belt, and put the bed in the low position.
- Stand facing the patient with a wide base of support. Place your foot closest to the head of the bed forward of the other foot.
- Position your hands on each side of the gait transfer belt.
- Rock onto your back foot as you move the patient into a sitting position, and pivot to bring the patient's legs over the side of the bed.
- Stay with the patient as he dangles.

Procedure 31-2C: Transferring a Patient from Bed to Chair

- Instruct the patient to wear nonskid footwear (slippers or shoes).
- Place the bed in the low position, and lock the wheels.
- Assist the patient to dangle at the side of the bed (see Procedure 31-2B).
- Brace your feet and knees against the patient. Bend your hips and knees, and hold onto the transfer belt.
- If two nurses are available to assist with the transfer, one nurse should be on each side of the patient.
- Instruct the patient to place her arms around you between your shoulders and waist. (The location depends on the height of the patient and the nurses.)
- Ask the patient to stand as you move to an upright position by straightening your legs and hips.
- Instruct the patient to pivot and turn with you toward the chair.
- Ask the patient to flex her hips and knees as she lowers herself to the chair. Guide her motion while maintaining a firm hold on her.
- If the chair is a wheelchair, the wheels must be in the locked position.

Equipment

- Nonlatex gloves, if you may be exposed to body fluids
- Transfer board (for transferring from bed to stretcher, and sometimes bed to chair)
- Pull or lift (draw) sheet (for transfers)
- Gait transfer belt (for dangling and transferring from bed to chair)

Delegation

You may ask nursing assistive personnel (NAP) to dangle, transfer a patient from bed to stretcher, or transfer a patient from bed to chair. Ensure that the NAP has the necessary skills and that the patient's condition is stable. Inform the NAP of any special considerations when dangling or transferring the patient and evaluate the patient after transfer.

Pre-Procedure Assessment

- Assess for any restrictions in movement or position by asking the patient and checking the physician's orders.
- Observe for the presence of equipment such as IV lines, drains, or catheters.

- Assess possible side effects of medications (e.g., dizziness and sedation). Assess the patient's level of consciousness, ability to follow directions, and ability to assist with the move.
- Assess the physical size of the patient and your own strength and ability to move the patient.
- Before transferring a patient to a chair, assess the patient's tolerance of dangling.

The preceding assessments inform you about activity tolerance, readiness to get out of bed, and ability to participate in the transfer. They help you determine how many assistants you need, the appropriate transfer device, and how to proceed with the move while preventing injury and dislodging of equipment.

- Assess vital signs, and monitor for postural hypotension.

If the patient is at risk for postural hypotension, you may need to allow additional time for the patient to change position.

- Assess the patient's level of comfort using a standardized pain scale.

If the patient is experiencing pain, you may need to administer an analgesic before moving.

(continued on next page)

Procedure 31-2 ■ Transferring Patients (continued)

■ Procedure 31-2A Transferring a Patient from Bed to Stretcher

➤ When performing the procedure, always identify your patient according to agency policy and be attentive to standard precautions, hand hygiene, patient safety and privacy, body mechanics, and documentation.

Procedure Steps

1. Lock the wheels on the bed. Position the bed so that it is flat (if the patient can tolerate being supine) and at the height of the stretcher.
Locking the wheels ensures client safety during the transfer. Having the bed flat helps prevent injury to staff, because the patient is easier to move.

2. Lower the siderails, and position at least one nurse on each side of the bed. Move the patient to the side of the bed where the stretcher will be placed by rolling up the drawsheet close to the patient's body and pulling it toward the designated side. Align the patient's legs and head with her trunk.
Positions patient to enable nurses to move her to the stretcher.

3. Position the stretcher next to the bed. Lock the stretcher wheels.
Locking the wheels keeps the stretcher from moving during the transfer; prevents falls.

4. Place the transfer board against the patient's back.
  a. Place a friction-reducing device, such as a transfer roller sheet, over the transfer board. (You can improvise this device by placing a clean, unused plastic bag or plastic film under the drawsheet.)
  b. The nurse on the side opposite the stretcher uses the drawsheet to turn the patient away from the stretcher, while the other nurse places the transfer board against the patient's back halfway between bed and stretcher. Turn the patient to her back and onto the transfer board.

Safely positions the transfer board under the patient, without friction. ▼

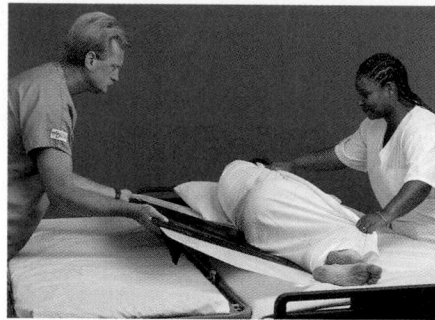

5. Ensure the patient's feet and shoulder are over the edge of the transfer board.
To prevent injury to the patient from the edge of the board.

6. Have the patient raise her head if able. Use the drawsheet to slide her across the transfer board onto the stretcher.
Using a transfer board and transfer roller sheet facilitates the move to stretcher; prevents friction on patient's skin. ▼

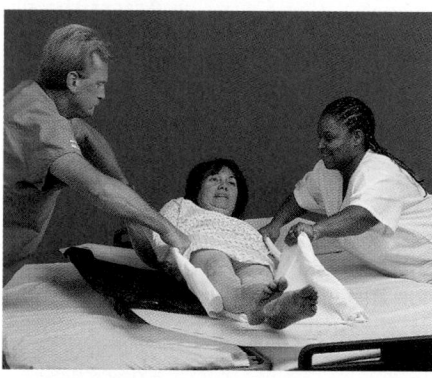

7. Use the drawsheet to turn the patient away from the bed; remove the board and roller sheet.

8. Reposition the patient on the stretcher for comfort and alignment.
Provides support and maintains proper alignment.

9. Provide a blanket, if needed for warmth or privacy.

10. Fasten safety belts, and raise the siderails on the stretcher.
Prevents falls.

Procedure Variation
Transferring a Patient from Bed to Stretcher with a Slipsheet

Note: A slipsheet may be used instead of a transfer board. A slipsheet is a large, low-friction fabric that facilitates transfer.

11. Lock the bed. Position the bed so that it is flat (if the patient can tolerate being supine) and at the height of the stretcher.
Ensures patient safety during the transfer. Helps prevent injury to staff because the patient is easier to move if the bed is flat.

12. With the drawsheet, turn the patient to the side opposite where the stretcher will be placed. Position the midline of the slipsheet under the patient. Roll the remaining half tightly, and tuck it under the patient.

13. Turn the patient to the opposite side, and pull the slipsheet through from under the patient.

14. Place the patient supine, and lower the siderail on the side where the stretcher will be placed.

15. Move the stretcher next to the bed and lock the wheels on the stretcher.

16. Position at least two nurses on the far side of the stretcher. Using the slipsheet, pull the patient onto the stretcher. ▼

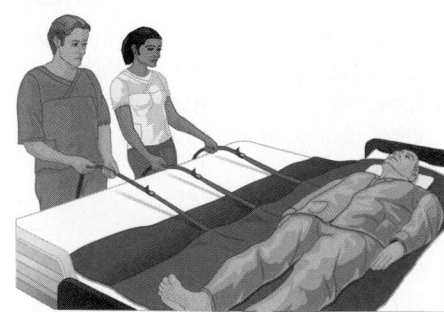

■ **Procedure 31-2B** **Dangling a Patient at the Side of the Bed**

➤ When performing the procedure, always identify your patient according to agency policy and be attentive to standard precautions, hand hygiene, patient safety and privacy, body mechanics, and documentation.

Procedure Steps

1. Lock the bed wheels. Place the patient in a supine position, and raise the head of the bed to 90°. Keep the siderail elevated on the side opposite where you are standing.
Locking the wheels prevents the bed from moving as you move the patient. Raising the head of the bed prepares the patient to be dangled and requires less effort from you to help the patient sit erect.

2. Apply a gait transfer belt to the patient at waist level. Place the bed in the low position.
Ensures patient safety and proper body mechanics.

3. Instruct the patient to bend his knees and turn the patient onto his side, if possible, keeping knees flexed.
Prepares the patient to be able to dangle his legs over side of bed.

4. Stand on the side of the bed, facing the patient and using a wide base of support. Place your foot closest to the head of the bed forward of the other foot. Lean forward, bending at the hips,

with your knees flexed. Instruct the patient to use his arm to push off the bed.
Allows you to maintain proper body mechanics and prevents injury. ▼

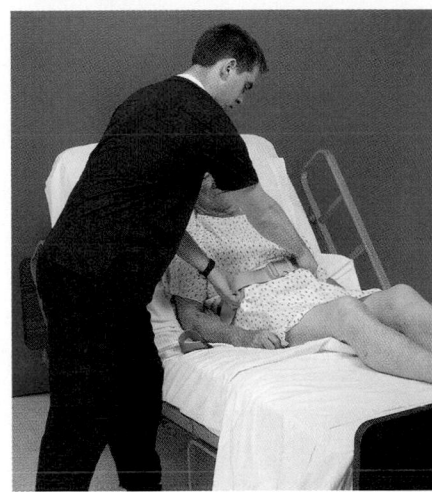

5. Position your hands on each side of the gait transfer belt.

6. Rock onto your back foot as you assist the patient toward you with the gait transfer belt, thereby moving the patient into a sitting position at the side of the bed.

Uses your body weight as leverage to reposition the patient, preventing injury to your back. ▼

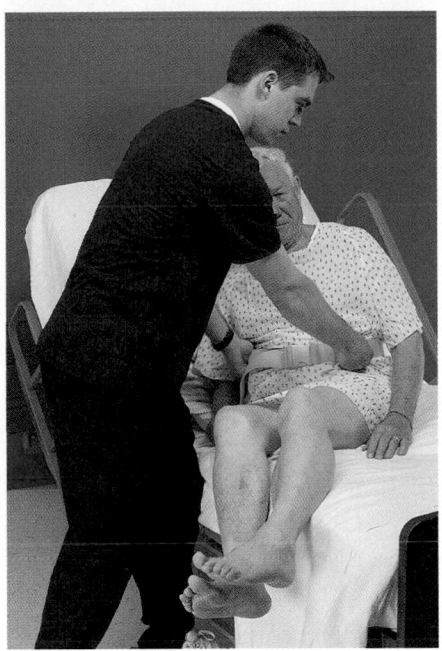

7. Stay with the patient as he dangles. Reassess comfort level and for dizziness.
Helps prevent falls.

■ **Procedure 31-2C** **Transferring a Patient from Bed to Chair**

➤ When performing the procedure, always identify your patient according to agency policy and be attentive to standard precautions, hand hygiene, patient safety and privacy, body mechanics, and documentation.

Procedure Steps

1. Position the chair next to the bed. If possible, lock the chair.
Prevents the chair from moving during transfer. Ensures patient safety.

2. Put nonskid footwear on the patient.
Prevents the patient from slipping during transfer.

3. Place the bed in a low position, and lock the bed.

Prevents the bed from moving during the transfer. Low position allows patient to place feet firmly on the floor.

4. Assist the patient to dangle at the side of the bed (see Procedure 31-2B). Be sure the patient doesn't need support before releasing him.

5. Apply a transfer belt.
Facilitates transfer of the patient to the chair and helps prevent back injury to the nurse.

6. Stand toward the bed, facing the patient. Brace your feet and knees against the patient. Pay particular attention to any known weakness. Bend your hips and knees, and, keeping your back straight, hold onto the transfer belt on both sides. If two nurses are available to assist with the transfer, one nurse should be on each side of the patient.
Bracing provides stability. Bending the hips and knees allows you to use the major muscle groups and limit the risk of

(continued on next page)

Procedure 31-2 ▪ **Transferring Patients** (continued)

injury. Lifting the patient at waist level prevents injury to the arm or shoulder. ▼

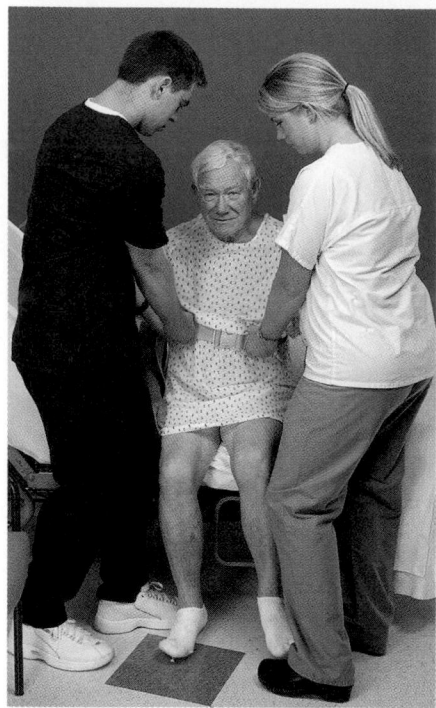

7. Instruct the patient to place his arms around you between the shoulders and waist (the location depends on your height and the height of the patient).
Having the patient hold you on your trunk prevents injury to your neck.

8. Ask the patient to stand as you move to an upright position by straightening your legs and hips.
Straightening your thighs and hips uses your large muscle groups and prevents injury to your back.

9. Allow the patient to steady himself for a moment.

Provides the patient an opportunity to rest before further movement. Allows you to evaluate his tolerance to activity and ability to maintain an upright posture before continuing.

10. Instruct the patient to pivot and turn with you toward the chair.
Pivoting helps prevent twisting and straining the patient's back muscles.

11. Assist the patient to position himself in front of the chair. Have the patient flex his hips and knees, and as he lowers himself to the chair, reach for arms of the chair. Guide his motion while maintaining a firm hold on him and keeping your back straight.
Maintains good body mechanics and balance and ensures patient safety. ▼

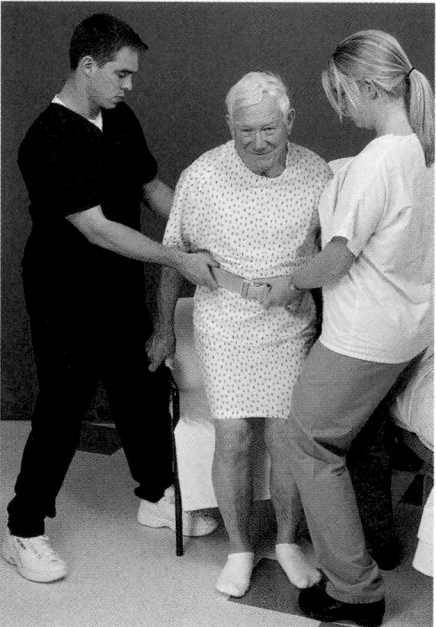

12. Assist the patient to a comfortable position in the chair.

13. Provide a blanket if needed for warmth or privacy.

14. Place the call light in reach of the patient or position the patient where he can be seen by staff members at all times.

What if . . .

▪ **The patient is obese?**

If the patient is obese or unable to assist, use a full body sling that allows the patient to assume a seated position. You may also use a powered standing assist lift, if one is available.

▪ **The patient has had hip surgery (replacement or fracture repair).**

When assisting the patient out of bed, raise the bed to a higher position, allowing the patient to exit the bed without acute hip flexion.
To avoid hip dislocation

▪ **The patient becomes dizzy during the transfer?**

Return the patient to recumbent position and assess his vital signs.

▪ **The patient has a weaker side, for example, from a CVA or surgical procedure?**

Instruct the patient to exit the bed from his unaffected side. Stand on the patient's weaker side.
The stronger side should lead a transfer.

Evaluation

▪ Assess the level of patient participation in the transfer.
▪ Assess the patient's comfort level during the transfer and in the new position.
▪ Assess proper body position and alignment after his position change.
▪ Assess the patient's vital signs for postural hypotension after dangling or transferring to a chair.

Patient Teaching

▪ Explain the importance of frequent position changes and getting out of bed to avoid complications of immobility.

Home Care

▪ Instruct the family member or caregiver in the proper technique for assisting the client to dangle at the bedside or transfer to a chair.
▪ Provide instruction in the importance of changing position and maintaining proper body alignment.

Documentation

Patients are usually moved to a stretcher for transport to a test or procedure. The movement is a routine aspect of care and is not documented. When dangling or transferring a patient to a chair, document in the nursing notes how much assistance was required, the use of assistive devices, any problems with positioning the patient, how long the patient was out of bed, and how the patient tolerated the activity.

Sample documentation:

10/04/11 1100 *Pt assisted to dangle at the side of the bed for 5 minutes. Pt experienced some initial feelings of vertigo with BP 108/60, P 110, RR 28. After 5 minutes BP 126/72, P 90, RR 24. Pt assisted back to bed.* ———————————— *S. Jones, RN*

11/11/11 0630 *Pt dangled at side of bed and assisted to chair with minimal assistance. Able to sit up for 90 minutes with no pallor and no change in vital signs.* ————— *B. Bowen, RN*

Practice Resources

Collins, J. W., Nelson, A., & Sublet, V. (2006); Kjellberg, K., Lagerstrom, M., & Hagberg, M. (2004); National Institute for Occupational Safety and Health (2009); Nelson, A., Lloyd, J., Menzel, N., & Gross, C. (2003); Nelson, A., Pragala, G., & Menzel, N. (2004); Trinkoff, A. M., Brady, B., & Nielsen, K. (2003).

Thinking About the Procedure

 Go to the *Fundamentals of Nursing Skills Videos*, **Transferring Patients: Bed to Stretcher.**

I. What kind of friction-reducing device do the nurses in the video use to transfer the patient from the bed to the stretcher?

Transferring Patients: Bed to Chair

I. For those who can assist in transferring from the bed to the chair, how should the patient hold on to the nurse?

 For suggested responses, go to Chapter 31, **Thinking About the Procedure Suggested Responses (Procedure 31-2),** on the Student Resource Disk or DavisPlus at http://davisplus.fadavis.com/Wilkinson2

Procedure 31-3 ☐ Assisting with Ambulation

➤ For steps to follow in *all* procedures, refer to the Universal Steps for All Procedures found on the inside back cover of Volume 2.

Critical Aspects

- Instruct the patient to wear nonskid footwear.
- Place the bed in low position, and lock the wheels.
- Assist the patient to dangle at the side of the bed.
- If two nurses are available to assist with the transfer, one nurse should be on each side of the patient.
- Brace your feet and knees against the patient. Bend your hips and knees, and hold onto the transfer belt. Pay attention to any known weakness.
- Instruct the patient to place her arms around you between your shoulders and waist (the location depends on the height of the patient and the nurses). Ask the patient to stand as you move to an upright position by straightening your legs and hips.
- Allow the patient to steady herself for a moment.
- *One nurse:* Stand at the patient's side, placing both hands on the transfer belt. If the patient has weakness on one side, position yourself on the weaker side.
- *Two nurses:* One nurse is on each side of the patient, grasping the transfer belt.
- Slowly guide the patient forward. Observe for signs of fatigue or dizziness.
- If the patient has an IV pole, ask the patient to hold onto the pole on the side where you are standing. Assist the patient to advance the pole as you ambulate together.

(continued on next page)

Procedure 31-3 ■ **Assisting with Ambulation** (continued)

Equipment

■ Nonlatex gloves, if you may be exposed to body fluids
■ Transfer belt
■ Nonskid footwear

Delegation

You may ask nursing assistive personnel (NAP) to assist with ambulation. Ensure that the NAP has the necessary skills and that the patient's condition is stable. Inform the NAP of any special considerations when assisting a patient with ambulation and evaluate the patient after the activity.

Pre-Procedure Assessment

■ Assess for any restrictions in movement or position by asking the patient and checking the physician's orders.
■ Observe for the presence of equipment such as IV lines, drains, or catheters.
■ Assess possible side effects of medications (e.g., dizziness and sedation).
■ Assess the patient's level of consciousness, ability to follow directions, and ability to assist with the move
■ Assess the physical size of the patient and your own strength and ability to move the patient.

■ Assess the patient's tolerance when dangling before beginning to ambulate.

The preceding assessments inform you about activity tolerance, readiness to get out of bed, and ability to participate in the transfer. They help you determine how many assistants you need, the appropriate transfer device, and how to proceed with the move while preventing injury and dislodging of equipment.

■ Assess vital signs, and monitor for postural hypotension.

If the patient is at risk for postural hypotension, you may need to allow additional time for the patient to change position and plan for adequate help.

■ Assess the patient's level of comfort using a standardized pain scale.

If the patient is uncomfortable, you may need to administer an analgesic before moving.

■ Assess for factors that may increase the risk of falls (elderly, muscle weakness, chronic disease, gait disturbance).

Identifies patients at risk.

■ Procedure 31-3A **Assisting with Ambulation (One Nurse)**

➤ When performing the procedure, always identify your patient according to agency policy and be attentive to standard precautions, hand hygiene, patient safety and privacy, body mechanics, and documentation.

Procedure Steps

1. Put nonskid footwear on the patient.
Prevents the patient from slipping while transferring and ambulating.

2. Place the bed in a low position, and lock the bed.
Prevents the bed from moving during transfer. Makes it easier for the patient's feet to reach the floor.

3. Apply the transfer belt.
Allows you to safely support the patient during the transfer and ambulation.

4. Assist the patient to dangle at the side of the bed (see Procedure 31-2B, if you need to review).

5. Face the patient. Brace your feet and knees against the patient's feet and knees. Pay particular attention to any known weakness. Bend your hips and knees, and hold onto the transfer belt.
Bracing provides stability of the patient's legs. Bending the hips and knees allows you to use the major muscle groups and limit injury. Lifting at the patient's waist level prevents injury to his arm or shoulder.

6. Instruct the patient to place his arms around you between the shoulders and waist (the location depends on your height and the height of the patient). Ask the patient to stand as you move to an upright position by straightening your legs and hips.

Having the patient hold you on your trunk prevents injury to your neck. Straightening your thighs and hips uses your large muscle groups and promotes good body mechanics.

7. Allow the patient to steady himself for a moment.
Allows the patient an opportunity to rest before further movement and to regain equilibrium before walking.

8. Stand at the patient's side, placing both hands on the transfer belt. If the patient is weak on one side, position yourself on the weaker side.
By standing on the weaker side, the patient is freer to reach with the stronger arm and grip wall or bed rails with his strong-side hand, and use the stronger side for strength and balance.

This position also keeps you clear of a cane or other assistive device, which would be used on the strong side, and allows you to support the weaker side to prevent the patient from falling. ▼

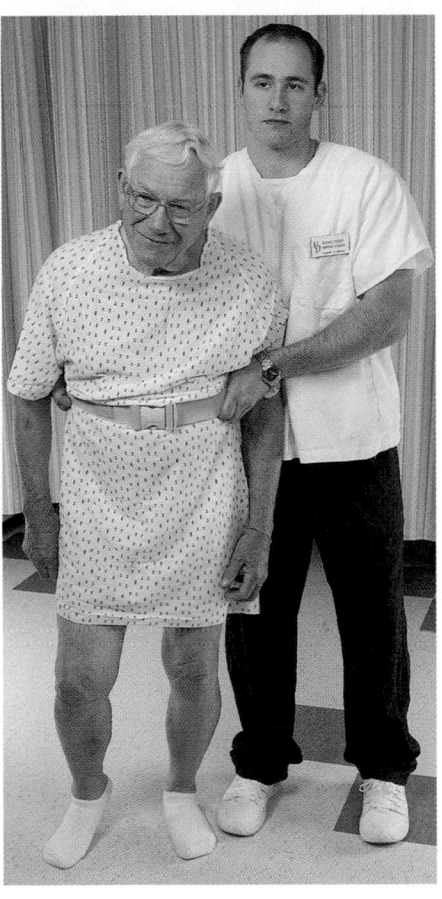

9. Slowly guide the patient forward. Observe for signs of fatigue or dizziness.
Helps prevent falls.

10. If the patient has an IV pole, ask him to hold on to the pole on the side where you are standing. Assist the patient to advance the pole as you ambulate. Be sure the patient does not rely on the pole for support.
Provides a grip for the patient and positions the IV pole near you so that you can assist the patient to move the pole. ➤

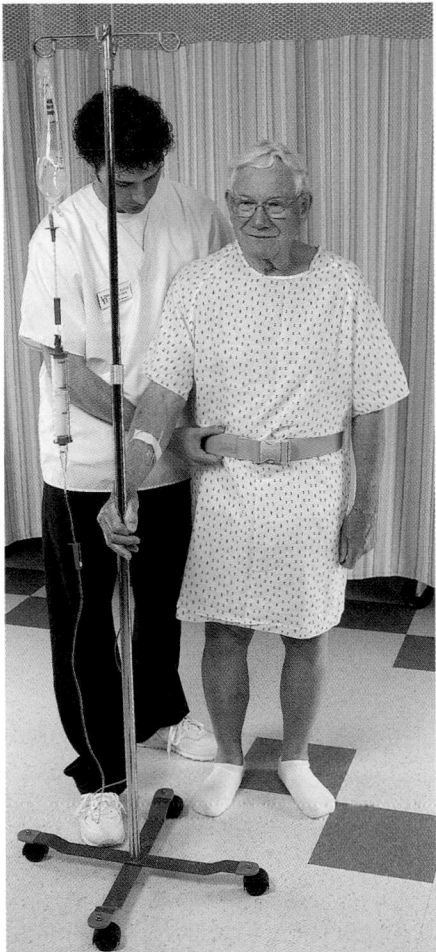

■ Procedure 31-3B Assisting with Ambulation (Two Nurses)

➤ When performing the procedure, always identify your patient according to agency policy and be attentive to standard precautions, hand hygiene, patient safety and privacy, body mechanics, and documentation.

Procedure Steps

1. Put nonskid footwear on the patient.
Prevents the patient from slipping during the transfer and ambulation.

2. Place the bed in low position, and lock the bed.
Prevents the bed from moving during transfer and prevents the patient from falling.

3. Apply the transfer belt.
Allows you to support client during transfer and ambulation.

4. Assist the patient to dangle at the side of the bed (see Procedure 31-2B, as needed).

5. Each nurse should stand facing the patient on opposite sides of the patient. Brace your feet and knees against the patient, paying particular

attention to any known weakness. Bend from the hips and knees and hold onto the transfer belt.
Bracing provides stability. Bending the hips and knees allows you to use the major muscle groups and limit injury. Lifting at the patient's waist level prevents injury to his arm or shoulder.

6. Instruct the patient to place his arms around each of you between the shoulders and waist (the location

(continued on next page)

Procedure 31-3 ■ Assisting with Ambulation (continued)

depends on your height and the height of the patient). Ask the patient to stand as each of you move to an upright position by straightening your legs and hips.

7. Allow the patient to steady himself for a moment.

Allows the patient an opportunity to rest before further movement and to regain equilibrium. Allows you to evaluate the patient's tolerance to activity and ability to maintain an upright posture before ambulating.

8. Each nurse stands at the patient's sides, grasping hold of the transfer belt. If no belt is available, the nurses grasp each other's arms at the patient's waist.

Helps patient maintain an erect posture. ➤

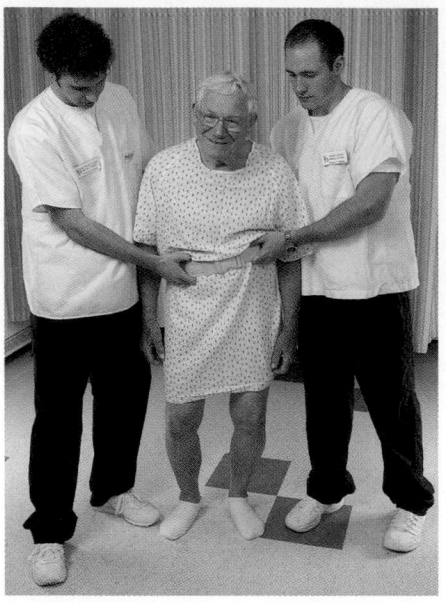

9. Slowly guide the patient forward. Observe for signs of fatigue or dizziness. Ensures client safety.

10. If the patient has an IV pole, one nurse advances the IV pole along the side of the patient by holding the pole with the outside hand. Remind the patient not to use the IV pole for support.

Positions the IV pole out of the path of the patient. Because the IV pole is on rollers, it will not support the patient if he starts to fall.

What if . . .

■ **The patient has a weaker side (i.e., CVA)?**

If the patient has weakness on one side, provide additional support but allow him to use that side as he is able.

This will force him to use his weaker side.

Evaluation

- Assess the level of patient participation in the transfer.
- Assess patient comfort with ambulation.
- Assess posture and base of support.
- Assess vital signs for postural hypotension.

Patient Teaching

- Instruct the patient to inform you if he feels dizzy or weak.
- Explain the importance of ambulation to prevent complications of immobility.

Home Care

- Teach family members or caregivers how to assist the client with ambulation.
- Provide instruction on importance of ambulation.

Documentation

Document in the nursing notes how much assistance was required, any problems with ambulation, and the distance walked.

Sample documentation:

| 11/11/11 | 0630 | Pt assisted to ambulate to doorway in room. Required minimal assistance from one nurse. Placed in chair for 30 minutes and then assisted back to bed. Required maximum assist from two nurses to return to bed. —————— B. Bowen, RN |

Practice Resources
Rutledge, D., & Matteucce, R. (2008).

Thinking About the Procedure

Go to the *Fundamentals of Nursing Skills Videos*, **Dangling and Ambulation: One Nurse Assist.**

1. How does the patient steady herself before dangling?

Go to the *Fundamentals of Nursing Skills Videos*, **Dangling and Ambulation: Two Nurse Assist.**

1. What does the nurse do with the transfer belt to keep it from becoming looser?

2. What could nurses do to assist the patient who requires assistance with ambulation if no transfer belt is available?

 For suggested responses, go to Chapter 31, **Thinking About the Procedure Suggested Responses (Procedure 31-3),** on the Student Resource Disk or DavisPlus at http://davisplus.fadavis.com/Wilkinson2

Clinical Insights

Clinical Insight 31-1 ▶ Applying Principles of Body Mechanics

✚ Principles of body mechanics are the rules that enable you to move your body without causing injury. Use the following guidelines to decrease the risk of back and other injuries. Teach them to your patients as well. Remember that the ANA states you should use mechanical equipment for lifting and transferring whenever possible and not rely on body mechanics alone to prevent injury.

■ **Assess patient dependency levels** and select equipment after determining the patient's ability to assist in the transfer. You will also want to be aware of the patient's strength and ability to bear weight. Height and weight of the patient factor into how you transfer the patient safely.

Transferring Patients According to Dependency Level

PATIENT LEVEL OF DEPENDENCE	ASSISTIVE DEVICE
Complete dependence (immobile; no assistance)	Mechanical lift with full sling
Extensive dependence (holds on to device but with minimal strength)	Mechanical lift with full sling or stand/assist lift
Moderate dependence (no patient assist for lifting from floor)	Mechanical lift with full sling, or if transfer is manual, more than one helper might be needed
Patient assists with limited mobility.	Transfer belt or gait belt
Limited dependence	Stand/assist lift or friction-reducing device

Adapted from American Nurses Association (ANA). (2006). Preventing back injuries: Safe patient handling and movement. Retrieved from http://www.nursingworld.org/MainMenuCategories/OccupationalandEnvironmental/occupationalhealth/OccupationalResources/PreventingBackInjuries.aspx

■ **Use a wide base of support** (feet spread apart).
■ **Minimize bending and twisting**. These movements increase the stress on the back. Instead, face the object or person, and bend at the hips or squat.
■ **Squat to lift heavy objects from the floor.** (Squatting lowers your center of gravity.) Push against the strong hip and thigh muscles to raise yourself to a standing position. Avoid bending at the waist.
■ **Use the muscles in your legs** as the power for lifting. Bend your knees, keep your back straight, and lift smoothly. Repeat the same movements for setting the object down.
■ **Keep objects close to your body** when you lift, move, or carry them. The closer an object is to the center of gravity, the greater the stability and the less strain on the back.
■ **Use both hands and arms** when you lift, move, or carry heavy objects.
■ **Raise the height of the bed and over-the-bed table to waist level** when you are working with a patient.
■ **When possible, keep your elbows bent** when you carry an object.
■ **Do not stand on tiptoes to reach an object**. If you must use a ladder or stepstool to reach an object, make sure it is stable and adequate to position your body close to the object.
■ **Push, slide, or pull heavy objects** whenever possible rather than lifting.
■ **Maintain a good grip on the patient or object** you are moving before attempting to move it.
■ **Work with smooth and even movements.** Avoid sudden or jerky motions.
■ **Get help to move a heavy object or patient**. Assess the object or patient you are going to lift. If you have any doubt that you can do it by yourself, get help from a co-worker.
■ **Use assistive devices at all times** to limit the risk of back and musculoskeletal injury.
■ **Maintain competency** in using all assistive and transfer devices.

Clinical Insight 31-2 ▶ Using Common Positioning Devices

Applying a Trochanter Roll

Trochanter rolls prevent external hip rotation when the patient is in a supine position.

- Fold a towel or bath blanket lengthwise.
- Roll the towel or bath blanket tightly.
- Invert the roll. Turning the patient to one side, place the bath blanket or towel under the patient's hip and thigh. Repeat on the other side if needed.
- Roll the sheet or towel under until it is snug against the patient's hip and thigh.

The patient's weight should keep the roll from moving and help to prevent external (outward) rotation of the hips.

- Make sure the roll does not extend as far as the knee. To avoid nerve compression and palsy that can lead to footdrop.
- Alternately, you can place the patient on a sheet that has been folded so that the top edge is at the top of the hips, and the lower edge is about one-third the way down the thighs. Then place the rolled towels under the sheet and roll the sheet under tightly.

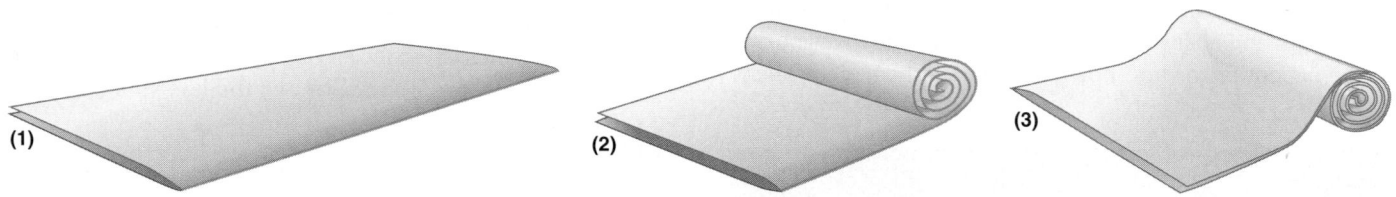

(1)   (2)   (3)

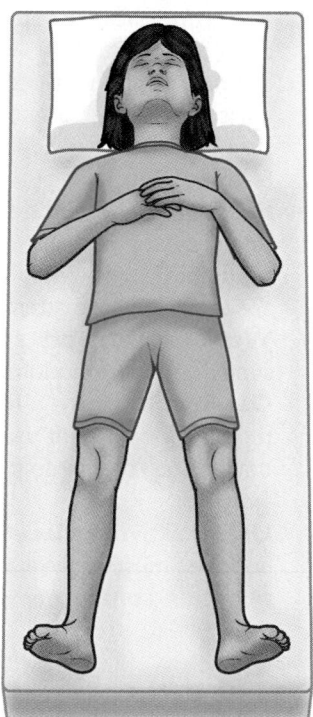

External rotation can occur without a trochanter roll.

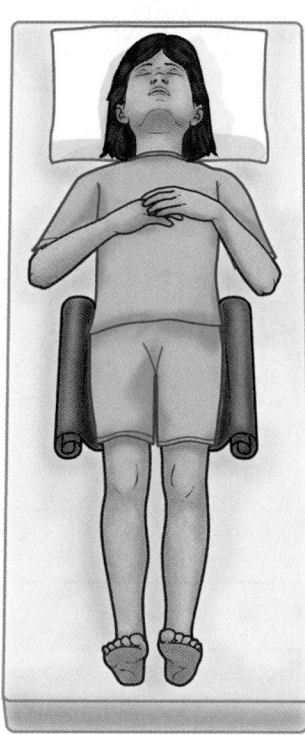

Proper alignment using a trochanter roll.

To see a nurse using a trochanter roll,

 Go to the *Fundamentals of Nursing Skills Videos*, **Activity and Exercise: Trochanter Roll.**

Applying Hand Rolls

▪ Place a rolled up washcloth or commercial hand roll in the patient's palm.

The roll maintains neutral position.

▪ Secure the strap, if present.
▪ Roll soft gauze around the hand and secure with nonallergenic, adhesive tape.

Wrapping the roll in gauze keeps it from falling out of the patient's hand.

▪ Place another roll in the patient's other hand, if needed.

Hand rolls help prevent hand contractures.

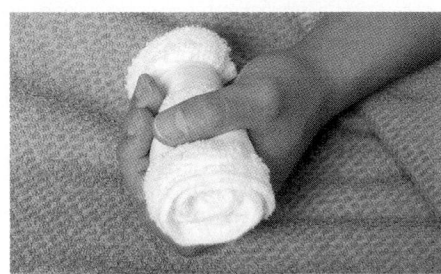

Applying Cradle Boots

Cradle boots prevent foot drop, hip rotation, and pressure on bony prominences, which lead to skin breakdown.

▪ Open the slit on the top surface of the boot.
▪ Place the patient's heel in the round cut-out for the heel. If the patient is positioned on her side, you may put the boot on the bottom foot.
▪ Support the flexed top foot with a pillow.
▪ Apply the boot to the other foot, as needed.
▪ Position the patient's legs in neutral alignment with slight flexion.

Neutral positioning prevents strain on hip ligaments.

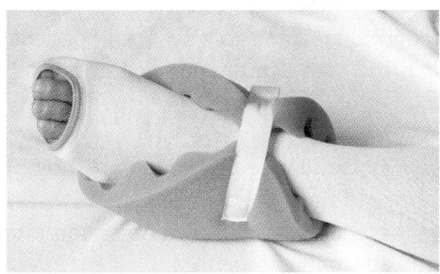

Applying Hip Abduction Pillow

Hip abduction pillows prevent internal hip rotation and hip adduction when the patient is in a supine position.

▪ Place the wedge-shaped, spongy pillow between the patient's legs when she is lying on her back.
▪ Slide it toward the groin so it touches the legs all along the inside of the thigh.
▪ Place both upper legs in the pillow's lateral indentations.
▪ Secure the straps to prevent the pillow from slipping down the mattress.

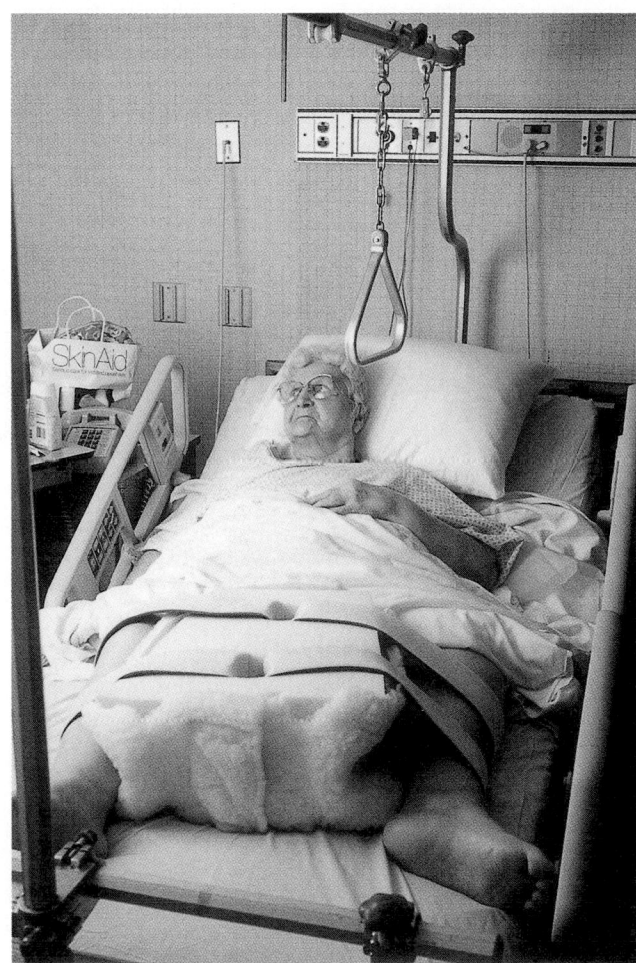

Clinical Insight 31-3 ▶ Performing Passive Range-of-Motion Exercises

Passive range of motion (PROM) is the movement of the joints through their full range of motion by another person. Nurses frequently perform PROM to maintain joint mobility.

▪ **Explain the purpose of PROM.** You may also wish to teach family members and caregivers about the importance of ROM exercises and enlist their help in exercising the patient when they visit.

▪ **Observe the patient as you perform PROM.** You may need to perform the exercises in several short segments if the patient tires easily or experiences discomfort.

▪ **Support the patient's limb** above and below the joint that is to be exercised.

▪ **Move the joint in a slow, smooth, rhythmic manner.** Avoid fast movements; they may cause muscle spasm.

▪ **Never force a joint.** Some patients may have limited ROM. Move each joint to the point of resistance. This should not be painful.

▪ **Perform PROM** at least twice daily. Move each joint through ROM three to five times with each session. Consider incorporating PROM into care activities, for example, while bathing or turning the patient.

▪ **Return the joint to a neutral position** when exercise is complete.

▪ **Encourage active exercise** whenever possible.

Thinking About the Procedure

To see a nurse using a performing passive range-of-motion exercises,

 Go to the *Fundamentals of Nursing Skills Videos*, **Activity and Exercise: Passive Range-of-Motion Exercises.**

Clinical Insight 31-4 ▶ Assisting with Physical Conditioning Exercises to Prepare for Ambulation

Patients who have been confined to bed for more than a week or who have sustained major injury require conditioning before they are able to resume walking. Conditioning exercises include the following.

Quadriceps and Gluteal Drills

▪ Ask the patient to tighten her thigh muscles by pushing downward with her knees and flexing her feet. Each leg may be done separately if moving both is contraindicated.

▪ Ask the patient to hold the position for a count of 5 and then relax.

▪ Repeat this process two to three times per hour during the waking hours.

▪ To exercise the gluteal muscles, ask the patient to pinch her buttocks together.

▪ Do this exercise when the patient exercises her quadriceps muscles.

▪ Instruct the patient not to hold her breath as she exercises.

Arm Exercises

▪ Install a trapeze bar on the patient's bed. Ask the patient to do pull-ups on the bar from a lying position. This exercises the biceps muscles.

▪ To exercise the triceps muscles, ask the patient to lift his upper body off the mattress by firmly pressing down with the palms.

▪ The patient can also do push-ups from a seated position at the side of the bed or from a stationary chair or wheelchair.

Dangling

▪ Dangling is a seated position at the side of the bed, feet resting on the floor.

▪ Provide a footstool if the patient's feet do not reach the floor.

▪ Assess for light-headedness or postural hypotension.

▪ Do not progress to ambulation until the patient is comfortable and stable in the dangling position.

Daily Activities

▪ Encourage your patient to be active in bed by repositioning and turning herself.

▪ Encourage the patient to get out of bed and into a chair before attempting to walk.

▪ Encourage the patient to perform as much of her activities of daily living (ADLs) as possible.

▪ ADLs exercise many of the muscle groups used in ambulation.

To see a nurse using a performing passive range-of-motion exercises,

 Go to the *Fundamentals of Nursing Skills Videos*, **Activity and Exercise: Physical Conditioning Exercises: Quadriceps, Gluteal, Arm, and Dangling.**

Clinical Insight 31-5 ▸ Sizing Walking Aids

Sizing Canes

- Ask the patient to stand erect, and place the cane tip 20 cm (4 in.) to the side of the foot.
- The top of the cane should reach the top of the hip joint so that the patient can hold the cane with her elbow flexed 30°.

Sizing Walkers

- Ask the patient to stand erect, holding onto the walker.
- The walker should extend from the floor to the hip joint so that the patient can comfortably hold the walker with 30° flexion of the elbow.

Sizing Crutches

To measure a patient for an axillary crutch, follow these guidelines:

- Ask the patient to lie down wearing the nonskid shoes that will use when walking.
- Measure the distance between the heel and the anterior fold of the axilla, then add 2.5 cm (1 in.).
- Select a crutch that can be adjusted to this height.
- Have the patient stand, and position the crutch tip 10 to 15 cm (4 to 6 inches) to the side of the heel. Adjust the axillary crutch pad three fingerbreadths below the axilla.
- Adjust the handgrips so that the patient can comfortably grasp the bar while the elbow is slightly flexed. The patient's axilla should not rest on the crutchpad.

Clinical Insight 31-6 ▸ Teaching Patients to Use Canes, Walkers, and Crutches

Canes

After ensuring the cane is the proper size (refer to Clinical Insight 31-5), instruct the patient to do the following:

- Hold the cane on the stronger side.
- Distribute weight evenly between the feet and cane.
- Advance the cane and weaker leg simultaneously, then bring the stronger leg through.
- Avoid leaning over or on the cane.
- Maintain the integrity of the rubber tip for traction.

Walkers

After ensuring the walker is the proper size (refer to Clinical Insight 31-5), instruct the patient to:

- Stand between the back legs of the walker. Do not stand too far behind the walker.
- Pick up the walker, and advance it as you step ahead. Do not advance it so far as to lose balance.
- If one leg is weaker, move it forward as the walker moves forward.
- Pick up, rather than slide, the walker (unless it has wheels).

Crutches

After ensuring the crutches are the proper size (refer to Clinical Insight 31-5), do the following:

- When first teaching crutch walking, instruct the patient to stand near a wall with a chair behind him. Help the patient to stand and grip the crutches. Ask the patient to sway from side to side on the crutches to become accustomed to weight bearing by the arms.
- *Tripod position* is the basic crutch gait standing position. Place crutches 15 cm (6 in.) in front of the feet, with the crutch point 15 cm from the patient's center. In this position, a triangle is formed by the crutches and the body.
- Five crutch gaits exist (see accompanying chart): 2-point gait, 3-point gait, 4-point gait, swing-to gait, and swing-through gait.
- To teach the patient how to go up and down stairs, instruct him to lead with the unaffected leg when going up the stairs and to lead with the affected leg coming down the stairs.

(continued on next page)

Clinical Insight 31-6 ➤ **Teaching Patients to Use Canes, Walkers, and Crutches** (continued)

◆ Navigating stairs with crutches can be dangerous. When possible, have the patient practice this technique before discharge. When having a patient practice, the nurse should always stand below the patient on the stairs to prevent falling.

Note: Read this table from bottom to top.

2-Point gait	3-Point gait	4-Point gait	Swing to	Swing through
• Partial weight bearing, both feet; faster, but less support than a 4-point gait	• Non-weight bearing; faster than a 4-point gait; can use with walker	• Partial weight bearing, both feet; patient must shift weight constantly	• Weight bearing, both feet; can use with walker	• Weight bearing; requires the most coordination and balance
4. Advance right foot and left crutch	**4.** Advance right foot	**4.** Advance right foot	**4.** Lift both feet; swing them forward, landing feet next to the crutches	**4.** Lift both feet; swing them forward, landing feet in front of the crutches
3. Advance left foot and right crutch	**3.** Advance left foot and both crutches	**3.** Advance left crutch	**3.** Advance both crutches	**3.** Advance both crutches
2. Advance right foot and left crutch	**2.** Advance right foot	**2.** Advance left foot	**2.** Lift both feet; swing them forward, landing feet next to the crutches	**2.** Lift both feet; swing them forward, landing feet in front of the crutches
1. Advance left foot and right crutch	**1.** Advance left foot and both crutches	**1.** Advance right crutch	**1.** Advance both crutches	**1.** Advance both crutches
Tripod position	Tripod position	Tripod position	Tripod position	Tripod position

Crutch gaits. The shaded area represents weight bearing. The arrow shows movement.

Clinical Insight 31-7 ▶ Teaching Care of a Cast at Home

- Always keep the cast clean and dry.
- Before bathing, cover the cast with a plastic bag and tape the opening shut or use a special cast cover with Velcro straps. Do not place the cast into water unless it is made of water-repellent material. Keep in mind that waterproof casts are not for all types of fractures. They can't be used for recently manipulated fractures or when skin pins are used.
- If the cast gets wet enough that the skin gets wet under the cast, it may break down and infection may occur. Dry it immediately with a blow dryer on the cool setting. Be careful—skin can be burned using the hot setting. If you have any trouble getting the cast dry, the cast may need to be replaced. Call the healthcare provider if the cast doesn't dry properly.
- Sweating under the cast enough to make it damp may cause mold or mildew to develop. Call the healthcare provider if you notice odor coming from the cast.
- ◆ Never put anything inside the cast. Do not try to scratch the skin under the cast with any sharp objects, such as a hanger or pencil. This may break the skin under the cast and cause it to become infected. Do not use powders, ointments, or lotions inside the cast.
- Sometimes when swelling goes down, the cast can become loose and rub on the skin. If this is the case,

advise your patient to call the primary provider to look at the cast.
- Check the circulation by gently squeezing a finger or toe below the cast. It should blanch (turn lighter) and quickly return to a pink color. The fingers and toes should be warm to the touch, able to move freely, and not tingling or numb.
- Do not trim the cast or break off any rough edges. This may weaken or break the cast. If a fiberglass cast has a rough edge, use a metal file to smooth it or call the healthcare provider.
- A sling may be needed for support if the cast is on the hand, wrist, arm, or elbow. It is helpful to wrap soft sheepskin or padding behind the neck to protect the skin and make it feel more comfortable.
- If the cast is on the foot or leg, do not walk on or put any weight on the injured leg, unless the doctor allows it.
- If the primary provider allows walking on the cast, be sure to wear the cast boot. The boot is to reduce wear and tear on the bottom and has a tread to prevent slipping and falling.
- Crutches may be needed to walk if a cast is on the foot, ankle, or leg. Make sure the crutches are adjusted properly before leaving the hospital or the doctor's office.

Assessment Guidelines and Tools

Suggested History Questions for Assessing Activity and Exercise

Usual Activity

Describe your typical daily activity level.

If the patient has very restricted activity, ask the following questions:

Are you able to care for yourself in regard to hygiene, dressing, toileting, and getting out of bed?

If the patient has ADL limitations: Who helps you with these daily activities?

If the patient does not indicate restricted activity, ask the following questions:

What is your usual form of exercise?

How often do you exercise?

How long are your exercise sessions?

How long have you been engaged in this type of activity?

What types of exercise or sports have you participated in in the past?

Describe your activity level over the last 10 years.

Are you exercising more or less than in the past?

What factors have changed your activity level?

Fitness Goals

What aspects of exercise do you enjoy? What aspects of exercise do you dislike?

What do you think are the benefits of exercise?

How do you schedule your exercise?

What motivates you to exercise?

What are your current fitness goals?

Mobility Concerns

Do you have any pain or discomfort with activity?

Do you avoid any activities because of pain, discomfort, shortness of breath, or chest pain?

Continued

Suggested History Questions for Assessing Activity and Exercise—cont'd

If you answered "yes" to either question, describe the following:

> Type of problem
>
> Onset of concern
>
> Frequency of problem
>
> Activities that trigger and relieve
>
> Severity and type of symptoms
>
> Effect of problem on day-to-day activities
>
> Treatments used to alleviate and how they worked

Underlying Health Concerns

Do you have any healthcare problem that affects your ability to engage in activity or exercise?

If so, describe the problem and the effect.

What medications do you take?

Have you ever been told you have a bone problem? If so, what was the nature of the problem?

Have you ever experienced a fracture, strain, or sprain? If so, where was the problem? When did it occur? How did it occur?

Have you ever had weakness of the muscles or problems coordinating movement?

Do you have any cardiac or respiratory problems that affect your ability to perform activities?

Have you ever experienced anxiety or depression that affected your ability to participate in activities?

Lifestyle

What kind of work do you do?

Describe your typical work activities.

How many hours per week do you work?

What other commitments do you have (school, family, other obligations)?

External Factors

Are there any restrictions in your home that limit your ability to be active?

Do you feel you need an assistive device?

Are you comfortable exercising outside your home or in your neighborhood?

Focused Physical Assessments for Activity and Body Alignment

With the patient standing, observe from the anterior, posterior, and lateral views. Check for the following:
Shoulders and hips are level.

> Toes are pointed forward.
>
> The spine is straight, with no abnormal curvatures noted.
>
> The posture is not slumped.

Ask the patient to sit down; observe as he does so.

> Does he have difficulty lowering his torso?
>
> Can he control the movement?
>
> Is he able to get into this position with ease?
>
> When he sits, does he slump?

If the patient cannot stand or sit, assess his alignment in bed. Look for ability to move in bed, as well as the posture the patient maintains.

Joint Function

Assessing joint function includes inspection and palpation of the joints and assessment of range of motion.

Begin your assessment at the neck and systematically work your way through each of the joints.

At each joint observe for swelling, erythema, asymmetry, or obvious deformity.

Compare the size of the muscles above and below the joint and on each side of the body.

Palpate the joint for temperature and crepitus. Warmth over a joint indicates inflammation or infection. Be sure to compare body temperature over several joints and right to left. **Crepitus** is a grating sensation when the joint is moved. It can often be heard as well as felt. Crepitus is associated with degenerative joint disease or arthritic changes in the joint.

As you palpate the joint, move it through its range of motion.

Muscle Strength

Assess muscle strength by having the patient push and then pull against your hands.

Start at the neck, and test the strength of all major joints' range of motion.

To see a nurse using a performing passive range-of-motion exercises,

 Go to the *Fundamentals of Nursing Skills Videos,* **Activity & Exercise: Passive Range-of-Motion Exercises.**

Gait

Gait is divided into two phases: stance and swing.

Stance—In the stance phase, the heel of one foot strikes the ground while the opposite foot pushes off and leaves the ground.

Swing—In the swing phase, the leg from behind moves in front of the body. When the right leg is in stance mode, the left leg is in swing mode.

You must observe the patient walking. Normal gait includes the following features:

> Head is erect, gaze forward.
>
> Heel strikes the ground before the toe.
>
> Opposite arm moves forward at the same time.
>
> Feet are dorsiflexed in the swing phase.
>
> Gait is coordinated and rhythmic.
>
> Weight is evenly distributed, with minimal swing from side to side.
>
> Movement starts and stops with ease.
>
> Movement is at a moderate pace.

If the patient uses an assistive device, such as a cane, crutch, or walker, pay attention to how he uses it. Ask the patient to ambulate a short distance with and without the device to determine if the device is actually providing stability.

Suggested History Questions for Assessing Activity and Exercise—cont'd

Activity Tolerance

Assess and record vital signs before having the patient engage in 3 minutes of activity.

Select an activity appropriate for the patient. For example, if the patient uses a walker, ask the patient to walk down the hallway. For a patient without obvious health limitations, consider asking her to run in place for 3 minutes.

Observe the patient throughout the exercise. If she shows any signs of distress, stop the exercise, immediately take a set of vital signs, and repeat the vital signs every minute until they have returned to baseline.

If the patient can exercise continuously for 3 minutes, assess the patient at the end of the 3-minute period and at 1-minute intervals. Note the change in heart rate, blood pressure, and respiratory rate.

 This type of approach is not appropriate for patients who easily become short of breath, develop chest pain, or are very unsteady on their feet. Instead, for example, limit your assessment to determining the amount of assistance the patient needs to turn in bed or get out of bed.

As you observe the patient, compare muscle mass on the right and left sides. If you notice an obvious discrepancy in size, measure the circumference of the limbs and compare.

Muscle Mass and Strength

To assess strength, ask the patient to push against your hand with the hands and feet. Once again, compare both sides.

For guidelines for assessing mobility in the home,

VOL 1 Go to Chapter 31, **Home Care Box: Home Assessment for a Patient with Mobility Concerns,** in Volume 1.

Tables

Range of Motion at the Joints

JOINT	NORMAL RANGE	ILLUSTRATION
Neck (Pivot Joint) *Flexion*—Move the head from upright midline position to the chin, resting the head on the chest.	45° from midline	
Extension—Move the head from flexed to upright midline position.	45° from midline	
Hyperextension—Move the head from upright midline position to as far back as possible.	10°	
Lateral flexion—Tilt the head laterally from midline position toward the shoulder.	40° from midline	
Rotation—Rotate the head in a circular motion from upright midline position to as far right or left as possible.	180°	

Continued

Range of Motion at the Joints—cont'd

JOINT	NORMAL RANGE	ILLUSTRATION
Shoulder (Ball-and-Socket Joint)		
Flexion—Raise the arm from a neutral position at the side to alongside the head.	180°	
Extension—Move the arm from flexed to a neutral position at the side of the body.	180°	
Hyperextension—Move the arm, keeping the elbow straight, from a neutral position at the side of the bed to behind the body.	45°–60°	
Abduction—Raise the arm laterally from a neutral position at the side of the body to a position at the side of the head, palm facing outward.	180°	
Adduction—Move the arm downward from a position beside the head to across the front of the body as far as possible.	230°–320°	
Circumduction—Circle the arm from the shoulder.	360°	
External rotation—Keeping arm held out to the side at shoulder level and bent to a right angle, fingers pointing down, move the arm upward so that the fingers point upward and are above the shoulder.	90°	
Internal rotation—Move the arm forward and down to return to the starting position, fingers pointing down.	90°	
Elbow (Hinge Joint)		
Flexion—Bend at the elbow to move the forearm from a straightened position up toward the shoulder.	150°	
Extension—Straighten the arm by bringing the lower arm forward and down.	150°	

Range of Motion at the Joints—cont'd

JOINT	NORMAL RANGE	ILLUSTRATION
Rotation (for supination)—With the arm at the side, elbow bent, move the hand and forearm so that the palm is facing upward.	70°–90°	
Rotation (for pronation)—With the arm at the side, elbow bent, move the hand and forearm so that the palm is facing downward.	70°–90°	
Wrist (Condyloid Joint)		
Flexion—Bend the fingers of the hand toward the inner aspect of the forearm.	80°–90°	
Extension—Straighten the wrist so that it is on the same plane as the forearm.	80°–90°	
Hyperextension—Bend the wrist as far back as possible toward the outer aspect of the forearm.	70°–90°	
Abduction (radial flexion)—With the hand supinated, bend each wrist laterally toward the thumb side.	0–20°	
Adduction (ulnar flexion)—With the hand supinated, bend each wrist laterally toward the fifth finger side.	30°–50°	
Hands and Fingers (Condyloid Joints; Interphalangeal Joints are Hinge)		
Flexion—Bend the fingers into a fist.	90°	
Extension—Straighten the fingers.	90°	
Hyperextension—Bend the fingers back.	30°	

Continued

Range of Motion at the Joints—cont'd

JOINT	NORMAL RANGE	ILLUSTRATION
Abduction—Spread the fingers apart.	20°	
Adduction—Bring the fingers together.	20°	
Thumb (Saddle Joint)		
Flexion—Move the thumb across the palm of the hand toward the fifth finger.	90°	
Extension—Move the thumb laterally away from the fingers.	90°	
Opposition—Touch the thumb to the top of each finger of the same hand.	N/A	
Hip (Ball-and-Socket Joint)		
Flexion—Move the leg forward and up.	Knee extended 90°	
Extension—Move the leg back down beside the other.	Knee flexed 120°	
Hyperextension—Move the leg back behind the body.	30–50°	

Range of Motion at the Joints—cont'd

JOINT	NORMAL RANGE	ILLUSTRATION
Abduction—Move the leg laterally. *Adduction*—Sweep the leg inward across the midline.	45–50° 20–30° beyond the other leg	
Circumduction—Circle the leg, keeping the knee straight.	360°	
Internal rotation—Turn the foot and leg inward toward the other leg. *External rotation*—Turn the foot and leg outward, pointing the toes as far as possible away from the other leg.	90° 90°	
Knee (Hinge Joint) *Flexion*—Bend at the knee, bringing the heel back toward the buttocks. *Extension*—Straighten the knee, returning the leg to its original position.	120°–130° 120°–130°	
Ankle (Hinge Joint) *Extension (plantar flexion)*—Point the toes and foot downward. *Flexion (dorsiflexion)*—Pull the toes and foot upward.	45°–50° 20°	

Continued

Range of Motion at the Joints—cont'd

JOINT	NORMAL RANGE	ILLUSTRATION
Foot (Gliding Joint)		
Eversion—Turn the sole of the foot laterally.	5°	
Inversion—Turn the sole of the foot medially.	5°	
Toes (Hinge, Except Intertarsal Joints, Which are Gliding Joints)		
Flexion—Curl the toes downward.	35°–60°	
Extension—Straighten the toes.	35°–60°	
Abduction—Spread the toes apart.	0–15°	
Adduction—Bring the toes together.	0–15°	
Trunk		
Flexion—At the waist, bend forward toward the toes.	70°–90°	
Extension—Straighten the trunk from the flexed position.	70°–90°	
Hyperextension—Bend the trunk backward.	20°–30°	
Lateral flexion—Bend the trunk to the side.	20°–40°	

Range of Motion at the Joints—cont'd

JOINT	NORMAL RANGE	ILLUSTRATION
Rotation—Turn the upper body from side to side (twist at the waist).	30°–45°	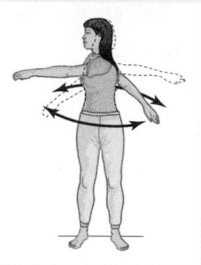

NANDA-I Diagnoses for Activity and Exercise Problems

NURSING DIAGNOSIS	DEFINING CHARACTERISTICS	ETIOLOGIES
Activity Intolerance – A state in which a patient has insufficient physical or psychological energy to carry out daily activities	*Subjective*: fatigue, weakness, discomfort on exertion, dyspnea, and verbalization of no interest in activity *Objective*: changes in heart rate, blood pressure disproportionate to activity, dysrhythmias or evidence of ischemia on electrocardiogram (ECG), and pallor or cyanosis with activity	Conditions that affect tissue oxygenation (e.g., chronic obstructive pulmonary disease or cardiac disease) Conditions that produce fatigue, such as depression, prolonged immobility, bed rest, and sedentary lifestyle
Impaired Physical Mobility – Limitation of independent purposeful movement of the body (specify level of independence using a standardized functional scale)	*Subjective*: pain or discomfort with movement, exertional dyspnea *Objective*: limited ROM, limitations in fine- or gross-motor movement, lack of coordination with movement, unstable gait, decreased reaction time, postural instability, slowed movement, and difficulty performing ADLs	Neuromuscular, sensoriperceptual, or musculoskeletal impairment, malnutrition, obesity, deconditioning due to sedentary lifestyle, lack of knowledge about the importance of activity and exercise for maintenance of health, anxiety, cognitive impairment, discomfort, limited cardiovascular endurance, malnutrition, medications, pain, prescribed movement restrictions

Note: Impaired Physical Mobility is a broad, general diagnosis. Use the following, more descriptive diagnoses when the patient has specific deficits:

Impaired Bed Mobility	Impaired Walking	Sedentary Lifestyle
Impaired Wheelchair Mobility	Impaired Transfer Ability	

Note: Mobility problems may also be the etiology of other diagnoses. The following are examples:

- *Risk for Ineffective Peripheral Tissue Perfusion* (specify) r/t blood flow compromised by reduced mobility
- *Risk for Disuse Syndrome* occurs when there is a risk for deterioration of body systems due to musculoskeletal inactivity. Risk factors include prescribed bed rest, severe pain, altered level of consciousness, mechanical immobilization (traction), and paralysis.
- *Acute Pain* r/t musculoskeletal injury
- *Ineffective Health Maintenance* r/t prescribed bed rest
- *Risk for Injury* r/t unsteady gait
- *Self-Care Deficit (Bathing/Hygiene, Feeding, Dressing/Grooming, Toileting)* r/t Impaired Physical Mobility

Selected NOC Outcomes for Energy Maintenance and Mobility

CLASS: ENERGY MAINTENANCE	CLASS: MOBILITY
Activity Tolerance	Ambulation
Endurance	Ambulation: Wheelchair
Energy Conservation	Balance
Fatigue Level	Body Positioning: Self-Initiated
Psychomotor Energy	Coordinated Movement
Rest	Immobility Consequences: Physiological
Sleep	Immobility Consequences: Psycho-Cognitive
	Joint Movement
	Joint Movement: Ankle, Elbow, Fingers, Hip, Knee, Neck, Shoulder, Spine, Wrist (specify)
	Joint Movement: Passive
	Mobility
	Skeletal Function
	Transfer Performance

Source: Moorhead, S., Johnson, M., Maas, M., et al. (Eds.). (2008). *Nursing outcomes classification (NOC)* (4th ed.). St. Louis, MO: C.V. Mosby. Used with permission.

Selected NIC Interventions for Activity and Exercise Management and Immobility Management

CLASS: ACTIVITY AND EXERCISE MANAGEMENT	CLASS: IMMOBILITY MANAGEMENT
Body Mechanics Promotion	Bed Rest Care
Energy Management	Cast Care: Maintenance
Exercise Promotion	Cast Care: Wet
Exercise Promotion: Strength Training	Physical Restraint
Exercise Promotion: Stretching	Positioning
Exercise Therapy: Ambulation	Positioning: Wheelchair
Exercise Therapy: Balance	Self-Care Assistance: Transfer
Exercise Therapy: Joint Mobility	Splinting
Exercise Therapy: Muscle Control	Traction/Immobilization Care
Teaching: Prescribed Activity/Exercise	Transfer

Source: Bulechek, G., Butcher, H., & Dochterman, J. (Eds.). (2008). *Nursing interventions classification (NIC)* (5th ed.). St. Louis, MO: C.V. Mosby. Used with permission.

THINKING CRITICALLY ABOUT ACTIVITY AND EXERCISE

The exercises in the following sections allow you to practice the kind of thinking you will use as a full-spectrum nurse. Because these are critical-thinking questions, there is usually no single right answer. We do not provide answers for these questions because it is more important for you to think about the questions than to arrive at the "right" answer. These questions are designed to improve your thinking more than to "cover content." Discuss answers with your peers—discussion can stimulate critical thinking. If you have difficulty with any of these questions, consult with your instructor.

Applying the Full-Spectrum Nursing Model

PATIENT SITUATION

Mr. Ronald Ornduff is a 72-year-old retired man who lives with his wife in a one-story home. He has excellent general health with no significant health problems. Ronald typically walks with a moderate to fairly vigorous pace in his neighborhood or at the mall in the winter. He belongs to a health club and works out two or three times a week, walking on the treadmill or using the weight machines or taking a basic conditioning class. Mr. Ornduff considers himself fit and of an acceptable weight for his age. When going outdoors to pick up the morning paper, he slipped on a patch of ice and fell. You are now caring for him 2 days after hip surgery. He is experiencing pain and seems fearful his injury could be the beginning of a decline in his health.

THINKING

1. *Theoretical Knowledge:*

   a. Based on Mr. Ornduff's age, physical condition, and activity level, make a rough estimate of the number of minutes/week of physical activity he should have after he recovers from surgery and resumes full mobility. What are the benefits of this physical activity?

   b. As a nurse planning the care for a patient after hip surgery, what complications of immobility can occur?

2. *Critical Thinking (Considering Alternatives):* What are some possible barriers for an older adult's participating in physical activity? What might you teach your patient to do to overcome those barriers?

DOING

3. *Practical Knowledge:*

   a. How might you position your patient after hip surgery?

   b. What equipment would you need to position your patient after surgery? Is there anything you can set up that will help your patient move around in bed when he can tolerate it?

   c. What type of physical activity would you recommend Mr. Ornduff incorporate into his exercise plan after he experiences full recovery from his surgery? What benefit will these exercises provide?

4. *Nursing Process (Diagnosis):* Write at least two nursing diagnoses for Mr. Ornduff. Use just the data provided in the situation. Assume he is 2 days post-op.

CARING

5. *Self-Knowledge*: What would you be feeling if you were in Mr. Ornduff's situation of being physically fit one day and suffering pain and immobility the next?

6. *Ethical Knowledge*: What are one or two things you would do to help Mr. Ornduff feel cared for and cared about?

Critical Thinking and Clinical Reasoning

1. In Volume 1, you were introduced ("Meet Your Patient") to Helen Jillian, a 72-year-old woman with hypertension, high cholesterol levels, and chest pain. She is 61 inches tall and weighs 290 pounds. Ms Jillian is admitted to the hospital for another episode of chest pain. You are assigned to care for her. Her physician has ordered her to be out of bed in the chair at least twice daily and to ambulate every day. How will you safely move this patient from bed to chair and assist her with ambulation? Work through that decision by answering the following questions.

   a. What aspects of this situation require the most careful attention (what are the risks; what could go wrong)?

   b. What steps can you take to prevent those difficulties?

2. Ms Jillian is refusing to get out of bed. "I'm sick," she tells you. "If you make me get out of bed, I'll probably have chest pain." How would you respond to this statement?

3. Vince Fulk is an 85-year-old man who sustained a massive cerebrovascular accident. He is unresponsive and immobile. What activity or mobility interventions should you incorporate into his plan of care? What is your rationale for these interventions?

4. For each of the following concepts, use critical thinking to describe how or why it is important to nursing, patient care, or activity and exercise. Note that these are *not* to be merely definitions.

   Body mechanics   Activity tolerance
   Exercise   Assistive devices
   Immobility

What Are the Main Points in This Chapter?

➤ The skeletal system includes bones, cartilage, ligaments, and tendons. The skeleton forms the framework of the body and protects the internal organs.

➤ Movement depends on the interaction between the skeleton and the muscles. The ligaments, tendons, and cartilage serve as the interface between these two systems.

➤ Contraction of skeletal muscles causes the muscles to shorten, thus causing the bones to move at the joints.

➤ There are four natural curves to the spine. Proper posture maintains these natural curves.

➤ For your body to be balanced, your line of gravity must pass through your center of gravity, and your center of gravity must be close to your base of support.

In the human body, the center of gravity is below the umbilicus at the top of the pelvis. The feet provide the base of support.

➤ Range of motion (ROM) is the maximum movement possible at a joint. Active range of motion is defined as the movement of the joint through the entire ROM by the individual.

➤ Principles of body mechanics are the rules that allow you to move your body without causing injury.

➤ The U.S. Department of Health and Human Services recommends 150 minutes per week of moderate-intensity, or 75 minutes per week of vigorous-intensity aerobic physical activity, or an equivalent combination of moderate- and vigorous-intensity aerobic physical activity.

➤ A well-rounded exercise program focuses on flexibility, resistance training, and aerobic conditioning.

➤ Regular physical activity each week, sustained for months and years, can produce long-term health benefits. Strong evidence links regular physical activity with a lower risk for early death, heart disease, stroke, type 2 diabetes, hypertension, colon and breast cancers, and depression.

➤ Together with a healthy diet, regular physical activity also aids in weight management, better heart and lung function and muscular fitness, fall prevention, and improved memory and mental clarity in older adults.

➤ People who are physically active tend to feel better and have more energy. Sleep quality is improved. And, overall, for many people, physical activity promotes a sense of optimism and positive self-esteem.

➤ Factors that influence activity and exercise level include developmental stage, health concerns, nutrition, lifestyle, attitudes, and external factors.

➤ Severe illness associated with prolonged immobilization causes physiological changes in almost every body system.

➤ A nursing history focused on activity and exercise assesses usual activity, fitness goals, mobility concerns, underlying health concerns, lifestyle, and external factors.

➤ Physical assessment that is focused on activity and exercise examines the musculoskeletal system and activity tolerance. Important data include vital signs, height, weight, body mass index, body alignment, joint function, gait, and activity tolerance.

➤ Patients require a change of position at least every 2 hours to prevent skin breakdown, muscle discomfort, damage to superficial nerves and blood vessels, or contractures.

➤ Range-of-motion exercises maintain joint mobility and limit the complications of immobility.

➤ Patients who have been confined to bed for more than a week or who have sustained major injury require conditioning before they are able to resume walking.

➤ Canes, braces, walkers, and crutches are available to assist a patient to walk. These aids promote stability and independence.

For practice questions for this chapter,

Go to **NCLEX-Style Chapter Quiz,** on the Student Resource Disk or DavisPlus at http://davisplus.fadavis.com/Wilkinson2

To practice documentation for a patient experiencing mobility problems activity and exercise,

Go to **Practice Documentation,** on the Student Resource Disk or DavisPlus at http://davisplus.fadavis.com/Wilkinson2

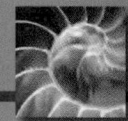

Knowledge Map

Positioning Patients:

Why: prevents skin breakdown; contractions; discomfort

Ways to position:
- Fowlers
- Lateral
- Prone
- Sims
- Supine

Positioning devices:
- Adjustable beds; siderails
- Pillows
- Trapeze; footboard/foot cradle

Moving Patients:

In bed:
Moving up in bed; turning; logrolling for spinal surgery/injury

Transfer out of bed: to stretcher or wheelchair

Assistive devices:
- Transfer board
- Mechanical lift
- Transfer roller or belt

Promoting Activity:

Performing range of motion:
- Active
- Passive

Assisting with ambulation:
- Assess readiness; patient condition
- Obtain assistance/equipment
- Physical conditioning prior to

Ambulation aids:
- Cane
- Walker
- Braces
- Crutches

Principles Guiding Care

- Use lifting devices
- Get adequate help
- Use good body mechanics
- Assess pt size/restrictions
- Control pt pain; explain activity interventions
- Avoid friction

Eliminating

Activity and Exercise

Types:
- Isometric
- Isokinetic
- Aerobic
- Anaerobic

Promoting

Programs:
- Flexibility training
- Resistance training
- Aerobic conditioning

Hazards of Immobility:
- Muscle atrophy; stiff joints
- Decreased respiration depth; pooling secretions; pneumonia/atelectasis
- Venous pooling; clotting; orthostatic hypotension
- Glucose intolerance; reduced muscle mass; stress response
- Constipation; flatus; ileus
- Urinary stasis; calculi
- Depression; anxiety; sleep disturbances; apathy

ACTIVITY   **EXERCISE**

Bones, Muscles, & Neurological Control

Diseases Affecting   **Body Mechanics**

Factors Affecting

MOBILITY

Specific Diseases:
- M/S: hip dysplasia, scoliosis
- Bone formation: OI
- Joint Mobility: arthritis
- Bone integrity: osteoporosis/osteomyelitis
- Trauma
- Neuro: SCI, MS

- Developmental stage
- Nutritional status
- Lifestyle
- Stress
- Environmental/socioeconomic factors

Components:
- Body alignment: posture; proper spinal curve position
- Balance: via alignment; line of gravity through center of gravity
- Coordination: neuromuscular pairing for smooth movement
- Joint mobility: ROM

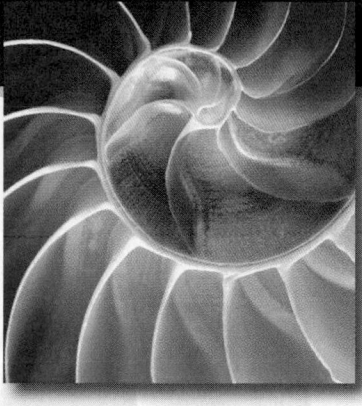

CHAPTER 32

Sexual Health

For a podcast of an overview of this chapter,

 Go to Student Resources, **Podcast – Chapter Overviews, Chapter 32,** on DavisPlus at http://davisplus.fadavis.com/ Wilkinson2

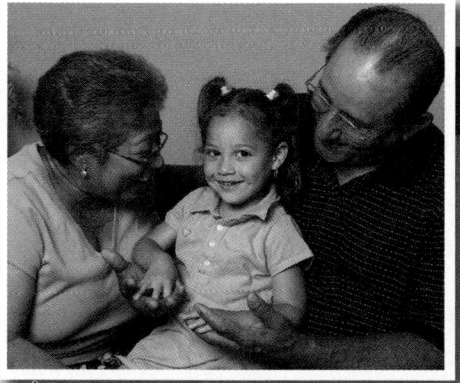

Caring for the Garcias

The exercises in the following section allow you to practice the kind of thinking you will use as a full-spectrum nurse. Because these are critical-thinking questions, there is usually no single right answer. We do not provide answers for these questions because it is more important for you to think about the questions than to arrive at the "right" answer. These questions are designed to improve your thinking more than to "cover content." Discuss answers with your peers— discussion can stimulate critical thinking. If you have difficulty with any of these questions, consult with your instructor.

As you may recall, Joe and Flordelisa Garcia are raising their 3-year-old granddaughter, Bettina. Bettina has made friends with Lili, another little girl at preschool. Bettina has asked whether they can play together.

Flordelisa works at the preschool and knows Lili and her family. She is unsure whether she should allow her granddaughter to play with Lili because Flordelisa is uncomfortable with Lili's family. Lili was conceived via artificial insemination and is being raised by a lesbian couple. Her parents are open about the relationship and shared the conception information with Flordelisa voluntarily.

A. Flordelisa calls the clinic to speak with you. She explains the situation and asks you whether you think it would be a problem to allow the girls to play together. She is concerned that being around this family may be a bad influence on Bettina. How would you respond?

B. Flordelisa remains concerned and presses you for more information. She is concerned that Bettina's interest in Lili may indicate that Bettina has homosexual tendencies. How would you address her concerns?

C. Flordelisa admits that Joe does not agree with her. "He told me that sexual orientation is genetic." How would you react to this statement?

Practical **Knowledge**
knowing how

In this section you will find guidelines to assist you in assessing and planning care related to patients' sexual health.

Clinical Insights

Clinical Insight 32-1 ▶ **Providing Care After Sexual Assault**

- **Carefully collect information about the incident** and document findings in a fact-based manner, following your institution's protocol.
- **Be sensitive to the victim's fear, anxiety, and guilt** related to the event.
  Open discussion without communicating judgment or disapproval helps with fact finding for better care.
- **Assess the victim's emotional status,** including sexual identity, stress disorder, and risks for suicide and self-harm. Also discuss the potential for sexual and physical violence, including violence within relationships.
- When collecting a nursing history for people with disabilities, be sure to **screen for sexual violence**.
- **Administer prophylactic treatment** for sexually transmitted infections, such as chlamydia and gonorrhea, to patients who have been assaulted (vaginally, anally, or orally). If there is a significant risk for HIV, prophylaxis may be prescribed within 72 hours of exposure.
- **Administer vaccines to prevent hepatitis B and human papillovirus (HPV),** as prescribed and according to your agency's policy.

- **Administer emergency pregnancy prevention** (e.g., the "morning after" pill) to patients who have been vaginally assaulted even if penetration is uncertain, according to your agency's policy.
- **Document pregnancy status** with a urine or blood sample.
- Advise the female victim who has had vaginal penetration to **obtain pregnancy testing** again 2 weeks after the event. The victim should receive follow-up care within 1 week after the event to assess for healing of injuries and presence of sexually transmitted infection.
- **Know the current reporting requirements** for sexual assault in your state. Some states require reporting assault of children and adolescents, even if they do not consent to the reporting.
- **Be familiar with support services** available in your community for victims of abuse. Consider referring the victim to a sexual assault center for support, counseling, and additional information.
  Because of the long-term psychological and emotional consequences of sexual assault, most victims benefit from counseling.

Clinical Insight 32-2 ▶ **Guidelines for Taking a Sexual History**

1. **Provide privacy.**
   - Usually it is not enough merely to pull the curtains around the bed. Ask others to leave the room who could overhear private conversation behind the curtain.
   - Talk to the client alone.
   - In some situations it is good to also talk to the partners as a unit, with the consent of both of course.
2. **Protect confidentiality.** Assure your client that information will not be shared with others unless directly related to planning or delivering healthcare.
3. **Be relaxed in your approach,** and allow the client time to answer your questions fully. Your manner and attitude are critical.
4. **Make eye contact.** Do not act embarrassed or allow your body language to show your discomfort.
5. **Avoid communication stoppers,** such as:
   - "I'm only asking you these questions because I have to."
   - "I know that you probably won't want to tell me but ..."
   - "You're not having any sexual problems, are you?"

6. **Consider a more inviting opening,** such as:
   - "Many people are embarrassed when asked questions about their sexuality, but whatever you tell me will remain confidential."
   - "Many people hesitate to talk about sexual problems. However, your sexual health is important to your overall health, and I would like to ask you a few questions about that."
7. **Be aware of verbal and nonverbal cues** that indicate concerns. Many people will cloak their concerns in comments such as, "I suppose that I won't need to worry about sexy lingerie any longer," or "Sex is for the young. I just have to accept that I'm sick and older now." Be careful your response to such statements does not either negate or validate your patient's identity as a sexual being. Follow up with comments that encourage the client to provide more details (see Chapter 18 if you would like to review communication techniques).
8. **Realize the client may be embarrassed.** If the client is uncomfortable discussing topics about his own sexual health, reassure him by letting him know that

some information, because of its private nature, may be difficult to discuss but important.

9. **Encourage your client to use terminology that he is comfortable with.**
10. **Help the client feel comfortable.** Consider statements such as the following:
    - "Most people wonder how this surgery (or illness) may affect their sexual functioning."
    - "Whenever these medications are suggested, there are questions about sexual side effects."

- "Have you thought about the kinds of adaptations you may have to make in your sex life after this surgery/treatment/illness?"
11. **Begin with a less sensitive topic,** such as "How is your relationship with your partner (spouse)?" Then you can move into more sensitive areas: "Many older women have some vaginal dryness that creates discomfort during intercourse. Do you have any concerns about this?"

Clinical Insight 32-3 ▶ Teaching Your Patient to Use a Condom

Using Male Condoms

The male condom is a sheath that covers the penis during sexual activity.
- Put the condom on before the penis touches the vagina, mouth, or anus.
- Inspect the package to ensure that the condom has not been damaged.
- Open the package without tearing the condom.
- Squeeze out the air at the tip of the condom, and unroll it over the erect penis, leaving some space at the tip to collect the ejaculate.
- After sex, to avoid breaking the condom, hold the condom at the rim as the penis is withdrawn. Wash your hands.
- Use a new condom if you want to have sex again.

Using Female Condoms

The female condom is a plastic pouch that fits inside the vagina so that all vaginal tissue is protected from contact with the penis. The condom is inserted with the inner ring placed high in the vagina near the cervix and the outer ring on the labia.
- Insert the condom before the penis touches the vagina.
- Inspect the package to ensure that the condom has not been damaged.

- Open the package without tearing the condom.
- Put the inner ring and pouch inside the vagina.
- Push the inner ring as far into the vagina as it will go.
- Ensure that the outer ring stays outside the vagina.
- If needed, add lubricant to the inside of the condom.
- After sex, gently pull out the condom and discard.

Do
- Use latex condoms unless you or your partner are allergic to latex, or use polyurethane condoms.
- Treat condoms gently, and keep them out of the sun.
- Use only water-based lubricants to reduce friction and prevent tearing.
- Check the expiration date of the condom and packaging. Old condoms may be brittle and more likely to break.

Don't
- Don't store condoms in your wallet or other place where body heat can break down the latex.
- Don't use fingernails or teeth to open the condom wrapper; doing so can tear the condom.
- Don't reuse a condom.
- Don't use lotions or oils with condoms; these may cause breakage.

Assessment Guidelines and Tools

Guidelines and Questions for Taking a Sexual History

Topics to Include in a Sexual History

The topics to include in the sexual history depend on the nature of the patient's concern. The following topics are most commonly included in a sexual history.
- Reproductive history
- Sexual self-concept
- History of sexually transmitted infections
- History of sexual dysfunction
- Present sexual functioning
- Other factors that affect sexuality, such as medications and diseases
- Signs or symptoms of sexual abuse (see Procedure 9-1)

- Knowledge level about sex, reproduction, and contraception

Tailor your assessment to meet the client's needs. For example, Frank Thanee ("Meet Your Patients") is concerned about his family's reaction to his lifestyle and sexual orientation. In his situation, you would focus your assessment on his sexual self-concept, family relationships, present sexual functioning, and specific concerns about his heart and the impending family visit.

Sexual Health History: Questions to Ask

Women

Menstrual Cycle
- How old were you when you started your menstrual periods?

Continued

Guidelines and Questions for Taking a Sexual History—cont'd

- When was your last menstrual period?
- How often are your periods? How would you describe the flow? How long does your period last?
- Do you have any problems with your periods, such as cramping, breast pain, or heavy flow?
- Does your menstrual period ever prevent you from going to work or school or doing the activities you enjoy?
- What products do you use during your period, such as tampons and pads? Do you ever use douches, either during your period or at other times?

Cancer Screening

- When was your last Pap smear?
- Have you received a vaccine for HPV?
- Have you ever had an abnormal Pap smear? If so, how was it treated?
- Do you examine your breasts? If so, how often?
- Have you noticed asymmetry, lumps, or masses in your breasts? If so, describe them and show me where they are.
- When was your last mammogram? What were the results?
- Is there any history of breast cancer in your family?

Child-Bearing History

- How many living children do you have?
- How many times have you been pregnant?
- Have you ever had a miscarriage? An abortion?
- How many of your births were preterm (prior to 38 weeks)? Term?

Sexual Activity

- How often do you typically have sexual intercourse per month?
- Are you satisfied with the frequency or quality of sexual activity?
- Is there anything in your life that prevents you from sexual activity?
- Do you have any difficulty achieving orgasm?
- Is sexual intercourse ever painful for you?
- Are you sexually attracted to women? Have you had oral or genital sexual intercourse with women?

Men

Sexual Activity

- How many times a month do you typically have sexual intercourse?
- Do you have any difficulty achieving or maintaining an erection or orgasm?
- Are you satisfied with the firmness of your erection?
- Do you experience either premature ejaculation or have difficulty achieving sexual orgasm?
- Are you sexually attracted to men? Have you had oral or anal intercourse with men?

Cancer Screening

- Have you been taught to examine your testicles? Do you practice testicular self-exam?
- Is there a history of testicular cancer in your family?

Both Men and Women

Illnesses and Medications

- What types of illnesses have you been treated for in the past?
- Have you ever been hospitalized? Have you ever had surgery?
- What medications, herbal remedies, or over-the-counter medicines do you take?

Family Responsibilities

- Do you have children? If so, how many? How many are still at home? Dependent on you?
- Are you responsible for other children or adults? [This question may reveal whether the person continues to care for an adult disabled child or for grandchildren.]

Genitalia

- Have you noticed any redness, swelling, discharge, itching, or odor in your genital area?
- Have you noticed asymmetry, lumps, or masses in the genitals? If so, describe them and show me where they are.
- Have you ever been told you have a hernia?
- Have you ever had trauma to your genitals?
- Are you having any problems urinating?

Sexual Patterns

- Are you sexually active? If not, have you ever been?
- Do you have sex with men, women, or both?
- What types of sexual activity do you engage in? Oral, anal, or genital?
- How many partners do you currently have? How many partners have you had in the last 6 months?
- How would you describe your satisfaction with your current sexual relationship?
- What are your thoughts about how this procedure/illness may affect your sexual relationship?
- Have you experienced any recent changes in your sexual function—in your level of desire, your sexual activity, participation, or satisfaction?
- Do you have any concerns about your sexual function, including your level of desire, activity, participation, or satisfaction?

Contraception (as appropriate)

- Do you use birth control? If so, what type and how often?
- How satisfied are you with your method of contraception?

Sexually Transmitted Infections

- Have you ever been treated for an STI? If so, what type?
- Are you concerned about STIs or HIV?
- Do you take any precautions to avoid infections?

Abuse

- Have you ever been forced to have sex against your will?
- Have you ever been threatened or abused by a partner?
- Do you ever feel threatened by your partner?

For guidelines for your approach to taking a sexual history, see Clinical Insight 32-2.

Tables

Fertility Control Methods

FERTILITY CONTROL METHOD	ADVANTAGES	DISADVANTAGES
Abstinence—No sexual intercourse	100% effective Cost free	Lack of sexual expression May create stress in relationship.
Fertility awareness (natural family planning, rhythm method)—Intercourse only when a woman is thought to be in the infertile phase of her menstrual cycle	Cost free May be consistent with religious teachings No physical side effect	Requires cooperation of both partners. Menstrual cycle must be regular. Relatively high failure rate: Pregnancy may result. No protection against STIs
Withdrawal (coitus interruptus)—Removal of the penis from the vagina before ejaculation	Cost free	Requires discipline and mutual cooperation. Pre-ejaculatory fluid may contain sperm. Relatively high failure rate; pregnancy may result No protection against STIs
Male and female condoms	Obtained without a prescription Relatively inexpensive Protects against STIs	Must be put on before penetration; therefore, may diminish spontaneity of intercourse. May decrease sensation for both partners Cannot use certain types of condoms if either partner has latex allergy
Spermicides—Jelly, creams, or foams placed in the vagina	Obtained without a prescription More effective when used with a barrier (condom)	Significant pregnancy rate when used without a barrier (condom) No protection against STIs
Contraceptive sponge	May offer some protection against STIs Can be inserted into the vagina up to 24 hours before intercourse Inexpensive	Not fully effective against pregnancy
Vaginal ring	Highly effective in preventing pregnancy Does not have to be inserted before each act of intercourse—can be left in place for weeks to months, depending on the type.	Requires a prescription because it is a hormonal method. Similar risks as birth control pills Costs similar to or greater than those of birth control pills Correct insertion is key factor in effectiveness of the method.
Oral contraceptives (birth control pills)	Very effective Do not interfere with intercourse. Regulate menstrual flow. Decrease menstrual cramps.	Require a healthcare visit and prescription Significant cost Must be taken as prescribed to be effective Drug interactions No protection against STIs Carry some undesirable side effects Contraindicated for some women (e.g., those who smoke, who have significant varicose veins)
Depo-Provera injections	Last 3 months Highly effective Do not interfere with intercourse	Require a healthcare provider visit Amenorrhea (may be seen as an advantage) No protection against STIs

Continued

Fertility Control Methods—cont'd

FERTILITY CONTROL METHOD	ADVANTAGES	DISADVANTAGES
Intrauterine device (IUD)—A small piece of plastic that also may contain metal or a hormone: placed through the cervix into the uterus by a healthcare provider	Highly effective May remain in place for years Does not interfere with intercourse	Increased risk of pelvic inflammatory disease (PID) Must be inserted by a healthcare provider Increased menstrual flow and cramping No protection against STIs
Diaphragm—Latex dome-shaped cup with a flexible rim that is inserted in the vagina and fits over the cervix	Few side effects Quite effective if used properly with spermicide	Must be inserted prior to intercourse, thereby compromising spontaneity Must be removed about 6 hours after intercourse Must be used with a spermicide Increased risk of urinary tract infection (UTI) No protection against STIs
Hormonal implant—Small rod(s) containing hormones that are inserted under the skin, usually in the back of upper arm	One of the safest and most effective forms of birth control available (The World Health Organization). Users do not have to think about your birth control every day or for every sexual intercourse. Periods are fewer and lighter for most women. Effective for 3 years Can be removed at any time Does not contain estrogen	No protection against STIs May be able to see the rod if the woman is very thin A small number of women have longer and heavier periods with breakthrough bleeding. Maybe limited availability More expensive than some other birth control methods
Female sterilization (tubal ligation)	Effective Long-term cost-effectiveness May be reversible	Surgical procedure May not be reversible No protection against STIs
Male sterilization (vasectomy)	Effective Long-term cost-effectiveness Does not interfere with sexual performance May be reversible in some cases	Usually not reversible Psychological effects No protection against STIs

Standardized Language

Examples of NOC Outcomes and Goals for Sexuality Problems

NANDA-I DIAGNOSIS	NOC OUTCOMES	EXAMPLES OF GOALS USING NOC INDICATORS
Ineffective Sexuality Patterns	Abuse Recovery: Sexual	(3, moderate) Demonstrates evidence of appropriate same-sex relationships
	Body Image	(4, often positive) Satisfaction with body function
	Child Development: Adolescence (12–17 years)	(4, often demonstrated) Expresses comfort with own sexual identity
	Child Development: Middle Childhood (6–11 years)	(4, often demonstrated) Identifies with same-sex peer group
	Role Performance	(3, moderately adequate) Performance of intimate role behaviors
	Self-Esteem	(4, often positive) Description of self
	Sexual Identity	(4, often demonstrated) Challenges negative images of sexual self

Examples of NOC Outcomes and Goals for Sexuality Problems—cont'd

NANDA-I DIAGNOSIS	NOC OUTCOMES	EXAMPLES OF GOALS USING NOC INDICATORS
Sexual Dysfunction	Abuse Recovery: Sexual	(4, substantial) Evidence of appropriate opposite-sex relationships
	Physical Aging	(3, moderate deviation from normal range) Sexual functioning
	Risk Control: Sexually Transmitted Diseases	(4, often demonstrated) Notifies sexual partner(s) in event of STD infection.
	Sexual Functioning	(4, often demonstrated) Sustains arousal through orgasm

Source: Moorhead, S., Johnson, M., Maas, M., et al. (Eds.). (2008). *Nursing outcomes classification (NOC)* (4th ed.). St. Louis, MO: C.V. Mosby. Used with permission.

Examples of NIC Interventions and Nursing Activities for Sexuality Problems

NANDA-I DIAGNOSIS	NIC INTERVENTIONS	EXAMPLES OF NURSING ACTIVITIES (NIC)
Ineffective Sexuality Patterns	Body Image Enhancement	Instruct children about the functions of the various body parts, as appropriate.
	Coping Enhancement	
	Counseling	Assist the patient in developing an objective appraisal of the event.
		Demonstrate empathy, warmth, and genuineness.
	Family Planning: Contraception	Explain reasons for most unplanned pregnancies.
	Role Enhancement	Encourage patient to identify a realistic description of change in role.
	Self-Esteem Enhancement	Explore previous achievements.
	Sexual Counseling	Preface questions about sexuality with a statement that tells the patient that many people experience sexual difficulties.
	Teaching: Safe Sex	Discuss abstinence as a means of birth control, as appropriate.
Sexual Dysfunction	Abuse Protection Support	Refer adult(s) to shelters for abused spouses, as appropriate.
	Behavior Management: Sexual	Identify sexual behaviors that are unacceptable, given the particular setting and patient population.
	Coping Enhancement	Explore with the patient previous methods of dealing with life problems.
	Counseling	Encourage expression of feelings.
	Infection Protection	Teach patient and family members how to avoid infections.
	Risk Identification	Determine compliance with medical and nursing treatments.
	Sexual Counseling	Begin with the least sensitive topics and proceed to the more sensitive.
	Teaching: Safe Sex	Discuss with patient ways to convince partners to use condoms.
	Teaching: Sexuality	Discuss peer and social pressure in relation to sexual activity.

Source: Bulechek, G., Butcher, H., & Dochterman, J. (Eds.). (2008). *Nursing Interventions Classification (NIC)* (5th ed.). St. Louis, MO: C.V. Mosby. Used with permission.

THINKING CRITICALLY ABOUT SEXUAL HEALTH

The exercises in the following sections allow you to practice the kind of thinking you will use as a full-spectrum nurse. Because these are critical-thinking questions, there is usually no single right answer. We do not provide answers for these questions because it is more important for you to think about the questions than to arrive at the "right" answer. These questions are designed to improve your thinking more than to "cover content." Discuss answers with your peers—discussion can stimulate critical thinking. If you have difficulty with any of these questions, consult with your instructor.

Applying the Full-Spectrum Nursing Model

PATIENT SITUATION

Debra is perimenopausal at age 52, and her husband Roberto is 59. She has been feeling tired in the afternoon and moody at times. At her annual women's health visit, Debra tells you that she feels a lower level of sexual desire than she used to. Debra says, "I chalk it up to being very busy at work and yet still having so many demands on my time and energy with care of our three kids and housework." Debra is physically active, exercising four times a week, and is in good general health. She takes no medication and is within 15 pounds of her normal weight. Debra still has her period, but the flow is very heavy and cramping is more uncomfortable than it ever had been.

Recently, Debra has noticed that Roberto has been taking longer to achieve an erection, and his erection is not as firm as it used to be. His health is generally healthy except for high blood pressure and high blood cholesterol levels. He takes medication for both conditions.

THINKING

1. *Theoretical Knowledge (Factual Information):*

   a. What are the common physical and emotional manifestations occurring with perimenopause?

2. *Critical Thinking (Considering Alternatives, Deciding What to Do):*

   a. How would you respond to Debra when she asks for information and support regarding her husband's erectile dysfunction?

   b. Debra asks you if her desire for sexual intimacy will continue to decline after she goes through "the change of life". Describe in detail what you would tell her.

DOING

3. *Practical Knowledge:*

   a. What general topics would you explore with Debra to assess her sexual history?

   b. What questions would you ask Roberto to assess his sexual history?

CARING

4. *Self-Knowledge:* What might you be feeling if you were in Debra's situation?

5. *Ethical Knowledge:* What are one or two things you would do to help Debra and Roberto feel cared for and cared about?

Critical Thinking and Clinical Reasoning

1. A 34-year-old married woman is admitted to the hospital following an alleged rape. You are caring for her the next day. She will remain hospitalized for several days because of a head injury she suffered during the rape.

   a. How can you best approach this woman to establish a positive rapport?

  b. What fears are this patient likely to express?

  c. The patient's spouse is coming to visit. What concerns do you think that he may have?

  d. You begin to feel overwhelmed by this couple's emotions and questions. What can you do to help provide this couple with optimal care?

2. Your 26-year-old male client recently had a spinal cord injury. The doctors have talked to him about the possibility of regaining motor function and perhaps being able to walk again after intense therapy. What he now seems to be most concerned about is his relationship with his 25-year-old fiancée.

  a. What aspects of their relationship do you think he is concerned about?

  b. Do you have enough theoretical and patient information regarding his injury to answer all of his concerns?

  c. As you consider some of the changes in sexual functioning that may follow a spinal cord injury, what suggestions might you share with him?

  d. What clues might you get that would indicate that talking to the fiancée may be appropriate?

3. You are seeing Jessica, a 14-year-old girl, at the clinic. Her throat culture is positive for gonorrhea. The girl's mother has gone down to the coffee shop. The doctor has left a prescription for antibiotics. You are left to take care of the discharge from the clinic.

  a. How would you explain the culture results to Jessica?

  b. Jessica tells you that she cannot possibly have a sexually transmitted infection (STI) because she has not had sexual intercourse. How would you respond?

  c. Jessica tells you that she has had oral sex with her boyfriend, but no one else. What education regarding STIs and antibiotics would be appropriate?

  d. What information would you give the mother when she returns?

4. A 45-year-old married man with young children has just been informed that he is HIV positive. He is shocked by the news. He admits he had an extramarital relationship with a man 7 years ago.

  a. What concerns is he likely to have? As his nurse, what biases do you have that you will have to put aside to help him?

  b. What theoretical knowledge would you need at a later time to help him deal with questions about sexual activity?

  c. What patient information would you need to help him deal with questions about sexual activity?

5. Review the following scenarios from "Meet Your Patients" in Volume 1.

  Two days after undergoing a fine-needle aspiration to evaluate a small breast mass, Jocelyn Carter's surgeon informed her that the mass was malignant. He recommended a mastectomy (removal of the breast). Today, she arrives alone at the surgery registration area at 0600. You ask how she is feeling, and she tells you that the last week has been a whirlwind of activity. "I had to arrange child care, cancel a business trip, and organize the house so that I could take a few days off to have the surgery. My husband is working overseas this fall, so he couldn't be here to help me. Honestly, I don't know how I'm feeling. I haven't had time to think about it." A few minutes later, as she waits in the surgery holding area, she begins to cry. You hold her hand and ask whether she would like to talk. She asks you, "Do you think my husband will still want me? I'm afraid he will be turned off when he looks at me now."

Gabriel Thomas comes to the outpatient clinic complaining of a throbbing headache for the last 3 days. He explains that he has tried several over-the-counter medicines and has had no relief. You check his blood pressure, and measure the reading at 240/130 mm Hg. When you ask whether he has ever been treated for high blood pressure, he replies, "Are you another one of these people trying to get me to take drugs that will ruin my sex life?"

Frank Thanee, who has heart disease, had a mitral valve replacement 3 days ago. He has been transferred to the cardiology floor for an additional day of hospitalization. His partner, Greg, has spent the last 3 days at the hospital and has just left to check on the apartment and feed their cat. Frank confides that he is worried about his parents' expected visit. "I've never been able to tell them about Greg. They wouldn't be able to understand it, never mind approve. I don't know how to handle this. What do you think I should do?"

a. Write etiologies for each of the patients. The nursing diagnosis label is provided for you in each case.

Jocelyn Carter—Ineffective Sexuality Patterns

Gabriel Thomas—Ineffective Sexuality Patterns

Frank Thanee—Sexual Dysfunction

b. For each of the patients, instead of the sexuality diagnosis, identify another nursing diagnosis label that you should explore to see whether it fits the situation better. Consult a nursing diagnosis handbook, as needed.

Jocelyn Carter:

Gabriel Thomas:

Frank Thanee:

6. For each of the following concepts, use critical thinking to describe how or why it is important to nursing, patient care, or sexual health. Note that these are *not* to be merely definitions.

Sexual health   Sexual expression
Gender   Sexually transmitted infections
Sexual orientation   Fertility control

What Are the Main Points in This Chapter?

➤ Sexuality is a broad and complex aspect of the self, with physical, emotional, social, and spiritual dimensions.

➤ Sexuality involves how we feel about ourselves as individuals and how we interact with others and our environment.

➤ Gender, gender roles, gender identity, and sexual orientation contribute to expression of our sexuality throughout the life cycle.

➤ There are both typical and atypical forms of sexual expression.

➤ Culture, religion, lifestyle, sexual knowledge, and physical health all influence our attitudes toward sexuality, sexual behaviors, and intimate relationships.

➤ Sexual victimization is a societal and healthcare concern.

➤ Physical and psychological health status affects sexuality and sexual functioning.

➤ Sexual health is challenged by high-risk sexual behaviors, sexually transmitted infections (STI), negative interpersonal relationships, and sexual dysfunctions.

➤ Four phases of the sexual response cycle are excitement, plateau, orgasm, and resolution.

➤ A sexual history is a component of the nursing assessment.

➤ There are strategies you can use to help you gain comfort and competence in collecting sexual data.

➤ The PLISSIT model was developed as a guideline for counseling for sexual problems: Permission, Limited Information, Specific Suggestions, and Intensive Therapy.

➤ Sexual well-being may be enhanced through nursing interventions such as counseling for sexual problems; dealing with inappropriate sexual behavior; and teaching about body function and reproduction, self-care, contraception, and prevention of STIs.

For practice questions for this chapter,

Go to **NCLEX-Style Chapter Quiz,** on the Student Resource Disk or DavisPlus at http://davisplus.fadavis.com/Wilkinson2

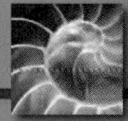

Knowledge Map

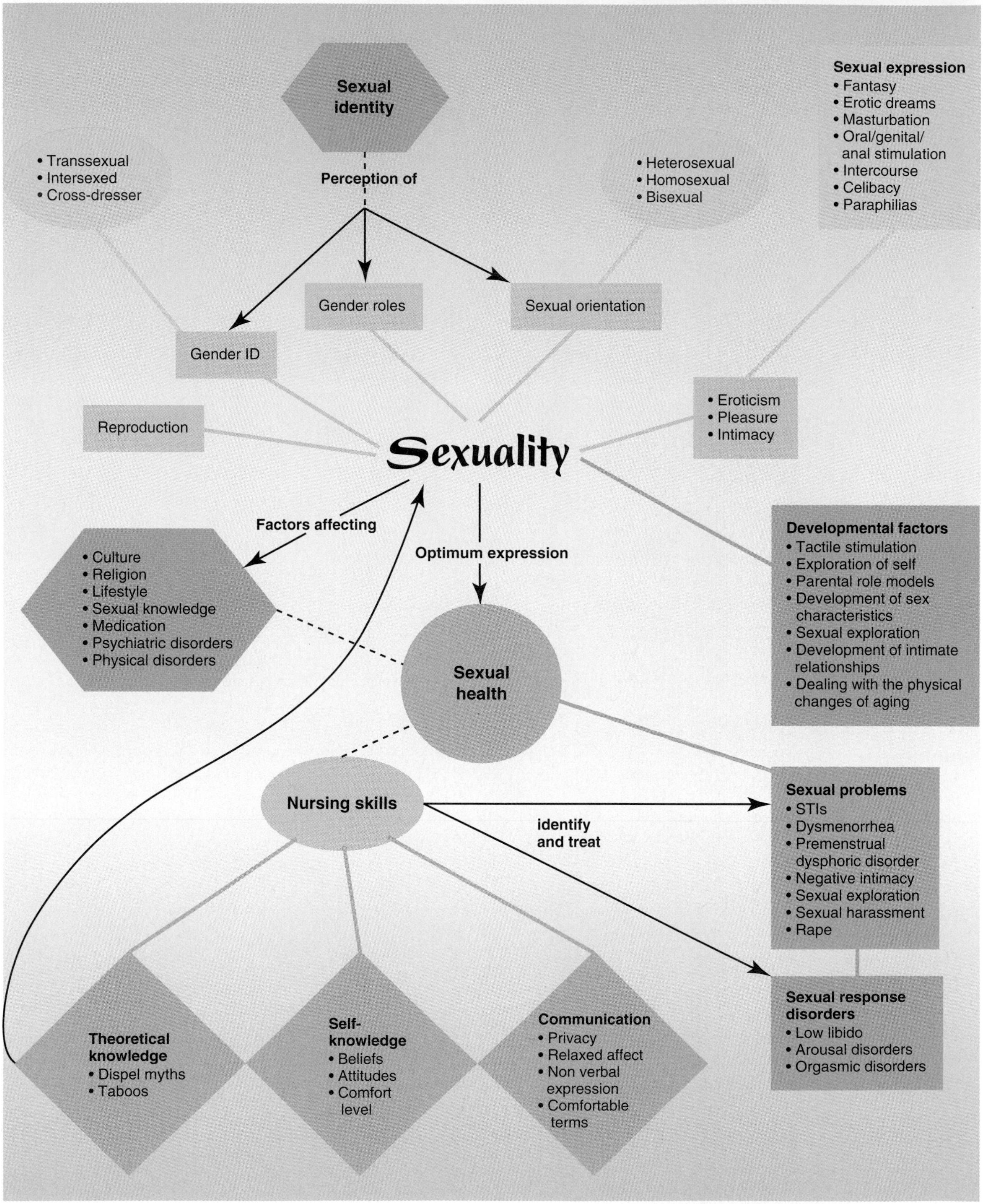

Sexual identity

• Transsexual
• Intersexed
• Cross-dresser

Perception of

• Heterosexual
• Homosexual
• Bisexual

Sexual expression
• Fantasy
• Erotic dreams
• Masturbation
• Oral/genital/
  anal stimulation
• Intercourse
• Celibacy
• Paraphilias

Gender roles

Sexual orientation

Gender ID

Reproduction

• Eroticism
• Pleasure
• Intimacy

Sexuality

Factors affecting

• Culture
• Religion
• Lifestyle
• Sexual knowledge
• Medication
• Psychiatric disorders
• Physical disorders

Optimum expression

Developmental factors
• Tactile stimulation
• Exploration of self
• Parental role models
• Development of sex
  characteristics
• Sexual exploration
• Development of intimate
  relationships
• Dealing with the physical
  changes of aging

Sexual health

Nursing skills

identify and treat

Sexual problems
• STIs
• Dysmenorrhea
• Premenstrual
  dysphoric disorder
• Negative intimacy
• Sexual exploration
• Sexual harassment
• Rape

Theoretical knowledge
• Dispel myths
• Taboos

Self-knowledge
• Beliefs
• Attitudes
• Comfort
  level

Communication
• Privacy
• Relaxed affect
• Non verbal
  expression
• Comfortable
  terms

Sexual response disorders
• Low libido
• Arousal disorders
• Orgasmic disorders

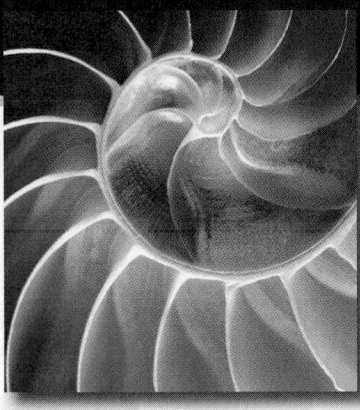

CHAPTER 33

Sleep & Rest

For a podcast of an overview of this chapter,

 Go to Student Resources, **Podcast – Chapter Overviews, Chapter 33,** on DavisPlus at http://davisplus.fadavis.com/ Wilkinson2

Caring for the Garcias

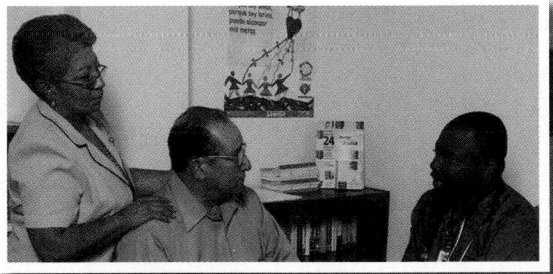

The exercises in the following section allow you to practice the kind of thinking you will use as a full-spectrum nurse. Because these are critical-thinking questions, there is usually no single right answer. We do not provide answers for these questions because it is more important for you to think about the questions than to arrive at the "right" answer. These questions are designed to improve your thinking more than to "cover content." Discuss answers with your peers— discussion can stimulate critical thinking. If you have difficulty with any of these questions, consult with your instructor.

Flordelisa Garcia arrives at the clinic accompanied by her husband, Joe. She appears very tired. Joe tells you that she has been sleeping poorly. "She worries so much. She worries about Bettina, our grandchild. She worries about our kids. Now she's worried about my mother. When we were going through that mammogram scare, she was even worse!"

Mrs. Garcia shrugs her shoulders. "I can't help it. I'm like that. I've always been a worrier. But it's gotten worse lately. Now I worry and get so emotional. I lie in bed thinking about all this stuff and end up in tears. Then, when I finally get to sleep, I wake up covered with sweat. I've tried extra soy for hot flashes, melatonin from the health food store, herbal tea, and even Benadryl—but nothing seems to work. I'm so tired. But when I get up, I have to deal with all these little kids at work. They're bouncing all over the place and noisy. I just get so short-tempered with them. That's not like me. I can't take this anymore."

A. *Patient data:* Clearly Mrs. Garcia has a sleep problem. Underline the data that are defining characteristics (symptoms) of a sleep problem.

B. *Patient data:* Which data suggest ideas about the etiologies (causes) of Mrs. Garcia's sleep problem?

C. Nursing diagnosis: Two NANDA-I sleep-related nursing diagnoses are Sleep Deprivation and Disturbed Sleep Pattern. You have already identified the patient's defining characteristics. Now, what *knowledge* do you need to decide which of these NANDA-I labels to use?

(continued on next page)

Caring for the Garcias (continued)

D. How could you obtain this knowledge?

E. Sleep Deprivation is defined as "prolonged periods of time without sleep" and Disturbed Sleep Pattern is defined as "time-limited disruption of sleep." Can you

make the diagnoses on the basis of this knowledge? Why or why not?

F. Following are some of the defining characteristics for these two nursing diagnoses:

Disturbed Sleep Pattern	**Sleep Deprivation**
Verbal complaints of not feeling well rested	Daytime drowsiness
Dissatisfaction with sleep	Decreased ability to function
Change in normal sleep pattern	Agitation
Decreased ability to function	Irritability
Reports being awakened	Hallucinations
Reports no difficulty falling asleep	Anxiety
	Inability to concentrate
	Apathy
	Slowed reactions
	Combativeness
	Fatigue
	Fleeting nystagmus
	Hand tremors
	Heightened sensitivity to pain
	Lethargy, listlessness, malaise
	Perceptual disorders (e.g., disturbed body sensation, delusions, feeling afloat)
	Restlessness
	Transient paranoia

Certainly there is some overlap between the two sets of symptoms. Nevertheless, which set seems to be a better fit for Mrs. Garcia? Why?

G. Write a nursing diagnosis for Mrs. Garcia.

Practical **Knowledge**
knowing how

This section will help you learn to give a back massage, assist you in obtaining a sleep history, and provide standardized language to use in planning care for clients with sleep problems.

Procedures

In the not-so-distant past, a relaxing back massage was a part of the evening care routine for every hospitalized patient. In this era of cost containment, this sleep enhancer has become a "nice but not essential" procedure in most agencies. Massage has therapeutic benefits, however. It promotes circulation, physical and emotional comfort, and sleep. Furthermore, it is an independent nursing activity for which you do not need a medical prescription (except in very rare circumstances). Try to offer a back rub whenever you can, and teach and encourage nursing assistive personnel (NAP) to do so as well. Refer to the following procedure.

Procedure 33–1 ▢ Giving a Back Massage

➤ For steps to follow in *all* procedures, refer to the Universal Steps for All Procedures found on the inside back cover of Volume 2.

Critical Aspects

- Warm the lotion.
- Raise the bed to working height.
- Position the patient comfortably on her side or prone.
- Place lotion on your hands.
- Rub down the length and then up the sides of the back.
- Never rub directly over the spine.
- Apply gentle thumb pressure on either side of the spine at midback, pushing outward for about 2.5 cm (1 in.) along the trapezius muscle.
- Always apply pressure away from the spine, not toward it.
- Go to the spots that felt the tightest or that the patient states are tight. Work in small circles, using gentle thumb pressure.
- Gently shake the scapula.
- Apply horizontal strokes across the scapula, using your thumb.
- Apply pressure in circles using the heels of your hands down both sides of the spine.
- Apply horizontal strokes using the heels of your hands across the latissimus dorsi muscle.
- Gently rub your hands up either side of the spine from the base of the back to the base of the neck, and then down the sides of the back.

Equipment
Skin care lotion

Delegation
You can delegate back massage to the NAP if the patient's condition and the NAP's skills allow. However, giving the

back rub yourself provides an excellent opportunity to assess the patient, develop rapport, and provide emotional support.

Pre-Procedure Assessment
Check the skin for reddened areas or skin breakdown.

➤ When performing the procedure, always identify your patient according to agency policy and be attentive to standard precautions, hand hygiene, patient safety and privacy, body mechanics, and documentation.

Procedure Steps

1. Warm the lotion by placing the bottle in warm water.
Cold lotion can cause muscle contraction; warming the lotion helps relax the muscles.

2. Raise the bed to working height.
Prevents back strain of the nurse.

3. Position the patient comfortably on her side or prone.
  a. Untie the patient's gown, and expose her back.
  b. Raise the siderail on the opposite side of the bed.
Siderails prevent the patient from falling off the bed when you turn her toward the side of the bed away from you.

  c. Wash the patient's back with warm water, if needed.
Warm water will help relax the muscles while removing any sweat and soiling.

4. Place lotion on your hands.
Placing the lotion directly on the back may cause the patient's muscles to tighten.

5. Place your hands on either side of the spine at the base of the neck. Using gentle, continuous pressure, rub down the length and then up the sides of the back.
  a. Repeat this motion several times.
  b. Never rub directly over the spine.

The spine is a vulnerable area. ▼

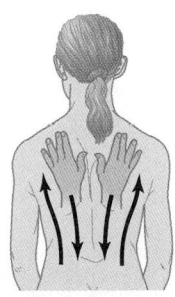

6. Apply gentle thumb pressure (using the fleshy part of your thumbs) on either side of the spine at the midback, pushing outward for about 2.5 cm (1 in.).
  a. Repeat from the midback to the base of the neck in a series of small, outward strokes.

(continued on next page)

Procedure 33-1 ■ **Giving a Back Massage** (continued)

Strokes should be along the muscle length and not across the muscle to help stretch and relax it.

b. Ask the patient whether the amount of pressure is comfortable. Be careful not to cause the patient discomfort, which might cause further muscle tightness.

c. Always apply pressure away from the spine, not toward it.
This gently stretches the muscles and helps prevent placing pressure on the spine.

d. If you are unable to massage both sides at the same time, work on one side and then the other.
Work as symmetrically as possible to increase muscle relaxation. ▼

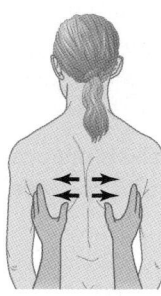

7. Now go to the spots that felt the tightest or that the patient states are tight. Work in small circles, using gentle thumb pressure.
Small circular movements can help release muscle "knots" and relax tightened muscles. ▼

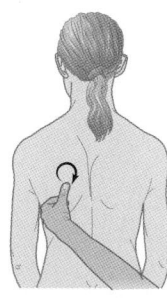

8. Gently shake the scapula. Place your palm on one scapula, and gently shake it by quickly moving your palm back and forth. Repeat on the other side.
Movement of the scapula decreases when muscles tighten; gently vibrating the scapula helps loosen the muscles. ▼

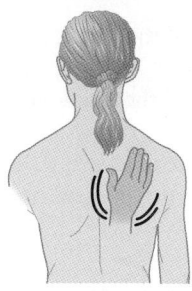

9. Apply horizontal strokes across the scapula, using your thumb. Using horizontal strokes from near the spine across the bottom of the scapula, push out all the way across the scapula from the spine. Move up and repeat until you have covered the entire scapula and top of the shoulder. Repeat on the other side.
This movement helps loosen the trapezius muscle. ▼

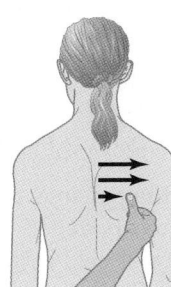

10. If you find tender spots, use the fleshy parts of your fingers in a small circular motion.

11. Apply pressure in circles using the heels of your hands down both sides of the spine. Beginning at the

upper shoulder and working down to the lower back, apply pressure in medium-sized circles down the sides of the spine with the heels of your hands. Be cautious not to apply too much pressure. Assess patient for comfort.
The circular motion helps relax tightened areas in the paraspinal muscles. ▼

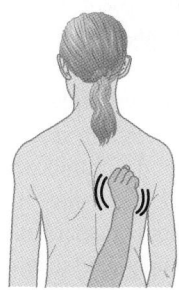

12. Apply horizontal strokes using the heels of your hands across the latissimus dorsi muscle. Using horizontal strokes from near the spine below the scapula, push out from the spine across to the ribs, and work down across the lower back with the heels of your hands.
This movement helps relax the latissimus dorsi muscle.

13. Gently rub your hands up either side of the spine from the base of the back to the base of the neck and then down the sides of the back. Repeat several times.
Long strokes help increase circulation and promote relaxation of the back muscles.

Note: If you are unable to do a complete back massage, ask the patient where she is most uncomfortable, and massage those areas. If the patient has general tightness, use the long strokes down each side of the spine and back up the sides.

Evaluation

■ Assess the patient's report of comfort, relaxation, and how soon she falls asleep.

Documentation

This is a routine aspect of care and is usually documented on a flowsheet.

Thinking About the Procedure

 Go to the *Fundamentals of Nursing Skills Videos*, **Hygiene: Back Massage.**

1. What does the nurse do between the bed bath and back massage?

2. What does the narrator say the benefit of the back rub is to this patient in bed?

 For suggested responses, go to Chapter 33, **Thinking About the Procedure Suggested Responses (Procedure 33-1),** on the Student Resource Disk or DavisPlus at http://davisplus.fadavis.com/Wilkinson2

Assessment Guidelines and Tools

This section will assist you in screening for sleep problems.

Questions for a Sleep History

A brief assessment for all patients should include questions about the following:

Usual Sleeping Pattern

- When do you go to sleep and wake up?
- How many hours do you sleep?
- Do you have a regular sleep schedule?
- How would you rate the quality of your sleep on a scale of 1 to 10, with 10 meaning "great"?
- Do you take a nap? If you do, for how long?
- How often do you waken during sleep, for example, to go to the bathroom?
- Do you feel adequately rested when you wake up?

Sleeping Environment

- Would you like a night-light?
- What room temperature do you prefer?
- What noise level do you prefer (for example, radio, television, absolute quiet)?

Bedtime Routines/Rituals

- What do you typically do in the hour before bedtime?
- What do you do to help you fall asleep?

Sleep Aids

- Do you need a special pillow or positioning aid?
- Do you take any sleep medications or other drugs, natural sleep aids, or homeopathic remedies that may affect sleep?

Sleep Changes or Problems

- Have your sleep patterns changed? If so, how?
- How often do you experience difficulty falling asleep? Staying asleep?
- Do you currently, or have you in the past, ever experienced a sleep disorder (e.g., narcolepsy, insomnia)?
- Do you remember your dreams after you wake? Do you ever have night terrors? Do you sleepwalk?
- Do you ever experience an unpleasant creeping feeling, crawling, or tingling, relieved only by moving the legs at night?
- Do you snore? Does your own snoring or grunting ever wake you or anyone in the room?
- Do you wear a cap at night? Do you require oxygen at night? Or any other medical aid or therapy while you sleep?
- Do you grind your teeth while you sleep? Do you wear a dental appliance to prevent grinding?
- Do you experience any kind of pain that makes it difficult for you to fall asleep or stay asleep?
- Is there anything that I have not asked that might help you sleep while you are in the hospital (having surgery, receiving home care)?

If the client reports experiencing satisfactory sleep, that is an adequate assessment, and you merely need to support her usual sleep patterns and rituals. When you suspect a sleep problem, you will perform a more in-depth assessment, such as a detailed sleep history or sleep diary.

Sleep Diary

A sleep diary provides specific information on the patient's sleep–wakefulness patterns over a long period. The diary is usually kept for 14 days and may include the following.

1. Time you went to bed:_____
2. What did you eat or drink just before bedtime? _____
3. What mental and physical activities did you engage in the 2 to 3 hours before bedtime?_____
4. Were you worried or anxious about anything when you went to bed?_____
5. Approximate time you fell asleep:_____

6. Times you woke during the night:_____
7. Times you fell back to sleep:_____
8. Time you woke up:_____
9. Sleep medications you have taken:_____
10. Any repeated doses? _____ Times:_____
11. Episodes of "disorientation":_____
12. Frequency of pain medication taken and times:_____
13. Did you feel refreshed in the morning?_____

Standardized Language

Selected NOC Outcomes and NIC Interventions for Sleep Diagnoses

NURSING DIAGNOSIS	NOC OUTCOMES	NIC INTERVENTIONS
Readiness for Enhanced Sleep	Rest	Environmental Management: Comfort
	Sleep	Sleep Enhancement
	Personal Well-Being	
Disturbed Sleep Pattern	Rest	Coping Enhancement
	Sleep	Energy Management
	Personal Well-Being	Environmental Management: Comfort
		Simple Relaxation Therapy
		Sleep Enhancement
Sleep Deprivation	Rest	Coping Enhancement
	Sleep	Energy Management
	Symptom Severity	Environmental Management: Comfort
		Simple Relaxation Therapy
		Sleep Enhancement
Insomnia	NOC outcomes and NIC interventions have not yet been linked to Insomnia. However, those for other sleep diagnoses may be useful.	

Sources: Bulechek, G., Butcher, H., & Dochterman, J. (Eds.). (2008). *Nursing interventions classification (NIC)* (5th ed.). St. Louis, MO: C.V. Mosby; Johnson, M., Bulechek, G., Butcher, H., et al. (2006). *NANDA, NOC, and NIC linkages* (2nd ed.). St. Louis, MO: C.V. Mosby; Moorhead, S., Johnson, M., & Maas, M., et al. (Eds.). (2008). *Nursing outcomes classification (NOC)* (4th ed.). St. Louis, MO: C.V. Mosby. Used with permission.

THINKING CRITICALLY ABOUT SLEEP AND REST

The exercises in the following sections allow you to practice the kind of thinking you will use as a full-spectrum nurse. Because these are critical-thinking questions, there is usually no single right answer. We do not provide answers for these questions because it is more important for you to think about the questions than to arrive at the "right" answer. These questions are designed to improve your thinking more than to "cover content." Discuss answers with your peers—discussion can stimulate critical thinking. If you have difficulty with any of these questions, consult with your instructor.

Applying the Full-Spectrum Nursing Model

PATIENT SITUATION

A 43-year-old healthy woman, Maria Lupe, is being seen for her annual women's health visit. She tells you she lies awake in bed for hours before falling asleep at night. Sometimes she falls asleep OK but will wake up and then have trouble going back to sleep. After feeling like she was awake nearly all night, Maria wakes in the morning feeling exhausted. She tells you she feels tired all the time and can't seem to get things done during her time off because of her fatigue. Maria admits to feeling irritable with her co-workers and children. Because of her lack of rest, she doesn't have the desire to do things socially anymore.

THINKING

1. *Theoretical Knowledge:*

   The NANDA-I definition and defining characteristics of Insomnia differ slightly from the medical diagnosis of insomnia.

   a. What is insomnia, as defined medically (e.g., by the National Sleep Foundation)?

   b. What other health conditions might a medical diagnosis of insomnia be confused with?

   c. What factors either lead to or aggravate insomnia, as described medically?

2. *Critical Thinking (Contextual Awareness):*

   a. Obviously Maria has trouble sleeping. Based on the data you have, do you consider her difficulty sleeping significant enough to require consultation with her primary healthcare provider? Explain your thinking.

DOING

3. *Nursing Process (Assessments):*

   a. When conducting a sleep history for Maria, what questions would you ask her in order to (1) describe more fully her sleeping problem and (2) identify the cause of her sleeping problem?

   b. What would you suggest Maria do to help you gain more information about her sleeping problem?

4. *Nursing Process (Nursing Diagnosis):*

   Based on the data in the Patient Situation, would you use a nursing diagnosis of Sleep Deprivation or Insomnia for Maria? Explain your thinking. Use a nursing diagnosis handbook, as needed, to compare the defining characteristics of the two diagnoses.

5. *Nursing Process (Interventions):*

   How might you help your patient manage her Insomnia other than using prescription medication? What might you suggest?

CARING

6. *Self-Knowledge:*

   a. Have you ever had trouble falling or staying asleep? How did you feel at the time and in the morning? Describe your experience.

   b. How might you provide better emotional care and support to your patient after recalling your own episodes of sleeping difficulty?

Critical Thinking and Clinical Reasoning

1. You are a nurse working on a psychiatric unit. You are assigned to Sheryl, a 23-year-old woman with the diagnosis of anorexia nervosa (a life-threatening eating disorder characterized by an intense fear of weight gain and extremely restrictive food intake). Sheryl attends therapy each day, seems to be taking her medications, and is eating the required amount of food at each meal. But she continues to lose weight. The nurse working the night shift reports that Sheryl is unable to sleep at night; seems frightened, almost panicky; paces the hall; and cries. Sheryl is unwilling to talk about her inability to sleep, but you read in her chart that she was sexually abused during the night while she was in a foster home. As you are straightening up in her room, you find several of Sheryl's sleeping pills. Sheryl walks into the room and begs you to be her friend and not to tell anyone. She promises to take her pills that night.

   a. What do you think may be contributing to Sheryl's inability to sleep? Explain your reasoning.

   b. How do you feel about keeping Sheryl's secret? Why might you want to tell other caregivers about the sleeping pills? What reasons can you think of for *not* telling?

   c. For you to deal effectively with Sheryl's sleep problem, what theoretical knowledge would you need?

   d. Now assess your current theoretical knowledge. Do you need more knowledge about certain topics to help Sheryl? If so, where can you find out what you need to know?

2. Imagine that you are a registered nurse at a local nursing home. Gwen, a 74-year-old woman, has captured your heart. Gwen has severe rheumatoid arthritis with pain and joint deformities, so she cannot ambulate or perform activities of daily living independently. Gwen's family visits every weekend, and they always bring cookies or candy, usually chocolate. Gwen likes to eat these treats just before bedtime, right after her bedtime medications. She receives a stool softener, a sleeping pill, and a pain pill for her arthritis. Lately she has been awakening at least twice each night, seeming quite confused. She tells the day shift nurse that she needs another sleeping pill at bedtime because "I'm not sleeping as well as I used to, because I have to get up so many times to go to the bathroom." She also seems more sluggish than usual during the day. You will need to integrate all available information. Don't worry if you do not know much about arthritis or if there are other things you have not yet studied. Just try to reason out the questions based on the knowledge you *do* have.

   a. If you have not yet studied arthritis and urinary elimination, you may lack some theoretical knowledge you need to answer the following questions. What information do you need? Where would you go to get it?

   b. What are some reasons that Gwen might be awakening?

   c. What might be causing her confusion at night?

   d. Should you address the problem of having chocolate before bed? Why or why not?

   e. List as many different interventions as you can that you might use to address the problem of eating sweets before bed.

f. Consider the consequences. How might her family react if you suggest that they bring something besides sweets?

g. What teaching might you do with the family?

3. You are a home health nurse. One of your patients is a 55-year-old man named Grant. He is homebound because of complications of diabetes. He states that he sleeps during the day, taking several naps. His chief complaint today is a pain in his left foot. There are books about alternative medicine and bottles of vitamins and minerals all over the house. He believes he can cure his diabetes with herbs. He refuses to take any medications that are prescribed for him by his physician.

a. Do you have enough information to conclude that Grant has a sleep problem? Explain your answer.

b. Examine the patient situation (context). What factors lead you to suspect that Grant may not be sleeping enough at night?

c. What would you do to find out whether Grant is getting enough sleep?

d. Imagine how you would feel about Grant's decision to forgo his medication and use herbal treatments.

e. What personal values and biases do you have that will affect the way you respond to Grant?

4. For each of the following concepts, use critical thinking to describe how or why it is important to nursing, patient care, or sleep and rest. Note that these are *not* to be merely definitions.

Sleep

Rest

Theoretical knowledge about
   the physiology of sleep

Circadian rhythm

Stages of sleep (e.g., REM sleep)

Sleep apnea

Sedatives

Sleep diary

What Are the Main Points in This Chapter?

➤ Sleep is a basic physiological need.

➤ Sleep and rest promote physical, mental, and spiritual well-being by restoring energy and reducing body demands while the body repairs itself.

➤ Illness can interfere with the ability to sleep and rest; conversely, people who suffer from sleep disorders have an increased susceptibility to illnesses.

➤ The hypothalamus and various neurotransmitters are involved in the physiology of sleep.

➤ Circadian rhythm is a biorhythm that is influenced by both internal and external stimuli, especially the light–dark patterns of day and night.

➤ The brain waves produced during REM sleep are similar to those of alert wakefulness. REM is characterized by rapid eye movements and dreaming.

➤ Duration of sleep varies according to age.

➤ Factors affecting sleep include developmental needs and stressors, work, exercise, foods, other lifestyle factors, use of medications, illness, pain, and the environment.

➤ Common sleep disorders include insomnia, sleep apnea, and narcolepsy.

➤ It is important to obtain information about the patient's usual sleep patterns and rituals; this may require use of a sleep diary.

➤ Nursing interventions to promote sleep include scheduling nursing care, creating a restful environment, and supporting bedtime rituals and routines.

➤ Pain is one of the main deterrents to sleep.

➤ Sleep medications, as a rule, should be used only as a temporary measure.

➤ Teaching patients and their families about the importance of rest and sleep is an important health promotion intervention.

For practice questions for this chapter,

Go to **NCLEX-Style Chapter Quiz,** on the Student Resource Disk or DavisPlus at http://davisplus.fadavis.com/Wilkinson2

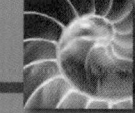 # Knowledge Map

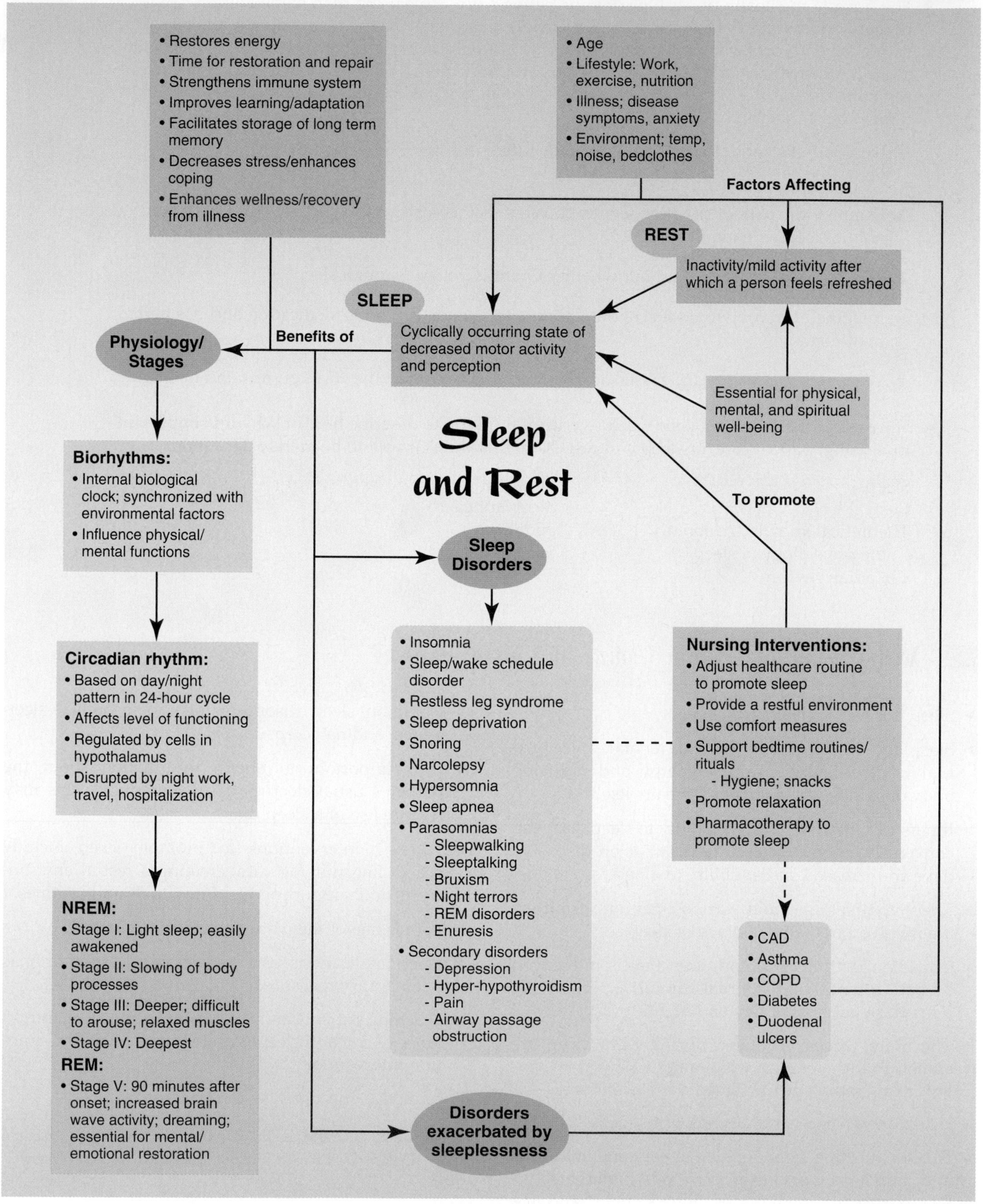

- Restores energy
- Time for restoration and repair
- Strengthens immune system
- Improves learning/adaptation
- Facilitates storage of long term memory
- Decreases stress/enhances coping
- Enhances wellness/recovery from illness

- Age
- Lifestyle: Work, exercise, nutrition
- Illness; disease symptoms, anxiety
- Environment; temp, noise, bedclothes

Factors Affecting

REST

Inactivity/mild activity after which a person feels refreshed

SLEEP

Cyclically occurring state of decreased motor activity and perception

Benefits of

Physiology/ Stages

Essential for physical, mental, and spiritual well-being

Sleep and Rest

To promote

Biorhythms:
- Internal biological clock; synchronized with environmental factors
- Influence physical/ mental functions

Sleep Disorders

Circadian rhythm:
- Based on day/night pattern in 24-hour cycle
- Affects level of functioning
- Regulated by cells in hypothalamus
- Disrupted by night work, travel, hospitalization

- Insomnia
- Sleep/wake schedule disorder
- Restless leg syndrome
- Sleep deprivation
- Snoring
- Narcolepsy
- Hypersomnia
- Sleep apnea
- Parasomnias
  - Sleepwalking
  - Sleeptalking
  - Bruxism
  - Night terrors
  - REM disorders
  - Enuresis
- Secondary disorders
  - Depression
  - Hyper-hypothyroidism
  - Pain
  - Airway passage obstruction

Nursing Interventions:
- Adjust healthcare routine to promote sleep
- Provide a restful environment
- Use comfort measures
- Support bedtime routines/ rituals
  - Hygiene; snacks
- Promote relaxation
- Pharmacotherapy to promote sleep

NREM:
- Stage I: Light sleep; easily awakened
- Stage II: Slowing of body processes
- Stage III: Deeper; difficult to arouse; relaxed muscles
- Stage IV: Deepest

REM:
- Stage V: 90 minutes after onset; increased brain wave activity; dreaming; essential for mental/ emotional restoration

- CAD
- Asthma
- COPD
- Diabetes
- Duodenal ulcers

Disorders exacerbated by sleeplessness

CHAPTER 34

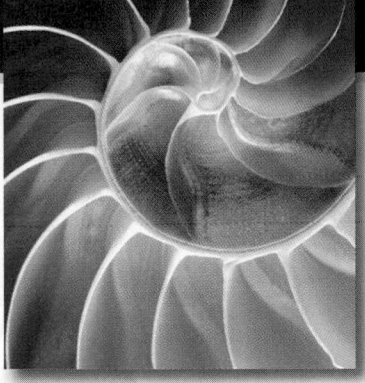

Skin Integrity & Wound Healing

For a podcast of an overview of this chapter,

 Go to Student Resources, **Podcast – Chapter Overviews, Chapter 34,** on DavisPlus at http://davisplus.fadavis.com/ Wilkinson2

Caring for the Garcias

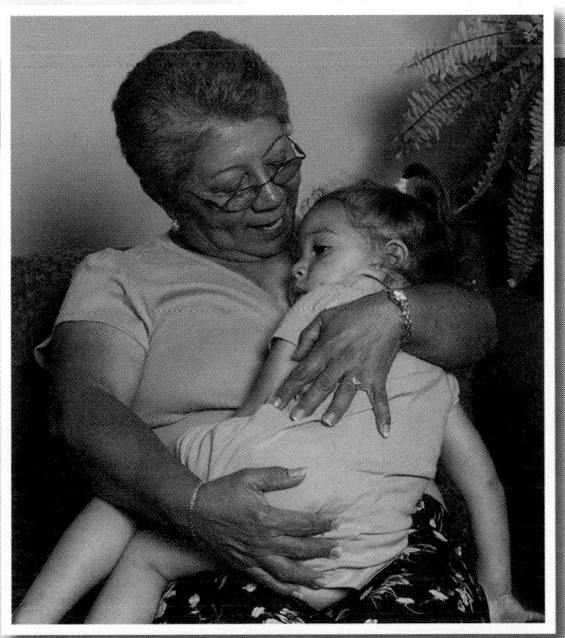

The exercises in the following section allow you to practice the kind of thinking you will use as a full-spectrum nurse. Because these are critical-thinking questions, there is usually no single right answer. We do not provide answers for these questions because it is more important for you to think about the questions than to arrive at the "right" answer. These questions are designed to improve your thinking more than to "cover content." Discuss answers with your peers— discussion can stimulate critical thinking. If you have difficulty with any of these questions, consult with your instructor.

Bettina Sanford, Joe and Flordelisa Garcia's 3-year-old grandchild, fell at the neighborhood playground. She has abrasions on her knees, a deep puncture wound on her left hand, and a laceration on her scalp. Mr. and Mrs. Garcia bring her to the clinic for assessment. She is crying loudly and moving all extremities. No treatment has been given.

A. What should be your first course of action?

B. What kind of care will Bettina need at the clinic?

C. You determine that the scalp laceration will need to be sutured. What actions should you take to prepare Bettina for the suturing?

D. One week later Bettina arrives at the clinic with her grandmother to have the sutures removed. The scalp laceration is dried and healed. When you inspect her other wounds, you notice that her left knee is erythematous, warm and painful to touch, and draining a moderate amount of purulent drainage. What assessment questions should you ask?

(continued on next page)

Caring for the Garcias (continued)

e. Flordelisa Garcia tells you that Bettina would not allow her to clean or dress the abraded knees. You cleanse the knee and remove several small pieces of gravel from the wound bed. The wound is yellow and malodorous. What kind of care will Flordelisa need to provide to Bettina to heal the left knee?

Practical **Knowledge**
knowing how

Procedures

As a nurse, you will care for many patients who have wounds or who are at risk for impaired skin integrity. You will need practical knowledge of wound assessment and wound care.

All wounds require a focused assessment. Assessment frequency depends on the condition of the wound, the work setting, the patient's overall condition and underlying disease process, the type of wound, and the type of treatment used for the wound. If you are providing wound care, you will assess the wound with every treatment.

Specific nursing interventions directed at maintaining skin integrity or healing wounds focus on providing wound care and applying heat and cold therapies. In this section, you will find procedures for obtaining wound cultures, cleansing wounds, and dressing wounds, for placing and removing wound closures, caring for wound drains, and applying binders and bandages, as well as clinical insights for applying local heat and cold therapy.

Procedure 34-1 ▢ Obtaining a Wound Culture by Swab

➤ For steps to follow in *all* procedures, refer to the Universal Steps for All Procedures found on the inside back cover of Volume 2.

Note: This procedure uses modified sterile technique because wound care is now usually performed using a clean approach rather than sterile technique.

Critical Aspects

- Position the patient for easy access to the wound and in a manner that will allow the irrigation solution to flow freely from the wound with the assistance of gravity.
- Don protective equipment: gown, face shield, and clean procedure gloves.
- Remove the soiled dressing and dispose of gloves and dressing.
- Don clean gloves, and fill a 35-mL syringe with attached 19-gauge angiocatheter with 0.9% (normal) saline solution.
- Holding the angiocatheter tip 2 cm from the wound bed, gently irrigate the wound (superior to inferior).
- Press the culture swab against an area of red granulating tissue, and rotate.
- Reinsert the swab into the culturette tube, label the tube, and transport it to the lab.

Equipment

- Three pairs of clean procedure gloves
- Culturette tube
- Sterile 4 in. × 4 in. gauze in an impermeable tray or separate 4 × 4 packs and an impermeable barrier
- Sterile 0.9% (normal) saline solution for irrigation, warmed to body temperature when possible
Cold solution lowers the temperature of the wound bed and slows the healing process.
- 35-mL syringe

- 19-gauge angiocatheter
- Gown and face shield
- Emesis basin
- Water-resistant disposable drapes

Delegation

This is an invasive procedure that requires knowledge of wound healing. It should be performed by a licensed nurse. Do not delegate this skill to nursing assistive personnel (NAP).

Pre-Procedure Assessments

Note: If the wound is covered when you begin, you will make these assessments when you remove the soiled dressing *and* after cleansing the wound.

■ **Assess for pain.**

Wounds may be very painful, and wound irrigation may increase pain. Provide prescribed pain medication 30 minutes before performing the procedure, if indicated.

■ **Determine whether the wound requires sterile, modified sterile, or clean technique.**

Sterile technique is used for acute surgical wounds and for wounds that have undergone recent sharp débridement, or when the physician prescribes it. Chronic wounds are colonized with baceria and may be cared for using clean technique, as in this procedure. To perform sterile wound irrigation, see Procedure 34-3.

■ **Assess the amount and type of tissue present in the wound bed.**

Granulating tissue is beefy red with a velvety appearance. It appears with the growth of new blood vessels and connective tissue. Pale pink tissue may indicate compromised blood supply to the wound bed. Necrotic tissue, which is black, brown, or yellow in appearance, is nonviable, and inhibits healing. Only red granulating tissue should be swabbed for a culture.

■ **Assess the type and amount of exudate.**

Exudate may be a sign of infection.

■ **Assess the wound for odor.**

A foul odor may indicate infection. Cleanse wounds before you assess for odor, because some dressings interact with wound drainage to produce an odor.

■ **Assess the tissue surrounding the wound edge.**

Surrounding tissue that is red, warm, and/or edematous may indicate infection.

> When performing the procedure, always identify your patient according to agency policy and be attentive to standard precautions, hand hygiene, patient safety and privacy, body mechanics, and documentation.

Procedure Steps

1. Place the patient in a comfortable position that provides easy access to the wound and will allow the irrigation solution to flow freely from the wound, with the assistance of gravity. Position a water-resistant disposable drape to protect the bedding from any possible runoff.

2. After washing and drying hands, apply a gown, face shield, and clean gloves.

Protects against splattering that may occur during wound irrigation.

3. Remove the soiled dressing. Dispose of gloves and soiled dressing in a biohazard bag.

Soiled dressings contain contaminants and should be treated as biohazardous waste.

4. Apply clean procedure gloves.

5. Place an emesis basin at the bottom of the wound to collect irrigation runoff. Avoid touching the wound with the basin.

Prevents contamination of wound from the emesis basin; protects linens from runoff.

6. Using a 19-gauge angiocatheter, remove the metal stylet needle and dispose into a sharps container. Attach the angiocatheter to a 35-mL syringe and fill with normal saline irrigation solution.

Prevents contamination and needlestick injury. A 19-gauge angiocatheter with a 35-mL syringe provides 8 psi (pounds per square inch) of pressure and is effective for removing bacteria, necrotic tissue, exudate, and/or metabolic wastes.

Note: This procedure follows guidelines established by the Agency for Healthcare Research Quality (AHRQ). Commercial irrigation kits containing a piston tip syringe may also be used. Their use is discussed in Procedure 34-3.

7. Holding the angiocatheter tip 2 cm from the wound bed; gently irrigate the wound with a back-and-forth motion, moving from the superior aspect to the inferior aspect.

Irrigating from top to bottom prevents flow of contaminated solution over the cleansed area. ▼

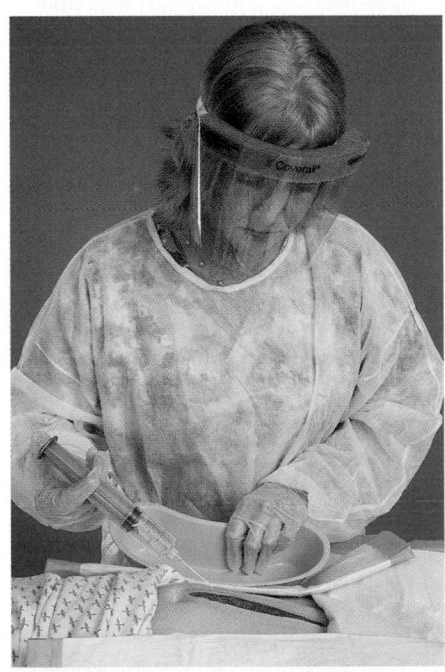

8. Dispose of the syringe and angiocatheter in the sharps container, and gloves in the biohazardous waste receptacle.

(continued on next page)

Procedure 34-1 ■ Obtaining a Wound Culture by Swab (continued)

Disposal into appropriate receptacles prevents contamination and needlestick injury.

9. Obtain a culturette tube, and twist the top of the tube to loosen the swab.

10. Apply clean procedure gloves, and locate an area of red, granulating tissue in the wound bed.

11. Withdraw the swab from the culturette tube. Press the swab against the granulating area with sufficient pressure to express fluid from the wound tissue, and rotate the swab.

    a. Do not allow the swab to touch anything other than the granulating area of the wound.

    b. Do not swab culture areas where slough or eschar is present.
These are areas of avascular or necrotic tissue and are contaminated with bacteria. Swab cultures detect only surface bacteria and are not a reliable means for diagnosing wound infection.

    c. Do not roll the swab around in a pool of exudative material.
Pus is a collection of white blood cells that have already done their work, and includes the microorganisms that have already died. Obtaining a culture from this material would not produce reliable culture result. The culture specimen must be of "tissue" or "tissue" fluid, not surface fluid or exudate. ▼

12. Carefully insert the swab back into the culturette tube, making sure it does not make contact with the opening of the tube upon reinsertion. Twist the cap to secure the tube.
Decreases risk of contamination; ensures that any microorganisms that grow in the culture are from the wound and were not introduced from the environment.

13. Crush the ampule of culture medium at the bottom of the tube. (*Note:* Inspect the culture tube to determine whether this step is required.)
The ampule contains medium for growth of microorganisms.

14. Label the culturette tube with the patient's name, birthdate, source of specimen, and date and time of collection.
Labeling ensures obtaining the results for the correct patient.

15. Transport the specimen for culture to the lab.

16. Apply a clean dressing to the wound as ordered.

What if . . .

■ **You determined this wound requires sterile technique?**

After removal of soiled dressing, apply sterile gloves for irrigating, obtaining culture, and applying new sterile dressing.

Sterile technique is used for acute surgical wounds and for wounds that have undergone recent, sharp débridement, or when the provider prescribes it.

■ **The culture tube is not sent to the lab within 72 hours?**

If the culture swab is not sent to the lab within 48 to 72 hours, it must be discarded. Be sure to check the policy within your institution.

The swab culture needs to be exposed to ideal laboratory conditions to allow microbial growth. If the culture sits on the unit too long, the culture medium might not produce reliable results. Most swab transport systems are validated for 48 to 72 hours after collection. However, if bacteria are suspected, the quicker the specimen is sent to the lab, the better.

■ **The wound care and culture supplies are kept on a common treatment cart?**

Common treatment carts should be left in the hall and not taken into individual rooms.

When a mobile cart is rolled into a room, it is a source for possible cross-contamination.

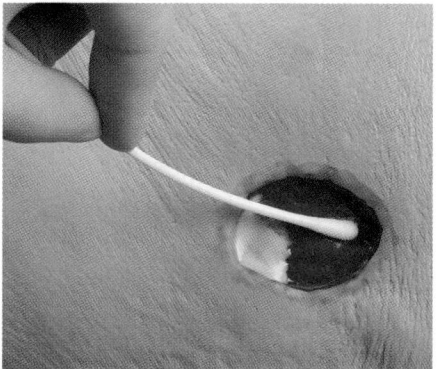

Evaluation

■ Assess patient's pain level. Medicate according to prescriptions.
■ Monitor lab reports for results of the swab culture.

Documentation

Document the following information (some agencies use a wound/skin flowsheet):
■ Appearance and location of the wound and surrounding tissue. Note type, consistency and amount of exudate, and odor, if present, after irrigation.
■ Patient's pain level before you obtained the culture
■ If the patient was medicated for pain, document the drug and dose used, time given, and patient response.
■ Method by which the wound was cleansed before you obtained the swab culture
■ Description of the area where the culture was obtained
■ Dressing reapplied to wound, if applicable
■ Education provided to the patient

Sample EHR documentation:

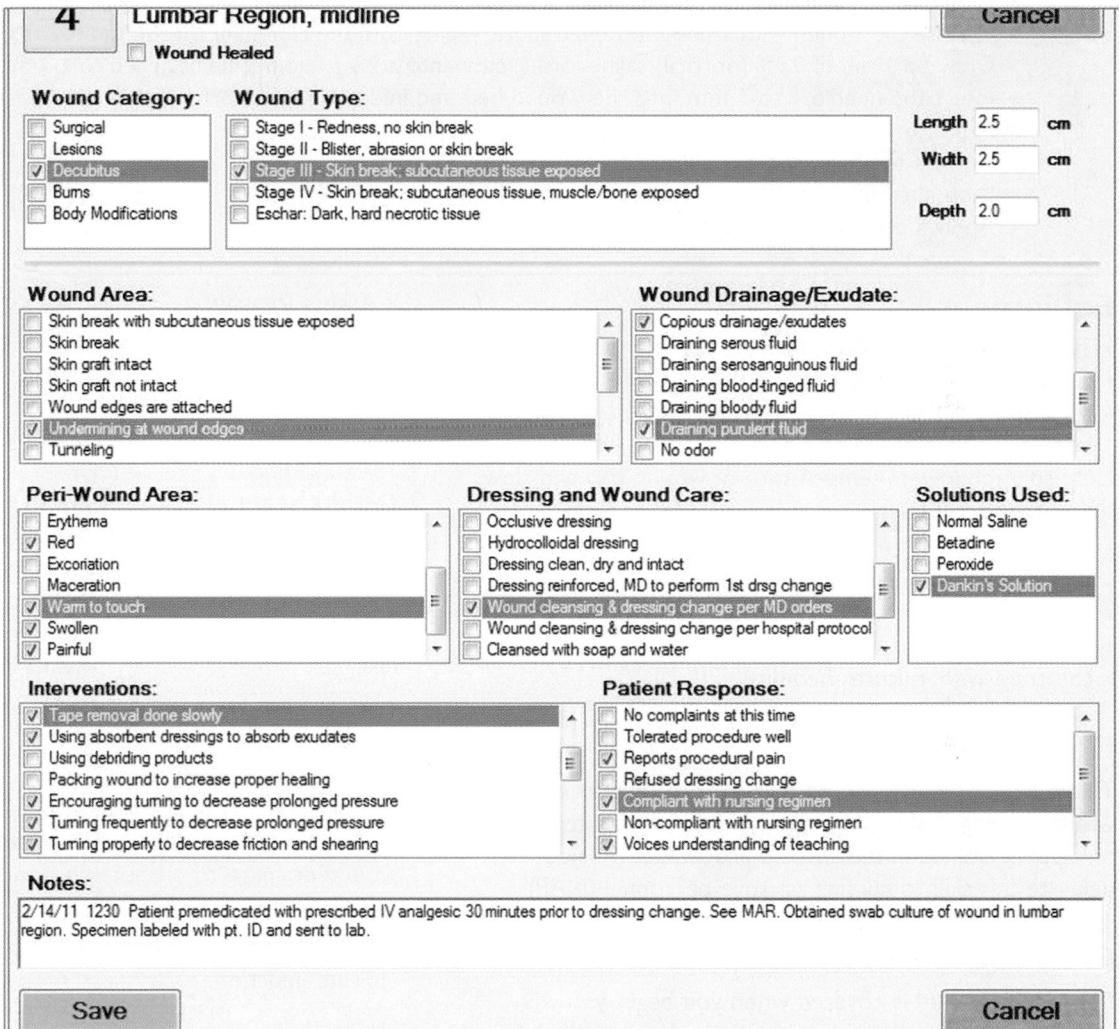

Practice Resources

Moore, Z., & Cowman, S. (2007); National Guideline Clearinghouse (2006, Dec, revised 2008 Dec); National Pressure Ulcer Advisory Panel (2007d).

Procedure 34-2 ▪ Obtaining a Needle Aspiration Culture from a Wound

➤ For steps to follow in *all* procedures, refer to the Universal Steps for All Procedures found on the inside back cover of Volume 2.

Note: This procedure uses modified sterile technique because wound care is now usually performed using a clean approach rather than sterile technique.

Critical Aspects

- Administer pain medication 30 minutes before the procedure, if necessary.
- Cleanse the wound with saline-moistened gauze, wiping from the center of the wound toward the edge.
- Draw up 1 mL of 0.9% (normal) saline for injection into a 22-gauge needle attached to a 3-mL syringe.
- Insert the needle 1 to 2 mm into the wound bed, and inject 1 mL of normal saline.
- Aspirate 1 mL of fluid from the wound bed.
- Express the fluid into the culture tube.
- Label the culture tube, and transport it to the lab.
- Apply a clean dressing to the wound as ordered.

Equipment

- Two pairs of clean procedure gloves
- Gown and face shield
- 0.9% (normal) saline solution for irrigation, warmed to body temperature when possible

Cold solution lowers temperature of wound bed and slows the healing process.

- Sterile 4 in. × 4 in. gauze pads in an impermeable tray
- Vial of 0.9% (normal) saline for injection
- 22-gauge needle
- 3-mL syringe
- Lab tube with culture medium

Delegation

This is an invasive procedure that requires knowledge of wound healing. It should be performed by a registered nurse or an LPN trained in the correct procedure. Do not delegate this skill to nursing assistive personnel (NAP).

Pre-Procedure Assessments

Note: If the wound is covered when you begin, you will make these assessments when you remove the soiled dressing *and* after cleansing the wound.

- Assess for pain.

Wounds may be painful, and wound irrigation may increase pain. Provide prescribed pain medication 30 minutes before performing the procedure, as indicated.

- Assess the amount and type of tissue present in the wound bed.

Granulating tissue is beefy red with a velvety appearance. It appears with the growth of new blood vessels and connective tissue. Pale pink tissue may indicate compromised blood supply to the wound bed. Necrotic tissue, which is black, brown, or yellow in appearance, is nonviable and inhibits healing.

- Assess the type and amount of exudate.

Exudate may be a sign of infection.

- Assess the wound for odor.

A foul odor may indicate infection. Cleanse wounds before you assess for odor, because some dressings interact with wound drainage to produce an odor.

- Assess the tissue surrounding the wound edge.

Surrounding tissue that is red, warm, and/or edematous may indicate infection.

➤ When performing the procedure, always identify your patient according to agency policy and be attentive to standard precautions, hand hygiene, patient safety and privacy, body mechanics, and documentation.

Procedure Steps

1. Position the patient so the wound is easily accessible. Position a water-resistant disposable drape under the patient to collect fluid runoff.

A drape protects the linens.

2. After washing and drying your hands, apply a gown, face shield, and clean gloves.

Protects you from splattering of contaminated bodily fluid or drainage.

3. Remove the soiled dressing. Dispose of gloves and soiled dressing in a biohazardous waste bag.

Soiled dressings contain wound exudate, blood, or debris and should be treated as biohazardous waste.

4. Open a tray of sterile 4 in. × 4 in. gauze. Moisten the gauze with normal saline solution for irrigation.

The sterile container tray is impermeable.

5. Attach a 22-gauge needle to a 3-mL syringe, and aspirate 1 mL of sterile normal saline from the vial. Cap the needle, using a one-handed technique (see Procedure 23–10), and place the syringe on the bedside table.
Maintains sterility and prevents needlestick injury.

6. Apply sterile gloves.
Reduces the incidence of introducing microorganisms into the wound to be cultured.

7. Gently cleanse the wound with the saline-moistened gauze by lightly wiping a section of the wound from the center toward the wound edge. Discard the gauze in a biohazard receptacle, and repeat in the next section using a new piece of gauze with each wiping pass.
Removes surface bacteria and exudate. ▼

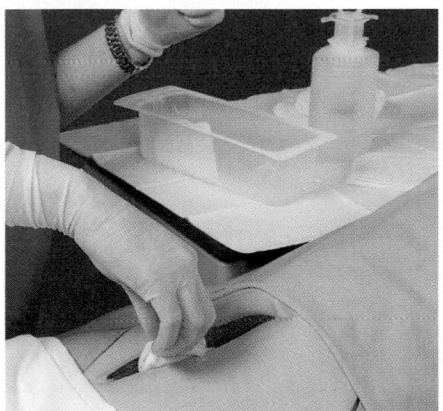

8. Uncap the syringe from the bedside table, and insert the needle 1 to 2 mm into the wound bed. Inject 1 mL of normal saline into the wound tissue.
Allows for an adequate amount of culture fluid to be aspirated. ▼

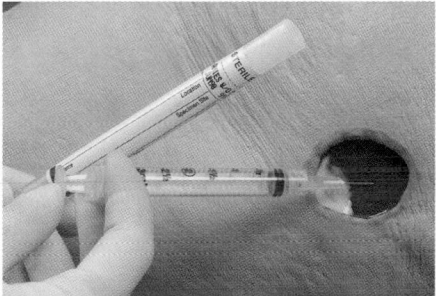

9. Pull back on the syringe plunger to aspirate approximately 0.5 to 1.0 mL of fluid into the barrel of the syringe. Remove the needle from the wound bed after you have collected the aspirate.
This method assesses for bacteria within the tissue, rather than surface colonization.

10. Place the collected fluid into a culture tube containing culture medium.
Culture medium supports the growth of microorganisms. ▼

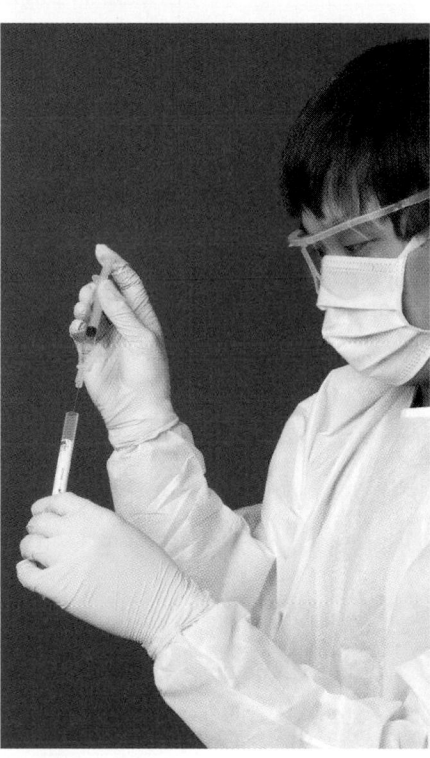

11. Label the culture tube with the patient's name, birthdate, source of specimen, and date and time of collection. (A label may be supplied with the culture kit.)
Labeling ensures obtaining culture results for the correct patient.

12. Transport the specimen for culture to the lab.

13. Apply a clean dressing to the wound as ordered.

What if. . .

■ **The wound is covered in eschar or slough?**

Since only red granulating tissue is appropriate for culture, you would need to consult the primary care provider.

■ **The wound had deep tunneling or sinus tracts?**

These types of wounds may provide an oxygen-depleted environment that could allow proliferation of anaerobic microbes. You may need to culture this type of wound for both aerobic and anaerobic microorganisms.

■ **The wound covers a large surface area?**

Large wounds should have separate cultures taken from different areas of the wound bed.

(continued on next page)

Procedure 34-2 ▪ **Obtaining a Needle Aspiration Culture from a Wound** (continued)

Evaluation

- Determine whether the patient remains comfortable. If not, medicate as prescribed.
- Monitor the wound bed at the puncture site for evidence of bleeding.
- Monitor lab reports for results of the aspirate culture.

Documentation

Document the following information (many agencies use a wound/skin flowsheet):

- Appearance and location of the wound and surrounding tissue. Note type, consistency and amount of exudate, and odor, if present, after irrigation.
- Length, width, and depth of wound when the patient's condition changes or at regular intervals
- The patient's pain level before and after you obtained the culture
- If the patient was medicated for pain, document the drug and dose used, time given, and patient response.
- Method by which the wound was cleansed before you obtained the aspiration culture
- Description of the area where the culture was obtained
- Dressing reapplied to wound, if applicable
- Education provided to patient

Sample documentation:

> 09/14/12   1620   *Patient reports tenderness at the wound site at the right lateral edge of abdominal incision approximately 9 days post-op. Incision well approximated except for 2 cm area with malodorous exudate with purulent material noted. Surrounding skin tissue slightly edematous with erythema. Wound cleansed with saline soaked gauze q 6 hours per surgeon's prescription. Fine needle aspiration with 22-gauge needle inserted at a 60° angle into the wound bed. No bleeding noted at the puncture site. Aspirated 0.7 mL purulent exudate. Sent for culture. Wound redressed with hydrocolloid dressing. Patient tolerated procedure with report of minimal pain.*——————— *S. Burback, RN*

Practice Resources

Myers, B. A. (2008); National Guideline Clearinghouse (2006, Dec, revised 2008 Dec); National Pressure Ulcer Advisory Panel (2007d); Sussman, C., & Bates-Jensen, B. M. (2007).

Procedure 34-3 ▪ **Performing a Sterile Wound Irrigation**

➤ For steps to follow in *all* procedures, refer to the Universal Steps for All Procedures found on the inside back cover of Volume 2.

Critical Aspects

- Administer pain medication 30 minutes before the procedure, if necessary.
- Position the patient for easy access to the wound and in a manner that will allow the irrigation solution to flow freely from the wound with the assistance of gravity.
- Don protective equipment: gown, face shield, and clean gloves.
- Remove the soiled dressing, and dispose of gloves.
- Set up a sterile field with a sterile irrigation kit or a 35-mL syringe and a 19-gauge angiocatheter (needle removed), dressing supplies, and irrigation solution.
- Wearing sterile gloves, fill either the syringe and angiocatheter or the piston-tip syringe with irrigation solution.
- Holding the syringe 2 cm (¾ to 1 in.) from the wound bed, gently irrigate the wound with a back-and-forth motion, moving from the superior aspect to the inferior aspect.
- Dry the tissue surrounding the wound with sterile gauze.
- Apply a new dressing as ordered.
- Dispose of used equipment and soiled dressings in a biohazardous waste container.
- Reposition the patient.

Equipment

- Clean gloves
- Sterile gloves
- Gown and face shield
- Water-resistant, disposable drapes
- Tepid (body temperature) irrigation solution
- Cold solution lowers temperature of wound bed and slows the healing process.
- Sterile gauze
- Dressing supplies
- Biohazardous waste container
- Sterile impermeable barrier
- Sterile bowl

For Step 10A Variation:

- Sterile emesis basin
- 35-mL syringe
- 19-gauge angiocatheter (needle removed)

For Step 10B Variation:

- Sterile commercial irrigation kit containing a sterile basin and piston-tip syringe

Delegation

This is an invasive, sterile procedure that requires nursing assessment, judgment, evaluation, and teaching during the procedure. It requires knowledge of wound healing and should be performed by a registered nurse. Do not delegate this skill to nursing assistive personnel (NAP).

Pre-Procedure Assessments

Note: If the wound is covered when you begin, you will make these assessments when you remove the soiled dressing *and* after cleansing the wound.

- Assess the amount and type of tissue present in the wound bed.

Granulating tissue is beefy red with a velvety appearance. It appears with the growth of new blood vessels and connective tissue. Pale pink tissue may indicate a delay in wound healing due to compromised blood supply to the wound bed or lack of proper nutrition. Necrotic tissue, which is black, brown, or yellow in appearance, is nonviable and inhibits healing and is a source of bacterial growth.

- **Determine whether the wound requires sterile, modified sterile, or clean technique for irrigation.**

Irrigation helps wounds to heal because it removes bacteria, old drainage, and necrotic tissue from the wound bed. Sterile technique is used for acute surgical wounds, for wounds that have undergone recent sharp débridement, or when the primary care provider has ordered it. Chronic wounds are colonized with bacteria and may be irrigated with clean technique. Irrigation using clean technique is presented in steps 1 through 7 of Procedure 34-1.

- Assess the wound for signs of infection (erythema, induration, amount and type of drainage).

Exudate may be a sign of infection. Infected wounds require higher flow pressures for irrigation.

- Assess the wound for odor.

A foul odor may indicate infection. Cleanse wounds before you assess for odor, because some dressings interact with wound drainage to produce an odor.

- Assess the tissue surrounding the wound edge.

Surrounding tissue that is red, warm, and/or edematous may indicate infection. Tissue that is macerated (white and moist) indicates too much fluid is being held against the skin, usually from saturated dressings.

- Assess for pain.

Wound irrigation may be very painful.

> When performing the procedure, always identify your patient according to agency policy and be attentive to standard precautions, hand hygiene, patient safety and privacy, body mechanics, and documentation.

Procedure Steps

1. Administer pain medication 30 minutes before the treatment, if necessary.

2. Place the patient in a comfortable position that provides easy access to the wound and will allow the irrigation solution to flow freely from the wound, with the assistance of gravity. Position a water-resistant disposable drape to protect the bedding from any possible runoff.

3. After washing and drying your hands, apply a gown, face shield, and clean gloves.

Personal protective equipment (PPE) provides a barrier against splattering that commonly occurs during wound irrigation.

4. Remove the soiled dressing. Dispose of gloves and soiled dressing in a biohazard bag.

Soiled dressings contain body fluids and other contaminants and should be treated as biohazardous waste.

5. Set up a sterile field on a clean, dry surface. Add the following supplies to the field based on the type of irrigation to be performed:

Sterile gauze
Sterile bowl
Dressing supplies
A sterile commercial irrigation kit, *or* a 19-gauge angiocatheter, 35-mL syringe, and sterile emesis basin.

Setting up a sterile field at bedside provides easy access to equipment for irrigation and reduces the risk for contamination when retrieving supplies after getting started. ▼

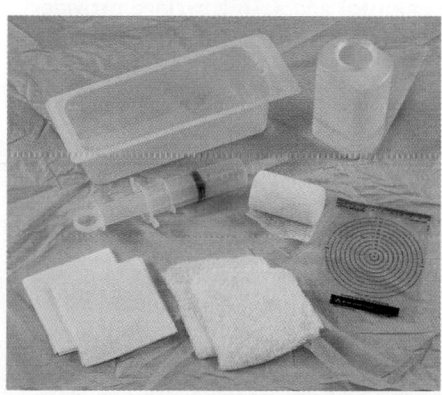

(continued on next page)

Procedure 34-3 ■ **Performing a Sterile Wound Irrigation** (continued)

6. Select irrigation solution based on the wound assessment, goals of therapy and primary care provider's orders. Running water is the solution of choice unless the patient is immunocompromised. ✚ Do not use povidone-iodine (Betadine), if the patient has an iodine allergy.

Common antiseptic solutions can be more harmful to healing tissues than to bacteria. Though effective in some conditions and against limited bacteria, hydrogen peroxide, acetic acid, povidone-iodine, and sodium hypochlorite solutions, in standard dilutions, are all toxic to fibroblasts and white blood cells Commercial wound-cleansing solutions also contain antimicrobial ingredients that can damage wound cells.

7. Pour the tepid (room temperature) irrigation solution into the sterile bowl.
Local cooling of wound tissues impairs healing. This can occur if you irrigate with refrigerated solutions and change dressings frequently.

8. Don sterile gloves.
Gloving maintains sterile technique.

9. Place the sterile basin at the bottom of the wound to collect irrigation runoff.

10. Fill the irrigation syringe.

Step 10 Variation. Using an Angiocatheter
a. Attach the 19-gauge angiocatheter (with needle removed) to the 35 mL syringe, and fill with the irrigation solution.
A 19-gauge angiocatheter (with needle removed) and 35-mL syringe provides 8 psi of pressure and is effective for removing bacteria, necrotic tissue, exudate, and/or metabolic wastes.

Step 10 Variation. Using a Piston-Tip Syringe
b. Fill a piston-tip syringe with irrigation solution.

11. Holding the angiocatheter tip or syringe tip 2 cm from the wound bed, gently irrigate the wound with a back-and-forth motion, moving from the superior aspect to the inferior aspect.
Irrigating from top to bottom prevents flow of contaminated solution over cleansed area. Irrigating a clean, noninfected wound with gentle low-pressure (8 psi) reduces disruption of the healthy, healing tissue. Irrigating an infected wound, with higher flow (but < 15 psi) selectively débrides necrotic tissue while protecting healthy tissue. ▼

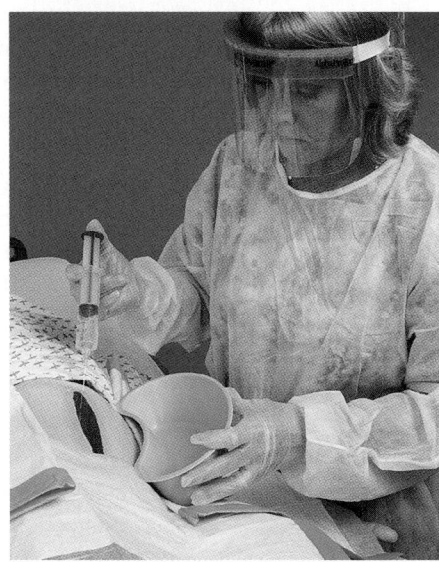

a. Ensure any undermining or tunnelling is irrigated as well.
b. Repeat the irrigation until the solution returns clear.
Flushing removes exudate, debris, and some surface bacteria.

12. Remove the basin or sterile container from the base of the wound.

13. Pat the skin surrounding the wound dry with sterile gauze, beginning at the top of the wound and working downward.
Moisture on the surrounding tissue may lead to maceration and further breakdown of the wound margins.

14. Dress the wound as prescribed.

15. Consider applying a waterproof skin protectant around the wound if drainage is heavy.
Wound drainage contains irritating chemicals that can damage healthy tissues, especially at the wound edge and surrounding skin. Solutions used to keep the wound bed moist can also macerate or damage healthy skin if allowed to remain on intact skin.

16. Dispose of the contaminated irrigation fluid in a biohazardous receptacle.
Contaminated fluid should be disposed of as biohazardous waste.

17. Remove soiled drapes from the patient area.

18. Remove your gloves, face shield, and gown. Dispose of these items appropriately.
Contaminants from the irrigation may be present on these items, and they should also be considered biohazardous.

19. Reposition the patient to a comfortable position.

20. Wash your hands.
Hand hygiene prevents cross-contamination.

What if. . .

■ **The client has a wound covering a large area of the body?**

A general rule is that the larger the wound, the more solution needed to clean it.

Remember that the purpose of cleansing a wound is to remove bacteria and debris by flushing the wound.

■ **Peroxide or another antiseptic solution is prescribed?**

First, identify the reason that the solution was ordered for the wound type. Then identify the length of time it is to be used. Weigh the benefit of using the solution with the potential risks to healing tissues. Finally, discuss any concerns with the primary care provider.

✚ Peroxide is indicated more for acute, traumatic wounds to remove dirt and other debris. Peroxide and other commercial antiseptics can damage fibroblasts, and cause air embolism if used to forcefully irrigate or pack a tunneling wound. Fibroblasts produce collagen, the major structural protein of skin and healing tissues.

Evaluation

- Determine whether the patient remains comfortable. If not, medicate according to prescriptions.
- Reassess the wound at regular intervals.

Patient Teaching

- Answer any questions the patient may have.
- Teach the patient about the expected healing process.
- Inform the patient and caregiver about signs and symptoms of infection and the need to report these findings.

Home Care

- Wound irrigation is commonly done in the home. In most cases, clean technique is used in the home setting.
- Irrigation solutions, such as saline, can be made and stored up to 7 days if refrigerated.
- Review with the family proper disposal of contaminated supplies.

Documentation

Document the following information (many agencies use a wound/skin flowsheet):

- Appearance and location of the wound, size, tissue in wound base, periwound tissue, type and amount of exudate, and odor, if present, after irrigation
- The patient's pain level. If the patient was medicated for pain, document the drug and dose used, time given, and patient response.
- Method by which the wound was cleansed
- Dressing reapplied to the wound, if applicable
- Education provided to the patient

Sample documentation:

> *02/22/12 0800 Dressing change to sacral wound using modified sterile technique due to saturation of old dressing with serous drainage. Patient premedicated with Lortab 5 mg PO 30 minutes prior to dressing change. Wound irrigated with normal saline using 19-gauge needle-less angiocatheter and 35-cc syringe. Wound re-packed with saline-moistened fluffed gauze and ABD to cover. Healing Stage IV pressure ulcer with 100% granulation tissue to the wound bed; 4 X 3.5 cm, with 1 cm of undermining at 6:00; copious serous drainage though no odor was noted. Periwound is slightly macerated; therefore zinc-based barrier cream applied for protection. Patient reported no pain with procedure. Will continue to monitor and change dressing as needed.* ——— L. Syzmanski, RN

Practice Resources

Bergstrom, N., Bennett, M. A., Carlson, C., et al. (1994); Hess, C. T. (2007); Myers, B. A. (2008); Rolstad, B. S., & Ovington, L. G. (2007); Stotts, N. A., & Gunningberg, L. (2007).

Procedure 34-4 ■ Taping a Dressing

➤ For steps to follow in *all* procedures, refer to the Universal Steps for All Procedures found on the inside back cover of Volume 2.

Note: This procedure uses clean technique because wound care is now usually performed using a clean, rather than sterile, technique.

Critical Aspects

- Place the patient in a comfortable position that provides easy access to the wound.
- Ensure skin surrounding the dressing is clean and dry.
- Choose a tape that is appropriate for the dressing.
- Place tape parallel to the incision.
- Tear strips that extend ½ inch beyond the dressing.
- Apply tape without pulling or stretching.
- Smooth tape in place by gently stroking the surface to maximize adhesion.

Equipment

- Procedure gloves
- Tape (cloth, plastic, foam, silk-like, etc.)

Delegation

As a nurse, you are responsible for assessing the wound and evaluating interventions. However, this procedure may be delegated to nursing assistive personnel (NAP).

(continued on next page)

Procedure 34-4 ■ **Taping a Dressing** (continued)

Pre-Procedure Assessments

■ **Assess the degree of importance of the dressing.**
The more critical the dressing, the more adhesion required.

■ **Assess the characteristics the dressing material, weight and conformability, and the device or tubing to be held.**
Heavier dressings require higher adhesion. Bulky dressings may need high conformability or greater adhesion.

■ **Assess the skin surface (i.e., dry, damp, diaphoretic, oily, hairy, edematous, fragile, or impaired skin integrity).**
Fragile skin may require less adhesion while damp or oily skim may require higher adhesion.

■ **Assess the anticipated wear time.**
Tape adhesion gets stronger over time. Breathable tapes can be used longer. Occlusive plastic tapes build up moisture and are used when adhesion is intended for a shorter period of time.

■ **Assess the patient's history and current medical conditions.**
Review allergies or sensitivities to tapes. Review medical conditions that be may affected by adhesives.

■ **Assess for activity level of the patient and the anticipated length of time the dressing will be needed.**
The more active the patient, the more adhesion required.

➤ When performing the procedure, always identify your patient according to agency policy and be attentive to standard precautions, hand hygiene, patient safety and privacy, body mechanics, and documentation.

Procedure Steps

1. Wash your hands. Don gloves.

2. Choose the type of tape based on wound size, location, amount of drainage or edema, frequency of dressing changes, patient's activity level, and type of dressings used.
Tapes come in many different adhesive types and backings. Select the tape based on individual characteristics.

 a. Choose tape of the width that is appropriate for the size of the dressing. The larger the dressing, the wider the tape needed for securing.
For example, a large abdominal dressing may require 3-inch tape, whereas a small incision on an extremity may need only ½-inch tape.

 b. Choose a tape that stretches if the area is at risk for distention, edema, hematoma formation, or movement.
Skin distention under tape may cause blistering or skin tears.

3. Tear strips that extend ½ inch beyond the dressing.
To anchor the dressing to the skin.

4. Place the tape perpendicular to the incision.
Fewer skin tension injuries occur with taping perpendicular to the incision.

 a. When taping over joints, apply the tape at a right angle to the direction of joint movement, or at a right angle to a body crease. For example, tape a shoulder or knee horizontally, not lengthwise.
 b. Apply tape with an even amount tension on both sides, being careful not to pull at the edges.
This reduces the risk of skin damage.

5. Smooth tape in place by gently stroking the surface to maximize adhesion.

6. Replace tape if site becomes edematous, or the skin is not intact.

What if. . .

■ **The tape will not adhere to the patient's skin due to excess hair?**
Remove the hair with clippers or scissors. Do not shave the site with a razor.
 Shaving can cause nicks or abrasions to the skin that could become a portal of entry for bacteria.

■ **The patient's skin is diaphoretic or excessively oily?**
Cleanse the skin with soap and water before the dressing change. You may use polymer skin barriers to place a seal over the skin and allow the tape adhesive to adhere.

■ **The patient has fragile skin (e.g., older adult)?**
Use skin sealant preparations under adhesives. Use the least adhesive product possible for the need.
 The junction between the epidermis and dermis on the older adult is not as strong as in a younger person.

■ **The patient is allergic to tape adhesives?**
Use hypoallergenic products.
 Circular wraps, ace bandages, or other such products may be used to secure dressings.

Evaluation

- Verify type of tape that is appropriate for the patient and dressing.
- Note whether the tape adheres comfortably to the skin.
- Ensure that the patient verbalized understanding of the treatment.
- Inspect the dressing daily for intactness, edema, or hematoma.

Patient Teaching

- Teach the patient about the expected healing process.
- Educate the patient about the purpose of the procedure.
- Instruct the patient to keep the dressing dry.

Documentation

Document the following information (many agencies use a wound/skin flowsheet):

- Type of dressing and tape applied
- Location and characteristics of wound
- Education given to patient

Sample documentation:

> 02/16/12   0900   *Dressing applied to left hip incision using conformable cloth tape. Wound edges are well approximated with no drainage noted. Periwound skin is dry and intact, without erythema, induration, or odor. Wound cleaned with normal saline using sterile technique. Educated patient on the purpose of the dressing and expected outcomes. Will continue to monitor.* ——————— *B. Hopkins, RN*

Practice Resources

3M (2004); Association of periOperative Registered Nurses (2008); Fletcher, R. K. (1999).

Procedure 34-5   Removing and Applying Dry Dressings

➤ For steps to follow in *all* procedures, refer to the Universal Steps for All Procedures found on the inside back cover of Volume 2.

Note: This procedure uses clean technique because wound care is now usually performed using clean rather than sterile technique.

Critical Aspects

- Administer pain medication 30 minutes before the procedure, if necessary.
- Place the patient in a comfortable position that provides easy access to the wound.
- Wearing clean gloves, remove the soiled dressing and discard it in a biohazard receptacle.
- Change gloves.
- Cleanse the wound with saline-moistened gauze.
- Assess the wound for location, appearance, odor, and drainage.
- Don clean procedure gloves and apply a dry dressing.
- Secure the dressing with tape.

Equipment

- Three pairs of clean nonsterile gloves
- Sterile normal saline solution for irrigation, warmed to body temperature when possible

Cold solution lowers the temperature of wound bed and slows the healing process.

- Tray of sterile 4 in. × 4 in. gauze
- Sterile gauze for dressings
- Tape

Delegation

This procedure requires knowledge of wound healing. It should be performed by a registered nurse. Do not delegate this skill.

Pre-Procedure Assessments

Note: When you begin, the wound will likely be covered with a dressing. You will make these assessments when you remove the soiled dressing *and* after cleansing the wound.

- Assess for pain at least 30 minutes before performing the procedure.

Wounds may be very painful. Provide pain medication 30 minutes before performing the procedure if needed, to allow the medication time to be distributed in target tissues. Changes in the quality or severity of pain are some symptoms linked with infection.

- Assess the type and amount of exudate.

Exudate may be a sign of infection.

(continued on next page)

Procedure 34-5 ■ Removing and Applying Dry Dressings (continued)

■ Assess the wound for odor.
A foul odor may indicate infection. Clean wounds before you assess for odor, because some dressings interact with wound drainage to produce an odor.

■ Assess the tissue surrounding the wound edge.
Surrounding tissue that is red, warm, and/or edematous may indicate infection.

■ Determine the type of dressing needed.
The type of dressing depends on the characteristics of the wound and the goal of treatment. Dry dressings are appropriate when there is no need to keep the wound bed moist, such as a wound healing by primary intention or a wound covered by eschar.

➤ When performing the procedure, always identify your patient according to agency policy and be attentive to standard precautions, hand hygiene, patient safety and privacy, body mechanics, and documentation.

Procedure Steps for Removing the Dressing

1. Place the patient in a comfortable position that provides easy access to the wound.
Provides for patient comfort and proper nurse body mechanics during dressing change.

2. Wash your hands, and apply clean nonsterile gloves.
Handwashing is one of the most important measures for preventing infection transmission.

3. Gently loosen the edges of the tape of the old dressing at an angle parallel to the skin. Hold that edge with one hand and gently raise the edge until it is taut, but not pulling on the skin. Using your other hand, push down on the exposed skin at the point where the tape and skin meet. Push the skin off of the tape.
The pull–push method will help prevent skin stripping from the adhesive and reduce discomfort and skin trauma as you remove the tape.

4. Beginning at the edges of the dressing, lift the dressing toward the center of the wound. If the dressing sticks, moisten it with normal saline before removing it completely.
Moistening the dressing decreases the risk of bleeding and/or removal of granulating tissue.

5. Assess the type and amount of drainage on the soiled dressing.
Allows for evaluation of wound healing. Purulent drainage is an indication of infection.

6. Dispose of the soiled dressing and gloves in a biohazard receptacle.
Soiled dressings contain bodily fluids and other contaminants and should be disposed of as biohazardous waste.

7. Remove the cover of a tray of sterile 4 in. × 4 in. gauze. Moisten the gauze with sterile saline.
The sterile container tray is impermeable and allows you to moisten the gauze while maintaining sterility. Gauze will not shed fibers into the wound (as do cotton balls). Fibers and any other foreign bodies in a wound promote inflammation and delay healing.

8. Apply clean nonsterile gloves.

9. Gather a gauze pad by pulling the four corners up toward the middle. Use the center ball of the gauze to cleanse the wound.
Forming a ball with the gauze pads prevents contamination of gloved hands during cleansing.

10. Gently cleanse the wound with the saline-moistened gauze by lightly wiping a section of the wound. Wipe from the center toward the wound edge or from top to bottom or dirty to clean, depending on the wound. Repeat as needed, discarding the gauze in a biohazard receptacle, using a new piece of gauze with each wiping pass.
Removes surface bacteria and exudate. Prevents transfer of microorganisms from the surrounding skin into the wound.

11. Discard the gloves and soiled gauze into a biohazard bag.

12. Reassess wound for size, color of tissue present, amount and type of exudate, and odor.

Procedure Steps for Applying Dry Dressing

13. Wash your hands, or use an antiseptic handrub at the bedside.

14. Open sterile gauze packages on a clean, dry surface.
Maintains sterility of gauze. ▼

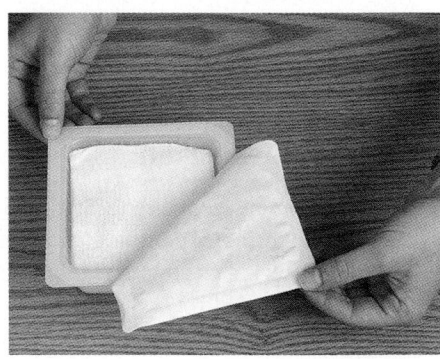

15. Apply clean nonsterile gloves.

16. Apply a layer of dry dressings over the wound. If drainage is expected, use an additional layer of dressings.
The first layer serves as a wick for drainage. A second layer is needed if increased absorption is required.

17. Place strips of tape at the ends of the dressing and evenly spaced over the remainder of the dressing. Use strips that are sufficiently long to secure the dressing in place. Tape the dressing around all edges, "window paning," if appropriate.

Edges remain taped down and dressing stays intact. ▼

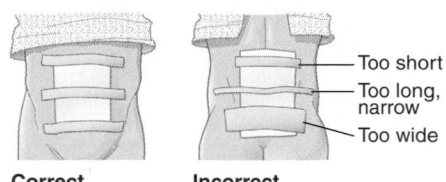

Correct   **Incorrect**

Too short
Too long, narrow
Too wide

18. Remove gloves, turning them inside out, and discard them in a biohazard receptacle.

19. Assist the patient to a comfortable position.

What if . . .

■ **Signs of infection are noted with wound assessment?**

Notify the primary care provider. Cultures, wound care interventions, and potentially even antibiotics may be required.

■ **The wound is not approximated?**

Place the patient in a supine position, apply Steri-Strips™, and cover with sterile saline dressings. Notify primary care provider.

This could indicate wound dehiscence.

■ **The skin surrounding the incision is not intact?**

Clean the area with sterile saline, dry thoroughly, and apply protective moisture barrier dressing. Consider using Montgomery straps.

Montgomery straps are useful when dressings must be changed frequently because they do not cause trauma to the skin.

■ **A drain or drainage tube is present?**

Always clean the drain site after cleaning the primary incision site.

Reduces the risk of cross contamination.

Evaluation

■ Determine whether the dressing is clean, dry, and intact.
■ Verify that the patient experienced minimal discomfort during the procedure.

Patient Teaching

■ Teach the patient about the expected healing process.
■ Inform the patient and caregiver about the signs and symptoms of infection and the need to report these findings.

Home Care

■ Help the client to store dressings appropriately to keep them clean, for example, in a plastic container with a lid.
■ Teach the client or caregivers to dispose of contaminated dressings and gloves by double-bagging them in moisture-proof bags (e.g., plastic grocery bags).
■ Advise the client and family whether they can get the wound wet (e.g., during bathing). If it must be kept dry, demonstrate how to cover it with a waterproof barrier (e.g., a plastic bag).

Documentation

Document the following information (many agencies use a wound/skin flowsheet):
■ Appearance and location of the wound, type and amount of exudate, and odor, if present, after cleansing

■ The patient's pain level before the procedure. If the patient was medicated for pain, document the drug and dose used, time given, and patient response.
■ Method of cleansing the wound
■ Type of dressing applied to the wound
■ Education provided to the patient

Sample documentation:

> 09/27/12 1500   *Pt. with no c/o pain. Gauze dressing removed from lateral aspect of right forearm without difficulty. No drainage noted on gauze. Surrounding skin intact. Abrasion on right, lateral forearm cleansed with normal saline. Sterile gauze dressing reapplied to wound and anchored with cloth tape. Pt. instructed to report any changes noted at wound site, such as bleeding, drainage, or increase in pain.* ——— *D. Enferma, RN*

Practice Resources
Atiyeh, B. S., & Hayek, S. N. (2004); Dunaway, E., & Goldrick, B. A. (2007); The Joanna Briggs Institute (2002); National Pressure Ulcer Advisory Panel (2007d).

Thinking About the Procedure

 Go to the *Fundamentals of Nursing Skills Videos*, **Wound Care: Dressings: Dry.**

1. What kind of personal protective equipment did the nurse don to protect herself from infection when changing the patient's bandage?

2. What should the nurse do to remove the dressing if it sticks to the wound?

 For suggested responses, go to Chapter 34, **Thinking About the Procedure Suggested Responses (Procedure 34-5),** on the Student Resource Disk or DavisPlus at http://davisplus.fadavis.com/Wilkinson2

Procedure 34-6   Removing and Applying Wet-to-Damp Dressings

➤ For steps to follow in *all* procedures, refer to the Universal Steps for All Procedures found on the inside back cover of Volume 2.

Note: This procedure uses clean technique because wound care is now usually done using a clean or modified sterile approach rather than sterile technique. However, sterile technique is recommended for wounds that have recently had sharp débridement, have a drain, or are fresh surgical wounds.

Critical Aspects

- Assess for pain, and medicate 30 minutes before procedure, if necessary.
- Place the patient in a comfortable position that provides easy access to the wound.
- Wearing clean gloves, remove the soiled dressing and discard it in a biohazard receptacle.
- Change gloves and cleanse the wound with saline-moistened gauze.
- Assess the wound for location, appearance, odor, and drainage.
- Don clean gloves and apply a single layer of moist, fine-mesh gauze to the wound. Be sure to place gauze in all depressions of the wound.
- Apply a secondary moist layer over the first layer. Repeat this process until the wound is filled with moistened sterile gauze.
- Cover the moistened gauze with a surgical pad.
- Secure the dressing with tape or Montgomery straps.

Equipment

- Three pairs of clean nonsterile gloves
- Sterile solution for irrigation, warmed to body temperature when possible

Cold solution reduces the temperature of wound bed and slows the healing process.

- Water-resistant disposable drapes
- Sterile fine-mesh gauze in a tray for dressing
- Surgipad
- Tape or Montgomery straps

Delegation

This is an invasive procedure that requires knowledge of wound healing. It should be performed by a registered nurse. Do not delegate this skill to nursing assistive personnel (NAP).

Pre-Procedure Assessment

Note: When you begin, the wound will likely be covered with a dressing. You will make these assessments when you remove the soiled dressing *and* after cleansing the wound.

- Assess the amount and type of tissue present in the wound bed.

Granulating tissue is beefy red with a velvety appearance. It appears with the growth of new blood vessels and connective tissue. Pale pink tissue may indicate compromised blood supply to the wound bed. Necrotic tissue, which is black, brown, or yellow in appearance, is nonviable and inhibits healing.

- Assess the type and amount of exudate.

Exudate may be a sign of infection.

- Assess the wound for odor.

A foul odor may indicate infection. Clean wounds before you assess for odor, because some dressings interact with wound drainage to produce an odor.

- Assess the tissue surrounding the wound edge.

Surrounding tissue that is red, warm, and/or edematous may indicate infection.

- Assess for pain.

Wounds may be very painful. Assess for pain and provide prescribed pain medication 30 minutes before performing procedure, if needed. A change in the quality or intensity of pain may be a sign of infection.

➤ When performing the procedure, always identify your patient according to agency policy and be attentive to standard precautions, hand hygiene, patient safety and privacy, body mechanics, and documentation.

Procedure Steps for Removing the Wet-to-Damp Dressing

1. Place the patient in a comfortable position that provides easy access to the wound.

Provides for patient comfort during dressing change.

2. Wash your hands, and apply clean gloves.

Handwashing complies with standard precautions, helping to prevent transfer of pathogens.

3. Gently loosen the edges of the tape of the old dressing. Hold that edge with one hand and gently raise the edge until it is taut, but not pulling on the skin. Using your other hand, push down on the exposed skin at the point where the tape and skin meet. Push the skin off of the tape.

The pull–push method will help prevent skin stripping from the adhesive and reduce discomfort and skin trauma as you remove the tape.

4. Beginning with the top layer, lift the dressing from the corner toward the center of the wound. If the dressing sticks, moisten it with normal saline or tap water before completely removing it. Remove first from one side of the wound, first toward the wound, and then from the other side. Continue to remove layers until you have removed the entire dressing.

Moistening the dressing decreases the risk of bleeding and/or removal of granulating tissue. ▼

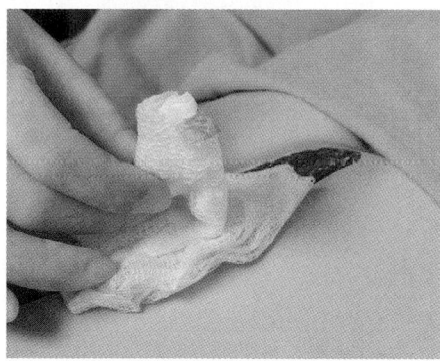

5. Assess the type and amount of drainage present on the soiled dressing.

Type of drainage is an indication of the stage of healing. Purulent drainage is an indication of infection.

6. Dispose of the soiled dressing and gloves in a biohazard container. Wash your hands.

Soiled dressings contain body fluids contaminants and should be disposed of as biohazardous waste.

7. Remove the cover of a tray of sterile 4 in. × 4 in. gauze. Moisten the gauze with sterile saline or water.

The sterile container tray is impermeable and allows you to

moisten the gauze while maintaining sterility.

8. Apply clean procedure gloves.

Avoids introducing microorganisms into the wound.

9. Gather a gauze pad by pulling the four corners up toward the middle. Use the center of the gauze to cleanse the wound.

Prevents contamination of your gloves during wound cleansing.

10. Gently cleanse the wound with the saline- or water-moistened gauze by lightly wiping a section of the wound from the center toward the wound edge. Discard the gauze in a biohazard receptacle, and repeat in the next section using a new piece of gauze with each wiping pass.

Removes surface bacteria and exudate. Prevents transfer of microorganisms from the skin to the wound.

11. Assess the wound for location, amount of tissue present, exudate, and odor.

Allows for determination of most effective treatment and type of dressing.

12. Discard the gloves and soiled gauze into a biohazard bag.

Soiled gauze contains contaminants and should be disposed of as biohazardous waste.

Procedure Steps for Applying a Wet-to-Damp Dressing

13. Open a sterile gauze pack tray and a surgipad. The amount of gauze you use depends on the size of the wound.

Maintains sterile field and supplies.

14. Moisten sterile gauze with saline solution or water for irrigation.

15. Apply clean gloves.

16. Squeeze out excess moisture from the gauze. Apply a single layer

of moist, fine-mesh gauze to the wound. Be sure to place gauze in all depressions or crevices of the wound. You may need to use forceps or a cotton applicator to ensure that you fill deep depressions or sinus tracts with gauze.

Maintains a moist environment for the wound bed. ▼

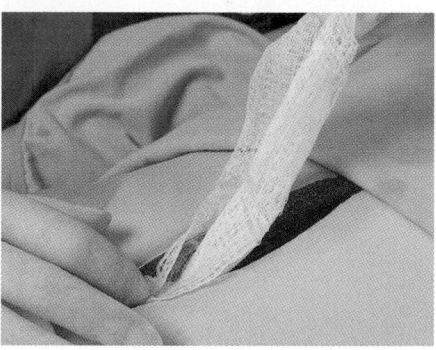

17. Apply a secondary moist layer over the first layer. Repeat this process until the wound is completely filled with moistened sterile gauze— but do not tightly *pack* the gauze into the wound. Do not extend the moist dressing onto the surrounding skin.

Packing the gauze can restrict blood flow to the area. Moist dressing on the surrounding skin can cause maceration.

18. Cover the moistened gauze with a surgipad.

Protects the wound from external contaminants. ▼

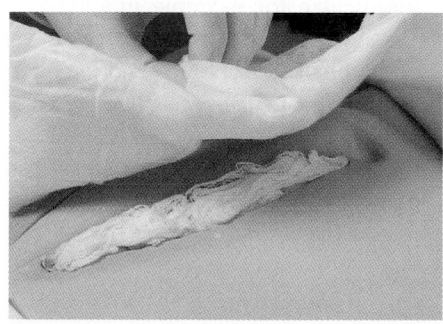

19. Secure the dressing with tape or Montgomery straps.

Montgomery straps are useful when dressings must be frequently changed

(continued on next page)

Procedure 34-6 ■ Removing and Applying Wet-to-Damp Dressings (continued)

because they do not cause trauma to the skin. ▼

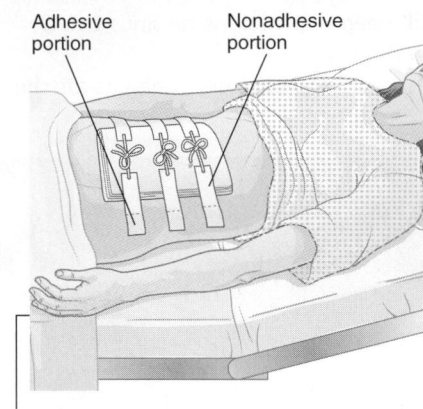

Adhesive portion   Nonadhesive portion

Montgomery straps

20. Dispose of gloves and materials in the biohazard waste receptacle.

21. Assist the patient to a comfortable position.

What if . . .

■ **Gauze becomes dry between dressing changes?**

Moisten with sterile saline before removing dressings, change dressing more frequently, and consider using a semi-occlusive dressing.

A moistened dressing, prevents débridement of granulating tissue, maintains a moist environment, and prevents

tissue injury. Dressings that become too dry will injure healthy tissue and impair healing.

■ **The patient has multiple wounds?**

The most infected wound should be treated last and change your gloves in between wound dressing changes.

The risk of cross contamination is reduced when moving from clean to dirty and with fresh gloves.

Evaluation

■ Verify that the patient experiences minimal discomfort with the procedure.
■ Note whether the patient verbalizes understanding of the procedure.

Patient Teaching

■ Teach the patient about the expected healing process.
■ Inform the patient and caregiver about signs and symptoms of infection and the need to report these findings.

Home Care

■ Help the client store dressings appropriately to keep them clean, for example, in a plastic container with a lid.
■ Teach the client or caregivers to dispose of contaminated dressings and gloves by double-bagging them in moisture-proof bags (e.g., plastic grocery bags).
■ Advise the client and family whether they can get the wound wet (e.g., during bathing). If it must be kept dry, demonstrate how to cover it with a waterproof barrier (e.g., a plastic bag).

Documentation

Document the following information (many agencies use a wound/skin flowsheet):
■ Appearance and location of the wound, type and amount of exudate, and odor, if present, after cleansing

■ The patient's pain level before and after the procedure
■ Pain medication given including the dose, time, your name, and the patient's response.
■ Method of cleansing the wound
■ Type of dressing applied to the wound
■ Education provided to the patient

Sample documentation:

> 08/03/12   2100   100% red granulating tissue noted in wound bed of stage IV pressure ulcer on sacrum. No tunneling or undermining observed. Minimal amount of serosanguineous drainage on old dressing. Wound cleansed with normal saline prior to application of new dressing. Wet-to-damp dressing applied. Pt. tolerated procedure well, with no verbalization of pain throughout procedure. Pt. placed on 2-hour turn schedule and educated on pressure relief. Pt. verbalizes understanding. ——
> —————————————— W. Earl, RN

Practice Resources

Atiyeh, B. S., & Hayek, S. N. (2004); Dunaway, E., & Goldrick, B. A. (2007); The Joanna Briggs Institute (2002); National Pressure Ulcer Advisory Panel (2007d).

Thinking About the Procedure

 Go to the *Fundamentals of Nursing Skills Videos,* **Wound Care: Dressings: Wet-to-Damp.**

1. Did the nurse use clean or sterile technique for the dressing change?

2. Where is the patient's wound located? And how did the nurse protect his privacy when changing a wound dressing?

 For suggested responses, go to Chapter 34, **Thinking About the Procedure Suggested Responses (Procedure 34-6),** on the Student Resource Disk or DavisPlus at http://davisplus.fadavis.com/Wilkinson2

Procedure 34-7 ☐ Applying a Negative Pressure Wound Therapy (NPWT) Device

➤ For steps to follow in *all* procedures, refer to the Universal Steps for All Procedures found on the inside back cover of Volume 2.

Critical Aspects

- Administer an analgesic if needed.
- Select an appropriate dressing, per NPWT unit, to fill the entire wound cavity.
- Obtain a suction pump unit as ordered.
- Prepare a sterile field for supplies.
- Don sterile gloves for new surgical wounds, or clean gloves for chronic wounds.
- Irrigate the wound.
- Apply appropriate dressing per NPWT unit.

Procedure 34-7A: Open-Pore Reticulated Polyurethane Foam (i.e., Vacuum-Assisted Closure Therapy [V.A.C.®], patented by KCI)
- Cut the foam to fill the wound cavity.
- Do not place foam into blind/unexplored tunnels.
- Do not allow foam dressing to overlap onto healthy skin.

Procedure 34-7B: Nonadherent Antimicrobial Gauze Dressing Application (i.e., Chariker–Jeter Method)
- Measure the length of the drain.
- Moisten gauze.
- Sandwich the drain in the moistened gauze and place in the wound base.
- Tuck gauze into any undermining areas to ensure contact with the wound bed.
- Apply a strip or dollop of ostomy paste 1 cm from wound edge and secure the drain as needed.

For Both Types of Dressing
- Connect tubing attached to the dressing to the evacuation tubing going to the collection system.
- Position the tubing and connector away from bony prominences and skin creases.
- Ensure clamps are open on all tubing.
- Turn on the pump and set to prescribed settings.
- Listen for audible leaks and observe for dressing collapse or pruning.
- Change canister once a week or sooner if it fills.

Equipment

- Suction unit (pump)
- Collection canister with connecting tubings
- Appropriate dressing per manufacturer unit
- Semipermeable transparent adhesive dressing
- Skin preparation product or sealant (skin prep)
- Sterile 4 in. × 4 in. gauze
- Clean procedure gloves
- Two pairs of sterile gloves (if using sterile technique)
- Sterile scissors (if using sterile technique)
- Waterproof pad
- Bath blanket

- Goggles or safety glasses, mask, and protective gown
- 10–20 mL irrigation syringe
- Normal saline for irrigation
- Emesis basis
- Biohazard bag for contaminated materials

Procedure 34-7A: Vacuum-Assisted Closure (V.A.C.) Therapy
- GranuFoam (black), white or silver foam dressing
- Therapeutic regulated accurate care (TRAC) pad

Procedure 34-7B: Chariker–Jeter Dressing Application
- Fenestrated drain
- Ostomy paste

(continued on next page)

Procedure 34-7 ■ **Applying a Negative Pressure Wound Therapy (NPWT) Device** (continued)

Delegation

As a nurse, you are responsible for assessing the wound and evaluating interventions. You should not delegate application of a negative pressure wound therapy device to a NAP. However, you may ask the NAP to report to you any changes in the wound dressing, pressure in the unit, or alarms.

Pre-Procedure Assessments

■ **Assess the type of wound to be treated with negative pressure.**
Negative pressure wound therapy is used to promote wound healing by secondary or tertiary intention in acute, chronic, traumatic, and dehisced wounds; partial-thickness burns; or flaps and grafts. NPWT will prepare the wound bed for closure, reduce edema, promote granulation formation, and remove exudate and infective material.

■ **Determine if there is any contraindication to use of a NPWT:** nonenteric or unexplored fistulas; necrotic tissue with eschar; untreated osteomyelitis; malignancy in the wound or in exposed blood vessels, anastomotic sites, organs, or nerves.

■ **Assess patients for active or prolonged bleeding;** patients who are on anticoagulant therapy or platelet aggregation inhibitors; or patients with infected, damaged, irradiated, or sutured blood vessels.
Patients who are at increased risk for bleeding should be closely monitored. These conditions could be fatal if negative pressure is applied and bleeding is uncontrolled (exsanguination could occur). Notify the primary care provider of these conditions.

■ **Assess the wound for bone fragments or sharp edges.**
When NPWT is activated, mechanical stress is placed upon the wound. Sharp edges or bone may puncture protective barriers, vessels, or organs, causing injury, and bleeding, if uncontrolled, could be fatal.

■ **Assess the wound for infection.**
Monitor infected wounds closely, as they may require more frequent dressing changes than noninfected wounds.

■ **Assess the wound for size** (length, width, and depth in centimeters); location and depth of undermining or tunneling; amount, character, and odor of drainage; type and percentage of tissue present in wound bed (granulation, slough, fibrin, necrotic); and periwound condition (i.e., intact, denuded, erythema, induration, or maceration).
If no response or improvement in the wound condition occurs in 2 weeks, use of NPWT should be reevaluated.

■ **Assess the patient's nutritional status.**
Adequate protein stores are needed for wounds to heal. Evaluate the patient's albumin or prealbumin level before initiating therapy, as NPWT may deplete these levels and prevent healing.

■ **Assess for pain.**
Wound care is very painful. Wound pain that is inadequately treated can lead to wound bed hypoxia that impairs wound healing and increases infection rates. Wound pain also negatively affects the patient's quality of life.

➤ When performing the procedure, always identify your patient according to agency policy and be attentive to standard precautions, hand hygiene, patient safety and privacy, body mechanics, and documentation.

➤ *Note:* The success of NPWT can depend on the training and expertise of the clinician. Allow adequate time for this procedure. Experienced nurses need at least 15 to 30 minutes. You will need more time if problems arise, and even more if you are a novice.

➤ *Note:* This procedure assumes you are performing the initial application of V.A.C. therapy. If you are changing the dressing, first read "What If. . ." near the end of this procedcure.

Procedure Steps

1. Consider administering pain medication before initiating negative pressure wound therapy. Allow sufficient time for the medication to take effect.

2. Select the appropriate dressing (per NPWT system used) to fill the entire wound cavity.
Dressings should be placed directly against the wound surface to allow for equal suction/pressure throughout the wound bed.

3. Obtain suction pump unit as prescribed.
Negative pressure wound therapy is provided by several different manufacturers. Use the unit and dressing method that is approved by your facility.

a. Place the suction unit upright on a level surface.
b. Remove the canister from the sterile package and insert it into the pump.
c. Connect the tubing to the canister.

d. Ensure the opposite end of the tubing remains clean before connecting with the tubing from the dressing.
e. You may place the suction unit at the end of the bed or hang it on an IV pole.
f. Do not place the unit on the floor. Ensure the unit is not knocked over, as drainage from the canister can back up and contaminate the pump's filter, blocking suction.

4. Place the waterproof bag or trash receptacle so you can reach it easily during the procedure.
Convenient placement facilitates access to safe disposal of the dressing into a trash receptacle for biohazardous waste.

5. Assist the patient to a comfortable position that allows for easy access to the wound.
Facilitates access to the wound site with less contamination and promotes good body mechanics for the nurse.

6. Expose the wound area and drape the patient (use a bath blanket if needed) to expose only the wound area.
Draping provides privacy and emotional comfort.

7. Place a waterproof pad as needed.
An underpad protects the linens from moisture and drainage.

8. Prepare a sterile or clean field and add all supplies: gloves, scissors, irrigation supplies, gauze pad, selected wound dressings, tubing, and/or connectors.

9. Don sterile or clean procedure gloves. Use gown and protective eyewear.
Using sterile/aseptic versus clean technique is based on the wound type, physician preference, or facility protocol. A safe rule to follow is to use sterile gloves for a fresh noninfected wound; clean gloves for other wounds.

10. Irrigate the wound with 10 to 30 mL of normal saline or other prescribed solution before all dressing changes. Use a 35-mL syringe and a 19-gauge angiocatheter (needle removed) to direct the flow of the irrigant from the clean end toward the dirty end of the wound
Irrigation facilitates loosening of adherent tissue and removes debris and exudate while adhering to infection control principles of clean-to-dirty.

11. Remove the excess solution from the wound. Clean and dry periwound skin with sterile gauze sponge, as needed. Consider a skin protectant around the wound edges.
Excess moisture predisposes skin to maceration and possible damage. Applying a skin protectant can assist the drape in sticking to the skin, and protecting the skin when the drape is removed (i.e., from stripping of skin by the adhesive).

12. Remove soiled gloves and don new nonsterile ones for the procedure.
Change gloves during patient care if the hands will move from a contaminated body site (e.g., perineal area or wound) to a clean body site.

13. To apply appropriate dressing per preferred negative pressure wound therapy unit, follow Procedure 34-7A or 34-7B.

■ Procedure 34-7A Open-Pore Reticulated Polyurethane Foam Therapy (i.e., Vacuum-Assisted Closure [V.A.C.])

➤ When performing the procedure, always identify your patient according to agency policy and be attentive to standard precautions, hand hygiene, patient safety and privacy, body mechanics, and documentation.

Begin with Procedure steps 1 through 13, at the beginning of Procedure 34-7. Then proceed as follows.

1. Select the appropriate foam dressing: black, white, or silver.
Black foam is sufficient for most wounds unless individual patient circumstances require white or silver. White foam is denser and will limit granulation formation. It may be used for painful or superficial wounds, tunneling/sinus tracts/undermining, or where granulation tissue growth needs to be limited. Silver dressings may act as a barrier to bacterial penetration in the wound bed. Silver may eradicate biofilms of colonized bacteria.

2. Cut the foam dressing to the appropriate size to fill the wound cavity. Do not cut the foam dressing over the wound. Rub the cut edges to remove any loose pieces.
If you cut the foam over the wound, particles may fall into the wound and create irritation. ▼

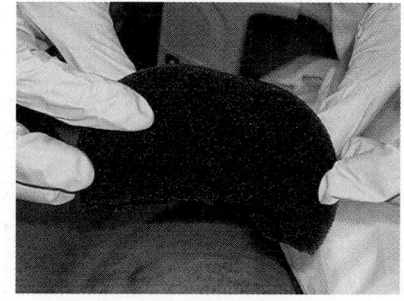

3. Gently place the foam dressing into the cavity without overlapping onto intact skin. Do not overfill the cavity or pack into deep crevices.
  a. Do not place foam into blind/unexplored tunnels.
Forcing foam dressings into any area may damage tissue, alter the delivery of negative pressure, or hinder exudates or foam removal.

  b. Do not allow foam dressing to overlap onto healthy skin.
Foam dressing becomes very wet during therapy and will macerate and damage intact skin.

  c. If you use more than one piece, note the total number of pieces that were placed into the wound so you can document them on the transparent dressing and in the patient record.
An accurate record of the number of foam pieces is necessary to prevent retained material within the wound.

4. Apply a liquid skin preparation product to periwound, if needed.
Skin preps can protect the periwound skin from excess fluid, adhesive stripping, or other damage.

(continued on next page)

Procedure 34-7 ■ Applying a Negative Pressure Wound Therapy (NPWT) Device (continued)

5. Apply transparent film/drape 3 to 5 cm (1 to 2 in.) from wound margins without pulling, stretching, or wrinkling the drape. Do not push down or compress foam while placing drape.
The occlusive dressing creates a seal to help create negative pressure within the wound. Tension from pulling, stretching, or wrinkling the dressing may lead to tissue injury. More pressure will be placed on the wound bed than necessary if you have flattened the foam before turning on the suction unit.

6. Avoid placing dressings that wrap all the way around an extremity. If necessary, place several smaller pieces of drape rather than one continuous piece.
When pressure is applied, a circumferential dressing may interfere with circulation, if wrapped too tightly.

7. Identify a site over the dressing for the suction track tubing apparatus.

8. Pinch up a piece of drape and cut at least a 2-cm round hole. Do not make a slit or X, as this may close off under pressure. ▼

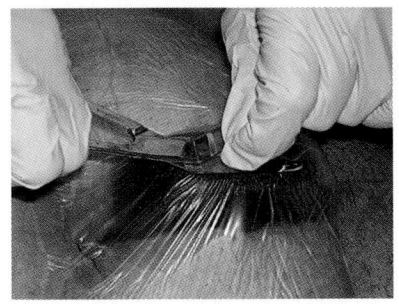

9. Place the track adhesive and suction device directly over the hole in the drape and apply gentle pressure to secure.
Negative pressure removes excess wound exudate from the wound bed. ▼

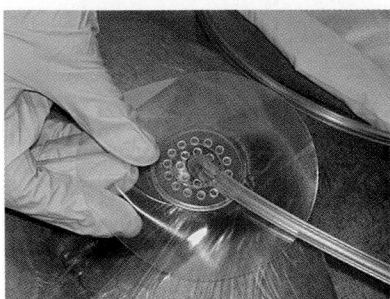

10. Connect suction track tubing to the canister tubing and open clamps.
The canister is attached to a vacuum pump that provides either continuous or intermittent negative pressure, adjusted for the type of wound. Pressure is applied in the range of –5 to –125 mm Hg (adjustable pressures, depending on the particular device used).
Suction draws excess exudate away from the wound and into an evacuation container.

11. Connect tubing from the dressing to the suction track tubing going to the collection canister.
Allows for collection and measurement of drainage.

12. Position the tubing and connector away from bony prominences and skin creases.
Prevents pressure injury to the skin.

13. Ensure clamps are open on all tubing.

14. Turn on power to the pump and set to the prescribed therapy settings to initiate therapy.
Therapy should be maintained for at least 22 out of 24 hours daily. Alternate wound care should be considered if vacuum cannot be tolerated for this length of time.

15. Listen for audible leaks and observe dressing collapse or wrinkling as pressure is applied to the wound bed.
With an adequate seal, the dressing will collapse almost immediately. Any leak (i.e., between the dressing and drape, around tubing, at skin crevices, or at tubing connection sites) will prevent collapse. ▼

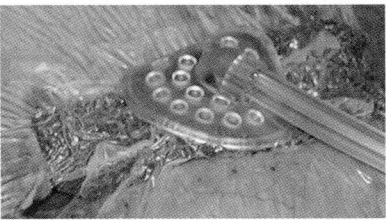

16. Change the canister at least once a week or when it is filled. Write the date on the canister.
This will help to know when it was changed last as well as how often it is being changed for fluid loss.

■ Procedure 34-7B Gauze Dressing Application (i.e., Chariker–Jeter Method)

➤ When performing the procedure, always identify your patient according to agency policy and be attentive to standard precautions, hand hygiene, patient safety and privacy, body mechanics, and documentation.

Begin with Procedure steps 1 through 13, at the beginning of Procedure 34-7. Then proceed as follows.

1. Measure the length of drain from wound margin, starting with the first hole perforation and pull back 1 cm.

2. Moisten gauze with normal saline.

3. Wrap or "sandwich" the drain in the moistened gauze and place in the wound base. Tuck gauze into any undermining areas to ensure contact with the wound bed.

4. Apply a strip or dollop of ostomy paste 1 cm from the wound edge and secure the drain as needed.

Paste is occlusive and will help maintain a seal between the drain and the transparent film dressing. Paste that is too close to the wound edge can get sucked into the drain, and occlude pressure.

5. Apply liquid skin preparation product to periwound, if needed. Extra drape, hydrocolloid, or transparent dressing may be used to protect fragile skin.

Skin preps can protect the periwound skin from excess fluid, adhesive stripping, or other damage.

6. Apply transparent film approximately 1.0 to 2.5 cm (½ to 1 in.) beyond the wound margin to intact skin. Pinch the film around the drain tubing to ensure a tight seal.

7. Avoid wrapping dressings around an extremity. If necessary, place several smaller pieces of drape rather than one continuous piece.

When pressure is applied, a circumferential dressing may interfere with circulation.

8. Attach filter tubing to the canister spout.

9. Connect tubing from the dressing to the evacuation tubing going to the collection canister.

Allows for collection and measurement of drainage.

10. Position the tubing and connector away from bony prominences and skin creases.

Prevents pressure injury to the skin. ▼

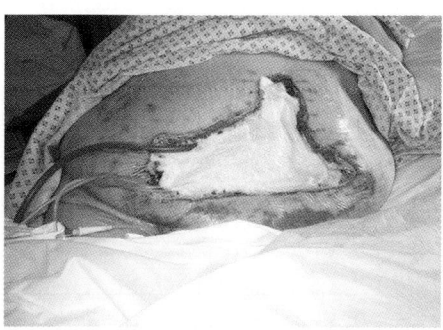

11. Ensure clamps are open on all tubing.

12. Turn on power to pump and set to the prescribed therapy settings to initiate therapy.

Therapy should be maintained for at least 22 out of 24 hours daily. Alternate wound care should be considered suction cannot be tolerated for this length of time.

13. Listen for audible leaks and observe dressing collapse as pressure is applied to the wound bed.

With an adequate seal, the dressing will collapse almost immediately. Any leak

(i.e., between the dressing and drape, around tubing, at skin crevices, or at tubing connection sites) will prevent collapse.

14. Change the canister at least once a week or when it is filled. Write the date on the canister.

This will help to know when it was changed last as well as how often it is being changed for fluid loss.

What if...

■ **You are changing the dressing instead of applying it for the first time.**

Follow the procedure steps below. *Note:* Dressings should be changed every 48 to 72 hours.

Dressings left in the wound longer than the recommended time frame can become difficult to remove if tissue grows into the foam, or can lead to infection or other adverse events.

  a. Evaluate the need for analgesia.
  b. Turn the suction pump unit off during the procedure.
  c. Place a waterproof, biohazard pad under the body part requiring the dressing change.
  d. Perform hand hygiene and don sterile or clean gloves as appropriate.
  e. Remove the transparent dressing, using a push–pull method to gently pull up drape while pushing it slowly from the skin. Separating the drape from the skin in this manner will decrease the risk of tape stripping.
  f. Gently remove gauze or foam dressing. If dressing is difficult to remove, instill normal saline onto the dressing for 15 to 30 minutes.

Dressing removal can damage new granulation tissue if tissue has grown into the dressing.

  ✥ g. Count all pieces of gauze or foam dressing that were removed to ensure none remain in the wound bed. Ensure no dressing is left in tunneled or undermined areas.

Dressings are not bioabsorbable and can abscess if left in the wound.

  h. Discard soiled dressings in a biohazardous waste receptacle.
  i. Start at the beginning of Procedure 34-7 and perform steps 1 through 13. Then, as instructed in step 13, follow either Procedure 34-7A or 34-7B.

■ **After 2 weeks, you see that the wound is not improving?**

Consult with the primary provider or a wound care specialist. Average length of therapy is usually 4 to 6 weeks. Therapy should be discontinued if the wound shows no improvement in 1 to 2 consecutive weeks, the patient is unwilling or unable to follow the medical plan, or the goal of therapy has been met.

The longer a wound is open, the longer it takes to heal, and places the patient at risk for complications. A steady decrease in wound size should be seen every week. If NPWT is not effective, alternate wound care should be evaluated.

■ **You cannot find or remove a piece of foam?**

Notify the provider, as this may necessitate surgery.

The material could be retained in the patient and create an inflammatory response.

■ **There is a foul odor when the dressing is removed?**

Clean the wound with normal saline to ensure odor is not eminating from the soiled dressing. If other signs of infection are present (i.e., fever, tenderness, redness, swelling, purulent drainage), notify the provider.

■ **Suction cannot be maintained?**

Identify why the seal cannot be maintained. If the wound is very near the coccyx and gluteal fold, use a dollop of paste to help fill in the crack and maintain a seal. If the skin around the wound is moist, adhesive drape will not adhere to skin. Use a skin prep product or drape to protect the skin. If the tube is pulling away from the dressing or tension is being placed on the tube, anchor it with additional drape or tape several centimetres from the dressing or wound.

(continued on next page)

Procedure 34-7 ■ Applying a Negative Pressure Wound Therapy (NPWT) Device (continued)

■ **The canister is filling with blood?**

Immediately discontinue negative pressure therapy. The gauze or foam dressing will not stop the bleeding, so take measures to control bleeding (i.e., hold pressure on wound). Do not remove dressing until the treating primary care provider is consulted.

■ **Dressing does not collapse or the alarm sounds?**

a. Press firmly around the transparent dressing to seal.

b. Verify the machine is turned on, and all clamps are open and tubing is not kinked.

c. Check tubing and drape for leaks. Listen for leaks with a stethoscope or by moving your hand around the wound margins while applying slight pressure.

d. Additional small pieces of transparent dressing may be used to seal around hardware, skin fold, or creases.

e. Do not place multiple layers of drape or adhesive dressing.

Several layers may decrease the dressing's moisture vapor transmission rate, increasing the risk of maceration.

f. Never leave foam in place without an adequate seal for more than 2 hours. If an adequate seal cannot be achieved in that time, remove the foam and apply a saline moistened gauze dressing.

Evaluation

- Note the patient's response to the procedure.
- Continue to monitor wound healing and changes in periwound tissues.
- Monitor dressing every 2 hours to ensure it is firm and collapsed in the wound bed while therapy is on.
- Monitor the seal of the dressing, and pressure settings.
- Monitor for brisk or bright bleeding, evisceration or dehiscence, and symptoms of infection.

These must be reported to the provider.

Home Care

- Refer the client to a home health agency for wound care.
- In limited circumstances, some clients or caregivers may be able to perform dressing changes. Determine their ability to perform dressing changes teach and demonstrate as needed.
- Instruct the client or family to visually check the dressing every 2 hours to ensure it is firm and collapsed in the wound bed.
- Review safety labeling, alarms, and pump instructions.
- Review conditions in which to seek medical care: bleeding, infection, unresolved alarms, or loss of suction.
- Review proper disposal of contaminated supplies.

Documentation

Document the following information:
- Date and time of dressing change
- Wound assessment: location of the wound, size (length, width, diameter), undermining or tunneling, amount and character of drainage, odor, wound bed including type and percentage of tissue seen, and periwound appearance
- Evaluation of therapy with evidence of healing
- Treatment selected: type of NPWT, type of gauze or foam, number of pieces placed in the wound
- Treatment settings: pressures, intermittent vs. continuous, or variable pressures
- Patient response to dressing change

11/25/11   0900   *Patient reported pain of 5 on a scale of 1 to 10. Analgesic given IV. See MAR. Two pieces of black foam removed. Wound cleaned with normal saline irrigation and two pieces of black foam replaced to obliterate undermining using modified sterile technique. Activated negative pressure wound therapy unit to 125 mm Hg intermittent pressure. Abdominal wound is 3 X 2 X 2 cm with 1 cm undermining at 12:00. The wound bed is 100% granular. Periwound skin is intact without erythema or induration. Serous drainage without odor is noted in the canister, 15 cc this shift. After dressing change, client rated pain in wound area as 2 on a scale of 1 to 10. Plan: continue dressing change every 48 hours. —*

— *L. Opperta, RN*

Sample documentation for Procedure 34-7A: Vacuum-Assisted Closure (V.A.C.) Therapy

05/13/11   0915   Patient reported pain of 5
on a scale of 1 to 10. Administered hydro-
codone 5.0 mg PO at 0815, before initiation of
negative wound pressure therapy. Stage 4
pressure ulcer to coccyx has been surgically
debrided. Wound is 4 X 6 X 2 cm with no appre-
ciated undermining. Wound bed is now clean of
necrotic tissue, with 100% pink tissue noted.
Periwound has 1 cm of erythema to wound
edges, but with scant nonmalodorus, sero-
sangenous drainage. Using sterile technique, a
moistened saline gauze was applied to wound
bed with fenestrated drain. Ostomy paste was
applied at wound edge to assist in seal. Pump
was activated to 80 mm Hg continuous pressure. Patient rated pain in wound area as a 2
post procedure. Plan: Begin dressing changes
every 48 hours. ————— L. Opperta, RN

*Sample documentation for Procedure 34-7B: Chariker-Jeter
Dressing Application*

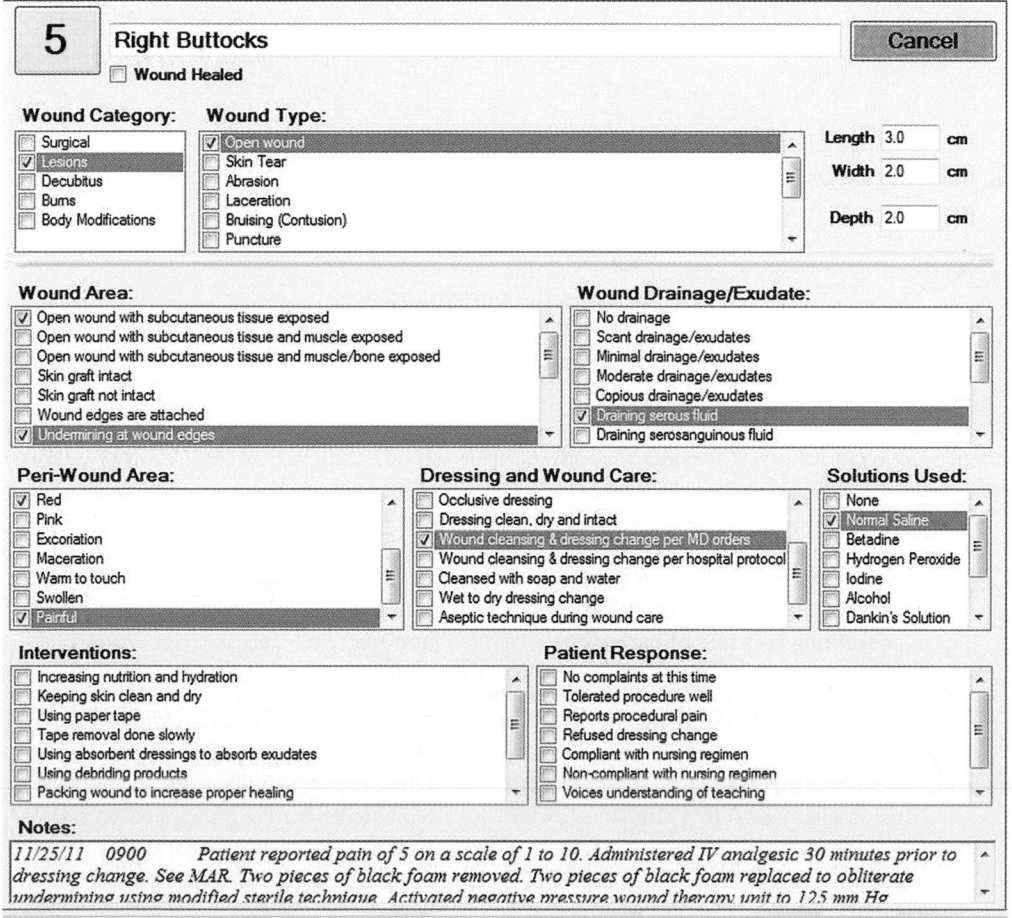

Sample EHR documentation

Practice Resources

Armstrong, D. G., Attinger, C. E., Boulton, A. J., et al. (2004); Chariker, M. (2009); Kinetic Concepts Incorporated (2007, 2008); Krasner, D. L., Shapshak, D., & Hopf, H. W. (2007); Medica-Rents Co. (2008); National Guideline Clearinghouse (2006 Dec; revised 2008 Dec); Samson, D., Lefevre, F., & Aronson, N. (2004); Siegel, J. D., Rhinehart, E., Jackson, M., et al. (2007); Sullivan, N., Snyder, D. L., Tipton, K., et al. (2009).

Procedure 34-8   Applying and Removing a Transparent Film Dressing

➤ For steps to follow in *all* procedures, refer to the Universal Steps for All Procedures found on the inside back cover of Volume 2.

Critical Aspects

- Place the patient in a comfortable position that provides easy access to the wound.
- Remove the soiled dressing, if necessary.
- Cleanse the surrounding skin and wound.
- Assess the condition of the wound.
- Apply the transparent film dressing to the wound by removing the center backing and holding the dressing firmly by the edges.
- Remove the edge liners.

Equipment

- Clean nonsterile gloves
- Sterile gauze
- Normal saline solution or specified cleansing agent, warmed to body temperature when possible

Cold solution lowers the temperature of the wound bed and slows the healing process.

- Scissors (if needed)
- Liquid skin preparation (if needed)
- Transparent film dressing (e.g., Op-Site, Tegaderm, Bio-Occlusive)

Delegation

Because assessment of the wound and knowledge of clean technique are important, you should not delegate this procedure to a NAP.

Pre-Procedure Assessment

- Assess the area to determine whether a transparent film dressing is appropriate.

Transparent film dressings are indicated as primary dressings (dressings that touch the wound or area to be treated) to protect high-risk intact skin; for superficial or partial-thickness wounds that have little to no drainage (i.e., stage I or II pressure ulcers); and to assist in debriding eschar by autolysis. Films may be used as a secondary dressing to protect other types of dressings from bodily fluids (i.e., wounds near the perineum).

- Assess the wound to determine if use of a transparent film is contraindicated.

Films are contraindicated in third-degree burns, arterial ulcers, and infected wounds. Films should not be used to fill dead space.

- Determine the size of the wound.

Film dressings are available in many sizes. Select the appropriate size based on wound measurements, allowing for a 2.5 cm (1 in.) perimeter of intact skin around the wound for the adhesive to stick.

- Assess the periwound area.

Film dressings should be attached to intact skin. The adhesive is not waterproof and will not adhere to wet or moist skin.

➤ When performing the procedure, always identify your patient according to agency policy and be attentive to standard precautions, hand hygiene, patient safety and privacy, body mechanics, and documentation.

Procedure Steps

1. Place the patient in a comfortable position that provides easy access to the wound.

Procedure Steps for Applying the Dressing

2. If a dressing is present, wash your hands, apply clean nonsterile gloves, and remove the old dressing.

3. Dispose of the soiled dressing and gloves in the biohazard waste receptacle.
Observe universal precautions, preventing transfer of pathogens.

4. Apply clean gloves, and cleanse the skin surrounding the wound with normal saline or a mild cleansing agent. Be sure to rinse the skin well if you use a cleanser. Allow the skin to dry.
Cleansing prepares the skin for application of the dressing. Skin must be dry for the dressing to adhere.

5. Cleanse the wound as ordered or according to agency procedure.
Cleansing of wounds removes bacteria and necrotic debris from wound beds.

6. Consider placing a skin barrier around the wound before transparent film dressing application.
Skin sealants may be applied to skin before tape to protect fragile skin from tears or epidermal stripping.

7. Remove the center backing liner from the transparent film dressing. ▼

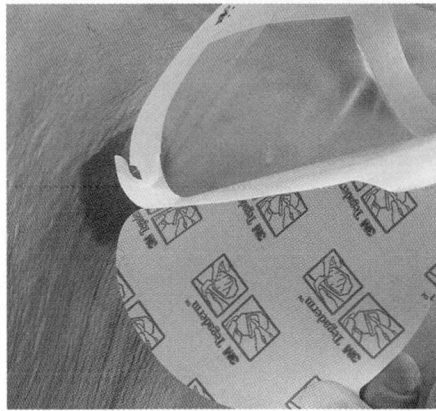

8. Holding the dressing by the edges, apply the transparent film to the wound without stretching or pulling the dressing or the skin.
This reduces the risk of skin damage to skin.

9. Remove the edging liner from the dressing.

10. Gently smooth and secure the dressing to skin.
Allows the dressing to adhere fully to the patient's skin.

11. Dispose of soiled equipment, and remove your gloves.

Procedure Steps for Removing the Dressing

Transparent film dressings are typically changed every 3 days. Change dressing sooner if drainage extends beyond the edges of the wound onto periwound skin. To remove the dressing, do the following:
- Grasp one edge of the film dressing.
- Gently lift the edge.
- Stabilize the skin underneath the elevated edge with your finger.
Stabilizing the skin as the adhesive is taken off will prevent epidermal stripping.

- With the other hand, slowly peel the dressing back over itself, "low and slow," in the direction of hair growth.
Removing the dressing at an angle will increase the risk of pulling on the epidermis and causing mechanical trauma.

- As dressing is removed, keep moving your finger as necessary to avoid newly exposed skin.

What if . . .

- **The adhesive will not adhere to the patient's skin due to excess hair?**

Hair may be removed with clippers/scissors. Do not shave the site with a razor.

Shaving can cause nicks or abrasions to the skin that could become a portal of entry for bacteria.

- **The patient's skin is diaphoretic or excessively oily?**

Cleanse the skin with soap and water before the dressing change. Also, polymer skin barriers may be used to place a seal over the skin and allow the tape adhesive to adhere.

- **The patient has fragile skin (i.e., elderly patient)?**

Skin sealant preparations may be used under adhesives.

The junction between the epidermis and dermis on the older adult is not as strong as with a younger person. Less pressure or tension is needed to break those bonds and cause skin damage.

- **The dressing sticks to itself before it can be applied?**

If a small portion of the dressing is stuck to itself, gently stretch or pull the edges in opposite directions. If a large portion is involved, throw the dressing away and start over.

Transparent dressings can be difficult to apply because they are polyurethane sheets coated on one side with an acrylic, hypoallergenic adhesive and are flimsy in nature, making them clumsy to work with at times.

- **Purulent-appearing fluid has collected underneath the film dressing?**

This does not necessarily mean the wound is infected. Remove the dressing and clean the wound per policy. Select an alternate dressing that will be more absorptive.

Because films do not have absorptive capabilities, any drainage produced by the wound will pool underneath.

Evaluation

- Verify the transparent film dressing is appropriate for the wound.
- Determine whether the dressing adheres comfortably to skin.
- Ensure that patient verbalizes understanding of treatment.

Patient Teaching

- Teach the patient about the expected healing process.
- Teaching the patient about the use of transparent film dressings.
- Inform the patient and caregiver about signs and symptoms of infection and the need to report these findings.

Documentation

Document the following information (many agencies use a wound/skin flowsheet):
- Wound assessment: location of the wound, size (length × width × diameter) undermining or tunneling, amount and character of drainage, odor, wound bed including type and percentage of tissue seen, and periwound appearance
- Appearance and location of the wound, type and amount of exudate, and odor, if present, after cleansing
- The patient's pain level before the procedure. If the patient was medicated for pain, document the drug and dose used, time given, and the patient's response to analgesia.
- Method of cleansing the wound and surrounding skin
- Type of dressing applied to the wound
- Education provided to the patient

(continued on next page)

Procedure 34-8 ■ **Applying and Removing a Transparent Film Dressing** (continued)

Sample documentation:

> 02/19/12 1400   *Transparent film dressing*
> *applied to stage 1 pressure ulcer on left lateral*
> *heel, 1 X 1 cm. Area is nonblanchable and painful*
> *to the touch. Cleaned with normal saline before*
> *dressing application. Heel protectors placed*
> *bilaterally to keep heels suspended off of the*
> *bed. Discussed pressure ulcer formation with*
> *patient and the need to keep pressure off of*
> *the area. Will continue to assist patient in*
> *turning every 2 hours.——— M.K. Leonard, RN*

Practice Resources

3M (2004); Association of periOperative Registered Nurses (2008); Bryant, R. A., & Nix, D. P. (2006).

Procedure 34-9   Applying a Hydrating Dressing (Hydrocolloid or Hydrogel)

➤ For steps to follow in *all* procedures, refer to the Universal Steps for All Procedures found on the inside back cover of Volume 2.

Critical Aspects

- Place the patient in a comfortable position.
- Remove the soiled dressing, if necessary.
- Cleanse the wound, if necessary.
- Assess the wound, or other area where hydrocolloid dressing will be applied, for size, location, appearance, exudate, odor, and signs and symptoms of infection.
- Clip the hair around the wound if necessary.
- Apply the hydrating dressing.

Equipment

- Clean nonsterile gloves
- Hydrating dressing 3 to 4 cm (1.5 in.) larger than the wound
- Moisture-proof bag
  Obtain the following items, only if needed:
- Sterile normal saline solution or tap water according to agency policy or as prescribed for irrigation, warmed to body temperature when possible
  Cold solution lowers the temperature of wound bed and slows the healing process.
- Emesis basin
- Sterile gauze for cleansing
- Disposable clippers or scissors (to trim hair or dressing)
- Skin prep
- Measuring device
- Tape

Delegation

This procedure requires knowledge of wound healing, dressings, and infection control and prevention. You should not delegate this procedure to a NAP.

Pre-Procedure Assessments

- Assess the area to determine whether a hydrating dressing is appropriate.
  Hydrating dressings are appropriate for wounds with minimal drainage. These dressings autolytically débride necrotic tissue from the wound bed. They may also be used to protect skin at risk for breakdown.

- Determine the size of the wound.
  Allows you to select a dressing of the appropriate size. Choosing a dressing size that extends beyond the ulcer ensures complete coverage.

➤ When performing the procedure, always identify your patient according to agency policy and be attentive to standard precautions, hand hygiene, patient safety and privacy, body mechanics, and documentation.

Procedure Steps

1. Place the patient in a comfortable position that provides easy access to the wound.
Provides for patient comfort and proper nurse body mechanics during dressing change.

2. If a dressing is present, wash your hands, apply clean nonsterile gloves, and remove the old dressing.
Prevents transfer of pathogens.

3. Dispose of the soiled dressing and gloves in the biohazard waste receptacle.
Dressings may contain body fluids and other contaminants, so they must be disposed of moisture-proof containers.

4. Wash your hands. Apply clean gloves, and cleanse the skin surrounding the wound with normal saline or a mild cleansing agent. Be sure to rinse the skin well if you use a cleanser. Allow the skin to dry. Do not attempt to remove residue that is left on the skin from the old dressing.
Cleansing and drying prepare the skin for application of the dressing. Removing residue irritates the surrounding skin.

5. Apply skin prep to the area covered by tape.
Skin prep protects intact skin from breakdown from tape removal.

6. Cleanse the wound as directed. Wound cleansing may be performed with clean or sterile technique, depending on the type of wound.
Cleansing the wound removes microbes and necrotic debris from wound bed. Studies show using saline or tap water are both similarly effective for cleansing.

7. Remove soiled gloves, and assess the condition of the wound. Note the size, location, type of tissue present, amount of exudate, and odor.
Granulating tissue is beefy red with a velvety appearance. It appears with the growth of new blood vessels and connective tissue. Pale pink tissue may indicate compromised blood supply to the wound bed. Necrotic tissue, which is black, brown, or yellow in appearance, is nonviable and inhibits healing. A hydrocolloid dressing will interact with wound drainage to produce a thick, yellow gel that may have a foul odor. Clean the wound before assessing for exudate and odor.

8. With the backing still intact, cut the hydrating dressing, if necessary, to the desired shape and size. Size the hydrocolloid dressing so it will extend 3 to 4 cm (1.5 in.) beyond the wound margin on all sides and cover all areas of non intact skin.
Provides complete coverage of the wound.

9. Apply clean gloves, and remove the backing of the hydrocolloid dressing, starting at one edge. Place the exposed adhesive portion on the patient's skin. Position the dressing to cover the wound. ▼

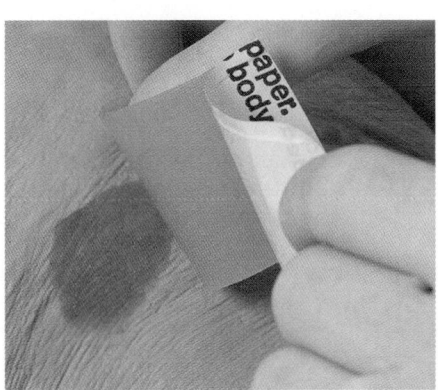

10. Gradually peel away the remaining liner, and smooth the hydrocolloid dressing onto the skin by placing your hand on top of dressing and holding in place for 1 minute.
Warmth helps the dressing adhere to the skin. ▼

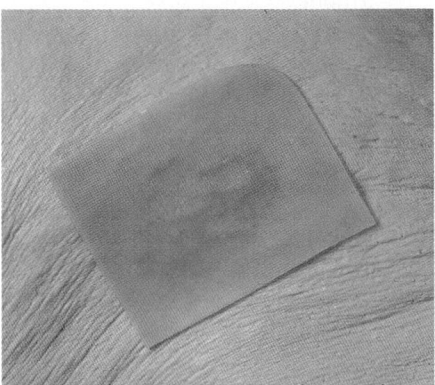

11. Assist the patient to a comfortable position, and remove your gloves. Wash your hands.

What if . . .

■ **Signs of infection are noted?**
Notify primary care provider. Cultures may be prescribed. A different type of dressing may be prescribed, as well.

■ **The surrounding skin is not intact?**
Choose a larger size hydrocolloid dressing to cover the nonintact area. Document your observations and report new findings to the primary care provider.

(continued on next page)

Procedure 34-9 ■ **Applying a Hydrating Dressing (Hydrocolloid or Hydrogel)** (continued)

Evaluation

- Verify that a hydrocolloid dressing is still appropriate for the wound.
- Note whether the dressing adheres comfortably to the skin.
- Ensure the patient verbalizes understanding of treatment.
- Inspect the dressing daily. Change it if it becomes dislodged, leaks, or wrinkles or if it develops an odor.

Patient Teaching

- Teach the patient about the expected healing process.
- Inform the patient and caregiver about signs and symptoms of infection and the need to report these findings.

Home Care

- Hydrating dressings may be required in the home setting. Teach caregivers to use the appropriate size and change the dressing if it begins to leak, develops an odor, or begins to separate from the skin.

Documentation

Document the following information. (Many agencies use wound care flowsheets.)

- Appearance and location of the wound, type and amount of exudate, and odor, if present, after cleansing. Include wound measurements, if taken, and condition of surrounding skin.

- The patient's pain level before the procedure. If the patient was medicated for pain, document the drug and dose used, time given, and patient response.
- Method of cleansing the wound and surrounding skin
- Type of dressing applied to the wound
- Use of skin prep
- Education provided to the patient

Sample documentation:

11/19/12   1730   Pt. medicated with ibuprofen 600 mg by mouth for mild wound pain post-op. Pain rated as a 2 out of 10 at this time. Soiled hydrocolloid dressing removed from shear injury to left mid-scapular area. Shear cleansed with normal saline and gauze. After cleansing, shear is 3.5 X 4 cm and covered with a 100% yellow slough. Moderate amount of serous drainage with no odor noted. Hydrocolloid reapplied as prescribed. Pt. with no complaints of pain. Educated patient about autolytic action of hydrocolloid, plan of care, and expected outcomes.———— S. Terril, RN

Practice Resources

Atiyeh, B. S., & Hayek, S. N. (2004); Dunaway, E., & Goldrick, B. A. (2007); The Joanna Briggs Institute (2002).

Thinking About the Procedure

 Go to the *Fundamentals of Nursing Skills Videos,* **Wound Care: Dressings: Hydrocolloid.**

1. Did the nurse place a pad under the patient when changing the dressing? Why or why not?

2. What kind of wound is the nurse dressing with the hydrocolloid dressing in this demonstration?

 For suggested responses, go to Chapter 34, **Thinking About the Procedure Suggested Responses (Procedure 34-9),** on the Student Resource Disk or DavisPlus at http://davisplus.fadavis.com/Wilkinson2

Procedure 34-10 Placing Skin Closures

➤ For steps to follow in *all* procedures, refer to the Universal Steps for All Procedures found on the inside back cover of Volume 2.

Critical Aspects

- Place the patient in a comfortable position that provides easy access to the wound.
- Cleanse the surrounding skin and wound.
- Assess the wound and determine the size and type of skin closure needed.
- Peel the skin closure from the card at a 90° angle.
- Place closures across the wound without tension, starting at the middle of the wound.
- Place closures 3 mm ($\frac{1}{8}$ in.) apart along the entire wound.

Equipment

- Adhesive skin closures
- Tincture of benzoin
- Forceps
- Normal saline
- Gauze
- Gloves (sterile if indicated)

Delegation

This procedure itself may be delegated to a NAP unless it is a new wound requiring sterile technique. Assessment of the incision line or wound is a licensed professional's responsibility and should not be delegated.

Pre-Procedure Assessment

- Assess the type of wound to be closed.

Adhesive closures are frequently used to keep surgical incisions well approximated. They may be used in conjunction with staples or sutures or following early staple/suture removal. Closures may be used to approximate the edges of lacerations or skin tears.

- Assess the wound for skin edge approximation.

Wounds that are gaping or appear to have undermining should not be closed using adhesive closures.

- Assess the wound for drainage, amount, type, and odor.

Wounds that are draining heavily might not be suitable for Steri-Strips™ because the adhesive would not stick to the skin.

- Assess the periwound area or surrounding skin. Assessment should include skin color, texture, temperature, and integrity of the surrounding skin. Look for maceration (caused by heavy drainage), excoriation (from caustic effluent), stripping (from inappropriate adhesive removal), pustules, papules, or lesions.

Adhesive closures should be placed only on intact skin.

- Assess the length of the wound, the location (over a joint), or if edema may occur, to determine the size of the skin closure used. Consider elastic skin closures if distention or movement is anticipated.

Closures come in several different lengths, widths, and flexibility capabilities to meet elasticity and conformability needs.

➤ When performing the procedure, always identify your patient according to agency policy and be attentive to standard precautions, hand hygiene, patient safety and privacy, body mechanics, and documentation.

Procedure Steps

1. Don clean nonsterile gloves.
Gloving prevents cross-contamination.

2. Cleanse the skin at least 5 cm (2 in.) around the wound with a saline-moistened gauze. Pat the skin dry, allowing it to dry thoroughly.
The skin surrounding the wound must be clean and dry in order for the strips to adhere.

3. Apply tincture of benzoin, and allow it to dry (or follow agency procedures). Avoid benzoin on fragile skin.
Benzoin enhances adhesion of the strips.

4. Do not allow benzoin to contact the wound.
It may impair healing.

5. Peel back package tabs to access the adhesive closures.

6. Remove the card from the package using modified sterile technique as necessary.
Careful technique should be followed when applying to a surgical wound to minimize contamination and promote healing.

7. Grasp end of skin closure with forceps or gloved hand and peel strip from the card at a 90° angle.

Closures lifted at a lesser angle or directly back on themselves may "curl," complicating handling.

8. Starting at the middle of the wound, apply strips across the wound, drawing the wound edges together. Apply closures without tension; do not stretch or strap closures.
   a. Apply half of the closure to the wound margin and press firmly in place.
   b. Using fingers or forceps, ensure skin edges are approximated.
   c. Press free half firmly on the other side of the wound.

(continued on next page)

Procedure 34-10 ■ **Placing Skin Closures** (continued)

d. Place the strips so that they extend at least 2 to 3 cm (¾ to 1 in.) on either side of the wound to ensure closure.

e. Place the wound closure strips 3 mm (1 in.) apart along the wound. ▼

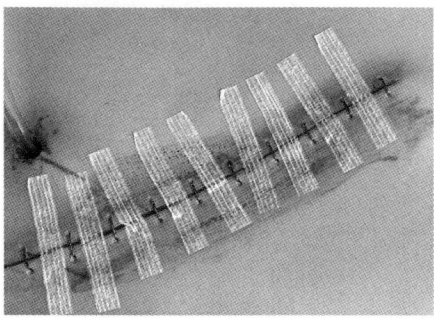

What if . . .

■ **A flap of skin rolls up on the edges?**

Cleanse the wound with normal saline and reapproximate the edges of the skin flap with the intact epidermis. Apply skin closures across the flap.

Elderly or immature skin can experience delayed wound healing.

■ **The skin around the wound is swollen?**

Apply skin closures without tension, and reapply as swelling increases.

This prevents pulling on the skin that can delay healing or disrupt the approximated borders of the wound, which is more likely to lead to scarring.

■ **Edges are not accurately approximated or tension has been placed on the skin?**

Remove the closure over the affected area, peeling each side toward the wound, and reapply.

Use of adhesive products can cause superficial skin damage if the skin is stretched during application or with edema formation. Tension blisters are the most common problem associated with taping.

Patient Evaluation

■ Verify that skin closures are appropriate for the wound.

■ Note whether the closures adhere comfortably to the skin.

■ Ensure the patient verbalized understanding of the treatment.

■ Inspect the wound daily. Lifted closure edges may be trimmed or closures replaced if less than half of the strip remains.

Patient Teaching

■ Teach the patient about the expected healing process.

■ Inform the patient or caregiver about signs and symptoms of infection and the need to report these findings.

■ Instruct patients not to pull or tug on the strips.

Improper removal may damage the underlying skin or the wound itself.

■ Instruct patients that they do not need to keep the strips dry.

They can bathe and shower as directed by the healthcare provider.

■ Instruct the patient that adhesive strips are often kept in place until they begin to separate from the skin on their own.

Documentation

Document the following information. (Many agencies use specialized wound care flowsheets.)

■ Appearance and location of the wound, type and amount of exudates, and odor, if present, after cleansing

■ The patient's level of pain before the procedure. If the patient was medicated for pain, document the drug and dose used, time given, and the patient response to analgesia.

■ Method of cleansing the wound and surrounding skin

■ Type of skin closures applied

■ Education provided to the patient

Sample documentation:

> 02/08/12 2100   Skin closures applied to midline abdominal incision following staple removal. Wound edges are well approximated with no drainage noted. Periwound skin is dry and intact, without erythema, induration, or odor. Wound cleansed with normal saline using sterile technique. Due to the length of the wound and moderate size of the abdominal drape, ½ inch X 4 inch skin closures applied without tension. Educated patient on the purpose of the closures and expected outcomes. Will continue to monitor. ————
> ———————————————— S. Wong, RN

Practice Resources

3M (2004); Bryant, R. A., & Clark, A. (2006).

Thinking About the Procedure

 Go to the *Fundamentals of Nursing Skills Videos*, **Wound Care: Steri–Strips.**

I. How are the skin closure strips positioned on the patient's wound?

 For suggested responses, go to Chapter 34, **Thinking About the Procedure Suggested Responses (Procedure 34-10),** on the Student Resource Disk or DavisPlus at http://davisplus.fadavis.com/Wilkinson2

Procedure 34-11 ◾ Applying Binders

➤ For steps to follow in *all* procedures, refer to the Universal Steps for All Procedures found on the inside back cover of Volume 2.

Critical Aspects

- Choose a binder of the correct type and size for the intended purpose.
- Make sure the binder is positioned properly to provide support but not compromise circulation or impair breathing.
- Pad any pressure areas or skin abrasions.
- *Abdominal binder:* Remove every 2 hours, and assess the underlying skin and dressings. Fasten from the bottom up.
- *Triangular strap binder:* Position the patient's arm across the chest with elbow flexed slightly. Place one end of the triangle over the shoulder of the uninjured arm, and allow the triangle to fall open so that the elbow of the injured arm is at the apex of the triangle.
- *T-binders:* T-binders come in two types—those for females have a perineal strap; those for males have a split in the perineal strap.

Equipment

- Abdominal binder, triangular arm binder, or T-binder
- Clean nonsterile gloves
- Measuring tape

Delegation

This procedure itself may be delegated to a NAP. Assessment of the incision line or wound is a licensed professional's responsibility and should not be delegated.

Pre-Procedure Assessments

- Assess the condition of the wound (if one is present). Note the amount and type of drainage. A wound must be dressed before it is bandaged; if there is a significant amount of exudate, you will need to apply a secondary dressing.
- Assess for pain, and check the circulation of the underlying body parts before and after applying the binder. Look for cool, pale, or cyanotic skin, tingling, and numbness.
- Determine whether the client or family has the skills to reapply the binder when necessary.

➤ When performing the procedure, always identify your patient according to agency policy and be attentive to standard precautions, hand hygiene, patient safety and privacy, body mechanics, and documentation.

➤ Observe the following guidelines, regardless of the type of binder you use:

Procedure Steps

I. Choose a binder of the proper size.

2. Wash hands. Don gloves.

3. Thoroughly clean and dry the part to be covered.
Moisture contributes to skin breakdown.

4. Place the body part in its natural, comfortable position (e.g., with the joint slightly flexed), whenever possible.
This prevents strain on ligaments and muscles.

5. Pad between skin surfaces (e.g., under the axilla) and over bony prominences.
This prevents pressure and abrasion of the skin.

6. Fasten from the bottom up, especially for abdominal binders.
Fastening from the bottom up gives upward support.

◆ Make sure the binder is secured with enough pressure to provide the needed support and control bleeding, but not so tightly as to compromise circulation or impair breathing.

(continued on next page)

Procedure 34-11 ■ **Applying Binders** (continued)

7. Change binders whenever they become soiled or wet.

Proceed to step 8, 14, or 20, depending on the type of binder you are using.

Procedure Variation
Applying an Abdominal Binder

8. Measure the patient for the abdominal binder.
  a. Place the patient in supine position.
  b. With a measuring tape, encircle the abdomen at the level of the umbilicus. Note the measurement. This is the length of the binder. ▼

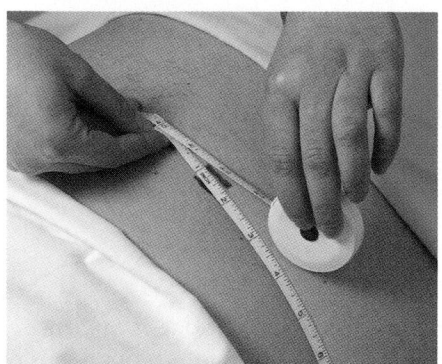

  c. Measure the distance from the costal margin to the top of the iliac crests. This is the width of the binder.
  d. Dispose of gloves and measuring tape, and wash your hands.
  e. Based on the measurements, obtain an abdominal binder.

9. Assist the patient to roll to one side. Roll one end of the binder to the center mark. Place the rolled section of the abdominal binder underneath the patient. Position the binder appropriately between the costal margin and iliac crest.

10. Make sure the binder does not slip upward or downward.
If the binder is positioned too high, it could impair lung expansion and gas exchange. If it is positioned too low, the binder will not provide adequate support.

11. Assist the patient to turn to the other side as you unroll the binder from underneath him.

✚ Pad any pressure areas or skin abrasions to avoid pressure injury.

12. With your dominant hand, grasp the end of the binder on the side furthest from you, and steadily pull toward the center of the patient's abdomen. With your nondominant hand, grasp the end of binder closest to you, and pull toward the center. Overlap the ends of the binder so that the hook and loop fasteners (e.g., Velcro®) meet. ▼

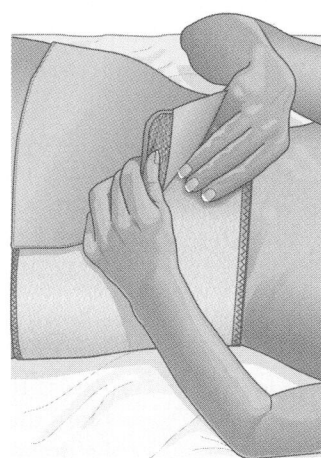

13. Remove the abdominal binder every 2 hours, and assess the underlying skin and dressings. Change wound dressings if they are soiled, or as prescribed.

Procedure Variation
Applying a Triangular Arm Binder

A triangular arm binder or sling is used to support the upper extremities. Obtain a commercial sling (consisting of a sleeve for the arm and a strap to go around the neck) or a triangular piece of fabric. To form a splint from a triangular cloth, follow these steps:

14. Ask the patient to place the affected arm in a natural position across the chest, elbow flexed slightly.
Slight flexion prevents swelling of the hand and relieves pressure on the shoulder.

15. Place one end of the triangle over the shoulder of the uninjured arm, and allow the triangle to fall open so that the elbow of the injured arm is at the apex of the triangle.

16. Move the sling behind the injured arm.

17. Pull up the lower corner of the triangle over the injured arm to the shoulder of the injured arm.

18. Tie the sling with a square knot at the neck on the side of the arm requiring support.
A square not will not slip and is easy to untie.

19. Adjust the injured arm within the sling.
To ensure patient comfort. ▼

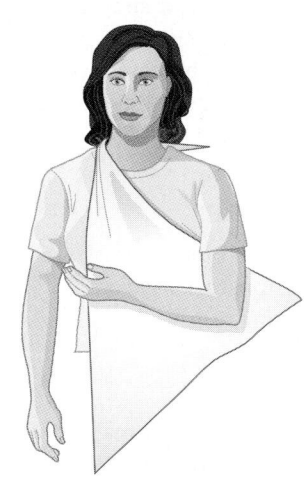

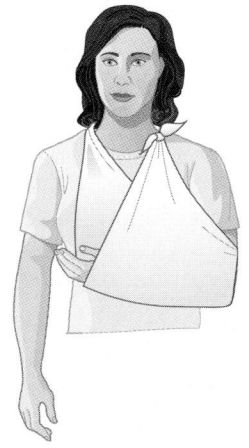

Procedure Variation
Applying a T-Binder

A T-binder is used to secure dressings or pads in the perineal area. A single T-binder is often used for women.

A double T-binder is most commonly used for men. To apply a T-binder, follow these steps:

20. Position the waist tails under the patient at the natural waistline. Bring the right and left tails together, and secure them at the waist with pins or clips. ▼

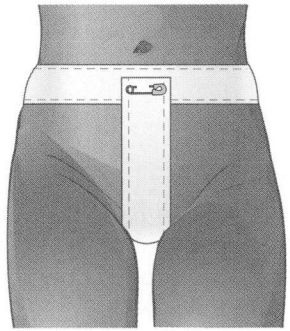

21. For a single T-binder, bring the center tail up between the legs of the patient. Secure the tail at the waist with pins or clips.

22. For a double T-binder, bring the tails up on either side of the penis. Secure the tail at the waist with pins or clips. ▼

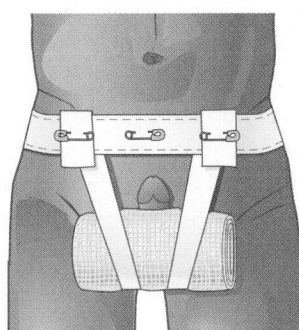

23. Fasten the ties at the waist using pins or clips.

What if . . .

■ **The patient is obese?**

Obtain the appropriate size binder before applying. Do not try to position a binder that is too small for the patient.

A poorly fitting binder can constrict circulation, cause pressure points that can injure the skin, and can restrict movement of the chest for adequate breathing. A binder that is too tight is uncomfortable and it will not provide the proper support of an incision or wound needed for healing.

Evaluation

■ Evaluate whether the patient's physical condition has changed since using the binder.
■ Assess circulation to be sure the binder is not securely too tightly. Check color, warmth, tingling, sensation, and capillary refill.
■ Assess the depth of breathing to be sure the binder is not restricting ventilation.
■ Check the skin under the binder to be sure there are no areas of irritation, pressure, or skin abrasion.
■ Assess incisions or wounds under the binder to be sure they are are not bleeding and are healing properly.
■ Monitor comfort regularly.
■ Assess the client's ability to perform ADLs while wearing the binder.

Home Care

■ Teach the client and/or caregiver how to apply the binder in the proper position, snugly but not too tightly.
■ Teach the family to inspect the site under the binder to be sure the skin is not pinched or with other points of pressure. This is especially crucial for older adults.
■ Clean binders in warm, soapy water when soiled. Use a mesh laundry bag to keep the Velcro® straps from catching other clothing in the washer. Air dry thoroughly. Clients should have two binders at home—a clean one to wear while the other is laundered.
■ Apply and remove binder to promote comfort and ensure good circulation. This also allows the patient and caregiver to inspect any incision or wound underneath.
■ Binders for children at home could be decorated with permanent marking pens.
■ Allow children to help with applying and removing the binder.

Documentation

Document the following information. (Many agencies use specialized wound care flowsheets.)

■ Appearance and location of the wound or incision under the binder, type and amount of exudates, and odor, if present, after cleansing
■ The patient's level of pain before and after the procedure. If the patient was medicated for pain, document the drug and dose used, time given, and patient response.
■ Type of binder applied
■ Date and time the binder was applied and removed
■ Any change in the appearance of the wound or skin in contact with the binder
■ Education provided to the patient

Sample documentation:

01/23/12 1240   Abdominal binder applied. Vertical abd incision with dressing dry and intact. No sign of active bleeding or wound drainage noted. Oral pain medication given approximately 60 minutes before applying binder (see MAR). Patient reported no pain, discomfort, or pressure points after application of abd binder. Patient instructed to report if the binder feels too tight or too loose.
— C. Marano, RN

Procedure 34-12 ☐ **Applying Bandages**

➤ For steps to follow in *all* procedures, refer to the Universal Steps for All Procedures found on the inside back cover of Volume 2.

Critical Aspects

- Bandage the body part in its natural position.
- Work from distal to proximal position.
- Choose a bandage of the proper width.
- Clean the wound (if present).
- Apply primary dressing as prescribed.
- Apply bandage as needed to secure primary dressing.

Equipment

- Appropriate bandage dressing
- Clean procedure gloves (2 pairs)
- Gauze sponges
- Normal saline
- Primary dressing (as prescribed)
- Scissors
- Tape or metal closures

Delegation

This procedure itself may be delegated to a NAP who has the appropriate training. Assessment of the incision line or wound is a licensed professional's responsibility and should not be delegated.

Pre-Procedure Assessment

- Determine the body part or area to be bandaged.
This allows you to choose the correct width of gauze or elastic bandage to use.

- Assess the condition of the wound (if one is present). Assess the wound for size (length, width, and depth in centimeters); location and depth of undermining or tunneling; amount, character and odor of drainage; type and percentage of tissue present in wound bed (granulation, slough, fibrin, necrotic); and periwound condition (intact, denuded, erythema, induration, or maceration)
Wound dressings should be chosen based on the characteristics of the wound.

- Assess for pain, and check the circulation of the underlying body parts before and after applying the bandage. Look for cool, pale, or cyanotic skin, tingling, and numbness.
Circulation to an extremity can be compromised if the bandage is too tight or the extremity swells after application.

- Determine whether the client or family has the skills to reapply the bandage when necessary.
Teaching might be needed for home care.

➤ When performing the procedure, always identify your patient according to agency policy and be attentive to standard precautions, hand hygiene, patient safety and privacy, body mechanics, and documentation.

Procedure Steps

Observe the following guidelines, regardless of the type of bandage you use:

1. Choose a bandage of the proper width. For example, use a 2.5-cm (1-in.) wide bandage for a finger, a 5-cm (2-in.) wide bandage for an arm, and a wider bandage for a leg.
This prevents pressure and abrasion of the skin.

2. Thoroughly clean and dry the part to be covered. Use a nontoxic cleansing solution, such as normal saline.

Cleaning the wound removes debris, exudates, and bacteria. Drainage and moisture on the skin contribute to irritation.

3. Remove excess fluid by gently patting the wound and surrounding skin with gauze sponge.
Drainage and moisture contribute to skin breakdown.

4. Stand facing the patient.
In this position you can wrap the bandage evenly in the proper direction.

5. Bandage the body part in a comfortable position (e.g., with the joint slightly flexed), whenever possible.

This prevents strain on ligaments and muscles. Movement of the extremity (extension) may cause skin damage if the bandage is too tight or the extremity is not properly positioned.

6. Always work from distal to proximal (or peripheral to central).
This improves venous return and helps to prevent edema.

7. If a wound is present, apply a primary dressing, as prescribed, over the wound.
A primary dressing is any dressing that is placed first in the wound bed. It provides exudates absorption, holds medications in place, provides

antimicrobial coverage, or maintains a moist wound bed.

8. Apply the bandage with enough pressure to provide the needed support, but do not bandage too tightly. Make sure circulation to the area is not interrupted.

9. If possible, leave the fingers (if you are bandaging an arm) or toes (if you are bandaging a leg or foot) exposed so that you can assess the circulation to the extremity. Begin the wrap along the pad of the foot or hand, just under the first bend of the toes or fingers (metatarsal or metacarpal joints).

10. Begin the wrap with the bandage against the skin. Unwind the bandage as if rolling it over the extremity. This helps to keep the bandage snug against the skin.

11. Pad bony prominences before bandaging if there are pressure concerns.

12. Change bandages whenever they become soiled or wet from external sources (stool, urine, etc.) and internal sources (drainage that has wicked on the outer surface of the bandage). Wound drainage contains chemicals, enzymes, and bacteria that can damage fragile healing tissues.

13. After bandaging, assess circulation and comfort regularly.

Proceed to step 14, 16, 19, 25, or 28, depending on the type of bandaging you are using.

Procedure Variation
Circular Turns

Use this technique to wrap a finger or toe, or as an anchor at the beginning and end of another wrapping technique.

14. With one hand, hold one end of the bandage in place. With the other hand, encircle the body part two times with the bandage—the second wrap should partially cover the first wrap.

Continue to wrap the body part by overlapping two-thirds of the width of the bandage.

15. If circular turns are not being combined with another technique, secure the bandage with tape or metal clips when you are finished. ▼

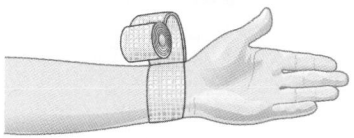

Procedure Variation
Spiral Turns

Spiral turns are a variation of the circular turn technique. Spiral turns are most commonly used to wrap an extremity.

16. Anchor the bandage by making two circular turns—the second wrap completely covering the first one.

17. Continue to wrap the extremity by encircling the body part with each turn angled at approximately 30° so that you are overlapping the preceding wrap by two-thirds the width of the bandage.

18. Complete the wrap by making two circular turns and securing the bandage with tape or metal clips. ▼

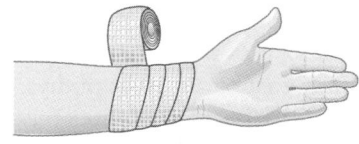

Procedure Variation
Spiral Reverse Turns

Spiral reverse turns are used to bandage cylindrical body parts that are not uniform in size.

19. Anchor the bandage by making two circular turns.

20. Bring the next wrap up at a 30° angle.

21. Place the thumb of your nondominant hand on the wrap to hold the bandage. ▼

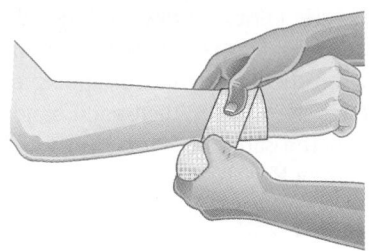

22. Fold the bandage back on itself, and continue to wrap at a 30° angle in the opposite direction. ▼

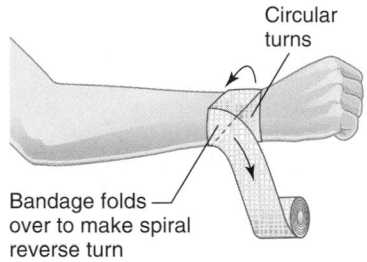

Circular turns

Bandage folds over to make spiral reverse turn

23. Continue to wrap the bandage, overlapping each turn by two-thirds. Align each bandage turn at the same position on the extremity. ▼

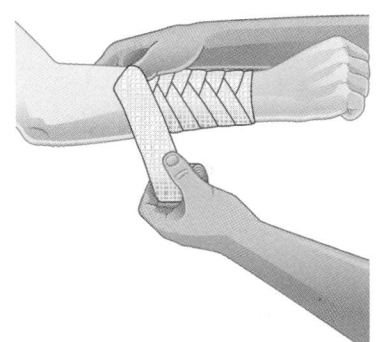

24. Complete the wrap by making two circular turns and securing the bandage with tape or metal clips.

Procedure Variation
Figure-8 Turns

The figure-8 wrap is used on joints (e.g., ankle, elbow).

25. Anchor the bandage by making two circular turns.

(continued on next page)

Procedure 34-12 ■ **Applying Bandages** (continued)

26. Wrap the bandage by ascending above the joint and descending below the joint to form a figure 8. Continue to wrap the bandage, overlapping each turn by two-thirds. Align each bandage turn at the same position on the extremity. ▼

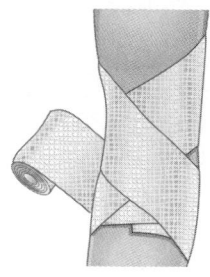

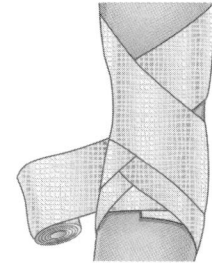

27. Complete the wrap by making two circular turns and securing the bandage with tape or metal clips.

Procedure Variation
Recurrent Turns

28. Anchor the bandage by making two circular turns.

29. Fold the bandage back on itself; hold it against the body part with one hand. With the other hand, make a half turn perpendicular to the circle turns

and central to the distal end being bandaged. ▼

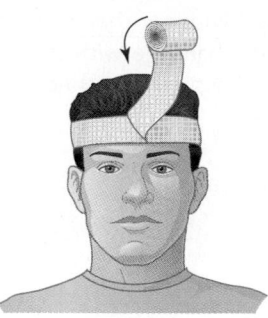

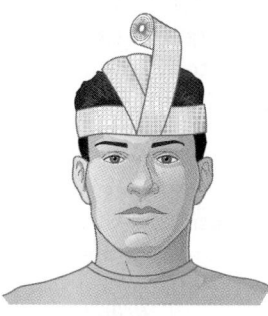

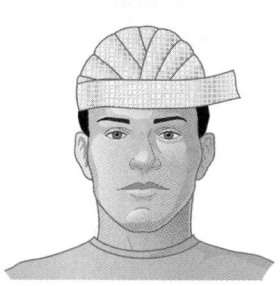

30. Hold the central turn with one hand, and fold the bandage back on itself; bring it over the distal end of the body part to the right of the center, overlapping the center turn by two-thirds the width of the bandage.

31. Next, hold the bandage at the center with one hand as you bring the bandage back over the end to the left of center. Continue holding and folding the bandage back on itself, alternating right and left until the body part is covered. Overlap by two-thirds the bandage width with each turn.

32. Start and return each turn to the midline or center of the body part, and angle it slightly more each time to continue covering the body part.

33. Complete the bandage by making two circular turns and securing the bandage with tape or metal clips.

What if . . .

■ **Drainage breaks through the outer bandage more frequently than expected?**

Determine the cause of the drainage if possible (i.e., is it blood or serum?). Increased drainage may be a sign of infection and should be evaluated. The dressing change frequency may need to be increased or an alternate dressing with a higher degree of exudate absorption may be needed.

Wound exudates can harm healing tissues. Dressings that are saturated should be changed as soon as possible to prevent prolonged moisture exposure or maceration.

Patient Teaching

■ Teach the patient about the expected healing process.
■ Inform the patient and caregiver about signs and symptoms of infection and the need to report these findings.
■ Instruct the patient and family about signs of circulation problems and how to remove bandage if needed.

Home Care

■ Refer the client to a home health agency for wound care.
■ Some clients or caregivers may be able to perform dressing changes. Determine the client and/or caregiver's ability to perform dressing changes; teach and demonstrate as needed.

Documentation

Many agencies use wound care flowsheets.
■ Appearance and location of the wound, type and amount of exudates, and odor, if present, after cleansing.
■ Level of pain before the procedure. If the patient was medicated for pain, document the drug and dose used, time given, and patient response.
■ Method of cleansing the wound and surrounding skin, if performed
■ Application of primary and secondary dressings
■ Education provided to the patient

Sample EHR documentation:

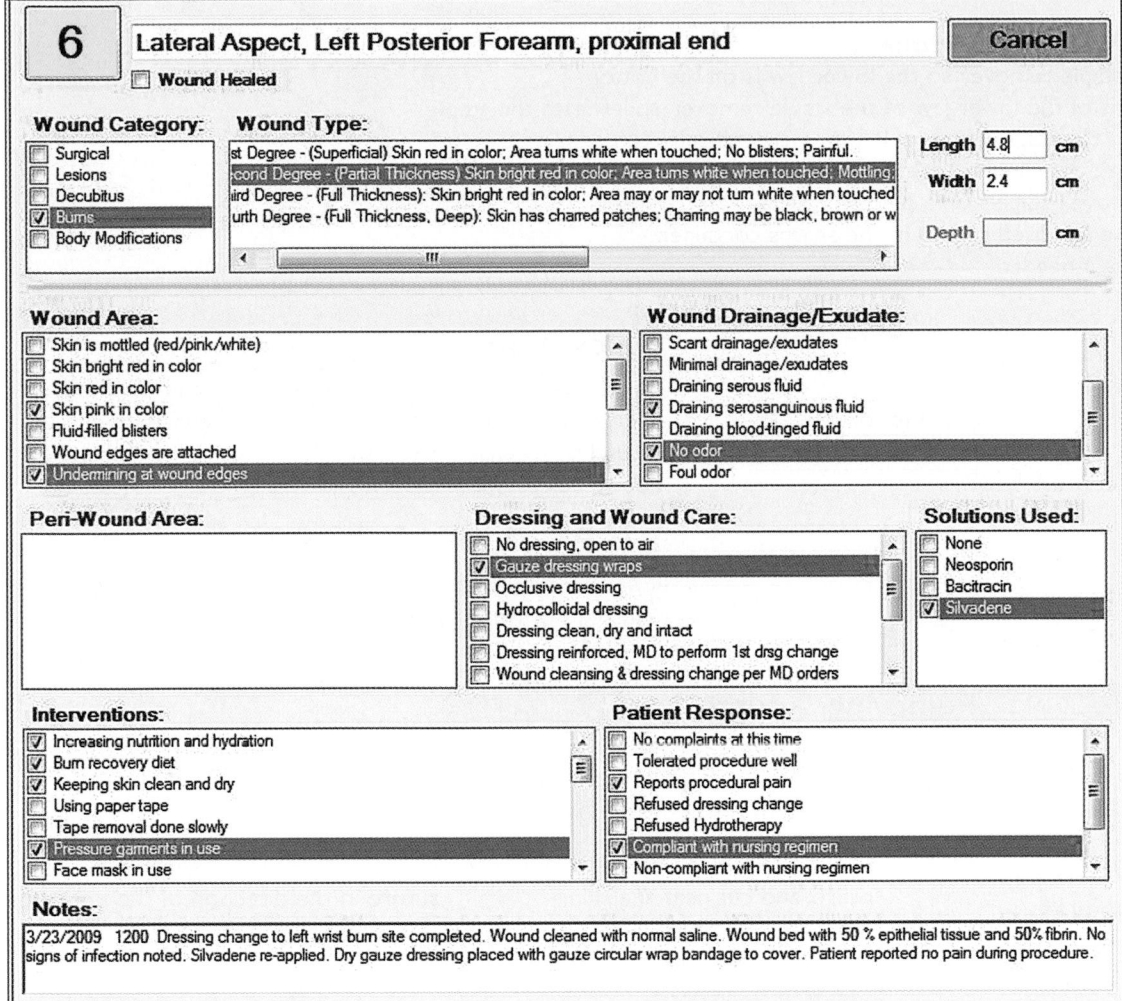

Practice Resources

Bergeron, J. D., Bizjak, G., Le Badour, G., et al. (2009); Rolstad, B. S., & Ovington, L. G. (2007).

Thinking About the Procedure

 Go to the *Fundamentals of Nursing Skills Videos,* **Wound Care: Bandaging with Circular and Spiral Turns.**

1. Name three tips the nurse suggested for bandaging using circular and spiral turns?

 For suggested responses, go to Chapter 34, **Thinking About the Procedure Suggested Responses (Procedure 34-12),** on the Student Resource Disk or DavisPlus at http://davisplus.fadavis.com/Wilkinson2

Procedure 34-13   Removing Sutures and Staples

> For steps to follow in *all* procedures, refer to the Universal Steps for All Procedures found on the inside back cover of Volume 2.

Critical Aspects

Procedure 34-13A: Suture Removal
- Place the patient in a comfortable position that provides easy access to the wound.
- Use the forceps to pick up one end of the suture. Slide the small scissors around the suture, and cut near the skin.
- With the forceps, gently pull the suture in the direction of the knotted side to remove it.

(continued on next page)

Procedure 34-13 ■ Removing Sutures and Staples (continued)

Procedure 34-13B: Staple Removal
- Position the staple remover so the lower jaw is on the bottom.
- Place both tips of the lower jaw of the staple remover underneath the staple.
- Lift slightly on the staple ensuring it stays perpendicular to the skin.
- Gently squeeze the handles together and lift the staple straight up.
- Place the removed staples on a piece of gauze.
- Dispose of the removed staples in the sharps container.
- Apply dressing if needed.

Equipment
- Nonsterile procedure gloves
- Suture removal kit or sterile scissors and forceps (Procedure 34-13A)
- Staple remover (Procedure 34-13B)
- Gauze

Delegation
This procedure itself may be delegated to a NAP who has been trained in the skill. Assessment of the incision line or wound is a licensed professional's responsibility and should not be delegated.

Pre-Procedure Assessment
- Assess staples to ensure none have rotated or turned instead of lying flat along the incision.

■ Procedure 34-13A Removing Sutures

➤ When performing the procedure, always identify your patient according to agency policy and be attentive to standard precautions, hand hygiene, patient safety and privacy, body mechanics, and documentation.

Procedure Steps

1. Obtain a suture removal kit.

2. Use the forceps to pick up one end of the suture. ▼

3. Slide the small scissors around the suture, and cut near the skin.
This helps you avoid pulling the exposed portion of the suture through the underlying tissue.

4. With the forceps, gently pull the suture in the direction of the knotted side to remove it. ▼

Suture types

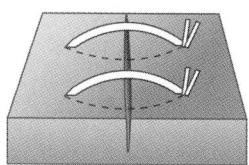

Plain interrupted

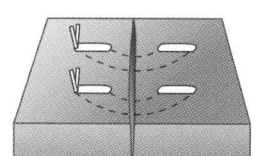

Mattress interrupted

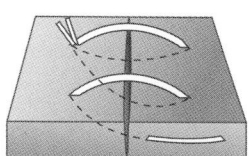

Plain continuous

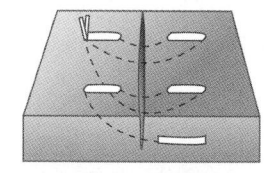

Mattress continuous

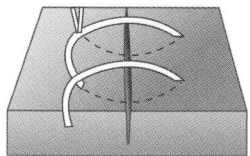

Blanket continuous

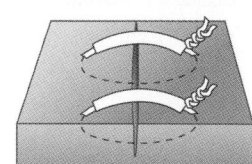

Retention

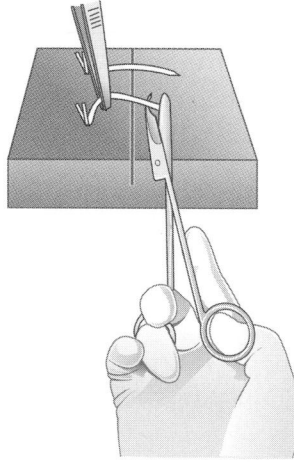

Removing interrupted sutures

5. Apply dressing if needed.

6. Remove gloves and perform hand hygiene.

■ Procedure 34-13B Removing Staples

1. Wash hands. Don gloves.

2. After cleansing the wound or incision, position the staple remover so that the lower jaw is on the bottom.

3. Place both tips of the lower jaw of the remover under the staple. ▼

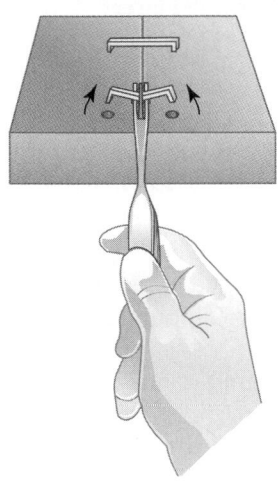

Removing staples

4. Ensure the staple is perpendicular to the plane of the skin. If not, reposition the staple with the tips of the lower jaw and apply gentle pressure, causing it to straighten the ends for easier removal.

5. Lift slightly on the staple ensuring that it stays perpendicular to the skin.

6. Continue to lift slightly as you gently squeeze the handles together to close.
This spreads the ends of the staples apart, freeing them from the skin.

7. Lift the reshaped staple straight up from the skin.

8. Remove every other staple, and check the tension on the wound.

9. If there is no significant pull on the wound, remove the remaining staples.

10. Place the removed staples on a piece of gauze.
Staples are small and can be easily lost. Keeping them in one place prevents this.

11. Apply dressing if needed.

12. Dispose of the removed staples in the sharps container.
Ends of the staples are sharp and should be handled with care.

13. Remove gloves and wash hands.

What if . . .

■ **A staple gets stuck?**

Gently manipulate the staple with the remover until it is perpendicular to the skin.

When the skin is stapled, the edges of the staple are crimped to hold the incision together. To be removed, those edges must be reshaped and straightened. If one edge of the staple is reshaped and the other is not, it can be painful to remove if not further manipulated.

■ **The incision needs a dressing once the staples or sutures have been removed?**

New surgical incisions should be covered with a sterile dressing the first 24 to 48 hours, but not necessarily after that time. Apply a dressing if you are concerned about soiling or per your institution's policy.

In a healing incision, epithelial resurfacing is complete in 24 to 48 hours. Though only a few cells thick, this epithelium is enough to keep the wound closed and provide a bacterial barrier.

Evaluation

- Note whether the incision is well approximated after the procedure.
- Ensure that the patient verbalized understanding of the treatment.
- Inspect the wound daily.

Patient Teaching

- Instruct the client of signs and symptoms of wound infections (i.e., redness, drainage) and the need to report these findings.
- Instruct the client that he may be able to shower once sutures or staples are removed, if approved by the provider.

Documentation

Document the following information. (Many agencies use wound care flowsheets.)
- Appearance and location of the wound, type and amount of exudates, and odor, if present, after cleansing
- The patient's level of pain before and after the procedure. If the patient was medicated for pain,

document the drug and dose used, time given, and patient response.
- Method of cleansing the wound and surrounding skin, if performed
- Removal of staples or sutures
- Education provided to the patient

Sample documentation:

02/23/12 1100   *Staples removed from*
abdominal midline incision. Incision edges well
approximated without erythema, drainage, or
swelling. Dry dressing applied. Patient
tolerated the procedure without discomfort.
Discussed purpose of staple removal with
patient. Will continue to monitor wound daily.—
                                    M. Daley, RN

Practice Resources
Autio, L., & Olsen, K. K. (2002).

Procedure 34-14 ☐ Shortening a Wound Drain

➤ For steps to follow in *all* procedures, refer to the Universal Steps for All Procedures found on the inside back cover of Volume 2.

Critical Aspects

- Before shortening a wound drain, make sure it is secured tightly.
- Firmly grasp the full width of the drain at the level of the skin and pull it out by the prescribed amount (e.g., 6 mm [¼ in.]).
- Insert a sterile safety pin through the drain at the level of the skin. Hold the drain tightly, and insert the pin above your fingers.
- Using sterile scissors, cut the drain a little above the safety pin.

Equipment

- Nonsterile procedure gloves
- Sterile gloves
- Sterile scissors
- Two safety pins or other clips (sterile)
- Sterile gauze

Delegation

This procedure may be delegated to a NAP who has been appropriately trained in the skill. Assessment of the incision line or wound is a licensed professional's responsibility and should not be delegated.

Pre-Procedure Assessment

- Inspect the site around the drain, noting skin excoriation, tenderness, erythema, warmth to the touch, and drainage seeping from the wound.

Could indicate a wound infection or irritation of the drain at the skin site. Excoriation can be the result of seeping drainage around the tube (e.g., if the tube diameter is not sufficient size to handle drainage output) or more likely, an obstruction within the tubing.

- Assess the characteristics of the drainage, including color, volume drainage, presence of blood, odor, pus, and any change in the type or amount of drainage through the tubing.

A sudden decrease in drainage might indicate a blocked drain. Presence of fresh blood might be a sign of irritation within the wound. Pus and odor in the drainage could indicate wound infection.

- Check the suction apparatus to be sure it is functioning properly.

A self-suction apparatus might need to be recompressed from time to time to maintain effective vacuum. Electric suction units can fail, delivering too much suction, which can lead to injury. Too little suction can contribute to insufficient drainage, which can lead to pressure on sutures if present, or cause the wound to become infected or heal more slowly.

➤ When performing the procedure, always identify your patient according to agency policy and be attentive to standard precautions, hand hygiene, patient safety and privacy, body mechanics, and documentation.

Procedure Steps

1. After donning procedure gloves, remove wound dressings.

2. Remove soiled gloves and discard in a moisture-proof biohazard collection container.

3. Open sterile supplies (scissors, etc.).

4. Don sterile gloves; use sterile scissors to cut halfway through a sterile gauze dressing (for later use), or use a sterile precut drain dressing.

5. If the drain is sutured in place, use sterile scissors to cut the suture.

6. Firmly grasp the full width of the drain at the level of the skin and pull it out by the prescribed amount (e.g., 6 mm [¼ in.]).

7. Insert a sterile safety pin through the drain at the level of the skin. Hold the drain tightly, and insert the pin above your fingers.
This will keep from sticking the client or your fingers. The pin keeps the drain from disappearing into the wound. ▼

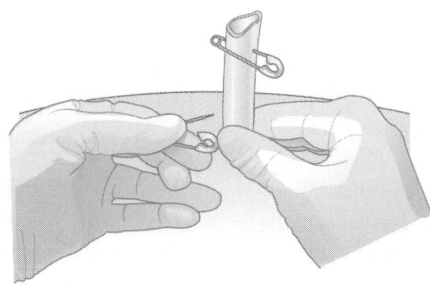

8. Using sterile scissors, cut off the drain at about 2.5 cm (1 in.) above the skin. ▼

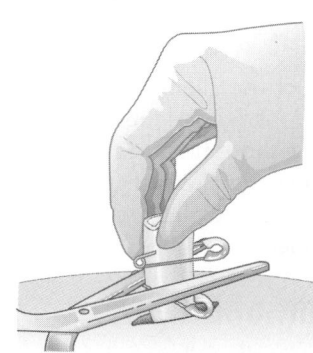

9. Cleanse the wound, using sterile gauze swabs and the prescribed cleaning solution. In some situations,

you may use sterile forceps to manipulate the swabs.

10. Apply precut sterile gauze around the drain; then redress the wound. ▼

11. Remove gloves and discard in a biohazard container. Wash your hands.

12. Leave the patient in a safe and comfortable position.

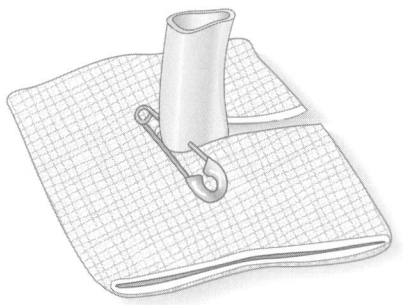

What if...

■ **You shorten the drain too much?**
Immediately notify the surgeon who placed the drain.

The drain will need to be evaluated to be sure it remains intact, which it mostly likely will. Drainage tubing is secured under the skin surface and will probably not be dislodged with shortening.

Patient Evaluation

■ Assess the local area of skin around the drain after manipulating it.
■ Note the patency of the drain after shortening it.
■ Be sure the drain is secure after shortening.
■ Evaluate for complications occurring related to shortening procedure.

Patient Teaching

■ Patients should not shorten their own drains. Consult a healthcare provider if concerned about the length of tubing or drains.

Documentation

■ Record the intervention.
■ Note the amount and characteristics of the drainage.
■ Document the appearance of the wound.
■ Note any complications that occur with shortening a drain (e.g., manipulation of tubing causes bleeding or drainage at the site).

Sample EHR documentation

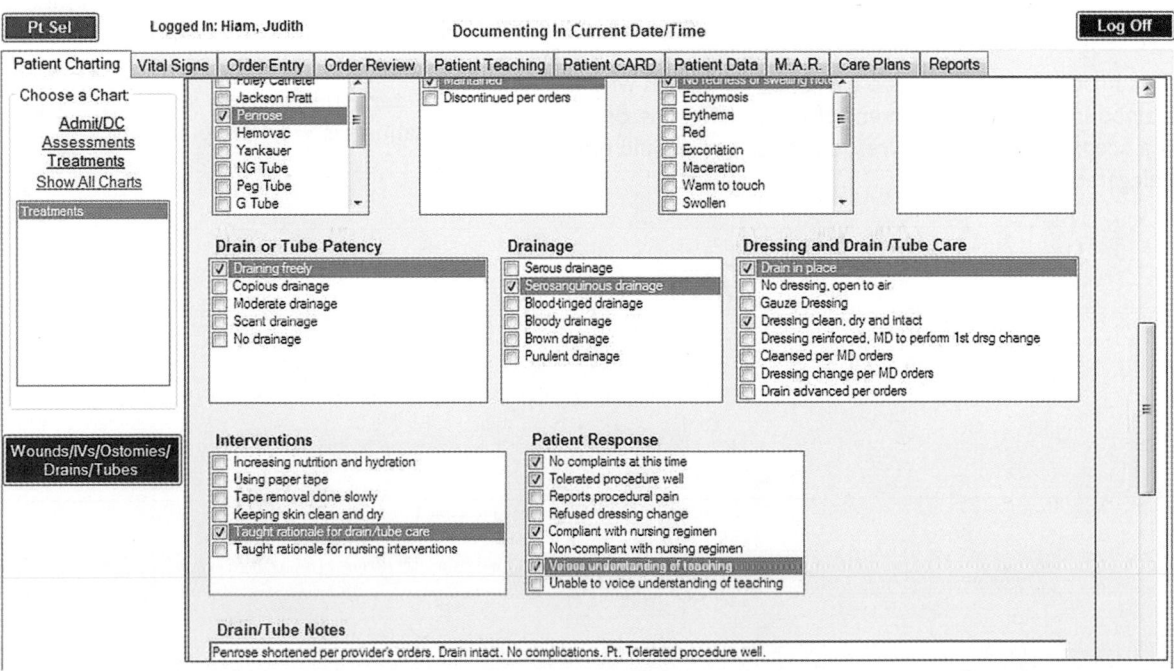

(continued on next page)

Procedure 34-14 ■ **Shortening a Wound Drain** (continued)

Thinking About the Procedure

 Go to the *Fundamentals of Nursing Skills Videos*, **Wound Care: Wound Drainage Systems, Penrose.**

1. In what manner does the nurse clean around the penrose drainage tubing?

2. Where is the drain positioned when redressing the wound?

 For suggested responses, go to Chapter 34, **Thinking About the Procedure Suggested Responses (Procedure 34-14),** on the Student Resource Disk or DavisPlus at http://davisplus.fadavis.com/Wilkinson2

Procedure 34-15   **Emptying a Closed-Wound Drainage System**

➤ For steps to follow in *all* procedures, refer to the Universal Steps for All Procedures found on the inside back cover of Volume 2.

Critical Aspects

- Don personal protective equipment as needed, including nonsterile procedure gloves, gown, and eyewear.
- Properly dispose of contaminated items into designated biohazard waste receptacles.
- Measure drainage and report excess volume to the primary care provider.

Equipment

- Drainage container with graduated markings
- Nonsterile procedure gloves
- Disposal sink for biomaterial
- Biohazard disposal receptacle

Delegation

This procedure itself may be delegated to a NAP who is trained in the skill. Assessment of the incision line or wound is a licensed professional's responsibility and should not be delegated.

Pre-Procedure Assessment

- Assess the appearance of the drainage tube site and sutures, if in place.
- Inspect for warmth, edema, redness, or pus where tubing penetrates the skin.
- Check to be sure the closed-wound drainage system is securely fastened at the connections and within the wound.
- Determine whether suction (electric, portable, or manual) is working properly.

➤ When performing the procedure, always identify your patient according to agency policy and be attentive to standard precautions, hand hygiene, patient safety and privacy, body mechanics, and documentation.

Procedure Steps

1. Read the instructions about the drainage device.

Procedures vary among manufacturers and different systems.

2. Don procedure gloves and goggles or mask.

3. Unpin the drainage device from the patient's gown.

The drainage device is often pinned to the patient's gown to prevent it from dislodging.

4. Open the drainage port, and empty the drainage into a small graduated container. ▼

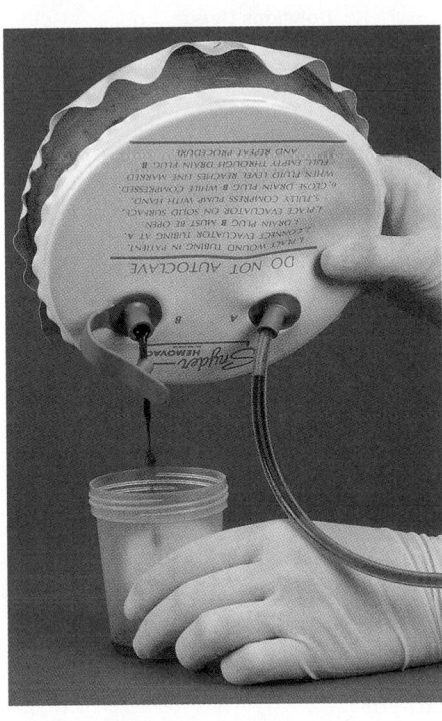

5. With the port still open, place the collection device on a firm, flat surface (e.g., the overbed table).

6. Use the palm of one hand to press down on the device and eject air from it. Do not stand directly over the air vent. Do not touch the drainage port.

It can splash or bubble.

7. Use the other hand to scrub the port and plug with an alcohol-based antiseptic or povidone iodine swab (Betadine), if the patient is not allergic to iodine. ▼

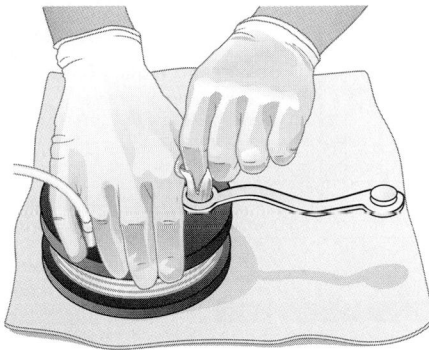

8. Continuing to press down on the device, replace the plug in the port. Do not touch the open port or the part of the plug that goes into the port.

This will create a constant, negative pressure vacuum to facilitate suction.

9. Repin the drainage device to the patient's gown.

Pinning keeps it secure and prevents it from accidentally dislodging.

10. Measure the drainage in the graduated container; discard drainage in the disposable container for biohazardous material. Wash the graduated container. Do not stand in front of an air vent while doing so.

Forced air in the room can cause the drainage to splash or bubble, introducing biohazard into the environmental air.

11. Remove your gloves. Perform hand hygiene.

12. Document in the patient's record.

What if . . .

■ **The wound drainage spills?**

Don procedure gloves. Wipe up the spilled biomaterial (patient body fluid). Dispose of contaminated materials in a biohazard waste receptacle.

Proper handling of contaminated biomaterials is important to prevent transmission of infectious organisms.

Home Care

■ Teach family members who are emptying drainage systems at home to wear gloves and avoid touching the drainage port.

Documentation

■ Note the date and time the drainage system is emptied.
■ Record the volume lost. Report excess fluid loss to the primary care provider.
■ Describe the appearance of drainage, including presence of blood or purulent material.

(continued on next page)

Procedure 34-15 ■ **Emptying a Closed-Wound Drainage System** (continued)

Sample EHR documentation:

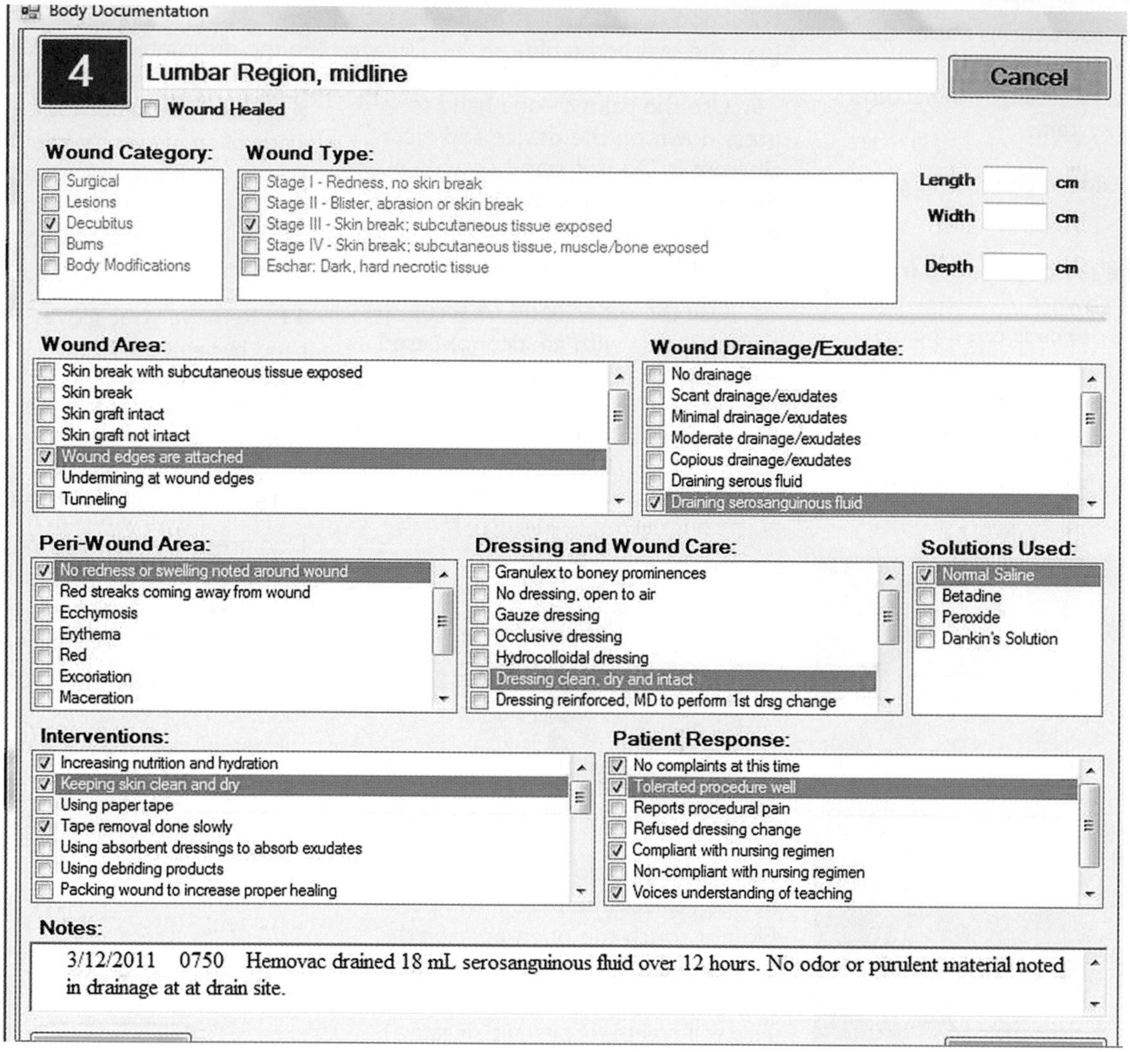

Body Documentation

4 | **Lumbar Region, midline** | **Cancel**

☐ Wound Healed

Wound Category:
- ☐ Surgical
- ☐ Lesions
- ☑ Decubitus
- ☐ Bums
- ☐ Body Modifications

Wound Type:
- ☐ Stage I - Redness, no skin break
- ☐ Stage II - Blister, abrasion or skin break
- ☑ Stage III - Skin break; subcutaneous tissue exposed
- ☐ Stage IV - Skin break; subcutaneous tissue, muscle/bone exposed
- ☐ Eschar: Dark, hard necrotic tissue

Length ____ cm
Width ____ cm
Depth ____ cm

Wound Area:
- ☐ Skin break with subcutaneous tissue exposed
- ☐ Skin break
- ☐ Skin graft intact
- ☐ Skin graft not intact
- ☑ Wound edges are attached
- ☐ Undermining at wound edges
- ☐ Tunneling

Wound Drainage/Exudate:
- ☐ No drainage
- ☐ Scant drainage/exudates
- ☐ Minimal drainage/exudates
- ☐ Moderate drainage/exudates
- ☐ Copious drainage/exudates
- ☐ Draining serous fluid
- ☑ Draining serosanguinous fluid

Peri-Wound Area:
- ☑ No redness or swelling noted around wound
- ☐ Red streaks coming away from wound
- ☐ Ecchymosis
- ☐ Erythema
- ☐ Red
- ☐ Excoriation
- ☐ Maceration

Dressing and Wound Care:
- ☐ Granulex to boney prominences
- ☐ No dressing, open to air
- ☐ Gauze dressing
- ☐ Occlusive dressing
- ☐ Hydrocolloidal dressing
- ☑ Dressing clean, dry and intact
- ☐ Dressing reinforced, MD to perform 1st drsg change

Solutions Used:
- ☑ Normal Saline
- ☐ Betadine
- ☐ Peroxide
- ☐ Dankin's Solution

Interventions:
- ☑ Increasing nutrition and hydration
- ☑ Keeping skin clean and dry
- ☐ Using paper tape
- ☑ Tape removal done slowly
- ☐ Using absorbent dressings to absorb exudates
- ☐ Using debriding products
- ☐ Packing wound to increase proper healing

Patient Response:
- ☑ No complaints at this time
- ☑ Tolerated procedure well
- ☐ Reports procedural pain
- ☐ Refused dressing change
- ☑ Compliant with nursing regimen
- ☐ Non-compliant with nursing regimen
- ☑ Voices understanding of teaching

Notes:

3/12/2011   0750   Hemovac drained 18 mL serosanguinous fluid over 12 hours. No odor or purulent material noted in drainage at at drain site.

Thinking About the Procedure

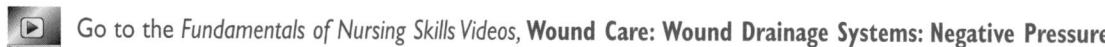 Go to the *Fundamentals of Nursing Skills Videos,* **Wound Care: Wound Drainage Systems: Negative Pressure.**

1. What does the nurse empty the wound drainage into? Where is the drainage discarded?

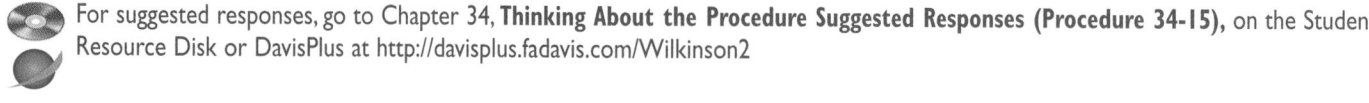 For suggested responses, go to Chapter 34, **Thinking About the Procedure Suggested Responses (Procedure 34-15),** on the Student Resource Disk or DavisPlus at http://davisplus.fadavis.com/Wilkinson2

Clinical Insights

Clinical Insight 34-1 ▶ **Applying Local Heat Therapy**

Preparation

■ Determine whether there are any contraindications to the treatment, such as impaired circulation, bleeding, wound complications, or inability to tolerate the treatment.

■ Explain the application and rationale to the client.

Moist Heat (Irrigations, Compresses, Hot Soaks)

If skin is intact:

■ Soak a washcloth or towel in warm water (105° to 115°F [40° to 46°C]), and wring out the excess before applying to the skin. Reapply and change water frequently to maintain a constant temperature.

For open areas, use a compress, a soak, or a bath:

■ To make a compress, soak gauze in the heated solution (105° to 115°F [40° to 46°C]), and then apply it to the wound. Usually, you will use sterile gloves, gauze, and solution.

■ Reapply compresses or towels, and change the water frequently to maintain a constant temperature.
Heat disperses quickly.

■ **For a soak** you will need to immerse the affected area. Sterilized tubs are often used for this procedure.

■ **A sitz bath** soaks the client's perineal area. A special tub or chair may be used. Because of infection control concerns, disposable sitz baths are preferred. Check that the water temperature is from 105° to 110°F (40° to 43°C). Instruct the client to soak for 15 minutes.

Dry Heat (Electric Heating Pads, Disposable Hot Packs, Hot Water Bags)

Aquathermia pads (also called K-pads) are plastic or vinyl pads that circulate water in the interior.

■ Connect the pad via tubing to the electric heating unit, which constantly exchanges water that has been heated to the specified temperature.

■ Fill the reservoir about two-thirds full of distilled water.

■ Set the temperature control to 98° to 105°F (37° to 40.5°C).

■ Cover the pad, and apply it to the body part.
To prevent tissue injury.

Disposable hot packs and hot water bags or bottles:

■ Use water that is 115° to 125°F (46° to 52°C).

■ Fill the bag about two-thirds full of warm tap water, expel the air from the bag, and close the top.

■ Tip the bag upside down to test for leaking.

■ Wrap the bag in a towel, and place it on the client.
Never place a heat source directly on the client's skin. Burns can occur.

Electric heating pads:

■ Be sure that the body part is dry or that the pad has a waterproof cover.

✚ **Safety Precautions for Electric Heating Pads**

■ Do not use pins (e.g., to hold a cover in place) or other sharp objects on the pad.
The pin could go through a wire and cause an electric shock.

■ Tell the client to report any discomfort during the treatment

■ Measure water temperature with a bath thermometer.

■ For home use, warn the client about the danger of burns from high settings. Use pads with a switch that the client cannot turn up.

■ Avoid direct contact with the heating device. Cover the heat source with a washcloth, towel, or fitted sleeve.

■ Do not place the heating device (pad, bag) under the client; place it over the body part.
This helps prevent burns.

■ Apply heat intermittently, leaving it on for no more than 15 minutes at a time in an area.
This helps prevent tissue injury (e.g., burns, impaired circulation). It also makes the therapy more effective by preventing rebound phenomenon: At the time the heat reaches maximum therapeutic effect, the opposite effect (vasoconstriction) begins.

■ Check the skin frequently for extreme redness or blistering.

■ Assess for hypotension and faintness. If they occur, discontinue the treatment. Have the client lie down for several minutes. When the faint feeling passes, assist the client to sit up slowly. Recheck the blood pressure (BP) when the client is in the sitting position. If the BP remains low, encourage the client to remain seated. If the client is ambulatory, have her dangle her feet for several minutes before she gets up.

Clinical Insight 34-2 ▶ **Applying Local Cold Therapy**

Preparation

- Determine whether there are any contraindications to the treatment, such as impaired circulation, bleeding, wound complications, or inability to tolerate the treatment.
- Explain the application and rationale to the client.
- Assess for indications for cold application (e.g., fever above 104°F [40°C]). Measure the client's temperature.

Cooling Baths

A cooling bath is often used to treat a high fever (above 104°F [40°C]). It promotes heat loss through conduction and vaporization.

- Prepare a pan of water with a temperature from 65° to 90°F (18° to 32°C).
- You may add a fan to increase heat loss if the temperature is markedly elevated.
- Slowly sponge the face, arms, legs, back, and buttocks with the cool water. Do not dry the areas; cover with a damp towel.
- Take about 30 minutes to complete the bath.

Cooling the body too rapidly will cause shivering, which will increase heat production.

- You may also place ice bags or cold packs on the forehead and in the axillae and the groin.
- Assess the client constantly during a cooling bath.

If the client begins to shiver, his temperature may actually rise.

Cold Compresses

- Apply a cool, damp cloth or towel to the body part.
- Renew the compress or cloth frequently.

The temperature of the compress or cloth will rapidly rise toward body temperature.

Ice Collars, Ice Bags, Commercially Prepared Cold Packs, Aquapads

- You can make an ice bag out of a procedure glove or small plastic bag by filling it with ice chips and tying a knot in the top.
- Fill the ice bag with ice chips or an alcohol-based solution.
- Cover ice bags or packs with a towel or soft cover.
- Apply to the skin for a maximum of 15 minutes, then remove. You may reapply the cold pack in 1 hour.

◆ Safety Precautions for Cooling Devices

- Measure water temperature with a bath thermometer.
- Tell the client to report any discomfort during the treatment.
- Avoid direct contact with the cooling device. Cover the cold pack with a washcloth, towel, or fitted sleeve.
- Apply cold intermittently, leaving it on for no more than 15 minutes at a time in an area.

This helps prevent tissue injury (e.g., impaired circulation). It also makes the therapy more effective by preventing rebound phenomenon: At the time the cold reaches maximum therapeutic effect, the opposite effect (vasodilation) begins.

- Observe for tissue damage: bluish purple mottled appearance of the skin, numbness, and sometimes blisters and pain.
- Monitor for elevated blood pressure.

Assessment Guidelines and Tools

History Questions for Skin and Wound Assessment

- What is your typical activity level?
- Do you ever use a wheelchair or mobile device to get around? Do you require assistance to get out of bed or a chair?
- Tell me about your usual diet.
- How much liquid do you drink each day?
- Do you have any areas of numbness and tingling?
- Have you had any recent changes in your skin?
- Do you have any sores or open areas? If so, how long have you had the wound?
- Have you ever had difficulty with wound healing?

- What kinds of healthcare problems have you been experiencing?
- What medications—prescribed, herbal, or over-the-counter—are you taking?
- What is your typical hygiene routine?
- Do you ever lose control of your bladder or bowels?
- Do you smoke?
- How much time do you spend outdoors?
- Do you have diabetes? If so, how often do you check your feet? How often do you see a podiatrist? What is your average blood sugar?

Physical Examination: Wound Assessment

All Wounds

Assess all wounds for the following:

Location

Describe the location of the wound in anatomical terms. For example, you would describe an incision from cardiac surgery as a midsternal incision extending from the manubrium to the xiphoid process.

Size

- Measure the length and width of the wound in centimeters.
- To measure wound depth, gently insert a sterile cotton tip applicator into the deepest part of the wound. Measure the applicator from the skin level to the tip.
- If possible, use photo documentation, indicating the dimensions on the photo. This is especially useful in the case of a wound with an irregular border.

Appearance

Your description of the appearance of the wound should be very detailed. You must describe:

- **Type of wound** (open or closed)
- **If the wound is sutured,** examine the closure. Are the wound edges approximated? Is there tension on any aspect of the wound? Are the stitches intact?
- **The color of the wound.** Redness and inflammation for the first 2 to 3 days is normal, but erythema or swelling beyond that time may indicate infection.
- **Condition of the wound bed (in an open wound).** A beefy red, moist appearance is evidence of healing. A pale color or dry texture indicates a delay in healing.
- **Examine for necrosis, slough, and eschar.** Examine for a tunnel or sinus tract in the wound bed; if there is one, inspect and probe it for depth and characteristics.
- **The skin surrounding the wound.** Observe for skin discoloration, hematoma, or additional injury to the surrounding tissue. Observe for maceration, tunneling, crepitus, blistering, or erythema. Examine the edges of the wound for epithelial tissue and contraction. Look for undermining beneath the wound margins.

Drainage

- **Presence of drainage or exudate.** Describe the color, consistency, amount, and odor.

- **Assess the quantity of wound drainage** by weighing dressings before they are applied and again when they have been removed. The change in weight reflects the amount of drainage that they have absorbed.
- **If a drain is present,** measure the amount of fluid in the collection container.
- **Odor** may indicate fistula formation or contamination with bacteria. If a new odor develops, assess carefully for presence of a fistula.

Patient Responses

Ask your patients about pain, discomfort, or itching related to the wound or wound care.

Assessing an Untreated Wound

Your assessment should determine what, if any, additional professional support is necessary. Assess the following same aspects as for treated wounds above: location, size, appearance, description of drainage, condition of wound margins, condition of surrounding skin, and effect of the wound on the patient. In addition, assess the following:

- **Bleeding.** If bleeding is profuse, apply direct pressure to the site. If bleeding continues after you apply pressure for 5 minutes or if blood is spurting from the wound, call the physician immediately.
- **Severity of the wound.** A gaping wound, or a deep wound with fat, fascia, or muscle exposed, will need additional care.
- **Last tetanus immunization.** Immunization should be given if (1) the last immunization was 10 years ago or longer, (2) the wound is contaminated with dirt or debris and the tetanus injection was given more than 5 years ago, or (3) it is uncertain when the patient last received an immunization.
- **Whether the wound was caused by a bite.** Determine whether the wound was caused by any type of bite, animal or human. A deep bite wound usually requires additional observation and/or antibiotics.
- **Pain.** Assess for pain. Any wound causing severe pain requires a comprehensive evaluation.
- **Numbness or loss of movement.** If any deficit is detected, the patient will need immediate evaluation.
- **Presence of chronic medical conditions.** Examples include diabetes, malnutrition, immunocompromise, or a bleeding disorder. Patients with conditions that affect wound healing will need ongoing evaluation.

The Braden Scale for Predicting Pressure Sore Risk

BRADEN SCALE FOR PREDICTING PRESSURE SORE RISK

Patient's Name _____   Evaluator's Name _____   Date of Assessment _____

	1	2	3	4
SENSORY PERCEPTION ability to respond meaningfully to pressure-related discomfort	**1. Completely Limited** Unresponsive (does not moan, flinch, or grasp) to painful stimuli, due to diminished level of consciousness or sedation. OR limited ability to feel pain over most of body.	**2. Very Limited** Responds only to painful stimuli. Cannot communicate discomfort except by moaning or restlessness OR has a sensory impairment which limits the ability to feel pain or discomfort over ½ of body.	**3. Slightly Limited** Responds to verbal commands, but cannot always communicate discomfort or the need to be turned. OR has some sensory impairment which limits ability to feel pain or discomfort in 1 or 2 extremities.	**4. No Impairment** Responds to verbal commands. Has no sensory deficit which would limit ability to feel or voice pain or discomfort.
MOISTURE degree to which skin is exposed to moisture	**1. Constantly Moist** Skin is kept moist almost constantly by perspiration, urine, etc. Dampness is detected every time patient is moved or turned.	**2. Very Moist** Skin is often, but not always moist. Linen must be changed at least once a shift.	**3. Occasionally Moist:** Skin is occasionally moist, requiring an extra linen change approximately once a day.	**4. Rarely Moist** Skin is usually dry, linen only requires changing at routine intervals.
ACTIVITY degree of physical activity	**1. Bedfast** Confined to bed.	**2. Chairfast** Ability to walk severely limited or non-existent. Cannot bear own weight and/or must be assisted into chair or wheelchair.	**3. Walks Occasionally** Walks occasionally during day, but for very short distances, with or without assistance. Spends majority of each shift in bed or chair.	**4. Walks Frequently** Walks outside room at least twice a day and inside room at least once every two hours during waking hours.
MOBILITY ability to change and control body position	**1. Completely Immobile** Does not make even slight changes in body or extremity position without assistance.	**2. Very Limited** Makes occasional slight changes in body or extremity position but unable to make frequent or significant changes independently.	**3. Slightly Limited** Makes frequent though slight changes in body or extremity position independently.	**4. No Limitation** Makes major and frequent changes in position without assistance.
NUTRITION usual food intake pattern	**1. Very Poor** Never eats a complete meal. Rarely eats more than ½ of any food offered. Eats 2 servings or less of protein (meat or dairy products) per day. Takes fluids poorly. Does not take a liquid dietary supplement OR is NPO and/or maintained on clear liquids or IVs for more than 5 days.	**2. Probably Inadequate** Rarely eats a complete meal and generally eats only about ½ of any food offered. Protein intake includes only 3 servings of meat or dairy products per day. Occasionally will take a dietary supplement. OR receives less than optimum amount of liquid diet or tube feeding.	**3. Adequate** Eats over half of most meals. Eats a total of 4 servings of protein (meat, dairy products per day. Occasionally will refuse a meal, but will usually take a supplement when offered OR is on a tube feeding or TPN regimen which probably meets most of nutritional needs.	**4. Excellent** Eats most of every meal. Never refuses a meal. Usually eats a total of 4 or more servings of meat and dairy products. Occasionally eats between meals. Does not require supplementation.

FRICTION & SHEAR	1. Problem	2. Potential Problem	3. No Apparent Problem				
	Requires moderate to maximum assistance in moving. Complete lifting without sliding against sheets is impossible. Frequently slides down in bed or chair, requiring frequent repositioning with maximum assistance. Spasticity, contractures or agitation leads to almost constant friction.	Moves feebly or requires minimum assistance. During a move skin probably slides to some extent against sheets, chair, restraints or other devices. Maintains relatively good position in chair or bed most of the time but occasionally slides down.	Moves in bed and in chair independently and has sufficient muscle strength to lift up completely during move. Maintains good position in bed or chair.				
							Total Score

Source: U.S. Department of Health and Human Services. (1992). *Clinical practice guideline. Pressure ulcers in adults: Prediction and prevention.* PPPPUA Publication No. 92-0047. Rockville, MD: Public Health Service, pp. 16–17. Copyright © Barbara Braden and Nancy Bergstrcm, 1988. Reprinted with permission.

The Norton Scale for Assessing Risk
of Pressure Ulcers

Norton Scale for Assessing Risk of Pressure Ulcers

	Physical Condition	Mental Condition	Activity	Mobility	Incontinent	
	Good 4 Fair 3 Poor 2 Very bad 1	Alert 4 Apathetic 3 Confused 2 Stupor 1	Ambulant 4 Walk/help 3 Chair-bound 2 Bed 1	Full 4 Slightly limited 3 Very limited 2 Immobile 1	Not 4 Occasional 3 Usually/urine 2 Doubly 1	Total Score
Name/Date						

The Norton Scale uses five criteria to assess patients' risk for pressure ulcers. Scores of 14 or less indicate liability to ulcers; scores of <12 indicate very high risk.

Source: Norton, D., McLaren, R., & Exton-Smith, A. N. (1975). *An investigation of geriatric nursing problems in hospitals.* Edinburgh, UK: Churchill Livingstone. Used with permission.

The PUSH Tool for Evaluation of Pressure Ulcers

PUSH Tool - Version 3.0

Patient Name:_____   Patient ID#:_____

Ulcer Location: _____   Date:_____

DIRECTIONS:
Observe and measure the pressure ulcer. Categorize the ulcer with respect to surface area, exudate, and type of wound tissue. Record a sub-score for each of these ulcer characteristics. Add the sub-scores to obtain the total score. A comparison of total scores measured over time provides an indication of the improvement or deterioration in pressure ulcer healing.

	0	1	2	3	4	5	Subscore
Length x Width	$0\ cm^2$	$<0.3\ cm^2$	$0.3 - 0.6\ cm^2$	$0.7 - 1.0\ cm^2$	$1.1 - 2.0\ cm^2$	$2.1 - 3.0\ cm^2$	
		6	7	8	9	10	
		$3.1 - 4.0\ cm^2$	$4.1 - 8.0\ cm^2$	$8.1 - 12.0\ cm^2$	$12.1 - 24.0\ cm^2$	$> 24\ cm^2$	
	0	1	2	3			Subscore
Exudate Amount	None	Light	Moderate	Heavy			
	0	1	2	3	4		Subscore
Tissue Type	Closed	Epithelial Tissue	Granulation Tissue	Slough	Necrotic Tissue		
							Total Score

Length x Width: Measure the greatest length (head to toe) and the greatest width (side to side) using a centimeter ruler. Multiply these two measurements (length • width) to obtain an estimate of surface area in square centimeters (cm^2). **Caveat:** Do not guess! Always use a centimeter ruler and always use the same method each time the ulcer is measured.

Exudate Amount: Estimate the amount of exudate (drainage) present after removal of the dressing and before applying any topical agent to the ulcer. Estimate the exudate (drainage) as none, light, moderate, or heavy.

Tissue Type: This refers to the types of tissue that are present in the wound (ulcer) bed. Score as a "4" if there is any necrotic tissue present. Score as a "3" if there is any amount of slough present and necrotic tissue is absent. Score as a "2" if the wound is clean and contains granulation tissue. A superficial wound that is reepithelializing is scored as a "1". When the wound is closed, score as a "0".

> **4 - Necrotic Tissue (Eschar):** black, brown, or tan tissue that adheres firmly to the wound bed or ulcer edges and may be either firmer or softer than surrounding skin.
> **3 - Slough:** yellow or white tissue that adheres to the ulcer bed in strings or thick clumps, or is mucinous.
> **2 - Granulation Tissue:** pink or beefy red tissue with a shiny, moist, granular appearance.
> **1 - Epithelial Tissue:** for superficial ulcers, new pink or shiny tissue (skin) that grows in from the edges or as islands on the ulcer surface.
> **0 - Closed/Resurfaced:** the wound is completely covered with epithelium (new skin).

Note: Refer to the NPUAP Website (www.npuap.org) for further information regarding development and use of the PUSH Tool.

Version 3.0: 9/15/98
© National Pressure Ulcer Advisory Panel

PRESSURE ULCER HEALING CHART
(use a separate page for each pressure ulcer)

Patient Name:_____   Patient ID#:_____

Ulcer Location: _____   Date:_____

Directions: Observe and measure pressure ulcers at regular intervals using the PUSH Tool. Date and record PUSH Sub-scale and Total Scores on the Pressure Ulcer Healing Record below.

PRESSURE ULCER HEALING RECORD

DATE													
Length × Width													
Exudate Amount													
Tissue Type													
Total Score													

Graph the PUSH Total Score on the Pressure Ulcer Healing Graph below.

PUSH Total Score	PRESSURE ULCER HEALING GRAPH												
17													
16													
15													
14													
13													
12													
11													
10													
9													
8													
7													
6													
5													
4													
3													
2													
1													
Healed 0													
DATE:													

Version 3.0: 9/15/98
© National Pressure Ulcer Advisory Panel

Source: National Pressure Ulcer Advisory Panel. (2002). Retrieved from http://www.npuap.org/push3-0.htm.

Diagnostic Testing

Diagnostic Testing

Tests for Assessing Wounds

Test	Normal Range	Comments
Leukocyte (WBC) count	4500–11,000/mm^3	Usually done as a part of a complete blood count (CBC) but may be ordered as an independent test. WBCs may increase when a wound develops; continued elevation may signal infection. A low WBC count may delay wound healing.
		Leukocytes are responsible for an inflammatory reaction at the wound site, phagocytosis of bacteria and cellular debris, and the creation of antibodies.
Serum protein	6.0–8.0 g/dL	Low serum levels indicate limited nutritional stores that delay wound healing or place the patient at high risk for pressure ulcers.
Serum albumin	3.4–4.8 g/dL	
Serum prealbumin	12–42 mg/dL	Serum protein may be monitored as an indicator of the ability to heal a wound or prevent a pressure ulcer. Serum protein and albumin levels are closely related. However, both fluctuate slowly. A more accurate measure of a patient's immediate protein stores is reflected in prealbumin level.
Erythrocyte sedimentation rate (ESR)	< 50 years old: 0–15 mm/hr; > 50 years old: 0–20 mm/hr	In the presence of an inflammatory and necrotic process, blood proteins are altered. This test indicates if the RBCs stick together, become heavier, and settle at the bottom of a lab tube when held vertically.
Coagulation studies: Partial thromboplastin time, activated (aPTT)	Varies with respect to equipment and reagents used. Critical values: > 70 seconds or < 53 seconds	Prolonged coagulation times may result in excessive blood loss or ongoing bleeding in the wound bed. Shortened coagulation times increase the risk for blood clot formation problems, such as deep vein thrombosis, pulmonary embolus, or stroke.
Prothrombin time (clotting time)	Critical values: > 20 seconds (uncoagulated) or 3 times normal control (anticoagulated)	Altered coagulation may result from anticoagulant medications, a concurrent illness, trauma, or reaction to transfusions.
International normalized ratio (INR)	< 2.0 for patients not receiving anticoagulation therapy; 2.0–3.0 for those receiving coagulation therapy	A standardized test to evaluate clotting times, considered the gold standard.
Wound cultures	Negative; no growth of pathogens	Wound cultures may be prescribed to determine the types of bacteria present in the wound. Cultures may be obtained by swab, aspiration, or tissue biopsy. A positive culture may not indicate an infection as chronic wounds are colonized with bacteria.
Tissue biopsy	Negative; no growth of pathogens	Wounds are not considered infected unless the bacteria count exceeds 100,000 organisms per gram of tissue. Exception: The presence of beta-hemolytic streptococci in any number indicates infection.

Standardized Language

Selected Standardized Outcomes and Interventions for Skin and Wound Diagnoses

PATIENT SITUATION (DATA/DEFINING CHARACTERISTICS)	NANDA-I DIAGNOSIS	NOC OUTCOMES	SELECTED INDICATORS	SELECTED NIC INTERVENTIONS AND SPECIFIC ACTIVITIES
Mrs. Whitefeather is 95 years old. She has cancer and has stopped eating and become very thin. Recently she has become too weak to move about in bed without help. However, her skin is intact with no redness, even over her bony prominences. She has a very low score on the Braden pressure ulcer assessment scale.	Risk for Impaired Skin Integrity	Tissue Integrity: Skin & Mucous Membranes Other outcomes: Immobility Consequences: Physiological Nutritional Status: Food & Fluid Intake Nutritional Status: Nutrient Intake	(5—Not compromised) Hydration Tissue perfusion Skin integrity (5—None) Erythema Blanching Skin lesions	**Bed Rest Care** ▪ Keep bed linen clean, dry, and wrinkle free. ▪ Facilitate small shifts of body weight. **Pressure Ulcer Prevention** ▪ Monitor any reddened areas closely. ▪ Turn every 1–2 hours, as appropriate. ▪ Turn with care (e.g., avoid shearing) to prevent injury to fragile skin. ▪ Post a turning schedule at the bedside, as appropriate. ▪ Avoid massaging over bony prominences. ▪ Utilize specialty beds and mattresses, as appropriate. ▪ Avoid use of "donut" type devices in the sacral area. *Other Interventions* ▪ Nutrition Management ▪ Positioning ▪ Pressure Management ▪ Skin Surveillance
Eddie Allen is 4 years old. He has a severe case of poison ivy, which has made blisters on his skin. He has been scratching and has bleeding, excoriated areas over his limbs, face, and trunk.	Impaired Skin Integrity	Tissue Integrity: Skin & Mucous Membranes *Other outcomes:* Infection Immune Hypersensitivity Response	(4—Mildly compromised) Skin integrity (4—Mild) Skin lesions Erythema (3—moderate) Itching Localized inflammatory response	**Wound Care** ▪ Monitor characteristics of the wound, including drainage, color, size, and odor. ▪ Cleanse with normal saline or a nontoxic cleanser, as appropriate. ▪ Apply an appropriate ointment to the skin/lesion, as appropriate. ▪ Instruct the child and family member(s) about wound care procedures and signs of infection. *Other Interventions* ▪ Pruritus ▪ Management ▪ Skin Surveillance ▪ Wound Irrigation

Selected Standardized Outcomes and Interventions for Skin and Wound Diagnoses—cont'd

PATIENT SITUATION (DATA/DEFINING CHARACTERISTICS)	NANDA-I DIAGNOSIS	NOC OUTCOMES	SELECTED INDICATORS	SELECTED NIC INTERVENTIONS AND SPECIFIC ACTIVITIES
Allie Newton has a stage II pressure ulcer on her left heel.	Impaired Tissue Integrity	Wound Healing: Secondary Intention *Other outcomes:* Tissue Integrity: Skin & Mucous Membranes	(4—Substantial) Granulation Decreased wound size (4—Limited) Purulent drainage Surrounding skin erythema Wound inflammation Foul wound odor	**Pressure Ulcer Care** ■ Débride the ulcer, as needed. ■ Cleanse the ulcer with the appropriate nontoxic solution, working in a circular motion from the center. ■ Cleanse the skin around the ulcer with mild soap and water. ■ Monitor for infection in the wound. ■ Position every 1–2 hours to avoid prolonged pressure. ***Other Interventions*** ■ Wound Care ■ Pressure Management ■ Infection Protection ■ Medication ■ Administration

Sources: NANDA International. (2009). *Nursing diagnoses: Definitions and classification 2009–2011.* Philadelphia: Author; Johnson, M., Bulechek, G., Butcher, H., et al. (2006). *NANDA, NOC, and NIC linkages* (2nd ed.). St. Louis, MO: C. V. Mosby; Moorhead, S., Johnson, M., Maas, M., et al. (Eds.). (2008). *Nursing outcomes classification (NOC)* (4th ed.). St. Louis, MO: C. V. Mosby; and Bulechek, G., Butcher, H., & Dochtermann, J. (Eds.). (2008). *Nursing interventions classification (NIC)* (5th ed.). St. Louis, MO: C. V. Mosby. Used with permission.

THINKING CRITICALLY ABOUT SKIN INTEGRITY AND WOUND HEALING

The exercises in the following sections allow you to practice the kind of thinking you will use as a full-spectrum nurse. Because these are critical-thinking questions, there is usually no single right answer. We do not provide answers for these questions because it is more important for you to think about the questions than to arrive at the "right" answer. These questions are designed to improve your thinking more than to "cover content." Discuss answers with your peers—discussion can stimulate critical thinking. If you have difficulty with any of these questions, consult with your instructor.

Applying the Full-Spectrum Nursing Model

PATIENT SITUATION

A 66-year-old obese man with diabetes and hypertension, Tio Santos, is being seen for a wound on his right foot that doesn't seem to be healing. He injured his foot when repairing drywall at home. He is otherwise relatively sedentary at home. The wound is oozing, swollen, tender, and warm to the touch. Tio is now running a low-grade fever of 100.4°F at home. He tells you his foot is very painful, especially with any weight-bearing, and throbs when sitting or lying still. You measure the wound bed to be 6 cm × 4 cm and note purulent exudate at the distal edge. He is referred to an outpatient wound care center for treatment.

THINKING

1. *Theoretical Knowledge:*

   a. What is the Braden Scale and why might it be used for Mr. Santos?

   b. What risk factors for delayed wound healing does Mr. Santos have?

2. *Critical Thinking (Considering Alternatives, Deciding What to Do):*

   a. To care for Mr. Santos' wound, should you use sterile gloves, clean nonsterile gloves, or no gloves? Explain your thinking.

DOING

3. *Practical Knowledge (Assessment):*

   a. What symptoms of infection does Mr. Santos have?

   b. To be certain the wound is infected, what would you need to know or do?

CARING

4. *Self-Knowledge:* Use your imagination. Imagine you have had a wound on your foot for 6 weeks. It has not healed and you have all Mr. Santos' symptoms and, in fact, are in his situation. What would be the most troublesome symptom in your daily life? What would worry you the most?

Critical Thinking and Clinical Reasoning

1. You are caring for a 22-year-old man who is paralyzed from the waist down secondary to an automobile accident. He has been admitted to the hospital with a urinary tract infection manifested by a fever of 102°F (39°C) and lethargy. His family reports he has been withdrawn and sits in his wheelchair watching TV all day long.

   a. What risk factors does this patient have for skin breakdown?

b. What locations of his body should you be most concerned about in regard to pressure ulcer formation?

c. What actions should you take to decrease the risk of pressure ulcers in this man? What further information do you need?

2. A 63-year-old man is admitted to your unit after an emergency appendectomy. His appendix was ruptured, and the surgeon has left the wound open to heal by secondary intention. A Jackson–Pratt drain is in place in the wound bed. A moderate amount of purosanguineous drainage is visible in the drain. The surgeon has ordered saline-moistened gauze packing every 4 hours.

a. What actions should you take as you prepare to do the first dressing change?

b. How will you secure the dressing?

3. For the following patients, write a NANDA-I diagnosis related to skin integrity. Include problem, etiology, and defining characteristics. If you do not have enough data for one of those components, state what additional data you need.

a. Mrs. Whitefeather is 95 years old. She has cancer, and she has stopped eating and become very thin. Recently she has become too weak to move about in bed without help. However, her skin is intact with no redness, even over her bony prominences. She has a very low score on the Braden pressure ulcer assessment scale.

b. Eddie Allen is 4 years old. He has a severe case of poison ivy, which has made blisters on his skin. He has been scratching his "itchies" and has bleeding, excoriated areas over his limbs, face, and trunk.

c. Allie Newton has a stage II pressure ulcer on her left heel.

4. For each of the following concepts, use critical thinking to describe how or why it is important to nursing, patient care, or skin integrity and wound healing. Note that these are *not* to be merely definitions.

Shearing   Wound assessment
Friction   Preventing pressure ulcers
Pressure   Dressing changes

What Are the Main Points in This Chapter?

➤ The layers of the skin are the epidermis (outermost), the dermis, and the subcutaneous layer (innermost).

➤ The major functions of the skin are protection of the internal organs, unique identification of an individual, thermoregulation, metabolism of nutrients and metabolic waste products, and sensation.

➤ Age, mobility, nutrition, hydration, moisture underlying conditions, medications, contamination or infection, diminished sensation, cognitive impairment, hygiene, and lifestyle are factors that influence the ability to maintain intact skin and heal wounds.

➤ If there are no breaks in the skin a wound is described as *closed*. A wound is considered *open* if there is a break in the skin or mucous membranes.

➤ Acute wounds may be intentional (e.g., surgical incisions) or unintentional (e.g., from trauma) and are expected to be of short duration.

➤ Wounds that exceed the anticipated length of recovery are classified as chronic wounds. Chronic wounds include pressure, arterial, venous, and diabetic ulcers. A chronic wound may linger for months or years.

➤ *Clean wounds* are uninfected wounds with minimal inflammation. *Clean-contaminated wounds* are surgical incisions that enter the gastrointestinal, respiratory, or genitourinary tracts. *Contaminated wounds* include open, traumatic wounds or surgical incisions in which a major break in asepsis occurred. *Infected wounds* are wounds with evidence of infection, such as presence of microorganisms.

➤ A wound that involves minimal or no tissue loss and has wound edges that approximate heals by primary intention.

➤ A wound that involves extensive tissue loss and has margins that cannot be approximated, or is infected, heals by secondary intention. The wound is left open and allowed to heal from the inner layer to the surface.

➤ Tertiary intention healing, or delayed primary closure, occurs when two surfaces of granulation tissue are brought together. Initially the wound is allowed to heal by secondary intention. The length of time for secondary healing varies but is usually less than 1 week.

➤ Healing occurs in three stages: inflammatory, proliferative, and maturation. The *inflammatory phase* lasts from 1 to 5 days and consists of two major processes: hemostasis and inflammation. *The proliferative phase* occurs from days 5 to 21. It is characterized by cell development aimed at filling the wound defect and resurfacing the skin. The *maturation phase* is the final phase of the healing process. It begins in the second or third week and continues until the wound is completely healed.

➤ Wound closure methods include adhesive strips (Steri-Strips™), absorbent sutures, surgical staples, and surgical glue.

➤ Drainage is the flow of fluids from a wound or cavity. It is often referred to as *exudate* (fluid that oozes as a result of inflammation).

➤ Complications of wound healing include hemorrhage, infection, dehiscence, evisceration, and fistula formation.

➤ Pressure ulcers are caused by unrelieved pressure that compromises blood flow to tissue, resulting in ischemia in the underlying tissue.

➤ A stage I pressure ulcer is an area of persistent redness.

➤ Stage II pressure ulcers involve partial-thickness skin loss of the epidermis, dermis, or both.

➤ A stage III pressure ulcer is characterized by full-thickness skin loss involving damage or necrosis of subcutaneous tissue, which may extend down to, but

not through, the underlying fascia. The ulcer appears as a deep crater.

➤ Stage IV pressure ulcers involve full-thickness skin loss with extensive destruction; tissue necrosis; or damage to muscle, bone, or support structures. Undermining and sinus tracts (blind tracts underneath the epidermis) are common.

➤ Factors contributing to pressure ulcers are those that alter the skin and tissue integrity and blood supply (e.g., aging, low blood pressure, neurological injury, poor nutrition, edema, and fever).

➤ Extrinsic factors include friction and shearing, and exposure to moisture and pressure.

➤ Not all lower extremity ulcers are related to pressure. Some are caused by poor circulation and perfusion, such as venous stasis ulcers, diabetic foot ulcers, and arterial ulcers.

➤ An eschar is a black leathery covering of necrotic tissue. An ulcer covered by an eschar cannot be classified because it is impossible to determine the depth.

➤ The Braden and Norton scales evaluate risk for problems with skin integrity.

➤ When assessing a wound, note the following: the type of wound, color of the wound and surrounding skin, condition of the wound bed, drainage and odor, and level of pain associated with the wound or wound care.

➤ Preventing pressure ulcers focuses on skin care, nutrition, turning and positioning, using therapeutic mattresses and cushions, and patient/family teaching.

➤ Five types of débridement are sharp, mechanical, enzymatic, autolytic, and biotherapy (maggot débridement).

➤ Wound care therapies to promote healing might include negative pressure wound therapy (NPWT), electrical stimulation, tissue growth factors, ultrasound, bioengineered skin substitutes, and surgical options.

➤ Primary dressings are ones that are placed in the wound bed and actually touch the wound. A secondary dressing is one that covers or holds a primary dressing in place. Many dressings can act as both.

➤ Types of wound dressings are absorption, alginate, antimicrobial, collagen, gauze, FOAM dressings, hydrocolloid, hydrogel, skin sealants, and moisture barriers.

➤ Ideal wound irrigation pressures range from 4 to 15 psi. Current recommendations are to use a 35-mL syringe attached to a 19-gauge angiocatheter. This will deliver the solution at approximately 8 psi.

➤ Heat application promotes vasodilatation, increases tissue metabolism, increases capillary permeability, reduces blood viscosity, and reduces muscle tension.

➤ The application of cold causes vasoconstriction, local anesthesia, reduced cell metabolism, increased blood viscosity, and decreased muscle tension.

For practice questions for this chapter,

 Go to **NCLEX-Style Chapter Quiz,** on the Student Resource Disk or DavisPlus at http://davisplus.fadavis.com/Wilkinson2

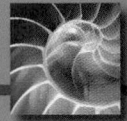

Knowledge Map

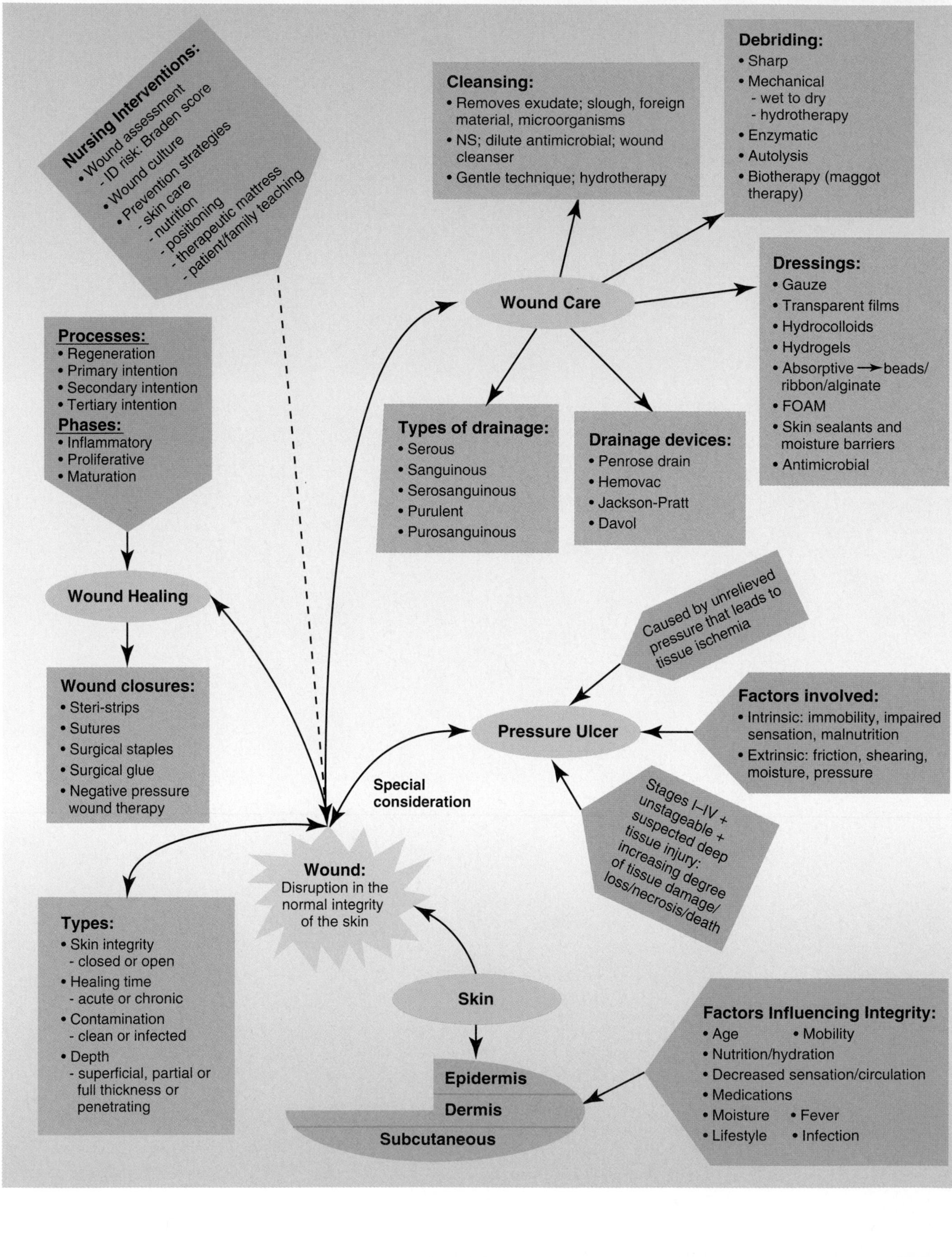

Nursing Interventions:
• Wound assessment
  - ID risk: Braden score
  - Wound culture
• Prevention strategies
  - skin care
  - nutrition
  - positioning
  - therapeutic mattress
  - patient/family teaching

Cleansing:
• Removes exudate; slough, foreign material, microorganisms
• NS; dilute antimicrobial; wound cleanser
• Gentle technique; hydrotherapy

Debriding:
• Sharp
• Mechanical
  - wet to dry
  - hydrotherapy
• Enzymatic
• Autolysis
• Biotherapy (maggot therapy)

Processes:
• Regeneration
• Primary intention
• Secondary intention
• Tertiary intention

Phases:
• Inflammatory
• Proliferative
• Maturation

Wound Care

Dressings:
• Gauze
• Transparent films
• Hydrocolloids
• Hydrogels
• Absorptive → beads/ribbon/alginate
• FOAM
• Skin sealants and moisture barriers
• Antimicrobial

Types of drainage:
• Serous
• Sanguinous
• Serosanguinous
• Purulent
• Purosanguinous

Drainage devices:
• Penrose drain
• Hemovac
• Jackson-Pratt
• Davol

Wound Healing

Wound closures:
• Steri-strips
• Sutures
• Surgical staples
• Surgical glue
• Negative pressure wound therapy

Caused by unrelieved pressure that leads to tissue ischemia

Pressure Ulcer

Factors involved:
• Intrinsic: immobility, impaired sensation, malnutrition
• Extrinsic: friction, shearing, moisture, pressure

Stages I–IV + unstageable + suspected deep tissue injury: increasing degree of tissue damage/loss/necrosis/death

Special consideration

Wound:
Disruption in the normal integrity of the skin

Types:
• Skin integrity
  - closed or open
• Healing time
  - acute or chronic
• Contamination
  - clean or infected
• Depth
  - superficial, partial or full thickness or penetrating

Skin

Epidermis

Dermis

Subcutaneous

Factors Influencing Integrity:
• Age   • Mobility
• Nutrition/hydration
• Decreased sensation/circulation
• Medications
• Moisture   • Fever
• Lifestyle   • Infection

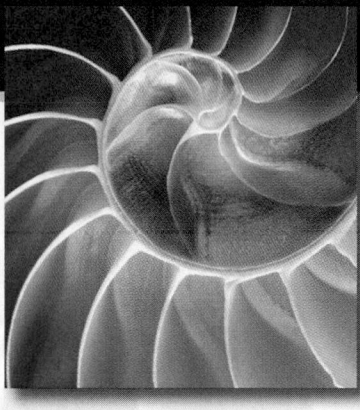
Oxygenation

For a podcast of an overview of this chapter,

 Go to Student Resources, **Podcast – Chapter Overviews, Chapter 35,** on DavisPlus at http://davisplus.fadavis.com/ Wilkinson2

Caring for the Garcias

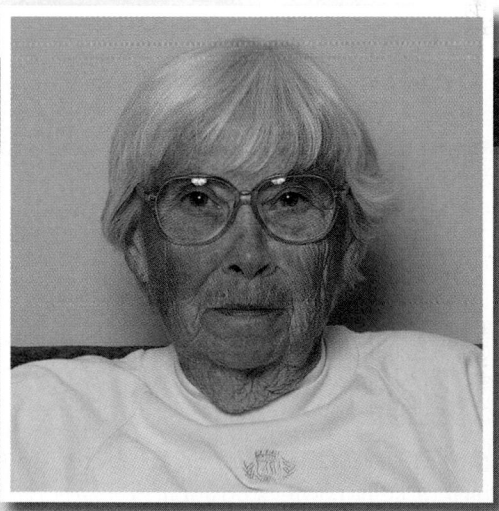

The exercises in the following section allow you to practice the kind of thinking you will use as a full-spectrum nurse. Because these are critical-thinking questions, there is usually no single right answer. We do not provide answers for these questions because it is more important for you to think about the questions than to arrive at the "right" answer. These questions are designed to improve your thinking more than to "cover content." Discuss answers with your peers—discussion can stimulate critical thinking. If you have difficulty with any of these questions, consult with your instructor.

Katherine Garcia, Joe's 76-year-old mother, has been complaining of fatigue and a persistent cough for approximately 2 weeks. Joe scheduled an appointment for his mother at the family clinic. You are the nurse at the clinic. Katherine appears disheveled. Her clothes are mismatched and rumpled, and her hair is tousled.

Normally she appears at the clinic dressed neatly and wearing makeup. She has a hard time signing in at the desk and tells the receptionist she has a 1:00 P.M. appointment, but it is 9:00 A.M. Katherine's vital signs are as follows: BP, 142/90 mm Hg; pulse, 94 beats/min and regular; respirations 24 breaths/min and labored; temperature, 99.6°F (37.5°C) oral.

A. What additional assessment data would be useful to gather at this time?

B. During her visit at the clinic, you notice that Katherine is very confused. Her weight has dropped 7 pounds

since her visit last month, her mucous membranes are dry, and she is dyspneic with any activity. Katherine is diagnosed with pneumonia. Because of her rapid decline, she is admitted to the hospital to receive antibiotics administered intravenously. At the hospital, *(continued on next page)*

Caring for the Garcias (continued)

her initial pulse oximetry reading is 90%, and she is unable to cough up secretions. Write the most appropriate nursing diagnosis to focus interventions for Katherine.

C. What actions should you anticipate taking?

D. The hospitalist (hospital-based physician) writes prescriptions for IV fluids, antibiotics, suction prn, and continuous pulse oximetry. What additional prescriptions will you need to provide care for Katherine? What therapy would you suggest?

E. Katherine requires suctioning to help remove secretions. She has a weak cough and crackles and rhonchi throughout all lung fields. There are few secretions in her oropharynx, and she bites down on the catheter. What technique would you use to suction her? Explain your choice.

F. After 4 days in the hospital, Katherine is discharged to home. She asks the hospital nurse, "What can I do to make sure I never get that sick again?" How would you answer this question?

Practical **Knowledge**
knowing how

Procedures

In this section you will find the procedures necessary for supporting oxygenation. As you perform the procedures, apply the theoretical knowledge you obtained in Volume 1. The registered nurse is responsible for assessing patients' oxygenation and their responses to procedures. Some, but not all, of the procedures in this section can be delegated to qualified nursing assistive personnel (NAPs). Refer to the delegation notes in the procedures and to agency policies.

Procedure 35-1 ☐ **Collecting a Sputum Specimen**

➤ For steps to follow in *all* procedures, refer to the Universal Steps for All Procedures found on the inside back cover of Volume 2.

Critical Aspects

Procedure 35-1A: Obtaining an Expectorated Specimen
- Use high or semi-Fowler's position.
- Caution the patient not to touch the inside of the sterile container or lid.
- Instruct the patient to breathe deeply for three or four breaths, cough deeply, then expectorate in the container.
- Label the specimen container with patient's name, test name, and collection date and time.
- Place the specimen in a plastic bag with a biohazard label. Follow agency policy.
- Send the specimen to the laboratory immediately. If specimen transport is delayed, consult the lab; refrigeration may be required.

Procedure 35-1B: Obtaining a Specimen by Suction
- Position in high or semi-Fowler's position.
- Don protective eyewear.
- Attach the suction tubing to the male adapter of the inline sputum specimen container.
- Don sterile gloves.
- Attach the sterile suction catheter to the rubber tubing on the inline sputum specimen container.
- Lubricate the suction catheter with sterile saline solution.
- Insert the tip of the suction catheter through the nasopharynx, endotracheal tube, or tracheostomy tube. Advance into the trachea
- When the patient begins coughing, apply suction for 5 to 10 seconds to collect the specimen.
- If an adequate specimen is not obtained, allow the patient to rest for 1 or 2 minutes, and then repeat the procedure. Administer oxygen at this time, if indicated.

- When an adequate specimen is collected, discontinue suction, and gently remove the suction catheter.
- Label the specimen container.
- Place the specimen in a plastic bag with a biohazard label.
- Send the specimen to the laboratory immediately. If specimen transport is delayed, consult the lab; refrigeration may be required.

Equipment

Procedure 35-1A: Obtaining an Expectorated Specimen

- Sterile specimen container with lid
- Procedure gloves
- Glass of water
- Emesis basin
- Tissues
- Pillow (if abdominal or chest incision is present)
- Patient identification label
- Completed laboratory requisition form
- Small plastic bag with a biohazard label for delivering the specimen to the laboratory (or container designated by the agency)

Procedure 35-1B: Obtaining a Specimen by Suction

- Sterile suction catheter or sterile suction kit
- Suction device (portable or wall)
- Sterile gloves
- Protective eyewear
- Inline sputum specimen container or trap
- Sterile saline solution
- Patient identification label
- Completed laboratory requisition form
- Small plastic bag with a biohazard label for delivering the specimen to the laboratory (or container designated by the agency)
- Oxygen therapy equipment, if indicated
- Linen-saver pad or towel

Delegation

You can delegate collection of an expectorated sputum specimen to a NAP who has been adequately trained in performing the skill. Assess the patient's respiratory status first; if the patient's condition is unstable, do not delegate the procedure. Do not delegate obtaining a specimen by tracheal suctioning.

Pre-Procedure Assessment

- Assess the patient's comprehension of the procedure.
Understanding allays anxiety and promotes cooperation.

- Assess respiratory status, including breath sounds; respiratory rate, depth, and pattern; skin and nail bed color; and tissue perfusion.
You may need to delay sputum collection if the patient is in respiratory distress.

- Assess ability to deep-breathe, cough, and expectorate.
If the patient is unable to deep-breathe, cough, and expectorate, suctioning may be necessary to obtain an adequate sputum specimen.

 - Check when the patient last ate or had a tube feeding, especially for a specimen obtained by suction.
Specimen collection should be delayed for 1 to 2 hours after eating because the procedure may cause vomiting, which creates a risk for aspiration of stomach contents.

- If suctioning is required to obtain the specimen, check for factors such as anticoagulant therapy, bleeding disorders, or low platelet count.
These factors place the patient at risk for bleeding when the suction catheter is introduced.

➤ When performing the procedure, always identify your patient according to agency policy and be attentive to standard precautions, hand hygiene, patient safety and privacy, body mechanics, and documentation.

Procedure Steps

1. Verify the medical prescription for type of sputum analysis.
The type of sputum specimen determines the number of specimens required and the time of day the specimen should be collected. For example, specimens to confirm tuberculosis typically require three consecutive morning samples.

2. Position the patient according to the required specimen collection technique.

a. For an expectorated specimen, assist the patient to high or semi-Fowler's position or to a sitting position at the edge of the bed.
b. For a suctioned specimen, position the patient in high or semi-Fowler's position.
These positions facilitate insertion of the suction catheter and the ability to cough. They also promote lung expansion, and prevent aspiration should the patient vomit during the procedure.

3. Drape a towel or linen-saver pad over the patient's chest. Ask the patient to rinse his mouth and gargle with water.
A towel or pad protects the patient's gown from soiling during specimen collection. Rinsing the mouth removes flora that may contaminate the specimen; however, evidence is not conclusive on this point.

4. If the patient has an abdominal or chest incision, have the patient splint the incision with a pillow.
Splinting the incision decreases discomfort when the patient coughs.

(continued on next page)

Procedure 35-1 ■ **Collecting a Sputum Specimen** (continued)

■ *Procedure 35-1A* **Collecting an Expectorated Specimen**

Procedure Steps

Follow steps 1 through 4, above.

5. Provide the patient with the specimen container. Advise the patient to avoid touching the inside of the container. If you must hold the container for the patient, first don procedure gloves.
The inside of the container should remain sterile. Wear gloves because you may come in contact with secretions or airborne bacteria when the patient coughs and expectorates. ▼

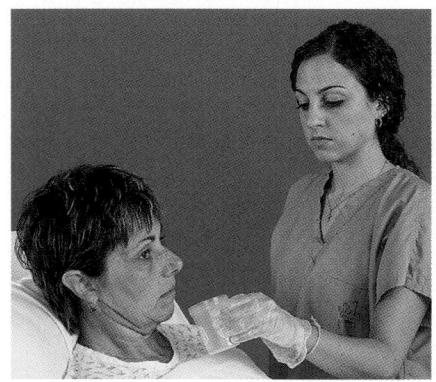

6. Ask the patient to breathe deeply for three or four breaths, and then ask him after a full inhalation to hold his breath and then cough.
Deep breathing opens airways and stimulates the cough reflex. Coughing after a full inhalation creates enough force to mobilize secretions through the airways and into the pharynx.

7. Instruct the patient to expectorate the secretions directly into the specimen container.
Prevents specimen contamination from outside organisms.

8. Tell the patient to repeat deep breathing and coughing until an adequate sample is obtained.
Typically 5 to 10 mL of sputum is required to ensure adequate sputum analysis.

9. Don procedure gloves, if you are not already wearing them; and cover the specimen container with the lid immediately after the specimen is collected.
Gloves protect you in the event the patient's coughing has contaminated the outside of the container. Covering the container immediately prevents spread of microorganisms.

10. Label the specimen container with a patient identification label that contains the name of the test and collection date and time.
Correctly identifying the specimen ensures accurate diagnosis and treatment.

11. Place the specimen in a plastic bag labeled with a biohazard label. Attach a completed laboratory requisition form.
Placing the specimen in a plastic bag protects healthcare workers from exposure to microorganisms. Completing the laboratory requisition form ensures proper processing of the specimen.

12. Send the specimen to the laboratory immediately, or refrigerate it if transport might be delayed.
If bacterial cultures are delayed, contaminating organisms may grow, producing false culture results and possibly inappropriate treatment.

■ *Procedure 35-1B* **Collecting a Suctioned Specimen**

Procedure Steps

Follow steps 1 through 4, on the preceding page.

5. Administer oxygen to the patient, if indicated.
Suctioning may cause hypoxemia; providing oxygen prevents hypoxemia.

6. Prepare the suction device, and make sure it is functioning properly.
Adequate suction is necessary to mobilize secretions.

7. Don protective eyewear.
Protects your eyes from splattering of secretions during suctioning.

8. Attach the suction tubing to the male adapter of the inline sputum specimen container. ▼

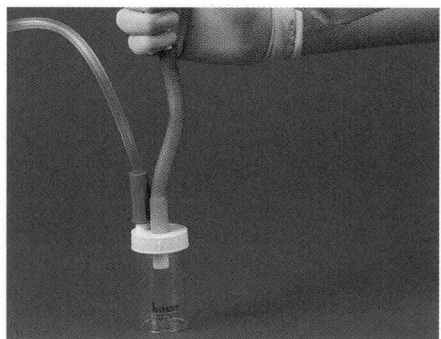

9. Don sterile gloves.
Protects the patient's sterile airways from contamination by outside organisms.

10. Attach the sterile suction catheter to the flexible tubing on the sputum specimen container. The hand that touches the specimen container is no longer sterile.
Ensures that the sputum specimen goes directly into the specimen container instead of the suction tubing. ▼

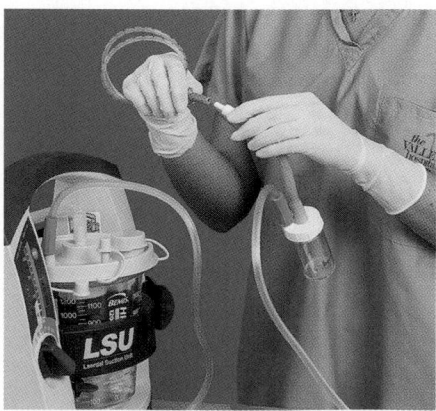

11. Lubricate the suction catheter with sterile saline solution.
Lubrication eases insertion and prevents trauma to mucosa.

12. Insert the tip of the suction catheter gently through the nasopharynx, endotracheal tube, or tracheostomy tube. Advance the tip into the trachea (see Procedure 35-8 or Procedure 35-9).
Gently inserting the suction catheter prevents airway trauma.

13. When the patient begins coughing, apply suction by placing your finger over the suction control port for 5 to 10 seconds to collect the specimen.
Applying suction for longer than 10 seconds can cause hypoxia.

14. If an adequate specimen (5 to 10 mL) is not obtained, allow the patient to rest for 1 or 2 minutes, and then repeat the procedure. Administer oxygen to the patient at this time, if indicated.
Allowing the patient to rest and administering oxygen prevent hypoxia. You must assess your patient continually during this procedure to ensure patient safety and respiratory status.

15. When you have collected an adequate specimen, discontinue suction, then gently remove the suction catheter.
Applying suction during catheter removal can damage the airway mucosa.

16. Remove the suction catheter from the specimen container, and dispose of the catheter in the appropriate container.
Disposal of contaminated supplies prevents the spread of infection.

17. Remove the suction tubing from the specimen container, and connect the rubber tubing on the specimen container to the plastic adapter. ▼

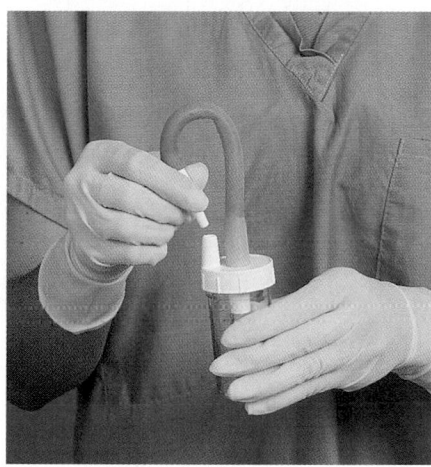

18. If sputum comes in contact with the outside of the specimen container, clean the outside with a disinfectant, according to agency policy.

Prevents spread of infection to staff members who must handle the specimen.

19. After the patient expectorates, offer tissues and provide mouth care.
Mouth care promotes patient comfort.

20. Label the specimen container with a patient identification label that contains the name of the test and collection date and time.
Correctly identifying the specimen ensures accurate diagnosis and treatment.

21. Place the specimen in a plastic bag affixed with a biohazard label. Attach a completed laboratory requisition form.
Placing the specimen in a plastic bag protects healthcare workers from exposure to microorganisms. Completing the laboratory requisition form ensures proper processing of the specimen.

22. Send the specimen to the laboratory immediately, or refrigerate it if transport might be delayed.
If bacterial cultures are delayed, contaminating organisms may grow, producing false culture results and possibly inappropriate treatment.

Evaluation

- Evaluate the patient's respiratory status during and after the procedure, especially if suctioning was necessary.
- Examine the color, consistency, and odor of the sputum specimen.
- Promptly report laboratory results to the primary care provider.
- Evaluate the patient's understanding of the procedure and test results.

Patient Teaching

- Explain proper collection techniques to avoid specimen contamination.
- Show the patient proper coughing techniques to ensure an adequate specimen.
- Explain the importance of avoiding mouthwash before the procedure, as it may alter laboratory results.

- If the patient has an incision, show him how to splint his incision to avoid discomfort during coughing and expectoration.

Home Care

Explain how to collect an expectorated sputum specimen and the importance of sending the specimen to the laboratory immediately after collection.

Documentation

- Record the date and time the specimen was collected, the method of collection, and the type of specimen ordered.
- Note the amount, color, consistency, and odor of the specimen.
- Document the patient's tolerance of the procedure.

(continued on next page)

Procedure 35-1 ■ Collecting a Sputum Specimen (continued)

Sample documentation:

> 06/05/11 2100   Expectorated specimen collected for culture and sensitivity. Specimen contained 10 mL of thick, green, sweet-smelling sputum. Patient tolerated procedure with no dyspnea, distress, or signs of hypoxia. Specimen sent to the lab immediately after collection.————————S. Ryan, RN

Sample documentation:

> 06/05/11 0700   Patient suctioned via tracheostomy, sputum specimen obtained and sent for acid fast bacillus (AFB) analysis. Specimen contained 15 mL of yellow, tenacious, odorless sputum. Patient became short of breath with suctioning. 100% O_2 administered via tracheostomy hood for 10 minutes after suctioning. Shortness of breath abated with treatment. O_2 returned to 40%.————————S. Ryan, RN

Practice Resources

California Department of Public Health (2007); Ontario Agency for Health Protection and Promotion (2008); Texas Department of State Health Services, Laboratory Services Section Home (2009).

Procedure 35-2   Monitoring Pulse Oximetry (Arterial Oxygen Saturation)

➤ For steps to follow in *all* procedures, refer to the Universal Steps for All Procedures found on the inside back cover of Volume 2.

Critical Aspects

- Choose a sensor that is appropriate for the patient's age, size, and weight and for the desired location.
- Attach the probe sensor to the site. Photodetector and light-emitting diodes on the probe sensor should face each other.
- Connect the sensor probe to the oximeter, and turn it on.
- Read the Sao_2 measurement on the digital display when it reaches a constant value.
- Set and turn on the alarm limits for Sao_2 and pulse rate, according to the manufacturer's instructions, patient condition, and agency policy if continuous monitoring is necessary.
- When monitoring is no longer needed, remove the probe sensor, and turn off the oximeter.

Equipment

- Nail polish remover, if necessary
- Oximeter
- Oximeter probe sensor appropriate for patient age, size, weight, and for the desired location

Delegation

Because it is noninvasive and simple to perform, the RN can delegate application of the pulse oximeter probe and measurement of arterial oxygen saturation (Sao_2) to a NAP or LPN who is adequately trained to perform the skill. Inform the NAP or LPN how often to take measurements, and instruct them to notify you immediately if Sao_2 falls below 95%. Although this procedure can be delegated, it is the responsibility of the RN to interpret the results, assess the patient, and notify the primary care provider.

Pre-Procedure Assessment

- Assess the patient's need for Sao_2 monitoring: risk factors, such as heart or pulmonary disease; low hemoglobin level; confusion, decreased level of consciousness, or respiratory distress.

Sao_2 monitoring helps detect oxygenation problems early. Monitoring is especially important in patients at risk, such as those with heart and pulmonary disease, those recovering from anesthesia, and those who are ventilator-dependent. Patients with underlying pulmonary disease may be accustomed to low oxygen saturation levels, so you may need to adjust the lower limit alarm and, if you have delegated the procedure, the level for notification for these patients.

- Assess the patient's respiratory status, including breath sounds; respiratory rate, depth, and pattern; tissue perfusion; Sao_2; and skin and nail bed color.

Assessment findings may suggest a decrease in oxygen saturation and validate oximetry readings.

- Determine the optimal location for the oximeter probe sensor, for example, the fingertip, earlobe, forehead, or bridge of the nose. Check the capillary refill and pulse at the pulse closest to the site.

To ensure accurate monitoring, choose a site that has adequate circulation, is free of artificial nails, and contains no moisture. Clinical Insight 35-2 offers suggestions on site placement based on patient factors.

- Assess for factors that may interfere with pulse oximetry measurement, such as hypotension, hypothermia, and tremors.

The sensor requires adequate circulation to recognize hemoglobin molecules that absorb the emitted light. Tremors may produce artifact that may be misinterpreted by the oximeter, causing false readings.

- Check patient history for allergy to adhesive.

An allergic reaction may occur if an adhesive-backed disposable probe sensor is used in a patient with a history of allergy to adhesives.

➤ When performing the procedure, always identify your patient according to agency policy and be attentive to standard precautions, hand hygiene, patient safety and privacy, body mechanics, and documentation.

➤ *Note:* This procedure explains how to apply a pulse oximeter. Refer to Clinical Insight 35-2 for tips for obtaining accurate pulse oximetry readings.

Procedure Steps

1. Choose a sensor appropriate for the patient's age, size, and weight and for the desired location. If the patient is allergic to adhesive, use a clip-on probe sensor. Use a nasal sensor if the patient's peripheral circulation is compromised.

An appropriate type of sensor is more comfortable for the patient and ensures accurate readings.

2. Prepare the site by cleansing and drying it. If the finger is the desired location, remove nail polish or an acrylic nail, if present.

Dirt and skin oils on the site can interfere with passage of light waves. Nail polish or acrylic nails may interfere with signal transmission, causing inaccurate Sao_2 measurement. However, a recent study found that nail polish did not cause a clinically significant change in readings in *healthy* people (Rodden, Spicer, Spicer, et al., 2007).

3. Remove the protective backing if you are using a disposable probe sensor that contains adhesive.

4. Attach the probe sensor to the chosen site. Make sure the photodetector and light-emitting diodes on the probe sensor face each other. Most probe sensors contain markings to facilitate correct placement.

Step 4 Variation. Clip-on Probe Sensor

If you are using a clip-on probe sensor, warn the patient that he may feel a pinching sensation.

Choose the site based on the status of circulation to the extremity and patient movement. Inadequate circulation to the site and artifact caused by motion may alter Sao_2 results. The photodetector and light-emitting diodes must be properly placed to ensure accurate readings.

5. Connect the sensor probe to the oximeter and turn it on. Check the pulse rate displayed on the oximeter to see whether it correlates with the patient's radial pulse. (Be sure the pulse oximeter is plugged in to an electrical socket).

Correlation between the oximeter pulse display and the patient's radial pulse confirms accurate readings.

6. Read the Sao_2 measurement on the digital display when it reaches a constant value, usually in 10 to 30 seconds, but may take up to 2 minutes.

The oximeter requires time to detect the pulse, calculate oxygen saturation, and register an accurate reading. ▼

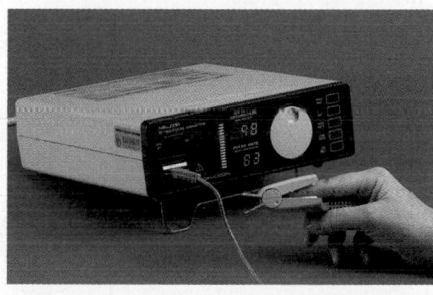

7. Set and turn on the alarm limits for Sao_2 and pulse rate, according to

the manufacturer's instructions, patient condition, and agency policy if continuous monitoring is necessary. Alarms must be set at appropriate levels to signify when Sao_2 or pulse rate falls below predetermined levels. Alarms help ensure prompt recognition and treatment of hypoxia.

8. Obtain readings as prescribed or indicated by the patient's respiratory status.

Some agencies require a prescription for pulse oximetry to ensure reimbursement.

9. Rotate the site if continuous monitoring is indicated.

Step 9 Variation. Adhesive Probe Sensor

Rotate the site every 4 hours.

Step 9 Variation. Clip-on Probe Sensor

Rotate the site every 2 hours.

Probe sensors and prolonged pressure may irritate the skin; rotating the site prevents skin breakdown.

10. Remove the probe sensor, and turn off the oximeter when monitoring is no longer necessary.

Some oximeters are battery powered; leaving them on after use depletes the battery.

(continued on next page)

Procedure 35-2 ■ Monitoring Pulse Oximetry (Arterial Oxygen Saturation) (continued)

Evaluation

- Evaluate the patient's understanding of the procedure and the obtained values.
- Compare pulse oximetry results with the patient's clinical presentation.
- Evaluate the effectiveness of therapy by comparing Sao$_2$ results before, during, and after treatment.
- Assess the site every 4 hours if you are using an adhesive probe sensor or every 2 hours if you are using a clip-on probe sensor.

Skin breakdown may occur if continuous monitoring is instituted. Assessment also confirms that the sensor is still in place.

Patient Teaching

- Demonstrate the procedure to the patient and caregiver, especially if the patient will be continuing pulse oximetry at home.
- Explain to the patient and caregiver the significance of Sao$_2$ results.
- Discuss the signs and symptoms of hypoxia (confusion, restlessness, shortness of breath, dyspnea, cyanosis, and somnolence) with the patient and caregiver.

Sample EHR documentation:

Note: Because this isn't the entire computer screen, the image does not show the patient's name, the date, or the nurse's name.

Home Care

- Explain where to obtain a pulse oximeter.
- Discuss normal Sao$_2$ results with the client and caregiver, and tell them when to notify the primary provider of abnormal results or signs and symptoms of hypoxia.
- Help the client identify risk factors that decrease Sao$_2$ levels.

Documentation

- Record the date and time of each pulse oximetry reading obtained. Most agencies use a flowsheet if frequent monitoring is necessary.
- Document whether readings are intermittent or continuous.
- If readings are continuous, record alarm parameters.
- Chart the patient's vital signs and Sao$_2$ results, and indicate whether the patient is breathing room air or receiving oxygen therapy. For oxygen therapy, note the oxygen concentration and the mode of delivery.
- Document acute decreases in Sao$_2$, any precipitating factors, treatment interventions, and the patient's response.

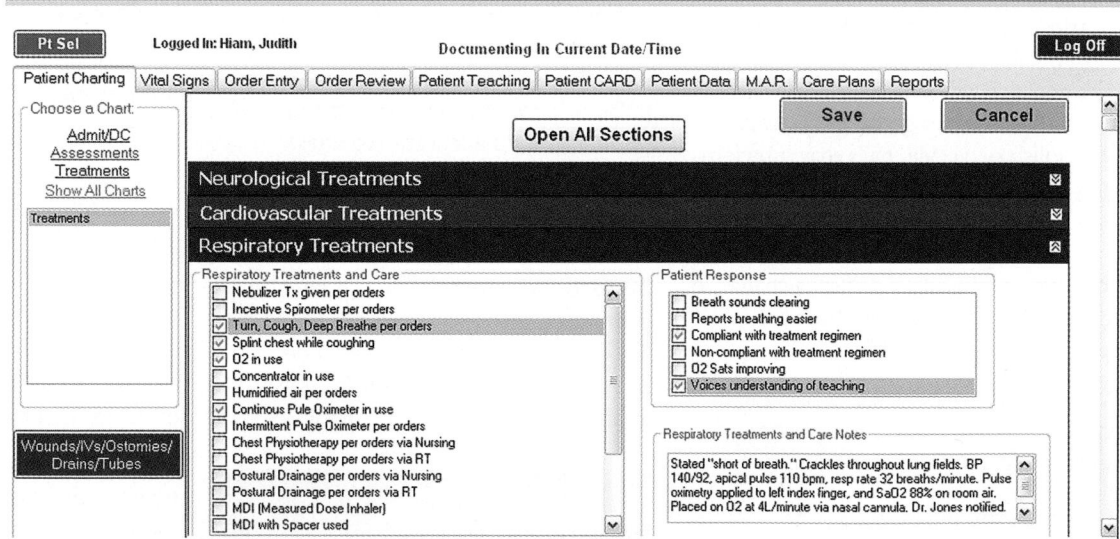

Practice Resources

American Association of Critical-Care Nurses (2005); Hill, E., & Stoneham, M. (2000); Rajkumar, A., Karmarkar, A., & Knott, J. (2006); Rodden, A., Spicer, L., Diaz, V., et al. (2007).

Thinking About the Procedure

 Go to the *Fundamentals of Nursing Skills Videos,* **Oxygenation: Pulse Oximetry.**

1. Based on the type of sensor used, would you infer that the patient's peripheral circulation was adequate or inadequate?

2. Which kind of sensor did the nurse use: clip-on or adhesive?

3. What did the nurse do after reading the Sao$_2$ measurement on the pulse oximeter?

 For suggested responses, go to Chapter 35, **Thinking About the Procedure Suggested Responses (Procedure 35-2),** on the Student Resource Disk or DavisPlus at http://davisplus.fadavis.com/Wilkinson2

Procedure 35-3   Performing Cardiac Monitoring

➤ For steps to follow in *all* procedures, refer to the Universal Steps for All Procedures found on the inside back cover of Volume 2.

Critical Aspects

- Identify electrode sites based on the monitoring system and the patient's anatomy.
- With an alcohol pad, clean the areas for electrode placement; allow to dry.
- Connect lead wires to the electrodes.
- Apply the electrodes, pressing firmly.
- If the patient's chest is very hairy, shave small areas for the electrodes.
- Check the ECG tracing on the monitor. If necessary, adjust the gain to increase the waveform size.
- Set the upper and lower heart rate alarm limits and turn them on.
- Obtain a rhythm strip by pressing the "record" button.

Equipment

- Alcohol pads
- Gauze dressing
- Washcloth
- Shaving supplies or scissors, if necessary
- Disposable electrodes

For hardwire monitoring, add:

- Cardiac monitor
- Cable with lead wires
- Safety pin
- 1-inch tape

For telemetry, add:

- Transmitter with lead wires (with a new battery inserted before each use)
- Pouch to carry transmitter

Delegation

You should not delegate this procedure to the LPN or NAP because it requires knowledge of anatomy, physiology, and advanced assessment techniques.

Pre-Procedure Assessment

- Assess cardiovascular status, including heart sounds, pulse rate, and blood pressure, and check for the presence of pain.
- Assess skin integrity of the chest before applying electrodes.

Skin lesions contraindicate the application of leads to the affected area.

- Assess for history of dysrhythmias.

Early recognition of dysrhythmias allows for prompt treatment, which improves patient outcomes.

➤ When performing the procedure, always identify your patient according to agency policy and be attentive to standard precautions, hand hygiene, patient safety and privacy, body mechanics, and documentation.

Procedure Steps

1. Prepare the monitoring equipment.

Step 1 Variation. Hardwire Monitoring

  a. Plug the cardiac monitor into an electrical outlet, and turn it on.

Allows the monitor to warm up while you prepare the patient for monitoring.

  b. Connect the cable with lead wires into the monitor.

The cable and lead wires must be properly connected to the monitor to obtain an accurate ECG tracing. Most are color coded.

Step 1 Variation. Telemetry Monitoring

  c. Insert a new battery into the transmitter.

A new battery should be inserted with each use to ensure transmitter function.

(continued on next page)

Procedure 35-3 ■ **Performing Cardiac Monitoring** (continued)

d. Turn on the transmitter.
Tests the unit to make sure that the battery is functional.

e. Connect the lead wires to the transmitter, if they are not permanently attached. Be sure to attach each one to its correct outlet.
The lead wires must be properly connected to the transmitter to obtain an accurate ECG tracing.

2. Expose the patient's chest, and identify electrode sites based on the monitoring system being used and the patient's anatomy. Gently rub the placement sites with a washcloth or gauze pad until the skin reddens slightly. The monitoring system will dictate lead placement. Sites over soft tissues or close to bone provide accurate waveforms; sites over bony prominences, thick muscles, and skinfolds can produce artifact. ▼

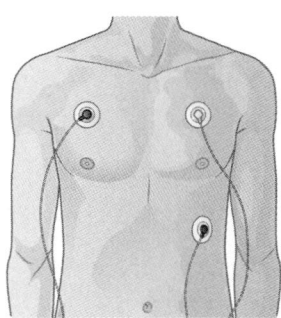

3. If the patient's chest has dense hair, shave or clip the hair with scissors at each electrode site.
Hair may interfere with electrical contact, preventing accurate ECG waveform transmission.

4. With an alcohol pad, clean the areas chosen for electrode placement, and allow them to dry.
Alcohol removes oil on the skin that may prevent the electrodes from adhering.

5. Remove the electrode backing, and make sure the gel is moist. Discard the electrode if the gel is dry. The number of electrodes needed will depend on the monitoring system being used. It will be three to five electrodes.
A dry electrode will not conduct electrical activity.

6. Attach the lead wires to the electrodes by snapping or clipping them in place.

7. Apply the electrode to the site by pressing it firmly. Repeat with the remaining electrodes.
Pressing the electrode firmly creates a tight seal, which ensures electrical contact.

8. Secure the monitoring equipment.

Step 8 Variation. Hardwire Monitoring
a. Wrap a piece of 1-inch tape around the cable, and secure it to the patient's gown with a safety pin.
Secures the cable so leads are not disconnected with patient movement.

Step 8 Variation. Telemetry Monitoring
b. Place the transmitter in the pouch, and tie the pouch strings around the patient's neck. Place the transmitter into the patient's robe or gown pocket if a pouch is not available.
Allows the patient independence with ambulation.

9. Check the patient's ECG tracing on the monitor. If necessary, adjust the gain on the monitor to increase the waveform size.
The ECG tracing should be of adequate size to accurately assess all of the waveform components.

Step 9 Variation. Telemetry Monitoring
You may need to call a monitoring room to verify ECG tracing and rhythm.

10. Set the upper and lower heart rate alarm limits according to agency policy or patient condition, and turn them on.

11. Obtain a rhythm strip by pressing the "record" button.
You must obtain a rhythm strip to document the patient's cardiac rhythm. ▼

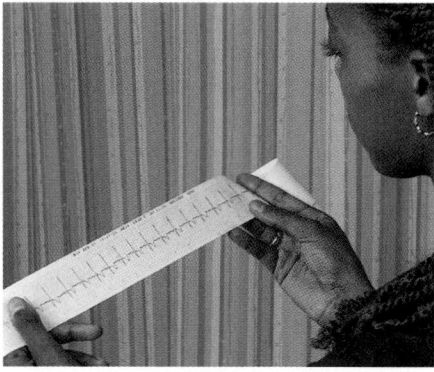

Step 11 Variation. Hardwire Monitoring
a. Press the "record" button on the bedside monitor.
The "record" button, located on the monitor at the bedside, allows you to print a rhythm strip immediately when cardiac symptoms occur.

Step 11 Variation. Telemetry Monitoring
b. Press the "record" button on the transmitter of the telemetry unit, or call the monitoring room to have the ECG trip printed.
The "record" button on the telemetry transmitter allows you or the patient to print a rhythm strip immediately when cardiac symptoms occur.

12. Interpret the rhythm strip, and mount it appropriately (e.g., with transparent tape) in the patient's chart. *Provides a permanent record of the patient's heart activity; identifies abnormalities in the patient's rhythm.*

What if. . .

■ **The patient is diaphoretic?**

Remove electrodes, clean the area with alcohol, allow the area to dry, and then reapply electrodes.

Clean, dry skin is necessary for an accurate ECG tracing.

■ **The patient is receiving a cardiac medication?**

Print a strip before giving medication and after giving medication. You may also need to call the telemetry station to have the ECG monitored.

To assess and monitor effects of medication.

■ **You are not getting a good reading on the monitor?**

Recheck the leads; replace leads or move leads if necessary.

New leads might be needed for accurate ECG tracing.

Evaluation

■ Evaluate changes in the patient's cardiac rhythm.
■ Check skin integrity, and replace the electrodes at least every 24 hours.

Avoids skin irritation at the electrode sites. In addition, the gel begins to dry, so replacement ensures an adequate waveform.

Patient Teaching

■ Explain the rationale for cardiac monitoring.
■ Teach the patient that if he experiences symptoms (e.g., shortness of breath, chest pain, dizziness, palpitations) he should notify the nurse immediately so a rhythm strip can be recorded.
■ Tell the patient being monitored by telemetry to remove the transmitter before showering. Ask the patient to inform you before removing it.
■ Discuss home telemetry monitoring with the patient and caregiver if the patient requires telemetry monitoring after discharge.

Home Care

■ Evaluate the client's and caregiver's ability to continue telemetry monitoring at home with help from an outside agency.

■ Help the client and caregiver arrange for home telemetry monitoring by contacting the monitoring agency.
■ Explain to the caregiver and patient that the emergency medical service will be notified by the monitoring agency if a dysrhythmia develops.
■ Instruct the caregiver and patient about proper lead placement and the need to rotate electrode sites to prevent skin breakdown.
■ Allow the caregiver and client time for questions and to verbalize concerns.

Documentation

■ Document the date and time that monitoring was instituted.
■ Note the monitoring lead selected.
■ Document a rhythm strip every 8 hours and with changes in the patient's condition according to agency policy. Label the rhythm strip (if the monitor does not label it for you) with the date, time, patient's name, and room number. Indicate on the strip when symptoms and treatment interventions occurred.
■ Document the patient's response to treatment.

(continued on next page)

Procedure 35-3 ■ **Performing Cardiac Monitoring** (continued)

Sample EHR documentation:

Note: Because this isn't the entire computer screen, the image does not show the patient's name, the date, or the nurse's name.

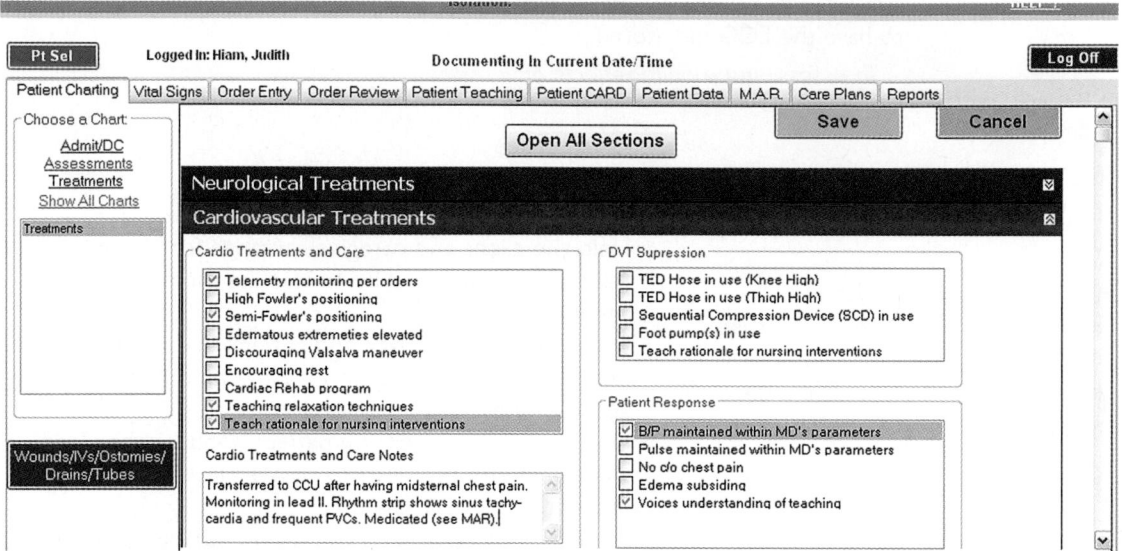

Practice Resources

Hazinski, M., Nadkarni, V., Hickey, R., et al. (2005); Hill, E., & Stoneham, M. (2000); Kligfield, P., Leonard, S., Bailey, J., et al. (2007).

Procedure 35-4 □ **Performing Percussion, Vibration, and Postural Drainage**

➤ For steps to follow in *all* procedures, refer to the Universal Steps for All Procedures found on the inside back cover of Volume 2.

Critical Aspects

- Help the patient assume the appropriate position based on the lung field that requires drainage.
- Keep the patient in the desired position for 10 to 15 minutes.
- Using cupped hands, perform percussion over the affected lung area for 1 to 3 minutes while the patient is in the desired drainage position.
- Next, perform vibration.
- Assist the patient to sit up. Ask him to cough at the end of a deep inspiration to clear the airways of secretions.
- Repeat postural drainage, percussion, and vibration for each lung field that requires treatment. The entire treatment should not exceed 60 minutes.
- Provide mouth care.

Equipment

- Bed capable of being placed in the Trendelenburg position
- Pillows
- Patient gown
- Facial tissues
- Emesis basin
- Sputum specimen container, if needed
- Suction equipment, if needed
- Stethoscope

Delegation

You should assess the patient to determine the need for the procedure and to evaluate whether the patient can tolerate the procedure. You should perform the initial procedure, but you can delegate subsequent treatments to a respiratory therapist or NAP who is adequately trained. Instruct the respiratory therapist or NAP to report any changes in the patient's condition immediately. The RN is responsible for ongoing assessment and monitoring of airway clearance and respiratory status.

Pre-Procedure Assessment

■ Check the patient's chest x-ray results.
Identifies which lung fields require treatment.

■ Assess the patient's respiratory status, including respiratory rate, depth, and rhythm; breath sounds; color; and pulse oximetry results.
Determines the need for and effectiveness of percussion, vibration, and postural drainage.

■ Determine when the patient has last eaten.
Postural drainage should not be performed for at least 2 hours after meals to prevent nausea, vomiting, and aspiration.

■ Assess the patient for dysrhythmias, coagulopathy (a defect in blood clotting), hypertension, and pain or tenderness in the chest area being treated.
If any of these are present, the procedure should be avoided because it might worsen these conditions.

➤ When performing the procedure, always identify your patient according to agency policy and be attentive to standard precautions, hand hygiene, patient safety and privacy, body mechanics, and documentation.

Procedure Steps

1. Help the patient assume the appropriate position, based on the lung field that requires drainage.
Helps mobilize secretions in the affected lung field by gravity.

a. **Apical areas of the upper lobes.** Ask the patient sit at the edge of the bed, if possible. If needed, place a pillow at the base of the spine for support. If the patient is not able to sit at the edge of the bed, place him in high-Fowler's position.▼

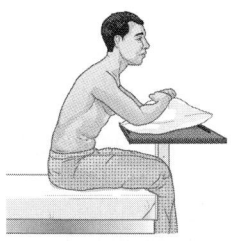

b. **Posterior section of the upper lobes.** Position supine with a pillow under the hips and knees flexed. Have the patient rotate slightly away from the side that requires drainage.▼

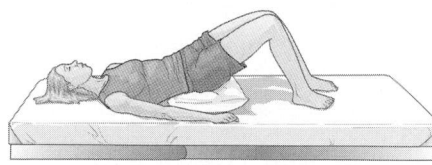

c. **Middle or lower lobes.** Place the bed in the Trendelenburg position. Position the patient in Sims' position. To drain the left lung, position the patient on his right side. For the right lung, position the patient on his left side.▼

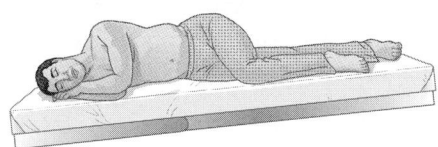

d. **Posterior lower lobes.** Keeping the bed flat, position the patient prone with a pillow under her stomach.▼

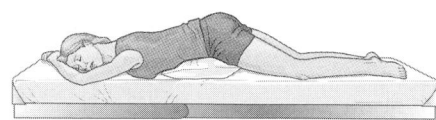

2. Have the patient remain in the desired position for 10 to 15 minutes, if tolerated.
Allows adequate drainage of secretions by gravity from the desired lung field.

3. Perform percussion over the affected lung area while the patient is in the desired drainage position.
Loosens and mobilizes secretions.

a. Instruct the patient to breathe deeply and slowly.
Relaxation helps the patient tolerate the procedure.

b. Place a towel over the patient's skin or cover with the patient's gown the area to be percussed.
Protects the skin and promotes patient privacy and comfort.

◆ c. Avoid clapping over bony prominences, female breasts, or tender areas of the chest.
Percussing over these areas may cause discomfort and compromise tissue integrity.

d. Cup your hands, keeping your fingers flexed and your thumbs pressed against your index fingers.
Cupping your hands promotes patient comfort during percussion.

e. Place your cupped hands over the lung area that requires drainage.

f. Percuss the lung area for 1 to 3 minutes by alternately striking your cupped hands rhythmically against the patient.▼

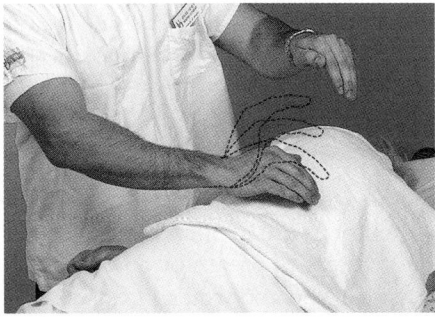

4. Perform vibrations while the patient remains in the desired drainage position.▼

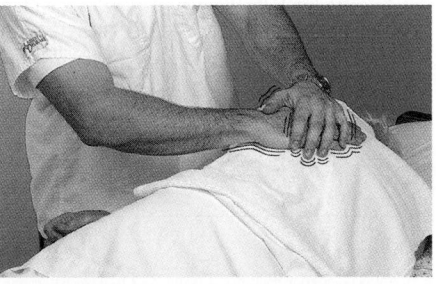

a. Place the flat surface of one hand over the lung area that requires vibration. Place your other hand on top of that hand at a right angle.
Using the flat surfaces of the hands provides a large surface area to

(continued on next page)

Procedure 35-4 ■ **Performing Percussion, Vibration, and Postural Drainage** (continued)

transmit vibrations through the chest. Placing one hand on top of the other provides better leverage for vibrating.

　　b. Instruct the patient to inhale slowly and deeply.
Promotes relaxation and lung expansion.

　　c. Instruct the patient to make an "fff" or "sss" sound as she exhales.
　　d. As the patient exhales, press your fingers and palms firmly against her chest wall.

Vibrating during exhalation enhances the downward movement of the rib cage that occurs during exhalation.

　　e. Push down, and gently vibrate with your hands over the lung area.
Vibration helps mobilize secretions.

　　f. Continue performing vibrations for three exhalations.

5. After performing postural drainage, percussion, and vibration, allow the patient to sit up. Ask her to cough at the end of a deep inspiration. Suction the patient if she is unable to

expectorate secretions. If a sputum specimen is needed, collect it in a specimen container.
Coughing helps clear the airway of secretions.

6. Repeat steps 1 through 5 for each lung field that requires treatment. The entire treatment should not exceed 60 minutes.
Treating for longer than 60 minutes fatigues the patient.

7. Provide mouth care.
Cleanses the mouth of secretions and promotes patient comfort.

Evaluation

- Evaluate the effectiveness of percussion, vibration, and postural drainage.
- Auscultate breath sounds every 2 to 4 hours, as indicated.
- Monitor pulse oximetry and arterial blood gas results.
- Evaluate the need for further treatment with percussion, vibration, and postural drainage.

Patient Teaching

- Demonstrate percussion, vibration, and postural drainage if the patient will be continuing it at home.
- Reinforce the importance of immediately reporting shortness of breath or any difficulty breathing.
- Explain the importance of drinking fluids to help thin and mobilize secretions.
- Explain coughing and deep-breathing exercises.

Home Care

- Explain to the family and caregiver how to perform percussion, vibration, and postural drainage if the client requires continued treatment at home.
- Be sure the client/family/caregiver knows how often the procedure should be done. There should be a prescription from the primary care provider.

- Explain the goal of the treatments and why they are important.
- Most clients will not have a bed that can be placed in the Trendelenburg position. Teach the client and caregivers how to position the client with hips elevated on pillows, higher than the chest, or, if the client is able, to assume a knee–chest position.
- Provide the client and caregiver with contact information of healthcare personnel who can be reached for advice or emergencies.

Documentation

- Document the date and time you performed percussion, vibration, and postural drainage.
- Note the positions used for postural drainage and the length of time the patient maintained each position.
- Note the locations in which you performed percussion and vibration.
- Document the patient's tolerance of the procedure, as well as any complications and the nursing interventions you used to treat the complication.
- Document the amount, color, odor, and consistency of sputum you obtained during the procedure and whether you sent a sputum specimen to the lab.

Sample EHR documentation:

Note: Because this isn't the entire computer screen, the image does not show the patient's name, the date, or the nurse's name.

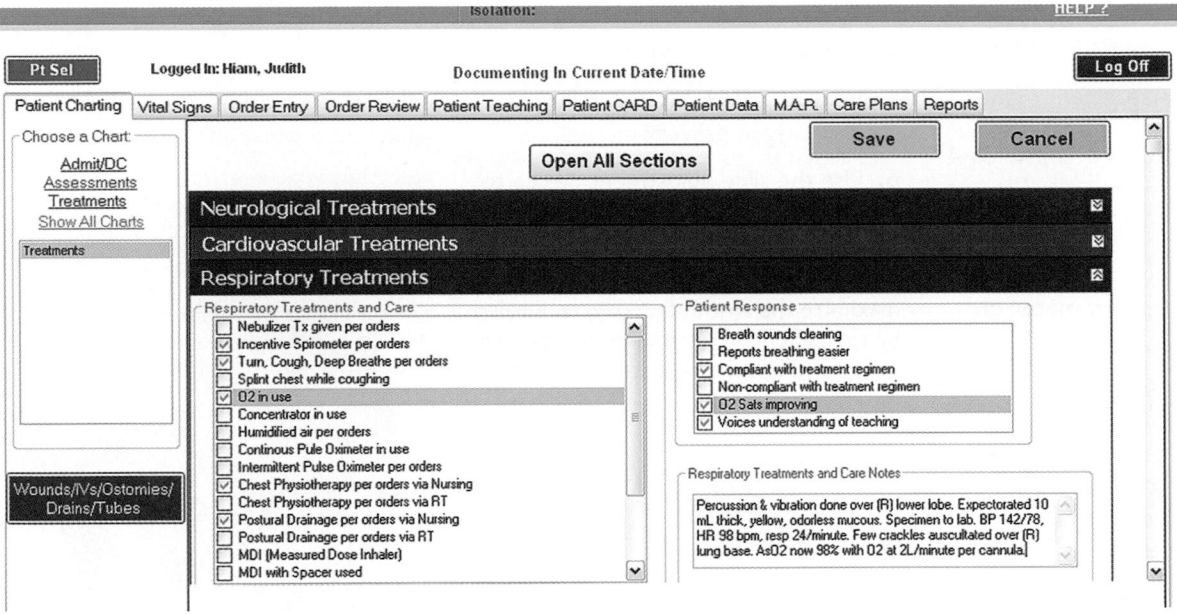

Practice Resources

No author (2007). *Best practices: Evidence-based nursing procedures* (2nd ed.).

Procedure 35-5 ☐ **Administering Oxygen**

➤ For steps to follow in *all* procedures, refer to the Universal Steps for All Procedures found on the inside back cover of Volume 2.

Critical Aspects

- Attach the flow meter to the oxygen source.
- Assemble and apply the oxygen equipment according to the device prescribed (nasal cannula, face mask, or face tent).
- Turn on the oxygen using the flow meter, and adjust according to the prescribed flow rate.
- Double check that the oxygen equipment is set up correctly and functioning properly.
- Assess the patient's respiratory status before you leave the bedside.

Equipment

- Oxygen source
- Flow meter
- Oxygen tubing
- Nasal cannula, oxygen mask, or face tent
- Prefilled humidification device

Delegation

The RN is responsible for assessing respiratory function and initiating oxygen therapy. However, you may delegate reapplication of oxygen therapy to appropriately trained assistive personnel when necessary.

Pre-Procedure Assessment

- Assess the patient's understanding of oxygen therapy.
- Assessment of the patient's respiratory status; includes respiratory rate, depth, and rhythm; breath sounds; color; capillary refill and pulse oximetry results.
  Respiratory assessment determines the need for further treatment and effectiveness of oxygen therapy.
- Assess nares for patency (if a nasal cannula is being used) and behind the ears for signs of skin breakdown.

(continued on next page)

Procedure 35-5 ▪ **Administering Oxygen** (continued)

➤ When performing the procedure, always identify your patient according to agency policy and be attentive to standard precautions, hand hygiene, patient safety and privacy, body mechanics, and documentation.

➤ *Note:* Oxygen requires a medical prescription. In an emergency, place oxygen on the patient to prevent respiratory distress, then notify the primary care provider for a prescription.

Procedure Steps

✚ Also use Clinical Insight 35-4: Oxygen Therapy Safety Precautions.

1. Attach the flow meter to the wall oxygen source (the green meter on the wall).

Step I Variation. Portable Oxygen Tank

Attach the flow meter to the tank if it is not already connected. Once tubing is attached to the portable tank, check the amount of oxygen in the tank by looking at the meter.
The flow meter regulates the amount of oxygen delivered per minute.

2. Assemble the oxygen equipment. (See the table at the end of this procedure for various oxygen delivery devices.)

3. Attach the humidifier to the flow meter. The humidifier is simply a small plastic container containing normal saline. If you are not using a humidifier, attach the adapter to the flow meter.
The humidifier adds moisture in with the oxygen, which can dry the nasal or oral cavity.

Procedure Variation A. Nasal Cannula

Follow steps 1 through 3.

4. Attach the nasal cannula tubing to the humidifier or the adapter.

5. Place the nasal prongs in the patient's nares—prongs curved downward—and then place the tubing around each ear.

Properly positions the device for optimal oxygen delivery.

6. Use the slide adjustment device to tighten the cannula in place under the patient's chin.
The nasal cannula must fit securely to maximize the amount of oxygen inhaled by the patient. A good fit minimizes the amount of oxygen lost around the prongs. ▼

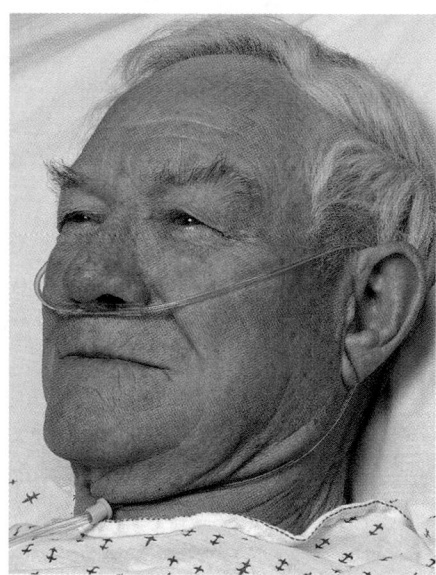

Go to step 11.

Procedure Variation B. Face Mask

Follow steps 1 through 3.

7. Gently place the face mask on the patient's face, applying it from the bridge of the nose to under the chin.

8. Secure the elastic band around the back of the patient's head. Make sure the mask fits snugly but comfortably.
The mask must fit snugly so that oxygen cannot escape around the

edges of the mask. If the mask is too tight, it may cause skin breakdown. ▼

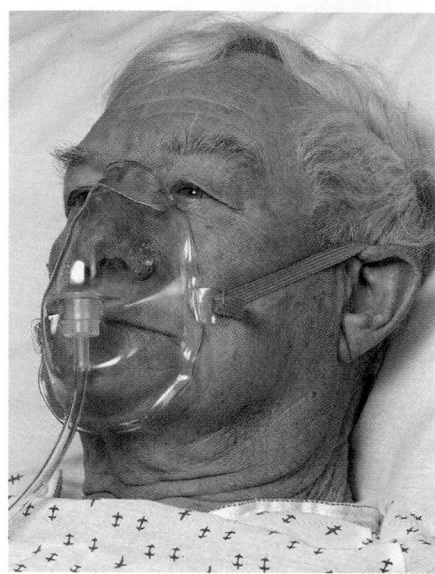

Go to step 11.

Procedure Variation C. Face Tent

Follow steps 1 through 3.

9. Gently place the face tent in front of the patient's face, making sure that it fits under the chin.

10. Secure the elastic band around the back of the patient's head.
The elastic band must go around the back of the patient's head to keep the face mask in place. ▼

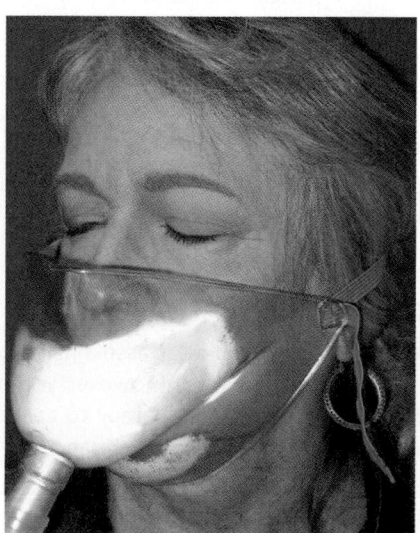

11. Turn on the oxygen at the flow meter, and adjust to the prescribed flow rate.

Ensures that the oxygen is delivered at the prescribed rate. Oxygen delivered at an incorrect rate can cause patient injury.

13. Assess the patient's respiratory status before leaving the bedside. To be certain it is safe to leave the patient.

12. Double check that the oxygen equipment is set up correctly and functioning properly.

Evaluation

- Assess respiratory rate, depth, and effort.
- Auscultate breath sounds before leaving the bedside, then monitor every 2 to 4 hours, and as indicated.
- Monitor pulse oximetry until respiratory status improves.
- Monitor arterial blood gas results if prescribed.
- Evaluate for skin breakdown, paying close attention to areas behind the ears, cheekbones, and under the chin—areas that are in contact with the oxygen delivery system.
- Notify the primary provider of respiratory status, oxygen, and response and any additional prescriptions needed.

Patient Teaching

- Demonstrate oxygen administration to the patient and caregiver if the patient will be continuing oxygen therapy at home. Allow for time to answer questions, and return demonstration of attaching and placing oxygen on.
- Explain the importance of immediately reporting shortness of breath or any difficulty breathing to the nursing staff before discharge. If the patient is at home, he will need to report the difficulty to the home health and/or primary care provider, and, if needed, to call 911.

Home Care

- Explain to the family and caregiver where to obtain oxygen equipment and what services are available. Make sure they choose a supplier who has 24-hour emergency services.

- Instruct the client and caregiver about oxygen therapy and its use, as well as safety measures that they must institute. Safety measures include keeping oxygen away from items that may cause ignition such as lighters, cigarettes, fire places, heaters, etc.
- To demonstrate the oxygen is on, client can hold nasal prongs on the side of the cheek to feel air flow or over a glass of water to see air moving water.
- Teach the client and caregiver to clean the nasal cannula or face mask with soap and warm water when it becomes soiled. The mask needs to air dry.
- Provide the client and caregiver with contact information of healthcare personnel who can be reached for advice or emergencies.
- In the home, liquid oxygen and oxygen concentrators are more commonly used than portable oxygen tanks. Liquid oxygen may be kept in small, portable containers; an oxygen concentrator removes nitrogen from room air and concentrates O_2. It requires a battery pack or electrical outlet for power. Oxygen concentrators can deliver a flow of 6 to 8 L/min.

Documentation

- Document the date, time, and reason oxygen therapy was initiated.
- Note the type of oxygen delivery system used, the amount of oxygen administered, and the patient's response to oxygen therapy.
- Document vital signs, pulse oximetry values, breath sounds, skin color, and respiratory effort.

(continued on next page)

Procedure 35-5 ■ **Administering Oxygen** (continued)

Sample EHR documentation:

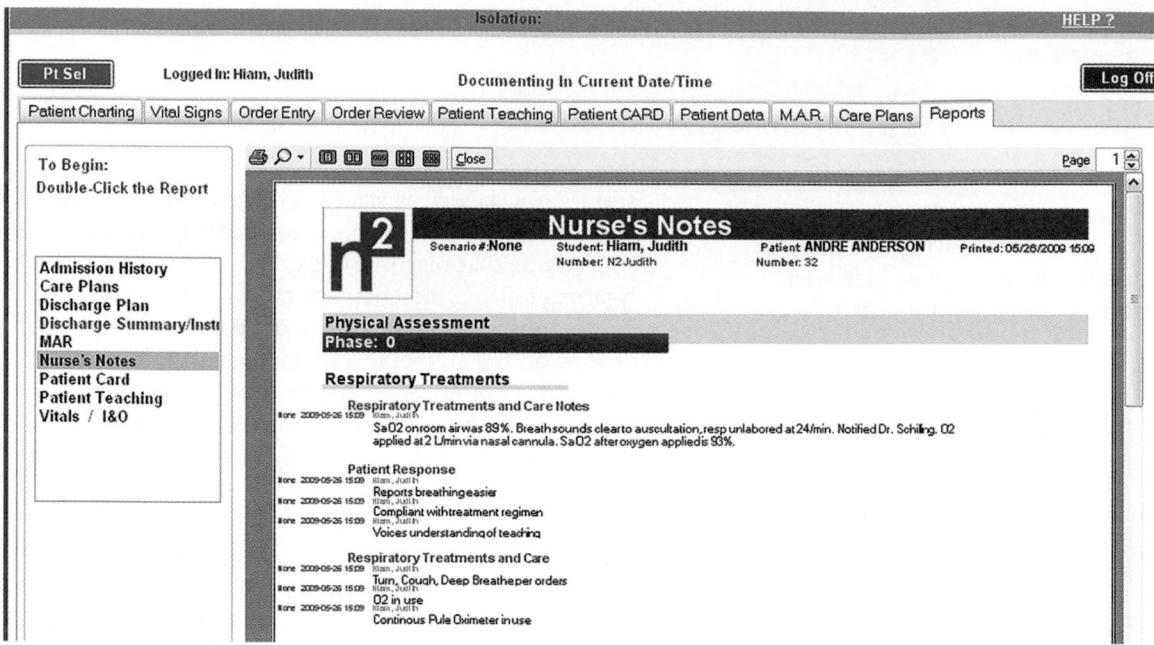

Sample documentation:

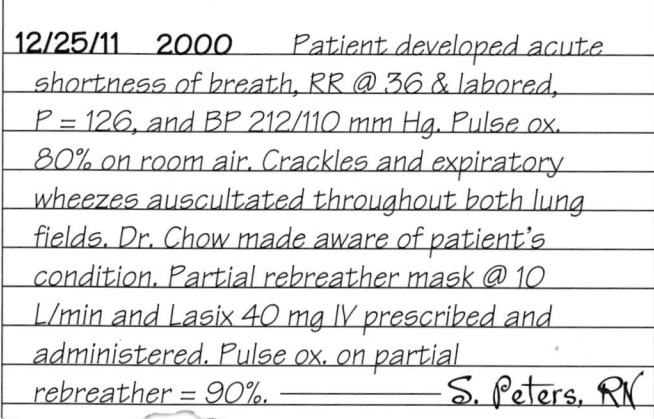

12/25/11   2000   *Patient developed acute shortness of breath, RR @ 36 & labored, P = 126, and BP 212/110 mm Hg. Pulse ox. 80% on room air. Crackles and expiratory wheezes auscultated throughout both lung fields. Dr. Chow made aware of patient's condition. Partial rebreather mask @ 10 L/min and Lasix 40 mg IV prescribed and administered. Pulse ox. on partial rebreather = 90%. ———————— S. Peters, RN*

Practice Resources

No author. (2007). *Best practices: Evidence-based nursing procedures* (2nd ed.).

Oxygen Delivery Systems

DELIVERY METHOD	F$_{IO_2}$	DISCUSSION	NURSING RESPONSIBILITIES
Nasal cannula	1 L/min = 24% 2 L/min = 28% 3 L/min = 32% 4 L/min = 36% 5 L/min = 40% 6 L/min = 44%	■ Relatively comfortable. ■ Patients can eat, talk, and cough with a nasal cannula in place. ■ Works best if the patient breathes through his nose.	■ Check frequently that the prongs are in the patient's nose. ■ Assess for dryness of the nasal mucosa. ■ Humidify flow at rates above 3 L/min (flow rates > 3 L/min are drying). ■ Encourage the patient to take slow, deep breaths, so he will inhale more oxygen and less room air.

Oxygen Delivery Systems—cont'd

DELIVERY METHOD	FIO₂	DISCUSSION	NURSING RESPONSIBILITIES
Simple face mask: A clear, flexible mask that covers the nose and mouth and delivers oxygen flow into the mask.	5–10 L/min = 40%–60% FIO_2	■ Requires flow rates greater than 5 L/min to prevent accumulation and rebreathing of exhaled CO_2 from within the mask. ■ Masks are not easily tolerated because they fit tightly and keep heat from radiating from the face, making patients feel hot. ■ Talking is muffled by the mask, and it must be removed for the patient to eat or drink.	■ Place face mask securely over the mouth and nose. ■ Elastic straps fit around the head to hold the mask in place. Place the straps well above the ears to prevent skin irritation and breakdown. ■ Place gauze or other soft material beneath the straps to prevent irritation. ■ Check the skin around the mask frequently. ■ Check the skin over the ears where the mask strap rubs. ■ Encourage the patient to take slow, deep breaths, so he will inhale more oxygen and less room air.
Partial rebreather mask: Uses the reservoir bag to capture some exhaled gas for rebreathing	6–15 L/min = 50%–90% FIO_2	■ Allows higher FIO_2 levels to be delivered because O_2 is collected in the reservoir bag for inhalation. ■ Exhalation ports allow most exhaled air to escape. ■ Several types are available. ■ Can deliver an FIO_2 above 50% at flow rates of 6–15 L/min. ■ Patient rebreathes some exhaled air along with O_2.	■ Maintain the flow at a high enough rate to prevent the reservoir bag from collapsing during inhalation. ■ Encourage the patient to take slow, deep breaths, so he will inhale more oxygen and less room air.
Nonrebreather mask: A type of reservoir bag mask; a valve keeps exhaled air from entering the reservoir bag.	6–15 L/min = 70%–100% FIO_2	■ Contains only O_2, which allows higher FIO_2 delivery. An FIO_2 of 60–100% can be delivered at flow rates of 6–15 L/min. ■ This mask is the only external device capable of delivering an FIO_2 of 100% (in practice, it is rare to achieve a concentration over 75% because the mask does not seal perfectly with the face).	■ Maintain the flow at a rate high enough to keep the reservoir at least one-third to one-half full during inhalation. ■ Be sure the mask fits snugly so the patient will breathe in less room air.

(continued on next page)

Procedure 35-5 ▪ **Administering Oxygen** (continued)

Oxygen Delivery Systems—cont'd

DELIVERY METHOD	FIO_2	DISCUSSION	NURSING RESPONSIBILITIES
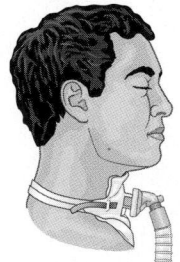 **Venturi mask:** A cone-shaped adapter that serves as a mixing valve to control the amount of O_2 and room air that flows through the mask.	24%–50% FIO_2	▪ The cone-shaped adapter at the base of the mask allows a precise FIO_2 to be delivered. This is very useful for patients with chronic lung disease. ▪ Exhalation ports keep CO_2 buildup to a minimum.	▪ The adapter indicates the required oxygen flow rate needed to deliver the desired FIO_2. Ensure that flow is set at the rate specified to deliver the FIO_2 desired.
Face tent: A large, open plastic mask that fits under the chin. It is open at the top and is held in place with an elastic band around the head.	8–12 L/min = 30%–55% FIO_2	▪ Less reliable than a face mask for delivering precise FIO_2 levels. ▪ Allows moderate- to high-density aerosol delivery for humidification. ▪ Patients who feel claustrophobic in a face mask often tolerate a face tent.	▪ Check the skin over the ears where the mask strap rubs.
Tracheostomy collar: A small, cup-shaped device that fits over the tracheostomy opening and is held in place with elastic straps around the neck.	4–10 L/min = 24%–100%	▪ It is possible to deliver both high FIO_2 and high humidity with a tracheostomy collar. ▪ Large-bore tubing is used to deliver humidification to the trachea; however, water frequently condenses inside the tubing and can be accidentally drained into the tracheostomy. Usually, a water trap of some sort is placed in the tubing to prevent this problem.	▪ Watch for water accumulation in the tubing.

Oxygen Delivery Systems—cont'd

DELIVERY METHOD	F$_{IO_2}$	DISCUSSION	NURSING RESPONSIBILITIES
T-piece: A T-shaped plastic piece; the bottom of the T fits directly and tightly onto the tracheostomy tube.	4–10 L/min = 24%– 100% F$_{IO_2}$	■ Oxygen and humidity are delivered into one side of the T and exhaled through the other side.	■ Take care that the oxygen delivery tubing does not pull on the T-piece, which can dislodge the tracheostomy tube and create an airway emergency.

Thinking About the Procedure

Go to the *Fundamentals of Nursing Skills Videos,* **Oxygenation: Administration, Cannula.**

1. Does the nurse wear gloves for this procedure? What do you think is the reason for that?

Go to the *Fundamentals of Nursing Skills Videos,* **Oxygenation: Administration, Face Mask.**

2. Why does the nurse not attach a humidifier to the oxygen delivery system?

Go to the *Fundamentals of Nursing Skills Videos,* **Oxygenation: Administration, Face Tent.**

3. Compare this procedure to **Administering Oxygen by Cannula.** Both procedures attach a humidifier to the flow meter. But what is different in the tubing that delivers the oxygen to the patient?

For suggested responses, go to Chapter 35, **Thinking About the Procedure Suggested Responses (Procedure 35-5),** on the Student Resource Disk or DavisPlus at http://davisplus.fadavis.com/Wilkinson2

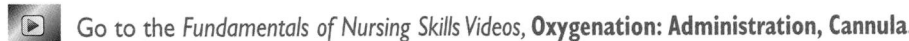

Procedure 35-6   Performing Tracheostomy Care

➤ For steps to follow in *all* procedures, refer to the Universal Steps for All Procedures found on the inside back cover of Volume 2.

Critical Aspects

- Position the patient in a semi-Fowler's position.
- Don gown, eye protection, and sterile gloves.
- Suction the tracheostomy.
- Remove soiled dressing; remove gloves; wash hands.
- Set up the sterile field and prepare the equipment, keeping supplies sterile.
- Don sterile gloves (procedure gloves for modified sterile technique)
- Remove the oxygen source if the patient is receiving supplemental oxygen, and attach to the outer cannula if possible. If not possible, clean and return the inner cannula before proceeding.
- Remove the inner cannula with your nondominant hand, and dispose of it or clean it (if reusable).
- Clean the stoma under the faceplate with the applicators saturated with normal saline or tap water.
- Clean the top surface of the faceplate and the skin around it with the normal saline-saturated gauze pads and applicators. (Use wash cloth and tap water for modified sterile technique.)
- Dry the skin around the faceplate and stoma with dry sterile gauze.
- With the help of an assistant, remove soiled tracheostomy ties.
- Ask the patient to flex his neck, and apply new tracheostomy ties.
- Insert a precut, sterile tracheostomy dressing under the faceplate and new ties.

(continued on next page)

Procedure 35-6 ■ **Performing Tracheostomy Care** (continued)

Equipment

- Tracheostomy suction equipment (see Procedure 35-7)
- Tracheostomy care kit or the following sterile supplies: several cotton-tipped applicators, two basins, a brush, sterile 4 in. × 4 in. gauze pads, sterile precut tracheostomy dressing
- Two pairs of sterile gloves (for modified sterile technique, use procedure gloves)
- Disposable inner cannula that is the same size as the tracheostomy, if available. Most tracheostomy tubes have disposable inner cannulas.
- Normal saline solution (for modified sterile technique, you can use tap water if agency policy allows)
- Hydrogen peroxide for cleaning of reusable inner cannula only
- Roll of twill tape or hook and loop fastener (Velcro®) tracheostomy holder
- Bandage scissors
- Towel or linen-saver pad
- Overbed table
- Face shield
- Protective gown
- For modified sterile technique: mild soap and two clean washcloths

✚ Use only the sterile precut dressing, or open and refold a 4 in. × 4 in. gauze pad into a V-shape. Do not cut 4 in. × 4 in. gauze, and do not use cotton-filled gauze squares. The patient may aspirate the cotton or gauze fibers.

Delegation

In acute care settings and with new tracheostomies, you should not delegate this procedure to the NAP. For long-standing and well-healed tracheostomies, you can safely delegate care to a NAP or LPN who is adequately trained to perform the skill. This varies by state. In some states only RNs can perform tracheostomy care. If you are not familiar with your state's nurse practice act, contact your state board of nursing.

Pre-Procedure Assessment

- Assess the patient's respiratory status, including respiratory rate, depth, and rhythm; breath sounds; color; and pulse oximetry results.

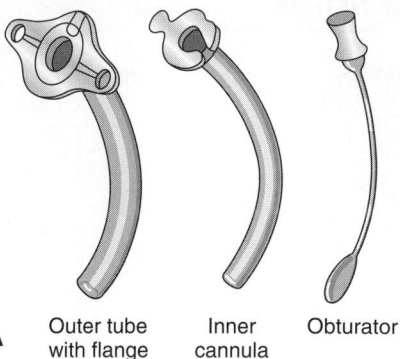

A   Outer tube with flange   Inner cannula   Obturator

a, **Nondisposable tracheostomy equipment**

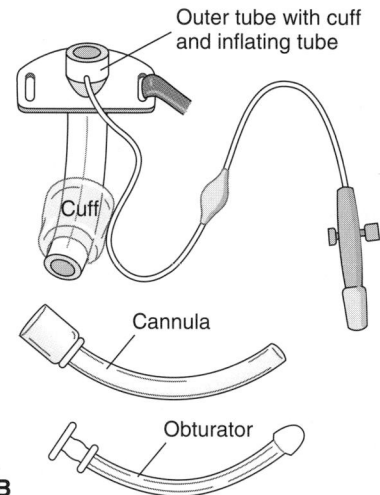

Outer tube with cuff and inflating tube

Cuff

Cannula

Obturator

B

b, **Disposable tracheostomy equipment**

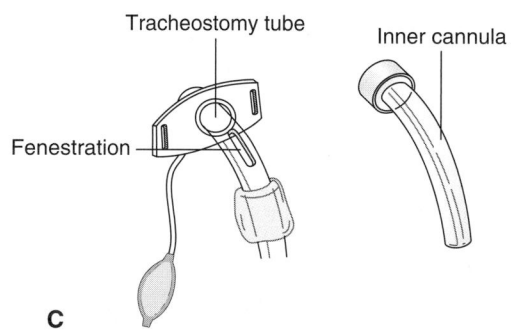

Tracheostomy tube

Inner cannula

Fenestration

C

c, **Fenestrated tracheostomy equipment**

Helps determine whether the patient can tolerate tracheostomy care.

- Assess the tracheostomy site for drainage, redness, or swelling.

Drainage, redness, or swelling may indicate infection.

- Determine when the patient last ate.

It is best to schedule this procedure at least 3 hours after a meal to decrease the risk of the patient vomiting and aspirating stomach contents.

■ Procedure 35-6A Tracheostomy Care Using Sterile Technique*

If you wish to use modified sterile technique, when you see a step with an asterisk (*), go to the same step number in Procedure 35-6B. The basic differences are that you will use nonsterile procedure gloves and tap water.

➤ When performing the procedure, always identify your patient according to agency policy and be attentive to standard precautions, hand hygiene, patient safety and privacy, body mechanics, and documentation.

Procedure Steps

1. Position the patient in semi-Fowler's position, and place a towel or linen-saver pad over the patient's chest.
A semi-Fowler's position promotes lung expansion and prevents back strain for the nurse. A towel or linen-saver pad prevents soiling of the patient's gown.

*2. Don sterile gloves, gown, and face shield or mask.

Step 2 Variation. One Sterile Glove

Alternatively, you may put a sterile glove on your dominant hand and a clean glove on your other hand.

3. Suction the tracheostomy (see Procedure 35-7 or 35-8).
Suctioning clears the tracheostomy of secretions that could occlude the outer cannula after the inner cannula is removed for care.

Step 3 Variation. Passy–Muir Valve

Remove the Passy–Muir valve before suctioning the patient to prepare for trach care

(A Passy–Muir Valve is a device that is used to enable the patient with a tracheostomy to speak. It is attached to the end of the inner cannula at the tracheostomy site.)

4. Remove and discard the soiled tracheostomy dressing in the appropriate receptacle, and then remove and discard your gloves. Wash your hands.

5. Place the tracheostomy care equipment on the overbed table, and prepare the equipment, using sterile technique.
Helps maintain sterility during tracheostomy care. Preparing the equipment before beginning care ensures efficiency.

*a. Disposable inner cannula– Pour sterile normal saline solution into the two sterile containers.
b. Resuable inner cannula–Pour hydrogen peroxide into one of the sterile solution containers, and pour normal saline solution into the other one.
If the inner cannula is not disposable, use hydrogen peroxide to clean only the inner cannula. Use the normal saline to rinse the inner cannula and clean the faceplate and tracheostomy site.

*c. (c through g apply to both types of cannula) Open two 4 in. × 4 in. gauze packages. Wet the gauze in one package with normal saline solution, and keep the second package dry.
You will use the second package of gauze to dry the skin around the tracheostomy site after cleaning.

*d. Open one cotton-tipped applicator package. Wet the applicators with normal saline solution.
Prepares the applicators for cleaning the exposed surface of the outer cannula and the stoma site located under the faceplate of the tracheostomy tube, respectively.

e. Open the package containing a new disposable inner cannula, if available.
Allows for quick replacement of the inner cannula.

f. Open the package of Velcro® tracheostomy ties, or cut a length of twill tape long enough to go around the patient's neck two times. Make sure to cut end of the tape on an angle.
Allows for quick stabilization of the tracheostomy tube, preventing dislodgement. Cutting the twill tape on an angle allows for easy insertion through the faceplate eyelets.

g. Position a biohazard bag within reach.
This allows you to dispose of contaminated supplies safely as you use them without leaving the patient or interrupting the procedure.

*6. Don sterile gloves (or a sterile glove on your dominant hand and a clean glove on your nondominant hand); keep the glove on your dominant hand sterile. Handle the sterile supplies with the dominant hand only.

7. For patients receiving oxygen: With your nondominant (nonsterile) hand, remove the oxygen or humidification source. Attach the oxygen source to the outer cannula, if possible. If not possible, have the respiratory therapist set up oxygen blow-by to use while you are cleaning the reusable inner cannula.

(continued on next page)

Procedure 35-6 ■ **Performing Tracheostomy Care** (continued)

Prevents oxygen desaturation in the patient during the procedure.

8. Unlock and remove the inner cannula with your nondominant hand, and care for it accordingly.

Step 8 Variation. Disposable Inner Cannula

a. Dispose of the inner cannula in the biohazard receptacle according to agency policy. You should never clean and reuse a disposable inner cannula.

Prevents contamination by bacteria contained in the inner cannula.

b. With your dominant hand, insert the new inner cannula into the patient's tracheostomy in the direction of the curvature. Following the manufacturer's instructions, lock the inner cannula in place securely to prevent it from dislodging. Remember to keep your dominant hand sterile.

Step 8 Variation. Reusable Inner Cannula

c. If a reusable inner cannula was used, place the inner cannula into the basin filled with hydrogen peroxide.

Hydrogen peroxide helps loosen tenacious (sticky) secretions.

d. Pick up the reusable inner cannula from the container of hydrogen peroxide with your nonsterile hand, and scrub it with the sterile nylon brush, using your sterile dominant hand. ▼

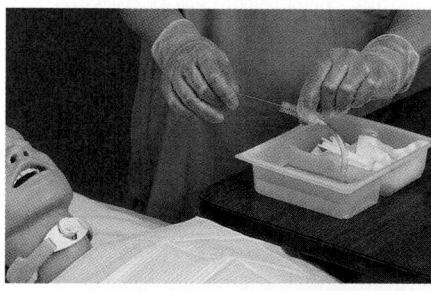

*e. Immerse the inner cannula in the container of sterile normal saline solution, and agitate it until it is rinsed thoroughly.

Immersing the inner cannula in normal saline solution and agitating it removes the hydrogen peroxide (which can cause tissue irritation) and debris from the inner cannula.

*f. Tap the inner cannula against the side of the container.

Removes excess fluid so the patient does not aspirate it when you reinsert the cannula.

g. With your dominant hand, reinsert the inner cannula into the patient's tracheostomy in the direction of the curvature. Following the manufacturer's instructions, lock the inner cannula in place securely to prevent it from dislodging. Remember to keep your dominant hand sterile.

Step 8 Variation. Passy–Muir Valve

h. Swish the Passy–Muir valve (PMV) in warm tap water with mild soap.
i. Rinse the PMV thoroughly in warm tap water.
j. DO NOT use hot water, peroxide, bleach, vinegar, alcohol, brushes, or Q-tips® to clean PMV, as this could damage the valve.
k. Shake the PMV to remove excess fluid. If you are going to store the valve, be sure to air-dry the valve before placing it in a storage container.

Removes moisture, which can promote bacterial growth.

l. Set the PMV aside on clean surface to be replaced when the inner cannula is replaced.

Step 8 Variation. For Patients Receiving Oxygen

m. Remove the humidification or oxygen source from the outer cannula, if indicated, using your nondominant hand.
n. Reinsert the inner cannula into the patient's tracheostomy in the direction of the curvature.
o. Following the manufacturer's instructions, lock the inner cannula in place securely. Remember to keep dominant hand sterile.

p. Lock the inner cannula in place securely to prevent it from dislodging.
q. Reattach the humidification or oxygen source, if indicated.

Provides the patient with needed humidity or oxygen and prevents oxygen desaturation.

*9. Clean the stoma under the faceplate with cotton-tipped applicators saturated with normal saline solution, using a circular motion from the stoma site outward. Use each applicator only once, and then discard it.

Prevents contamination of the cleaned area. ▼

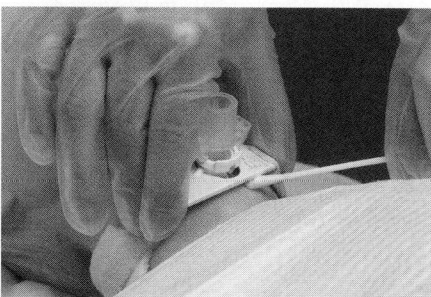

*10. Clean the top surface of the faceplate and the skin around it with the gauze pads saturated with normal saline solution. Use each gauze pad only once, and then discard it.

Removes secretions that provide a prime medium for microbial growth; prevents contamination of cleaned areas.

11. Dry the skin and outer cannula surfaces by patting them lightly with the remaining dry gauze pad.

Clean, dry skin is needed to aviod skin breakdown and removes moisture, which can promote bacterial growth around the stoma site.

✚ *12. Seek assistance from another staff member to help with changing the tracheostomy stabilizers.

Prevents accidental dislodging should the patient begin coughing during the procedure.

13. Remove soiled tracheostomy stabilizers.

Step 13 Variation. Removing a Soiled Velcro® Tracheostomy Holder

   a. With an assistant stabilizing the tracheostomy tube, disengage the Velcro® on both sides of the soiled holder, and remove it gently from the eyes of the faceplate. Discard the Velcro® holder in the nearest biohazard receptacle.

Removing the soiled holder promotes hygiene and prevents the spread of infection.

Step 13 Variation. Removing Soiled Twill Tape Tracheostomy Ties

   b. With an assistant stabilizing the tracheostomy tube, cut the soiled tracheostomy ties using bandage scissors. *Do not* cut the tube of the tracheostomy balloon (if you do, the tracheostomy tube must be replaced). Remove the ties gently from the eyes of the faceplate, and discard them in the nearest biohazard receptacle.

The tracheostomy balloon helps stabilize the tracheostomy in the trachea and prevents an air leak. Cutting the tube to the balloon prevents the balloon from holding air. Removing the soiled holder promotes hygiene and prevents the spread of infection.

14. Ask the patient to flex his neck, or, if he is unable, ask the assistant to hold the patient's head forward, and apply new tracheostomy ties.

Flexing the neck provides the same neck circumference as when the patient coughs and thus helps keep you from placing the tracheostomy stabilizers in such a way that they would be excessively tight.

Step 14 Variation. Using a Velcro® Tracheostomy Holder

   a. Unfasten the Velcro®. Thread one end of the tracheostomy holder through the eyelet of the faceplate, and fasten the Velcro®.

   b. Bring the holder around the back of the patient's neck.

The holder must be placed around the patient's neck to adequately secure the tracheostomy.

   c. Thread the remaining end of the tracheostomy holder through the empty eyelet of the faceplate and fasten the Velcro®, making sure that the holder fits securely. ▼

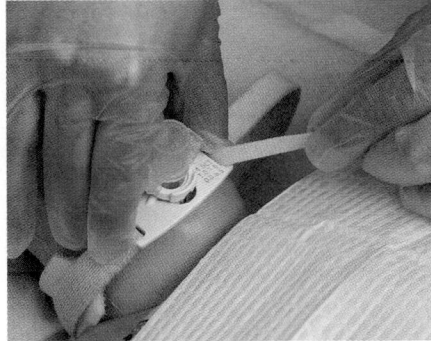

   d. Place one finger under the holder to make sure that the holder is securing the tracheostomy effectively but isn't too tight.

Securing the tracheostomy too tightly might place pressure on the jugular veins; interfere with coughing; or cause necrosis at the tracheostomy insertion site.

Step 14 Variation. Using Twill Tape

   e. Thread one end of the twill tape into one of the eyelets on the tracheostomy faceplate.

   f. Continue to thread the twill tape through the eyelet, bringing both ends of the tape together.

   g. Bring both ends of the twill tape around the back of the patient's neck.

The twill tape must be placed around the patient's neck to adequately secure the tracheostomy.

   h. Thread the end of the twill tape that is closest to the patient's neck through the back of the eyelet on the faceplate.

   i. Have your assistant place one finger under the twill tape while you tie the two ends together in a square knot.

Ensures you do not secure the tracheostomy too tightly.

   j. Place one finger under the holder to make sure that the holder is securing the tracheostomy effectively but isn't too tight.

Securing the tracheostomy too tightly might place pressure on the jugular veins; interfere with coughing; or cause necrosis at the tracheostomy insertion site.

15. Insert a precut, sterile tracheostomy dressing under the faceplate and new tracheostomy stabilizers or fold a 4 in. × 4 in. gauze pad into a V shape (below). ▼

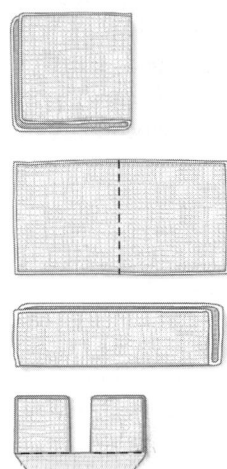

The new dressing absorbs secretions and prevents skin breakdown under the faceplate. Never cut the gauze to make a dressing because lint and fibers from the cut edge could enter the trachea and cause respiratory distress. ▼

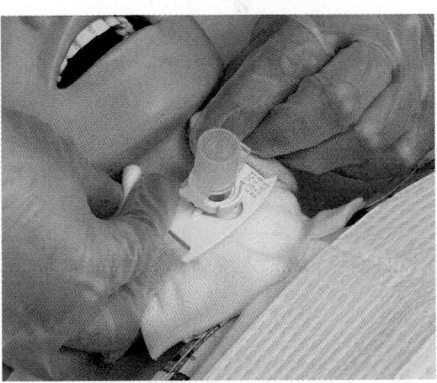

16. Dispose of the used equipment in the appropriate biohazard receptacle according to agency policy.

Properly disposing of used equipment prevents cross-contamination.

What if. . .

■ **Your patient begins coughing?**

   a. If the tracheostomy is still secured with ties or Velcro® holder, wait to continue tracheostomy care until coughing has ended.

(continued on next page)

Procedure 35-6 ■ **Performing Tracheostomy Care** (continued)

b. If tracheostomy is unsecured, stabilize the tube so that it does not become dislodged being careful not to press to hard on the site. Continue with tracheostomy care when the patient finishes coughing.

Pressing too hard at the tracheostomy site will stimulate the coughing reflex.

c. If coughing continues, suspend tracheostomy care and suction the patient to remove any retained secretions.

Retained secretions may cause increased airway irritation and coughing. Removing these secretions will reduce this irritation.

■ **You do not have an assistant to hold the cannula in place while you replace the soiled tracheostomy ties?**

✚ Never cut the soiled tape before applying the clean tape. Always place the new tape/holders, be certain the tracheostomy is secured, and then cut off the soiled tape or holder.

■ **The tracheostomy tube becomes dislodged?**

a. To prevent this, plan ahead and always have another staff member with you to secure the tracheostomy tube while you change the tracheostomy ties or Velcro® holder.

b. If the tracheostomy tube slips out slightly but is still in the trachea site, gently push it back into the stoma and secure it.

The pilot balloon will help to keep the tracheostomy tube from completely dislodging.

c. If the tracheostomy tube becomes completely dislodged, stay with the patient and ask your assistant to call for the respiratory therapist or trained person in your facility to insert a new tracheostomy tube.

■ **At step 9, there are crusts around the stoma when you are cleaning the stoma?**

Remove the crusts with a cotton-tipped swab soaked in hydrogen peroxide; then rinse with a swab soaked in normal saline (or tap water in modified sterile technique). Have the patient hold his breath while you remove crusts so he does not inhale them.

■ *Procedure 35-6B* **Tracheostomy Care Using Modified Sterile Technique**

➤ When performing the procedure, always identify your patient according to agency policy and be attentive to standard precautions, hand hygiene, patient safety and privacy, body mechanics, and documentation.

Procedure Steps
Follow Procedure 35-6A, except:

*2. Don clean gloves.

*5a. Pour tap water or sterile normal saline (per agency policy) into the two sterile containers.

*5c. Instead of sterile gauze, you may wet one washcloth with tap water (or saline) and keep the second washcloth dry.

*5d. Open one cotton-tipped applicator package. Wet the applicators with tap water or normal saline solution.

*6. Don clean gloves.

*8e. Hold the inner cannula under running tap water briefly (or place it in the normal saline) and agitate it until it is rinsed thoroughly.

Rinsing the inner cannula in tap water and agitating it removes the hydrogen peroxide (which can cause tissue irritation) and debris from the inner cannula.

*8f. Tap the inner cannula against the side of the container if using saline. If using running tap water, shake the cannula to remove water.

Tapping the inner cannula against the side of the container removes excess fluid so the patient does not aspirate it when you reinsert the cannula.

*9. Clean the stoma under the faceplate with the cotton-tipped applicators saturated with tap water or normal saline solution, using a circular motion from the stoma site outward. Use each applicator only once, and then discard it.

Prevents contamination of the cleaned area.

*10. Clean the top surface of the faceplate and the skin around it with a washcloth the saturated with tap water (or normal saline solution). Or you can use the gauze pads if they are contained in the tracheostomy kit.

Removes secretions that provide a prime medium for microbial growth; prevents contamination of cleaned areas.

*11. Dry the skin and outer cannula surfaces by patting them lightly with the remaining dry washcloth. Or you can use the gauze pads if they are contained in the tracheostomy kit.

Helps prevent skin breakdown and removes moisture, which can promote bacterial growth around the stoma site.

Evaluation

- Assess the area around the stoma site for signs of skin breakdown.
- Evaluate the patient's tolerance of the procedure. Note whether there were any signs of respiratory distress.

Patient Teaching

- Explain to the patient and his family that bloody secretions are normal for 2 to 3 days after tracheostomy tube insertion or for 24 hours after a tracheostomy tube change.
- Tell the patient and/or family to inform the nurse immediately if the tracheostomy tube becomes dislodged.
- Teach tracheostomy care to the patient and caregiver if the tracheostomy is expected to remain long term.

Home Care

- Clean technique can be used for tracheostomy care if the tracheostomy is more than 1 month old.
- Instruct the client and caregiver about home oxygen therapy and suctioning, if necessary.
- Demonstrate tracheostomy care to the caregiver, and ask for a return demonstration.
- Provide the client and caregiver with information about where to obtain tracheostomy care supplies.
- Supply the client and caregiver with contact information of healthcare personnel who can be reached for advice or emergencies.

Sample documentation:

Note: Because this isn't the entire computer screen, the image may not show all the information you would need to record about the patient.

- Recommend ways of adding moisture to the air, with a goal of maintaining a relative humidity of 50% (e.g., a large humidifier, house plants, wearing damp gauze over the stoma, closing the bathroom door and turning on the hot water to fill the room with steam).
- The stoma should be cleaned at least twice daily, using clean technique (or more often, depending on the amount of secretions).
- Stress good handwashing before and after doing any part of tracheostomy care.
- Remind client and caregiver not to use cotton or gauze. These can leave fibers that may get into the airway and increase the incidence of infection.

Documentation

- Document the date and time that you performed tracheostomy care.
- Note the color, amount, consistency, and odor of secretions.
- Note the condition of the stoma and skin around the stoma site; note the presence of drainage, redness, or swelling.
- Document respiratory status, including respiratory rate, depth, and pattern; skin color; and breath sounds.
- Note the patient's tolerance of the procedure.
- If problems arose, document any interventions that were necessary.

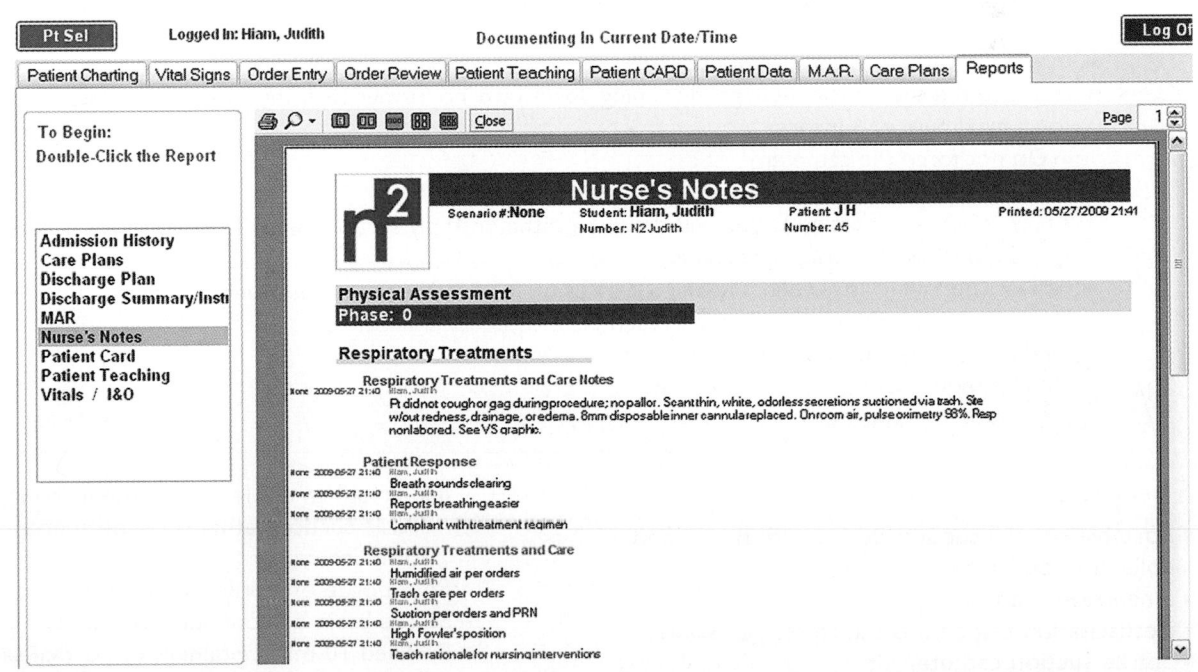

Practice Resources

American Thoracic Society and the Infectious Diseases Society of America (2005); Barnett, M. (2005); Johnston, J., Davis, S., & Sherman, J. (n.d.); Lewarski, J. (2005); Pierson, D., Epstein, S., Durbin, C. Jr., et al. (2005); Siegel, J., Rhinehart, E., Jackson, M., et al. (2007); Tablan, O., Anderson, L., Besser, R., et al. (2004).

(continued on next page)

Procedure 35-6 ■ Performing Tracheostomy Care (continued)

Thinking About the Procedure

 Go to the *Fundamentals of Nursing Skills Videos,* **Oxygenation: Tracheostomy Care (Modified Sterile Technique) – Disposable Inner Cannula, Dressing, & Stabilizer Change; Cleansing the Passy–Muir Valve.**

1. Where does the nurse place the biohazard container?

2. What kind of gloves does the nurse wear to remove the soiled dressing and the Passy-Muir valve?

3. When is the first time the nurse changes her gloves?

 For suggested responses, go to Chapter 35, **Thinking About the Procedure Suggested Responses (Procedure 35-6),** on the Student Resource Disk or DavisPlus at http://davisplus.fadavis.com/Wilkinson2

Procedure 35-7   Performing Tracheostomy or Endotracheal Suctioning (Open System)

➤ For steps to follow in *all* procedures, refer to the Universal Steps for All Procedures found on the inside back cover of Volume 2.

Critical Aspects

- Suction only when necessary.
- Use a suction catheter that is no more than half the internal diameter of the airway tube.
- Position the patient in semi-Fowler's position.
- Adjust the suction regulator according to agency policy, using the lowest possible suction pressure.
  Adults: 100 to 150 mm Hg
  Children: 100 to 120 mm Hg
  Infants: 50 to 95 mm Hg
- Don sterile gloves. (Dominant hand is sterile; nondominant is unsterile.)
- Using your dominant hand, attach the suction catheter to the connecting tubing.
- Hyperoxygenate the patient.
- Insert the catheter gently, without suction.
- Advance the suction catheter, gently aiming downward, no further than the carina tracheae
  (or a maximum of 6 inches).
  - Do not force the catheter.
  - Do not apply suction as you enter the airway.
- Apply continuous suction as you withdraw the catheter. Apply suction for no longer than 15 seconds.
- Avoid saline lavage during suctioning.
- Repeat suctioning as needed, allowing intervals of at least 30 seconds between suctioning.
  Hyperoxygenate the patient between each pass.
- Replace the oxygen source when finished.
- Provide mouth care.
- Reposition the patient.

Equipment

- Portable or wall suction device with tubing and a collection canister
- Linen-saver pad or towel
- Resuscitation bag connected to oxygen source
- Sterile suction catheter kit:
  Adults: 12 to 18 Fr
  Children: 8 to 10 Fr
  Infants: 5 to 8 F

If a kit isn't available, collect the following: sterile gloves, sterile suction catheter of the appropriate size, and a sterile container.
- Pour-bottle of sterile, normal saline solution
- Sterile basin or container for fluids
- Prefilled 10-mL containers of normal saline solution
- Face shield or goggles
- Sterile gloves (or procedure gloves; follow agency policy)
- Protective gown

Delegation

Typically you should not delegate tracheostomy or endotracheal suctioning to an LPN or NAP, because both procedures require professional-level theoretical knowledge, assessment skills, and problem solving ability. However, if the patient has a permanent tracheostomy tube in place and the patient will require long-term care, care can be delegated to trained personnel. Refer to individual state board of nursing for rules on delegating this procedure.

Pre-Procedure Assessment

■ Assess the patient's respiratory status, including respiratory rate, depth, and rhythm; breath sounds; color; and pulse oximetry results.

■ Assess for signs that indicate the need for suctioning: restlessness, cyanosis, labored respirations, decreased oxygen saturation, increased heart and respiratory rates, visible secretions in the airway, increased peak airway pressures on the ventilator, decreasing Sao_2 or PaO_2, and the presence of adventitious breath sounds during auscultation.
These assessments help determine whether the patient requires suctioning. Suctioning should be performed only when necessary to prevent unnecessary oxygen desaturation and tissue trauma.

> When performing the procedure, always identify your patient according to agency policy and be attentive to standard precautions, hand hygiene, patient safety and privacy, body mechanics, and documentation.

Procedure Steps

1. Position the patient in semi-Fowler's position, unless contraindicated.
Promotes lung expansion and oxygenation.

2. Place the linen-saver pad or towel on the patient's chest.
Prevents soiling of the patient's gown during suctioning.

3. Put on a face shield or goggles and a gown.
Protects you from contamination with secretions that may splash during suctioning.

4. Turn on the wall suction or portable suction machine, and adjust the pressure regulator according to agency policy, using the lowest possible suction pressure. Typically, this is:
  Adults: 100 to 150 mm Hg
  Children: 100 to 120 mm Hg
  Infants: 50 to 95 mm Hg
Choosing the appropriate pressure prevents tissue trauma and ensures successful suctioning. Higher pressures are associated with hypoxemia, tissue trauma, and atelectasis, yet do not improve removal of secretions

5. Don a nonsterile glove and face shield or goggles. Test the suction equipment by occluding the connection tubing. Remove and discard the glove. Perform hand hygiene.
Ensures proper functioning before you insert suction catheter.

6. Open the suction catheter kit or (if a kit isn't available) the gathered equipment.
Sterile technique is necessary to avoid contaminating the upper airway when you introduce the suction catheter.

7. Pour sterile saline into the sterile container, using your nondominant hand.
Sterile saline is used to clear the suction catheter of secretions after suctioning.

8. Don sterile gloves; consider your dominant hand sterile and your nondominant hand nonsterile.
Keeping your dominant hand sterile prevents contamination of the suction catheter.

Step 8 Variation. Modified Sterile Procedure

  a. Some guidelines allow for clean procedure gloves; follow agency policy. Consider your dominant hand clean and your nondominant hand contaminated.

9. Pick up the suction catheter with your dominant hand, and attach it to the connection tubing. Do not touch the connection tubing with your sterile glove.
Prepares the suction catheter for use.

10. Put the tip of the suction catheter into the sterile container of normal saline solution, and suction a small amount of normal saline solution through the suction catheter. Apply

suction by placing a finger over the suction control port of the suction catheter.
Lubricates the catheter and helps ensure that the suction equipment is functioning properly.

11. If the patient is receiving oxygen, hyperoxygenate the patient according to agency policy. If the patient does not require oxygen, you do not need to hyperoxygenate.
Helps prevent hypoxia and related complications (cardiac arrhythmias, seizures, arrest) during suctioning. Suctioning clears secretions, but it also removes oxygen from airways.

Step 11 Variation. Patient Requiring Mechanical Ventilation

  a. Press the 100% O_2 button on the ventilator. Some agencies require the nurse to manually hyperoxygenate the patient; follow agency policy.
Ventilators typically have a button that allows you to hyperoxygenate the patient for a total of 2 minutes. Once this time period elapses, the ventilator automatically resumes its previous settings.

Step 11 Variation. Patient Not Requiring Mechanical Ventilation

  b. You will require the assistance of a second provider so that you can maintain sterile technique while suctioning.
  c. Have your partner attach the resuscitation bag to the
(continued on next page)

Procedure 35-7 ■ Performing Tracheostomy or Endotracheal Suctioning (Open System) (continued)

tracheostomy or endotracheal tube, and hyperoxygenate the patient by compressing the resuscitation bag three to five times as the patient inhales. Remove the resuscitation bag, and place it next to the patient when you are finished.
You must perform hyperoxygenation manually if the patient does not require mechanical ventilation. ▼

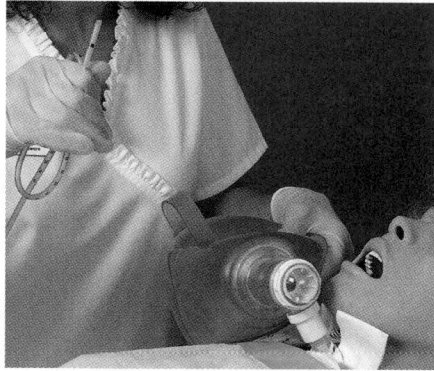

12. Perform suctioning.
a. Lubricate the suction catheter tip with the normal saline solution.
Lubrication eases passage of the suction catheter through the endotracheal tube or tracheostomy tube.

b. Using your dominant hand, gently but quickly insert the suction catheter into the endotracheal tube or tracheostomy tube. ▼

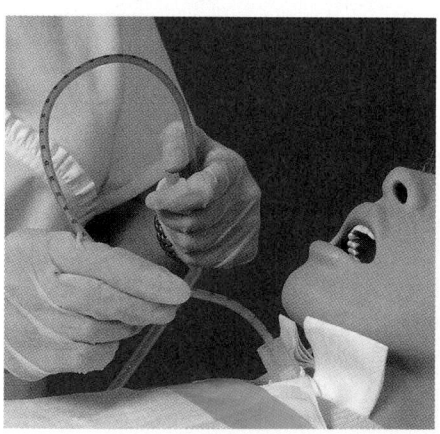

◆ c. Advance the suction catheter, with suction off, gently aiming downward, and being careful not to force the catheter. Insert to the premeasured length: no farther than the **carina tracheae** (the ridge at the lower end of the trachea that separates the openings of the two mainstem bronchi); do not insert more than 6 inches (15 cm).
Premeasure the catheter insertion distance for 0.5 to 1 cm (¼ to ½ in.) past the distal end of the endotracheal tube (ETT); the ETT normally sits between 3 and 7 cm (1 to 2¾ in.) above the carina. Forcing the catheter during insertion may cause tissue trauma.

d. Apply suction while you withdraw the catheter; rotate the catheter (roll it between your thumb and forefinger) as you remove it. Make sure to apply suction for no longer than 15 seconds.
Applying suction for longer than 15 seconds causes hypoxia and may cause tissue trauma.

13. Repeat suctioning as needed.
Several passes with the suction catheter may be needed to clear the airway of secretions.

a. Allow at least 30-second intervals between suctioning.
b. Make sure to hyperoxygenate the patient between each pass.
c. Limit total suctioning time to 5 minutes.

14. Replace the oxygen source, if it was removed during suctioning.
The oxygen source must be replaced to prevent hypoxia.

15. Coil the suction catheter in your dominant hand (alternatively, wrap it around your dominant hand). Pull the sterile glove off over the coiled catheter. Discard the glove containing

the catheter in a fluid-resistant receptacle designated by your agency.
Coiling the catheter inside the glove prevents contaminating the environment with secretions.

16. Don clean procedure gloves and provide mouth care.
Clears the mouth of secretions and bacteria, which place the patient at risk for hospital-acquired pneumonia.

17. Using your nondominant hand, clear the connecting tubing of secretions by placing the tip into the container of sterile saline.
Prepares the tubing for later reuse.

18. Turn off the oxygen and suction units.

19. Reposition the patient.
Repositioning promotes comfort and prevents skin breakdown.

What if . . .

■ **The patient has a cuffed tracheostomy tube?**

Check to see that it is properly inflated before suctioning. Usually this is 20 to 25 mm Hg or less, but follow the manufacturer's instructions and use a cuff manometer. See Clinical Insight 35-5 to learn how to check cuff inflation.

Evaluation

- Assess the color, amount, and consistency of secretions.
- Evaluate the patient's tolerance of the procedure. Note whether there were signs of respiratory distress during the procedure.
- Evaluate the effectiveness of the procedure by comparing breath sounds, vital signs, and pulse oximetry before and after suctioning.

Patient Teaching

- Teach the patient and caregiver how to perform suctioning if the patient will be discharged with an artificial airway. Make sure they can successfully provide a return demonstration.
- Teach the caregiver strategies for managing the patient's airway at home.

Home Care

- Instruct the family and caregiver where to obtain suction equipment.

- Provide contact information of healthcare personnel who can be reached for advice or emergencies.
- Provide information about home oxygen therapy.
- Guidelines recommend clean technique for home care, and for repeated catheter use as long as the catheter is still clear.
- Teach the family and caregiver how to clean catheters for reuse (soak in hot, soapy water; rinse inside and out with clean water; air dry; store in a dry container).

Documentation

- Document the date, time, and reason you performed suctioning.
- Note the size of the suction catheter you used.
- Note the amount, color, consistency, and odor of secretions.
- Document the patient's respiratory status before and after the procedure.
- Document the patient's tolerance of the procedure.
- Document any complications that occurred as a result of the procedure, and document interventions you made in response.

Sample documentation:

Note: Because this isn't the entire computer screen, the image may not show all the information you would need to record about the patient.

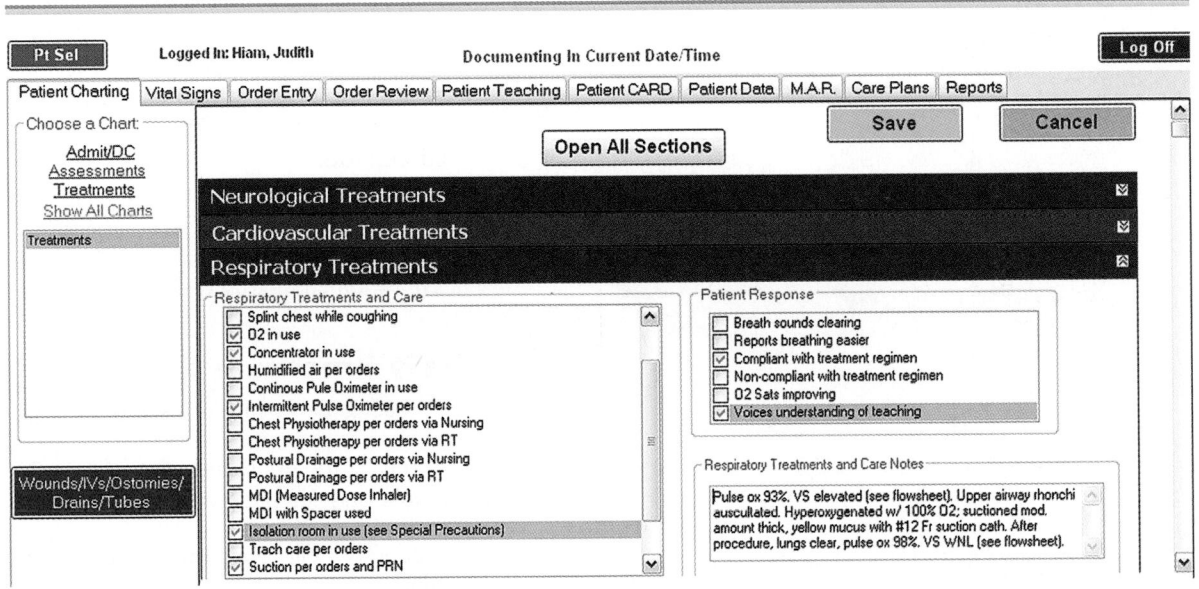

Practice Resources

Johnston, J., Davis, S., & Sherman, J. (n.d.); Kuriakose, A. (2008); Morrow, B., & Argent, A. (2008); Rauen, C., Chulay, M., Bridges, E., et al. (2008); Tablan, O., Anderson, L., Besser, R., et al. (2004); Thompson, L. (2000).

Thinking About the Procedure

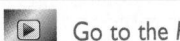 Go to the *Fundamentals of Nursing Skills Videos,* **Oxygenation: Suctioning: Tracheostomy, Open System.**

1. What personal protective equipment did this nurse use?

2. What did the nurse do right after she donned the one clean procedure glove?

3. Did the nurse wear gloves to pour the sterile saline into the sterile container? Why (or why not?)

 For suggested responses, go to Chapter 35, **Thinking About the Procedure Suggested Responses (Procedure 35-7),** on the Student Resource Disk or DavisPlus at http://davisplus.fadavis.com/Wilkinson2

Procedure 35-8 ☐ Performing Tracheostomy or Endotracheal Suctioning (Inline Closed System)

➤ For steps to follow in *all* procedures, refer to the Universal Steps for All Procedures found on the inside back cover of Volume 2.

Critical Aspects

- Position the patient in semi-Fowler's position unless contraindicated.
- Adjust suction regulator according to guidelines or agency policy.
- Hyperoxygenate the patient according to agency policy.
- Insert the suction catheter gently, with suction off.
- Advance the suction catheter gently, aiming downward, no further than the carina trachea (premeasure). Do not force the catheter.
- Do not apply suction as you enter the airway.
- Apply continuous suction as you withdraw the catheter, but for no longer than 15 seconds.
- Avoid saline lavage during suctioning.
- Repeat suctioning as needed, allowing intervals of at least 30 seconds between suctioning. Make sure to hyperoxygenate the patient between each pass.
- Withdraw the suction catheter completely into the sleeve, until you see the indicator line.
- Use normal saline to clear secretions from the catheter.
- Lock the suction regulator port.
- Provide mouth care.
- Reposition the patient.

Equipment

For the once-a-day steps:
- Procedure gloves
- Inline suction catheter

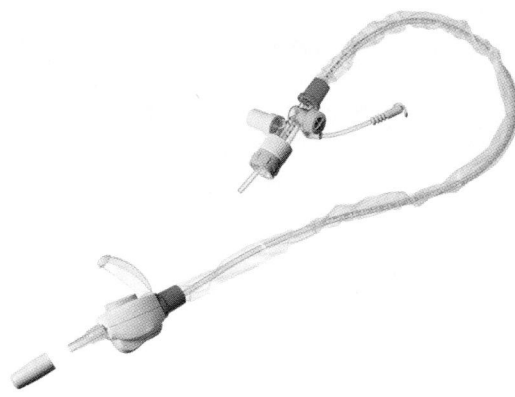

When suctioning:
- Sterile normal saline

Delegation

Typically you should not delegate tracheostomy or endotracheal suctioning to an LPN or NAP, because both procedures require professional-level theoretical knowledge, assessment skills, and problem solving ability. Refer to the individual state board of nursing for rules on delegating this procedure.

Pre-Procedure Assessment

- Assess respiratory status, including respiratory rate, depth, and rhythm; breath sounds; color; and pulse oximetry results.

- Assess for signs that indicate the need for suctioning: restlessness, cyanosis, labored respirations, decreased oxygen saturation, increased heart and respiratory rates, visible secretions in the airway, and the presence of adventitious breath sounds during auscultation.

These assessments help determine whether the patient requires suctioning. Suctioning should be performed only when necessary to prevent unnecessary oxygen desaturation and tissue trauma.

Daily Procedure Steps

You need to perform these steps only once per day:

1. Prepare the equipment. An inline suction unit is available only for patients using a mechanical ventilator.

2. Open the inline suction catheter package, using sterile technique.

3. Remove the adapter on the ventilator tubing.

4. Attach the inline suction catheter equipment to the ventilator tubing.

5. Reconnect the adapter on the ventilator tubing.

6. Attach the other end of the inline suction catheter to the connection tubing placed to suction.

➤ When performing the procedure, always identify your patient according to agency policy and be attentive to standard precautions, hand hygiene, patient safety and privacy, body mechanics, and documentation.

Suctioning Procedure Steps

1. Place the patient in semi-Fowler's position, unless contraindicated, and don clean procedure gloves. Place a linen-saver pad or towel on the patient's chest.
The suction catheter is contained within a sterile unit. You do not need to wear sterile gloves.

2. If a lock is present on the suction control port, unlock it.

3. Turn on the wall suction or portable suction machine, and adjust the pressure regulator according to agency policy or provider's prescription.
Choosing the appropriate pressure prevents tissue trauma and ensures successful suctioning.

4. Pick up the catheter with your dominant hand and use your nondominant hand for the suction port.
Using the dominant hand improves dexterity.

5. Unlock the inline catheter and gently insert the suction catheter into the airway by maneuvering the catheter within the sterile sleeve. ▼

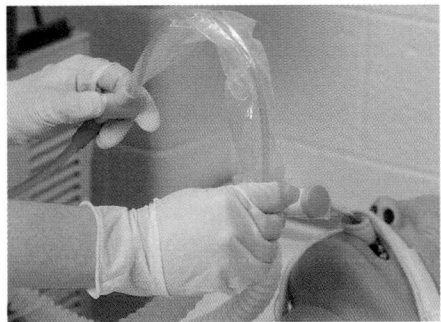

6. Advance the suction catheter into the airway, being careful not to force the catheter. Ask the patient to take slow, deep breaths if she can cooperate. Advance the catheter to the predetermined and premarked distance. Do not apply suction while advancing.
Forcing the catheter during insertion may cause airway trauma.

7. Apply suction by depressing the button over the suction control port as you withdraw the catheter. Make sure to apply suction for no longer than 15 seconds.
Applying suction for longer than 15 seconds causes hypoxia and may cause tissue trauma.

8. Withdraw the inline suction catheter completely into the sleeve. The indicator line on the catheter should appear through the sleeve.
The indicator line is a safety mechanism designed to make sure the suction catheter is withdrawn completely to prevent airway obstruction.

9. Attach the prefilled, 10-mL container of normal saline solution to the saline port located on the inline equipment.
Provides a flush solution to clear the suction catheter of secretions.

10. Squeeze the 10-mL container of normal saline solution while applying suction.
Clears the catheter of secretions, preparing the catheter for repeat use. If

allowed to remain in the catheter or suction line, secretions may dry and harden, reducing line suction efficiency.

11. Lock the suction regulator port.
Prevents you from inadvertently applying suction.

What if . . .

■ **The patient experiences a dysrhythmia?**

Abort the procedure and hyperoxygenate the patient. If a further attempt at suctioning promotes a dysrhythmia, notify the medical care provider.

For Evaluation, Patient Teaching, and Documentation, see Procedure 35-7. Typically, you would not be doing inline suctioning in the home.

Practice Resources
Kuriakose, A. (2008); Morrow, B., & Argent, A. (2008); National Institutes of Health (2000).

Procedure 35-9   Performing Orotracheal and Nasotracheal Suctioning (Open System)

➤ For steps to follow in *all* procedures, refer to the Universal Steps for All Procedures found on the inside back cover of Volume 2.

Critical Aspects

■ Position the patient in semi-Fowler's position.
■ Adjust suction pressure according to guidelines or agency policy (typically 100 to 150 mm Hg for adults, 100 to 120 mm Hg for children, 80 to 100 mm Hg for infants, and 60 to 80 mm Hg for neonates).
■ Prepare the suction equipment. For the nasotracheal (NT) approach, open the water-soluble lubricant.
■ Don sterile glove(s).

(continued on next page)

Procedure 35-9 ■ **Performing Orotracheal and Nasotracheal Suctioning (Open System)** (continued)

- Use protective eye equipment and gown.
- Pick up the suction catheter with your dominant hand, and attach it to the connection tubing.
- Approximate the depth the suction catheter should be inserted.
- Preoxygenate, if indicated.
- Lubricate (for NT approach) and insert the catheter, and advance it to the pharynx as the patient inhales.
- Advance the catheter from pharynx to the trachea by advancing it to the trachea when the patient inhales.
- Apply suction (no longer than 15 seconds) while you withdraw the catheter, using a continuous rotating motion.
- Withdraw the catheter and clear it with sterile saline.
- Repeat lubrication and suctioning as needed, allowing intervals of at least 30 seconds between suctioning.
- Replace the oxygen source.
- Coil the suction catheter in your dominant hand. Pull the sterile glove off over the coiled catheter. Discard in a biohazard receptacle.
- Make sure new suction supplies are readily available for future suctioning.
- Provide mouth care.

Equipment

- Portable or wall suction device with connection tubing and a collection canister
- Linen-saver pad or towel
- Sterile, flexible, multiple-eyed suction catheter kit (12 to 18 Fr for adults, 8 to 10 Fr for children, and 5 to 8 Fr for infants). If a kit isn't available, collect the following: sterile gloves, sterile suction catheter of the appropriate size, and a sterile container
- Sterile gloves
- Pour-bottle of sterile water or normal saline solution
- Sterile basin or other container for fluids
- Face shield or goggles and gown
- Water-soluble lubricant for NT suctioning
- Sputum trap, if a specimen is needed
- Nasopharyngeal airway when frequent NT suctioning is required
- Resuscitation bag with mask

Delegation

You should not delegate orotracheal and nasotracheal suctioning to an LPN or NAP, because these procedures require theoretical knowledge, assessment skills, and problem-solving ability.

Pre-Procedure Assessment

- Assess respiratory status, including respiratory rate, depth, and rhythm; breath sounds; skin color; and pulse oximetry results.
- Assess for signs that indicate the need for suctioning: gurgling sounds during respiration, restlessness, labored respirations, decreased oxygen saturation, increased heart and respiratory rates, and the presence of adventitious breath sounds during auscultation.

The preceding assessments help determine whether the patient requires suctioning. Suctioning removes oxygen from airways an can cause tissue trauma. It should be done only when essential (i.e., only when less invasive techniques have proved unsuccessful and when the secretions are causing physiological deterioration and/or distress).

- Assess the effectiveness of the cough.

➤ When performing the procedure, always identify your patient according to agency policy and be attentive to standard precautions, hand hygiene, patient safety and privacy, body mechanics, and documentation.

Procedure Steps

1. Position the patient.

Step 1 Variation. Orotracheal Suctioning

a. Position the patient in semi-Fowler's position, with the head turned to face you.

Step 1 Variation. Nasotracheal Suctioning

b. Position the patient in semi-Fowler's position, with his neck hyperextended, unless contraindicated.

Hyperextending the neck makes it easier to insert the suction catheter.

Upright position helps to prevent back strain.

2. Place the linen-saver pad or towel on the patient's chest.

Prevents soiling of the patient's gown during suctioning.

3. Put on a face shield or goggles and gown.

Protects you from contamination with secretions that may splash during suctioning.

4. Turn on the wall suction or portable suction machine, and adjust the pressure regulator according to agency policy. Guidelines from American Association for Respiratory Care (AARC) specify:

Adults: 100 to 150 mm Hg
Children: 100 to 120 mm Hg
Infants: 80 to 100 mm Hg
Neonates: 60 to 80 mm Hg

The suction regulator must be set appropriately to prevent tissue trauma and hypoxia and yet remove secretions effectively.

5. Don a procedure glove and test the suction equipment by occluding the connection tubing. Discard the glove and perform hand hygiene.
Testing the equipment ensures proper functioning before you insert the catheter in the patient's airway.

6. Open the suction catheter kit or, if a kit isn't available, the gathered equipment.

Nasal approach: If you are using the nasal approach, open the water-soluble lubricant and, preferably, a nasopharyngeal airway.

7. Don sterile gloves. Alternatively, put a sterile glove on your dominant hand and a clean procedure glove on your nondominant hand. Consider your dominant hand sterile and your nondominant hand nonsterile.
Keeping the dominant hand sterile prevents contaminating the upper airways with a nonsterile suction catheter. This is a modified sterile suction technique because the catheter enters the trachea via nose or the mouth—which are not sterile. However, take care to keep the catheter free from other contaminants.

8. Pour sterile saline into the sterile container, using your nondominant hand.
Sterile saline will be used to clear the suction catheter of secretions after suctioning.

9. Pick up the suction catheter with your dominant hand, and attach it to

the connection tubing, maintaining sterility of your hand and the catheter.
Prepares the suction catheter for use.

10. Put the tip of the suction catheter into the sterile container of normal saline solution, and suction a small amount of normal saline solution through the suction catheter. Apply suction by placing a finger over the suction control port of the suction catheter.
Lubricates the catheter and helps ensure that the suction equipment is functioning properly.

11. Ask the patient to take several slow, deep breaths.
Taking several slow deep breaths promotes relaxation and helps hyperoxygenate the patient before suctioning.

12. Using your nondominant hand, remove the oxygen delivery device, if present.

Step 12 Variation. Oral Approach, Patient Receiving Nasal Oxygen
a. If the patient is receiving nasal oxygen and you are doing orotracheal suctioning, you do not need to remove the oxygen source.

Step 12 Variation. Nasal Approach, Patient Receiving Nasal Oxygen
b. Remove the nasal oxygen and place the nasal cannula in the patient's mouth. See Procedure 35-5.
Placing the cannula in the patient's mouth makes it easier to access the nares for suctioning while still delivery oxygen to the patient (orally).

13. Premeasure to approximate the depth you should insert the suction catheter. For adults, insert the catheter about 15 cm (6 in.) for an oral approach and 20 cm (8 in.) for a nasal approach. Be careful not to contaminate the catheter while you measure.
Inserting the suction catheter the proper distance prevents trauma at the carina and ensures suctioning of the full length of the trachea.

Step 13 Variation. Oral Approach
a. Measure the distance between the edge of the patient's mouth to the tip of the ear lobe and down to the bottom of the neck. ▼

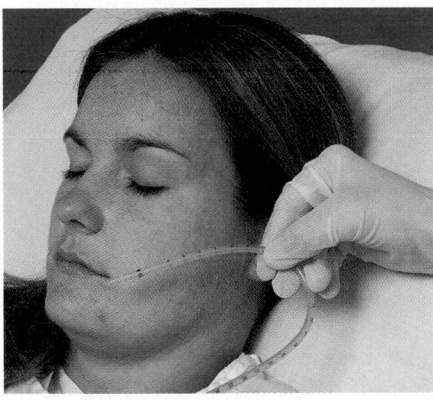

Step 13 Variation. Nasal Approach
b. Measure the distance from the tip of the nose to the tip of the ear lobe and down to the bottom of the neck.

14. Lubricate and insert the suction catheter.
Lubrication makes it easier to pass a suction catheter through the nares.

Step 14 Variation. Orotracheal Suctioning
a. Lubricate the suction catheter tip with normal saline solution.
b. Using your dominant hand, gently but quickly insert the suction catheter along the side of the patient's mouth into the oropharynx.
Quick insertion along the side of the mouth prevents gagging.

c. When the patient inhales, advance the suction catheter to the predetermined distance, being careful not to force the catheter.
Advancing the suction catheter when the patient inhales ensures that the catheter enters the trachea rather than the esophagus. Forcing the catheter during insertion may cause tissue trauma.

Step 14 Variation. Nasotracheal Suctioning
d. Lubricate the catheter tip with the water-soluble lubricant.
Water-soluble lubricant is preferred because it will dissolve if it accidentally

(continued on next page)

Procedure 35-9 ■ **Performing Orotracheal and Nasotracheal Suctioning (Open System)** (continued)

enters the lungs, whereas an oil-based lubricant (e.g., petroleum jelly) won't dissolve in the respiratory tract and causes complications if it enters the lungs.

e. Using your dominant hand, gently but quickly insert the suction catheter into the naris and down to the pharynx. When the patient inhales, advance the suction catheter, gently aiming downward to the predetermined distance, being careful not to force the catheter.

Ensures that the catheter enters the trachea. Forcing the catheter during insertion may cause tissue trauma.

15. Place a finger (e.g., your thumb) over the suction control port of the catheter.

✦ Apply suction while you withdraw the catheter, using a continuous rotating motion. Apply suction for no longer than 15 seconds.

Using a continuous rotating motion and suctioning while withdrawing the catheter prevents trauma to any one area of the airway. Limiting suctioning to less than 15 seconds prevents hypoxia. ▼

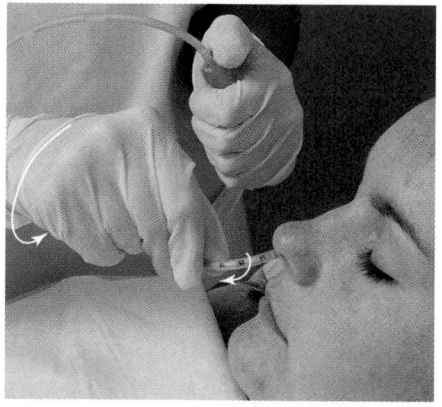

16. After you withdraw the catheter, clear it by placing the tip of the catheter into the container of sterile saline and applying suction.

Ensures patency of the catheter for repeat suctioning. ▼

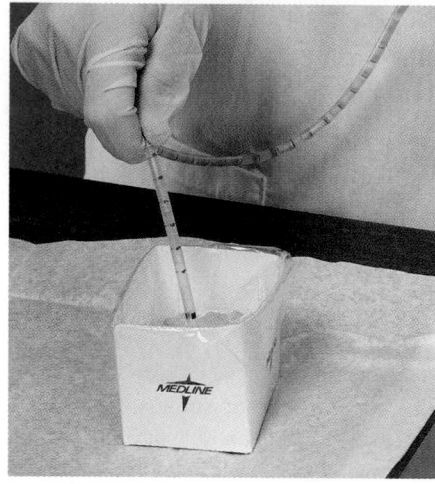

17. Lubricate the catheter, and repeat suctioning as needed, allowing intervals of at least 30 seconds between suctioning. Reapply oxygen between suctioning efforts, if required. Several passes with the suction catheter may be needed to clear the airway of secretions. Total suctioning time should be limited to 5 minutes, however, to prevent trauma and hypoxia.

18. Replace the oxygen source.
Prevents hypoxia.

19. Coil the suction catheter in your dominant hand (alternatively, wrap it around your dominant hand). Hold the catheter while you pull the sterile glove off over it. Discard the glove containing the catheter in a biohazard receptacle (e.g., bag) designated by your agency.

Coiling the catheter inside the glove and using a biohazard receptacle prevent contaminating the environment with secretions.

20. Using your nondominant hand, clear the connecting tubing of secretions by placing the tip into the container of sterile saline.
Ensures patency and prepares the equipment for future use.

21. Dispose of equipment, and make sure new suction supplies are readily available for future suctioning.
The patient may require suctioning at any time, so equipment must be readily available.

22. Provide mouth care.
Promotes patient comfort and clears the mouth of any secretions the patient may have expectorated.

23. Position the patient in a comfortable position, and allow him to rest.
Comfort and rest help the patient recover from the stress of suctioning.

What if . . .

■ **The patient's oxygen saturation is less than 94%, or if he is in any distress?**

Administer supplemental oxygen before, during, and after suctioning. Notify the patient's primary provider if the patient does not respond to additional oxygen.

Evaluation

■ Assess the color, consistency, and amount of secretions.
■ Evaluate the patient's tolerance of the procedure. Note whether there were signs of respiratory distress during the procedure.
■ Evaluate the effectiveness of the procedure by comparing breath sounds, vital signs, and pulse oximetry or blood gas data before and after the procedure.

Patient Teaching

■ Explain the importance of administering supplemental oxygen or of taking several deep breaths before suctioning.

- Inform the patient that coughing typically increases with suctioning.
- Demonstrate orotracheal or nasotracheal suctioning to the caregiver, and ask for a return demonstration if suctioning will be required at home.

Home Care

- Instruct the family and caregiver about where to obtain suction equipment.
- Provide the client and caregiver with contact information of healthcare personnel who can be reached for advice or emergencies.
- Explain that the procedure can be performed using clean technique instead of sterile technique in the home.
- Instruct the caregiver that suction catheters can be cleaned for reuse by washing them with soapy water and then boiling them for 10 minutes. After they are cleaned, rinse the catheters with normal saline solution or tap water.
- Change the secretion collection container every 24 hours, or clean it according to home care agency guidelines every 24 hours.

Documentation

- Document the date, time, and reason you performed suctioning.
- Note the suction technique you used and the catheter size.
- Note the color, consistency, and odor of secretions.
- Document the patient's respiratory status before and after the procedure.
- Document the patient's tolerance of the procedure and any complications that occurred as a result of the procedure.
- Document any interventions you performed to address complications that occurred.

Sample EHR documentation:

Note: Because this isn't the entire computer screen, the image may not show all the information you would need to record about the patient.

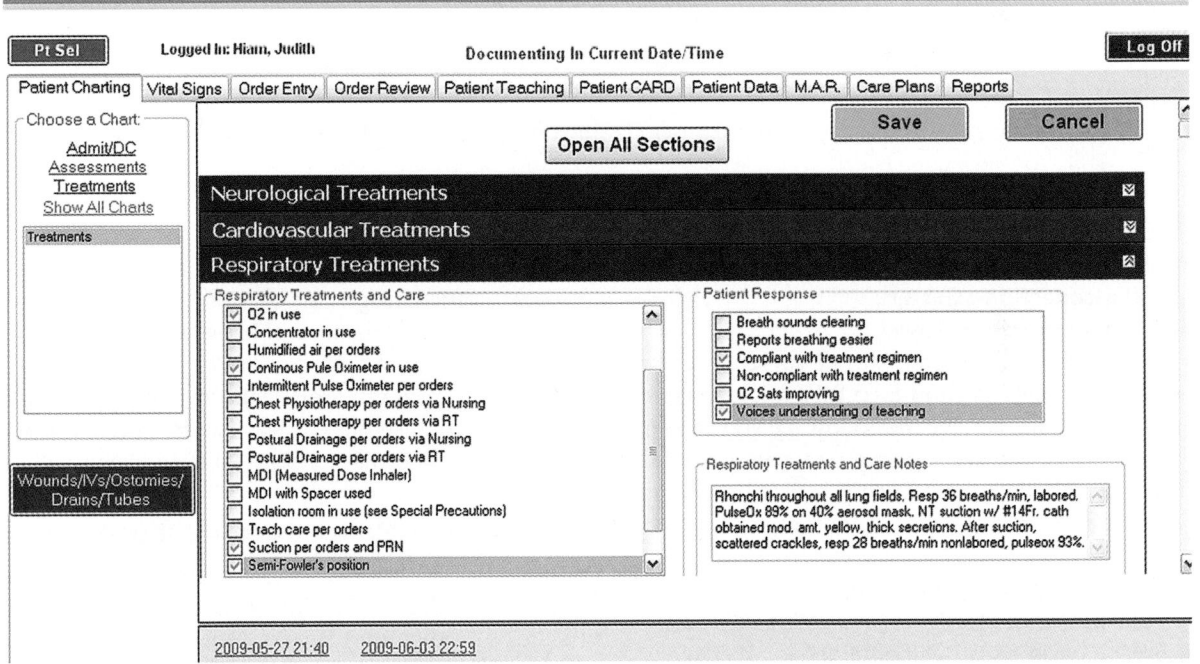

Practice Resources

American Association for Respiratory Care (2004a); American Thoracic Society and the Infectious Diseases Society of America (2005); Centers for Disease Control and Prevention (2004).

Thinking About the Procedure

 Go to the *Fundamentals of Nursing Skills Videos*, **Oxygenation: Suctioning, Inline Closed System.**

1. This procedure in your text describes oro- and nasotracheal suctioning by the open method. The DVD shows orotracheal suctioning using the closed method. Why do you think the closed method was used for this patient?

 For suggested responses, go to Chapter 35, **Thinking About the Procedure Suggested Responses (Procedure 35-9),** on the Student Resource Disk or DavisPlus at http://davisplus.fadavis.com/Wilkinson2

Procedure 35-10   **Performing Upper Airway Suctioning**

➤ For steps to follow in *all* procedures, refer to the Universal Steps for All Procedures found on the inside back cover of Volume 2.

Critical Aspects

- Position the patient in a semi-Fowler's position.
  Oropharyngeal: Patient's face turned toward you
  Nasopharyngeal: Neck hyperextended
- Adjust the suction regulator according to agency policy (typically 100 to 120 mm Hg for adults, 95 to 110 mm Hg for children, and 50 to 95 mm Hg for infants).
- If using the nasal approach, open the water-soluble lubricant.
- Don procedure gloves.
- Using your dominant hand, attach the suction catheter to the connection tubing.
- Approximate the depth the suction catheter should be inserted.
- Remove the oxygen delivery device, if necessary.
- If the oxygen saturation is less than 94%, or if patient is distress, administer supplemental oxygen before, during, and after suctioning.
- Lubricate and insert the suction catheter.
- Gently advance the catheter the premeasured distance into the pharynx.
- Engage the suction and apply it while you withdraw the catheter, using a continuous rotating motion.
- Clear the catheter with sterile saline.
- Lubricate the catheter, and repeat suctioning as needed, allowing 20-second intervals between suctioning.

Note: Upper airway suctioning may be done via the oropharyngeal or nasopharyngeal route. However, nasal suction is usually required to improve oxygenation only in infants because most adult airway obstruction occurs in the mouth and oropharynx.

✚ Vigorous nasal suction can induce epistaxis (nosebleed) and further complicate an already difficult airway.

Equipment

- Portable or wall suction device with connection tubing and a collection canister
- Linen-saver pad or towel
- Sterile suction catheter kit (12 to 18 Fr for adults, 8 to 10 Fr for children, and 5 to 8 Fr for infants). If a kit isn't available, collect the following: sterile suction catheter of the appropriate size, and a sterile container. If you plan to suction both the oropharynx and the nasopharynx, you need a separate sterile catheter for each.
- Yankauer device can be used for oropharyngeal suction.
- Pour-bottle of sterile normal saline solution
- Sterile basin or other container for fluids
- Face shield or goggles and gown
- Procedure gloves
- Water-soluble lubricant for nasopharyngeal suctioning
- Sputum trap, if a specimen is needed
- Biohazard bag

Delegation

Do not delegate oropharyngeal and nasopharyngeal suctioning to an LPN or NAP, because these procedures require theoretical knowledge, assessment skills, and problem-solving ability. However, the NAP (and the client or family) can use a Yankauer tube to suction the oral cavity because there is less risk for trauma to mucosa than with oro- or nasopharyngeal suctioning.

Pre-Procedure Assessment

- Assess respiratory status, including respiratory rate, depth, and rhythm; breath sounds; color; and pulse oximetry results. Note signs that indicate the need for suctioning: restlessness, cyanosis, labored respirations, decreased oxygen saturation, increased heart and respiratory rates, visible secretions in the airway, and the presence of adventitious breath sounds during auscultation.

You must be certain the patient requires suctioning. Suctioning should be performed only when necessary to prevent unnecessary oxygen desaturation and tissue trauma.

➤ When performing the procedure, always identify your patient according to agency policy and be attentive to standard precautions, hand hygiene, patient safety and privacy, body mechanics, and documentation.

➤ *Note:* This procedure describes modified sterile technique: sterile supplies with clean procedure gloves. The patient's oropharynx and nasopharynx are not sterile. However, you should keep the suction catheter free from other contaminants as much as possible. Some facilities do use sterile gloves for this procedure.

Procedure Steps

1. Position the patient. Explain that suctioning may stimulate coughing or gagging, but that coughing helps mobilize secretions.

Step 1 Variation. Oropharyngeal Suctioning

Position the patient in a semi-Fowler's or high Fowler's position, with his head turned toward you.

This position facilitates insertion of the suction catheter and prevents straining your back. It also promotes lung expansion and effective coughing.

Step 1 Variation. Nasopharyngeal Suctioning

Position the patient in semi-Fowler's or high Fowler's position with his neck hyperextended, unless contraindicated.

2. Place the linen-saver pad or towel on the patient's chest.

Prevents soiling of the patient's gown during suctioning.

3. Put on a face shield or goggles and gown.

Protects you from contamination with secretions that may splash during suctioning. Not all guidelines specify wearing a gown for this procedure.

4. Turn on the wall suction or portable suction machine, and adjust the pressure regulator according to agency policy, typically:

    Adults: 100 to 150 mm Hg
    Children: 100 to 120 mm Hg
    Infants: 50 to 95 mm Hg

The suction regulator must be set appropriately to prevent tissue trauma and hypoxia and to function effectively to remove secretions. Higher pressures are associated with hypoxemia, tissue trauma, and atelectasis, yet do not improve removal of secretions.

5. Test the suction equipment by occluding the connection tubing.

Testing the equipment ensures proper functioning before use.

6. Open the suction catheter kit or the gathered equipment. If you are using the nasal approach, open the water-soluble lubricant.

7. Don procedure gloves; consider (and keep) your dominant hand clean; consider your nondominant hand to be contaminated.

This is not a sterile suction procedure but care should be taken to keep the suction catheter free from other contaminants. Keeping the dominant hand clean prevents contaminating the upper airways with an unclean suction catheter.

8. Pour sterile saline into the sterile container, using your nondominant hand.

Sterile saline is necessary to clear the suction catheter of secretions after suctioning. The outside of the saline container is not sterile; it would contaminate your dominant hand.

9. Pick up the suction catheter with your dominant hand, and use your other hand to hold the connection tubing (to suction) while you attach it.

10. Put the tip of the suction catheter into the sterile container of normal saline solution, and suction a small amount of normal saline solution through the suction catheter. Apply suction by placing a finger over the suction control port. When using a Yankauer-type device, the suction is continuous and there is no port to occlude.

Ensures that the suction equipment is functioning properly. If you need to see a Yankauer device,

VOL 1   Go to **Figure 35-14,** in Volume 1.

11. Approximate the depth to which you will insert the suction catheter.

Step 11 Variation. Oropharyngeal Suctioning

Measure the distance between the edge of the patient's mouth and the tip of the patient's ear lobe.

Determines the proper distance you should insert the suction catheter for oropharyngeal suctioning.

Step 11 Variation. Nasopharyngeal Suctioning

Measure the distance between the tip of the patient's nose and the tip of the patient's ear lobe.

Helps determine the correct distance you should insert the suction catheter for nasopharyngeal suctioning.

12. Using your nondominant hand, remove the oxygen delivery device, if present. Have the patient take several slow, deep breaths. You do not need to remove the oxygen delivery device if the patient is on nasal oxygen and you are suctioning the oropharynx. Deep breathing helps to hyperoxygenate the patient and helps prevent hypoxia during suctioning.

13. Lubricate and insert the suction catheter.

Step 13 Variation. Oropharyngeal Suctioning

    a. Lubricate the catheter tip with the normal saline solution.
    b. Using your dominant hand, gently but quickly insert the suction catheter along the side of the patient's mouth into the oropharynx.

Inserting the suction catheter along the side of the mouth prevents gagging. ▼

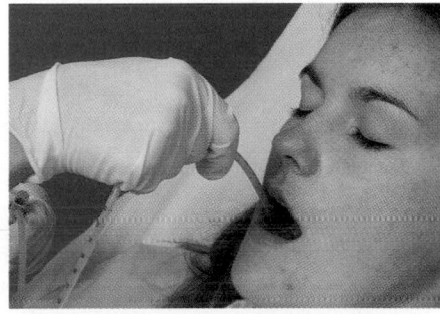

    c. Advance the suction catheter quickly to the premeasured distance—usually 7.5 to 10 cm (3 to 4 in.) in the adult—being careful not to force the catheter.

(continued on next page)

Procedure 35-10 ■ **Performing Upper Airway Suctioning** (continued)

Ensures that the suction catheter will reach the pharynx. Forcing the catheter during insertion may cause tissue trauma.

Step 13 Variation.
Nasopharyngeal Suctioning

d. Lubricate the catheter tip with the water-soluble lubricant.

Eases passage of the suction catheter through the naris. Water-soluble lubricant is preferred because it will dissolve if it accidentally enters the lungs, whereas an oil-based lubricant (e.g., petroleum jelly or lotion) will not dissolve in the respiratory tract and causes complications if it enters the lungs.

e. Using your dominant hand, gently but quickly insert the suction catheter into the naris.

Prevents trauma to the naris. ▼

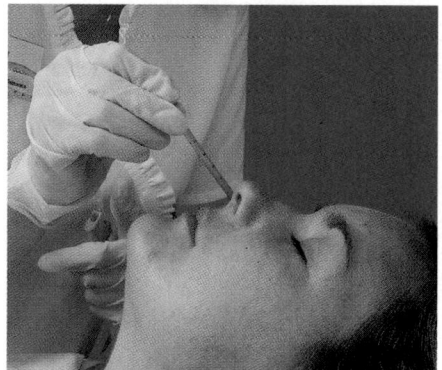

f. Advance the suction catheter, aiming downward to the premeasured distance—usually 13 to 15 cm (5 to 6 in.) in the adult—and being careful not to force the catheter. If you meet resistance, you may need to try the other naris.

Advancing the suction catheter the premeasured distance ensures that the

suction catheter will reach the pharynx. Forcing the catheter during insertion may cause tissue trauma.

14. Place a finger (e.g., your thumb) over the suction control port of the suction catheter, and start suctioning the patient. Apply suction while you withdraw the catheter, using a continuous rotating motion.

◆ Limit suctioning to 10 to 15 seconds.
Using a continuous rotating motion while withdrawing the catheter prevents trauma to any one area of the airway. Limiting suctioning to less than 10 to 15 seconds prevents hypoxia.

15. After you withdraw the catheter, clear it by placing the tip of the catheter into the container of sterile saline and applying suction.
Ensures patency of the catheter for repeat suctioning.

16. Lubricate the catheter, and repeat suctioning as needed, allowing at least 20-second intervals between suctioning.
Several passes with the suction catheter may be needed to clear the airway of secretions. The total suctioning time should be limited to 5 minutes, however, to prevent hypoxia and trauma to the mucosal membranes.

Step 16 Variation.
Nasopharyngeal Suctioning
Each time you repeat suction, alternate nares.
Alternating nares prevents trauma that would occur if you used only one naris.

17. Coil the suction catheter in your dominant hand. Pull the sterile glove off over the coiled catheter. (Alternatively, wrap the catheter

around your dominant, gloved hand, and hold the catheter as you remove the glove over it.) Discard the glove containing the catheter in a biohazard receptacle designated by your agency.
Coiling the catheter inside the glove prevents contamination with secretions.

18. Using your nondominant hand, clear the connecting tubing of secretions by placing the tip into the container of sterile saline.
Ensures patency and prepares the equipment for future use.

19. Dispose of equipment in biohazard waste container/bag, and make sure new suction supplies are readily available for future suctioning needs.
The patient may require suctioning at any time, so equipment must be readily available.

20. Provide mouth care.
Promotes patient comfort and clears the mouth of any secretions the patient may have expectorated.

21. Discard your other glove and remaining supplies.

22. Position the patient in a comfortable position, and allow him to rest.
Promoting comfort and allowing for a period of rest helps the patient recover from suctioning, which may be very tiring.

What if . . .

■ **The patient's oxygen saturation is less than 94%, or if he is in any distress?**
You may need to administer supplemental oxygen before, during, and after suctioning. See Procedure 35-5.

Evaluation

■ Assess the color, consistency, and amount of secretions.
■ Evaluate the patient's tolerance of the procedure. Note whether there were signs of respiratory distress during the procedure.
■ Evaluate the effectiveness of the procedure by comparing breath sounds, vital signs, and pulse oximetry before and after the procedure.

Patient Teaching

■ Explain the importance of administering supplemental oxygen to the patient before suctioning.
■ Inform the patient that coughing typically increases with suctioning.
■ Demonstrate oropharyngeal or nasopharyngeal suctioning to the caregiver, and ask for a return demonstration if suctioning will be required at home.

Home Care

- Instruct the family and caregiver where to obtain suction equipment.
- Provide the client and caregiver with contact information for healthcare personnel who can be reached for advice or emergencies.
- Explain that the procedure can be performed using clean technique instead of sterile technique in the home setting.
- Instruct the caregiver that suction catheters can be cleaned for reuse by washing them with soapy water and then boiling them for 10 minutes. After they are cleaned, rinse the catheters with normal saline solution or tap water.
- Change the secretion collection container every 24 hours, or clean it according to home care agency guidelines every 24 hours.

Documentation

- Document the date, time, and reason you performed suctioning.
- Note the suction technique you used and the catheter size.
- Note color, consistency, and odor of secretions.
- Document the patient's respiratory status before and after the procedure.
- Document the patient's tolerance of the procedure and any complications that occurred as a result of the procedure, with resulting interventions.

Thinking About the Procedure

 Go to the *Fundamentals of Nursing Skills Videos,* **Oxygenation: Suctioning, Nasopharyngeal, Open System.**

1. In what position did the nurse place this patient?

2. What did the nurse use to lubricate the suction catheter?

 For suggested responses, go to Chapter 35, **Thinking About the Procedure Suggested Responses (Procedure 35-10),** on the Student Resource Disk or DavisPlus at http://davisplus.fadavis.com/Wilkinson2

Sample documentation:

> 02/08/12 2100   *Skin closures applied to midline abdominal incision following staple removal. Wound edges are well approximated with no drainage noted. Periwound skin is dry and intact, without erythema, induration, or odor. Wound cleansed with normal saline using sterile technique. Due to the length of the wound and moderate size of the abdominal drape, 1/2 inch X 4 inch skin closures applied without tension. Educated patient on the purpose of the closures and expected outcomes. Will continue to monitor.*
> — *S. Wong, RN*

Practice Resources

Birmingham East and North Primary Care Trust (2006); Centers for Disease Control and Prevention (2004); Roberts, J. (2004); Siegel, J., Rhinehart, E., Jackson, M., et al. (2007); Tablan, O., Anderson, L., Besser, R., et al. (2004); Vandenberg, J., Lutz, R., & Vinson, D. (1999); Vandenberg, J., & Vinson, D. (1999).

Procedure 35-11   Caring for a Patient Requiring Mechanical Ventilation

➤ For steps to follow in *all* procedures, refer to the Universal Steps for All Procedures found on the inside back cover of Volume 2.

Critical Aspects

- Prepare the resuscitation bag; keep it at the bedside.
- Wear protective eye covering and gown.
- Respiratory therapists are responsible for setting up mechanical ventilation in most agencies. If you must assume the responsibility, refer to the manufacturer's instructions.
  1. Verify ventilator settings with the medical prescription.
  2. Make sure the ventilator alarm limits are set appropriately.

(continued on next page)

Procedure 35-11 ■ **Caring for a Patient Requiring Mechanical Ventilation** (continued)

3. Don gloves.

4. Attach the ventilator tubing to the endotracheal tube or tracheostomy tube.

5. Secure the ventilator tubing.

6. Attach capnography device, if available.

7. Prepare the inline suctioning equipment.

After the initial ventilator setup:

- Check arterial blood gases (ABGs) and respiratory status about 30 minutes after setup.
- Maintain the patient in a semirecumbent position (head of bed at 30° to 45°).
- Check the ventilator tubing frequently for condensation.
  - Drain the condensate into a collection device, or briefly disconnect the patient from the ventilator and empty the tubing into a waste receptacle, according to agency policy.
  - Never drain the condensate into the humidifier.
- Provide the patient with an alternative form of communication.
- Check ventilator and humidifier settings regularly.
- Check the inline thermometer.
- Give sedatives or antianxiety drugs as needed.
- Reposition the patient regularly (every 1 to 2 hours), being careful not to pull on the ventilator tubing.
- Moisten the lips with a cool, damp cloth and water-based lubricant.
- Provide frequent antiseptic oral care.
- Ensure that the call light is always within reach, and answer call light and ventilator alarms promptly.
- Monitor the tracheostomy tube for proper cuff inflation.
- Monitor for gastric distention.

Ventilator Terminology

TERM	EXPLANATION
F_{IO_2}	Fraction of inspired oxygen
Modes of ventilation	Describes the setting on the ventilator which assists the patient to breathe. Can be controlled (CMV), intermittent mandatory (IMV), or synchronized intermittent mandatory (SIMV).
Tidal volume	Amount of air delivered from the ventilator with each breath
Assist-control mode—also known as continuous mechanical ventilation (CMV)	The preset number of breaths per minute delivered by the machine. If the patient is able to initiate breaths, the machine will deliver a breath when the patient begins to inspire. If the patient is unable to breathe on his own, the machine will deliver the preset number of breaths in a rhythmic fashion.
Intermittent mandatory ventilation	A ventilator setting that delivers a minimum number of breaths per minute if the patient does not ventilate independently.
Synchronized intermittent mandatory ventilation (SIMV)	A ventilator setting that delivers a minimum number of ventilations per minute if the patient does not ventilate independently. The ventilator breaths are synchronized with the patient's breaths. This mode is used for weaning patients from the ventilator.
Pressure support	Provides positive pressure on inspiration to decrease the workload of breathing.
Continuous positive airway pressure (CPAP)	Provides positive pressure during inspiration and expiration to keep alveoli open in a spontaneously breathing patient.
Positive end expiratory pressure (PEEP)	Provides positive pressure on expiration to keep airways open for patients on CMV or SIMV mode ventilation.

Equipment

- Two oxygen sources
- Air source that provides 50 psi
- Mechanical ventilator
- Resuscitation bag with oxygen connection tubing
- Humidification device
- Ventilator tubing, connectors, and adaptors
- Condensation collection device
- Pulse oximetry device
- Procedure gloves, protective gown, and eye covering
- Sterile gloves, if you will perform suctioning
- Suction equipment (possibly)
- Sterile water for the humidifier
- Inline thermometer

Delegation

Care of a mechanically ventilated patient requires advanced knowledge of pulmonary anatomy and physiology and, therefore, should not be delegated to assistive personnel.

Pre-Procedure Assessment

- Review the patient's health record to make sure that mechanical ventilation is included in the options outlined in his advance directive.

Mechanical ventilation may be a care option that the patient does not wish to pursue. If a patient who does not wish to be ventilated mechanically is currently on a ventilator, consult your hospital ethics committee.

- If the patient's condition allows, assess his understanding of mechanical ventilation therapy.

Understanding helps allay the patient's anxiety and promotes cooperation.

- Assess the patient's respiratory status, including respiratory rate, depth, and rhythm; breath sounds; color; and pulse oximetry results.

Confirms the need for mechanical ventilation.

- Blood will probably be drawn for an ABG analysis

To establish a baseline.

➤ When performing the procedure, always identify your patient according to agency policy and be attentive to standard precautions, hand hygiene, patient safety and privacy, body mechanics, and documentation.

Procedure Steps

Initial Ventilator Setup

1. Prepare the resuscitation bag.

The resuscitation bag should be readily available to provide ventilation in the event of an emergency. ▼

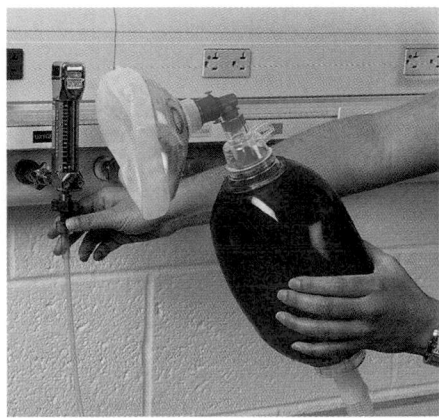

a. Attach a flow meter to one of the oxygen sources.

The flow meter helps regulate oxygen delivery.

b. Attach an adapter to the flow meter, and connect the oxygen tubing to the adapter.
c. Turn on the oxygen, and adjust the flow rate.

The flow meter adjusts the oxygen flow.

2. Respiratory therapists are responsible for setting up mechanical

ventilation in most agencies. If you must assume the responsibility, refer to the manufacturer's instructions.

The respiratory therapist is specially trained to set up mechanical ventilation equipment.

3. Plug the ventilator into a grounded electrical outlet and turn it on.

4. Verify ventilator settings and adjust as medically prescribed.

Ventilator settings must be individualized according to the patient's need for respiratory support. Incorrect settings may cause harm (e.g., hypoxia or barotrauma) to the patient. ▼

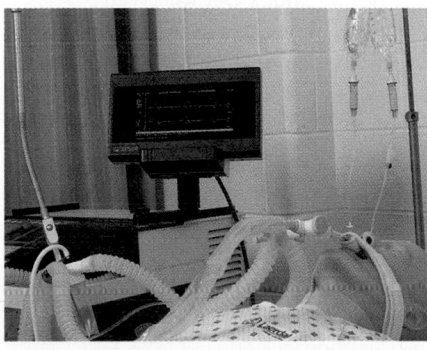

5. Make sure that ventilator alarm limits are set appropriately.

Alarm limits that are not set appropriately could result in harm to the patient.

6. Make sure the humidifier is filled with sterile distilled water.

7. Don gloves, gown, and eye protection if you have not already done so.

8. Attach the ventilator tubing to the endotracheal tube or tracheostomy tube.

9. Place the ventilator tubing in the securing device.

Prevents dislodging the endotracheal tube or tracheostomy when the patient moves.

10. Attach a capnographic device, if available.

To measure levels of carbon dioxide. These data are used to confirm placement of the endotracheal tube and disconnection from or malfunction of the ventilator. Oxygen levels alone are not sufficient for the ventilated patient.

11. Prepare the inline (closed) suction equipment (see Procedure 35-8).

Suctioning equipment should be readily available when the patient requires suctioning. Closed catheters are recommended to prevent ventilator-associated pneumonia.

(continued on next page)

Procedure 35-11 ■ **Caring for a Patient Requiring Mechanical Ventilation** (continued)

After Initial Ventilator Setup

12. Check respiratory status and ABGs again about 30 minutes after setup. Also check whenever there are changes in the ventilator settings and as the patient's condition indicates.
To be certain the patient is being adequately ventilated and not experiencing oxygen toxicity

13. Check the ventilator tubing frequently for condensation. Drain the fluid into a collection device, or briefly disconnect the patient from the ventilator and empty the tubing into a waste receptacle, according to agency policy.

✦ Never drain the fluid into the humidifier.
Condensation in the ventilator tubing can cause resistance to airflow. Moreover, the patient can aspirate it. The fluid should not be drained into the humidifier because the patient's secretions may have contaminated it. ▼

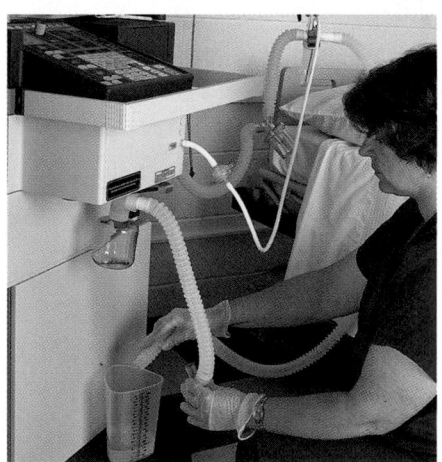

✦ **14.** Maintain the patient in a semirecumbent position (head of bed elevated 30 to 45°). This is extremely important.
To promote lung expansion, reduce gastric reflux, and prevent ventilator-associated pneumonia.

15. Check ventilator and humidifier settings regularly.

16. Check the inline thermometer.
To ensure that the air being delivered to the patient is close to the body temperature to prevent scalding of the mucosal tissue or instead, cooling the patient (core temperature).

17. Provide the patient with an alternative form of communication, such as a letter board or white board.
The patient on a mechanical ventilator is unable to speak, which can produce extreme anxiety. An alternative method of communication must be offered so the patient can express her needs and concerns.

18. Reposition the patient regularly (every 1 to 2 hours), being careful not to pull on the ventilator tubing.
Repositioning protects skin integrity. However, pulling on the tubing creates pain. Patient comfort promotes relaxation, which improves the effectiveness of the ventilator.

19. Keep the patient's lips moistened with a cool, damp cloth and water-based lubricant; and provide regular antiseptic oral care. A recommended regimen includes the following:
■ Brush the teeth twice a day.
■ Use a soft toothbrush.
■ Moisturize oral mucosa and lips every 2 to 4 hours.
■ Use a chlorhexidine gluconate (0.12%) rinse twice a day during the

perioperative period for patients who undergo cardiac surgery (adult patients).
■ Use mouthwash twice a day for adult patients. (AACN, 2007)
Mouth care provides comfort and preserves integrity of the mucous membranes. Patients being mechanically ventilated, even for a short period, are at high risk for developing ventilator-associated pneumonia (VAP). VAP is not uncommon, and it is associated with high mortality rates. This regimen is thought to help prevent VAP.

20. Make sure the call light is always within reach, and answer call light and ventilator alarms promptly.
Provides the patient with immediate access to help if a breathing problem occurs; reassures the patient and thus relieves anxiety.

21. Monitor the tracheostomy tube for proper cuff inflation (usually 20 to 25 mm Hg); see Clinical Insight 35-5.

22. Check for gastric distention and take measures to prevent aspiration.
Aspiration creates high risk for pneumonia.

23. Clean, disinfect, or change ventilator tubing and equipment according to agency policy.
There is not good evidence to indicate how often this should be. Research so far indicates that tubing and equipment should not be routinely changed for infection control purposes.

24. Give sedatives or antianxiety drugs as prescribed.

Evaluation

■ After mechanical ventilation is instituted, assess for chest expansion and auscultate for bilateral breath sounds.
■ Evaluate the patient's tolerance of mechanical ventilation. Verify that the patient is being adequately ventilated and that she is breathing in synchrony with the ventilator.

■ Auscultate breath sounds every 2 to 4 hours, according to agency policy.
■ When monitoring vital signs, count spontaneous breaths as well as those delivered by the ventilator.
■ Monitor continuous pulse oximetry, capnography, and ABGs.

Patient Teaching

- Explain mechanical ventilation to the patient and her family. Include information about the alarms they will hear.
- Demonstrate an alternative form of communication to the patient and family.
- When appropriate, explain the weaning process to the patient and family.
- If the patient requires mechanical ventilation after discharge, make arrangements for a home ventilator, and teach the patient and caregiver how to use it.

Home Care

- Consult with your facility discharge planning program and/or case management for discharge plans.
- Explain to the family and caregiver where to obtain a home ventilator, resuscitation bag, and oxygen equipment and what services are available. Make sure they choose a supplier who has 24-hour emergency services available.
- Help the client and caregiver devise a backup plan for ventilating the client in the event of a power failure.
- Tell the caregiver to notify the utility company and area emergency personnel that the client is being maintained on a ventilator at home.
- Instruct the client and caregiver about oxygen therapy and its use as well as safety measures that they must institute.
- Teach the client and caregiver to clean the ventilator tubing with soap and warm water when it becomes soiled.
- Provide the client and caregiver with contact information of healthcare personnel who can be reached for advice or emergencies.

Documentation

- Document the date and time mechanical ventilation was initiated.
- Note the type of ventilator used and the prescribed settings used.
- Document the client's response to mechanical ventilation, including vital signs, breath sounds, ease of breathing, pulse oximetry, intake and output, skin color, and ABG and chest x-ray results.

Sample documentation:

02/26/11 0800   Patient found difficult to arouse. Dr. Henry made aware. ABG obtained, results included: pH 7.28; PCO_2 78 mm Hg; PO_2 48 mm Hg. Dr. Henry in to evaluate patient, anesthesia called to intubate patient. Patient medicated with Versed 5 mg IV and intubated orally with a 7.5 Fr. ET tube. Patient placed on mechanical ventilator: TV 700 mL; FiO_2 80%, and RR 14. Portable chest x-ray confirms ideal placement of endotracheal tube as well as white-out of both lung fields. Arterial blood gases to be obtained in 30 minutes. Pulse oximetry 90% since being placed on ventilator.
————————————————— L. Biello, RN

Practice Resources

American Association of Critical-Care Nurses (AACN) (2007, 2008a); Bozyk, P., & Hyzy, R. (2008); Coffin, W., Klompas, M., Classen, D., et al. (2008); Munro, C., Grap, M., Jones, D., et al. (2009); Tablan, O., Anderson, L., Besser, R., et al. (2004); Thille, A., Rodriguez, P., Cabello, F., et al. (2006).

Procedure 35-12 ▪ Setting Up Disposable Chest Drainage Systems

➤ For steps to follow in *all* procedures, refer to the Universal Steps for All Procedures found on the inside back cover of Volume 2.

Critical Aspects

- Obtain and prepare the prescribed drainage system.
- Position the patient according to the indicated insertion site.
- Set up the sterile field and supplies you will need for dressing the insertion site.
- Don mask, gown, and sterile gloves.
- As soon as the chest tube is inserted, attach it to the drainage system.
- Turn on the wall (or other) suction source (usually −80 mm H_2O).
- Set the prescribed chest drainage unit (CDU) suction level.
- Don a clean pair of sterile gloves.
- Using sterile technique, wrap petroleum gauze around the chest tube at the insertion site, and dress the site with two precut sterile drain dressings covered by a large drainage dressing (e.g., ABD).
- Apply an occlusive dressing over the insertion site (e.g., with 2-inch silk tape); cover the dressing completely. Date, time, and initial the dressing.

(continued on next page)

Procedure 35-12 ■ **Setting Up Disposable Chest Drainage Systems** (continued)

- Using the spiral taping technique, wrap 1-inch silk tape around the connections. Wrap from top to bottom and bottom to top. (Or use locking connections, if furnished with the CDU.)
- With an 8-inch-long piece of 2-inch tape, secure the top end of the drainage tube to the chest tube dressing.
- Make sure the tubing lies with no kinks and no dependent areas, in a straight line to the CDU.
- Prepare the patient for a portable chest x-ray exam.
- Keep emergency supplies at the bedside in the event of tube dislodgement or system failure.
- Maintain the chest tube and drainage system by preventing kinks, ensuring patency of the air vent, and keeping the system below the level of the chest tube.
- Keep the head of the bed always elevated to at least 30°.

Equipment

- Two disposable drainage systems
- Chest tube insertion kit (common tube size for adults is 36 Fr). Should contain povidone-iodine, local anesthetic, syringe, needles, drapes, scalpel, suture.
- 5-in-1 or Y-connector for two chest tubes, if not contained in insertion kit
- Sterile water (for water-seal system)
- Two rubber-tipped hemostats
- Sterile gloves
- Masks and sterile gowns
- Sterile 4 in. × 4 in. gauze dressings
- Sterile, precut drain dressings
- Petroleum gauze dressings
- Large drainage dressings (e.g., ABD)
- 2-inch silk tape
- 1-inch silk tape or nylon banding system
For securing tube connections.

For disposable dry-seal systems:
- 50-mL syringe and 45 mL of sterile water or saline. Some dry-seal CDUs include these.

Delegation

Some agencies permit only registered nurses in the critical care units to perform dressing changes. The physician must perform dressing changes on other units. You should not delegate this procedure, because it requires advanced knowledge of pulmonary anatomy and physiology. As needed, teach the LPN and NAP how to safely provide care for the patient with chest tubes. Instruct them to notify a registered nurse immediately if the chest drainage system becomes disconnected, the chest tube becomes dislodged, sudden bleeding occurs, or the patient develops respiratory distress.

Pre-Procedure Assessment

- Ensure that the patient has venous access.
- Assess vital signs.
- Assess the level of consciousness, orientation, responsiveness, anxiety, and restlessness.
These can indicate hypoxemia.

- Assess the patient's knowledge of chest tube therapy.
Understanding helps allay fears and anxiety.

- Assess cardiac and respiratory status, including respiratory rate, depth, and rhythm; breath sounds; skin color; pulse oximetry and arterial blood gas results.
Provides a baseline for comparison after chest tube insertion. Evaluates chest tube functioning afterward.

- Assess type, color, and amount of chest tube drainage.
Confirms chest tube patency and determines whether bleeding is present.

- Assess for the presence of crepitus and drainage around the chest tube insertion site.
Crepitus is a sign that air is leaking into the subcutaneous tissues. Drainage is a sign that fluid is leaking around the insertion site. Both may indicate a compromise in tube patency.

- Check the disposable chest drainage system for the presence of an air leak.
An air leak indicates that air is leaking from the chest and a tight seal has not yet formed over the site of injury.

➤ When performing the procedure, always identify your patient according to agency policy and be attentive to standard precautions, hand hygiene, patient safety and privacy, body mechanics, and documentation.

Procedure Steps

1. Obtain and prepare the prescribed chest drainage unit (CDU). ▼

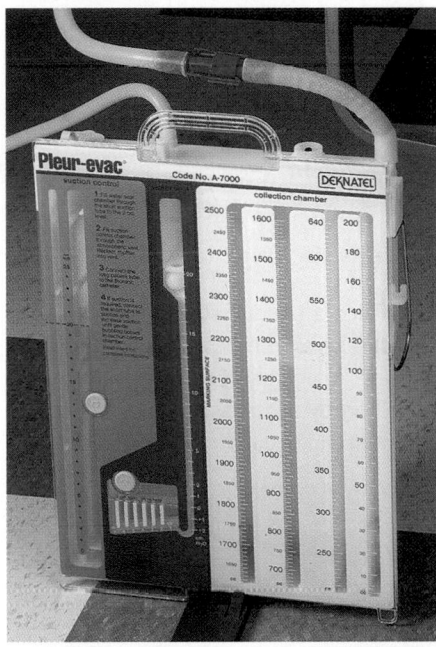

Disposable water-seal system

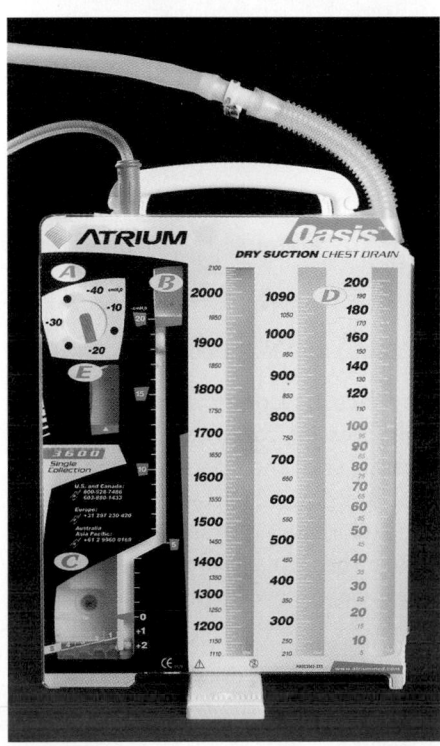

Disposable dry-seal system

Procedure Variation. Disposable Water-Seal CDU Without Suction

2. Remove the cover on the water-seal chamber, and, using the funnel provided, fill the second (water-seal) chamber with sterile water or normal saline. Fill the chamber to the 2-cm mark, or as indicated. (Note that some systems come prefilled.)

The water-seal chamber allows air to exit from the pleural space during exhalation and prevents air from entering the pleural space during inspiration.

3. Place the chest drainage unit (CDU) upright, usually on the floor, and at least 30 cm (1 ft) below the patient's chest level.

4. Replace the cover on the water-seal chamber.

Protects the chamber from contamination.

Go to step 13.

Procedure Variation. Disposable Water-Seal CDU with Suction

5. Remove the cover on the water-seal chamber, and, using the funnel provided, fill the water-seal chamber (second chamber) with sterile water or normal saline to the 2-cm mark. (Note that some systems come prefilled.)

The water-seal chamber allows air to exit from the pleural space during exhalation and prevents air from entering the pleural space during inspiration.

6. Add sterile water or normal saline solution to the suction control chamber. Add the amount specified by the clinician's order, typically 20 cm (7 in.). Place the CDU upright, usually on the floor, and at least 30 cm (1 ft) below the patient's chest level.

Suction is regulated by the height of fluid in the suction control chamber.

7. Attach the tubing from the suction control chamber to the suction source tubing. Turn on the wall (or other) suction source. A wall suction of −80 cm H_2O is common. ▼

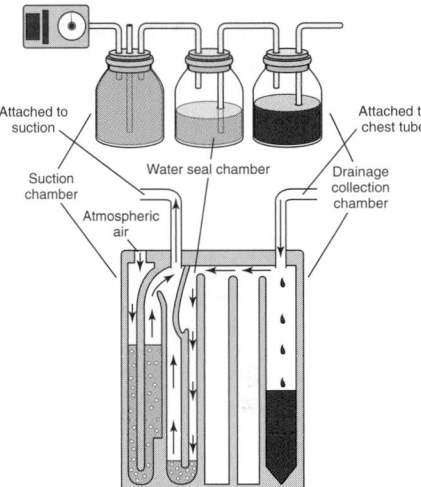

Comparison of glass bottles and disposable CDUs

Go to step 13.

Procedure Variation. Disposable Dry-Seal CDU with Suction

8. Remove the nonsterile outer protective bag and the sterile inner wrapper following agency policy.

9. Place the CDU upright, usually on the floor, and at least 30 cm (1 ft) below the patient's chest level. Some CDUs have hangers for hanging at the bedside.

10. If suction will be required, attach the tubing from the suction control chamber to the connecting tubing attached to the suction source.

11. Fill a syringe with 45 mL of sterile water or saline (follow agency policy and the manufacturer's

(continued on next page)

Procedure 35-12 ■ **Setting Up Disposable Chest Drainage Systems** (continued)

recommendation for type of fluid), or use the small bottle of sterile fluid in the CDU package. Fill the air leak monitor on the CDU by injecting the fluid via the needleless injection port on the back until it reaches the fill line.

Once filled, the water may become colored for improved visibility of air leaks. Bubbles in this section of the CDU indicate an air leak.

Go to step 13.

Procedure Variation. Heimlich Valve

12. When a patient has little or no drainage and does not require suction, the chest tube may be connected to a Heimlich valve instead of a CDU. These valves are attached to the end of the chest tube and allow one-way flow of air out of the chest tube. They contain "flutter" leaflets that allow air to exit but not reenter the pleural space. These valves can also be used for emergency transport until a chest drainage system is available.

Note: Steps 13 through 31 apply to all variations.

13. Position the patient according to the indicated insertion site.

A chest tube to remove air is usually inserted in the second intercostal space at the midclavicular line. If the chest tube is indicated for fluid drainage, the physician typically inserts the tube on the midaxillary line in the 5th or 6th intercostal space.

14. Open the chest tube insertion tray and set up the sterile field. Using sterile technique, drop any necessary supplies on the field (e.g., 4 in. × 4 in. gauze pads, petroleum gauze, syringes).

15. Don a mask, gown, and sterile gloves, and organize the supplies you will need for dressing the chest tube insertion site.

Protective clothing prevents contamination of the surgical site and protects you from splashing.

16. Provide support to the patient while the physician prepares the sterile field, anesthetizes the patient, and inserts and sutures the chest tube.

17. As soon as the chest tube is inserted, attach it to the CDU tubing, using a connector.

Usually the nurse holds the nonsterile tubing that leads to the collection chamber and the physician attaches the sterile chest tube to it. Immediately attaching the chest tube to the drainage system prevents air from entering the pleural cavity.

18. If suction is prescribed, adjust the CDU suction to the level the clinician specifies, usually –20 cm H_2O. Also adjust the wall (or other) suction source, usually to –80 cm H_2O.

Step 18 Variation. Water-Seal Drainage Unit

Adjust the suction source (e.g., wall suction) until gentle bubbling occurs in the suction control chamber. When the tube is functioning properly, the height of the fluid level in the drainage tube fluctuates with the respiratory cycle.

Note: Increasing suction at the suction source increases airflow through the system and creates more bubbling, but it does not increase the amount of suction placed on the chest cavity.

Step 18 Variation. Dry-Seal Drainage Unit

Adjust the CDU suction (e.g., to –20 cm H_2O) by turning the suction control dial on the CDU. Adjust the wall (or portable) suction pressure to –80 mm Hg or greater until the display on the suction-control chamber confirms adequate suction.

Step 18 Variation. Suction is Not Prescribed.

Leave the suction tubing on the drainage system open to maintain negative pressure. Follow the manufacturer's directions on the CDU, as models will differ.

19. When the chest tube is functioning properly, the clinician will

suture it in place. Then don a new pair of sterile gloves. Using sterile technique, wrap petroleum gauze around the chest tube at the insertion site. (Note: Sometimes the physician dresses the site.)

Petroleum gauze creates a seal that prevents air from leaking around the site. However, continued use of petroleum gauze or ointments can macerate the skin, so they should be used with caution.

20. Place a precut, sterile split-drain dressing over the petroleum gauze. Absorbs drainage from the insertion site, thereby reducing skin irritation and possible breakdown. ▼

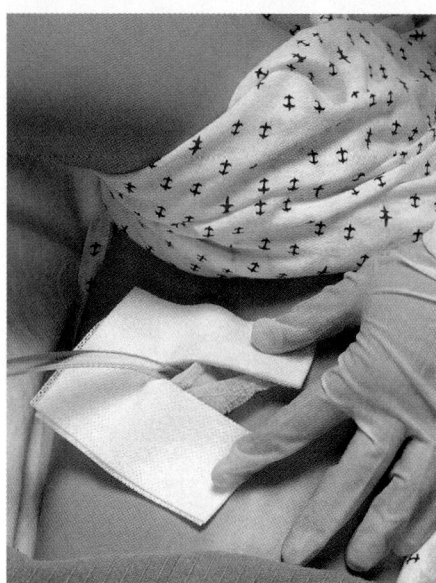

21. Place a second sterile, precut drain dressing over the first drain dressing with the opening facing in the opposite direction from the first. The second drain dressing helps secure the first drain dressing and provides reinforcement against drainage.

22. Place a large drainage dressing (e.g., ABD) over the two precut drain dressings. The large drainage dressing covers the insertion site, protecting it from outside sources of infection.

23. Secure the dressing in place (e.g., with 2-inch silk tape), making sure to cover the dressing completely.

Creates an occlusive dressing that protects the chest tube from becoming dislodged and provides a seal over the insertion site, protecting it from outside sources of infection.

24. Date, time, and initial the dressing. Informs other staff members when the dressing change was completed and by whom.

✚ **25.** Using the spiral taping technique, wrap 1-inch silk tape around the chest tube, starting above the connector and continuing below the connector. Reverse your wrapping by taping back up the tubing (using the spiral technique) until the wrapping is above the connector. The CDU may come with locking connections or bands; if so, use those.
Ensures a tight connection between the two tubings, thereby preventing an air leak at the connection site. ▼

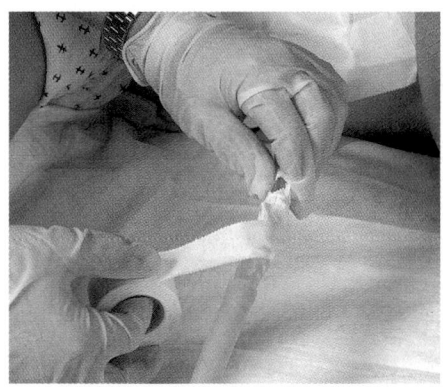

26. Cut an 8-inch-long piece of 2-inch tape. Loop one end around the top portion of the drainage tube, and secure the remaining end of the tape to the chest tube dressing.
Prevents pulling at the chest tube site when the patient moves.

27. Make sure the drainage tubing lies with no kinks from the chest tube to the drainage chamber.
Facilitates drainage and prevents fluid from accumulating in the pleural cavity. ▼

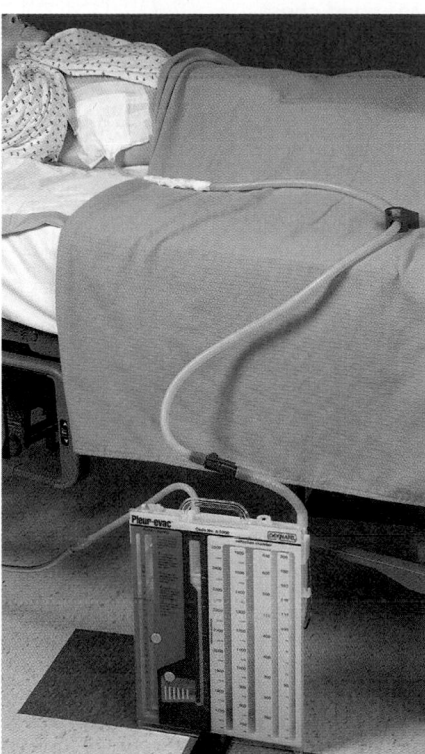

28. Prepare the patient for a portable chest x-ray exam.
A chest x-ray exam should be performed after the chest tube is inserted to ensure proper placement.

✚ **29.** Institute safety measures.
a. Place two rubber-tipped clamps at the patient's bedside for special situations.
Rubber-tip clamps are used to clamp the chest tube to check for an air leak, to change the drainage system, and to assess whether the chest tube can be safely removed.

b. Place a petroleum gauze dressing at the bedside in case the chest tube becomes dislodged.
If the tube becomes dislodged, place a petroleum gauze dressing over the insertion site to prevent air from entering the pleural cavity.

c. Keep a spare disposable drainage system at the patient's bedside.
To use in case the drainage system in use is accidentally upended or the drainage collection chamber becomes filled. ▼

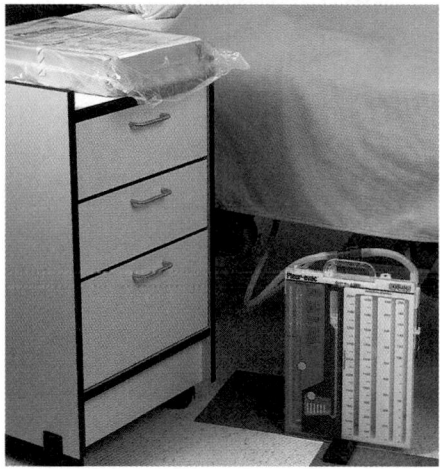

30. Position the patient for comfort, as indicated, but with the head of the bed elevated to at least 30°.
■ If the patient received a chest tube to relieve a pneumothorax, the preferred position is semi-Fowler's position.
■ If the chest tube was inserted to promote fluid drainage, high-Fowler's position is recommended.

31. Maintain patency of the chest tube and drainage system. See Clinical Insight 35-6.

Management of Chest Tubes

For monitoring and managing chest tubes, refer to Clinical Insight 35-6.

Evaluation

■ Evaluate the patient's tolerance to the chest tube insertion. Determine whether the patient's respiratory status has changed.
■ Auscultate breath sounds every 2 hours.

■ Check chest drainage every 15 minutes for the first 2 hours, and then check as prescribed.
■ Monitor the chest tube insertion site for drainage and subcutaneous emphysema at least every 4 hours.
■ Monitor intake and output (I&O) every 8 hours.
■ Check laboratory values to evaluate blood loss and oxygenation.
■ For more details about monitoring chest drainage, see Clinical Insight 35-6.

(continued on next page)

Procedure 35–12 ■ **Setting Up Disposable Chest Drainage**
                    Systems (continued)

Patient Teaching

■ Teach the patient and family about chest tube insertion.
■ Explain the importance of immediately reporting chest pain, shortness of breath, or tube dislodgement.

Home Care

■ Explain to the client and caregiver how to care for the chest tube at home.
■ Provide the client and caregiver with contact information should problems with the chest tube arise.

Documentation

■ Assessment findings before, during, and after chest tube insertion (e.g., vital signs, breath sounds, cardiac status, pulse oximetry)

■ Date and time of the chest tube insertion
■ Name of the clinician who performed the procedure
■ The location of the insertion site, the size of the chest tube, the type of drainage system, and the amount of suction applied, if any
■ Any medications the patient received during the procedure
■ Color and amount of drainage
■ Chest tube output on the intake and output portion of the flowsheet (in most agencies)
■ Patient's tolerance to the procedure
■ Presence of subcutaneous emphysema or air leak, if any
■ Complications and any interventions preformed as a result of the complications
■ Chest x-ray findings

Sample EHR documentation:

Note: Because this isn't the entire computer screen, the image does not show the patient's name or the nurse's name.

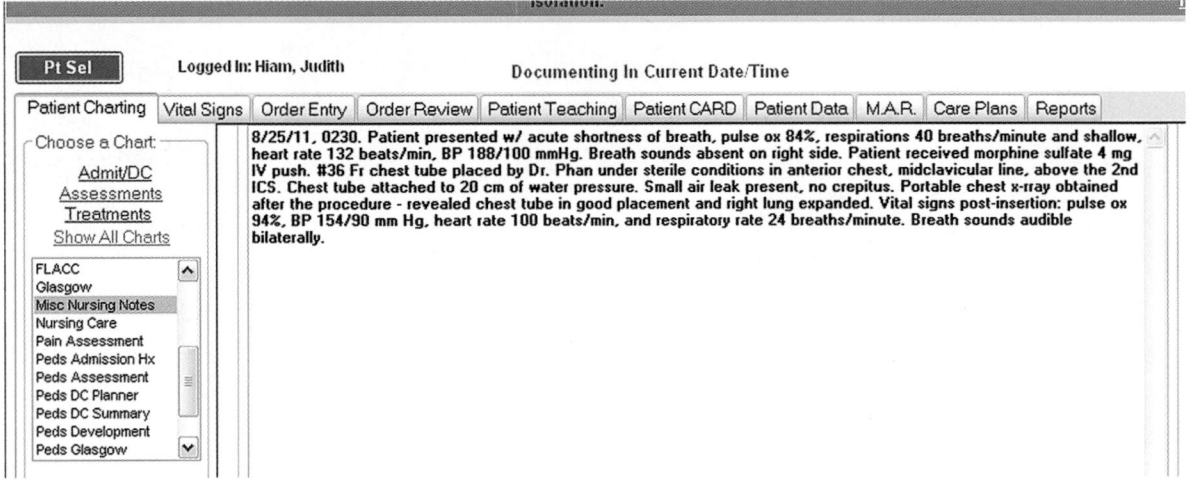

Practice Resources

Lazzara, D. (2002); Siegel, J., Rhinehart, E., Jackson, M., et al. (2007); Roman, M., & Mercado, D. (2006); Tablan, O., Anderson, L., Besser, R., et al. (2004).

Thinking About the Procedure

 Go to the *Fundamentals of Nursing Skills Videos,* **Oxygenation: Chest Tube Care.**

1. What kind of a chest drainage unit was used in this DVD?

2. What is the first type of dressing the nurse used at the chest tube site?

3. How many sterile precut drain dressings did the nurse use?

 For suggested responses, go to Chapter 35, **Thinking About the Procedure Suggested Responses (Procedure 35-12),** on the Student Resource Disk or DavisPlus at http://davisplus.fadavis.com/Wilkinson2

Procedure 35-13 □ Inserting an Oropharyngeal Airway

➤ For steps to follow in *all* procedures, refer to the Universal Steps for All Procedures found on the inside back cover of Volume 2.

Critical Aspects

- You will need a variety of sizes of airway, procedure gloves, tongue blade, suction equipment, and possibly a handheld resuscitation bag and oxygen source.
- Measured on the outside of the cheek, the airway should extend from the front teeth to the end of the jaw line.
- Clear the mouth of debris and secretions. Suction if needed.
- Position patient in supine or semi-Fowler's position, neck hyperextended.
- Hold the tongue down with a tongue blade, as needed, and insert the airway in the upside-down position.
- Rotate the airway 180° and continue inserting until the front flange is flush with the lips.
- Keep the patient's head slightly tilted and chin elevated.
- Verify airway patency by auscultating breath sounds.
- Do not tape the airway in place.
- Keep suction available at the bedside.
- Suction the oropharynx as needed.

◆ The American Heart Association guidelines (2005) direct that you should insert an oropharyngeal airway only if you are trained in its use.

Equipment

- Oral airways in a variety of sizes
- Tongue blade
- Procedure gloves
- Suction equipment
- Resuscitation bag and oxygen source (depending on the patient's status)
- Padded tongue blade

Delegation

You should not delegate this procedure because it requires specialized knowledge, training, and assessment skills.

Pre-Procedure Assessments

- Determine the appropriate airway size by placing the airway on the outside of the patient's cheek. The length of the airway should extend from the front teeth to the end of the jaw line.
- Assess respiratory status (e.g., breath sounds, respiratory rate and effort, skin color, pulse oximetry findings).
  Findings confirm the need for the airway and provide a baseline for evaluating the effectiveness of the intervention.
- Assess for contraindications (e.g., patient is conscious or semiconscious; patient has loose teeth or recent oral surgery)
  An oropharyngeal airway may stimulate the gag reflex, causing vomiting or laryngospasm in a conscious patient.

➤ When performing the procedure, always identify your patient according to agency policy and be attentive to standard precautions, hand hygiene, patient safety and privacy, body mechanics, and documentation.

Procedure Steps

1. Wash your hands, and don clean procedure gloves.
Helps prevent transfer of microorganisms from the patient.

2. Explain the procedure to the patient, even if he appears to be unresponsive.
Recall that hearing is the last sense lost, so the patient may be able to hear you. Information may help relieve the patient's anxiety, if present.

3. Clear the mouth of any debris or secretions. You may need to suction the mouth.

4. Place the patient in supine or semi-Fowler's position. Hyperextend the neck, unless contraindicated.
Mild hyperextension allows the airway to slide naturally toward the pharynx.

5. Gently open the mouth. Remove dentures, if present.
Dentures may cause further airway obstruction.

Step 5 Variation. Tongue Blade Technique
Open the patient's mouth and use the blade to depress the tongue.

Step 5 Variation. Crossed Fingers Technique
Place your thumb on the lower teeth. Cross your index finger over your thumb and place the finger on the upper teeth. Push the teeth apart.

6. You may need to hold the tongue down with a tongue blade as you insert the airway.

(continued on next page)

Procedure 35-13 ■ Inserting an Oropharyngeal Airway (continued)

7. Insert the airway into the mouth in the upside-down position (inner curve of the C faces upward toward the nose).
Prevents pushing the tongue toward the pharynx. ▼

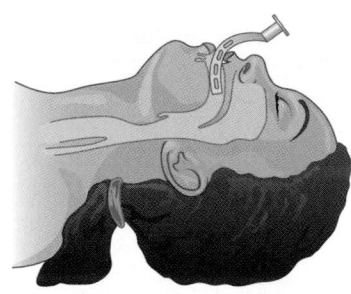

8. As the airway approaches the posterior wall of the pharynx, rotate the airway 180° so that the ends of the C turn downward over the back

of the tongue. Continue to insert the airway until the front flange is flush with the lips. ▼

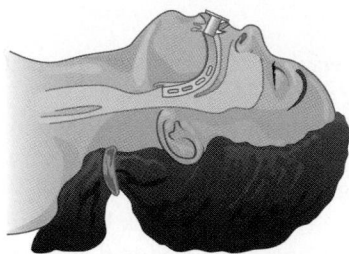

9. Keep the patient's head tilted slightly back and the chin elevated.
This position helps the oropharygeal airway function optimally.

10. Do not tape the airway in place.
You may need to remove the airway quickly for suctioning. Untaping would

delay airway removal, increasing the risk of aspiration.

11. Position the patient on her side.
To minimize the risk of aspiration

12. Provide oral hygiene at least every 2 to 4 hours. Remove and cleanse the airway at that time; use hydrogen peroxide and then rinse with water.

What if. . .

■ **After inserting the airway, respirations are absent or inadequate?**

Use a mouth-to-mask technique, a hand-held resuscitation bag, or an oxygen-powered breathing device to ventilate the patient. Have someone call for help.

Evaluation

■ After inserting the airway, verify patency by auscultating for bilateral breath sounds.
■ Check for bleeding or tooth damage in the mouth.
May be caused by airway insertion, especially if it must be done rapidly.

■ Check to be certain the patient's lips and tongue are not caught between the teeth and the airway.
Prevents trauma to the soft tissues.

■ Monitor the airway position frequently.
Ensures correct placement.

■ Continually reassess the need for the airway. Remove it when the patient begins to cough or gag.
■ Frequently assess oral mucous membranes when you remove the airway for care.
Prolonged airway use can cause tissue irritation or ulceration.

■ Keep suction available at the bedside. Suction the oropharynx as needed by inserting the suction catheter alongside the airway.

Documentation

Document the following:
■ Date and time of airway insertion
■ Type and size of airway (oropharyngeal or nasopharyngeal)
■ Assessments before and after the procedure, including breath sounds and focused respiratory assessment
■ Any suctioning performed
■ Patient's tolerance of the procedure
■ Adverse reactions and interventions taken

Practice Resources

American Association for Respiratory Care (2004b); American Heart Association (2005).

Procedure 35-14   Inserting a Nasopharyngeal Airway

➤ For steps to follow in *all* procedures, refer to the Universal Steps for All Procedures found on the inside back cover of Volume 2.

Critical Aspects

■ You will need a correctly sized nasopharyngeal airway, procedure gloves, tongue blade, water-soluble lubricant, suction equipment, and possibly a handheld resuscitation bag and oxygen source.
■ Measured on the outside of the cheek, the airway should extend from the tip of the nose to the earlobe. It should be slightly smaller than the nares.
■ Position the patient in supine or semi-Fowler's position, neck hyperextended.
■ Lubricate the airway with water-soluble lubricant.

- Advance the airway through the naris until the outer flange rests on the nostril. Do not force.
- Visually inspect the top of the posterior pharynx; only the tip of the tube should be visible.
- Use your finger to check for air exchange at the naris.
- Auscultate the lungs bilaterally.
- Keep suction available at the bedside.
- Suction as needed.

✠ The American Heart Association guidelines (2005) direct that you should insert an oropharyngeal airway only if you are trained in its use.

Equipment

- Nasopharyngeal airway of the correct size
- Tongue blade
- Procedure gloves
- Water-soluble lubricant
- Penlight
- Suction equipment
- Resuscitation bag and oxygen source (depending on the patient's status)

Delegation

You should not delegate this procedure because it requires specialized knowledge, training, and assessment skills. Commonly, this procedure is performed by a respiratory therapist.

Pre-Procedure Assessments

- Determine the appropriate airway size: (1) Measure the diameter of the patient's nostril and use an airway that is slightly smaller than that; and (2) Measure the distance from the tip of the patient's nose to the earlobe, and use an airway about 2.5 cm (1 in.) longer than that measurement. Airways are sized by their internal diameter. Generally, the larger the internal diameter, the longer the tube. Airways are available in a variety of pediatric and adult sizes.
  Small adult: 6 to 7 mm
  Medium adult: 7 to 8 mm
  Large adult: 8 to 9 mm
- Assess respiratory status (e.g., breath sounds, respiratory rate and effort, skin color, pulse oximetry findings).
Findings confirm the need for the airway and provide a baseline for evaluating the effectiveness of the intervention.
- Assess for contraindications (e.g., anticoagulant therapy, hemorrhagic disorder, nasopharyngeal deformity, sepsis)
Up to 30% of patients experience airway bleeding after insertion of a nasopharyngeal airway.

➤ When performing the procedure, always identify your patient according to agency policy and be attentive to standard precautions, hand hygiene, patient safety and privacy, body mechanics, and documentation.

Procedure Steps

1. Don procedure gloves.
Helps prevent transfer of microorganisms from the patient.

2. Position the patient supine or in semi-Fowler's position. Explain the procedure to the patient.
A semi-Fowler's position facilitates airway insertions. Explaining may alleviate anxiety, enabling the patient to cooperate more with the procedure.

3. Validate that the airway size is correct. Hold the airway next to the patient's face. The length of the airway should extend from the nares to the end of the jawline below the ear.

4. Lubricate the airway with water-soluble lubricant.
Prevents trauma to mucosa during insertion.

5. Tilt the patient's head backward to hyperextend the neck. Then push up the tip of the nose and gently insert the tip of the airway into the nose.

6. Advance the airway along the floor of the nostril into the posterior pharynx behind the tongue—until the outer flange rests on the nostril. If you meet resistance, rotate the tube slightly to enhance passage. Do not force against resistance.
Forcing the tube can cause tissue trauma and airway kinking.

7. Have the patient open her mouth. Depress the tongue with a tongue blade and inspect the pharynx for proper placement of the tube tip. Use a penlight, if necessary, for better visualization.
When the tube is fully inserted, the outer flange of the tube should rest on the nostril, and only the tip of the tube should be visible at the top of the posterior pharynx. ▼

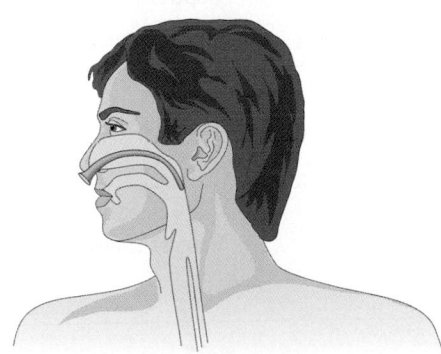

8. Check for correct placement and function: Close the patient's mouth, and place your finger close to the tube's opening to feel for air exchange.

9. Auscultate the lungs for the presence of bilateral breath sounds.

(continued on next page)

Procedure 35-14 ■ Inserting a Nasopharyngeal Airway (continued)

10. Remove the airway at least every 8 hours to check nasal mucous membranes for ulceration or irritation. Clean the airway at this time: Place in a basin, rinse with hydrogen peroxide, then rinse with water. Use a pipe cleaner to remove secretions, if necessary. Reinsert the airway in the other nostril.

To avoid skin and mucous membrane irritation and breakdown and to prevent infection

What if. . .

■ **After you insert the airway, the patient coughs, gags, vomits, or has laryngospasm?**

The tube may be too long. If the tip extends beyond the top of the posterior pharynx, remove it and insert a shorter one.

Evaluation

■ Provide frequent oral and nares care; assess the skin around the nostril.
■ Assess respiratory rate and effort.
■ Assess breath sounds.
■ Observe for bleeding of nasal mucosa; suction as necessary.
■ If the patient is receiving artificial ventilation, monitor for gastric distention and hypoventilation.

Documentation

Document the following:
■ Date and time of airway insertion

■ Type and size of airway (oropharyngeal or nasopharyngeal)
■ Assessments before and after the procedure, including breath sounds, focused respiratory assessment, and condition of the mucous membranes
■ Any suctioning performed
■ Patient's tolerance of the procedure
■ Adverse reactions and interventions taken
■ Removal of the airway, cleaning, and replacement in the other nostril

Practice Resources

American Association for Respiratory Care (2004a,b); American Heart Association (2005); Roberts, K., Whalley, H., & Bleetman, A. (2005).

Clinical Insights

Clinical Insight 35-1 ▶ Assessing Breathing Patterns

Type	Description	Illustration	Discussion
Eupnea	Normal respirations, with equal rate and depth		Rate is about 12–20 breaths/min.
Bradypnea	Slow respirations, < 10 breaths/min		May cause poor gas exchange. Caused by sedative and opioid medications and neuromuscular dysfunction.
Tachypnea	Fast respirations, > 24 breaths/min, usually shallow		Generally caused by hypoxemia or increased oxygen demand (e.g., exercise); however, respirations that are rapid but shallow draw limited air into the alveoli and may result in hypoventilation.
Kussmaul's respirations	Respirations that are regular but abnormally deep and increased in rate		A compensatory mechanism for metabolic disorders that lower blood pH, as well as a form of hyperventilation caused by fear, anxiety, or panic.

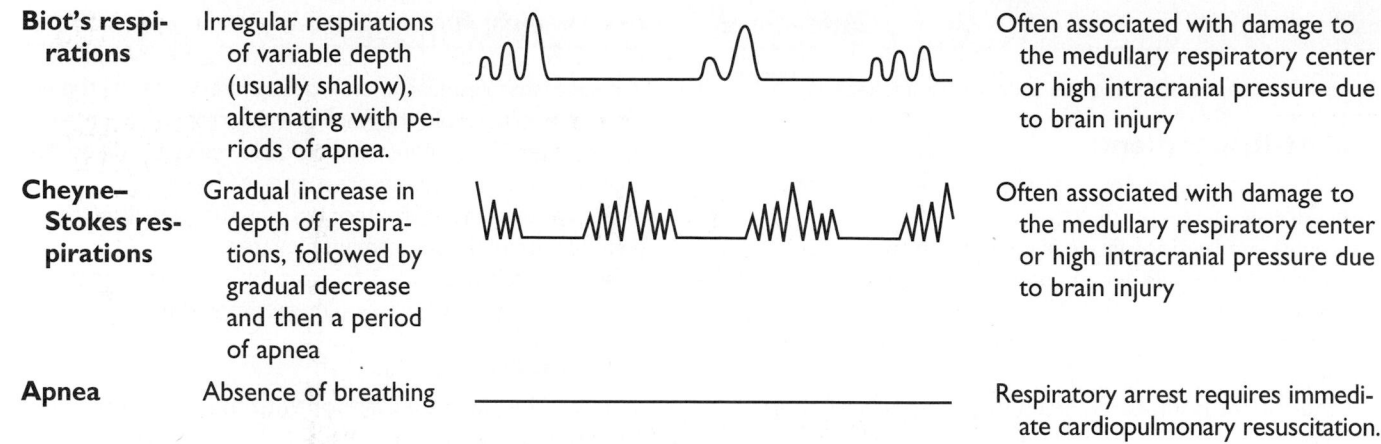

Biot's respirations	Irregular respirations of variable depth (usually shallow), alternating with periods of apnea.		Often associated with damage to the medullary respiratory center or high intracranial pressure due to brain injury
Cheyne–Stokes respirations	Gradual increase in depth of respirations, followed by gradual decrease and then a period of apnea		Often associated with damage to the medullary respiratory center or high intracranial pressure due to brain injury
Apnea	Absence of breathing		Respiratory arrest requires immediate cardiopulmonary resuscitation.

Most irregular breathing patterns are due to brain injury or the effects of drugs on the brain.

Clinical Insight 35-2 ▶ Tips for Obtaining Accurate Pulse Oximetry Readings

Pulse oximetry may be continuous or intermittent. Frequency of measurement depends on the clinical condition of the patient. Pulse oximetry is a valuable assessment tool. However, the following factors can interfere with the accuracy of the readings.

Patient Movement. A fingernail bed is the most common site to place the probe. A tremor, twitch, shivering, or movement in bed can make pulse oximetry readings inaccurate. If the patient is unable to cooperate or control his movement, try using an ear probe or nasal sensor.

Acrylic Fingernails and Nail Polish. If the patient has acrylic nails, place the probe on a toe or earlobe. Many facilities stock individually packaged nail polish remover pads to remove nail polish before placing the probe.
Nail polish or acrylic nails may interfere with signal transmission, causing inaccurate SaO_2 measurement. However, a recent study found that nail polish did not cause a clinically significant change in readings in *healthy* people (Rodden, Spicer, Spicer, et al., 2007).

Dirt and Skin Oils Dirt and oils on the site can interfere with passage of light waves.

Poor Perfusion. A low reading may result from poor perfusion of the area where the probe is placed.
■ A bent elbow, for example, may cause a slight decrease in circulation to the fingernail bed. If SaO_2 results are crucial to the patient's plan of care, use the earlobe to minimize the effect of movement on the reading.

■ Vasoconstriction due to cool extremities may also limit circulation. Keep the extremities warm to obtain a more accurate reading.
■ If poor perfusion is related to a disease process, use the earlobe or nose as the monitoring site.

Lighting. Bright fluorescent lighting may influence the accuracy of the reading. Dim the lights or cover the probe with bed covers or a towel to reduce error.

Anemia, Carbon Monoxide, Intravascular Dyes, and Dark Skin Color. These must be considered when interpreting oximetry readings. Because these factors cannot be controlled, watch for trend changes in the readings.

Equipment Function. Look for a displayed waveform; a reading is meaningless without the waveform. If there is a weak signal or no signal, check the patient's vital signs. If vital signs are satisfactory, check the circulation to the site. If that is satisfactory, check equipment connections.

Accuracy of the Reading. If there is an instantaneous change in saturation (e.g., from 99% to 82%), suspect an error. This is not physiologically possible. For any suspected inaccuracy, check the reading using the equipment on a healthy person. If it seems accurate, check the patient's medications and check for history of circulatory disorders; also check items listed above. When in doubt, rely on your clinical judgment more than the reading from the machine.

⊕ Clinical Insight 35-3 ▶ Guidelines for Preventing Aspiration

To prevent aspiration, use the following guidelines.

For At-Risk Patients

▪ Position the unconscious patient on his side to protect the airway.
▪ Request medications in elixir or liquid form.
▪ Break or crush pills, when appropriate, before you administer them.
▪ Keep a suction setup available for routine and emergency use.
▪ If the patient is intubated, keep the endotracheal or tracheostomy cuff inflated, and suction above the cuff before deflating the cuff.
▪ Do not offer food or fluids if the patient is heavily sedated or in the initial recovery phase of anesthesia.

Enteral Feedings

▪ Check the placement of the nasogastric tube before you administer enteral feedings.

▪ Check gastric residual volume before administering the next enteral feeding. Hold the feeding if the residual volume is high. (*Note:* The amount of acceptable residual volume depends on the amount and frequency of feedings.)
▪ If the patient is receiving continuous tube feedings, the head of the bed must remain elevated.
▪ Also see Procedure 26-3 for step-by-step instructions for administering feedings through gastric and enteric tubes.

Oral Feedings

▪ Position the patient upright or with the head of the bed elevated for feedings or meal.
▪ Be sure the head of bed remains elevated for at least 30 minutes after each feeding or meal.
▪ Offer small, frequent meals.
▪ Avoid thin liquids, or use thickening agents.
▪ Offer foods or liquids that can be formed into a bolus before they are swallowed.
▪ Cut food into small pieces.

⊕ Clinical Insight 35-4 ▶ Oxygen Therapy Safety Precautions

▪ Post signs indicating that oxygen is in use.
▪ Do not permit smoking near oxygen delivery systems.
▪ Ensure that three-pronged plugs are used for electrical devices (to prevent sparks).
▪ Allow no open flames (e.g., candles) near oxygen.
▪ Avoid electrical equipment with frayed wires or loose connections.

▪ Avoid using petroleum products, aerosol products, and products containing acetone where oxygen is in use. (These are flammable substances that are easily ignited.)
▪ Secure oxygen tanks to rigid stands.
▪ Secure portable oxygen cylinders in holders or carriers provided.

⊕ Clinical Insight 35-5 ▶ Caring for Patients with Endotracheal Airways

The following are activities associated with the care of all types of endotracheal airways.

▪ ◆ Have emergency equipment, including a duplicate tracheostomy kit, extra cannula, and suction set-up immediately available for reintubation if the tube should become dislodged.
▪ **Keep an extra cannula at the bedside,** as patients may accidentally decannulate.
▪ **Secure the endotracheal tube** with ties, Velcro® tapes, or a commercial holder to prevent accidental displacement.

▪ **Provide tracheostomy care every 4 to 8 hours** (Dennis-Rouse & Davidson, 2008).
▪ **Change the endotracheal or tracheostomy ties every 24 hours.**
▪ **Secure the orotracheal tube** to the opposite side of the mouth with each change of tape or ties to prevent skin erosion and breakdown.
▪ **Inspect skin around the tube** or tracheal stoma for redness, swelling, drainage, or irritation at least every 8 hours.
▪ **Provide skin care** around the tube and tape or holder at least daily.

▪ **Perform regular oral care.**
▪ **Inflate the cuff of the tube with a minimal occlusive volume and monitor cuff pressures** to prevent pressure necrosis inside the trachea. (This is a joint responsibility with the respiratory therapist.) Maximum acceptable tube cuff pressure is 25 mm Hg. The following is a method for checking for minimal occluding volume:
  1. Place stethoscope on patient's neck over the carotid pulse.
  2. Attach a 10-mL syringe to the pilot balloon of the inflated cuff.
  3. Remove air from the cuff—(1 mL at a time) until you hear a slight leak at the peak of inspiration.
  4. When you hear the leak, inject 1 mL of air back into the cuff.
▪ **Monitor and document cuff pressure** once per shift and when the tube is changed or repositioned.
▪ **Note the centimeter reference marking** on the endotracheal tube to monitor for possible displacement.
▪ **Minimize pulling and traction** on the artificial airway by supporting all tubing connected to the airway and using flexible catheter mounts and swivels.

- If the patient is conscious, **remind him not to pull on the airway.**
- **Use a bite block** between the teeth to prevent the patient from occluding an orotracheal tube.
- **Provide 100% humidification** of inspired air. Check the oxygen setup regularly.

- **Routine saline instillation** to thin secretions is no longer recommended.
- **Ensure adequate hydration** with oral or IV fluids to keep the mucosa moist and thin secretions.
- **Suction the airway** when secretions collect. Remember, the patient probably can't cough effectively to clear secretions.

Clinical Insight 35-6 ▸ Managing Chest Tubes

Monitor Breathing, Gas Exchange, and Drainage

- Frequently assess breathing patterns, breathing effort, and breath sounds.
- Assess mental status, heart rate and rhythm, and pulse oximetry readings.

These reflect adequacy of oxygenation.

- Monitor character, color, and amount of chest drainage. Immediately report sudden or large increases in drainage or new onset of bright red blood, along with an assessment of the patient's condition at that time.

Drainage is usually greatest when the chest tube is initially inserted and decreases as the lung reexpands. The chest drainage unit (CDU) must be replaced when the drainage compartment is almost full.

Prevent complications or intervene if they occur.

- Observe the dressing at least every 4 hours.
  - Make sure that the chest dressing around the tube insertion site is occlusive (e.g., not wet or loose). Usually, petroleum gauze is wrapped around the insertion site to ensure occlusion.
  - Inspect for excessive, abnormal, or foul-smelling drainage.

This may indicate hemorrhage or infection.

- Palpate around the dressing for **subcutaneous emphysema** (air in the subcutaneous tissues).

This may be caused by an incomplete seal at the chest tube insertion site.

- Assess for pain; medicate as needed.
- Reposition the patient every 2 hours and use pillows to keep the patient's weight off the chest tube.

To prevent occlusion of the tube, to promote drainage, and to preserve skin integrity.

- Encourage the patient to use the arm on the affected side. Assist with range-of-motion exercises, if necessary.

To maintain joint mobility.

- ✚ A **tension pneumothorax** is a life-threatening complication of chest drainage. It occurs when positive pressure builds up in the pleural space and pushes the lungs, great vessels, and heart toward the other side of the chest. If a patient with a chest drainage system becomes acutely short of breath, immediately check for occlusion of the system. Relieve the occlusion to prevent pressure build-up.

- **Recollapse of the lung** can occur because of loss of negative pressure within the system. This is commonly caused by air leaks, disconnections, or breaks or cracks of the bottles or chambers. If any of these occur, immediately place the disconnected end nearest the patient into a bottle of sterile water or saline.

- ✚ Do not clamp the chest tube. Clamp chest tubes only for changing the drainage system. Limit the clamp time and monitor respiratory status constantly until the clamp is removed.

Clamping can rapidly lead to a tension pneumothorax.

- ✚ If the tube is accidentally pulled out, immediately cover the wound with a dry sterile dressing. Listen for air leaking out of the site. If you can hear air, tape the dressing loosely so that you do not occlude the site.

If air cannot escape from the chest, a tension pneumothorax will occur, eventually compromising cardiovascular function.

Promote Lung Reexpansion.

- Encourage the patient to be as active as his condition permits.

Chest drainage systems are bulky, but with disposable systems, some patients can still get out of bed and ambulate. Most patients will need assistance from one or two staff members to protect and monitor the system and the patient.

- Instruct the patient to perform deep-breathing and coughing every 2 hours, unless contraindicated. Assist the patient to sit upright and splint the chest with a pillow or the hands, and provide analgesia as needed.

These interventions help to minimize discomfort.

Key Points for Managing a One-Bottle System

- Keep the intake tube below the fluid level in the drainage bottle to prevent drawing air into the pleural space with inhalation.
- Maintain the tubing about 2 cm below the water level. As tubing length below the water increases, more effort is required to exhale.

(continued on next page)

Clinical Insight 35-6 ➤ **Managing Chest Tubes** (continued)

■ Take precautions to see that the bottle is not accidentally tipped over, uncovering the long vent tube and allowing air to enter the pleural space.

Maintain the drainage system.

For All Types of CDUs:

■ Make sure the drainage system is located below the insertion site.

If the drainage system is located above the insertion site, fluid may flow back into the pleural cavity, compromising the patient's respiratory status.

■ Regularly inspect tubing to ensure that connections are air-tight, tubing is not kinked or occluded.

Kinks in the drainage tubing increase pressure in the pleural cavity and prevent fluid drainage.

■ Monitor drainage.

Blood or purulent matter can occlude the tubing.

■ Inspect the air vent in the drainage system to make sure it is patent.

The air vent must remain patent to allow air to escape. If air builds up in the pleural cavity, pneumothorax may occur.

■ Monitor to ensure the system is maintaining consistent negative pressure levels.

■ ✚ Do not "milk" or strip the tubing.

Doing so can create excess negative pressure and damage lung tissue.

■ Most systems will have some type of check system to ensure that the system is operating correctly. Always be sure to verify operation through the users' manual or with the product's vendor.

■ To transport or ambulate a patient: (a) keep the CDU upright below chest level; (b) disconnect the CDU from suction source and make sure the air vent is open.

Water-Seal Drainage Systems:

■ Take precautions that the CDU is not tipped over (e.g., tape it to the floor).

■ Observe for **tidaling**, which indicates fluctuations in the water-seal chamber's fluid level that correspond with

respiration. The level will increase on inspiration and decrease on exhalation. This will be opposite for a patient on a mechanical ventilator.

■ Bubbling in the bottom of the water-seal chamber indicates an air leak. When this occurs, check for poor tubing connections. A small amount of bubbling right after insertion or with exhalation or cough is normal.

■ Check the water in the suction control chamber; replace as needed.

The water can evaporate.

■ ✚ If the chest tube disconnects from the drainage unit, establish a temporary water seal by immersing the open end of the chest tube in a bottle of sterile water to a depth of 2 cm until a new system can be connected. Cleanse the end of the patient connector on the drain system with alcohol and reconnect it if it has not been contaminated. If the patient connector on the drain system is contaminated, you must initiate a new CDU.

Dry-Seal Drainage Systems:

■ Inspect the air vent in the drainage system to make sure it is patent.

The air vent must remain patent to allow air to escape. If air builds up in the pleural cavity, pneumothorax may occur.

■ Check the indicators on the CDU to be certain suction is operating properly.

A dry chest drainage system doesn't use water in the suction chamber. A dynamic automatic control valve (ACV) is located inside the regulator, which continuously balances the forces of suction and the atmosphere. The ACV responds and adjusts to changes in patient air leaks and fluctuations in suction source vacuum to deliver accurate suction to the patient. Pressure can be set from -10 cm H_2O to -40 cm H_2O by adjusting the rotary dry suction dial.

■ Observe for bubbling. If the water in a dry-seal CDU is bubbling, it means there is an air leak.

Assessment Guidelines and Tools

Focused Assessment: Oxygenation

Part I. Questions to Assess Risk for Impaired Oxygenation

Demographic Data

■ What is your age?

■ Where do you live?

■ What is your occupation?

Health History

■ What healthcare problems are you currently being treated for?

■ Have you ever been hospitalized or had surgery? If so, when and for what reason?

■ Do you have a history of allergies or asthma?

■ What medications do you currently take?

■ What over-the-counter medications or alternative treatments do you use? What do you use them for?

Respiratory History

■ Have you ever been diagnosed with a respiratory problem? If so, what was the diagnosis? When was the diagnosis made?

Focused Assessment: Oxygenation—cont'd

- Have you noticed any changes in your breathing?
- How often do you cough?
- When you do cough, is it productive?
- What do the secretions you cough up look like and smell like?
- How much sputum do you produce?
- How do you treat your cough? What effect did it have?
- Do you ever wheeze or feel short of breath?
- What causes you to wheeze or feel short of breath?
- Do body positions affect your breathing pattern?
- What position do you lie in when you sleep? Do you use more than one pillow?
- Do you ever wake up short of breath?

Cardiovascular History

- Have you ever been diagnosed with a heart or circulatory problem?
- Have you ever been told you have high blood pressure or a heart murmur?
- Do you experience cold hands and feet frequently?
- Have you ever had chest pain? If so, describe the circumstances.
- How was the chest pain treated?
- What measures do you take to relieve or prevent the pain?
- Do you easily become fatigued or feel your heart rate is very rapid?

Environmental History

- Are there pets in the house?
- What response, if any, do you have to pets, dust, pollen, or plants?
- Are you exposed to smoke or fumes in the home and workplace?
- Are you exposed to respiratory irritants such as asbestos, chemicals, coal dust, fungus, molds, or soot in the home or workplace?
- What type of heating, air conditioning, or air filtering system do you have in the home or workplace?

Lifestyle

- What is your current stress level? What are your major sources of stress?
- What is you usual diet? Is your current diet typical, or have you recently changed your eating habits?
- What is your usual activity level?
- What level of activity makes you feel short of breath?
- Do you smoke now, or have you ever smoked?

- If you smoke, how many packs per day and for how many years have you smoked?
- Do you smoke marijuana or use other substances?

Part II. Focused Physical Examination

Pulmonary System

- **Inspect** to observe respiratory patterns, signs of respiratory distress, chest structures and movement, skin and mucous membrane color, presence or absence of edema, sputum characteristics, and overall general appearance.
- **Palpate** skin temperature and areas of tenderness.
- **Percuss** over the lung fields (for consolidation or excess air pockets).
- **Auscultate** breath sounds and vascular sounds.
- **Assess breathing patterns:** eupnea, tachypnea, bradypnea, apnea, Kussmaul's breathing, Biot's breathing, and Cheyne–Stokes respirations.
- **Assess cough and related symptoms:**

  Nasal congestion, sneezing, water eyes, and nasal discharge suggest allergies.

  Fever, chest congestion, noisy breath sounds, sputum production suggest an upper respiratory tract infection (URI).

  Dyspnea, chest tightness, and wheezing suggest airway obstruction (e.g., asthma).
- **Assess sputum:** appearance, color, odor, amount, and timing.
- **Obtain sputum samples** as needed.
- **Assess respiratory effort.** Breathing should be effortless. Observe for shortness of breath, dyspnea, nasal flaring, head bobbing, retractions, use of accessory muscles during inspiration, grunting, needing to sit upright to breathe, paroxysmal nocturnal dyspnea, conversational dyspnea, stridor, and wheezing.

Cardiovascular System

- **Inspect the neck** for carotid and jugular pulsations. Palpate each carotid separately. Auscultate the carotid arteries and jugular veins for bruits and hums.
- **Inspect the precordium** for pulsations. Palpate for pulsations, lifts, heaves, and thrills. Auscultate for heart sounds.
- Also review Procedure 19-13: Assessing the Heart and Vascular System.
- **Assess peripheral circulation:** Palpate peripheral pulses, assess skin color and temperature, note hair distribution on extremities. Inspect for skin ulcers and edema of the feet and ankles.
- **Inspect** for venous valve competence.
- **Perform the capillary refill test** anywhere you note signs of diminished blood flow.

Diagnostic Testing

Lung Volumes and Capacities

The norms presented in this table are based on averages for a young adult man.

Title	Definition	Significance
Tidal volume (V_T)	The amount of air moved into and out of the lungs with each normal breath. Normally around 500 mL.	In a healthy state, V_T increases when oxygen demand increases. Diseases that restrict lung inflation, create muscular weakness, or paralyze the diaphragm limit the ability of the body to increase tidal volume. When such disorders become severe, V_T will fall too low to support even resting oxygen demands.
Inspiratory reserve volume (IRV)	The maximum amount of air that can be inhaled above and beyond the normal tidal volume. Ranges from 2000 to 3000 mL.	IRV determines how much the tidal volume can increase when oxygen demands increase.
Expiratory reserve volume (ERV)	The maximum extra amount of air that can be forcefully exhaled after the end of a normal tidal expiration. Ranges from 1000 to 1500 mL.	Some diseases (e.g., emphysema) cause collapse of alveoli and airways, which traps extra air in the lungs. This "trapped" air cannot be exhaled and lowers ERV.
Residual volume (RV)	The amount of air remaining in the lungs after the most forceful exhalation. Ranges from 1000 to 1500 mL.	Diseases that reduce ERV lead to an increase in RV. As more air is trapped in the lungs and cannot be exhaled even with forceful attempts (ERV), it becomes part of the residual volume that is never completely exhaled.
Inspiratory capacity (IC)	The combination of the tidal volume and inspiratory reserve volume (V_T + IRV). Ranges from 2500 to 3500 mL.	This is the amount of air that can be inhaled with maximum effort. It reflects the capacity one has to inhale deeply.
Functional residual capacity (FRC)	The combination of expiratory reserve volume and residual volume (ERV + RV). Ranges from 2000 to 3000 mL. Exhalation of additional air requires effort to force more air out.	This is the amount of air that stays in the lungs at the end of a normal passive quiet exhalation. Disorders that cause air trapping increase the FRC.
Vital capacity (VC)	The combination of inspiratory reserve volume and expiratory reserve volume (IRV + ERV). Ranges from 3000 to 4500 mL.	This is the maximum amount of air that can be forcefully exhaled after filling the lungs to their maximum level with the deepest possible inspiratory effort.

Tests Related to Oxygenation

Test	Purpose
Angiogram	A contrast dye is injected into a vein, and serial films are taken to assess patency of the vessels.
Arterial blood gases (ABG)	An analysis of arterial blood that evaluates the effectiveness of gas exchange
Bronchoscopy	Insertion of a flexible endoscope to examine the larynx, trachea, and bronchial tree
Cardiac catheterization	A catheter is passed into the heart to assess pressures, blood flow, and the size and patency of chambers.
Chest x-ray study (CXR)	Provides an anterior–posterior or lateral view of the heart and lungs, shows tissue density (e.g., to evaluate size, masses, fluid).
Creatine kinase-MB (CK-MB)	The MB isoenzyme is present only in the heart muscle. A serum measurement of the MB band is used to detect a myocardial infarction (MI). Levels rise with an acute MI.

Diagnostic Testing

Echocardiogram	An ultrasound evaluation of the heart that examines heart function and blood flow
Electrocardiogram (ECG)	Electrodes placed on the extremities and chest wall conduct electrical activity from the heart. ECG illustrates heart rate, rhythm, and size and helps evaluate heart damage.
Hemoglobin (Hgb)	A serum measurement that affects the oxygen-carrying capacity of the blood. May be measured separately or as part of a complete blood count.
Holter monitor	A continuous ECG tracing used to correlate symptoms and cardiac activity. Typically the tracing lasts 48 hours to 7 days.
Pulmonary function studies	A series of tests to detect lung volume and capacity
Sputum culture	A microscopic evaluation of the sputum
Technetium scan	Technetium-99m sestamibi is injected intravenously. Approximately 90 to 120 minutes later, the heart is scanned. Areas of myocardial damage appear as "hot spots" on the scan.
Thoracentesis	Insertion of a large-bore needle through the chest wall into the pleural space to obtain fluid specimens, to instill medication, or to drain accumulations of fluid.
Throat culture	A swab of the pharynx or tonsils is performed to assess pathogens present in the pharynx.
Treadmill test	Evaluates the effect of exercise on the heart and circulation via continuous ECG and vital sign monitoring during exercise.
Troponin	A serum evaluation of a complex of proteins is used to detect myocardial infarction (MI). Levels of these contractile proteins remain elevated for up to 7 days after MI.
Ventilation–perfusion scan	Used to assess for pulmonary embolus, this scan entails injection of a radioactive substance that allows blood flow to the lungs to be evaluated. A second substance is inhaled that maps out oxygen distribution in the lungs.
White blood cell (WBC) count	A serum measure to assess for the presence of infection.

Diagnostic Testing

Reading a Tuberculin Skin Test Result

Size of Induration	Considered Positive For
> 5 mm	➤ People who have had recent close contact with someone with active TB
	➤ People who have HIV or risk factors for HIV
	➤ People with previous history of TB
> 10 mm	➤ IV drug users known to be HIV-negative
	➤ People with medical conditions that increase the risk of progressing from latent TB to active TB (e.g., diabetes mellitus, use of steroids, chronic renal failure, some malignancies)
	➤ Residents and employees of high-risk congregate settings: prisons, skilled nursing facilities (SNFs) and other long-term facilities, healthcare facilities, and homeless shelters
	➤ Foreign-born persons recently arrived (i.e., within the last 5 years) from countries having a high incidence of TB
	➤ Low-income groups
	➤ Children younger than 4 years of age or exposed to adults in high-risk categories
> 15 mm	➤ People who do not meet any of the above criteria

Diagnostic Testing

Arterial Blood Gas Values: Evaluating Adequacy of Oxygenation

Sao$_2$	Arterial Po$_2$	Comment
95%–100%	80–100 mm Hg	Normal arterial values in healthy people.
90%	60 mm Hg	PO$_2$ > 60 mm Hg is required to sustain life and activity. This level is **not** normal in healthy people.
75%	40 mm Hg	Normal venous values; a **life-threatening arterial value** in anyone.

Standardized Language

Nursing Diagnoses Associated with Impaired Ventilation and Gas Exchange

NURSING DIAGNOSIS	DEFINITION AND/OR DISCUSSION
Ineffective Airway Clearance	The inability to maintain a clear airway. The main mechanism for keeping airways open is a strong cough that moves secretions into the throat to be expectorated or swallowed. Patient may have weak cough, adventitious breath, copious secretions, and signs of hypoxia.
Risk for Aspiration	Should be used when there is a risk for gastrointestinal or oropharyngeal secretions, solids, or fluids entering into tracheobronchial passages (e.g., for patients who have had head or neck surgery, who have a reduced level of consciousness, impaired swallowing, or are receiving tube feedings).
Ineffective Breathing Pattern	Used to describe inadequate ventilation, such as hypoventilation, hyperventilation, tachypnea, or bradypnea. Patient may have abnormal respiratory rate, depth, or pattern; dyspnea, orthopnea, and other signs of difficulty breathing.
Impaired Gas Exchange	This is the appropriate diagnosis if the patient is adequately ventilating but diffusion across the alveolar–capillary membrane is impaired. The NANDA-I definition specifies "excess or deficit in oxygenation and/or CO$_2$ elimination at the alveolar-capillary membrane" (NANDA International, 2009, p. 112). Although ABG analysis is the most accurate way to detect Impaired Gas Exchange, you will be called on to assess adequacy of gas exchange without having this information available. Patient will show signs of hypoxia (e.g., confusion, nasal flaring, pallor, abnormal blood gases, diaphoresis, headache upon awakening).
Impaired Spontaneous Ventilation	Describes a condition in which a patient, as a result of decreased energy reserves, is unable to maintain breathing adequate to support life. This situation requires collaborative emergency intervention, including resuscitation and mechanical ventilation. You will see increased P$_{CO_2}$, decreased Po$_2$, decreased Sao$_2$, dyspnea, apprehension, restlessness, increased metabolic heart rate, and decreased tidal volume.
Dysfunctional Ventilatory Weaning Response (DVWR)	Represents a specific situation in which a patient who is being mechanically ventilated cannot adjust to lower levels of ventilator support, prolonging the ventilatory weaning process. Etiologies may be psychological (e.g., anxiety), situational (e.g., low nurse-to-patient ratio), or physiological (e.g., uncontrolled pain). You will see deterioration in ABG levels, increases in heart and respiratory rates, and increase in BP; as well as adventitious breath sounds, pallor and cyanosis. Specific symptoms of hypoxia depend on whether the DVWR is mild, moderate, or severe.

Source: NANDA International (2009). *NANDA nursing diagnoses: Definitions and classifications. 2009–2011.* Philadelphia: Wiley-Blackwell. Used with permission.

Nursing Diagnoses Associated with Impaired Circulation

NURSING DIAGNOSIS	DEFINITION AND/OR DISCUSSION
Decreased Cardiac Output	Inadequate blood pumped by the heart to meet metabolic demands of the body. Symptoms vary depending on whether the problem is one of preload or afterload, but are likely to include changes in heart rate and rhythm, palpitations, ECG changes, anxiety, fluid retention, oliguria, weak peripheral pulses, hypotension, adventitious lung sounds, and symptoms of hypoxia and hypoxemia.
Risk for Ineffective Cardiac Tissue Perfusion	Risk for a decrease in cardiac (coronary) circulation. Risk factors are too numerous to list, but some examples are: taking birth control pills, drug abuse, family history of coronary artery disease, diabetes mellitus, and lack of knowledge of modifiable risk factors such as smoking, sedentary lifestyle, and obesity.
Risk for Ineffective Cerebral, Gastrointestinal, or Renal Perfusion (Specify)	At risk for decrease in circulation to the organ. Risk factors are numerous and depend on the specified organ. For example, some risk factors for Ineffective Gastrointestinal Perfusion are abdominal aortic aneurysm, acute GI bleeding, and liver dysfunction. Risk factors for Ineffective Renal Perfusion include diabetes mellitus, renal artery stenosis, and malignancy. Risk factors for Ineffective Cerebral Tissue Perfusion include atrial fibrillation, brain tumor, and carotid stenosis. Cardiac or circulatory problems present a risk for ineffective perfusion of all organs.
Ineffective Peripheral Tissue Perfusion	Decrease in blood circulation to the periphery that may compromise health. Symptoms (defining characteristics) of Ineffective Peripheral tissue will be different depending on whether the etiology is arterial or venous. Look for such symptoms as absent or weak pulses, claudication, pale and shiny skin, edema, numbness or pain in the extremity, and delayed wound healing.

Source: NANDA International. (2009). *NANDA nursing diagnoses: Definitions and classifications 2009–2011.* Philadelphia: Wiley-Blackwell. Used with permission.

Examples of NOC Outcomes and NIC Interventions Linked to Oxygenation Diagnoses

Nursing Diagnoses Related to Pulmonary Functioning

NURSING DIAGNOSIS	NOC OUTCOMES	NIC INTERVENTIONS
Ineffective Airway Clearance	Respiratory Status: Airway Patency	Airway Management Airway Suctioning Cough Enhancement Respiratory Monitoring
Ineffective Breathing Pattern	Respiratory Status: Ventilation Vital Signs	Airway Management Vital Signs Monitoring
Impaired Gas Exchange	Respiratory Status: Gas Exchange Vital Signs	Airway Management Oxygen Therapy Respiratory Monitoring
Risk for Aspiration	Aspiration Prevention Respiratory Status: Ventilation Swallowing Status	Aspiration Precautions Swallowing Therapy Vomiting Management

Nursing Diagnoses Related to Circulation

NURSING DIAGNOSIS	NOC OUTCOMES	NIC INTERVENTIONS
Activity Intolerance (could also be related to Pulmonary Functioning)	Activity Tolerance Energy Management Self-Care: Activities of Daily Living (ADL)	Energy Conservation Exercise Promotion: Strength Training Self-Care Assistance

Continued

Examples of NOC Outcomes and NIC Interventions Linked to Oxygenation Diagnoses—cont'd

NURSING DIAGNOSIS	NOC OUTCOMES	NIC INTERVENTIONS
Decreased Cardiac Output	Blood Loss Severity	Bleeding Reduction
	Cardiac Pump Effectiveness	Cardiac Care
	Circulation Status	Cerebral Perfusion Promotion
	Tissue Perfusion: Cardiac	Circulatory Care: Arterial or Venous Insufficiency
	Tissue Perfusion: Abdominal, Cerebral, Pulmonary, Peripheral	Hemodynamic Regulation
	Vital Signs	Hemorrhage Control
		Intravenous Therapy
		Shock Management
Ineffective Peripheral Tissue Perfusion	Circulation Status	Circulatory Care (Arterial and Venous Insufficiency)
	Fluid Overload Severity	Fluid Management
	Sensory Function: Cutaneous	Peripheral Sensation Management
	Tissue Integrity: Skin & Mucous Membranes	Skin Surveillance
Risk for Ineffective Cerebral, Gastrointestinal, or Renal Perfusion	Circulation Status	Cerebral Perfusion Promotion
	Electrolyte & Acid/Base Balance	Neurologic Monitoring
	Cognition	Hypovolemia Management
	Fluid Balance	Fluid/Electrolyte Management
	Neurological Status: Consciousness	Circulatory Care (Arterial and Venous Insufficiency)
	Kidney Function	Circulatory Precautions
	Tissue Perfusion: Abdominal Organs	Hemodialysis Therapy

Source: Johnson, M., Bulechek, G., Butcher, H., et al. (2006). *NANDA, NOC, and NIC linkages.* St. Louis, MO: C.V. Mosby: Bulechek, G., Butcher, H., & Dochterman, J. (Eds.). (2008). *Nursing interventions classification (NIC)* (5th ed.). St. Louis, MO: C.V. Mosby; Moorhead, S., Johnson, M., Maas, M., et al. (Eds.). (2008). *Nursing outcomes classification (NOC)* (4th ed.). St. Louis, MO: C.V. Mosby. Used with permission.

THINKING CRITICALLY ABOUT OXYGENATION

The exercises in the following sections allow you to practice the kind of thinking you will use as a full-spectrum nurse. Because these are critical-thinking questions, there is usually no single right answer. We do not provide answers for these questions because it is more important for you to think about the questions than to arrive at the "right" answer. These questions are designed to improve your thinking more than to "cover content." Discuss answers with your peers—discussion can stimulate critical thinking. If you have difficulty with any of these questions, consult with your instructor.

Applying the Full-Spectrum Nursing Model

PATIENT SITUATION

Haley, a 15-year-old female high-school student, was admitted to the hospital with shortness of breath and right-sided chest pain when breathing. She states that she has had "the flu" for 3 days. She has a history of asthma since age 6, and smokes a half pack of cigarettes a day. Both her parents are heavy smokers, as well. An IV was initiated, and she is receiving 800 mg of vancomycin (an antibiotic) intravenously every 12 hours. She is not on oxygen therapy, but receives 10 incentive spirometer treatments per hour while awake. Her heart rate is 80 beats/minute, respiratory rate 24 breaths/min, and blood pressure 110/70 mm Hg. Her skin is pale but warm, and capillary refill time is 2 seconds. She has no clubbing of the fingers. She is urinating approximately 400 mL of clear yellow urine every 8 hours and maintaining a normal bowel elimination pattern. Laboratory results are:

Red blood cell count (RBCs): 3.56×10^6 (3.56 million/mm^3)

White blood cell count (WBCs): 11,800/mm^3

Hemoglobin: 11.2 g/dL

Hematocrit: 32.7%

Haley says, "I feel really tired, and too weak to even pick up a glass of water." Her cough produces white, thick sputum. Sputum culture on admission confirms a diagnosis of streptococcal pneumonia. (Case adapted from C. Green, 2000, pp. 233–234.)

THINKING

1. *Theoretical Knowledge*:

   a. According to the Centers for Disease Control and Prevention, should Haley have received a pneumonia immunization? Why or why not?

   b. What is clubbing of the fingers? You may wish to refer to Chapter 19 for review, or to a medical–surgical nursing text.

2. *Critical Thinking (Analyzing Assumptions)*:

   Why is it a positive finding for Haley that she does not have clubbed fingers?

DOING

3. *Practical Knowledge*:

   Twenty-four hours after the antibiotics were started, Haley's respiratory status becomes worse. She says, "It's so hard to breathe." It is decided to begin administering oxygen. Another sputum culture is prescribed. You are to collect a sputum specimen from the patient.

   a. What position should Haley assume for this procedure?

   b. What kind of protective clothing do you need for this procedure?

c. You remove the lid from the specimen container. When you hand it to Haley, she touches the inside of the container with her fingers. What should you do?

d. What would you tell Haley to do in order to expectorate the sputum specimen?

4. *Nursing Process (Implementation)*:

In the admission data, what important information is missing with regard to her respiratory status?

CARING

5. *Self-Knowledge*:

Describe one or two patient care experiences you might draw upon to help you in caring for Haley. In what ways were those patients similar to Haley, and how might that help you?

6. *Ethical Knowledge*:

After you finish collecting the sputum specimen, what do you think Haley's biggest concern is right now?

Critical Thinking and Clinical Reasoning

1. Recall the four patients discussed in the "Meet Your Patients" scenario:

- Mary is a 4-year-old girl with a history of asthma. Her mother, Ms Green, has brought her in for an "asthma attack." Mary is sitting in her mother's lap and breathing rapidly through an open mouth. She has a cough that sounds congested and wheezy. The physician has already prescribed a nebulized treatment containing albuterol (Proventil) and ipratropium bromide (Atrovent).
- Mr. Chu is a 78-year-old man complaining of cough, sore throat, fatigue, and weakness. His BP is 166/82, pulse is 90 beats/min, respirations are 26 breaths/min, and temperature is 100.4°F (38.0°C).
- William is a 19-year-old man who has had a sudden onset of right-sided chest pain and shortness of breath. His chest x-ray film revealed a right pneumothorax, and he is currently receiving 35% oxygen by face mask while waiting for an ambulance to transport him to the hospital for further evaluation.
- Ms Saunders is a 45-year-old homemaker. She says she has been extremely tired, easily becomes short of breath, and is unable to complete her chores without frequent rest breaks. She is pale and seems tired. Her vital signs are as follows: BP, 136/78 mm Hg; pulse, 86 beats/min; respirations, 24 breaths/min and unlabored; temperature, 98.4°F (36.7°C); and pulse oximetry 98% on room air. She is now waiting for her lab results, which include a complete blood count (CBC).

a. Which patients are experiencing problems with ventilation? Explain your answer.

b. Which patient appears to be experiencing problems with hypoxia? Does the problem appear to be related to oxygenation or perfusion? Explain your answers.

c. Mr. Chu has smoked two packs of cigarettes per day for 50 years. ABGs reveal a low Po_2 and a high PCO_2 consistent with chronic lung disease. He is diagnosed with an acute exacerbation of chronic bronchitis. He is placed on oral antibiotics and long-acting bronchodilators by metered-dose inhaler (MDI). What teaching could you offer to help Mr. Chu mobilize and expectorate secretions?

d. Mary receives her nebulizer treatment and markedly improves. The physician has prescribed a variety of take-home medications that you must teach her mother about. The treatment plan includes a protocol based on peak expiratory flow monitoring. Discuss how you might involve Mary in her own care.

  e. William's chest x-ray film reveals a spontaneous pneumothorax. There is no apparent fluid in the pleural space. What chest tube systems can be used to treat his pneumothorax? Explain your thinking.

  f. Ms Saunders is diagnosed with severe anemia. She is hospitalized because her hemoglobin is 5.9 g/dL. How will this affect her oxygenation? What interventions would improve her fatigue?

2. You are caring for a 68-year-old woman on the night shift. Earlier today she had an abdominal hysterectomy under general anesthesia. You note that her respiratory rate has steadily risen from 16 to 26 breaths/min and that she has developed a mild, nonproductive cough. When you listen to her chest, you hear crackles throughout. She has a 40 pack-year cigarette smoking history. Identify an appropriate nursing diagnosis for this patient. Explain the reasons for your choice.

3. For each of the following concepts, use critical thinking to describe how or why it is important to nursing, patient care, or oxygenation. Note that these are *not* to be merely definitions.

Ventilation	Hypoventilation
Gas exchange	Hyperventilation
Artificial airways	Perfusion
Suctioning	Supplemental oxygen
Negative pressure in the chest	Pulse oximetry

What Are the Main Points in This Chapter?

➤ The structures of the airways, lungs, chest cavity, heart, and blood vessels function together to supply oxygen to the tissues; thus, abnormalities in any of these structures can interfere with tissue oxygenation.

➤ Developmental stage, environment, individual characteristics, lifestyle, medications, and pathological factors can interfere with ventilation, circulation, or gas exchange, leading to problems with tissue oxygenation.

➤ A health assessment related to oxygenation includes assessment of ventilation (breathing), circulation (blood flow), and gas exchange (exchange of oxygen and carbon dioxide). The length and focus of the assessment varies with the purpose and urgency of the clinical situation.

➤ A physical examination related to adequacy of oxygenation includes observations of adequacy of breathing, circulation, and gas exchange.

➤ Pulse oximetry and arterial blood gases are used to monitor oxygen saturation.

➤ Small changes in oxygen saturation are associated with large shifts in the amount of oxygen available to the tissues and organs.

➤ Interventions to promote optimal respiratory function include deep regular breathing, flu and pneumonia immunizations for at-risk individuals, frequent position changes, incentive spirometry, and preventing aspiration.

➤ Deep breathing, coughing exercises, and hydration promote deep inhalation and forceful expulsion of secretions.

➤ Supplemental oxygen is used to prevent hypoxemia. It may be delivered by a variety of methods.

➤ Artificial airways provide an open airway for patients who cannot maintain their own airway. The most common artificial airways are oropharyngeal, nasopharyngeal, and endotracheal.

➤ Airways can be suctioned to remove secretions and maintain patency. Signs that indicate the need for suctioning include gurgling sounds during respiration, restlessness, labored respirations, decreased oxygen saturation, increased heart and respiratory rates, and the presence of adventitious breath sounds during auscultation.

➤ Mechanical ventilation with a positive pressure ventilator requires the patient to have an artificial airway.

➤ Chest tubes remove air or fluid from the pleural space so that the lungs can fully expand. Chest tubes should be clamped only for changing the drainage system; clamping can lead to tension pneumothorax.

➤ Respiratory medications promote ventilation and oxygenation by their effects on the respiratory system. The major types of respiratory medicines include bronchodilators, corticosteroids, cough preparations, decongestants, antihistamines, and mucolytics.

➤ Cardiovascular function is influenced by developmental stage, environment, lifestyle, substance abuse, medications, and pathophysiological conditions such as heart failure, coronary artery disease, and peripheral vascular disorders.

➤ The purposes of cardiac monitoring are to identify the patient's baseline rhythm and rate, recognize significant changes in the baseline rhythm and rate, and recognize life-threatening dysrhythmias that require immediate intervention.

➤ Promoting circulation ensures that oxygenated blood reaches tissues and organs and venous blood returns to the heart. Activities that promote venous return and prevent clot formation assist with circulation.

➤ Cardiovascular drugs are used to enhance cardiac output, thus providing increased blood flow and oxygenation to organs and tissues. They include vasodilators, beta-adrenergic blocking agents, diuretics, and positive inotropes.

For practice questions for this chapter,

 Go to **NCLEX-Style Chapter Quiz,** on the Student Resource Disk or DavisPlus at http://davisplus.fadavis.com/Wilkinson2

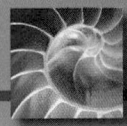 # Knowledge Map

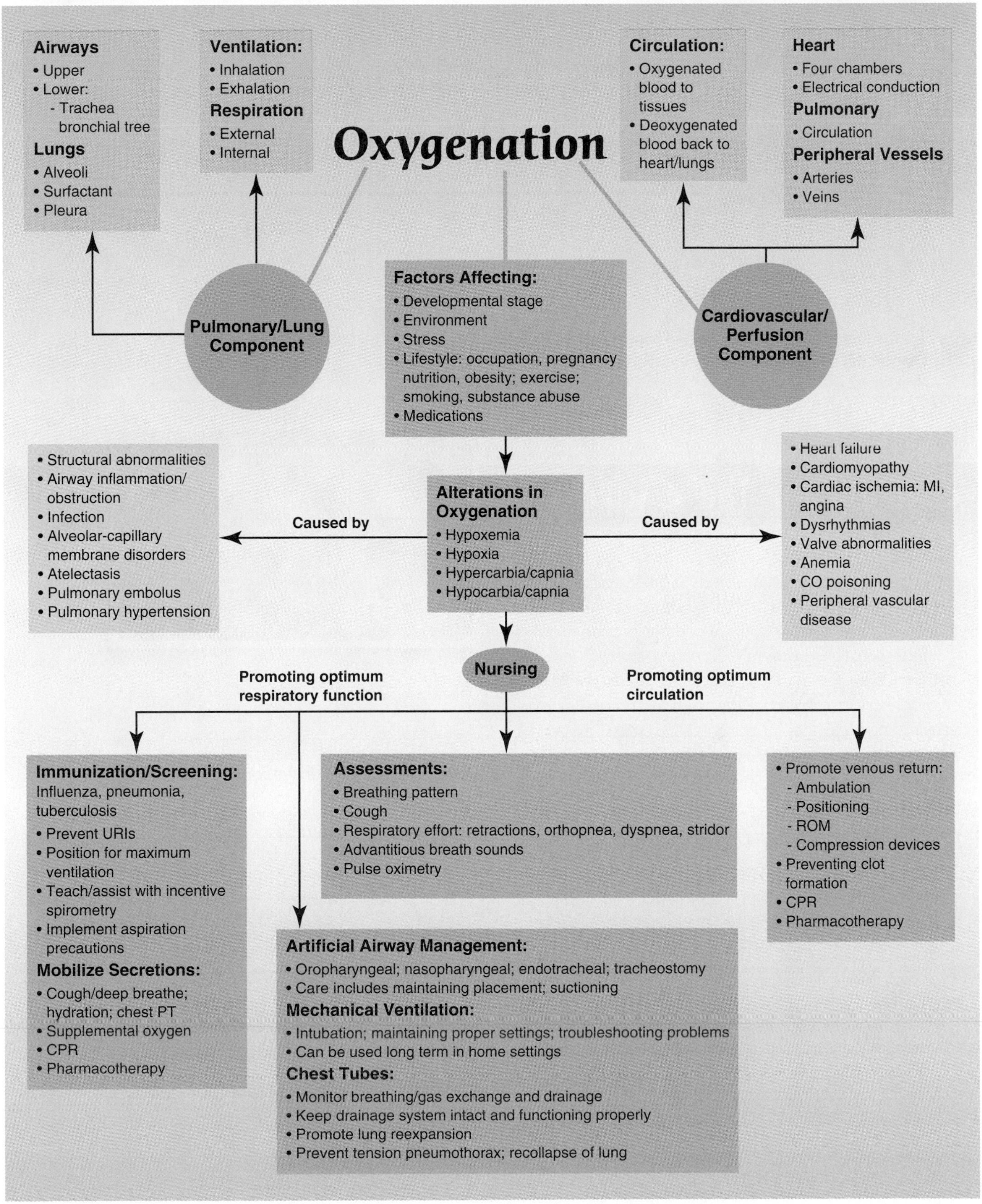

Oxygenation

Airways
- Upper
- Lower:
  - Trachea bronchial tree

Lungs
- Alveoli
- Surfactant
- Pleura

Ventilation:
- Inhalation
- Exhalation

Respiration
- External
- Internal

Circulation:
- Oxygenated blood to tissues
- Deoxygenated blood back to heart/lungs

Heart
- Four chambers
- Electrical conduction

Pulmonary
- Circulation

Peripheral Vessels
- Arteries
- Veins

Pulmonary/Lung Component

Cardiovascular/Perfusion Component

Factors Affecting:
- Developmental stage
- Environment
- Stress
- Lifestyle: occupation, pregnancy nutrition, obesity; exercise; smoking, substance abuse
- Medications

- Structural abnormalities
- Airway inflammation/obstruction
- Infection
- Alveolar-capillary membrane disorders
- Atelectasis
- Pulmonary embolus
- Pulmonary hypertension

Caused by

Alterations in Oxygenation
- Hypoxemia
- Hypoxia
- Hypercarbia/capnia
- Hypocarbia/capnia

Caused by

- Heart failure
- Cardiomyopathy
- Cardiac ischemia: MI, angina
- Dysrhythmias
- Valve abnormalities
- Anemia
- CO poisoning
- Peripheral vascular disease

Nursing

Promoting optimum respiratory function

Promoting optimum circulation

Immunization/Screening:
Influenza, pneumonia, tuberculosis
- Prevent URIs
- Position for maximum ventilation
- Teach/assist with incentive spirometry
- Implement aspiration precautions

Mobilize Secretions:
- Cough/deep breathe; hydration; chest PT
- Supplemental oxygen
- CPR
- Pharmacotherapy

Assessments:
- Breathing pattern
- Cough
- Respiratory effort: retractions, orthopnea, dyspnea, stridor
- Advantitious breath sounds
- Pulse oximetry

Artificial Airway Management:
- Oropharyngeal; nasopharyngeal; endotracheal; tracheostomy
- Care includes maintaining placement; suctioning

Mechanical Ventilation:
- Intubation; maintaining proper settings; troubleshooting problems
- Can be used long term in home settings

Chest Tubes:
- Monitor breathing/gas exchange and drainage
- Keep drainage system intact and functioning properly
- Promote lung reexpansion
- Prevent tension pneumothorax; recollapse of lung

- Promote venous return:
  - Ambulation
  - Positioning
  - ROM
  - Compression devices
- Preventing clot formation
- CPR
- Pharmacotherapy

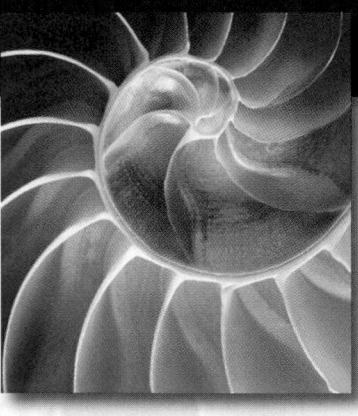

CHAPTER 36

Fluids, Electrolytes, & Acid–Base Balance

For a podcast of an overview of this chapter,

 Go to Student Resources, **Podcast – Chapter Overviews, Chapter 36,** on DavisPlus at http://davisplus.fadavis.com/Wilkinson2

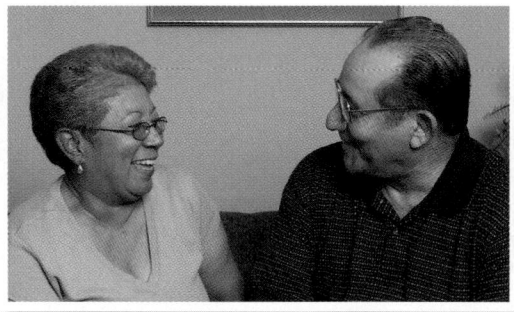

Caring for the Garcias

The exercises in the following section allow you to practice the kind of thinking you will use as a full-spectrum nurse. Because these are critical-thinking questions, there is usually no single right answer. We do not provide answers for these questions because it is more important for you to think about the questions than to arrive at the "right" answer. These questions are designed to improve your thinking more than to "cover content." Discuss answers with your peers—discussion can stimulate critical thinking. If you have difficulty with any of these questions, consult with your instructor.

Joseph Garcia has been prescribed the following medicines:

lisinopril (Prinivil) 20 mg PO daily
hydrochlorothiazide (Diuril) 25 mg PO daily in the a.m.
metformin (Glucophage) 500 mg PO before breakfast and lunch

Today he had blood drawn for analysis. Following are the electrolyte panel results.

Sodium	136 mEq/L
Potassium	3.0 mEq/L
Chloride	96 mEq/L
Bicarbonate	24 mEq/L
BUN	18 mg/dL
Creatinine	0.8 mg/dL

A. Review the lab results. Compare Joe's lab work with the established norms for these values. Based on the lab results, what kind of assessment questions would be appropriate to ask Joe?

B. Use your pharmacology text to review Joe's medications. Which, if any, of these medicines might be contributing to Joe's lab results?

C. What teaching would be appropriate for Joe?

Practical **Knowledge**
knowing why

To prevent, identify, and treat fluid, electrolyte, and acid–base problems, you will need to be skilled at initiating and managing intravenous infusions of fluids and blood, performing focused history and physical assessments, and interpreting arterial blood gas (ABG) values.

Procedures

Procedure 36-1 ☐ **Initiating a Peripheral Intravenous Infusion**

➤ For steps to follow in *all* procedures, refer to the Universal Steps for All Procedures found on the inside back cover of Volume 2.

Critical Aspects

- Prepare the intravenous solution and administration set, including extension tubing and volume-control device if used.
- Apply the tourniquet.
- Locate a vein. As a rule, select the most distal vein in an upper extremity.
- Don clean nonsterile gloves and cleanse the site. Allow the antiseptic to dry on the skin.
- Use your nondominant hand to stabilize the vein.
- Inform the patient that you are about to insert the catheter.
- Hold the catheter bevel up at a 30° to 45° angle and pierce the skin.
- Lower the catheter so that it is parallel to the skin, and advance the catheter.
- Watch for a flashback of blood; continue inserting the catheter. Remove (or retract) the needle when the catheter has been advanced at least halfway.
- While holding the catheter in place with one hand, release the tourniquet with your other hand.
- Connect the IV administration set or extension tubing to the IV catheter.
- Adjust the flow rate according to the prescriber's order.
- Secure the connection, stabilize the catheter, and apply dressing to the IV insertion site.
- Secure the tubing by looping and taping it to the skin.
- Label the dressing, tubing, and IV solution. Apply a time tape.
- Place an arm board as needed.

Equipment

- IV solution
- Administration set or IV lock and injection caps. (For a glass solution container, use vented tubing; for a plastic container you may use either vented or nonvented tubing.)
- Extension tubing with or without saline lock, possibly
- Appropriately sized intravenous (IV) catheter
- Prefilled syringe to prime extension tubing.
- Clean, unsterile gloves
- Scissors
- Antiseptic swabs that contain solutions such as chlorhexidine (preferred by the CDC, 2002) or 70% alcohol wipes. Some agencies still use 2% tincture of iodine or 10% povidone-iodine, sometimes in combination with.
- Tourniquet (non-latex, if available)
- Sterile manufactured catheter stabilization device; or ½-inch tape.

- 2-in. × 2-in. sterile gauze, and/or transparent semipermeable occlusive dressing
- 1-inch nonallergenic tape, preferably clear
- Labels, time tape
- Linen-saver pad
- Arm board, if necessary

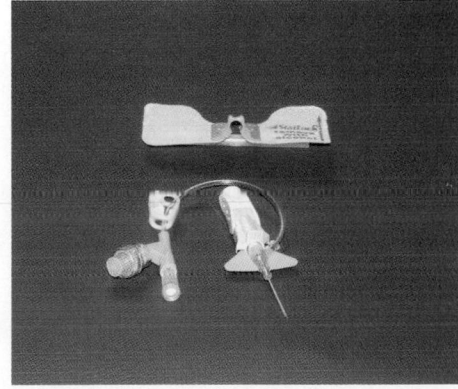

Catheter stabilization devices

(continued on next page)

Procedure 36-1 ■ Initiating a Peripheral Intravenous Infusion (continued)

Delegation

In some states and agencies you can delegate peripheral IV catheter insertion to a licensed practical nurse (LPN) who is adequately trained in the skill.

Pre-Procedure Assessment

■ Assess the patient's need for IV therapy by checking vital signs, laboratory values, urine output, skin turgor, breath sounds, and the condition of mucous membranes.

Notify the primary care provider of any situations that may contraindicate administering the prescribed fluids to the patient.

■ Assess for allergy to tape.
■ Assess the veins on the arms and hands for a potential insertion site.

Preferred sites are the upper extremities because of better blood flow, easier access, and less potential for complications than in other locations. Consider the best most distal sites first.

■ Check the medical record for factors such as anticoagulant therapy, bleeding disorders, or low platelet count.

These factors place the patient at risk for bleeding during IV catheter insertion.

➤ When performing the procedure, always identify your patient according to agency policy and be attentive to standard precautions, hand hygiene, patient safety and privacy, body mechanics, and documentation.

Procedure Steps

✚ *Note*: Maintain scrupulous aseptic technique throughout this procedure.

Any microorganisms introduced can cause infection at the site, which could quickly migrate into the bloodstream and cause sepsis.

1. Place the patient in a comfortable position and the bed at a comfortable working height and supplies within reach. Explain the procedure to the patient.

A comfortable position for the patient and the nurse will make the procedure safer, easier, and decrease the risk for the nurse to develop back problems from improper body mechanics.

2. Prepare the intravenous solution and administration set or IV lock solution.

   a. Following the "rights" of medication administration, check the IV solution to make sure that you have the proper solution with the prescribed additives.

IV solution is considered medication, and you should check it carefully to avoid administration and compatibility errors.

   b. Check the expiration date on the IV solution.

Do not use IV solution after the expiration date.

   c. Check the IV solution for discoloration or particulate matter.

Solutions that are discolored or contain particulate matter may be contaminated and should not be used.

   d. Label the IV solution container with the patient's name, date, and your initials. Place a time tape on the solution container with the prescribed infusion rate, time the infusion begins, and the time it is to be completed.

Policies govern when IV systems need to be changed, including solution containers, administration sets, dressings, and IV catheters to avoid complications such as infection. Although not all agencies require a time tape, labeling infusion rates on the solution containers in this manner will

alert others and makes it easy to see at a glance whether the solution is infusing on time.▼

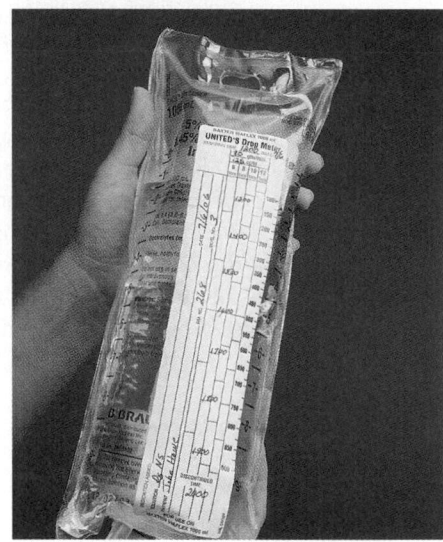

   e. Take the administration set from the package and close the roller clamp by rolling it downward. Label the tubing with the date and time.

Close the roller clamp so that fluid does not flow through inadvertently after the bag is spiked.

   f. Remove the protective cover from the solution container port.

g. Remove the protective cover from the spike on the IV administration set, making sure the spike remains sterile. Place the spike into the port of the solution container.▼

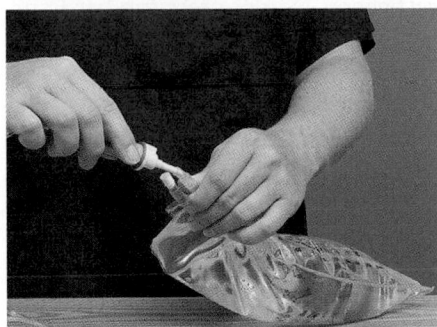

Step 2(g) Variation. Glass Bottle

If the solution is contained in a glass bottle, clean the rubber stopper on the top of the bottle with an alcohol pad. Then insert the spike of the administration set through the black rubber stopper.

h. Be certain the tubing is clamped. Hang the IV solution container on an IV pole.

Clamping prevents leakage of fluid.

i. Lightly compress the drip chamber, and allow it to fill up halfway.

Overfilling the drip chamber will impair your ability to see the drips and adequately regulate the IV flow rate.▼

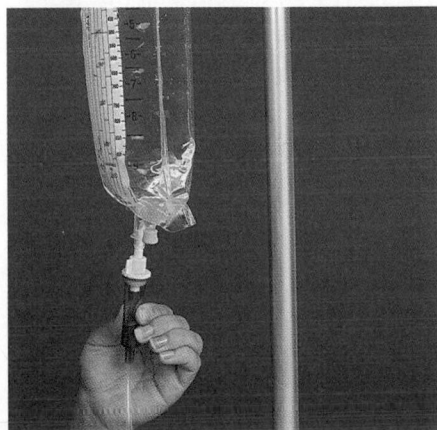

Step 2(i) Variation. No Extension Tubing

Prime the tubing by opening the roller clamp and allowing the fluid to slowly fill the tubing. When tubing is filled, close the clamp.

Step 2(i) Variation. Extension Tubing

If you are using extension tubing, either attach it to the end of the administration set now and prime it with the rest of the IV line, or prime it separately, as follows:

(1) Scrub the injection port, if there is one, of the extension tubing with an alcohol pad and let it dry.

(2) Attach a flush syringe filled with normal saline to the injection port or to the non-Luer-lock end and slowly push the fluid through the tubing until completely primed. (Consult packaging instructions for the amount of saline needed to flush the tubing.)

(3) Leave flush syringe attached to the extension tubing.

IV extension tubing makes it easier to convert an IV to a saline lock without disturbing the IV dressing and catheter. Manipulation of the IV catheter increases the risk of complications such as phlebitis, inflammation, infection, and infiltration.

j. Inspect the tubing for air. If air bubbles remain in the tubing, flick the tubing with a fingertip to mobilize them into the drip chamber. Recap end of tubing firmly.

Air in the tubing creates the potential for air embolism.

3. Place a linen-saver pad under the patient's arm.

A pad protects the bed from soiling during venipuncture.

4. Place the patient's arm in a dependent position.

Gravity helps fill and dilate the vein, making venipuncture easier.

5. Apply a tourniquet 10 to 20 cm (4 to 8 in.) above the selected site. Palpate the radial pulse. If no pulse is present, loosen the tourniquet, and reapply it with less tension.

Occluding the arterial flow diminishes venous filling, making venipuncture difficult.

6. Locate a vein for inserting the IV catheter. Select the best most distal vein on the hand or arm. Check with the medical provider before using an arm or hand that contains a dialysis

graft or fistula, or the affected arm of a patient who has undergone a mastectomy. See Clinical Insight 36-4 for more guidelines.

Choose the most distal veins on the hand or arm so that you can perform subsequent venipunctures proximal to the previous site. This preserves veins for long-term therapy and prevents extravasation of fluid and medicines.

7. Palpate the vein and press it downward, making sure that it rebounds quickly. If the vein is not adequately dilated, ask the patient to open and close his fist; apply heat (e.g., a warm towel, a warming mitt); lightly tap the vein site; or stroke the extremity from distal to proximal, beginning below the selected venipuncture site. If available in your agency, use an infrared or other visualization device to assist in locating a vein.

Maneuvers such as these also help bring blood to the local area to dilate the vein, making venipuncture easier.

8. Loosen the tourniquet. If excessive hair is present at the venipuncture site, clip it with a scissor. Loosen the tourniquet to restore blood flow and allow for patient comfort while preparing for venipuncture. Clipping the hair helps the dressings to adhere after catheter insertion. Shaving is not recommended because it may abrade the skin, providing a portal of entry for pathogens.

9. Don clean nonsterile gloves. Provides protection from inadvertent exposure to blood. Note that some nurses don gloves routinely, even when preparing supplies and equipment. However, there is no risk for coming in contact with body fluids before this step, so strictly speaking, CDC standard precautions require gloves only from this step forward.

10. Select an appropriate IV catheter based on the size of the vein, the solution to be infused, and the expected duration of therapy. Using aseptic technique, open the package. Reduces the risk of extravasation and phlebitis. Always use the smallest diameter and shortest catheter that

(continued on next page)

Procedure 36-1 ■ Initiating a Peripheral Intravenous Infusion (continued)

will deliver the desired solution flow. For most adults this will be a 20 to 24 gauge to minimize venous irritation and promote blood flow around the catheter. Aseptic handling reduces the risk of infection.

11. Gently reapply the tourniquet and scrub the site, using an antiseptic swab that contains chlorhexidine gluconate (preferred, [CDC, 2002]); if this is not available, use 70% alcohol wipes. Cleanse for 30 seconds, using friction. (Some agencies still use 2% tincture of iodine, 10% povidone-iodine. If using either of these, start at the site and work outward 2 to 3 inches.)

Removes microorganisms from the skin so that they do not enter the venous system during venipuncture. Working "clean to dirty," or from the venipuncture site outward, avoids moving microorganisms toward the puncture site. ▼

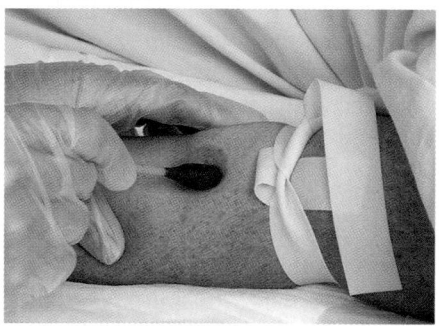

Step 11 Variation. Patient is an infant younger than 2 months old.
Proceed as in step 11, preceding, but do not use chlorhexidine to cleanse the site. Use another recommended antiseptic.

12. Allow the antiseptic to air-dry on the skin. Do not fan.
Increases the antiseptic's effectiveness; promotes patient comfort on puncture of the skin; promotes adherence of dressing.

13. Inform the patient that you are about to insert the catheter and that it may be uncomfortable.
Keeping the patient informed promotes cooperation and lessens anxiety.

14. Pick up the catheter and inspect the tip for integrity.
There should be no burrs (rough spots, ridges) on the needle or peeling of the catheter material.

Step 14 Variation. Wing-Tipped Catheter (Butterfly)
Grasp the catheter by the wings, using the thumb and forefinger of your dominant hand and making sure that the bevel is up. Remove the protective cap from the needle.
Stabilizes the catheter for insertion. Inserting the needle bevel up makes it less likely that you will pierce both vein walls (go "through" the vein) as well as making piercing the skin less painful for the patient. ▼

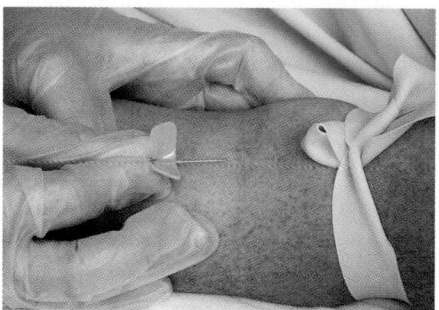

Step 14 Variation. Over-the-Needle Catheter
Grasp the catheter by the hub, using the thumb and forefinger of your dominant hand and making sure that the bevel is up.
For both variations, inserting the needle with the bevel up makes it less likely that you will pierce both vein walls (go "through" the vein) as well as making piercing the skin less painful for the patient. ▼

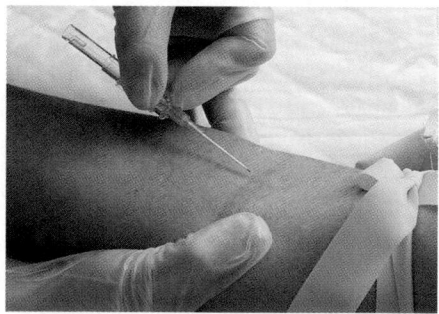

15. Using your nondominant hand, stabilize the vein by continuously pulling the skin taut below the puncture area (pull downward toward the hand or fingers). Do not press too hard, and make sure not to contaminate the insertion site.
Stabilizing the vein eases insertion and prevents damage to the underside of the vein as well as preventing the vein from rolling. Pressing too hard compresses blood flow in the vein and causes it to collapse. ▼

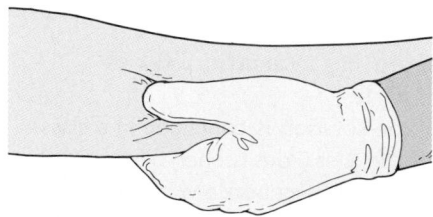

16. Holding the catheter at a 30° to 45° angle, pierce the skin directly over the vein. Penetrate all layers of the vein with one quick, smooth motion.
Holding the catheter at a 30° to 45° angle allows you to pierce the skin without inadvertently passing through the vein, and allows backflow of blood into the catheter.

17. Watch closely for a flashback of blood into the chamber of the catheter or the tubing of the winged catheter.
The flashback of blood indicates that the vein has been cannulated, but only by the needle when using an over-the-needle catheter.

18. Lower the angle of the catheter and needle to skin level and advance them into the vein.

Step 18 Variation. Wing-Tipped Catheter
Fully advance the catheter.

Step 18 Variation. Over-the-Needle Catheter
Still maintaining traction on the skin with your nondominant hand, hold the catheter hub with your thumb and middle finger, and use your index finger to advance the catheter to at least half of its length before you begin withdrawing the needle. When a steady

backflow of blood occurs, partially withdraw the needle while advancing the catheter fully into the vein. Withdrawing the needle too early will result in the catheter not fully entering the vein, only the needle. There will be no bleeding from the catheter and infiltration will occur when starting the IV solution. The patient will also complain of pain. ▼

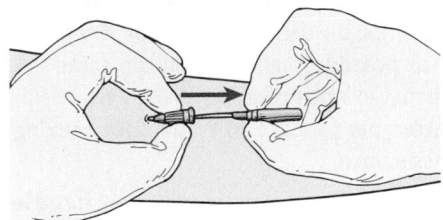

19. While holding the catheter in place with one hand, release the tourniquet and remove or retract the needle. For an over-the-needle catheter, hold the catheter in place by placing light pressure on the catheter, away from the hub and venipuncture site. For a winged needle, place a finger lightly on the same area plus a finger further along the vein away from the needle so the needle does not go through the vein.

✚ Never attempt to reinsert the needle after it is withdrawn. This can damage the catheter and even cause bits of it to break off within the vein.

Releasing the tourniquet restores full circulation to the patient's extremity and prevents injury. Placing light pressure on the catheter or vein minimizes bleeding from the catheter or needle while you complete the procedure.

20. Quickly connect the administration set to the IV catheter, using aseptic technique.
Done quickly and with aseptic technique to minimize bleeding and prevent infection. ▼

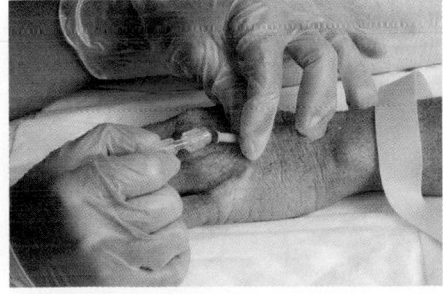

Step 20 Variation. Saline Lock
If using extension tubing with a saline lock, once connected, flush with normal saline and then disconnect the flush. A common amount is 1 to 2 mL, but tubing varies, so check package instructions for the exact amount needed.
Flushing the catheter both clears it and keeps it sterile.

21. While still stabilizing the catheter, slowly open the roller clamp. Observe that flow is achieved. Adjust the drip to the prescribed flow rate.

22. Secure the connection between the tubing and the catheter. Many sets have Luer-lock connections, so no further securing is needed. If not using Luer-lock tubing, clasping devices and threaded devices can be used. Do not use tape.
Secure the connection to prevent separation of tubing from the hub.

✚ Taping is not recommended because the junction is not visible under tape; therefore, the tubing could separate from the catheter without being discovered, possibly leading to air embolism, bleeding, or infection.

23. Stabilize the catheter. Use an agency-approved device. Catheter stabilization devices include manufactured devices (such as StatLok®), or tape.

Step 23 Variation. Stabilizing with Tape
If using tape, place a narrow (¼ in.) strip of tape under the catheter hub and crisscross the ends over the hub to form a chevron. Apply tape only to the catheter hub, not to the catheter itself, and do not apply tape directly to the site where the catheter enters the skin.
Luer locks are designed to prevent accidental disengagement of tubing and catheter; they do not stabilize the catheter. Catheter stabilization is important to minimize catheter movement and help prevent complications such as phlebitis, inflammation, infiltration, and infection.

24. Dress the site, following agency policy. If needed, clean the site with an antiseptic swab and allow it to dry before applying the dressing.

Step 24 Variation. Transparent Dressing
 a. Open the package containing the dressing. Remove the protective backing from the dressing, making sure not to touch the sterile surface.
 b. Cover the insertion site and the hub or winged portion of the catheter with the dressing. Do not cover the junction with the administration tubing.
 c. Gently pinch the transparent dressing around the catheter hub to secure the hub further. Smooth the remainder of the dressing so that it adheres to the skin. ▼

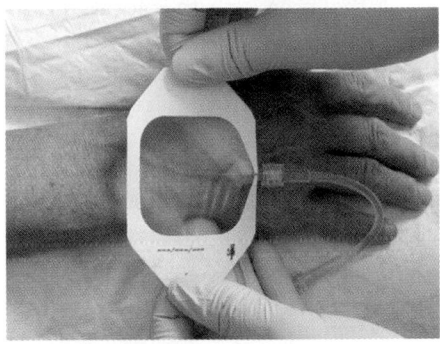

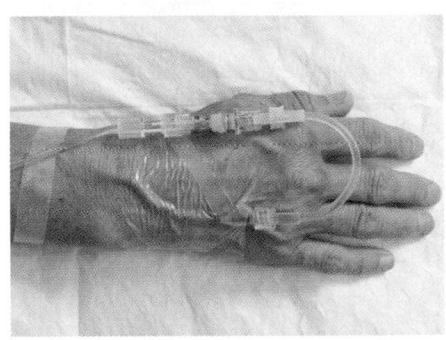

Step 24 Variation. Gauze Dressing
 a. Fold a 2 in. × 2 in. sterile gauze dressing in half, cover it with 1-inch tape (about 3 in. long).
 b. Place under the tubing/hub junction and press down on the tape.
Raises hub off the skin and prevents pressure on the skin.

 c. Place a sterile gauze pad over the insertion site and catheter hub—but not over the catheter–hub junction.
 d. Secure all edges with tape.
(continued on next page)

Procedure 36-1 ■ Initiating a Peripheral Intravenous Infusion (continued)

25. Label the dressing with the date and time of insertion, catheter size, and your initials.
A label lets nurses see at a glance how long the dressing has been in place.

26. Secure the IV administration tubing by looping and taping the tubing to the skin.
Looping the tubing supplies slack to prevent the IV catheter from becoming dislodged as well as decreases movement of the catheter decreasing the risk of phlebitis, inflammation and infiltration.

27. If the insertion site is located near a joint, place an arm board under the joint, and secure it with tape.
Using an arm board stabilizes the joint and helps prevent the catheter from becoming dislodged. However, avoid inserting an IV near a joint when possible, as there is increased potential for movement of the IV catheter, leading to an increased risk of complications. IVs placed in the antecubital fossa are difficult to assess for infiltration. Armboards are not widely used because of the high acuity of inpatients, many of whom have central lines instead of peripheral IVs.

28. Dispose of all supplies, including sharps, into appropriate receptacles; raise the siderail; lower the bed; and

be sure the patient call system is within reach. Wash your hands.
Prevent infection and ensure patient and staff safety.

What if . . .

■ **The patient is an older adult?**
Do not scrub skin too vigorously.
This can damage fragile surface tissue, creating a portal for pathogens.

Use a softer tourniquet and do not apply tightly; for well-dilated veins do not use one at all.
This increases the risk of rupture of fragile veins.

Use the smallest catheter possible to meet the infusion needs.
Insert the needle at an almost flat angle (10° to 20°).
In most older adults, veins are close to the skin surface.

Before penetrating the skin, apply traction to the vein below the insertion site.
Insert the catheter on top of the vein; do not use the side access technique.
If bleeding occurs, hold gentle pressure longer than for younger patients.
A clot may take longer to form.

■ ◆ **The patient is allergic to iodine or shellfish?**
Use 70% alcohol or chlorhexidine for 30 seconds to cleanse the site, not povidone-iodine or iodine.

■ **You are not successful with the first venipuncture attempt?**
Use a new cannula and make a second attempt on the other arm; or if that is not possible, higher up on the same arm. Do not make more than two attempts to start an IV without seeking assistance.

■ ◆ **When you insert the needle and catheter and connect the tubing, you see bright red blood quickly appear and start to advance up the tubing?**
You may have inadvertently entered an artery. If this occurs, remove the catheter and apply direct pressure for at least 5 minutes. Notify the primary care provider. Monitor the extremity distal to the insertion site for pulses, color, and temperature.

Evaluation

■ Monitor the IV site and flow rate regularly (many agency standards require hourly) while IV fluid is infusing. Check for signs of infiltration, inflammation, and phlebitis.

■ Monitor the patient's tolerance of IV therapy by auscultating breath sounds and monitoring vital signs, urine output, laboratory values, and neck vein distention. Report to the primary provider any signs of fluid overload, such as crackles, edema, shortness of breath, diminished urine output, increased blood pressure, increased heart rate with bounding pulse, and distended neck veins. Fluid overload can lead to pulmonary edema and heart failure.

Patient Teaching

■ Instruct the patient about IV therapy.

■ ◆ Teach the patient the importance of notifying staff immediately if the catheter or administration set becomes dislodged; the insertion site becomes tender, red, or swollen; or if the patient notices moisture or fluid leakage.

■ ◆ Explain the desired and adverse effects of IV therapy, and tell the patient to notify staff if he develops discomfort or breathing difficulty.

■ Teach the patient measures to avoid dislodging the catheter.

Home Care

- Explain home IV therapy to the client and caregiver, and teach them how to identify complications.
- Provide the client with the name and phone numbers of people to contact in case problems arise with the catheter site or if there is a change in level of comfort.

Documentation

- Date and time of insertion, gauge and type of catheter, number of attempts, and location of the insertion site
- Tourniquet use (or nonuse)
- Blood return in catheter; whether the IV flushes, type and amount of flush solution used
- Dressing and tape type used
- Method of securing or stabilizing the IV line
- Type and rate of the IV fluid infusing
- Patient's tolerance of the procedure, any adverse reactions to the insertion or IV therapy, and the interventions required
- Patient teaching
- Often, IV care is documented on a flowsheet. Fluids infused are documented on the I&O record as well.

Sample documentation:

06/07/11 0200 20-gauge, winged catheter inserted in cephalic vein, with tourniquet, without difficulty on first attempt. Obtained blood return, catheter flushed easily. Dressed site with a transparent, semipermeable dressing and clear tape. Catheter stabilized with fixation device. 1 L of D5/0.9% NSS hung at 125 mL/hour. Patient tolerated venipuncture without difficulty. Instructed to notify nursing staff immediately if pain or swelling occurs at the site. Also instructed about precautions to take to avoid dislodging IV catheter and importance of notifying staff immediately should catheter become dislodged.————
————————————— S. Siminez, RN

Practice Resources

Association of periOperative Registered Nurses (AORN, 2009); Betsy Lehman Centre for Patient Safety and Medical Error Reduction, JSI Research and Training Institute, Inc. (2008); Centers for Disease Control and Prevention (CDC, 2002); Gorski, L. (2007a); Infusion Nurses Society (INS, 2006b); The Joanna Briggs Institute (2008); Oncology Nursing Society (ONS, 2004); Smith, B., & Royer, T. (2007); Uslusoy, E., & Mete, S. (2008).

Thinking About the Procedure

 Go to the *Fundamentals of Nursing Skills Videos*, **Medications, Intravenous: Peripheral IV: Initiating and Regulating.**

1. Describe how the nurse secures the connection between the IV tubing and the catheter.

2. When does the nurse put on her clean nonsterile gloves? In what step of Procedure 36-1 are you instructed to don your gloves? Either way is acceptable. Which way would you prefer to do it? Explain why.

 For suggested responses, go to Chapter 36, **Thinking About the Procedure Suggested Responses (Procedure 36-1),** on the Student Resource Disk or DavisPlus at http://davisplus.fadavis.com/Wilkinson2

Procedure 36-2 □ Regulating the IV Flow Rate

➤ For steps to follow in *all* procedures, refer to the Universal Steps for All Procedures found on the inside back cover of Volume 2.

Critical Aspects

- When hanging a new container of IV solution:
  - Check the solution to make sure that you have the proper IV fluid with the prescribed additives.
  - Apply a time tape to the IV solution container. Mark the time the infusion was started.
  - Open the roller clamp so that IV fluid begins to flow.
- Verify the prescribed infusion rate.
- Calculate the drip rate.

(continued on next page)

Procedure 36-2 ■ **Regulating the IV Flow Rate** (continued)

- Hold a watch beside the drip chamber; count the number of drops for 1 minute.
- Adjust the roller clamp, increasing or decreasing the flow until you achieve the prescribed drip rate.
- Monitor the manually regulated infusion rates closely for the first 15 minutes after you begin the infusion; then monitor the rate hourly.

Equipment

- IV solution hanging on an IV pole and attached to an administration set
- Watch with a second hand or digital seconds
- Time tape

Delegation

Refer to your state nurse practice act and agency policy regarding delegation of this task to an LPN.

Pre-Procedure Assessment

- Assess the IV catheter for patency and date of insertion before starting the infusion and then regularly (many agencies specify hourly) while the IV fluid infuses.

Decreases risk of complications related to incorrect infusion rate, expired infusion solution, tubing, or catheter dwell time.

- Assess the IV site for signs of phlebitis, infiltration, infection, or inflammation.

You must change the IV catheter before regulating the flow rate if any of these complications occur.

- Confirm the patient's need for IV therapy by verifying the order and checking laboratory values, urine output, vital signs, and breath sounds.

Ensures that the patient still needs IV fluids and that the solution is correct. Laboratory values and assessment findings monitor the IV treatment plan. IV therapy creates a risk for fluid overload.

➤ When performing the procedure, always identify your patient according to agency policy and be attentive to standard precautions, hand hygiene, patient safety and privacy, body mechanics, and documentation.

Procedure Steps

1. Follow all the "checks" and "rights" of medication administration, including verifying the prescription. Check the solution to make sure that you have the proper IV fluid hanging with the prescribed additives, and that there is no discoloration of or particles or crystallization in the fluid. Also verify the infusion rate.

IV solution is considered medication, and you should check it carefully to avoid administration and compatibility errors. Do not simply pull a bag of fluid from a shelf assuming that the shelf is labeled properly, as bags are often misplaced and this is a potential source of error.

Note: If you are using a volume-control pump, you can omit steps 2, 3, and 4.

2. Calculate the hourly rate if it is not specified in the order. Divide the volume to be infused by the number of hours it is to be infused. For example, if the physician prescribes

1000 mL to run over 4 hours, the infusion rate is 250 mL/hr.

You must carefully calculate the infusion rate to ensure that the patient receives the correct volume of fluid.

3. Calculate the drip rate by multiplying the number of milliliters to be infused in 60 minutes by the drop factor in drops/per milliliter; then divide by 60 minutes:

$$\frac{\text{Hourly rate in mL} \times (\text{drops/mL})}{60 \text{ minutes}} = \text{drip rate}$$

For example, an hourly rate of 100 mL multiplied by 15 drops/mL and divided by 60 minutes equals 25. Therefore, the drip rate equals 25 drops per minute.

Each administration set has a drip factor that is determined by the manufacturer. The **drip factor** is the number of drops necessary to deliver 1 mL of solution. Microdrip tubing has a drip factor of 60 drops/mL; blood administration tubing typically has a drip factor of 10 drops/mL; macrodrip tubing has a drip factor of 15 drops/mL.

Most IV solutions are delivered via a volume-control pump; however, there may be instances in which you will need to perform these calculations.

4. Verify your calculations.

To prevent dosage errors, either have a second person verify your calculations or check them a second time yourself.

5. When hanging a new bag, apply a time tape to the IV solution container next to the volume markings. Mark the time tape with the time that the infusion was started. Continue to mark 1-hour intervals on the time tape until you reach the bottom of the container.

The time tape allows all nurses to accurately monitor the rate of administration.

6. Open the roller clamp so that IV fluid begins to flow (when hanging a new bag).

The roller clamp must be opened to allow the flow of fluid.

7. Set the rate.

Step 7 Variation. Gravity Drip

Using a watch placed next to the drip chamber, count the number of drops entering the drip chamber in 1 minute. Adjust the roller clamp by increasing or decreasing the flow until you achieve the prescribed drip rate.

Timing the drip rate for 1 minute helps to accurately achieve the correct drip rate and having the watch next to what you are counting will ensure that you do not miss seeing any drops. ▼

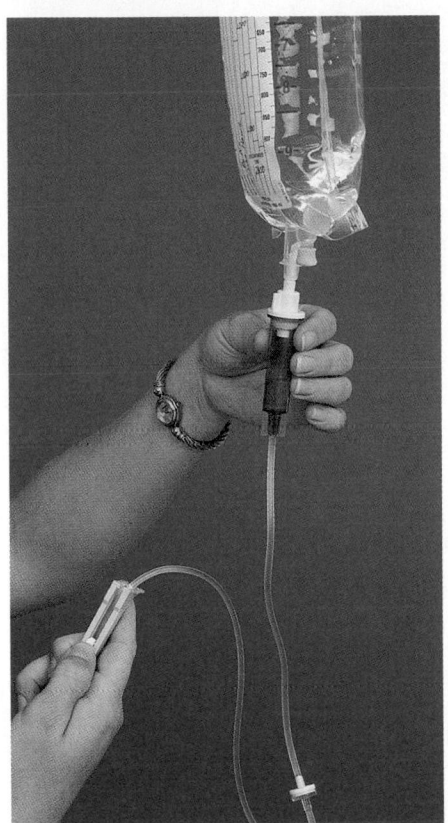

Step 7 Variation. Volume-Control Pump

Program the ordered rate into the pump.

IV solution is considered a medication and must infuse at the prescribed rate.

8. Monitor manually regulated infusion rates closely for the 15 minutes after you begin an infusion; then monitor it regularly by counting drops per minute or reading the numbers on the pump.

Changes in the patient's position may speed up or slow down the infusion rate; frequent monitoring of the infusion rate ensures that the correct volume of fluid infuses over the correct length of time.

What if...

- **The prescription for the IV flow rate changes?**

Recalculate the new flow rate and adjust the drops/minute to obtain the desired new flow rate. Also, remove the old time tape and place a new time tape with the new rate of infusion.

- **When you check the rate, you discover that the IV has been running too slowly for the past hour?**

Adjust to the correct rate, but do not attempt to catch up by adjusting the flow to a rate higher than prescribed. Too rapid IV infusion can lead to fluid overload for patients with congestive heart failure or other cardiopulmonary problems.

- **When you check the rate, you discover that the IV has been running too fast for the past hour?**

Slow the rate and assess the patient for signs of fluid volume excess.

Evaluation

- Evaluate the patient's response to IV therapy by checking for signs of excessive or deficient fluid volume.
- Evaluate the IV site for signs of infiltration, inflammation, infection, and phlebitis.
- Check laboratory studies to help evaluate the effectiveness of IV therapy.
- Monitor for correct IV rate at least hourly.
- Evaluate the tubing for kinks, patient lying on the tubing.

  Kinked tubing will interfere with the flow rate.

Patient Teaching

- Explain the desired and adverse effects of IV therapy.
- Discuss the importance of notifying staff immediately if the catheter or administration set becomes dislodged; if the insertion site becomes tender, red, or swollen; if the patient notices moisture or fluid leakage; or if he has difficulty breathing.
- Teach safety measures if the patient is permitted to ambulate while the IV is infusing.

(continued on next page)

Procedure 36-2 ■ Regulating the IV Flow Rate (continued)

Home Care

- Explain home IV therapy to the client and caregiver, and teach them how to identify complications.
- Provide the client and caregiver with the name and phone numbers of people to contact in case problems arise with the catheter, insertion site, or level of comfort.

Documentation

- Date and time the infusion was started
- Type of IV fluid, rate of infusion, and IV catheter site
- Whether rate is manual or pump controlled
- Patient's tolerance of IV therapy, any complications, and the interventions taken
- Document the volume infused on the I&O record. Often IV care is documented on a flowsheet.

Sample documentation:

09/18/11   1500   An infusion of D₅1/2 NS was started through a 20-gauge catheter, located in the right forearm at a rate of 100 mL/hr. No redness, swelling, or discomfort present at the site. Patient's lungs are clear to auscultation. Urine output greater than 30 mL/hour; see I & O sheet. Patient NPO for a CT scan of the abdomen. Tolerating IV fluid without difficulty. ————
                                                S. Chen, RN

Practice Resources

Infusion Nurses Society (INS, 2006a, 2006b); Oncology Nursing Society (ONS, 2004); Phillips, L. (2010).

Thinking About the Procedure

 Go to the *Fundamentals of Nursing Skills Videos,* **Medications, Intravenous: Peripheral IV: Initiating and Regulating.**

1. Near the very end of the procedure, the nurse times the IV drip rate. Is the IV running by pump or by gravity?

2. What kind of administration set is hanging, macrodrip or microdrip?

3. Aside from the fact that the drops are difficult to see, why can you not count the drip rate accurately from the DVD?

 For suggested responses, go to Chapter 36, **Thinking About the Procedure Suggested Responses (Procedure 36-2),** on the Student Resource Disk or DavisPlus at http://davisplus.fadavis.com/Wilkinson2

Procedure 36-3 ■ Setting Up and Using Volume-Control Pumps

➤ For steps to follow in *all* procedures, refer to the Universal Steps for All Procedures found on the inside back cover of Volume 2.

Critical Aspects

- Calculate the infusion rate.
- Attach the volume-control pump to the IV pole, and plug it into the nearest electrical outlet.
- Take the administration set from the package, close the clamp, and spike the port of the solution container.
- Label the tubing and solution container.
- Hang the solution container on the IV pole.
- Place the electronic eye on the drip chamber, if there is one. If not consult the manufacturer's instructions.
- Prime the administration tubing then close the clamp.
- Turn on the pump, and load the administration tubing into the pump.
- Program the pump with the hourly infusion rate, total hours, and the volume to be infused.
- Apply clean nonsterile gloves.
- Cleanse the injection port and check the IV site for patency.
- Connect the tubing adapter to the injection port.
- Unclamp the administration set tubing, and press the start button.
- Make sure that the alarms are turned on and audible.
- Check the pump regularly to make sure that the correct volume is infusing.
- At the end of your shift (or at the specified time), clear the pump and record the volume.

Equipment

- Nonsterile gloves
- Alcohol wipes or chlorhexidine/alcohol antiseptic product
- Volume-control pump
- Administration set appropriate for the pump
- IV pole
- IV fluid or medicated solution
- Tape for IV fluid solution time tape

Delegation

You can delegate the task of setting up a volume-control pump to an LPN who is specially trained in IV therapy if covered by the agency's policy and procedure. Do not delegate this task to a nursing assistive personnel (NAP). Do, however, instruct the NAP to notify you of any pump alarms that sound.

Pre-Procedure Assessment

- Confirm the patient's need for IV therapy by checking vital signs, laboratory values, urine output, skin turgor, breath sounds, and the moisture of mucous membranes.

Following laboratory values and assessment findings monitors the IV treatment plan. IV therapy creates a risk for fluid overload and electrolyte imbalance.

- Assess the existing IV catheter for patency.

Occlusion of the IV catheter prevents the infusion of IV fluid. If not patent, you will need to change the IV.

- Assess the IV site hourly for signs of phlebitis, infiltration, infection and inflammation.

Complications of IV therapy retard the therapeutic benefit of the fluids as well as increase medical concerns, and treatment cost for the patient. You must change the IV if any of these complications occur.

➤ When performing the procedure, always identify your patient according to agency policy and be attentive to standard precautions, hand hygiene, patient safety and privacy, body mechanics, and documentation.

Procedure Steps

1. Calculate the infusion rate by dividing the volume to be infused by the number of hours it is to be infused. For example, if the order states 1000 mL to run over 8 hours, divide 1000 mL by 8 hours to determine the infusion rate of 125 mL/hr.

This is to ensure that the patient receives the correct dose. Pumps are usually programmed in milliliters per hour instead of drops per minute.

2. Verify your calculations.

To prevent dosage errors, either ask a second person verify your calculations or check them a second time yourself.

3. Attach the pump to the IV pole, and plug it into the nearest electrical outlet.

✚ Check to be sure that the infusion pump has a safety sticker on it and that the cord and plug are intact.

Volume-control pumps need regular maintenance checks. Using an electrical outlet saves battery power if needed for transport or electrical outage. As with gravity flow, the IV solution container needs to remain above the pump to prevent occlusion

and for proper drainage of the container. ▼

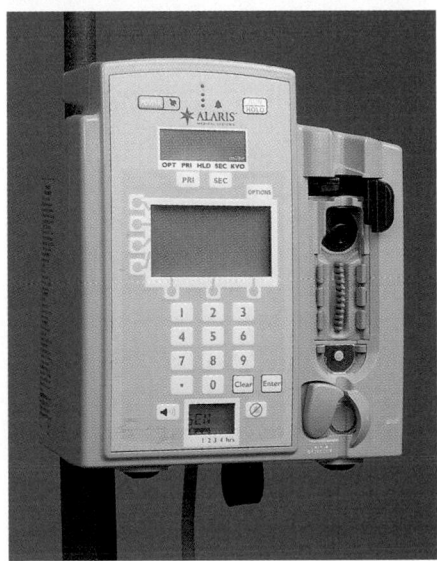

4. Take the administration set from the package, and close the clamp on the administration set.

Close the clamp to prevent inadvertent loss of fluid.

5. If a filter is required, attach it to the end of the administration set.

Filters are sometimes used to filter minute particles from the solution.

6. Remove the protective covers, and spike the port of the solution container with the administration set, maintaining sterility. Label the IV tubing and solution container with

the date and time, and place a time tape on the solution container. Hang the container on the IV pole.

Labeling the administration set with the date and time informs the nursing staff when the administration set should be changed. The time tape allows you, and other nurses, to see at a glance whether the correct volume is infusing.

7. Compress the drip chamber of the administration set, and allow it to fill halfway. Consult the manufacturer's instructions for setup, as pumps differ. (On older gravity pumps, place the electronic eye on the drip chamber between the fluid level and the origin of the drop.)

Prepares the administration set for priming and prevents air from entering the tubing with the solution. Infusion pumps compress the tubing to move fluid; they measure the amount internally. On older gravity-type pumps, an electronic eye counts the number of drops to ensure the proper rate.

8. Prime the administration set with fluid by opening the roller clamp and allowing the fluid to flow slowly through the tubing. Close the clamp.

Priming removes air from the tubing to prevent air embolus.

9. Inspect the tubing for the presence of air. If air bubbles remain in the tubing, flick the tubing with a fingertip

(continued on next page)

Procedure 36-3 ■ **Setting Up and Using Volume-Control Pumps** (continued)

to mobilize the bubbles into the drip chamber.
Air bubbles in the administration tubing interrupt flow and they can cause air emboli, which can be dangerous to the patient if they accumulate in the circulation.

10. Turn on the pump, and load the administration tubing into the pump according to the manufacturer's instructions.
This process differs among manufacturers. ▼

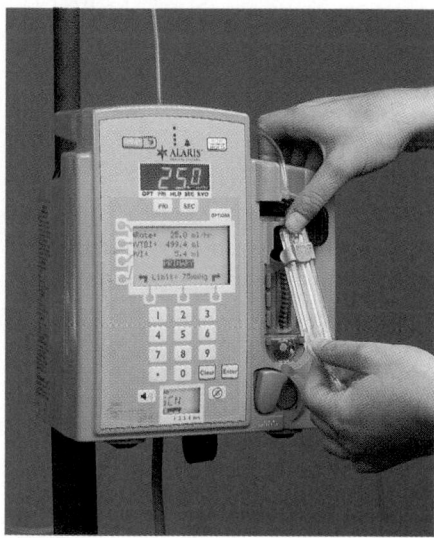

11. Program the pump with the prescribed information: total hours, infusion rate (hourly rate) and the volume to be infused (usually the total amount in the IV bag). *Note:* Some pumps have only total hours and

volume to infuse and do not have a calculation-of-rate feature. ▼

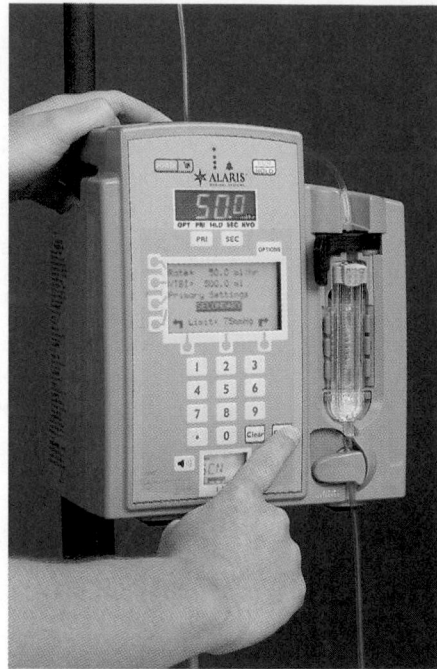

12. Apply clean nonsterile gloves, check the IV site for patency, and scrub all surfaces of the injection port or needleless connector, including the threads, with an antiseptic pad for at least 15 seconds. Allow it to dry.
Clean nonsterile gloves protect from exposure to body fluids when you connect the tubing to the IV catheter or port. Scrubbing the port helps prevent infection.

13. Connect the administration set adapter to the injection port, keeping the connecting ends sterile.
Aseptic technique decreases the risk for contamination.

14. Unclamp the administration set tubing (open the roller clamp all the way), and press the start button on the pump.
Allows the IV fluid to flow through the administration set.

15. Make sure that the alarms are turned on and audible.
The alarms must be functioning so that the pump can alert you of problems, such as kinks, air in the tubing, or catheter occlusion. Do not depend on the pump alarms to indicate IV patency. Pumps can infuse fluid, even if the line is clogged or infiltrated into the surrounding tissue.

16. Check the pump regularly (often this is hourly) to make sure the correct volume is infusing.
Infusion pumps sometimes malfunction, so frequent monitoring is essential.

17. At the end of your shift (or at the time specified by your healthcare facility), clear the pump of the volume infused and record the volume on the patient's I&O form.
Clearing the pump of the volume infused during your shift helps the oncoming shift accurately monitor the fluid infused during their shift.

What if. . .

■ **In later evaluation you find the IV free flowing and not running via the pump setting?**

Immediately slow the IV fluid down. At the same time, begin assessing the patient: vital signs, mental awareness, lung sounds, pulse oximetry. Depending on the type of fluid running, you may need to make other assessments as well. Calculate the amount of IV fluid actually infused compared to the prescribed amount. Notify the provider and write out an occurrence report. If the pump is malfunctioning, notify biomedical engineering so they can repair it. Manufacturers sometimes recall certain pump models due to malfunctioning.

Evaluation

■ Monitor the correct functioning of the pump regularly, perhaps hourly.

Patient Teaching

■ Explain use of the IV infusion pump to the patient.
■ Teach the patient the importance of notifying staff immediately if the infusion pump alarm sounds, the

catheter or administration set becomes dislodged, the insertion site becomes tender, red, or swollen, or the dressing becomes wet.
■ Teach the patient safety measures if he is able to ambulate while the infusion pump is in use.

Home Care

■ Explain home IV infusion pump use to the client and caregiver, and teach them how to identify complications.

Most home infusion pumps are smaller than institutional pumps.

■ Provide the client with the name and phone numbers of people to contact in case problems arise with the catheter, insertion site, IV infusion pump, or other equipment.

Documentation

■ Type and volume of IV fluid infusing, along with the infusion rate
■ Use of the infusion pump, and patient's tolerance of IV therapy
■ Any complications of IV therapy and the interventions taken
■ Document volume infused on the patient's I&O record and/or an IV flowsheet.

Sample documentation:

07/26/11   0600   *Patient admitted from the ED with dehydration. NSS infusing at 250 mL/hr via infusion pump through an 18-gauge catheter. No signs of infiltration. No tenderness, redness, or swelling at the insertion site. Temp 102.6°F orally, HR 118 beats/minute, RR 24 breaths/minute, and BP 90/46.* —————————— *R. Brill, RN*

Practice Resources
Phillips, L. (2010).

Thinking About the Procedure

 Go to the *Fundamentals of Nursing Skills Videos,* **Medications, Intravenous: Infusion Pump.**

1. When did the nurse spike the IV bag with the administration set: before or after hanging the bag on the IV pole?

2. When does the procedure in this book tell you to spike the bag?

3. Do you think it makes any difference which is done first? Explain your thinking.

 For suggested responses, go to Chapter 36, **Thinking About the Procedure Suggested Responses (Procedure 36-3),** on the Student Resource Disk or DavisPlus at http://davisplus.fadavis.com/Wilkinson2

Procedure 36-4 ☐ Changing IV Solutions and Tubing

➤ For steps to follow in *all* procedures, refer to the Universal Steps for All Procedures found on the inside back cover of Volume 2.

Critical Aspects

Procedure 36-4A: Changing the IV Solution
■ Prepare and label your next container of IV solution at least 1 hour before the present infusion is scheduled to finish.
■ Close the roller clamp on the infusing (empty) administration set.
■ Remove the old IV solution container from the IV pole. Remove the spike from the bag, keeping the spike sterile.
■ Spike the new IV solution container.
■ Hang the new IV solution, and clear the tubing of air.
■ Adjust the drip rate.
■ Place a time tape on the new IV solution container. Mark the times.

Procedure 36-4B: Changing the IV Solution and Tubing
■ Prepare and hang the new IV solution and tubing.
■ Close the roller clamp on the old administration set.
■ Wearing clean nonsterile gloves, stabilize the IV catheter while applying pressure over the vein just above the insertion site.
■ Disconnect the used tubing.
■ Remove the protective cover from the distal end of the new administration set.
■ Stabilize the IV catheter while applying pressure over the vein just above the insertion site and connect the new tubing.

(continued on next page)

Procedure 36-4 ■ **Changing IV Solutions and Tubing** (continued)

- Disengage the old tubing from the IV catheter and insert the new tubing.
- Adjust the drip rate.
- Cleanse the IV site.
- Resecure the IV catheter and tubing connection; loop and tape the tubing.
- Label tubing and solution with date, initials, rate, and time tape.

Equipment

- Nonsterile gloves
- Administration set
- IV solution
- IV pole
- Antiseptic swabs that contain solutions such as 70% alcohol or 2% chlorhexidine (chlorhexidine is not recommended in infants younger than age 2 months). You may use iodine-based products if alcohol or chlorhexidine are contraindicated and the patient is not allergic to iodine.
- 1-inch nonallergenic tape
- Time tape
- Watch with a second hand or digital seconds

Delegation

You can delegate the tasks of changing IV solutions and tubing to an LPN who is specially trained in IV therapy. The task should not be delegated to a NAP. Do, however, instruct the NAP to notify you of any problems that occur with IV therapy, such as the disconnecting of the administration set; catheter dislodging; or complaints of pain, swelling, or redness at the insertion site.

Pre-Procedure Assessments

- Assess the IV catheter for patency before changing the solution container or administration set.
- Assess the IV site for signs of phlebitis, infiltration, infection, or inflammation.

If any of these complications exist, the current IV will need to be discontinued and a new IV started.

- Check IV catheter insertion date.

IV catheters are replaced per agency guidelines, which are based on the Centers for Disease Control (CDC) recommendations of changing a peripheral IV site every 72 to 96 hours.

■ Procedure 36-4A   **Changing the IV Solution**

➤ When performing the procedure, always identify your patient according to agency policy and be attentive to standard precautions, hand hygiene, patient safety and privacy, body mechanics, and documentation.

Procedure Steps

1. Following the "rights" of medication administration, prepare and label your next container of IV solution at least 1 hour before the present infusion is scheduled to finish.

Preparing the next IV solution container reduces the risk of the present container running dry and thereby causing clots to form that would occlude the catheter.

2. Close the roller clamp on the administration set.

Prevents air from entering the tubing while the IV solution container is being changed.

3. Wearing clean nonsterile gloves, remove the old IV solution container from the IV pole. Remove the spike

from the bag, keeping the spike sterile.

The spike must remain sterile to prevent contamination of the new IV fluid. Clean nonsterile gloves protect you from exposure to body fluids.

4. Remove the protective cover from the new IV solution container port.

5. Place the spike into the port of the new solution container.

Step 5 Variation. Glass Bottle

If the solution is contained in a glass IV bottle, first scrub the rubber stopper on the top of the bottle with an antiseptic pad; then, insert the spike of the administration set through the black rubber stopper.

Cleansing the stopper removes particulate matter and microbes.

6. Hang the IV solution container on the IV pole.

Allows the fluid to infuse by gravity.

7. Inspect the tubing to be sure that it is free of air bubbles and the drip chamber remains half-filled. Flick the tubing with a finger to mobilize the bubbles into the drip chamber.

Prevents air from entering the system as the new solution is hung. If the drip chamber becomes too full, it will be difficult to impossible to count the drip rate properly and regulate the IV.

8. Open the roller clamp and adjust the drip rate, as prescribed.

IV solution is considered a medication and must infuse at the prescribed rate for therapeutic effect and to prevent fluid overload.

9. If practiced within your agency, affix the time tape to the new IV solution container. Mark the tape with the time the infusion was started, and continue to mark 1-hour intervals on the time tape until you reach the bottom of the container.
The time tape allows you and other nurses to monitor the rate of administration accurately.

10. Dispose of used supplies into appropriate receptacles, according to agency policy in line with CDC guidelines.

■ **Procedure 36-4B** **Changing the IV Administration Tubing and Solution**

➤ When performing the procedure, always identify your patient according to agency policy and be attentive to standard precautions, hand hygiene, patient safety and privacy, body mechanics, and documentation.

Procedure Steps

1. Prepare the IV solution and tubing as you would when initiating a new IV. (See Procedure 36-1, step 2.)

2. Hang the new administration set on the IV pole.

3. Close the roller clamp on the old administration set.
Stops the flow of fluid from the old container.

4. Disconnect the old tubing:
   a. Wearing clean nonsterile gloves, place a sterile swab under the catheter hub.
The swab absorbs any leakage from the catheter hub when you disconnect the tubing.

   b. Apply pressure to the vein about 3 inches above the insertion site, using the fourth or fifth finger of your nondominant hand. Hold the catheter hub firmly with the thumb and index finger of that hand, but do not apply downward pressure.
This prevents blood from leaking out of the catheter during the tubing change. Holding the hub firmly keeps the catheter from moving about and traumatizing the vein.

   c. Then carefully remove the device securing the connection between the catheter and tubing. This may be as simple as unscrewing a Luer lock. The connection should not be covered by tape, but if it is, remove it so you can access the connection.

5. Remove the protective cover from the distal end of the new administration set.

Cover keeps the distal end sterile until you are ready to connect it to the IV catheter.

6. Continue to stabilize the IV catheter with your nondominant hand while applying pressure over the vein. ▼

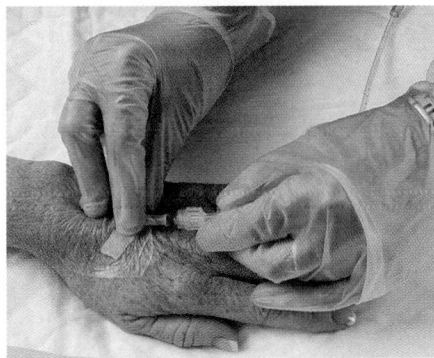

7. Gently disengage the used tubing from the IV catheter, and place it in a basin or other receptacle. Quickly insert the new tubing into the catheter hub.
IV tubing should be changed every 72 to 96 hours, depending on agency policy and solution. Certain solutions require more frequent, every 24 to 48 hours, tubing changes. Change it quickly to prevent microorganisms from entering the IV catheter.

8. Open the roller clamp on the new administration set, and allow the IV solution to infuse.
Allowing the solution to infuse clears the IV catheter of blood, preventing catheter occlusion.

9. Program and turn on the volume-control pump. Or, for a gravity drip, use the roller clamp to adjust the flow to the prescribed rate.
IV solution is considered a medication and must infuse at the prescribed rate.

10. Cleanse the IV site and secure the IV catheter and tubing connection.
Removes microorganisms and media for growth; helps preserve the integrity of the intact line; and prevents air and microorganisms from entering the line.

11. Loop and tape tubing to patient's skin.
Helps minimize catheter movement, which contributes to phlebitis.

12. Label tubing and solution with date, initials, rate, and time tape.
Alerts staff to when tubing and solution was changed and to when they will need to be changed again to decrease the incidence of infection.

13. Dispose of used supplies into appropriate receptacles according to agency policy in line with CDC guidelines.

What if . . .

■ **The drip chamber becomes too full (over half) so that drops cannot be adequately counted?**
Close the roller clamp, invert the bag or bottle, and squeeze the excess fluid back into the bag/bottle.

■ **The tubing will not separate from the catheter connection when you attempt to disconnect it?**
If the lock does not twist off, gently try using a hemostat ("mosquito" clamp) to twist the lock. Do not lock the hemostat; merely use it lightly as a grip. After the lock is off, if the tubing will not separate, use the hemostat to gently twist the tubing back and forth. If the catheter needs to be stabilized, wear a sterile glove or use a sterile hemostat.

(continued on next page)

Procedure 36-4 ■ **Changing IV Solutions and Tubing** (continued)

Evaluation

- Evaluate the IV insertion site for signs of infiltration, inflammation, infection, and phlebitis.
- Evaluate the effectiveness of IV therapy by assessing the patient's hydration status or expected effect of the intravenous medication/solution.
- Evaluate proper IV rate regularly (usually hourly).

Patient Teaching

- Discuss the importance of notifying staff immediately if the catheter or administration set becomes dislodged; if the insertion site becomes tender; red, or swollen; or if the IV dressing becomes wet.

Home Care

- Explain home IV therapy to the client and caregiver; teach them how to identify complications.
- Obtain a return demonstration to ensure the caregiver is able to perform fluid and tubing, changes when necessary.

Documentation

- Fluid and tubing changes are usually documented on a flowsheet.
- Document the date and time the IV fluid and tubing were changed; type of IV fluid and rate of infusion; as well as the location and condition of the IV catheter insertion site.
- Any complications of IV therapy and the interventions taken.

Sample documentation:

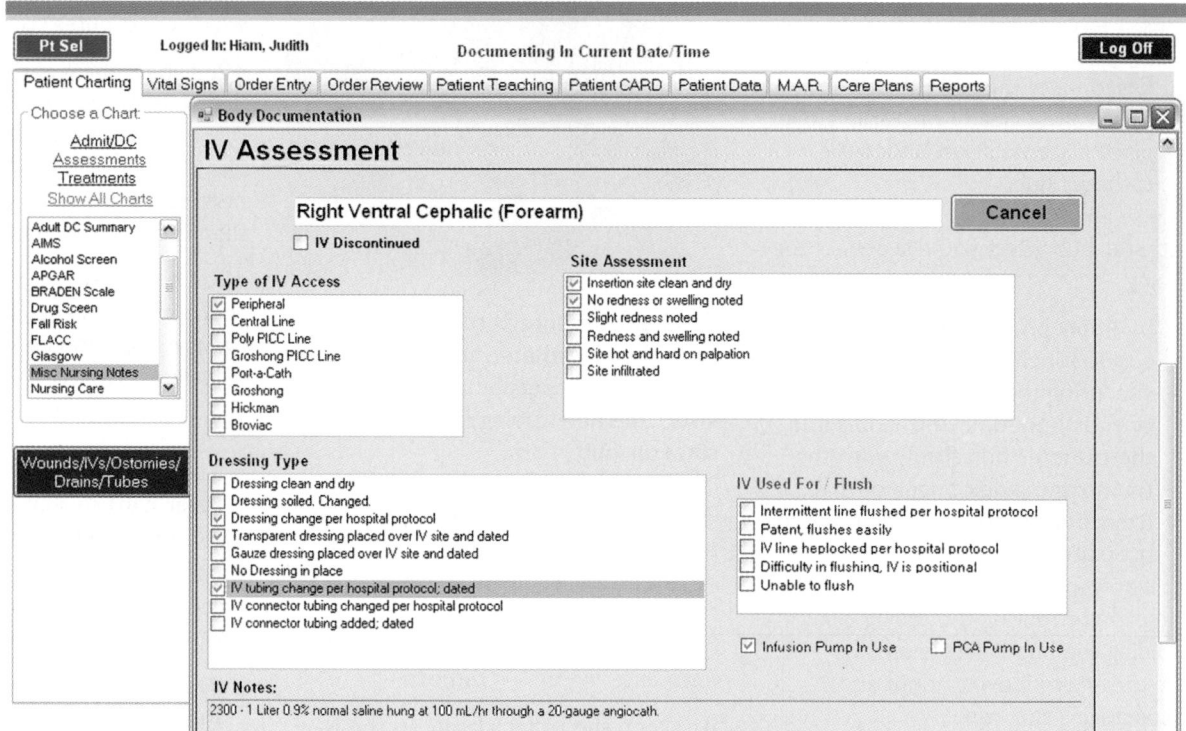

Practice Resources

Centers for Disease Control and Prevention (CDC, 2002); Gillies, D., Wallen, M., Morrison, A. L., et al. (2005); Infusion Nurses Society (INS, 2006a, 2006b); Oncology Nursing Society (ONS, 2004).

Procedure 36-5 ☐ Changing IV Dressings

➤ For steps to follow in *all* procedures, refer to the Universal Steps for All Procedures found on the inside back cover of Volume 2. For this procedure, also refer to Clinical Insights 20-3, 20-4, 20-5, and 20-7 if you need to review information about medical and surgical asepsis.

Critical Aspects

Procedure 36-5A: Peripheral IV Dressings
- Wearing clean nonsterile gloves, stabilize the catheter with your nondominant hand, and carefully remove the dressing.
- Inspect the insertion site.
- Don clean gloves. Cleanse the insertion site, following the manufacturer's guidelines for product use.
- Allow the antiseptic to dry on the skin.
- Don clean nonsterile gloves.
- Apply a new sterile catheter stabilization device and dressing.
- Secure the connection between the catheter and the tubing.
- Loop and tape the tubing to the patient's skin.
- Label the dressing with the date and time of insertion, catheter size, the date the dressing was changed, and your initials.

Procedure 36-5B: Central Line Dressings
- Obtain sterile central line dressing kit and mask for the patient. If there is no kit, you will need at least a mask, sterile gloves, antiseptic solution, dressing, and tape.
- Place the patient in a comfortable position. Some guidelines advise semi-Fowler's.
- Ask the patient to turn his head to the opposite side if unable to tolerate a mask.
- Don mask and clean nonsterile gloves.
- Carefully remove the old dressing and stabilization device.
- Inspect the site for signs of complications.
- Remove and discard gloves and soiled dressing. Wash hands.
- Set up a sterile field and arrange your supplies.
- Don sterile gloves contained in the kit.
- Scrub the site, using swabs contained in kit.
- Scrub the catheter, hubs, extension tails, and sutures (if any) with an antiseptic swab for at least 15 seconds.
- Allow the site to dry.
- Apply dressing that comes in the kit.
- Apply the new catheter stabilization device, if one is used.
- Remove the drape, if one was used.
- Loop the catheter gently and secure it with tape to the skin. Avoid securing it to the dressing.
- Label the dressing with the date changed, time, and your initials.

Equipment

Peripheral IV Dressings

- Clean nonsterile gloves
- Sterile transparent semipermeable dressing or dressing specified by institution
- Antiseptic swabs: alcohol or chlorhexidine (*Note:* Use iodine-based products only if the preferred antiseptics cannot be used. Chlorhexidine is not recommended in infants younger than age 2 months.)
- 1-inch nonallergenic tape or manufactured stabilization device

Central Line Dressings

- Clean nonsterile gloves
- Central line dressing kit. It should include sterile gloves, a mask, a sterile transparent semipermeable dressing, sterile tape, an antimicrobial agent, and a sterile catheter

stabilization device. If it does not, obtain them. *Note:* It is acceptable to povidone-iodine followed by alcohol as the antimicrobial if the preferred chlorhexidine is contraindicated.
- A sponge containing the antimicrobial agent chlorhexidine gluconate may be used as a part of the dressing, as well.

To reduce the risk for catheter-related infection (Timsit, Schwebel, Boudma, et al., 2009).

- Mask for patient (possibly)

Note: Some institutions do not include this in their procedure and a few patients cannot tolerate wearing a mask.

Delegation

You can delegate the tasks of changing dressings to an LPN who is specially trained in IV therapy. The task should not be delegated to a NAP. Do, however, instruct the NAP to notify

(continued on next page)

Procedure 36-5 ■ **Changing IV Dressings** (continued)

you of any problems that occur with dressing such as soiling, blood, leakage, or loosening.

Pre-Procedure Assessments

For Peripheral Catheters

■ Assess the IV catheter for patency before changing the dressing.
Ensure that the IV is still working properly.

■ Assess the IV site for signs of phlebitis, infiltration, infection, or inflammation.

If any of these complications exist, the current IV will need to be discontinued and a new IV started.

■ Assess for allergy to tape.
■ Assess IV catheter start date.

IV catheters are replaced per agency guidelines which are based on the Centers for Disease Control (CDC) recommendations of changing a peripheral IV site every 72 to 96 hours. Changing more often than recommended actually increases the risk of infection.

■ Procedure 36-5A **Peripheral IV Dressings**

➤ When performing the procedure, always identify your patient according to agency policy and be attentive to standard precautions, hand hygiene, patient safety and privacy, body mechanics, and documentation.

➤ *Note:* This procedure is usually performed at the same time the IV tubing is changed because the old dressing may need to be removed to do that. Most dressings may remain in place for 72 to 96 hours and are changed when the insertion site is rotated. However, dressings should be changed at other times if they become soiled or dislodged. Gauze dressings must be changed every 48 hours.

Procedure Steps

1. Wearing clean nonsterile gloves, stabilize the catheter with your nondominant hand, avoiding direct pressure on the catheter/hub junction, and carefully remove and discard the dressing and the catheter stabilization device. *Note:* If the catheter has an extended dwell time, sterile gloves are required for this step.
Remove the dressing gently to avoid dislodging the catheter.

2. Inspect the insertion site. Look for erythema, drainage, and note any tenderness.
If signs of infection, phlebitis, or infiltration are present, you must remove the IV catheter.

3. Don a clean pair of nonsterile gloves.

4. Cleanse the insertion site, and then allow the antiseptic to dry on the skin. Do not fan.

Step 4 Variation. Using Chlorhexidine
Apply using a back-and-forth motion and friction for at least 30 seconds. (Avoid using chlorhexidine in infants younger than age 2 months)

Step 4 Variation. Using Alcohol or 2% Tincture of Iodine
Using a circular motion, start at the insertion site and work outward 2 to 3 inches. Do not "go back over" any cleansed area.
Removes microorganisms from the skin to minimize the risk of their entering the venipuncture site. Allowing the antiseptic to dry increases the effectiveness of the antiseptic.

5. Change procedure gloves and apply a new sterile catheter stabilization device and dressing. For illustrations, see Procedure 36-1.

Step 5 Variation. Transparent Dressing
a. Open the package containing the sterile, semipermeable, transparent dressing. Remove the protective backing from the dressing, making sure not to touch the sterile surface.
b. Cover the insertion site and the hub or winged portion of the catheter with the dressing. Do not cover the junction with the tubing of the administration set.
c. Gently pinch the transparent dressing around the catheter hub to secure the hub. Smooth the

remainder of the dressing so that it adheres to the skin.
Pinching the dressing around the hub prevents pressure of the hub on the underlying skin.

Step 5 Variation. Gauze Dressing
d. Fold a 2 in. × 2 in. sterile gauze dressing in half, cover it with 1-inch tape (about 3 inches long).
e. Place under the tubing/hub junction and press down on the tape.
Raises hub off the skin and prevents pressure on the skin.

f. Place a sterile gauze pad over the insertion site and catheter hub—but not over the catheter/hub junction
g. Secure all edges with tape.

6. Secure the connection between the catheter and the tubing, but do not cover the catheter-tubing junction with tape.
Securing the connection helps maintain a closed system and prevent entry of microorganisms. You should not cover the junction with tape because removing the tape may interfere your ability to disconnect the tubing from the hub quickly, should you need to do so. Removing tape requires much

manipulation; the more the catheter is manipulated, the higher the risk for infection.

7. Secure the IV administration tubing by looping and taping the tubing to the skin.
Looping the tubing supplies slack to prevent the IV catheter from becoming dislodged.

8. Label the dressing with the date and time of insertion, catheter size,

and the date the dressing was changed and your initials.
Peripheral IV catheters should be replaced every 72 to 96 hours to prevent phlebitis. Labeling the dressing with the date and time of insertion helps communicate to other nurses when to change catheters. Gauze dressings covering the insertion site should be changed every 48 hours to inspect for signs of complications.

9. Discard all supplies in the appropriate containers according to agency policy in line with CDC guidelines.

What if...

■ **The patient is immunocompromised? Or the peripheral midline catheter must be in the same site for an extended time?**

Use sterile gloves and a mask when changing the dressing and giving site care.

Thinking About the Procedure

 Go to the *Fundamentals of Nursing Skills Videos,* **Medications, Intravenous: Peripheral IV: Dressing Change.**

1. At what point in the procedure did the nurse don clean nonsterile gloves? That is, what does she do before donning the gloves, and what does she do immediately after?

 For suggested responses, go to Chapter 36, **Thinking About the Procedure Suggested Responses (Procedure 36-5A),** on the Student Resource Disk or DavisPlus at http://davisplus.fadavis.com/Wilkinson2

■ Procedure 36-5B **Central Line Dressings**

➤ When performing the procedure, always identify your patient according to agency policy and be attentive to standard precautions, hand hygiene, patient safety and privacy, body mechanics, and documentation.

➤ *Note:* This procedure focuses on dressing change. Refer to Clinical Insight 36-5 for assessments and maintenance of CVCs.

Procedure Steps

1. Obtain sterile central line dressing kit (or equivalent supplies if there is no kit) and mask for the patient, if one is needed.
Because central lines have direct access to the central circulation, the risk of systemic infection is greater. Therefore, the procedure uses aseptic technique. All supplies must be sterile.

2. Place the patient in a semi-Fowler's position, if tolerated. Lower the siderail and adjust the bed to working height.
Semi-Fowler's position and bed adjustments facilitate site cleansing and dressing application and reduce strain on the nurse's back.

3. Explain the procedure and ask the patient to turn his head to the opposite side from the insertion site. If he cannot cooperate, place a mask on the patient.
Explanation may reduce anxiety and enhance cooperation; turning helps prevent contamination of the insertion site.

4. Put on mask and clean nonsterile gloves and carefully remove the old dressing and catheter stabilization device if present.

5. Inspect the site for signs and symptoms of infection and other complications.
If a complication is suspected, notify the person who placed the central line.

6. Remove and discard your gloves, along with the soiled dressing. Wash your hands.

7. Set up a sterile field and arrange and open the dressing kit and supplies.

8. Put on sterile gloves contained in the kit.
To prevent contamination of the insertion site and the sterile supplies.

9. Scrub the insertion site and surrounding skin with an antiseptic swab.

Step 9 Variation. Using Chlorhexidine
Use a back-and-forth motion with friction and scrub for at least 30 seconds.

Step 9 Variation. Using Povidone-Iodine and Alcohol
The kit should contain three swabs of each. Beginning with a povidone-iodine swabs, start at the insertion site and work outward several inches ("dirty to clean"). Repeat with the other two povidone-iodine swabs. Then, using the same method, cleans with the three alcohol swabs. With each swab, do not "go back over" an area you have just cleaned with that swab.
To rid the site of any potential infectious microorganisms, working "from clean to contaminated."

10. Scrub the sutures (if any), and the catheter from insertion site to the hub or bifurcation, for at least 15 seconds with an alcohol swab or chlorhexidine/alcohol antiseptic product.

11. Allow the site to dry—do not fan.
Allows the antiseptic time to work completely and allows the dressing to stick properly. Povidone-iodine requires 1 minute to air-dry completely; chlorhexidine requires 30 seconds.

(continued on next page)

Procedure 36-5 ■ **Changing IV Dressings** (continued)

12. Apply the transparent dressing that comes in the kit.

Step 12 Variation. Gauze Under the Catheter Hub
You may first place a small piece of folded sterile gauze under the catheter hub.
To reduce pressure on the skin under the hub.

Step 12 Variation. Chlorhexidine Gluconate Sponge as Part of the Dressing
Apply the sponge directly over the catheter insertion site, ensuring that the sponge is in full contact with the skin. Then apply the transparent dressing over the sponge.

Reduces the risk for catheter-related infection, especially in units with high infection rates or in high-risk patients (Timsit, Schwebel, Boudma, et al., 2009).

13. Apply the new catheter stabilization device, if one is used.

14. Remove drape, if you used one.

15. Loop the catheter gently and secure it with tape to the skin. Avoid securing it to the dressing. Or, depending on type of CVC, place a piece of clear tape across the ends of the catheter lumens, near but not on the hubs.
Ensures that accidental tugging on the catheter does not accidentally dislodge

the catheter. Do not cover the hubs, as you may need to access them.

16. Label the dressing with the date changed, time, and your initials.
Alerts staff to when the next dressing change will be due.

17. Place the patient in a comfortable position, put siderail back up and be sure call light is accessible.

18. Dispose of supplies into the appropriate receptacles according to agency policy in line with CDC guidelines.

Evaluation

- Evaluate the IV insertion site and surrounding tissue for signs of infiltration, inflammation, infection, and phlebitis.
- Monitor the dressing for dampness, blood, soiling, or loosening.

If these occur, the dressing must be changed.

Patient Teaching

- Explain the importance of notifying staff if the IV dressing becomes soiled, dampened, or loosened.
- Remind the patient to notify staff immediately for bleeding, pain, or swelling around the catheter or dressing area or discomfort in the hand, arm, or shoulder on the same side as the catheter.

Home Care

- Explain home IV therapy to the client and caregiver; teach them how to identify complications.
- Obtain a return demonstration by the client or caregiver to ensure competent performance of fluid, tubing, and dressing changes when necessary.

Documentation

- Chart the date and time the dressing was changed. Document the location and condition of the IV catheter insertion site.
- Document any complications of IV therapy and the interventions taken.
- Document the dressing change on your IV record. Often, IV care is documented on a flowsheet.

Sample documentation:

07/17/11   2300   New transparent semipermeable dressing applied over PICC insertion site in left forearm. No redness, tenderness, swelling, or exudates at the site.
———————————— Mary Ramirez, RNC

Practice Resources

Centers for Disease Control and Prevention (CDC, 2002); Hadaway, L. (2010); Infusion Nurses Society (INS, 2006a, 2006b); The Joint Commission (2009); Oncology Nursing Society (ONS, 2004); Pronovost, P., Needham, D., & Berenholz, S. (2006); Pronovost, P., Goeschel, A., Colantuoi, E., et al. (2010); The Society for Healthcare Epidemiology of America (2008); Timsit, J-F., Schwebel, C., Boudma, L., et al. (2009); Wenzel, R., & Edmond, M. (2006).

Thinking About the Procedure

 Go to the *Fundamentals of Nursing Skills Videos,* **Medications, Intravenous: Central Venous Access Device: Dressing Change.**

1. What is the first piece of personal protective equipment the nurse puts on?

2. During the central line dressing change procedure, does the patient wear a mask or turn her head to help prevent contamination of the insertion site?

3. What does the nurse do immediately after donning the sterile gloves?

For suggested responses, go to Chapter 36, **Thinking About the Procedure Suggested Responses (Procedure 36-5B),** on the Student Resource Disk or DavisPlus at http://davisplus.fadavis.com/Wilkinson2

Procedure 36-6 ▪ Converting a Primary Line to a Heparin or Saline Lock

➤ For steps to follow in *all* procedures, refer to the Universal Steps for All Procedures found on the inside back cover of Volume 2.

Critical Aspects

- Don clean nonsterile gloves.
- Remove the IV lock from the package, and flush the adapter, according to agency policy.
- Remove the IV dressing and the tape that is securing the tubing.
- Close the roller clamp on the administration set.
- With your nondominant hand, apply pressure over the vein just above the insertion site; stabilize the catheter hub with your thumb and forefinger.
- Disengage the used tubing from the IV catheter.
- Quickly insert the lock adapter into the IV catheter and turn it to lock it in place.
- Scrub the adapter injection port for at least 15 seconds and flush the lock again.
- Apply a sterile transparent semipermeable dressing; do not cover the lock-hub connection.
- Label the dressing with date and initials.
- Discard used supplies.
- Maintain sterility of equipment throughout.

Equipment

- Clean nonsterile gloves
- Peripheral intermittent lock adapter
- Two syringes containing saline or dilute heparin solution
- Linen-saver pad
- Transparent semipermeable dressing
- Alcohol or chlorhexidine/alcohol or other antiseptic swab

Delegation

You can delegate the task of converting a primary IV line to an intermittent lock device to an LPN who is specially trained in IV therapy. The task should not be delegated to a NAP. However, you should instruct the NAP to notify you of any problems with the intermittent lock device, such as dislodging of the catheter or client complaints of pain, swelling, or redness at the insertion site.

Pre-Procedure Assessment

- Assess the patient's readiness to have the IV fluid discontinued (e.g., tolerating oral fluids, adequate urine output, and laboratory values within normal limits).

If the patient's condition indicates that he still requires IV fluids, notify the primary care provider and do not discontinue the IV line.

- Assess for allergy to tape.
- Assess the IV site for signs of phlebitis, infiltration, extravasation, or infection.

If complications are present or the IV has been in place longer than 72 to 96 hours, remove the IV catheter instead of converting it to an intermittent lock.

(continued on next page)

Procedure 36-6 ■ Converting a Primary Line to a Heparin or Saline Lock

(continued)

➤ When performing the procedure, always identify your patient according to agency policy and be attentive to standard precautions, hand hygiene, patient safety and privacy, body mechanics, and documentation.

➤ Maintain sterility of supplies and equipment (e.g., do not touch catheter opening or ends of the IV lock; keep flush syringe connector sterile).

Procedure Steps

1. Help the client assume a comfortable position that provides access to the IV site.
Promotes cooperation with the procedure and facilitates your ability to perform the procedure.

2. Lower siderails, raise bed to working height, and place linen-saver pad under extremity with the IV.
Protects linens from blood and fluid that might leak from the vessel during catheter removal and ensures good body mechanics.

3. Don clean nonsterile gloves. Remove the IV lock from the package and flush the adapter with the first syringe of saline or dilute heparin, according to agency policy. Place the lock back loosely inside the sterile package, keeping it sterile. **Continue with step 5.**
Removes air from the lock. ▼

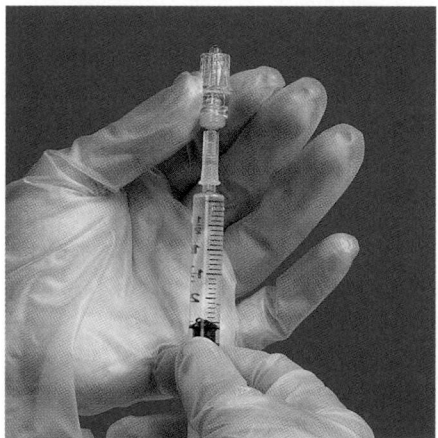

Procedure Variation:
Primary Tubing Set Up with Extension Tubing with a Lock

4. Merely discontinue the IV solution and disconnect the primary tubing from the extension tubing with lock.

Then, flush extension tubing per agency policy and skip to step 14.

5. Carefully remove the IV dressing and the tape that is securing the tubing.
Provides access to the IV catheter.

6. Close the roller clamp on the administration set.
Prevents loss of IV fluid during the procedure.

7. With the side of your nondominant hand, apply pressure over the vein just above the insertion site but not directly on the catheter–hub junction. At the same time, stabilize the catheter hub with your thumb and forefinger.
Applying pressure over the vein stops blood from flowing from the catheter as you change the administration tubing.

8. Gently disengage the used tubing from the IV catheter. If the tubing does not separate from the catheter, see "What If. . ." at the end of step 14.

9. Quickly insert the lock adapter into the IV catheter and turn it to lock it in place.
Insert the adapter quickly to prevent bleeding from the IV catheter. ▼

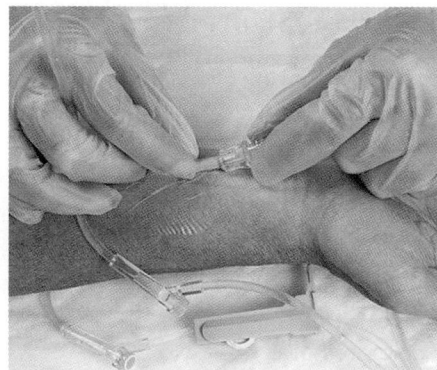

10. Scrub the injection port of the adapter with an antiseptic pad.
Cleaning the port with antiseptic helps prevent contamination by microorganisms when the adapter is flushed.

11. Insert the second syringe containing saline or dilute heparin into the injection port of the adapter. Flush the catheter using the method recommended in your agency.
Some experts recommend a turbulence (push-stop-push method) on the theory that turbulence ensures patency of the IV catheter by clearing the catheter and helping prevent reflux of blood back into the catheter. Others believe this method has undesired effects and recommend, instead, a steady, slow push. More evidence is needed to settle this question. In the meantime, follow agency policy regarding the flushing technique. ▼

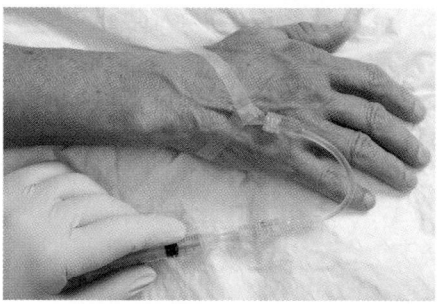

12. Using aseptic technique, cover the insertion site and catheter hub with a sterile transparent semipermeable dressing. Do not cover the junction of the catheter hub and the IV lock. See Procedure 36-5A for review of dressings.
Secures the IV catheter and prevents contamination of the site.

13. Label the dressing with the date changed and your initials.

14. Discard used supplies into appropriate receptacles according to agency policy in line with CDC guidelines.
Discarding used equipment properly keeps the healthcare environment safe.

What if. . .

- **At step 8, the tubing will not separate from the catheter?**

First, if it is a Luer-lock connection, be sure you have twisted the Luer lock "open." If so, place a hemostat ("mosquito" clamp) on the IV tubing and gently twist back and forth to loosen the connection. Then if the IV tubing still does not come loose, use the hemostat to gently twist the lock back and forth to loosen the connection. Do not lock the hemostat; merely use it lightly as a grip.

Use of hemostat may help loosen tubing from the catheter, but placement is critical so that the IV catheter and connector are not damaged.

- **At step 8, the IV catheter becomes dislodged while trying to disconnect the tubing?**

If you can see as much as three-fourths of the catheter emerging from the site, you must remove it and start a new IV at a different site.

Trying to re-advance the catheter might cause it to pierce through the vein as well as increase the risk of infection from reinserting a catheter that is no longer sterile. It also causes tissue trauma and increases the risk of phlebitis from catheter manipulation.

Evaluation

- Evaluate the patency of the catheter before each use according to institutional policy. Patency check and flushing are usually done every 8 to 24 hours.
- Evaluate the patient's tolerance to intermittent IV therapy.
- Evaluate the insertion site for signs of complications.

Patient Teaching

Explain the importance of notifying staff if the IV site becomes red, painful, or swollen; or if the dressing becomes soiled, damp, or loosened (indicating that the catheter has become dislodged or the connection is loose). Include the family in the teaching, as the patient may not be able to assess his own IV therapy.

Home Care

- Explain home use of the intermittent lock to the patient and caregiver. Teach them how to flush the catheter before and after administering prescribed medications.
- Provide the patient and caregiver with the name and phone numbers of people to contact in case problems arise with the catheter or insertion site.

Documentation

- Chart the date and time the IV line was converted to an intermittent lock device.
- Note the size and location of the catheter, as well as the type and amount of flush solution used.
- Record on the I&O record the amount of IV fluid infused.
- Document the condition of the IV site and any complications noted.
- Often, IV care is documented on a flowsheet or the electronic patient record.

Sample EHR documentation:

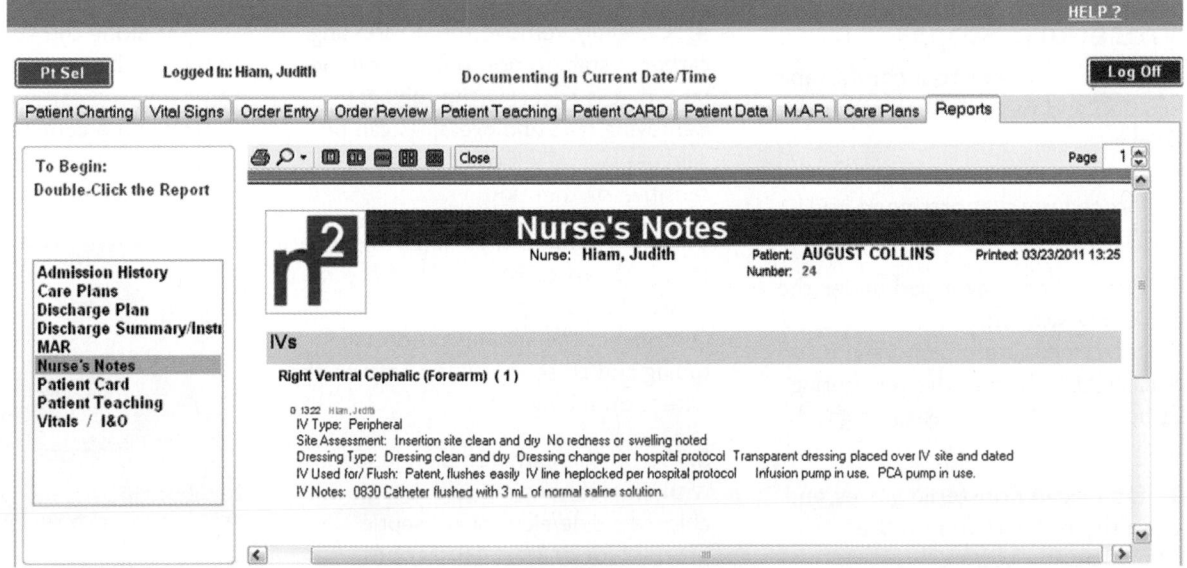

Practice Resources

Centers for Disease Control and Prevention (CDC, 2002); Hadaway, L. (2006, 2010); Infusion Nurses Society (INS, 2006b); Oncology Nursing Society (ONS, 2004).

Procedure 36-7 ■ Discontinuing a Peripheral IV

➤ For steps to follow in *all* procedures, refer to the Universal Steps for All Procedures found on the inside back cover of Volume 2.

Critical Aspects

- Place a linen-saver pad under the extremity with the IV catheter.
- Don clean nonsterile gloves, and close the roller clamp on the administration set.
- Carefully remove the IV dressing, catheter stabilizer, and tape securing the tubing.
- Cleanse the catheter-skin junction with an antiseptic pad.
- Place a sterile 2 in. × 2 in. gauze pad above the IV insertion site and gently remove the catheter. Do not press on the gauze pad while removing the catheter.
- Apply firm pressure with the gauze pad over the insertion site. Hold pressure for 1 to 3 minutes; hold longer if bleeding persists.
- Replace the soiled 2 in. × 2 in. gauze pad with a new sterile one. Secure it with tape or a transparent dressing.

Equipment

- Clean nonsterile gloves
- Sterile 2 in. × 2 in. gauze dressings
- 1-inch tape or transparent semipermeable dressing
- Linen-saver pad

Delegation

You can delegate the task of discontinuing an IV to an LPN who is specially trained in IV therapy. The task should not be delegated to a NAP. However, you should instruct the NAP to notify you of any bleeding from the insertion site.

Pre-Procedure Assessment

- Assess the patient's readiness to have the IV fluid discontinued and verify the order. For example, determine whether he is tolerating oral fluids and has adequate urine output and whether laboratory values are within normal limits.

If the patient's condition indicates that he still requires IV fluids, notify the physician and do not discontinue the IV line.

➤ When performing the procedure, always identify your patient according to agency policy and be attentive to standard precautions, hand hygiene, patient safety and privacy, body mechanics, and documentation.

Procedure Steps

1. Assist the client to a comfortable position and raise the bed to working height.
Helps ensure patient cooperation with the procedure; supports good body mechanics for the nurse.

2. Place a linen-saver pad under the extremity with the IV.
Protects linens from blood and fluid that might leak from the vein during catheter removal and ensures good body mechanics.

3. Don clean nonsterile gloves, and close the roller clamp on the administration set.
Closing the roller prevents IV fluid from spilling onto the bed or client during catheter removal. Procedure gloves protect you from body fluid exposure.

4. Carefully remove the IV dressing, catheter stabilization device, and the tape that is securing the tubing.
Removing tape and dressings can be painful especially if over hair or sensitive or thin skin.

Step 4 Variation. IV is running through an extension tubing or a saline lock.
Disconnect the administration set tubing and close the slide clamp on the extension tubing.

5. Scrub the catheter–skin junction with an alcohol prep pad or chlorhexidine/alcohol antiseptic product for at least 15 seconds.
Removes microorganisms from the skin entry site.

6. Apply a sterile 2 in. × 2 in. gauze pad above the IV insertion site and gently remove the catheter, directing it

straight along the vein. Do not press down on the gauze pad while removing the catheter.
Directing the catheter along the vein prevents vein injury while you are removing the catheter.▼

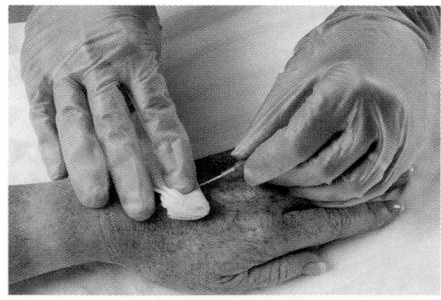

7. Immediately apply firm pressure with the gauze pad over the insertion site. Hold pressure for 1 to 3 minutes; hold longer if bleeding persists.
Holding pressure for 1 to 3 minutes typically stops bleeding by hastening clot formation.

8. Remove the soiled 2 in. × 2 in. gauze pad, and replace it with a sterile 2 × 2 gauze pad folded over to form a pressure dressing. Secure it with

1-inch tape or a transparent semipermeable dressing.
Protects the site from contamination.

9. Return the bed to a low position. Discard all supplies in the appropriate containers according to agency policy in line with CDC guidelines.

Evaluation

- Assess the integrity of the removed catheter; compare the length to the original insertion length to ensure the entire catheter is removed. If a catheter defect is noted, report to the manufacturer and regulatory agencies and complete an incident report according to agency policy.
- Evaluate the patient's response to oral fluids after IV therapy is discontinued.
- Monitor for changes in the patient's condition to assess whether IV therapy should be re-established.

Patient Teaching

- Instruct the client and family to notify staff if bleeding or discomfort occurs at the insertion site.
- Teach the importance of drinking adequate amounts fluid, within the prescribed plan of treatment, to prevent dehydration. (Some patients have fluid restrictions.)

Documentation

- Chart the date and time that IV therapy was discontinued.
- Note the condition of the site, including the presence of any complications. If complications are present, document your interventions, including physician notification.
- Often you will record this procedure on a flow sheet or in the electronic patient record.

Sample documentation:

12/25/11   2100   *RA#2, 22-gauge catheter discontinued. Site without redness, swelling, tenderness, or exudates. Pressure applied to site for 3 minutes. Bleeding stopped and sterile 2 × 2 gauze dressing applied. Informed patient to notify staff if bleeding or discomfort occurs.*
——————————————— *S. Horowitz, RN*

Practice Resources

Betsy Lehman Center for Patient Safety and Medical Error Reduction, JSI Research and Training Institute, Inc. (2008); Centers for Disease Control and Prevention (CDC, 2002); Infusion Nurses Society (INS, 2006a, 2006b); Oncology Nursing Society (ONS, 2004).

Thinking About the Procedure

Go to the *Fundamentals of Nursing Skills Videos*, **Medications, Intravenous: Peripheral IV: Discontinuing.**

1. Was this patient's IV being regulated by pump or by gravity?

2. Was the 2 in. × 2 in. gauze pad needed to absorb blood in this situation?

For suggested responses, go to Chapter 36, **Thinking About the Procedure Suggested Responses (Procedure 36-7),** on the Student Resource Disk or DavisPlus at http://davisplus.fadavis.com/Wilkinson2

Procedure 36-8 ▪ Administering a Blood Transfusion

➤ For steps to follow in *all* procedures, refer to the Universal Steps for All Procedures found on the inside back cover of Volume 2.

Critical Aspects

Procedure 36-8A: Administering Blood and Blood Products

- Verify that informed consent has been obtained.
- Verify the physician's order, noting the indication, and rate of infusion.
- Administer any prescribed pretransfusion medications.
- Obtain a blood administration set and 250 mL of IV normal saline solution.
- Obtain the blood product from the blood bank according to your institution's policy. Verify that the blood matches the order. Inspect it for abnormalities.
- With another qualified staff member and using two identifiers, verify the patient and blood product identification (e.g., date of birth, hospital identification number, blood type). Contact the blood bank immediately if there are discrepancies, and do not administer the blood product.
- Document on the blood bank form the date and time the transfusion is begun.
- Close all clamps on the blood administration set. Label the tubing.
- Hang the normal saline and prime the tubing.
- Gently invert the blood product container several times.
- Spike the blood product and hang the blood on the IV pole.
- Obtain a set of vital signs.
- Scrub the port with an alcohol swab or chlorhexidine/alcohol antiseptic product for at least 15 seconds before connecting to an existing line.
- Attach the administration set tubing to the IV catheter.
- Slowly open the roller clamp closest to the blood product. Infuse the first 50 mL slowly; if no reaction, set to the prescribed rate.
- Remain with the patient for the first 5 minutes. Measure vital signs in 5 minutes, 15 minutes, and 30 minutes; then hourly.
- Observe for and ask the patient to immediately report symptoms of transfusion reaction.
- When the blood has transfused, flush the line with the normal saline solution.
- Disconnect the tubing from the IV catheter, and dispose of the blood product container and tubing per agency policy.
- If a second unit of blood is to be transfused, the same administration set may be used.
- Administer any post-transfusion medications prescribed.

Procedure 36-8B: Managing a Transfusion Reaction

- If there are signs or symptoms of transfusion reaction, stop the transfusion immediately. Do not flush the tubing.
- Disconnect the administration set from the IV catheter.
- Call for help.
- Obtain vital signs, and auscultate heart and breath sounds.
- Maintain patency of the IV catheter by hanging a new infusion of normal saline solution, using new tubing.
- Notify the primary provider.
- Place the administration set and blood product container, with the blood bank form attached, inside a biohazard bag. Send the bag to the blood bank immediately.
- Obtain blood (in the extremity opposite the transfusion site) and urine specimens according to your institution's policy.
- Continue to monitor vital signs frequently.
- Administer medications, as prescribed.

Equipment

- Clean nonsterile gloves
- Blood product
- Normal saline IV solution, 250 mL

Normal saline solution is the only solution that is compatible with blood products; other IV solutions cause hemolysis of blood cells.

- Blood administration set (with a 200-micrometer filter and Luer-lock connection). If there is no filter on the tubing, you must attach one.
- IV pole
- Watch with a second hand or digital seconds
- Thermometer
- Blood pressure cuff with sphygmomanometer
- Stethoscope

Delegation

Do not delegate this procedure to the LPN or NAP, because blood product administration requires advanced assessment and critical-thinking skills. The LPN and NAP can assist by monitoring vital signs. Instruct both about the complications associated with blood product administration, and instruct them to inform you if any occur.

Pre-Procedure Assessment

- Confirm the patient's need for blood products by assessing vital signs, urine output, and laboratory studies.

Blood products may cause life-threatening complications; therefore, they should be administered only when needed.

- Check the patient's history for previous blood transfusions and reactions and verify the patient's blood type.

If the patient has a history of a blood transfusion reaction, precautions must be taken before she receives additional transfusions. For example, she may need premedication with acetaminophen, a corticosteroid, and diphenhydramine; specially treated blood products; and the use of a specialized administration set with greater filtering capabilities.

- Assess patency of the existing IV catheter, and make sure that it is the proper size for blood product administration.

Nurses often use a 20-gauge catheter for blood administration. However, for routine transfusion, a 22-gauge or even a 24-gauge catheter can be used. You would need an 18- or 20-gauge catheter when large amounts of blood must be transfused rapidly. The primary consideration should be the size of the patient's veins and not an arbitrary catheter size.

- Assess for allergy to tape.

■ Procedure 36-8A Administering Blood and Blood Products

➤ When performing the procedure, always identify your patient according to agency policy and be attentive to standard precautions, hand hygiene, patient safety and privacy, body mechanics, and documentation.

Procedure Steps

1. Verify that informed consent has been obtained.

Informed consent is required for blood product administration, as for any invasive or risk-bearing procedure.

2. Verify the medical order, noting the indication, rate of infusion, and any premedication prescriptions. Administer any pretransfusion medications as prescribed.

Verifying the orders helps prevent administration errors.

3. Obtain the blood product from the blood bank, according to your institution's policy. Wear clean nonsterile gloves whenever handling blood products.

Some blood banks require a pick-up slip that verifies the presence of a functioning IV catheter, signed informed consent, and an order, because blood must be discarded after it has been out of refrigeration for 30 minutes.

4. Verify that the blood product matches the order. Inspect the blood. If you note any abnormality, return it to the blood bank and obtain a new bag.

   a. Is the plasma pink?
Indicates hemolysis.

   b. Are the red cells red or are they purple or black?
Red is the normal color.

   c. Are any large clots visible?
There should be no clots.

   d. Is there any leakage?
There should be no leakage.

5. With another qualified staff member (as deemed by your institution), verify the patient and blood product identification.

Only one of the staff members is required by The Joint Commission to be qualified to administer blood products; however, agency policies may specify what those requirements are.

   a. Use two patient identifiers (e.g., ask the patient to tell you her full name and date of birth) and compare it to the name and date of birth located on the blood bank form and patient ID band.

Allowing the patient to confirm her identity and comparing the information against the blood bank form is a safety measure to ensure that the correct patient is receiving the correct blood product.

(continued on next page)

Procedure 36-8 ■ **Administering a Blood Transfusion** (continued)

b. Compare the patient name and hospital identification number on the patient's identification bracelet with the patient name and hospital identification number on the blood bank form attached to the blood product.

Verifies that the correct patient is receiving the correct blood product.

c. Compare the unit identification number located on the blood bank form with the identification number printed on the blood product container.

Verifies that the blood bank has dispensed the correct blood product. ▼

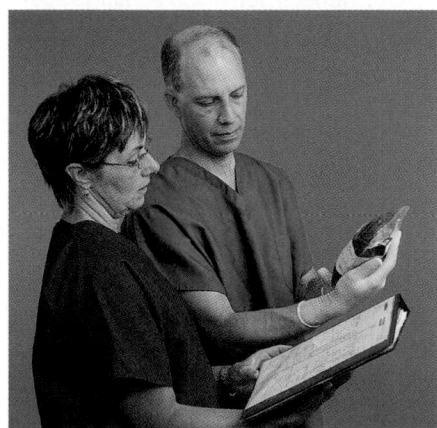

d. Compare the patient's blood type listed on the blood bank form with the blood type listed on the blood product container.

Verifies that the blood type of the product matches the patient's blood type.

e. If all verifications are in agreement, both staff members should sign the blood bank form attached to the blood product container.

✛ Contact the blood bank immediately if any discrepancies occur during the identification process. If there are any discrepancies, do not administer the blood product.

Signing the blood bank form confirms that the blood product was identified and verified by two qualified staff members.

f. Document on the blood bank form the date and time that the transfusion was begun.

Blood cannot be infused past the expiration time; documenting the start time alerts the nurse of the expiration time.

g. Make sure that the blood bank form remains attached to the blood product container until administration is complete.

Ensures product identity should a transfusion reaction occur.

6. Remove the blood administration set from the package, and label the tubing with the date and time. Then, close all clamps on the administration set.

Labeling the administration set with the date and time informs the nursing staff when the administration set should be changed.

7. Remove the protective covers from the normal saline solution container port and from one of the spikes located on the "Y" of the blood product administration set. Place the spike into the port of the solution container.

8. Hang the normal saline solution container on the IV pole. Refer to the photo in step 13.

Facilitates gravity flow.

9. Compress the drip chamber of the administration set, and allow it to fill halfway.

Prevents air from entering the tubing with the solution.

10. Open the roller clamp and prime the administration set tubing with normal saline.

Removes air from the tubing.

11. Close the roller clamp. Inspect the tubing for the presence of air. If air bubbles remain in the tubing, flick the tubing with a fingertip to mobilize the bubbles up into the drip chamber.

Air bubbles in the administration tubing can cause an air embolus.

12. Gently invert the blood product container several times.

Mixes the blood product with the preservatives that are added to the container.

13. Remove the protective covers from the blood spike on the blood tubing and the blood product port. Carefully spike the blood product container through the port.

Carefully spiking the blood product container prevents inadvertent puncturing of the container. ▼

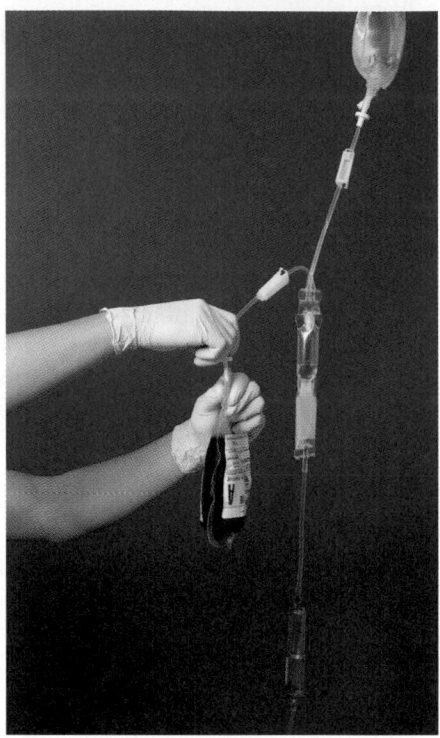

14. Hang the blood product container on the IV pole.

Enables the blood to flow by gravity.

15. Obtain and record the patient's vital signs, including temperature, pulse, and blood pressure, before beginning the transfusion.

Obtaining vital signs establishes a baseline to help monitor for transfusion reactions.

16. Using aseptic technique, attach the distal end of the administration set to the IV catheter.

Using aseptic technique prevents contamination of the IV catheter and administration set.

17. Slowly open the roller clamp closest to the blood product.

Allows the blood product to slowly fill that side of the "Y" of the administration set tubing.

18. Set the drip rate. Start the rate slowly until 50 mL have infused; if there is no reaction, set to prescribed rate.

A unit of blood cannot hang for more than 4 hours; otherwise, bacterial growth may occur.

Step 18 Variation. Volume-Control Infusion Pump
Program in the rate. Push "Start."

Step 18 Variation. Gravity Flow
Using the roller clamp, adjust the drip rate. (Keep in mind that blood administration sets have a drip factor of 10 drops/mL). *Note:* When using a 24-gauge needle, you will usually (but not always) use gravity infusion instead of a pump.

Forcing red blood cells through a smaller size catheter could result in some cell damage. Allowing the blood to flow by gravity allows time for the cells to change shape as they naturally do when flowing through small capillaries. However, certain models of infusion pumps have been approved that maintain a constant delivery of blood without significant hemolysis, even with small needle sizes (AABB, 2008b).

19. Remain with the patient during the first 5 minutes, and then obtain vital signs.

Most severe blood transfusion reactions occur during the transfusion of the initial 50 mL of blood.

20. Make sure that the patient's call bell or light is readily available, and have her alert you immediately of any signs or symptoms of a transfusion reaction, such as back pain, chills, itching, or shortness of breath.

To prevent serious complications, the patient should alert you immediately and the transfusion should be stopped.

21. Obtain vital signs again in 15 minutes (follow agency procedures), then again in 30 minutes, and then hourly while the transfusion infuses. Blood and blood product infusions must complete within 4 hours.

Frequent monitoring alerts you to detect early signs of transfusion reaction or fluid overload.

22. After the unit has infused, close the roller clamp to the blood product container, and open the roller clamp to the normal saline solution to flush the administration set with normal saline solution.

Flushing the tubing with normal saline solution clears the tubing of any blood and avoids wasting any of the blood product.

23. Close the roller clamp, and then disconnect the blood administration set from the IV catheter.

Disconnect the administration set if an additional unit of blood has not been prescribed.

24. If another unit of blood is required, you may hang the second unit with the same administration set. However, administration sets and add-on filters need to be changed every 4 hours.

The same administration set can be used for two units of blood or per agency policy.

25. Discard the empty blood container and administration set in the proper receptacle, according to your institution's policy.

Proper disposal of the blood container and administration set promotes a safer healthcare environment.

What if . . .

- **Two individuals are not available to verify that the blood and the patient are a match, and the blood must be hung now?**

In this instance, if it is available, an automated identification technology (e.g., bar coding) may be used in place of one of the individuals.

■ Procedure 36-8B Managing a Transfusion Reaction

➤ When performing the procedure, always identify your patient according to agency policy and be attentive to standard precautions, hand hygiene, patient safety and privacy, body mechanics, and documentation.

Procedure Steps

✚ **1.** If signs or symptoms of a transfusion reaction occur, stop the transfusion immediately. Do not flush the tubing.

Flushing the tubing causes the patient to receive the blood that remains in the tubing.

2. Disconnect the administration set from the IV catheter. Call for help. Obtain vital signs, and auscultate heart and breath sounds.

Severe transfusion reactions may cause respiratory distress and shock; early recognition and treatment improve patient outcomes.

3. Maintain patency of the IV catheter by hanging a new infusion of normal saline solution, using new tubing.

Maintaining a patent IV catheter with normal saline solution provides IV access in which emergency medication can be administered if necessary.

4. Notify the primary provider as soon as you have stopped the blood, assessed the patient, and hung the new normal saline solution.

5. Place the administration set and blood product container, with the blood bank form attached, inside a biohazard bag. Send the bag to the blood bank immediately.

The remainder of the blood must be sent to the blood bank, where it can be analyzed to help determine the cause of the reaction.

6. Obtain blood (in the extremity opposite the transfusion site) and urine specimens according to your institution's policy.

Blood banks typically require (1) a specimen for a type and crossmatch to

(continued on next page)

Procedure 36-8 ■ **Administering a Blood Transfusion** (continued)

compare with the pretransfusion type and crossmatch, (2) a specimen for free hemoglobin, and (3) a specimen for serum bilirubin level. A urine sample should also be sent to check for hemoglobinurinia, a sign of acute hemolytic reactions.

7. Continue to monitor vital signs frequently, at least every 15 minutes. To quickly detect worsening of the patient's condition

8. Administer medications, as prescribed.
Medications will vary depending on the type of transfusion reaction.

What if...

■ **At step 2, you do not have a new bag of normal saline to hang?**

Clamp the normal saline line until you can obtain a new bag of normal

saline, then disconnect the old normal saline. Do this as quickly as possible.
Preserves the patency of the IV catheter.

Evaluation

■ Evaluate the patient's response to the blood transfusion by checking for changes in blood pressure and oxygenation, improvement in color, or for signs of fluid overload.
■ Monitor for signs and symptoms of transfusion reaction.
■ Evaluate the IV insertion site for signs of infiltration, phlebitis, infection, or inflammation.
■ Check laboratory studies, such as complete blood count, to help evaluate the effectiveness of therapy and/or transfusion reaction.

Patient Teaching

■ Explain the signs and symptoms of transfusion reactions, and tell the client and family to notify staff immediately should they occur.
■ Warn the client or family to notify staff immediately if tenderness, redness, or swelling occurs at the IV catheter insertion site.
■ Explain the importance of notifying staff immediately if the administration set becomes disconnected from the IV catheter or the IV catheter becomes dislodged.

Documentation

■ Chart the date, time, and reason the transfusion was started.
■ Document transfusion vital signs according to institution policy (many institutions have a special form for transfusion vital signs).

■ Record the amount of blood transfused on the I&O record.
■ Chart any complications and the interventions taken.

Sample documentation:

10/22/11   0600   1 unit (250 ml) PRBCs was hung at 0300 and infused through LA#2, 20-gauge catheter for Hgb 8.3 mg/dL. Pretransfusion vital signs: T 98.9° F, BP 100/68 mm Hg, HR 114 beats/minute, and RR 22 breaths/minute. See frequent vital sign sheet for other transfusion vital signs. Breath sounds remained clear throughout the transfusion. No evidence of reaction. Post-transfusion lab due at 1200. —————————— L. Gilmore, RN

Practice Resources
AABB (2008b); Blest, A., Roberts, M., Murdock, J., et al. (2008); Finnish Medical Society Duodecim (2008); Infusion Nurses Society (INS, 2006a, 2006b); The Joint Commission (2009); Oncology Nursing Society (ONS, 2004).

Thinking About the Procedure

 Go to the *Fundamentals of Nursing Skills Videos,* **Oxygenation: Blood Transfusion.**

1. Where was the nurse when verifying the informed consent and the primary provider's prescription?

2. What size bag of normal saline did the nurse take into the room with her? What is the size usually used?

3. Why is it acceptable for the nurse, early in the DVD, to remove the blood product from the pneumatic tube system without wearing gloves?

4. What symptoms of transfusion reaction did the patient demonstrate (near the end of the DVD)?

 For suggested responses, go to Chapter 36, **Thinking About the Procedure Suggested Responses (Procedure 36-8),** on the Student Resource Disk or DavisPlus at http://davisplus.fadavis.com/Wilkinson2

Procedure 36-9 ▪ Assisting with Percutaneous Central Venous Catheter Placement

➤ For steps to follow in *all* procedures, refer to the Universal Steps for All Procedures found on the inside back cover of Volume 2.

Critical Aspects

- Perform meticulous hand hygiene.
- Use gowns and maximum barrier precautions.
- Obtain vital signs and verify informed consent.
- Gather and set up supplies and equipment.
- Prepare sterile field, and add supplies.
- Position the patient (Trendelenburg with a rolled towel between the shoulders).
- Offer mask, gown, and sterile gloves to physician.
- Don sterile gloves and mask (or follow agency policy).
- Prep an 8 × 10-inch area around the site, using applicators of 2% chlorhexidine gluconate in 70% alcohol, per agency guidelines.
- Place the large sterile drape to cover patient's head and chest.
- Have the patient turn his head opposite the direction of insertion.
- Observe while the physician inserts and sutures the catheter.
- Apply sterile transparent dressing, close any lumen clamps, and place tape across the lumens near the injection caps.
- Monitor for complications (especially respiratory distress).
- Obtain a chest x-ray.

Equipment

- Sterile gloves (two or three pairs)
- Masks, hats
- Barrier gowns
- 10-mL vials of normal saline (three or four)
- Syringes with 1-inch needle (two or three)
- 25-gauge ⅝-inch, and 18-gauge 1½-inch needles (two or three of each)
- Central venous catheter (CVC) kit containing: an introducer, antiseptic solution/swabs, sterile drapes, 10-mL syringe, 1% or 2% Xylocaine without epinephrine, suture, sterile scissors and needle holder, CVC kit (single- or multilumen)
- Injection caps
- Alcohol wipes

Delegation

Do not delegate this procedure because complex assessment and support skills are needed. The nurse must be alert to changes in the patient's condition and signs of developing complications. CVC placement at the bedside is associated with pneumothorax, hemothorax, cardiac tamponade, and air emboli.

Pre-Procedure Assessments

- Obtain baseline vital signs.
- Verify that informed consent has been given.
- Assess for allergy to tape.

(continued on next page)

Procedure 36-9 ■ **Assisting with Percutaneous Central Venous Catheter Placement** (continued)

➤ When performing the procedure, always identify your patient according to agency policy and be attentive to standard precautions, hand hygiene, patient safety and privacy, body mechanics, and documentation.

Procedure Steps

1. Explain the procedure to the patient.
To relieve anxiety and increase the patient's ability to cooperate with the procedure.

2. Gather supplies and perform hand hygiene.
Promotes efficiency; removes contaminants to help prevent infection.

3. Set up the sterile field and add supplies. Position the table so it is easily accessible by the physician or advanced practice nurse (APN) during the procedure.
Promotes efficiency and makes the procedure faster, and therefore less burdensome for the patient.

4. Position the patient to facilitate the procedure, usually in the Trendelenburg position with a rolled towel between the shoulders.
To prevent air embolism and dilate neck veins.

5. After the physician or advanced practice nurse (APN) performs hand hygiene, offer mask, gown, and sterile gloves (and possibly hat, depending on agency policy).
Maximum barrier precautions are required for central line placement.

6. Don mask and then sterile gloves.
To prevent contamination of sterile areas and of the insertion site as you cleanse it. Don mask first to keep gloves sterile.

7. Prep the marked site with 2% chlorhexidine gluconate in 70% alcohol applicators, using a friction scrub.
   a. Use a back-and-forth motion to scrub an area at least 20 to 25 cm (8 to 10 in.) in diameter. Do not go back over an area with the same applicator.
   b. Repeat with three applicators. Total scrub should take at least 30 seconds (2 minutes for a moist site such as the femoral vein).

   c. Allow site to air dry completely (about 2 minutes). Never wipe of blot dry.
Insertion kits and agency policies may vary. Follow agency policy. If it does not conform to evidence-based guidelines, work for policy change.

8. Drape the insertion site with a large sterile drape, exposing only the prepared skin area. Use other large drapes to cover the patient from head to toe. If your agency does not have a policy that the patient wears a mask, have the patient turn his head in the opposite direction of insertion.
Creates a sterile field and decreases the chance of contamination by the patient's exhalations. Turning the head to the opposite side also helps to make it easier to advance the catheter when it passes through the subclavian site.

9. Observe while the physician or APN performs the following steps:
   a. Anesthetizes the area with lidocaine.
   b. Primes the central venous catheter with saline.
   c. Performs venipuncture with the insertion needle (in the internal jugular or subclavian site). The femoral site may be used in emergencies, but it is associated with a higher rate of complications than other sites.
   d. Attaches a syringe to the needle and aspirates for blood.
To ensure the needle is in the vein.

   e. After obtaining blood return, removes syringe from the needle and inserts a guidewire through the needle.
The guidewire guides the flexible catheter into the vein.

   f. Aspirates all air out of the catheter lumens and then flushes them with normal saline.
To reduce the risk of air embolism.

   g. Places injection caps on each lumen.

To prevent blood loss and maintain sterility of the lumens

   h. Sutures the catheter in place.
To minimize movement and prevent catheter migration (in or out).

10. After the physician or APN is finished, apply sterile transparent dressing over the site.
Minimizes contamination of the site. The most common route of infection is via migration of skin organisms at the insertion site into the cutaneous catheter tract with colonization of the catheter tip. Transparent dressing allows for observation of the site without removing the dressing and manipulating the catheter.

11. If there are clamps on the lumens, close them.

12. Place tape over the lumens near the ends, but not on the injection caps.
To minimize movement of the catheter.

13. Remove sterile drape and assist the patient to a comfortable position.

14. Dispose of used supplies and equipment in the appropriate containers according to agency policy in line with CDC guidelines.

15. Remove and dispose of mask and gloves. Perform hand hygiene.
Observes standard precaution guidelines.

Guidelines
- The patient and all staff in the room should wear a mask.
- A health professional who has received appropriate education (e.g., a nurse) should observe the CVC insertion to ensure that aseptic technique is maintained.
- This person should stop the procedure if aseptic technique errors are made.
- A central line checklist should be used during the procedure. You may be responsible for auditing the procedure and completing the checklist.

What if . . .

■ **In step 8, a large sterile drape is not available.**

Use two small drapes to cover the patient from head to toe.

Evidence-based guidelines advise maximal barrier precautions for insertion of CVCs.

Evaluation

■ Obtain vital signs.
To assess for complications.

■ Auscultate the lungs and assess for respiratory distress, sharp chest pain, and coughing. Monitor for 24 hours for these signs.
To detect pneumothorax or cardiac tamponade.

■ Obtain a chest x-ray.
To verify correct location of catheter tip in the distal third of the superior vena cava, as well as absence of thorax and cardiac puncture.

■ Assess the patient daily to determine continuing need for the CVC.
Risk of infection is closely related to the length of time the CVC is in place.

■ For further evaluation and follow-up, refer to Clinical Insight 36-5, Caring for Patients with a Central Venous Access Device (CVAD) and Procedure 36-5B, Central Line Dressings.

Documentation

■ Date and time of catheter insertion
■ Catheter type and size
■ Site location
■ Assessments and interventions performed at insertion and immediately after
■ Patient's tolerance of procedure (subjective and objective data)
■ X-ray verification of catheter placement

Practice Resources

Betsy Lehman Center for Patient Safety and Medical Error Reduction, JSI Research and Training Institute, Inc. (2008); Infusion Nurses Society (INS, 2006a, 2006b); Institute for Healthcare Improvement (IHI, n.d.); The Joanna Briggs Institute (2008); Pronovost, P. J., Goeschel, C. A., Colantuoni, E., et al. (2010); Pronovost, P., Needham, D., Berenholtz, S., et al. (2006; corrected 2007); Rhoads, J., & Meeker, B. (2008); Riley, M-S (n.d.); The Society for Healthcare Epidemiology of America (2008); Wentzel, R. P., & Edmond, M. B. (2006).

Clinical Insights

Clinical Insight 36-1 ▶ Assessing for Trousseau's and Chvostek's Signs

Positive Trousseau's and Chvostek's signs are signs of hypocalcemia. To check for these signs, follow these instructions.

Trousseau's Sign

Inflate a blood pressure cuff above systolic pressure. Flexion of the wrist and hand constitutes a positive sign.

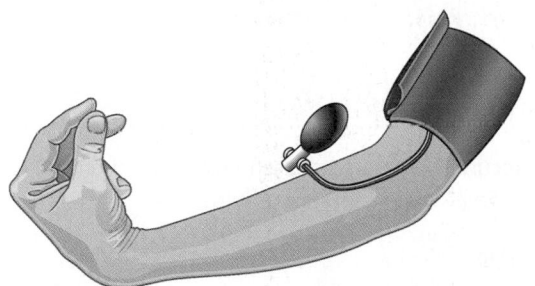

Chvostek's Sign

Tap the face in front of the ear and below the zygomatic bone (cheek bone). Facial twitching constitutes a positive sign.

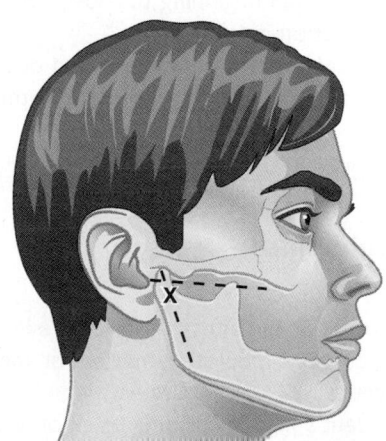

Clinical Insight 36-2 ▶ Interpreting Arterial Blood Gases

Use this table and the steps following to analyze ABG results. If you need further explanation,

 Go to Chapter 36, **Interpreting ABGs,** in Volume 1.

EXPLANATION OF CHANGES	ABG	NORMAL RANGE	ACIDOSIS	ALKALOSIS
Indicates acidosis, alkalosis, or normal acid–base balance	pH	7.35–7.45 (7.4 is "neutral")	Low	High
Carbon dioxide ("acid"). Signals respiratory cause.	Pco_2	35–45 mm Hg	High	Low
Sodium bicarbonate ("base"). Signals metabolic cause.	HCO_3^-	22–26 mEq/L	Low	High

Step 1: Examine the pH. (Is it acidotic, alkalotic, or normal?)

Step 2: Examine the Pco_2 and HCO_3. (Which value is responsible for the change in pH? Is it a respiratory or metabolic cause?)

　　a. Determine which one is abnormal.

　　b. Determine the direction of change (too high or too low). Is it acidosis or alkalosis?

Step 3: Determine whether there is compensation and if so, the degree of compensation.

- **No compensation**—If the pH and only one ABG component is abnormal, no compensation has occurred.
- **Partial compensation**—If the pH and one ABG component are abnormal, with the second ABG value starting to change and the pH beginning to move toward normal, partial compensation is taking place.
- **Full compensation**—Full compensation occurs when the pH returns to normal range and both other ABG

components are abnormal. The second ABG component (that originally had the normal values) has changed enough to return the pH to normal.

Example:

ABG values: pH = 7.30 Pco_2 = 50 mm Hg Hco_3 = 24 mEq/L

Step 1.　pH is low. Acidosis

Step 2a. Pco_2 is high; Hco_3^- is normal. A respiratory cause

Step 2b. pH is low (acidosis) and Pco_2 is high (acidosis).

Step 3.　pH is abnormal and only one other component is abnormal.

Answer: Respiratory acidosis with no compensation.

Clinical Insight 36-3 ▶ Guidelines for Measuring Intake and Output (I&O)

General Guidelines

Assessing

- Identify factors that can affect the patient's fluid intake or output (e.g., surgery, medical condition, or medications such as diuretics).
- Enlist the patient's help in keeping track of I&O if she is able.
- If you delegate the task of recording intake and output:
  - Be sure the assistive person understands its importance and knows how to perform the procedure correctly.
  - Be certain to evaluate the totals and the fluid sources. A patient or NAP can collect the data, but an RN must make the assessments.

- For accuracy, use a graduated container and hold it at eye level when measuring fluids.

Recording

- You will usually record measurements on a bedside I&O form and transfer the 8-hr total to a graphic sheet or the 24-hour I&O on the patient's record. You may sometimes need hourly measurements.
- Document your findings in milliliters (mL). Describe any fluid restrictions and the patient's compliance with them.

Measuring Intake

It is most accurate to premeasure fluids before they are consumed. However, if that is not possible, you can use the following estimates:

Record ice chips as fluid at half their volume (1 cup ice = ½ cup fluid)

1 oz = 30 mL

1 teaspoon = 5 mL

1 tablespoon = 15 mL

1 home measuring cup of fluid = 8 oz (240 mL)

1 pint of fluid = 16 oz (480 mL)

1 quart of fluid = 32 oz (960 mL)

Examples of fast food drinks:

Child size drink = 12 oz

Small drink = 16 oz

Medium drink = 21 oz

Large drink = 32 oz

Bowl (soup) = 180 mL

Creamer (small) = 30 mL

Custard cup = 100 mL

Drinking cup = 180 mL

Coffee mug = 240 mL

Gelatin cup = 100 mL

Ice cream serving = 120 mL

Juice glass = 120 mL

Paper cup, large = 200 mL

Paper cup, small = 120 mL

Water glass = 200 mL

Water pitcher = 1000 mL

Assessing

- Fluid intake includes the following:
  Oral fluids, including the liquid in prepared foods
  Soups
  Everything that melts into liquid at room temperature (e.g., gelatin, custard, ice cream, and ice)
  Liquid medications and fluids used to take pills or capsules
  IV fluids
  Enteral or parenteral nutrition fluids
  Instillations into the GI tract
  Bladder irrigations
- Measure oral fluids according to agency policy.
- For increased accuracy, use a graduated cup to measure and record fluid amounts before the patient consumes them. Subtract from the total any fluid that the patient throws away or saves for future consumption.
- Wash the measuring cup after each use, except after measuring water.

- Measure and teach the patient to measure and record the amount of fluid he drinks with each meal, with medicine, and between meals.
- In the home, cups come in many different sizes, so do the following:
  Use a measuring cup to measure how much the drinking cups and glasses hold.
  Use the same drinking cup or glass all of the time.
  Explain that the labels on cans and bottles will help to determine precise fluid amounts.

Recording

- At least every 8 hours, record the type and amount of all fluids the patient has received and indicate the route (oral, parenteral, rectal, or enteric tube).
- Record all forms of intake except blood and blood products

Measuring Output

Assessing

- Refer to Procedure 27-1 for a procedure for measuring urine.

Fluid output includes everything that leaves the body in fluid form: urine, watery stool, and vomitus, wound drainage, surgical drains, NG tubes, chest tubes, and any fluid aspirated from a body cavity.

- Use a calibrated container to measure fluids. Observe it at eye level and take the reading at the bottom of the fluid meniscus.
- Use a different graduated container for each patient; clean after use.
- Teach the patient to keep toilet paper out of the urine for accurate measurement.
- If irrigating an NG tube or the bladder, measure the amount instilled and subtract it from total output.
- You will need to empty wound drains or other devices to measure this volume.
- If a wound is draining but the fluid is not collected in a drainage device, you may measure the amount of fluid lost by weighing dressings before and after they are applied. If measuring the exact volume is not crucial, you may evaluate the degree of saturation of the dressing.

Recording

- Record the type, route, and amount of all fluids the patient loses.
- Insensible fluid losses can't be easily quantified. However, unusual losses (e.g., saturated dressing, excessive perspiration, rapid breathing patterns, and large burn areas) should be objectively described in narrative charting.

(continued on next page)

Clinical Insight 36-3 ▶ **Guidelines for Measuring Intake and Output (I&O)** (continued)

Tips for Analyzing I&O

- Measure and record all intake and output.
- Determine if output is more or less than intake.
- Evaluate trends over 24 to 48 hours.
- To identify problems, when evaluating total urine output, ask how many times the patient voided. For example, was a total of 300 obtained from 2 voids, or from 10 voids of 30 mL each?
- Evaluate patterns and values outside the normal range (e.g., frequent voiding, infrequent voiding), keeping in mind the normal range for 24-hour intake and output.

- The amount of output is important, but consider color, color changes, and odor too.
- Analyze intake and output holistically. Take into account the patient's usual pattern and amounts, age, medical problem, and type of surgical procedure.
- You must correlate I&O with daily weights to accurately determine overall fluid status (Pflaum, 1979, 2000, 2006).

Clinical Insight 36-4 ▶ **Guidelines for Selecting a Peripheral Venipuncture Site**

- As a general rule, select the most distal vein on an upper extremity.
- If available, use visualization technologies, such as portable ultrasound or imaging devices.

This minimizes the number of needlesticks the patient must undergo.

- For adults, you will usually use veins in the hand or arm; for infants, veins in the scalp or dorsum of the foot can also be used.
- If possible, select a vein on the patient's nondominant hand or arm.

Helps to preserve functional ability.

- Look for a vein that has a firm, round appearance with a relatively straight pathway. Do not use a red, hot, or hard vein.
- Avoid veins that are highly visible; they tend to roll.
- The cephalic vein of the arm is one of the best veins to use because it is relatively large, and the forearm provides a natural splint
- The dorsal veins of the hand are easy to access and are splinted by the metacarpals, but these veins are often quite small and fragile.

- Avoid the antecubital veins if possible. If the patient flexes her arm, the IV catheter may become displaced; so you would probably need to splint her elbow to prevent that. Furthermore, if a PICC line is needed at a later time, you will still have the antecubital veins available for it.
- For these situations, you need to use the largest vein available, keeping other selection criteria in mind:
  - Hypertonic solutions, viscous solutions, or irritating medications
  - Rapid rates (also require a larger IV catheter)
- Especially if the infusion is to be ongoing, begin the infusion with the best lowest vein and move proximal to the previous site (toward the heart) for subsequent insertions. Peripheral IV catheters are routinely changed every 72 to 96 hours. If you start the next IV below an already used site (i.e., to change the site or after a failed attempt at insertion), fluid may leak from the old site.
- Avoid areas where the vein crosses over joints. If you must use such an area, splint the joint to limit movement.

Splinting the joint helps preserve the vein for use, but it limits functional ability.

- Avoid areas with scarring, or with impaired circulation or neurological status (e.g., the affected arm following a mastectomy; an area with signs of infection, previous infiltration or thrombosis; an arm with an arteriovenous fistula [shunt for dialysis]; or the affected side after cerebrovascular accident [stroke]). If you must use such an area, first obtain a medical prescription.
- Do not use veins in the legs and feet unless there is no other option.

Peripheral circulation may not be adequate in the lower limbs, so there is increased danger of thrombus formation. In adults this location also interferes with mobility. Foot veins may be used for infants if the IV is taped securely.

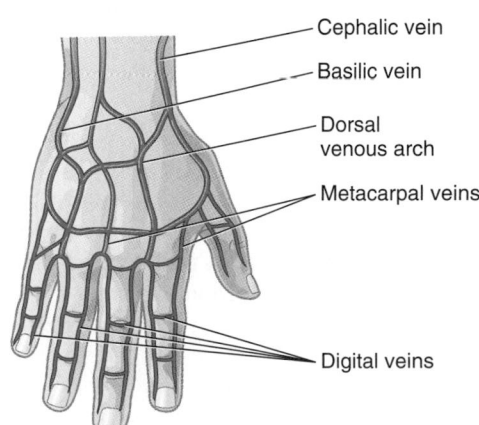

Cephalic vein

Basilic vein

Dorsal venous arch

Metacarpal veins

Digital veins

(a) Superficial veins of the hand

Clinical Insight 36-5 ▶ Caring for Patients with a Central Venous Access Device (CVAD)

Asepsis

■ Obviously, use good hand hygiene and follow agency protocols for site care.
To protect yourself and the patient.

■ Use strict aseptic technique when manipulating injection ports, catheter hub and extension legs, needleless connectors, insertion site, and dressing. This includes sterile gloves and supplies, mask, and in some agencies a mask for the patient.
To minimize line contamination and infection.

■ Scrub injection ports, extension legs, and catheter hubs vigorously for at least 15 seconds, preferably with 70% alcohol, or 2% chlorhexidine preparation before accessing them.

■ Appropriate antiseptics include alcohol and chlorhexidine gluconate. Do not use povidone-iodine and tincture of iodine to scrub ports unless there is some reason alcohol or CHG-alcohol combination products can't be used.

■ Do not apply acetone or acetone-based products to the skin before insertion of a catheter or during dressing changes.
These are organic solvents.

Assessments

■ Check the patient record for radiographic confirmation of correct tip location before beginning prescribed therapies.

■ Inspect catheter–skin junction sites through the transparent dressing and palpate for tenderness daily. Do not remove transparent dressing except when dressing change is required. If site is dressed with gauze, remove it to inspect the site.
A high-risk route of infection is via migration of skin organisms at the insertion site into the cutaneous catheter tract, with colonization of the catheter tip.

■ Observe for excessive bleeding at the insertion site.
You may need to obtain a prescription for a topical hemostatic agent and use with a pressure dressing.

■ If symptoms of infection occur (e.g., fever without obvious cause; redness, edema, induration, exudates or tenderness at the site), remove the dressing and inspect the site directly. Expect that blood cultures will be needed from both the peripheral site and the central catheter.

■ Be aware that risk of infection is higher with femoral catheters and with multilumen catheters.
Multilumen catheters require more manipulation, which encourages more colonization and bacterial growth within the catheter lumen.

■ Assess for compromised catheter integrity (wet dressing; kinked, cracked, or leaking external catheter).

■ Inspect catheter connections and pump function, including flow rate.

■ Observe for symptoms of catheter migration to the right atrium or ventricle (i.e., mid to lower sternal pain, dysrhythmias).

■ If there are signs of complications, notify the medical provider.

■ Assess the patient daily for indications that the CVC is still needed.
CVCs should be removed as soon as possible because the infection rate is closely related to the length of time the CVC is in place.

Interventions

■ The site should be covered with a semipermeable transparent dressing, the catheter secured with a sterile commercially manufactured stabilizer (instead of tape), and the lumens anchored near the ports with clear tape.

■ Keep dressings dry, intact, and air occlusive. Protocols generally require a dressing change every 5 to 7 days unless the integrity of the dressing is compromised (e.g., it is damp, loosened, or soiled) or if the site must be examined (e.g., because of pain or odor).

■ Perform site care with each dressing change. Cleanse the catheter–skin junction with an appropriate antiseptic solution, apply a sterile stabilizer, and a new sterile dressing.

■ Manipulate the catheter hub as little as possible.
To minimize catheter movement, phlebitis, and contamination of the line. Less catheter manipulation is associated with fewer bloodstream infections.

■ Flush catheters before and after any infusions or per agency protocol. This may be every 12 to 24 hours when not in use.
  ■ Flush volume should be twice the volume of the catheter and add-on devices (consult package label).
  ■ Use a syringe size recommended by the catheter manufacturer (10 mL is the smallest size recommended due to the pressure generated).
  ■ Type of flush solution depends on agency policy (saline versus heparin).
  ■ Use single-use, labeled syringes of flush solution.
To prevent cross-contamination.

■ If you have trouble flushing, the catheter may be kinked or malpositioned, the inline filter may be clogged, or a clamp may need to be released. You can correct these problems.

 Never flush against resistance.
The catheter might be clogged and you would risk dislodging a small clot. This could also rupture the catheter.

(continued on next page)

Clinical Insight 36-5 ▶ **Caring for Patients with a Central Venous Access Device (CVAD)** (continued)

▪ If the patient has a PICC line, take blood pressures on the alternate arm.

Using the arm with the PICC can cause bleeding at the site, thrombus formation, retrograde blood flow, and increased risk of catheter occlusion.

▪ If the patient is receiving parenteral nutrition, reserve and label one lumen just for that purpose.

Documentation

▪ Document routine assessments and the condition of the catheter–skin junction site. When site care is given, also document the patient's response and any actions taken to correct or prevent adverse reactions.

Related Information

For information about dressing changes, refer to Procedure 36-5B: Central Line Dressings.

For information about administering medications through a CVAD,

> Go to Chapter 23, **Procedure 23-18: Administering Medication Through a Central Venous Access Device.**

References

Betsy Lehman Center for Patient Safety and Medical Error Reduction, JSI Research and Training Institute, Inc. (2008). *Prevention and control of healthcare-associated infections in Massachusetts. Part 1: Final recommendations of the Expert Panel.* Boston, MA: Massachusetts Department of Public Health, pp. 69–82. In National Guideline Clearinghouse Brief Summary. Prevention of bloodstream infections. Retrieved March 2, 2009, from http://www.guideline.gov/summary/summary.aspx?doc_id=12922&nbr=006636&string=intravenous+AND+administration

Infusion Nurses Society. (2006a). *Policies and procedures for infusion nurses* (3rd ed.). Infusion Nurses Society Clinical Practice Committee. Norwood. MA: Author.

Infusion Nurses Society (INS). (2006b). Infusion nursing standards of practice. *Journal of Infusion Nursing, 29*(1S): S1–S92. Norwood, MA: Author.

Institute for Healthcare Improvement (n.d.). Implement the central line bundle. IHI. org [website]. Retrieved March 26, 2009, from http://www.ihi.org/IHI/Topics/CriticalCare/IntensiveCare/Changes/ImplementtheCentralLineBundle.htm

The Joanna Briggs Institute (2008). Management of peripheral intravascular devices. *Best Practice, 12*(5). Retrieved March 3, 2009, from http://www.joannabriggs.edu.au/pdf/BP_Book_Vol12_5.pdf

Marschall, J., Mermel, L., Classen, D., et al. (2008). Guideline Summary. Strategies to prevent central line-associated bloodstream infections in acute care hospitals. *Infection Control and Hospital Epidemiology, 29*(Suppl.1): S22–S30. In National Guideline Clearinghouse (NGC) [website]. Rockville, MD. Retrieved May 19, 2009, from http://www.guideline.gov/summary/summary.aspx?view_id=1&doc_id=13395

Rhoads, J., & Meeker, B. (2008). *Davis's guide to clinical nursing skills.* Philadelphia: F. A. Davis.

Riley, M-S. (n.d.). CE476. A lurking danger: A 'bundle' of safety measures available to fight central line infections. Nurse.com [website]. Retrieved March 26, 2009, from http://www.nurse.com/ce/course.html?CCID=4507&PageNum=3&Begin=9339

Clinical Insight 36-6 ▶ **Managing Infiltration and Extravasation**

▪ At the first sign or symptom of infiltration or extravasation, stop the IV. Symptoms include slowed or stopped flow, swelling, tenderness, pallor, hardness, and coolness at the site.

▪ The patient may report a burning sensation in the area.

For a Central Venous Catheter:

▪ Clamp and cap the catheter hub.
▪ Do not remove the catheter.
▪ Follow agency policy for flushing when you suspect infiltration or extravasation.
▪ If the patient has an implanted port, aspirate, remove the port access needle, and apply a dressing.
▪ Notify the provider who inserted the catheter, who may order an x-ray to help determine the cause of the problem.

For a Short Peripheral Catheter:

▪ Disconnect the tubing from the catheter hub; attach a 3- to 5-mL syringe and try to aspirate fluid from the catheter lumen. Use aseptic technique.
▪ Photograph the site to create a record of its condition, if agency policy allows.

▪ Wearing gloves, remove the catheter and hold a dry gauze pad over the site to stop the bleeding. Apply a dry dressing. Do not apply excessive pressure to the site.

▪ If you are to start a new IV, start it on the other arm, if possible. If it is not possible, start it in a more proximal location on the same arm.

▪ Measure the circumference of the arm and compare it with the opposite arm.

▪ Assess capillary refill, sensation, and motion distal to the infiltrated site.

▪ Apply cold or warm compresses depending on which fluid has escaped into the tissues.
  ▪ For alkaloids (e.g., vincristine) and epipodophyllotoxins (e.g., etoposide), use heat.
  ▪ For hypertonic fluids or medications, use cold.
  ▪ For isotonic or hypotonic fluids or medications, choose either heat or cold, or alternate them, based on patient comfort.

▪ Apply compresses for 15 to 30 minutes every 4 to 6 hours; continue for 24 to 48 hours.

▪ Estimate the volume of fluid that escaped into the tissues; notify the prescriber.

- Some medications leaked into the surrounding tissue can cause damage and even necrosis. For instance, when dopamine extravasates, you might need to give a prescribed amount of antidote (e.g., regitine injected subcutaneously) as well as hydrocortisone and an anti-inflammatory to minimize tissue damage. Be sure to check the protocol at your facility.
- Elevate the extremity and advise the patient to rest.
- Document all fluids and medications involved, equipment being used (e.g., pump), size and type of the catheter, description of the site (including location, size, and color),

methods used to assess the site before administering the fluids (e.g., aspiration), patient's signs and symptoms, interventions, notifications, and patient teaching.
- Complete an occurrence (or incident) report, as required by your facility.

References

Hadaway, L. (2007). Infiltration and extravasation, *American Journal of Nursing*, 107(8), 64–72.

Polovich, M., White, J., & Kelleher, L. (Eds.) (2006). Chemotherapy and biotherapy guidelines and recommendations for practice. *Journal of Infusion Nursing*, 29(1 Suppl), S1–S92.

Assessment Guidelines and Tools

The following questions and guidelines will help you obtain subjective and objective data about patients' fluid, electrolyte, and acid–base balance.

Focused Assessment for Fluids, Electrolytes, and Acid–Base Balance

Nursing History

Demographic Data

Age, gender, height, weight, body mass index (BMI)

Past Medical History

- Have you ever been hospitalized or had surgery? If so, when and for what reason?
- What healthcare problems are you currently being treated for?
- Have you ever been diagnosed with kidney disease, high blood pressure, diabetes, or thyroid or parathyroid problems?

Current Health Concerns

- What symptoms are you currently experiencing?
- Have you recently experienced any of the following symptoms?

Excessive thirst	Difficulty breathing
Fever	Swelling of your hands, feet, or ankles
Excessive perspiration	
Nausea, vomiting, or diarrhea	Dizziness or feeling faint
	Muscle weakness
Dry skin or mucous membranes	Excessive fatigue
	Numbness, tingling, or cramping sensations
Dark, concentrated urine	
Limited amounts of urine	

- Is your weight stable? Have you had any recent changes in your weight?
- Do you believe you have any problems with fluid loss?

Food and Fluid Intake

- How much fluid do you usually drink in a 24-hour period?
- Do you believe you drink adequate amounts of fluid?
- Describe your usual diet.
- Have you recently changed your diet or fluid intake?
- Are you following a special diet?
- Have you ever been placed on a restricted diet?
- Have you experienced any recent changes in your appetite or thirst?
- Do you salt your food?
- Do you ever use salt substitute?

Fluid Elimination

- How often do you urinate in a 24-hour period? Has that changed recently?
- How often do you get up during the night to urinate?
- Have you noticed any recent changes in the amount or appearance of your urine?
- How often do you experience vomiting, diarrhea, or constipation? Describe your experience.
- Do you have any wounds? If so, where are they, and how did they happen? What is the color of drainage and how much drainage are you experiencing?
- Do you have any breaks in your skin? If so, describe the problem, and show me the area.

Medications

- What prescribed medications do you currently take?
- What over-the-counter medications or alternative treatments do you use? What do you use them for?

Continued

Focused Assessment for Fluids, Electrolytes, and Acid–Base Balance—cont'd

- How often do you take laxatives or antacids?
- What vitamins, herbals, or supplements do you take?

Lifestyle

- What is your usual activity level?
- What type of exercise do you engage in? How often?
- How much fluid do you consume before, during, and after exercise?
- Do you drink alcohol? If so, how much do you consume in a day, week?
- Do you smoke? If so, how much? For how long?
- Do you use any illegal medications or drugs?

Physical Assessments

Skin

Assess the skin for color, temperature, moisture content, continuity, turgor, and edema.

- **Color and temperature** may be cues to the presence of fever and circulation status.
- **Moisture content** offers some indication of fluid status. A diaphoretic client is losing fluid at a faster rate than a client with dry skin. Dry, scaling skin may indicate a fluid deficit. Any breaks in the skin are potential areas for fluid loss.
- **Turgor** varies with age, weight, and skin condition but does offer information on fluid status. Pinch the skin over the sternum. Normally skin immediately returns to its usual position. In fluid volume deficit or malnutrition the skin may remain "tented" for a period of time before returning to its original position. You must, however, correlate skin turgor with context and other clinical signs. For example, the skin loses elasticity with aging, so clients older than age 65 often have decreased turgor, which is normal for them.
- **Edema** in dependent areas is a cue for fluid volume excess. In an ambulatory client, assess the lower extremities and hands. In a bedridden client, edema will shift as the client is turned.
- **To grade edema** (on a scale +1 to +4, +1 represents minimal edema and +4 represents the most severe edema),

 Go to Chapter 19, **Table 19-3,** in Volume 1.

Mucous Membranes

- Inspect the tongue and buccal mucosa. Mouth breathing alone usually does not change these areas.
- Dry, cracked, or dull mucous membranes are signs of fluid volume deficit.

Cardiovascular System

- **Assess vital signs** (see later section).
- If you suspect fluid volume deficit, assess for **orthostatic hypotension:**
  - **Assess blood pressure** while client is lying or sitting.

- Have the client rise to a seated or standing position, and reassess the blood pressure (BP).
  - A drop in systolic BP of > 15 mm Hg is a sign of orthostatic hypotension.
- **Check capillary refill.** Delayed capillary refill is a sign of fluid volume deficit; rapid capillary refill indicates adequate circulation and volume. If capillary refill is delayed, evaluate feet and hands bilaterally. Delays in just one area indicate impaired circulation to the extremity rather than volume changes.
- **Assess venous filling** by observing the jugular and hand veins. Flat jugular or hand veins indicate low fluid volume. Distended vessels are a sign of overload.

Respiratory System

- **Assess respiratory rate, depth, and pattern.** The respiratory system rapidly responds to changes in pH. Similarly, alterations in gas exchange at the alveolar–capillary membrane may trigger pH changes.
- **Assess breath sounds.** Crackles or moist rales may indicate fluid overload. Areas of consolidation indicate impaired gas exchange.

Neurological System

- Assess level of consciousness and orientation.
- Assess neuromuscular irritability.
- Assess energy level and fatigue.
- Assess reflexes.

For specific neurological cues to alterations in fluid, electrolyte, or acid–base balance,

 Go to Chapter 36, **Table 36-5: Electrolyte Imbalances,** and **Table 36-7: Acid–Base Imbalances,** in Volume 1.

Vital Signs

- **Temperature.** An elevated body temperature increases the loss of body fluids.

  In hypernatremia, body temperature elevates because less fluid is available for sweating.

  In uncomplicated fluid volume deficit, body temperature decreases.

- **Pulse:**
  - Tachycardia is an early sign of fluid volume deficit.
  - Pulse rate is affected by fluid status and some electrolytes (primarily sodium, potassium, calcium, and magnesium).
  - Dysrhythmias are seen with potassium and magnesium imbalances.

    The pulse volume is directly affected by fluid status. As fluid volume increases, the pulse volume also increases. Similarly, a drop in fluid volume leads to a drop in pulse volume.

- **Respiratory rate.** Alterations in respiratory rate may cause acid–base imbalances or be associated with compensation for a metabolic disorder.

Focused Assessment for Fluids, Electrolytes, and Acid–Base Balance—cont'd

- *Blood pressure:*
  - Blood pressure rises and falls with fluid volume.
  - Blood pressure is elevated by hypernatremia and fluid volume excess.
  - Respiratory acidosis causes increased heart rate, resulting in BP elevation.
  - High potassium intake may lower blood pressure.

Daily Weights
- Use the same balanced scale each day to monitor fluid status accurately.

- Weigh the client at the same time of day, making sure that the client is wearing the same amount of clothing.
- For clients undergoing hemodialysis (blood cleansing through an artificial kidney), weigh the client before and after dialysis treatments.
- You may institute weight monitoring as an independent nursing order.

Fluid Intake and Output
See table in Clinical Insight 36-3.

Diagnostic Testing

Assessing Fluid, Electrolyte, and Acid–Base Balance

Venous Blood Sample	Normal Ranges
Sodium	135–145 mEq/L
Potassium	3.5–5 mEq/L
Chloride	97–107 mEq/L
Bicarbonate	22-26 mEq/L
BUN	10–31 mg/dL
Creatinine	0.5-1.2 mg/dL
Serum osmolality	275–295 mOsm/kg
Urine osmolality	250–900 mOsm/kg
Hematocrit	43%–49% in men
	38%–44% in menstruating women

Freshly Voided Urine Sample

pH	5.0–9.0
Specific gravity	1.001–1.029

Arterial Blood Sample

pH	7.35–7.45
PCO_2	35–45 mm Hg
HCO_3^-	22–26 mEq/L

Diagnostic Testing

Standardized Language

NANDA-I Diagnoses Related to Fluid, Electrolyte, and Acid–Base Balance

NANDA-I LABEL AND DEFINITION	ETIOLOGIES OR RISK FACTORS	DEFINING CHARACTERISTICS
Deficient Fluid Volume Decreased intravascular, interstitial, and/or intracellular fluid. This refers to dehydration, water loss alone without change in sodium.	NANDA-I lists only active fluid volume loss and failure of regulatory mechanisms. The following adds inadequate intake: decreased fluid intake, fluid restrictions, inability to obtain or swallow fluids, abnormal fluid losses (e.g., through vomiting, diarrhea, or blood loss), increased need for fluids due to fever, extreme heat, or increased metabolic demands.	Dry mucous membranes, scant urine output, increased urine concentration, elevated hematocrit, thirst, weakness, weight loss, decreased skin and tongue turgor, decreased blood pressure (orthostatic blood pressure decline in systolic blood pressure by $\geq$ 20 mm Hg), elevated temperature, increased respirations pulse $\geq$ 100 beats/minute or pulse rate 10–20 beats/min greater than baseline (American Medical Directors Association, 2001, reviewed 2007)
Excess Fluid Volume Increased isotonic fluid retention	Compromised regulatory mechanism; excess fluid intake; excess sodium intake; limited fluid output (e.g., due to renal failure or low cardiac output)	Adventitious breath sounds (rales and crackles on auscultation); rapid respirations; pulmonary congestion; pleural effusion; orthopnea; dyspnea; altered electrolytes; anasarca, edema; increased BP; increased central venous pressure; jugular vein distention; pulmonary artery pressure changes; S_3 heart sound; bounding pulse volume; rapid weight gain; decreased hemoglobin and hematocrit; intake exceeds output; urine specific gravity changes; oliguria; azotemia; anxiety; changes in mental status; restlessness
Impaired Gas Exchange Excess or deficit in O_2 and/or CO_2 elimination at the alveolar–capillary membrane	Alveolar–capillary membrane changes; ventilation–perfusion problems. Impaired Gas Exchange limits the effectiveness of the carbonic acid–bicarbonate buffer system and alters serum pH.	Abnormal ABGs, abnormal breathing (e.g., rate, rhythm, depth); abnormal skin color; confusion; decreased CO_2; diaphoresis; dyspnea; headache upon awakening; hypercapnia; hypoxemia; hypoxia; irritability; nasal flaring; restlessness; somnolence; tachycardia; visual disturbances
Readiness for Enhanced Fluid Balance A pattern of equilibrium between fluid volume and chemical composition of body fluids that is sufficient for meeting physical needs and can be strengthened	None (wellness diagnosis)	Expresses willingness to enhance fluid balance; good tissue turgor; intake adequate for daily needs; moist mucous membranes; no evidence of edema; no excessive thirst; specific gravity within normal limits; stable weight; straw-colored urine; urine output appropriate for intake

NANDA-I Diagnoses Related to Fluid, Electrolyte, and Acid–Base Balance—cont'd

NANDA-I LABEL AND DEFINITION	ETIOLOGIES OR RISK FACTORS	DEFINING CHARACTERISTICS
Risk for Deficient Fluid Volume At risk for experiencing vascular, cellular, or intracellular dehydration	Deviations affecting access of fluids (e.g., Self-Care Deficit); deviations affecting intake (e.g., swallowing) or absorption of fluids; excessive losses (e.g., diarrhea, gastric suction, wounds); extremes of age; extremes of weight; factors affecting fluid needs (e.g., hypermetabolic state); deficient knowledge; use of diuretic medications	None (potential problem)
Risk for Electrolyte Imbalance At risk for change in serum electrolyte levels that may compromise health	Diarrhea, endocrine dysfunction, fluid imbalance (e.g., dehydration, water intoxication), impaired regulatory mechanisms (e.g., diabetes insipidus), renal dysfunction, treatment-related side effects (e.g., medications, drains), vomiting	None (potential problem)
Risk for Imbalanced Fluid Volume At risk for a decrease, increase, or rapid shift from one to the other of intravascular, interstitial, and/or intracellular fluid. This refers to body fluid loss, gain, or both.	Abdominal surgery; ascites, burns, intestinal obstruction, pancreatitis, receiving apheresis, sepsis, traumatic injury (e.g., fractured hip)	None (potential problem)
Risk for Vascular Trauma At risk for damage to a vein and its surrounding tissues related to the presence of a catheter and/or infused solutions	Catheter type, catheter width, inability to visualize the insertion site, inadequate catheter fixation, infusion rate, insertion site, length of insertion time, nature of solution (e.g., concentration, chemical irritant, temperature, pH)	None (potential problem)

Source: NANDA International (2009). *Nursing diagnoses definitions and classification 2009–2011.* Ames, IA: Wiley-Blackwell. Used with permission.

Selected NOC Outcomes, and Interventions for Fluid and Electrolyte Problems

NOC OUTCOMES	SELECTED INDICATORS
Electrolyte & Acid/Base Balance	Apical heart rate and rhythm
	Blood urea nitrogen
	Impaired cognition
	Muscle weakness
	Respiratory rate and rhythm
	Serum albumin, creatinine, bicarbonate
	Serum pH
	Serum sodium, potassium, chloride, calcium, magnesium
	Urine pH
	Urine specific gravity

Continued

Selected NOC Outcomes, and Interventions for Fluid and Electrolyte Problems—cont'd

NOC OUTCOMES	SELECTED INDICATORS
Fluid Balance	24-hr I&O balance
	Adventitious breath sounds
	Blood pressure, mean arterial pressure, central venous pressure, pulmonary wedge pressure
	Hematocrit
	Peripheral edema
	Skin turgor; soft, sunken eyeballs
	Stable body weight
	Thirst
	Urine specific gravity
Fluid Overload Severity	Ascites
	Decreased urine output
	Decreased specific gravity
	Hand edema
	Headache
	Leg edema
	Lethargy, confusion
	Periorbital edema
	Rales
Hydration	Fluid intake
	Decreased blood pressure
	Moist mucous membranes
	Rapid, thready pulse
	Skin turgor
	Thirst
	Urine output

NIC INTERVENTIONS	SELECTED ACTIVITIES
Acid–base Management*	Maintain patent IV access.
	Monitor ABGs and serum and urine electrolyte levels.
	Monitor respiratory pattern.
	Monitor for worsening electrolyte imbalance with correction of the acid–base imbalance.
	Reduce oxygen consumption (e.g., promote comfort, control fever, and reduce anxiety).
Acid–base Monitoring	Obtain blood for determination of ABG levels, ensuring adequate circulation to the extremity before and after blood withdrawal.
	Monitor for possible causes of HCO_3^- excess, such as vomiting, gastric suction, hyperaldosteronism, diuretic therapy, hypochloremia, and excessive ingestion of medications containing HCO_3^-.
	Monitor for possible causes of carbonic acid deficits and associated hyperventilation, such as pain, CNS lesions, fever, and mechanical ventilation.

Selected NOC Outcomes, and Interventions for Fluid and Electrolyte Problems—cont'd

NIC INTERVENTIONS	SELECTED ACTIVITIES
Electrolyte Management[†]	Place on cardiac monitor, as appropriate.
	Maintain patent IV access.
	Monitor for abnormal serum electrolyte levels, as available.
	Monitor for loss of electrolyte-rich fluids (e.g., nasogastric suction, ileostomy drainage, diarrhea, wound drainage, and diaphoresis).
Electrolyte Monitoring	Monitor for associated acid–base imbalances.
	Monitor for Chvostek's and/or Trousseau's sign.
	Monitor for signs and symptoms of specific electrolyte disorders [e.g., hyponatremia, hypernatremia].
	Monitor serum albumin and total protein levels, as indicated.
	Monitor the serum level of electrolytes.
Fluid Management	Give fluids as appropriate.
	Maintain accurate intake and output record.
	Monitor hydration status (e.g., moist mucous membranes, adequacy of pulses, and orthostatic blood pressure).
	Weigh daily and monitor trends.
Fluid/Electrolyte Management	Monitor for fluid loss (e.g., bleeding, vomiting, diarrhea, perspiration, and tachypnea).
	Monitor for signs and symptoms of fluid retention.
	Obtain laboratory specimens for monitoring of altered fluid or electrolyte levels (e.g., hematocrit, BUN, protein, sodium, and potassium levels).
	Restrict free water intake in the presence of dilutional hyponatremia with serum sodium level below 130 mEq/L.
Fluid Monitoring	Determine history of amount and type of fluid intake and elimination habits.
	Determine possible risk factors for fluid imbalance (e.g., hyperthermia, diuretic therapy, renal pathologies, cardiac failure, diaphoresis . . .).
	Monitor intake and output.
	Restrict and allocate fluid intake as appropriate.
Fluid Resuscitation	Collaborate with physicians to ensure administration of both crystalloids (e.g., normal saline and lactated Ringer's solution) and colloids (e.g., Hespan and Plasmanate).
	Obtain and maintain a large-bore IV.
Hemodialysis Therapy	Monitor clotting times and adjust heparin administration appropriately.
	Record baseline vital signs: weight, temperature, pulse, respirations, and blood pressure.
	Work collaboratively with patient to adjust diet regulations, fluid limitations, and medications to regulate fluid and electrolyte shifts between treatments.
Hypervolemia Management	Monitor changes in peripheral edema as appropriate.
	Monitor renal function (e.g., BUN and creatinine levels) if appropriate.
	Monitor respiratory pattern for symptoms of respiratory difficulty.
	Teach the patient the rationale for use of diuretic therapy.
	Weigh daily and monitor trends.

Continued

Selected NOC Outcomes, and Interventions for Fluid and Electrolyte Problems—cont'd

NIC INTERVENTIONS	SELECTED ACTIVITIES
Hypovolemia Management	Administer blood products (e.g., platelets and fresh frozen plasma) as appropriate.
	Administer hypotonic solutions (e.g., D_5W or 0.45% saline) for intracellular rehydration, if appropriate.
	Administer isotonic solutions (e.g., normal saline and lactated Ringer's solution) for extracellular rehydration, if appropriate.
	Combine crystalloid (e.g., normal saline and lactated Ringer's solution) and colloid (e.g., Hespan and Plasmanate) solutions for replacement of intravascular volume, as prescribed.
Intravenous Therapy	Administer IV fluids at room temperature, unless otherwise prescribed.
	Maintain strict aseptic technique.
	Perform IV site checks according to agency protocol.
	Perform IV site care according to agency protocol.

*There are specific interventions for each type of acid–base imbalance; for example, Acid–base Management: Metabolic Acidosis.

†There is a specific intervention for management of each individual electrolyte, for example, Electrolyte Management: Hypernatremia.

Sources: Bulechek, G., Butcher, H., & Dochterman, J. (Eds.). (2008). *Nursing interventions classification (NIC)* (5th ed.). St. Louis, MO: C.V. Mosby; Moorhead, S., Johnson, M., Maas, M., et al. (Eds.). (2008). *Nursing outcomes classification (NOC)* (4th ed.). St. Louis, MO: C.V. Mosby; NANDA International. (2009). *Nursing diagnoses: Definitions and classification 2009-2011.* Philadelphia: Author. Used with permission.

THINKING CRITICALLY ABOUT FLUIDS, ELECTROLYTES, AND ACID–BASE BALANCE

The exercises in the following sections allow you to practice the kind of thinking you will use as a full-spectrum nurse. Because these are critical-thinking questions, there is usually no single right answer. We do not provide answers for these questions because it is more important for you to think about the questions than to arrive at the "right" answer. These questions are designed to improve your thinking more than to "cover content." Discuss answers with your peers—discussion can stimulate critical thinking. If you have difficulty with any of these questions, consult with your instructor.

Applying the Full-Spectrum Nursing Model

PATIENT SITUATION

Darlene Malone, age 42, has been admitted to the emergency department with complaints of fatigue, extreme weakness, and heart palpitations. She says she has not seen a healthcare provider in nearly 10 years. Suddenly, she slumps and falls over. She is not breathing, has no pulse, and does not respond to verbal stimuli. She is resuscitated with CPR and IV epinephrine, and an endotracheal tube is placed. Stat lab results show a potassium level of 7 mEq/L, BUN of 102 mg/dL, and creatinine of 5 mg/dL. A physician diagnoses acute renal failure. Among other interventions, an IV is started to administer 10% calcium chloride solution, 1000 mg, by slow IV push to counteract the toxic effects of hyperkalemia on the cell membranes. The nurse used a 20-gauge over-the-needle catheter in Ms Malone's right cephalic vein, about 5 cm (2 in.) above her wrist.

THINKING

1. *Theoretical Knowledge*:

   a. Which lab results are abnormal? Are they high or low?

   b. Which lab results directly reflect her renal failure?

   c. What term correctly describes serum potassium of 7.7 mEq/L?

2. *Critical Thinking (Considering Alternatives)*:

   a. What do you think is causing Ms Malone to have hyperkalemia? You should be able to think this through and make a reasonable guess even if you have not studied pathophysiology.

   b. Ms Malone is to be given 50 mEq of sodium bicarbonate by slow IV push for an acid–base imbalance that is often associated with hyperkalemia. Which imbalance do you think would be treated with sodium bicarbonate: metabolic acidosis or metabolic alkalosis?

DOING

3. *Practical Knowledge*:

   a. When you prepare to administer the sodium bicarbonate (in question 2B), you notice that the IV infusion is barely flowing and that the insertion site is swollen and pale. What is the first thing you should do?

   b. You aspirate the catheter and do not obtain a blood return. Ms Malone absolutely must have this medication. Describe what you would do in the order you would do it.

4. *Nursing Process (Planning Goals)*: Choose the NOC outcome best suited to evaluating Ms Malone's hyperkalemia. Also choose three outcome indicators you could use to evaluate her goal achievement for that problem.

CARING

5. *Self-Knowledge*: Ms Malone will need dialysis to replace her inadequate renal function and control her serum potassium level. It is likely that her renal failure was brought on by years of illegal drug abuse. She has never held a full-time job and has not worked at all for the last 7 years. Her dialysis treatments will need to be paid for by Medicaid, which is funded by tax dollars. How do you feel about this—specifically, how do you feel about the issues of (a) a person's responsibility for her own health and (b) compassion for people who cannot afford to pay for healthcare? Focus on your own feelings, not on issues of what "should" be done.

Critical Thinking and Clinical Reasoning

1. Recall the "Meet Your Patients" scenario in Volume 1. When you review Jackson LaGuardia's chart to prepare for clinical day, you find that he is in the emergency department (ED) with four other members of the LaGuardia family. All of them have come to the ED complaining of nausea, vomiting, and diarrhea related to severe gastroenteritis, a viral intestinal disorder. The family members include the following:

   8-month-old Jason, grandson of Jackson

   26-year-old Susanna, Jackson's daughter and Jason's mother

   60-year-old Jackson

   58-year-old Gemma, Jackson's wife

   82-year-old Martha, Jackson's mother

   Jason, Jackson, and Martha are being admitted to the hospital. However, Susanna and Gemma have been asked to follow up tomorrow in the urgent care clinic. The following questions pertain to this scenario.

   a. Martha LaGuardia's orders call for lactated Ringer's solution with 20 mEq KCl per liter to infuse at 150 mL/hr. After 4 hours of infusion, Martha begins to complain of shortness of breath and develops a cough. What do you suspect may be happening? What actions should you take?

   b. What theoretical knowledge will you use in caring for Ms LaGuardia's immediate problem?

   c. Jason LaGuardia has been prescribed 250 mL of 0.9% saline solution over 8 hours. What type of equipment should you consider using?

   d. Calculate the drip rate for Jason's infusion if a gravity flow device is used. What further information do you need to perform this calculation?

   e. As you may recall, Jackson LaGuardia has end-stage renal disease. His lab work reveals a hemoglobin of 7.6 mg/dL and a hematocrit of 21%. He has been prescribed 2 units of packed red blood cells over 8 hours. Given his condition, for what fluid balance problem is he at risk? What additional parameters should you assess while he is receiving the transfusion?

2. You are asked to administer an antibiotic intravenously via piggyback. You are not familiar with the equipment that this facility uses. As a student, what approach should you take to solve this problem?

3. Identify techniques that you have observed that may contribute to contamination of an IV site.

4. Interpret the following ABG results. Explain your thinking.

    a. pH 7.47 P_{CO_2} 45 mm Hg HCO_3^- 32 mEq/L

    b. pH 7.32 P_{CO_2} 50 mm Hg HCO_3^- 25 mEq/L

    c. pH 7.30 P_{CO_2} 41 mm Hg HCO_3^- 18 mEq/L

    d. pH 7.45 P_{CO_2} 30 mm Hg HCO_3^- 22 mEq/L

5. For each of the following concepts, use critical thinking to describe how or why it is important to nursing, patient care or fluids, electrolytes, and acid–base balance. Note that these are not to be merely definitions.

Homeostasis	Acid–base imbalances
Selectively permeable membranes	Parenteral fluid and electrolyte
Fluid imbalance	replacement
Electrolyte imbalances	

▌ What Are the Main Points in This Chapter?

➤ Water is the largest single constituent of the body. Total body water content varies with age, gender, and the number of fat cells.

➤ Intracellular fluid (ICF) is contained within the cells. It is essential for cell function and metabolism and accounts for approximately 40% of body weight.

➤ Extracellular fluid (ECF) consists of three types of fluid: interstitial, intravascular, and transcellular fluid. ECF carries water, electrolytes, nutrients, and oxygen to the cells and removes the waste products of cell metabolism. ECF accounts for 20% of body weight.

➤ Electrolytes that carry a positive charge are called cations. They include sodium (Na^+), potassium (K^+), calcium (Ca^{2+}), and magnesium (Mg^{2+}). Electrolytes that carry a negative charge are called anions.

➤ Potassium and magnesium are the major cations in the ICF. Phosphate and sulfate are the major anions.

➤ The major electrolytes of ECF are sodium, chloride, and bicarbonate. Albumin is also present in the ECF.

➤ Osmosis is a mechanism to maintain homeostasis through the movement of water across a membrane from a less concentrated solution to a more concentrated solution.

➤ Diffusion is a passive process by which molecules move through a cell membrane from an area of higher concentration to an area of lower concentration.

➤ Filtration is the movement of both water and smaller particles from an area of high pressure to an area of low pressure.

➤ Active transport occurs when electrolytes move from an area of low concentration to an area of high concentration. Active transport requires energy expenditure for the movement to occur against a concentration gradient.

➤ General recommendations for total fluid intake are 2700 mL per day for women and 3700 mL per day for men.

➤ Fluid loss occurs throughout the day, creating a constant need to replenish fluid. Loss occurs through urine, skin, insensible losses, and feces. When the body is in a healthy state, fluid losses are equivalent to fluid intake.

➤ Sodium is the major cation in the ECF. Its function is to regulate fluid volume.

➤ Potassium is the major cation of the ICF. It is a key electrolyte in cellular metabolism.

➤ Calcium is a vital electrolyte responsible for bone health, neuromuscular function, and cardiac function, and it is an essential factor in blood clotting. Approximately 99% of body calcium is located in the bones and teeth. The remaining 1% circulates in the blood and is responsible for calcium's actions.

➤ Magnesium is a mineral used in more than 300 biochemical reactions in the body. As with calcium, only about 1% of magnesium is found in the blood. The remaining 99% is divided between the ICF and combined with calcium and phosphorus in bone.

➤ Chloride is the most abundant ion in the extracellular fluid. It is usually bound with other ions, especially sodium or potassium. Chloride works with sodium to regulate osmotic pressure between fluid

➤ compartments and assists in regulating acid–base balance through the bicarbonate buffer system.

➤ Phosphorus is the most abundant intracellular anion. Most phosphorus is found bound with calcium in teeth and bones. Phosphorus and calcium levels exist in an inverse relationship.

➤ Bicarbonate is present in intracellular and extracellular fluids. Extracellular bicarbonate levels, important in acid–base regulation, are regulated by the kidneys.

➤ The amount of acid or base present in a solution is measured as pH. The pH is reported on a scale of 1 to 14, with 1 to 6.9 being acidic, 7 neutral, and 7.1 to 14 basic, or alkaline.

➤ A buffer system consists of a weak acid and a weak base. These molecules react with strong acids or bases to keep them from altering the pH by either absorbing free hydrogen ions or releasing free hydrogen ions. The principal buffer system in the ECF is the carbonic acid (H_2CO_3) and sodium bicarbonate ($NaHCO_3^-$) system.

➤ When the serum pH is too acidic (pH is low), the lungs remove carbon dioxide through rapid, deep breathing. If the serum pH is too alkaline (pH is high), the lungs try to conserve carbon dioxide through shallow respirations.

➤ The kidneys affect pH by regulating the amount of bicarbonate (base) that is kept in the body.

➤ Fluid volume deficit occurs when there is a proportional loss of water and electrolytes from the ECF.

➤ Fluid volume excess involves excessive retention of sodium and water in the ECF.

➤ When the serum pH falls below 7.35, the patient is acidotic. When the serum pH increases above 7.45, the patient is alkalotic. Arterial blood gases (ABGs) are used to monitor acid–base balance.

➤ Physical assessment of a client's fluid, electrolyte, and acid–base balance includes examination of the skin, mucous membranes, cardiovascular and respiratory systems, and neurological status. Data are correlated with the nursing history and laboratory studies.

➤ Intake and output (I&O) are monitored to assess fluid status. To monitor, measure all fluids consumed and excreted in a 24-hour period.

➤ Tests used to monitor fluid, electrolyte, and acid–base balance include measurement of serum electrolytes and osmolality, complete blood count, urinalysis, and measurement of arterial blood gases.

➤ Nursing interventions for patients experiencing alterations in fluid, electrolyte, or acid–base balance address preventing imbalances, modifying oral intake, providing parenteral replacement, and transfusing blood products.

➤ Intravenous fluids are classified as isotonic, hypotonic, and hypertonic solutions, according to how they compare to the osmolality of blood serum.

➤ Vascular access devices may provide access to peripheral or central veins.

➤ Intravenous equipment consists of the IV catheter, an administration set, extension tubing, and the IV solution.

➤ Nurses are responsible for maintaining the correct rate of flow and for monitoring the client's response to the infusion.

➤ Calculate the drip rate by multiplying the number of milliliters to be infused in 60 minutes (hourly rate) by the drop factor in drops per milliliter and then dividing by 60 minutes. For example, an hourly rate of 100 mL multiplied by 15 drops/mL and divided by 60 minutes equals the drip rate. Therefore, the drip rate equals 25 drops per minute. Use this formula to calculate flow:

$$\frac{\text{Hourly rate in ml} \times (\text{drops/mL})}{60 \text{ minutes}} = \text{drip rate}$$

➤ Local complications at the IV site include infiltration, extravasation, infection, thrombus, and thrombophlebitis. Systemic complications include fluid volume excess, sepsis, and embolus. Systemic complications occur less frequently than local complications but may be life-threatening.

➤ Meticulous aseptic technique is required for initiation and care of intravenous infusions, especially when using central venous catheters, which are associated with higher bloodstream infection rates.

➤ Blood products are infused when the client has experienced significant blood loss, diminished oxygen-carrying capacity, or a deficiency in one of the blood components.

For practice questions for this chapter,

Go to **NCLEX-Style Chapter Quiz,** on the Student Resource Disk or DavisPlus at http://davisplus.fadavis.com/Wilkinson2

To practice documentation for an intravenous infusion,

Go to Chapter 36, **Practice Documentation,** on the Student Resource Disk or DavisPlus at http://davisplus.fadavis.com/Wilkinson2

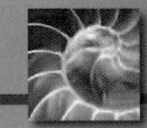 **Knowledge Map**

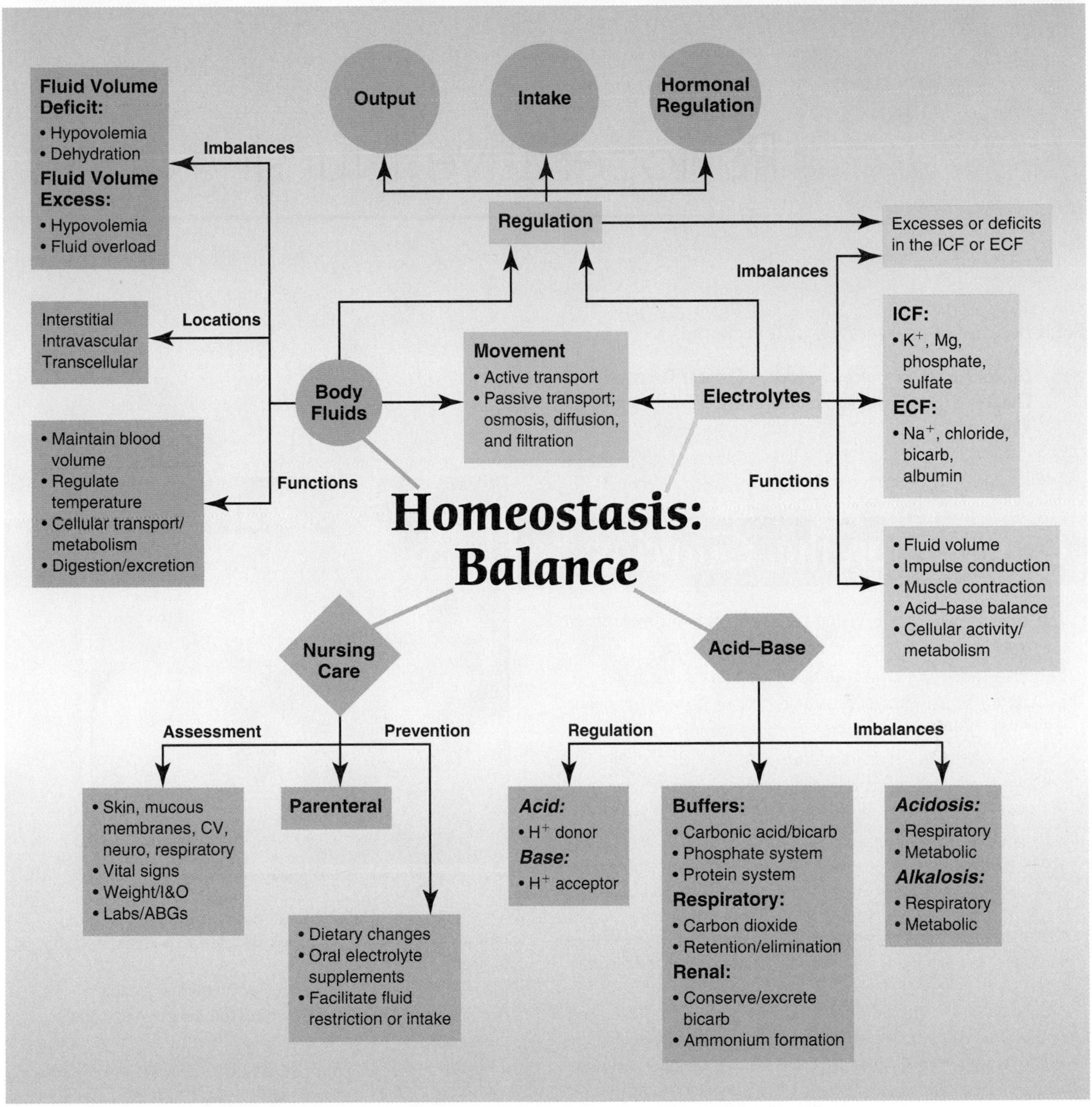

Output

Intake

Hormonal Regulation

Fluid Volume Deficit:
• Hypovolemia
• Dehydration
Fluid Volume Excess:
• Hypovolemia
• Fluid overload

Imbalances

Regulation ——— Excesses or deficits in the ICF or ECF

Imbalances

Interstitial
Intravascular
Transcellular

Locations

ICF:
• K$^+$, Mg, phosphate, sulfate
ECF:
• Na$^+$, chloride, bicarb, albumin

Movement
• Active transport
• Passive transport; osmosis, diffusion, and filtration

Body Fluids

Electrolytes

• Maintain blood volume
• Regulate temperature
• Cellular transport/ metabolism
• Digestion/excretion

Functions

Functions

• Fluid volume
• Impulse conduction
• Muscle contraction
• Acid–base balance
• Cellular activity/ metabolism

Homeostasis: Balance

Nursing Care

Acid–Base

Assessment

Prevention

Regulation

Imbalances

• Skin, mucous membranes, CV, neuro, respiratory
• Vital signs
• Weight/I&O
• Labs/ABGs

Parenteral

Acid:
• H$^+$ donor
Base:
• H$^+$ acceptor

Buffers:
• Carbonic acid/bicarb
• Phosphate system
• Protein system
Respiratory:
• Carbon dioxide
• Retention/elimination
Renal:
• Conserve/excrete bicarb
• Ammonium formation

Acidosis:
• Respiratory
• Metabolic
Alkalosis:
• Respiratory
• Metabolic

• Dietary changes
• Oral electrolyte supplements
• Facilitate fluid restriction or intake

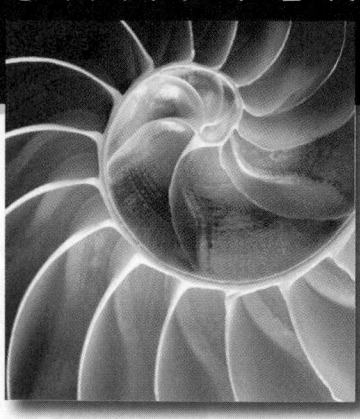

CHAPTER 37

Perioperative Nursing

For a podcast of an overview of this chapter,

 Go to Student Resources, **Podcast – Chapter Overviews, Chapter 37,** on DavisPlus at http://davisplus.fadavis.com/Wilkinson2

Caring for the Garcias

The exercises in the following section allow you to practice the kind of thinking you will use as a full-spectrum nurse. Because these are critical-thinking questions, there is usually no single right answer. We do not provide answers for these questions because it is more important for you to think about the questions than to arrive at the "right" answer. These questions are designed to improve your thinking more than to "cover content." Discuss answers with your peers—discussion can stimulate critical thinking. If you have difficulty with any of these questions, consult with your instructor.

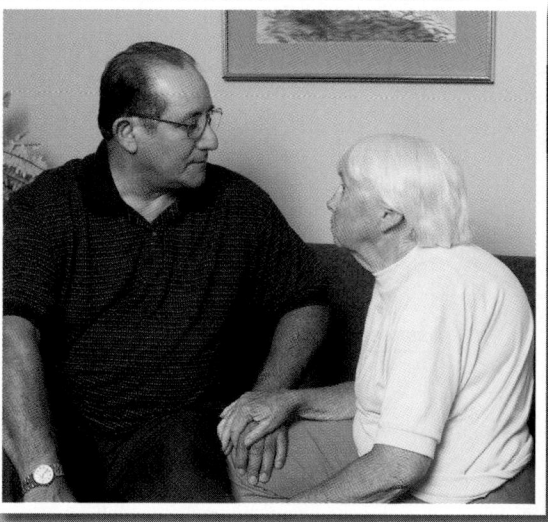

Katherine Garcia, the 76-year-old mother of Joe Garcia, has been experiencing blurred vision and decreased visual acuity. A local ophthalmologist diagnosed bilateral cataracts. The ophthalmologist has recommended cataract removal in the left eye, with insertion of an intraocular lens. He told Mrs. Garcia to schedule the surgery "at your convenience" and explained that the surgery would be performed on an outpatient basis. The ophthalmologist gave Mrs. Garcia a list of activities to prepare for the surgery, containing the following information:

■ Schedule a date for your surgery. My receptionist will set up a time for your surgery. All surgeries are

performed at Western Medical Center Same-Day Surgery Department.
■ Please arrange to be seen by your primary care provider 1 to 2 weeks prior to the surgery to receive clearance for surgery.
■ Make an appointment with the Preoperative Center at Western Medical Center Same-Day Surgery Department 1 to 2 days before surgery.
■ Arrange to have a ride to and from the surgery.

Caring for the Garcias (continued)

A. What preoperative testing is Mrs. Garcia likely to undergo? Explain your rationale.

B. The preoperative list states that the client must be seen by the primary care provider to receive clearance for surgery. Why is this an essential part of the preoperative period?

C. What theoretical knowledge do you need to perform preoperative teaching for Mrs. Garcia? How could you obtain that information? Be specific about your sources.

D. What content would you include in Mrs. Garcia's preoperative teaching?

E. The ophthalmologist has planned anesthesia via conscious sedation. What factors, if any, might keep Mrs. Garcia from receiving this form of anesthesia? What additional information do you need to answer this question?

Practical **Knowledge** **knowing** how

Perioperative care requires you to use the nursing process to ensure that the patient is in the best possible condition for surgery, is safe during surgery, and has the best possible outcomes postoperatively. Perioperative nursing care includes procedures and techniques designed for prevention and early detection of complications. Recall that full-spectrum nursing involves thinking, doing and caring—all are equally important, in perioperative as well as other settings.

Procedures

The procedures in this section will help you to prevent postoperative complications. Preoperative teaching of coughing, deep breathing, moving in bed, and leg exercises help to prevent thrombophlebitis, atelectasis, and pneumonia. Antiembolism stockings and sequential compression devices are designed to promote peripheral circulation and prevent thrombus formation. Gastrointestinal suction is used to relieve or prevent abdominal distention.

Procedure 37-1 | Teaching a Patient to Deep-Breathe, Cough, Move in Bed, and Perform Leg Exercises

➤ For steps to follow in *all* procedures, refer to the Universal Steps for All Procedures found on the inside back cover of Volume 2.

Critical Aspects

- Assess the patient's readiness to learn.
- Ensure that the patient is clear about the difference between coughing and merely clearing his throat.
- Demonstrate how to splint a chest or abdominal incision.
- Make sure the patient flexes her knees before turning on her side in bed.
- Use pillows to support the patient who is unable to maintain a side-lying position.
- Teach the patient to alternately flex and extend his knees.
- Teach the patient to alternately dorsiflex and plantar flex his feet.
- Teach the patient to rotate her ankles in a complete circle.

(continued on next page)

Procedure 37-1 ■ Teaching a Patient to Deep-Breathe, Cough, Move in Bed, and Perform Leg Exercises (continued)

Equipment

For teaching deep breathing and coughing:
- Folded blanket or a pillow (if teaching will include splinting of a surgical incision site)
- Tissues

For moving in bed:
- Small pillow or folded blanket
- Pillows

Delegation

You or another RN should perform the initial teaching. You may delegate reinforcement of the teaching to a licensed vocational nurse (LVN), licensed practical nurse (LPN), or nursing assistive personnel (NAP).

Pre-Procedure Assessments

- Assess the patient's cognitive level and level of consciousness.

Helps assess the patient's ability to understand and follow directions and select the appropriate teaching method.

- Assess the patient's pain level.

Even preoperatively, pain must be well controlled to ensure full patient participation.

- Determine whether the surgical procedure and/or a physical disability will limit the patient's participation.

For example, a fractured arm that has not yet been repaired will impair the patient's ability to hold a pillow for splinting.

- Determine whether the surgical procedure may entail special exercises or equipment. In addition, assess for any special equipment, such as braces, slings, or abductor wedges, that may be needed when turning a patient in bed.

Orthopedic surgeries involving the knee and hip often involve special exercises or equipment in the postoperative period. Consult the surgeon before teaching the patient any leg exercises. Spinal and neurological surgeries often limit movement in the postoperative period. For example, some spinal surgeries require the patient to logroll (move from head to toe as one unit). Some neurological procedures require limiting the amount of time the patient's head of bed is above 30°. Identify these restrictions preoperatively, and inform the patient and family about them during your teaching session.

- Assess the patient's belief about the ability of the surgical incision to remain intact.

If the patient believes that the incision will not stay together if he coughs or moves, compliance is likely to be low. This is a common fear among patients.

■ Procedure 37-1A Teaching a Patient to Deep Breathe and Cough

➤ When performing the procedure, always identify your patient according to agency policy and be attentive to standard precautions, hand hygiene, patient safety and privacy, body mechanics, and documentation.

Deep breathing and coughing expand the lungs, improve ventilation, promote gas exchange, and help prevent atelectasis and pneumonia. Coughing after deep breathing mobilizes secretions, which keeps airways and alveoli open and provides greater surface area for gas exchange.

Procedure Steps

1. Assist the patient to a Fowler's or semi-Fowler's position, with the shoulders relaxed.
Allows for best chest and lung expansion.

2. Assist the patient who will have a chest or abdominal incision to practice splinting the site with a folded blanket or pillow.

Counterpressure supports the incision and decreases pain.▼

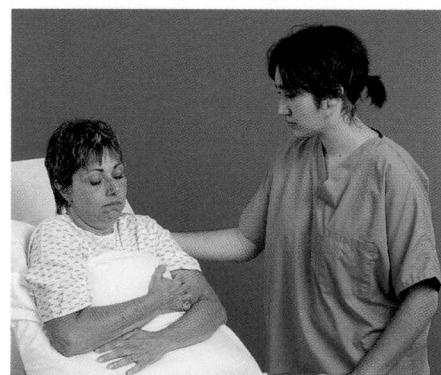

3. Teach the patient diaphragmatic/deep breathing. Tell the patient to:
   a. Place her hands anteriorly, along the lower end of the rib cage. The tips of the third fingers should touch at the midline.
   b. Slowly take a deep breath in through the nose. Tell the patient that she should feel her chest expanding as the diaphragm moves down.
   c. Hold her breath for 2 to 5 seconds.

Stimulates surfactant production and helps prevent alveolar collapse.

   d. Slowly and completely exhale the breath through her mouth.

4. Teach the patient to cough in conjunction with diaphragmatic breathing. Instruct her to:
   a. Complete two or three cycles of diaphragmatic breathing.
   b. On the next breath in, have the patient lean forward and cough rapidly, through an open mouth, using the muscles of the abdomen, thighs, and buttocks. Cough several times on that breath.

This information helps the patient to distinguish coughing from merely clearing her throat.

Step 4 Variation. Patient Experiencing Weakness

If the patient is too weak to perform this maneuver, have the patient inhale deeply, bend forward slightly, and perform three or four "huffs" against an open glottis to move secretions forward.

■ Procedure 37-1B Teaching a Patient to Move in Bed

➤ When performing the procedure, always identify your patient according to agency policy and be attentive to standard precautions, hand hygiene, patient safety and privacy, body mechanics, and documentation.

Moving in bed promotes blood circulation, stimulates respiratory function, and helps mobilize gas in the intestines.

Procedure Steps

1. Start with the patient in the supine position, bedrails up. Then instruct the patient as follows.

2. To turn to the left side: Bend the right leg, sliding the foot flat along the bed and flexing the knee.
Enables the patient to push herself over to the opposite side.

3. Reach the right arm across the chest, and grasp the opposite bedrail.
Helps the patient to turn, reduces the need to use the abdominal muscles for turning, and minimizes incision pain.

4. Breathe deeply, and practice splinting any potential abdominal or chest incisions. Assist the patient to practice as needed.
Facilitates comfort during movement.

5. Pull on the bedrail while pushing off with the right foot.
Assists patient to turn to the left. ▼

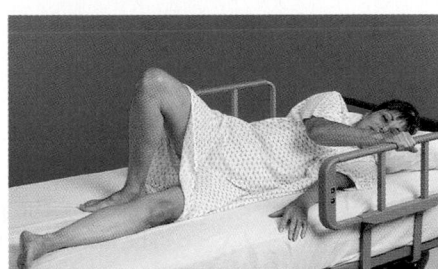

6. If the patient cannot maintain this position independently, place a folded pillow or blanket along her back for support.

7. Change positions every 2 hours, repeating the turning process with the opposite arm and leg. You will need to assist the patient who needs pillows placed for support.

■ Procedure 37-1C Teaching Leg Exercises

➤ When performing the procedure, always identify your patient according to agency policy and be attentive to standard precautions, hand hygiene, patient safety and privacy, body mechanics, and documentation.

Leg exercises flex and extend the leg muscles to increase peripheral circulation and help prevent thrombus formation. Thrombus formation is a common postoperative complication.

Procedure Steps

1. Instruct the patient to lie supine in the bed.
Note: These exercises can be done when the patient is up in a chair, but the effect will be diminished by the effects of gravity.

2. Perform ankle circles. Instruct patient to:
  a. Start with one foot in the dorsiflexed position.
  b. Slowly rotate the ankle clockwise.
  c. After three rotations, repeat the procedure in a counterclockwise direction.
  d. Repeat this exercise at least three times in each direction, then

switch and exercise the other ankle. ▼

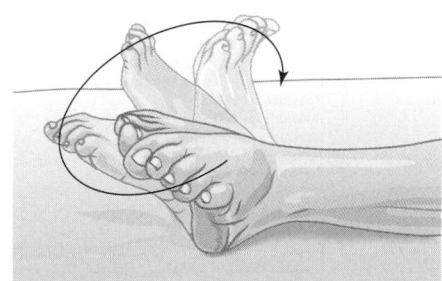

3. Perform ankle pumps. Instruct the patient to:
  a. Start with one foot, leg extended.
  b. Point the toe until her foot is plantar flexed.
  c. Pull the toes back toward her head until the foot is dorsiflexed; at the same time, press the back of the knee into the bed.
  d. Make sure she feels a pull, or a stretch, in the calf.

e. Repeat the alternation between plantar and dorsiflexion several times.
f. Repeat the cycle with the other foot.

4. Perform leg exercises. Instruct the patient to:
  a. Lie supine in the bed.
  b. Slowly begin bending the knee, sliding the sole of the foot along the bed until the knee is in a flexed position. ▼

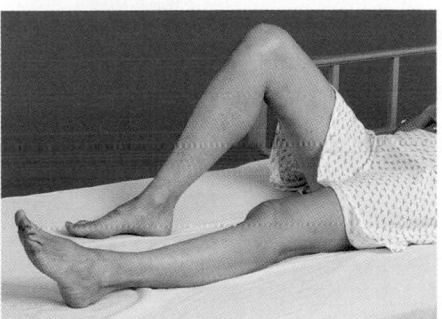

(continued on next page)

Procedure 37-1 ■ Teaching a Patient to Deep-Breathe, Cough, Move in Bed, and Perform Leg Exercises (continued)

c. Reverse the motion, extending the knee until the leg is once again flat on the bed.▼

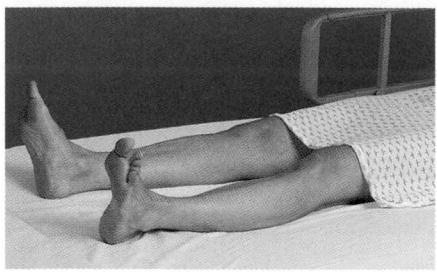

d. Repeat several times.
e. Repeat using the opposite leg.

What if . . .

■ **The patient has had knee, hip, or back surgery?**

Leg exercises may be contraindicated in patients having knee, hip, or back surgery. Check the surgeon's prescriptions and/or collaborate with the physical therapist.

■ **The patient has had nasal, ophthalmic, or neurological surgery?**

Coughing and deep-breathing exercises are contraindicated.

To avoid increasing intracranial pressure.

Evaluation

Make sure that the patient performs correctly a return demonstration of the procedures taught.

Documentation

In many healthcare facilities, checklists and charts have special areas in which to document patient teaching. Documentation should identify the person who completed the teaching, the person to whom the procedures were taught, what procedures were taught, and whether the patient understood the teaching. Also include the name and type of any printed materials given.

Sample electronic documentation:

Note that because this is just one screen of a documentation system, not all of the information is visible. For example, you cannot see the date or the name of the nurse.

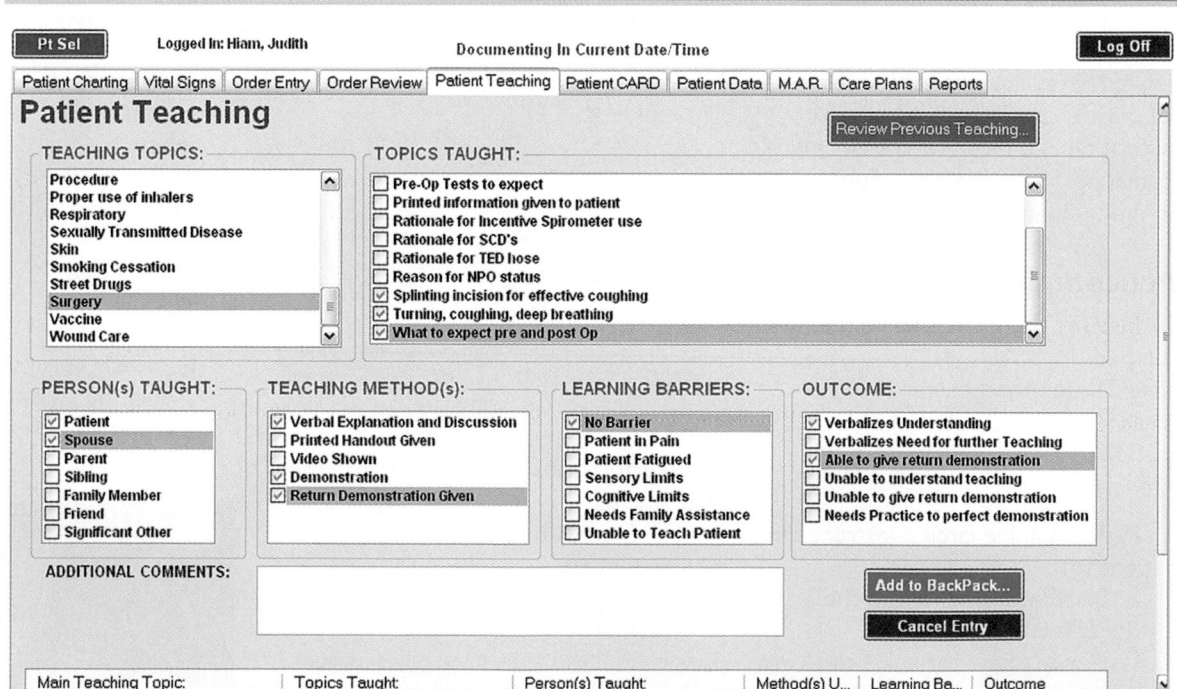

Practice Resources

No author. *Best practices* (2007).

Thinking About the Procedure

 Go to the *Fundamentals of Nursing Skills Videos*, **Perioperative Nursing: Teaching Coughing and Deep Breathing with Splinting.**

1. What position did the nurse use to teach coughing and deep breathing?

 Go to the *Fundamentals of Nursing Skills Videos*, **Perioperative Nursing: Teaching Leg Exercises.**

1. How was the patient positioned for the leg exercises?

2. Which exercise was taught first?

 Go to the *Fundamentals of Nursing Skills Videos*, **Perioperative Nursing: Teaching Moving in Bed.**

1. How did the nurse demonstrate the leg exercises to the patient?

For suggested responses for all three exercises, go to Chapter 37, **Thinking About the Procedure Suggested Responses (Procedure 37-1A, B, C),** on the Student Resource Disk or DavisPlus at http://davisplus.fadavis.com/Wilkinson2

Procedure 37-2 — Applying Antiembolism Stockings

➤ For steps to follow in *all* procedures, refer to the Universal Steps for All Procedures found on the inside back cover of Volume 2.

Critical Aspects

- Measure the patient's leg to ensure that you select stockings of the correct size.
- Inspect the legs and feet for edema, abrasions, lesions, open areas, and circulatory changes.
- Elevate the patient's legs for at least 15 minutes before applying stockings.
- Insert your hand and turn the stocking inside out to the level of the heel.
- Insert patient's foot into stocking. Gradually pull the remaining portion of the stocking up and over the leg.
  - Keep knee-high stockings 2.5 to 5 cm (1 to 2 in.) below the joint.
  - Do not apply thigh-high stockings if the thigh circumference is greater than 100 cm (25 in.).
- Make sure the stocking is free of wrinkles and is not rolled at the top or bunched.

Equipment
- Measuring tape
- Antiembolism stockings
- Washcloth and towel (if needed to cleanse legs)
- Talcum powder (optional: check manufacturer's recommendations)

Delegation
You can delegate application of antiembolism stockings to nursing assistive personnel who have been trained in the task. Instruct the NAP as follows:
- Report the presence of any abnormalities on the lower extremities, such as lesions, sores, or redness, before applying the stockings.
- Instruct the patient to maintain a recumbent position for at least 15 minutes before applying the stockings.

- Do not massage the legs.
- Make sure there are no wrinkles in the stockings once they have been applied.

Pre-Procedure Assessment
- Assess the level of consciousness and cognitive ability.
If the patient is unconscious or confused, you will need to call for assistance to hold and stabilize the lower extremities as you apply the stockings.

- Assess for signs and symptoms of severe peripheral arterial disease, such as weak or absent pulses, discoloration or cyanosis, or gangrene.
Antiembolism stockings should not be used in patients with any of these findings because they compress the vessels and, therefore, further impede the already compromised arterial flow.

(continued on next page)

Procedure 37-2 ■ **Applying Antiembolism Stockings** (continued)

■ Assess the condition of the skin. Note the presence of lesions, dermatitis, or major edema, as evidenced by shiny, taut skin.

If skin is overstretched by edema, antiembolism stockings may irritate or worsen skin conditions and cause skin breakdown.

■ Note the position of the patient and length of time the patient has been in that position.

Place the patient supine for at least 15 minutes before stocking application. This prevents trapping of pooled venous blood.

➤ When performing the procedure, always identify your patient according to agency policy and be attentive to standard precautions, hand hygiene, patient safety and privacy, body mechanics, and documentation.

➤ If possible, apply stockings in the morning, before the patient gets out of bed.

Prevents venous distention and edema that occur when the patient is sitting or standing.

Procedure Steps

1. Measure the patient's lower extremity.

Accurate measurement ensures that you order stockings of the proper size. Stockings must be sized correctly in order to apply the correct amounts of pressure at the ankle, mid-calf, and upper thigh. If they are not tight enough, they will not improve venous return effectively. If they are too tight, they may compress the veins and impair circulation to the skin. ▼

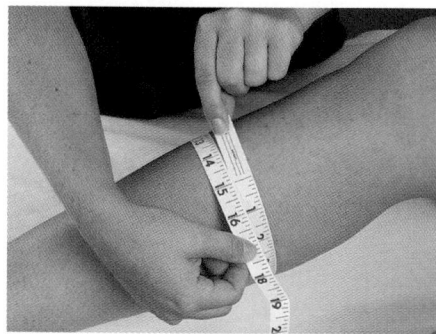

Step 1 Variation. Thigh-High Stockings

a. **Measure the circumference of the thigh at the widest section.**

The manufacturer of T.E.D.® brand stockings recommends that stockings not be applied if the thigh circumference exceeds 100 cm (25 inches).

b. **Measure the calf circumference at the widest section.**

c. **Measure the distance from the gluteal fold to the base of the heel.**

Step 1 Variation. Knee-High Stockings

a. **Measure the circumference of the calf at the widest section.**

b. **Measure the distance from the base of the heel to the middle of the knee joint.**

Evidence is not conclusive, but increasingly supports the use of knee-high instead of thigh-high hose.

2. Assist the patient to a supine position, and instruct him to maintain that position for at least 15 minutes before you apply the stockings.

Prevents trapping of pooled venous blood by the antiembolism stockings.

3. Cleanse the patient's legs and feet if necessary. Dry well.

Removing surface dirt and/or bacteria will decrease the likelihood of infection and odor.

4. Lightly dust the legs and feet with talcum powder if desired and if recommended by the manufacturer. Do not use powder if the patient is or is likely to become diaphoretic.

Powder eases the application of the stockings, but perspiration will cause the powder to clump.

5. Holding one stocking at the top cuff in your dominant hand, slide your nondominant arm down and into the stocking until your hand reaches the heel of the stocking.

6. Grasp the center of the heel with your hand inside the stocking, and then slowly turn the stocking inside out to the level of the heel with your other hand.

The elastic in the stockings is very strong; this method is the easiest way to fit it over the foot and calf. ▼

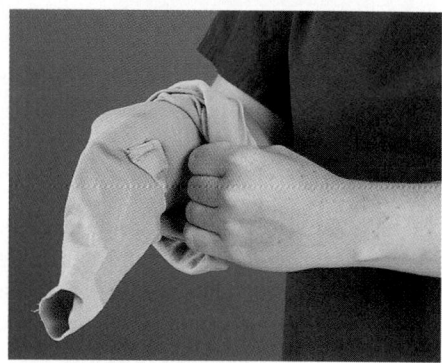

7. Ask the patient to point his toes as you grasp the turned foot of the stocking and ease it onto his foot and heel (like putting on a sock). Center the patient's heel in the heel of the stocking.

Ensures that the pressure of the stocking is over the correct anatomical areas.

8. Gradually pull the remainder of the stocking up and over the leg, turning it right side out as you proceed. Be certain the stocking is straight. ▼

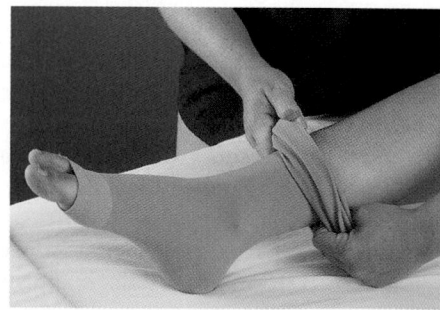

Step 8 Variation. Knee-High Stockings

a. **Pull up to 2.5 to 5 cm (1 to 2 in.) below the knee**

Step 8 Variation. Thigh-High Stockings

a. Pull up to the gluteal fold of the thigh, rotating inward so the gusset is centered over the femoral artery, slightly toward the inside of the leg.

Stockings apply varying amounts of compression between ankle, calf, and thigh areas. Keeping the stocking straight ensures that the pressure occurs over the correct areas.

9. Smooth out any excess material; keep stockings free of wrinkles and bunching.

Decreases the risk of skin breakdown and areas of inappropriate and potentially dangerous constriction.

10. When using stockings with closed toes, tug gently on the end of the stocking over the toes to create a small space between the end of the toes and the stocking.

Prevents compression of small vessels in the toes, which may impede circulation.

11. Repeat the procedure on the other leg.

12. Remove the stockings and bathe and dry the legs daily.

13. Launder the stockings at least every 3 days; dry them on a flat surface. Soiled stockings can irritate the skin; dry flat to prevent stretching.

What if. . .

■ **Both legs do not measure the same?**

Order two different sizes of stockings and use one from each package to make two pairs.

Evaluation

■ Evaluate patient comfort.

Severe, continuous discomfort may indicate that the stockings are the wrong size.

■ Check the stockings for wrinkles and/or rolling down at the top, especially when sitting.

Wrinkles and rolling down can cause skin breakdown and areas of constriction.

■ Evaluate and monitor skin condition.

Elastic stockings should be removed for 20 to 30 minutes every 8 to 12 hours to allow you to inspect the patient's skin and evaluate the adequacy of his circulation.

■ Evaluate the patient's ability to ambulate.

It is important to reduce the time the patient is immobile due to pain, sedation, mechanical ventilation, and so on.

■ Re-measure the legs regularly.

To prevent complications related to swelling and weight gain.

Home Care

■ Teach the client and/or caregiver to apply the stockings.
■ Encourage the client to have two pairs of stockings on hand so that one pair can be used while the other is being laundered.
■ Instruct the client to follow the manufacturer's directions for washing the stockings.
■ Teach the client not to roll down the tops of the stockings.

Documentation

■ Document leg measurements and size of the stockings used, to provide a baseline.
■ Document the time and date applied.
■ Note the condition of the skin, including any abnormalities.

Sample electronic documentation:

Note that because this is just one screen of a documentation system, not all of the information is visible. For example, you cannot see the date or the name of the nurse.

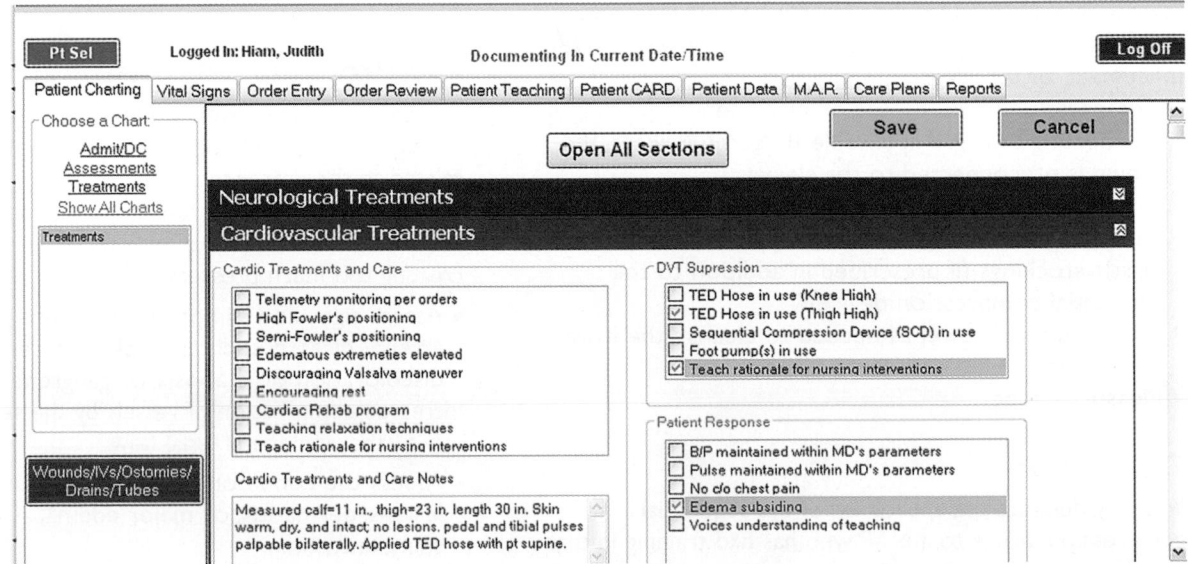

Practice Resources

American Association of Critical-Care Nurses (2005); The Joanna Briggs Institute (2008a); Winslow, E., & Brosz, D. (2008).

(continued on next page)

Procedure 37-2 ■ Applying Antiembolism Stockings (continued)

Thinking About the Procedure

 Go to the *Fundamentals of Nursing Skills Videos,* **Perioperative Nursing: Antiembolism Stockings.**

1. In what position did the nurse place the patient to measure leg length from the gluteal fold to the base of the heel?

2. How did the nurse position the patient to measure her leg length for knee-high stockings?

3. Did the nurse apply thigh-high or knee-high stockings?

 For suggested responses, go to Chapter 37, **Thinking About the Procedure Suggested Responses (Procedure 37-2),** on the Student Resource Disk or DavisPlus at http://davisplus.fadavis.com/Wilkinson2

Procedure 37-3 ☐ Applying Sequential Compression Devices

➤ For steps to follow in *all* procedures, refer to the Universal Steps for All Procedures found on the inside back cover of Volume 2.

Critical Aspects

- Determine whether elastic stockings are to be used concurrently with the sequential device. If so, apply them (see Procedure 37-2).
- Place the regulating pump for the sequential compression in a location that will ensure patient safety.
- Place the patient in a supine position.
- If you are using thigh-high compression sleeves or thigh-high pneumatic air stockings, measure the thigh.
- Place the lower extremity on the open sleeve, ensuring that the compression chambers are located over the correct anatomical structure (e.g., knee opening is at the level of the joint).
- Leave one to two fingerbreadths between the sleeve and the extremity.
- Set the regulating pump to the correct pressure, as prescribed.
- Instruct the patient to call for assistance in disconnecting the tubing from the sleeve.

Equipment

Note: Sequential compression devices may be referred to by several different brand names, including SCDS (sequential compression decompression stockings), Flowtrons, and PAS (pneumatic air stockings).

- Compression pump, motor, or machine
- Connecting tubing, if applicable (In some devices, the tubing is preconnected to the sleeves.)
- Compression sleeve (knee-high or thigh-high, depending on the order and the type of device)
- Elastic stockings (if prescribed in addition to the sequential compression device)
- Washcloth and towel as needed to cleanse the lower extremities
- Measuring tape

Delegation

You may delegate the application of the sequential compression device to a NAP who has had training in that task. Instruct the NAP to report any redness, irritation, or open areas on the lower extremities. Instruct the NAP to ensure that all cords and connecting tubing are in a place that will not create a fall risk for the patient or visitors.

SCDs should not be removed for long periods of time because they are needed to support the patient's peripheral circulation.

Pre-Procedure Assessment

- Assess cognitive level and level of consciousness.
Patients with altered cognition may be at higher risk for falls related to the presence of the connecting tubing and attachment to the compression pump. Patients who are unconscious will not be able to report a device that is creating too much pressure.

- Assess signs and symptoms of severe peripheral arterial disease, such as weak or absent pulses, discoloration or cyanosis, or gangrene.
Increased compression of vessels by the sequential device may further impede arterial flow.

- Assess the condition of the skin. Note the presence of lesions, dermatitis, or major edema, as evidenced by shiny, taut skin.
If skin is overstretched by edema, the sequential compression sleeve may irritate or worsen skin conditions and cause skin breakdown.

➤ When performing the procedure, always identify your patient according to agency policy and be attentive to standard precautions, hand hygiene, patient safety and privacy, body mechanics, and documentation.

Procedure Steps

1. Cleanse the lower extremities, if necessary.
Removing surface dirt and/or bacteria will decrease the likelihood of infection and odor.

2. If elastic stockings have been ordered in conjunction with the sequential compression device, apply them, following the steps in Procedure 37-2.

3. For thigh-high SCD sleeves, you must measure the thigh to ensure that the sleeves are of the proper size. Follow the manufacturer's instructions.

4. Place the patient in a supine position.
Prevents venous pooling. Allows for easier application of the compression sleeve.

5. ✚ Place the compression device pump in a location near an electrical outlet so that the cord will not pose a fall risk.

Plug it in. *Note:* Many compression pumps come equipped with hangers so you can hang the device at the bottom of the patient's bed.

6. Apply the compression sleeve. ▼

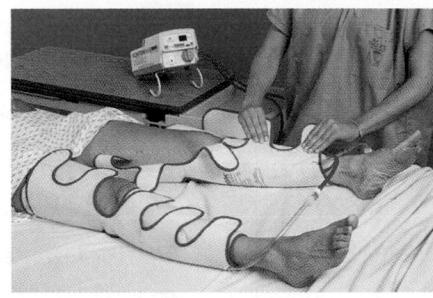

Step 6 Variation. For Flowtron Brand (available in knee-length only):
  a. Open the Velcro fasteners on the sleeve.
  b. Place the sleeve under the lower leg below the knee, with the "air bladder" side down on the bed.
  c. Bring the ends of the sleeve up, and wrap them around the lower leg, leaving one to two fingerbreadths of space between the leg and the sleeve.
Prevents excess pressure and overcompression.

Step 6 Variation. For SCDS/PAS Brands
  a. Open the Velcro® fasteners on the sleeve.

  b. Place the sleeve under the leg, ensuring that the fastener will close on the anterior surface. For thigh-high sleeves, place the opened sleeve under the leg, ensuring that the knee opening is at the level of the knee joint.
Ensures that compression occurs over the correct structures. Prevents restricted range of motion (ROM) of the knee joint.

  c. Bring the ends of the sleeve up, and wrap them around the leg, leaving one to two fingerbreadths of space between the leg and the sleeve.
Prevents excess pressure and overcompression.

7. Connect the sleeve to the compression pump.

8. Turn the pump on and, if applicable, set the compression pressure on the pump device to the manufacturer's recommended setting. *Note:* In some facilities, the compression pressure amount is preset and can be changed only by the central supply/equipment department.

Evaluation

After applying the device, make the following ongoing assessments:

■ Inflation and deflation of the sleeve
Ensures that the device is actually working.

■ Kinking or pinching of the connecting tubing
Would prevent correct inflation of sleeves and may cause overheating or malfunction of the unit.

■ Circulation, sensation, and motion of the foot, including skin color, pulses, temperature, capillary refill, motion, and sensation
■ Patient comfort
Increasing discomfort may indicate excess or incorrect pressure.

■ Skin condition. Remove the compression sleeves at intervals so that you can inspect skin and evaluate the adequacy of circulation. *Note:* If elastic stockings are being used in conjunction with the sequential compression device, follow the recommendations in Procedure 37-2.

■ Signs and symptoms of deep-vein thrombosis
Patients having sequential compression device therapy can still develop thrombi.

Patient Teaching

✚ Teach the patient to call for assistance when disconnecting the tubing from the compression pump in order to ambulate.
Prevents patient falls. The SCD tubing is a tripping hazard, and injuries from falls involving SCDs are likely to be more severe than injuries associated with general patient falls (Johnston & Davis, 2008).

Documentation

■ Document the date and time you applied the device.
■ Note the type and size (if applicable) of the compression sleeve used.
■ Document the skin condition, including any abnormalities.

(continued on next page)

Procedure 37-3 ■ **Applying Sequential Compression Devices** (continued)

Sample documentation:

11/11/11   1100   *Knee-high SCD applied per order. Skin warm, dry, and intact at time of application. Peripheral pulses palpable. Pt's wife instructed on use of SCD. Pt unresponsive. No evidence of discomfort, no grimace, or movement with application.* —————— S. Bee RN

Practice Resources

Berliner, E., Ozbilgin, B., & Zarin, D. (2003); Johnson, J., & Davis, M. (2008); Markel, D., & Morris, G. (2002).

Thinking About the Procedure

 Go to the *Fundamentals of Nursing Skills Videos,* **Perioperative Nursing: Sequential Compression Device.**

1. Where did the nurse place the compression pump?

2. What kind of compression sleeve was used: knee-high or thigh-high?

 For suggested responses, go to Chapter 37, **Thinking About the Procedure Suggested Responses (Procedure 37-3),** on the Student Resource Disk or DavisPlus at http://davisplus.fadavis.com/Wilkinson2

Procedure 37-4 ☐ **Managing Gastric Suction**

➤ For steps to follow in *all* procedures, refer to the Universal Steps for All Procedures found on the inside back cover of Volume 2.

Critical Aspects

Procedure 37-4A: Initial Equipment Set-Up
- Connect and secure the suction source, collection container, and drainage tubing.
- Don nonsterile gloves.
- Connect suction drainage tubing to nasogastric (NG) tubing.
- Secure the NG tube to the patient's nose and gown (if not already done).
- Turn on the suction.

Procedure 37-4B: Emptying the Suction Container
- Don nonsterile gloves.
- Turn off the suction; close the stopcock (or clamp the tubing).
- Empty the suction container and measure the contents.
- Empty and wash the graduated measuring container, if used.
- Cleanse the suction container port and close the stopper; place the container back in the holder.
- Turn on the suction and observe for proper functioning and tubing patency.

Procedure 37-4C: Irrigating the Nasogastric Tubing
- Prepare the irrigation set.
- Don nonsterile gloves.
- Check for NG tube placement.
- Fill the syringe with 30 to 50 mL of saline.
- Turn off the stopcock or clamp the NG tube.
- Disconnect the NG tube from drainage.
- Drain the suction tubing and turn off the suction source.
- Turn on the stopcock or unclamp the NG tube.
- Slowly instill and withdraw irrigant into the NG tube until fluid flows freely.
- Turn off the stopcock or reclamp the NG tube.

■ Reconnect the NG tube.
■ Turn on the stopcock or release the clamp.
Procedure 37-4D: Providing Comfort Measures
■ Don nonsterile gloves.
■ Provide mouth care.
■ Remove nasal secretions and apply water-soluble lubricant to nostrils.
■ Check that the tape or tube fixation device is secure.

Equipment

Procedure 37-4A Initial Equipment Set-Up
■ Nonsterile procedure gloves
■ Suction source (either a portable machine or piped-in wall source)
■ Suction container and tubing
■ Stopcock
To connect the NG tube to suction tubing.

Procedure 37-4B Emptying the Suction Container
■ Clean nonsterile procedure gloves
■ Graduated container
To measure gastric output when emptying the suction container. Not needed if suction canister is marked for measuring.
■ Alcohol wipes or chlorhexidine/alcohol antiseptic product

Procedure 37-4C Irrigating the Nasogastric Tubing
■ Nonsterile procedure gloves
■ Irrigating set (basin and bulb syringe or catheter-tipped syringe)
■ Normal saline irrigant (unless another irrigant is prescribed)
■ Linen-saver pads

Procedure 37-4D Comfort Measures
■ Nonsterile procedure gloves
■ Emesis basin, cup, and water for mouth care
■ Water-soluble lubricant
■ Cotton-tip applicators
■ Tissues or damp washcloth
Note: This procedure assumes a NG or other enteric tube is already in place and that its correct placement has already been verified. If you need to insert an NG tube or check placement, refer to Chapter 26. Tubes for gastric decompression are typically large-lumen tubes such as a

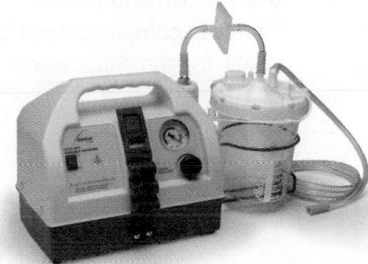

Portable suction source. (Courtesy of Allied Healthcare Products, St. Louis, MO.)

Salem sump or Levin tube. See the table at the end of this procedure for more information about tubes.

Delegation

As the registered nurse, you should do the initial set-up and any subsequent irrigation. You may delegate a NAP to empty and measure drainage and perform comfort measures. You must monitor equipment functioning and the patient's responses to the decompression. Instruct the NAP about observations that should be reported to you.

Pre-Procedure Assessments

■ Determine that the NG tube has been inserted and placement has been verified.
■ Verify the prescriber's order for type of tube and whether it is to be placed to suction or a drainage bag; also verify the type of suction to be used (low, high, continuous, intermittent).
■ Auscultate for bowel sounds.
■ Assess the patient's ability to cooperate with the procedure and understand explanations.
■ Refer to the Evaluation section of this procedure. This procedure assumes an NG tube is already in place, so assessments are ongoing.

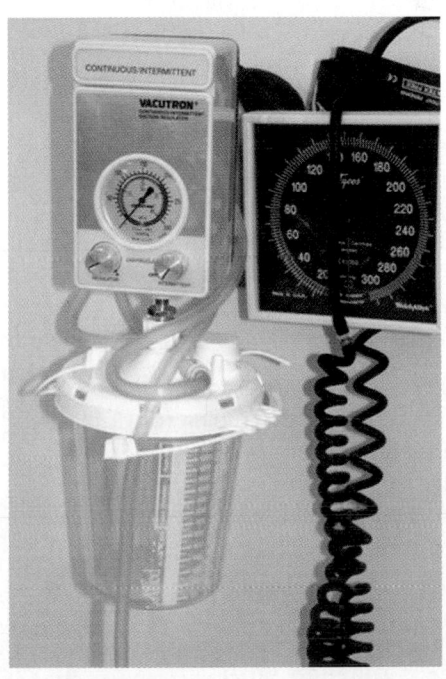

Wall suction unit.

(continued on next page)

Procedure 37-4 ■ **Managing Gastric Suction** (continued)

■ Procedure 37-4A Initial Equipment Set-Up

➤ When performing the procedure, always identify your patient according to agency policy and be attentive to standard precautions, hand hygiene, patient safety and privacy, body mechanics, and documentation.

Procedure Steps

1. Place the collection container in the holder (either on the portable suction machine or on the wall). Plug the power cord into a grounded outlet if using a portable suction machine.

2. Connect the short tubing between the container and the suction source. In some systems, the port will be marked "vacuum."

3. Connect the long suction tubing to the container (it may be marked "patient"); if available, connect a stopcock to the open end nearest the patient.

4. Don nonsterile procedure gloves.
Helps prevent transfer of microorganisms.

5. After the nasogastric (NG) tube has been inserted and placement verified, attach the end of the NG tube to the suction tubing.

See Chapter 26 to review importance of tube placement. You must be certain the NG tube is in the stomach, not in the esophagus or airways.

6. If using a Salem sump tube, instill 10 to 20 mL of air into the vent lumen to make sure it is patent. This should create a soft hissing sound.

7. Secure the NG tube to the client's nose and gown (see Chapter 26 to review).
Minimizes movement of the tube, helping to prevent irritation of the nares or other insertion site, as well as helping to keep the tube from migrating up out of the stomach.

8. Turn on the suction source to the prescribed amount. In an emergency, when there is no order, always use low suction. Open the stopcock—note the direction of the arrows.

9. Observe that drainage appears in the collection container.

It may take up to 5 minutes for air to be removed from the canister before the stomach contents will drain. ▼

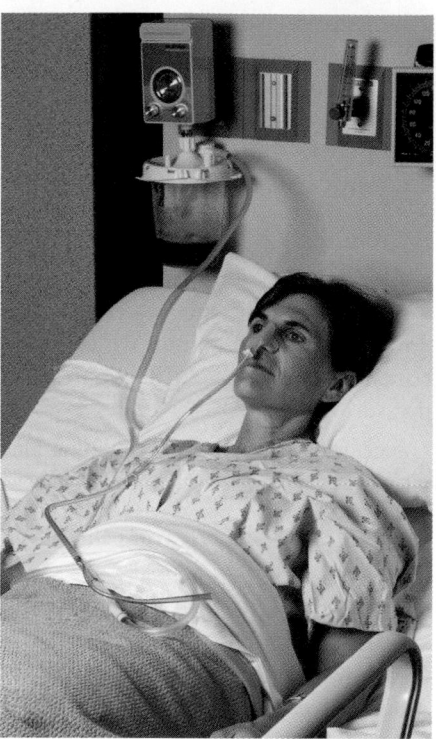

■ Procedure 37-4B Emptying the Suction Container

➤ When performing the procedure, always identify your patient according to agency policy and be attentive to standard precautions, hand hygiene, patient safety and privacy, body mechanics, and documentation.

1. Don clean nonsterile gloves.
Limits the transfer of microorganisms; protects your hands from contact with body secretions.

2. Turn off the suction source and close the stopcock on the tubing (or clamp the tubing, if there is no stopcock).
Prevents suction flow during emptying of the container.

3. Empty the suction canister.

Step 3 Variation. Suction container is marked with measurements.
Note the amount, color, and odor of the contents. Empty and rinse the container.

Step 3 Variation. Suction container is not marked incrementally.
Remove the cap from the lid of the suction container and pour the drainage into a graduated measuring container. Note color, odor, and amount.
A container with graduated markings enables you to monitor intake and output (I&O) accurately. Rinsing removes organic material that could be a reservoir for microorganisms.

4. Wipe the port of the suction container with an alcohol wipe. Place the suction container back in its holder and close the stopper on the lid.

5. Turn on the suction source to the prescribed amount. Turn on the stopcock (or unclamp the tubing), noting the direction of the arrows.

6. Observe for proper functioning of the suction and patency of the tubing.
Prevents complications that would result from malfunction.

7. Remove and discard gloves. Perform hand hygiene.

■ Procedure 37-4C Irrigating the Nasogastric Tubing

➤ When performing the procedure, always identify your patient according to agency policy and be attentive to standard precautions, hand hygiene, patient safety and privacy, body mechanics, and documentation.

1. Place a linen-saver pad on the bed under the NG tube.

2. Open the irrigation set and pour saline into the basin.
Water is not used because it may cause electrolyte imbalances.

3. Don clean procedure gloves.
Limits the transfer of microorganisms; protects your hands from contact with body secretions.

4. Check for correct placement of the NG tube (see Chapter 26 as needed).
Prevents accidental instillation of irrigant into the airways.

5. Fill the syringe with 30 to 50 mL of saline and lay it on the linen-saver pad.

6. Clamp the NG tube or turn off the stopcock connecting to the suction tubing. Disconnect the NG tube from the suction tubing.
Prevents backflow of drainage and soiling of linens and clothing.

7. Hold the drainage tubing up until suction clears it. Then lay it on the linen-saver pad or hook it over the suction machine.
Keeps secretions from soiling the bed linens or clothing.

8. Turn off the suction machine.

9. Unclamp the NG tube or turn on the stopcock.

10. Unpin the NG tube (or remove tape) from the patient's clothing.

11. With the syringe, instill the irrigant slowly into the NG tube. Do not force the solution. Be careful not to instill fluid into the air vent.
Clears the NG tube of gastric contents to keep it patent and helps keep the tube from adhering to the gastric mucosa. Partially digested food, clotted blood, or tissue debris may clog the tube and prevent effective drainage.

12. Lower the end of the NG tube and then release the syringe bulb (or pull back the plunger) to withdraw fluid. Instill and withdraw until fluid flows in and out freely.
Uses the force of gravity with negative pressure to withdraw instilled fluid and gastric contents.

Step 12 Variation. Double-Lumen NG Tube
Draw 30 mL of air into the syringe and inject it into the "pigtail" (the

smaller-bore tube). Follow agency policy for this.
This clears the air-vent tube of any secretions. It must be patent in order to equalize pressure and prevent gastric tissue trauma at the drainage ports. The air also keeps the tube from draining fluid out of the stomach by capillary action.

13. Reclamp the NG tube or turn off the stopcock.
Prevents backflow of drainage.

14. Reconnect the NG tube to the suction tube. Then release the clamp or turn on the stopcock.

15. Reattach the NG tube to the patient's clothing (with a pin or tape—see Chapter 26 as needed).
Prevents pulling on and irritating the patient's nostril.

16. Provide comfort measures (e.g., mouth care).

17. Remove and discard gloves. Perform hand hygiene.

■ Procedure 37-4D Providing Comfort Measures

➤ When performing the procedure, always identify your patient according to agency policy and be attentive to standard precautions, hand hygiene, patient safety and privacy, body mechanics, and documentation.

1. Don clean nonsterile procedure gloves.

2. Provide mouth care (see Procedures 22-6, 22-7, and 22-8 if you need to review). Use mouthwash as desired. Avoid using lemon-glycerine swabs. Apply water-soluble lubricant to the lips if they become dry and crusty.
The patient most likely has a dry mouth from not receiving oral intake and from mouth breathing. Lemon-glycerine swabs cause even more drying of tissues.

3. Remove nasal secretions with a tissue or a damp washcloth. Moisten a

cotton-tip applicator and wipe the inside of each nostril. If secretions are encrusted, moisten the applicator with hydrogen peroxide, then follow with an applicator moistened with water.
To soften, dissolve, and remove secretions and prevent tissue irritation.

4. Apply a small amount of water-soluble lubricant to the inside of each nostril.
Soothes and softens dried skin. Avoid petroleum-based lubricants, as complications may occur if they are inhaled.

5. Check that the tape or tube fixation device is secure. If it is not,

replace it (see Procedure 26-2 as needed).
Prevents irritation of the nasal skin and mucosa. Helps prevent migration of the NG tube from the stomach.

What if. . .

■ **Resistance is met when you irrigate the NG tube?**

Check the tubing for kinks or evidence of obstruction. Have the patient to turn to the left side.

Turning to one side changes the position of the distal tip of the NG tube.

(continued on next page)

Procedure 37-4 ■ **Managing Gastric Suction** (continued)

■ **The patient complains that the NG tube is pulling against her nostril?**

The tube may not be properly anchored to her clothing. Reattach the safety pin (or tape) closer to the nose so that there is more slack in the tube.

■ **The NG tube causes excoriation of the nares?**

Remove the tape or fixation device from the nose. Remove the residual adhesive from the skin. Apply skin sealant and anchor the tube so that the adhesive touches in a different place on the skin. Keep the excoriated areas clean and dry.

■ **The NG tube does not drain?**

Check tubing for kinks or blockage. Check the suction apparatus. If the collection container is higher than the patient's abdomen, lower it. If these aspects are working properly, irrigate the tube (see Procedure 37-4C, preceding). If the tube still is not draining and the patient is uncomfortable, document and notify the primary care provider. Encourage the patient to relax and breathe slowly through her nose. If the patient has abdominal distention, pain, or vomiting, notify the provider immediately.

If the container is too high, the negative pressure of low suction may not be enough to overcome the force of gravity. Abdominal distention, pain, or vomiting may mean the system is not working. Continued distention creates undue strain on the suture line. You should notify the care provider of these symptoms even when the mechanical aspects of the suction seem in working order.

Gastric Decompression Tubes				
TYPE	**LUMEN(S)**	**USE**	**MANAGEMENT**	**DISCUSSION**
Levin	1, unvented	Decompression, feedings, or irrigation	Use low intermittent suction; may require irrigation.	If the tube opening(s) rest(s) against the gastric mucosa, the suction may irritate or injure the tissue.
Salem Sump	2	Decompression, suction, gastric lavage	Vented. May use high continuous suction.	The air vent helps keep the tube away from the gastric mucosa during suction.
Sengsten–Blakemore	3	Decompression; treatment of active bleeding from esophageal or gastric varices	Use low intermittent suction.	Gastric or esophageal balloons hold the tube in place.
Cantor	1, unvented	Decompression	Use intermittent suction.	Distal end is weighted with a balloon. Used in bowel obstruction. Rarely used because of the hazard posed by the mercury in the weighted balloon.
Miller–Abbott	2	Decompression	Use intermittent suction	Distal end weighted with a balloon. Used in bowel obstruction. Rarely used because it contains mercury in the weighted balloon.
Ewald or other very large-bore tube	May be passed orally for emergency evacuation of stomach contents to prevent absorption of ingested medications, poisons, or products. A piston tip syringe is placed on the end of the tube for manual suction. Typically, the stomach is washed repeatedly with saline and all contents are withdrawn. Because of its large diameter, this type of tube is not tolerated by patients who are alert, and is not left in place after lavage is completed.			
Weighted Small-Bore Tubes (e.g., Keofeed)	For feedings only. Suction collapses the tube.			

Evaluation and Maintenance

■ Periodically assess placement of the tube by a combination of methods (i.e., checking pH of aspirate, by listening over the stomach with a stethoscope while injecting air into the tube, and by reviewing radiographic reports). See Chapter 26 for review, as needed.

■ Monitor patency of the tube and the effectiveness of the suction. Check tube connections.
■ Monitor patient comfort (e.g., sore throat).
The continuing presence of a tube in the nose and throat is bothersome to patients. The major nuisance is the pressure of the tube against the internal mucous membranes, irritating the nostril, pharynx, and esophagus.

- Auscultate for bowel sounds; turn off suction while auscultating.

Bowel sounds indicate the return of peristalsis and the success of gastric decompression. You may hear the sound of the suction apparatus and misinterpret it as bowel sounds.

- Monitor for gastric distention, vomiting, and abdominal pain.

These symptoms probably indicate the suction is not working effectively. See "What if...," preceding.

- Examine skin and mucous membranes around the insertion site (e.g., nares, abdomen).
- Follow agency policy or the primary care provider's prescription for irrigation of the gastric tube. It is common to irrigate with 30 to 60 mL of normal saline every 4 to 6 hours.
- Monitor the color of the drainage (should be green to gold). If there is blood in the drainage, notify the primary care provider.
- For clients undergoing prolonged GI suction, observe for signs and symptoms of hyponatremia and hypokalemia (i.e., fatigue, lethargy, confusion, seizures, muscle weakness, paresthesia, and cardiac dysrhythmias). Review lab results and report any symptoms to the primary care provider.
- Assess the patient's ability to move about in bed while attached to the suction source.

Sample electronic documentation:

Patient Teaching

- Instruct the patient to notify you of any discomfort, and to not tug on or try to reposition the NG tube if it becomes uncomfortable.
- Instruct the patient to notify you if feeling nauseated.

This could mean the tube is blocked and not draining effectively.

Home Care

Usually, gastric suction is performed in a hospital. If the client is to go home with gastric suction (e.g., a terminally ill person who has a bowel obstruction and wants to be in his or her own home), teach the family how to use the device before the person is discharged. Also arrange for home healthcare.

Documentation

- Record all drainage as output on the I&O record.
- Record the time, type, and volume of irrigations and the drainage returned.
- Be sure to include irrigation fluids as input on the I&O record.
- Note color, odor, and consistency of drainage.
- Document patient's emotional and physical responses to NG intubation.
- Document any evidence of tube or equipment malfunction.
- Document epigastric pain, discomfort, distention, or vomiting.

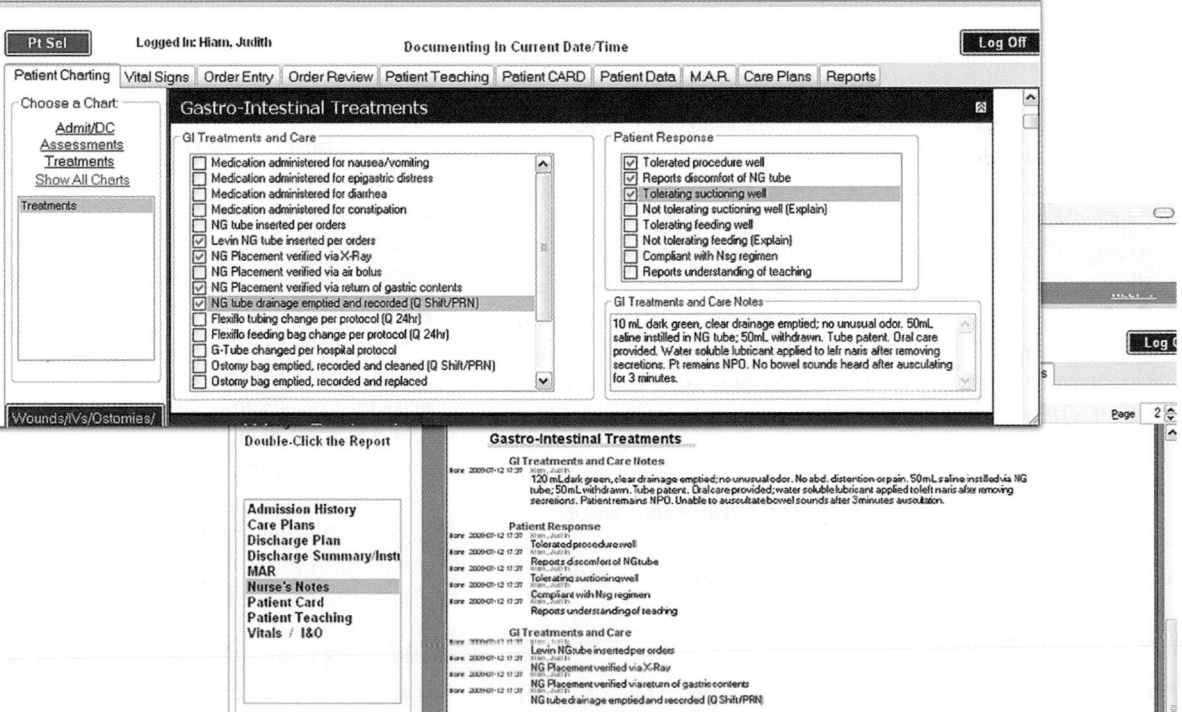

Practice Resources

No author. *Best practices* (2007); Allied Healthcare Products, Inc. (n.d.); Green, S., Harris, C., & Singer, J. (2008); Sarasota Memorial Hospital (2008).

(continued on next page)

Procedure 37-4 ■ **Managing Gastric Suction** (continued)

Thinking About the Procedure

 Go to the *Fundamentals of Nursing Skills Videos*, **Nutrition: Gastrointestinal Suction.**

1. What type of suction source was demonstrated in the DVD?

2. Why did the nurse not clamp the NG tube before disconnecting it from the suction tubing?

 For suggested responses, go to Chapter 37, **Thinking About the Procedure Suggested Responses (Procedure 37-4),** on the Student Resource Disk or DavisPlus at http://davisplus.fadavis.com/Wilkinson2

Clinical Insights

Clinical Insight 37-1 ▶ **Preoperative Teaching**

Explain what to expect before surgery.

- Explain the planned preoperative testing—lab tests, x-ray studies, ECG, and so on.
- Discuss skin preparation, including preoperative wash with an antibacterial product if this is included in the treatment plan.
- Discuss prescribed preoperative medications.
- Outline activities that will occur before surgery, such as insertion of an IV, placement of a urinary catheter, or cardiac monitoring.
- Review the preoperative restriction of fluid and food. Often the patient is to be NPO for at least 8 hours before the planned start of surgery. Some guidelines indicate that most children can drink clear liquids until 2 hours before surgery (The Joanna Briggs Institute, 2008).
- If the patient is having surgery on the gastrointestinal (GI) tract, an additional bowel prep may be ordered (e.g., a low-residue diet beginning 1 week before surgery, and a liquid diet for the 48 hours preceding surgery). Patients having GI surgery also may have enemas before surgery. (If you need to review special diets, refer to Chapter 26.)
- Explain the need to remove jewelry, makeup, hearing aids, glasses, contact lenses, and any removable dental prostheses before being transported to the operating suite. It is best to have a family member take valuable belongings home for safekeeping.
- Tell the patient that a member of the anesthesia team will speak with him about the proposed anesthesia before surgery.
- Give the patient and family a tentative schedule for the operative day, including the time to arrive at the hospital or surgery center.

Explain what to expect in the operative suite.

- Inform the patient and family where relatives may wait during surgery.
- Discuss the preoperative holding area and activities that may occur there.
- Describe the operating room and the activities that the patient may anticipate before the surgery.

- Explain that the anesthesiologist or nurse anesthetist will monitor the patient throughout the entire surgery and is responsible for keeping him comfortable with medications throughout the procedure.
- Describe the types of people who may be present in the operative suite. This is particularly important if the patient is not receiving a general anesthetic.

Explain what to expect after surgery.

- Explain that the patient will initially be cared for in the postanesthesia care unit. After a period of observation, he will be transferred to the surgical unit. Note that some patients may be transferred directly to a critical care unit after surgery. If this is expected, tell the patient and family about this preoperatively.
- Family may visit after the patient has been admitted and assessed on the surgical unit.
- Tell the patient what to expect in terms of dressings, equipment, and monitoring devices.
- Describe the types of assessments that will be performed.
- Explain that pain medication will be given to keep the patient comfortable. If he experiences pain, he should tell the nursing staff.
- Discuss the usual progression of recovery, including activity level, deep breathing, coughing, leg exercises, and dietary intake.
- Discuss the anticipated length of stay.
- Teach the importance of deep breathing and coughing, especially after general anesthesia. Demonstrate how to splint the incision to facilitate deep breathing and coughing.
- Teach the patient how to move into and out of bed after surgery.
- Teach and emphasize the importance of leg exercises to minimize the risk of thrombus formation. If decreased activity or prolonged bedrest is anticipated, explain the use of anitembolism stockings or sequential compression devices.

Note: If the patient is to be discharged the day of surgery, inform him in advance about what to wear to the facility, and explain that he must arrange for a responsible adult to drive her home.

Clinical Insight 37-2 ▶ **Preparing a Room for a Patient's Return from Surgery**

In many institutions, the patient is transported to surgery using the bed that is in his hospital room, so these steps may vary.

■ Put clean linens on the bed, including pads to protect the linen from drainage.

■ Fold the linens back to the end of the bed.

■ Raise the bed to stretcher height, and lock the wheels.

■ Move furniture and equipment so that the stretcher can be placed directly against the bed.

■ If needed, set up suction, oxygen, or other special equipment.

■ Place the following equipment in the room:
   Stethoscope, manometer, thermometer (to measure vital signs)
   IV pole
   Emesis basin
   Tissues
   A clean gown, washcloth, and towel
   Extra pillows for positioning the patient

Clinical Insight 37-3 ▶ **Creating an Operative Field**

■ A nonsterile team member (usually the circulating nurse) performs a surgical prep, using a scrub agent and "paint," to cleanse the operative site. Antiseptic agents must be FDA-approved and approved by the agency's infection control professional. Chlorhexidine and povidone-iodine solutions are most commonly used.

■ The area surrounding the operative site is then covered with sterile drapes so that only the operative area is exposed.

In the intraoperative period, sterile team members are the only persons allowed to enter the sterile field. The sterile field encompasses the patient and the area immediately surrounding the client. Creation of the sterile field proceeds as follows:

■ Don head covering and shoe covers before entering the surgical suite.

■ Perform a surgical scrub.

■ Don sterile gown, gloves, and other surgical attire (e.g., mask).

■ Cover the area surrounding the operative site with sterile drapes so that only the patient's operative area is exposed.

■ Place sterile draping over the remainder of the patient's body.

■ (In most cases) suspend a vertical drape at neck level so the client's head and airway are accessible to the anesthesiologist or nurse anesthetist (who is not sterile). For neurosurgery, even the head is draped, and the anesthesiologist or nurse anesthetist sits to the side of the head.

Assessment Guidelines and Tools

Preoperative Assessment Topics

Include the following information in your preoperative assessment.

Health History—Discuss current and chronic health problems and prior hospitalizations or surgeries.

Physical Status—Identify any mobility concerns, and determine whether the client uses hearing aids, glasses, or contact lenses. Identify risk factors for venous thromboembolism (Bartley, 2006):

■ Venous stasis (e.g., client on prolonged bed rest, lengthy surgery, varicose veins, and heart failure)

■ Vascular wall injury (e.g., surgery, IV catheter, irritating IV drugs, prior deep vein thrombus)

■ Hypercoagulability (e.g., estrogen therapy, oral contraceptive use, cancer, dehydration, pregnancy)

■ Older adults, especially those with other risk factors

Allergies—Check allergies to medications, food, tape, soaps, latex, or other substances.

Medications—Ask what prescribed medications and over-the-counter, herbal, or natural remedies the client takes (e.g., Echinacea, ephedra sinica, garlic, ginkgo biloba, ginseng, and St. John's wort). For more details about herbal products,

Mental Status—Note whether the client is able to respond to questions and offer a health history. Is he oriented? Does he appear anxious?

Knowledge—and understanding of the surgery and anesthesia. Ask the client to explain in his own words the planned surgery and postoperative course. Reinforce accurate statements, and correct any misconceptions.

Cultural and Spiritual Factors—Identify any cultural practices or spiritual beliefs that bring comfort to the client. Discuss how you can integrate these practices into the client's surgical experience.

Access to Social Resources—Identify the client's support network. Who is available to assist the client after surgery? Whom does the client rely on? Are those people aware of the client's upcoming surgery and condition?

Coping Strategies—Ask the client to identify the strategies he uses to cope with stress.

Use of Alcohol and Recreational Drugs—Inquire about the amount and frequency of alcohol use. Discuss the use of pain medications and recreational drugs. If the client uses these substances, identify the amount and frequency.

 Go to Chapter 37, **Tables, Boxes, Figures: ESG Box 37-1,** on the Student Resource Disk or DavisPlus at http:// davisplus.fadavis.com/Wilkinson2

AORN *SAMPLE* Preoperative Assessment Form **(Facility Name and Address)**	Addressograph

NOTE: *This record is a sample only. Clinical records should be customized to incorporate data fields that represent the setting, facility, procedure, and patient. Reproductions and variations are encouraged, provided credit is given to AORN.*

(Patient Information: name, age, gender, medical record number, date)

Date:_____

Structural Data:

Admitted via:
- ☐ Ambulatory   ☐ Wheelchair   ☐ Stretcher
- ☐ Other assistive devices:_____

Admitted from:
- ☐ Home   ☐ Transferring hospital
- ☐ Acute rehab facility   ☐ Extended/skilled care facility

Date of preoperative assessment:_____

Planned procedure:_____

Language(s) spoken: ☐ English ☐ Spanish ☐ Other:_____

☐ Patient's records, belongings, valuables secured (I115)
 Belonging inventory: ☐ Watch   ☐ Jewelry
  ☐ Contacts/glasses ☐ Dentures/partial(s) ☐ Hearing aid

Identity confirmed (I26): ☐ Yes   ☐ No

Advance directive signed: ☐ Yes   ☐ No
 Location:_____

Operative procedure, surgical site, and laterality verified (I143): ☐ Yes   ☐ No

Consent for planned procedures verified (I124): ☐ Yes   ☐ No

NPO status verified (I138): ☐ Yes   ☐ No
 Since: (date/time)_____

Preadmission testing
- ☐ CBC_____
- ☐ Potassium level_____
- ☐ CXR_____
- ☐ Type and cross
- ☐ Urinalysis_____
- ☐ EKG_____
- ☐ Pregnancy test:_____
-   # of units:_____

Nursing Data Elements:

General health status: (check when present)
- ☐ Diabetes   ☐ Cancer   ☐ Obesity   ☐ Pregnancy
- ☐ Hematologic disorders (anemia, sickle cell disease or conditions)

☐ **Vital signs:**
 Temperature:_____   Pulse:_____   BP:_____
 Respirations:_____   Height:_____   Weight:_____

☐ **Allergies verified (note type of reaction) (I123)**
 Latex allergy: ☐ Yes   ☐ No
 Medications: ☐ Yes:_____   ☐ No
  _____
  _____
 Food: ☐ Yes:_____   ☐ No
  _____

☐ **Daily medications** (prescription, OTC, vitamins, alternative medication, herbal remedies, chemotherapy):
 _____
 _____
 Medications taken day of surgery:_____

☐ Alcohol/Drug social use:_____

☐ **Neurologic assessment:** ☐ Alert and oriented
- ☐ Speech intact   ☐ Follows simple commands
- ☐ Risk of falls   ☐ History of seizures
 LOC: ☐ Alert/oriented ☐ Drowsy   ☐ Sedated
  ☐ Asleep   ☐ Unresponsive ☐ Disoriented
  ☐ Other:_____

☐ **Sensory assessment:**
- ☐ No limitations   ☐ Hearing impairment   ☐ Visual impairment

☐ **Cardiovascular assessment:**
- ☐ Pacemaker   ☐ Implanted defibrillator
- ☐ Chest pain
- ☐ Peripheral edema: Location:_____
- ☐ DVT/PE risk:
  ☐ None ☐ Low ☐ Med ☐ High
  _____
  _____

☐ **Respiratory assessment:**
- ☐ Tracheotomy
- ☐ Intubated
- ☐ Chest tube
 Respirations: ☐ Regular   ☐ Labored
 Smoking history ☐ Yes   ☐ No
  Packs/day:____ Years smoked:_____
  Quit date:_____
- ☐ Cough   ☐ Cold symptoms
- ☐ Current or recent respiratory infection
- ☐ Preexisting respiratory problems (specify):
  _____
  _____

☐ **Musculoskeletal assessment:**
- ☐ No limitations
- ☐ Paralysis
- ☐ Traction
- ☐ Limited ROM
- ☐ Amputation:_____
- ☐ Prosthesis:_____

Nursing Data Elements (continued):

☐ **Skin assessment:**
   ☐ Cool   ☐ Warm   ☐ Intact
   ☐ Dry   ☐ Moist
   ☐ Body jewelry removed
   ☐ Makeup removed
   ☐ Tattoos: _____
   ☐ Rash:_____
   ☐ Bruises:_____
   ☐ Wounds: _____
   ☐ Ostomy:_____
   ☐ Catheter/Drain: _____
   ☐ Venous access device: _____

☐ **Gastrointestinal assessment:**
Last bowel movement (date/time):_____
Usual diet: _____
_____

Recent unexplained weight loss
   ☐ Yes: Amount:_____ Time frame:_____
   ☐ No
Problems chewing or swallowing
   ☐ Yes   ☐ No
Special needs:
   ☐ Chewing   ☐ Swallowing
   ☐ Appetite   ☐ Diet preferences

☐ **Genitourinary/Gynecology assessment:**
   ☐ Voided on call to OR
     Time:_____ Amount:_____
   ☐ Urinary catheter: Amount in bag:_____
   ☐ Urinary incontinence

☐ **Psychosocial assessment:**
   ☐ Calm/relaxed   ☐ Anxious   ☐ Talkative
   ☐ Crying   ☐ Restless   ☐ Withdrawn
   ☐ Other:_____
   ☐ Concerns regarding surgery or hospitalization:
   _____
   ☐ Religious/cultural concerns/requests:
   _____
   ☐ Receives help from:
     ☐ Children   ☐ Support person
     ☐ Other (specify):
   _____
   ☐ Patient cares for:
     ☐ Children: Ages:_____
     ☐ Self   ☐ Spouse
     ☐ Other (specify):
   _____

☐ Determine level of knowledge (I135):
   ☐ Barriers to learning:_____
   ☐ Motivation to learn
     ☐ excellent   ☐ average   ☐ limited

☐ Abuse screening
Have you ever felt threatened verbally, emotionally, or physically in any of your relationships?
   ☐ Yes   ☐ No
Have you been hit, slapped, kicked, or otherwise physically hurt by an intimate partner?
   ☐ Yes   ☐ No
Are you afraid of your partner or anyone you live with?
   ☐ Yes   ☐ No
If yes, describe and make appropriate referral

☐ **Pain assessment**
   ☐ Instructed on use of pain scale
   ☐ Pain assessment (0-10): _____
     Location: _____

☐ **Discharge planning**
Will require assistance after discharge
   ☐ Yes   ☐ No
Discharge plan:
   ☐ Home
   ☐ Home nursing service
   ☐ Short-term care facility
   ☐ Extended care facility
   ☐ Other:_____

Individual who will escort patient home:
Name: _____
Phone number: _____
Relationship: _____

Comments:
_____
_____
_____
_____
_____

Preoperative nursing diagnoses
☐ Anxiety/fear (X4)
☐ Therapeutic regimen management ineffective (X33)
☐ Deficient knowledge (X30)
☐ Risk for injury (X29)
☐ Pain (X38)
☐ Other:_____

RN Signature:
X

Comments:

Example of a perioperative checklist. (*Source:* Reprinted with permission from AORN Perioperative Patient-Focused Model. Copyright AORN, Inc, 2170 Pakert Rd., Suite 300, Denver, CO 80231.)

Example of a Surgical Safety Checklist

World Health Organization	**SURGICAL SAFETY CHECKLIST** (FIRST EDITION)	

Before induction of anaesthesia ▶▶▶▶▶▶▶▶▶	Before skin incision ▶▶▶▶▶▶▶▶▶▶▶▶▶	Before patient leaves operating room
SIGN IN	**TIME OUT**	**SIGN OUT**
☐ **PATIENT HAS CONFIRMED** • IDENTITY • SITE • PROCEDURE • CONSENT	☐ **CONFIRM ALL TEAM MEMBERS HAVE INTRODUCED THEMSELVES BY NAME AND ROLE**	**NURSE VERBALLY CONFIRMS WITH THE TEAM:**
☐ **SITE MARKED/NOT APPLICABLE**	☐ **SURGEON, ANAESTHESIA PROFESSIONAL AND NURSE VERBALLY CONFIRM** • PATIENT • SITE • PROCEDURE	☐ **THE NAME OF THE PROCEDURE RECORDED** ☐ **THAT INSTRUMENT, SPONGE AND NEEDLE COUNTS ARE CORRECT (OR NOT APPLICABLE)**
☐ **ANAESTHESIA SAFETY CHECK COMPLETED**		
☐ **PULSE OXIMETER ON PATIENT AND FUNCTIONING**	**ANTICIPATED CRITICAL EVENTS**	☐ **HOW THE SPECIMEN IS LABELLED (INCLUDING PATIENT NAME)**
DOES PATIENT HAVE A:	☐ **SURGEON REVIEWS:** WHAT ARE THE CRITICAL OR UNEXPECTED STEPS, OPERATIVE DURATION, ANTICIPATED BLOOD LOSS?	☐ **WHETHER THERE ARE ANY EQUIPMENT PROBLEMS TO BE ADDRESSED**
KNOWN ALLERGY? ☐ NO ☐ YES	☐ **ANAESTHESIA TEAM REVIEWS:** ARE THERE ANY PATIENT-SPECIFIC CONCERNS?	☐ **SURGEON, ANAESTHESIA PROFESSIONAL AND NURSE REVIEW THE KEY CONCERNS FOR RECOVERY AND MANAGEMENT OF THIS PATIENT**
DIFFICULT AIRWAY/ASPIRATION RISK? ☐ NO ☐ YES, AND EQUIPMENT/ASSISTANCE AVAILABLE	☐ **NURSING TEAM REVIEWS:** HAS STERILITY (INCLUDING INDICATOR RESULTS) BEEN CONFIRMED? ARE THERE EQUIPMENT ISSUES OR ANY CONCERNS?	
RISK OF >500ML BLOOD LOSS (7ML/KG IN CHILDREN)? ☐ NO ☐ YES, AND ADEQUATE INTRAVENOUS ACCESS AND FLUIDS PLANNED	**HAS ANTIBIOTIC PROPHYLAXIS BEEN GIVEN WITHIN THE LAST 60 MINUTES?** ☐ YES ☐ NOT APPLICABLE	
	IS ESSENTIAL IMAGING DISPLAYED? ☐ YES ☐ NOT APPLICABLE	

THIS CHECKLIST IS NOT INTENDED TO BE COMPREHENSIVE. ADDITIONS AND MODIFICATIONS TO FIT LOCAL PRACTICE ARE ENCOURAGED.

World Health Organization's Surgical Safety Checklist. (*Source:* Reprinted with permission from the World Health Organization. Retrieved from http://www.who.int/patientsafety/safesurgery/tools_resources/SSSL_Checklist_finalJun08.pdf)

Intraoperative Care Questionnaire

- Common nursing interview questions include the following:
- What is your name?
- What type of surgery are you going to have today?
- Is someone here with you?
- Are you allergic to any medications, latex, or tape?
- When is the last time that you had anything to eat or drink?
- Do you have false teeth, contact lenses, or any other prostheses that need to be removed?

- Have you taken any medications today?
- Do you have any implants, such as metal plates or a pacemaker?
- Do you have any scratches, bruises, or other wounds on your body at this time?
- Are there any parts of your body that are painful, such as a stiff shoulder or leg?
- Also see the WHO Surgical Safety Checklist, preceding.

Postanesthesia Assessment: Essential Elements

The postanesthesia care nurse performs a quick, focused initial assessment of the surgical patient in the presence of the anesthesia provider and circulating RN. After that, the nurse assesses the patient every 5 to 15 minutes. The AORN (2009) has identified the essential elements of assessment in the PACU.

- *Vital signs*

  Blood pressure, cuff or arterial

  Respiratory rate, respiratory competence, and breath sounds

  Respiratory adequacy, including skin color and condition

  Temperature (record type of measurement used, for example, skin, tympanic, oral)

  Pulse (apical and peripheral)

  Oxygen saturation (e.g., pulse oximeter reading)

- *Peripheral circulation* (postoperative tissue perfusion), for example, peripheral pulses and sensation at extremities

- *Neurological status*, including pupil response and intracranial pressure (if indicated)

- *Mental status*: Level of consciousness, alertness, lucidity, orientation

- *Intravenous therapy*: Patency, location of sites, rates of solution(s), and/or blood products infusing

- *Allergies and sensitivities*

- *Pain*

- *Motor abilities*, including return of sensory and motor control in areas affected by local or regional anesthetics

- *Skin integrity*

- *Temperature regulation*

- *Positioning*

- *Surgical incision site,* including condition of suture line(s) if visible

- *Nausea and vomiting*

- *Fluid and electrolyte balance*

- *Safety needs* (e.g., siderails raised)

- *Central venous pressure (CVP), pulmonary wedge pressure*

- *Airway*: patency, presence of artificial airway, mechanical ventilator settings

- *Condition of dressing(s)*

- *Drainage*: Type, patency, and amount and type of drainage from dressings, tubes, and catheters

Diagnostic Testing

Common Preoperative Screening Tests

Test	Uses
Urinalysis	To detect urinary tract infections (UTIs) and the presence of glucose or protein in the urine, which may indicate poorly controlled diabetes or renal disease
Complete blood count (CBC)	To detect irregularities in hemoglobin (Hgb) and hematocrit (Hct). A low Hgb level is an indication of anemia, which may place the client at risk if significant blood loss occurs.
	Measures white blood cell (WBC) count as an indicator of immune function
	Measures platelet count, which affects clotting ability
ECG	To detect cardiac dysrhythmias (Electrocardiogram) and other cardiac pathology
Chest x-ray examination	To detect underlying pulmonary disease; also to reveal heart size, as an indicator of heart function
Blood type and crossmatch	To identify blood type in the event that blood transfusion becomes necessary
Serum electrolytes	To detect sodium, potassium, chloride, magnesium, calcium, and pH imbalances, which affect cardiac and other organ function and fluid balance
Fasting blood sugar	To detect diabetes or poorly controlled diabetes
Comprehensive metabolic panel	Includes electrolytes, blood glucose, liver function tests (ALT, AST), serum albumin and protein, and renal function tests (BUN and creatinine); used to detect underlying health problems that may affect surgical risk or outcome

Diagnostic Testing

Standardized Language

Preoperative Patients: Selected Standardized Nursing Diagnoses, Outcomes, and Interventions

NURSING DIAGNOSES	SELECTED NOC OUTCOMES AND GOALS USING NOC INDICATORS	SELECTED NIC INTERVENTIONS AND NURSING ACTIVITIES (SHADED ACTIVITIES ARE ROUTINE NURSING MEASURES FOR ALL PREOPERATIVE PATIENTS)
Anxiety related to change in health status	**NOC outcomes:** Anxiety Level Anxiety Self-Control **NOC goals:** Patient will exhibit: ■ (5) No restlessness ■ (4) Only mild muscle and facial tension ■ (4) Only mild difficulty concentrating ■ (5) No increased blood pressure, pulse rate, or respiratory rate ■ (5) No physical signs of anxiety such as: dilated pupils, sweating, and dizziness ■ (3) Moderate verbalized anxiety **Individualized goals:** ■ Identifies symptoms that are indicators of her anxiety. ■ Communicates need for assistance.	**Anxiety Reduction** ■ Use a calm, reassuring approach. ■ Explain all procedures, including sensations likely to be experienced during the surgical procedure. ■ Seek to understand the patient's perspective of the situation. ■ Provide accurate factual information about the surgery. **Calming Technique** ■ Maintain eye contact with patient. ■ Encourage slow, purposeful deep breathing. **Presence** ■ Stay with the patient and provide assurance of safety and security during periods of anxiety. ■ Listen to the patient's concerns. ■ Administer medications as appropriate to reduce anxiety.
Fear related to unknown outcome of surgery and fear of pain that may result	**NOC outcomes:** Fear Level Fear Self-Control **NOC goals:** ■ (5) Exhibits no restlessness or irritability. ■ (5) Reports no difficulty concentrating. ■ (5) No physical signs of fear: increased BP, radial pulse rate, respiratory rate, sweating, dilated pupils, pale skin ■ (5) No verbalized fear ■ (5) No crying **Individualized goals:** ■ Does not exhibit physical signs of fear (e.g., pupil dilation; dry mouth; increased BP, pulse and respiratory rate). ■ Reports understanding of pain control measures to be used during and after surgery.	**Anxiety Reduction** ■ (See Anxiety diagnosis) **Coping Enhancement** ■ Assist the patient in developing an objective appraisal of the event ■ Evaluate the patient's decision-making ability. ■ Encourage the use of spiritual resources, if desired. **Preparatory Sensory Information** ■ Identify the typical sensations (what will be seen, felt, smelled, tasted, heard) the majority of patients describe as associated with each aspect of the procedure/treatment. ■ Personalize the information by using personal pronouns. **Security Enhancement** ■ Explain all tests and procedures to the patient/family. ■ Assist the patient to use coping responses that have been successful in the past.

Preoperative Patients: Selected Standardized Nursing Diagnoses, Outcomes, and Interventions—cont'd

NURSING DIAGNOSES	SELECTED NOC OUTCOMES AND GOALS USING NOC INDICATORS	SELECTED NIC INTERVENTIONS AND NURSING ACTIVITIES (SHADED ACTIVITIES ARE ROUTINE NURSING MEASURES FOR ALL PREOPERATIVE PATIENTS)
Deficient Knowledge of preoperative procedures and postoperative expectations (may be the etiology of other problems, such as Ineffective Management of Therapeutic Regimen, or Risk for Infection)	**NOC outcomes:** Knowledge: Disease Process Knowledge: Treatment Procedure(s) **NOC goals:** Provides: ■ (3) Moderate description of specific disease process ■ (4) Substantial description of strategies to minimize disease progression ■ (4) Substantial description of signs and symptoms of disease complications **Individualized goals:** ■ Verbalizes rationale for pre- and postoperative interventions. ■ Describes or demonstrates. postoperative expectations (i.e., deep breathing, turning/position changes).	**Teaching: Preoperative** ■ Inform the patient/significant others how long surgery is expected to last. ■ Determine the patient's previous surgical experiences and level of knowledge related to surgery. ■ Provide time for the patient to ask questions and discuss concerns. ■ Describe preoperative routines (e.g., anesthesia, diet, bowel preparation, tests/labs, voiding, skin preparation, IV therapy, clothing, family waiting area, transportation to operating room). ■ Describe any preoperative medications, the effects these will have on the patient, and the rationale for using them. ■ Inform significant others of the place to wait for the results of the surgery. ■ Introduce the patient to perioperative staff as appropriate. ■ Discuss possible pain control measures. ■ Describe postoperative routines/equipment (e.g., medications, respiratory treatments, tubes, machines, support hose, surgical dressings, ambulation, diet, family visitation) and explain their purpose. ■ Instruct the patient in postoperative deep breathing exercises, splinting incision, coughing. ■ Reinforce information provided by other healthcare team members, as appropriate. ■ Include the family/significant others [in the teaching-learning process] as appropriate.
Disturbed Sleep Pattern related to anxiety about the upcoming surgery	**NOC outcome:** Sleep **NOC goals:** ■ (4) Mild interrupted sleep ■ (5) Hours of sleep (at least 5 hr/24 hr), not compromised ■ (4) Sleeps through the night consistently, mildly compromised. **Individualized goals:** ■ Reports minimal compromise in hours of sleep and sleep pattern. ■ No difficulty falling and staying asleep reported or observed	**Sleep Enhancement** ■ Determine the patient's usual sleep-activity pattern. ■ Determine effects of patient's current medications on sleep pattern. ■ Adjust environment (lighting, noise, temperature, etc.) to promote sleep. ■ Demonstrate and explain the procedure for progressive muscle relaxation. ■ Administer medication to promote sleep, as appropriate.

Sources: Bulechek, G. M., Butcher, H. K., & Dochterman, J. M. (Eds.). (2008). *Nursing interventions classification (NIC)* (5th ed.). St. Louis, MO: C.V. Mosby; Moorhead, S., Johnson, M., Maas, M., et al. (Eds.). (2008). *Nursing outcomes classification (NOC)* (4th ed.). St. Louis, MO: C.V. Mosby; NANDA International. (2009). *Nursing diagnoses: Definitions and classification 2009–2011*. Philadelphia: Author. Used with permission.

Intraoperative Patients: Selected Standardized Nursing Diagnoses, Outcomes, and Interventions

NURSING DIAGNOSES (NANDA-I) AND COLLABORATIVE PROBLEMS	NOC OUTCOMES AND INDICATORS	NIC INTERVENTIONS AND ACTIVITIES (NOTE: SHADED INTERVENTIONS ARE ROUTINELY PERFORMED FOR ALL SURGERY PATIENTS.)
Nursing diagnosis: Risk for Aspiration related to depressed respirations and reflexes secondary to anesthesia *Collaborative problem:* Potential Complication of anesthesia: aspiration	*NOC outcome:* Respiratory Status: Airway Patency *NOC goal:* (5) No choking or adventitious breath sounds	**Artificial Airway Management** ■ Institute endotracheal suctioning, as appropriate. **Aspiration Precautions** ■ Monitor pulmonary status. ■ Keep suction setup available. ■ Maintain an airway. **Sedation Management** ■ Ensure that emergency resuscitation equipment is readily available, specifically source to deliver 100% O_2, emergency medications, and a defibrillator. ■ Initiate an IV line. ■ Ensure availability of and administer antagonists as appropriate, per physician's order, or protocol **Vomiting Management** ■ Position to prevent aspiration.
Nursing diagnosis: Risk for Imbalanced Body Temperature related to exposure in cool environment and administration of cool IV fluids *Collaborative problem:* Potential Complication of surgery and anesthesia: hypothermia	*NOC outcome:* Thermoregulation *NOC goals:* ■ (5) No hyperthermia ■ (5) No hypothermia ■ (4) Mild increased (or decreased) skin temperature	**Temperature Regulation: Intraoperative** ■ Adjust operating room temperature for therapeutic effect. ■ Apply head covering ■ Cover exposed body parts. ■ Warm or cool all irrigating, IV, and skin preparation solutions, as appropriate. ■ Continuously monitor the patient's temperature. ■ Cover patient with heated blanket for transport to postanesthesia care unit. **Malignant Hyperthermia Precautions** ■ Maintain emergency equipment for malignant hyperthermia, per protocol, in operative areas. ■ Notify anesthesiologist and surgeon of patient history. ■ Provide a cooling blanket. **Vital Signs Monitoring** ■ Monitor blood pressure, pulse, temperature, and respiratory status, as appropriate. ■ Monitor skin color, temperature, and moistness.

Intraoperative Patients: Selected Standardized Nursing Diagnoses, Outcomes, and Interventions—cont'd

NURSING DIAGNOSES (NANDA-I) AND COLLABORATIVE PROBLEMS	NOC OUTCOMES AND INDICATORS	NIC INTERVENTIONS AND ACTIVITIES (NOTE: SHADED INTERVENTIONS ARE ROUTINELY PERFORMED FOR ALL SURGERY PATIENTS.)
Nursing diagnosis: Risk for Imbalanced Fluid Volume *Collaborative problem:* Potential complication of surgery: fluid and electrolyte imbalance (Clients undergoing surgery are at risk for vascular, cellular, and/or intracellular dehydration [Johnson, Holm, & Godshall, 2000]).	*NOC outcomes:* Blood Loss Severity Fluid Balance Urinary Elimination Vital Signs *NOC goals:* ■ (4) Systolic and diastolic blood pressures, mild deviation from normal range ■ (5) Mean arterial pressure not compromised ■ (5) Central venous pressure not compromised ■ (5) Pulmonary wedge pressure not compromised ■ (4) Peripheral pulses mildly compromised ■ (4) 24-hour intake and output balance mildly compromised ■ (5) Adventitious breath sounds not present ■ (5) Neck vein distension not present ■ (5) Peripheral edema not present	**Fluid Management** ■ Maintain accurate intake and output record. ■ Insert urinary catheter, if appropriate. ■ Administer IV therapy, as prescribed. ■ Monitor hemodynamic status, including CVP, MAP, PAP, and PCWP, if available. ■ Prepare for administration of blood products (e.g., check blood with patient identification and prepare infusion setup), as appropriate. **Fluid Monitoring** ■ Determine possible risk factors for fluid imbalance (e.g., renal pathologies, liver dysfunction . . .). ■ Monitor color, quantity, and specific gravity of urine. ■ Monitor for distended neck veins, crackles in the lungs, peripheral edema, and weight gain. ■ Monitor blood pressure, heart rate, and respiratory status. ■ Monitor serum and urine electrolyte values. **Intravenous (IV) Therapy** ■ Monitor IV flow rate and IV site during infusion. ■ Monitor for IV patency before administration of IV medication.
Nursing diagnosis: Risk for Latex Allergy Response; or Latex Allergy Response related to multiple previous exposures to latex	*NOC outcomes:* Immune Hypersensitivity Response Symptom Severity *NOC goals:* (5) No localized inflammatory responses (5) Respiratory, cardiac, renal, and neurological functions not compromised	**Latex Precautions (Intraoperative)** ■ Place allergy band on patient [if not already done preoperatively]. ■ Record allergy or risk in patient's medical record [or check to see that it was done]. ■ Post sign indicating latex precautions. ■ Survey environment and remove latex products. ■ Monitor latex-free environment. ■ Report information to physician, pharmacist, and other care providers, as indicated. **Preoperative Interventions** ■ Question patient or appropriate other about history of neural tube defect (e.g., spina bifida) or congenital urological condition (e.g., extrophy of the bladder). ■ Question patient or appropriate other about systemic reactions to natural rubber latex (e.g., facial or scleral edema, tearing eyes, urticaria, rhinitis, and wheezing). ■ Question patient or appropriate other about allergies to foods such as bananas, kiwi, avocado, mango, and chestnuts.

Continued

Intraoperative Patients: Selected Standardized Nursing Diagnoses, Outcomes, and Interventions—cont'd

NURSING DIAGNOSES (NANDA-I) AND COLLABORATIVE PROBLEMS	NOC OUTCOMES AND INDICATORS	NIC INTERVENTIONS AND ACTIVITIES (NOTE: SHADED INTERVENTIONS ARE ROUTINELY PERFORMED FOR ALL SURGERY PATIENTS.)
Nursing diagnosis: Risk for Perioperative Positioning Injury related to patient factors such as edema, emaciation, obesity, and sensory perceptual disturbances secondary to anesthesia *Collaborative problem:* Potential complication of surgery: neuromuscular, skeletal, or skin injury	*NOC outcomes:* Circulation Status Mobility Neurological Status Physical Injury Severity Tissue Perfusion: Peripheral *NOC goals:* ■ (4) Pao$_2$ mild deviation from normal range ■ (4) Paco$_2$ mild deviation from normal range ■ (4) Pallor and dependent rubor mild ■ (5) Joint movement not compromised ■ (5) Spinal sensory/motor function not compromised ■ (5) Central motor control not compromised ■ (5) No burns, bruises, extremity or back sprains, impaired mobility ■ (4) Capillary refill (fingers and toes) mild deviation from normal range ■ (5) No numbness ■ (5) All pulses no deviation from normal range ■ (5) Skin integrity not compromised	**Circulatory Precautions** ■ Perform a comprehensive appraisal of peripheral circulation (e.g., check peripheral pulses, edema, capillary refill, color, and temperature of extremity). **Positioning: Intraoperative** ■ Use assistive devices for immobilization. ■ Lock wheels of stretcher and operating room bed. ■ Use an adequate number of personnel to transfer patient. ■ Support the head and neck during transfer. ■ Immobilize or support any body part, as appropriate. ■ Maintain patient's proper body alignment. ■ Apply padding to bony prominences. ■ Apply safety strap and arm restraint, as needed. ■ Record position and devices used. **Surgical Precautions** ■ Verify surgical consent. ■ Verify surgical site. ■ Verify client's blood type. ■ Verify that there is blood on reserve. ■ Verify client's identity. ■ Verify patient's allergies. ■ Check ground isolation monitor. ■ Verify the correct functioning of equipment. ■ Check suction for adequate pressure and complete assembly of canisters, tubing, and catheters. ■ Count sponges, sharps, and instruments before, during, and after surgery, per agency policy; record results of counts. ■ Provide an electrosurgical unit, grounding pad, and active electrode, as appropriate. ■ Verify the integrity of electrical cords. ■ Verify the proper functioning of electrosurgical unit. ■ Verify that the client is not in contact with metal. ■ Check for the presence of implants, pacemakers, and metal prostheses pacemakers contraindicating use of electrosurgical cautery. ■ Verify the patient's skin integrity at site of [electrocautery] grounding pad. ■ Verify that skin prep solutions are non-flammable. ■ Adjust coagulation and cutting currents, as instructed by physician or per agency policy. ■ Inspect the patient's skin for injury [at conclusion of procedure]. ■ (non-NIC) Monitor sterile technique throughout procedure.

Sources: Bulechek, G. M., Butcher, H. K., & Dochterman, J. M. (Eds.). (2008). *Nursing interventions classification (NIC)* (5th ed.). St. Louis, MO: C.V. Mosby; Moorhead, S., Johnson, M., Maas, M., et al. (Eds.). (2008). *Nursing outcomes classification (NOC)* (4th ed.). St. Louis, MO: C.V. Mosby; NANDA International. (2009). *Nursing diagnoses: Definitions and classification 2009–2011.* Philadelphia: Author.

Selected Standardized Nursing Diagnoses, Outcomes, and Interventions for Postoperative Patients

NURSING DIAGNOSES	OUTCOMES AND GOALS	NURSING INTERVENTIONS AND ACTIVITIES
Activity Intolerance r/t pain and the surgical procedure and stressors of surgery	**NOC outcomes:** Activity Tolerance Endurance Energy Conservation Psychomotor Energy **NOC goals:** ■ O$_2$ saturation, heart rate, respiratory rate, systolic and diastolic blood pressure not compromised with activity ■ Ease of breathing with activity not compromised ■ Walking pace and distance not compromised ■ Ease of performing activities of daily living (ADLs) not compromised ■ Ability to speak with physical activity not compromised ■ Energy restored after rest, not compromised ■ Uses naps to restore energy, often demonstrated. ■ Exhibits concentration, consistently demonstrated.	**NIC interventions:** Activity Therapy Energy Management Exercise Promotion: Strength Training **Nursing activities:** ■ Collaborate with other disciplines to plan and monitor activity program as appropriate. ■ Assist to choose appropriate activities. ■ Assist to focus on strengths rather than weaknesses. ■ Assist to identify activity preferences. ■ Instruct the client and family how to perform desired activities. ■ Refer to community centers, programs as appropriate. ■ Arrange physical activities to reduce competition for oxygen supply to vital body functions (e.g., avoid activity immediately after meals). ■ Avoid care activities during scheduled rest periods. ■ Assist to sit on side of bed ("dangle"), if unable to transfer or walk. ■ Monitor location and nature of pain during activity. ■ Teach activity organization and time management techniques to prevent fatigue.
Acute Pain r/t (1) inflammation or injury in the surgical area, (2) abdominal distention secondary to decreased peristalsis, (3) muscle pain secondary to positioning and tension	**NOC outcomes:** Pain Level Pain Control **NOC goals:** ■ Consistently rates pain as controlled. ■ No moaning or crying ■ No facial expressions of pain ■ Describes causal factors. ■ Uses preventive measures. ■ Uses nonanalgesic relief measures. ■ Uses analgesics as recommended. ■ Reports changes in symptoms to a health professional. **Other goals:** No guarding of incision	**NIC interventions:** Analgesic Administration Pain Management Patient-Controlled Analgesia (PCA) Assistance **Nursing activities:** ■ Assess location, characteristics, onset, duration, frequency, quality, and intensity of pain and predisposing factors. ■ Observe for nonverbal discomfort cues. ■ Assure the client of analgesic availability. ■ Consider cultural influences of responses to pain. ■ Utilize developmentally appropriate assessment method. ■ Determine necessary frequency of pain assessment and formulate pain assessment plan. ■ Provide information about the pain, such as causes, anticipated duration. ■ Control environmental factors that may contribute to the client's response. ■ Provide information about the pain, such as causes of the pain, how long it will last, and anticipated discomforts from procedures (e.g., teach the client to splint incision when ambulating). ■ Provide optimal pain relief with analgesics as appropriate. ■ Implement PCA (patient-controlled analgesia) as appropriate. ■ Intervene before pain becomes severe. ■ Medicate before activity to increase participation. ■ Teach nonpharmacological pain relief measures (e.g., visualization, progressive muscle relaxation). ■ Utilize multidisciplinary approach to pain management.

Continued

Selected Standardized Nursing Diagnoses, Outcomes, and Interventions for Postoperative Patients—cont'd

NURSING DIAGNOSES	OUTCOMES AND GOALS	NURSING INTERVENTIONS AND ACTIVITIES
Anxiety r/t change in health status, hospital environment	**NOC outcomes:** Anxiety Level Anxiety Self-Control **NOC goals:** ■ Consistently uses effective coping strategies. ■ Often seeks information to reduce anxiety. ■ Consistently uses relaxation techniques to reduce anxiety. ■ Often maintains concentration. ■ Verbalizes that anxiety is mild. ■ Minimal restlessness, hand wringing, muscle tension, facial tension, difficulty concentrating. Minimal changes in vital signs; no dilated pupils, sweating or dizziness ■ Controls anxiety response consistently.	**NIC intervention:** Anxiety Reduction **Nursing activities:** ■ Use calm, reassuring approach. ■ Observe for verbal and nonverbal signs of anxiety. ■ Explain all procedures and activities. ■ Provide information concerning diagnosis, treatment, prognosis. ■ Administer back rub or neck rub as appropriate. ■ Listen attentively. ■ Create trusting atmosphere. ■ Assist the client to identify stressful situations. ■ Assist the client to recognize that she is anxious. ■ Assess the client's ability to make decisions. ■ Encourage verbalization of feelings, perceptions, and fears related to the surgical procedure. ■ Encourage family visits if these ease the client's stress. ■ Support use of appropriate defense mechanisms. ■ Instruct the client in use of relaxation techniques.
Nausea r/t manipulation of gastrointestinal tract, decreased peristalsis secondary to anesthesia	**NOC outcomes:** Nausea & Vomiting Control Nausea & Vomiting: Disruptive Effects Nausea & Vomiting Severity Nutritional Status: Food & Fluid Intake **NOC goals:** ■ No nausea, or intensity only mild ■ Reports nausea, retching, and vomiting controlled. ■ Mild or no intolerance of odors ■ Mild or no intolerance of movement ■ Recognizes onset of nausea. ■ Recognizes precipitating stimuli. ■ Frequency, intensity, and distress of nausea are mild. ■ Uses preventive measures often. ■ Only mild decrease in food and fluid intake ■ No weight loss ■ Reports bothersome side effects from antiemetics. ■ Reports failure of antiemetic treatment.	**NIC interventions:** Nausea Management Medication Management **Nursing activities:** ■ Provide information about the cause of nausea and vomiting and the expected duration. ■ Provide information about the goals, effects, and possible side effects of treatment with antiemetics. ■ Describe the limited role of administering parenteral fluids to prevent dehydration and to administer supplemental electrolytes (e.g., potassium). ■ Encourage to monitor own nausea experience, including use of a symptom diary. ■ Encourage to learn strategies for managing own nausea. ■ Perform complete assessment including frequency, duration, severity, and precipitating factors. ■ Observe for nonverbal cues of discomfort. ■ Evaluate past experiences with nausea. ■ Identify strategies that have been successful in relieving nausea. ■ Discuss relaxation and distraction techniques if anxiety is suspected of playing a role (e.g., guided imagery, self-hypnosis, biofeedback, music therapy). ■ Encourage frequent oral hygiene unless it stimulates nausea. Keep tissues and water to rinse the mouth nearby. ■ Give cold, clear, odorless foods, as appropriate. ■ Encourage the client to eat high-carbohydrate and low-fat foods and to eat small, frequent meals. ■ Drink cola, but not too cold; suck on an ice cube, sorbet, or a piece of frozen fruit. ■ Have the client sit in an upright position for 30 to 45 minutes after eating. ■ Control odors and unpleasant visual stimuli in the room. ■ Administer antiemetic medications. ■ Refer to a dietician as needed.

Selected Standardized Nursing Diagnoses, Outcomes, and Interventions for Postoperative Patients—cont'd

NURSING DIAGNOSES	OUTCOMES AND GOALS	NURSING INTERVENTIONS AND ACTIVITIES
Constipation r/t decreased activity, decreased food or fluid intake, decreased peristalsis secondary to anesthesia, pain medication	**NOC outcome:** Bowel Elimination **NOC goals:** ■ Elimination pattern not compromised ■ Reports ease of stool passage not compromised. ■ Bowel sounds not compromised ■ Muscle tone to evacuate stool not compromised ■ Passes soft, formed stool in amount appropriate for diet. ■ No pain with passage of stool **Other:** ■ Bloating not present	**NIC interventions:** Bowel Management Constipation/Impaction Management **Nursing activities:** ■ Monitor for signs and symptoms of constipation. ■ Note date of last bowel movement. ■ Monitor bowel sounds. ■ Monitor frequency, consistency, shape, volume, and color of bowel movements. ■ Teach the client about specific foods that assist promotion of bowel regularity. ■ Insert a rectal suppository, enema, or irrigation, as needed. ■ Evaluate medication profile for GI side effects (e.g., narcotic analgesics). ■ Give warm liquids after meals. ■ Instruct the client in foods high in fiber.
Urinary Retention r/t anesthesia, preoperative medications (anticholinergics), pain, fear, unfamiliar surroundings, client's position	**NOC outcome:** Urinary Elimination **NOC goals:** ■ Empties bladder completely. ■ Fluid intake not compromised ■ No hesitancy with urination **Other:** ■ Bladder not palpable ■ Reports subjective feeling of empty bladder. ■ 24-hour intake and output balanced	**NIC interventions:** Urinary Retention Care Urinary Catheterization **Nursing activities:** ■ Perform comprehensive urinary assessment (fluid intake, urinary output, voiding pattern, cognitive function, preexisting urinary problems). ■ Provide privacy for elimination. ■ Use power of suggestion (run water, flush toilet). ■ Provide ample time (at least 10 minutes) for client to empty bladder. ■ Use spirits of wintergreen in bedpan or urinal. ■ Insert urinary catheter as appropriate. ■ Use percussion and palpation to estimate degree of bladder distention. ■ Catheterize for post-voiding residual as appropriate.

Continued

Selected Standardized Nursing Diagnoses, Outcomes, and Interventions for Postoperative Patients—cont'd

NURSING DIAGNOSES	OUTCOMES AND GOALS	NURSING INTERVENTIONS AND ACTIVITIES
Delayed Surgical Recovery (etiologies will vary with pathology) (*Note:* This diagnosis is broad and encompasses some of the other diagnoses. If the client has Delayed Surgical Recovery, you will not, for example, need a diagnosis of Nausea on the plan of care.)	***NOC outcomes:*** Post-Procedure Recovery Wound Healing: Primary Intention Ambulation Blood Loss Severity Endurance Hydration Infection Severity Nausea & Vomiting Severity Pain Level ***NOC goals:*** ■ Systolic BP within 20 mm Hg of baseline ■ Ambulation tolerance in normal range ■ No nausea, vomiting, shivering ■ Only mild pain ***Other:*** ■ Ready for discharge within prescribed length of stay for surgery performed ■ No postoperative complications (e.g., bleeding, infection, delayed wound healing, pneumonia)	***NIC interventions:*** Embolus Precautions Exercise Therapy: Ambulation Incision Site Care Nutrition Management Pain Management Self-Care Assistance ***Nursing activities:*** ■ Monitor for postoperative complications. ■ Monitor the healing process in the incision site. ■ Provide incision care as needed. ■ Teach the client and family how to care for the incision. ■ Facilitate early ambulation postoperatively. ■ Encourage increased intake of protein, iron, and vitamin C, as appropriate. ■ Determine, in collaboration with the dietician as appropriate, number of calories and type of nutrients needed to meet nutrition requirements. ■ Select and implement a variety of measures (e.g., pharmacological, nonpharmacological, interpersonal) to facilitate pain relief, as appropriate. ■ Teach principles of pain management. ■ Encourage independence, but intervene when the client is unable to perform.

Sources: Bulechek, G. M., Butcher, H. K., & Dochterman, J. M. (Eds.). (2008). *Nursing interventions classification (NIC)* (5th ed.). St. Louis, MO: C.V. Mosby; Moorhead, S., Johnson, M., Maas, M., et al. (Eds.). (2008). *Nursing outcomes classification (NOC)* (4th ed.). St. Louis, MO: C.V. Mosby; NANDA International. (2009). *Nursing diagnoses: Definitions and classification 2009–2011.* Philadelphia: Author. Used with permission.

THINKING CRITICALLY ABOUT PERIOPERATIVE NURSING

The exercises in the following sections allow you to practice the kind of thinking you will use as a full-spectrum nurse. Because these are critical-thinking questions, there is usually no single right answer. We do not provide answers for these questions because it is more important for you to think about the questions than to arrive at the "right" answer. These questions are designed to improve your thinking more than to "cover content." Discuss answers with your peers—discussion can stimulate critical thinking. If you have difficulty with any of these questions, consult with your instructor.

▱ Applying the Full-Spectrum Nursing Model

PATIENT SITUATION

Recall Nishad Singh ("Meet Your Patient," in Volume 1). He is a 68-year-old man who came to the emergency department (ED) with sudden onset of rectal bleeding. He had been "tired and dragging for several months." The ED nurse identified nursing diagnoses of Mild Anxiety, Pain, and Risk for Bleeding. Preoperatively, his vital signs were as follow:

BP: 138/88 mm Hg

Pulse: 104 beats/min and regular; 120 beats/min; 134 beats/min

Respiratory rate: 20 breaths/min

Temperature: 36.7°C (98.0°F)

Oxygen saturation: 98%

Mr. Singh was admitted to the hospital, where he received An IV of 1000 mL of lactated Ringer's solution and a unit of packed red blood cells. He was to undergo emergency colon resection surgery; however, a left hemicolectomy including the sigmoid colon and the anus was required. He spent 4 hours in the PACU, until his vital signs stabilized. Mr. Singh now has a colostomy high in his descending colon, with a stoma on his left abdomen slightly superior to the level of his umbilicus. He also has an abdominal incision that was made for exploration. On the next day after the surgery, the surgeon informed Mr. Singh that he has widespread adencarcinoma (cancer) of the colon with metastasis to the liver. The nurse has identified these four nursing diagnoses (among others):

Deficient Knowledge (colostomy care) r/t lack of prior experience and no preparation prior to surgery

Fear r/t diagnosis of colon cancer, liver metastasis, and possible terminal illness

Pain secondary to surgical incision and manipulation of abdominal organs during the surgical procedure

Risk for Impaired Skin Integrity r/t irritation from fecal drainage and ostomy pouch

THINKING

1. *Theoretical Knowledge*:

   a. What is a left hemicolectomy? If you do not know the answer, consult an appropriate reference.

   b. What does "metastasis to the liver" mean? If you do not know the answer, consult an appropriate reference.

2. *Critical Thinking (Inquiry)*:

   a. Why might Mr. Singh have needed a colostomy instead of having his transverse colon reconnected to the remaining lower colon or rectum? State the reference you used to answer this question.

b. Why do you think Mr. Singh has a colostomy above the level of the umbilicus and not lower down in his abdomen? State the reference you used to answer this question.

DOING

3. *Practical Knowledge*: Mr. Singh returned from surgery with knee-high antiembolism stockings.

   a. You notice that the stockings have slid down and become wrinkled between his knees and ankles. After you straighten them and pull them up, the tops reach to about 7.6 cm (3 in.) below Mr. Singh's knees. What does this probably mean, and what should you do?

   b. Which of the following instructions should you give when delegating care of Mr. Singh's antiembolism stockings to the nursing assistant? (Mr. Singh's stockings have closed toes.)

   - Remove the stockings and bathe and dry the legs every 8 to 12 hours.
   - Massage the legs after removing Mr. Singh's stockings.
   - Before reapplying stockings, report the presence of any lesions, sores, or redness of the lower extremities.
   - Instruct the patient to remain supine for at least 15 minutes after removing the stockings.
   - Make sure there are no wrinkles in the stockings once they have been applied.
   - Tug gently on the end of the stocking to create a small space between the end of the toes and the stocking.

4. *Nursing Process (Nursing Diagnosis)*: List Mr. Singh's four nursing diagnoses in order of priority. List the highest priority first. Explain how you decided the priorities.

CARING

5. *Self-Knowledge*:

   a. If you were assigned to care for Mr. Singh today, what aspect of care would you feel best prepared to give? Explain your thinking.

   b. What aspect of Mr. Singh's care would you be most uncomfortable providing? Explain your thinking.

6. *Ethical Knowledge*: You want to provide culturally competent care. What is the first thing you will need to do in order to address Mr. Singh's cultural needs? Review Chapter 13 if you need to.

Critical Thinking and Clinical Reasoning

1. You are speaking with several classmates about an upcoming surgical rotation. During the rotation, you will have an opportunity to work with a circulating nurse and a scrub nurse. One of your classmates says that she is very nervous. "I don't know if I will be able to handle this rotation. I'm afraid I might not be able to watch the surgery. I've never really seen anything gross like that before." Another classmate confides that she is worried that she will contaminate everything and put the client at risk. What advice can you give them, and what actions can you take to prepare yourself for your experience in the OR?

2. You are working on a busy surgical unit on the evening shift. There is one NAP on the unit this evening. You are caring for the following clients:

   - Mr. Singh ("Meet Your Patient"), who underwent a colon resection and colostomy for colon cancer. He is now in postoperative day 2 and is complaining of chest pain and shortness of breath.
   - Ms Yasmin, a 52-year-old woman admitted to the unit from PACU 1 hour ago after total abdominal hysterectomy and bilateral salpingo-oophrectomy (TAH-BSO—removal of the uterus, ovaries, and fallopian tubes)
   - Steven Stellanski, a 16-year-old with trisomy 21 who underwent an emergency appendectomy early this morning.

The PACU calls to inform you that they are ready to transport Mrs. Bauer back to the unit. She is an 87-year-old woman from the local skilled nursing facility who underwent an extensive débridement of a stage IV pressure ulcer on the coccyx. The PACU nurse tells you Mrs. Bauer is confused and agitated and will need close monitoring.

   a. What problems do the admission of this new patient present for you? To answer this question, identify the priority nursing activity for each of the three patients you already have, as well as for Mrs. Bauer.

   b. How will you handle this situation? Identify three options, and explain their advantages and disadvantages.

3. You will be caring for a 23-year-old client who underwent emergency surgery after an automobile accident. He has had no preoperative teaching. What concerns does this raise for you? How will you address these concerns?

4. For each of the following concepts, use critical thinking to describe how or why it is important to nursing, patient care, or perioperative nursing. Note that these are not to be merely definitions.

Preoperative teaching
Preoperative physical preparation
Intraoperative safety measures

Anesthesia
Postoperative complications

■ What Are the Main Points in This Chapter?

➤ Perioperative nursing includes care of patients during the preoperative, intraoperative, and postoperative phases.

➤ Perioperative nursing requires the systematic integration and synthesis of the nursing process with established standards of practice.

➤ The Association of periOperative Registered Nurses (AORN) is one of the most highly organized and powerful specialty organizations within the profession of nursing. It is the organization that developed the standards of care that inform perioperative nursing and the standardized language, the Perioperative Nursing Data Set (PNDS).

➤ "Never events" are serious and costly errors resulting in severe consequences for the patient, and that are mostly preventable. Medicare will not reimburse institutions for care related to complications caused by never events.

➤ Surgical risk is associated with the type of surgery and the condition of the patient (e.g., age, general health, personal habits).

➤ During the preoperative period, it is essential to determine whether the client is physiologically, cognitively, and psychologically prepared for the intraoperative and postoperative phases of surgery.

➤ Preoperative care includes assessment, preoperative teaching, confirming that surgical consent has been obtained; preventing wrong patient, wrong site, wrong surgery; communicating with the surgical team; preparing the patient physically for surgery; and transferring the patient to the operative suite.

➤ The surgical consent form is a witnessed legal document that ensures that the surgical patient has given informed consent for the surgical procedure. The physician is legally responsible for obtaining informed consent; however, the nurse sometimes obtains the patient's signature on the form after verifying that the patient has been informed.

➤ A great deal of perioperative nursing care is standardized, aimed at preventing potential complications, and applicable to all patients having surgery.

➤ General anesthesia produces rapid unconsciousness and loss of sensation. Regional anesthesia produces loss of pain sensation without loss of consciousness.

➤ Intraoperative care includes skin preparation, positioning the patient for surgery, and protective measures to ensure patient safety during surgery.

➤ The PACU RN integrates knowledge of common complications of surgery, well-established nursing diagnoses for the postoperative client, and data from an individualized comprehensive postoperative assessment to plan and implement appropriate outcomes and interventions for the client during the postoperative stage.

➤ Assessments during postoperative recovery are the same as those performed in the PACU, but they can be performed less frequently.

➤ Antiembolism stockings and sequential compression devices may be used to help prevent thrombophlebitis.

➤ Incentive spirometry may be used to help prevent atelectasis and pneumonia.

➤ Gastrointestinal suction may be used for gastric decompression after certain surgeries to prevent gastric distention, which can increase respiratory complications, place a strain on suture lines, and interfere with wound closure.

For practice questions for this chapter,

 Go to **NCLEX-Style Chapter Quiz,** on the Student Resource Disk or DavisPlus at http://davisplus.fadavis.com/Wilkinson2

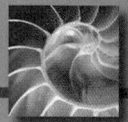

Knowledge Map

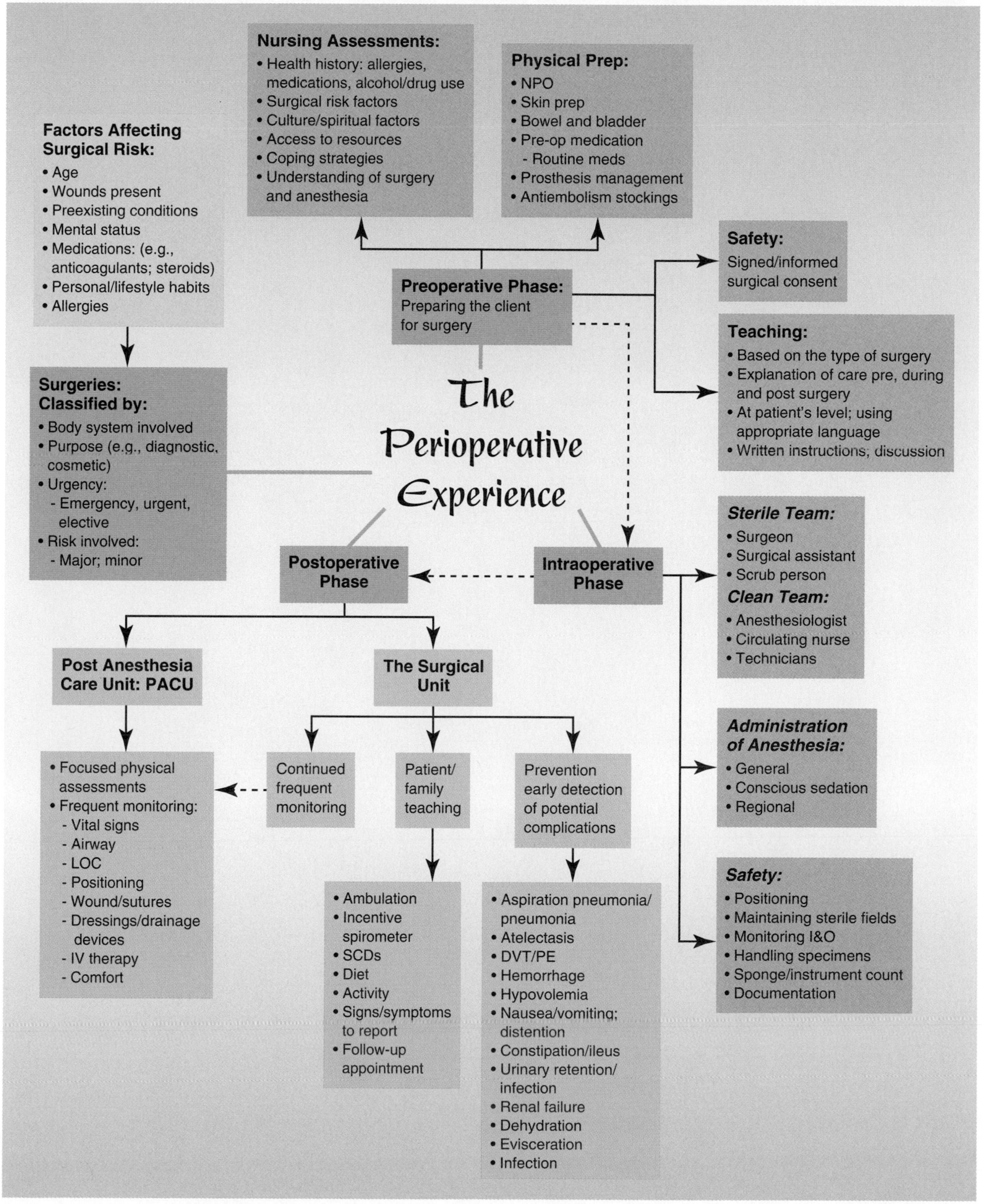

Nursing Assessments:
- Health history: allergies, medications, alcohol/drug use
- Surgical risk factors
- Culture/spiritual factors
- Access to resources
- Coping strategies
- Understanding of surgery and anesthesia

Physical Prep:
- NPO
- Skin prep
- Bowel and bladder
- Pre-op medication
  - Routine meds
- Prosthesis management
- Antiembolism stockings

Factors Affecting Surgical Risk:
- Age
- Wounds present
- Preexisting conditions
- Mental status
- Medications: (e.g., anticoagulants; steroids)
- Personal/lifestyle habits
- Allergies

Preoperative Phase:
Preparing the client for surgery

Safety:
Signed/informed surgical consent

Teaching:
- Based on the type of surgery
- Explanation of care pre, during and post surgery
- At patient's level; using appropriate language
- Written instructions; discussion

Surgeries: Classified by:
- Body system involved
- Purpose (e.g., diagnostic, cosmetic)
- Urgency:
  - Emergency, urgent, elective
- Risk involved:
  - Major; minor

The Perioperative Experience

Postoperative Phase

Intraoperative Phase

Sterile Team:
- Surgeon
- Surgical assistant
- Scrub person

Clean Team:
- Anesthesiologist
- Circulating nurse
- Technicians

Post Anesthesia Care Unit: PACU

The Surgical Unit

Continued frequent monitoring

Patient/ family teaching

Prevention early detection of potential complications

Administration of Anesthesia:
- General
- Conscious sedation
- Regional

- Focused physical assessments
- Frequent monitoring:
  - Vital signs
  - Airway
  - LOC
  - Positioning
  - Wound/sutures
  - Dressings/drainage devices
  - IV therapy
  - Comfort

- Ambulation
- Incentive spirometer
- SCDs
- Diet
- Activity
- Signs/symptoms to report
- Follow-up appointment

- Aspiration pneumonia/ pneumonia
- Atelectasis
- DVT/PE
- Hemorrhage
- Hypovolemia
- Nausea/vomiting; distention
- Constipation/ileus
- Urinary retention/ infection
- Renal failure
- Dehydration
- Evisceration
- Infection

Safety:
- Positioning
- Maintaining sterile fields
- Monitoring I&O
- Handling specimens
- Sponge/instrument count
- Documentation

Nursing Functions

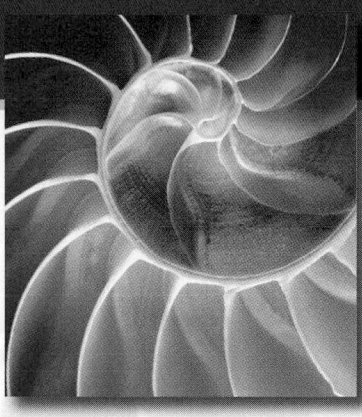

CHAPTER 38

Leading & Managing

For a podcast of an overview of this chapter,

 Go to Student Resources, **Podcast – Chapter Overviews, Chapter 38,** on DavisPlus at http://davisplus.fadavis.com/ Wilkinson2

Caring for the Garcias

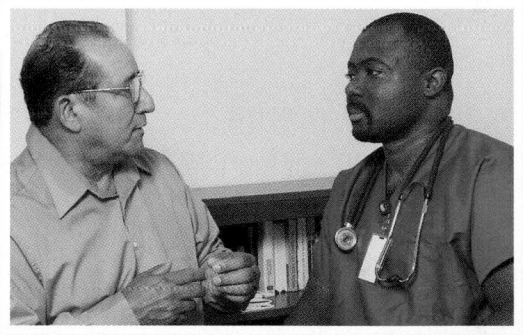

The exercises in the following section allow you to practice the kind of thinking you will use as a full-spectrum nurse. Because these are critical-thinking questions, there is usually no single right answer. We do not provide answers for these questions because it is more important for you to think about the questions than to arrive at the "right" answer. These questions are designed to improve your thinking more than to "cover content." Discuss answers with your peers—discussion can stimulate critical thinking. If you have difficulty with any of these questions, consult with your instructor.

Katherine Garcia, Joe's mother, is scheduled for out-patient cataract surgery later this week at the local hospital. Joe reports to the clinic wishing to discuss the plan for his mother's surgery "with whoever is the boss." Joe is concerned that his mother will not be staying at the hospital. "She's having surgery. I don't understand this! She's 76 years old. She's going to need help. This doesn't make sense. You have to change things. It won't be safe to do this as planned."

Joe tells you he has discussed his concerns with the ophthalmologist. He tells you that the ophthalmologist told him he was "overreacting. We always do it this way. You just don't understand."

Joe is visibly upset. He believes that his mother is receiving inadequate care. He appeals to you to help him take care of his mother. "This is where Mother gets her care. You know her. You have to change this."

Katherine has been seen at the family clinic several times over the last few years. She takes a medication for osteoporosis and has been counseled about the need for exercise and weight loss. She has also begun to experience problems with "accidents," that is, urine leakage. She has never had surgery in the past, and her only hospitalizations have been for childbirth. Katherine's husband recently passed away, and she has been living alone since then.

A. Devise a plan to resolve this conflict with Joe.

THINKING CRITICALLY ABOUT LEADING AND MANAGING

The exercises in the following sections allow you to practice the kind of thinking you will use as a full-spectrum nurse. Because these are critical-thinking questions, there is usually no single right answer. We do not provide answers for these questions because it is more important for you to think about the questions than to arrive at the "right" answer. These questions are designed to improve your thinking more than to "cover content." Discuss answers with your peers—discussion can stimulate critical thinking. If you have difficulty with any of these questions, consult with your instructor.

Applying the Full-Spectrum Nursing Model

ORGANIZATIONAL SITUATION

A small, not-for-profit hospice center in a small community has received a generous memorial gift from the family of a client who recently died. The family asked only that the money be "put to the best possible use." Everyone in the facility has an opinion about the best use for the money.

The administrator wants to renovate their old, run-down headquarters. The financial officer wants to put the money in the bank "for a rainy day." The chaplain wants to add a small chapel to the building. The nurses want to create a food bank to help the poorest of their clients. The social workers want to buy a van to transport clients to healthcare providers. The staff has agreed that all the ideas have merit and all the needs are important. Unfortunately, there is enough money to meet only one of them.

The more the staff members discuss how to use this gift, the more insistent each group becomes about defending its own idea. At the last meeting it is clear that some are becoming angry and frustrated. A shouting match even occurs between the administrator and the financial officer.

THINKING

1. *Theoretical Knowledge*:

   a. Which is appropriate at this point, a problem-solving approach or informal negotiation? Explain your answer.

DOING

2. *Practical Knowledge:*

   If you were to conduct the informal negotiation, list the steps of the plan you would follow.

CARING

3. *Self-Knowledge*:

   Which idea do you think has the most merit? Why did you select the one you did?

4. *Ethical Knowledge*:

   Which groups or individuals seem to demonstrate the value of caring for clients? Explain your thinking.

Critical Thinking and Clinical Reasoning

1. Identify a personal or professional change that you would like to see take place, and outline the steps needed to implement the change.

2. Eleanor, an LPN returning to school to obtain her associate's degree in nursing, is faced with a multitude of responsibilities. A wife, a mother of two toddlers, and a full-time staff member at a local hospital, Eleanor suddenly finds herself in a situation in which there just are not enough hours in a day. She is convinced that becoming a registered nurse is an impossible

goal. You are Eleanor's mentor. When you ask where she wants to be in 5 years, she answers, "At this moment, I think, on an island in Tahiti!"

   a. Help Eleanor develop a personal time inventory. To help her determine specifically what to include, make your own personal time inventory to share with her as an example.

   b. Once Eleanor has finished her time plan, how would you advise her to use it to make better use of her time? Make specific suggestions.

3. What strategies could you use to better manage your time?

4. Why is it important to learn good time management habits while you are a student?

5. This is your first semester in the nursing program. Although you have attended college to complete the prerequisite courses, this seems to be so different. All of a sudden, you have to attend clinical rotations in addition to classes. And you have to prepare ahead of time for the clinical experience, often even going to the hospital the night before to obtain information related to your patients. You feel like you are drowning! What can you do?

 Go to Chapter 38, **Table 38-4: Components of Time Management,** in Volume 1.

   Work through the table, asking yourself questions such as the following. Be very specific in your answers; give examples.

   a. *Prioritizing*

   - What tasks do you have to complete on a daily basis? Weekly? During the semester?
   - List the tasks in order of importance.
   - Which of the tasks do you have control over (e.g., scheduling a haircut or setting aside time to read the next assignment versus taking a test that is scheduled)?

   b. *Assigning priorities*: Assign priorities to the tasks you have identified.

   c. *Questioning effectiveness, efficiency*: Ask yourself, "How can I accomplish these tasks in the least amount of time but to the best of my ability?"

   d. *Rechecking*: Review your plan. Mentally and physically recheck the plan. Revise the plan as needed.

   e. *Self-reliance*: Carry out your plan. Use critical-thinking skills, and adapt the plan as needed so that you "go with the flow."

   f. *Treating*: Be good to yourself, but commit yourself to time management and excellence. How can you do that? What treats will you give yourself?

6. For each of the following concepts, use critical thinking to describe how or why it is important to nursing, patient care, or managing or leading. Note that these are *not* to be merely definitions.

Leadership skills	Time management
Management skills	Resolving conflicts
Becoming a mentor	Delegating appropriately
Being a mentee	Understanding the change process

What Are the Main Points in This Chapter?

➤ Leadership is the ability to influence other people.

➤ Transformational leaders communicate their vision in a way that reduces negativity and inspires commitment in people.

➤ Three common behavioral leadership styles are authoritarian, democratic, and laissez-faire.

➤ A manager is an employee of an organization who has power, authority, and responsibility for planning and directing the work of others.

➤ Effective managers possess a combination of qualities: leadership skills, clinical expertise, and business sense.

➤ A manager's activities are generally organizational, interpersonal, and informational.

➤ Not all leaders should be managers; but all managers should be leaders.

➤ It is never too early in your career to develop a SWOT or SOAR analysis. Throughout your nursing program, revisit the analysis, and update it as you gain new knowledge and skills.

➤ A mentor is a role model who develops the novice nurse to a professional by coaching, encouraging, supporting, and guiding him or her.

➤ Be mindful of nurses who demonstrate strong mentor qualities. Do not be afraid to ask for their support and guidance. Develop mentor qualities of your own, so you can also mentor a new student.

➤ At times throughout our nursing careers, we will all assume the role of follower.

➤ Followers need to be self-directing, actively participating experts who work on behalf of the organization.

➤ Sources of power include authority, reward, expertise, and coercion.

➤ Nurses have expertise power and authority over other healthcare workers. It is important that you understand your sources of power and use them wisely.

➤ Empowerment is the feeling of self-determination, competence, and recognition that your expertise and power within the healthcare system have meaning and positive impact.

➤ Evaluative feedback is a leadership responsibility that reinforces constructive and discourages undesirable behavior; provides recognition; and develops employee skills.

➤ Delegation of patient care tasks to other healthcare workers is one of the most important responsibilities of the registered nurse.

➤ Nurses must understand change and act as change agents within today's healthcare setting.

➤ Managing change involves recognizing and decreasing resistance.

➤ Conflict is inevitable, but it does not need to be destructive.

➤ One of a manager's responsibilities is to facilitate conflict resolution and, if necessary, function as an informal negotiator.

➤ Effective time management is essential to planning safe, effective patient care and demonstrating management skills.

➤ Time management includes goal setting and organizing and streamlining your work.

➤ Do not forget get rest and "time off" when managing time.

For practice questions for this chapter,

 Go to **NCLEX-Style Chapter Quiz,** on the Student Resource Disk or DavisPlus at http://davisplus.fadavis.com/Wilkinson2

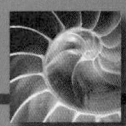

Knowledge Map

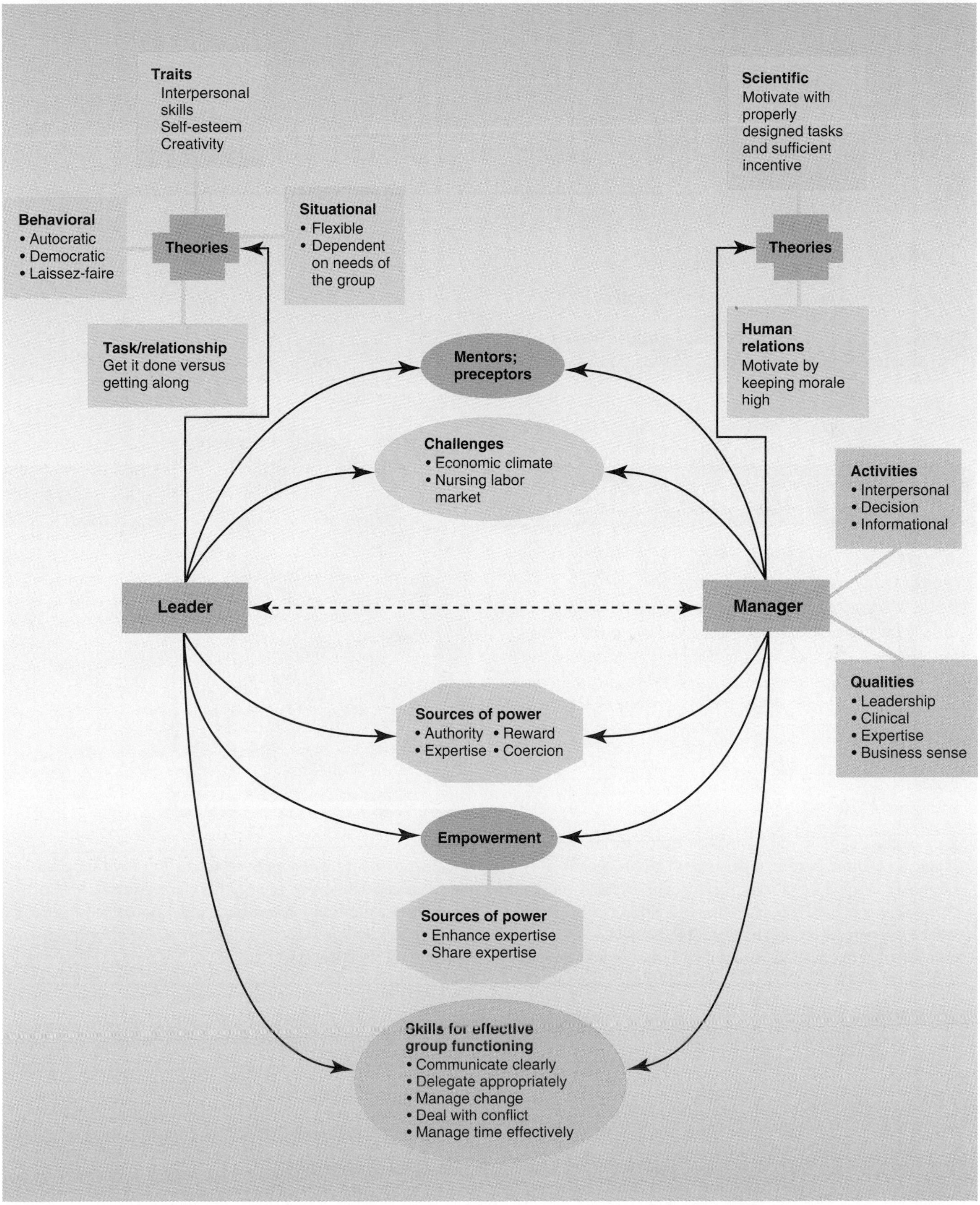

Traits
Interpersonal skills
Self-esteem
Creativity

Scientific
Motivate with properly designed tasks and sufficient incentive

Behavioral
• Autocratic
• Democratic
• Laissez-faire

Theories

Situational
• Flexible
• Dependent on needs of the group

Theories

Human relations
Motivate by keeping morale high

Task/relationship
Get it done versus getting along

Mentors; preceptors

Challenges
• Economic climate
• Nursing labor market

Activities
• Interpersonal
• Decision
• Informational

Leader ←------------------→ **Manager**

Qualities
• Leadership
• Clinical
• Expertise
• Business sense

Sources of power
• Authority   • Reward
• Expertise   • Coercion

Empowerment

Sources of power
• Enhance expertise
• Share expertise

Skills for effective group functioning
• Communicate clearly
• Delegate appropriately
• Manage change
• Deal with conflict
• Manage time effectively

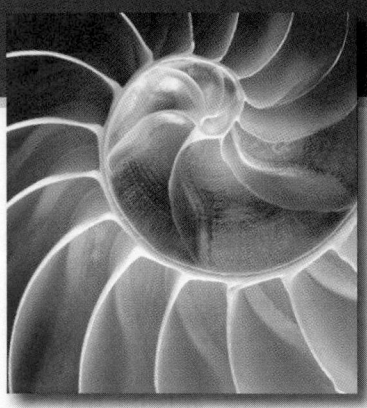

CHAPTER 39

Nursing Informatics

For a podcast of an overview of this chapter,

 Go to Student Resources, **Podcast – Chapter Overviews, Chapter 39,** on DavisPlus at http://davisplus.fadavis.com/ Wilkinson2

Caring for the Garcias

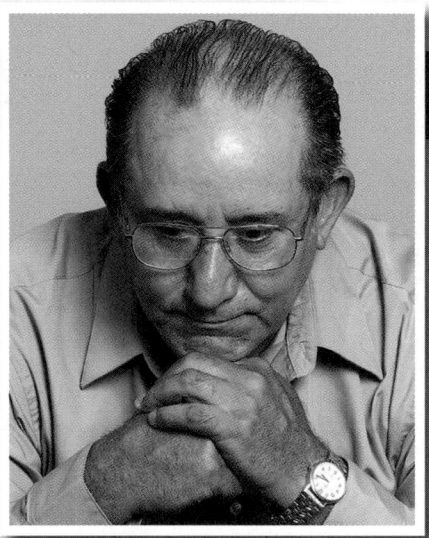

The exercises in the following section allow you to practice the kind of thinking you will use as a full-spectrum nurse. Because these are critical-thinking questions, there is usually no single right answer. We do not provide answers for these questions because it is more important for you to think about the questions than to arrive at the "right" answer. These questions are designed to improve your thinking more than to "cover content." Discuss answers with your peers—discussion can stimulate critical thinking. If you have difficulty with any of these questions, consult with your instructor.

Joe Garcia, a patient you have been caring for at the Family Medicine Center, has been devastated by his recent diagnoses of type 2 diabetes mellitus and hypertension. "Oh my, this is bad. This stuff kills you. I don't understand what I did to cause this," he sighs. He is having difficulty following his medication regimen and says he just doesn't understand what he is supposed to do. You have supplied him with information at each of his clinic visits as well as handouts, medication information, and a reminder sheet for his medicines. Joe asks you if there is any information available on the Internet.

A. What advice would you give him about looking up medical information on the Internet?

B. What sources would you recommend to Joe?

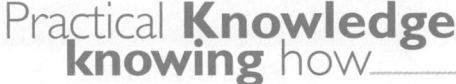

Standardized Language

American Nurses Association Recognized Languages for Nursing		
LANGUAGE	**DESCRIPTION**	**RECOGNITION DATE**
Diagnostic Related Group (DRG)	DRG is a classification system for most health conditions in order to establish a standardized reimbursement system for Medicare.	1983
NANDA International	2009-2011 Nursing Diagnoses Language includes 13 Domains with diagnostic labels with etiologies, risk factors, and defining characteristics.	1992
Nursing Interventions Classification (NIC)	The fifth edition contains 542 direct and indirect interventions assigned to one of seven domains and 30 classes. Each intervention includes a concept label, definition, and activities.	1992
Clinical Care Classification (CCC)	Developed by Virginia Saba, this language is used primarily by home health agencies and community settings. This language contains nursing diagnoses and interventions developed to code, index, classify, document, track, and analyze clinical care processes.	1992
Omaha System	This language also documents care in community and home care agencies. This system consists of 4 levels including 42 nursing diagnoses (patient assessment and problem classification), nursing interventions (delivery of care), and a problem-rating scale for outcomes.	1992
Nursing Outcomes Classification (NOC)	The fourth edition of NOC consists of 385 outcomes, including seven family unit and six community level outcomes. The NOC is a comprehensive standardized language designed to help clinicians evaluate the effectiveness of nursing interventions.	1997
Nursing Management Minimum Data Set (NMMDS)	This data set describes healthcare and nursing environment associated with the diagnosis, intervention, and outcome segments from the administrative, management, and resource management perspectives. It is composed of 17 data elements in 3 categories: environment, nurse resources, and financial resources.	1998
Patient Care Data Set (PCDS)	Judy Ozbolt developed this language, which is composed of a data dictionary, 363 nursing diagnoses, 1,357 patient care actions, and 311 patient care goals. The PCDS was developed for multidisciplinary use.	1998
Perioperative Nursing Data Set (PNDS)	The PNDS language describes perioperative nursing practice and consists of 64 nursing diagnoses, 127 nursing interventions, and 29 patient outcomes. This was the first nursing language developed by a nursing specialty.	1999
Statistical Nomenclature of Medicine Clinical Terminology (SNOMED CT)	SNOMED CT is a reference terminology that includes clinical concepts used to describe assessment, diagnosis, intervention, and outcome. Although it includes nursing concepts, it is not developed specifically for nursing, but rather for a broad spectrum of healthcare domains.	2002
Nursing Minimum Data Sets (NMDS)	This data collection establishes comparability of nursing data across population settings, geographic areas, and times. It describes the nursing care of patients or clients and their families in a variety of settings, both institutional and noninstitutional.	1999
International Classification for Nursing Practice (ICNP)	ICNP describes nursing practice in various clinical settings worldwide using common language. It includes nursing phenomena or diagnoses, outcomes, and actions.	2000

Continued

American Nurses Association Recognized Languages for Nursing—cont'd

LANGUAGE	DESCRIPTION	RECOGNITION DATE
ABCcodes	ABCcodes fit into existing data fields on insurance claim forms and in healthcare information systems. The design of ABCcodes supports more than 18 million code combinations to describe current and emerging alternative medicine, nursing, and other integrative healthcare practices. Approximately 4,327 codes have been assigned to date.	2000
Logical Observation Identifiers Names and Codes (LOINC®)	This is universal terminology for identifying laboratory results (e.g., hemoglobin) and other clinical observations (e.g., vital signs).	2002

THINKING CRITICALLY ABOUT NURSING INFORMATICS

The exercises in the following sections allow you to practice the kind of thinking you will use as a full-spectrum nurse. Because these are critical-thinking questions, there is usually no single right answer. We do not provide answers for these questions because it is more important for you to think about the questions than to arrive at the "right" answer. These questions are designed to improve your thinking more than to "cover content." Discuss answers with your peers—discussion can stimulate critical thinking. If you have difficulty with any of these questions, consult with your instructor.

Applying the Full-Spectrum Nursing Model

PATIENT SITUATION

Sarita, a nurse working in the surgical ICU, is ordering patient lab and recording patient information in the electronic health record (EHR). While at the computer terminal, the resident physician walks over to her and requests an update on the patient's condition. They go to the bedside to assess the patient's color and perfusion after surgery. The unit is very busy and another nurse, Janelle, needs to order a STAT x-ray using the central computer in the unit. When Sarita goes back to the computer screen to order lab work and finish her documentation, Janelle has stepped in and is now accessing another patient's record.

THINKING

1. *Theoretical Knowledge:*

  a. Name five benefits of using an electronic health record for storing and retrieving patient data in a busy critical care unit.

  b. List five potential areas of difficulty in using this same electronic health record.

2. *Critical Thinking (Considering Alternatives):*

  a. Brainstorm about possible solutions for dealing with bottlenecks among staff using a centralized computer.

DOING

3. *Practical Knowledge:*

  a. Where would you look to find out who accessed the patient record?

CARING

4. *Ethical Knowledge:*

  a. What violation has Sarita committed in this situation? What should she have done instead?

5. What is the nurse's responsibility in protecting patient information in the electronic record? What kinds of things should the nurse do?

6. *Self-Knowledge:*

  a. Have you ever been so busy that you feel like you just need to take a "necessary" shortcut to save time? Describe your experience.

Critical Thinking and Clinical Reasoning

1. Refer to the following table. For each of the uses listed, what kind of information do you think the database should provide? That is, what kind of data would you need? What kind of database would you use? For example, look at the first item under "In Nursing Practice" in column 1. For "Literature access and retrieval," you would use a database that contains information about journals, books, reports, and their content, perhaps CINAHL.

Work with your classmates. Share your knowledge and experience to answer these questions. Consult your instructor as needed.

USE	TYPE OF INFORMATION NEEDED
In Nursing Practice Literature access and retrieval (e.g., for evidence-based practice)	***Suggested response:*** CINAHL; information about books, journals, and their content; possibly the Internet
Care planning	***Clues:*** What information would you need for care planning? Where would you find it?
Client records (e.g., documenting, order entry, retrieving lab results)	
Telenursing (e.g., in home health)	
Case management	
In Nursing Education Literature access and retrieval	
Computer-assisted instruction (CAI) programs	
Classroom technology	
Distance learning	
Testing and grading	
Student records	
In Nursing Administration Quality assurance/improvement and utilization review	***Clues:*** What information would you need to evaluate the quality of care in your institution? Where would you find it?
Employee records (e.g., to track licenses, immunizations)	
Staffing patterns, hiring	
Buildings and facilities management	
Finance and budgets	
Accreditation reviews (e.g., monitoring quality control)	
In Nursing Research Literature review	
Data collection	
Data analysis (both qualitative and quantitative)	
Research dissemination	
Applying for grants	

2. Search for "online nursing journals" on the Internet. Make a list of nursing journals that provide full-text articles that are available on the Internet, and at no charge. Hint:

 Go to Chapter 39, **Resources for Caregivers and Health Professionals,** on the Student Resource Disk or DavisPlus at http://davisplus.fadavis.com/Wilkinson2

3. For each of the following concepts, use critical thinking to describe how or why it is important to nursing, patients, or nursing informatics. Note that these are *not* to be merely definitions.

Nursing informatics	Connectivity
Data	Listservs
Knowledge	Telehealth
Wisdom	Electronic health records
Evidence-based practice	Standardized nursing language
Computers	Literature databases
Hardware	The World Wide Web
Storage media	Evaluating Web sites

What Are the Main Points in This Chapter?

➤ Whatever their roles—staff nurse, administrator, educator, researcher, primary care provider—nurses use vast amounts of data, information, and knowledge in their daily work.

➤ Informatics is the processing and management of data, information, and knowledge necessary for making practice decisions.

➤ The nursing informatics specialist uses nursing science, computer science, and information science to manage and communicate data, information, knowledge, and wisdom in nursing practice.

➤ A computer has four main functions: input, processing, output, and storage.

➤ Connectivity is a term referring to the ways in which computers and other hardware communicate and share information.

➤ Some forms of electronic communication include telephone, videoconferencing, fax, e-mail, Listservs, and telehealth applications.

➤ Rogers' categories of adopters of innovation are innovators, early adopters, early majority, late majority, and laggards.

➤ Electronic health records (EHRs) enable an organization to replace its paper charts with electronic records, thereby increasing productivity and efficiency and facilitating research to improve healthcare.

➤ Standardized nursing languages facilitate the inclusion of nursing in the EHR and make visible nursing contributions to healthcare.

➤ It is important to use and protect passwords to protect the privacy of patient records.

➤ Evidence-based practice requires the ability to manage and process a great deal of information to identify a clinical problem, search the literature, evaluate the evidence, and decide on an intervention.

➤ Information taken from the Internet should be evaluated carefully; do not believe everything you see on the Internet.

➤ CINAHL and MEDLINE are two important databases to search for nursing literature.

For practice questions for this chapter,

 Go to **NCLEX-Style Chapter Quiz,** on the Student Resource Disk or DavisPlus at http://davisplus.fadavis.com/Wilkinson2

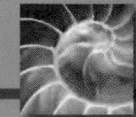

Knowledge Map

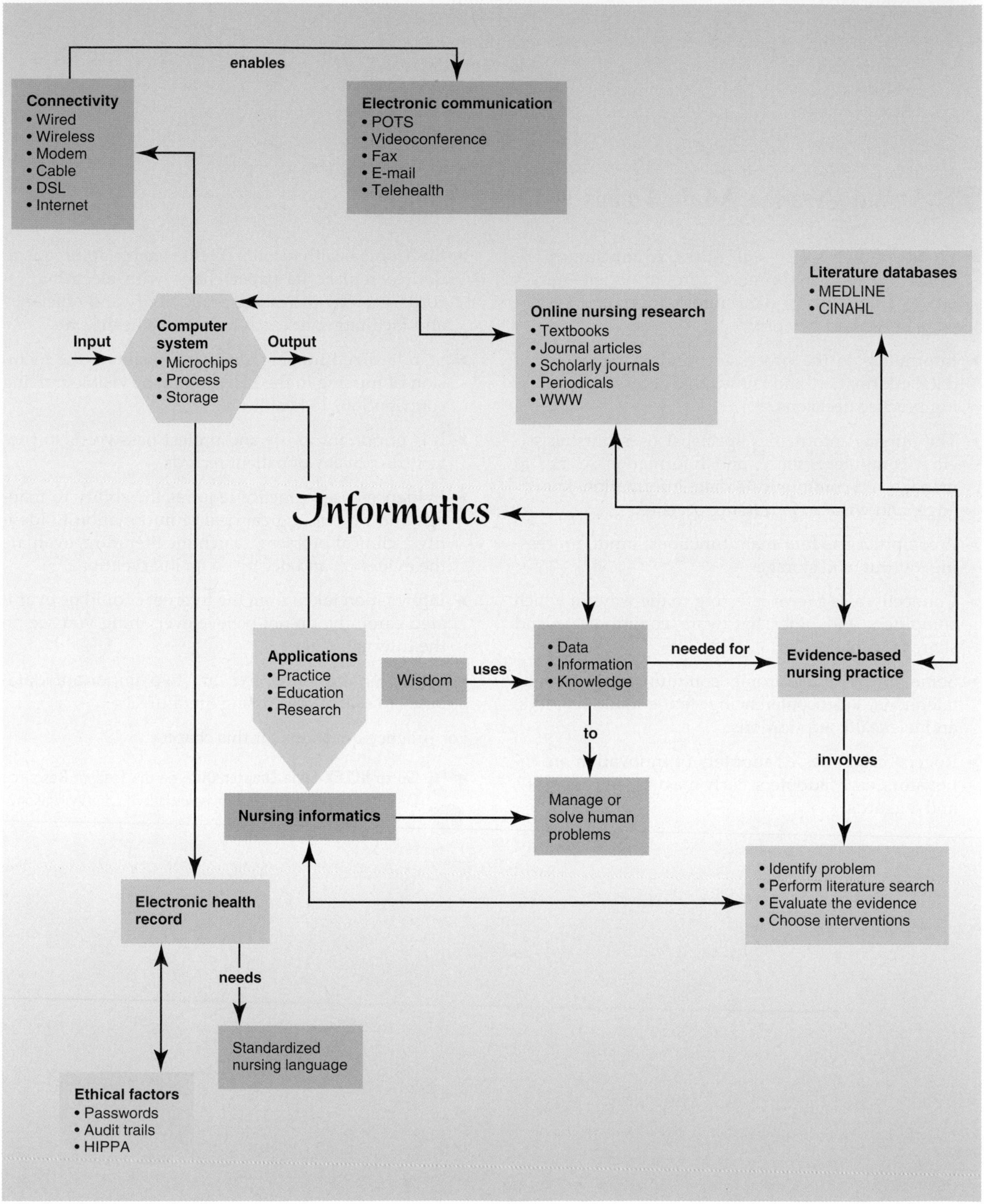

Connectivity
- Wired
- Wireless
- Modem
- Cable
- DSL
- Internet

enables

Electronic communication
- POTS
- Videoconference
- Fax
- E-mail
- Telehealth

Literature databases
- MEDLINE
- CINAHL

Input

Computer system
- Microchips
- Process
- Storage

Output

Online nursing research
- Textbooks
- Journal articles
- Scholarly journals
- Periodicals
- WWW

Informatics

Applications
- Practice
- Education
- Research

Wisdom uses

- Data
- Information
- Knowledge

needed for

Evidence-based nursing practice

to

Nursing informatics

Manage or solve human problems

involves

- Identify problem
- Perform literature search
- Evaluate the evidence
- Choose interventions

Electronic health record

needs

Standardized nursing language

Ethical factors
- Passwords
- Audit trails
- HIPPA

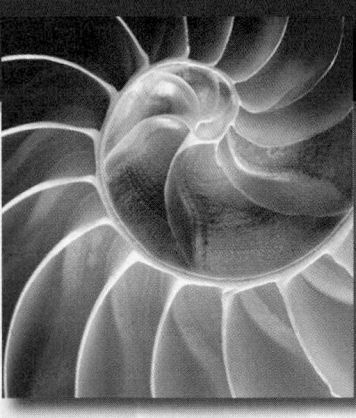

CHAPTER 40

Holistic Healing

For a podcast of an overview of this chapter,

Go to Student Resources, **Podcast – Chapter Overviews, Chapter 40,** on DavisPlus at http://davisplus.fadavis.com/ Wilkinson2

Caring for the Garcias

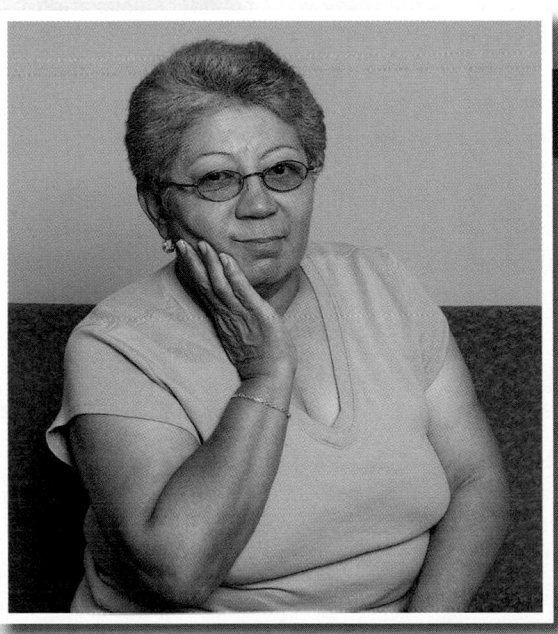

The exercises in the following section allow you to practice the kind of thinking you will use as a full-spectrum nurse. Because these are critical-thinking questions, there is usually no single right answer. We do not provide answers for these questions because it is more important for you to think about the questions than to arrive at the "right" answer. These questions are designed to improve your thinking more than to "cover content." Discuss answers with your peers— discussion can stimulate critical thinking. If you have difficulty with any of these questions, consult with your instructor.

Several months ago, Flordelisa Garcia had a complete physical examination with Jordan Miller, FNP. Flordelisa has been experiencing irregular menses, poor sleep, and hot flashes. Jordan explained that these were common complaints associated with menopause. Flordelisa has chosen to avoid hormone replacement therapy because of the controversy surrounding its use. Instead, she has been experimenting with complementary and alternative modality (CAM) therapies. Friends have suggested she try wild yam cream and a diet high in soy protein.

A. To know how to advise Flordelisa, what theoretical knowledge do you need?

B. Search the Internet and other CAM resources for information on these treatment modalities. What advice would you offer her about these modalities?

C. Flordelisa is also interested in CAM therapies for her husband, Joe. Several varieties of therapies and supplements are marketed for patients with hypertension and diabetes. Outline the approach you might take when working with Joe and Flordelisa to integrate their interest in CAM therapies with their conventional healthcare.

Practical **Knowledge**
knowing how

There are three very practical applications of complementary and alternative modalities (CAM) you can use in your practice:

1. You can, and should, facilitate communication about CAM between your patients and their healthcare providers.
2. You can use self-care practices to promote your own health and wholeness.
3. You can, with minimal training, use some of the less complex CAM therapies as independent nursing interventions.

Clinical Insights

In this section you will find techniques and guidelines for performing some of the less complex CAM therapies. All are NIC standardized interventions (Bulechek, Butcher, & Dochterman, 2008). You can learn to use most of the therapies by doing a little extra reading. For others, such as therapeutic touch, you will need to attend a workshop or find a mentor who will guide you in their use. None of the therapies included here requires credentialing or extensive training.

Clinical Insight 40-1 ▶ **Performing Autogenic Training**

Autogenic training is assisting with self-suggestions about feelings of heaviness and warmth for the purpose of inducing relaxation (Bulechek, Butcher, & Dochterman, 2008, p. 151). This is one of the many ways to induce relaxation. Follow these steps:

1. Seat the patient in a recumbent position or other meditative posture.
2. The goal is for the patient's body to feel warm, heavy, and relaxed.
3. Read a prepared script to the patient, pausing to give him enough time to repeat the script internally.
4. Use statements that elicit feelings of heaviness, lightness, or floating of specific body parts (e.g., "My arms and legs

are heavy," "My arms are warm," "My heartbeat is calm and regular," "My abdomen is warm," "My forehead is cool.")
5. Instruct the patient to repeat the statements to himself to elicit the feeling within the body part (e.g., say to the patient, "Repeat to yourself, 'My arm is getting heavy,' while you feel your arm growing heavy.")
6. Rehearse with the script for 15 to 20 minutes, one body part at a time.
7. After mastering heaviness sensations throughout his body, proceed to elicit feelings of warmth.

Clinical Insight 40-2 ▶ **Using Calming Technique**

Calming technique is "reducing anxiety in a patient experiencing acute distress" (Bulechek, Butcher, & Dochterman, 2008, p. 193). You do not need special preparation for this intervention; you are probably already doing it to some extent. The following are examples of nursing activities involved:

- Maintain eye contact.
- Maintain a calm, deliberate manner.
- Sit and talk with the patient.
- Encourage slow, purposeful deep breathing.

- Reassure the patient of her personal safety or security.
- Reduce or eliminate stimuli that create fear or anxiety.
- Use distraction as appropriate.
- Offer a back rub, as appropriate.
- Offer a warm bath or shower.
- Offer warm fluids or milk.
- Hold and comfort an infant or child.
- Speak softly or sing to an infant or child.
- Give a pacifier to an infant.

Clinical Insight 40-3 ▶ **Using Humor**

Humor is helping "the patient to perceive, appreciate, and express what is funny, amusing, or ludicrous in order to establish relationships, relieve tension, release anger, facilitate learning, or cope with painful feelings" (Bulechek, Butcher, & Dochterman, 2008, p. 409). Some healthcare agencies have created "humor rooms" for patients and staff, supplied with humorous books, videotapes, cartoons, and so on.

When using humor, you need to be aware of your feelings and those of others, as well as sensitive to cultural differences in what people see as funny.

- Determine the types of humor that the patient appreciates.
- Discuss with the patient advantages of laughter.
- Avoid content areas about which the patient is sensitive.

■ Make available a selection of humorous games, cartoons, jokes, videos, tapes, books, and so on.
■ Point out humorous incongruity in a situation.
■ Encourage visualization with humor (e.g., picture a forbidding authority figure dressed only in underwear).
■ Encourage silliness and playfulness.

■ Avoid using humor with patients who are cognitively impaired.
■ Respond positively to humor attempts that the patient makes.
■ Monitor patient response, and discontinue the humor strategy if it is ineffective.

Clinical Insight 40-4 ➤ **Facilitating Meditation**

Meditation facilitation consists of "facilitating a person to alter his/her level of awareness by focusing specifically on an image or thought" (Dochterman & Bulechek, 2008, p. 495). You will need some theoretical knowledge about meditation, but it is a simple, noninvasive technique that you can use at the bedside.
1. Prepare a quiet environment.
2. Instruct the patient to sit quietly and comfortably.
3. Instruct the patient to close his eyes, if he desires, and to relax all muscles and remain relaxed.

4. Help the patient to select a mental device to repeat during the procedure (e.g., repeating a word, such as "one").
5. Instruct the person to inhale, then say the word silently while breathing out through the nose.
6. Continue with the exercise, focusing on the mental device chosen, for as long as needed.
7. When finished, instruct the patient to sit quietly for several minutes with his eyes open.
8. Instruct the patient perform the procedure once or twice daily, but not within 2 hours after meals.

Clinical Insight 40-5 ➤ **Performing Simple Guided Imagery**

Guided imagery is "purposeful use of imagination to achieve a particular state, outcome, or action to direct attention away from undesirable sensations" (Dochterman & Bulechek, 2008, p. 382). This technique is useful for mild to moderate pain and anxiety. You do not need extensive training to use it. Commercial audiotapes are available to guide imagery, or you may guide the patient.
1. Instruct the patient assume a comfortable position, with eyes closed.
2. Arrange a quiet environment at a time when you will not be interrupted.
3. Ask the patient to describe an image he has experienced as pleasurable and relaxing, such as lying on a beach, watching a snowfall, floating on a raft, or watching the sun set.
4. Choose a scene that involves as many of the five senses as possible.
5. Use techniques (e.g., rhythmic breathing) to induce relaxation.
6. Using permissive directions, such as "perhaps," and "if you wish," or "you might like," ask the patient to travel

mentally to the scene and help him to describe the setting in detail.
7. Ask the patient to slowly experience the scene: How does it look, smell, sound, feel, taste?
8. Use words that convey pleasurable images (e.g., floating, melting, releasing).
9. Develop a cleansing or clearing portion of imagery (e.g., "all pain appears as red dust and washes downstream in a creek as you enter").
10. Assist the patient to develop a method of ending the imagery, such as counting slowly while breathing deeply and thinking about being relaxed, refreshed, and alert.
11. Encourage the patient to express his thoughts and feelings after the experience.
12. Prepare the patient for unexpected (but often therapeutic) experiences, such as crying.
13. Follow up to assess the effects of imagery and any resulting changes in sensation and perception.

Clinical Insight 40-6 ➤ **Performing Simple Massage**

Massage is "stimulation of the skin and underlying tissues with varying degrees of hand pressure to decrease pain, produce relaxation, and/or improve circulation" (Dochterman & Bulechek, 2008, p. 466). Unlike special massage techniques, simple massage does not require advanced training.
1. Determine the patient's degree of psychological comfort with touch.
2. Screen for contraindications (e.g., poor skin integrity, deep-vein thrombosis).

3. Prepare a warm, comfortable, quiet environment.
4. Apply moist heat before or during massage as indicated.
5. Drape to expose only the area to be massaged.
6. Use warm lotion, oil, or dry powder to reduce friction. Place no oils or lotion on the head or scalp.
7. Massage the hands or feet if other areas are inconvenient or uncomfortable for the patient.
8. Adapt the massage area, technique, and pressure to the patient's comfort and the purpose of the massage.

Clinical Insight 40-6 ▶ Performing Simple Massage (continued)

9. Encourage the patient to breathe deeply, relax, and concentrate on the good feelings of the massage.

10. Avoid lengthy conversation during the massage, unless you use it as a distraction technique.

 11. Do not massage over open lesions or tender skin areas.

12. When the message is completed, instruct the patient to rest until he is ready and then to move slowly.

Clinical Insight 40-7 ▶ Performing Simple Relaxation Therapy

Relaxation therapy is "use of techniques to encourage and elicit relaxation for the purpose of decreasing undesirable signs and symptoms such as pain, muscle tension, or anxiety" (Dochterman & Bulechek, 2008, p. 604). This technique does not require advanced training, but you will need to know various ways to induce relaxation (e.g., music therapy, meditation, and progressive muscle relaxation).

1. Explain to the patient the benefits of relaxation and the various types you can offer.
2. Provide a detailed description of the chosen relaxation intervention.
3. Instruct the patient to assume a comfortable position, with eyes closed.
4. Elicit behaviors that are conditioned to produce relaxation, such as deep breathing, yawning, abdominal breathing, or peaceful imaging.
5. Instruct the patient to relax and let the sensations happen.
6. Use low tone of voice and slow, rhythmical pace of words.

7. Demonstrate and practice the relaxation technique with the patient.
8. Encourage return demonstrations, if possible.
9. Encourage frequent repetition or practice of the technique(s) selected.

The following is an example of a relaxation technique you could use at steps 2 and 7.

- Ask the patient close her eyes and observe the breathing pattern at her nostrils, where air enters and leaves the body.
- Direct the patient to observe the sensation of the breath at the nostril, consistently staying with this focus point. Tell her that when a thought or feeling arises, she should simply return to breathing awareness.
- You can, at first, guide her breathing by saying, "Breathe in. Breathe out. Focus on the breath at your nostrils." Periodically say, "Focus on your breath at the end of your nose."

Clinical Insight 40-8 ▶ Performing Therapeutic Touch

Therapeutic touch (TT) is defined as "attuning to the universal healing field, seeing to act as an instrument for healing influence, and using the natural sensitivity of the hands to gently focus and direct the intervention process" (Dochterman & Bulechek, 2008, p. 751). It requires special training and practice (at least a one- or two-day workshop). If you have had some instruction and someone has demonstrated the technique to you, you may be able to use this intervention effectively. The following activities summarize it (some activities are from NIC, others are not).

1. **Center yourself.**
   To practice TT, you must establish and maintain a state of conscious awareness that fosters sensitivity to energy field phenomena. This state of awareness is developed by a meditative practice that TT practitioners call "centering"—a quiet focused state. Centering is simple and easy to learn and has an immediate calming affect. Do the following:
   - Sit in a quiet, comfortable place. Close your eyes and breathe deeply in and out.
   - Allow your muscles to progressively relax.
   - Concentrate on your breathing. Visualize taking in energy as you inhale and releasing tension as you exhale.

   - Focus on your breath, allow outside stimuli and thoughts to pass, and connect with your inner core of wholeness and stillness.
   - Then turn your attention to your professional role while concentrating on your breathing.
   - Approach your client with renewed focus and calm and intent to heal.

2. **Assess the patient's energy field:**
   - Once you have centered, focus on the intention to facilitate wholeness and healing at all levels of consciousness.
   - Place your hands 2.5 to 5 cm (1 to 2 in.) from the patient's body.
   - Begin the assessment of the energy field by moving your hands slowly and steadily over as much of the patient's body as possible, from head to toe and front to back.
   - Note the overall pattern of energy flow, especially any areas of disturbance, such as congestion or unevenness, which you may feel through very subtle cues in your hands. For example, some practitioners feel temperature change or tingling.

3. **Perform the TT treatment.**
   - Continue to focus on the intention to facilitate wholeness and healing at all levels of consciousness.

- Unruffle (smooth, clear) the field by sweeping away stagnant energy in sweeping motions from the midline toward the periphery.
- Repattern the field by transferring energy through yourself to the patient or by rebalancing the patient's energy from areas of congestion to areas of deficit.
- Focus intention on facilitating symmetry and healing in disturbed areas.
- Next, get the energy flowing. Begin by moving the hands in very gentle downward movements through the patient's energy field, thinking of the patient as a unitary whole and facilitating an open and balanced energy flow.

- Continue the treatment by very gently facilitating the flow of healing energy into areas of disturbance.

4. **Closure.**
   - Reassess the field continually to determine energy balance. Ask for feedback from the patient, and use your informed and intuitive judgment to know when to end the session.
   - Finish when you judge that the appropriate amount of change has taken place (i.e., for an infant, 1 to 2 minutes; for an adult, 5 to 7 minutes), keeping in mind the importance of being gentle.

THINKING CRITICALLY ABOUT HOLISTIC HEALING

The exercises in the following sections allow you to practice the kind of thinking you will use as a full-spectrum nurse. Because these are critical-thinking questions, there is usually no single right answer. We do not provide answers for these questions because it is more important for you to think about the questions than to arrive at the "right" answer. These questions are designed to improve your thinking more than to "cover content." Discuss answers with your peers—discussion can stimulate critical thinking. If you have difficulty with any of these questions, consult with your instructor.

Applying the Full-Spectrum Nursing Model

PATIENT SITUATION

Recall from Volume 1 that when Lisa put her hand on Mrs. Riddell's arm and said, "It must be very difficult for you," Mrs. Riddell reached for Lisa's hand and began sobbing, "I'm so afraid."

Just then the manager of the surgical unit walked in, speaking rapidly, "Lisa, you forgot to turn the call light off. Oh, Mrs. Riddell, you seem upset. Are you in pain?" Mrs. Riddell nodded her head yes. When the manager asked her to rate the pain on a scale of 1 to 10, Mrs. Riddell replied, "About a 5." The manager said, "Ms Jackson will check when you can have your next dose of pain medication."

Outside the room, Lisa explained to her manager that Mrs. Riddell was worried about her diagnosis. "First things first, Lisa, get the patient's pain under control," replied the manager. Lisa wanted to spend a few moments with the patient to allow her to express her feelings and concerns. She that it would be easier to relieve Mrs. Riddell's pain if it were not complicated by her anxious feelings. However, Lisa was new on the unit and decided to follow the manager's orders to address the physical pain.

When Lisa returned with the analgesic, Mrs. Riddell refused it. She was still tearful and distressed and said that she really just needed to have her bed straightened. Lisa closed the curtains and explained that she would get some fresh linens and help her get comfortable. The manager saw Lisa carrying linens, stopped her, and said, "We have nursing assistive personnel (NAPs) for bed changes, which frees you up to do the professional nursing care. There are two new patients being admitted, and I want you to learn the admission process." Lisa shared her concerns about Mrs. Riddell's psychosocial needs and explained that she wanted to help her relax and express her concerns. Lisa said, "She refused the pain medication, but I'd like to use therapeutic touch (an energy intervention) to treat her." The manager replied, "I wish we had more time to talk to patients and try new things, but we are short-staffed, and the admissions, charting, treatments, and other work, will never be done by the end of shift if we don't do first things first. I'm sorry to disillusion you, but welcome to the real world of nursing."

Lisa and Mrs. Riddell are experiencing some problems common to contemporary healthcare: inadequate staff, time, and resources for the care we know our patients deserve. Many patients and nurses feel caught in a model of sick care that emphasizes disease and fosters professional emotional neutrality.

THINKING

1. *Theoretical Knowledge:*

a. What do you know about the link between anxiety and pain?

b. What do you know about the effectiveness of therapeutic touch (TT) in relieving anxiety?

c. What do you know about the effectiveness of therapeutic touch (TT) in relieving pain?

2. *Critical Thinking (Deciding What to Do):* Based on your theoretical knowledge, if you were Lisa Jackson, the nurse, would you try using TT to relieve Mrs. Riddell's pain? Why or why not?

DOING

3. *Practical Knowledge*: If you were Mrs. Riddell's nurse and were preparing to use TT for her pain (assuming the manager had not objected), what is the first thing you should do, and how would you do it?

4. *Nursing Process (Assessment)*: After centering yourself, you begin the TT assessment. How do you do this, and what are you looking for?

CARING

5. *Ethical Knowledge*: What ethical concerns might you have about using TT to treat Mrs. Riddell's pain?

Critical Thinking and Clinical Reasoning

1. Recent health survey research indicates that U.S. healthcare consumers are increasing their use of complementary and alternative modalities (CAMs). Consumers often do not inform their primary care providers of such use. Use these findings to identify six implications for nursing practice.

2. As a nurse on a surgical day care unit, you notice how anxious patients are while they await surgery. Describe a simple relaxation technique that you could teach the patients.

3. Describe a simple imagery technique that could be used with all preoperative patients.

4. Patients who use alternative therapies may not disclose their use to conventional practitioners. Create three interview questions that would elicit this information.

5. How can you support a patient's placebo response to enhance healing?

6. What preliminary assessments and interventions should the nurse conduct before using aromatherapy with patients in a healthcare setting?

7. A NAP, Maggie, has been helping Janelle Hunt get settled into her room at a long-term care facility. Ms Hunt is very old and too frail to live alone, but she is mentally alert and competent. She says to Maggie, "I have brought my magnet mattress pad with me, and my special pillow. I have bad arthritis, and I have to have those on my bed." The NAP comes to you, visibly annoyed. "That new patient wants me to put her own special mattress on the bed. Now I ask you, what good would that thing do? It will be a pain to change the sheets with that thing on there, not to speak of what happens if she is incontinent on it. Do I really have to do that?" How would you respond to Maggie?

8. For each of the following concepts, use critical thinking to describe how or why it is important to nursing, patient care, or holistic healing. Note that these are *not* to be merely definitions.

Holistic care   Complementary treatment modality
Integrative care   American Holistic Nurses Association
Alternative treatment modality

What Are the Main Points in This Chapter?

➤ Holistic healthcare is founded on the belief that each person is a whole in constant interaction with the environment. There is no separation between body, mind, or spirit.

➤ The conventional medical approach is often referred to as *allopathy*, a term used to denote medical practice that is focused on counteracting symptoms.

➤ A complementary modality is one that is used in conjunction with traditional Western medical care.

➤ An alternative modality is one that is used instead of traditional Western medical care.

➤ Integrative healthcare refers to coordinated care that encompasses all treatments and health practices used by a patient.

➤ In holistic care, treatment outcomes are enhanced if both the practitioner and the patient believe that the treatment will be effective.

➤ Holism contends that all healing is self-healing.

➤ Absence of spirituality creates a sense of disconnection from one's true source, a loss of meaning to one's life, and a state of disease.

➤ Women, people with higher income levels, and people who have been hospitalized in the past year are more likely to use complementary and alternative modalities (CAMs).

➤ Alternative medical systems predate the traditional Western health system. They include ayurveda, traditional Chinese medicine, acupuncture, homeopathy, and naturopathy.

➤ Mind–body interventions target the mood and reaction to stress to enhance health. They include prayer, meditation, imagery, humor, music therapy, yoga, hypnosis, and biofeedback.

➤ They include dietary therapies, herbs and aromatherapy, and nonherbal dietary supplements (e.g., probiotics, vitamins, and hormones). These therapies are readily available and are often practiced in conjunction with traditional healthcare and other CAMs.

➤ Manipulative and body-based therapies focus on moving the body to improve health. They include chiropractic, massage, and osteopathy.

➤ Energy therapies manipulate the energy fields that surround the body. They are among the most widely used forms of CAM. They include therapeutic touch, t'ai chi and Qigong, Reiki, and magnet therapy.

➤ Holistic nursing practice is a theory-based, relationship-centered, potent solution to a number of problems facing contemporary nursing and healthcare.

➤ You should facilitate communication about CAM between patients and their health care providers.

➤ As a holistic healer, you should use self-care practices to promote your own health and wholeness.

➤ You should assess patients' use of CAM and integrate CAM into your nursing care as appropriate. Encourage practices that are effective but not harmful; "allow" practices that are safe, but not known to be effective; and discourage practices that are unsafe.

For practice questions for this chapter,

 Go to **NCLEX-Style Chapter Quiz,** on the Student Resource Disk or DavisPlus at http://davisplus.fadavis.com/Wilkinson2

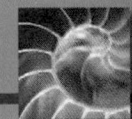

Knowledge Map

Related beliefs
- Uniqueness of the person
- Body, mind, and spirit connection
- Disease is due to multiple factors
- Health = balance
- Illness is opportunity for growth
- Recovery involves hope, faith, and will

Potential outcomes
- Enhanced resistance to illness
- Reduction of aggravating behaviors
- Lifestyle change
- Optimal wellness
- Placebo response

Holistic Health Care

Complementary modality
(used with traditional health care)

Alternative modality
(used instead of traditional health care)

Holistic nursing

Theorists
- Rogers
- Newman
- Watson

Concepts
- Meaning in disease
- Presence and intention
- Role modeling
- AHNA–practice support

Healing modalities
- Alternative medical systems
- Mind–body interventions
- Biological based treatments
- Manipulative and body-based methods
- Energy therapies

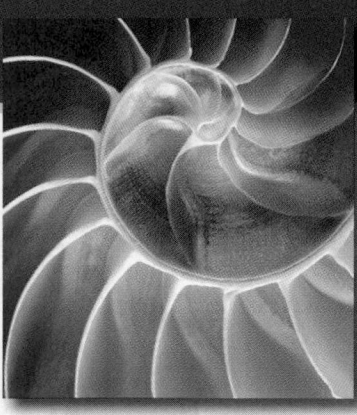

CHAPTER 41

Promoting Health

For a podcast of an overview of this chapter,

 Go to Student Resources, **Podcast – Chapter Overviews, Chapter 41,** on DavisPlus at http://davisplus.fadavis.com/Wilkinson2

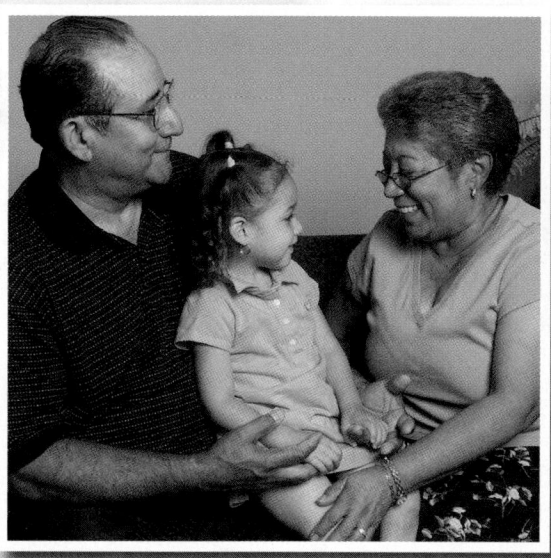

Caring for the Garcias

The exercises in the following section allow you to practice the kind of thinking you will use as a full-spectrum nurse. Because these are critical-thinking questions, there is usually no single right answer. We do not provide answers for these questions because it is more important for you to think about the questions than to arrive at the "right" answer. These questions are designed to improve your thinking more than to "cover content." Discuss answers with your peers—discussion can stimulate critical thinking. If you have difficulty with any of these questions, consult with your instructor.

Joe and Flordelisa Garcia; their 3-year-old granddaughter, Bettina; and Katherine, Joe's 76-year-old mother, are all patients at the Family Medicine Center. Jordan Miller, the family nurse practitioner at the center, asks you to devise a health promotion program for each member of the family.

A. What information should you gather before you begin?

B. How might you obtain this information?

C. How will the plans differ for each?

D. Review Meet the Garcias in the front of this volume. Also review the physical exam findings on Joe:

What health promotion strategies and health screenings should you recommend to Joe Garcia?

E. How would you begin to organize and prioritize a health promotion program for Joe?

F. Using therapeutic communication, give examples of appropriate questions to ask Joe about his health beliefs.

 Go to Chapter 19 in Volume 1.

Assessment Guidelines and Tools

Health Promotion: Physical Fitness Assessment

Cardiorespiratory Fitness

There are many different modes of testing, such as field tests (walking or running), motor-driven treadmills, stationary bicycles, and step testing.

- **Field tests** for running are good for children. A 9-year-old child should be able to complete a 1-mile run in approximately 10 minutes, and a 17-year-old boy should be able to complete a 1-mile run in approximately 7½ minutes (www.presidentschallenge.org).

- **The step test** is appropriate for most adults. Using a 12-inch bench, instruct the participant to step up and down at a rate of 24 steps per minute for 3 minutes. At the end of 3 minutes, he should check his heart rate. Stop testing immediately if the participant experiences any chest pain, shortness of breath, or light-headedness. Results depend on age and gender and are available below.

Step Test Evaluation Charts

3-Minute Step Heart Rate Test (Men)

Physical Condition	18–25 yrs	26–35 yrs	36–45 yrs	46–55 yrs	56–65 yrs	65+ yrs
Excellent	<79	<81	<83	<87	<86	<88
Good	79–89	81–89	83–96	87–97	86–97	88–96
Above average	90–99	90–99	97–103	98–105	98–103	97–103
Average	100–105	100–107	104–112	106–116	104–112	104–113
Below average	106–116	108–117	113–119	117–122	113–120	114–120
Poor	117–128	118–128	120–130	123–132	121–129	121–130
Very poor	>128	>128	>130	>132	>129	>130

3-Minute Step Test (Women)

Physical Condition	18–25 yrs	26–35 yrs	36–45 yrs	46–55 yrs	56–65 yrs	65+ yrs
Excellent	<85	<88	<90	<94	<95	<90
Good	85–98	88–99	90–102	94–104	95–104	90–102
Above average	99–108	100–111	103–110	105–115	105–112	103–115
Average	109–117	112–119	111–118	116–120	113–118	116–122
Below average	118–126	120–126	119–128	121–129	119–128	123–128
Poor	127–140	127–138	129–140	130–135	129–139	129–134
Very poor	>140	>138	>140	>135	>139	>134

Muscular Fitness

Muscle strength measures the amount of weight a muscle (or group of muscles) can move at one time. This is recorded as a ratio of weight pushed (or lifted) divided by body weight. For example, a woman weighing 150 pounds who is able to lift 86 pounds will have a ratio of 86 divided by 150, or 0.57.

- Instruct the participant warm up and stretch before the test. Weight benches are ideal sites for testing upper body and leg strength.

- Compare the ratio obtained to normative standards or to previous personal scores to evaluate improvement.

Muscle endurance refers to the ability of a muscle to perform repeated movements. The push-up or curl-up (crunch) test may be performed to evaluate endurance. Ask the participant to perform as many push-ups or curl-ups as possible without pausing. The number of repetitions is the score. Once again, compare scores to norms or previous performance.

Flexibility

Flexibility is the ability to move a joint through its range of motion. **The sit-and-reach test** evaluates low back and hip [trunk] flexion.

- Ask the participant sit on a floor mat with legs fully extended and feet flat against a box. Have her extend her arms and hands forward as far as possible and hold for a count of 3.

- Using a ruler, measure the distance in inches that the client can reach beyond the proximal edge of the box. If the client cannot reach the edge, measure the distance of the fingertips from the edge, and report it as a negative number.

Norms for trunk flexion vary among men and women. The desired range for men is 1 to +5 inches, and for women it is +2 to +6 inches (Pender, Murdaugh, & Parsons, 2002).

Lifestyle and Risk Assessment

Lifestyle refers to the manner in which a person conducts his life. You can gather this information by interview or by using a variety of questionnaires. A health risk appraisal (HRA) is a questionnaire that evaluates risk for disease based on current demographic data, lifestyle, and health behaviors. The following is an example of an HRA.

Name _____ Age _____ Gender _____

Health View

In general, would you say your present health is?

☐ Excellent

☐ Very good

☐ Good

☐ Fair

☐ Poor

General Practices

1. **Physical activity.** How many days each week do you get at least 30 minutes of physical activity, such as brisk walking, cycling, active gardening, active dance, swimming, jogging, or active sports? _____

2. **Strength exercises.** How many days each week do you do strength-building exercises, such as weight lifting or isometric exercises? _____

3. **Smoking status.** Indicate your present smoking status.

   ☐ Current smoker   ☐ Ex-smoker

   ☐ Nonsmoker, never smoked regularly.

Environmental smoke. Do you live with or work with smokers and breathe second-hand smoke regularly?

☐ Yes   ☐ No

4. **Alcohol.** How many drinks do you typically have on a day you drink? *One drink is a bottle or can of beer (12 oz), a glass of wine or wine cooler (3.5 oz), or a shot glass of liquor (1.5 oz).*

   ☐ Never drink.

   ☐ Have no more than one drink in a day.

   ☐ Have no more than two drinks in a day.

   ☐ Sometimes have three or four drinks in a day.

   ☐ Sometimes have five or more drinks in a day.

5. **Sleep.** How many hours of sleep do you usually get each night? _____

Eating Practices

6. **Breakfast.** How many days each week do you usually eat breakfast (more than just coffee and a roll)? _____

7. **Bread/grains.** How many servings of whole-grain breads and cereals do you eat daily? *One serving =1 slice bread, ½ cup dry cereal, ½ cup cooked oatmeal or other whole-grain cereal or brown rice.* _____

8. **Fruits and vegetables.** How many servings of fruits and vegetables do you eat daily? *One serving =1 medium fruit, 6 oz fruit or vegetable juice, 1 cup raw fruit or vegetables, ½ cup cooked fruit or vegetables.* _____

Legumes. How many times a week do you eat legumes (peas, beans, lentils, garbanzos)? *One serving = ½ cup cooked.* _____

9. **High-fat and high-cholesterol foods.** How often do you eat foods high in saturated fat and cholesterol (e.g., steak, hamburger, hot dog, sausage, bacon, cheese, fried chicken, French fries, ice cream, cheesecake, or other desserts)?

   ☐ Daily

   ☐ Eat these foods three or more times a week.

   ☐ Seldom or never eat these foods.

10. **Nuts/seeds.** How many servings of nuts do you usually eat each week? *One serving = 1 oz or a small handful, or 2 tablespoons of natural nut butter.* _____

Refined foods. How often do you eat highly refined foods (soda pop, snack foods, chips, refined cereals, pastry, candy)?

   ☐ Daily

   ☐ Eat these foods three or more times a week.

   ☐ Seldom or never eat refined foods.

Water. How many glasses (8 oz) of water do you typically drink each day? _____

11. **Weight.** How many pounds have you gained since you were 21 to 24 (enter 0 if you weigh the same, weigh less, or are younger than 21 years). _____

12. **Mental/Social Health**

Happiness. How happy have you been during the last month?

   ☐ Very happy

   ☐ Pretty happy

   ☐ Not too happy

   ☐ Very unhappy

Mood/feelings

1. During the past month, have you often been bothered by feeling down, depressed, or hopeless?

   ☐ Yes   ☐ No

2. During the past month, have you often been bothered by having little interest or pleasure in doing things?

   ☐ Yes   ☐ No

3. Have your feelings in the past month caused you significant distress or impaired your ability to function socially or at work (or school)?

   ☐ Yes   ☐ No

Stress and coping. How much of the time do you feel stressed out and unable to cope with life?

   ☐ Seldom or never

   ☐ Occasionally

   ☐ Much of the time

   ☐ Most of the time

Lifestyle and Risk Assessment—cont'd

13. Social Support

Support. Do you have family or friends you can get help from if needed?

☐ Yes ☐ No

Social Interaction. Do you have frequent social contact with family or friends?

☐ Yes ☐ No

14. Community

Do you meet regularly with a faith community or other group that gives you support, comfort, meaning, and direction in your life?

☐ Yes ☐ No

15. Safety

Seat belts. What percent of the time do you wear seat belts when riding in a car? _____

Smoke alarm. Do you have a working smoke alarm on each floor of your home, including the area in which you sleep?

☐ Yes ☐ No ☐ Don't know for sure.

Helmet. When biking or rollerblading, do you always wear a helmet and protective gear?

☐ Yes ☐ No

Substance use and driving. Do you ever drive soon after drinking alcohol or taking drugs or ride with someone who has been using illicit substances, including alcohol?

☐ Yes ☐ No

16. Safer Sex

Practice safer sex. Are you in a monogamous relationship?

☐ Yes ☐ No

Do you always use condoms, or abstain from sexual relations?

☐ Always ☐ Don't always practice safer sex

17. Preventive Exams

Do you keep current on recommended preventive exams (see list below) and immunizations?

☐ Yes ☐ No ☐ Don't know for sure.

Recommended Preventive Exams

- Periodic checkup, including blood pressure, height and weight, and cholesterol check as recommended by your doctor.
- Pap tests within last 1 to 3 years, for women 18 or older
- Mammogram within last 2 years, for women 40 or older
- Colorectal cancer screening for all persons 50 or older
- Prostate exam, for men 50 or older
- Flu and pneumonia immunizations, for everyone 65 or older

Height _____

Weight _____

Blood pressure _____

Blood cholesterol _____ (mg/dL)

——————————Scoring——————————

Your score is the number of good health indicators you meet out of the 17 possible listed (below) in this assessment. The higher your score, the healthier your lifestyle. The Average HealthStyle Score is 9.4

Health Indicator	Guidelines for Good Health
1. Physical activity	Get 30 or more minutes of physical activity most days of the week.
2. Strength training	Do strength-building exercises at least twice per week.
3. Not smoking	Avoid all tobacco use and frequent exposure to second-hand smoke.
4. Alcohol use	Alcohol is not recommended, but if you drink alcohol, limit to one to two drinks in a day.
5. Adequate rest	Get adequate rest, at least 7 to 8 hours of sleep daily for best health.
6. Breakfast daily	Eat a nutritious breakfast daily for optimal physical and mental performance.
7. Whole grains	Choose whole-grain breads and cereals, at least three or more servings/per day.
8. Fruits and vegetables	Eat at least five servings of fruits and vegetables daily.
9. Fats, cholesterol	Limit high-fat meats, whole milk, and butter. Vegetable oils are healthier than oils from animals.
10. Nuts	Nuts, such as almonds, contain healthy fats and protect against heart disease.
11. Healthy weight	Maintain a healthy weight by eating well and participating in regular, moderate-intensity physical activity.
12. Mental health	Develop effective coping skills, and maintain a happy, hopeful outlook.
13. Social support	Maintain good social support and frequent contact with family and friends.
14. Community	Participate regularly in a faith community or other group that provides meaning, direction, and support in your life.
15. Safety	Be safety conscious; wear safety belts in the car and helmets when biking.
16. Safer sex	Remain in a monogamous relationship, or always use condoms, or abstain.
17. Regular exams	Get regular exams, including age/gender recommended preventive exams.

Adapted from Hall, D. R. (2004). *Lifestyle check assessment.* Vanderbilt University Health and Wellness.

Life Stress Review

Daily hassles, life events, and other stressors trigger physiological responses that may, over time, induce illness (Selye, 1976; Rahe, 1974). You will find one type of life change events assessment tool in Chapter 25, Assessment Guidelines and Tools, The Holmes-Rahe Social Readjustment Scale. Alternatively, you might want to interview your patient to assess the following:

- His belief in his ability to control the experience (e.g., an impending decision, an illness)

- How deeply involved he feels in the activity that is producing stress (i.e., is it something he can change, or wants to change?)

- Whether he is able to view such a change as a challenge to grow

Standardized Language

Examples of NANDA-I Wellness Diagnoses

- Effective Breastfeeding
- Effective Therapeutic Regimen Management
- Health-Seeking Behaviors (specify)
- Readiness for Enhanced Communication
- Readiness for Enhanced Community Coping
- Readiness for Enhanced Coping
- Readiness for Enhanced Family Coping
- Readiness for Enhanced Family Processes
- Readiness for Enhanced Fluid Balance
- Readiness for Enhanced Knowledge (specify)

- Readiness for Enhanced Management of Therapeutic Regimen
- Readiness for Enhanced Nutrition
- Readiness for Enhanced Organized Infant Behavior
- Readiness for Enhanced Parenting
- Readiness for Enhanced Self-Concept
- Readiness for Enhanced Sleep
- Readiness for Enhanced Spiritual Well-Being
- Readiness for Enhanced Urinary Elimination

Source: NANDA International. (2009). *Nursing diagnosis: Definitions and classifications 2009–2011.* Philadelphia: Author. Used with permission.

Examples of NOC Standardized Health Promotion Outcomes

OUTCOME	DEFINITION*	EXAMPLES OF INDICATORS
Community Health Status	General state of well-being of a community or population	Prevalence of health promotion programs
Community Risk Control: Lead Exposure	Community actions to reduce lead exposure and poisoning	Organization of lead screening programs that include focus on preschools in neighborhoods with homes built before 1960.
Family Health Status	Overall health and social competence of family unit	Immunization of members
Health Beliefs	Personal convictions that influence health behaviors	Perceived importance of taking action
Health Beliefs: Perceived Ability to Perform	Personal conviction that one can carry out a given health behavior	Perception that health behavior is not too complex
Health Beliefs: Perceived Control	Personal conviction that one can influence a health outcome	Belief that own actions control health outcomes
Health Beliefs: Perceived Resources	Personal conviction that one has adequate means to carry out a health behavior	Perceived adequacy of time

Examples of NOC Standardized Health Promotion Outcomes—cont'd

OUTCOME	DEFINITION*	EXAMPLES OF INDICATORS
Health Beliefs: Perceived Threat	Personal conviction that a threatening health problem is serious and has potential negative consequences for lifestyle	Perceived threat to health
Health Orientation	Personal commitment to health behaviors as lifestyle priorities	Perception that health is a high priority in making lifestyle choices
Health Promoting Behavior	Personal actions to sustain or increase wellness	Balances activity and rest
Health Seeking Behavior	Personal actions to promote optimal wellness, recovery, and rehabilitation	Performs self-screening when indicated
Knowledge: Health Behavior	Extent of understanding conveyed about the promotion and protection of health	Strategies to manage stress
Knowledge: Health Promotion	Extent of understanding conveyed about information needed to obtain and maintain optimal health	Behaviors that promote health
Knowledge: Health Resources	Extent of understanding conveyed about relevant healthcare resources	Available community resources
Leisure Participation	Use of relaxing, interesting, and enjoyable activities to promote well-being	Participates in activities other than regular work
Personal Safety Behavior	Personal actions of an adult to control behaviors that can cause physical injury	Practices safe sexual behaviors
Physical Fitness	Performance of physical activities with vigor	Muscle strength Muscle endurance

*All of the outcomes in the Growth & Development class may be used (e.g., Child Development: Preschool; Physical Maturation: Female; Sexual Functioning).

Source: Moorhead, S., Johnson, M., Maas, M., et al. (Eds.). (2008). *Nursing outcomes classification (NOC)* (4th ed.). St. Louis, MO: C.V. Mosby. Used with permission.

Selected NIC Wellness Interventions

INTERVENTION	DEFINITION	EXAMPLES OF ACTIVITIES
Breast Examination	Performing activities to safeguard the health of the breasts and related areas	Advise regular mammograms as appropriate for age, condition and risk.
Community Health Development	Assisting members of a community to identify a community's health concerns, mobilize resources, and implement solutions	Identify health concerns, strengths, and priorities with community partners.
Environmental Management: Worker Safety	Monitoring and manipulation of the worksite environment to promote safety and health of workers	Identify applicable OSHA standards and worksite compliance with standards.
Environmental Risk Protection	Preventing and detecting disease and injury in populations at risk from environmental hazards	Monitor incidents of illness and injury related to environmental hazards.
Exercise Promotion	Facilitation of regular physical activity to maintain or advance to a higher level of fitness and health	Appraise individual's health beliefs about physical exercise.
Family Planning: Contraception	Facilitation of pregnancy prevention by providing information about the physiology of reproduction and methods to control conception	Determine ability and motivation of patient and partner to correctly and regularly use contraception.

Continued

Selected NIC Wellness Interventions—cont'd

INTERVENTION	DEFINITION	EXAMPLES OF ACTIVITIES
Health Education	Developing and providing instruction and learning experiences to facilitate voluntary adaptation of behavior conducive to health in individuals, families, groups, or communities	Target high-risk groups and age ranges that would benefit most from health education.
Health Policy Monitoring	Surveillance and influence of government and organization regulations, rules, and standards that affect nursing systems and practices to ensure quality care of patients	Compare requirements of policies and standards with current practices.
Health Screening	Detecting health risks or problems by means of history, examination, and other procedures	Complete appropriate Department of Health or other records for monitoring abnormal results, such as high blood pressure.
Health System Guidance	Facilitating a patient's location and use of appropriate health services	Inform the patient of accreditation and state health department requirements for judging the quality of a facility.
Immunization/ Vaccination Management	Monitoring immunization status, facilitating access to immunizations, and providing immunizations to prevent communicable disease	Determine immunization status at every health care visit (including emergency department and hospital admission), and provide immunizations as needed.
Oral Health Promotion	Promotion of oral hygiene and dental care for a patient with normal oral and dental health	Instruct and assist patient to perform oral hygiene after eating and as often as needed.
Parent Education: Childrearing Family	Assisting parents to understand and promote the physical, psychological, and social growth and development of their toddler, pre-school, or school-age child/children (also Parent Education: Adolescent and Parent Education: Infant)	Teach appropriate developmental tasks or goals for the child.
Patient Contracting	Negotiating and agreement with an individual that reinforces a specific behavior change	Encourage the individual to identify own goals, not those he/she believes the healthcare provider expects.
Program Development [Wellness]	Planning, implementing, and evaluating a coordinated set of activities designed to enhance wellness, or to prevent, reduce, or eliminate one or more health problems for a group or community	Assist the group or community in identifying significant health needs or problems.
Sleep Enhancement	Promoting restful sleep that meets body's needs for restoration	Determine patient's sleep/activity pattern.
Smoking Cessation Assistance	Helping another to stop smoking	Help patient identify reasons to quit and barriers to quitting.
Spiritual Growth Facilitation	Facilitation of growth in patient's capacity to identify, connect with, and call upon the source of meaning, purpose, comfort, strength, and hope in his/her life	Encourage conversation that assists the patient in sorting out spiritual concerns.
Sports-Injury Prevention: Youth	Reduce the risk of sports-related injury in young athletes	Monitor proper use and condition of safety equipment.
Substance Use Prevention	Prevention of an alcoholic or drug use lifestyle	Conduct programs in schools on the avoidance of drugs and alcohol as recreational activities.

Selected NIC Wellness Interventions—cont'd

INTERVENTION	DEFINITION	EXAMPLES OF ACTIVITIES
Teaching: Infant Nutrition Infant Safety Infant Stimulation Toddler Nutrition Toddler Safety Toilet Training	Providing education to parent(s) concerning topics relevant to growth, development, and safety of infants and toddlers.	Note: Teaching is integral to all health promotion/disease prevention activities, whether or not there is a special intervention label for the particular content.
Teaching: Safe Sex	Providing instructions concerning sexual protection during sexual activity	Create an accepting, nonjudgmental atmosphere.
Values Clarification	Assisting another to clarify her/his own values in order to facilitate effective decision making	Encourage consideration of values underlying choices and consequences of the choice.
Vehicle Safety Promotion	Assisting individuals, families, and communities to increase awareness of measures to reduce unintentional injuries in motorized and nonmotorized vehicles.	Educate about the importance of proper and regular use of protective devices to decrease risk of injury (e.g., car seats, seat belts, helmets).

Sources: Bulechek, G. M., Butcher, H. K., & Dochterman, J. M. (Eds.). (2008). *Nursing interventions classification (NIC)* (5th ed.). St. Louis, MO: C. V. Mosby. Used with permission.

THINKING CRITICALLY ABOUT PROMOTING HEALTH

The exercises in the following sections allow you to practice the kind of thinking you will use as a full-spectrum nurse. Because these are critical-thinking questions, there is usually no single right answer. We do not provide answers for these questions because it is more important for you to think *about the questions than to arrive at the "right" answer. These questions are designed to improve your thinking more than to "cover content." Discuss answers with your peers—discussion can stimulate critical thinking. If you have difficulty with any of these questions, consult with your instructor.*

Applying the Full-Spectrum Nursing Model

PATIENT SITUATION

Shandra Shane is a single 37-year-old woman with three children, ages 12, 15, and 17. She is raising the children on her own, although her sister occasionally helps with transportation or advice about disciplining her teenage daughters. Ms Shane is a night-shift worker at the hospital. Her typical schedule is 3 to 4 hours of sleep in the morning soon after she gets home and then a short nap in the early evening before going back to work. She smokes 1 to 1½ packs of cigarettes per day but tells you she has been trying to smoke less around her children. Her job stress is high, as the hospital is cutting back on the number of staff. Ms Shane also takes care of her elderly mother, who has Alzheimer's and lives with her. Ms Shane's outlet for stress is going out with friends and drinking beer on the weekend. She is seeking your professional guidance to lose some weight (about 60 pounds) and to feel more energetic.

THINKING

1. *Theoretical Knowledge:*

   List health behaviors that negatively influence health status.

2. *Critical Thinking (Contextual Awareness):*

   What factors in this situation would you consider threatening Ms Shane's health and could lead to disease later in life? Which diseases?

DOING

3. *Nursing Process (Planning/Intervention):*

   What suggestions might you make about Shandra's diet that could help her to lose weight? Why might these actions be effective for weight loss?

4. *Practical Knowledge*:

   What areas of her daily living other than her diet might you explore further and offer recommendations for improving to promote better health and prevent illness?

CARING

5. *Self-Knowledge*:

   Have you ever been in a situation where you felt stressed, tired, and wanting gratification offered by food, nicotine, or alcohol? Describe your experience.

6. *Ethical:*

   In what ways could you demonstrate genuine caring for Shandra?

Critical Thinking and Clinical Reasoning

1. While working in a physician's office, a 70-year-old woman is referred to you for counseling regarding health protection activities. She is hypertensive and obese.

   a. How does her age affect your assessments and communication?

   b. What type of learning aids might be needed?

   c. What health screenings are appropriate for this client?

2. Below is a group of clients who wish to enroll in a health promotion program.

   - Jennifer Kaska is 23 years old and was diagnosed with diabetes mellitus at the age of 12 years. She checks her blood sugar and administers insulin as needed. She runs 3 miles, 3 days per week.
   - Maurice Rosenthal is 47 years old with no known illness. He is 6 feet tall and weighs 240 pounds. His body mass index (BMI) is 33 kg/m², indicating obesity. He takes no routine medication, only acetaminophen for occasional headaches.
   - Clara Fenton is 83 years old and has been diagnosed with hypertension, emphysema, and osteoporosis. She takes ten prescription medications daily in addition to a multivitamin and an occasional laxative.

   Discuss the pros and cons of providing a group program that includes all three of these clients.

3. L. F. is a 50-year-old man with heart disease. He had coronary artery bypass surgery 1 month ago. He has stopped going to his prescribed cardiac rehabilitation program because of the distance he must travel to the rehabilitation center. Discuss at least two approaches for working with this client.

4. Cecelia Kent is 32 years old. She takes no medications and has annual physical exams. She walks 4 to 5 miles, 5 days per week, and lifts light weights two to three times per week. She eats a low-fat, low-salt, low-sugar diet. She has never smoked, and drinks only limited alcohol.

   a. She asks you to recommend further health promotion activities. How would you respond?

   b. How could you incorporate Cecelia into a health promotion class that includes Jennifer Kaska, Maurice Rosenthal, and Clara Fenton (from question 2)?

5. For each of the following concepts, use critical thinking to describe how or why it is important to nursing, patient care, or health promotion. Note that these are not to be merely definitions.

Health promotion	Hardiness
Illness prevention	Health screenings
Lifestyle	Health education

What Are the Main Points in This Chapter?

➤ Health promotion refers to helping clients develop an optimal state of health.

➤ Intention is the difference between health promotion and health protection (illness prevention).

➤ There are three levels of activities for health protection: primary, secondary, and tertiary prevention. *Primary interventions* are designed to prevent or slow the onset of disease. *Secondary interventions* are designed to detect illnesses in early stages. *Tertiary interventions* focus on stopping the disease from progressing and on rehabilitation.

➤ The Healthy People 2020 initiative is designed to achieve four overarching goals:

  ➤ Attain high quality, longer lives free of preventable disease, disability, injury, and premature death.

  ➤ Achieve health equity, eliminate disparities, and improve the health of all groups.

  ➤ Create social and physical environments that promote good health for all.

  ➤ Promote healthy development and healthy behaviors across every stage of life.

➤ Pender's Health Promotion Model (HPM) identifies three groups of variables that affect health behavior: (1) individual characteristics and experiences; (2) behavior-specific cognitions and affect; and (3) behavioral outcome.

➤ A wellness wheel identifies six dimensions of health: emotional, intellectual, physical, spiritual, social/family, and occupational.

➤ The transtheoretical model of change identifies four stages of change: contemplation, determination, action, and maintenance.

➤ Health promotion activities for all age groups include nutrition, exercise, safety concerns, changing unhealthy lifestyles, immunizations, and screenings.

➤ Health promotion activities may be conducted in acute care facilities, the workplace, local communities, or schools.

➤ A health promotion assessment involves obtaining a health history, physical examination, fitness assessment, lifestyle and risk appraisal, life stress review, assessment of healthcare beliefs, nutritional assessment, and screening activities.

➤ Health screening activities are designed to detect disease at an early stage so that treatment can begin before there is an opportunity for disease to spread or reduce the quality of life.

➤ Health screening activities vary based on developmental stage and identified risk factors.

➤ Nurses promote health through role models, counseling, health education, and providing and facilitating support.

For practice questions for this chapter,

 Go to **NCLEX-Style Chapter Quiz,** on the Student Resource Disk or DavisPlus at http://davisplus.fadavis.com/Wilkinson2

CarePlanning & MappingPractice

For Care Planning/Care Mapping practice,

 Go to Student Resources, **Care Planning & Care Mapping Practice,** at http://davisplus.fadavis.com/Wilkinson2

For Documentation practice,

 Go to Student Resources, **Documentation Practice,** on DavisPlus at http://davisplus.fadavis.com/Wilkinson2

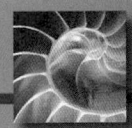

Knowledge Map

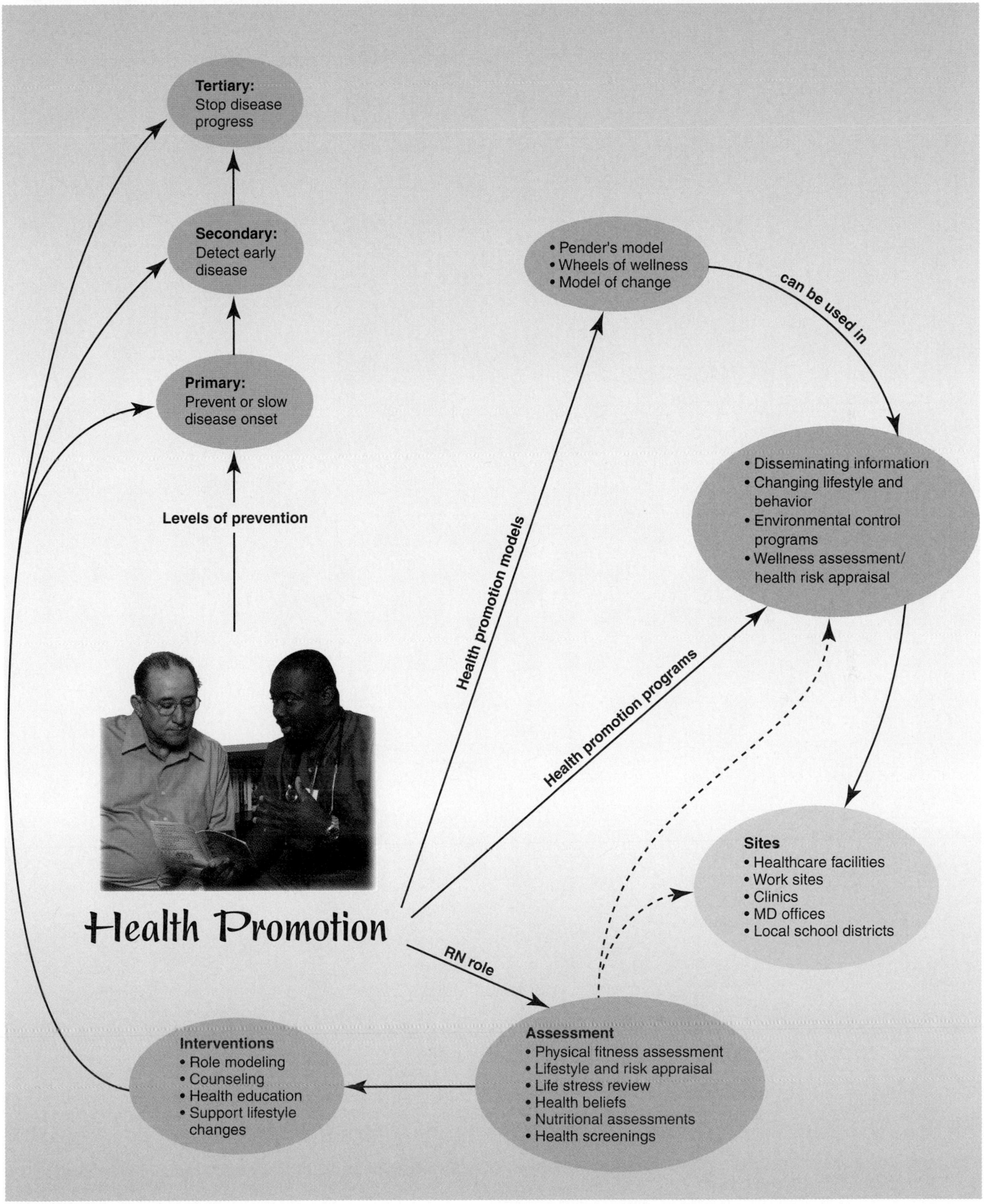

Tertiary:
Stop disease progress

Secondary:
Detect early disease

Primary:
Prevent or slow disease onset

Levels of prevention

• Pender's model
• Wheels of wellness
• Model of change

can be used in

Health promotion models

• Disseminating information
• Changing lifestyle and behavior
• Environmental control programs
• Wellness assessment/ health risk appraisal

Health promotion programs

Sites
• Healthcare facilities
• Work sites
• Clinics
• MD offices
• Local school districts

Health Promotion

RN role

Interventions
• Role modeling
• Counseling
• Health education
• Support lifestyle changes

Assessment
• Physical fitness assessment
• Lifestyle and risk appraisal
• Life stress review
• Health beliefs
• Nutritional assessments
• Health screenings

The Context for Nurses' Work

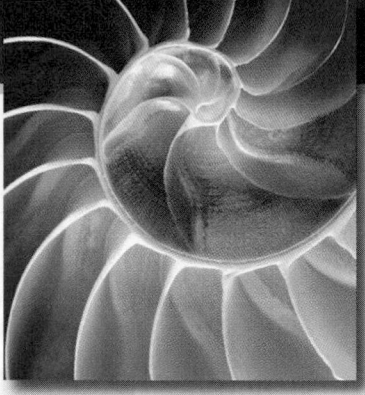

CHAPTER 42

Community Nursing

For a podcast of an overview of this chapter,

 Go to Student Resources, **Podcast – Chapter Overviews, Chapter 42,** on DavisPlus at http://davisplus.fadavis.com/ Wilkinson2

Caring for the Garcias

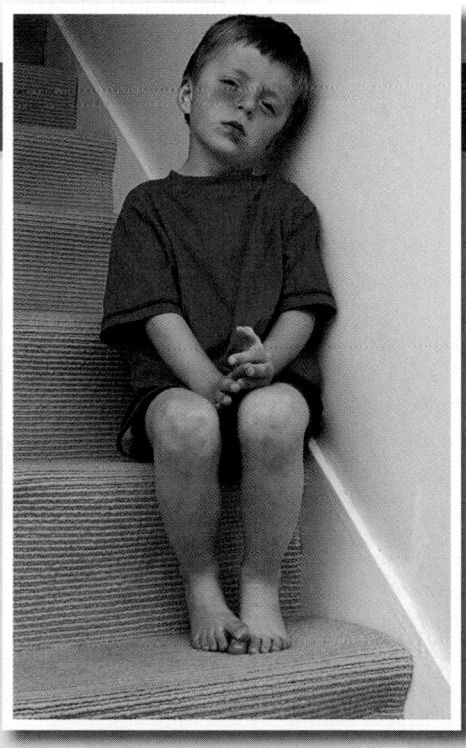

The exercises in the following section allow you to practice the kind of thinking you will use as a full-spectrum nurse. Because these are critical-thinking questions, there is usually no single right answer. We do not provide answers for these questions because it is more important for you to think about the questions than to arrive at the "right" answer. These questions are designed to improve your thinking more than to "cover content." Discuss answers with your peers— discussion can stimulate critical thinking. If you have difficulty with any of these questions, consult with your instructor.

Flordelisa Garcia works as preschool teacher in her community. Andre is a 4-year-old boy in her class. Over the last few months, she has noticed that Andre has many bruises in various stages of healing. He also seems withdrawn in the classroom and tends not to interact much with the other children. She is concerned that Andre might be experiencing child abuse, but she is reluctant to make that accusation, especially because her assistant doesn't seem to have noticed anything amiss.

Ms Garcia talks to her husband, Joe, about her concerns: "I'm worried about a child at school, but I'm afraid to say anything. What if I'm wrong? I'd probably lose my job. But if

I'm right and I don't say anything, I could still lose my job, and this boy could be hurt even worse." Joe suggests that she contact the clinic nurse at the Family Medicine Center for confidential advice on how to proceed.

A. Imagine that you are the clinic nurse. Use the full-spectrum nursing model to identify at least ten questions that you would need to answer to investigate Flordelisa's concerns further.

B. *Self-knowledge:* What personal values do you have that would affect the manner in which you handle this situation? Explain.

Caring for the Garcias (continued)

C. *Ethical knowledge:* What is the most important ethical issue in this situation? That is, what is the most important goal? Note that there may be several moral and legal issues, but you are being asked to identify the *most* important one. Note also that we are not asking you what the nurse *can* do, but rather what the nurse ideally *should* do.

D. You share the questions you have with Flordelisa. She believes that there is a real need to investigate child abuse. You advise her to call the local child protective services (CPS) agency. Based on your knowledge of community and public health nursing, what aspects of the community health role will the nurse from CPS use as she investigates this situation?

Practical **Knowledge**
knowing how

Practical knowledge in community nursing requires you to apply the nursing process to both individuals and groups.

Standardized Language

This section provides guidelines for using NANDA-I, NOC, NIC, and the Omaha System to develop problem statements, goals, and nursing orders to use in planning care for aggregates and communities.

Omaha Problem Classification Scheme

The Omaha System is a problem-solving model for community health practice, education, and research. The taxonomy consists of *diagnostic labels* organized into four *domains* (categories), along with two sets of *modifiers*. Within those domains, the system classifies 42 client problems or areas of concern. Refer to the accompanying box for the four Omaha categories, examples of diagnosis (problem) labels, and problem modifiers. As you can

see, the problem labels in the environment domain are especially useful in community nursing. For the complete problem classification scheme,

 Go to the **Omaha System** Web site at www.omahasystem. org

To create a diagnostic statement, choose an appropriate label, and add a modifier to it from each of the two sets in the accompanying box. For example, a group Environment diagnosis for workers in a meat-packing plant with lax safety standards might read *Deficit* in Group Workplace Safety. If only one worker were at risk (perhaps because of her inattention to safety rules), you could write *Potential Deficit in Individual* Workplace Safety.

Domain: Environment
Problems: Income, Sanitation, Residence, and Workplace Safety
Modifiers: (1) Health Promotion, Potential Deficit, or Deficit
          (2) Family, Individual, or Group
Diagnostic Statements:
    Deficit in Group Workplace Safety
    Potential Deficit in Individual Workplace Safety

Omaha System: Domains and Examples of Problem Labels

Environmental Domain—The material resources, physical surroundings, and substances both internal and external to the client, home, neighborhood, and broader community
  Problem (Diagnosis) Labels: Income, Sanitation, Residence, Neighborhood/Workplace Safety

Psychosocial Domain—Patterns of behavior, communication, relationships, and development.
  Problem (Diagnosis) Labels: Social Contact, Role Change, Interpersonal Relationships, Spirituality, Grief, Mental Health, Sexuality, Caretaking/Parenting, Neglect, Abuse

Physiological Domain—Functional status of processes that maintain life.
  Problem (Diagnosis) Labels: Hearing, Vision, Oral Health, Speech and Language, Pain, Respiration, Digestion-Hydration, Communicable/Infectious Condition

Health Related Behaviors Domain—Activities that maintain or promote wellness, promote recovery, or maximize rehabilitation potential.
  Problem (Diagnosis) Labels: Nutrition, Personal Hygiene, Prescribed Medication Regimen, Sleep and Rest Patterns, Family Planning, Physical Activity

Problem Modifiers

Set 1—Health Promotion, Potential Deficit, Deficit

Set 2—Family, Individual, Group*

---

*Martin and Scheet (1992, p. 67) suggest that *Group* be added to these modifiers.
Source: Martin, K. S., & Scheet, N. J. (1992). *The Omaha system: Applications for community health nursing.* Philadelphia: W. B. Saunders, pp. 67–74. Used with permission.

Using the NOC and Omaha Systems to Write Aggregate Goals

NOC Outcomes

NOC standardized outcomes in the Community Health domain include the following (Moorhead, Johnson, Maas, et al., 2008):

- Community Competence
- Community Disaster Readiness
- Community Disaster Response
- Community Health Status
- Community Health Status: Immunity
- Community Risk Control: Chronic Disease
- Community Risk Control: Communicable Disease
- Community Risk Control: Lead Exposure
- Community Risk Control: Violence
- Community Violence Level

You can use these NOC labels to write goals by adding the appropriate NOC indicators and scales (see the Standardized Language section of Chapter 5, in this volume).

Omaha System Outcomes

Using the Omaha System, you will develop goals/outcomes from the words in the nursing diagnosis. Recall that all nursing diagnoses are identified as either *individual*, *family*, or *group*, so a group nursing diagnosis will automatically indicate a group goal. For example, for the diagnosis Deficit in Group Workplace Safety, you would build the outcomes around the words "Group Workplace Safety." The Omaha system includes a five-point "Problem Rating Scale for Outcomes" (see the accompanying table) that describes what you expect to achieve in terms of the client's knowledge, behavior, and status.

Omaha Problem Rating Scale for Outcomes

CONCEPT	1	2	3	4	5
Knowledge The ability of the client to remember and interpret information	No knowledge	Minimal knowledge	Basic knowledge	Adequate knowledge	Superior knowledge
Behavior The client's observable responses, actions, or activities fitting the occasion or purpose	Never appropriate	Rarely appropriate	Inconsistently appropriate	Usually appropriate	Consistently appropriate
Status The condition of the client in relation to objective and subjective defining characteristics	Extreme signs/ symptoms	Severe signs/ symptoms	Moderate signs/ symptoms	Minimal signs/ symptoms	No signs/ symptoms

The Omaha System. (2009, May 11; updated). *Solving clinical data-information: Problem rating scale for outcomes.* Retrieved from http://www.omahasystem.org/problemratingscaleforoutcomes.html

Using the table, you would create expected outcomes by applying this scale to Group Workplace Safety, as follows:

Nursing Diagnosis: Deficit in Group Workplace Safety

Rating Scale Concept	Present Status, Before Interventions	Expected Outcome, After Interventions
Knowledge	(2) Minimal knowledge of workplace safety	(4) Adequate knowledge of workplace safety
Behavior	(2) Rarely appropriate safety behaviors	(4) Usually appropriate group safety behaviors
Status	(2) Severe signs/symptoms (e.g., frequent accidents or injuries)	(4) Minimal signs/symptoms (e.g., few accidents or injuries)

This means that after your interventions, you expect the group to have adequate knowledge of workplace safety, demonstrate usually appropriate behaviors (e.g., usually follow the safety rules), and demonstrate minimal accidents or injuries. To evaluate the client's progress, you would assign a scale number to the group's actual knowledge, behavior, and status *after interventions.*

Using the NIC and Omaha Interventions Labels

The NIC taxonomy includes 16 interventions specifically designed for community health (see NIC Community Health Classes and Interventions).

NIC Community Health Classes and Interventions

Class: Community Health Promotion—Interventions in that promote the health of the whole community

Interventions:

Case Management

Community Health Development

Fiscal Resource Management

Health Education

Health Policy Monitoring

Immunization/Vaccination Management

Program Development

Social Marketing

Class: Community Risk Management—Interventions that assist detecting or preventing health risks to the whole community

Interventions:

Bioterrorism Preparedness

Community Disaster Preparedness

Communicable Disease Management

Environmental Management: Community

Environmental Management: Worker Safety

Environmental Risk Protection

Health Screening

Risk Identification

Surveillance: Community

Vehicle Safety Promotion

Source: Bulechek, G. M., Butcher, H. K., & Dochterman, J. M. (Eds.). (2008). *Nursing interventions classification (NIC)* (5th ed.). St. Louis, MO: C.V. Mosby. Used with permission from Elsevier Science.

The Omaha taxonomy provides four "intervention categories" you can use in community-oriented nursing practice:

Health Teaching, Guidance and Counseling. These primary prevention activities include giving information, anticipating client problems, encouraging client action and responsibility for self-care, and assisting with coping, decision making, and problem solving. As a community-oriented nurse, you should spend most of your time offering this level of intervention.

Treatments and Procedures. These are secondary interventions directed toward preventing disease, identifying risk factors and early signs and symptoms, and decreasing or alleviating signs and symptoms.

Case Management. Case management is a tertiary intervention that includes coordination, advocacy, and referral. These activities involve facilitating service delivery on behalf of the client, communicating with health and human service providers, promoting assertive client communication, and guiding the client toward appropriate community resources.

Surveillance. These nursing activities include detection, measurement, critical analysis, and monitoring to indicate client status in relation to a given condition or phenomenon.

To write an intervention statement, you must combine one of those four "categories" of interventions with 63 "targets" (objects of the nursing interventions), such as bowel care and nutrition. Then you must add patient-specific information to individualize the nursing order. See the accompanying table for intervention categories, examples of targets, and intervention statements (nursing orders). To see the entire set of intervention targets,

 Go to the **Omaha System** Web site at www.omahasystem. org/shminter.htm

You will notice that the targets can be used for individuals as well as groups. It is the designation of the nursing diagnosis as *individual, family,* or *group* that determines this.

Omaha Intervention Categories and Examples of Targets

Categories	Examples of Targets
Categories	**Examples of Targets**
I. Health Teaching, Guidance, and Counseling	Anatomy/physiology
II. Treatments and Procedures	Behavior modification
III. Case Management	Communication
IV. Surveillance	Discipline
	Feeding procedures
	Homemaking
	Substance use
	Wellness

Examples of Aggregate Targets

Caretaking/parenting skills

Day-care/respite

Durable medical equipment

Education

Employment

Environment

Finances

Housing

Legal system

Transportation

Other community resource

Examples of Nursing Intervention Statements

Treatments and Procedures (II): Feeding procedures
(Demonstrate to Mrs. Adams how to feed Mr. Adams at
the next visit.)

Surveillance (IV): Feeding procedures (After teaching, observe
a feeding. Monitor for choking.)

Source: The Omaha System. (2009, May 11; updated). Solving the clinical data-information scheme: Intervention scheme. Retrieved from http://www.omahasystem.org/interventionscheme.html

THINKING CRITICALLY ABOUT COMMUNITY NURSING

The exercises in the following sections allow you to practice the kind of thinking you will use as a full-spectrum nurse. Because these are critical-thinking questions, there is usually no single right answer. We do not provide answers for these questions because it is more important for you to think about the questions than to arrive at the "right" answer. These questions are designed to improve your thinking more than to "cover content." Discuss answers with your peers—discussion can stimulate critical thinking. If you have difficulty with any of these questions, consult with your instructor.

Applying the Full-Spectrum Nursing Model

PATIENT SITUATION

Rachel, a freshman at State University, participated in a sorority rush activity during the second week of school. The event was attended by nearly 150 other freshman girls to socialize in the Student Union. About 2 or 3 days later, Rachel learned 6 of the students at the party tested positive for the H1N1 virus and displayed signs of illness. Cite the resources you used to answer the following questions. Be sure they are of professional quality.

THINKING

1. *Theoretical Knowledge*:

    a. What is another name for the H1N1 virus?

    b. Name 6 common outward signs of an H1N1 infection that you might see in a college student.

2. *Critical Thinking (Contextual Awareness)*:

    Why is it important to detect and treat H1N1 in a healthy population of young adults?

DOING

3. *Nursing Process (Assessment)*:

    How might you assess the extent of the problem of H1N1 illness within the campus community?

4. *Practical Knowledge*:

    a. As the Community Health nurse, you design a *primary* intervention program to prevent an outbreak of H1N1 virus on campus. What might you do for this program? What interventions would you likely implement to deliver a *secondary* intervention program?

    b. Or a *tertiary* program?

CARING

5. *Self-Knowledge*:

    How would you feel if you were one of the first-detected cases or H1N1 illness spread across the college campus?

▓▓ Critical Thinking and Clinical Reasoning

1. You are nearing completion of your fundamentals course. One night while you are preparing for your next clinical, the telephone rings. It is your neighbor, Tanya. Her 5-year-old daughter, Tiffany, attends kindergarten at the local public school. Tiffany came home with a letter from the school nurse stating that another child in the class was ill with H1N1 and that all the students in the class had been exposed to this flu virus.

   Tanya is concerned about the risks to Tiffany and the rest of the family. Tiffany was vaccinated against H1N1. Tanya is 8 months pregnant, and the family has no health insurance. She states that because you are a nursing student, she thought you might know what she should do or where she might go for assistance.

   What are the key pieces of information (both theoretical knowledge and patient data) you need to solve your neighbor's situation?

2. You are a nurse in a public health clinic providing routine childhood immunizations. A 16-year-old mother comes into the clinic requesting "shots" for her newborn baby as well as a birth control "shot." She indicates that she has no money to pay for the shots because her 20-year-old boyfriend gave her only enough to get to the clinic. Which of the following is your nursing priority for this situation? What will you do next? Explain *how* you have chosen your priority diagnosis. On what did you base your choice?

   ▪ Give the newborn the immunizations, and arrange for the client to meet with the social worker regarding securing healthcare coverage.
   ▪ Educate the mother about birth control.
   ▪ Take the client and child to a private room, and discuss the general health of the newborn and the plans for a healthcare provider to see the child. Also ask about the health needs of the mother.
   ▪ Ask the mother whether she is being abused and report the incident if so.

3. Your assignment is to conduct a community assessment of your neighborhood. How will your membership in the community affect your assessment? What activities could you delete from the assessment?

4. For each of the following concepts, use critical thinking and summarize how or why it is important to nursing, patient care, or community nursing. Note that these are *not* to be merely definitions.

Community	Primary intervention
Aggregates	Secondary intervention
Census tracts	Tertiary intervention
Vulnerable populations	Disaster preparedness
Healthy People 2020	Omaha system
Windshield survey	

What Are the Main Points in This Chapter?

➤ A community can be defined as a place with defined boundaries, a group of people with a common language, rituals, or customs.

➤ Each community determines the meaning of health and nursing activities to promote health.

➤ A vulnerable population is defined as an aggregate that is at increased risk of adverse health outcomes. Members of vulnerable groups have a higher probability of developing illness.

➤ The community nurse assesses three general dimensions of a community: structure, status, and process.

➤ Common practice areas for community-based nurses include schools, churches, prison systems, disaster relief services, occupational and public health clinics, and international relief organizations.

➤ Community health nursing focuses on the health of individuals, families, and groups and how their individual health affects the community as a whole.

➤ Public health nursing focuses on the community at large and the eventual effect of the community's health status on the health of individuals, families, and groups.

➤ Community-oriented nursing combines components of community and public health. Nurses practicing community-oriented nursing are fluid in their approach. Their focus is a comprehensive look at the individual, family, group, and community at large. Community-based nurses function as advocates, educators, collaborators, counselors, and effective communicators.

➤ Community-based nurses may provide care at three levels: primary (preventive), secondary (early detection and early treatment), and tertiary (halt disease progression). The focus is on primary prevention.

➤ The Omaha classification system is a commonly used documentation system for generating a care plan for a community or an individual within the community setting.

➤ A community health nurse might practice as a school nurse, public health nurse, parish or prison nurse, international health nurse, or disaster service.

For practice questions for this chapter,

 Go to **NCLEX-Style Chapter Quiz,** on the Student Resource Disk or DavisPlus at http://davisplus.fadavis.com/Wilkinson2

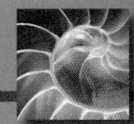

Knowledge Map

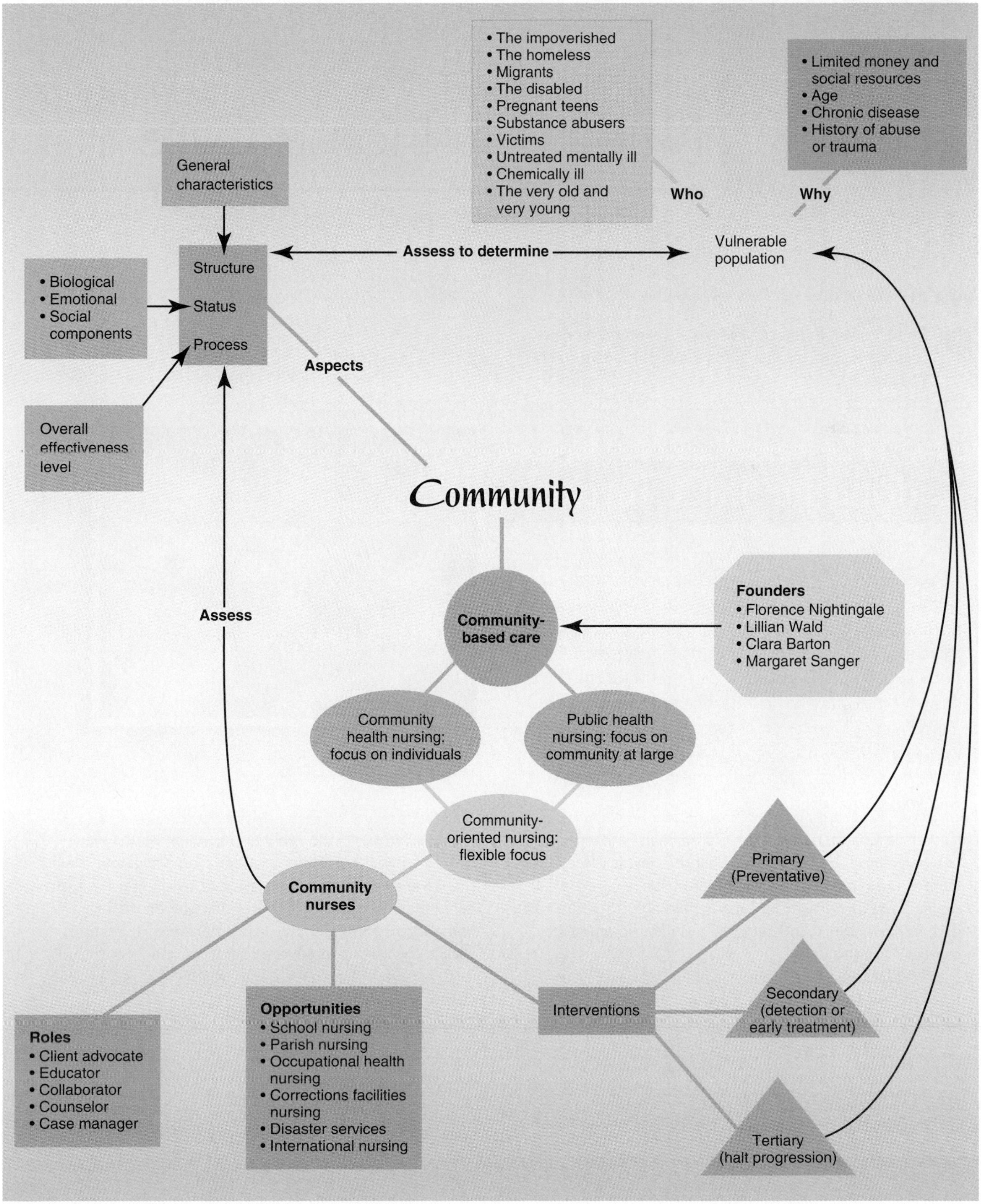

Community

General characteristics

- Biological
- Emotional
- Social components

Overall effectiveness level

Structure
Status
Process

Assess to determine

Aspects

Assess

Who

- The impoverished
- The homeless
- Migrants
- The disabled
- Pregnant teens
- Substance abusers
- Victims
- Untreated mentally ill
- Chemically ill
- The very old and very young

Why

- Limited money and social resources
- Age
- Chronic disease
- History of abuse or trauma

Vulnerable population

Community-based care

Founders
- Florence Nightingale
- Lillian Wald
- Clara Barton
- Margaret Sanger

Community health nursing: focus on individuals

Public health nursing: focus on community at large

Community-oriented nursing: flexible focus

Community nurses

Primary (Preventative)

Secondary (detection or early treatment)

Interventions

Roles
- Client advocate
- Educator
- Collaborator
- Counselor
- Case manager

Opportunities
- School nursing
- Parish nursing
- Occupational health nursing
- Corrections facilities nursing
- Disaster services
- International nursing

Tertiary (halt progression)

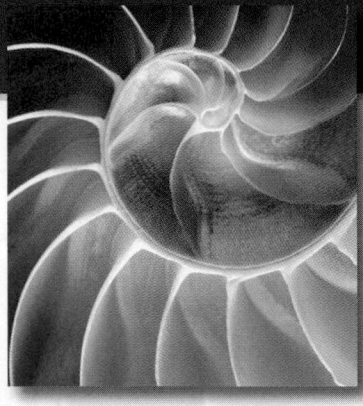
Nursing in Home Care

For a podcast of an overview of this chapter,

 Go to Student Resources, **Podcast – Chapter Overviews, Chapter 43,** on DavisPlus at http://davisplus.fadavis.com/ Wilkinson2

Caring for the Garcias

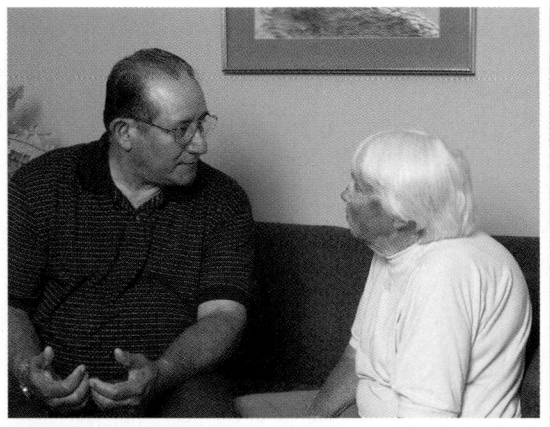

The exercises in the following section allow you to practice the kind of thinking you will use as a full-spectrum nurse. Because these are critical-thinking questions, there is usually no single right answer. We do not provide answers for these questions because it is more important for you to think about the questions than to arrive at the "right" answer. These questions are designed to improve your thinking more than to "cover content." Discuss answers with your peers—discussion can stimulate critical thinking. If you have difficulty with any of these questions, consult with your instructor.

Katherine Garcia, the 76-year-old mother of Joseph Garcia, has completed 2 weeks of physical therapy at Mercy Care Center (a skilled nursing facility) after her surgery to repair a fractured right hip. She is now able to get out of bed with assistance and requires a walker to ambulate even short distances.

Mrs. Garcia is very unhappy at Mercy Care Center. Some of her friends have entered nursing homes because of health problems, and two have died while at the facilities. Although she realizes that their deaths were related to health problems rather than placement issues, she is very nervous about staying at the center. At a care conference, her family requests that she be discharged home for ongoing therapy. It is determined that she is eligible for Medicare-covered services.

What type of home services will Mrs. Garcia probably need?

Practical **Knowledge**
knowing how

The clinical insights and standardized language tables in this section should be helpful to you when making a home visit.

Clinical Insights

Clinical Insight 43-1 ▶ **Conducting a Home Visit**

Before the Visit

- Gather information from the referral.
- Determine what supplies you will need; prepare them.
- Secure permission to visit and get directions to the home.
- Arrange time and date of visit with the client and/or family.
- Determine whether the client's health status has changed since the referral was made.
- On the way to the visit, make an environmental assessment; provide for your safety.

At the Visit

- Build trust: Introduce yourself; be respectful.
- Offer your card, to identify yourself and the agency.
- Provide information about client rights and financial policies of the agency.
- Assess the client, family, and surroundings.

- If this is an initial visit, verify or complete the date on the referral forms.
- Develop a plan with the client and family.
- Deliver skilled care.
- Identify need(s) for future services.
- Refer to appropriate departments and community services.

After the Visit

- Document assessments and care.
- Evaluate progress toward goals.
- Modify the plan as needed.
- Order supplies needed for the next visit.
- Make needed referrals and coordinate care among various services.
- Schedule the next visit.

Clinical Insight 43-2 ▶ **Infection Control in the Home**

The CDC has not yet developed guidelines for infection control in home care settings (Centers for Disease Control and Prevention, modified 2008), but the following suggestions can help you maintain infection control during a home visit.

Hand Hygiene

- Keep antibacterial cleanser and OSHA-approved protective equipment in your nursing bag.
- Perform hand hygiene using soap and warm water or an antibacterial hand-rub at the beginning and end of each visit and before and after any treatment.
- If the home conditions are very dirty or your hands become grossly soiled, wash your hands with soap and warm water as soon as possible after (if not during) the visit.

Supplies

- In homes that you know are not very clean, limit the supplies you bring into the home. For example, leave your nursing bag in the car, and bring only the supplies you need for the visit.
- Some infection control experts believe the "bag technique" (i.e., placing a newspaper under the nursing bag before placing it on a surface) is not routinely needed, but should be used when home conditions warrant.
- If necessary, use a 1:10 dilution of chlorine bleach in water to disinfect surfaces or equipment in the home. Some

equipment may need to be disinfected by boiling in a covered pan of water for 15 to 20 minutes. Do not boil plastic or rubber items.
- You can disinfect hard plastic items by wrapping them with a wet paper towel and placing them in a zippered plastic bag. Microwave the entire bag on high for 10 minutes.

Biohazard and Sharps Disposal

- Flush wound irrigation or potentially contaminated liquids down the toilet while wearing gloves and any other appropriate protective equipment.
- Double-bag dressings, equipment, or disposable supplies that have been contaminated with body secretions to prevent leakage. The bags should be labeled *Biohazard*.
- Carry small biohazard sharps containers. Place syringes and sharps in the container without recapping. If clients or family must use syringes or sharps, you may wish to leave a sharps container in the home. An alternative solution is to have them use a metal coffee can with lid or a thick plastic milk jug with lid.

Client Teaching

- Provide instruction on home cleanliness, hygiene, handwashing, food preparation, and instructions to avoid contact with persons who are ill, as needed.

(continued on next page)

Clinical Insight 43-2 ➤ **Infection Control in the Home** (continued)

■ If the client is immunocompromised, teach the signs and symptoms of infection and the process for immediate notification of the primary care provider.

Special Situations

■ If the patient has a multidrug-resistant infection or pulmonary tuberculosis, use appropriate barrier precautions. Leave reusable equipment (e.g., stethoscopes, blood pressure cuffs) in the home; and if possible, schedule these clients as the last appointment of the day.

Clinical Insight 43-3 ➤ **Safety Considerations in Home Care**

Before the Visit

Plan ahead. Know where you are headed. Use a map or global positioning system (GPS). Contact the client or family for directions if it is unclear where you are headed. File a visit plan with your office each day.

Dress in appropriate clothing as dictated by your agency. Wear a name tag clearly identifying you and the agency. Wear shoes that will allow you to run if necessary.

Carry a cell phone.

Do not carry a purse, multiple credit cards, or excess cash. Instead, use a waist or fanny pack and conceal it under clothing. In the pack, carry enough money for emergency transportation, telephone numbers for clients and home health agency, and emergency contact information.

Keep your car in good repair, and always have enough gasoline in the tank. Be prepared for inclement weather, and always carry an emergency car safety pack.

Do not get out of your car for any reason if driving in an area that might not be safe. Carjacking involves minor car impact ("fender bender") as a strategy to get a person to get out of the vehicle, leaving her vulnerable for attack, assault, or theft.

Observe your surroundings as you drive to the visit. Notice the location of emergency services, local gas stations, and public places if help is required.

Program 911 into your cell phone in case of an emergency. Carry mace or other items to aid in self-defense in case of situations in which you feel threatened.

Park as close to your destination as possible. If possible, park your car facing the direction you wish to go when you leave. Never enter dead end streets or alleys.

Check your surroundings before you leave your car. If you feel unsafe, leave the area immediately and call your office.

Lock the car. Leave no valuables in sight.

Prepare your bag while you are still in the car.

Carry your bag on one arm. In the opposite hand, carry your keys. Always have them ready. You may need them if you decide to exit quickly. Also, you can use keys to defend yourself by placing the pointed ends of the keys between your fingers.

Walk directly to the client's house. Walk in the middle of the sidewalk. Use common walkways. Avoid isolated and poorly lighted areas. Do not take shortcuts.

Knock or ring the doorbell before entering. Never enter without being invited. If there is no answer at the door, call the patient using your cell phone, or return to a secure public pay phone and dial the client.

If for any reason you feel that the neighborhood is unsafe, do not get out of the car. Instead, leave the neighborhood immediately and phone your agency.

At the Visit

Introduce yourself and clearly identify your agency. Show your name badge.

Sit where you have access to an exit. When you enter the home, observe all exits.

Notice who is present in the home. Request introductions. This information is useful for planning care as well as for ensuring safety.

Leave immediately if you suspect substance use, drug dealing, or drunken behavior.

Leave immediately if there is a violent domestic argument. Do not attempt to intervene. When you return to your car, use your cell phone to dial 911, or drive to a phone booth in a safe location and place the call.

Request that animals be kept in another room while you make your visit.

If weapons are visible, request that they be put away immediately. Leave the home if this request is not met.

If household members interfere with the visit, discuss the problem with the client. You may need to arrange a time to visit when they are not present.

After the Visit

Continue to observe the safety precautions you used when getting to the visit. Do not let down your guard as you return to your car.

If you are in an unsafe neighborhood or poorly lighted area, leave immediately and do not consult the map for directions to your next visit. Drive to a secure public location, and then consult the map.

Inform your agency if you believe the home or neighborhood is potentially hazardous.

Request a security escort service if future visits are required.

Document your assessments and the care delivered.

Report abuse if you suspect it in the home.

Other

The preceding tips focus on avoiding harm inflicted by others. However, you also need to protect yourself from infection and accidental injury, as you would in a hospital (see Clinical Insight 43-2). Use safe lifting techniques, and safe needle-handling techniques (see Chapters 23 and 31 if you need to review those). A small pilot study found that 13% of home healthcare nurses had experienced needlesticks in a 12-month period. Nurses attributed the sticks primarily to patient actions, followed by disposal-related activities (Gershon, Pogorzelska, Qureshi, et al., 2008).

Standardized Language

Clinical Care Classification: 21 Care Components (Version 2.0) Coded by Alphabetic Classes*

A	Activity Component	L	Respiratory Component
B	Bowel Gastric Component	M	Role Relationship Component
C	Cardiac Component	N	Safety Component
D	Cognitive Component	O	Self-Care Component
E	Coping Component	P	Self-Concept Component
F	Fluid Volume Component	Q	Sensory Component
G	Health Behavior Component	R	Skin Integrity Component
H	Medication Component	S	Tissue Perfusion Component
I	Metabolic Component	T	Urinary Elimination Component
J	Nutritional Component	U	Life Cycle Component
K	Physical Regulation Component		

---

*The Clinical Care Classification system is copyrighted, placed in public domain, and cannot be sold, but is available with written permission (Saba, V., 2007. *Clinical Care Classification (CCC) system manual.* New York: Springer Publishing Co., p. 162).

An Example of CCC Nursing Diagnoses and Interventions

A—ACTIVITY COMPONENT *(1 of 21 Care Components)*—A cluster of elements that involve the use of energy in carrying out musculoskeletal and bodily actions.

01 Activity Alteration *(Major Nursing Diagnosis)*—Change in or modification of energy used by the body.

Subcategories that provide greater definition of the problem (of "01 Activity Alteration")

01.1 Activity Intolerance

01.2 Activity Intolerance Risk

01.3 Diversional Activity Deficit

01.4 Fatigue

01.5 Physical Mobility Impairment

01.6 Sleep Pattern Disturbance

01.7 Sleep Deprivation

Actions performed to carry out physiological or psychological daily activities.

Example: Teach Passive Range of Motion

Source: Obtained from Saba, V. K. (n.d.). About. Clinical Care Classification System. Retrieved from http://sabacare.com/About/

THINKING CRITICALLY ABOUT NURSING IN HOME CARE

The exercises in the following sections allow you to practice the kind of thinking you will use as a full-spectrum nurse. Because these are critical-thinking questions, there is usually no single right answer. We do not provide answers for these questions because it is more important for you to think about the questions than to arrive at the "right" answer. These questions are designed to improve your thinking more than to "cover content." Discuss answers with your peers—discussion can stimulate critical thinking. If you have difficulty with any of these questions, consult with your instructor.

Applying the Full-Spectrum Nursing Model

PATIENT SITUATION

Recall the case of Flora Escobar in Volume 1. Flora is 78 years old. She lives at home with her 80-year-old husband, Roland. Until recently both have enjoyed good health. Roland suffered a cerebrovascular accident (CVA or stroke) 3 weeks ago. He was briefly hospitalized and then spent 2 weeks in a skilled nursing facility (SNF) for additional physical care and therapy. He returned home yesterday and will be followed by the local home health agency. You have been asked to make an initial visit today.

Mrs. Escobar greets you at the door. She is a petite woman who appears exhausted. She is wearing an apron over casual clothing. She opens the door with her left hand and carries a glass of water with her right. Her apron pockets are stuffed with pill bottles. The narrow hallway is partially blocked with a bedside commode, walker, and tray table. Mr. Escobar is in a hospital bed in the living room. He is a tall, stocky man who is sitting up in bed but is slumped and leaning to the left. He is wearing pajamas and a robe.

After you introduce yourself, you start with an open-ended question to build rapport: "How have things been going since you came home yesterday?" Mrs. Escobar slowly nods, sighs, and says, "I'm worried that I'm doing things wrong. I have such a hard time helping him to move. He is so much bigger than me, and I don't want to hurt him. He is frustrated with me, but he has difficulty talking and can't tell me what he needs." Tears fill Mrs. Escobar's eyes. Her husband turns away to avoid eye contact with you. To refocus their attention, you suggest that you go over some information and then begin to look at what additional services might be helpful.

THINKING

Both Mr. and Mrs. Escobar are in need of nursing interventions. However, this is your agency's first home visit to them, and you have other clients you must visit today, so you will need to prioritize.

1. *Theoretical Knowledge*:

   What *must* the home health nurse do on the initial visit to a client?

2. *Critical Thinking (Inquiry)*:

   In addition to completing your assessment and talking about a plan of care with the Escobars, what do you think is the single most important thing you can do for them today? Explain your thinking.

DOING

3. *Practical Knowledge*:

   When Mrs. Escobar meets you at the door and brings you into the living room, you notice a large German shepherd lying beside Mr. Escobar's bed. Mrs. Escobar says, "Stay, King"; and then to you, "Roland likes having him nearby." What should you do?

4. *Nursing Process*:

   a. *(Diagnosis)* Based on the information in the scenario, what nursing diagnoses might Mr. Escobar have? There may not be enough data to make definite diagnoses, but what probable diagnoses are there for which you would want to gather confirming data? Do not include potential diagnoses, such as Risk for Imbalanced Nutrition.

b. *(Implementation)*: Mr. Escobar has a potential problem, Risk for Falls. What are two interventions you would probably be able to do today to reduce his falls risk?

CARING

5. *Self-Knowledge*:

Describe an experience you have had with caregiving for a family member or friend. What feelings did you have? For example, did you feel satisfaction to be helping someone, frustration at a lack of cooperation, and so forth?

6. *Ethical Knowledge*:

The following are some nursing professional values:

Altruism—A concern for the welfare and well-being of others

Autonomy—The right to self-determination, to make independent choices and act on them

Human dignity—Respect for the inherent worth and uniqueness of individuals.

Name one thing you could do in caring for Mr. Escobar that would demonstrate each of these values.

Critical Thinking and Clinical Reasoning

1. As a beginning home health nurse, you have been assigned to visit the following clients today:

- Roland Escobar ("Meet Your Patient" in Volume 1), a 78-year-old man recovering from a CVA (stroke)
- Sally Littlemoon, a 48-year-old woman with diabetes mellitus, blindness, and lower extremity cellulitis (a skin infection)
- Beatrice Wayne, a 67-year-old woman who has undergone elective coronary artery bypass graft surgery (open heart surgery)
- Kent Churchill, an 80-year-old man with a recent hip fracture and surgical repair
- Ms Chana Padir, a 50-year-old woman with severe pain secondary to breast cancer with extensive metastases. She is receiving hospice care.

a. Explore some alternatives for your schedule. How would you prepare to make these five visits in one day? How would you determine how to arrange your schedule?

b. The report you receive from the home health supervisor includes the following information:

- Ms Littlemoon and Mr. Churchill require dressing changes.
- Mr. Escobar and Ms Wayne require teaching about their medications.
- Mr. Escobar, Ms Littlemoon, and Mr. Churchill require venipuncture for lab work.
- Ms Padir is having increasing pain.

(1) Based on this information, what else do you need to know and/or do before you begin your visits?
(2) What practical knowledge will you need to provide care for these clients?

c. How might the care you deliver to Ms Wayne differ from the care you give to Ms Padir? To answer the question, consider the context for each woman. How are their situations different?

d. When visiting Ms Padir, you realize that her husband and children are very fearful of her impending death. They seem overwhelmed by the care she requires.

(1) What values and beliefs do you have about death and dying that might influence your care of the Padir family? (Review Chapters 14 and 15 if you need to.)

(2) What must you consider in order to plan your interventions? How might you intervene?

e. When you arrive at the home of Ms Wayne, she is dressed and out of bed. She tells you she is able to get out of bed and walk about the house independently with very little pain. She can identify the medications she is receiving, their purpose, and their schedule for administration. Her chest wound is healing nicely, and her breath sounds are clear. She informs you that she is planning on going to her cabin in the mountains this upcoming weekend with her husband and children. What actions must you take with regard to continuing her home visits? Why? What rules/guidelines will influence your choice of action?

2. For each of the following concepts, use critical thinking to describe how or why it is important to nurses, patient care, or nursing in home care. Note that these are *not* to be merely definitions.

Delivering healthcare in the home setting
Skilled services
Caregiver Role Strain
Preparing for the home visit
Developing rapport at the home visit
Assessment of the home environment
Documentation of home health-care services
Clinical Care Classification system

What Are the Main Points in This Chapter?

➤ Home health nursing fosters client and family independence and promotes self-care.

➤ In the home setting, many factors, such as cleanliness and noise level, are not within the nurse's control. In addition, the home health nurse works without immediate on-site access to other healthcare professionals.

➤ Home health agencies may be public, voluntary, proprietary, or hospital-based agencies. They may provide direct or indirect care and may specialize in certain types of clients.

➤ As a full-spectrum nurse working in home healthcare, you will function in the following roles: communicator, direct care provider, client/family educator, client advocate, and care coordinator (case manager).

➤ Hospice nurses work in hospitals, special hospice facilities, or the homes of patients who are dying. The goal of their care is to provide comfort and manage symptoms.

➤ Home healthcare is reimbursed by Medicare, by Medicaid, by private insurance, and through direct payment from the client. Medicare and Medicaid are the largest payors.

➤ To be eligible for continuing care under Medicare and most private insurers, a client must be homebound and require skilled nursing care.

➤ Preparation for a home visit includes obtaining information from the referral, identifying the purpose of the visit, gathering required supplies, contacting the client to arrange the visit, and providing for your own safety.

➤ During a home visit, you will establish a rapport with the client and family, assess the needs of the client and caregivers, develop and discuss the plan of care and needed services with the client and caregivers, provide skilled care, and evaluate the need for continued services.

➤ Medicare requires specific client assessments using a form called the Outcome and Assessment Information Set (OASIS). It must be completed at the start of care, with each recertification (every 60 days), and at the termination of care.

➤ The Clinical Care Classification (CCC) system is a system of care and documentation used by most home care agencies.

➤ Interventions to reduce Caregiver Role Strain include providing emotional support and arranging additional home and community services to support the client and caregiver.

➤ As a nurse delivering home care, you will need to follow standard precautions but recognize how infection control techniques may be modified to the home environment.

➤ In addition to infection control, nursing interventions usually include assisting with medication management, assessing and supporting home safety, and providing caregiver support.

➤ After a home visit you must document care, coordinate services for the client, and prepare for future visits.

For practice questions for this chapter,

 Go to **NCLEX-Style Chapter Quiz,** on the Student Resource Disk or DavisPlus at http://davisplus.fadavis.com/Wilkinson2

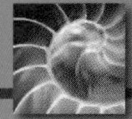

Knowledge Map

Increased prevalence due to:
• Reimbursement changes
• Population changes
• Decreasing length of stay

Home Care

Goals
• Promote self-care
• Promote independence
• Complete patient/family teaching

Providers
• Public agencies
• Voluntary agencies
• Proprietary organizations
• Hospital-based agencies
• Hospice organizations

Advantages
• Direct view of client environment
• Direct clues to client strength, resources, motivation

Challenges
• No control of environment
• No immediate assistance
• No stored client information on site
• No other healthcare team members

• Physicians
• Nurses
• Aides: PT/ST/OT/RT
• Nutritionists
• Social workers
• Pharmacists
• Chaplains

Nursing roles
• Provider
• Educator
• Advocate
• Care coordinator

Making a home visit
• Determine purpose
• Gather supplies
• Assess/address safety issues
• Develop rapport with client/family; show courtesy and respect
• Verify client data
• Provide care
• Document care

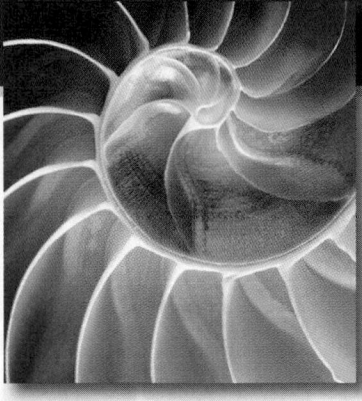

CHAPTER 44

Ethics & Values

For a podcast of an overview of this chapter,

 Go to Student Resources, **Podcast – Chapter Overviews, Chapter 44,** on DavisPlus at http://davisplus.fadavis.com/ Wilkinson2

Caring for the Garcias

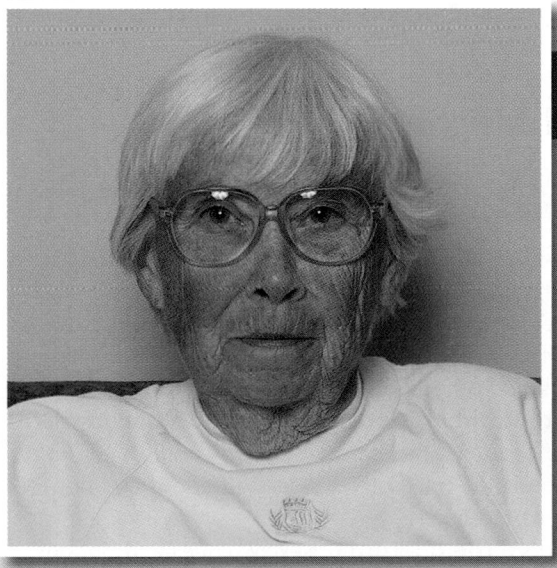

The exercises in the following section allow you to practice the kind of thinking you will use as a full-spectrum nurse. Because these are critical-thinking questions, there is usually no single right answer. We do not provide answers for these questions because it is more important for you to think about the questions than to arrive at the "right" answer. These questions are designed to improve your thinking more than to "cover content." Discuss answers with your peers—discussion can stimulate critical thinking. If you have difficulty with any of these questions, consult with your instructor.

Katherine Garcia, Joe's mother, has hypertension. She is forgetful about taking her medicines. Since her husband died, she has experienced periods of depression. When asked about her medicines she often replies, "It doesn't really matter since my husband died. If I die, what difference will it make?"

Katherine was scheduled to have lunch with friends but did not arrive. When her friends called the house, they got no answer. At the end of lunch, one of Katherine's friends decided to call Joe to inform him of her concerns about his mother. Joe found his mother unresponsive on the kitchen floor. He called 911, and she was brought to the hospital by ambulance. At the hospital, the emergency department (ED) doctor tells Joe that his mother has had a massive stroke brought on by uncontrolled hypertension.

He asks Joe whether Katherine has an advance directive or living will. Katherine has neither. The physician asks Joe to consider what level of care to offer his mother. He tells Joe that comprehensive treatment would include intubation, mechanical ventilation, and tube feeding support. He feels it is unlikely that she will experience significant recovery from this stroke.

Joe tells you, "I want everything done for my mother. I lost my father this year, and I'm not going to lose her, too." Flordelisa, Joe's wife, reminds you that Katherine has been depressed since her husband died and has expressed a desire to die. Because Joe and Flordelisa are not in agreement about the course of action, no decision is

(continued on next page)

Caring for the Garcias (continued)

communicated. Katherine's condition continues to deteriorate, and the ED physician feels he must intubate her, place her on a ventilator, and admit her to the ICU according to hospital protocol.

A. You are aware of Katherine's statements and her poor compliance with treatment. What, if any, concerns do you have about this course of action?

B. Katherine continues to decline. Joe is informed that the "only thing keeping his mother alive is the ventilator and IV medicines." Do you consider this heroic treatment?

C. How would you approach Joe to speak with him about how he is feeling?

D. Joe and Floredelisa have asked to meet with the team providing care to Katherine. They announce that they would like all the "heroic measures to end." They request that Katherine be allowed to die. Could you participate in this care? What actions would you be comfortable with? What actions would you be uncomfortable with?

Practical **Knowledge** **knowing** how

Practical knowledge in nursing ethics primarily involves communication and problem-solving skills. We have included one model of ethical decision-making, as well as guidelines for patient advocacy, for your quick reference in clinical situations.

Clinical Insights

Clinical Insight 44–1 ▶ Using the MORAL Model for Ethical Decision-Making

■ **M—Massage the dilemma.** Identify and define the issues in the dilemma. Consider the options of all the major players in the dilemma and their value systems. This includes patients, family members, nurses, physicians, religious representatives, and other interdisciplinary healthcare members.

■ **O—Outline the options.** Examine all the options, including those that are less realistic and conflicting. This stage is designed only for considering options and not for making final decisions.

■ **R—Resolve the dilemma.** Review issues and options, applying basic principles of ethics to each option. Decide the best option based on the views of all those concerned in the dilemma.

■ **A—Act by applying the chosen option.** This step is usually the most difficult because it requires actual

implementation, whereas the previous steps allow only for dialogue and discussion.

■ **L—Look back; reflect on the entire process.** Evaluate all steps, including the implementation. No process is complete without thorough evaluation. Ensure that those involved are able to follow through on the final option. If not, a second decision may be required and the process must begin again at the first step.

References

Tschundin, V. (2003). *Ethics in nursing: The caring relationship* (2nd ed.). Oxford: Butterworth & Heinemann.
Yoder-Wise, P. (2007). *Leading and managing in nursing* (4th ed.). St. Louis, MO: C. V. Mosby.

Clinical Insight 44-2 ▶ Guidelines for Advocacy

The following principles will help you to function effectively as an advocate.

- **Keep the moral principle of patient autonomy always in mind.**
- **Know and document the facts** of the case.
- **Know the arguments** of those who oppose the patient. **Use role playing** to develop a strategy for responding to the arguments.
- **Have a sound base of support for your actions.** Be familiar with any policies or laws that apply.
- **Form a coalition of allies,** if you can. Get consultation. Communicate, inform, and clarify their collaborative roles.
- **Intervene high enough in the hierarchy** to get the job done. If the difficulty is with a physician or an organizational policy, merely going to the charge nurse will not be enough. You will need to communicate with nurse administrators or other agency administrators.

- **Demonstrate to the system** how it is defeating its own goals (e.g., for patient care).
- **Avoid getting into a power struggle** if possible (use the preceding steps first). If you must, decide how far you need to go and whether you are willing to go that far. You will need to enlist people with more power in the system than you have (e.g., family members, physicians, administrators).
- **Be aware of client vulnerability.** When possible, avoid confrontation. If there is risk for the client (as in a power contest), be sure the client is aware of his risks and possible gains; then let him choose how far to take the situation.
- **Have alternative actions.** Assess risks realistically. Weigh them against potential gains.

THINKING CRITICALLY ABOUT ETHICS AND VALUES

The exercises in the following sections allow you to practice the kind of thinking you will use as a full-spectrum nurse. Because these are critical-thinking questions, there is usually no single right answer. We do not provide answers for these questions because it is more important for you to think about the questions than to arrive at the "right" answer. These questions are designed to improve your thinking more than to "cover content." Discuss answers with your peers—discussion can stimulate critical thinking. If you have difficulty with any of these questions, consult with your instructor.

Applying the Full-Spectrum Nursing Model

PRACTICE SITUATION

Read the following summary of the Kithari and Kirschner article:

Kothari, S., & Kirschner, K. (2006). Abandoning the Golden Rule: The problem with "putting ourselves in the patient's place." *Topics in Stroke Rehabilitation, 13*(4), 68–73.

A large body of evidence documents the difficulties healthcare professionals have in predicting what their patient believes or wishes. These difficulties extend from the predictions of:

- Very specific patient wishes, such as for life-sustaining therapies
- More global assessments of patients' lives as a whole (for instance, their quality of life)

One explanation for this phenomenon is that healthcare professionals, either consciously or unconsciously, adopt "Golden Rule thinking." This refers to our attempts to understand another person's situation by imagining what we would believe or want under similar circumstances, in other words, "putting ourselves in the patient's place."

Although Golden Rule thinking would seem to be a promising strategy, studies show that it actually results in inaccurate presumptions of patients' wishes or beliefs. These presumptions, in turn, have significant clinical and ethical implications. That is, they cause healthcare professionals and families to make decisions for the patient that are, in reality, *not* what the patient would want.

The thinking goes:

I should put myself in the patient's place.
If I were the patient, I would want X.
Therefore, the patient probably wants X.
Because the patient probably wants X, we will do X.

This thinking process can have different results: (1) The patient really does want X, so you have met his needs. (2) The patient really wanted Y, so you did not meet his needs.

THINKING

1. *Theoretical Knowledge*: What is the Golden Rule, or what does it say?

2. *Critical Thinking (Inquiry)*: What is one thing that could be done ahead of time to prevent the need for Golden Rule thinking? Explain why that would work.

DOING

3. *Nursing Process (Assessment)*: If you do not know what the patient would want, instead of thinking what *you* would want, how might you get an idea of what the patient might want?

CARING

4. *Self-Knowledge*: What is your earliest memory of being taught the Golden Rule?

5. *Ethical Knowledge*: Which moral principle does the Golden Rule seem to try to follow: autonomy, nonmaleficence/beneficence, fidelity, veracity, or justice?

Critical Thinking and Clinical Reasoning

1. Some examples of ethical issues you may encounter are end-of-life issues, abortion or other reproductive issues, breaches of patient confidentiality, and incompetent or illegal practices of colleagues. Stop for a moment and think about a time when you have witnessed an ethical challenge in the clinical area.

   a. Describe the situation.

   b. How well equipped did you feel to handle the situation?

   c. What guided your thoughts and actions?

2. At the beginning of this chapter in Volume 1, Alan ("Meet Your Patients"), a teenager, had been injured in a soccer game. Without a blood transfusion, he may die, but because his family is of the Jehovah's Witnesses faith, Alan's parents have refused to sign permission for his transfusion. Taking each of the abilities required for ethical agency, state whether or not you think these people have the abilities listed below: Alan, Alan's parents, the physician, the nurse. Explain your thinking. An ethical agent must be able to:

   a. Perceive the difference between good and evil, right and wrong.

      Alan

      Parents

      Physician/surgeon

      Nurse

   b. Understand abstract moral principles.

      Alan

      Parents

      Physician/surgeon

      Nurse

   c. Reason and apply moral principles to make decisions, weigh alternatives, and plan ways to achieve goals.

      Alan

      Parents

      Physician/surgeon

      Nurse

   d. Decide and choose freely.

      Alan

      Parents

      Physician/surgeon

      Nurse

   e. Act according to his choice; this assumes both the power and the capability to act.

      Alan

      Parents

      Physician/surgeon

      Nurse

3. Consider Alan's situation again. Analyze the situation (a) using a deontological framework and moral principles and then (b) using a utilitarian framework. Focus on this question: Is it ethical to try hard to influence the parents to consent to allow a blood transfusion?

   a. Deontology

   b. Utilitarianism

   c. Did you reach a different conclusion depending on the framework you selected?

4. You are a busy nurse caring for a caseload of eight patients. One patient is the mother of the hospital administrator. She had surgery 3 days ago and is progressing nicely, but she is very demanding and requires a great deal of assistance to be repositioned in bed and to move from bed to chair. She has frequent visitors, including children and young grandchildren. In the next room is a young Haitian woman whose bill is paid by Medicaid. She has a history of drug abuse and had surgery just this morning. She speaks little English and seems very anxious. She is experiencing nausea and pain and needs a transfusion of a unit of packed blood cells this evening. Her boyfriend is at the desk requesting to bring her 3-year-old daughter to the unit so that she may see her mother. The visiting policy says that children must be at least 12 years old to visit the unit. Consider what aspects of justice apply to this situation and how it might be most equitably handled. Focus on the principle of justice.

5. An example of the feminist ethical approach arises in deciding whether to allocate federal healthcare resources to younger people (e.g., education, day care, free immunizations) or to older adults (e.g., prescription drug insurance, long-term care). Feminist reasoning would be as follows:

   - In the United States, more older adults are women than men.
   - Older women tend to be poorer and are more likely to be alone than are men.
   - Therefore, if healthcare for older adults were to be rationed, it would negatively affect women more than men.
   - Therefore, it would be unfair and unethical to allocate more resources to younger people than to older adults.

   a. Analyze this decision using a deontological framework. Explain your reasoning, as was done above.

   b. Analyze this decision using a consequentialist framework. Explain your reasoning.

6. Deception can take different forms, from intentional lying to nondisclosure of information or partial disclosure of information. Think about your duty to tell the truth. Is there ever a time when being completely honest is not the best nursing intervention? Do you consider withholding information the same as lying?

7. Review the following scenario. Examine your self-knowledge, and work through the steps of the values clarification process (choosing, prizing, and acting). An older couple with no other children learn that their unborn child has Down syndrome (trisomy 21). The couple need to make a difficult decision because the mother is 18 weeks pregnant.

   a. How would you feel about this couple if they chose to have this child and insisted on doing everything possible to keep the baby alive even if it is born with severe handicaps?

   b. Do you think that your professional relationship with this couple would change if they chose to terminate the pregnancy?

   c. How can you help the couple clarify their values?

   (1) List alternatives.
   (2) Examine the possible consequences of the alternative choices.

(3) Choose freely.
(4) Feel good about the choice that has been made.
(5) Affirm the choice to others.
(6) Act on the choice.
(7) Act with a consistent pattern.

What Are the Main Points in This Chapter?

➤ Ethics is a formal process for deciding right and wrong conduct in situations where issues of values and morals arise.

➤ Nursing ethics refers to ethical questions that arise out of nursing practice.

➤ Morals are learned and internalized throughout the life span. Carol Gilligan proposed that moral development and reasoning are different among men and women.

➤ Ethical agency is the ability to make ethical choices and to be responsible for one's ethical actions. In practice, nurses sometimes make moral decisions that they are not able to carry out.

➤ Moral distress is the inability to carry out moral decisions.

➤ Whistleblowing occurs when a person identifies in the workplace an incompetent, unethical, or illegal situation or actions of others, and then appeals to someone who may have the power to stop it.

➤ Nursing ethics problems arise from technological advances, the needs of a multicultural population, cost containment efforts in healthcare, the nature of nursing work, and the nature of the nursing profession.

➤ Nurses have complex obligations and multiple complex relationships within healthcare organizations (e.g., with employers, physicians, patients, families, and other nurses).

➤ Ethical decisions are affected by a person's developmental stage, values, moral frameworks and principles, and professional guidelines.

➤ Attitudes are mental dispositions or feelings toward a person, object, or idea.

➤ A belief is something that one accepts as true.

➤ A value is a belief that you have about the worth of something; a value is highly prized and expressed through behaviors, feelings, and decisions.

➤ Values are transmitted through social interaction.

➤ Value neutrality means that we attempt to understand our own values regarding an issue and to know when to put them aside, if necessary, to become nonjudgmental.

➤ Six important moral principles are autonomy, nonmaleficence, beneficence, fidelity, veracity, and justice.

➤ Consequentialist theories are moral theories in which the rightness or wrongness of an action depends on the consequences of the act, rather than on the nature of the act itself.

➤ The principle of utility states that a "good" act is one that produces the greatest good for the greatest number of people.

➤ Deontological theories consider an action to be right or wrong independent of its consequences.

➤ Feminist ethics asserts that focusing on deontological principles distracts one from dealing with larger social issues and that objectivity is impossible.

➤ An ethics-of-care directs attention to a patient's specific situation viewed within the context of his or her life narrative. It emphasizes feelings, but not at the expense of some conventional ethical principles, such as autonomy, nonmaleficence, or beneficence.

➤ Nurses can obtain ethical guidance from professional codes of ethics, standards of practice, and the American Hospital Association's *Patient Care Partnership.*

➤ The principle of autonomy underlies informed consent—clients' right to decide for themselves whether or not they will agree to a proposed procedure or treatment.

➤ Specific ethical issues the nurse is likely to encounter may involve AIDS, abortion, allocation of resources, issues of confidentiality, end-of-life issues (e.g., advance directives, DNAR orders, life-sustaining treatments, informed consent, organ transplantation), and reproductive technologies.

➤ Values clarification is the process of becoming conscious of and naming one's values. Nurses can assist clients with values clarification.

➤ A full value must be chosen freely, cherished and made known to others, translated into behaviors, and integrated into lifestyles.

➤ Not all moral problems are dilemmas. A dilemma is a particular kind of moral problem: It is a painful situation in which a choice must be made between two equally undesirable actions. There is no clearly right or wrong option.

➤ One method of working through an ethical problem is to perform assessment and diagnosis, as in the nursing process; then use the mnemonic MORAL: **M**assage the dilemma, **O**utline the options, **R**esolve the dilemma, **A**ct by applying the chosen option, and **L**ook back and evaluate.

➤ A good compromise preserves the integrity of all parties when there is disagreement among them in a moral situation.

➤ Nurses should be patient advocates because (1) their professional role requires it, (2) they have special knowledge that the patient does not have, (3) they have a special relationship with patients, and (4) one aspect of the nursing role is to defend patient's autonomous decisions.

➤ The nurse's role as an advocate is to inform, support, and communicate.

For practice questions for this chapter,

Go to **NCLEX-Style Chapter Quiz,** on the Student Resource Disk or DavisPlus at http://davisplus.fadavis.com/Wilkinson2

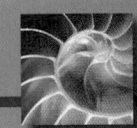

Knowledge Map

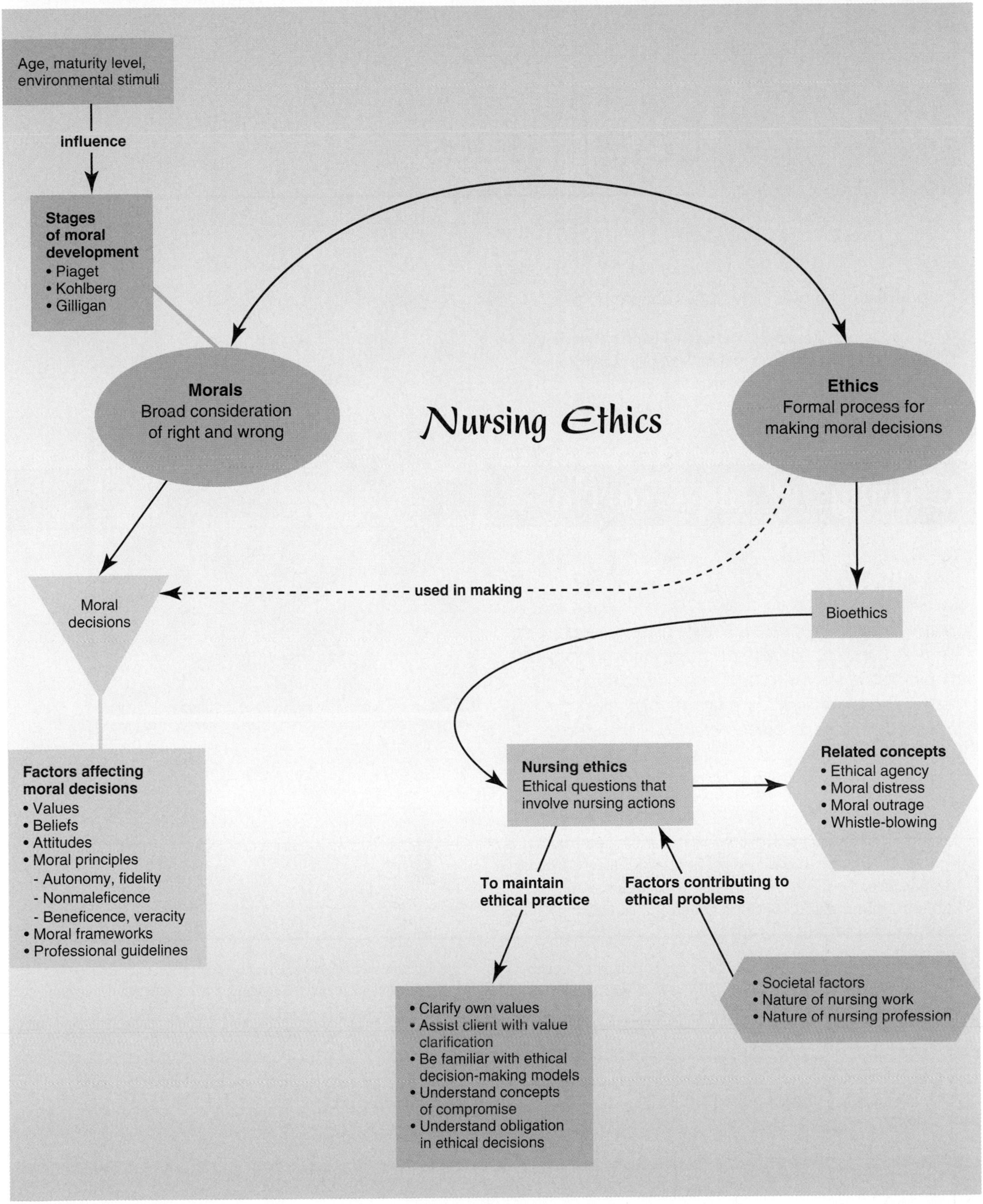

Age, maturity level, environmental stimuli

influence

Stages of moral development
• Piaget
• Kohlberg
• Gilligan

Morals
Broad consideration of right and wrong

Nursing Ethics

Ethics
Formal process for making moral decisions

Moral decisions

- - - **used in making** - - -

Bioethics

Factors affecting moral decisions
• Values
• Beliefs
• Attitudes
• Moral principles
  - Autonomy, fidelity
  - Nonmaleficence
  - Beneficence, veracity
• Moral frameworks
• Professional guidelines

Nursing ethics
Ethical questions that involve nursing actions

Related concepts
• Ethical agency
• Moral distress
• Moral outrage
• Whistle-blowing

To maintain ethical practice

Factors contributing to ethical problems

• Clarify own values
• Assist client with value clarification
• Be familiar with ethical decision-making models
• Understand concepts of compromise
• Understand obligation in ethical decisions

• Societal factors
• Nature of nursing work
• Nature of nursing profession

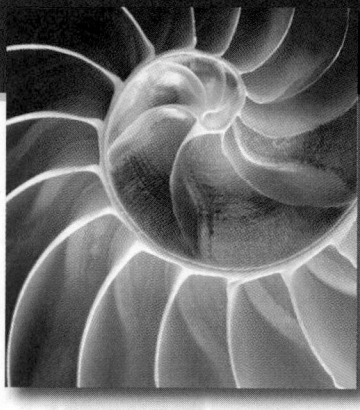

CHAPTER 45

Legal Issues

For a podcast of an overview of this chapter,

 Go to Student Resources, **Podcast – Chapter Overviews, Chapter 45,** on DavisPlus at http://davisplus.fadavis.com/Wilkinson2

Caring for the Garcias

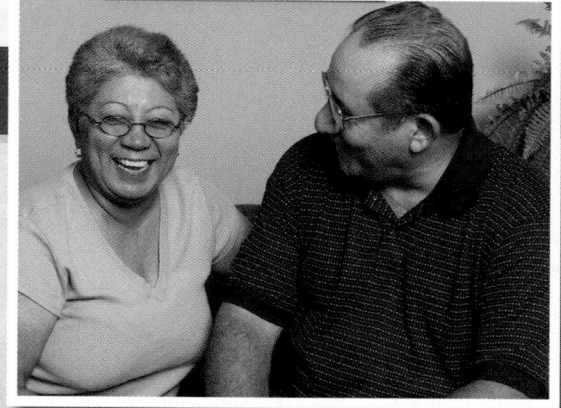

The exercises in the following section allow you to practice the kind of thinking you will use as a full-spectrum nurse. Because these are critical-thinking questions, there is usually no single right answer. We do not provide answers for these questions because it is more important for you to think about the questions than to arrive at the "right" answer. These questions are designed to improve your thinking more than to "cover content." Discuss answers with your peers—discussion can stimulate critical thinking. If you have difficulty with any of these questions, consult with your instructor.

Joe and Flordelisa Garcia have requested an appointment with you, the nurse at the Family Medicine Clinic, to discuss advance directives. Their experience with Joe's mother, Katherine, has created concerns about end-of-life care.

A. Joe asks you, "Do you think it's appropriate to create an advance directive at my age?" How would you respond?

B. Joe tells you that he believes in "natural death." He states, "I don't want extraordinary measures, and I never want to be resuscitated." Flordelisa responds that she is extremely uncomfortable with blanket statements about treatment. "If he got hit by a car or had some accident, I would want you to do everything in your power to treat him. I couldn't carry out his wishes," she states. What actions should you take to help Joe and Flordelisa resolve this discrepancy?

Practical **Knowledge**
knowing how

Clinical Insights

Clinical Insight 45-1 ▶ Tips for Avoiding Malpractice

- **Develop open, honest, respectful, caring relationships** with patients and families. Patients are less likely to sue if they feel that you were caring and professional. Angry patients who feel mistreated are more likely to bring suit.
- **Careful, thorough documentation** is the best defense if a lawsuit does occur:
  - Use and document all steps of the nursing process.
  - Be especially thorough when documenting care for patients who will not comply with treatments or who complain a lot.
  - Courts assume that if care is not documented, it was not given.
- **Know and follow applicable laws:** (1) federal and state laws, (2) your state's nurse practice act (perform only the activities within your scope of practice and competence).
- **Know and follow agency policies and procedures.**
- **Know and follow standards of care** set forth in the state nurse practice act, professional organizations, professional literature, agency policy, and so on.
- **Follow the "rights" of medication administration** (see Chapter 23).
- **Perform falls risk assessments,** document, and take measures to ensure patient safety.
- **Recognize "problem" patients.** Try to identify the basic problem or complaint and intervene to resolve it.
- **Follow medical orders,** but clarify them as needed. Do

not implement a questionable order or one you do not understand.
- **Don't blame or criticize other healthcare providers** in the presence of patients (e.g., "Sorry you didn't get your pain medication. The night shift was a little short-staffed last night.")
- **Maintain patient privacy and confidentiality.**
- **Don't make statements that may appear to be an admission of guilt** (e.g., "Omigosh, I forgot to shut off that IV!"). Errors should not be included on the patient's health record, but instead in an incident report.
- **Stay competent in your area of practice;** for example, attend continuing education and inservice programs to improve your knowledge and skills.
- **Don't accept a clinical assignment that you think you are not competent to perform.** Evaluate your assignment with your supervisor if there is a question.
- **Recognize significant assessment cues,** and notify primary care providers of changes in the patient's condition or patient complaints.
- **Document the time and content of telephone conversations with other healthcare providers.**
- **Send copies only,** never originals, of records and reports requested by other professionals.

Practice Resources
Aiken, T. (2004); Austin, S. (2008).

✚. Clinical Insight 45-2 ▶ Using Equipment Safely

The following will help you to ensure proper and safe use of equipment:
1. Obtain appropriate training on equipment use.
2. Follow the healthcare agency's protocols, policies, and procedures on the use of the equipment.
3. Follow the manufacturer's operating instructions.
4. Be sure medical equipment has been properly inspected.
5. Perform safety checks regularly and before use.
6. Position and use equipment properly during treatment.
7. Know how the equipment functions; be alert to signs that it is not working properly.
8. Make sure rooms are not cluttered with equipment.
9. Follow agency policies regarding equipment brought from the patient's home (e.g., hair dryers, electric shavers, radios); usually these should be inspected for proper grounding and safe cords.

Clinical Insight 45-3 ▶ Guidelines for Documenting Care

To be accurate and complete, your reporting and documentation of patient care must address the following:

1. Patient status (e.g., symptoms and responses to treatments)
2. The nursing care given
3. Physician, advance practice nurse, dentist, and podiatrist prescriptions
4. Medications and treatments
5. Patient responses
6. Consultations with other members of the healthcare team regarding patient status

You might find helpful the FACT mnemonic for documenting care. When documenting care, you must be:

Factual
Accurate
Complete
Timely

Another way to remember how to document is to use the 5 Cs.

Charting should be:

Complete
Clear
Correct
Comprehensive
Chronological

Reference

Helm, A. (2003). *Nursing malpractice: Sidestepping legal minefields.* Philadelphia: Lippincott, Williams & Wilkins, pp. 1–33.

THINKING CRITICALLY ABOUT LEGAL ISSUES

The exercises in the following sections allow you to practice the kind of thinking you will use as a full-spectrum nurse. Because these are critical-thinking questions, there is usually no single right answer. We do not provide answers for these questions because it is more important for you to think about the questions than to arrive at the "right" answer. These questions are designed to improve your thinking more than to "cover content." Discuss answers with your peers—discussion can stimulate critical thinking. If you have difficulty with any of these questions, consult with your instructor.

Applying the Full-Spectrum Nursing Model

PATIENT SITUATION

A nurse employed by a temporary agency is assigned to a neurology unit for a 12-hour shift. On arrival, she discovers that the registered nurse assigned for the shift called in sick, leaving her with two nursing assistive personnel (NAPs) to provide patient care and administer medication, including controlled substances. The nursing supervisor informs her that she will be responsible for the unit with 22 patients, 12 of whom are acutely ill and require close observation and frequent care. The nursing supervisor is not available to work on the unit and has no additional RNs to provide patient care. The nurse decides not to accept the assignment, to report the decision and reasons to her agency supervisor, and to leave the neuro unit immediately before starting the shift.

THINKING

1. *Theoretical Knowledge*:

   a. In addition to protecting her nursing license, what other factors should the nurse have considered in deciding whether to stay or leave the unit?

   b. Because the nurse decided not to accept the assignment, would this have been considered as abandonment?

   c. What standards, guidelines, and laws would apply to determine whether the nurse's behavior was in accordance with standards of practice?

2. *Critical Thinking (Contextual Awareness)*:

   a. Which statements in the ANA Bill of Rights for Nurses should the nurse have considered before deciding whether to accept the assignment?

   b. What factors in this situation could create legal problems for the nurse?

DOING

3. *Nursing Process (Planning/Intervention)*: The nurse's action (leaving the unit) might be viewed, under some laws in some situations, as abandonment of patients. What are some alternative actions the nurse might have taken to avoid that risk?

CARING

4. *Self-Knowledge*: Have you ever been in a situation where you felt a moral obligation to help out but yet knew you would be in over your head? Describe your experience.

5. *Ethical Knowledge*: In your opinion, did the nurse do the right thing when she decided not to accept the assignment and to leave the nursing unit immediately? Explain your thinking.

▓▓▓ Critical Thinking and Clinical Reasoning

1. Think about the "Meet Your Nurse Role Model" scenario you read at the beginning of the chapter in Volume 1. A nurse with 3 years' experience on a medical–surgical unit arrives to work and discovers that two of her colleagues called in sick, including the charge nurse. The nursing supervisor informs her that you will need to assume the charge nurse role, in addition to assuming care for three patients. Feeling frustrated, the nurse ponders whether she should just quit and find another job. She reasons that this is not the answer to resolve the situation, and accepts the assignment. Two hours into the shift, one of her patients began to experience complications requiring blood glucose checks every 2 hours and frequent monitoring. In addition, one of the nurses become ill and will be replaced by a float nurse from the labor and delivery unit. The nurse contacts the nursing supervisor and requests additional assistance, but is told no other nurse is available and she is involved with several emergency situations. The nurse begins to analyze this situation from a legal perspective to determine the best course of actions.

   Use the critical-thinking model to identify questions to ask yourself in reflecting and deciding what to do.

    Go to Chapter 2, **Table 2-2,** in Volume 1.

   a. What questions do you need to ask about context?

   b. What knowledge do you need to make an informed and credible decision?

   c. What questions do you need to ask about considering alternatives?

   d. What questions do you need to ask about analyzing your assumptions?

   e. What questions do you need to ask about reflecting and deciding?

2. Analyze this passage:

   The Health Care Quality Improvement Act of 1986 (HCQIA), implemented in 1990, created the National Practitioner Data Bank (NPDB). The NPDB collects and provides information related to (1) medical malpractice payments made on behalf of healthcare providers; (2) adverse actions taken against clinical privileges of physicians, osteopaths, and dentists; and (3) actions by professional societies adversely affecting membership. This law is designed to protect patients by providing knowledge of practitioners who have been sanctioned for not meeting legal standards of care in the past. Reporting of this information to the NPDB is mandatory, and failure to do so will result in fines and penalties (Fedorka & Resnick, 2000, pp. 105–106). (Note: This applies only to advanced practice nurses.)

   ■ How do you think the HCQIA functions?
   ■ What rights does it help protect?

3. Imagine that you are working in a large medical center in an area where there have been several robberies and assaults in the past 6 months, mostly late at night. Although the parking lot is nearly a block from the employees' exit and is not well lighted, there is only one security guard on duty outside the hospital after 10:00 P.M. Despite repeated requests from employees, all the way up the chain of command, no efforts are being made to improve lighting or to hire more security guards. What standards and laws might be helpful to the employees?

4. George Agnew, 75 years old, is admitted to the emergency department after being involved in a serious car accident. His wife is with him, and she is very upset—to the point of being hysterical. It is likely that Mr. Agnew will die, but physicians are considering whether he will need a ventilator in the next hour or so. You need to know Mr. Agnew's wishes on this issue, but he is not conscious. The charge nurse tells you not to ask Mrs. Agnew because it will just upset her more.

a. What is going on in the situation that may influence the outcome?

b. What factors may influence your behavior and others' behavior in this situation?

c. What values or biases do you have that influence your behavior in this situation?

d. Where might you get the information you need instead of asking Mrs. Agnew?

e. What would you do? What legal support, if any, do you have?

5. Compare and contrast the following definitions of practical nursing and professional nursing taken from the Nurse Practice Act in Missouri and then discuss the differences in the scope of practice for the LPN/LVN and the RN. Identify two tasks/responsibilities that only the RN can perform.

"Practical nursing," the performance for compensation of selected acts for the promotion of health and in the care of persons who are ill, injured, or experiencing alterations in normal health processes. Such performance requires substantial specialized skill, judgment and knowledge. All such nursing care shall be given under the direction of a person licensed by a state regulatory board to prescribe medications and treatments or under the direction of a registered professional nurse. For the purposes of this chapter, the term "direction" shall mean guidance or supervision provided by a person licensed by a state regulatory board to prescribe medications and treatments or a registered professional nurse, including, but not limited to, oral, written, or otherwise communicated orders or directives for patient care. When practical nursing care is delivered pursuant to the direction of a person licensed by a state regulatory board to prescribe medications and treatments or under the direction of a registered professional nurse, such care may be delivered by a licensed practical nurse without direct physical oversight; "Professional nursing," the performance for compensation of any act which requires substantial specialized education, judgment and skill based on knowledge and application of principles derived from the biological, physical, social and nursing sciences, including, but not limited to:

(a) Responsibility for the teaching of health care and the prevention of illness to the patient and his or her family;
(b) Assessment, nursing diagnosis, nursing care, and counsel of persons who are ill, injured or experiencing alterations in normal health processes;
(c) The administration of medications and treatments as prescribed by a person licensed by a state regulatory board to prescribe medications and treatments;
(d) The coordination and assistance in the delivery of a plan of health care with all members of a health team;
(e) The teaching and supervision of other persons in the performance of any of the foregoing.

(Missouri Revised Statutes, Chapter 335, Section 335.016, August 2008, retrieved on January 3, 2009 from: http://www.moga.mo.gov/statutes/C300-399/3350000016.HTM).

6. The patient was an older adult with various medical conditions and receiving multiple medications. The nurse determined the patient was a high fall risk, 8 on a scale of 0 to 10. The nurse decided to initiate the hospital's fall prevention plan, which meant raising the bed rails and placing restraints on the patient without physician's orders. Hospital policy, however, did require a nurse who initiated restraints on a patient for fall prevention to notify a physician or physician's assistant within 1 hour.

The next day another nurse, seeing that no orders for restraints had been received, removed the restraints. The patient was getting up out of bed on his own. His nursing neurological assessment showed signs of dementia and confusion. His oxygen saturation was low and his heartbeat was irregular. The physician was notified by phone but declined to order restraints. Later that evening the patient was found on the floor with a closed-head injury. He was transferred to a university hospital, where he died a few weeks later. The nurse was ruled not at fault.

Sturgill v. Ashe Memorial Hosp., __ S.E. 2d __, 2007 WL 3254411

(N.C. App., November 6, 2007).

Snyder, E. K. (2007, December). Fall: Patient not restrained, court does not fault nurses. *Legal Eagle Eye Newsletter for the Nursing Profession*, 15(12), 8.

1. In this case, in which the nurse was caring for a patient at high risk for fall but had no order to use restraints, what was the basis for the court's decision that the patient's death was not her fault?

2. What other action might the nurse have taken to prevent this patient's fall?

7. For each of the following concepts, use critical thinking to describe how or why it is important to nurses, patients, or legal issues. Note that these are *not* to be merely definitions.

Civil law
The U.S. Constitution Bill of Rights and
   the *Patient Care Partnership*
The ANA Code of Ethics; the ANA Standards of Practice; and the ANA Bill of Rights for Registered Nurses

Patient advocacy
Battery
Vicarious liability

▮ What Are the Main Points in This Chapter?

➤ The law is a binding practice, rule, or code of conduct that guides a community or society and is enforced by a controlling authority.

➤ Laws are primarily derived from four sources: (1) the Constitution, (2) statutes, (3) administrative bodies, and (4) the courts.

➤ The right of privacy comes from the Bill of Rights, Amendment I.

➤ A living will is prepared by an alert and oriented (competent) individual that gives directions to others about the person's wishes regarding life-prolonging treatments if the person becomes unable to make those decisions.

➤ A durable power of attorney for healthcare identifies a person who will make healthcare decisions in the event the patient is unable to do so.

➤ State laws affecting nursing practice include mandatory reporting laws, Good Samaritan laws, safe harbor laws, and institutional policies and procedures.

➤ The ANA Code of Ethics describes the standards of professional responsibility for nurses and provides insight into ethical and acceptable behavior.

➤ The ANA Bill of Rights identifies the rights nurses should expect from their workplace and work environment that are necessary for sound professional practice.

➤ A primary function of the medical malpractice system is to encourage healthcare providers to adhere to standards of practice and perform their responsibilities in a competent manner.

➤ Nurse Practice Acts are established by state boards of nursing to govern the practice of nursing.

➤ In most states, nurses are obligated legally to report suspected or actual patient abuse and also to report impaired health professionals and certain communicable diseases.

➤ State boards of nursing, under the state's nurse practice act, are responsible for licensing, credentialing, and disciplinary procedures involving nurses and nursing. They do not manage day-to-day oversight.

➤ Standards of care look to what a reasonable and prudent nurse would do in the same or similar situation.

➤ Criminal law deals with wrongs or offenses against society. Civil law deals with wrongs to individuals.

➤ Intentional torts include assault, battery, false imprisonment, fraud, and invasion of privacy.

➤ Quasi-intentional torts involve those actions that injure a person's reputation.

➤ Nonintentional torts that involve healthcare professionals are negligence or malpractice.

➤ Negligence is a wrong committed against an individual by one who has failed to use ordinary care.

➤ Malpractice is negligence committed against an individual by a licensed professional involving a duty, breach of that duty, an injury, and damages.

➤ Litigation is the formal process where the legal issues, rights, and duties between the parties are heard and decided. The stages include: (1) pleading and pretrial motions, (2) discovery, (3) alternative dispute resolution, (4) trial, and (5) appeal.

➤ Malpractice claims, in general, result from failure to maintain the standard of practice, including failure to assess, diagnose, plan, implement, and evaluate patient responses to care.

➤ Nurses can help reduce their legal risks by developing open, honest, respectful, caring relationships with patients and families and observing standards of care.

➤ You may witness a patient's signature on a consent form, but you are not legally responsible for explaining the treatments and options, nor for evaluating whether the provider has adequately explained them.

For practice questions for this chapter,

 Go to **NCLEX-Style Chapter Quiz,** on the Student Resource Disk or DavisPlus at http://davisplus.fadavis.com/Wilkinson2

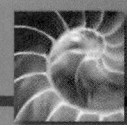

Knowledge Map

State laws
- Mandatory reporting
- Good Samaritan
- Nurse Practice Acts
  - Credentialing
  - Licensing
  - Discipline

Standards of practice
- What a reasonable and prudent nurse would do
- Mandatory = Nurse Practice Act
- Voluntary = ANA

Federal laws
- Bill of Rights
- EMTALA
- ADA
- Patient Self-Determination Act
- HIPAA

Other guidelines
- Agency policies and procedures
- Nursing Code of Ethics
- Patient Care Partnership
- ANA Bill of Rights for Nurses

Laws and Regulations

Criminal law

Civil law

Contract law

Tort law

- Misdemeanor
- Felony

- Negligence
- Malpractice

Types of torts
Quasi-intentional:
- Defamation
- Slander
- Libel

Intentional:
- Assault and battery
- False imprisonment
- Fraud
- Invasion of privacy

Common nursing malpractice claims
Failure to:
- Assess and diagnose
- Plan
- Implement plan
- Evaluate

How to avoid →
- Observe standards of care
- Avoid medication/treatment errors
- Report/document
- Obtain informed consent
- Attend to safety
- Maintain confidentiality
- Provide education
- Delegate correctly
- Observe boundaries

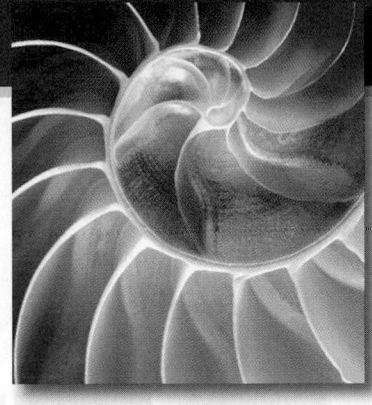

Credits

Note: Unless cited below, text credits appear within the text.

Chapter 3

Nursing Admission Data Form: From North Broward Hospital District, Ft. Lauderdale, FL.

Patient Assessment Tool: Lawton Instrumental Activities of Daily Living: From Lawton, M. P., & Brody, E. M. (1960). Assessment of older people: Self-maintaining and instrumental activities of daily living. *The Gerontologist*, 9, 179–186. Copyright © by the Gerontological Society of America. Used by permission of the publisher.

Chapter 5

Discharge Planning Form: Courtesy of Shawnee Mission Health System, Shawnee Mission, KS.

Standardized Language, NOC Measurement Scales: From Moorhead, S., Johnson, M., Maas, M., & Swanson, E. (2008). *Nursing outcomes classification* (4th ed.). St. Louis, MO: Mosby/Elsevier.

Chapter 6

Caring for the Garcias: From Per-Se Technologies, 2840 Mount Wilkinson Highway, Atlanta, GA. Used with permission.

Chapter 7

Unnumbered Figure: From Wilkinson, J. (2007). *Nursing process and critical thinking* (4th ed.). Upper Saddle River, NJ: Prentice-Hall.

The Five Rights of Delegation: From National Council of State Boards of Nursing (1995). Delegation: Concepts and decision-making process. National Council Position Paper. Chicago: Author.

Delegation Decision-Making Grid: Used by permission from the National Council of State Boards of Nursing (NCSBN), Chicago, IL (1997). Retrieved February 1, 2008 from the NCSBN Web site.

Evaluation Checklist: From Wilkinson, J. (2007). *Nursing process and critical thinking* (4th ed., pp. 424–427). Upper Saddle River, NJ: Prentice-Hall.

Chapter 9

Procedure 1, Step 3b, Body: Adapted from Child Protection and the Dental Team commissioned by the UK Department of Health.

Chapter 10

Discharge/Assessment/Instructions: From Fisherman's Hospital, Marathon, FL. Used with permission.

Patient Education Form: From Fisherman's Hospital, Marathon, FL. Used with permission.

Chapter 11

Depression Assessment Guide: © Pfizer, Inc. All rights reserved. Reproduced with permission.

Chapter 15

Do Not Resuscitate Orders: Courtesy of St. Joseph's Hospital Center.

Standard Nursing Language: From Moorhead, S., Johnson, M., Maas, M. L., & Seanson, E. (Eds.). (2008). *Nursing outcomes classification* (NOC) (5th ed.). St. Louis, MO: C. V. Mosby; Bulechek, G. M., Bulechek, H. K., & Dochterman, J. M. (Eds.) (2008). *Nursing interventions classification* (NIC) (5th ed.). St. Louis, MO: C. V. Mosby.

Chapter 16

Adult Admission History: Courtesy of Cerner Corporation.

Unnumbered Figure: Courtesy of Teton Valley Hospital, Driggs, ID.

Chapter 19

Abnormal Atlas:

Alopecia areata, Cyanosis, Fungal infection, Half-and-half nails, Herpes simplex, Kyphosis, Lordosis, Locations of direct and indirect hernias, Propulsive gait, Ringworm, Scissors gait, Scoliosis, Spastic gait, Steppage gait, Vitiligo, Waddling gait, Locations of direct and indirect hernias, Herpes simplex, Petechiae, Venous star: From Dillon, P. (2007). *Nursing health assessment* (2nd ed.). Philadelphia: F. A. Davis.

Capillary hemangioma, Port-wine stain, Syphilitic chancre, Vesicles (blisters): From Goldsmith, L. A., Lazarus, G. S., & Tharp, M. D. (1997). *Adult and pediatric dermatology: A color guide to diagnosis and treatment*. Philadelphia: F. A. Davis.

Degenerative joint disease: Courtesy of MCP–Hahnemann University Department of Dermatology, Philadelphia, 2007.

Gingival recession: Courtesy of Robert A. Levine, D.D.S. and Sheryl Radin, D.D.S., Pediatric Dentistry.

Jaundice: From Chapman, L., & Durham, R. (2009). *Maternal-newborn nursing: The critical components of nursing care*. Philadelphia: F. A. Davis.

Leukoplakia and cancer of the tongue: Courtesy of Tina S. Liang, D.M.D.

Pediculosis, Pterygium, Subconjuntival hemorrhage: Courtesy of Will's Eye Institute, Philadelphia.

Enlarged tonsil with exudates: Courtesy of SIU BIOMED, CMSP Clearing House 071-2786.

Black hairy tongue, Genital warts, Herpes vulvovaginitis, Heberden's nodes, Rheumatoid arthritis, Syphilitic chancre, and Herpes vulvovaginitis: Courtesy of MCP–Hahnemann University Department of Dermatology.

Clinical Insight 19-1a and b, Clinical Insight 19-3, Collecting (all figures), Procedure 19-6 (Steps 4a through 5f, Steps 6e(2) through Step8e[2]), Procedure 19-7 (Step1ai through Step 3e2, Step 5 through 6c), Procedure 19-10 (all figures), Procedure 19-1, 2, 5, 6, 7, and 9, Procedure 19-13 (all figures), Procedure 19-14 (Bimanual and One Hand, Steps 6 and 7), Procedure 19-15 (Steps 1 through 6, Step 9, What if), Procedure 19-16 (Steps 11 through 24), Procedure 19-17 (Steps 5 through 7), Procedure 19-18 (Maturation Status in Females Stage B1–B4, Steps 2 and 3), Procedure 19-19 (Equipment a, Steps 6e(2) through 8e(2), Procedure 19-7 Step1ai through Step 3e(2): From Dillon, P. (2007). *Nursing health assessment* (2nd ed.). Philadelphia: F. A. Davis.

Describing Skin Lesions, Procedure 19-8 (Step 2b, Step 4d, Step 5 b and c), Procedure 19-9 (Step 2b 1 and 2), Procedure 19-11 (Step4 a, b, and c), Procedure 19-14 (Step 5), Procedure 19-15

(Step 8, all figures), Procedure 19-19 (part 2, Step 1 and 7, Part 4, Step 1, Part 5 Steps 2 and 4): From Dillon, P. (2003). *Nursing health assessment* (1st ed.). Philadelphia: F. A. Davis.

Procedure 19-7, Step 3f(1, 2, and 3): Courtesy of Ann Marie Ramsay, RN, MSN, CPNO, Section of Pediatric Otolaryngology, University of Michigan, Ann Arbor.

Procedure 19-9 (Step 4/1): From CMSP.

Procedure 19-9 (Step 4/2): Courtesy of MCP–Hahnemann University Department of Dermatology, Philadelphia.

Procedure 19-12 (Step 2b), Procedure 6 (Step 3): From Scanlon, V. C., & Sanders, T. (2007). *Essentials of anatomy and physiology* (5th ed.). Philadelphia: F. A. Davis.

Procedure 19-17 (Tanner Staging and Maturation Status in Females Stage P1 through P5): From Tanner, J. M. (1962). *Growth at adolescence* (2nd ed.). Oxford: Blackwell Scientific Publications.

Chapter 20

Procedure 20-2, Step 1(e): Courtesy of Moldex-Metric, Inc. Culver City, CA. www.moldex.com

Chapter 21

Procedure 21-1, Steps 1c and 1d: Courtesy of Smart Caregiver Corporation.

Chapter 22

Procedure 22-8: Courtesy of Sage Products, Inc., Cary, IL.

Procedure 22-9, Equipment, Step 10, Home Care and Documentation: Courtesy of EZ Access, Auburn, WA.

Chapter 23

Procedure 23-10, Equipment 1: Courtesy of Edward Lin, MD, Ingenious Technologies Corporation. Training video link: http://ingenious.com/NS/ns.htm

Chapter 25

Holmes-Rahe Social Readjustment Scale: From Holmes, T., & Rahe, R. (1967). Social readjustment rating scale. *Journal of Psychosomatic Research*, 11(2), 213–218. Reprinted with permission from Elsevier.

Chapter 26

Assessment: References: Guigoz, Y. (2006). The Mini-Nutritional Assessment (MNA®) Review of the literature—What does it tell us? *Journal of Nutrition, Health, and Aging, 10*, 466–487; Rubenstein L., Harker J., Salva A., et al. (2001).

Screening for Undernutrition in Geriatric Practice: Developing the Short-Form Mini Nutritional Assessment (MNA-SF). *Journal of Gerontology, 56A*, M366–377; Vellas, B., Villars, H., Abellan, G., et al. (2006). Overview of the MNA® - Its History and Challenges. *Journal of Nutrition, Health, and Aging, 10*, 456–465.

Clinical Assessment 26-2 a and b: From Lutz, C., & Przytulski, K. (2006). *Nutrition and diet therapy* (4th ed.). Philadelphia, F. A. Davis.

Procedure 26-2 (Step 11): From Scanlon, V. C., & Sanders, T. (2007). *Essentials of anatomy and physiology* (5th ed.). Philadelphia: F. A. Davis.

Procedure 26-2, Step 20g: Courtesy Dale Medical Products, Plainville, MA.

Procedure 26-5 (Equipment): Permission for use granted by Cook Medical Incorporated, Bloomington, IN.

Chapter 27

Guidelines: From Dillon, P. (2007). *Nursing health assessment* (2nd ed.). Philadelphia: F. A. Davis.

Chapter 28

Procedure 28-6 (Equipment): From Williams, L., & Hopper, P. (2003). *Understanding medical surgical nursing* (2nd ed.). Philadelphia: F. A. Davis.

Procedure 28-8B (Step 8 and Step 11): Courtesy of Hollister Incorporated, Libertyville, IL.

Procedure 28-8 (Documentation): Courtesy of Nurse 2.

Procedure 28-8 (Equipment and Step 11): Courtesy of Hollister Incorporated, Libertyville, IL.

Chapter 30

Wong FACES Scale: From Hockenberry, M. J., & Wilson, D. (2009). *Wong's essentials of pediatric nursing* (8th ed.). St. Louis, MO: C. V. Mosby. Used with permission.

Chapter 31

Clinical Insight 31-2 (Unnumbered figure) and Procedure 31-1A (Step 4): From Williams, L., & Hopper, P. (2003). *Understanding medical surgical nursing* (2nd ed.). Philadelphia: F. A. Davis.

Chapter 34

Unnumbered Figure: From Department of Health and Human Services (1992). Clinical Practice Guideline. Pressure ulcers in adults. Prediction and prevention PPPUA. Publication No. 92-0047. Rockville, MD: Public Health Service, pp. 16–17.

Copyright Barbara Braden and Nancy Bergstrom, 1988. Reprinted with permission.

Unnumbered Figure: From Norton, D., McLaren, R., & Exton-Smith, A. N. (1975). An investigation of geriatric nursing problems in hospitals. Edinburgh, UK: Churchill University. Used with permission.

Unnumbered Figure: From National Pressure Ulcer Advisory Panel. (2002). Retrieved from http://www.npuap.org/push3-0.htm

Procedure 34-7A (Steps 2, 8, 10, and 15): From Rhoads, J., & Meeker, B. J. (2008). *Davis's guide to clinical nursing skills*. Philadelphia: F. A. Davis.

Procedure 34-7B (Step 10): Courtesy of Talley Group Limited, Hampshire, England.

Table 34-2 (Unnumbered figure): Courtesy of Wound Educators. www.woundeducators.com

Chapter 35

Procedure 8 (Equipment): © 2009 Unomedical, Skillman, NJ.

Chapter 36

Procedure 36-1 (Steps 15 and 18): From Rhoads, J., & Meeker, B. J. (2008). *Davis's guide to clinical nursing skills*. Philadelphia: F. A. Davis.

Chapter 37

AORN Preoperative Checklist: Used with permission from AORN, Inc. Copyright © 2009 AORN, Inc. Denver, CO. All rights reserved.

World Health Organization Surgical Safety Checklist: Reprinted with permission from the World Health Organization.

Procedure 37-4 (Portable Suction Source): Gomco ® Model 3005 Portable Aspirator. Courtesy of Allied Healthcare Products, St. Louis, MO.

Chapter 42

Meet the Garcias: © istockphoto.com/agostinosangel

Chapter 43

Standardized Language (CCC Care Components): From the Clinical Care Classification System, Dr. Virginia K. Saba.

Chapter 45

Clinical Insight 45-3: Helm, A. (2003). *Nursing malpractice: Sidestepping legal minefields*. Philadelphia: Lippincott Williams & Wilkins.

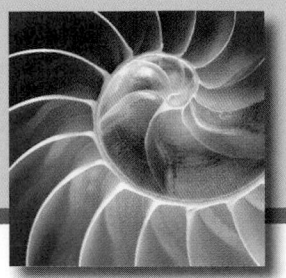

Bibliography

Caveat: As you know, web addresses change frequently. The URLs in this Bibliography were checked in 2010; however, many will likely not be working over time. When you find a non-working URL, try truncating the address back to the main page (e.g., for http://www.guideline.gov/content.aspx?id=14174, cut it down to http://www.guideline.gov), then browse for the article on that web site. Or, you can search for the author name and/or article title and year on Google or your preferred search engine.

Chapter 1

Aiken, L., Clarke, S., Sloane, D., et al. (2002). Hospital nurse staffing and patient mortality, nurse burnout, and job dissatisfaction. *JAMA, 288*, 1987–1993.

Alberta Association of Registered Nurses. (1998). *Bylaws.* Edmonton, AB: Author.

American Association for the History of Nursing. (2001). *Nursing history in the curriculum: Preparing nurses for the 21st century.* Philadelphia: Author.

American College of Nurse Practitioners. (ACNP). (2007). What is the difference between a skilled nursing facility and a nursing facility? Retrieved December 7, 2007, from http://www.acnpweb.org/i4a/pages/Index.cfm?pageID=3433%20American%20College%20of%20Nurse%20Practioners

American Hospital Association. (2007). *Hospital Statistics, 2007.* Chicago: Author.

American Nurses Association (ANA). (1980). *Nursing's social policy statement.* Washington, DC: Author.

American Nurses Association (ANA). (1991). *Nursing's agenda for health care reform.* Kansas City, MO: Author.

American Nurses Association (ANA). (1995). *Nursing's social policy statement.* Washington, DC: Author.

American Nurses Association (ANA). (1998a). *Managed care: Challenges and opportunities for nursing.* Retrieved October 4, 2008, from http://www.nursingworld.org/readroom/fsmgdcar.htm

American Nurses Association (ANA). (1998b). *Standards of clinical nursing practice* (2nd ed.). Washington, DC: American Nurses Publishing.

American Nurses Association (ANA). (2001). Code of ethics for nurses. Working draft#10A. Washington, DC: Author. Retrieved October 5, 2008, from http://nursingworld.org/ethics/chcode10.htm#9_1

American Nurses Association (ANA). (2003). *Nursing's social policy statement.* Washington, DC: Author.

American Nurses Association (ANA). (2004). *Standards of clinical nursing practice* (3rd ed.). Washington, DC: American Nurses Publishing.

American Nurses Association (ANA). (2005). ANA's health care agenda 2005. Retrieved December 8, 2007, from http://www.nursingworld.org/MainMenuCategories/HealthcareandPolicyIssues/Reports/HealthCareAgenda.aspx

American Nurses Association (ANA). (2008). Health system reform agenda. Silver Spring, MD: Author. Retrieved November 1, 2009, from http://www.nursingworld.org/HSRA08.

American Public Health Association (APHA). (1996). The definition and role of public health nursing: A statement of the APHA public health nursing section. Washington, DC: Author. Retrieved December 28, 2007, from http://www.dhss.missouri.gov/LPHA/PHNursing/DefinitionPHN_%20R_04.htm

Anthony, M., Standing, T., & Hertz, J. (2001). Nurses' beliefs about their abilities to delegate within changing models of care. *Journal of Continuing Education in Nursing, 32*(5), 210–215.

Article 54-02 (2003). North Dakota Article 54–02. Nurse Licensure. Retrieved December 15, 2007, from http://www.legis.nd.gov/information/acdata/pdf/54-02-01.pdf

Association for Registered Nurses in Newfoundland and Labrador. (2007). Standards for nursing practice. St. Johns, NL: Author. Retrieved December 1, 2007, from http://www.arnnl.nf.ca/PDF/Standards_for_Nursing_Practice_April_07.pdf

Bannock, G., Baxter, R., & Davis, E. (2003) *Dictionary of economics.* New York: Bloomberg Press.

Benner, P. (1984). *From novice to expert: Excellence and power in clinical nursing practice.* Menlo Park, CA: Addison-Wesley.

Benner, P., & Wrubel, J. (1989). *The primacy of caring.* Menlo Park, CA: Addison-Wesley.

Beverage, P. A. (2004). How LPNs can be part of the solution. *North Carolina Medical Journal, 65*(2), 96–97.

Bodenheimer, T. S., & Grumbach, K. (2005). *Understanding health policy: A clinical approach* (4th ed.). Stamford, CT: Appleton and Lange.

Bright, M. A. (2002). *Holistic health and healing.* Philadelphia: F. A. Davis.

Brush, B. L., & Capezuti, E. (2001). Historical analysis of siderail use in American hospitals. *Journal of Nursing Scholarship, 33*(4), 381–385.

Brush, B., Lynaugh, G., Boschman, A., et al. (1999). *Nurses of all nations: A history of the International Council of Nurses, 1899–1999.* Hagerstown, MD: Lippincott Williams & Wilkins.

Buerhaus, P. I. (1997). How changes in payment systems are affecting nurses. In: J. C. McCloskey & H. K. Grace (Eds.), *Current issues in nursing* (5th ed.). St. Louis, MO: C.V. Mosby.

Bureau of Labor Statistics, U.S. Department of Labor. (last modified August 4, 2006). *Occupational outlook handbook, 2006–2007 edition: Licensed practical and licensed vocational nurses.* Retrieved November 8, 2007, from http://www.bls.gov/oco/ocos102.htm

Bureau of Labor Statistics, U.S. Department of Labor. (2006). *Occupational outlook handbook, 2006–2007 edition: Registered nurses.* Retrieved November 8, 2007, from http://www.bls.gov/oco/ocos083.htm

Canadian Institute for Health Information (CIHI). (2006). Regulated nursing workforce: Highlights from the regulated nursing workforce in Canada, 2006. Ottawa: CIHI. Retrieved December 1, 2007, from http://www.cihi.ca/cihiweb/dispPage.jsp?cw_page=PG_970_E&cw_topic=970&cw_rel=AR_1173_E

Canadian Nurses Association (CNA). (1987). *A definition of nursing practice. Standards for nursing practice.* Ottawa: Author.

Canadian Nurses Association (CNA). (1993). *The scope of nursing practice: A review of issues and trends.* Ottawa: Author.

Capezuti, E. E., Wagner, L., Brush, B., et al. (2007). Consequences of an intervention to reduce restrictive side rail use in nursing homes. *Journal of the American Geriatrics Society, 55*(3), 334–341.

Carnegie, M. E. (1995). *The path we tread: Blacks in nursing 1854–1994* (3rd ed.). New York: National League for Nursing.

Centers for Disease Control and Prevention (CDC), National Center for Health Statistics. (2007). Early release of selected estimates based on data from the 2006 National Health Interview Survey (released June 25, 2007). Retrieved December 8, 2007, from http://www.cdc.gov/nchs/about/major/nhis/released200706.htm#1

Centers for Disease Control and Prevention (CDC), National Center for Health Statistics. (2004). Nursing home care. Retrieved December 8, 2007, from http://www.cdc.gov.nchs/fastats/nursing.htm

Chambers, P. (1958). *A doctor alone: A biography of Elizabeth Blackwell, the first woman doctor.* London: Abelard-Schuman.

Christy, T. (1975). The methodology of historical research: A brief foundation. *Nursing Research, 24*(3), 189–192.

College & Association of Registered Nurses of Alberta. (2005). Nursing practice standards. Retrieved November 8, 2007, from https://www.nurses.ab.ca/Carna-Admin/Uploads/Nursing%20Practice%20Standards.pdf

College of Nurses of Ontario. (1996). *Professional standards for registered nurses and Registered practical nurses in Ontario.* Toronto: Author.

College of Registered Nurses of Nova Scotia. (2004). Standards for nursing practice. Halifax, NS: Author. Retrieved November 4, 2007, from http://www.crnns.ca/documents/standards2004.pdf

Critical Care (2007, July 21). Low hospital staff levels increase infection rates. Adapted by *Science Daily* from materials retrieved from *Critical Care.* Retrieved December 8, 2007, from http://www.sciencedaily.com/releases/2007/07/070719115825.htm

Cronenwett, L., Sherwood, G., Barnsteiner, J., et al. (2007). Quality and safety education for nurses. *Nursing Outlook, 55*(3), 122–131.

Curran, C. (1997). The future of academic health centers in a cost-driven market. In: J. C. McCloskey & H. K. Grace (Eds.), *Current issues in nursing* (5th ed.). St. Louis, MO: C. V. Mosby.

D'Antonio, P., Baer, E., Lynaugh, J., et al. (2006). *Nurses' work.* New York: Springer.

Darcé, K. (2007, November). Are retail clinics a healthy choice? Outlets opening in county could fill niche; physicians warn of drawbacks. *The San Diego Union-Tribune.* Retrieved November 8, 2007, from http://www.signonsandiego.com/news/business/20071107-9999-1n7clinics.html

Dietz, L. D., & Lehozky, A. R. (1967). *History and modern nursing.* Philadelphia: F.A. Davis.

Disch, J., Bellman, G., & Ingbar, D. (2001). Medical directors as partners in creating healthy work environments. *AACN Clinical Issues, 12*(3), 366–377.

Dock, L. L., & Stewart, I. M. (1938). *A short history of nursing* (4th ed.). New York: Putnam.

Donahue, M. P. (1985). *Nursing: The finest art. An illustrated history.* St. Louis, MO: C. V. Mosby.

Donaldson, S. K., & Crowley, D. (1978). The discipline of nursing. *Nursing Outlook, 26*(2), 113–120.

Dossey, B., Selanders, L., Beck, D., et al. (2005). *Florence Nightingale today: Healing, leadership, global action.* Washington, DC: Nursesbooks.org

Fuchs, V. R. (1998). *The future of health policy.* Cambridge, MA: Harvard University Press.

Griffin, G. J., & Griffin, J. K. (1973). *History & trends of professional nursing* (7th ed.). St. Louis, MO: C.V. Mosby.

Hadley, F., Graham, K., & Flannery, M. (2004). Workforce management, objective A: Workload measurement tools. Retrieved December 1, 2007, from http://www.cna-aiic.ca/CNA/documents/pdf/publications/Workload_Measurement_Tools_e.pdf

Health Care Financing Agency. (1998). National health expenditures projections:1998–2008.www.hcfa.gov/stats/nhe%2Dproj/proj1998/hilites.htm

Health Resources and Services Administration. (2004). Supply, demand, and use of licensed practical nurses. Washington, DC: U.S. Department of Health and Human Services, Bureau of Health Professions. Retrieved December 1, 2007, from http://bhpr.hrsa.gov/healthworkforce/reports/nursing/lpn/c7.htm

Health Resources and Services Administration. (2004). The registered nurse population: Findings from the March 2004 national sample survey of registered nurses. Washington, DC: U.S. Department of Health and Human Services, Bureau of Health Professions. Retrieved December 1, 2007, from http://bhpr.hrsa.gov/healthworkforce/rnsurvey04/

Henderson, V. (1966). *The nature of nursing.* New York: Macmillan.

Hicks, L. L., & Boles, K. E. (1984). Why health economics? *Nursing Economic$, 2*(3), 175–180.

Hobbs, F. (2001). The elderly population. U.S. Census Bureau. Retrieved December 7, 2007, from http://www.census.gov/population/www/pop-profile/elderpop.html

Huntington, J. A. (1997). Glossary for managed care. *Online Journal of Issues in Nursing.* www.nursingworld/ojin/tpc2_gls.htm

International Council of Nurses. (2007). ICN definition of nursing. Retrieved December 1, 2007, from http://www.icn.ch/definition.htm

Jameton, A. (1984). *Nursing practice: The ethical issues.* Englewood Cliffs, NJ: Prentice-Hall.

The Joint Commission (TJC). (2006). *2006 Hospital accreditation standards.* Retrieved December 1, 2007, from http://www.jointcommission.org/NR/rdonlyres/F42AF828–7248–48C0–B4E6–BA18E719A87C/0/06_hap_accred_stds.pdf

Jonas, S., & Kovner, A. R. (2005). *Health care delivery in the U.S.* (8th ed.). New York: Springer.

Kalisch, B., & Kalisch, P. (1995). *The advance of American nursing* (3rd ed.). Philadelphia: J. B. Lippincott.

Kane, R., Shamliyan, T., Mueller, C., et al. (2007). The association of registered nurse staffing levels and patient outcomes: Systematic review and meta-analysis. *Medical Care, 45*(12), 1195–1204.

Landon, B., Normand, S., Lessler, A., et al. (2006). Quality of care for the treatment of acute medical conditions in U.S. hospitals. *Archives of Internal Medicine, 166,* 2511–2517.

Laugesen, M., & Rice, T. (2003). Is the doctor in? The evolving role of organized medicine in health policy. *Journal of Health Politics, Policy and Law, 28*(2–3), 289–316.

Mahaffey, E. H. (2002). The relevance of associate degree nursing education: Past, present, future. *Online Journal of Issues in Nursing, 7*(2), 3.

Meadus, R. J. (2000). Men in nursing: Barriers to recruitment. *Nursing Forum, 35*(3), 5.

Meleis, A. I. (1991). *Theoretical nursing: Development and progress.* Philadelphia: J. B. Lippincott.

National Association for Practical Nursing Education and Service, Inc. (2004). Licensed practical/vocational nurses standards of practice. Retrieved December 6, 2007, from http://www.napnes.org/about/standards.pdf

National League for Nursing. (2008). *Nursing data review 2005–2006.* New York: Author.

Nelson, M. (2002). Education for professional nursing practice: Looking backward into the future. *Online Journal of Issues in Nursing, 7*(2).

Nightingale, F. (1860). *Notes on nursing: What it is, and what it is not.* New York: D. Appleton and Company.

Nightingale, F. (1876). *Notes on Nursing for the Labouring Classes.* London: Harrison.

Northwest Territories Registered Nurses Association. (2006). Standards of practice for registered nurses. Retrieved December 1, 2007, from http://www.rnantnu.ca/Portals/0/Documents/Standards_Nrsing_Prac_2006.pdf

Nothrup, D. T., Tschanz, C. L., Olynyk, K. L. S., et al. (2004). Nursing: Whose discipline is it anyway? *Nursing Science Quarterly, 17*(1), 55–62.

Nurses Association of New Brunswick. (2005). Standards of practice for registered nurses. Fredericton, NB: Author. Retrieved November 5, 2007, from http://www.nanb.nb.ca/pdf_e/Publications/General_Publications/StandardsofRegisteredNursesE.pdf

Nurseweek. CE requirements by state. Copyright 2007 Gannett Healthcare Group. Retrieved December 7, 2007, from http://www.nurse.com/ce/Requirements.html

Office of National Cost Estimates. (2000). Revisions to the national health accounts and methodology. *Health Care Financing Review*, 11(4), 42–54. HCFA Pub. No. 03298. Office of Research and Demonstrations. Health Care Financing Administration. Washington, DC: U.S. Government Printing Office.

Parse, R. R. (1999). Nursing: The discipline and the profession. *Nursing Science Quarterly*, 12(4), 275–276.

Pew Health Professions Commission. (1995). *Critical challenges: Revitalizing the health professions for the twenty-first century* (3rd report). Durham, NC: Author.

Pew Health Professions Commission. (1998). *Twenty-one competencies for the twenty-first century.* Durham, NC: Author.

Potera, C. (2007). In the news. Infections and deaths down, quality up. *American Journal of Nursing*, 107(4), 19.

Pullen, R. L., Jr. (2006). Why choose nursing education? *Men in Nursing*, 1(5), 36–39.

Quadagno, J. S. (2004). Physician sovereignty and the purchasers' revolt. *Journal of Health Politics, Policy and Law*, 29(4), 815–834.

Rasmussen, E. (2001). Picture imperfect. *Nurseweek*, May 7, 2001, pp. 1–3.

Registered Nurses Association of British Columbia. (2003). Standards for registered nursing practice in British Columbia. *Nursing BC*, October 2003. Retrieved November 5, 2007, from http://findarticles.com/p/articles/mi_qa3916/is_200310/ai_n9318871

Registered Nurses Association of the Northwest Territories and Nunavut. (2006). Standards of nursing practice for registered nurses. Yellowknife, NT: Author. Retrieved November 1, 2007, from http://www.rnantnu.ca/Portals/0/Documents/Standards_Nrsing_Prac_2006.pdf

Registered Nurses Association of Nova Scotia. (2004). Standards for nursing practice. Halifax, NS: Author. Retrieved October 30, 2007, from http://www.crnns.ca/documents/standards2004.pdf

Reverby, S. (1987). *Ordered to care: The dilemma of American nursing 1850–1945.* New York: Cambridge University Press.

Rockwell, L. H., Jr. (1994). The American Medical Association: A sordid history. Retrieved December 5, 2007, from http://www.healthelivingnews.com/articles/american_medical_association_sorbid_history.html

Rosenberg, C. (1987). *The care of strangers.* New York: Basic Books.

Safriet, B. J. (1994). Impediments to progress in healthcare work-force policy: License and practice laws. *Inquiry*, 31(3), 310–317.

Schorr, T., & Kennedy, M. S. (1999). *100 years of American nursing: Celebrating a century of caring.* Hagerstown, MD: Lippincott Williams & Wilkins.

Shapiro, S. E. (2002). Viewpoint: In favor of the bachelor's degree. *AJN*, 102(10), 11.

Starr, P. (1982). *The social transformation of American medicine.* New York: Basic Books.

Sterchi, S. (2007, July). Perceptions that affect physician-nurse collaboration in the perioperative setting. *AORN Journal.* Retrieved November 6, 2007, from http://findarticles.com/p/articles/mi_m0FSL/is_1_86/ai_n19448209/pg_1

Stewart, I. M., & Austin, A. L. (1962). *A history of nursing* (5th ed.). New York: G. P. Putnam's Sons.

Takase, M., Kershaw, E., & Burt, L. (2002). Does public image of nurses matter? *Journal of Professional Nursing*, 18(4), 196–205.

Thomka, L. A. (2001). Graduate nurses' experiences of interactions with professional nursing staff during transition to the professional role. *Journal of Continuing Education in Nursing*, 32(1),15–19.

Tourangeau, A., Doran, D., Hall, L., et al. (2007). Impact of hospital nursing care on 30-day mortality for acute medical patients. *Journal of Advanced Nursing*, 57(1), 32–44.

U.S. Census Bureau (last modified May 31, 2007). U.S. interim projections by age, sex, race, and Hispanic origin. Summary tables. Retrieved December 7, 2007, from http://www.census.gov/ipc/www/usinterimproj/

U.S. Census Bureau (2008). U.S. Census Bureau News. Released May 1, 2008. Retrieved June 26, 2008, from http://www.census.gov/Press-Release/www/releases/archives/population/011910.html

U.S. Department of Commerce, International Trade Administration. (2002). Health and medical services. In *U.S. Industrial Outlook 2002.* Washington, DC: Author.

U.S. Department of Health and Human Services (USDHHS). (2003). *Healthy People 2010.* Retrieved June 7, 2008, from http://dhhs.gov

U.S. Department of Health and Human Services (USDHHS). (2007). Annual update of the HHS poverty guidelines. Retrieved June 30, 2008, from http://aspe.hhs.gov/poverty/07poverty.shtml

Venes, D. (2009). *Taber's cyclopedic medical dictionary* (21st ed.). Philadelphia: F. A. Davis.

Watson, J. (1981). Socialization of the nursing student in a professional nursing education programme. *Nursing Papers*, 13, 19–24.

White, W. D. (1990). The "corporatization" of U.S. hospitals: What can we learn from the nineteenth century industrial experience?" *International Journal of Health Services*, 20, 85–113.

Wilkinson, J. M. (1996). The C word: A curriculum for the future. *N&HC: Perspectives on Community*, 17(2), 72–77.

World Health Organization (WHO). (1984). Health promotion: A discussion document on the concepts and principles. Geneva, Switzerland: Author.

World Health Organization (WHO). (2007). Frequently Asked Questions. *Preamble to the Constitution of the World Health Organization* as adopted by the International Health Conference, New York, June 19–July 22, 1946; signed on July 22 by the representatives of 62 States (Official Records of the World Health Organization, no. 2, p. 100) and entered into force on April 7, 1948. Retrieved November 8, 2007, from http://www.who.int/suggestions/faq/en/

Zwarenstein, M., & Reeves, S. (2002). Working together but apart: Barriers and routes to nurse-physician collaboration. *Joint Commission Journal of Quality Improvement*, 28(5).

Chapter 2

Alberta Association of Registered Nurses. (2003). *Nursing: Scope and standards of practice.* Retrieved January 12, 2007, from http://www.nurses.ab.ca/Carna-Admin/Uploads/Nursing%20Practice%20Standards_1.pdf

American Nurses Association (ANA). (2010). *Nursing: Scope and standards of practice* (2nd ed.). Public Comment draft, January 2010. Silver Spring, MD: Nursebooks.org Retrieved February 1, 2010, from http://www.nursingworld.org/DocumentVault/NursingPractice/Draft-Nursing-Scope-Standards-2nd-Ed.aspx

American Philosophical Association. (1990). *Executive summary of: Critical thinking: A statement of expert consensus for purposes of educational assessment.* Millbrae, CA: The California Academic Press.

Assessment Technologies Institute. (2003). Critical thinking assessment developmental and statistical manual. Overland Park, KS: Assessment Technologies Institute.

Broadbear, J. T., & Keyser, B. B. (2000). An approach to teaching for critical thinking in health education. *Journal of School Health*, 70(8), 322–326.

Brookfield, S. D. (1991). *Developing critical thinkers.* San Francisco: Jossey-Bass.

Burton, A. J. (2000). Reflection: Nursing's practice and education panacea? *Journal of Advanced Nursing*, 31I(5), 1009–1017.

Canadian Nurses Association (CNA). (1987). *CNA: A definition of nursing practice: Standards for nursing practice.* Ottawa: Author.

Daly, W. M. (2001). The development of an alternative method in the assessment of critical thinking as an outcome of nursing education. *Journal of Advanced Nursing*, 36(1), 120–130.

Ellis, E. B., & Miller, D. A. (2004). Infusing critical thinking into health education. *Academic Exchange Quarterly.* Retrieved January 13, 2008, from http://goliath.ecnext.com/coms2/gi_0199–3541166/Infusing-critical-thinking-into-health.html

Ennis, R. H. (2006). A Super-streamlined conception of critical thinking. Retrieved January 13, 2008, from http://faculty.ed.uluc.edu/rhennis/

Facione, P. A., & Facione, N. C. (2007). *Thinking and reasoning in human decision making: The method of argument and heuristic analysis.* Millbrae, CA: The California Academic Press LLC.

Frauman, A. C., & Skelly, A. H. (1999). Evolution of the nursing process. *Clinical Excellence in Nursing Practice, 3*(4), 238–244.

Girot, E. A. (2000). Graduate nurses: Critical thinkers or better decision makers? *Journal of Advanced Nursing, 31*(2), 288–297.

Greenwood, J. (2000). Critical thinking and nursing scripts: The case for the development of both. *Journal of Advanced Nursing, 31*(2), 428–436.

Haladyna, T. M. (2004). *Developing & validating multiple choice test items.* New York: Routledge.

Heaslip, P. (1992). Creating the thinking practitioner: Critical thinking in clinical practice. Unpublished manuscript. (ERIC Document Reproduction Service No. ED 354 822).

Hicks, F. D. (2001). Research issues. Critical thinking: Toward a nursing science perspective. *Nursing Science Quarterly, 14*(1), 14–21.

Johns, C., & Freshwater, D. (2005). *Transforming nursing through reflective practice.* Malden, MA: Blackwell.

Lipe, S., & Beasley, S. (2003). *Critical thinking in nursing: A cognitive skills workbook.* Philadelphia: Lippincott Williams & Wilkins.

McDonald, M. E. (2002). *Systematic assessment of learning outcomes: Developing multiple-choice exams.* Boston: Jones and Bartlett.

Miller, L., & Connelly, M. (1996). *Critical thinking core concepts.* (Critical Thinking Across The Curriculum Project). Lee's Summit, Missouri: Longview Community College.

Moore, B. N., & Parker, R. (2009). *Critical thinking* (9th ed.). Columbus, OH: McGraw-Hill.

NANDA International. (2007). *NANDA nursing diagnoses: definitions & classification, 2005–2007.* Philadelphia: Author.

Parker, R. (2005). *Critical thinking* (8th ed.). Columbus, OH: McGraw-Hill.

Paul, R. W. (1990). *Critical thinking.* Rohnert Park, CA: The Center for Critical Thinking and Moral Critique, Sonoma State University.

Paul, R. W. (1993). *Critical thinking: What every person needs to survive in a rapidly changing world* (3rd ed.). Santa Rosa, CA: Foundation for Critical Thinking.

Paul, R. W., & Elder, L. (2002). *Critical thinking: Tools for taking charge of your professional and personal life.* Upper Saddle River, NJ: Financial Times Prentice-Hall.

Paul, R. W., Ennis, R. H., & Norris, S. (1996). In: B. Fowler, *Critical thinking definitions.* (Critical Thinking Across The Curriculum Project). Lee's Summit, Missouri: Longview Community College.

Profetto-McGrath, J., Hesketh, K. L., Lang, S., et al. (2003). A study of critical thinking and research utilization among nurses. *Western Journal of Nursing Research, 25*(3), 322–337.

Raingruber, B., & Haffer, A. (2001). *Using your head to land on your feet.* Philadelphia: F. A. Davis.

Registered Nurses Association of British Columbia. (2003). *Standards for nursing practice in British Colombia.* Retrieved October 30, 2007, from http://findarticles.com/p/articles/mi_qa3916/is_200310/ai_n9318871

Simpson, E., & Courtney, M. D. (2002). Critical thinking in nursing education: A literature review. *International Journal of Nursing Practice, 8*(April), 89–98.

Smith, K. V., & Godfrey, N. S. (2002). Being a good nurse and doing the right thing: A qualitative study. *Nursing Ethics, 9*(3), 301–312.

Smith-Blair, N., & Neighbors, M. (2000). Use of the Critical Thinking Disposition Inventory in critical care orientation. *Journal of Continuing Education in Nursing, 31*(6), 251–256.

Stahl, N., & Stahl, R. (1991). We can agree after all! Achieving consensus for a critical thinking component of a gifted program using the Delphi Technique. *Roeper Review, 14*(2), 79–88.

Swanson, K. M. (1990). Providing care in the NICU: Sometimes an act of love. *Advances in Nursing, 13*, 60–73.

Taft, S. H., & White, J. (2007). Ethics education: Using inductive reasoning to develop individual, group, organizational, and global perspectives. *Journal of Management Education, 31*(5), 614–646.

Tanner, C. A. (2000). Critical thinking: Beyond nursing process. *Journal of Nursing Education, 39*(8), 338–339.

Wilkinson, J. M. (2007). *Nursing process & critical thinking* (4th ed.). Upper Saddle River, NJ, Prentice-Hall.

Chapter 3

Acute Pain Management Guideline Panel (1992). *Acute pain management in adults: operative procedures, quick reference guide for clinicians* (AHCPR Publication No. 92-0019). Rockdale, MD: Author.

American Nurses Association (ANA). (2001) *Code of Ethics for Nurses – Provisions* [Electronic version, page updated 2008]. Retrieved February 20, 2008, from http://nursingworld.org/MainMenuCategories/ThePracticeofProfessionalNursing/EthicsStandards.aspx

American Nurses Association (ANA). (2010). *Nursing: Scope and standards of practice* (2nd ed.). Public Comment draft, January 2010. Silver Spring, MD: Nursebooks.org Retrieved February 1, 2010, from http://www.nursingworld.org/DocumentVault/NursingPractice/Draft-Nursing-Scope-Standards-2nd-Ed.aspx

Carnevali, D. L., & Thomas, M. D. (1993). *Diagnostic reasoning and treatment decision making in nursing.* Philadelphia: J. B. Lippincott.

College & Association of Registered Nurses of Alberta. (2003). *Nursing practice: Professional conduct: Nursing practice standards.* Retrieved January 17, 2008, from https://www.nurses.ab.ca/Carna-Admin/Uploads/Nursing%20Practice%20Standards_1.pdf

Cronenwett, L., Sherwood, G., Barnsteiner, J., et al. (2007). Quality and safety education for nurses. *Nursing Outlook, 55*(3), 122–131.

Dochterman, J. M., & Jones, D. A. (Eds.). (2003). Unifying nursing languages: The harmonization of NANDA, NIC, and NOC. Washington, DC: American Nurses Association, Nursesbooks.org

Galanti, G. A. (2004). *Caring for patients from different cultures* (3rd ed.). Philadelphia: University of Pennsylvania Press.

Giger, J. N., & Davidhizar, R. E. (2008). *Transcultural nursing: Assessment and intervention* (5th ed.). St. Louis, MO: C. V. Mosby.

Gordon, M. (1994). *Analysis/ Nursing Diagnosis: Process and application* (3rd ed., p. 70). St. Louis, MO: C. V. Mosby.

Gorman, L. M., Raines, M. L., & Sultan, D. F. (2008). *Psychosocial nursing for general patient care* (3rd ed.). Philadelphia: F. A. Davis.

Graf, C. (2008). How to try this: The Lawton Instrumental Activities of Daily Living Scale. *American Journal of Nursing, 108*(4), 52–62.

The Joint Commission (TJC). (2008). *Hospital accreditation standards.* Oakbrook Terrace, IL: Author.

Karnofsky, D. A., & Burchenal, J. H. (1949). The clinical evaluation of chemotherapeutic agents in cancer. In: C. M. MacLeod (Ed.), *Evaluation of chemotherapeutic agents.* New York: Columbia University Press. (Classic) Retrieved January 18, 2008, from http://www.acsu.buffalo.edu/~drstall/assessmenttools.html, last updated November 13, 2006.

Katz, S., Ford, A. B., Moskowitz, R. W., et al. (1963). Studies of illness in the aged. The Index of the ADL: A standardized measure of biological and psychosocial function. *JAMA, 185*, 914–919.

Lawton, M. P. (1969). *Lawton instrumental activities of daily living.* The Philadelphia Geriatric Center, Philadelphia. Retrieved January 18, 2008, from http://www.acsu.buffalo.edu/~drstall/assessmenttools.html, last updated November 13, 2006.

Maslow, A. (1970). *Motivation and personality* (2nd ed.). New York: Harper & Row.

Maslow, A., & Lowery, R. (Eds.). (1998). *Toward a psychology of being* (3rd ed.). New York: Wiley & Sons.

McCaffery, M., & Pasero, C. (1999). *Pain clinical manual* (2nd ed.). St. Louis, MO: C. V. Mosby.

NANDA International. (2007). *Nursing diagnoses: definitions & classification 2007–2008.* Philadelphia: NANDA International.

National Council of State Boards of Nursing (NCSBN). (1997). Delegation decision-making grid. Retrieved March 6, 2003, from http://nursingworld.org/snas/ia/grid.htm

National Council of State Boards of Nursing (NCSBN). (2007). *Model nursing practice act.* Retrieved January 18, 2008, from https://www.ncsbn.org/312.htm

Orem, D. (1991). *Nursing: Concepts of practice* (4th ed., p. 126). St. Louis, MO: C. V. Mosby-Year Book.

Pender, N. J., Murdaugh, C. L., & Parsons, M. A. (2006). *Health promotion in nursing practice* (5th ed.). Upper Saddle River, NJ: Prentice-Hall.

Purnell, L. D., & Paulanka, B. J. (2008). *Transcultural health care: A culturally competent approach* (3rd ed.). Philadelphia: F. A. Davis.

Roy, C., & Andrews, H. (1991). *The Roy adaptation model: The definitive statement* (pp. 15–17). Norwalk, CT: Appleton & Lange.

Spector, R. E. (2003). *Cultural diversity in health and illness* (6th ed.). Upper Saddle River, NJ: Prentice-Hall.

Spector, R. E. (2004). Cultural care: Guides to heritage assessment and health traditions (3rd ed.). Upper Saddle River, NJ: Prentice-Hall.

Stewart, M. J. (1993). *Integrating social support in nursing*. Newbury Park, CA: Sage.

Wallace, M., & Shelkey, M. (2007). Katz index of independence in activities of daily living (ADL). *Try This: Best Practices in Nursing Care to Older Adults*. Issue No. 2. From The Hartford Institute of Geriatric Nursing, New York University, College of Nursing. Retrieved January 18, 2008, from http://www.hartfordign.org/publications/trythis//issue02.pdf

Wilkinson, J. M. (2007). *Nursing process & critical thinking* (4th ed.). Upper Saddle River, NJ: Prentice-Hall.

Williams, S. R., & Schlenker, E. D. (2003). *Essentials of nutrition and diet therapy* (8th ed.). St. Louis, MO: C. V. Mosby.

Chapter 4

Abdellah, F. (1957). Methods of identifying covert aspects of nursing problems. *Nursing Research, 6*(1), 4–23.

American Medical Association (AMA). (2010). *Current procedural terminology: CPT 2010. Professional edition.* Chicago: Author.

American Nurses Association (ANA). (1980). *ANA social policy statement.* Washington, DC: Author.

American Nurses Association (ANA). (2003b). *Nursing's social policy statement* (2nd ed.). Washington, DC: Author.

American Nurses Association (ANA). (2006). ANA recognized terminologies and data element sets. Nursing Practice Information Infrastructure. Retrieved March 14, 2008, from http://nursingworld.org/npii/terminologies.htm

American Nurses Association (ANA). (2010). *Nursing: Scope and standards of practice* (2nd ed.). Public Comment draft, January 2010. Silver Spring, MD: Nursebooks.org Retrieved February 1, 2010, from http://www.nursingworld.org/DocumentVault/Nursing-Practice/Draft-Nursing-Scope-Standards-2nd-Ed.aspx

American Philosophical Association (1990). Executive summary of: Critical thinking: A statement of expert consensus for purposes of educational assessment. Millbrae, CA: The California Academic Press.

American Psychiatric Association. (2000). *Diagnostic and statistical manual of mental disorders.* Arlington, VA: American Psychiatric Publishing.

Barton, A. J., Gilbert, L., Erickson, V., et al. (2003, May/June). A guide to assist nurse practitioners with standardized nursing language. *CIN: Computers, Informatics, Nursing, 21*(3), 128–133.

Bates, D. W., Ebell, M., Gotlieb, E., et al. (2003). A proposal for electronic medical records in U.S. primary care. *Journal of the American Medical Informatics Association, 10*(1), 1–10.

Beyea, S. (2000, May). Standardized nursing vocabularies and the perioperative nursing data set: Making clinical practice count. *CIN plus, 3(2)*, 1, 5, 6.

Beyea, S. (1999, November). Standardized language-making nursing practice count. *AORN Journal, 70*(5), 831–832, 834, 837, 838.

Carpenito, L. J. (2006). *Nursing diagnosis: Application to clinical practice* (11th ed.). Philadelphia: J. B. Lippincott.

College & Association of Registered Nurses of Alberta. (2005). *Nursing practice standards.* Retrieved December 8, 2007, from https://www.nurses.ab.ca/Carna-Admin/Uploads/Nursing%20Practice%20Standards.pdf

Cosgrove, L. (2006). When labels mask oppression: Implications for teaching psychiatric taxonomy to mental health counselors. *Journal of Mental Health Counseling, 27*(4), 283–296.

Craft-Rosenberg, M. (1999). NDEC guidelines for development and evaluation of diagnoses. *Nursing Diagnosis, 10*(2), 84–85.

Delaney, C., Herr, K., Maas, M., et al. (2000). Reliability of nursing diagnoses documented in a computerized nursing information system. *Nursing Diagnosis, 11*(3), 121–134.

Fry, V. (1953). The creative approach to nursing. *American Journal of Nursing 98*(6), 44–47.

Gebbie, K. (1976). Development of a taxonomy of nursing diagnosis. In: J. Walter, J. Walter, D. P. Pardee, & D. M. Molbo, *Dynamics of problem-oriented approaches: Patient care and documentation.* Philadelphia: J. B. Lippincott.

Gordon, M. (1994). *Nursing diagnosis: Process and application* (3rd ed.). St. Louis, MO: C. V. Mosby.

Green, P. M., & Slade, D. S. (2001). Environmental nursing diagnoses for aggregates and community. *Nursing Diagnosis, 12*(1), 5–13.

Henderson, V. (1964). The nature of nursing. *American Journal of Nursing, 64*(8), 62–68.

International Council of Nurses. (2005). *International classification for nursing practice.* ISBN: 92-95040-36-8 ICNP® version 1.0. Geneva, Switzerland: ICN

Johnson, M. (2002, January/March). Criteria for standardized nursing language. *Outcomes Management, 6*(1),1–3.

Johnson, M., Bulechek, G., Dochterman, J. M., et al. (2006). *Nursing diagnoses, outcomes, and interventions: NANDA, NOC, and NIC linkage* (2nd ed.). St. Louis, MO: C. V. Mosby.

Lunney, M. (2008). Critical need to address accuracy of nurses' diagnoses. *Online Journal of Issues in Nursing, 13.*

Maslow, A. H. (1970). *Motivation and personality* (2nd ed.). New York: Harper & Row.

Maslow, A. (1971). *The farther reaches of human nature.* New York: The Viking Press.

Maslow, A., & Lowery, R. (Eds.). (1998). *Toward a psychology of being* (3rd ed.). New York: Wiley & Sons.

Müller-Staub, M., Lavin, M. A., Needham, I., et al. (2006). Nursing diagnoses, interventions and outcomes—application and impact on nursing practice: Systematic review. *Journal of Advanced Nursing, 56*(5j), 514–531.

NANDA International. (2009). *NANDA Nursing diagnoses: definitions & classification 2009–2011.* Philadelphia: NANDA International,

Nurses Association of New Brunswick. (2005). *Standards of practice for registered nurses.* Fredericton, NB: Author. Retrieved December 8, 2007, from http://www.nanb.nb.ca/pdf_e/Publications/General_Publications/StandardsofRegisteredNursesE.pdf

Ollson, P. T., & Gardulf, A. (2006). Nurses and head nurses views of nursing diagnoses at a geriatric clinic. *Journal of Clinical Nursing, 15*(10), 1338–1339.

Parris, K. M., Place, P. J., Orellana, E., et al. (1999). Integrating nursing diagnoses, interventions, and outcomes in public health nursing practice. *Nursing Diagnosis, 10*(2), 49–56.

Smith, H. K., & Donald, J. G. (2002, April). Thinking processes used by nurses in clinical decision making. *Journal of Nursing Education. 41*(4), 145–153.

Wilkinson, J. M. (2007). *Nursing process and critical thinking* (4th ed.). Upper Saddle River, NJ: Prentice-Hall.

World Health Organization (WHO). (1992). *Manual of the international classification of diseases and related health problems* (10th rev. ed.). Geneva, Switzerland: WHO.

Chapter 5

Agency for Health Care Policy and Research. (1993). *Clinical practice guideline development, AHCPR program note.* AHCPR Publication Number 93–0023. Last modified July 31, 1995. Washington, DC: Author.

Agency for Health Care Policy and Research. (1998). Invitation to submit guidelines to the National Guideline Clearinghouse™. *Federal Register, 63*(70), 18027. Retrieved March 12, 2008, from http://www.ahrq.gov/fund/ngcguidl.htm

American Medical Association (AMA). (2008). *CPT® 2008 professional edition.* Chicago: AMA Press.

American Nurses Association (ANA). (2010). *Nursing: Scope and standards of practice* (2nd ed.). Public Comment draft, January 2010. Silver Spring, MD: Nursebooks.org Retrieved February 1, 2010, from http://www.nursingworld.org/DocumentVault/NursingPractice/Draft-Nursing-Scope-Standards-2nd-Ed.aspx

American Nurses Association (ANA). (2006). *ANA recognized terminologies and data element sets.* Retrieved March 13, 2008, from http://www.nursingworld.org/npli/terminologies.htm

American Nurses Association (ANA)/Nursing Information & Data Set Evaluation Center. (2008). Nursing Information & Data Set Evaluation Center, American Nurses Association, Nursing World. Retrieved March 12, 2008, from http://www.nursingworld.org/MainMenuCategories/ThePracticeofProfessionalNursing/DocInfo/NIDSEC.aspx

Beyea, S. (2000). Standardized nursing vocabularies and the perioperative nursing data set: Making clinical practice count. *Computers in Nursing, 3*(2), 1, 5, 6.

Bonaiuto, M. M. (2007). School nurse case management: Achieving health and educational outcomes. *Journal of School Nursing, 23*(4), 202–209.

Bulechek, G., Butcher, H., & Dochterman, J. M. (2008). *Nursing intervention classification (NIC)* (5th ed.). St. Louis, MO: C. V. Mosby.

Bull, M. J., Hansen, H. E., & Gross, C. R. (2000). Differences in family caregiver outcomes by their level of involvement in discharge planning. *Applied Nursing Research, 13*(2), 76–82.

College & Association of Registered Nurses of Alberta. (2005). Nursing practice standards. 11620 168th Street, Edmonton, AB, Canada, T5M 4A6.

College of Registered Nurses of Nova Scotia. (2003). Standards for nursing practice. 600-1894 Barrington Street, Halifax, NS, Canada.

Greenwald, J. L., Denham, C. R., & Jack, B. W. (2007). The hospital discharge: A review of a high risk care transition with highlights of a reengineered discharge process. *Journal of Patient Safety, 3*(2), 97–106.

Harris, B. L. (1990). Becoming deprofessionalized: One aspect of the staff nurse's perspective on computer-mediated nursing care plans. *Advances in Nursing Science, 13*(2), 63–74.

Head, B., Maas, M., & Johnson, M. (1997). Outcomes for home and community nursing in integrated delivery systems. *Caring, 16*(1), 50–56.

Healthy People 2020. (2010). Washington, DC: U.S. Department of Health and Human Services. Retrieved January 10, 2010, from http://www.healthypeople.gov/hp2020/Objectives/framework.aspx

Hunt, S. (2008). Data management in home care: Using data to drive acute care hospitalization. *Home Health Care Management & Practice, 20*(2), 175–179.

Johnson, M., Bulechek, G., Butcher, H., et al. (2006). *Nursing diagnoses, outcomes, and interventions: NANDA, NOC, and NIC linkage* (2nd ed.). St. Louis, MO: C. V. Mosby.

Malijanian, R., Effken, J. A., & Kaerhle, P. (2000). Design and implementation of an outcomes management model. *Outcomes Management for Nursing Practice, 4*(1), 19–25.

Martin, K. (2005). *The Omaha System: A key to practice, documentation, and information managementt* (2nd ed.). Philadelphia: W. B. Saunders.

McCloskey, J. C., & Bulechek, G. M. (Eds.). (1992). *Nursing interventions classification (NIC).* St. Louis, MO: C. V. Mosby.

Moorhead, S., Johnson, M., Maas, M., et al. (2008). *Nursing outcomes classification* (4th ed.). St. Louis, MO: C. V. Mosby/Elsevier.

Mueller, A., Johnston, M., & Bligh, D. (2001). Mind-mapped care plans, a remarkable alternative to traditional nursing care plans. *Nurse Educator, 26*(2), 75–80.

Mueller, A., Johnston, M., & Bligh, D. (2002). Viewpoint: Joining mind mapping and care planning to enhance student critical thinking and achieve holistic nursing care. *Nursing Diagnosis: The International Journal of Nursing Language and Classification, 13*(1), 24–27.

Nolan, S. (2008). Nursing M&M reviews: Learning from our outcomes. *RN, 71*(1), 36–40.

NSW Department of Health. (2007). Policy directive. Discharge planning: Responsive standards (revised November 2007). Retrieved March 10, 2008, from http://www.health.nsw.gov.qu/policies

Parlocha, P. K., & Henry, S. G. (1998). The usefulness of the Georgetown Home Health Care Classification system for coding patient problems and nursing interventions in psychiatric home care. *Computers in Nursing, 16*(1), 45–52.

A practical guide to improving patient outcomes. (2000). *Orthopedic Nursing, 19*(Supplement), 22–28.

Rutherford, M. A. (1998). Standardized nursing language: What does it mean for nursing practice? *Online Journal of Issues in Nursing, 3*(2). Retrieved March 13, 2008, from http://www.nursingworld.org/SpecialPages/Search.aspx?SearchMode=1&SearchPhrase=nidsec

Saba, V. K. (1995). Home Health Care Classifications (HHCCs): Nursing diagnoses and nursing interventions. In: *An emerging framework: Data system advances for clinical nursing practice.* ANA Publication No. NP-94. Washington, DC: American Nurses Association (ANA). Retrieved September 1, 2002, from http://www.sabacare.com/nursinginterventions.html

Saba, V. K. (1997). Why the Home Health Care Classification is a recognized nursing nomenclature. *Computers in Nursing, 15*(92), 69–76.

Saba, V. K. (2003). Clinical Care Classification System. Retrieved November 27, 2004, from http://www.sabacare.com

Schuster, P. M. (2000). Concept mapping: Reducing clinical care plan paperwork and increasing learning. *Nurse Educator, 24*(2), 76–81.

Schuster, P. (2008). *Concept mapping: A critical-thinking approach to care planning* (2nd ed.). Philadelphia: F. A. Davis.

Simpson, R. (1998). Setting the informatics standards: An overview of NDISEC's information systems evaluation criteria. *Nursing Economic$,* (September–October), 279–281.

Van Walraven, C., Seth, R., Austin, P. C., et al. (2002). Effect of discharge summary availability during post-discharge visits on hospital readmission. *Journal of General Internal Medicine, 17*(3), 186–192.

Walker, C., Hogstel, M., & Curry, L. (2007). Hospital discharge of older adults. *American Journal of Nursing, 107*(6), 60–71.

Wilkinson, J. M. (2007). *Nursing process & critical thinking* (4th ed.). Upper Saddle River, NJ: Prentice-Hall.

Zander, K. (1998). Historical development of outcomes-based care delivery. *Critical Care Nursing Clinics of North America, 10*(1), 1.

Chapter 6

Acton, G. J., & Winter, M. A. (2002). Interventions for family members caring for an elder with dementia. *Annual Review of Nursing Research, 20,* 149–179.

Agency for Healthcare Research and Quality (2002, August 30). Clinical practice guideline: Pressure ulcers in adults: Prediction and prevention. Skin care and early treatment. Retrieved January 24, 2008, from http://hstat.nlm.nih.gov/hq/Hquest/screen/TextBrowse/t/1030737344857/s/58838

American Medical Association (AMA). (2008). *CPT ® 2008 professional edition.* Chicago: AMA Press.

American Nurses Association/Nursing Information & Data Set Evaluation Center. (2002, January 23). Recognized languages for nursing. Retrieved January 18, 2010, from http://nursingworld.org/MainMenuCategories/ThePracticeofProfessionalNursing/NursingStandards/DocumentationInformatics/NIDSEC/RecognizedLanguagesforursing.aspx

American Nurses Association (ANA). (2010). *Nursing: Scope and standards of practice* (2nd ed.). Public Comment draft, January 2010. Silver Spring, MD: Nursebooks.org Retrieved February 1, 2010, from http://www.nursingworld.org/DocumentVault/NursingPractice/Draft-Nursing-Scope-Standards-2nd-Ed.aspx

Barton, M. B., Miller, T., Wolff, T., et al. (2007). How to read the new recommendation statement: methods update from the U.S. Preventive Services Task Force. Originally published in *Annals of Internal Medicine, 147,* 123–127. Agency for Healthcare Research and Quality, Rockville, MD. http://www.ahrq.gov/clinic/uspstf07/methods/methupd.htm

Bowker, G. C., Star, S. L., & Spasser, M. A. (2001, March). Classifying nursing work. *Online Journal of Issues in Nursing*. Retrieved January 18, 2010, from http://www.nursingworld.org/MainMenuCategories/ANAMarketplace/ANAPeriodicals/OJIN/TableofContents/Volume62001/No2May01/ArticlePreviousTopic/ClassifyingNursingWork.aspx

Bulechek, G. M., Butcher, H. K., & Dochterman, J. C. (2008). *Nursing interventions classification (NIC)* (5th ed.). St. Louis, MO: C. V. Mosby.

Burgener, S. C., & Twigg, P. (2002). Interventions for persons with irreversible dementia. *Annual Review of Nursing Research, 20,* 89–124.

College & Association of Registered Nurses of Alberta. (2003). *Nursing practice standards.* Edmonton, AB: Author.

College of Registered Nurses of Nova Scotia. (2003). *Standards for nursing practice.* Halifax, NS: Author.

Cronenwett, L., Sherwood, G., Barnsteiner, J., et al. (2007). Quality and safety education for nurses. *Nursing Outlook, 55*(3), 122–131. Retrieved February 1, 2008, from http://qsen.org/competencydomains/

Cronenwett, L. R. (2002). Research, practice and policy: Issues in evidence based care. *Online Journal of Issues in Nursing, (7)*2. Retrieved March 23, 2008, from http://www.nursingworld.org/ojin

Dicenso, A., Guyatt, G., & Ciliska, D. (2005). *Evidence-based nursing: A guide to clinical practice.* St. Louis, MO: Elsevier/Mosby.

Evidence-based guidelines. (2002). *Evidence-Based Practice, 5*(2), 12, insert 2p.

Fain, J. A. (2003). *Reading, understanding, and applying nursing research: A text and workbook* (2nd ed.). Philadelphia: F. A. Davis.

Frisch, N. C. (May 31, 2001). Nursing as a context for alternative/complementary modalities. *Online Journal of Issues in Nursing, 6*(2), Manuscript 2, p. 2. Retrieved March 23, 2008, from http://www.nursingworld.org/ojin.

Griens, A. M. G., Goossen, W. T. F., & Van der Kloot, W. S. (2001). Exploring the Nursing Minimum Data Set for the Netherlands using multidimensional scaling techniques. *Journal of Advanced Nursing, 36*(1), 89–101.

Harris, R. M. (1998, June 10). Advanced nursing practice in the 21st Century: Do we want to be right or do we want to win? *Online Journal of Issues in Nursing, 3*(1). Retrieved March 23, 2008, from http://www.nursingworld.org/ojin/

Institute of Medicine. (1992). Guidelines for clinical practice: From development to use. In: M. J. Field & K. N. Lohr (Eds.). Washington, DC: National Academies Press.

International Council of Nurses (ICN). (2005). *ICNP version 1.0.* Geneva, Switzerland. Author. Retrieved March 23, 2008, from http://www.icn.ch/icnp_v1.htm

Iowa Intervention Project. (2001). Determining cost of nursing interventions: A beginning. . . Iowa Intervention Project. *Nursing Economics, 19*(4), 146–160.

Johnson, M., Bulechek, G., Dochterman, J. M., et al. (2006). *Nursing diagnoses, outcomes, and interventions: NANDA, NOC, and NIC linkages* (2nd ed.). St. Louis, MO: C. V. Mosby.

Kajermo, K. N., Unden, M., Gardule, A., et al. (2008). Predictors of nurses' perceptions of barriers to research utilization. *Journal of Nursing Management, 16*(3), 305–314.

Lavin, M. A., Meyer, G., Krieger, M., et al. (2002). Viewpoint. Essential differences between evidence-based nursing and evidence-based medicine. *International Journal of Nursing Terminologies and Classifications, 13*(3), 101–106.

Marchionni, C., & Ritchie, J. (2008). Organizational factors that support the implementation of a nursing Best Practice Guideline. *Journal of Nursing Management, 16*(3), 266–274.

Martin, K. (2005). *The Omaha System: A key to practice, documentation, and information management* (2nd ed.). Philadelphia: W. B. Saunders.

Martin, K. S., & Scheet, N. J. (1992). *The Omaha system: Applications for community health nursing.* Philadelphia: W. B. Saunders. Also available at http://www.omahasystem.org/shminter.htm (Retrieved January 24, 2008).

McCloskey, J. C., & Bulechek, G. M. (Eds.). (1992). *Nursing interventions classification (NIC).* St. Louis, MO: C. V. Mosby.

National Guideline Clearinghouse, Agency for Healthcare Research and Quality (AHRQ), U.S. Department of Health and Human Services. Retrieved January 24, 2008, from http://www.guideline.gov/

Newman, D., & Palmer, M. (Eds.). (2003, March). State of the science on urinary incontinence. *American Journal of Nursing, 103*(3), 2–53 Supplement.

No author. (2001). Standardized treatment cuts pneumonia deaths: Guidelines also help lower admission rates. *Quality Improvement/Total Quality Management, 11*I(6), 65–67.

No author. (2002). Evidence-based guidelines. *Evidence Based Practice, 5*(2), 12, insert 2p.

No author. (2007). Topical skin care in aged care facilities. *Best Practice Information Sheet, 11*(3). The Joanna Briggs Institute. Retrieved January 24, 2010, from http://www.joannabriggs.edu.au/pdf/BPISEng_11_3.pdf

Nursing Practice Information Infrastructure. (2007, last updated May 11, 2006). ANA recognized terminologies and data element sets. Retrieved March 23, 2008, from http://nursingworld.org/npii/terminologies.htm

O'Connor, N. A., Kershat, W., & Hameister, A. D. (2001). Documenting patterns of nursing interventions. *Journal of Nursing Measurement, 9*(1), 73–90.

Parlocha, P. K., & Chafetz, L. (1999). Planning home care for elderly patients with major depressive disorder: Limits of diagnosis-based critical paths. *Home Health Care Management and Practice 11*(4), 27–37.

Parris, K. M., Place, P. J., & Orellana, E. (1999). Integrating nursing diagnoses, interventions, and outcomes in public health nursing practice. *Nursing Diagnosis 10*(2), 49–56.

Pravikoff, D. S., Pierce, S., & Tanner, A. (2003). Are nurses ready for evidence-based practice? *American Journal of Nursing, 103*(5), 95–96.

Reed, D., Titler, M. G., Dochterman, J. M., et al. (2007). Measuring the dose of nursing interventions. *International Journal of Nursing Terminologies and Classifications, 18*(4), 121–130.

Rew, L. (2000). Possible outcomes of holistic nursing interventions. *Journal of Holistic Nursing, 18*(4), 307–309.

Saba, V. K. (1995). Home Health Care Classifications (HHCCs): Nursing diagnoses and nursing interventions. In: *An emerging framework: Data system advances for clinical nursing practice.* ANA Publication No. NP-94. Washington, DC: American Nurses Association (ANA). Also available at http://www.sabacare.com/interventions/ (Retrieved January 24, 2008).

Saba, V. K. (2006). *Clinical care classification system manual: A guide to nursing documentation.* New York: Springer

Titler, M. G., Mentes, J. C., Rakel, B. A., et al. (1999). From book to bedside: Putting evidence to use in the care of the elderly. *Joint Commission Journal of Quality Improvement, 25,* 545–556.

Venes, D. (2009). *Taber's cyclopedic medical dictionary* (21st ed.). Philadelphia: F. A. Davis.

Wilkinson, J. M. (2007). *Nursing process & critical thinking.* (4th ed.) Upper Saddle River, NJ: Prentice-Hall.

Chapter 7

American Nurses Association (ANA). (1992). Position statements. Registered nurse education relating to the utilization of unlicensed assistive personnel. Retrieved January 24, 2008, from http://nursingworld.org/readroom/position/uap/uapuse.htm.

American Nurses Association (ANA). (1996). *Registered professional nurses and unlicensed assistive personnel* (2nd ed.). Washington, DC: Author.

American Nurses Association (ANA). (1999). *Nursing quality indicators: Guide for implementation* (2nd ed.). Washington, DC: Author.

American Nurses Association (ANA). (2001). *Code of ethics for nurses with interpretive statements.* Washington, DC: Author.

American Nurses Association (ANA). (2010). *Nursing: Scope and standards of practice* (2nd ed). Public Comment draft, January 2010. Silver Spring, MD: Nursebooks.org

American Nurses Association (ANA). (2005). *Principles for delegation.* Retrieved February 1, 2008, from http://www.safestaffing-saveslives.org/WhatisSafeStaffing/SafeStaffingPrinciples/PrinciplesofDelegation.aspx

American Nurses Association (ANA). (2007). Revised position statement: Registered nurses utilization of nursing assistive personnel in all settings. Retrieved March 1, 2008, from http://www.nursingworld.org/MainMenuCategories/HealthcareandPolicy-Issues/ANAPositionStatements/uap/UnlicensedAssistivePersonnel.aspx

American Nurses Association (ANA) and the National Council of State Boards of Nursing (NCSBN). (2006). Joint statement on delegation. American Nurses Association (ANA) and the National Council of State Boards of Nursing (NCSBN). Retrieved February 1, 2008, from https://www.ncsbn.org/joint_statement.pdf

Ayers, D. M. M., & Montgomery, M. (2008). Delegating the "right" way. *Nursing2008, 38*(4), 57–58.

(2001). Baldridge criteria spur ongoing change. *QI/TQM, 11*(8), 89.

(2002). Baldridge National Quality Program. *Health care criteria for performance excellence.* Retrieved January 24, 2008, from http://www.quality.nist.gov/

Barter, M. (1999). Delegation and supervision outside the hospital. *AJN, 99*(7), 24A-24B, 24D.

Basco, A. (2008). Overcoming the myths surrounding adherence. *The Clinical Advisor, 11*(10), 74, 76–78.

Batsie, C. (1999). Patient call system provides efficient delegation. *Nursing Management 30*(1), 50.

Bentley, J. (2001). Promoting patient partnership in wound care. *British Journal of Community Nursing, 6*(10), 493–494, 496, 498, 500.

Bulechek, G. M., Butcher, H. K., & Dochterman, J. M. (2008). *Nursing interventions classification (NIC).* St. Louis, MO: C. V. Mosby.

College & Association of Registered Nurses of Alberta (2003). *Nursing practice standards.* Edmonton, AB: Author.

College of Registered Nurses of Nova Scotia. (2003). *Standards for nursing practice.* Halifax, NS: Author.

Cronenwett, L., Sherwood, G., Barnsteiner, J., et al. (2007). Quality and safety education for nurses. *Nursing Outlook, 55*(3), 122–131.

Davidson, S. G., & Scott, R. (1999). Professional practice: Thinking critically about delegation. *AJN, 99*(6), 61–62.

Dickens, G., Stubbs, J., & Haw, C. (2008). Delegation of medication administration: An exploratory study. *Nursing Standard, 22*(22), 35–40.

Dowding, D. (2001). Examining the effects that manipulating information given in the change of shift report has on nurses' care planning ability. *Journal of Advanced Nursing, 33*(6), 836–846.

Elliott, K. (2001). Implementing nursing clinical indicators. *Professional Nurse, 16*(6), 1158–1161.

Fisher, M. (2000). Do you have delegation savvy? *Nursing 2000, 30*(12), 58–59.

Gibberd, R., Pathmeswaran, A., & Burtenshaw, K. (2000). Using clinical indicators to identify areas for quality improvement. *Journal of Quality in Clinical Practice, 20*I(4), 136–144.

Gould, D., Gammon, J., Donnelly, M., et al. (2000). Improving hand hygiene in community healthcare settings: The impact of research and clinical collaboration. *Journal of Clinical Nursing, 9*(1), 95–102.

Hamill, C. T., & Luchok, J. (1999). Commission/URAC. Best practices: A necessity in modern health care. *Case Manager, 10*(5), 23–25

Hopkins, D. L. (2002). Evaluating the knowledge deficits of registered nurses responsible for supervising nursing assistants. A learning needs assessment tool. *Journal of Nurses Staff Development, 18*(3), 152–156.

ISO. (2002). ISO 9000: A system-oriented approach to quality management. *QI-TQM, 12*i(1), 1–5.

Johnson, K., Hallsey, D., Meredith, R. L., et al. (2006). A nurse-driven system for improving patient quality outcomes. *Journal of Nursing Care Quality, 21*(2), 168–175.

The Joint Commission (TJC). (2008). *Hospital Accreditation Standards: Accreditation policies, standards, elements of performance, scoring.* Oakbrook Terrace, IL: Author.

Kleinman, C. S., & Saccomano, S. J. (2006). Registered nurses and unlicensed assistive personnel: An uneasy alliance. *The Journal of Continuing Education in Nursing, 37*(4), 162–170.

Kummeth, P., de Ruiter, H., & Capelle, S. (2001). Developing a nursing assistant model: Having the right person perform the right job. *MedSurg Nursing, 10*(5), 255–263.

London, F. (1998). Improving compliance. What you can do. *RN, 61*(1), 43–46.

Malloch, K. (1999). The Performance Measurement Matrix: A framework to optimize decision making. *Journal of Nursing Care Quality 13*(3), 1–12.

Meyer, G. S., & Massagli, M. P. (2001). The forgotten component of the quality triad: Can we still learn something from "structure"? *Joint Commission Journal on Quality Improvement, 27*(9), 484–493.

National Council of State Boards of Nursing (NCSBN). (1995a). *Delegation: Concepts and decision-making process.* National Council Position Paper. Chicago: Author. Retrieved April 10, 2008, from http://www.ncsbn.org/files/files/publications/positions/Delegation

National Council of State Boards of Nursing (NCSBN). (1997a). Delegation decision-making grid. NCSBN. Retrieved April 10, 2008, from http://www.ncsbn.org/files/uap/delegationgrid.pdf

National Council of State Boards of Nursing (NCSBN). (1997b). Delegation decision-making tree. Retrieved April 10, 2008, from http://www.ncsbn.org/files/uap/delegationtree.pdf

National Council of State Boards of Nursing (NCSBN). (1997c). The five rights of delegation. Retrieved April 10, 2008, from http://www.ncsbn.org/files/uap/fiverights.pdf

Nurses Association of New Brunswick. (2005). *Standards of practice for registered nurses.* Fredericton, NB: Author.

Oermann, M., & Huber, D. (1999). Patient outcomes: A measure of nursing's value. *American Journal of Nursing, 99*(9), 40–48.

Page, C. K. (1999). Performance improvement integration: A whole systems approach. *Journal of Nursing Care Quality, 13*(3), 59–70.

Parsons, L. C. (1999). Building RN confidence for delegation decision-making skills in practice. *Journal for Nurses in Staff Development, 15*(6), 263–269.

Pelletier, L. R. (2000). Error-free healthcare: Mission possible! *Journal for Healthcare Quality, 22*(2), 2, 9.

Pelletier, L. R., Beaudin, C. L., & van Leeuwen, D. (1999). The use of a prioritization matrix to preserve quality resources. *Journal for Healthcare Quality, 21*(5), 36–38.

Poole, L. (2001). PEPP: Collaborating to improve quality. *Journal of the American Health Information Management Association, 72*(4), 43–47.

Rantz, M. J., Popejoy, L., Petroski, G. F., et al. (2001). Randomized clinical trial of a quality improvement intervention in nursing homes. *The Gerontologist, 41*(4), 525.

Reinhard, S. C., Young, H. M., Kane, R. A., et al. (2006). Nurse delegation of medication administration for older adults in assisted living. *Nursing Outlook, 54*(2), 74–80.

Spencer, S. A. (2001). Education, training, and use of unlicensed assistive personnel in critical care. *Critical Care Nursing Clinics of North America, 13*(1), 105–118.

Thomas, L. (1999). Is delegation the answer? *Elder Care, 11*(4), 1

Wilkinson, J. (2007). *Nursing process & critical thinking* (4th ed.). Upper Saddle River, NJ: Prentice-Hall.

Wilson, L. (2000). "Quality is everyone's business": Why this approach will not work in hospitals. *Journal of Quality in Clinical Practice, 20*(4), 131–135.

Woodring, B. C. (2000). If you have taught—have the child and family learned? *Pediatric Nursing, 26*(5), 505–509.

Chapter 8

Abdellah, F. G., Beland, I. L., Martin, A., et al. (1960). *Patient-centered approaches to nursing.* New York: Macmillan.

American Nurses Association (ANA). (1981). *Guidelines for the investigative functions of nurses.* Washington, DC: Author.

American Nurses Association (ANA). (1994). Position statement: Education for participation in nursing research—4/94. © 1997. Retrieved March 2, 2008, from http://nursingworld.org/MainMenuCategories/HealthcareandPolicyIssues/ANAPositionStatements/Archives/rseducat14484.aspx

American Nurses Association (ANA). (2010). *Nursing: Scope and standards of practice* (2nd ed.). Public Comment draft, January 2010. Silver Spring, MD: Nursebooks.org

American Nurses Association Commission on Nursing Research. (1980). Generating a scientific basis for nursing practice: Research priorities for the 1980's. *Nursing Research*, 29, 219.

Anderson, M. A. (2005). *Nursing leadership, management, and professional practice for the LPN/LVN: In nursing school and beyond* (3rd ed.). Philadelphia: F. A Davis.

Ball, J., & Bindler, R. (2007). *Pediatric nursing: Caring for children* (4th ed.). Upper Saddle River, NJ: Prentice-Hall.

Benner, P. (1984). *From novice to expert. Excellence and power in clinical nursing practice*. Menlo Park, CA: Addison-Wesley.

Benner, P., & Wrubel, J. (1989). *The primacy of caring: Stress and coping in health and illness*. Menlo Park, CA: Addison-Wesley.

Brockopp, D. Y., & Hastongs-Tolsma, M. T. (2003). *Fundamentals of nursing research* (3rd ed.). Sudbury, MA: Jones and Bartlett.

Brown, S. S. (1992). Meta-analysis of diabetes patient education research: Variation in intervention effects across studies. *Research in Nursing and Health*, 16(6), 409–419.

Bulechek, G. M., Butcher, H. K., & Dochterman, J. M. (2008). *Nursing interventions classification (NIC)* (5th ed.). St. Louis, MO: C. V. Mosby.

Burns, N., & Grove, S. K. (2003). *The practice of nursing research: Conduct, critique, and utilization* (4th ed.). Philadelphia: W. B. Saunders.

Carniah, S. (1997). Utilization of nursing research in practice and application: Strategies to raise research awareness amongst nurse practitioners: A model for success. *Journal of Advanced Nursing*, 26(6), 1193–1202

Center for Evidence Based Medicine. Asking focused clinical questions. Page last edited, April 7, 2009. Retrieved February 19, 2008, from http://www.cebm.net/index.aspx?o=1036

Chinn, P. L., & Kramer, M. K. (2007). *Theory and nursing: Integrated knowledge development* (7th ed.). St. Louis, MO: C. V. Mosby.

Code of Federal Regulations. (2005). Title 45 Public Welfare, Part 46, Protection of Human Subjects. Last updated July 30, 2007. Retrieved February 9, 2008, from http://www.hhs.gov/ohrp/humansubjects/guidance/45cfr46.htm

Cook, P. R., & Cullen, J. A. (2003). Caring as an imperative for nursing education. *Nursing Education Perspectives*, 24(4), 293–297.

Cronenwett, L., Sherwood, G., Barnsteiner, J., et al. (2007). Quality and safety education for nurses. *Nursing Outlook*, 55(3), 122–131. Retrieved February 1, 2008, from http://qsen.org/competencies/php/

Dossey, B. M. (1999). *Florence Nightingale: Mystic, visionary, healer*. Springhouse, PA: Springhouse Corporation.

Fain, J. A. (2009). *Reading, understanding, and applying nursing research: A text and workbook* (3rd ed.). Philadelphia: F. A. Davis.

Feil, N. (2003). *V/F validation*. (revised edition). Cincinnati, OH: Feil Productions. Also available from http://www.edwardfeilproductions.com/catalogue.html#books

Flaskerud, J. H., & Halloran, E. J. (1980). Areas of agreement in nursing theory development. *Advances in Nursing Science*, 3(1), 1–7.

Goode, C., Butcher, L., Cipperley, J., et al. (1996). *Research utilization: A study guide* (2nd ed.). Ida Grove, IA: Horn Video Productions.

Haller, K. B., Reynolds, M. A., & Horsley, J. A. (1979). Developing research-based innovation protocols: Process, criteria and issues. *Research in Nursing and Health*, 2, 45–51.

Harvey, G., Loftus-Hills, A., Rycroft-Malone, J., et al. (2002). Getting evidence into practice: The role and function of facilitation. *Journal of Advanced Nursing*, 37(6), 577–588.

Henderson, V. (1966). *The nature of nursing*. New York: Macmillan.

Horsley, J. A., Crane, J., & Bingle, J. D. (1978). Research utilization as an organizational process. *Journal of Nursing Administration*, July, 4–6.

Horsley, J. A., Crane J., Crabtree, M. K., et al. (1983). *Using research to improve practice*. Orlando, FL: Grune & Stratton.

International Consortium of Parse Scholars (n.d.). Retrieved July 18, 2003, from http://www.humanbecoming.org/

Johnson, D. E. (1968). Theory in nursing: Borrowed and unique. *Nursing Research*, 11, 206.

Johnson, D. E. (1980). The behavioral system for nursing. In: J. P. Riehl & C. Roy (Eds.), *Conceptual models for nursing practice* (2nd ed., pp. 207–216). New York: Appleton-Century-Crofts.

King, I. M. (1971). *Toward a theory for nursing: General concepts of human behavior*. New York: John Wiley & Sons.

Kolcaba, K. Y. (1994). A theory of holistic comfort for nursing. *Journal of Advanced Nursing*, 19, 1178–1184.

Leininger, M. M. (1978). *Transcultural nursing: Concepts, theories and practices*. New York: John Wiley & Sons.

Leininger, M. M. (1984). *Care: The essence of nursing and health*. Thorofare, NJ: Charles B. Slack.

Levine, M. E. (1967). The four conservation principles of nursing. *Nursing Forum*, 6, 45–59.

Levine, M. E. (1969). *Introduction to clinical nursing*. Philadelphia: F. A. Davis.

Marriner-Tomey, A., & Raile-Alligood, M. (2006) *Nursing theorists and their work* (6th ed.). St. Louis, MO: C. V. Mosby.

Maslow, A. H. (1970). *Motivation and personality* (2nd ed.). New York: Harper & Row.

Maslow, A. (1971). *The farther reaches of human nature*. New York: The Viking Press.

Maslow, A., & Lowery, R. (Eds.). (1998). *Toward a psychology of being* (3rd ed.). New York: Wiley & Sons.

Mayo, A. (1997). Orem's Self-Care Model: A Professional Nursing Practice Model. http://members.aol.com/annmrn/nursing_portfolio_I_index.html. Accessed July 16, 2003.

McCalla, C. (1998) University of Western Ontario Faculty of Nursing, Hildegard Peplau Nursing Theorist Home Page. Retrieved February 10, 2008, from http://publish.uwo.ca/~cforchuk/peplau/1981–1999.html

Merskey, H., & Bogduk, N. (1994). *Classification of chronic pain: descriptions of chronic pain syndromes and definitions of pain terms*. Seattle: IASP (International Association for the Study of Pain) Press.

National Heart, Lung, and Blood Institute; National Institutes of Health. (2002). *Framingham Heart Study*. Available at http://www.nhlbi.nih.gov/about/framingham/index.html. Updated September 20, 2007. Retrieved February 8, 2008.

National Heart, Lung, and Blood Institute; National Institutes of Health, U.S. Department of Health and Human Services (2006). *Your guide to lowering your blood pressure with DASH*. Retrieved February 14, 2008, from http://emall.nhlbihin.net/product2.asp?source=&sku=06-4082

National Institutes of Health (NIH). (n.d.). Nuremberg Code: Directives for human experimentation. *Regulations and ethical guidelines*. Office of Human Subjects Research. Retrieved February 20, 2008, from http://ohsr.od.nih.gov/guidelines/nuremberg.html

National Institutes of Health (NIH). (2002). The NIH Almanac—Organization. National Institute of Nursing Research. Retrieved February 10, 2008, from http://nih.gov/about/almanac/organization/NINR.htm

National Institutes of Health, Office of Human Subjects Research. (2008). Directives for Human Experimentation. Nuremberg Code. Reprinted from *Trials of War Criminals before the Nuremberg military tribunals under Control Council Las No. 10, Vol. 2*, pp. 181.182. Washington, DC: U.S. Government Printing Office, (1949). Retrieved February 9, 2008, from http://ohsr.od.nih.gov/guidelines/nuremberg.html

National Institute of Nursing Research (NINR). (2003a). 2004 Areas of Research Opportunity. Retrieved February 15, 2008, from http://www.nih.gov/ninr/research/dea/2004AoRO.html

National Institute of Nursing Research (NINR). (2003b). Research Themes for the Future. Retrieved February 15, 2008, from http://www.nih.gov/ninr/research/dea/PARFApage.html

Neuman, B. M., & Young, R. J. (1972). A model for teaching total person approach to patient problems. *Nursing Research*, 21, 264–269.

Neumann College (2000). Academics. Division of Nursing & Health Sciences. Neuman Systems Model. Retrieved February 10, 2008, from http://www.neumann.edu/academics/undergrad/nursing/model.asp

Newman, M. (n.d.). Health As Expanding Consciousness. Retrieved February 1, 2008, from http://www.healthasexpandingconsciousness.org/

Nieswiadomy, R. M. (2008). *Foundations of nursing research*. (5th ed.). Upper Saddle River, NJ: Prentice-Hall.

Nightingale, F. (1859/1992). *Notes on nursing: What it is and what it is not*. Philadelphia: J. B. Lippincott.

NurseScribe©. (2003). Nursing Theory Page. Available at http://www.enursescribe.com/nurse_theorists.htm. Updated July 16, 2003. Accessed July 16, 2003.

Orlando, I. J. (1961). *The dynamic nurse-patient relationship: Function, process, and principles*. New York: G. P. Putnam's Sons.

Parker, M. (2001). *Nursing theories and nursing practice*. Philadelphia: F. A. Davis.

Pender, N. J., Murdaugh, C. L., & Parsons, M. A. (2006). *Health promotion in nursing practice* (5th ed.). Upper Saddle River, NJ: Prentice-Hall.

Peplau, H. E. (1952). *Interpersonal relations in nursing*. New York: G. P. Putnam's Sons.

Pettengill, M. M., Gillies, D. A., & Clark, C. C. (1994). Factors encouraging and discouraging the use of nursing research findings. *Journal of Nursing Scholarship, 26*(2), 143–148.

Polit, D. F., & Beck, C. T. (2007). *Nursing research: Generating and assessing evidence* (8th ed.). Philadelphia: Lippincott Williams & Wilkins.

Rigdon, I. S., Clayton, B. D., & Dimond, M. (1987). Toward a theory of helpfulness for the elderly bereaved: An invitation to a new life. *Advances In Nursing Science, 9*(2), 32–43.

Rogers, M. (1970). *An introduction to the theoretical basis of nursing*. Philadelphia: F. A. Davis.

Roy, C. (2003). Boston College. The Roy Adaptation Model. Retrieved February 3, 2008, from http://www.bc.edu/schools/son/faculty/featured/theorist/Roy_Adaptation_Model.html

Selye, H. (1993). *Neuroendocrinology and stress*. New York: New York Academy of Science.

Straus, S. E., Richardson, W. S., Glasziou, P., et al. (2005). *Evidence-based medicine: How to practice and teach EBM* (3rd ed.). Edinburgh: Churchill Livingston.

Sullivan, D. T., & Warren, J. (2007). Quality and safety education for nurses. *Nursing Outlook, 55*(3), 122–131. Retrieved February 1, 2008, from http://qsen.org/competencydomains/

Transcultural Nursing Society. (1998–2003). Theories and Models. Retrieved February 10, 2008, from http://www.tcns.org/Theories.html

University of Kentucky, The Nun Study. Retrieved March 20, 2008, from http://www.mc.uky.edu/nunnet/Public.htm

University of Kentucky Chandler Medical Center. (1999). University of Kentucky. The Nun Study. Retrieved February 12, 2008, from http://www.nunstudy.org.

University of Southern California, Health Sciences, Los Angeles. Evidence Based Decision Making, Asking a Good Question (PICO). Site updated July, 2007. Retrieved February 19, 2008, from http://www.usc.edu/hsc/ebnet/ebframe/PICO.htm

Von Bertalanffy, L. (1976). *General system theory: Foundations, development and applications* (rev. ed.). New York: George Braziller.

Watson, J. (1988). *Nursing: Human science and human care. A theory of nursing*. New York: National League for Nursing Press. Pub. No. 15–2236.

Watson, J. (2000). University of Colorado Health Sciences Center, School of Nursing. Watson's Caring Theory. Retrieved February 2, 2008, from http://www.ucdenver.edu/academics/colleges/nursing/caring/Pages/Caring.aspx

Watson, J. (2008). Theory evolution: Watson's Caring Theory. University of Colorado Health Sciences Center School of Nursing, Denver, CO. Retrieved February 3, 2008, from http://www2.uchsc.edu/son/caring/content/evolution.asp

Wiedenbach, E. (1964). *Clinical nursing: A helping art*. New York: Springer Publishing Co., Inc.

Wilson, H. S. (1993). *Introducing research in nursing* (2nd ed.). Redwood City, CA: Addison-Wesley Nursing.

Yura, H., & Torres, G. (1975). *Today's conceptual frameworks with the baccalaureate nursing programs*. NLN Pub. No. 15-1558. New York: National League for Nursing.

Chapter 9

AARP Public Policy Institute. (2005). Beyond 50.5, a report to the nation on livable communities: creating environments for successful aging. Washington, DC: AARP.

About Teen Depression (n.d.). A fact sheet. Educational web site sponsored by CRC Health Group. Retrieved March 29, 2008, from http://www.about-teen-depression.com/teen-depression.html.

Advisory Committee on Immunization Practices (ACIP). (2008). Prevention and control of influenza. Recommendations of the Advisory Committee on Immunization Practices (ACPI), 2007. *MMWR Recommendations and Reports, 57*(RR07), 1–60. Retrieved August 18, 2008, from http://www.cdc.gov/mmwr/preview/mmwrhtml/rr5707a1.htm

Alley, D., Liebig, P., Pynoos, J., et al. (2007). Creating elder-friendly communities: Preparations for an aging society. *Journal of Gerontological Social Work, 49*(1/2), 1–18.

Al Omari, H., Kramer, K., Hronek, C., et al. (2005) The Wheat Valley assisted living culture: Rituals and rules. *Journal of Gerontological Nursing, 31*(1), 9–16.

Alzheimer's Association. (2008). Risk factors. Retrieved November 2, 2008, from http://www.alz.org/alzheimers_disease_causes_risk_factors.asp

American Academy of Family Physicians (AAFP). (2006). Toilet training your child. (Written by familydoctor.org editorial staff.) Retrieved March 26, 2008, from http://familydoctor.org/online/famdocen/home/children/parents/toilet/179.html

American Academy of Pediatrics (AAP). (2006). Policy statement. Active healthy living: Prevention of childhood obesity through increased physical activity. *Pediatrics, 117*(5), 1834–1842.

American Academy of Pediatrics (AAP). (2008). Car safety seats: A guide for families 2008. Retrieved March 26, 2008, from http://www.aap.org/family/carseatguide.htm

American Cancer Society (ACS). (2007). Detailed guide: Breast cancer. Can breast cancer be found early? Retrieved March 28, 2008, from http://www.cancer.org/docroot/CRI/content/CRI_2_4_3X_Can_breast_cancer_be_found_early_5.asp

American Cancer Society (2009a). American Cancer Society guidelines for the early detection of cancer. Retrieved December 13, 2009, from http://www.cancer.org/docroot/PED/content/PED_2_3X_ACS_Cancer_Detection_Guidelines_36.asp?sitearea+PED

American Cancer Society (2009b). Detailed guide. Breast cancer: Can breast cancer be found early? Retrieved September 2, 2009, from http://www.cancer.org/docroot/CRI/content/CRI_2_4_3X_Can_breast_cancer_be_found_early_5.asp?mav=cri

The American College of Obstetricians and Gynecologists (ACOG) (2003, Reaffirmed 2006). Breast cancer screening. Washington, DC: ACOG. ACOG practice bulletin No 42. Retrieved May 14, 2010, from http://www.guideline.gov/content.aspx?id=3990&search=breast+cancer+screening

The American College of Obstetricians and Gynecologists (ACOG) (2009). Interpreting the U. S. preventive services task force breast cancer screening recommendations for the general population. Retrieved December 13, 2009, from http://www.acog.org/from_home/Misc/uspstfinterpretation.cfm

American Heart Association (AHA). (2008a). Overweight in children. Retrieved March 27, 2008, from http://www.americanheart.org/presenter.jhtml?identifier=4670

American Heart Association (AHA). (2008b). Overweight, obese women improve quality of life with 10 to 30 minutes of exercise. Retrieved April 18, 2008, from http://americanheart.mediaroom.com/index.php?s=43&item=364

American Lung Association (ALA). (2007). Smoking and teens fact sheet. Retrieved March 29, 2008, from http://www.lungusa.org/site/pp.asp?c=dvLUK9O0E&b=39871

APGAR. (n.d., last updated November 14, 2007). Medline Plus, U.S. National Library of Medicine, National Institutes of Health. Retrieved March 27, 2008, from http://www.gov/medlineplus/ency/article/003402.htm#top

Assisted Living Quality Coalition. (1998). *Assisted living quality initiative: Building a structure that promotes quality.* Washington, DC: Author.

Badgwell, B., Giordano, S., Duan, Z., et al. (2008). Mammography before diagnosis among women age 80 years and older with breast cancer. *Journal of Clinical Oncology, 26*(15), 2482–2488.

Balkaya, N., Memis, S., & Demirkiran, F. (2007). The effects of breast self-exam education on the performance of nursing and midwifery students: A 6-month follow-up study. *Journal of Cancer Education, 22*(2), 77–79.

Bartali, B., Semba, R., Frongillo, E., et al. (2006). Low micronutrient levels as a predictor of incident disability in older women. *Archives of Internal Medicine, 166*(21), 2335–2340.

Bellavance, A., & Freter, K. (2008). Helping stop domestic violence. *The Clinical Advisor, 1*(2), 134.

Blustein, J., & Weiss, L. J. (1998). The use of mammography by women aged 75 and older: Factors related to health, functioning, and age. *Journal of the American Geriatric Society, 46,* 941–946.

Brazelton, T., & Nugent, J. (1996). *Neonatal behavioral assessment scale* (3rd ed.). London: MacKeith.

Breast cancer screening in older women (reviewed and updated in 2005). American Geriatrics Society. Retrieved May 4, 2010, from http://www.americangeriatrics.org/education/cp_index.shtml

Breheny, M., & Stephens, C. (2007). Individual responsibility and social constraint: The construction of adolescent motherhood in social science research. *Culture, Health & Sexuality, 9*(4), 333–346.

Broderick, P. (1998). Pediatric vision screening for the family physician. (Includes American Academy of Pediatrics Vision Screening Guidelines). *American Family Physician, 58*(3). Retrieved March 27, 2008, from http://www.aafp.org/afp/980901ap/broderic.html

Brodowski, M. L., Nolan, C. M., Gaudiosi, J. A., et al. (2008, April 4). Nonfatal maltreatment of infants-United States, October 2005–September 2006. *Morbidity and Mortality Weekly Report, 57*(13), 336–339.

Bureau of Justice Statistics. (2007, last revised July 11, 2007). Homicide trends in the U.S., Intimate homicide. U.S. Department of Justice, Office of Justice Programs. Retrieved March 15, 2008, from http://www.ojp.usdoj.gov/bjs/homicide/intimates.htm

Centers for Disease Control and Prevention (CDC). (n.d.). Genital herpes–CDC Fact Sheet. Retrieved April 15, 2008, from http://www.cdc.gov/STD/herpes/STDFact-Herpes.htm#common (last reviewed and modified January 4, 2008).

Centers for Disease Control and Prevention (CDC). (n.d., last updated May 22, 2007). Nutrition for everyone. Bone health. Retrieved March 28, 2008, from http://www.cdc.gov/nccdphp/dnpa/nutrition/nutrition_for_everyone/bonehealth/

Centers for Disease Control and Prevention (CDC). (2001a). Prevalence of overweight and obesity among adults: United States, 1999–200. Retrieved March 15, 2008, from http://www.cdc.gov/nccdphp/dnpa/obesity/trend

Centers for Disease Control and Prevention (CDC). (2001b). Youth risk behavior surveillance system: Alcohol/other drug use. Retrieved October 1, 2003, from http://www.cdc.gov/GraphV

Centers for Disease Control and Prevention (CDC). (2002a). Child passenger safety. Retrieved April 25, 2003, from http://www.cdc.gov/safeusa/move/childpassenger.htm

Centers for Disease Control and Prevention (CDC). (2002b). Infant mortality statistics from the 1999 period linked birth/infant death data set. *National Vital Statistics Reports, 50*(4). Retrieved March 26, 2008, from http://www.cdc.gov/nchs/fastats/infant_health.htm

Centers for Disease Control and Prevention (CDC). (2005a). 10 Leading causes of unintentional injury deaths, United States, 2005; and WISQARS injury mortality reports, 1999–2005. (Last reviewed January 23, 2008). *National Center for Injury Prevention and Control.*

Retrieved March 28, 2008, from http://webappa.cdc.gov/sasweb/ncipc/mortrate10_sy.html

Centers for Disease Control and Prevention (CDC). (2005b). Sexual behavior and selected health measures: Men and women 15–44 years of age, United States, 2002. *Advance Data from Vital and Health Statistics,* #362(September 15). Retrieved March 28, 2008, from http://www.cdc.gov/nchs/data/ad/ad362.pdf

Center for Disease Control and Prevention (CDC). (2005c). Table 7. Deaths and death rates for the 10 leading causes of death in specified age groups: United States, preliminary 2005. Retrieved October 30, 2008, from http://www.cdc.gov/nchs/data/hestat/preliminarydeaths05_tables.pdf#A

Centers for Disease Control and Prevention (CDC). (2006, December 12). The state of childhood asthma, United States, 1980–2005. Advance Data from Vital and Health Statistics, 381. Retrieved March 28, 2008, from http://www.cdc.gov/nchs/data/ad/ad381.pdf

Centers for Disease Control and Prevention (CDC). (2007a). Summary health statistics for U.S. children: National health interview survey, 2006. *Vital and Health Statistics,* Series 10(234). Retrieved March 28, 2008, from http://www.cdc.gov/nchs/data/series/sr_10/sr10_234.pdf

Centers for Disease Control and Prevention (CDC). (2007b). Adolescent reproductive health home. Teen pregnancy. Retrieved March 29, 2008, from http://www.cdc.gov/reproductivehealth/AdolescentReproHealth/

Centers for Disease Control and Prevention (CDC). (2008). HIV/AIDS in the United States. Department of Health and Human Services. Retrieved March 26, 2008, from http://www.cdc.gov/vaccines/recs/schedules

Centers for Disease Control and Prevention (CDC). (2009). 2009 Child & adolescent immunization schedules. Department of Health and Human Services. Retrieved January 7, 2009, from http://www.cdc.gov/vaccines/recs/schedules/child-schedule.htm#printable

Cherkas, L., Hunkin, J., Kato, B., et al. (2008). The association between physical activity in leisure time and leukocyte telomere length. *Archives of Internal Medicine, 168*(2), 154–158.

Child Trends Data Bank. (2007). Condom use. Retrieved March 29, 2008, from http://www.childtrendsdatabank.org/indicators/28CondomUse.cfm

Coyne, I. (2006). Children's experiences of hospitalization. *Journal of Child Health Care, 10,* 326–336.

Denver II. (1990). Available for purchase from Denver Developmental Materials, Inc., Denver, CO. Retrieved March 26, 2008, from http://www.denverii.com/home.html

Eaton, D. K., Kann, L., Kinchen, S., et al. (2006). Youth risk behavior surveillance—United States, 2005. *Morbidity and Mortality Weekly Report, 55*(SS05), 1–108.

Erikson, E. H. (1963). *Childhood and society* (2nd ed.). New York: W. W. Norton.

Ertel, K., Glymour, M., & Berkman, L. F. (2008). Effects of social integration on preserving memory function in a nationally representative US elderly population. *American Journal of Public Health, 98*(7), 1215–1220.

Faber, M., Bosscher, R., Paw, M., et al. (2006). Effects of exercise programs on falls and mobility in frail and pre-frail older adults: A multicenter randomized controlled trial. *Archives of Physical Medicine and Rehabilitation, 87*(7), 885–896.

Federal Interagency Forum on Aging Related Statistics. (2008). Older Americans 2008: Key indicators of well-being. Retrieved October 30, 2008, from http://agingstats.gov/agingstatsdotnet/Main_Site/Data/Data_2008.aspx

Ferenczy, A. (1995). Viral testing for genital human papillomavirus infections: Recent progress and clinical potentials. *Journal of Gynecologic Cancer, 5,* 321–328.

Flaherty, J., Morley, J., Murphy, D., et al. (2002). The development of outpatient clinical glidepaths. *Journal of the American Geriatrics Society, 50,* 1886–1901.

Folstein, M. F., Folstein, S., & McHugh P. R. (1975). Mini mental state: A practical method for grading the cognitive state of patients for the clinician. *Journal of Psychiatric Research*, *12*, 189–198.

Fowler, J. W. (1981). *Stages of faith: The psychology of human development and the quest for meaning*. New York: Harper & Row.

Frailty in older adults. (2006). JAMA patient page. JAMA, *296*(18). Retrieved December 13, 2008, from http://jama. ama-assn.org/cgi/content/full/296/18/2280?maxtoshow5& HITS510&hits510&RESULTFORMAT5&fulltext5patient1page 1frail&searchid51&FIRSTINDEX50&resourcetype5HWCIT

Freud, A. (1966). *The ego and the mechanisms of defense*. New York: International Universities Press.

Futterman, M. (2008). Over 80, it's anyone's race. *The Wall Street Journal*, W1, W4.

Garofalo, R., Herrick, A., Mustanski, B. S., et al. (2007). Tip of the iceberg: Young men who have sex with men, the Internet, and HIV risk. *American Journal of Public Health*, *97*(6), 1113–1117.

Gavin, L., MacKay, A., Brown, K., et al. (2009). Sexual and reproductive health of persons aged 10–24 years—United States, 2002–2007. *MMWR Surveillance Summaries*, *58*(SS06), 1–58.

Gilligan, C. (1982). *In a different voice: Psychological theory and women's development*. Cambridge, MA: Harvard University Press.

Gilligan, C. (1993). *In a different voice: Psychological theory and women's development*. Cambridge, MA: Harvard University Press.

Graf, C. (2008). The Lawton instrumental activities of daily living scale. *American Journal of Nursing*, *108*(4), 52–61.

Green, B. B., & Taplin, S. H. (2003). Breast cancer screening controversies. *The Journal of the American Board of Family Practice*, *16*, 233–241.

Guide to Clinical Preventive Services. (2008). AHRQ Publication No. 08–05122, September 2008. Agency for Healthcare Research and Quality, Rockville, MD. Retrieved September 30, 2008, from http://www.ahrq.gov/clinic/pocketgd.htm

Hackshaw, A. K., & Paul, E. A. (2003). Breast self-examination and death from breast cancer: A meta-analysis. *British Journal of Cancer*, *88*, 1047–1053.

Havighurst, J. (1963). Successful aging. In: R. H. Williams, C. Tibbitts, & W. Donahue (Eds). *Processes of aging*. New York: Atherton Press.

Havighurst, R. J. (1971). *Developmental tasks and education* (3rd ed.). New York: Longman.

He, F. J., Marrero, N. M., & MacGregor, G. A. (2008). Salt intake is related to soft drink consumption in children and adolescents. *Hypertension*, *51*, 629–634.

Hockenberry, M., & Wilson, D. (2007). *Wong's nursing care of infants and children* (8th ed.). St. Louis, MO: C. V. Mosby.

Houser, A., Fox-Grage, W., & Gibson, M. J. (2009). *Across the states: Profiles of long term care and independent living* (8th ed.). Washington, DC: AARP Public Policy Institute.

Hussey, J. M., Chang, J. J., & Kotch, J. B. (2006). Child maltreatment in the United States: Prevalence, risk factors, and adolescent health consequences. *Pediatrics*, *118*(3), 933–942.

Kammerling, S. (2002). Airbags and children: Making correct choices in child passenger restraints. *Maternal Child Nursing*, *27*(5), 264–273.

Knutson, D., & Steiner, E. (2007). Screening for breast cancer: Current recommendations and future directions. *American Family Physician*, *75*(11), 1660–1666.

Kohlberg, L. (1968). Moral development. In: *International encyclopedia of social science*. New York: Macmillan.

Kohlberg, L. (1981). *Essays on moral development*, Volumes 1–3. San Francisco: Harper & Row.

Kösters, J. P., & Gøtzsche, P. C. (2004). Regular self-examination or clinical examination for early detection of breast cancer. *Evidence Based Nursing*, *7*(1), 15.

Kulig, J. W. (2005). Tobacco, alcohol and other drugs: The role of the pediatrician in prevention, identification and management of substance abuse. *Pediatrics*, *115*, 816–821.

Kung, H-C., Hoyert, D. L., Xu J., et al. (2008, April 24). [US Department of Health and Human Services, Centers for Disease Control and Prevention] Deaths: Final Data for 2005. *National Vital Statistics Reports*, *56*(10), 1–121. Retrieved from http://www.cdc.gov/nchs/data/nvsr/nvsr56/nvsr56_10.pdf

Laumann, E. O., Leitsch, S. A., & Waite, L. J. (2008). Elder mistreatment in the United States: Prevalence estimates from a nationally representative study. *Journal of Gerontology: Social Sciences*, *63B*(4), S248–S254.

Leckie, T. (2004). Normal temperature in the elderly. *SpR Emergency Medicine*. *BestBETs*. Retrieved December 11, 2008, from http://www.bestbets.org/bets/bet.php?id=00774

Lippert, J., Shea, J., & Seagrave, M. (2008). Anorexia nervosa: Dying to be thin. *The Clinical Advisor*, *11*(1), 67–70.

Macko, R., Benvenuti, F., Stanhope, S., et al. (2008). Adaptive physical activity improves mobility function and quality of life in chronic hemiparesis. *Journal of Rehabilitation Research and Development*, *45*(2), 323–328.

MADD (n.d.). Statistics. (site of Mothers Against Drunk Driving). Retrieved March 29, 2008, from http://www.madd.org/Drunk-Driving/Drunk-Driving/Statistics/AllStats.aspx

Martin, F. C., & Brighton, P. (2008). Frailty: Different tools for different purposes? *Age and Ageing*, *37*, 129–131.

McFarlane, J. H., & Miller, A. (2005). Promoting community protection of adolescents. Juvenile Rights Project, Inc. Retrieved March 29, 2008, from http://www.jrplaw.org/Documents/CJA%20final%20part%201.pdf

Miller, J. L., & Silverstein, J. H. (2007). Management approaches for pediatric obesity. *Nature Clinical Practice Endocrinology & Metabolism*, *312*, 810–818. Retrieved March 28, 2008, from http://www.medscape.com/viewarticle/565533

Molzahn, A. (2007). Spirituality in later life. *Journal of Gerontological Nursing*, *33*(1), 32–39.

Morbidity and Mortality Weekly Report (2008a). Nonfatal maltreatment of infants—United States, October 2005–September 2006. *57*(13), 336–339. Retrieved December 12, 2008, from http://www.cdc.gov/mmwr/preview/mmwrhtml/mm5713a2.htm#top

Morbidity and Mortality Weekly Report. (2008b). Recommended immunization schedules for persons aged 0–18 years–United States, 2008. 57: Q1. Retrieved April 21, 2008, from http://www.cdc.gov/mmwr/preview/mmwrhtml/mm5701a8.htm

Mosher, W., Chandra, A., & Jones, J. (2005). Sexual behavior and selected health measures: Men and women 15–44 years of age, United States 2002. *Advance Data from Vital and Health Statistics*, 362. Centers for Disease Control and Prevention (CDC). Division of Vital Statistics. Retrieved December 12, 2008, from http://www.cdc.gov/nchs/products/pubs/pubd/ad/361–370/ad362.htm

National Campaign to Prevent Teen Pregnancy. (2002). United States birth rates for teens 15–19. Retrieved September 22, 2002, from http://www.teenpregnancy.org

National Cancer Institute (NCI). (2008). Breast cancer screening (PDQ®). Retrieved August 28, 2008, from http://www.cancer.gov/cancertopics/pdq/screening/breast/HealthProfessional/page10

National Cancer Institute (NCI). (2005, last updated November 1, 2007). What you need to know about breast cancer: Risk factors. Retrieved April 18, 2008, from http://www.cancer.gov/cancertopics/wyntk/breast/page4

National Cancer Institute (NCI). (2007). The prostate-specific antigen (PSA) test: Questions and answers. U.S. National Institutes of Health. Retrieved April 18, 2008, from http://www.cancer.gov/cancertopics/factsheet/Detection/PSA

National Center for Health Statistics (NCHS). (n.d.). Prevalence of overweight among children and adolescents: United States 1999–2002. Last reviewed January 11, 2007. Retrieved March 27, 2008, from http://www.cdc.gov/nchs/products/pubs/pubd/hestats/overwght99.htm

National Center for Health Statistics (NCHS). (2005). Leading causes of death—older teens. Retrieved March 28, 2008, from http://www.statisticstop10.com/Causes_of_Death_Older_Teens.html

National Center for Health Statistics (NCHS). (2007a). *National Vital Statistics Reports*, *56*(7). Retrieved April 15, 2008, from http://www.cdc.gov/nchs/pressroom/07newsreleases/teen-birth.htm

National Center for Health Statistics (NCHS). (2007b). New CDC study finds no increase in obesity among adults; but levels still high. Retrieved April 18, 2008, from http://www.cdc.gov/nchs/pressroom/07newsreleases/obesity.htm

National Center for Health Statistics (NCHS). (2009). Health, United States, 2008. With Chartbook. Hyattsville, MD. Retrieved February 20, 2009, from http://www.cdc.gov/nchs/data/hus/hus08.pdf

National Center for Injury Prevention and Control (NCIPC). (2003). Fatal firearm injuries in the United States, 1993–1998. Violence surveillance summary series, No. 3. Retrieved April 6, 2008, from http://www.cdc.gov/mmwr/preview/mmwrhtml/ss5002a1.htm

National Guideline Clearinghouse (NGC). (2004). Screening for family and intimate partner violence: Recommendation statement. Retrieved March 25, 2008, from http://www.guideline.gov/summary/summary.aspx?doc_id=4427&nbr=003341&string=%22screening+for+family%22+and+intimate

National Guideline Clearinghouse (NGC). (2007). Evidence-based practice guideline. Exercise promotion: Walking in elders. Iowa City, IA: University of Iowa Gerontological Nursing Interventions Research Center, Research Dissemination Core.

National Guideline Clearinghouse (NGC). (2008). Dementia and movement disorders. Complete summary. Retrieved December 12, 2008, from http://www.guideline.gov/summary/summary.aspx?ss=15&doc_id=11600&nbr=6012

National Institutes of Health (NIH). (2008). NIH News. WHI follow up study confirms health risks of long-term combination hormone therapy outweigh benefits for postmenopausal women. U.S. Department of Health and Human Services. Retrieved April 18, 2008, from http://www.nih.gov/news/health/mar2008/nhlbi-04.htm

The National Women's Health Information Center (2006). Pap test. Retrieved Marcy 28, 2008, from http://www.4women.gov/FAQ/pap.htm#pap04

The Obesity Society. (2008). Childhood overweight. Retrieved March 29, 2008, from http://www.obesity.org/information/childhood_overweight.asp

Office of Minority Health. (2004). Highlights in minority health: What is the burden of intimate partner violence in the United States? Centers for Disease Control and Prevention (CDC). Retrieved March 15, 2008, from http://www.cdc.gov/OMH/Highlights/2004/HOct04.htm

Perls, T. (2006). The different paths to 100. American Journal of Clinical Nutrition, 83(Supplement): 484S-487S.

Perls, T., Silver, M. H., & Lauerman, J. F. (1999). Living to 100: Lessons in living to your maximum potential at any age. New York: Basic Books.

Piaget, J. (1952). The origins of intelligence in children. New York: International Universities Press.

Piper, E. (2002). Faith development: A critique of Fowler's model and a proposed alternative. The Journal of Liberal Religion, 3(1), 2–8.

Polan, E., & Taylor, D. (2007). Journey across the life span: Human development and health promotion (3rd ed.). Philadelphia: F. A. Davis.

Remez, L. (2000). Oral sex among adolescents: Is it sex or is it abstinence? Family Planning Perspectives, 32, 298–304.

Rockwood, K. (2005). What would make a definition of frailty successful? Age and Ageing, 34, 432–434.

Rosolowich, V. (2006). Breast self-examination. Journal of Obstetrics and Gynaecology Canada, 28, 728–730.

Sadock, B., & Sadock, V. (2007). Kaplan & Sadock's synopsis of psychiatry (10th ed.). Philadelphia: Lippincott Williams & Wilkins.

Schnitzer, P. G., & Ewigman, B. G. (2005). Child deaths resulting from inflicted injuries: Household risk factors and perpetrator characteristics. Pediatrics, 116(5), e687–693.

Schnitzer, P. G., & Ewigman, B. G. (2008). Household composition and fatal unintentional injuries related to child maltreatment. Journal of Nursing Scholarship, 40(1), 91–97.

Shephard, R. J. (2008, April). Maximal oxygen intake and independence in old age. British Journal of Sports Medicine, 10. Retrieved December 12, 2008, from http://bjsm.bmj.com/cgi/content/abstract/bjsm.2007.044800v1

Smith, C. A., Ireland, T. O., & Thronberry, T. P. (2005). Adolescent maltreatment and its impact on young adult antisocial behavior. Child Abuse & Neglect, 29(10), 1099–1119.

Smith, R., Cokkinides, V., & Eyre, H.; American Cancer Society. (2003). American Cancer Society guidelines for the early detection of cancer. CA-Ca-A Cancer Journal for Clinicians, 53, 27–43.

Snowdon, D. A. (2003). Healthy aging and dementia: Findings from the Nun study. Annals of Internal Medicine, 139(5 Pt 2), 450–454.

Substance Abuse and Mental Health Services Administration (SAMHSA), Office of Applied Studies, Department of Health and Human Services. (2006). Results from the 2005 national survey on drug use and health: National findings. Retrieved March 28, 2008, from http://www.drugabusestatistics.samhsa.gov/NSDUH/2k5NSDUH/2k5results.htm

Tanner, J. (1962). Growth at adolescence (2nd ed.). Oxford: Blackwell.

Task force says men age 75 and older should not be screened for prostate cancer. Press Release, August 4, 2008. Agency for Healthcare Research and Quality, Rockville, MD. Retrieved from http://www.ahrq.gov/news/press/pr2008/tfproscanpr.htm

Taylor, R. W., McAuley, K. A., Barbezat, W., et al. (2007). APPLE project: 2-y findings of a community-based obesity prevention program in primary school age children. American Journal of Clinical Nutrition, 86(3), 735–742.

Theodore, A. D., Chang, J. J., Runyan, D. K., et al. (2005). Epidemiologic features of the physical and sexual maltreatment of children in the Carolinas. Pediatrics, 115(3), e331–337.

Tomita, M., Mann, W., Stanton, K., et al. (2007). Use of currently available smart home technology by frail elders. Process and outcomes. Topics in Geriatric Rehabilitation, 23(1), 24–34.

Townsend, M. (2009). Psychiatric mental health nursing: Concepts of care (6th ed.). Philadelphia: F. A. Davis.

U.S. Census Bureau. (2005). Median age of the total population: 2005. 2005 American Community Survey. Washington, DC: Author. Retrieved November 4, 2008, from http://factfinder.census.gov/servlet/GRTTable?_bm=y&-_box_head_nbr=R0101&-ds_name=ACS_2005_EST_G00_&-_lang=en&-format=US-30

U.S. Census Bureau. (2006, last modified December 1). National Populations Estimates for the 2000s. Washington, DC: Author. Retrieved November 7, 2008, from http://www.census.gov/population/www/projections/usinterimproj/

U.S. Census Bureau. (2007). American Community Survey 2006. Washington, DC. Author. Retrieved October 30, 2008, from http://www.census.gov/Press-Release/www/releases/archives/american_community_survey_acs/010709.html

U.S. Census Bureau. (2008). 2008 National population projections. Washington, DC: Author. Retrieved November 7, 2008, from http://www.census.gov/population/www/projections/2008projections.html

U.S. Census Bureau. (2009). Facts for features. Older Americans month: May 2009. U.S. Census Bureau News, March 3, 2009. Washington, DC: U.S. Department of Commerce. Retrieved March 9, 2009, from http://www.census.gov/Press-Release/www/releases/archives/facts_for_features_special_editions/013384.html

U.S. Department of Health and Human Services (USDHHS). (2005). U.S. Surgeon general gives tips to parents on teenagers. News Release. USDHHS. Retrieved April 10, 2008, from http://www.surgeongeneral.gov/pressreleases/sg12302005.html

U.S. Department of Health and Human Services (USDHHS). (2008). Physical activity guidelines for Americans. At-a-glance: A fact sheet for professionals. Retrieved November 3, 2008, from http://www.health.gov/paguidelines/factsheetprof.aspx

U.S. Department of Health and Human Services (USDHHS). (2010). Maternal, infant and child health. Healthy People 2020 (goals for public comment). Retrieved May 20, 2010, from http://www.healthypeople.gov/hp2020/Objectives/TopicArea.aspx?id=32&TopicArea=Maternal%2c+Infant+and+Child+Health

U.S. Environmental Protection Agency (EPA). (last updated February 19, 2008). Asthma. Indoor environmental asthma triggers. Retrieved March 28, 2008, from http://www.epa.gov/asthma/triggers.html

U.S. Preventive Services Task Force (USPSTF). (2002). Screening for breast cancer: Systematic evidence review. Rockville, MD: Agency for Healthcare Research and Quality. Retrieved April 15, 2008, from http://www.cdc.gov/cancer/breast/basic_info/screening.htm. Last updated October 16, 2006.

U.S. Preventive Services Task Force (USPSTF). (January, 2003). Screening for cervical cancer. Topic Page. Rockville, MD: Agency for Healthcare Research and Quality. Retrieved December 13, 2009, from http://www.ahrq.gov/clinic/uspstf/uspscerv.htm

U.S. Preventive Services Task Force (USPSTF). (2003). Screening for cervical cancer. What's new from the USPSTF. Retrieved December 12, 2008, from http://www.ahrq.gov/clinic/3rduspstf/cervcan/cervcanwh.htm

U.S. Preventive Services Task Force (USPSTF). (2004a). Screening for family and intimate partner violence: Recommendation statement. National Guideline Clearinghouse (NGC). Retrieved April 18, 2008, from http://www.guideline.gov/summary/summary.aspx?doc_id=4427&nbr=003341&string=abuse

U.S. Preventive Services Task Force (USPSTF). (2004b). Screening for testicular cancer: Recommendation statement. Rockville, MD: Agency for Healthcare Research and Quality. Retrieved February 12, 2010, from http://www.ahrq.gov/clinic/3rduspstf/testicular/testiculrs.htm

U.S. Preventive Services Task Force (USPSTF). (2008). Screening for prostate cancer: Recommendation statement. Rockville, MD: Agency for Healthcare Research and Quality. Retrieved January 5, 2010, from http://www.ahrq.gov/clinic/uspstf08/prostate/prostaters.htm

U.S. Preventive Services Task Force (USPSTF). (2009a). The guide to clinical preventive services, 2009: Recommendation statement. Rockville, MD: Agency for Healthcare Research and Quality. Retrieved December 13, 2009, from http://www.ahrq.gov/clinic/pocketgd09/pocketgd09.pdf

U.S. Preventive Services Task Force (USPSTF). (2009b). Screening for breast cancer: Clinical summary. Rockville, MD: Agency for Healthcare Research and Quality. Retrieved December 13, 2009, from http://www.ahrq.gov/clinic/uspstf09/breastcancer/brcansum.htm

U.S. Preventive Services Task Force (USPSTF). (2009c). Screening for breast cancer. Topic Page. Rockville, MD: Agency for Healthcare Research and Quality. Retrieved April 20, 2010, from http://www.ahrq.gov/clinic/uspstf/uspsbrca.htm

Uphold, C. R., & Grahan, M.V. (2004). Clinical guidelines in family practice. Gainsville, FL: Barmarrae Books.

Villareal, D., Banks, M., Sinacore, D., et al. (2006). Effect of weight loss and exercise on frailty in obese older adults. Archives of Internal Medicine, 166(8), 860–866.

Waldrop, J. (2008). Stopping childhood obesity before it begins. The Clinical Advisor, 11(1), 35–36, 39–41.

Wallace, M., & Shelkey, M. (2008). Monitoring functional status in hospitalized older adults. American Journal of Nursing, 108(4), 64–72.

Waugh, D. (1978). Moral development: Theory and process. In: Teaching and evaluating the affective domain in nursing programs (pp. 17–30). Thorofare, NJ: Charles B. Slack.

Whitaker, R. C., Phillips, S. M., Orzol, S. M., et al. (2007). The association between maltreatment and obesity among preschool children. Child Abuse & Neglect, 31(11–12), 1187–1199.

Wilkinson, J. (2009). Nursing diagnosis handbook (9th ed.). Upper Saddle River, NJ: Prentice-Hall.

Williams, K. N., Herman, R., Gajewski, B., et al. (2008). Elderspeak communication: Impact on dementia care. American Journal of Alzheimer's Disease & Other Dementias, Online First, published on June 30, 2008 as doi:10.1177/1533317508318472.

Wilson, D. M., & Palha, P. (2007). A systematic review of published research articles on health promotion at retirement. Journal of Nursing Scholarship, Fourth Quarter, 330–337.

Women's Health Initiative. (n.d.). The estrogen-plus-progestin study. National Heart, Lung, and Blood Institute, National Institutes of Health. Retrieved April 18, 2008, from http://www.nhlbi.nih.gov/whi/estro_pro.htm

Woodhouse, K. W., & O'Mahony, M. S. (1997). Frailty and ageing. Age and Ageing, 26, 245–46.

Yang, Y. (2008). Social inequalities in happiness. American Sociological Review, 73(2), 204–226.

Zimmerman, S., & Sloane, P. D. (2007). Improving practice through research in and about assisted living: Definition and classification of assisted living. The Gerontologist, 47(Special issue III), 33–39.

Chapter 10

Agency for Healthcare Research and Quality (2009). Press release. Educating patients before they leave the hospital reduces readmissions, emergency department visits and saves money. Retrieved Feburary 4, 2009, from http://www.ahrq.gov/news/press/pr2009/redpr.htm

Albom, M. (1997). Tuesdays with Morrie. New York: Doubleday.

American Medical Association (AMA). (2007). Evidence-based principles of discharge and discharge criteria. Report 4 of the Council on Scientific Affairs (A-96). Retrieved February 22, 2008, from http://www.ama-assn.org/ama/pub/category/print/13663.html

Benner, P., & Wrubel, J. (1989). The primacy of caring. Menlo Park, CA: Addison-Wesley.

Bettelheim, B. (1979). Surviving and other essays. New York: Alfred A. Knopf.

Centers for Disease Control and Prevention (CDC) (n.d.). Quick Facts: Economic and Health Burden of Chronic Disease. Chronic Disease Prevention. NCCDPHP Office of Communication. Retrieved March 1, 2008, from http://www.cdc.gov/nccdphp/press

Centers for Disease Control and Prevention (CDC). (n.d.). Death Rates for Major Chronic Diseases, by Race and Ethnicity, United States, 1998. Retrieved March 1, 2008 from http://www.cdc.gov/nccdphp/upo/overview.htm

Centers for Disease Control and Prevention (CDC). (2001). Prevalence of self-reported arthritis or chronic joint symptoms among adults—United States, 2001. Morbidity and Mortality Weekly Report 51(42), 948. October 2002. Retrieved March 1, 2008, from http://www.cdc.gov/mmwr/preview/mmwrhtml/ mm5142a2.htm

Centers for Disease Control and Prevention (CDC). (2005). Unintentional non-fire-related carbon monoxide exposure—United States, 2001–2003. Morbidity and Mortality Weekly Report, 54(2), 36–39. Retrieved March 1, 2008, from http://www.cdc.gov/mmwrhtml/mm540212.htm

Centers for Disease Control and Prevention (CDC). (2006). Cigarette smoking: Related mortality. Updated September 2006. Retrieved March 1, 2008, from http://www.cdc.gov/tobacco/data_statistics/Factsheets/cig_smoking_mort.htm

Centers for Medicare & Medicaid Services (CMS). (2007, May 8). Medicare Program; Inpatient rehabilitation facility prospective payment system for FY 2008. Federal Register, 72(88), 26230.

Cheng, N. (1986). Life and death in Shanghai. New York: Grove Press.

Cockerham, W. (2000). Medical sociology. Upper Saddle River, NJ: Prentice-Hall.

Cousins, N. (1979). Anatomy of an illness. New York: W. W. Norton.

Department of Health. (2003). Discharge from hospital pathway, process and practice. National Health Service, United Kingdom. Retrieved March 3, 2008, from http://www.dh.gov.uk/en/Publicationsandstatistics/Publications/PublicationsPolicyAndGuidance/DH_4003252

Dossey, B. M., & Keegan, L. (2009). Holistic nursing: A handbook for practice (5th ed.). Sudbury, MA: Jones and Bartlett.

Dossey, L. (2003). Healing beyond the body: Medicine and the infinite reach of the mind. Boston: Shambala Publications.

Drummond-Dye, R. (2007, December). Medicare focuses on home health policies. PT Magazine. Retrieved March 2, 2008, from the

American Physical Therapy Association, http://www.apta.org/AM/Template.cfm?Section=Home&TEMPLATE=/CM/HTML-Display.cfm&CONTENTID=45281

Dudas, V. (2001). The impact of follow-up telephone calls to patients after hospitalization. *The American Journal of Medicine*, 111(9), 26–30.

Dunn, H. L. (1959). High level wellness for man and society. *American Journal of Public Health*, 49(6), 786–788.

Eliasson, B. (2003). Cigarette smoking and diabetes. *Progress in Cardiovascular Diseases*, 45(5), 405–413.

Ellis, B. H., Shannon, E. D., Cox, J. K., et al. (2004). Chronic conditions: Results of the Medicare Health Outcomes Survey, 1998–2000. *Health Care Financing Review* (Summer, 2004). Retrieved March 1, 2008, from http://findarticles.com/p/articles/mi_m0795/is_4_25/ai_n6332418

Frankl, V. (1959, 1962, 1984). *Man's search for meaning*. New York: Washington Square Press.

Frankl, V. (2004). *Man's search for meaning*. London: Rider.

Glod, C. A. (1998). *Contemporary psychiatric-mental health nursing: The brain-behavior connection*. Philadelphia: F. A. Davis.

Godress, J., Ozgul, S., Owen, C., et al. (2005). Grief experiences of parents whose children suffer from mental illness. *Australian and New Zealand Journal of Psychiatry*, 39, 88–94.

Gonzales, S. (1991). One woman's story of rape. *The Kansas City Star*, August 4, pp. A1, A16, A17.

Greenwald, J. L., Denham, C. R., & Jack, B. W. (2007). The hospital discharge: A review of a high risk care transition with highlights of a reengineered discharge process. *Journal of Patient Safety*, 3(2), 97–106.

Joint Commission on Accreditation of Healthcare Organizations (JCAHO). (2000). *Pain assessment and management: An organizational approach*. Library of Congress Catalog Number: 00–102701.

The Joint Commission (TJC). (2008a). *2008 Hospital accreditation standards* (pp. 216–218, 366–367). Oakbrook Terrace, IL: Author.

The Joint Commission (TJC). (2008b). 2008 National patient safety goals. Retrieved February 22, 2008, from http://www.jcaho.org/PatientSafety/

Kapleau, P. (1997). *The Zen of living and dying*. Boston: Shambhala Publications.

Kokanovic, R., Petersen, A., & Klimidis, S. (2006). "Nobody can help me. . . I am living through it alone": Experiences of caring for people diagnosed with mental illness in ethno-cultural and linguistic minority communities. *Journal of Immigrant and Minority Health*, 8(2), 125–135.

Krishnamurti, J. (1956). *Commentaries on living*. Ojai, CA: Krishnamurti Foundation of America.

Lewis, C. S. (1961). *A grief observed*. London: Faber and Faber.

Lifton, R., & Olson, E. (1974). *Living and dying*. New York: Praeger Publishers.

Lusseyran, J. (1987). *And there was light*. (E. R. Cameron, Trans.). New York: Parabola Books.

Makaryus, A. N., & Friedman, E. A. (2005). Patients' understanding of their discharge treatment plans and diagnosis at discharge. *Mayo Clinic Proceedings*, 80, 991–994.

McFetridge, B., Gillesxpie, M., Goode, D., & Melby, V. (2007). *Nursing in Critical Care*, 12(6), 261–269.

Moltmann, J. (1983). *The power of the powerless*. San Francisco: Harper & Row.

Myers, J., Sweeney, T., & Witmer, J. (2000). The wheel of wellness counseling for wellness: A holistic model for treatment planning. *Journal of Counseling & Development*, 78(3), 251–267.

National Institute of Mental Health. (2003). Older adults: Depression and suicide facts, 2003. Retrieved March 1, 2008, from http://www.nimh.nih.gov/publicat/elderlydepsuicide.cfm

Naylor, M., Brooten, D., Jones, R., et al. (1994). Comprehensive discharge planning for the hospitalized elderly. A randomized clinical trial. *Annals of Internal Medicine*, 120, 999–1006.

Neuman, B. (1995). The Neuman systems model. In: B. Neuman, *The Neuman systems model* (3rd ed.). Norwalk, CT: Appleton and Lange.

Neuman, B. (2002). The Neuman systems model. In: B. Neuman, *The Neuman systems model* (4th ed.). Norwalk, CT: Appleton and Lange.

Neuman, B., & Fawcett, J. (2002). *The Neuman systems model* (4th ed.). Upper Saddle River, NJ: Prentice-Hall.

New South Wales Department of Health. (2007). *Policy directive: Discharge planning: Responsive standards* (revised November 2007). North Sydney, NSW: Author.

Nightingale, F. (1859/1992). *Notes on nursing: What it is, and what it is not*. Philadelphia: Lippincott.

The Ottawa Charter for Health Promotion. (1986). First International Conference on Health Promotion, Ottawa, 21 November 1986. World Health Organization (WHO). Retrieved February 29, 2008, from http://www.who.int/healthpromotion/conferences/previous/ottawa/en/

Parsons, T. (1975). The sick role and role of the physician reconsidered. *Milbank Memorial Fund Quarterly*, 53, 257–278.

Phillips, C. O., Wright, W. M., Kern, D. E., et al. (2004). Comprehensive discharge planning with postdischarge support for older patients with congestive heart failure—a meta-analysis. *JAMA*, 291, 1358–1367.

Reeve, C. (1998). *Still me*. New York: Random House.

Roper, C., & Happell, B. (2007). Reflection without shame—reflection without blame: Towards a more collaborative understanding between mental health consumers and nurses. *Journal of Psychiatric and Mental Health Nursing*, 14, 85–91.

Seigel, B. (1986). *Love, medicine and miracles*. New York: Harper & Row.

Sheinfeld-Gorin, S., & Arnold, J. (2006). *Health promotion in practice*. San Francisco: Jossey-Bass (John Wiley & Sons).

Smith, P. (1992). *Living the disrupted life: A symphony of survival*. University of Kansas: unpublished dissertation.

Stuck, A. E., Walthert, J. M., Nikolaus, T., et al. (1999). Risk factors for functional status decline in community living elderly people: A systematic literature review. *Social Science and Medicine*, 48(4), 445–469.

Suchman, E. A. (1972). Stages of illness and medical care. In: E. G. Jaco (Ed.), *Patients, physicians, and illness* (2nd ed.). New York: Free Press.

Thompson, J., & Manore, M. (2009). *Nutrition: An applied approach* (2nd ed.). San Francisco: Benajmin/Cummings.

Valladares, A. (2001). *Against all hope: A memoir of life in Castro's gulag*. San Francisco: Encounter Books.

Vanauken, S. (1977). *A severe mercy*. New York: Bantam Books.

Watson, J. (1979). *Nursing: The philosophy and science of caring*. Boston: Little, Brown and Company, 2nd printing 1985. Boulder, CO: University Press of Colorado.

Wilber, K. (2000). *Grace and grit: Spirituality and healing in the life and death of Treya Killam Wilber* (rev. ed.). Boston: Shambhala Publications.

World Health Organization (WHO). (1948). Preamble to the Constitution of the World Health Organization as adopted by the International Health Conference, New York, June 19–22, 1946 and entered into force on April 7, 1948.

Young, J. T. (2004). Illness behaviour: A selective review and synthesis. *Sociology of Health & Illness*, 26(1), 1–31.

Zwicker, D., & Picariello, G. (2003). Discharge planning for the older adult. In: M. Mezey, T. Fulmer, I. Abraham, & D. A. Zwicker (Eds.). *Geriatric nursing protocols for best practice* (2nd ed., pp. 292–316). New York: Springer.

Chapter 11

Albom, M. (1997). *Tuesdays with Morrie*. New York: Doubleday.

Allen, J., Murray, M., & Simmons, K. (2005). *How to succeed with developing resilience*. Carleton South, Victoria: Curriculum Corporation.

American Psychiatric Association (APA). (2000). *Diagnostic and statistical manual of mental disorders* (4th ed., text rev.). Washington, DC: Author. Also available from http://www.psychiatryonline.com/

Anandarajah, G., & Hight, I. (2001). Spirituality and medical practice: Using the HOPE questions as a practical tool for spiritual assessment. *American Family Physician, 63*, 81–88.

Association of Saskatchewan Home Economists. (n.d.). Help your child develop a positive body image. Retrieved March 26, 2008, from http://www.homefamily.net/index.php?/categories/results/help_your_child_develop_a_positive_body_image1

Balon, R. (2001). Anxiety across the life span: Epidemiological evidence and treatment data. *Depression and Anxiety, 13*(4), 184–189.

Barker, P. J. (2004). *Assessment in psychiatric and mental health nursing* (2nd ed.). Cheltenham, UK: Nelson Thomes.

Bigler, M., Neimeyer, G. J., & Brown, E. (2001). The divided self revisited: Effects of self-concept clarity and self-concept differentiation on psychological adjustment. *Journal of Social and Clinical Psychology, 20*(3), 396–415.

Blanchflower, D. B., & Oswald, A. J. (2008), Is well-being U-shaped over the life cycle? *Social Science & Medicine, 66*, 1733–1749.

Bourne, E. J. (2005). *The anxiety and phobia workbook* (4th ed.). Oakland, CA: New Harbinger Publications.

Bracken, B. A. (Ed.). (1996). *Handbook of self-concept*. New York: John Wiley & Sons.

Branden, N. (1994). *Six pillars of self-esteem*. New York: Bantam.

Branden, N. (2001). *The psychology of self-esteem: A revolutionary approach to self-understanding that launched a new era in modern psychology* (32nd Anniversary Edition). Danvers, MA: Jossey-Bass.

Brigham and Women's Hospital (2001). *Psychosocial approaches to deeply disturbed persons*. Boston: Author.

Brody, D., & Serby, M. (2007). Taking steps to head off serious depression. *The Clinical Advisor, 19*(1), 42, 45–46, 50.

Bulechek, G. M., Butcher, H. K., & Dochterman, J. M. (Eds.). (2008). Nursing interventions classification (NIC). St. Louis, MO: C. V. Mosby.

Center for Food Safety and Applied Nutrition. U.S. Food and Drug Administration (2002, March 25). Consumer Advisory. Kava-containing dietary supplements may be associated with severe liver injury. Retrieved March 20, 2008, from http://www.cfsan.fda.gov/%7Edms/addskava.html

Centers for Disease Control and Prevention (CDC). (2002). Hepatic toxicity possibly associated with kava-containing products—United States, Germany, and Switzerland, 1999–2002, *Morbidity and Mortality Weekly Report, 51*(47), 1065–1067. Retrieved March 20, 2008, from http://www.cdc.gov/mmwr/PDF/wk/mm5147.pdf

Centers for Disease Control and Prevention (CDC). (2007). Suicide. Facts at a glance. Retrieved March 20, 2008, from http://www.cdc.gov/ncipc/dvp/Suicide/SuicideDataSheet.pdf

Chen, T. M., Huang, F. Y., Chang, C., et al. (2006). Using the PHQ-9 for depression screening and treatment monitoring for Chinese Americans in primary care. *Psychiatric Services, 57*, 976–981.

Cheung, Y. B., Law, C. K., Chan, B., et al. (2006). Suicidal ideation and suicidal attempts in a population-based study of Chinese people: Risk attributable to hopelessness, depression, and social factors. *Journal of Affective Disorders, 90*(2–3), 193–199.

Clark, M. M., Croghan, I. T., Reading, S., et al. (2005). The relationship of body image dissatisfaction to cigarette smoking in college students. *Body Image, 2*(3), 263–270.

Coopersmith, S. (1967). *The antecedents of self-esteem*. San Francisco: W. H. Freeman.

Dickstein, E. (1977). Self and self-esteem: Theoretical foundations and their implications for research. *Human Development, 20*, 129–140.

Drench, M. E., Sharby, N., Noonan, A., et al. (2006). *Psychosocial aspects of healthcare* (2nd ed.). Upper Saddle River, NJ: Prentice-Hall.

Edwards, N. (2003). Differentiating the three D's: Delirium, dementia, and depression. *MedSurg Nursing*. Retrieved March 18, 2008, from http://findarticles.com/p/articles/mi_m0FSS/is_6_12/ai_n18616788

Ellemers, N., Spears, R., & Doosje, B. (2002). Self and social identity. *Annual Review of Psychology, 53*, 161–186.

Erikson, E. (1963). *Childhood and society* (2nd ed.). New York: W. W. Norton.

Fortinash, K. M., & Worret, P. A. (2008). *Psychiatric mental health nursing* (4th ed.). St. Louis, MO: Mosby/Elsevier.

Gazmararian, J., Baker, D., Parker, R., et al. (2000). A multivariate analysis of factors associated with depression: Evaluating the role of health literacy as a potential contributor. *Archives of Internal Medicine, 160*(21), 3307–3314.

Ghosh, T. B., & Victor, B. S. (1994). Suicide. In: R. E. Hales, S. C. Yudofsky, & J. A. Talbott (Eds.). *The American Psychiatric Press textbook of psychiatry* (2nd ed.). Washington, DC: American Psychiatric Press.

Goldston, D. B., Reboussin, B. A., & Daniel, S. S. (2006). Predictors of Suicide Attempts: State and Trait Components. *Journal of Abnormal Psychology, 115*(4), 842–849.

Gorman, L. M., & Sultan, D. E. (2008). *Psychosocial nursing for general patient care* (3rd ed.). Philadelphia: F. A. Davis.

Greenberg, S. A. (2007). The Geriatric Depression Scale: Short Form. *American Journal of Nursing, 107*(10), 60–70.

Gregory, J. (1996). *The psychosocial education of nurses: The interpersonal dimension*. Aldershot, Hampshire, England: Avebury Ashgate Publishing.

Hammen, C. (2005). Stress and Depression. *Annual Review of Clinical Psychology, 56*(1), 293–319.

Hattie, J. (1992). *Self concept*. Hillsdale, NJ: Erlbaum Bacon.

Hentz, P. (2008). Separating anxiety from physical illness. *The Clinical Advisor, 11*(3), 82–85.

Hewitt, M. E., Herdman, R., & Holland, J. C. (2004). *Meeting psychosocial needs of women with breast cancer*. Washington, DC: National Academies Press.

Hillman, J. (1975). *Re-visioning psychology*. New York: Harper & Row.

Himmelhoch, J., Levine, J., & Gershon, S. (2001). Historical overview of the relationship between anxiety disorders and affective disorders. *Depression and Anxiety, 14*, 53–66.

Howarth, D., Heath, J., & Snope, F. (1999). Beyond the Folstein: Dementia in primary care. *Primary Care: Clinics in Office Practice, 26*, 299–314.

Hulisz, D. T. (2008). Top herbal products: Efficacy and safety concerns. Medscape Nurses. ©2007. Retrieved March 20, 2008, from http://www.medscape.com/;/viewarticle/568235

Institute for Clinical Systems Improvement (ICSI). (2008). *Major depression in adults in primary care*. Bloomington, MN: Author.

International Society for Mental Health Online (ISMHO). (last updated September 2004). All about depression. Retrieved March 20, 2008, from http://www.allaboutdepression.com/gen_01.html#3

Jamison, K. R. (1997). *An unquiet mind: A memoir of moods and madness*. London: Picador.

Johnson, M., Bulechek, G., Dochterman, J., et al. (2006). *NANDA, NOC, and NIC linkages: Nursing diagnoses, outcomes, and interventions* (2nd ed.). St. Louis, MO: C. V. Mosby.

Khouzam, H. R., Tan, D. T., & Gill, T. S. (2007). *Handbook of emergency psychiatry*. St. Louis, MO: C. V. Mosby.

Kleinman, A., & Good, B. (1985). *Culture and depression*. Berkeley, CA: University of California Press.

Kroenke, K., Spitzer, R. L., & Williams, J. B. W. (2001). The PHQ-9. Validity of a brief depression severity measure. *Journal of General Internal Medicine, 16*(9), 606–613.

Kurlowicz, L. H. (2008). Depression. In: E. Capezuti, D. Zwicker, M. Mezey, & T. Fulmer (Eds.), *Evidence-based geriatric nursing protocols for best practice* (3rd ed., pp. 57–82). New York: Springer.

Levine, J., Cole, D. P., Chengappa, R., et al. (2001). Anxiety disorders and major depression, together or apart. *Depression and Anxiety, 14*, 94–104.

Marsh, H. W. (1988). *Self-description questionnaire I*. San Antonio, TX: Psychological Corporation.

Marsh, H. W. (1989). *Self-description questionnaire III (SDQIII) manual*. Sydney, Australia: University of Western Sydney.

Marsh, H. W. (1991). *Self-description questionnaire II: Manual and research monograph*. San Antonio, TX: Psychological Corporation.

Maslow, A. (1968). *Toward a psychology of being* (2nd ed.). New York: Van Nostrand-Reinhold.

Maybury, B. C. (2008, March 10). Suicide prevention: Every nurse's responsibility. Nurse.com Retrieved January 22, 2010, from http://news.nurse.com/apps/pbcs.dll/article?AID=200880305017

McCabe, M. P., Ricciardelli, L. A., Sitaram, G., et al. (2006). Accuracy of body size estimation: Role of biopsychosocial variables. *Body Image, 3*(2), 163–171.

Mead, M. (1934). *Mind, self and society.* Chicago: University of Chicago Press.

Menninger, K. (1963). *The vital balance.* New York: Viking Press.

Moorhead, S., Johnson, M., Maas, M. L., et al. (Eds.). (2008). *Nursing outcomes classification (NOC)* (4th ed.). St. Louis, MO: C. V. Mosby.

Morris, C. G., & Maisto, A. A. (2001). *Psychology: An Introduction* (11th ed.). Upper Saddle River, NJ: Pearson Higher Education.

Moser, D. K. (2007). "The rust of life": Impact of anxiety on cardiac patients. *American Journal of Critical Care, 16*, 361–369.

Murdock, M. (1990). *The heroine's journey.* Boston: Shambhala Publications.

NANDA International. (2009). *Nursing diagnoses: Definitions and classification 2009–2011.* Philadelphia: Author.

National Guideline Clearinghouse (NGC). (2006). Major depression in adults in primary care. Retrieved March 22, 2008, from http://www.guideline.gov/summary/summary.aspx?doc_id=10866&nbr=005679&string=%22Major+depression%2c+panic+disorder%22+and+%22generalized+anxiety+disorder+in+adults+in+primary+care%22

National Guideline Clearinghouse (NGC). (2008a). Assessing cognitive function. In: *Evidence-based geriatric nursing protocols for best practice.* Retrieved September 1, 2008, from http://www.guideline.gov/summary/summary.aspx?view_id=1&doc_id=12266

National Guideline Clearinghouse (NGC). (2008b). Delirium: Prevention, early recognition, and treatment. In: *Evidence-based geriatric nursing protocols for best practice.* Retrieved September 1, 2008, from http://www.guideline.gov/summary/summary.aspx?view_id=1&doc_id=12261

National Guideline Clearinghouse (NGC). (2008c). Depression. In: *Evidence-based geriatric nursing protocols for best practice.* Retrieved September 1, 2008, from http://www.guideline.gov/summary/summary.aspx?view_id=1&doc_id=12260

National Institute of Mental Health (NIMH). Older adults: Depression and suicide fact sheet. Revised April 2007. NIH Publication No. 4593. http://www.nimh.nih.gov/publicat/elderlydepsuicide.cfm

National Institute of Mental Health (NIMH). Suicide in the U.S.: Statistics and prevention (Page last reviewed March 20, 2008). Retrieved March 22, 2008, from http://www.nimh.nih.gov/health/publications/suicide-in-the-us-statistics-and-prevention.shtml

Newell, R., & Gournay, K. (Eds.). (2000). *Mental health nursing: An evidence-based approach.* London: Churchill Livingstone.

Parker, G. (2005). *Dealing with depression: A commonsense guide to mood disorders* (2nd ed.). Australia: Allen & Unwin.

Pekrun, R. (2004). Self-concepts: Educational Aspects. *International Encyclopedia of the Social & Behavioral Sciences,* 13799–13803.

Peplau, H. (1963). A working definition of anxiety. In: S. Burd & M. Marshall (Eds.), *Some clinical approaches to psychiatric nursing.* New York: Macmillan.

Pleis, J. R., & Lethbridge-Cejku, M. (2006). Summary health statistics for U.S. Adults: National health interview survey, 2005. *Vital and Health Statistics, Series 10* (232), December 2006. Centers for Disease Control. Retrieved March 17, 2008, from http://www.cdc.gov/nchs/data/series/sr_10/sr10_232.pdf

Reeve, C. (1998). *Still me.* New York: Random House.

Richardson, S. (2003). Delirium: Assessment and treatment of the elderly patient. *The American Journal for Nurse Practitioners, 7*(1), 9–15.

Schwartz, M. B., & Brownell, K. D. (2004). Obesity and body image. *Body Image, 1*(1), 3–56.

Schwartz, T. L., & Peterson, T. J. (Eds.). (2006). *Depression: Treatment strategies and management.* New York: Taylor & Francis.

Sheikh, J. I., & Yesavage, J., A. (1986). Geriatric Depression Scale (GDS): Recent evidence and development of a shorter version. In: *Clinical gerontology: A guide to assessment and intervention* (pp. 165–173). New York: The Haworth Press. Also available at http://www.stanford.edu/~yesavage/GDS.html (Retrieved March 18, 2008).

Shen, B. J., Avivi, Y. E., Todaro, J. F., et al. (2008). Anxiety characteristics independently and prospectively predict myocardial infarction in men. The unique contribution of anxiety among psychologic factors. *Journal of the American College of Cardiology, 51,* 113–119.

Sleeth, D. B. (2006). The self and the integral interface: Toward a new understanding of the whole person. *The Humanistic Psychologist, 34*(3), 243–261.

Sleeth, D. B. (2007a). The self system: Toward a new understanding of the whole person (part 2). *The Humanistic Psychologist, 35*(1), 27–43.

Sleeth, D. B. (2007b). The self system: Toward a new understanding of the whole person (Part 3). *The Humanistic Psychologist, 35*(1), 56–66.

Stanley, M., Blair, K. A., & Beare, P. G. (2005). *Gerontological nursing* (3rd ed.). Philadelphia: F. A. Davis.

Stein, K. F., & Corte, C. (2007). Identity impairment and the eating disorders: content and organization of the self-concept in women with anorexia nervosa and bulimia nervosa. *European Eating Disorders Review, 15*(1), 58–69

Steptoe, A. (Ed.). (2007). *Depression and physical illness.* New York: Cambridge University Press.

Stice, E., & Shaw, H. (2003). Prospective relations of body image, eating, and affective disturbances to smoking onset in adolescent girls: How Virginia slims. *Journal of Consulting and Clinical Psychology, 71*(1), 129–135.

Stokes, R., & Frederick-Recascino, C. (2003). Women's perceived body image: Relations with personal happiness. *Journal of Women & Aging, 15*(1), 17–29.

Stuart, G. W., & Laraia, M. T. (2001). *Principles and practice of psychiatric nursing* (7th ed.). St. Louis, MO: C. V. Mosby.

Therapeutic Goods Administration. (2005). Kava fact sheet. Retrieved March 22, 2008, from http://www.tga.health.gov.au/cm/kavafs0504.htm

Thombs, B. D., Haines, J. M., Bresnick, M. G., et al. (2007). Depression in burn reconstruction patients: symptom prevalence and association with body image dissatisfaction and physical function. *General Hospital Psychiatry, 29*(1), 14–20

Thombs, B. D., Notes, L. D., Lawrence, J. W., et al. (2008). From survival to socialization: A longitudinal study of body image in survivors of severe burn injury. *Journal of Psychosomatic Research, 64*(2), 205–212.

Townsend, M. C. (2008). *Essentials of psychiatric mental health nursing* (4th ed.). Philadelphia: F. A. Davis.

U.S. Preventive Services Task Force (USPSTF). (2002). Screening for depression: Recommendations and rationale. *Annals of Internal Medicine, 136*(10), 760–764.

U.S. Preventive Services Task Force (USPSTF). (2004). Screening for suicide risk. Retrieved March 18, 2008, from http://www.ahrq.gov/clinic/uspstf/uspssuic.htm

Videbeck, S. L. (2006). *Psychiatric mental health nursing* (3rd ed.). Philadelphia: Lippincott.

Wingood, G. M., DiClemente, R. J., Harrington, K., et al. (2002). Body image and African American females' sexual health. *Journal of Women's Health and Gender Based Medicine, 11*(5), 433–439.

Yaghmale, F., Khalafi, A., Majd, H. A., et al. (2008). Correlation between self-concept and health status aspects in haemodialysis patients at selected hospitals affiliated to Shaheed Beheshti University of Medical Sciences. *Journal of Research in Nursing, 13*(3), 198–205.

Zigmond, A. S., & Snaith, R. P. (1983). The hospital anxiety and depression scale. *Acta Psychiatrica Scandinavica, 67,* 361–370.

Chapter 12

American Medical Association (AMA). (2007). AMA health policy publishes new proposal for expanding health insurance coverage. Retrieved February 7, 2008, from http://www.ama-assn.org/ama/pub/category/3373.html

Centers for Disease Control and Prevention (CDC). (2009a). Understanding child maltreatment. Retrieved December 4, 2009, from http://www.cdc.gov/ViolencePrevention/childmaltreatment/

Centers for Disease Control and Prevention (CDC). (2009b). Child maltreatment prevention program: Program activities guide. Retrieved December 4, 2009, from http://www.cdc.gov/violenceprevention/pub/PreventingCM.html

Centers for Disease Control and Prevention (CDC). (2005). Burden of chronic disease on minority racial populations and women. Retrieved December 4, 2009, from http://www.cdc.gov/nccdphp/overview.htm#4

Child Welfare Information Gateway. (2007). Child abuse and neglect statistics. Retrieved December 13, 2008, from http://www.childwelfare.gov/systemwide/statistics/can.cfm

DeNavas-Walt, C. B., Proctor, B. D., & Lee, C. H. (2006). Income, Poverty, and Health Insurance Coverage in the United States: 2005 U.S. Census Bureau.

Dochterman, J. M., & Bulechek, G. M. (Eds.). (2004). *Nursing interventions classification (NIC)* (4th ed.). St. Louis, MO: C. V. Mosby.

Friedman, M. M., Bowden, V. R., & Jones, E. G. (2003). *Family nursing: Research, theory, and practice* (5th ed.). Upper Saddle River, NJ: Prentice-Hall.

Gillis, C. L., Highley, B. L., Roberts, B. M., et al. (1989). *Toward a science of family nursing*. Menlo Park, CA: Addison-Wesley.

Hanna, D. R., & Roy, C. (2001). Roy adaptation model and perspective on the family. *Nursing Science Quarterly*, 14(1), 9–12.

Harmon, S. M., Gedaly-Duff, V., & Kaakinen, J. R. (2005). *Family health care nursing: Theory, practice & research* (3rd ed.). Philadelphia: F. A. Davis.

Hill, R., & Hansen, D. (1960). The identification of conceptual frameworks utilized in family study. *Marriage and Family Living*, 22(4), 299–311.

Huges, M. E., Waite, L. J., LaPierre, T. A., et al. (2007). All in the family: The impact of caring for grandchildren on grandparents' health. *The Journals of Gerontology Series B: Psychological Sciences and Social Sciences*, 62, S108–19.

Johnson, B. S. (2000). Mothers' perceptions of parenting children with disabilities. *Maternal Child Nursing: American Journal of Maternal-Child Nursing*, 25(3), 127–132.

Johnson, M., Bulechek, G., Butcher, H., et al. (2006). *NANDA, NOC, and NIC linkages*. St. Louis, MO: C. V. Mosby.

Leder, S., Grinstead, L. N., & Torres, E. (2007). Grandparents raising grandchildren: Stressors, social support, and health outcomes. *Journal of Family Nursing*, 13(3), 333–352.

Martin, J. A., Brady, E. H., Sutton, D. P., et al. (2007). Births: Final data for 2005, National Vital Statistics Report. Retrieved December 5, 2009, from http://www.cdc.gov/nchs/fastats/prenatal.htm

Mather, M., Rivers, K., & Jacobsen, L. (2005). The American community survey. *Population Bulletin*, 60(3), 3–20.

McGoldrick, M., & Carter, E. (1985). The stages of the family life cycle. In: J. Henslin (Ed.), *Marriage and family in a changing society*. New York: Free Press.

Moorhead, S., Johnson, M., & Maas, M. (Eds.). (2008). *Nursing outcomes classification (NOC)* (4th ed.). St. Louis, MO: C. V. Mosby.

Parsons, T., & Bales, R. F. (1955). *Family socialization and interaction process*. New York: Free Press.

Population Reference Bureau. (2003). What is a marriage? What is a household? Retrieved December 5, 2009, from http://www.prb.org/Articles/2003/WhatsaHouseholdWhatsaFamily.aspx

Population Reference Bureau. (2006). Families, fathers, and demographic change. Retrieved December 5, 2009, from http://www.prb.org/Articles/2006/FamiliesFathersandDemographicChange.aspx

Primeau, L. (2000). Divisions of household work, routines, and child care occupations in families. *Journal of Occupational Science*, 7(1), 19–28.

Qureshi, N., Wilson, B., Santaguida, P., et al. (2009, August). NIH State-of-the-Science Conference: Family history and improving health. *Evidence Report/Technology Assessment No. 186*. (Prepared by the McMaster University Evidence-based Practice Center, under Contract No. 290-2007-10060-I.) AHRQ Publication No. 09–E016. Rockville, MD: Agency for Healthcare Research and Quality. Retrieved September 17, 2009, from http://www.ahrq.gov/clinic/tp/famhimptp.htm

Rehabilitation and Training Research Center on Disability Demographics Statistics. (2007). *The 2006 annual disability status report*. Ithaca, NY: Cornell University.

Schwartz, A. N. (1979). Psychological dependency: An emphasis on the later years. In: P. Ragan (Ed.), *Aging parents*. Los Angeles: Andrus Gerontology Center, University of Southern California.

U.S. Census Bureau. (2006). Households by size: 1960 to present and households by type: 1940 to present. Table HH1. Retrieved December 5, 2009, from http://www.census.gov/population/socdemo/hh-fam/hh1.pdf

U.S. Census Bureau. (2007; updated August 27, 2008). America's families and living arrangements: 2006. Current Population Reports P20–553: Table HH-1. Retrieved December 5, 2009, from http://www.census.gov/population/www/socdemo/hh-fam/cps2006.html

U.S. Census Bureau. (2009, September). America's families and living arrangements: 2007. Current Population Reports P20-561. Retreived January 27, 2010, from http://www.census.gov/population/www/socdemo/hh-fam.html

Winstead-Fry, P. (2000). Rogers' conceptual system and family nursing. *Nursing Science Quarterly*, 13(4), 278–280.

Wright, L. M., & Leahey, M. (1984). *Nurses and families: A guide to family assessment and intervention*. Philadelphia: F. A. Davis.

Chapter 13

Agency for Healthcare Research and Quality (2003). National healthcare disparities report, 2003. Rockville, MD. Current as of August 2007. Retrieved August 1, 2008, from http://www.ahrq.gov/qual/nhdr03/nhdr03.htm

American Nurses Association (ANA). (1997). *Position statements: Cultural diversity in nursing practice*. Retrieved January 12, 2003, from http://www.nursingworld.org/readroom/position/ethics/etcldv.htm

American Nurses Association (ANA). (2010). *Nursing: Scope and standards of practice* (2nd ed.). Public Comment draft, January 2010. Silver Spring, MD: Nursebooks.org Retrieved February 1, 2010, from http://www.nursingworld.org/DocumentVault/NursingPractice/Draft-Nursing-Scope-Standards-2nd-Ed.aspx

Andrews, M. M., & Boyle, J. S. (2007). *Transcultural concepts in nursing care* (5th ed.). Philadelphia: Lippincott Williams & Wilkins.

Broome, B. (2006). Culture 101. *Urologic Nursing*, 26(6), 486–489.

Bulechek, G. M., Butcher, H. K., & Dochterman, J. M. (Eds.). (2008). *Nursing interventions classification (NIC)* (5th ed.). St. Louis, MO: C. V. Mosby.

Burns, T., Catty, J., Becker, T., et al. (2007). The effectiveness of supported employment for people with severe mental illness: A randomized controlled trial. *Lancet*, 370(9593), 1146–1152.

Calvillo, E. R., & Flaskerud, J. H. (1993). Evaluation of the pain response by Mexican American and Anglo American women and their nurses. *Journal of Advanced Nursing*, 18(3), 451–459.

Campinha-Bacote, J. (2003). Many faces: Addressing diversity in health care. *Online Journal of Issues in Nursing*, 8(1), Figure 3. Retrieved February 25, 2008, from http://nursingworld.org/MainMenuCategories/ANAMarketplace/ANAPeriodicals/OJIN/TableofContents.aspx

Campinha-Bacote, J. (2007). Cultural competence in nursing curricula: How are we doing 20 years later? Presented November 9, 2007, at the National Organization for Associate Degree Nursing 2007 Annual Convention, Las Vegas, NV.

Canadian Census. (2007a). Ethnic diversity and immigration. Statistics Canada. Last modified September 7, 2007. Retrieved February 22, 2008, from http://www41.statcan.ca/2007/30000/ceb30000_000_e.htm

Canadian Census. (2007b, last modified September 7, 2007). Population. Statistics Canada. Retrieved February 22, 2008, from http://www41.statcan.ca/2007/3867/ceb3867_000_e.htm

Carballeira, N. (1997). The LIVE and LEARN model for cultural competent family services. *Continuum*, 7–12.

Cloyes, K. (2007). Prisoners signify: A political discourse analysis of mental illness in a prison control unit. *Nursing Inquiry, 14*(3), 202–211.

Cronenwett, L., Sherwood, G., Barnsteiner, J., et al. (2007). Quality and safety education for nurses. *Nursing Outlook, 55*(3), 122–131.

Cross, T., Bazron, B., Dennis, K., & Issacs, M. (1989). *Towards a culturally competent system of care: Vol. I.* Washington, DC: Georgetown University Child Development Center, CASSP Technical Center.

Developing *Healthy People 2020.* (2008). Phase I report: Recommendations for the framework and format of *Healthy People 2020.* The Secretary's Advisory Committee on National Health Promotion and Disease Prevention Objectives for 2020. Retrieved December 12, 2009, from http://www.healthypeople.gov/hp2020/advisory/PhaseI/default.htm

Dozier, W. L. (2003). Race: Anthropologists say divisions were made by man. *The Gazette.* Retrieved August 5, 2003, from http://www.gazette.net/200018/frederickcty/state/10106–1.html

Eggenbereger, S. K., Grassley, J., & Restrepo, E. (2006). Competent nursing care: Listening to the voices of Mexican-American Women. *Online Journal of Issues in Nursing, 11*(3), 7.

Fitzpatrick, J. J., Nyamathi, A., & Koniak-Griffin, D. (2007). *Annual review of nursing research,* Vol. 25: *Vulnerable populations.* New York: Springer.

Geissler, E. M. (1991). Transcultural nursing and nursing diagnosis. *Nursing and Health Care, 12*(4), 190–203.

George, T. B. (2000). Defining care in the culture of the chronically mentally ill living in the community. *Journal of Transcultural Nursing, 11*(2), 102–110.

Giger, J. N., & Davidhizar, R. (2002). The Giger and Davidhizar transcultural assessment model. *Journal of Transcultural Nursing, 13*(3), 185–188.

Giger, J. N., & Davidhizar, R. (2008). *Transcultural nursing: Assessment and intervention* (5th ed.). St. Louis, MO: C. V. Mosby.

Graham-Garcia, J., Raines, T. L., Andrews, J. O., et al. (2001). Race, ethnicity, and geography: Disparities in heart disease in woman of color. *Journal of Transcultural Nursing, 12*(1), 56–67.

Hagman, L. W. (2004). New Mexico nurses' cultural self-efficacy: A pilot study. *Journal of Cultural Diversity, 11*(4), 146–149.

Jackson, A. K. (2007). Cultural competence in health visiting practice: A baseline survey. *Community Practitioner, 80*(2), 17–22.

Kardong-Edgren, S., Bond, M. L., Schlosser, S., et al. (2005). Cultural attitudes, knowledge, and skills of nursing faculty toward patients from four diverse cultures. *Journal of Professional Nursing, 21*(3), 175–182.

Kleinman, A., & Benson, P. (2006). Anthropology in the clinic: The problem of cultural competency and how to fix it. *PLoS Medicine 3*(10), e294 doi:10.1371/journal.pmed.0030294. Retrieved February 24, 2008, from http://medicine.plosjournals.org/perlserv/?request=get-document&doi=10.1317/journal.pmed.0030294&ct=1

Lavoie, M., & Shyu, Y. L. (2007). Nursing, healthcare, and culture: Views from Canada and Taiwan for the year 2050. Interview by Jacqueline Fawcett. *Nursing Science Quarterly, 20*(1), 51–55.

Leininger, M. (1978). *Transcultural nursing: Concepts, theories, and practices.* New York: John Wiley & Sons.

Leininger, M. (Ed.). (1991). *Culture care diversity and universality: A theory of nursing.* New York: National League for Nursing Press.

Leininger, M. (2002). Founder's focus: Linguistic clichés and buzzwords in the culture of nursing. *Journal of Transcultural Nursing, 13*(4), 334.

Leininger, M. (2007). Theoretical questions and concerns: Response from the Theory of Culture Care Diversity and Universality perspective. *Nursing Science Quarterly, 20*(1), 9–13.

Leininger, M. M., & McFarland, M. R. (2002). *Transcultural nursing: Concepts, theories, research and practices.* (3rd ed.). New York: McGraw-Hill.

Leininger, M. M., & McFarland, M. R. (2006). *Culture care diversity and universality: A worldwide nursing theory.* Sudbury, MA: Jones and Bartlett.

Leppa, C. (2000). Transcultural communication within the health care subculture. In: J. Luckmann (Ed.), *Transcultural communication in health care* (pp. 74–83). Clifton Park, NY: Thomson Delmar Learning.

Lipson, J., & Meleis, A. (1985). Culturally appropriate care: The case of immigrants. *Topics in Clinical Nursing, 7*(3), 48–56.

Logan, D. M. (2007). Culturally and linguistically appropriate services: An overview of policy and safe acute care nursing practice in the United States. *Gastroenterology Nursing, 30*(1), 29–35.

Lustig, M. W., & Koester, J. (2003). *Intercultural competence: Interpersonal communication across cultures* (4th ed.). Boston: Pearson Education.

Marks, B. (2007). Cultural competence revisited: Nursing students with disabilities. *Journal of Nursing Education, 46*(2), 70–74.

Mechanic, D. (1963). Religion, religiosity, and illness behavior: The special case of the Jews. *Human Organization, 22,* 202–208.

Michel, C., & Bellegarde-Smith, P. (2006). *Voudo in Haitian life and culture: Invisible powers.* New York: Palgrave Macmillan.

Munoz, C., & Luckmann, J. (2004). *Transcultural communication in health care* (2nd ed.). Clifton Park, NY: Thomson Delmar Learning.

Office of Minority Health & Health Disparities (OMHD). (2001). National standards for culturally and linguistically appropriate services in health care. Washington, DC: U.S. Department of Health and Human Services. Retrieved February 25, 2008, from http://www.omhrc.gov/CLAS

Office of Minority Health & Health Disparities (OMHD). (2007). About minority health. Last modified June 6, 2007. Retrieved February 28, 2008, from http://www.cdc.gov/omhd/AMH/AMH.htm

Proposed Healthy People 2020 objectives   List for public comment. U. S. Department of Health and Human Services. Retrieved January 22, 2010, from http://www.healthypeople.gov/hp2020/Objectives/TopicAreas.aspx

Purnell, L. (2000). A description of the Purnell model for cultural competence. *Journal of Transcultural Nursing, 11,* 40–46.

Purnell, L. (2002). The Purnell model for cultural competence. *Journal of Transcultural Nursing, 13*(3), 193–196.

Purnell, L. D., & Paulanka, B. J. (2008). *Transcultural health nursing: A culturally competent approach* (3rd ed.). Philadelphia: F. A. Davis.

Robichaux, C., Dittmar, V., & Clark, A. P. (2005). Are we providing culturally competent care? *Clinical Nurse Specialist, 19*(1), 11–14.

The Secretary's Advisory Committee on National Health Promotion and Disease Prevention Objectives for 2020. (2008). Developing *Healthy People 2020.* Phase I report: Recommendations for the framework and format of *Healthy People 2020.* Retrieved December 12, 2009, from http://www.healthypeople.gov/hp2020/advisory/PhaseI/default.htm

Spector, R. E. (2002). Cultural diversity in health and illness. *Journal of Transcultural Nursing, 13*(3), 197–199.

Spector, R. E. (2004). *Cultural diversity in health and illness* (6th ed.). Upper Saddle River, NJ: Prentice-Hall.

Strickland, O. L., Giger, J. N., Nelson, M. A., et al. (2007). The relationships among stress, coping, social support, and weight class in premenopausal African American women at risk for coronary heart disease. *Journal of Cardiovascular Nursing, 22*(4), 272–278.

Suchman, E. A. (1964). Sociomedical variations among ethnic groups. *American Journal of Sociology, 70,* 319–331.

Suchman, E. A. (1965). Social patterns of illness and medical care. *Journal of Health and Human Behavior, 6,* 2–16.

Suzuki, L. A., & Ponterotto, J. G. (2007). *Handbook of multicultural assessment: Clinical, psychological, and educational applications* (3rd ed.). San Francisco: Jossey-Bass.

Swanson, E. (2006). Culturally competent care for older adults: We are making progress. *Journal of Gerontological Nursing, 32*(10), 4.

Taylor, R. (2005). Addressing barriers to cultural competence. *Journal for Nurses in Staff Development, 21*(4), 135–142.

Trask, B. S., & Hamon, R. R. (2007). *Cultural diversity and families: Expanding perspectives.* Thousand Oaks, CA: Sage Publications.

U.S. Census Bureau. 2010 census constituent FAQs. Retrieved January 30, 2010, from http://2010.census.gov/partners/pdf/ConstituentFAQ.pdf

U.S. Census Bureau (n.d.). Fact sheet: United States 2006 American community survey data profile highlights. Retrieved February 22, 2008, from http://factfinder.census.gov/home/saff/main.html?_lang=en

U.S. Census Bureau (2000). QT-P55. Race alone or in combination: 2000. Retrieved February 22, 2008, from http://factfinder.census.gov/home/saff/main.html?_lang=en

U.S. Census Bureau. (2004). *Table 1a. Projected Population of the United States, by Race and Hispanic Origin: 2000 to 2050.* Retrieved February 22, 2008, from http://www.census.gov/ipc/www/usinterimproj/

U.S. Census Bureau. (2005). Race and Hispanic origin in 2005. Retrieved February 22, 2008, from http://www.census.gov/population/pop-profile/dynamic/RACEHO.pdf

U.S. Census Bureau (2006). Nation's population one-third minority. Released May 10, 2006. Retrieved February 22, 2008, from http://www.census.gov/Press-Release/www/releases/archives/population/006808.html

U.S. Census Bureau. (2007). Minority population tops 100 million. Released May 17, 2007. Retrieved February 22, 2008, from http://www.census.gov/Press-Release/www/releases/archives/population/010048.html

U.S. Census Bureau. (2008). *State and County QuickFacts. Race.* Source: 2000 Census of Population, Public Law 94–171 Redistricting Data File. Updated every 10 years. Retrieved February 24, 2008, from http://quickfacts.census.gov/qfd/meta/long_68184.htm

U.S. Census Bureau. (2010). The questions on the form. Retrieved April 22, 2010, from http://2010.census.gov/2010census/how/interactive-form.php

U.S. Census Bureau News. (August 14, 2008). Washington, DC: U.S. Department of Commerce. Retrieved August 22, 2008, from http://www.census.gov/Press-Release/www/releases/archives/population/012496.html

U.S. Department of Health and Human Services, OPHS, Office of Minority Health. (2001). National standards for culturally and linguistically appropriate services in health care: Executive summary. Washington, DC: Author. Retrieved February 26, 2008, from http://www.haa.omhrc.gov/templates/content.aspx?iD=2806. Page last modified April 12, 2007.

Urban Indian Health Commission. (2007). Invisible tribes: Urban Indians and their health in a changing world. Robert Wood Johnson Foundation report. Retrieved February 26, 2008, from http://www.rwjf.org/files/research/ulhc2007report.pdf

Wells, M. (2000). Beyond cultural competence: A model for individual and institutional cultural development. *Journal of Community Health Nursing, 17*(4), 189–199.

Wilkinson, J. M. (2007). *Nursing process & critical thinking* (4th ed.). Upper Saddle River, NJ: Pearson/Prentice-Hall.

Zambrana, R. E., Molnar, C., Munoz, H. B., & Lopez, D. S. (2004). Cultural competency as it intersects with racial/ethnic, linguistic, and class disparities in managed healthcare organizations. *The American Journal of Managed Care,* September. Special Issue. Pages SP037–SP044. Retrieved February 24, 2008, from http://www.ajmc.com/Article.cfm?Menu=1&ID=2687

Zborowski, M. (1952). Cultural components in responses to pain. *Journal of Social Issues, 8,* 16–30.

Zborowski, M. (1969). *People in pain.* San Francisco: Jossey-Bass.

Zola, I. K. (1966, October). Culture and symptoms: An analysis of patients presenting complaints. *American Sociological Review, 31,* 615–630.

Chapter 14

Ameling, A. (2000). Prayer: An ancient healing practice becomes new again. *Holistic Nursing Practice, 14*(3), 40–48.

American Nurses Association (ANA). (2004). *Code for nurses.* Washington, DC: American Nurses Publishing.

American Psychiatric Association (APA). (2000). *Diagnostic and statistical manual of mental disorders, Text Revision, DSM-IV-TR* (4th ed.). Washington, DC: Author.

Andrews, M. M., & Boyle, J. S. (2007). *Transcultural concepts in nursing care* (5th ed.). Philadelphia: Lippincott.

Aspen Reference Group. (2002). *Palliative care: Patient and family counseling manual* (2nd ed.). Clifton Park, NY: Thomson Delmar Learning.

Aukst-Margetic, B., & Margetic, B. (2005). Religiosity and health outcomes: A review of literature. *Collegium Antropologicum, 29,* 365–371.

Bates, M. S. (1996). *Biocultural dimensions of chronic pain.* Albany, NY: SUNY Press.

Beck, S. E., & Goldberg, E. K. (1996). Jewish beliefs, values and practices: Implications for culturally sensitive nursing care. *Advance Practice Nursing Quarterly, 2*(2), 15–22.

Beckman, S., Boxley-Harges, S., Bruick-Sorge, C., et al. (2007). Five strategies that heighten nurses' awareness of spirituality to impact client care. *Holistic Nursing Practice, 21*(3), 135–139.

Benson, H., Dusek, J. A., Sherwood, J. B., et al. (2006). Study of the therapeutic effects of intercessory prayer (STEP) in cardiac bypass patients: A multicenter randomized trial of uncertainty and certainty of receiving intercessory prayer. *American Heart Journal, 151*(4), 934–942.

Bodhi, B. (2007). The Buddhist way of life on the eightfold path. Hindu Website. Retrieved April 26, 2008, from http://www.hinduwebsite.com/buddhism/eightfoldpath.asp

Book of common prayer. (1979). New York: Oxford University Press.

Boyd, D. (1974). *Rolling thunder.* New York: Random House.

Bradshaw, A. (1996). The legacy of Nightingale . . . spiritual care. *Nursing Times, 92*(6), 42–43.

Brown-Saltzman, K. (1997). Replenishing the spirit by meditative prayer and guided imagery. *Seminars in Oncology Nursing, 13*(4), 255–259.

Brussat, F., & Brussat, M. A. (1996). *Spiritual literacy: Reading the sacred in everyday life.* New York: Simon & Schuster.

Bulechek, G. M., Butcher, H. K., & Dochterman, J. M. (Eds.) (2008). *Nursing interventions classification (NIC).* St. Louis, MO: C. V. Mosby.

Byrne, M. (2002). Spirituality in palliative care: What language do we need? *International Journal of Palliative Nursing, 8*(2), 67–74.

Campbell, A. (2006). Spiritual care for sick children of five world faiths. *Paediatric Nursing, 18*(10), 22–25.

Carpenter, K., Girvin, L., Kitner, W. L., et al. (2008). Spirituality: A dimension of holistic critical care nursing. *Dimensions of Critical Care Nursing, 27*(1), 16–20.

Carson, J. W., Keefe, F. J., Lynch, T. R., et al. (2005). Loving-kindness meditation for chronic low back pain: Results from a pilot trial. *Journal of Holistic Nursing, 23*(3), 287–304.

Cavendish, R., Konecny, L., Mitzeliotis, C., et al. (2003). Spiritual care interventions of nurses using Nursing Interventions Classification (NIC) labels. *International Journal of Nursing Terminologies and Classifications, 14*(4), 113–124.

Cavendish, R., Luise, B., Horne, K., et al. (2000). Opportunities for enhanced spirituality relevant to well adults. *Nursing Diagnosis: International Journal of Nursing Language and Classification, 11*(4), 151–163.

Cenkner, W. (1990). Hinduism. In: J. A. Komonchak, M. Collins, & D. A. Lane (Eds.), *The new dictionary of theology* (pp. 466–469). Collegeville, MN: Liturgical Press.

(2007). *The Collected Works of Florence Nightingale.* University of Guelph, Ontario, Canada. Retrieved April 22, 2008, from http://www.sociology.uoguelph.ca/fnightingale

Cotton, S., Zebracki, K., Rosenthal, S. L., et al. (2006). Religion/spirituality and adolescent health outcomes: A review. *Journal of Adolescent Health, 38*(4), 472–480.

Dickenson, C. (1975). The search for spiritual meaning. *American Journal of Nursing, 75*(10), 1789–1793.

DiJoseph, J., & Cavendish, R. (2005). Expanding the dialogue on prayer relevant to holistic care. *Holistic Nursing Practice, 19,* 147–155.

Dombeck, M. (1997). Healing the fractured self. In: M. S. Roach (Ed.), *Caring from the heart: The convergence of caring and spirituality* (pp. 50–67). Mahwah, NJ: Paulis & Press.

Donahue, M. P. (1985). *Nursing: The finest art. An illustrated history.* St. Louis, MO: C. V. Mosby.

Dunn, K., & Horgas, A. (2000). The prevalence of prayer as a spiritual self-care modality in elders. *Journal of Holistic Nursing, 18*(4), 337–351.

Elfried, S. (1998). Helping patients find meaning: A caring response to suffering. *International Journal for Human Caring, 2*(1), 33–39.

Elliott, B. A., Gessert, C. E., & Peden-McAlpine, C. (2007). Decision making by families of older adults with advanced cognitive impairment: Spirituality and meaning. *Journal of Gerontological Nursing, 33*(8), 49–55.

Emblen, J., & Pesut, B. (2001). Strengthening transcendent meaning. A model for the spiritual nursing care of patients experiencing suffering. *Journal of Holistic Nursing, 19*(1), 42–56.

Esposito, J. L. (1990). Islam. In: J. A. Komonchak, M. Collins, & D. A. Lane (Eds.), *The new dictionary of theology* (pp. 527–529). Collegeville, MN: Liturgical Press.

Fox, M. (1983). *Meditations with Meister Eckhart.* Santa Fe, NM: Bear & Company.

George, L. K., Ellison, C. G., & Larson, D. B. (2002). Exploring the relationships between religious involvement and health. *Psychological Inquiry, 13,* 190–200.

Gowri, A., & Hight, E. (2001). Spirituality and medical practice: Using the HOPE questions as a practical tool for spiritual assessment. *American Family Physician, 63,* 81–88.

Grant, D. (2004). Spiritual interventions: How, when, and why nurses use them. *Holistic Nursing Practice, 18,* 36–41.

Hamptom, J. S., & Weinert, C. (2006). An exploration of spirituality in rural women with chronic illness. *Holistic Nursing Practice, 20I*(1), 27–33.

Harris, W., Gowda, M., Kilb, J., et al. (1999). A randomized, controlled trial of the effects of remote, intercessory prayer on outcomes in patients admitted to the coronary care unit. *Archives of Internal Medicine, 159*(19), 2273–2278.

Harrison, M. O., Edwards, C. L., Koenig, H. G., et al. (2005). Religiosity, spirituality, and pain in patients with sickle cell disease. *Journal of Nervous and Mental Disorders, 193,* 250–257.

Hermann, C. P. (2006). Development and testing of the spiritual needs inventory for patients near the end of life. *Oncology Nursing Forum, 33,* 737–744.

Highfield, M. E. F. (1992). Spiritual healing of oncology patients: Nurse and patient perspectives. *Cancer Nursing, 15*(1), 1–8.

Highfield, M. E. F. (2000). Providing spiritual care to patients with cancer. *Clinical Journal of Oncology Nursing, 4*(3), 115–120.

Highfield, M. E. F., & Cason, C. (1983). Spiritual needs of patients: Are they recognized? *Cancer Nursing, 6*(3), 187–192.

Hill, P. C., & Pargament, K. I. (2003). Advances in the conceptualization and measurement of religion and spirituality: Implications for physical and mental health research. *American Psychologist, 58*(1), 64–74.

Humphreys, J. (2000). Spirituality and distress in sheltered battered women. *Journal of Nursing Scholarship, 32*(3), 273–278.

Hungelmann, J., Kenkel-Rossi, E., Klassen, L., et al. (1996). Focus on spiritual well-being: Harmonious interconnectedness of mind-body-spirit—use of the JAREL spiritual well-being scale. *Geriatric Nursing, 17*(6), 262.

Johnson, C. (2001). An Islamic understanding of health care: What can it teach us? *Accident and Emergency Nursing, 9*(1), 38–45.

The Joint Commission (TJC). (2008). *2008 hospital accreditation standards.* Oakbrook Terrace, IL: Author.

Keddington, R. K. (2007). Caring for members of the church of Jesus Christ of Latter-Day Saints (Mormons) in the emergency department. *Journal of Emergency Nursing, 33*(3), 252–256.

Keegan, L. (2000). A comparison of the use of alternative therapies among Mexican Americans and Anglo-Americans in the Texas Rio Grande Valley. *Journal of Holistic Nursing, 18*(3), 280–295.

Kinney, A., Emery, G., Dudley, W., et al. (2002). Screening behaviors among African American women at high risk for breast cancer: Do beliefs about God matter? *Oncology Nursing Forum, 29*(5), 835–843.

Kirkwood, N. A. (2005). *A hospital handbook on multiculturalism* (rev. ed.). Harrisburg, PA: Morehouse Publishing.

Kluckhohn, C., & Leighton, D. (1962). *The Navajo.* Garden City, NY: Doubleday.

Knierim, T. (last updated March, 2008). The noble eightfold path. Retrieved April 26, 2008, from http://www.thebigview.com/buddhism/eightfoldpath.html

Koenig, H. G., McCollough, M. E., & Larson, D. B. (2001). *Handbook of religions and health.* New York: Oxford University Press.

Krishnamurti, J. (1989). *Think on these things.* New York: Harper Perennial.

Lane, J. (1987). The care of the human spirit. *Journal of Professional Nursing, 3*(6), 332–337.

Larson, D. B., Swyers, J. P., & McCollough, M. E. (1998). Scientific research on spirituality and health: A report based on the Scientific Progress in Spirituality Conferences. Bethesda, MD: National Institute for Health Care Research.

le Gallez, P., Dimmock, S., & Bird, H. (2000). Spiritual healing as adjunct therapy for rheumatoid arhtritis. *British Journal of Nursing, 9*(11), 695–700.

Leininger, M. (1997). Transcultural spirituality: A comparative care and health focus. In: M. S. Roach (Ed.), *Caring from the heart: The convergence of caring and spirituality* (pp. 99–118). Mahwah, NJ: Paulis & Press.

Levoy, G. (1997). *Callings: Finding and following an authentic life.* New York: Harmony Books.

Lewis, C. S. (1961). *A grief observed.* New York: Seabury Press.

Lo, R. (2003). The use of prayer in spiritual care. *Australian Journal of Holistic Nursing, 10*(1), 22–29.

Macquarrie, J. (1977). *Principles of Christian theology* (2nd ed.). New York: Scribner.

Macrae, J. (1995). Nightingale's spiritual philosophy and its significance for modern nursing. *Image: Journal of Nursing Scholarship, 27*(1), 8–10.

Marler, K. I., & Hadaway, C. K. (2002). "Being religious" or "being spiritual" in America: A zero-sum proposition? *Journal for the Scientific Study of Religion, 41,* 289–300.

Matthews, D., Marlowe, S., & MacNutt, F. (2000). Effects of intercessory prayer on patients with rheumatoid arthritis. *Southern Medical Journal 93*(12), 1177–1186.

Matthews, W., Conti, J., & Sireci, S. (2001). The effects of intercessory prayer, positive visualization, and expectancy on the well-being of kidney dialysis patients. *Alternative Therapies in Health and Medicine, 7*(5), 42–52.

McCaffrey, A. M., Eisenberg, D. M., Legedza, A. T. R., et al. (2004). Prayer for health concerns: Results of a national survey on prevalence and patterns of use. *Archives of Internal Medicine, 164*(8), 858–862.

McCollough, M. E., Hoyt, W. T., Larson, D. B., et al. (2000). Religious involvement and mortality: A meta-analytic review. *Health Psychology, 19,* 211–222.

McEwen, M. (2005). Spiritual nursing care. *Holistic Nursing Practice, 19,* 161–168.

McSherry, W., Cash, K., & Ross, L. (2004). Meaning of spirituality: Implications practice. *Journal of Clinical Nursing, 13,* 934–941.

McSherry, W., & Watson, R. (2002), Spirituality in nursing care: Evidence of a gap between theory and practice. *Journal of Clinical Nursing 2002, 11,* 843–844.

Millspaugh, C. D. (2005). Assessment and response to spiritual pain: Part II. *Journal of Palliative Medicine, 8*(6), 1110–1117.

Moberg, D. (1982). Spiritual well-being of the dying. In: G. Lesnoff-Carabaglia (Ed.), *Aging and the human condition.* Springfield, IL: Human Sciences Press.

Molzahn, A. E. (2007). Spirituality in later life: Effect on quality of life. *Gerontological Nursing, 33*(1), 32–39.

Money, M. (2001). Shamanism as a healing paradigm for complementary therapy. *Complementary Therapy and Nurse Midwifery, 7*(3), 126–131.

Moorhead, S., Johnson, M., & Maas, M. L., et al. (Eds.). (2008). *Nursing outcomes classification (NOC)* (4th ed.). St. Louis, MO: C. V. Mosby.

NANDA International. (2009). *Nursing diagnoses: Definitions and classification 2009–2011.* Philadelphia: Author.

Narayanasamy, A. (2003). Spiritual coping mechanisms in chronically ill patients. *British Journal of Nursing, 11*(22), 1461–1470.

National Guideline Clearinghouse (NGC). (2005). Promoting spirituality in the older adult. Retrieved April 26, 2008, from http://www.guidelines.gov/summary/summary.aspx?docJ_id=6830&nbr=004197&string=nursing

Newlin, K., Knafl, K., & Melkus, G. (2002). African-American spirituality: A concept analysis. *ANS Advances in Nursing Science, 25*(2), 57–70.

O'Brien, M. E. (1999). *Spirituality in nursing: Standing on holy ground.* Sudbury, MA: Jones and Bartlett.

Olson, T. (2003). Buddhism, behavior change, and OCD. *Journal of Holistic Nursing, 21*(2), 149–162.

Oxtoby, W. G., & Segal, A. G. (2007). *A concise introduction to world religions.* Cary, NC: Oxford University Press.

Palmer, R. F., Katerndahl, D., & Morgan-Kidd, J. (2004). A randomized trial of the effects of remote intercessory prayer: Interactions with personal beliefs on problem-specific outcomes and functional status. *The Journal of Alternative and Complementary Medicine, 10*(3), 438–448.

Partridge, C. H. (2005). *Introduction to world religions.* Minneapolis, MN: Fortress Press

Pawlikowski, J. (1990). Judaism. In: J. Komonchak, M. Collins, & D. A. Lane (Eds.), *The new dictionary of theology* (pp. 543–548). Collegeville, MN: Liturgical Press.

Plante, T. G., & Sherman A. C. (Eds.). (2001). *Faith and health: Psychological perspectives.* New York: Guilford Press.

Reeve, C. (1998). *Still me.* New York: Random House.

Reeve, C. (2002). *Nothing is impossible: Reflections on a new life.* New York: Random House.

Roberts, L., Ahmed, I., & Hall, S. (2000). Intercessory prayer for the alleviation of ill health. *Cochrane Database of Systematic Reviews,* Issue 2, Art. No.: CD000368.

Robinson-Smith, G. (2002). Prayer after stroke: Its relationship to quality of life. *Journal of Holistic Nursing, 20*(4), 352–366.

Ross, R., Sawatphanait, W., & Tatirat, S. (2007). Finding peace (Kwam Sa-ngob Jai): A Buddhist way to live with HIV. *Journal of Holistic Nursing, 25*(4), 228–235.

Ryan, P. (1992). Perception of the most helpful nursing behaviors in a home-care hospice setting: Care-givers and nurses. *American Journal of Hospice and Palliative Care, 9*(5), 22–31.

Satterly, L. (2001). Guilt, shame, and religious and spiritual pain. *Holistic Nursing Practice, 15*(2), 30–39.

Sawatzky, R., & Pesut, B. (2005). Attributes of spiritual care in nursing practice. *Journal of Holistic Nursing, 23*, 19–33.

Seybold, K. S., & Hill, P. C. (2001). The role of religion and spirituality in mental and physical health. *Current Directions in Psychological Science, 10*, 21–24.

Shelley, J., Miller, A., & Fish, S. (1995). Praying with patients: Why, when and how. *Journal of Christian Nursing, 12*(1), 9–13, 28.

Simpson, R. (2002). Healing health care, healing nursing in the 21st century. *Nursing Administration Quarterly, 26*(5), 94–98.

Smith, A. R. (2007). Using the synergy model to provide spiritual nursing care in critical care settings. *Critical Care Nurse, 26*, 41–47.

Sodestrom, K., & Martin, I. M. (1987). Patients' spiritual coping strategies: A study of nurse and patient perspectives. *Oncology Nursing Forum, 14*(2), 41–46.

Sparber, A., Bauer, L., Curt, G., et al. (2000). Use of complementary medicine by adult patients participating in cancer clinical trials. *Oncology Nursing Forum, 27*(6), 887–888.

Speck, P. (2005). The evidence base for spiritual care. *Nursing Management, 12*, 28–31.

Stiles, M. (1990). The shining stranger: Nurse-family spiritual relationship. *Cancer Nursing, 13*(4), 235–245.

Sumner, C. (1998). Recognizing and responding to spiritual distress. *American Journal of Nursing, 98* (Nurse Practice Extra Edition), 26–31.

Taylor, E., & Outlaw, F. (2002). Use of prayer among persons with cancer. *Holistic Nursing Practice, 16*(3), 46–60.

Terkel, S. (2003). *Hope dies last: Keeping the faith in difficult times.* New York: New Press.

Tinley, S. T., & Kinney, A. Y. (2007). Three philosophical approaches to the study of spirituality. *Advances in Nursing Science, 30*(1), 71–80.

Todd, K. (1996). Pain assessment and ethnicity. *Annals of Emergency Medicine, 27*(4), 421–423.

Van Dover, L., & Bacon, J. (2001). Spiritual care in nursing practice: A close-up view. *Nursing Forum, 36*(1), 18–30.

Wachholtz, A. B., Pearce, M. J., & Koenig, H. (2007). Exploring the relationship between spirituality, coping, and pain. *Journal of Behavioral Medicine, 30*, 311–318.

Widerquist, J. G. (1992). The spirituality of Florence Nightingale. *Nursing Research, 41*(1), 49–55.

Wilkinson, J. M., & Ahern, N. R. (2009). *Prentice-Hall nursing diagnosis handbook* (9th ed.). Upper Saddle River, NJ: Prentice-Hall.

Wright, L. M. (2005). *Spirituality, suffering, and illness. Ideas for healing.* Philadelphia: F. A. Davis.

Wright, M. C. (2002). The essence of spiritual care: A phenomenological enquiry. *Palliative Medicine, 16*(2), 125–132.

Wright, S. G. (2002). Examining the impact of spirituality on nurses and health-care provision. *Professional Nurse, 17*(12), 709–711.

Zborowski, M. (1952). Cultural components in responses to pain. *Journal of Social Issues, 8*, 16–30.

Chapter 15

Ahrens, T., Yancey, V., & Kollef, M. (2003). Improving family communications at the end of life: Implications for length of stay in the intensive care unit and resource use. *American Journal of Critical Care, 12*(4), 317–324.

American Association of Colleges of Nurses (AACN). (2004). *Peaceful death: Recommended competencies and curricular guides to end-of-life care.* (Report from the Robert Wood Johnson End-of-Life Care Roundtable). Washington, DC: Author. Retrieved May 7, 2008, from http://www.aacn.nche.edu/publications/deathfin.htm

American Nurses Association (ANA). (1994a). Position statement: Active euthanasia. Washington, DC: Author. Retrieved May 5, 2008, from http://www.nursingworld.org/MainMenuCategories/HealthcareandPolicyIssues/ANAPositionStatements/EthicsandHumanRights/prteteuth14450.aspx

American Nurses Association (ANA). (1994b). Position statement: Assisted suicide. Washington, DC: Author. Retrieved May 5, 2008, from http://www.nursingworld.org/MainMenuCategories/HealthcareandPolicyIssues/ANAPositionStatements/EthicsandHumanRights/prtetsuic14456.aspx

American Nurses Association (ANA). (2003). Position statement: Pain Management and Control of Distressing Symptoms in Dying Patients. http://www.nursingworld.org/MainMenuCategories/HealthcareandPolicyIssues/ANAPositionStatements/EthicsandHumanRights/etpain14426.aspx

American Nurses Association (ANA). (2004). Position statement: Nursing care and do-not-resuscitate decisions. Washington, DC: Author. Retrieved May 2, 2008, from http://www.nursingworld.org/MainMenuCategories/HealthcareandPolicyIssues/ANAPositionStatements/EthicsandHumanRights/dnr0414405.aspx

Banura, D., Fender, M., Roesler, M., et al. (2001). Culturally congruent end-of-life care for Jewish patients and their families. *Journal of Transcultural Nursing, 12*(3), 211, 220.

Bednash, G., & Ferrell, B. (2000). *The end-of life nursing education consortium (2000). The ELNEC curriculum.* Washington, DC: American Association of Colleges of Nursing and City of Hope National Medical Center.

Bowlby, J. (1982). *Attachment and loss.* 3 vols. New York: Basic Books.

Boyle, D. K., Miller, P. A., & Forbes-Thompson, S. A. (2005). Communication and end-of-life care in the intensive care unit. Patient, family, and clinician outcomes. *Critical Care Nursing Quarterly, 28*(4), 302–316.

Boyle, J. S., Bunting, S. M., Hodnicki, D. R., et al. (2001). Critical thinking in African American mothers who care for adult children with HIV: A cultural analysis. *Journal of Transcultural Nursing, 12*(3), 193–202.

Briggs, D. A., & Pehrsson, D-E. (2008). Use of bibliotherapy in the treatment of grief and loss: A guide to current counseling practices. *Theory, Research & Practice, 71*, 32–42.

Brosche, T. A. (2007). A grief team within a healthcare system. *Dimensions of Critical Care Nursing, 26*(1), 21–28.

Bulechek, G., Butcher, H., & Dochterman, J. M. (2008). *Nursing interventions classification (NIC)* (5th ed.). St. Louis, MO: C. V. Mosby.

Campbell, C. L. (2007). Respect for persons. *Journal of Hospice & Palliative Nursing, 9*(2), 74–78.

College of American Pathologists (last updated 2007). Autopsy. Postmortem flow chart. College of American Pathologists, Autopsy Colmmittee. Retrieved August 21, 2009, from http://capstaging.cap.org/apps/docs/committees/autopsy/POSTMORTEM_FLOW_CHART.pdf

Corr, C., Nabe, C., & Corr, D. (2003). *Death and dying—Life and living.* Belmont, CA: Thomson-Wadsworth Press.

Davis, C., Wortman, C., Lehman, D., et al. (2000) Searching for meaning in loss: Are clinical assumptions correct? *Death Studies, 24*, 497–540.

DeSpelder, L., & Strickland, A. (1996). *The last dance.* Mountain View, CA: Mayfield.

Doka, K. (1989). *Disenfranchised grief: Recognizing hidden sorrow.* New York: Lexington Books.

Doka, K. (1998). *Living with grief: Who we are, how we grieve.* Washington, DC: Hospice Foundation of America

Duffy, S., Jackson, F., Schim, S., et al. (2006). Cultural concepts at the end of life. *Nursing Older People, 18*(8), 10–14.

Egan, K. A., & Arnold, R. L. (2003). Grief and bereavement care. *American Journal of Nursing, 103*(9), 42–52.

Eisenhandler, S. A. (2004). The arts of consolation: Commemoration and folkways of faith. *Generations, 28*(2), 37.

Emanuel, L., Ferris, F., von Gunten, C., et al. (2008). The last hours of living: Practical advice for clinicians CME/CE. From L. Emanuel, F. Ferris, C. von Gunten, et al. (2005), EPEC™-O: Education in Palliative and End-of-life Care for Oncology. (Module 6: Last Hours of Living © The EPEC Project™, Chicago, IL). Major funding provided by the National Cancer Institute; Supplementemental funding provided by the Lance Armstrong Foundation. Retrieved August 30, 2008, from http://www.medscape.com/viewarticle/542262

Engel, G. L. (1961). Is grief a disease: A challenge for medical research. *Psychosomatic Medicine, XXIII*(1), 18–22.

Engel, G. L. (1964). Grief and grieving. *American Journal of Nursing, 64*, 93–98.

Erikson, E. (1963). *Childhood and society* (2nd ed.). London: Faber and Faber.

Erikson, E. (1968). *Identity, youth and crises.* New York: Norton.

Fallowfield, L., Jenkins, V., & Beveridge, H. (2002). Truth may hurt but deceit hurts more: Communication in palliative care. *Palliative Medicine, 16*(4), 297–303.

Ferrell, B., & Coyle, N. (2002). An overview of palliative care nursing. *American Journal of Nursing, 102*(5), 26–32.

Ferrell, B., & Coyle, N. (Eds.). (2005). *Textbook of palliative care nursing* (2nd ed.). Oxford: Oxford University Press.

Ferrell, B., & Coyle, N. (2008). *The nature of suffering and the goals of nursing.* Oxford: Oxford University Press.

Ferrell, B., Grant, M., & Virani, R. (1999). Strengthening nursing education to improve end-of-life care. *Nursing Outlook, 47*(6), 252.

Ferszt, G. G., & Leveillee, M. (2006). How do you distinguish between grief and depression? *Nursing2006, 36*(9), 60–61.

Fessick, S. (2007). The use of a staff retreat with a grief counselor for inpatient medical oncology nurses to assist with bereavement and coping. *Oncology Nursing Forum, 34*(2), 529.

Florczak, K. L. (2008). The persistent yet ever changing nature of grieving a loss. *Nursing Science Quarterly, 21*(1), 7–11.

Furman, J. (2002). What you should know about chronic grief: Learn to deal with your own lingering emotions when a patient dies. *Nursing, 32*(2), 56.

Gambles, M., Crooke, M., & Wilkinson, S. (2002). Evaluation of a hospice based reflexology service: A qualitative audit of patient perceptions. *European Journal of Oncology Nursing, 6*(1), 37–44.

Goldsmith, B., Morrison, R. S., Vanderwerker, L. C., et al. (2008). Elevated rates of prolonged grief disorder in African Americans. *Death Studies, 32*, 352–365.

Griffie, J., Nelson-Marten, P., & Muchka, S. (2004). Acknowledging the "elephant": Communication in palliative care. *American Journal of Nursing, 104*(1), 48–58.

Hall, P., Shcroder, C., & Weaver, L. (2002). The last 48 hours of life in long-term care: A focused chart audit. *Journal of the American Geriatrics Society, 50*(3), 501–506.

Hancock, K., Clayton, J., Parker, S., et al. (2007). Truth-telling in discussing prognosis in advanced life-limiting illnesses: A systematic review. *Palliative Medicine, 21*, 507–517.

Harvey, J. (2001). Debunking myths about post-mortem care. *Nursing2001, 31*(7), 44–45.

Hospice Association of America (1994). All about hospice: A consumer's guide. Retrieved May 6, 2008, from http://www.nahc.org/HAA/guide.html

Howard, S. (1989, January). How do I ask? Requesting tissue or organ donations from bereaved families. *Nursing, 89*, 70–73.

Hudson, P. L. (2006). How well do family caregivers cope after caring for a relative with advanced disease and how can health professionals enhance their support? *Journal of Palliative Medicine, 9*(3), 694–703.

Johnson, M., Bulechek, G., Butcher, H., et al. (2006). *Nursing diagnoses, outcomes, and interventions: NANDA, NOC, and NIC linkages* (2nd ed.). St. Louis, MO: C. V. Mosby.

Johnstone, P., Polston, G., Niemtzow, R., et al. (2002). Integration of acupuncture into the oncology clinic. *Palliative Medicine, 16*(3), 235–239.

The Joint Commission (TJC). (2008). *Hospital accreditation standards.* Oakbrook Terrace, IL: Author.

Karnes, B. (1995). *Gone from my sight: The dying experience.* Stillwell, KS: Barbara Karnes Books.

Kouch, M. (2006). Managing symptoms for a "good death." *Nursing2006, 36*(11), 58–63.

Kruse, B. (2004). The meaning of letting go: The lived experience for caregivers of persons at the end of life. *Journal of Hospice and Palliative Nursing, 6*(4), 215–222.

Kübler-Ross, E. (1969). *On death and dying.* New York: Macmillan.

Kurtz, S. F., Strong, C. W., & Gerasimow, D. (2007, February). The 2006 Revised Uniform Anatomical Gift Act—A law to save lives. *Health Law Analysis.* Retrieved May 5, 2008, from http://www.anatomicalgiftact.org/Uploads/kurtzarticle.pdf

Lindemann, E. (1944). Symptomatology and management of acute grief. *American Journal of Psychiatry, 101*, 141–148.

Manzanec, P., & Tyler, M. K. (2003). Cultural considerations in end-of-life care. *American Journal of Nursing, 103*(3), 50–59.

Matzo, M., & Sherman, D. (2006). *Palliative care nursing* (2nd ed.). New York: Springer.

Matzo, M., Sherman, D., Sheehan, D., et al. (2003). Teaching strategies from the ELNEC curriculum. *Nursing Education Perspectives, 1*(24), 176–183.

Moorhead, S., Johnson, M., Maas, M., et al. (2007). *Nursing outcomes classification (NOC)* (4th ed.). St. Louis, MO: C. V. Mosby.

NANDA International. (2009). *NANDA nursing diagnoses: Definitions and classification 2009–2011.* Philadelphia: Author.

National Conference of Commissioners on Uniform State Laws (2006). Revised Uniform Anatomical Gift Act (2006). Retrieved May 5, 2008, from http://www.anatomicalgiftact.org/DesktopDefault.aspx?tabindex=0&tabid=1

National Guideline Clearinghouse (NGC). (2005). Promoting spirituality in the older adult. Retrieved April 26, 2008, from http://www.guidelines.gov/summary/summary.aspx?docJ_id=6830&nbr=004197&string=nursing

National Hospice and Palliative Care Organization (NHPCO). (2007). NHPCO facts and figures: Hospice care in America. Retrieved May 2, 2008, from http://www.nhpco.org/files/public/Statistics_Research/NHPCO_facts-and-figures_Nov2007.pdf

No author. (2007). *Best practices: Evidence-based nursing procedures* (2nd ed.). Philadelphia: Lippincott Williams & Wilkins.

Norton, S., & Bowers, B. (2002). Working toward consensus: Providers' strategies to shift patients from curative to palliative treatment choices. *Research in Nursing and Health, 24*(4), 258–269.

O'Connor, L., & Lunney, M. (1998). Care of the caregiver—Family member with a chronic illness. *Nursing Diagnosis, 9*(4), 152.

Parkes, C. M. (2001). *Bereavement: Studies of grief in adult life* (3rd ed.). New York: Routledge.

Pilkington, F. B. (2008). Expanding nursing perspectives on loss and grieving. *Nursing Science Quarterly, 21*(1), 6–7.

Pitorak, E. (2003). Care at the time of death. *American Journal of Nursing, 103*(7), 42–52.

Poor, B., & Poirrier, G. (2001). *End of life nursing care.* Boston: Jones & Bartlett and the National League for Nursing.

President's Commission for the Study of Ethical Problems in Medicine and Biomedical and Behavioral Research. (1981). *Defining death: A report on the medical, legal, and ethical issues in the determination of death.* Washington, DC: U.S. Government Printing Office.

Purnell, L. D., & Paulanka, B. J. (2008). *Transcultural health care: A culturally competent approach* (3rd ed.). Philadelphia: F. A. Davis.

Qaseem, A., Snow, V., Shekelle, P., et al. (2008). Evidence-based interventions to improve the palliative care of pain, dyspnea, and depression at the end of life: A clinical practice guideline from the American College of Physicians. *Annals of Internal Medicine, 148*(2), 141–146.

Rando, T. (1984). *Grief, dying and death: Clinical interventions for caregivers.* Champaign, IL: Research Press.

Rando, T. (1986). *Loss and anticipatory grief.* Lexington, MA: Lexington Books.

Rando, T. (1991). *How to go on living when someone you love dies.* New York: Bantam.

Rando, T. (1993). *Treatment of complicated mourning.* Champaign, IL: Research Press.

Rando, T. (2000). *Clinical dimensions of anticipatory mourning: Theory and practice in working with the dying, their loved ones, and their caregivers.* Champaign, IL: Research Press.

Rodriguez, K. L., Barnato, A. E., & Arnold, R. M. (2007). Perceptions and utilization of palliative care services in acute care hospitals. *Journal of Palliative Medicine, 10*(1), 99–110.

Schneider, J. (1984). *Stress, loss, and grief.* Baltimore: University Park Press.

Schwartz, J. (2003). Understanding and responding to patients' requests for assistance in dying. *Journal of Nursing Scholarship, 35*(4), 377–383.

Shahar, D., Schultz, R., Shahar, A., et al. (2001). The effect of widowhood on weight change, dietary intake, and eating behavior in the elderly population. *Journal of Aging and Health, 13*, 186–199.

Shear, K., Frank, E., Houck, P. R., et al. (2005). Treatment of complicated grief. A randomized controlled trial. *JAMA, 293*(21), 2601–2608.

Sloman, R. (2002). Relaxation and imagery for anxiety and depression control in community patients with advanced cancer. *Cancer Nursing, 25*(6), 432–435.

Steinhauser, K., Christakis, N., Clipp, E., et al. (2001). Preparing for the end of life: Preferences of patients, families, physicians, and other care providers. *Journal of Pain and Symptom Management, 22*(3), 727–737.

Sulmasy, D. (2001). Addressing the religious and spiritual needs of dying patients. *Western Journal of Medicine, 175*, 251–254.

Teno, J. M., Casey, V. A., Welch, L. C., et al. (2001). Patient-focused, family-centered end-of-life medical care: Views of the guidelines and bereaved family members. *Journal of Pain and Symptom Management, 22*, 738–751.

Thompson, E., & Reilly, D. (2002). The homeopathic approach to symptom control in the cancer patient: A prospective observational study. *Palliative Medicine, 16*(3), 227–233.

Tilden, V. (2000). Advance directives: Meaningful existence and appropriate care at the end of life. *American Journal of Nursing, 100*(12), 49, 51.

Traylor, E., Hayslip, B., Kaminski, P. L., et al. (2003). Relationships between grief and family system characteristics: A cross lagged longitudinal analysis. *Death Studies, 27*(7), 575–601.

Verheijde, J. L., Rady, M. Y., & McGregor, J. L. (2007). The United States Revised Uniform Anatomical Gift Act (2006), New challenges to balancing patient rights and physician responsibilities. *Philosophy, Ethics, and Humanities in Medicine.* Retrieved May 5, 2008, from http://www.pubmedcentral.nih.gov/articlerender.fcgi?artid=2001294

Von Gunten, C. F., Ferris, F. D., & Emanuel, L. L. (2000). Ensuring competency in end-of-life care: Communication and relational skills. *JAMA, 284*(23), 3051–3057.

Wildiers, H., & Menten, J. (2002). Death rattle: Prevalence, prevention and treatment. *Journal of Pain and Symptom Management, 23*(4), 310–317.

Worden, J. W. (2002). *Grief counseling and grief therapy: A handbook for the mental health practitioner* (3rd ed.). New York: Springer.

Chapter 16

Allred, S., Smith, K., & Flowers, L. (2004). Electronic implementation of national nursing standards—NANDA, NOC, and NIC as an effective teaching tool. *Journal of Healthcare Information Management, 18*(4), 56–60.

American Nurses Association (ANA). (2010). *Nursing: Scope and standards of practice* (2nd ed.). Public Comment draft, January 2010. Silver Spring, MD: Nursebooks.org Retrieved February 1, 2010, from http://www.nursingworld.org/DocumentVault/NursingPractice/Draft-Nursing-Scope-Standards-2nd-Ed.aspx

American Nurses Association (ANA). (2005). Principles for documentation. Retrieved December 6, 2008, from http://nursingworld.org/MainMenuCategories/ThePracticeofProfessionalNursing/DocInfo/PrinciplesforDocumentation.aspx

American Nurses Association (ANA). (2008). The nursing process: A common thread amongst all nurses. From ANA, Considering Nursing? Retrieved August 5, 2008, from http://www.nursingworld.org/EspeciallyForYou/StudentNurses/Thenursingprocess.aspx

AMNews. (2007, March 19). Hospital EMR not widespread yet. Retrieved August 10, 2008, from http://www.ama-assn.org/amednews/2007/03/19/bicb0319.htm

Austin, S. (January 2006). Ladies and gentleman of the jury, I present….. the nursing documentation. *Nursing Center CE Connection.* Retrieved August 10, 2008, from http://www.nursingcenter.com/prodev/ce_article.asp?tid=622257

Ball, M., Weaver, C., & Abbott, P. (2003). Enabling technologies promise to revitalize the role of nursing in an era of patient safety. *International Journal of Medical Informatics, 69*, 29–38.

Chard, R. (2008). Clinical issues: Using appropriate abbreviations in perioperative nursing. *AORN Journal, 87*(4), 820–822.

Chart Smart: The A-to-Z guide to better nursing documentation (2006) (2nd ed.). Springhouse, PA: Lippincott Williams & Wilkins.

College of Nurses of Ontario. (2005). Documentation. Toronto: Author. Retrieved August 5, 2008, from http://www.cno.org/docs/prac/41001_documentation.pdf

Committee on Quality Health Care in America, Institute of Medicine. (2000). In: L. Kohn, J. Corrigan, & M. Donaldson (Eds.), *To err is human: Building a safer health system.* Washington, DC: Institute of Medicine National Academy Press.

Committee on Quality of Healthcare in America, Institute of Medicine. (2001). *Crossing the quality chasm: A new health system for the 21st century.* Washington, DC: Institute of Medicine National Academy Press.

Complete guide to documentation. (2007). Philadelphia: Lippincott Williams & Wilkins.

Currie, J. (2002). Improving the efficiency of patient handover. *Emergency Nurse, 10*(3), 24–28.

Curtis, C. (2007, August 19). Electronic health records: Nursing evaluation of electronic documentation systems. Retrieved August 5, 2008, from http://healthfieldmedicare.suite101.com/article.cfm/electronic_health_records

Dumple, H., James, M., & Phillips, T. (1999, June/July). Charting by exception. *California Nurse*, 9–10.

Fitzpatrick, J., & Wallace, M. (Eds.) (2006). *Encyclopedia of nursing research*. New York: Springer.

Green, S. (2008, May–June). Interdisciplinary collaboration and the electronic medical record. *Pediatric Nursing*. Retrieved August 4, 2008, from http://www.pediatricnursing.net/ce/2010/Article34225229.pdf

Gugerty, B., Maranda, M., Beachley, M., et al. (May, 2007). Challenges and opportunities in documentation of the nursing care of patients. Retrieved July 28, 2008, from http://www.mbon.org/commission2/documenation_challenges.pdf

Haig, K., Sutton, S., & Whittington, J. (2006). SBAR: A shared mental model for improving communication between clinicians. *Joint Commission Journal of Quality and Patient Safety*, 32(3), 167–175.

Handling verbal orders safely: Learn how to instill a measure of safety into those "whispering down the lane" verbal orders. (2001). *Nursing*, 31(12), 43.

Hansen, D. (2008, January 7). Congress considers mandate for Medicare e-prescribing. Amednews.com. Retrieved August 26, 2008, at http://www.ama-assn.org/amednews/2008/01/07/gvsb0107.htm

Hays, M. (2003). The phenomenal shift report: A paradox. *Journal for Nurses in Staff Development*, 19(1), 25–33.

Hing, E., Burt, C. & Woodwell, D. (2006, October 26). Electronic medical record use by office-based physicians and their practices: United States, 2006. Number 393. Washington, DC: Centers for Disease Control Advance Data from Vital Health Statistics.

How do medical-surgical nurses spend their time? *Permanence Journal*, 12, 25–34.

Institute for Safe Medication Practices. (2004). ISMP's list of error-prone abbreviations, symbols, and dose designations. Retrieved September 30, 2008, from http://www.ismp.org/Tools/errorproneabbreviations/pdf

The Joint Commission (TJC). (2008a). Hospital Accreditation Program. 2009 chapter: National patient safety goals. Retrieved July 1, 2008, from http://www.jointcommission.org/NR/rdonlyres/31666E86–E7F4–423E-9BE8–F05BD1CB0AA8/0/09_NPSG_HAP.pdf

The Joint Commission (TJC). (2008b). *2008 hospital accreditation standards* (pp. 116–117). Oakbrook Terrace, IL: Author.

The Joint Commission (TJC). (2008c). The official "do not use" list. Retrieved August 27, 2008, from http://www.jointcommission.org/PatientSafety/DoNotUseList/. Also available in .pdf format.

Kaiser Permanente of Colorado. (unknown). SBAR technique for communication. Institute for Healthcare Improvement. Retrieved August 16, 2008, from http://www.ihi.org/IHI/Topics/PatientSafety/SafetyGeneral/Tools/SBARTechniqueforCommunicationASituationalBriefingModel.htm

Keenan, G. M. (1999). Use of standardized nursing language will make nursing visible. *Michigan Nurse*, 72(2), 12–15.

Keenan, G., Yakel, E., Tschannen, D., et al. (2008, April). Documentation and the nurse care planning process. In: R. Hughes (Ed.), *Patient safety and quality: A handbook for nurses*. Agency for Healthcare Research and Quality. Retrieved July 20, 2008, from http://www.ahrq.gov/qual/nurseshdbk/docs/KeenanG_DNCPP.pdf

Kossman, S., & Scheidenhelm, S. (2008). Nurses' perceptions of the impact of electronic health records on work and patient outcomes. *CIN: Computers, Informatics, Nursing*, 26(2), 69–77.

Lampe, S. (1985). Focus charting: Streamlining documentation. *Nurse Manager*, 16(7), 43–46.

Langowski, C. (2005). The times they are a changing: Effects of online nursing documentation systems. *Quality Management in Health Care*, 14(2), 121–125.

Legal questions. (2002). *Nursing*, 32(1), 66.

Lipe, S., & Beasley, S. (2003). *Critical thinking in nursing: A cognitive skills workbook*. Philadelphia: Lippincott Williams & Wilkins.

Martin, A., Hinds, C., & Felix, M. (1999). Documentation practices of nurses in long-term care. *Journal of Clinical Nursing*, 8, 345–352.

McCain, C. (2008). The right mix to support electronic medical record training. *Journal for Nurses in Staff Development*, 24(4), 151–154.

McFetridge, B., Gillespie, M., Goode, D., et al. (2007). An exploration of the handover process of critically ill patients between nursing staff from the emergency department and the intensive care unit. *Nursing in Critical Care*, 12(6), 261–268.

McKay, C., & Crippen, L. (2008). Collaboration through clinical integration. *Nursing Administration Quarterly*, 32(2), 109–116.

Melnyk, B., & Fineout-Overholt, E. (2005). *Evidence-based practice in nursing & healthcare: A guide to best practice*. Philadelphia: Lippincott Williams & Wilkins.

Moody, L., Slocomb, E., Berg, B., et al. (2004). Electronic health records documentation in nursing: Nurses' perceptions, attitudes, and preferences. *Computers, Informatics, Nursing*, 22(6), 337–344.

No author. (2005). Do's and don'ts of nursing documentation. Medi-Smart. Retrieved August 16, 2008, from http://www.medi-smart.com/documentation.htm

No author. (2006). Medical policy documentation guidelines. Ohio Bureau of Workman's Compensation. Retrieved August 16, 2008, from http://www.ohiobwc.com/provider/services/meddocument-policy.asp

No author. (2008). Thorough documentation, accurate assessments add up to improvement. *Hospital Home Health*, 25(4), 37–39.

Nursing know-how: Charting patient care. (2008). Philadelphia: Lippincott Williams & Wilkins.

Pearson, A. (2003). The role of documentation in making nursing work visible. *International Journal of Nursing Practice*, 9(5), 280–284.

Pope, B., Rodzen, L., & Spross, G. (2007). Raising the SBAR: How better communication improves patient outcomes. *Nursing2008*, 38(3), 41–43.

Robert Wood Johnson Foundation. (2009). Charting nursing's future. Addressing the quality and safety gap—Part I: Case studies in transforming hospital nursing and building cultures of safety. Retrieved August 3, 2009, from http://www.rwjf.org/humancapital/product.jsp?id=45629

Saba, V. (2006). *Clinical care classification (CCC) system manual: A guide to nursing documentation*. New York: Springer.

Schroeder, S. (2006). Picking up the PACE: A new template for shift report. *Nursing 2006*, 36(10), 22–23.

Smith, C., & Haque, S. (2006) Paper versus electronic documentation in complex chronic illness: A comparison. *AMIA Annual Symposium Proceedings, 2006*, 734–738. PMCID: PMC1839347. Retrieved August 16, 2008, from http://www.pubmedcentral.nih.gov/articlerender.fcgi?artid=1839347

Smith, K., Smith, V., Krugman, M., et al. (2005). Evaluating the impact of computerized clinical documentation. *CIN: Computers, Informatics, Nursing*, 23(3), 132–138.

Smith, L. (2002). How to chart by exception. *Nursing*, 32(9), 30.

Springhouse. (2006). Chart smart: *The A-Z guide to better nursing documentation* (2nd ed.). Philadelphia: Lippincott Williams & Wilkins.

Springhouse. (2007). *Complete guide to documentation*. Philadelphia: Lippincott Williams & Wilkins.

Squires, A. (2003). Documenting surgical incision care. *Nursing*, 33(1), 74.

Thorough documentation, accurate assessments add up to improvement (2008). *Hospital Home Health*, 25(4), 37–39.

Triplett, L. (2002). Electronic supportive documentation: Welcome to the future. *Nursing Home Long Term Management*, 51(12), 40–41.

Trossman, S. (2002). The documentation dilemma. *Tar Heel Nurse*, 64(3), 10.

University of North Texas Regulatory Compliance Office. (2004, Spring). *Clinical documentation & compliance manual: A guide to documentation, coding, and billing of medical services for compliance*. University of North Texas Health Science Center, Office of Regulatory Compliance. Retrieved August 16, 2007, from http://www.hsc.unt.edu/policies/QuAssure/Clinical%20Documentation&ComplianceManual042704.pdf

U.S. Department of Health & Human Services. (2003). General overview of standards for privacy of individually identifiable health information [45 CFR Part 160 and Subparts A and E of Part 164].

Retrieved September 27, 2008, from http://www.hhs.gov/ocr/hipaa/guidelines/overview.pdf

Von Krogh, G., & Naden, D. (2008). Implementation of a documentation model comprising nursing terminologies – theoretical and methodological issues. *Journal of Nursing Management, 16*(3), 275–283.

Waggoner, M., & Grindel, M. (1999). Oasis: Measuring outcomes in home care. *Medsurg Nursing, 8*(3), 214–216.

Weaver, C., Warren, J., & Delaney, C. (2005, December). Bedside, classroom, and bench: Collaborative strategies to generate evidence-based knowledge for nursing practice. *International Journal of Medical Informatics, 74*(11–12), 989–999.

Yen, P., & Gorman, P. (2005). Usability testing of a digital pen and paper system in nursing documentation. AMIA Annual Symposium Proceedings Archive, American Medical Informatics Association. Retrieved August 30, 2008, from http://www.pubmedcentral.nih.gov/articlerender.fcgi?artid=1560675

Chapter 17

Adiyaman, A., Tosun, N., Elving, L. D., et al. (2007). The effect of crossing legs on blood pressure. *Blood Pressure Monitoring, 12*(3), 189–193.

American Association of Critical-Care Nurses (AACCN). (2006). *AACN Practice Alert. Noninvasive blood pressure monitoring.* Retrieved May 22, 2008, from http://www.aacn.org/AACN/practiceAlert.nsf/vwdoc/pa2

American Heart Association (AHA). (n.d.). *Blood pressure.* Retrieved May 22, 2008, from http://www.americanheart.org/presenter.jhtml?identifier=4473

American Heart Association (AHA). (n.d.). *Blood pressure—Buying and caring for home equipment.* Retrieved May 22, 2008, from http://www.americanheart.org/presenter.jhtml?identifier=4495

American Heart Association (AHA). (n.d.). High blood pressure, factors that contribute to. Retrieved May 22, 2008, from http://www.americanheart.org/presenter.jhtml?identifier=4650

American Heart Association (AHA). (n.d.). Blood pressure statistics. Retrieved May 22, 2008, from http://www.americanheart.org/presenter.jhtml?identifier=4621

American Heart Association (AHA). (2005). AHA scientific statement. Recommendations for blood pressure measurement in humans and experimental animals. Part 1: Blood pressure measurement in humans: A statement for professionals from the subcommittee of professional and public education of the American Heart Association Council on High Blood Pressure Research. *Hypertension, 45,* 142. Also available, retrieved August 28, 2008, from http://hyper.ahajournals.org/cgi/content/full/45/1/142

American Heart Association (AHA). (2008). Hypertension: Ambulatory blood pressure monitoring in children and adolescents: Recommendations for standard assessment. *Hypertension, 5a3,* 433–451. Retrieved August 28, 2008, from http://hyper.ahajournals.org/cgi/content/full/52/3/433

American Nurses Association (ANA). (2004). *Nursing: scope and standards of practice* (3rd ed.). Washington, DC: Author.

Bernard, L., Kereveur, A., Durand, D., et al. (1999). Bacterial contamination of hospital physicians' stethoscopes. *Infection Control and Hospital Epidemiology, 20,* 626–628.

Best practices: Evidence-based nursing procedures (2nd ed., pp. 59–62). Philadelphia: Lippincott Williams & Wilkins.

Blazys, D. (2000). Does taking an orthostatic blood pressure include taking the pulse? *Journal of Emergency Nursing, 26*(5), 479–480.

Brasel, K. J., Guse, C., Gentilello, L. M., et al. (2007). Heart rate: Is it truly a vital sign? *Journal of Trauma, 62*(4), 812–817.

British Hypertension Society, Hypertension Influence Team. (2006). *Let's do it well.* Retrieved May 24, 2008, from http://www.bhsoc.org/

Centers for Disease Control and Prevention (CDC). (2005). Disinfection and sterilization of patient-care equipment, 1985. (updated 2005). Retrieved May 20, 2009, from http://www.cdc.gov/ncidod/dhqp/disinfection.html

Centers for Disease Control and Prevention (CDC). (2007a). National health and nutrition examination survey (NHANES). *Physician examination procedures manual.* Retrieved May 22, 2009, from http://www.cdc.gov/nchs/nhanes.htm

Centers for Disease Control and Prevention (CDC). (2007b). Guideline for isolation precautions: Preventing transmission of infectious agents in healthcare settings. Standard precautions. Atlanta, GA: Author. Retrieved May 20, 2008, from http://www.cdc.gov/ncidod/dhqp/gl_isolation.html

Centers for Disease Control and Prevention (CDC). (2009). May is high blood pressure education month. Retrieved May 23, 2009, from http://www.cdc.gov/Features/HighBloodPressure/

Clark, A. P., Guiliano, K., & Chen, H. M. (2006). Pulse oximetry revisited: "But his O_2 sat was normal." *Clinical Nurse Specialist, 20*(6), 268–262.

De Curtis, M., Calzolari, F., Marciano, A., et al. (2008). Comparison between rectal and infrared skin temperature in the newborn. *Archives of Disease in Childhood – Fetal and Neonatal Edition, 93,* F55–F57.

Fallis, W. M., Hamelin, K., Wang, X., et al. (2006). A multimethod approach to evaluate chemical dot thermometers for oral temperature measurement. *Journal of Nursing Measurement, 14*(3), 151–162.

Farnell, S., Maxwell, L., Tan, S., et al. (2005). Temperature measurement: Comparison of non-invasive methods used in adult critical care. *Journal of Clinical Nursing, 14*(8), 1026–1027.

Funk, K. L., Elmer, P. J., Stevens, V. J., et al. (2008). PREMIER-A trial of lifestyle interventions for blood pressure control: Intervention design and rationale. *Health Promotion Practice, 9*(3), 271–280.

Gomolin, I. H., Aung, M. M., Wolf-Klein, G., et al. (2005). Older is colder: Temperature range and variation in older people. *Journal of the American Geriatrics Society, 53*(12), 2170–2172.

Goodrich, C. (2006). Continuous central venous oximetry monitoring, *Critical Care Nursing Clinics of North America, 18*(2), 203–209.

Guiliano, K. K., & Liu, L. M. (2006). Knowledge of pulse oximetry among critical care nurses. *Dimensions of Critical Care Nursing, 25*(1), 44–49.

Gyi, A. A. (2007). Evidence summary: Vital signs. JBI Evidence Summary, #ES6699. Retrieved May 30, 2008, from http://www.jbiconnect.org/connect/docs/cis/es_html_viewer.php?SID=6699&lang=en&region=AU

Hausfater, P., Zhao, Y., Defrenne, S., et al. (2008). Cutaneous infrared thermometry for detecting febrile patients. *Emerging Infectious Diseases, 14*(8), 1255–1258.

Heusch, A. I., & McCarthy, P. W. (2005). The patient: A novel source of error in clinical temperature measurement using infrared aural thermometry. *Journal of Alternative & Complementary Medicine, 11*(3), 473–476.

High, K., Bradley, S., Gravenstein, S., et al. (2009). Clinical practice guideline for the evaluation of fever and infection in older adult residents of long-term care facilities: 2008 update by the Infectious Diseases Society of America. In: National Guideline Clearinghouse (NGC) [Web site]. Rockville, MD. Retrieved August 31, 2009, from http://www.guideline.gov/summary/summary.aspx?view_id=1&doc_id=14177

Holcomb, S. S. (2007). Guide to care for patients: Blood pressure. *The Nurse Practitioner, 32*(8), 9–10.

Hwu, Y. J., Coates, V. E., & Lin, F. Y. (2000). A study of the effectiveness of different measuring times and counting methods of human radial pulse rates. *Journal of Clinical Nursing, 9*(1), 146–152.

Jensen, B. N., Jensen, F. S., Madsen, S. N., et al. (2000). Accuracy of digital tympanic, oral, axillary, and rectal thermometers compared with standard rectal mercury thermometers. *European Journal of Surgery, 166*(11), 848–851.

Jevon, P., Ewens, B., & Lowe, R. (2000). Practical procedures for nurses. Measuring apex and radial pulse. *Nursing Times, 96*(50), 43–44.

Jianhua, L., Qi, Z., & Hui, G. (2007). The influence of long duration of isometric contraction on blood pressure. *Journal of Physical Therapy Science, 19*(2), 111–115.

Johnson, M., Bulechek, G., Butcher, H., et al. (2006). *Nursing diagnoses, outcomes, and interventions: NANDA, NIC, and NOC linkages* (2nd ed.). St. Louis, MO: C. V. Mosby.

Joint National Committee on Prevention, Detection, Evaluation, and Treatment of High Blood Pressure. (2003). *JNC 7 Complete Report. The seventh report of the Joint National Committee on Prevention, Detection, Evaluation, and Treatment of High Blood Pressure.* Bethesda, MD: National Institutes of Health. Retrieved August 22, 2009, from http://www.nhlbi.nih.gov/guidelines/hypertension/index.htm

Kaplan, N., Mendis, S., Poulter, N., et al. (2003). 2003 World Health Organization (WHO)/International Society of Hypertension (ISH) statement on management of hypertension. World Health Organization, International Society of Hypertension Writing Group. *Journal of Hypertension, 21,* 1983–1992. Retrieved May 22, 2008, from http://www.who.int/cardiovascular_diseases/guidelines/hypertension_guidelines.pdf

Kawabe, H., & Saito, I. (2007). Which measurement of home blood pressure should be used for clinical evaluation when multiple measurements are made? *Journal of Hypertension, 25*(7), 1369–1374.

Kelechi, T. J., Michel, Y., & Wiseman, J. (2006). Are infrared and thermistor thermometers interchangeable for measuring localized skin temperature? *Journal of Nursing Measurement, 14*(1), 19–30.

Kelly, G. (2006). Body temperature variability (Part 1), A review of the history of body temperature and its variability due to site selection, biological rhythms, fitness, and aging. *Alternative Medicine Review, 11*(4), 278–293.

Kennedy, K. J., Dreimanis, D. E., Beckingham, W. D., et al. (2003). Letters. *Staphylococcus aureus* and stethoscopes. *The Medical Journal of Australia, 178*(9), 468.

Kennedy, S. (2007). Detecting changes in the respiratory status of ward patients. *Nursing Standard, 21*(49), 42–46.

Khorshid, L., Eser, I., Zaybak, A., et al. (2006). Comparing mercury-in-glass, tympanic and disposable thermometers in measuring body temperature in healthy young people. *Journal of Clinical Nursing, 15*(10), 1343–1345.

Lance, R., Link, M. E., Padua, M., et al. (2000). Comparison of different methods of obtaining orthostatic vital signs. *Clinical Nursing Research, 9*(4), 479–491.

Latman, N. S., Hans, P., Nicholson, L., et al. (2001). Evaluation of clinical thermometers for accuracy and reliability. *Biomedical Instrumentation and Technology, 35*(4), 259–265.

Lawson, L., Bridges, E. J., Ballou, I., et al. (2007). Accuracy and precision of noninvasive temperature measurement in adult intensive care patients. *American Journal of Critical Care, 16*(5), 485–496.

Lewis, A. M. N. (2007). Heatstroke in older adults. *American Journal of Nursing, 107*(6), 52–56.

Lockwood, C., Conroy-Hiller, T., & Page, T. (2004). Vital signs. JBI Database of Systematic Reviews, ID #SR0115. Retrieved May 22, 2008, from http://www.jbiconnect.org/connect/docs/jbi/members/connect-getpdfphp?pdf_file=25_2004_VitalSigns.pdf

Ma, G., Sabin, N., & Dawes, M. A. (2008). A comparison of blood pressure measurement over a sleeved arm versus a bare arm. *Canadian Medical Association Journal, 178*(5), 585–589.

Mackowiak, P. A. (1998). Concepts of fever. *Archives of Internal Medicine, 158*(17), 1870–1881.

Mackowiak, P. A., Wasserman, S. S., & Levine, M. M. (1992). A critical appraisal of 98.6 degrees F, the upper limit of the normal body temperature, and other legacies of Carl Reinhold August Wunderlich. *JAMA, 268*(12), 1578–1580.

Markides, G. A., Omorphos, S., Kotoulas, C., et al. (2007). Evaluation of a wireless ingestible temperature probe in cardiac surgery. *Thoracic & Cardiovascular Surgeon, 55*(7), 442–446.

McCance, K. L., & Huether, S. E. (2006). *Pathophysiology: The biologic basis for disease in adults and children* (5th ed.). St. Louis, MO: C. V. Mosby.

McKay, D. W. (2008). Measuring blood pressure: A call to bare arms? *Canadian Medical Association Journal, 178*(5), 591–592.

Moore, T. (2007). Respiratory assessment in adults. *Nursing Standard, 21*(49), 48–56.

NANDA International (2007). *Nursing diagnoses: Definitions and classification 2007–2009.* Philadelphia: Author.

National Guideline Clearinghouse (NGC). (2005). Recommendations for blood pressure measurement in humans and experimental animals: Part 1: Blood pressure measurement in humans: A statement for professionals from the subcommittee of Professional and Public Education of the American Heart Association Council on High Blood Pressure Research. Page last modified May 19, 2008. Retrieved May 22, 2008, from http://www.ngc.gov/summary/summary.aspx?doc_id=6527&nbr=004093&string=Standard+AND+blood+AND+pressure+AND+measurement

National Guideline Clearinghouse (NGC). (2007). Guideline summary: 2007 guidelines for the management of arterial hypertension. In: National Guideline Clearinghouse (NGC) [Web site]. Rockville, MD. Retrieved May 22, 2008, from http://www.guideline.gov/summary/summary.aspx?doc_id=10952

National Guideline Clearinghouse (NGC). (2008). Guideline summary: Hypertension diagnosis and treatment. In: National Guideline Clearinghouse (NGC) [Web site]. Rockville, MD. Retrieved May 22, 2009, from http://www.guideline.gov/summary/summary.aspx?view_id=1&doc_id=13481

National Heart Lung and Blood Institute (NHLBI). (2007). *A pocket guide to blood pressure measurement in children.* From the National High Blood Pressure Education Program Working Group on High Blood Pressure in Children and Adolescents. National Institutes of Health. Retrieved May 24, 2008, from http://www.nhlbi.nih.gov/health/public/heart/hbp/bp_child_pocket/bp_child_pocket.pdf

Northeast Waste Management Officials' Association (NEWMOA). (n.d.). P2RX Topic Hubs. Mercury-thermometers table of contents. Retrieved May 16, 2008, from http://www.newmoa.org/prevention/topichub/toc.cfm?hub=101&subsec=7&nav=7&CFID=18246819&CFTOKEN=28863840

Oikawa, T., Obara, T., Ohkubo, T., et al. (2006). Characteristics of resistant hypertension determined by self-measured blood pressure at home and office blood pressure measurements. *Journal of Hypertension, 24*(9), 1737–1743.

Padfield, P. L., & Parati, G. (2007). Home blood pressure monitoring in clinical practice: How many measurements and when? *Journal of Hypertension, 25*(7), 1337–1339.

Perk, G., Stessman, J., Ginsberg, G., et al. (2003). Sex differences in the effect of heart rate on mortality in the elderly. *Journal of the American Geriatrics Society, 51*(9), 1260–1264.

Perloff, D., Grim, C., Flack, J., et al. (1993). Human blood pressure determination by sphygmomanometry. AHA Medical/Scientific Statement, Product Code: 88:2460–2467. Dallas: American Heart Association.

Popov, T. A., Dunev, S., Kralimarkova, T. Z., et al. (2007). Evaluation of a simple, potentially individual device for exhaled breath temperatures. *Respiratory Medicine, 101*(10), 2044–2050.

Quatrara, B., Coffman, Z., Jenkins, T., et al. (2007). The effect of respiratory rate and ingestion of hot and cold beverages on the accuracy of oral temperatures measured by electronic thermometers. *MedSurg Nursing, 16*(2), 105–108.

Rabinowitz, R. P., Cookson, S. T., Wasserman, S. S., et al. (1996). Effects of anatomic site, oral stimulation, and body position on estimates of body temperature. *Archives of Internal Medicine, 156*(7), 777–780.

Rajkumar, A., Karmarkar, A., & Knott, J. (2006). Pulse oximetry: An overview. *Journal of Perioperative Practice, 16*(10), 502–504.

Rhinehart, E. (2001). Infection control in home care. *Emerging Infectious Diseases, 7*(2). Retrieved May 20, 2008, from http://www.cdc.gov/ncidod/eid/vol7no2/rhinehart.htm

Robinson, J. L., Jou, H., & Spady, D. W. (2005). Accuracy of parents in measuring body temperature with a tympanic thermometer. *Family Practice, 6*(1), 3.

Rodden, A. M., Spicer, L., Diaz, V. A., et al. (2007). Does fingernail polish affect pulse oximeter readings? *Intensive & Critical Care Nursing, 23*(1), 51–55.

Roubsanthisuk, W., Wongsurin, U., Saravbich, S., et al. (2007). Blood pressure determination by traditionally trained personnel is less reliable and tends to underestimate the severity of moderate to severe hypertension. *Blood Pressure Monitoring, 12*(2), 61–68.

Roumie, C. L., Elasy, T. A., Greevy, R., et al. (2006). Improving blood pressure control through provider education, provider alerts, and patient education: a cluster randomized trial. *Annals of Internal Medicine, 145*(3), 165–175.

Roy, R., Boucher, J. P., & Comtois, A. S. (2006). Validity of infrared thermal measurements of segmental paraspinal skin surface temperature. *Journal of Manipulative & Physiological Therapeutics*, 29(2), 150–155.

Rutala, W. A., & Weber, D. J. (2004). Disinfection and sterilization in health care facilities: What clinicians need to know. *Clinical Infectious Diseases*, 39, 702–709.

Scanlon, V. C., & Sanders, T. (2007). *Essentials of anatomy and physiology* (5th ed.). Philadelphia, F. A. Davis.

Scisney-Matlock, M., Watkins, K. W., & Colling, K. B. (2001). The interaction of age and cognitive representations in predicting blood pressure. *Western Journal of Nursing Research*, 23(5), 476–489.

Siegel, J. D., Rhinehart, E., Jackson, M., et al. (2006). Healthcare Infection Control Practices Advisory Committee. Management of multidrug-resistant organisms in healthcare settings. Atlanta, GA: Centers for Disease Control & Prevention. Retrieved May 20, 2008, from http://www.guideline.gov/search/searchresults.aspx?Type=3&txtSearch=stethoscopes+cleaning&num=20

Siegel, J. D., Rhinehart, E., Jackson, M., et al. (2007). Healthcare Infection Control Practices Advisory Committee. Guideline for isolation precautions: Preventing transmission of infectious agents in healthcare settings, 2007. Standard precautions. Atlanta, GA: Centers for Disease Control & Prevention. Retrieved May 20, 2008, from http://www.guideline.gov/summary/summary.aspx?doc_id=10764&nbr=005592&string=stethoscopes+AND+cleaning

Smeltzer, S., Bare, B., Hinkle, J., et al. (2008). *Brunner & Suddarth's textbook of medical-surgical nursing* (11th ed.). Philadelphia: Wolters Kluwer/Lippincott Williams & Wilkins.

Smith, J. E. (2005). Cooling methods used in the treatment of exertional heat illness. *British Journal of Sports Medicine*, 39(8), 503–507.

St. John, R. E., & Thomson, P. D. (1999). Noninvasive respiratory monitoring. *Critical Care Nursing Clinics of North America*, 11(4), 423–435.

Sund-Levander, M., Forsberg, C., & Wahren, L. K. (2002). Normal oral, rectal, tympanic and axillary body temperature in adult men and women: A systematic literature review. *Scandinavian Journal of Caring Sciences*, 16(2), 122–128.

Sund-Levander, M., Grodzinsky, E., Loyd, D., et al. (2004). Errors in body temperature assessment related to individual variation, measuring technique and equipment. *International Journal of Nursing Practice*, 10(5), 216–223.

Terry, P. D., Abramson, J. L., & Neaton, J. D. (2007). Effects of BP & risk from death of elevated BP. *Journal of Epidemiology*, 165(3), 294–301.

Therapeutic Research Center (2007). Thermometer comparison. *Healthcare professional information*, 23(231006). Stockton, CA: Author. Retrieved June 1, 2008, from http://www.pharmacistsletter.com

Thomas, S. A., Liehr, P., DeKeywer, F., et al. (2002). A review of nursing research on blood pressure. *Journal of Nursing Scholarship*, 34(4), 313–321.

Trim, J. (2005). Monitoring pulse. *Nursing Times*, 101(21), 30–31.

U.S. Environmental Protection Agency (EPA). (2001). Memorandum of understanding between the American Hospital Association & the U.S. Environmental Protection Agency. Retrieved May 16, 2008, from http://www.h2e-online.org/docs/h2emou101501.pdf

Van den Bruel, A., Aertgeerts, B., De Boeck, C., et al. (2005). Measuring the body temperature: How accurate is the TempaDot? *Technology & Health Care*, 13(2), 97–106.

Van der Velde, N., van den Meiracker, A. H., Stricker, B. H. C., et al. (2007). Using a finger manometer to take orthostatic BP readings. *Blood Pressure Monitoring*, 12(3), 167–171.

Van Rijn, M. J., Schut, A. F. C., Aulchenko, Y. S., et al. (2007). Heritability of blood pressure traits and the genetic contribution to blood pressure variance explained by four blood-pressure related genes. *Journal of Hypertension*, 25(3), 565–570.

Vara-Gonzalez, L., Alonso, S. A., Fernandex, R. M. G., et al. (2006). Reproducibility of postural changes of blood pressure in hypertensive elderly patients in primary care. *Blood Pressure Monitoring*, 11(1), 17–20.

Vital Signs. (1999). *Best Practice*, 3(3), 1–6. Retrieved May 18, 2008, from http://www.joannabriggs.edu.au/pdf/BPISEng_3_3.pdf

Walters, T. P. (2007). Pulse oximetry knowledge and its effects on clinical practice. *British Journal of Nursing*, 16(21), 1332–1340.

Wang, X., Poole, J. C., Treiber, F. A., et al. (2006). Ethnic and gender differences in ambulatory blood pressure trajectories: Results from a 15-year longitudinal study in youth and young adults. *Circulation*, 114(25), 2780–2787.

Weir, M. R. (2007). The drug link behind secondary hypertension. *The Clinical Advisor*, 10(10), 66, 69–71.

Wister, A., Loewen, N., Kennedy-Symonds, H., et al. (2007). One-year follow-up of a therapeutic lifestyle intervention targeting cardiovascular disease risk. *Canadian Medical Association Journal*, 177(8), 859–865.

Woodrow, P., May, V., Buras-Rees, S., et al. (2006). Comparing no-touch and tympanic thermometer temperature recordings. *British Journal of Nursing*, 15(18), 1012–1016.

Wunderlich, C. A. (1871). *On the temperature in diseases* (2nd ed.). Translated by W. Bathurst Woodman. London: The New Sydenham Society. Retrieved May 14, 2008, from Google Book Search, http://books.google.com/books?hl=en&lr=&id=3-wHAAAAIAAJ&oi=fnd&pg=PA1&dq=wunderlich+temperature&ots=97uPlXqxky&sig=NmJTwucR4Q0Bep7MfFxfvGAoDUE#PPR10,M1

Chapter 18

Adams-Wendling, L., & Pimple, C. (2007, June). Nursing management of hearing impairment in nursing facility residents. Iowa City (IA): University of Iowa Gerontological Nursing Interventions Research Center. Research Dissemination Core, 56 p. Brief Summary of Guideline, National Guideline Clearinghouse. Retrieved June 9, 2008, from http://www.guideline.gov/summary/summary.aspx?doc_id=11053&nbr=005832&string=hearing

Alberti, R. E., & Emmons, M. (2001) *Your perfect right? Assertiveness and equality in your life and relationships* (8th ed.). Atascadero, CA: Impact Publishers.

American Association of Critical-Care Nurses (AACN). (2005). *AACN standards for establishing and sustaining healthy work environment: A journey to excellence.* Aliso Viejo, CA: Author.

American Nurses Association (ANA). (2010). *Nursing: Scope and standards of practice* (2nd ed.). Public Comment draft, January 2010. Silver Spring, MD: Nursebooks.org Retrieved February 1, 2010, from http://www.nursingworld.org/DocumentVault/NursingPractice/Draft-Nursing-Scope-Standards-2nd-Ed.aspx

Ammentorp, J., Sabroe, S., Kofoed, P. E., et al. (2007). The effect of training in communication skills on medical doctors' and nurses' self-efficacy: A randomized controlled trial. *Patient Education and Counseling*, 66(3), 270–277.

Apker, J., Propp, K. M., Ford, W. S. Z., et al. (2006). Collaboration, credibility, compassion, and coordination: Professional nurse communication skill sets in health care team interactions. *Journal of Professional Nursing*, 22(3), 180–189.

Avila, D. L., & Combs, A. W. (1985). *Helping relationships and the helping professions: Past, present, and future.* Boston: Allyn & Bacon.

Badzek, L. (2006). Nursing's ethical commitment to effective patient communication: A patient-centered approach to communication improves care. *American Nurse Today*, 1(1), 68–70.

Baker, L. H., Reifsteck, S. W., & Mann, W. R. (2003). Connected: Communication skills for nurses using the electronic medical record. *Nursing Economics*, 21(2), 85–88.

Beyea, S. (2004). Improving verbal communication in clinical care. *AORN Journal*, 1053–1057.

Black-Schaffer, R. M. (2002). Communication among levels of care for stroke patients. *Topics in Stroke Rehabilitation*, 9(3), 26–28.

Bruderle, E. (last updated February 10, 2003). Communication in nursing. Retrieved June 1, 2008, from http://www06.homepage.villanova.edu/elizabeth.bruderle/1103/communication.htm

Buckman, R. (2002). Communication and emotions. *British Medical Journal, 325*(7366), 672.

Carroll, H. (2003). Improving patients' health: Words matter. *Patient Care Manager, 19*(7), 1–2.

Cronenwett, L., Sherwood, G., Barnsteiner, J., et al. (2007). Quality and safety education for nurses. *Nursing Outlook, 55*(3), 122–131.

Dickerson, S. S., Stone, V. I., Panchura, C., et al. (2002). The meaning of communication. Experiences with augmentive communication devices. *Rehabilitation Nursing, 27*(6), 215–220.

Edwards, N., Peterson, W. E., & Davies, B. L. (2006). Evaluation of a multiple component intervention to support the implementation of a 'Therapeutic Relationships' best practice guideline on nurses' communication skills. *Patient Education and Counseling, 63*(1–2), 3–11.

Haig, K. M., Sutton, S., & Whittington, J. (2006). National Patient Safety Goals. SBAR: A shared mental model for improving communication between clinicians. *Joint Commission Journal on Quality and Patient Safety, 32*(3), 167–175

Hall, E. T. (1992). *The hidden dimension.* Gloucester, MA: Peter Smith.

Hebert, B. (2006). Family matters. Spanish health information resources for nurses. *Pediatric Nursing, 32*(4), 350–353.

Hopkins, L. (2005, January 19). Assertive Communication - 6 tips for effective use. Retrieved June 7, 2008, from http://ezinearticles.com/?Assertive-Communication—6–Tips-For-Effective-Use&id=10259

Hughes, J. P. (2003). Confidentiality. Careless comments: Communicating respect. *Nursing, 33*(7), 81.

James, B. (2007, October). Evidence summary: Dementia: Communication. *The Joanna Briggs Institute.* Retrieved June 9, 2008, from http://www.jbiconnect.org/connect/docs/cis/es_html_viewer.php?SID=6787&lang=en&region=AU

Jayasekara, R. (2009, August). Evidence summary: Dementia: Communication Skills for Staff. *The Joanna Briggs Institute.* Retrieved June 9, 2008, from http://www.jbiconnect.org/connect/docs/cis/es_html_viewer.php?SID=6786&lang=en&region=AU

The Joint Commission (TJC). (2006). *National Patient Safety Goals. 2006 critical access hospital and hospital national patient safety goals.* Retrieved June 6, 2008, from http://www.jointcommission.org/PatientSafety/NationalPatientSafetyGoals/06_npsgs.htm

The Joint Commission (TJC). (2008a). *Hospital accreditation standards: Accreditation policies, standards, elements of performance, scoring.* Oakbrook Terrace, IL: Author.

The Joint Commission (TJC). (2008b). *2009 Chapter: National patient safety goals* (pre-publication version). Retrieved July 2, 2008, from http://www.jointcommission.org/AccreditationPrograms/

Karhila, P., Kettunen, T., Poskiparta, M., et al. (2003). Negotiation in type 2 diabetes counseling: From problem recognition to mutual acceptance during lifestyle counseling. *Qualitative Health Research, 13*(9), 1205–1224.

Kettunen, T., Poskiparta, M., & Gerlander, M. (2002). Nurse-patient power relationship: Preliminary evidence of patients' power messages. *Patient Education Counseling, 47*(2), 101–113.

Kevan, F. (2003). Challenging behavior and communication difficulties. *Journal of Learning Disabilities, 31*(2), 12–16.

Lee, T. T. (2007). Nurses' experiences using a nursing information system: Early stage of technology implementation. *Computers, Informatics, Nursing, 25*(5), 294–300.

Leininger, M. M., & MacFarland, M. R. (2002). *Transcultural nursing: Concepts, theories, research, and practices* (3rd ed.). New York: McGraw-Hill.

Lindeke, L. L., & Sieckert, A. M. (2005). Nurse-physician workplace collaboration. *Online Journal of Issues in Nursing, 10*(1). Retrieved June 6, 2008, from http://www.medscape.com/viewarticle/499268_1

McAleer, M. (2006). Communicating effectively with deaf patients. *Nursing Standard, 20*(19), 18–24.

McGilton, K., Irwin-Robinson, H., Boscart, V., et al. (2006). Communication enhancement: Nurse and patient satisfaction outcomes in a complex continuing care facility. *Journal of Advanced Nursing, 54*(1), 35–44.

Miller, C. A. (2008). How to try this. Communication difficulties in hospitalized older adults with dementia. *American Journal of Nursing, 108*(3), 58–62.

Mitchell, A. M., Sakraida, T. J., Dysart-Gale, D., et al. (2006). Nurses' narratives of end-or-life care. *Journal of Hospice and Palliative Nursing, 8*(4), 210–221.

Moffat, M., Cleland, J., van der Molen, T., et al. (2007). Poor communication may impair optimal asthma care: A qualitative study. *Family Practice, 24*(1), 65–70.

Morello, R., Jean, A., Alix, M., et al. (2007). A scale to measure pain in non-verbally communicating older patients: The EPCA-2 study of its psychometric properties. *Pain, 133*(1–3), 87–98.

Patak, L., Gawlinski, A., Fung, N. I., et al. (2006). Communication boards in critical care: Patients' views. *Applied Nursing Research, 19*(4), 182–190.

Pope, B. B., Rodzen, L., & Spross, G. (2008). Raising the SBAR: How better communication improves patient outcomes. *Nursing2008, 38*(3), 41–43.

Poskiparta, M., Liimatainen, L., Kettunen, T., et al. (2001). From nurse-centered health counseling to empowermental health counseling. *Patient Education Counseling, 45*(1), 69 79.

Pullen, R. L. (2007). Tips for communicating with a patient from another culture. *Nursing2007, 37*(10), 48–49.

Stein, L., Watts, D., & Howell, T. (1990). Sounding board: The doctor-nurse game revisited. *New England Journal of Medicine, 322*(8), 546–549.

Stewart, L. A. (2002). The importance of effective communication during a labor action. *Patient Care Staff Report, 2*(5), 7–9

Tannen, D. (2001). *You just don't understand: Women and men in conversation.* New York: HarperCollins.

Thornby, D. (2006). Beginning the journey to skilled communication. *AACN Advanced Critical Care, 17*(3), 266–271.

Trueman, I., & Parker, J. (2006). Exploring community nurses' perceptions of life review in palliative care. *Journal of Clinical Nursing, 15*(2), 197–207.

Trummer, U. F., Mueller, U. O., Nowak, P., et al. (2006). Does physician-patient communication that aims at empowering patients improve clinical outcome: A case study. *Patient Education and Counseling, 61*(2), 299–306.

Venes, D. (2009). *Taber's cyclopedic medical dictionary* (21st ed.). Philadelphia, F. A. Davis.

Williams, K., Herman, R., Gajewski, B., et al. (2009). Elderspeak communication: Impact on dementia care. *American Journal of Alzheimer's Disease and other Dementias, 24*, 11–20.

Williams, K., Kemper, S., & Hummer, L. (2004). Enhancing communication with older adults: Overcoming elderspeak. *Journal of Gerontological Nursing, 30*(10), 17–25.

Young, J., Siffleet, J., Nikoletti, S., et al. (2006). Use of a behavioural pain scale to assess pain in ventilated, unconscious and/or sedated patients. *Intensive & Critical Care Nursing, 22*(1), 32–39.

Zapka, J., Hennessy, W., Carter, R. E., et al. (2006). End-of-life communication and hospital nurses: An educational pilot. *Journal of Cardiovascular Nursing, 21*(3), 223–231.

Chapter 19

American Cancer Society (2009). American Cancer Society guidelines for the early detection of cancer. Retrieved December 13, 2009, from http://www.cancer.org/docroot/PED/content/PED_2_3X_ACS_Cancer_Detection_Guidelines_36.asp?sitearea+PED

American Cancer Society. (2009). Detailed guide. Breast cancer: Can breast cancer be found early? Retrieved September 2, 2009, from http://www.cancer.org/docroot/CRI/content/CRI_2_4_3X_Can_breast_cancer_be_found_early_5.asp

American Cancer Society. (2009). How to perform a breast self-exam. Retrieved April 8, 2009, from http://www.cancer.org/docroot/CRI/content/CRI_2_6x_How_to_perform_a_breast_self_exam_5.asp

The American College of Obstetricians and Gynecologists (ACOG). (2007). ACOG news release. ACOG co-sponsors National Breast Cancer Awareness Month in October. Retrieved August 28, 2008, from http://www.acog.org/from_home/publications/press_releases/nr10–01–07–3.cfm

The American College of Obstetricians and Gynecologists (ACOG). (2003). ACOG news release. Cervical cancer screening: Testing can start later and occur less often under new ACOG recommendations. Retrieved July 1, 2008, from http://www.acog.org/from_home/publications/press_releases/nr07–31–03–1.cfm

The American College of Obstetricians and Gynecologists (ACOG) (2009). Interpreting the U.S. Preventive Services Task Force breast cancer screening recommendations for the general population. Retrieved December 13, 2009, from http://www.acog.org/from_home/Misc/uspstfinterpretation.cfm

Anderson, B., Kelly, A. M., Kerr, D., et al. (2008). Impact of patient and environmental factors on capillary refill time in adults. *American Journal of Emergency Medicine, 26*(1), 62–65.

Balkaya, N. A., Memis, S., & Demirkiran, F. (2007). The effects of breast self-exam education on the performance of nursing and midwifery students: A 6–month follow-up study. *Journal of Cancer Education, 22*(2), 77–79.

Bickley, L. S., & Szilagyi, P. G. (2007). *Bates' guide to physical examination and history taking* (9th ed.). Philadelphia: Lippincott Williams & Wilkins.

Blustein, J., & Weiss. L. J. (1998). The use of mammography by women aged 75 and older: Factors related to health, functioning, and age. *Journal of the American Geriatric Society, 46*, 941–946.

Breast cancer screening in older women (reviewed and updated in 2005). American Geriatrics Society. Retrieved May 4, 2010, from http://www.americangeriatrics.org/education/cp_index.shtml

Centers for Disease Control and Prevention (CDC). (n.d.). Glasgow Coma Scale. Last reviewed June 23, 2006. Retrieved June 29, 2008, from http://www.bt.cdc.gov/masscasualties/gscale.asp

Centers for Disease Control and Prevention (CDC). (2005). Disinfection and sterilization of patient-care equipment, 1985. (Updated 2005). Retrieved May 20, 2008, from http://cdc.gov/ncidod/dhqp/disinfection.html

Demirkiran, F., Balkaya, N. A., Memis, S., et al. (2007). How do nurses and teachers perform breast self-examination: Are they reliable sources of information? *BMC Public Health, 7*(147), 96

Dillon, P. M. (2007). *Nursing health assessment: A critical thinking, case studies approach* (2nd ed.). Philadelphia: F. A. Davis.

Flaherty, J., Morley, J., Murphy, D., et al. (2002). The development of outpatient clinical glidepaths. *Journal of the American Geriatrics Society, 50*, 1886–1901.

Fulmer, T. (1991). The geriatric nurse specialist role: A new model. *Nursing Management, 22*(3), 91–93.

Fulmer, T. (2007). How to try this. Fulmer SPICES. *American Journal of Nursing, 107*(10), 40–49.

Goldsmith, L. A., Lazarus, G. S., & Tharp, M. D. (1997). *Adult and pediatric dermatology: A color guide to diagnosis and treatment.* Philadelphia: F. A. Davis.

Goroll, A., & Mulley, A. (2006). *Primary care medicine* (5th ed.). Philadelphia: Lippincott, Williams & Wilkins.

Green, B., & Taplin, S. (2003). Breast cancer screening controversies. *Journal of the American Board of Family Practice, 16*(3), 233–241.

Habif, T. (2005). *Skin disease: Textbook & CD-ROM PDA software.* St. Louis, MO: C. V. Mosby.

Hackshaw, A., & Paul, E. (2003). Breast self-examination and death from breast cancer: A meta-analysis. *British Journal of Cancer, 88*(7), 1047–1053.

Hockenberry, M. J., & Wilson, J. (2008). *Wong's essentials of pediatric nursing* (8th ed.). St. Louis, MO: C. V. Mosby.

Inouye, S., van Dyck, C., Alessi, C., et al. (1990). Clarifying confusion: The confusion assessment method. *Annals of Internal Medicine, 113*(12), 941–948.

Kennedy, K. J., Dreimanis, D. E., Beckingham, W. D., et al. (2003). Letters. *Staphylococcus aureus* and stethoscopes. *The Medical Journal of Australia, 178*(9), 468.

Knutson, D., & Steiner, E. (2007). Screening for breast cancer: Current recommendations and future directions. *American Family Physician, 75*(11), 1660–1666.

Kösters, J., & Gøtzsche, P. (2003). Regular self-examination or clinical examination for early detection of breast cancer. *Cochrane Database of Systematic Reviews*, Issue 2. Art. No.: CD003373.

Martin, L. (2007). Cyanosis. *eMedicine from WebMD*. Last updated January 17, 2007. Retrieved June 20, 2008, from http://www.emedicine.com/med/topic3002.htm

McDonald, S., Saslow, D., & Alciati, M. H. (2004). Performance and reporting of clinical breast examination: A review of the literature. *CA: A Cancer Journal for Clinicians, 54*(6), 345–361.

National Cancer Institute (NCI). (2008). Breast cancer screening (PDQ®). Retrieved August 28, 2008, from http://www.cancer.gov/cancertopics/pdq/screening/breast/HealthProfessional/page10

National Guideline Clearinghouse (NGC). (2006). VA/DoD clinical practice guideline for screening and management of overweight and obesity. Management of Overweight and Obesity Working Group. Washington, DC: Department of Veterans Affairs, Department of Defense. Retrieved June 22, 2008, from http://www.guideline/gov/summary/summary.aspx?doc_id=10714&nbr=j005577&string=body+mass+AND+index

National Heart Lung and Blood Institute (NHLBI), Obesity Education Initiative (n.d.). Body mass index table. Retrieved June 22, 2008, from http://www.nhlbi.nih.gov/guidelines/obesity/bmi_tbl.htm

National Heart, Lung, and Blood Institute (NHLBI). (2001). ATP III guidelines at-a-glance quick desk reference. National Cholesterol Education Program, National Institutes of Health, U.S. Department of Health and Human Services, NIH Publication No. 01–3305. Retrieved June 10, 2008, from http://www.nhlbi.nih.gov/guidelines/cholesterol/atglance.pdf

Oleske, D. M., Galvez, A., Cobleigh, M. A., et al. (2007). Are tri-ethnic low-income women with breast cancer effective teachers of the importance of breast cancer screening to their first-degree relatives? Results from a randomized clinical trial. *Breast Journal, 13*(1), 19–27.

Pocket guide to staying healthy at 50+. (2003). Rockville, MD: Agency for Healthcare Research and Quality. AHRQ Publication No. 04–IP001–A. Retrieved June 22, 2008, from http://www.ahrq.gov/ppip/50plus/

Purnell, L., & Paulanka, B. (2008). *Transcultural health care: A culturally competent approach* (3rd ed.). Philadelphia: F. A. Davis.

Rauen, C., Chulay, M., Bridges, E., et al. (2008). Seven evidence-based practice habits: Putting some sacred cows out to pasture. *Critical Care Nurse, 28*(2), 98–124.

Rosolowich, V. (2006). Breast self-examination. *Journal of Obstetrics & Gynaecolocy Canada: JOGC, 28*(8), 728–730.

Rowley, G., & Fielding, K. (1991). Reliability and accuracy of the Glasgow Coma Scale with experienced and inexperienced users. *Lancet, 337*, 55–538.

Rutala, W. A., & Weber, D. J. (2004). Disinfection and sterilization in health care facilities: What clinicians need to know. *Clinical Infectious Diseases, 39*, 702–709.

Scanlon, V. C., & Sanders, T. (2007). *Essentials of anatomy and physiology* (5th ed.). Philadelphia: F. A. Davis.

Sloane, P. D., Slatt, L. M., Ebell, M. H., et al. (2007). *Essentials of family medicine* (5th ed.). Philadelphia: Lippincott.

Smith, R., Cokkinides, V., & Eyre, H.; American Cancer Society. (2003). American Cancer Society guidelines for the early detection of cancer. *CA-Ca-A Cancer Journal for Clinicians, 53*, 27–43.

Soyer, M. T., Ciceklioglu, M., & Ceber, E. (2007). Breast cancer awareness and practice of breast self-examination among primary health care nurses: Influencing factors and effects of an in-service education. *Journal of Clinical Nursing, 16*(4), 707–715.

Tanner, J. (1962). *Growth at adolescence* (2nd ed.). Oxford: Blackwell Scientific.

Tarrant, M. (2006). Why are we still promoting breast self-examination? *International Journal of Nursing Studies, 43*(4), 519–520.

Teasdale, G., & Jennett, B. (1974). Assessment of coma and impaired consciousness. *Lancet* 1974, 81–84.

Teasdale, G., Kril-Jones, R., & van der Sande, J. (1978). Observer variability in assessing impaired consciousness and coma. *Journal of Neurology, Neurosurgery, and Psychiatry, 41*, 603–610.

U.S. Preventive Services Task Force (USPSTF). (January, 2003). Screening for cervical cancer. Topic Page. Rockville, MD: Agency for Healthcare Research and Quality. Retrieved December 13, 2009, from http://www.ahrq.gov/clinic/uspstf/uspscerv.htm

U.S. Preventive Services Task Force (USPSTF). (2004). Screening for testicular cancer. Recommendation statement. Rockville, MD: Agency for Healthcare Research and Quality. Retrieved December 9, 2009, from http://www.ahrq.gov/clinic/3rduspstf/testicular/testiculrs.htm

U.S. Preventive Services Task Force (USPSTF). (2008). Screening for prostate cancer. Rockville, MD: Agency for Healthcare Research and Quality. Retrieved December 9, 2009, from http://www.ahrq.gov/CLINIC/uspstf/uspsprca.htm

U.S. Preventive Services Task Force (USPSTF). (2009a). The guide to clinical preventive services. Rockville, MD: Agency for Healthcare Research and Quality. Retrieved October 6, 2009, from http://www.ahrq.gov.clinic/pocketgd09/pocketgd09.pdf

U.S. Preventive Services Task Force (USPSTF). (2009b). Screening for breast cancer: Clinical summary. Rockville, MD: Agency for Healthcare Research and Quality. Retrieved December 13, 2009, from http://www.ahrq.gov/clinic/uspstf09/breastcancer/brcansum.htm

Van Leeuwen, A. M., Kranpitz, T. R., & Smith, L. S. (2007). *Davis's comprehensive handbook of laboratory and diagnostic tests: With nursing implications* (2nd ed.). Philadelphia: F. A. Davis.

Venes, D. (Ed.). (2009). *Taber's cyclopedic medical dictionary* (21st ed.). Philadelphia: F. A. Davis.

Weiss, N. S. (2003). Breast cancer mortality in relation to clinical breast examination and breast self-examination. *Breast Journal, 9* (Supplement 2), S86–89.

Yifan Xue. (2007). Dehydration: Assessment. Evidence Summaries—Joanna Briggs Institute. Retrieved June 22, 2008, from http://www.jbiconnect.org/connect/docs/cis/es_html_viewer.php?SID=5104&lang=en&region=AU

Chapter 20

Adams, K., & Corrigan, J. M. (Eds.). (2003). *Priority areas for national action: Transforming health care quality.* Washington, DC: National Academies Press. Also available at http://www.nap.edu/books/0309085438/html/

Agency for Healthcare Research and Quality. (2009). Health care-associated infections. Retrieved August 21, 2009, from http://www.ahrq.gov/qual/hais.htm

Allegranzi, B., Storr, J., Dziekan, G., et al. (2007). The first global patient safety challenge: "Clean care is safer care": From launch to current progress and achievements. *Journal of Hospital Infection, 65*(52), 115–123.

American Heart Association (AHA). (2008). Hypertension: Ambulatory blood pressure monitoring in children and adolescents: Recommendations for standard assessment. *Hypertension, 5a3,* 433–451. Retrieved August 28, 2008, from http://hyper.ahajournals.org/cgi/content/full/52/3/433

American Institute of Architects. (2006). Guidelines for design and construction of hospital and health care facilities. *American Institute of Architects.* Washington, DC: American Institute of Architects Press.

American Nurses Association (ANA). (2010). *Nursing: Scope and standards of practice* (2nd ed.). Public Comment draft, January 2010. Silver Spring, MD: Nursebooks.org Retrieved February 1, 2010, from http://www.nursingworld.org/DocumentVault/NursingPractice/Draft-Nursing-Scope-Standards-2nd-Ed.aspx

The Association of periOperative Registered Nurses (AORN). Recommended Practices Committee. (2004). Recommended practices for surgical hand: Antisepsis/hand scrubs. *AORN Journal, 79*(2), 416–431.

The Association of periOperative Registered Nurses (AORN). (2005a). Recommended practices for surgical attire. In: *Standards, recommended practices, and guidelines* (pp. 377–385). Denver: Author.

The Association of periOperative Registered Nurses (AORN). (2005b). Recommended practices for surgical hand antisepsis/hand scrubs. In: *Standards, recommended practices, and guidelines* (pp. 299–305). Denver: Author.

The Association of periOperative Registered Nurses (AORN). (2006). Recommended practices for maintaining a sterile field. In: *Standards, recommended practices, and guidelines* (pp. 402–416). Denver: AORN, Inc.

The Association of periOperative Registered Nurses (AORN). (2007). Recommended practices for prevention of transmissible infections in the perioperative practice setting. *AORN, 85*(2), 383–384, 386–390, 392–396.

Association for Professionals in Infection Control and Epidemiology (APIC). (2007a). Guide to the elimination of methicillin-resistant *Staphylococcus aureus* (MRSA) transmission in hospital settings. Washington, DC. Retrieved August 8, 2008, from http://www.ihatoday.org/issues/quality/apicguide.pdf

Association for Professionals in Infection Control and Epidemiology (APIC). (2007b). U.S. funds work on drugs for plague, tularemia, anthrax. Retrieved August 8, 2008, from http://id-center.apic.org/apic/bt/tularemia/news/oct1607nano.html

Aumeran, C., Paillard, C., Robin, F., et al. (2007). *Pseudomonas aeruginosa* and *Pseudomonas putida* outbreak associated with contaminated water outlets in an oncohaematology paediatric unit. *Journal of Hospital Infection, 65*(1), 47–53.

Bauman, R. W., Machunis-Masuoka, E., & Tizard, I. R. (2006). *Microbiology: Alternate edition with disease by body system..* San Francisco: Benjamin Cummings.

Bearman, G. M. L., Marra, A. R., & Sessler, C. N., et al. (2007). A controlled trial of universal gloving versus contact precautions for preventing the transmission of multidrug-resistant organisms. *American Journal of Infection Control, 35*(10), 650–655.

Best practices: Evidence-based nursing procedures (2nd ed.). (2007). Philadelphia: Lippincott Williams & Wilkins.

Blom, A. W., Gozzard, C., Heal, J., et al. (2002). Bacterial strike-through of re-usable surgical drapes: The effect of different wetting agents. *Journal of Hospital Infection, 52*(1), 52–55.

Boyce, J. M., & Pittet, D. (2002, October 25). Guideline for hand hygiene in health-care settings. Recommendations of the Healthcare Infection Control Practices Advisory Committee, & the HICPAC/SHEA/APIC/IDSA Hand Hygiene Task Force. *Morbidity and Mortality Weekly Report, 51*(RR16), 1–44.

Braunschweig, C., Gomez, S., & Sheean, P. M. (2000). Impact of declines in nutritional status on outcomes in adult patients hospitalized for more than 7 days. *Journal of the American Dietetic Association, 100*(11), 1316–1324.

Bulechek, G. M., Butcher, H. K., & Dochterman, J. M. (2008). *Nursing interventions classification (NIC)* (5th ed.). St. Louis, MO: C. V. Mosby.

Calfee, D., Salgado, C., Classen, D., et al. (2008). Guideline Summary. Strategies to prevent transmission of methicillin-resistant *Staphylococcus aureus* in acute care hospitals. *Infection Control and Hospital Epidemiology, 29*(Supplement1), S62–S80. In: National Guideline Clearinghouse (NGC) [Web site]. Rockville, MD. Retrieved May 18, 2009, from http://www.guideline.gov/summary/summary.aspx?view_id=1&doc_id=13397

Calil, R., Marba, S. T., von Nowakonski, A., et al. (2001). Reduction in colonization and nosocomial infection by multiresistant bacteria in a neonatal unit after institution of educational measures and restriction in the use of cephalosporins. *American Journal of Infection Control, 29*(3), 133–138.

Capitano, B., Leshem, O. A., Nightingale, C. H., et al. (2003). Cost effect of managing methicillin-resistant *Staphylococcus aureus* in a long-term care facility. *Journal of the American Geriatrics Society, 51*(1), 10–16.

Carbon monoxide poisoning (2006). Centers for Disease Control and Prevention (CDC). Retrieved August 23, 2008, from http://www.cdc.gov/co/pdfs/faqs.pdf

Carling, P. C., Parry, M. F., & Von Beheren, S. M. for the Healthcare Environmental Hygiene Study Group (2008). Identifying opportunities to enhance environmental cleaning in 23 acute care hospitals. *Infection Control & Hospital Epidemiology, 29*(1), 1–7.

Carling, P. C., Von Beheren, S., & Kim, S., et al. for the Healthcare Environmental Hygiene Study Group (2008). Intensive care unit environmental cleaning: An evaluation in sixteen hospitals using a novel assessment tool. *Journal of Hospital Infection, 68*(1), 39–44.

Castella, A., Charrier, L., Di Legami, V., et al. (2006). Surgical site infection surveillance: Analysis of adherence to recommendations for routine infection control practices. *Infection Control & Hospital Epidemiology, 27*(8), 835–840.

Centers for Disease Control and Prevention (CDC). (n.d.). Tips for adult patients to prevent antimicrobial resistance. From the Campaign to Prevent Antimicrobial Resistance in Healthcare Settings, CDC, Department of Health and Human Services. Last reviewed April 15, 2004. Retrieved August 4, 2008, from http://www.cdc.gov/drugresistance/healthcare/tools.htm#tips

Centers for Disease Control and Prevention (CDC), National Center for Infectious Diseases (n.d.). *Streptococcus pneumoniae.* Retrieved July 31, 2008, from http://www.cdc.gov/ncidod/aip/research/spn.html#refs

Centers for Disease Control and Prevention (CDC). (last updated August 31, 2000). Multidrug-resistant organisms in non-hospital healthcare settings.

Centers for Disease Control and Prevention (CDC). (2002). Guidelines for hand hygiene in health-care settings, Recommendations and reports, *Morbidity and Mortality Weekly Report, 51*(RR-16). Accessed November 2, 2008, from http://www.cdc.gov/mmwr/preview/mmwrhtml/rr5116a1.htm

Centers for Disease Control and Prevention (CDC). (2004). Interim recommendations for infection control in health-care facilities caring for patients with known or suspected Avian influenza. Retrieved August 8, 2008, from http://www.cdc.gov/flu/avian/professional/pdf/infectcontrol.pdf

Centers for Disease Control and Prevention (CDC). (2005). Community-associated MRSA information for clinicians. Retrieved July 29, 2008 from http://www.cdc.gov/ncidod/dhqp/ar_mrsa_ca_clinicians.html

Centers for Disease Control and Prevention (CDC). (last updated 2007). Living with HIV/AIDS. Brochure. Retrieved December 12, 2008, from http://www.cdc.gov/hiv/resources/brochures/livingwithhiv.htm#q3

Centers for Disease Control and Prevention (CDC). (2008a). Vancomycin resistant enterococci (VRE). Retrieved August 7, 2008, from http://www.cdc.gov/ncidod/dhqp/ar_VRE_publicFAQ.html

Centers for Disease Control and Prevention (CDC), Division of Healthcare Quality Promotion. (2008b). Protocol: Multidrug-resistant organism (MDRO) and *Clostridium difficile*-associated disease (CDAD) module. Patient Safety Component. *The National Healthcare Safety Network (NHSN) Manual.* Retrieved July 31, 2008, from http://www.cdc.gov/ncidod/dhqp/pdf/nhsn/MDRO_CDAD_Protocol_v4REV.pdf

Centers for Disease Control and Prevention (CDC). (2008c). Guideline for disinfection and sterilization in healthcare facilities, 2008. Infection Control Practices Advisory Committee (HICPAC). Retrieved January 6, 2009, from http://www.cdc.gov/ncidod/dhqp/pdf/guidelines/Disinfection_Nov_2008.pdf

Centers for Disease Control and Prevention (CDC). (2009a). CDC estimates of 2009 H1N1 influenza cases, hospitalizations and deaths in the United States, April–November 14, 2009. Retrieved December 17, 2009, from http://www.cdc.gov/h1n1flu/estimates_2009_h1n1.htm

Centers for Disease Control and Prevention (CDC). (2009b). 2009 H1N1 and seasonal flu: What you should know about flu antiviral drugs. Retrieved December 17, 2009, from http://www.cdc.gov/H1N1flu/antivirals/geninfo.htm#box

Cloud, J., & Kelly, C. P. (2007). Update on *Clostridium difficile* associated disease. *Current Opinion in Gastroenterology, 23*(1), 4–9.

Cousins, N. (1979). *Anatomy of an illness.* New York: Bantam.

Croenenwett, L., Sherwood, G., Barnsteiner, J., et al. (2007). Quality and safety education for nurses. *Nursing Outlook, 55*(3), 122–131.

Daugherty, E. L. (2008). Health care worker protection in mass casualty respiratory failure: Infection control, decontamination, and personal protective equipment. *Respiratory Care, 53*(2), 212–214.

Davey, V. (2007). Disaster care. Questions and answers on pandemic influenza. *American Journal of Nursing, 107*(7), 50–57.

Davidson, S. J., & Malkary, G. (2008, January 9). Dangerous devices. *Most Wired Magazine.* Retrieved August 10, 2008, from http://www.hhnmostwired.com/hhnmostwired_app/jsp/articledisplay.jsp?dcrpath=HHNMOSTWIRED/Article/data/Fall2007/080109MW_Online_Davidson&domain=HHNMOSTWIRED

De Gialluly, C., Morange, V., de Gialluly, E., et al. (2006). Blood pressure cuff as a potential vector of pathogenic microorganisms: A prospective study in a teaching hospital. *Infection Control and Hospital Epidemiology, 27,* 940–943.

Diaz, M. H., Silkaitis, C., & Malczynski, M., et al. (2008). Contamination of examination gloves in patient rooms and implications for transmission of antimicrobial-resistant microorganisms. *Infection Control & Hospital Epidemiology, 29*(1), 63–65.

Digison, M. B. (2007). A review of antiseptic agents for preoperative skin preparation. *Plastic Surgical Nursing, 27*(4), 185–189.

Dubberke, E. R., Reske, K. A., Noble-Wang, J., et al. (2007). Prevalance of *Clostridium difficile* environmental contamination and strain variability in multiple health care facilities. *Journal of Infection Control, 35*(5), 315–318.

Elixhauser, A., & Steiner, C. (2007). Statistical brief #35. Infections with methicillin-resistant *Staphylococcus aureus (MRSA)* in U.S. hospitals, 1993–2005. *Healthcare Cost and Utilization Project.* Retrieved July 29, 2008, from http://www.hcup-us.ahrq.gov/reports/statbriefs/sb35.jsp

Emergency Preparedness & Response: Emergency preparedness and you (n.d.). Centers for Disease Control and Prevention. Retrieved August 8, 2008, from http://emergency.cdc.gov/preparedness/

English, J. F., Cundiff, M. Y., Malone, J. D., Pfeiffer, J. A., & APIC Bioterrorism Task Force. (1999). *Bioterrorism readiness plan: A template for healthcare facilities.* Retrieved August 8, 2008, from http://www.cdc.gov/ncidod/dhqp/pdf/bt/13apr99APIC-CDCBioterrorism.PDF

Fouad, F. M., Mamer, O., Sauriol, F., et al. (2004). Cardiac heart disease in the era of sucrose polyester, *Helicobacter pylori* and *Chlamydia pneumoniae. Medical Hypotheses, 62*(2), 257–267.

Franco, G. P., de Barros, A. L., Nogueira-Martins, L. A., et al. (2003). Stress influence on genesis, onset and maintenance of cardiovascular diseases: Literature review. *Journal of Advanced Nursing, 43*(6), 548–554.

Gammon, J., Morgan-Samuel, H., & Gould, D. (2008). A review of the evidence for suboptimal compliance of healthcare practitioners to standard/universal infection control precautions. *Journal of Clinical Nursing, 17*(2), 157–167.

Ganczak, M., & Szych, Z. (2007). Surgical nurses and compliance with personal protective equipment. *Journal of Hospital Infection, 66*(4), 346–351.

Gould, D. J., Hewitt-Taylor, J., Drey, N. S., et al. (2007). The Clean YourHandsCampaign: Critiquing policy and evidence base. *Journal of Hospital Infection, 65*(2), 95–101.

Goyal, P., Kalek, S. C., Chaudhry, R., et al. (2007). Association of common chronic infections with coronary artery disease in patients without any conventional risk factors. *Indian Journal of Medical Research, 125*(2), 112–114.

Guyton, A., & Hall, J. (2005). *Textbook of medical physiology* (11th ed.). Philadelphia: W. B. Saunders.

Haas, J. P., & Larson, E. L. (2008). Compliance with hand hygiene guidelines. Where are we in 2008? *American Journal of Nursing, 108*(8), 41–45.

Halcomb, E. J., Griffiths, R., & Fernandez, R. (2008a). Evidence Synthesis. Role of MRSA reservoirs in the acute care setting. *International Journal of Evidence Based Healthcare, 6*(2), 50–62.

Halcomb, E. J., Griffiths, R., & Fernandez, R. (2008b). Evidence Synthesis. The role of patient isolation and compliance with isolation practices in the control of nosocomial MRSA in acute care. *International Journal of Evidence Based Healthcare, 6*(2), 206–213

High, K., Bradley, S., Gravenstein, S., et al. (2009). Clinical practice guideline for the evaluation of fever and infection in older adult residents of long-term care facilities: 2008 update by the Infectious Diseases Society of America. In: National Guideline Clearinghouse (NGC) [Web site]. Rockville, MD. Retrieved August 31, 2009, from http://www.guideline.gov/summary/summary.aspx?view_id=1&doc_id=14177

Hinkin, J., Gammon, J., & Cutter, J. (2008). Review of personal protection equipment used in practice. *British Journal of Community Nursing, 13*(1), 14–19.

Holcomb, S. S. (2008). MRSA infections. *Nursing2008, 38*(6), 33.

Humphreys, H. (2007). Control and prevention of healthcare-associated tuberculosis: The role of respiratory isolation and personal respiratory protection. *Journal of Hospital Infection, 66*(1), 1–5.

Institute for Healthcare Improvement (n.d.[a]). Protecting 5 million lives from harm. Retrieved July 29, 2008, from http://www.ihi.org/IHI/Programs/Campaign/

Institute for Healthcare Improvement (n.d.[b]). Reduce methicillin-resistant *Staphylococcus aureus (MRSA)* infection. Retrieved July 29, 2008, from http://www.ihi.org/IHI/Programs/Campaign/MRSA–Infection.htm

Jamulitrat, S., Narong, M. N., & Thongpiyapoom, S. (2002). Trauma severity scoring systems as predictors of nosocomial infection. *Infection Control & Hospital Epidemiology, 23*(5), 268–273.

Johnson, M., Bulechek, G., Butcher, H., et al. (2006). *NANDA, NOC, and NIC linkages* (2nd ed.). St. Louis, MO: C. V. Mosby.

The Joint Commission (TJC). (2008a). *2008 hospital accreditation standards.* Oakbrook Terrace, IL: Author.

The Joint Commission (TJC). (2008b). *Hospital Accreditation Program. 2009 chapter: National patient safety goals.* Retrieved July 1, 2008, from http://www.jointcommission.org/NR/rdonlyres/31666E86–E7F4–423E-9BE8–F05BD1CB0AA8/0/09_NPSG_HAP.pdf

Kayabas, U., Bayraktar, M., Otlu, B., et al. (2008). An outbreak of *Pseudomonas aeruginosa* because of inadequate disinfection procedures in a urology unit: A pulsed-field gel electrophoresis-based epidemiologic study. *American Journal of Infection Control, 36*(1), 33–38.

Kerwat, K., & Wulf, H. (2008). Hospital hygiene—clothing in hospitals: Protection for staff and patients. *Anasthesiologie, Intensivmedizin, Notfallmedizin, Schmerztherapie, 43*(3), 214–215.

Klein, E., Smith, D. L., & Laxminarayan, R. (2007). Hospitalizations and deaths caused by methicillin-resistant *Staphylococcus aureus,* United States, 1999–2005. *Emerging Infectious Diseases, 13*(12), 1840–1846.

Klevens, R. M., Morrison, M. A., & Nadle, J., et al. (2007). Invasive methicillin-resistant *Staphylococcus aureus* infections in the United States. *JAMA, 298*(15), 1763–1771.

Larson, E., Girard, R., & Pessoa-Silva, C. L., et al. (2006) Skin reactions related to hand hygiene and selection of hand hygiene products. *Association for Professionals in Infection Control and Epidemiology, 34,* 627–635.

Larson, E. L., Quiros, D., & Lin, S. X. (2007). Dissemination of the CDC's Hand Hygiene Guideline and impact on infection rates. *American Journal of Infection Control, 35*(10), 666–675.

Lashley, F. R. (2006). Emerging infectious diseases at the beginning of the 21st century. *Online Journal of Issues in Nursing, 11*(1). Retrieved July 22, 2008, from http://nursingworld.org/MainMenuCategories/ANAMarketplace/ANAPeriodicals/OJIN/TableofContents/Volume112006/No1Jan31/tpc29_116054.aspx#Smolinski

Lazarus, R., Kleinman, K., Dashevsky, I., et al. (2002, August). Use of automated ambulatory-care encounter records for detection of acute illness clusters, including potential bioterrorism events. *Emerging infectious diseases* [serial online]. Retrieved March 24, 2003, from http://www.cdc.gov/ncidod/EID/vol8no8/02–0239.htm

Loh, W., Ng, W., & Holton, J. (2000). Bacterial flora on the white coats of medical students. *Journal of Hospital Infection, 45*(1), 65–68.

Manges, A. R., Perdreau-Remington, F., Solberg, O., et al. (2005). Multidrug-resistant *Escherichia coli* clonal groups causing community-acquired bloodstream infections. *Journal of Infection, 53*(1), 25–29.

McKibben, L., Horan, T., & Tokars, M. D. (2005). Guidance on public reporting of healthcare-associated infections: Recommendations of the Healthcare Infection Control Practices Advisory Committee. *American Journal of Medical Quality, 33*(4), 217–226. Retrieved July 9, 2008, from http://www.cdc.gov/ncidod/hlp/PublicReportingGuide.pdf

Minnesota Department of Health (n.d.). Components of personal protective equipment. Retrieved May 7, 2010, from http://www.health.state.mn.us/divs/idepc/dtopics/infectioncontrol/ppe/comp/index.html

Moorhead, S., Johnson, M., Maas, M. L., et al. (2008). *Nursing outcomes classification (NOC)* (4th ed.). St. Louis, MO: C. V. Mosby.

Munoz, P., Hortal, J., Giannella, M., et al. (2008). Nasal carriage of *S. aureus* increases the risk of surgical site infection after major heart surgery. *Journal of Hospital Infection, 68*(1), 25–31.

NANDA International. (2009). *Nursing diagnoses: Definitions & classification 2009–2011.* Philadelphia: Author.

Nasraway, S. A., Jr. (2007). "Search and destroy" for methicillin-resistant *Staphylococcus aureus* in the intensive care unit: Should this now be the standard of care? *Critical Care Medicine, 35*(2), 642–644.

National Institute of Allergy and Infectious Diseases (NIAID). (2001). *Microbes in sickness and health.* Washington, DC: National Institutes of Health.

Nordman, P., Naas, T., Fortineau, M., et al. (2007). Superbugs in the coming new decade; multidrug resistance and prospects for treatment of *Staphylococcus aureus, Enterococcus spp.,* and *Pseudomonas aeruginosa* in 2010. *Current Opinion in Microbiology, 10*(5), 436–440.

Novoa, A. M., Pi-Sunyer, T., Sala, M., et al. (2007). Evaluation of hand hygiene adherence in a tertiary hospital. *American Journal of Infection Control, 35*(10), 676–683.

Occupational Safety & Health Administration. U.S. Department of Labor. (n.d.). Bloodborne pathogens and needlestick prevention. Post-exposure evaluation. Retrieved November 8, 2008, from http://www.osha.gov/SLTC/bloodbornepathogens/postexposure.html

Ott, S. J., El Mokhtari, N. E., Musfeldt, M., et al. (2006). Detection of diverse bacterial signatures in atherosclerotic lesions of patients with coronary heart disease. *Circulation, 113*(7), 929–937.

Owens, R. D., Jr., Donskey, C. J., Gaynes, R. P., et al. (2008). Antimicrobial-associated risk factors for *Clostridium difficile* infection. *Clinical Infectious Diseases, 46*(Supplement 1), S19–31.

Patel, S. (2006). Principles of appropriate use of disposable gloves. *Nursing Times, 102*(24), 44–45.

Pellowe, C. M. (2007). New guidelines for prevention of HCAIs in acute care. *Nursing Times, 103*(26), 28–29.

Perry, C., Marshall, R., & Jones, E. (2001). Bacterial contamination of uniforms. *Journal of Hospital Infection, 48*(3), 238–241.

Pitout, J. D. D., & Laupland, K. B. (2008). Extended-spectrum B-lactamase-producing Enterobacteriaceae: An emerging public-health concern. *The Lancet Infectious Diseases, 8,* 159–166.

Pratt, R. J., Pellowe, C. M., Wilson, J. A., et al. (2007). Epic2: National evidence-based guidelines for preventing healthcare-associated infections in NHS hospitals in England. *Journal of Hospital Infection, 65*(Supplement 1), S1–64.

Price, M. F., Dao-Tran, T., Garey, K. W., et al. (2007). Epidemiology and incidence of *Clostridium difficile*-associated diarrhoeae diagnosed upon admission to a university hospital. *Journal of Hospital Infection, 65*(1), 42–46.

Protecting 5 million lives from harm (n.d.). The Institute for Healthcare Improvement. Retrieved August 8, 2008, from http://www.ihi.org/IHI/Programs/Campaign/Campaign.htm?TabId=6

Randle, J., & Fleming, K. (2006). The risk of infection from toys in the intensive care setting. *Nursing Standard, 20*(40), 50–54.

Raskind, C. H., Worley, S., Vinski, J., et al. (2007). Hand hygiene compliance rates after an educational intervention in a neonatal intensive care unit. *Infection Control & Hospital Epidemiology, 28*(9), 1096–1098.

Reduce methicillin-resistant *Staphylococcus aureus (MRSA) infection.* Institute for Healthcare Improvement. (n.d.). Retrieved August 8, 2008, from http://www.ihi.org/IHI/Programs/Campaign/MRSA–Infection.htm

Rice, L. B. (2001). Emergence of vancomycin-resistant enterococci. *Emerging Infectious Diseases, 7*(2), 183–187.

Robicsek, A., Beaumont, J. L., Beaumont, S. M., et al. (2008). Universal surveillance for methicillin-resistant *Staphylococcus aureus* in 3 affiliated hospitals. *Annals of Internal Medicine, 148*(6), 409–418.

Rupp, M. E., Fitzgerald, T., Puumala, S., et al. (2008). Prospective, controlled, cross-over trial of alcohol-based hand gel in critical care units. *Infection Control and Hospital Epidemiology, 29*(1), 8–15.

Sax, H., Perneger, T., Hugonnet, S., et al. (2005). Knowledge of standard and isolation precautions in a large teaching hospital. *Infection Control & Hospital Epidemiology, 26*(3), 298–304.

Schneider, R., Alexander, C., Staggers, F., et al. (2005). Long-term effects of stress reduction on mortality in persons ≤ 55 years of age with systemic hypertension. *The American Journal of Cardiology, 95*(9), 1060–1064.

Siegel, J. D., Rhinehart, E., Jackson, M., et al. (2006). *Management of multidrug-resistant organisms in healthcare settings.* Retrieved July 7, 2008, from http://www.cdc.gov/ncidod/dhqp/pdf/ar/mdroGuideline2006.pdf

Siegel, J. D., Rhinehart, E., Jackson, M., et al. (2007). *2007 Guideline for isolation precautions: Preventing transmission of infectious agents in the healthcare setting.* Retrieved February 8, 2010, from http://www.cdc.gov/ncidod/dhqp/pdf/guidelines/Isolation2007.pdf

Siegel, J. H., & Korniewicz, D. M. (2007). Keeping patients safe: An interventional hand hygiene study at an oncology center. *Clinical Journal of Oncology Nursing, 11*(5), 643–646.

Smith, G., Vijaykrishna, D., Bahl, J., et al. (2009). Origins and evolutionary genomics of the 2009 swine-origin H1N1 influenza A epidemic. *Nature, 459,* 1122–1125.

Society of Gastroenterology Nurses and Associates, Inc. (2006). Standards of infection control in reprocessing of flexible gastrointestinal endoscopes. *Gastroenterology Nursing, 29*(2), 142–148.

Spahr, A., Klein, E., Khuseyinova, N., et al. (2006). Periodontal infections and coronary heart disease. *Archives of Internal Medicine, 166*(5), 554–559.

Spak, C. W. (2007). How worried should you be about XDR TB? *The Clinical Advisor, 10*(10), 25–26, 29.

Springer, R. (2008). Laundering scrubs. *Plastic Surgical Nursing, 28*(1), 45–46.

Tablan, O. C., Anderson, L. J., Besser, R., et al. (2004). Guidelines for preventing health-care-associated pneumonia, 2003. *Morbidity and Mortality Weekly Report, 53*(RR03), 1–36.

Todd, B. (2007). Emerging infections. Extensively drug-resistant tuberculosis. *American Journal of Nursing, 107*(6), 29–31.

U.S. Department of Labor. (n.d.). *Occupational Safety and Health Standards: General description and discussion of the levels of protection and protective gear.* 1910.120 App B. Retrieved November 1, 2008, from http://www.osha.gov/pls/oshaweb/owadisp.show_document?p_table=STANDARDS&p_id=9767

U.S. Department of Labor. (n.d.). (Lack of) personal protective equipment. *Occupational Safety and Health Standards.* 1910.1030(d)(3)(xii). Retrieved May 5, 2010, from http://www.osha.gov/SLTC/etools/hospital/hazards/ppe/ppe.html

Vajani, M., Annest, J. L., Ballesteros, M., et al. (2005). Unintentional non-fire-related carbon monoxide exposures — United States, 2001–2003. *Morbidity and Mortality Weekly Report, 54*(2), 36–39.

Vandenberghe, A., Laterre, P., Goenen, M., et al. (2002). Surveillance of hospital-acquired infections in an intensive care department—the benefit of the full-time presence of an infection control nurse. *Journal of Hospital Infection, 52*(1), 56–59.

Veneema, T. G., & Tõke, J. (2006). Early detection and surveillance for biopreparedness and emerging infectious diseases. *Online Journal of Issues in Nursing, 11*(1). Retrieved July 29, 2008, from http://www.nursingworld.org/MainMenuCategories/ANAMarketplace/ANAPeriodicals/OJIN/TableofContents/Volume112006/No1Jan31/tpc29_2c16059.aspx

Vonesch, N., Tomao, P., DiRenzi, S., et al. (2006). Biosafety in laboratories concerning exposure to biological agents. *Giornale Italiano di Medicina del Lavoro Ed Ergonomia, 28*(4), 444–456.

Ward, D. J. (2007). Hand adornment and infection control. *British Journal of Nursing, 16*(11), 654–656.

Weber, D. J., Sickbert-Bennett, E., Brown, E. E., et al. (2007). Compliance with isolation precautions at a university hospital. *Infection Control & Hospital Epidemiology, 28*(3), 358–361.

Weinstein, R. S., & Alibek, K. (2003). *Biological and chemical terrorism: A guide for healthcare providers and first responders.* New York: Thieme.

Whyte, J. (2008). MRSA: Not a new crisis. *The Clinical Advisor, 11*(1), 100.

World Health Organization (WHO). (2007). *Epidemic and pandemic alert and response (EPR): avian influenza.* World Health Organization (WHO). Retrieved July 29, 2008, from http://www.who.int/csr/disease/avian_influenza/en/index.html

World Health Organization (WHO). (2008). *The world health report 2007—A safer future: Global public health security in the 21st century.* Retrieved August 1, 2008, from http://www.who.int/whr/2007/en/index.html

Yamamoto, L., & Marten, M. (2007). Protecting patients from harm: Listen up, MRSA the bug stops here. *Nursing2007, 37*(12), 50–55

Yokoe, D., & Classen, D. (2008). Supplement article: Introduction. Improving patient safety through infection control: A new healthcare imperative. *Infection Control & Hospital Epidemiology, 29*(Supplement 1), S3–S11. Retrieved October 10, 2008, from http://www.journals.uchicago.edu/doi/abs/10.1086/591063

Yokoe, D. S., Mermel, L. A., Anderson, D. J., et al. (2008). Supplement article: Executive summary. A compendium of strategies to prevent healthcare-associated infections in acute care hospitals. *Infection Control & Hospital Epidemiology, 29*(Supplement 1), S12–S21. Retrieved October 10, 2008, from http://www.journals.uchicago.edu/doi/pdf/10.1086/591060

Zitella, L. J., Friese, C. R., Hauser, J., et al. (2006). Putting evidence into practice: Prevention of infection. *Clinical Journal of Oncology Nursing, 10*(6), 739–750.

Chapter 21

(2009). QuickStats: Motor-vehicle traffic and poisoning death rates, by age—United States, 2005–2006. *MMWR Weekly, 58*(27), 753. Retrieved July 16, 2009, from http://www.cdc.gov/mmwr/preview/mmwrhtml/mm5827a7.htm?s_cid=mm5827a7_e

Ackley, B., & Ladwig, G. (2008). *Nursing diagnosis handbook* (8th ed.). St. Louis, MO: C. V. Mosby.

Adams, P., Barnes, P., & Vickerie, J. (2008). Summary health statistics for the U.S. population: National Health Interview Survey, 2007. *Vital Health Statistics 2008, 10*(238). Retrieved August 13, 2009, from http://www.cdc.gov/nchs/data/series/sr_10/sr10_238.pdf

AHI of Indiana Inc. (n.d.). A vital sign for safety. The AHI fall prevention program with the Hendrich II fall risk model©. Retrieved October 25, 2008, from http://www.ahincorp.com/hfrm/index.php#

Akyol, A. D. (2007). Falls in the elderly: What can be done? *International Nursing Review, 54*(2), 191–196.

Alden, N. E., Bessey, P. Q., Rabbits, A., et al. (2007). Tap water scalds among seniors and the elderly: Socio-economics and implications for prevention. *Burns, 33*(5), 666–669.

American Academy of Neurology (AAN). (2008a, February). Get Up and Go Test. Retrieved October 27, 2008, from http://www.aan.com/practice/guideline/uploads/273.pdf

American Academy of Neurology (AAN). (2008b, February). Get Up and Go Test. Retrieved October 27, 2008, from http://www.aan.com/practice/guideline/uploads/274.pdf

American Academy of Pediatrics (AAP). (2009). *Car safety seats: A guide for families 2009.* Retrieved August 26, 2008, from http://www.aap.org/family/Carseatguide.htm

American Academy of Pediatrics Committee on Injury, Violence, and Poison Prevention. (2003). Poison treatment in the home. *Pediatrics, 112*(5), 1182–1185.

American Heart Association (AHA). (2008). Relief of choking in children. Retrieved August 25, 2008, from http://www.american-heart.org/presenter.jhtml?identifier=3025002

American Nurses Association (ANA). (2002). *Needlestick prevention guide*. Retrieved November 1, 2008, from http://www.nursingworld.org/MainMenuCategories/OccupationalandEnvironmental/occupationalhealth/SafeNeedles/NeedlestickPrevention.aspx

American Nurses Association (ANA). (2003). ANA launches "Handle with Care" ergonomics campaign (September 17, 2003). Press release. Retrieved October 25, 2008, from http://www.nursingworld.org/MainMenuCategories/OccupationalandEnvironmental/occupationalhealth/handlewithcare/HandleWCarePressRelease.aspx

American Nurses Association (ANA). (2007). Health care worker safety. *Nursing's legislative and regulatory initiatives for the 110th Congress: Workplace health and safety*. Retrieved October 25, 2008, from http://www.nursingworld.org/MainMenuCategories/ThePracticeofProfessionalNursing/workplace/Workplace.aspx

American Nurses Association (ANA). (2008). *ANA's health system reform agenda*. Retrieved August 20, 2008, from http://www.nursingworld.org/MainMenuCategories/HealthcareandPolicyIssues/HSR.aspx

American Red Cross (2007). Be Red Cross ready. Conscious choking. Retrieved February 9, 2010, from http://www.redcross.org/flash/brr/English-html/conscious-choking.asp

American Red Cross. (2008). Re: Question re choking. Personal communication, August 26, 2008, from A. Adorante, Director of Preparedness, Health & Safety Services, American Red Cross, Kansas City, KS. (adorantea@usa.redcross.org)

Anonymous. (2005). Patient education. How to stay safe in a lightning storm. *RN, 68*(5), 47.

Association of Poison Control Centers. (n.d.). *Poison proof your home*. Retrieved August 20, 2008, from http://www.aapcc.org/dnn/PoisoningPrevention/PoisonProofYourHome/tabid/118/Default.asp

Berg, J., McConnell, R., Milam, J., et al. (2008). Rodent allergen in Los Angeles inner city homes of children with asthma. *Journal of Urban Health, 85*(1), 52–61.

Bertera, E., & Bertera, R. (2008). Fear of falling and activity avoidance in a national sample of older adults in the United States. *Health & Social Work, 33*(1), 54–62.

Brush, B., & Capezuti, E. (2001). Historical analysis of siderail use in American hospitals. *Journal of Gerontological Nursing, 25*, 26–34.

Bulechek, G., Butcher, H., & Dochterman, J. (Eds.). (2008). *Nursing interventions classification (NIC)* (5th ed.). St. Louis, MO: C. V. Mosby.

Bureau of Labor Statistics. (2006). Economic news release. Nonfatal occupational injuries and illnesses requiring days away from work, 2006. Retrieved October 25, 2008, from http://www.bls.gov/news.release/osh2.nr0.htm

Capezuti, E., Wagner, L., Brush, B., et al. (2007). Consequences of an intervention to reduce restrictive side rail use in nursing homes. *Journal of the American Geriatrics Society, 55*(3), 334–342.

Centers for Disease Control and Prevention (CDC). (n.d.). Accidents or unintentional injuries. FastStats. Retrieved July 16, 2009, from http://www.cdc.gov/nchs/fastats/acc-inj.htm

Centers for Disease Control and Prevention (CDC). (n.d., last modified March 13, 2008). Poisoning in the United States: Fact sheet. Retrieved August 20, 2008, from http://www.cdc.gov/ncipc/factsheets/poisoning.htm

Centers for Disease Control & Prevention (CDC). (n.d.). Sharps injury prevention workbook. Retrieved November 2, 2008, from http://www.cdc.gov/sharpssafety/pdf/workbookcomplete.pdf

Centers for Disease Control and Prevention (CDC). (n.d., last modified April 25, 2008). Falls among older adults: An overview. Retrieved August 25, 2008, from http://www.cdc.gov/ncipc/factsheets/adultfalls.htm

Centers for Disease Control and Prevention (CDC). (2004, last modified 2008). Downloadable leading causes charts. Retrieved August 20, 2008, from http://www.cdc.gov/ncipc/osp/charts.htm

Centers for Disease Control and Prevention (CDC). (2005). Foodborne illness. Frequently asked questions. Retrieved August 26, 2008, from http://www.cdc.gov/ncidod/dbmd/diseaseinfo/files/foodborne_illness_FAQ.pdf

Centers for Disease Control and Prevention (CDC), National Center for Injury Prevention and Control (2006a). Child passenger safety: Fact sheet. Retrieved August 26, 2008, from http://www.cdc.gov/ncipc/factsheets/childpas.htm

Centers for Disease Control and Prevention (CDC), National Center for Injury Prevention and Control. Web-based Injury Statistics Query and Reporting System (WISQARS) [online]. (2006b) [cited January 15, 2007]. Retrieved August 25, 2008, from http://www.cdc.gov/ncipc/wisqars

Centers for Disease Control and Prevention (CDC). (2006c). Measures to prevent bites from mosquitoes, ticks, fleas and other insects and arthropods. Retrieved August 29, 2008, from http://www.cdc.gov/travel/contentMosquitoTick.aspx

Centers for Disease Control and Prevention (CDC), National Center for Injury Prevention and Control. (2007). National child passenger safety week, September 16–22, 2007. Last updated May, 2008. Retrieved August 26, 2008, from http://www.cdc.gov/ncipc/duip/spotlite/chldseat.htm

Centers for Disease Control and Prevention (CDC), National Center for Injury Prevention and Control. (2008). Preventing falls: How to develop community-based fall prevention programs for older adults. Retrieved August 26, 2008, from http://www.cdc.gov/ncipc/preventingfalls/CDC_Guide.pdf

Centers for Medicare & Medicaid Services. (2006a). Press Release. Eliminating serious, preventable, and costly medical errors—never events. Department of Health & Human Services. Retrieved August 20, 2008, from http://www.cms.hhs.gov/apps/media/press/release.asp?Counter=1863

Centers for Medicare and Medicaid Services, Department of Health and Human Services. (2006b, December 8). Medicare and Medicaid Programs; Hospital Conditions of Participation: Patients' Rights; Final Rule. Retrieved October 8, 2008, from http://www.cms.hhs.gov/CFCsAndCoPs/downloads/finalpatientrightsrule.pdf

Centers for Medicare and Medicaid Services. (2008). Press release. Medicare and Medicaid move aggressively to encourage greater patient safety in hospitals and reduce never events. CMS Office of Public Affairs, July 31, 2008. Retrieved October 20, 2008, from http://www.cms.hhs.gov/apps/media/press/release.asp?Counter=3219&intNumPerPage=10&checkDate=&checkKey=&srchType=1&numDays=3500&srchOpt=0&srchData=&keywordType=All&chkNewsType=1%2C+2%2C+3%2C+4%2C+5&intPage=&showAll=&pYear=&year=&desc=&cboOrder=date

Clarkson, T., & Magos, L. (2006). The toxicology of mercury and its chemical compounds. *Critical Reviews in Toxicology, 36*(8), 609–662.

Cleveland, L., Minter, M., Cobb, K., et al. (2008). Lead hazards for pregnant women and children: Part 1. *American Journal of Nursing, 108*(10), 40–50.

Committee on Quality of Health Care in America. (1999). In: L.T. Kohn, J. M. Corrigon, & M. S. Donaldson (Eds.), *To err is human: Building a safer health system*. Washington, DC: The National Academies Press, National Academy of Sciences.

Condon, M., & Brannen, L. (2006). Mercury elimination update: New policies—and persistence—help create alternatives and safer facilities. *American Journal of Nursing, 106*(3), 88.

Cote, V. (2004). Are your residents safe in their beds? *Director, 12*(3), 166, 168.

Cronenwett, L., Sherwood, G., Barnsteiner, J., et al. (2007). Quality and safety education for nurses. *Nursing Outlook, 55*(3), 122–131.

Delahanty, K., & Myers, F. III (2007). Infection control survey report. *Nursing 2007, 37*(6), 28–38.

Deshpande, N., Metter, E., Bandinelli, S., et al. (2008a). Psychological, physical, and sensory correlates of fear of falling and consequent activity restriction in the elderly: The InCHIANTI study. *American Journal of Physical Medicine & Rehabilitation, 87*(5), 354–362.

Deshpande, N., Metter, E., Lauretani, F., et al. (2008b). Activity restriction induced by fear of falling and objective and subjective measures of physical function: A prospective cohort study. *Journal of the American Geriatrics Society, 56*(4), 615–620.

Doenges, M., Moorhouse, M., & Geissler-Murr, A. (2005). *Nursing diagnosis manual*. Philadelphia: F. A. Davis.

Eaton, D. K., Kann, L., Kinchen, S., et al. (2006). Youth risk behavior surveillance—United States, 2005. *Morbidity and Mortality Weekly Report, 55*(SS05), 1–108.

ECRI Institute. (2007). Mercury reduction and elimination in healthcare facilities proven a success. *Healthcare Hazard Management Monitor, 20*(12), 1–8

Evans, L., & Cotter, V. (2008). Avoiding restraints in patients with dementia. *American Journal of Nursing, 108*(3), 40–50.

Evergreen Industries & Obviously Enterprises. (2006). The Internet Consumer Recycling Guide. The world's shortest comprehensive recycling guide. Retrieved August 29, 2008, from http://www.obviously.COM/recycle/guides/shortest.html

FAQs for the 2007 National Patient Safety Goals (updated January 2007). Retrieved October 10, 2008, from http://www.jointcommission.org/NR/rdonlyres/D4844675–25D7–4B5B-A47D-C549D939F9E5/0/07_NPSG_FAQs_9.pdf

Federwisch, A. (2005, February 28). Back to basics. *NurseWeek.* Retrieved October 25, 2008, from http://www.nurseweek.com/news/Features/05–02/BackPain.asp

First aid tips. (n.d.). American Association of Poison Control Centers. Retrieved August 20, 2008, from http://www.aapcc.org/dnn/FirstAid/tabid/115/Default.aspx

Flores, N. (2008). Dealing with an angry patient. *Nursing2008, 38*(5), 30–31.

Fonad, E., Wahlin, T., Winblad, B., et al. (2008). Falls and fall risk among nursing home residents. *Journal of Clinical Nursing, 17*(1), 126–134.

Forbis, S. G., McAllister, T. R., Monk, S. M., et al. (2007). Children and firearms in the home: A Southwestern Ohio Ambulatory Research Network (SOAR-Net) study. *Journal of the American Board of Family Medicine: JABFM, 20*(4), 385–391.

Gates, S., Fisher, J., Cooke, M., et al. (2008). Multifactorial assessment and targeted intervention for preventing falls and injuries among older people in community and emergency care settings: Systematic review and meta-analysis. *BMJ, 336*, 130–133.

Gerber, L. (2007). Tips for keeping home care patients fall-free. Nurse.com, November 19. Retrieved August 16, 2008, from http://include.nurse.com/apps/pbcs.dll/article?AID=/20071119/PA02/711190342&SearchID=73327064206539

Gray, L., McReynolds, T., & Jordan, Z. (2008). Falls prevention in a secured dementia unit. *PACEsetterS, 5*(2), 14–15.

Gray-Micelli, D. (2008). Preventing falls in acute care. In: E. Capezuti, D. Zwicker, M. Mezey, et al. (Eds.), *Evidence-based geriatric nursing protocols for best practices* (3rd ed., pp. 161–198). New York: Springer.

Gross, A., Miltenberger, R., Knudson, P., et al. (2007). Preliminary evaluation of a parent training program to prevent gun play. *Journal of Applied Behavior Analysis, 40*(4), 691–695.

Grossman, V. (2003). Gang members in the ED. *American Journal of Nursing, 103*(2), 52–53.

Han, R. K., Ungar, W. J., & Macarthur, C. (2007). Cost-effectiveness analysis of a proposed public health legislative/educational strategy to reduce tap water scald injuries in children. *Injury Prevention, 13*(4), 248–253.

Health Care Financing Administration. (2000, June). Quality of care-standards. Hospital conditions of patients' rights: Interpretive guidelines. Retrieved November 10, 2002, from http://www.hcfa.gov/quality/4b2htm

Hendrich, A. (2007). How to try this. Predicting patient falls. *American Journal of Nursing, 107*(11), 50–59.

Hill, K. D., Moore, K. J., Dorevitch, M. I., et al. (2008). Effectiveness of falls clinics: an evaluation of outcomes and client adherence to recommended interventions. *Journal of the American Geriatrics Society, 56*(4), 600–608.

Hizel, S., Ozcebe, H., Sanli, C., et al. (2008). Children and firearms in Turkish homes. *Child: Care, Health & Development, 34*(1), 32–34.

Injury Center, Centers for Disease Control and Prevention (CDC). (n.d., last updated March, 2008). *Tips to prevent poisonings.* Retrieved August 20, 2008, from http://www.cdc.gov/ncipc/factsheets/poisonprevention.htm

Institute for Clinical Systems Improvement (ICSI). (2008). Prevention of falls (acute care). Health care protocol. Bloomington (MN): ICSI. In: National Guideline Clearinghouse (NGC) [Web site]. Rockville, MD. Retrieved August 24, 2009, from http://www.guideline.gov/summary/summary.aspx?view_id=1&doc_id=13697

Johnson, C. L., DeMass, S. L., & Markle-Elder, S. (2007). A national solution to patient handling injuries. Findings from a UAN survey highlight the need for legislation. *American Journal of Nursing, 107*(9), 73–75.

Johnson, M., Bulechek, G., Butcher, H., et al. (2006). *NANDA, NOC, and NIC linkages* (2nd ed.). St. Louis, MO: C. V. Mosby.

The Joint Commission (TJC). (2000, July 12). Sentinel event alert. Retrieved October 10, 2008, from http://www.jointcommission.org/SentinelEvents/SentinelEventAlert/sea_14.htm

The Joint Commission (TJC). (2005). Restraint and seclusion. Retrieved October 23, 2008, from http://www.jointcommission.org/AccreditationPrograms/BehavioralHealthCare/Standards/FAQs/Provision+of+Care+Treatment+and+Services/Restraint+and+Seclusion/Restraint_Seclusion.htm

The Joint Commission (TJC). (2008a). 2009 National patient safety goals. Retrieved August 20, 2008, from http://www.jointcommission.org/PatientSafety/NationalPatientSafetyGoals/

The Joint Commission (TJC). (2008b). *2008 Hospital accreditation standards.* Oakbrook Terrace, IL: Author.

Karch, D. L., Lubell, K. M., Friday, J., et al. (2008). Surveillance for violent deaths—National Violent Death Reporting System, 16 states, 2005. *Morbidity & Mortality Weekly Report. Surveillance Summaries, 57*(3), 1–45.

Kenny, R., Rubenstein, L., Martin, F., et al. (2001). (American Geriatrics Society (AGS) Panel on Falls in Older Persons). Special series: Clinical practice. Guideline for the prevention of falls in older persons. *Journal of the American Geriatrics Society, 49*(5), 644–672.

Kerrison, S., & Chapman, R. (2007). What general emergency nurses want to know about mental health patients presenting to their emergency department. *Accident & Emergency Nursing, 15*(1), 48–55.

Keskin, D., Borman, P., Ersoz, M., et al. (2008). The risk factors related to falling in elderly females. *Geriatric Nursing, 29*(1), 58–63.

Kielb, C., Hurlock-Chorostecki, C., & Sipprell, D. (2005). Can minimal patient restraint be safely implemented in the intensive care unit? *Dynamics, 16*(1), 16–19.

Kondro W. (2007). Mercury disposal sole health concern with fluorescent lights. *Canadian Medical Association Journal, 177*(2), 136–137.

Krieger, J., & Higgins, D. (2002). Housing and health: Time again for public health action. *American Journal of Public Health, 92*(5), 758–768.

Kurtzman, E. T., & Buerhaus, P. I. (2008). New Medicare payment rules: Danger or opportunity for nursing? *American Journal of Nursing, 108*(6), 30–35.

Leahy, N. E., Hyden, P. J., Bessey, P. Q., et al. (2007). The impact of a legislative intervention to reduce tap water scald burns in an urban community. *Journal of Burn Care & Research, 28*(6), 805–810.

leBel, J., & Goldstein, R. (2005). Special section on seclusion and restraint: The economic cost of using restraint and the value added by restraint reduction or elimination. *Psychiatric Services, 56*, 1109–1114.

Lewis, S., Heitkemper, M., Dirksen, S., et al. (2007). *Medical surgical nursing: Assessment and management of clinical problems* (7th ed.). St. Louis, MO: C. V. Mosby/Elsevier.

Lopes, M. I. L., Miranda, P. J., & Sarinho, E. (2006). Use of the skin prick test and specific immunoglobulin E for the diagnosis of cockroach allergy. *Journal of Pediatrics, 82*(3), 204–209.

Manoguerra, A. S., Cobaugh, D. J., & the Members of the Guidelines for the Management of Poisonings Consensus Panel. (2004). Guideline on the use of ipecac syrup in the out-of-hospital management of ingested poisons. In: *Guidelines for the management of poisonings.* Washington, DC: American Association of Poison Control Centers.

MayoClinic.com (2009). Choking: First aid. Retrieved February 9, 2010, from http://www.mayoclinic.com/health/first-aid-choking/fa00025

Medline Plus. A service of the U.S. National Library of Medicine and the National Institutes of Health. (n.d.). Food poisoning. *Medical encyclopedia*. Last updated May, 2006. Retrieved August 26, 2008, from http://www.nlm.nih.gov/medlineplus/ency/article/001652. htm#top

Miniño, A. M., Heron, M. P., Murphy, S. L., et al. (2007). Deaths: Final data for 2004. *National Vital Statistics Reports*, 55(19). Hyattsville, MD: National Center for Health Statistics.

Moorhead, S., Johnson, M., Maas, M., et al. (Eds.). (2008). *Nursing outcomes classification (NOC)* (4th ed.). St. Louis, MO: C. V. Mosby.

Morse, J. (1997). *Preventing patient falls*. Thousand Oaks, CA: Sage.

Morse, J. (2001). Preventing falls in the elderly. *Reflections on Nursing Leadership*, First Quarter, 26–27.

NANDA International. (2009). *NANDA nursing diagnoses: Definitions and classification 2009–2011*. Ames, IA: Wiley-Blackwell.

National Ag Safety Database (NASD). (2003a). Protect your children from poisons at home. Retrieved November 2, 2008, from http://www.cdc.gov/nasd/documents/d0001501–d001600/d001584/d0001584.html

National Ag Safety Database (NASD). (2003b). Home safety 1, 2, and 3. Retrieved November 2, 2008, from http://www.cdc.gov/nasd/docs/d001501–d001600/d001509/1.html

National Cancer Institute (n.d.). Factsheet. Secondhand smoke: Questions and answers. Retrieved August 29, 2008, from http://www.cancer.gov/cancertopics/factsheet/Tobacco/ETS

National Center for Injury Prevention and Control, Centers for Disease Control and Prevention (CDC). (2007). *Injury—A risk at any stage of life*. Retrieved August 20, 2008, from http://www.cdc.gov/ncipc/fact_book/factbook.htm

National Fire Protection Association. (2008, August). News Release: NFPA report finds smoking is leading factor in home fires involving oxygen administration equipment. Retrieved August 25, 2008, from http://www.nfpa.org/newsReleaseDetails.asp?categoryID=488&itemID=40199

National Guideline Clearinghouse (NGC). (2005, November). Changing the practice of physical restraint use in acute care. Retrieved October 9, 2008, from http://www.guideline.gov/summary/summary.aspx?doc_id=8626&nbr=004806&string=changing+AND+practice+AND+physical

National Guideline Clearinghouse (NGC). (2006). Guideline synthesis: Prevention of falls in the elderly. Revised 2008. Retrieved October 7, 2008, from http://www.guideline.gov/Compare/comparison.aspx?file=FALLPREVENTION3.inc

National Institute on Aging (2006, October). *NIH Senior Health*. Falls and older adults. Retrieved August 25, 2008, from http://nihseniorhealth.gov/falls/homesafety/01.html

National Institute for Occupational Safety and Health (NIOSH). (n.d.). Safer medical device implementation in health care facilities. Centers for Disease Control and Prevention, Department of Health and Human Services. Retrieved August 26, 2008, from http://www.cdc.gov/niosh/topics/bbp/safer/

National Institute for Occupational Safety and Health (NIOSH). (2003). *Protect your family: Reduce contamination at home*. DHHS (NIOSH) Publication No. 97-125. Retrieved August 23, 2008, from http://www.cdc.gov/niosh/thttext.html

National Institute for Occupational Safety and Health (NIOSH). (2004). *Worker health chartbook 2004*. NIOSH Publication No. 2004–146. Centers for Disease Control and Prevention, Department of Health and Human Services. Retrieved August 26, 2008, from http://www.cdc.gov/niosh/docs/2004–146/

National Quality Forum (NQF). (2009). *Safe practices for better healthcare—2009 update*. Washington, DC, National Quality Forum. Retrieved March 10, 2009, from http://www.qualityforum.org

The National Rifle Association Headquarters. (2008). Education & training programs. NRA gun safety rules. Retrieved August 25, 2008, from http://www.nrahq.org/education/guide.asp

National Safety Council (n.d.). Baby-proofing your home. Retrieved August 25, 2008, from http://www.nsc.org/resources/factsheets/hl/baby_proofing.aspx

National Safety Council. (2005). News release. Costs of preventable injuries "crippling" families, businesses, health care system,

National Safety Council warns. Retrieved August 25, 2008, from http://nsc.org/news/nr060105.aspx

National Safety Council. (2008a). Report on injuries in America. Retrieved August 18, 2007, from http://www.nsc.org/lrs/injuriesinamerica08.aspx

National Safety Council. (2008b). Trends in unintentional poisoning deaths and death rates. Centers for Medicare & Medicaid Services, Department of Health & Human Services. Retrieved August 18, 2008, from http://www.nsc.org/resources/issues/poisonpretips/poison_trends.aspx

O'Keefe, L. (2009). Keep your toddler in a rear-facing car seat until age 2 (not 1). *AAP News*, 30(4), 12. In: *NeoReviewsPlus*, American Academy of Pediatrics [Web site]. Retrieved July 15, 2009, from http://aapnews.aappublications.org/cgi/content/full/30/4/12–a

Oliver, D. (2007). Older people who fall: Why they matter and what you can do. *British Journal of Community Nursing*, 12(11), 500–507.

Overview of the 100,000 lives campaign. (n.d.). Institute for Healthcare Improvement. Retrieved October 20, 2008, from http://www.ihi.org/IHI/Programs/Campaign/100kCampaignOverviewArchive.htm

Rhodes, K. V., & Iwashyna, T. J. (2007). Child injury risks are close to home: Parent psychosocial factors associated with child safety. *Maternal & Child Health Journal*, 11(3), 269–275.

Sclafani, M., Humphrey, F., Repko, S., et al. (2008). Reducing patient restraints: a pilot approach using clinical case review. *Perspectives in Psychiatric Care*, 44(1), 32–39.

Shever, L., Titler, M., Kerr, P., et al. (2008). The effect of high nursing surveillance on hospital cost. *Journal of Nursing Scholarship*, 40(2), 161–169.

Smart Disposal. (2008). A prescription for a healthy planet. Retrieved August 23, 2008, from http://www.smarxtdisposal.net/about.html

Stevens, J., & Sogolow, E. (2008). Preventing falls: What works. Atlanta, GA: Centers for Disease Control and Prevention, National Center for Injury Prevention and Control. Retrieved August 26, 2008, from http://www.cdc.gov/ncipc/preventingfalls/CDCCompendium_030508.pdf

Talerico, K., & Capezuti, E. (2001). Myths and facts about side rails. *American Journal of Nursing*, 101(7), 43–48.

Taschner, M. (2008). Responding to a fire emergency, *Nursing2008*, 38(5), 44–47.

Tilly, J., & Reed, P. (2008). Falls, wandering, and physical restraints: A review of interventions for individuals with dementia in assisted living and nursing homes. *Alzheimer's Care Today*, 9(1), 45–50.

Tommasini, C., Talamini, R., Bidoli, E., et al. (2008). Risk factors of falls in elderly population in acute care hospitals and nursing homes in north Italy: A retrospective study. *Journal of Nursing Care Quality*, 23(1), 43–49.

U.S. Department of Health and Human Services (USDHHS). (2006). *The health consequences of involuntary exposure to tobacco smoke: A report of the Surgeon General*. Rockville, MD: Centers for Disease Control and Prevention (CDC), Coordinating Center for Health Promotion, National Center for Chronic Disease Prevention and Health Promotion, Office of Smoking and Health.

U.S. Department of Health and Human Services (USDHHS). (2000). *Healthy people 2010*. (conference edition, in two volumes). Washington, DC: Author.

U.S. Department of Labor, Occupational Safety and Health Administration (OSHA). (n.d.). Hospital e-Tool – HealthCare Wide Hazards Module. Mercury. Retrieved October 25, 2008, from http://www.osha.gov/SLTC/etools/hospital/hazards/mercury/mercury.html

U.S. Department of Labor, Occupational Safety and Health Administration (OSHA). (n.d.). Bloodborne pathogens and needlestick prevention. OSHA standards. Retrieved October 25, 2008, from http://www.osha.gov/SLTC/bloodbornepathogens/standards.html (Last updated September 17, 2007).

U.S. Department of Labor, Occupational Safety and Health Administration (OSHA). (1991). Federal Register: Occupational exposure to bloodborne pathogens. Final rule. 29 CFR Part 1910.1030. *Federal Register*, 56, 235.

U.S. Department of Labor, Occupational Safety and Health Administration (OSHA). (2001). Enforcement procedures for the occupational exposure to bloodborne pathogens CPL 02-02-069. Retrieved November 2, 2008, from http://www.osha.gov/pls/oshaweb/owadisp.show_document?p_table=DIRECTIVES&p_id=2570

U.S. Environmental Protection Agency (EPA). (n.d.). Table of products that may contain mercury and recommended management options. Retrieved October 20, 2008, from http://www.epa.gov/epawaste/hazard/tsd/mercury/con-prod.htm

U.S. Environmental Protection Agency (EPA). (1996). Solid Waste and Emergency Response (5305W). The consumer's handbook for reducing solid waste. EPA publication # 530–K-96–003. Retrieved January 30, 2009, from http://www.epa.gov/waste/wycd/catbook/index.htm

U.S. Environmental Protection Agency (EPA). (2002a). Eliminating mercury in hospitals. Environmental best practices for health care facilities. Retrieved August 29, 2008, from http://www.epa.gov/region09/waste/p2/projects/hospital/mercury.pdf

U.S. Environmental Protection Agency (EPA). (2002b). Software for environmental awareness: Mercury in medical facilities. Retrieved September 26, 2002, from http://www.epa.gov/seahome/mercury.html

U.S. Environmental Protection Agency (EPA). (2003, January 6). Wastes: your home and community. Retrieved February 13, 2003, from http://www.epa.gov/ epaoswer/osw/citizens.htm

U.S. Environmental Protection Agency (EPA). (2005). Fact sheet: Mercury-containing equipment classified as universal waste. Retrieved October 20, 2008, from http://www.epa.gov/osw/hazard/recycling/electron/mce-fs.pdf

U.S. Environmental Protection Agency (EPA). (2007). Methods of mosquito control. Retrieved August 29, 2008, from http://www.epa.gov/pesticides/health/mosquitoes/mosquito.htm

U.S. Environmental Protection Agency (EPA). (2008). Wastes. Retrieved August 29, 2008, from http://www.epa.gov/epawaste/

U.S. Food and Drug Administration (FDA). (2007a). Food safety for you! Retrieved August 28, 2008, from http://www.foodsafety.gov/~dms/ftt-411.html

U.S. Food and Drug Administration (FDA). (2007b, December 4). Public Health Notification from FDA: Vail products enclosed bed systems. Retrieved October 8, 2008, from http://www.fda.gov/cdrh/safety/120407–vail.html

U.S. Food and Drug Administration (FDA), Center for Food Safety and Applied Nutrition (n.d.). Last updated March 17, 2004. Consumer advice on food safety, nutrition, and cosmetics. Retrieved July 11, 2004, from http://www.fda.gov

Walker, B. Jr., & Mouton, C. P. (2008). Environmental influences on cardiovascular health. Journal of the National Medical Association, 100(1), 98–102.

Weber, V., White, A., & McIlvried, R. (2008). An electronic medical record (EMR)-based intervention to reduce polypharmacy and falls in an ambulatory rural elderly population. Journal of General Internal Medicine, 23(4), 399–404.

Wijlhuizen, G., de Jong, R., & Hopman-Rock, M. (2007). Older persons afraid of falling reduce physical activity to prevent outdoor falls. Preventive Medicine, 44(3), 260–264.

Wilburn, S. (2004). Needlestick and sharps injury prevention. Online Journal of Issues in Nursing, 9(3), 104.

Wilkinson, J., & Ahern, N. (2009). Prentice-Hall nursing diagnosis handbook (9th ed.). Upper Saddle River, NJ: Prentice-Hall.

Winfield, R. D., Chen, M. K., Langham, M. R., et al. (2008). Ashes, embers, and coals: Significant sources of burn-related morbidity in children. Journal of Burn Care & Research, 29(1), 109–113.

World Health Organization (WHO). (1997). The world health report 1997: Conquering suffering, enriching humanity. Geneva, Switzerland: Author.

Worthington, K. (2001). Take-home toxins. American Journal of Nursing, 101(9), 88.

Zafren, K., Durrer, B., Herry, J., et al. (2005). Lightning injuries: Prevention and on-site treatment in mountains and remote areas. Resuscitation, 65(3), 369–372.

Chapter 22

AARP. (2007). Consumer guide to hearing aids. Washington, DC: AARP. Retrieved December 20, 2008 at http://www.aarphealthcare.com/Learn/Docs/HearingGuide.pdf

American Academy of Orthopedic Surgeons (AAOS). (2001). 85% of women changed shoe-wear habits due to foot problems. Newswise. Retrieved September 1, 2004, from http:www.newswise.com/articles/view/26033/

American Association of Critical-Care Nurses (AACN). (2007). AACN practice alert. Oral care in the critically ill. Retrieved December 18, 2008, from http://classic.aacn.org/AACN/practiceAlert.nsf/Files/OC/$file/Oral%20Care%20in%20the%20Critically%20Ill%20.pdf

American Dental Association (ADA). (n.d.). Cleaning your teeth and gums (oral hygiene). Retrieved December 20, 2008, from http://www.ada.org/public/topics/cleaning.asp

American Nurses Association (ANA). (2003). ANA launches "Handle with Care" ergonomics campaign (September 17, 2003). Press release. Retrieved October 25, 2004, from http://nursingworld.org/MainMenuCategories/OccupationalandEnvironmental/occupationalhealth/handlewithcare/HandleWCarePressRelease.aspx

Bausch & Lomb. (2008). Official Home Page. Retrieved January 5, 2009, from http://www.bausch.com

Bausch & Lomb. (2009). Inserting and removing your GP contact lenses. Retrieved January 5, 2009, from http://www.bausch.com/en_US/consumer/visioncare/product/rgpinsert.aspx

Berry, A. (2007). Consensus based clinical guideline for the provision of oral care for the critically ill adult. Intensive Care Coordination & Monitoring Unit. Retrieved November 21, 2008, from http://intensivecare.hsnet.nsw.gov.au/current/system/files/8++Final+oral+guideline+December+5_1.pdf

Best practices: Evidence-based nursing procedures (2008) (pp. 117–124). Philadelphia: Lippincott Williams & Wilkins.

Birch, S., & Coggins, T. (2003). No-rinse, one-step bed bath: The effects on the occurrence of skin tears in a long-term care setting. Ostomy Wound Management, 49(1), 64–67.

Bliss, D., Zehrer, C., Savik, K., et al. (2006). Incontinence-associated skin damage in nursing home residents: A secondary analysis of a prospective multicenter study. Ostomy and Wound Management, 52(12), 46–55.

Bloomfield, J., Pegram, A., & Jones, A. (2008). Recommended procedure for bedmaking in hospital. Nursing Standard, 22(23), 41–44.

Brawley, E. C. (2002). Bathing environments: How to improve the bathing experience. Alzheimer's Care Quarterly, 3(1), 38–41.

Bulechek, G., Butcher, H., & Dochterman, J. (Eds.). (2008). Nursing interventions classification (NIC) (5th ed.). St. Louis, MO: C. V. Mosby.

Cason, C., Tyner, T., Saunders, S., et al. (2007). Nurses' implementation of guidelines for ventilator-associated pneumonia from the Centers for Disease Control and Prevention (CDC). American Journal of Critical Care, 16(1), 28–38.

Centers for Disease Control and Prevention (CDC). (2002). Guideline for hand hygiene in health-care settings. Morbidity and Mortality Weekly Report, RR-26, 1–47. Retrieved December 22, 2008, from http://www.cdc.gov/handhygiene/

Chalmers, J. (2005). Oral hygiene care for residents with dementia: A literature review. Journal of Advanced Nursing, 52(4), 410–419.

Chu, J. (2004). Customary vs disposable baths. American Journal of Nursing, 104(9), 72.

Collins, J., Nelson, A., & Sublet, V. (2006). Safe lifting and movement of nursing home residents. National Institute for Occupational Safety and Health. Retrieved November 18, 2008.

Coughlan, M., & Healy, C. (2008). Nursing care, education and support for patients with neutropenia. Nursing Standard, 22(46), 35–41

Deaf and Hard of Hearing Services Metro. (n.d.). Care and troubleshooting of hearing aids. St. Paul, MN: Minnesota Department of Human Services. Retrieved December 20, 2008, from http://www.dhs.state.mn.us/main/dhs_id_018642.pdf

Department of Veteran Affairs. (n.d.). Your VA Hearing Aid. Retrieved December 20, 2008 at http://www.ncrar.research.va.gov/ForVets/documents/HearingAidbook.pdf

Downey, L., & Lloyd, H. (2008). Bed bathing patients in hospital. *Nursing Standard*, 22(34), 35–40.

Duffin, C. (2008). Dive into the pool of knowledge. *Nursing Older People*, 20(8), 9–10.

Erikson Labs Northwest. (2007). Prosthetic care. Retrieved January 5, 2009, from http://www.ericksonlabs.com/artificial-eye-care.html

EZ-Shampoo Instructions for use. (2005). EZ-Access, a division of Homecare Products, Inc., 1704 B Street N.W., Suite 110, Auburn, WA 98001–1650. Retrieved January 5, 2009, from http://www.ezaccess.com/dealers/Instr_Sheets/EZ-SHAMPOO_IS.pdf

Flori, L. (2007). Don't throw in the towel: Tips for bathing a patient who has dementia. *Nursing2007*, 37(7), 22–23.

Frazer, C., Frazer, R., & Byron, R. (2009). Prevent infections with good denture care. *Nursing 2009*, 39(8), 50–53.

George, M., & Naik, A. (2006). Clinician's role in the treatment of bathing disability. *Geriatrics Aging*, 9(9), 642–645.

Gray, M., Bliss, D., Doughty, D., et al. (2007). Incontinence-associated dermatitis: A consensus. *Journal of Wound, Ostomy and Continence Nursing*, 34(1), 45–54.

Haas, J., & Larson, E. (2008). Compliance with hand hygiene guidelines. *American Journal of Nursing*, 108(8), 40–44.

Harris D., Eilers J., Harriman, A., et al. (2008). Putting evidence into practice: Evidence-based interventions for the management of oral mucositis. *Clinical Journal of Oncology Nursing*, 12(1), 141–152.

Hayward, M., & Tindale, R. (2008). Knowing your "dydoe" from your "madonna": An emergency nurse guide to body piercing. *Emergency Nurse*, 15(10), 26–36.

Holman, C., Roberts, S., & Nicol, M. (2005). Promoting healthy sight and eye care. *Nursing Older People*, 17(1), 37–38.

Hospital Info. (2008). Artificial eye service (ocular prosthetics). Norfolk and Norwich University Hospitals, NHS Foundation Trust. Retrieved December 30, 2008, from http://www.nnuh.nhs.uk/Dept.asp?ID=517&q=prosthetic,eye

Human, L., & Bell, J. (2007). Oral hygiene in critically ill patients. *SAJCC*, 23(2), 61–65. Retrieved October 22, 2008, from http://www.sajcc.org.za/index.php/SAJCC/article/viewFile/24/27

The Joanna Briggs Institute. (2004). Oral hygiene care for adults with dementia in residential aged care facilities. *Best Practice*, 8(4), 1–6. ISSN 1329-1874. Retrieved December 21, 2008, from http://www.joannabriggs.edu.au/pdf/BPISEng_8_4.pdf

The Joanna Briggs Institute. (2007). Topical skin care in aged care facilities. *Best Practice*, 11(3), 1–3.

Katz, S., Down, T., Cash, H., et al. (1970). Progress in the development of the Index of ADL. *The Gerontologist*, 10(1), 20–30. Copyright © The Gerontological Society of America. Retrieved November 18, 2008, from http://www.consultgerirn.org/uploads/File/trythis/issue02.pdf

Kennard, C. (2006). Caregiver tips: Washing and bathing someone with Alzheimer's disease. Retrieved December 16, 2008, from http://alzheimers.about.com/od/practicalcare/a/Wash_Bath.htm

Kleinpell, R. M. (2010). Can we discard the traditional soap-and-basin bath? *Medscape Nurses*. Retrieved May 25, 2010, from http://www.medscape.com/viewarticle/7119552

Kovach, C. R., & Meyer-Arnold, E. A. (1996). Coping with conflicting agendas: The bathing experience of cognitively impaired older adults. *Scholarly Inquiry in Nursing Practice*, 10(1), 23–36.

Larson, E., Ciliberti T., Chantler, C., et al. (2004). Comparison of traditional and disposable bed baths in critically ill patients. *American Journal of Critical Care*, 13(3), 235–241.

Lentz, J. (2003). Daily baths: Torment or comfort at end of life? *Journal of Hospice and Palliative Nursing*, 5(1), 34–40.

Lucas, L. J., & Matthews-Flint, L. J. (2001). Sound advice about hearing aids. *Nursing2001*, 2, 59–61.

Massachusetts Eye and Ear Infirmary (last updated January 5, 2009). Contact lens options. Retrieved January 5, 2009, from http://www.masseyeandear.org/specialties/ophthalmology/contact-lens/about/

McKeighen, R. J., Mehmert, P. A., & Dickel, C. A. (June, 2008). Bathing/hygiene self-care deficit: Defining characteristics and related factors across age groups and diagnosis-related groups in an acute care setting. *International Journal of Nursing Terminologies and Classifications*, 1(4), 155–161.

McNeill, H. E. (2000). Biting back at poor oral hygiene. *Intensive and Critical Care Nursing*, 16(6), 367–372.

Meade, C., Bursell, A., & Ketelsen, L. (2007). Effects of nursing rounds: On patients' call light use, satisfaction, and safety. *American Journal of Nursing*, 107(2), 58–70; quiz 70–71.

Moorhead, S., Johnson, M., & Maas, M., et al. (Eds.). (2008). *Nursing outcomes classification (NOC)* (4th ed.). St. Louis, MO: C. V. Mosby.

NANDA International. (2009). *NANDA nursing diagnoses: Definitions and classification, 2009–2011*. Oxford: Wiley-Blackwell.

National Collaborating Centre for Primary Care. (2004). Clinical guidelines for type 2 diabetes. Prevention and management of foot problems. London (UK): National Institute for Clinical Excellence (NICE); 2004 June. 104 pp. Retrieved October 27, 2008 from National Guideline Clearinghouse http://www.guidelines.gov/summary/summary.aspx?_id=5062&nbr=003546&string=prevention+and!%22management+of+foot+problems%22

National Collaborating Centre for Primary Care. (2006). Postnatal care. Routine postnatal care of women and their babies. London (UK): Royal College of General Practitioners. Retrieved October 27, 2008, from http://www.guidelines.gov/summary/summary.aspx?doc_id=9630&nbr=005150&string=routine+AND+postnatal+ANDcare

National Guideline Clearinghouse (NGC). (2005a). Nursing management of oral hygiene. Retrieved December 21, 2008, from http://www.guideline.gov/summary/summary.aspx?doc_id=7153&nbr=004285&string=nursing+AND+management+AND+oral+AND+hygiene

National Guideline Clearinghouse (NGC). (2005b). Registered Nurses Association of Ontario (RNAO). Risk assessment & prevention of pressure ulcers. Toronto (ON): Registered Nurses Association of Ontario. Retrieved December 2, 2008, from http://www.guidelines.gov/summary/summary.aspx?doc_id=7006&nbr=004215&string=P...

National Institute on Deafness and Other Communication Disorders (NIDCD). (2007). NIDCD fact sheet: hearing aids. Retrieved December 20, 2008, from http://www.nidcd.nih.gov/staticresources/health/hearing/HearingAids07.pdf

Nelson, A., Lloyd, J., Menzel, N., et al. (2003). Preventing nursing back injuries: redesigning patient handling tasks. *Journal of the American Association of Occupational Health Nurses*, 51(3), 126–134.

Nelson, A., Pragala, G., & Menzel, N. (2003). Myths and facts about back injuries in nursing. *American Journal of Nursing*, 103(2), 32–40.

Neppelenbroek, K., Pavarina, A., Spolidorio, D., et al. (2008). Effectiveness of microwave disinfection of complete dentures on the treatment of *Candida*-related denture stomatitis. *Journal of Oral Rehabilitation*, 35(11), 836–846.

Nightingale, F. (1860). *Notes on nursing: What it is and what it is not*. New York: D. Appleton and Co. Reprint, 1969. New York: Dover Publications.

O'Flynn, J. (2007). Prospective sampling of patient bath basins in acute care setting: Qualitative evaluation of bacterial colonization. *American Journal of Infection Control*, 35(5), E50–51.

Pappas, P., Rex, J., Sobel, J., et al. (2009). Guidelines for treatment of candidiasis: 2009 update by the Infectious Diseases Society of America. *Clinical Infectious Disease*, 38(2), 161–189. Retrieved November 4, 2008, from National Guideline Clearinghouse http://www.guidelines.gov/content.aspx?id=14174

Peters, R. (n.d.). Artificial eyes of glass and plastic and suggestions regarding their care. Center for Ocular Prosthetics. Retrieved January 2, 2009, from http://www.artificialeyesplastic.com/new-eye-care.htm

Plummer, E., & Albert, S. (2008). Diabetic foot care management in the elderly. *Clinics in Geriatric Medicine*, 24(3), 551–567, viii.

Procter & Gamble. (n.d.). 7 Tips for the Best Shave Ever (n.d.). Cincinnati, OH: Author. Retrieved December 24, 2008, from http://www.gillettefusion.com/us/custom/en_US/tips.html

Procter & Gamble. (2008). How to shave. Trim and shape. Retrieved January 5, 2009, from http://www.gillette.com/en-US/#/home/

Rader, J., Barrick, A., Hoeffer, B., et al. (2006). The bathing of older adults with dementia. *American Journal of Nursing, 106*(4), 40–48.

Ramponi, D. R. (2001). Eye on contact lens removal. *Nursing 31*(8), 56–57.

Rasin, J., & Barrick, A. L. (2004). Bathing patients with dementia. *American Journal of Nursing, 104*(3), 30–33.

Robles, R., Corcoles, G., Torres, L., et al. (2002). Frequency of the adverse events during the hygiene of the critical patients [Spanish]. *Enfermia Intensiva, 13*(2), 47–56.

Rose, M., & Drake, D. (2008). Best practices for skin care of the morbidly obese. *Bariatric Nursing and Surgical Patient Care, 3*(2), 129–134.

Schwartz, M. (2000). The oral health of the long-term care patient. *Annals of Long Term Care, 8*(12), 41–46.

Sehulster, L., & Chinn, R. (2003). Guidelines for environmental infection control in health-care facilities. Recommendations of CDC and the Healthcare Infection Control Practices Advisory Committee (HICPAC). *Morbidity and Mortality Weekly Report, 52*(RR-10), 1–42.

Shiomori, T., Miyamoto, H., Makishima, K., et al. (2002). Evaluation of bedmaking-related airborne and surface methicillin-resistant *Staphylococcus aureus* contamination. *Journal of Hospital Infection, 50*(1), 30–35.

Siegel, J., Rhinehart, E., Jackson, M., Chiarello, L., & the Healthcare Infection Control Practices Advisory Committee (2007). *2007 Guideline for isolation precautions: Preventing transmission of infectious agents in the healthcare setting.* Retrieved July 6, 2008, from http://www.cdc.gov/ncidod/dhqp/gl_isolation.html

Slot, D., Dörfer, C., & Van der Weijden, G. (2008). The efficacy of interdental brushes on plaque and parameters of periodontal inflammation: A systematic review. *International Journal of Dental Hygiene, 26*(4), 253–264.

Sommer, S. K., & Sommer, N. W. (2002). When your patient is hearing impaired. *RN, 65*(12), 23–32.

Spector, R. (2009). *Cultural diversity in health and illness* (7th ed.). Upper Saddle River, NJ: Prentice-Hall Health.

Stern, C. (2007). Evidence summary: Older adults: Bathing & skin care. The Joanna Briggs Institute. Retrieved December 18, 2008, from http://www.jbiconnect.org/connect/docs/cis/es_html_viewer.php?SID=6298&lang=en&region=AU

Thiru-Chelvam. B. (2004). Bathing persons with dementia. Iowa City, IA: University of Iowa Gerontological Nursing Interventions Research Center, Research Dissemination Core. Retrieved from National Guideline Clearinghouse, October 21, 2008, from http://www.guidelines.gov/summary/summary.aspx?doc_id=6220&nbr=003991&string+

Thompson Healthcare, Inc. (2008). How to shampoo the hair of a person in bed. Retrieved December 20, 2008, from http://www.drugs.com/cg/how-to-shampoo-the-hair-of-a-person-in-bed.html

Trinkoff, A., Brady, B., & Nielsen, K. (2003). Workplace Prevention and Musculoskeletal Injuries in Nurses. *Journal of the Association of Occupational Health Professionals in Healthcare, 23*(4), 26–30.

Video: How to Shave (n.d.). Retrieved December 24, 2008, from http://www.gillette.com/en-US/#/grooming/howtoshave/en-US/index.shtml/

Walton, J. C., Miller, J., & Tordecilla, L. (2001). Elder assessment and care. *MEDSURG Nursing, 10*(1), 37–44.

Warshaw, E., Nix, D., Kula, J., et al. (2002). Clinical and cost effectiveness of a cleanser protectant lotion for treatment of perineal skin breakdown in low-risk patients with incontinence. *Ostomy and Wound Management, 48*(6), 44–51. Retrieved November 18, 2008, from https://docline.gov/docline/requests/receipt/receipt.cfm?Program=Doc&type=n&t=0.155594086426

Watando, A., Ebihara, S., Ebihara, T., et al. (2004). Daily oral care and cough reflex sensitivity in elderly nursing home patients. *Chest, 126*(4), 1066–1070.

Wilkinson, J. M., & Ahern, N. (2009). *Nursing diagnosis handbook with NIC interventions and NOC outcomes* (9th ed.). Upper Saddle River, NJ: Prentice-Hall Health.

Chapter 23

Abrams, A. C., Smith, S. P., & Lammon, C. B. (2006). *The clinical drug therapy: Rationales for nursing practice.* Philadelphia: Lippincott Williams & Wilkins.

Ahlin, C., Klane-Soderlvist, B., Brundin, S., et al. (2006). Implementation of a written protocol for management of central venous access devices: A theoretical and practical education, including bedside examination. *Journal of Infusion Nursing, 29*(5), 253–259.

American Academy of Family Physicians (AAFP). (2006). Nasal sprays: How to use them correctly. *Family Doctor.* Retrieved December 5, 2009, from http://familydoctor.org/online/famdocen/home/common/allergies/treatment/104.html

American Academy of Family Physicians (AAFP). (2006). Metered-dose inhaler: How to use it correctly. *Family Doctor.* Retrieved December 5, 2009, from http://familydoctor.org/online/famdocen/home/common/asthma/medications/040.html

American Society of Health-System Pharmacists, Inc. (2001). How to use rectal suppositories properly. Retrieved December 6, 2009, from http://www.safemedication.com/safemed/MedicationTipsTools/HowtoAdminister/HowtoUseRectalSuppositoriesProperly.aspx

Aschenbrenner, D., & Venable, S. (2008). *Drug therapy in nursing.* Philadelphia: Lippincott Williams & Wilkins.

Azar-Cavanagh, M., Burdt, P., & Green-McKenzie, J. (2007). Effect of the introduction of an engineered sharps injury prevention device on the percutaneous injury rate. *Infection Control & Hospital Epidemiology, 28*(2), 165–170.

Beers, M. H., Berkow, R., & Jones, T. V. (Eds.). (2006a). Drug therapy and the elderly. *The Merck manual of diagnosis and therapy* (18th ed.). Whitehouse Station, NJ: Merck.

Beers, M. H., Berkow, R., & Jones, T. V. (Eds.). (2006b). Drug toxicity. *The Merck manual of diagnosis and therapy* (18th ed.). Whitehouse Station, NJ: Merck.

Beers, M. H., Berkow, R., & Jones, T. V. (Eds.). (2006c). Factors affecting drug response. *The Merck manual of diagnosis and therapy* (17th ed.). Whitehouse Station, NJ: Merck.

Best practices: Evidence-based nursing procedures (2008). (pp. 117–124). Philadelphia: Lippincott Williams & Wilkins.

Bollinger, M. B. (2005). How do patients determine that their metered-dose inhaler is empty? *Pediatrics, 116,* 563–564. Retrieved September 14, 2008, from http://www.pediatrics.org/cgi/content/full/116/2/S1/563–a

Bradshaw, A. Dip, N., & Price, L. (2006). Rectal suppository insertion: the reliability of the evidence as a basis for nursing practice. *Journal of Clinical Nursing, 16*(1), 98–103.

Brock, T. P., Wessell, A. M., Williams, D. M., et al. (2004). Accuracy of float testing for metered-dose inhaler canisters. *Journal of the American Pharmaceutical Association, 42*(4), 582–586.

Bulecheck, G., Butcher G., & Dochterman, J. (Eds.). (2007). *Nursing interventions classification (NIC)* (5th ed.). St Louis, MO: C. V. Mosby.

Caesar, B. R., & Hutchinson, B. (2006). Doing it better: Reducing medication errors by using applied technology. *Nursing, 26*(8), 24–25.

Catalano, K., & Fickenscher, K. (2008). Complying with the 2008 national patient safety goals, *AORN Journal, 87*(3), 547–556.

Cescon, D. W., & Etchells, E. (2008). Barcoded medication administration: a last line of defense. *JAMA, 299*(18), 2200–2202.

Chalupka, S. M., Markkanen, P., Galligan, C., et al. (2008). Sharps injuries and bloodborne pathogen exposures in home health care. *AAOHN Journal, 56*(1), 15–29.

Chan, H. (2001). Effects of injection duration on site-pain intensity and bruising associated with subcutaneous heparin. *Journal of Clinical Nursing, 25*(6), 882–892.

Cocoman, A., & Barron, C. (2008). Administering subcutaneous injections to children: what does the evidence say? *Journal of Children's and Young People's Nursing, 2*(2), 84–89.

Cook, I. F. (2006). Optimal technique for intramuscular injection of infants and toddlers. *Medical Journal of Australia, 183*(2), 60–63.

Curren, A., & Munday, L. (2008). *Math for meds: Dosage and solutions* (10th ed.). Clifton Park, NY: Thomson Delmar Learning.

Deglin, J. H., & Hazard, A. (2008). *Davis' drug guide for nurses* (11th ed.). Philadelphia: F. A. Davis.

Disease Control and Epidemiology, Health and Community Services, Government of Newfoundland and Labrador. (2006). Tuberculosis screening and testing program. Retrieved August 10, 2008, from http://www.health.gov.nl.ca/health/publications/immunization/pdf/7section.pdf

Floyd, S., & Meyer, A. (2007). Intramuscular injections—what's best practice? *Nursing, 13*(6), 20–2.

Gaga, D., & Howard, S. (2002). Fatigue among clinicians and the safety of patients. *New England Journal of Medicine, 347,* 1249–1255.

Gahart, B., & Nazareno, A. (2007). *2008 Intravenous medications: A handbook for nurses and health professions.* St. Louis, MO: C. V. Mosby.

Glazer, G. (2002). Medication administration interventions that must be performed by a registered nurse. *Online Journal of Issues in Nursing, 7*(2), 4.

Gommans, J. M., McIntosh, P., Bee, S., et al. (2008). Improving the quality of written prescriptions in a general hospital: The influence of 10 years of serial audits and targeted interventions. *Internal Medicine Journal, 38*(4), 243–248.

Greenway, K. (2004). Using the ventral gluteal site for intramuscular injection. *Nursing Standard, 18*(29), 39–42.

Hadaway, L. (2008). Targeting therapy with central venous access devices. *Nursing2008, 38*(6), 34–41.

Haines, T., & Stringer, B. (2007). Could the death of a BC or nurse have been prevented by using the hands-free technique? *Canadian Operating Room Nursing Journal, 25*(4), 8, 10–11, 19–20.

Hitchen L. (2008). Frequent interruptions linked to drug errors. *BMJ, 336*(7654), 1155.

Hockenberry-Eaton, M. J., & Tashiro, J. (2005). *Wong's essentials of pediatric nursing* (8th ed.). St. Louis, MO: C. V. Mosby.

Howard, A., Mercer, P., Nataraj, H. C., et al. (1997). Bevel-down superior to bevel-up in intradermal skin testing. *Annals of Allergy, Asthma, & Immunology, 78,* 594–596.

Hughes, R., & Ortiz, E. (2005). Medication errors. *American Journal of Nursing,* Supplement, 14–24.

Hunter, J. (2008). Intramuscular injection techniques. *Nursing Standard, 22*(24), 35–40.

Infusion Nurses Society (INS). (2006a). *Infusion nursing standards of practice.* Norwood, MA: Gardner Foundation.

Infusion Nurses Society (INS). (2006b). Infusion nursing standards of practice. *Journal of Infusion in Nursing, 29*(1S), S1–9.

Ipp, M., Taddio, A., Sam, J., et al. (2006). Needle aspiration and intramuscular vaccination. *Archives of Pediatric Adolescent Medicine, 160*(4), 451.

Ipp, M., Taddio, A., Sam, J., et al. (2007). Vaccine-related pain: Randomized controlled trial of two injection techniques. *Archives of Disease in Childhood, 92*(12), 1105–1108.

The Joanna Briggs Institute. (2005). Strategies to reduce medication errors with reference to older adults. *Best Practice, 9*(4), 1–6.

The Joint Commission (TJC). (2006). Using medication reconciliation to prevent errors. *Sentinel Event Alert,* 35.

The Joint Commission (TJC). (2007). *2008 hospital accreditation standards* (2nd ed.). Oakbrook Terrace, IL: Author.

The Joint Commission (TJC). (2008). Preventing pediatric medication errors. *Sentinel Event Alert,* 39. Retrieved December 6, 2009, from http://www.jointcommission.org/SentinelEvents/SentinelEventAlert/sea_39.htm

Karch, A. M. (2008). Make the right connection: verify that tubing is correct. *American Journal of Nursing, 108*(3), 72.

Karch, A. M., & Karch, F. E. (2003). Practice errors: Not so fast! IV push drugs can be dangerous when given too rapidly. *American Journal of Nursing, 103*(8), 71.

Article I. Kroger A. T., Atkinson, W. L., Marcuse, E. K., Pickering, L. K., & Advisory Committee on Immunization Practices (ACIP) Centers for Disease Control and Prevention (CDC). (2006). General recommendations on immunization: Recommendations of the Advisory Committee on Immunization Practices (ACIP). *MMWR, 55*(RR-15), 1–48. Retrieved August 8, 2008, from http://www.cdc.gov/mmwr/preview/mmwrhtml/rr5515a1.htm

Article II. Lacy, C., Armstrong, L., & Goldman, M. (2008). *Drug information handbook 2008–2009.* (17th ed.). Chicago, IL: Lexi-Comp.

Lapum, J. L. (2006). Patency of arterial catheters with heparinized solutions versus non-heparinized solutions: A review of the literature. *Canadian Journal of Cardiovascular Nursing, 16*(2), 64–70.

Lassetter, J. H., & Warnick, M. L. (2003). Medical errors, drug-related problems, and medication errors: A literature review on quality of care and cost issues. *Journal of Nursing Care Quality, 18*(3), 175–183.

Lavery, I., & Smith, E. (2008). Peripheral vascular access devices: risk prevention and management. *British Journal of Nursing, 16*(22), 1378, 1380, 1382–1383.

LeDuc, K. (1997). Efficacy of normal saline solution versus heparin solution for maintaining patency of peripheral intravenous catheters in children. *Journal of Emergency Nursing, 23*(4), 306–309.

Lehne, R. A. (2006). *Pharmacology for nursing care* (6th ed.). St. Louis, MO: Elsevier/Mosby.

LeMone, P., & Burke, K. (2007). *Medical-surgical nursing: Critical thinking in client care* (4th ed.). Upper Saddle River, NJ: Prentice-Hall.

Levine, A., & Brennan, A. P. (2007). Diabetes under control. Rethinking sliding-scale insulin: One hospital's efforts in the ICU and elsewhere. *American Journal of Nursing, 107*(10), 74–79.

Lilley, L., Harrington S., & Snyder, J. S. (2007). *Pharmacology and the nursing process* (5th ed.). St. Louis, MO: C. V. Mosby.

Martinez De Castillo, S., Castillo, S., & Werner-McCullough, M. (2007). *Calculating drug dosages* (2nd ed.). Philadelphia: F. A. Davis.

McConnell, E. A. (2002). Administering medication through a gastrostomy tube. *Nursing, 32*(12), 22.

Mok, E., Kwong, T. K., Chan, Y., et al. (2007). A randomized controlled trial for maintaining peripheral intravenous lock in children. *International Journal of Nursing Practice, 13*(1), 33 45.

Moorhead, S., Johnson, M., & Maas, M. (2007). *Nursing outcomes classification (NOC)* (4th ed.). St. Louis, MO: C. V. Mosby.

Morrison-Karch, A., & Karch, A. (2007). *Focus on nursing pharmacology* (4th ed.). Philadelphia: Lippincott Williams & Wilkins.

Mudge, B., Forcier, D., & Slarrert, M. J. (1998). Patency of 24-gauge peripheral intermittent infusion devices: A comparison of heparin and saline flush solutions. *Pediatric Nursing, 24*(2), 142–149.

National Center for HIV, STD, and TB Prevention, Division of Tuberculosis Elimination. Mantoux tuberculosis skin test facilitator guide. (2008). Part one: Administering the Mantoux tuberculin skin test. Retrieved December 5, 2009, from http://www.cdc.gov/tb/education/Mantoux/part1.htm

Nicholl, L. H., & Hesby, A. (2002). Intramuscular injection: An integrative research review and guideline for evidence-based practice. *Applied Nursing Research, 15*(3), 149–162.

Nisbet, A. C. (2006). Intramuscular injections in the increasingly obese population: Retrospective study. *BMJ, 332,* 637–638; Retrieved November 12, 2008, from http://www.bmj.com/cgi/reprint/332/7542/637

Ozel, A., Yavuz, H., & Erkul, I. (1995). Gangrene after penicillin injection: A case report. *The Turkish Journal of Pediatrics, 37*(1), 567–571.

Paparella, S. (2008). Choosing the right strategy for medication error reduction: Part I. *Journal of Emergency Nursing, 34*(2), 145–146.

Pape, T. M. (2003). Applying airline safety practices to medication administration. *MedSurg Nursing, 12*(2), 77–94.

Perhats, C., Valdez, A. M., & St. Mars, T. (2008). Promoting safer medication use among older adults. *Journal of Emergency Nursing, 34*(2), 156–158.

Phillips, D. (2010). *Manual of IV therapeutics* (5th ed.). Philadelphia: F. A. Davis.

Phillips, N., & Nay, R. N. (2007). Nursing administration of medication via enteral tubes in adults: A systematic review. *International Journal of Evidence-Based Healthcare, 5*(3), 324–353.

Phillips, N., & Nay, R. N. (2008). A systematic review of nursing administration of medication via enteral tubes in adults. *Journal of Clinical Nursing, 17*(17), 2257–2265.

Picone, D. M., Titler, M. G., Dochterman, J., et al. (2008). Predictors of medication errors among elderly, hospitalized patients. *American Journal of Medical Quality, 23*(2), 115–127.

Polifroni, E., McNulty, J., & Allchin, N. (2003). Medication errors: More basic than a system issue. *Journal of Nursing Education, 42*(10), 41.

Preston, S. T. (2004). Glass contamination in parenterally administered medication. *Journal of Advanced Nursing, 48*(3), 266–270.

Preventing pediatric medication errors. (2008). *Sentinel Event Alert, 39,* 1–4.

Pullen, R. L. (2005). Administering medication by the Z-track method. *Nursing, 35*(7), 24.

Ram, F. S. F., Brocklebank, D. M., White, J., et al. (2002). Pressurized metered dose inhalers versus all other hand-held inhaler devices to deliver beta-2 agonist bronchodilators for non-acute asthma. *Cochrane Database of Systematic Reviews* 2002, Issue 2. Art. No.: CD002158. DOI: 10.1002/14651858.CD002158, Retrieved December 6, 2009, from http://www.cochrane.org/reviews/en/ab002158.html

Rantahal, J., Ramlaskhan, S., & Singh, K. (2006). Sciatic nerve injury following intramuscular injection: A case report and review of the literature. *Journal of Neuroscience Nursing, 38*(4), 238–240.

Rochon, P. A. (2006). *Drug prescribing for older adults.* Waltham, MA: UpToDate, Inc.

Rosenthal, K. (2003). Keeping I.V. therapy safe with needleless systems. *Nursing,* Supplement, 16–18, 20. Retrieved December 7, 2009, from http://findarticles.com/p/articles/mi_qa3689/is_200310/ai_n9308529?tag=artBody;col1

Rothschild, J. M., Landrigan, C. P., Cronin, J. W., et al. (2006). The critical care safety study: The incidence and nature of adverse events and serious medical errors in intensive. *Critical Care Medicine, 33*(8), 1694–1700.

Rowan, N. (2006, September). Insulin (subcutaneous). Evidence summaries - *Joanna Briggs Institute,* p. 1. Retrieved September 11, 2008, from ProQuest Nursing & Allied Health Source database. (Document ID: 1446922971).

Roy, V., Gupta, P., & Srivastava, S. (2005). Medication errors: Causes & prevention. *Health Administrator, XIX*(1), 60–64.

Rushing, J. (2008). Administering enoxaparin injection. *Nursing2008, 38*(3), 19.

Santell, J. P., & Heath, W. M. (2008). Paying attention to anticoagulant medication errors: What have we learned? USP Center for the Advancement of Patient Safety CAPSLink. Retrieved December 6, 2009, from http://www.usp.org/pdf/EN/patientSafety/capsLink2008–01–01.pdf

Skokal, W. (2000). IV push at home? *RN, 63*(20), 26–29.

Smith, B., & Royer, T. I. (2007). New standards for improving peripheral IV catheter securement. *Nursing, 37*(3), 72–74.

Smith, L. I., & Smith, E. (2008). Peripheral vascular access devices: risk prevention and management. *British Journal of Nursing, 16*(22), 1378, 1380, 1382–1383.

Talbert, J. L., Haslam, R. H., & Haller, J. A. (1967). Gangrene of the foot following intramuscular injection in the lateral thigh: A case report with recommendations for prevention. *The Journal of Pediatrics, 70*(1), 110–114.

Tarnow, K., & King, N. (2004). Intradermal injections: Traditional bevel up versus bevel down. *Applied Nursing Research, 17*(4), 275–282.

Taylor, J. L., Loan, L. A., Blackburn, S., et al. (2008). Medication administration variances before and after implementation of computerized physician order entry in a neonatal intensive care unit. *Pediatrics, 121*(1), 123–128.

Thompson, C. A. (2005). Technology hasn't eliminated medication errors yet. *American Journal of Health-System Pharmacy, 62*(3), 243, 245.

Trinkoff, A. M., Le, R., Geiger-Brown, J., et al. (2007). Work schedule, needle use, and needlestick injuries among registered nurses. *Infection Control & Hospital Epidemiology, 28*(2), 156–164.

Umpierrez, G. E., Palacio, A., & Smiley, D. (2007). Sliding scale insulin use: Myth or insanity? *American Journal of Medicine, 20*(7), 563–567.

U.S. Department of Health and Human Services (USDHHS), Centers for Disease Control and Prevention, National Immunization Program. (2002). General recommendations on immunizations. *Morbidity and Mortality Weekly Report,* 51(RR02), 1–36. Retrieved December 6, 2009, from http://www.cdc.gov/mmwr/preview/mmwrhtml/rr5102a1.htm

U.S. Department of Health and Human Services (USDHHS), Division of Healthcare Quality Promotion (DHQP). (1991, last updated November, 2008). Regulations (Standards - 29 CFR) Bloodborne pathogens—1910.1030. Retrieved December 14, 2009, from http://www.osha.gov/pls/oshaweb/owadisp.show_document?p_table=STANDARDS&p_id=10051

U.S. Department of Health and Human Services (USDHHS), Division of Healthcare Quality Promotion (DHQP). (2008). A patient safety threat—syringe reuse. Retrieved December 7, 2009, from http://www.cdc.gov/ncidod/dhqp/about.html

U.S. Department of Health and Human Services (USDHHS), National Institute for Occupational Safety and Health (NIOSH). (n.d.). What every worker should know—How to protect yourself from needlestick injuries. Publication No. 2000–135. Retrieved December 5, 2009, from http://www.cdc.gov/niosh/docs/2000–135/

U.S. Department of Health and Human Services (USDHHS), National Institute for Occupational Safety and Health (NIOSH). (1999). Preventing needlestick injuries in health care settings. Publication No. 2000–108. Retrieved December 5, 2009, from http://www.cdc.gov/niosh/docs/2000–108/

U.S. Department of Labor, Occupational Safety & Health Administration (OSHA). (2007). Hospital eTool—Healthcare wide hazards module: Needlesticks/sharps injuries. Retrieved December 5, 2009, from http://www.osha.gov/SLTC/etools/hospital/hazards/sharps/sharps.html

U.S. Food and Drug Administration, Center of Evaluation and Research. (2008). Metered-dose inhalers (MDI). Retrieved December 5, 2009, from http://www.fda.gov/Drugs/DrugSafety/InformationbyDrugClass/ucm063054.htm

U.S. Food and Drug Administration: Center for Drug Evaluation and Research. (2009). FDA 101: Medications errors. Retrieved December 5, 2009, from http://www.fda.gov/ForConsumers/ConsumerUpdates/ucm048644.htm

Varkey, P., Cunnigham, J., & Bisping, D. S. (2007). Improving medication reconciliation in the outpatient setting. *Joint Commission Journal of Patient Safety, 33*(5), 286–292. Retrieved December 8, 2009, from http://www.ihi.org/ihi/gateway.aspx?target=http%3a%2f%2fwww.ncbi.nlm.nih.gov%2fentrez%2fquery.fcgi%3fdb%3dpubmed%26amp%3bcmd%3dRetrieve%26amp%3bdopt%3dAbstractPlus%26amp%3blist_uids%3d17503684%26amp%3bquery_hl%3d1%26amp%3bitool%3dpubmed_docsum

Ward, K. R., & Koemer, D. K. (2008). Sink or swim: The Titanic: Medication administration fair. *Journal of Continuing Education in Nursing, 39*(4), 179–184.

Wood, D. (2007). Speedy shots equal less pain: Canadian study calls for rapid injections in young children. *Nursing Spectrum—DC, Maryland & Virginia Edition, 17*(22), 12–12. Retrieved September 11, 2008, from CINAHL database.

World Health Organization (WHO), Department of Essential Health Technologies. (n.d.). Guiding principles to ensure injection device security. Retrieved December 5, 2009, from http://www.who.int/injection_safety/WHOGuidPrinciplesInjEquipFinal.pdf

Wright, D. (2002). Swallowing difficulties protocol: Medication administration. *Nursing Standard, 17*(14/15), 43.

Wynaden, D., Landsborough, I., McGowan, S., et al. (2006). Best practice guidelines for the administration of intramuscular injections in the mental health setting. *International Journal of Mental Health Nursing, 15*(3), 195–200.

Zaybak, A., & Khorshid, L. (2008). Study on the effect of the duration of subcutaneous heparin injection on bruising and pain. *Journal of Clinical Nursing, 17*(3), 378–385.

Zwicker, D., & Fulmer, T. (2008). Reducing adverse drug events. In: E. Capezuti, D. Zwicker, M. Mezey, & T. Fulmer (Eds.), *Evidence-based geriatric nursing protocols for best practice* (3rd ed.). New York: Springer.

Chapter 24

American Hospital Association. (1992). *A patient's bill of rights.* Chicago, IL: Author. Retrieved December 5, 2009, from http://www.patienttalk.info/AHA-Patient_Bill_of_Rights.htm

American Hospital Association. (2003). *The patient care partnership.* Chicago, IL: Author. Retrieved December 8, 2009, from http://www.aha.org/aha/issues/Communicating-With-Patients/pt-care-partnership.html

American Nurses Association (ANA). (2001). *Code of ethics for nurses with interpretive statements.* Washington, DC: American Nurses Publishing. Retrieved December 8, 2009, from http://www.nursingworld.org/MainMenuCategories/ThePracticeofProfessionalNursing/EthicsStandards/CodeofEthics.aspx

American Nurses Association (ANA). (2010). *Nursing: Scope and standards of practice* (2nd ed). Public Comment draft, January 2010. Silver Spring, MD: Nursebooks.org Retrieved February 1, 2010, from http://www.nursingworld.org/DocumentVault/NursingPractice/Draft-Nursing-Scope-Standards-2nd-Ed.aspx

Anderson, A. S., & Klemm, P. (2008). The Internet: Friend or foe when providing patient education? *Clinical Journal of Oncology Nursing, 12*(1), 55–63.

Bader, J. L., & Stickman-Stein, N. (2003). Evaluation of new multimedia format for cancer communications. *Journal of Medical Internet Research, 5*(3), e16. Retrieved February 15, 2010, from http://www.jmir.org/2003/3/e16/

Bastable, S. B. (2008). Nurse as educator: *Principles of teaching and learning for nursing practice* (3rd ed.). Boston: Jones and Bartlett.

Bietz, J. M., & Snarponis, A. (2006). Strategies for online teaching and learning: Lessons learned. *Nurse Educator, 31*(1), 20–25.

Bloom B. S., & Krathwohl, D. R. (1956). Taxonomy of educational objectives: The classification of educational goals. *Handbook I: Cognitive domain.* New York: Longmans, Green.

Bloom, B. S., Mesia, B. B., & Krathwohl, D. R. (1964). Taxonomy of educational objectives (Vol. 1: *The Affective Domain* and Vol. 2: *The Cognitive Domain*). New York: David McKay.

Bremner, M. N., Aduddell, K., Bennett, D. N., et al. (2006). The use of human patient simulators. *Nurse Educator, 31*(4), 170–174.

Bulechek, G., Butcher, H., & Dochterman, J. M. (2008). *Nursing interventions classification (NIC)* (5th ed.). St. Louis, MO: C. V. Mosby.

Cangelosi, P. R., & Sorrell, J. N. (2008). Storytelling as an educational strategy for older adults with chronic illness. *Journal of Psychosocial Nursing & Mental Health Services, 46*(7), 19–22. Retrieved September 25, 2008, from Research Library database. (Document ID: 1518641321).

Caruana, E. (2007, August). Patient information (pre-operative): Knowledge retention. *Evidence Summaries – Joanna Briggs Institute.* Retrieved September 25, 2008, from ProQuest Nursing & Allied Health Source database. (Document ID: 1451740781).

Christman, L. (2000). Patient and family education in managed care and beyond: Seizing the teachable moment. *Nursing Administration Quarterly, 25*(1), 155–156.

Clarke Tasker, V. A., & Wade, R. (2002, May–June). What we thought we knew: African American males' perception of prostate cancer and screening methods [electronic version]. *Association of Black Nursing Faculty Journal, 13*(3), 56–60.

The Communication Initiative (TCI). (2003, July 29). Health belief model. Retrieved April 20, 2004, from http://www.comminit.com/ctheories/sid-8180.html

Dept of Health and Human Services, The Secretary's Advisory Committee on National Health Promotion and Disease Prevention Objectives for 2020 (2009). Proposed objectives for Healthy People 2020: Draft for public comment. Washington, DC: U.S. Government Printing Office; 82. Retrieved February 19, 2010, from http://www.healthypeople.gov/HP2020/

Dept of Health and Human Services, The Secretary's Advisory Committee on National Health Promotion and Disease Prevention Objectives for 2020 (2008). Phase I report: Recommendations for the framework and format of Healthy People 2020. Washington, DC: U.S. Government Printing Office.

Fenner, P. C. (2002). Understanding the role of practice in learning for geriatric individuals. *Topics in Geriatric Rehabilitation, 17*(4), 11–32.

Friberg, F., Bergh, A., & Lepp, M. (2006). In search of details of patient teaching in nursing documentation—an analysis of patient records in a medical ward in Sweden. *Issues in Clinical Nursing, 15*(12), 1550–1558.

Friesen, P., Pepler, C., & Hunter, P. (2002). Interactive family learning following a cancer diagnosis. *Oncology Nursing Forum, 29*(6), 981–987.

Greenawald, D. A. (2008, July). LIVE! from the Sim Lab: Broadcasting a simulated patient-care scenario as a teaching-learning strategy in a nursing fundamentals clinical lab. *Clinical Simulation in Nursing, 4*(2), e11–14.

Grimes, V. (2002, March–April). Comparing the effect of a skills checklist on teaching time required to achieve independence in administration of infusion medication. *Journal of Infusion Nursing, 25*(2), 109–120.

Henderson, A., & Zernike, W. (2001). A study of the impact of discharge information for surgical patients. *Journal of Advanced Nursing, 35*(3), 435–441.

Henneman, E. A., Cunningham, H., Roche, J. P., & Curnin, M. E. (2007). Human patient simulation: Teaching students to provide safe care. *Nurse Educator, 32*(5), 212–217.

Henning, J. E., Nielson, L.E., & Hauschildt, J. A. (2006). Implementing case study methodology in critical care nursing: A discourse analysis. *Nurse Educator, 31*(4), 153–158.

Henry, P. R. (2006). Making groups work in the classroom. *Nurse Educator, 31*(1), 26–30.

Hilgenberg, C., & Schlickau, J. (2002). Building transcultural knowledge through intercollegiate collaboration. *Journal of Transcultural Nursing, 13*(3), 241–247.

Hill, C. M. (2006). Integrating clinical experiences into the concept mapping process. *Nurse Educator, 31*(1), 26–29.

Hohler, S. E. (2004). Tips for better patient teaching. *Nursing2004, 34*(7), 7–8.

Holmes, T., & Rahe, R. (1967). The social readjustment and rating scale. *Journal of Psychosomatic Research, 11*, 213–218.

Janda, M., Stanek, C., Newman, B., et al. (2002). Impact of videotaped information on frequency and confidence of breast self-examination. *Breast Cancer Research and Treatment, 73*(1), 37–43.

The Joint Commission (TJC). (2008a). *Accreditation manual for hospitals 2009.* Chicago: Author.

The Joint Commission (TJC). (2008b). What did the doctor say?: Improving health literacy to protect patient safety. Retrieved December 7, 2009, from http://www.jointcommission.org/NR/rdonlyres/D5248B2E-E7E6-4121-8874-99C7B4888301/0/improving_health_literacy.pdf

The Joint Commission (TJC). (2009). The Joint Commission 2009 requirements that support effective communication, cultural competence, and patient-centered care Hospital Accreditation Program (HAP). Retrieved February 20, 2010, from http://www.jointcommission.org/.../PDF32009HAPSupportingStds.pdf

Karten, C. (2007). Easy to write? Creating easy-to-read patient education materials. *Clinical Journal of Oncological Nursing, 11*(4), 506–510.

Knowles, M. S. (1990). *The adult learner: A neglected species* (4th ed.). Houston: Gulf Publishing.

Lazarus, H. (1999). *Stress and emotion: A new synthesis.* New York: Springer.

Lazarus, H., & Folkman, S. (1948). *Stress appraisal and coping.* New York: Springer.

Lee, D. S., & Lee, S. S. (2000). Pre-operative teaching: How does a group of nurses do it? *Contemporary Nurse, 9*(1), 80–88.

Leininger, M. (1994). Transcultural nursing education: A worldwide imperative. *Nursing & Health Care, 15*(5), 254–257.

London, F. (1999). *No time to teach.* Philadelphia: J. B. Lippincott.

Marchese, K. (2006). Using Peplau's Theory of Interpersonal Relations to guide the education of patients undergoing urinary diversions. *Urologic Nursing, 26*(5), 363–371.

Marcum, J., Ridenour, G., Hammons, M., et al. (2002). A study of professional nurses' perceptions of patient education. *The Journal of Continuing Education in Nursing, 33*(3), 112–121.

Mayer, G. G. (2002). Writing easy-to-read teaching aids. *Nursing, 32*(3), 48–49.

McCaffery, M. (2002). Teaching your patient to use a pain rating scale. *Nursing, 32*(8), 17–20.

Monat, A., & Lazarus, R. (Eds.) (1991). *Stress and coping* (3rd ed.). St. Louis, MO: C. V. Mosby.

Moorhead, S., Johnson, M., Maas, M., et al. (Eds.). (2008). *Nursing outcomes classification (NOC)* (4th ed.). St. Louis, MO: C. V. Mosby.

Muilenburg, L.Y., & Bergeb, Z. L. (2005). Student barriers to online learning: A factor analytic study. *Distance Education, 26*(1), 1475–1498.

NANDA International. (2009). *NANDA nursing diagnoses: Definitions and classification 2009–2011*. Philadelphia: Author.

National Network of Libraries of Medicine. (2008). Health literacy. Retrieved September 19, 2008, from http://nnlm.gov/outreach/consumer/hlthlit.html

Nightingale, F. (1860/1992). *Notes on nursing: What it is and what it is not.* Philadelphia: Lippincott.

Oermann, M., Masserang, M., Maxey, M., et al. (2002). Clinic visit and waiting: Patient education and satisfaction. *MedSurg Nursing, 11*(5), 247–257.

Osborne, H. (2004). *Health literacy from A to Z: Practical ways to communicate your health message.* Boston: Jones and Bartlett.

Palmer, M. H., Kowlowitz, V., Campbell, J., et al. (2008). Using clinical simulations in geriatric nursing continuing education. *Nursing Outlook, 56(4),* 159–166.

PEW Health Professions Commission. (1998). Recreating health professional practice for a new century: Fourth report. San Francisco: UCSF Center for the Health Professions.

Piaget, J. (1966). *Origins of intelligence in children.* New York: W. W. Norton.

Rankin, S. H., Stallings, K. D., & London, F. (2004). *Patient education in health and illness.* Philadelphia: Lippincott Williams & Wilkins.

Roberts, D. (2004). Advocacy through patient teaching. *MedSurg Nursing, 13*(6), 363, 382.

Schrecengost, A. (2001). Do humorous preoperative teaching strategies work? *AORN Journal, 74*(5), 683–689.

Selye, H. (1974). *Stress without distress.* Philadelphia: J. B. Lippincott.

Selye, H. (1976). *The stress of life* (rev. ed.). New York: McGraw-Hill.

U.S. Department of Education, Institute of Education Sciences, National Center for Education Statistics. (2005). National assessment of adult literacy. Retrieved January 24, 2009, from http://nces.ed.gov/programs/coe/2007/section2/table.asp?tableID=692

U.S. Department of Health and Human Services (USDHHS), Health Resources and Services Association. (unknown). Health literacy. Retrieved September 19, 2008, from http://hrsa.gov/healthliteracy/

Valente, S. M. (2007). Oncology nurses' teaching and support for suicidal patients. *Journal of Psychosocial Oncology, 25*(1), 121–137.

Wayman, K. I., Yaeger, K. A., Sharek, P. J., et al. (2007). Simulation-based medical error disclosure training for pediatric healthcare professionals. *Journal for Healthcare Quality: Official Publication of the National Association for Healthcare Quality, 29*(4), 12–19.

Wehrli, G., & Nyquist, J. G. (2003). Teaching strategies/methodologies: Advantages, disadvantages /cautions, keys to success. *Creating an Educational Curriculum for Learners at Any Level AABB Conference.*

Wiljer, D., & Catton, P. (2003). Multimedia formats for patient education and health communication: Does user preference matter? *Journal of Medical Internet Research, 5*(3),e19.

Wykurz, G., & Kelly, D. (2002). Developing the role of patients as teachers: Literature review. *BMJ, 325*(7368), 818–821.

Chapter 25

Alford, L. (2007). Findings of interest from immunology and psychoneuroimmunology. *Manual Therapy, 12*(2), 176–180.

American Psychiatric Association (APA). (1994). *Diagnostic and statistical manual of mental disorders* (4th ed.). Washington, DC: Author.

Argentero, P., Dell'Olivo, B., & Ferretti, M. (2008). Staff burnout and patient satisfaction with the quality of dialysis care. *American Journal of Kidney Diseases, 51*(1), 80–92.

Badger, J. (2008). Critical care nurse intern program: Addressing psychological reactions related to critical care nursing. *Critical Care Nursing Quarterly, 31*(2), 184–187.

Bennett, M., & Lengacher, C. (2007). Humor and laughter may influence health: IV. Humor and immune function. *Evidence-Based Complementary and Alternative Medicine*, obtained from *eCAM 2007*, doi:10.1093/ecam/nem149, retrieved January 9, 2009, from http://ecam.oxfordjournals.org.cgi/reprint/nem149v1

Benson, H. (1976). *The relaxation response.* New York: Avon Books.

Bisson, J., & Andrew, M. (2007). Psychological treatment of posttraumatic stress disorder (PTSD). *Cochrane Database of Systematic Reviews*, Issue 3. Art. No.: CD003388.

Brammer, L. M., & MacDonald, G. (2003). *The helping relationship: Process and skills* (8th ed.). Old Tappan, NJ: Pearson.

Brennan, B. (1987). *Hands of light: A guide to healing through the human energy field.* New York: Bantam Books.

Bulechek, F., Butcher, H., & Dochterman, J. (2008). *Nursing interventions classification (NIC).* (5th ed.). St. Louis, MO: C. V. Mosby.

Collins, B., & Clancy, C. (2008). Limiting nurse overtime, and promoting other good working conditions influences patient safety. *Journal of Nursing Care Quality, 23*(2), 97–100.

Cousins, N. (1979). *Anatomy of an illness.* New York: Bantam Books.

Davidson, R., Kabat-Zinn, J., Schumacher, J., et al. (2003). Alterations in brain and immune function produced by mindfulness meditation. *Psychosomatic Medicine, 65*, 564–570.

Davies, W. (2008). Mindful meditation: Healing burnout in critical care nursing. *Holistic Nursing Practice, 22*(1), 32–36.

deKloet, E., Karst, H., & Joels, M. (2008). Corticosteroid hormones in the central stress response: Quick-and-slow. *Frontiers in Neuroendocrinology, 29*(2), 268–272.

Donahue, M., Piazza, I., Griffin, M., et al. (2008). The relationship between nurses' perceptions of empowerment and patient satisfaction. *Applied Nursing Research, 21*(1), 2–7.

Dowben, J., Grant, J., & Keltner, N. (2007). Psychobiological substrates of posttraumatic stress disorder: part II. *Perspectives in Psychiatric Care, 43*(3), 146–149.

du Pré, A. (1998). *Humor and the healing arts.* Mahwah, NJ: Lawrence Erlbaum.

Franco, G. P., de Barros, A. L., Nogueira-Martins, L. A., et al. (2003). Stress influence on genesis, onset and maintenance of cardiovascular diseases: Literature review. *Journal of Advanced Nursing, 43*(6), 548–554.

Gardner, J., Thomas-Hawkins, C., Fogg, L., et al. (2007). The relationships between nurses' perceptions of the hemodialysis unit work environment and nurse turnover, patient satisfaction, and hospitalizations. *Nephrology Nursing Journal: Journal of the American Nephrology Nurses' Association, 34*(3), 271–281; quiz 282.

Gonzalez, L., & Lengacher, C. (2007). Coping with breast cancer: A qualitative analysis of reflective journals. *Issues in Mental Health Nursing, 28*(5), 489–510.

Hall, L., Doran, D., & Pink, L. (2008). Outcomes of interventions to improve hospital nursing work environments. *The Journal of Nursing Administration, 38*(1), 40–46.

Hegge, M., & Larson, V. (2008). Stressors and coping strategies of students in accelerated baccalaureate nursing programs. *Nurse Educator, 33*(1), 26–30.

Holmes, T., & Rahe, R. (1967). The social readjustment and rating scale. *Journal of Psychosomatic Research, 11*, 213–218.

Hughes, F., Grigg, M., Fritsch, K., et al. (2007). Psychosocial response in emergency situations—the nurse's role. *International Nursing Review, 54*(1), 19–27.

Irwin, M. (2008). Human psychoneuroimmunology: 20 years of discovery. *Brain, Behavior, & Immunity, 22*(2), 129–139.

Joels, M., Krugers, H., & Karast, H. (2007). Stress-induced changes in hippocampal function. *Progress in Brain Research, 167,* 3–15.

Johnson, M., Bulechek, G., Butcher, H., et al. (2006). *Nursing diagnoses, outcomes & interventions: NANDA, NOC, and NIC linkages* (2nd ed.). St. Louis, MO: C. V. Mosby.

Johnson, P. (2002). The use of humor and its influences on spirituality and coping in breast cancer survivors. *Oncology Nursing Forum, 29*(4), 691–695.

Keegan, L. (2003). Therapies to reduce stress and anxiety. *Critical Care Nursing Clinics of North America, 15*(3), 321–327.

Krieger, D. (1993). *Accepting your power to heal*. Santa Fe, NM: Bear & Company.

Lardy, S. (2008). Decompress to fight disease. *Advance for Nurse Practitioners, 16*(8), 49–52.

Lazarus, R. (1999). *Stress and emotion: A new synthesis*. New York: Springer.

Lazarus, R., & Folkman, S. (1984). *Stress appraisal and coping*. New York: Springer.

Leach, S. (2006). Aromatherapy massage: An essential service? *Practising Midwife, 9*(3), 34–35.

Maddi, S. (1987). Hardiness training at Illinois Bell Telephone. In: J. P. Opatz (Ed.), *Health promotion evaluation* (pp. 1101–1115). Stevens Point, WI: National Wellness Institute.

Maddi, S. (2002). The story of hardiness: Twenty years of theorizing, research and practice. *Consulting Psychology Journal, 54*, 173–185.

Maville, J., Bowen, J., & Genham, G. (2008). Effect of healing touch on stress perception and biological correlates. *Holistic Nursing Practice, 22*(2), 103–110.

McCance, K., & Huether, S. (2008). *Pathophysiology: The biologic basis for disease in adults and children* (5th ed.). St. Louis, MO: C. V. Mosby.

Mitchel, A. M., Kameg, K., & Sakraida, T. J. (2003). Post-traumatic stress: Clinical implications. *Disaster Management Response, 1*(1), 14–18.

Monat, A., & Lazarus, R. (Eds.) (1991). *Stress and coping* (3rd ed.). St. Louis, MO: C. V. Mosby.

Moorhead, S., Johnson, M., & Maas, M., et al. (Eds.). (2008). *Nursing outcomes classification (NOC)* (4th ed.). St. Louis, MO: C. V. Mosby.

Morgan, P., Fogel, J., Rose, L., et al. (2005). African American couples merging strengths to successfully cope with breast cancer. *Oncology Nursing Forum, 32*(5), 979–987.

Morse, D. (2007). Use of humor to reduce stress and pain and enhance healing in the dental setting. *Journal of the NJ Dental Association, 78*(4), 32–36.

NANDA International. (2009). *Nursing diagnoses: Definitions and classification 2009–2011*. Oxford: Wiley-Blackwell.

Nassau, J., Tien, K., & Fritz, G. (2008). Review of the literature: Integrating psychoneuroimmunology into pediatric chronic illness interventions. *Journal of Pediatric Psychology, 33*(2), 195–207.

Neeb, K. (2006). *Fundamentals of mental health nursing* (3rd ed.). Philadelphia: F. A. Davis.

Olson, R. (2003). Definitions of biofeedback. In: M. S. Schwartz & F. Andrasik (Eds.), *Biofeedback: A practitioner's guide* (3rd ed.). New York: Guilford Press.

Pemberton, E., & Turpin, P. (2008). The effect of essential oils on work-related stress in intensive care unit nurses. *Holistic Nursing Practice, 22*(2), 97–102.

Pervanidou, P., & Chrousos, G. (2007). Post-traumatic stress disorder in children and adolescents: From Sigmund Freud's "trauma" to psychopathology and the (dys)metabolic syndrome. *Hormone & Metabolic Research, 39*(6), 413–419.

Quick, J., Saleh, K., Sime, W., et al. (2006). Symposium: Stress management skills for strong leadership: Is it worth dying for? *The Journal of Bone & Joint Surgery, 88–A*(1), 217–225.

Rankin, M., Carretta, C., & Jaroszynski, A. (2008). Nursing care of posttraumatic stress disorder after anesthesia awareness. *Plastic Surgical Nursing, 28*(1), 35–40.

Rice, E., Rady, M., Hamrick, A., et al. (2008). Determinants of moral distress in medical and surgical nurses at an adult acute tertiary care hospital. *Journal of Nursing Management, 16*(3), 360–373.

Robinson, F. P., Mathews, H. L., & Witek-Janusek, L. (2000). Stress reduction and HIV disease: A review of intervention studies using a psychoneuroimmunology framework. *Journal of the Association of Nurses in AIDS Care, 11*(2), 87–96.

Selye, H. (1974). *Stress without distress*. Philadelphia: J. B. Lippincott.

Selye, H. (1976). *The stress of life* (rev. ed.). New York: McGraw-Hill.

Slattery, D., & Neumann, I. (2008). No stress please! Mechanisms of stress hyporesponsiveness of the maternal brain. *Journal of Physiology, 586*(2), 377–385.

Sloan, E., Capitanio, J., & Cole, S. (2008). Stress-induced remodeling of lymphoid innervation. *Brain, Behavior, & Immunity, 22*(1), 15–21.

Sneed, N. V., Olson, M., Bubolz, B., et al. (2001). Influences of a relaxation intervention on perceived stress and power spectral analysis of heart rate variability. *Progress in Cardiovascular Nursing, 16*(2), 57–64, 79.

Stephenson, P. (2006). Before the teaching begins: Managing patient anxiety prior to providing education. *Clinical Journal of Oncology Nursing, 10*(2), 241–245.

Stuart, B., & Sundeen, S. (2009). *Nurse-client interaction: Implementing the nursing process* (6th ed.). St. Louis, MO: C. V. Mosby.

Substance Abuse and Mental Health Services Administration. Division of Population Surveys. Office of Applied Studies (2007). *Results from the 2006 national survey on drug use and health: National findings*. Rockville, MD: U.S. Department of Health and Human Services, 2007. DHHS Publication No. SMA 07–4293. Retrieved May 15, 2009, from http://www.oas.samhsa.gov/NSDUH/2k6NSDUH/2k6Results.pdf

Sullivan, M., Hawes, K., Winchester, S., et al. (2008). Developmental origins theory from prematurity to adult disease. *JOGNN Journal of Obstetric, Gynecologic, & Neonatal Nursing, 37*(2), 158–164.

Thompson, A., & Page, L. (2007). Psychotherapies for hypochondriasis. *Cochrane Database of Systematic Reviews*, Issue 4. Art. No.: CD006520.

Thompson, J., & Manore, M. (2008). *Nutrition and health: An applied approach* (2nd ed.). San Francisco: Benjamin Cummings.

Townsend, M. C. (2009). *Psychiatric mental health nursing* (6th ed.). Philadelphia: F. A. Davis.

U.S. Department of Health and Human Services (USDHHS). (2000). *Healthy People 2010*. Washington, DC: Author.

Vahey, D., Aiken, L., Sloane, D., et al. (2004). Nurse burnout and patient satisfaction. *Medical Care, 42*(2, Supplement), II57–66.

Vaillant, G. E., Bond, M., & Vaillant, C. O. (1986). An empirically validated hierarchy of defense mechanisms. *Archives of General Psychiatry, 73*, 786–794.

Weeks, R. (2007). Integration of behavioural techniques into clinical practice. *Neurological Sciences, 28*(Supplement 2), S84–88.

Wilkinson, J., & Ahern, N. (2009). *Prentice-Hall nursing diagnosis handbook* (9th ed.). Upper Saddle River, NJ: Prentice-Hall.

Yang, K-P, & Huang, C-K. (2005). The effects of staff nurses' morale on patient satisfaction. *Journal of Nursing Research: JNR, 13*(2), 141–152.

Chapter 26

Agency for Healthcare Research and Quality (2003). Routine Vitamin Supplementation to Prevent Cancer and Cardiovascular Disease. What's New from the USPSTF. AHRQ Publication No. APPIP03–0012, June 2003. Agency for Healthcare Research and Quality, Rockville, MD. http://www.ahrq.gov/clinic/3rduspstf/vitamins/vitaminswh.htm

Aghdassi, E., Royall, D., & Allard, J. (1999). Oxidative stress in smokers supplemented with vitamin C. *International Journal of Vitamin and Nutrition Research, 69*, 45.

Amella, E. (2007). Eating and feeding issues in older adults with dementia: Part II: Interventions. *Try this: Best practices in nursing care for hospitalized older adults with dementia*, D11.2. The John A. Hartford Institute for Geriatric Nursing and the Alzheimer's Association. Retrieved February 18, 2009, from http://www.hartfordign.org.

American Academy of Pediatrics (AAP). (2006). Policy statement. Dietary recommendations for children and adolescents: A guide for practitioners. *Pediatrics, 117*(2), 544–559.

American Academy of Pediatrics (AAP). (2007). Low-iron and non-DHA/ARA formulas being discontinued. *AAP News, 28*(1), 20062378. Retrieved February 20, 2009, from http://aapnews.aap-publications.org/cgi/content/full/e2007238v1

American Association of Critical-Care Nurses (AACCN). (2005a). Practice alert. Verification of feeding tube placement. Retrieved January 16, 2009, from http://www.aacn.org/WD/Practice/Docs/Verification_of_Feeding_Tube_Placement_05–2005.pdf

American Association of Critical-Care Nurses (AACCN). (2005b). Practice alert. Dye in enteral feeding. Retrieved April 16, 2009, from http://www.aacn.org/WD/Practice/Docs/Dye_in_Enteral_Feeding_4–2005.pdf

American College of Sports Medicine. (2009, February). Appropriate physical activity intervention strategies for weight loss and prevention of weight regain for adults. Position Stand. Medicine & Science in Sports & Exercise, Retrieved February 13, 2009, from http://www.acsm-msse.org/pt/pt-core/template-journal/msse/media/0209.pdf

American Diabetes Association. (n.d.). Managing diabetes. Checking blood glucose. Retrieved March 9, 2009, from http://www.diabetes.org/for-parents-and-kids/diabetes-care/CheckingBG.jsp

American Diabetes Association. (2006). Clinical practice recommendations 2006. Diabetes Care, 29(Suppl)(1), S47.

American Dietetic Association. (2006, May). Adult weight management evidence based nutrition practice guideline. Chicago, IL: American Dietetic Association (ADA). In: Guideline Summary. National Guideline Clearinghouse (NGC) [Web site]. Rockville, MD. Retrieved February 15, 2009, from http://www.guideline.gov/summary/summary.aspx?doc_id=12820

American Gastrointestinal Association. (1995). American Gastroenterological Association medical position statement: Guidelines for the use of enteral nutrition. Retrieved February 17, 2009, from http://www3.us.elsevierhealth.com/gastro/policy/v108n4p1280.html

American Heart Association (AHA). (n.d.[a]). AHA recommendation. Retrieved February 5, 2009, from http://www.americanheart.org/presenter.jhtml?identifier=4582

American Heart Association (AHA). (n.d.[b]). Fat substitutes. Retrieved February 15, 2009, from http://www.americanheart.org/presenter.jhtml?identifier=4633

American Heart Association (AHA). (last revised 2008). Consumer FAQ – "Better" fats (monounsaturated and polyunsaturated fats). Retrieved February 6, 2009, from http://www.americanheart.org/presenter.jhtml?identifier=3046644

American Society for Parenteral and Enteral Nutrition (A.S.P.E.N.) and Nestlé HealthCare Nutrition. (2008). Be A. L. E. R. T. poster. Retrieved February 2, 2009, from http://www.nutritioncare.org/WorkArea/showcontent.aspx?id=2968

American Society for Parenteral and Enteral Nutrition (A.S.P.E.N.) Board of Directors (2009a). Clinical guidelines for the use of parenteral and enteral nutrition in adult and pediatric patients, 2009. Journal of Parenteral and Enteral Nutrition, 33(3), 255–259. Retrieved June 2, 2009, from http://online.sagepub.com/cgi/searchresults?src=selected&andorexactfulltext=and&journal_set=sppen&fulltext=guidelines+for+the+use+of+parenteral

American Society for Parenteral and Enteral Nutrition (A.S.P.E.N.). (2009b). Special report: Enteral nutrition practice recommendations. Journal of Parenteral and Enteral Nutrition, 20(10). Retrieved February 2, 2009, from http://www.nutritioncare.org/wcontent.aspx?id=2078

A.S.P.E.N. Board of Directors and Task Force on Parenteral Nutrition Standardization (2007). A.S.P.E.N. statement on parenteral nutrition standardization. Journal of Parenteral and Enteral Nutrition, 31(5), 441–448.

Baath, C., Hall-Lord, M., Idvall, E., et al. (2008). Interrater reliability using Modified Norton Scale, Pressure Ulcer Card, Short Form-Mini Nutritional Assessment by registered and enrolled nurses in clinical practice. Journal of Clinical Nursing, 17(5), 618–626.

Barberger-Gateau, P., Raffaitin, C., Letenneur, L., et al. (2007). Dietary patterns and risk of dementia. The three-city cohort study. Neurology, 69, 1921–1930.

Barbosa-Silva, M., & Barrios, A. (2006). Indications and limitations of the use of subjective global assessment in clinical practice: An update. Current Opinion in Clinical Nutrition & Metabolic Care, 9(3), 263–269.

Barclay, L., & Lie, D. (2008). Calcium may improve bone mineral density in men. Medscape Medical News. Medscape Nurses. Retrieved February 14, 2009, from http://www.medscape.com/viewarticle/583343. Also published in 2008 in Archives of Internal Medicine, 168, 2276–2282.

Barone, L., Milosavljevic, M., & Gazibarich, B. (2003). Assessing the older person: Is the MNA a more appropriate nutritional assessment tool than the SGA? Journal of Nutritional Health Aging, 7(1), 13–17.

Berkowitz, B., & Borchard, M. (2009). Advocating for the prevention of childhood obesity: A call to action for nursing. Online Journal of Issues in Nursing, 14(1), Manuscript 2. Retrieved February 23, 2009, from http://www.nursingworld.org/MainMenuCategories/ANA-Marketplace/ANAPeriodicals/OJIN/TableofContents/Vol142009/No1Jan09/Prevention-of-Childhood-Obesity.aspx

Best practices. (2007). (2nd ed.). Philadelphia: Lippincott Williams & Wilkins.

Blewett, H., Cicalo, H., Holland, M., et al. (2008). The immunological components of human milk. Advances in Food & Nutrition Research, 54, 45–80.

Bourgault, A., Weaver, I., Swartz, S., et al. (2007). Development of evidence-based guidelines and critical care nurses' knowledge of enteral feeding. Critical Care Nurse, 27(4), 17–22, 25–29; quiz 30.

Brody, J. (2008). Health. Sorting out coffee's contradictions. The New York Times, August 5, 2008. Retrieved February 15, 2009, from http://www.nytimes.com/2008/08/05/health/05brod.html?_r=science&oref=slogin

Bulechek, G., Butcher, H., & Dochterman, J. (2007). Nursing interventions classification (NIC). (5th ed.). St. Louis, MO: C. V. Mosby.

Burns, S. M., Carpenter, R., Blevins, C., et al. (2006). Detection of inadvertent airway intubation during gastric tube insertion: Capnometry versus a colorimetric carbon dioxide detector. [Electronic version]. American Journal of Critical Care, 15(2), 188–195.

Callen, B., & Wells, T. (2005). Screening for nutritional risk in community-dwelling old-old. Public Health Nursing, 22(2), 138–146.

Centers for Disease Control and Prevention (CDC). (2005). Recommended infection-control and safe injection practices to prevent patient-to-patient transmission of bloodborne pathogens. Diabetes care procedures & techniques. MMWR, 54(09), 220–223. Retrieved January 16, 2009, from http://www.cdc.gov/hepatitis/Populations/PDFs/diabetes_handout.pdf

Centers for Disease Control and Prevention (CDC). (2008). Overweight and obesity. Obesity prevalence. Retrieved February 8, 2009, from http://www.cdc.gov/nccdphp/dnpa/obesity/childhood/prevalence.htm

Centers for Disease Control and Prevention (CDC). (2009). Application of lower sodium intake recommendations to adults—United States, 1999–2006. MMWR, 58(11), 281–283. Retrieved March 26, from http://www.cdc.gov/mmwr/preview/mmwrhtml/mm5811a2.htm

Christopher, D. (2006). Antioxidant intake and risk of osteoporotic hip fracture in Utah: An effect modified by smoking status. American Journal of Epidemiology, 163(1), 9–17.

Clark, R., Birks, J., Nexo, E., et al. (2007). Low vitamin B_{12} status and risk of cognitive decline in older adults. American Journal of Clinical Nutrition, 86(5), 1384–1391.

Clarke, S. (2008). Drug administration via nasogastric tube. [Electronic version]. Paediatric Nursing, 20(7), 32.

Cullen, L., Taylor, D., Taylor, S., et al. (2004). Nebulized lidocaine decreases the discomfort of nasogastric tube insertion: A randomized, double-blind trial. Annals of Emergency Medicine, 44(2), 131–137.

DeLegge, M. (2008). Enteral feeding. Current Opinion in Gastroenterology, 24(2), 184–189.

Department of Internal Medicine, Faculty of Medicine and Health Sciences, United Arab Emirates University. (2008). Dietary intake of older patients in hospital and at home: the validity of patient kept food diaries. Journal of Nutrition, Health & Aging, 12(2), 102–106.

Detsky, A., McLaughlin, J., Baker, J., et al. (1987). What is subjective global assessment? Journal of Parenteral and Enteral Nutrition, 11(1), 813–817.

DiMaria-Ghalili, R. (2008). Nutrition. In: E. Capezuti, D. Zwicker, M. Mezey, et al. (Eds.). *Evidence-based geriatric nursing protocols for best practice* (3rd ed., pp. 353–367). New York: Springer.

DiMaria-Ghalili, R., & Guenter, P. (2008). The mini nutritional assessment. *American Journal of Nursing, 108*(2), 50–59; quiz 60.

Earley, T. (2005). NT clinical. Using pH testing to confirm nasogastric tube position. [Electronic version]. *Nursing Times, 101*(38), 24–26.

Ebersole, P., Hess, P., Touhy, T., et al. (2005). *Gerontological nursing & healthy aging* (2nd ed.). Philadelphia: Elsevier Health Sciences.

Editorial Board Palliative Care. (2006, January 12). Practice guidelines: nausea and vomiting. Utrecht, The Netherlands: Association of Comprehensive Cancer Centres (ACCC). Guideline summary: Nausea and vomiting. In: National Guideline Clearinghouse (NGC) [Web site]. Rockville, MD. Retrieved February 14, 2009, from http://www.ngc.gov/summary/summary.aspx?doc_id=11793&nbr=006067&string=nausea+and+vomiting

Elpern, E., Killeen, K., Talla, E., et al. (2007). Capnometry and air insufflations for assessing initial placement of gastric tubes. [Electronic version]. *American Journal of Critical Care, 16*(6), 544–550.

Food and Nutrition Board, National Academy of Science, Institute of Medicine. (2002/2005). *Dietary reference intakes: Macronutrients.* Retrieved January 19, 2009, from http://www.iom.edu/Object.File/Master/7/300/0.pdf

Freer, Y., & Lyon, A. (2006). Risk management, or just a different risk? [Electronic version]. *Archives of Diseases in Childhood, 91*(5), F327–F329.

Freisling, H., & Elmadfa, I. (2008). Food frequency index as a measure of diet quality in non-frail older adults. *Annals of Nutrition & Metabolism, 52*(Supplement 1), 43–46.

Friedman, N., & Zeiger, R. (2005). The role of breast-feeding in the development of allergies and asthma. *Journal of Allergy and Clinical Immunology, 115*(8), 1238–1248.

Fritz, K., & Elmadfa, I. (2008). Quality of nutrition of elderly with different degrees of dependency: Elderly living in private homes. *Annals of Nutrition & Metabolism, 52*(Supplement 1), 47–50.

Fulbrook, P., Bongers, A., & Albarran, J. (2007). A European survey of enteral nutrition practices and procedures in adult intensive care units. *Journal of Clinical Nursing, 16*(11), 2132–2141.

GlaxoSmithKline (last updated 2008). Diabetes.com. How to test your blood sugar. Retrieved September 1, 2008, from http://www.diabetes.com/blood-sugar-control-matters/low-blood-sugar.html

Glucose monitoring. A guide to checking your blood sugar. (2008). *Advance for Nurse Practitioners, 16*(12), 28.

Griffiths, R., Thompson, D., Chau, J., et al. (2006). Systematic reviews. Insertion and management of nasogastric tubes for adults. The Joanna Briggs Institute. Retrieved January 15, 2009, from http://www.joannabriggs.edu.au/protocols/protnasotube.php

Guedon, C. (2000). Enteral nutrition: Techniques and indications. [Electronic version]. *Annales De Médecine Interne, 151*(8), 658–663.

Guenter, P., Hicks, R., Simmons, D., et al. (2008). Enteral feeding misconnections: A consortium position statement. *The Joint Commission Journal on Quality and Patient Safety, 34*(50), 285–292. Retrieved February 2, 2009, from http://www.premierinc.com/quality-safety/tools-services/safety/topics/tubing-misconnections/downloads/S5-JQPS-05-08-guenter.pdf

Guigoz, Y. (2006). The Mini-Nutritional Assessment (MNA®) Review of the Literature - What does it tell us? *Journal of Nutrition, Health, and Aging, 10,* 466–487.

Guyton, A. C., & Hall, J. E. (2000). *Textbook of medical physiology* (10th ed.). Philadelphia: W. B. Saunders.

Health Canada. (2007). Canada's food guide for healthy eating. Retrieved February 7, 2009, from http://www.hc-sc.gc.ca/fn-an/food-guide-aliment/order-commander/eating_well_bien_manger-eng.php#1

Heird, W. (2007). Progress in promoting breast-feeding, combating malnutrition, and composition and use of infant formula, 1981–2006. *Journal of Nutrition, 137*(2), 499S-502S.

Henderson, G., Fahey, T., & McGuire, W. (2007). Nutrient-enriched formula versus standard term formula for preterm infants following hospital discharge. [update of Cochrane Database Syst Rev. 2005;(2),CD004696; PMID: 15846728]. *Cochrane Database of Systematic Reviews,* Issue 4. Art. No. CD004696.

Hoffman, D., Ziebler, E., Mitmesser, S., et al. (2008). Soy-based infant formula supplemented with DHA and ARA supports growth and increases circulating levels of these fatty acids in infants. *Lipids, 43*(1), 29–35.

Hollis, J., Gullion, C., Stevens, V., et al. and Weight Loss Maintenance Trial Research Group (2008). Weight loss during the intensive intervention phase of the weight-loss maintenance trial. *American Journal of Preventive Medicine, 35*(2), 118–126.

Honenyard, D. (2008). Dietary strategies for preventing cancer. *The Clinical Advisor, 11*(3), 23–25, 29–30.

Hopkins, D., Emmett, P., Steer, C., et al. (2007). Infant feeding in the second 6 months of life related to iron status: An observational study. *Archives of Disease in Childhood, 92*(10), 850–854.

Horodynski, M., Olson, B., Arndt, M., et al. (2007). Low-income mothers' decisions regarding when and why to introduce solid foods to their infants: Influencing factors. *Journal of Community Health Nursing, 24*(2), 101–118.

Infusion Nurses Society (INS). (2006a). *Policies and procedures for infusion nurses* (3rd ed.). Infusion Nurses Society Clinical Practice Committee. Norwood, MA: Author.

Infusion Nurses Society (INS). (2006b). Infusion nursing standards of practice. *Journal of Infusion Nursing, 29*(1S). ISSN 1533-1458. Norwood, MA: Author.

Institute of Medicine. (2000). Dietary intakes of vitamin C, vitamin E, selenium, and carotenoids. *Pharmacist's Letter, 16*(5), 26–27. Washington, DC: The National Academy Press.

The Joanna Briggs Institute. (2007a). Effective dietary interventions for overweight and obese children. *Best Practice, 11*(1), 69–72.

The Joanna Briggs Institute. (2007b). Effectiveness of interventions for undernourished older inpatients in the hospital setting. *Best Practice, 11*(2), 1–4.

Jockers, B. (2007). Vitamin D sufficiency: An approach to disease prevention. *The American Journal for Nurse Practitioners, 11*(10), 43–50.

The Joint Commission (TJC). (2006). Sentinel event alert: Tubing misconnections—a persistent and potentially deadly occurrence. Retrieved February 2, 2009, from http://www.premierinc.com/quality-safety/tools-services/safety/topics/tubing-misconnections/downloads/jcaho-sentinel-event-issue-36.pdf

The Joint Commission (TJC). (2007). Avoiding catheter and tubing mis-connections. *Patient Safety Solutions, 1*(7), Retrieved February 2, 2009, from http://www.premierinc.com/quality-safety/tools-services/safety/topics/tubing-misconnections/downloads/PS-Solution7.pdf

The Joint Commission (TJC). (2008). *2008 Hospital accreditation standards.* Oakbrook Terrace, IL: Author.

Kaushik, N., Pietraszewski, M., Holst, J., et al. (2005). Enteral feeding without pancreatic stimulation. [Electronic version]. *Pancreas, 31*(4), 353–359.

Kazal, L. (2002). Prevention of iron deficiency in infants and toddlers. *American Family Physician, 66,* 1217–1224, 1227. Retrieved March 9, 2009, from http://www.aafp.org/afp//AFPprinter/20021001/1217.html

Kendrick, S., & Day, C. (2007). A coffee with your brandy, Sir? *Journal of Hepatology, 46*(5), 980–982.

Kidd, P. S., & Wagner, K. D. (2005). *High acuity nursing* (4th ed.). Upper Saddle River, NJ: Prentice-Hall.

Knutson, K., Spiegel, K., Penev, P., et al. (2007). The metabolic consequences of sleep deprivation. *Sleep Medicine Reviews, 11*(3), 163–178.

Kubrak, C., & Jensen, L. (2007). Critical evaluation of nutrition screening tools recommended for oncology patients. *Cancer Nursing, 30*(5), E1–6.

Kumaniyika, S. (2008). Environmental influences on childhood obesity: Ethnic and cultural influences in context. *Physiology & Behavior, 94*(1), 61–70.

Leydon, N., & Dahl, W. (2008). Improving the nutritional status of elderly residents of long-term care homes. *Journal of Health Services & Research Policy, 13*(Supplement 1), 25–29.

Lormer, M., Parkes, G., & Sanderson, J. (2008). Review article: Lactose intolerance in clinical practice—Myths and realities. *Alimentary Pharmacology & Therapeutics, 27*(2), 93–103.

Lutz, C., & Przytulski, K. (2006). *Nutrition and diet therapy* (4th ed.). Philadelphia: F. A. Davis.

MacLeod, J., Lefton, J., Houghton, D., et al. (2007). Prospective randomized control trial of intermittent versus continuous gastric feeds for critically ill trauma patients. *Journal of Trauma-Injury Infection & Critical Care, 63*(1), 57–61.

Madsen, D., Sebolt, T., Cullen, L., et al. (2005). Listening to bowel sounds: An evidence-based practice project. [Electronic version]. *American Journal of Nursing, 105*(12), 40–50.

Marion County Children's Alliance. (n.d.) 5-2-1-0 brochure. Retrieved February 15, 2009, from http://www.mcchildrensalliance.com/newsletter/5210.pdf

May, S. (2007). Testing nasogastric tube positioning in the critically ill: Exploring the evidence. [Electronic version]. *British Journal of Nursing, 16*(7), 414–418.

Mayo Clinic Staff. (2008). Weight loss: 6 strategies for success. Retrieved February 15, 2009, from http://www.mayoclinic.com/health/weight-loss/HQ01625

Messina, V., Melina, V., & Mangels, R. (2003). A new food guide for North American vegetarians. *Canadian Journal of Dietetic Practice and Research, 64*, 82–86.

Metheney, N. (2006). Preventing respiratory complications of tube feedings: Evidence based practice. *American Journal of Critical Care, 16*, 360–369. Retrieved January 15, 2009, from http://ajcc.aacnjournals.org/cgi/content/full/15/4/360

Metheney, N., Smith, L., Wehrle, M., et al. (1998b). pH, color, and feeding tubes. *RN, 61*(1), 25–27.

Metheney, N., Wehrle, A., Wiersema, L., et al. (1998a). Testing feeding tube placement: Auscultation vs. pH method. *American Journal of Nursing, 98*(5), 37–42.

Mitrou, P., Kipnis, V., Thiébaut, A., et al. (2007). Mediterranean dietary pattern and prediction of all-cause mortality in a US population. *Archives of Internal Medicine, 167*(22), 2461–2468.

Modified MyPyramid for Older Adults. (2007). Tufts University, Gerald J. and Dorothy R. Friedman School of Nutrition Science and Policy. Retrieved February 7, 2009, from http://nutrition.tufts.edu/1197972031385/Nutrition-Page-nl2w_1198058402614.html

Moorhead, S., Johnson, M., Maas, M., et al. (2007). *Nursing outcomes classification (NOC)* (4th ed.). St. Louis, MO: C. V. Mosby.

Murphy, M. C., & Brooks, C. N. (2000). The use of the Mini Nutritional Assessment tool in elderly orthopedic patients. *European Journal of Clinical Nutrition, 54*(7), 555–562.

Murphy, S. (2008). Using DRIs for dietary assessment. *Asia Pacific Journal of Clinical Nutrition, 17*(Supplement 1), 299–301.

NANDA International. (2009). *Nursing diagnoses: Definitions and classification 2009–2011.* Ames, IA: Wiley-Blackwell.

National Association of Anorexia Nervosa and Associated Disorders. (n.d.). Eating disorders and the internet. Retrieved February 8, 2009, from http://www.anad.org/621734/240600.html

National Center for Health Statistics (2008a [reviewed]). Faststats A to Z. Overweight. In: Centers for Disease Control [Web site]. Retrieved February 23, 2009, from http://www.cdc.gov/nchs/fastats/overwt.htm

National Center for Health Statistics. (2008b). Prevalence of overweight and obesity among adults: United States, 2003–2004. Centers for Disease Control. Retrieved February 22, 2010, from http://www.cdc.gov/nchs/data/hestat/overweight/overweight_adult.pdf

National Digestive Diseases Information Clearinghouse (NDDIC). (2006). Lactose intolerance. National Institute of Diabetes and Digestive and Kidney Diseases, National Institutes of Health. Retrieved February 8, 2009, from http://digestive.niddk.nih.gov/ddiseases/pubs/lactoseintolerance/#cause

National Guideline Clearinghouse (NGC). (n.d.). Brief summary: Mealtime difficulties. In: Evidence-based geriatric nursing protocols for best practice. National Guideline Clearinghouse (NGC) [Web site]. Rockville, MD. Retrieved February 16, 2009, from http://www.guideline.gov/summary/summary.aspx?doc_id=12267&nbr=006351&string=mealtime+AND+difficulties

National Guideline Clearinghouse (NGC). (n.d.). Brief Summary: Treatment of obesity. In: National Guideline Clearinghouse (NGC) [Web site]. Rockville, MD. Retrieved February 2, 2009, from http://www.guideline.gov/summary/summary.aspx?view_id=1&doc_id=12802

National Guideline Clearinghouse (NGC). (n.d.). Complete Summary: Evidence-based guidelines for nutritional support of the critically ill: Results of a bi-national guideline development conference. In: National Guideline Clearinghouse (NGC) [Web site]. Rockville, MD. Retrieved February 17, 2009, from http://www.guideline.gov/summary/summary.aspx?ss=15&doc_id=8012&nbr=4499

National Guideline Clearinghouse (NGC). (2001). [Reviewed 2006]). Brief summary: Altered nutritional status. In: National Guideline Clearinghouse (NGC) [Web site]. Rockville, MD. Retrieved February 21, 2009, from http://www.guidelines.gov/summary/summary.aspx?doc_id=3304&nbr=002530&string=enteral+AND+feedings

National Guideline Clearinghouse (NGC). (2005a). Complete Guideline Summary: Nutritional management in long-term care: Development of a clinical guideline. National Guideline Clearinghouse (NGC) [Web site]. Rockville, MD. Retrieved February 18, 2009, from http://www.ngc.gov/summary/summary.aspx?ss=15&doc_id=5235&nbr=3577

National Guideline Clearinghouse (NGC). (2005b). Guideline summary: Evidence-based guidelines for nutritional support of the critically ill: Results of a Bi-National Guideline Development Conference (2005). National Guideline Clearinghouse (NGC) [Web site]. Rockville, MD. Retrieved March 6, 2009, from http://www.guideline.gov/summary/summary.aspx?ss=15&doc_id=8012&nbr=4499

National Guideline Clearinghouse (NGC). (2006). Brief Guideline Summary: Nutrition support in adults: Oral nutrition support, enteral tube feeding and parenteral nutrition. National Guideline Clearinghouse (NGC) [Web site]. Rockville, MD. Retrieved February 18, 2009, from http://www.guideline.gov/summary/summary.aspx?doc_id=8739&nbr=004851&string=parenteral+AND+nutrition+AND+guide

National Guideline Clearinghouse (NGC). (2008a). Brief Guideline Summary: Parenteral nutrition administration. In: Safe practices for parenteral nutrition. National Guideline Clearinghouse (NGC) [Web site]. Rockville, MD. Retrieved February 18, 2009, from http://www.guideline.gov/summary/summary.aspx?view_id=1&doc_id=12513

National Guideline Clearinghouse (NGC). (2008b). Brief Guideline Summary: Prevention of bloodstream infections. In: Prevention and control of healthcare-associated infections in Massachusetts. National Guideline Clearinghouse (NGC) [Web site]. Rockville, MD. Retrieved March 9, 2009, from http://www.guideline.gov/summary/summary.aspx?doc_id=12922&nbr=006636&string=intravenous+AND+administration

National Guideline Clearinghouse (NGC). (2009, April). Guideline summary: Screening for osteoporosis in the adult U.S. population: ACPM position statement on preventive practice. In: National Guideline Clearinghouse (NGC) [Web site]. Rockville, MD. Retrieved September 18, 2010, from http://www.guideline.gov/summary/summary.aspx?view_id=1&doc_id=15270

National Health Service: National Patient Safety Agency. (2007). Patient safety alert: Promoting safer measurement and administration of liquid medicines via oral and other enteral routes. Retrieved February 2, 2009, from http://www.premierinc.com/quality-safety/tools-services/safety/topics/tubing-misconnections/downloads/Oral-medicines-alert.pdf

National Heart, Lung and Blood Institute (NHLBI). (n.d.). Body mass index table. Retrieved February 8, 2009, from http://www.nhlbi.nih.gov/guidelines/obesity/bmi_tbl.htm

National Heart, Lung and Blood Institute (NHLBI). (n.d.). Classification of overweight and obesity by BMI, waist circumference, and associated risks. Retrieved February 8, 2009, from http://www.nhlbi.nih.gov/health/public/heart/obesity/lose_wt/bmi_dis.htm

National Heart, Lung and Blood Institute (NHLBI). (1998). Clinical guidelines on the identification, evaluation, and treatment of overweight and obesity in adults: The evidence report. Washington, DC: U.S. Department of Health & Human Services. Retrieved February 8, 2009, from http://www.nhlbi.nih.gov/guidelines/obesity/ob_gdlns.htm

National Institutes of Health (NIH). (2002/2005). Nutrient recommendation: Dietary Reference Intakes (DRI) and Recommended Dietary Allowances (RDA). Office of Dietary Supplements, National Institutes of Health. Retrieved January 19, 2009, from http://ods.od.nih.gov/Health_information/Dietary_Reference_Intakes.aspx

Neuhauser, L., Rothschild, R., & Rodriguez, F. (2007). MyPyramid.gov: Assessment of literacy, cultural and linguistic factors in the USDA food pyramid [Web site]. *Journal of Nutrition Education & Behavior, 39*(4), 219–225.

Newman, A. (2009, January 31). Obesity in older adults. *OJIN, 14*(1), Manuscript 3. Retrieved February 23, 2009, from http://www.nursingworld.org/MainMenuCategories/ANAMarketplace/ANAPeriodicals/OJIN/TableofContents/Vol142009/No1Jan09/Obesity-in-Older-Adults.aspx

Noel, M., & Reddy, M. (2005). Nutrition and aging. *Primary Care: Clinics in Office Practice, 32*(3), 659–669.

Nunwa, A. (2005). Adult enteral nutrition guidelines. Harrow, Middlesex, England. The Burdett Institute of Gastrointestinal Nursing, St. Mark's Hospital.

Nutrition Screening Initiative. (2003). *Determine your nutritional health.* Washington, DC: National Council on Aging.

Owen, C., Martin, R., Whincup, P., et al. (2007). Does breastfeeding influence risk of type 2 diabetes in later life? A quantitative analysis of published evidence. *American Journal of Clinical Nutrition, 84*(5), 1045–1054.

Pai, M. P., & Paloucek, F. P. (2000). The origin of the "ideal" body weight equations. *Annals of Pharmacotherapy, 34,* 1066–1069.

Patras, A., & Brozenec, S. (1984). Gastrointestinal assessment: Identifying significant problems. [Electronic version]. *AORN Journal, 40*(5), 726–731.

Peter, S., & Gill, F. (2009). Development of a clinical practice guideline for testing nasogastric tube placement. [Electronic version]. *Journal for Specialists in Pediatric Nursing, 14*(1), 3–11.

Pi-Sunyer, F. (2007). Getting patients to stay off the fat track. *The Clinical Advisor, 10*(9), 64, 68.

Preston, A., Rodriguez, C., Rivera, C., et al. (2003). Influence of environmental tobacco smoke on vitamin C status in children. *American Journal of Clinical Nutrition, 77*(1), 167–172.

Rauen, C., Chulay, M., Bridges, E., et al. (2008). Seven evidence-based practice habits: Putting some sacred cows out to pasture. *Critical Care Nurse, 28*(3), 98–124.

Rosenbauer, J., Herzig, P., & Giani, G. (2008). Early infant feeding and risk of type 1 diabetes mellitus—A nationwide population-based case-control study in pre-school children. *Diabetes/Metabolism Research Reviews, 24*(3), 211–222.

Rosenbauer, J., Herzig, P., Kaiser, P., et al. (2007). Early nutrition and risk of type 1 diabetes mellitus—A nationwide case-control study in preschool children. *Experimental & Clinical Endocrinology & Diabetes, 115*(8), 502–508.

Rubenstein L., Harker J., Salva A., et al. (2001). Screening for Undernutrition in Geriatric Practice: Developing the Short-Form Mini Nutritional Assessment (MNA-SF). *Journal of Gerontology, 56A,* M366–377.

Russell, R., Rasmussen, H., & Lichtenstein, A. (1999). Modified food guide pyramid for people over seventy years of age. *Journal of Nutrition, 129*(3), 751–753.

Schardt, D. (2008). Caffeine. The good, the bad, and the maybe. *Nutrition Action Health Letter,* March. Center for Science in the Public Interest. Retrieved February 15, 2009, from http://www.cspinet.org/nah/02_08/caffeine.pdf

Schlenker, E., & Roth, S. (2006). *Williams' essentials of nutrition & diet therapy* (9th ed.). St. Louis, MO: C. V. Mosby.

Schmiedling, N., Waldman, R., & Desaulles, C. (1997). Nasogastric tubes: Insertion, placement, and removal in adult patients. [Electronic version]. *Gastroenterological Nursing, 20*(1), 15–19.

Sebastian, R., Cleveland, L., & Goldman, J. (2008). Effect of snacking frequency on adolescents' dietary intakes and meeting national recommendations. *Journal of Adolescent Health, 42*(5), 503–511.

Severson, K., & Burke, C. (2003). *The trans fat solution: Cooking and shopping to eliminate the deadliest fat from your diet.* Berkeley, CA: Ten Speed Press.

Shaw, A., Fulton, L., Davis, C., et al. (n.d.). *Using the Food Guide Pyramid: A resource for nutrition educators.* U.S. Department of Agriculture Food, Nutrition, and Consumer Services. Retrieved February 7, 2009, from http://www.cnpp.usda.gov/Publications/MyPyramid/OriginalFoodGuidePyramids/FGP/FGPResourceForEducators.pdf#xml=http://65.216.150.153/texis/search/pdfhi.txt?query=SERVING+SIZE&pr=MyPyramid&sufs=2&order=r&cq=&id=4592b7130

Shlamovitz, G. Z., & Shah, N. R. (2008). Nasogastric tube. *Emedicine.* Retrieved September 6, 2008, from http://www.emedicine.com/proc/TOPIC80925.HTM#section~References

Sitzman, K. (2006). The new food pyramid. *AAOHN Journal, 54*(1), 48.

Sofi, F., Conti, A., Gori, A., et al. (2007). Coffee consumption and risk of coronary heart disease: A meta-analysis. *Nutrition, Metabolism and Cardiovascular Diseases, 17*(3), 209–223.

Sorokin, R., & Gottlieb, J. (2006). Enhancing patient safety during feeding-tube insertion: A review of more than 2000 insertions. *Journal of Parenteral and Enteral Nutrition, 30*(5), 440–445.

Speroni, K., Earley, C., & Atherton, M. (2007). Evaluating the effectiveness of the Kids Living FitTM Program: A comparative study. *The Journal of School Nursing, 23*(6), 329–336.

Stock, A., Gilbertson, H., & Babl, F. E. (2008). Confirming nasogastric tube position in the emergency department: pH testing is reliable. [Electronic version]. *Pediatric Emergency Care, 24*(12), 805–809.

Swinburn, B., Sacks, G., Lo, S., et al. (2009). Estimating the changes in energy flux that characterize the rise in obesity prevalence. *American Journal of Clinical Nutrition, 89*(6), 1723–1728.

Task Force for the Revision of Safe Practices for Parenteral Nutrition. (2004). Safe practices for parenteral nutrition. *Journal of Parenteral and Enteral Nutrition, 28*(6), S39–S70.

Thomas, J., Isenring, E., & Kellet, E. (2007). Nutritional status and length of stay in patients admitted to an Acute Assessment Unit. *Journal of Human Nutrition & Dietetics, 20*(4), 320–328.

Thompson, J., & Manore, M. (2008). *Nutrition: An applied approach* (2nd ed.). San Francisco: Benjamin Cummings.

Toladelli, R., Bankhead, R., Boullata, J., et al. (2004). *Clinical nutrition: Enteral and tube feeding.* Philadelphia: W. B. Saunders.

Truby, H., Baiic, S., deLooy, A., et al. (2006). Randomised controlled trial of four commercial weight loss programmes in the UK: Initial findings from the BBC "diet trials." *BMJ, 332,* 1309–1314.

U.S. Department of Agriculture (USDA), Food and Nutrition Center (2002–2005). *Dietary Guidance. DRI Tables. Dietary Reference Intakes: Macronutrients.* National Academy of Sciences. Institute of Medicine. Food and Nutrition Board. Retrieved January 19, 2009, from http://fnic.nal.usda.gov/nal_display/index.php?info_center=4&tax_level=3&tax_subject=256&topic_id=1342&level3_id=5140

U.S. Department of Agriculture (USDA). (2005). MyPyramid: Steps to a healthier you. Retrieved February 7, 2009, from http://www.mypyramid.gov/pyramid/index.html

U.S. Department of Agriculture (USDA). Food and Nutrition Service (2008a). Supplemental nutrition assistance program (SNAP). Retrieved February 14, 2009, from http://www.fns.usda.gov/FSP/

U.S. Department of Agriculture (USDA), Food and Nutrition Service (2008b). National school lunch program. Retrieved February 14, 2009, from http://www.fns.usda.gov/cnd/Lunch/AboutLunch/NSLPFactSheet.pdf

U.S. Department of Health and Human Services (USDHHS). (2000). Nutrition and overweight. *Healthy People 2010: Understanding and improving health* (2nd ed.). Washington, DC: U.S. Government Printing Office. Retrieved February 14, 2009, from http://www.healthypeople.gov/Document/HTML/Volume2/19Nutrition.htm

U.S. Department of Health and Human Services (USDHHS) and U.S. Department of Agriculture. *Dietary guidelines for Americans, 2005* (6th ed.). Washington, DC: U.S. Government Printing Office. Retrieved February 6, 2009, from http://www.healthierus.gov/dietaryguidelines/

U.S. Department of Health and Human Services (USDHHS). (2008). *2008 Physical activity guidelines for Americans.* ODPHP Publication No. U0036. In: USDHHS, Office of Disease Prevention and Health Promotion [Web site]. Retrieved February 14, 2009, from http://www.health.gov/paguidelines/guidelines/default.aspx

U.S. Department of Health and Human Services (USDHHS). (2010a). Developing *Healthy People 2020* objectives. Nutrition and weight status [for comment]. Washington, DC: U.S. Government Printing Office. Retrieved January 20, 2010, from http://www.healthypeople.gov/HP2020/Objectives/ViewObjective.aspx?Id=328&TopicArea=Nutrition+and+Weight+Status&Objective=HP2010+19-13&TopicAreaId=35

U.S. Department of Health and Human Services (USDHHS). (2010b). *Healthy People 2020.* Proposed *Healthy People 2020* objectives—list for public comment. Retrieved February 22, 2010, from http://www.healthypeople.gov/hp2020/Objectives/TopicAreas.aspx

U.S. Food and Drug Administration (FDA). (2003). Examples of revised Nutrition Facts panel listing trans fat. Center for Food Safety and Applied Nutrition. Retrieved February 21, 2009, from http://www.cfsan.fda.gov/~dms/labtr.html

U.S. Food and Drug Administration (FDA). (2004). How to understand and use the nutrition facts label. Center for Food Safety and Applied Nutrition. Updated 2003 and 2004. Retrieved February 7, 2009, from http://www.cfsan.fda.gov/~dms/foodlab.html

U.S. Food and Drug Administration (FDA). (2005). Luer lock misconnections can be deadly. Retrieved February 2, 2009, from http://www.premierinc.com/quality-safety/tools-services/safety/topics/tubing-misconnections/downloads/fda-luer-lock-misconnections.pdf

U.S. Food and Drug Administration (2007a). Food labeling and nutrition. Center for Food Safety and Applied Nutrition. Retrieved February 21, 2009, from http://www.cfsan.fda.gov/label.html

U.S. Food and Drug Administration (FDA). (2007b). Continuous 7–day glucose monitoring system. Consumer update. Retrieved January 16, 2009, from http://www.fda.gov/consumer/updates/glucose060407.html

U.S. Preventive Services Task Force (USPSTF). (2009). Folic acid for the prevention of neural tube defects. Clinical summary of U.S. Preventive Services Task Force recommendation. Agency for Healthcare Research and Quality. Retrieved May 13, 2009, from http://www.ahrq.gov/clinic/uspstf09/folicacid/folicsum.htm

Van Dam, R., & Hu, F. (2005). Coffee consumption and risk of type 2 diabetes: A systematic review. *JAMA, 294*(1), 97–104.

Van Leeuwen, A., Kranpitz, R., & Smith, L. (2006). *Davis's comprehensive handbook of laboratory and diagnostic tests with nursing implications* (2nd ed.). Philadelphia: F. A. Davis.

Vegetarian Diet Information. (2003–2008). U.S. Vegetarian Dietary Guideline. Retrieved January 29, 2009, from http://www.vegetarian-diet.info/vegetarian-dietary-guidelines.htm

Vegetarian Diet Pyramid© 1998–2009. Mayo Foundation for Medical Education and Research (MFMER), with permission. Retrieved October 13, 2009, from http://www.mayoclinic.com/health/medical/IM02769

Vegetarian Food Pyramid Guidelines. (n.d.). Retrieved January 29, 2009, from http://www.vegetarian-diet.info/vegetarian-food-pyramid.htm

Vellas, B., Guigoz, Y., Garry, P. J., et al. (1999). The Mini Nutritional Assessment (MNA) and its use in grading the nutritional status of elderly patients. *Nutrition, 15*(2), 116–122.

Vellas, B., Villars, H., Abellan, G., et al. (2006). Overview of the MNA® - Its History and Challenges. *Journal of Nutrition, Health, and Aging, 10,* 456–465.

Wagner, C., Greer, F. & the Section on Breastfeeding and Committee on Nutrition. (2008). Prevention of rickets and vitamin D deficiency in infants, children, and adolescents. *Pediatrics, 122*(5), 1142–1152. Retrieved February 6, 2009, from http://aappolicy.aappublications.org/cgi/content/full/pediatrics;122/5/1142

Wiegand, D., & Carlson, K. (Eds.) (2005). *AACN procedure manual for critical care* (5th ed.). St. Louis, MO: Elsevier Saunders.

Wilkinson, J. M., & Ahern, N. (2009). *Prentice-Hall nursing diagnosis handbook with NIC interventions and NOC outcomes* (9th ed.). Upper Saddle River, NJ: Prentice-Hall Health.

Winkelmeyer, W., Stampfer, M., Willett, W., et al. (2005). Habitual caffeine intake and the risk of hypertension in women. *JAMA, 294*(18), 2273–2386.

Winkler, M. (2005). Invited commentary: Improving safety and reducing harm associated with specialized nutrition support. *Nutrition in Clinical Practice, 20,* 595–596.

Wolfe, T., Fosnocht, D., & Linscott, M. (2000). Atomized lidocaine as topical anesthesia for nasogastric tube placement: A randomized, double-blind, placebo-controlled trial. *Annals of Emergency Medicine, 35*(5), 421–425.

World Health Organization (WHO). (2006a). BMI classification. Global database on body mass index. Retrieved February 8, 2009, from http://www.who.int/bmi/index.jsp?introPage=intro_3.html

World Health Organization (WHO). (2006b). WHO child growth standards length/height-for-age, weight-for-age, weight-for-length, weight-for-height and body mass index-for-age. Retrieved March 1, 2009, from http://www.who.int/childgrowth/standards/Technical_report.pdf

Young, J., Shand, B., McGregor, P., et al. (2007). Comparative effects of enzogenol and vitamin C supplementation versus vitamin C alone on endothelial function and biochemical markers of oxidative stress and inflammation in chronic smokers. *Free Radical Research, 40*(1), 85–94.

Chapter 27

Agency for Health Care Research and Quality: National Guideline Clearinghouse. (2006). Guideline synthesis: Evaluation and management of urinary incontinence. Retrieved February 23, 2010, from http://www.guideline.gov/Compare/comparison.aspx?file=INCONTINENCE1.inc

Beers, M. H., Jones, T. V., Berkwits, M., et al. (2000, updated 2006). *The Merck manual of geriatrics* (3rd ed.). Philadelphia: F.A. Davis. Retrieved May 18, 2009, from http://www.merck.com/mkgr/mmg/sec12/ch97/ch97b.jsp

Best practices: Evidence-based nursing procedures. (2008). (pp. 117–124). Philadelphia: Lippincott, Williams & Wilkins.

Bulechek, G., Butcher, H., & Dochterman, J. (2007). *Nursing interventions classification (NIC).* (5th ed.). St. Louis, MO: C. V. Mosby.

Burgio, K. L., Goode, P., Urban, M., et al. (2007). Postoperative biofeedback assisted behavioral training to decrease prostatectomy incontinence: A randomized, controlled trial. *Journal of Urology, 175*(1), 196–210.

Dillon, P. M. (2007). *Nursing health assessment: A critical thinking, case studies approach* (2nd ed.). Philadelphia: F. A. Davis.

Dingwall, L. (2008). Promoting social continence using incontinence management products. *British Journal of Nursing, 17*(9), S12–19.

Dougherty, M. C., Dwyer, J. W., Pendergast, J. F., et al. (2002). Urinary incontinence in older rural women. *Research in Nursing & Health, 25,* 3–13.

Dowling-Castronovo, A., & Bradway, C. (2003, updated 2008, January). Urinary incontinence. In: M. Mezey, T. Fulmer, I. Abraham, & D. A. Zwicker (Ed.), *Geriatric nursing protocols for best practice* (pp. 83–98). New York: Springer. Retrieved February 23, 2010, from http://consultgerirn.org/topics/urinary_incontinence/want_to_know_more

Dowling-Castronovo, A., & Bradway, C. (2008). Urinary incontinence (UI) in older adults admitted to acute care. In: E. Capezuti, D. Zwicker, M. Mezey, et al. (Eds.), *Evidence-based geriatric nursing protocols for best practice* (3rd ed., pp. 309–336). New York: Springer. Retrieved on February 21, 2010, from http://www.guideline.gov/summary/summary.aspx?doc_id=13163

Ellsworth, P., & Caldamone, A. (2008). Pediatric voiding dysfunction: current evaluation and management. *Urologic Nursing, 28*(4), 249–258, 283.

Engberg, S. J., Bender, M. A., & Stilley, C. S. (2003). Bladder matters: Kegels and communication. *American Journal of Nursing, 103*(7), 93–94.

Fantl, J. A., Newman, D. K., Colling, J., et al. (1996, January). Managing acute and chronic urinary incontinence. Clinical Practice Guideline. *Quick Reference Guide for Clinicians*, No. 2, 1996 Update. Rockville, MD: U.S. Department of Health and Human Services, Public Health Service, Agency for Health Care Policy and Research. AHCPR Pub. No. 96–0686.

Finnish Medical Society. (2008, August). Urinary incontinence in women. In: *EBM Guidelines. Evidence-Based Medicine* [Internet]. Helsinki, Finland: Wiley Interscience. In: Guideline Summary (releases 2009, January). National Guideline Clearinghouse (NCG) [Web site]. Rockville, MD. Retrieved December 9, 2009, from http://www.guideline.gov/summary/summary.aspx?doc_id=9926

Fultz, N. H., & Herzog, A. R. (2001). Self-reported social and emotional impact of urinary incontinence. *Journal of the American Geriatric Society, 49*(7), 892–899.

Gamiero, M. O., Gamiero, E. H., Gamiero, F. O., et al. (2010, January). Vaginal weight cone versus assisted pelvic floor muscle training in the treatment of female urinary incontinence. A prospective, single-blind, randomized trial. *International Urogynecology Journal*. Retrieved February 22, 2010, from http://www.springerlink.com/content/f30811hl28g8733t/

Grabe, M., Bishop, M. C., Bjerklund-Johansen, T. E., et al. (2008, March). Catheter-associated urinary tract infections. In: Guidelines on the management of urinary and male genital tract infections. ARNHEM, Netherlands: European Association of Urology. In: Guideline Summary. National Guideline Clearinghouse (NGC) [Web site]. Rockville, MD. Retrieved March 15, 2009, from http://www.guideline.gov/summary/summary.aspx?view_id=1&doc_id=12583

Gray, M., Ratliff, C., & Donovan, A. (2002). Tender mercies: Providing skin care for an incontinent patient. *Nursing, 32*(7), 51–54.

Griffith, R., & Fernandez, R. (2007, republished 2009, January). Strategies for the removal of short-term indwelling urethral catheters in adults. *Cochrane Database of Systematic Reviews*, Issue 2. Art. No.: CD004011. DOI: 10.1002/14651858.CD004011.pub3. Retrieved on December 7, 2009, from http://www.cochrane.org/reviews/en/ab004011.html

Hartmann, K. E., McPheeters, M. L., Biller, D. H., et al. (2009, August). Treatment of overactive bladder in women. Evidence Report/Technology Assessment No. 187 (Prepared by the Vanderbilt Evidence-based Practice Center under Contract No. 290-2007-10065-I.) AHRQ Publication No. 09-E017. Rockville, MD: Agency for Healthcare Research and Quality. Retrieved December 7, 2009, from http://www.ahrq.gov/CLINIC/tp/bladdertp.htm

Hay-Smith, J. (2000, November/December). Pelvic floor re-education. *Evidence Based Medicine, 5*, 183.

Hooten, T. M., Bradley, S. F., Cardenas, D. D., et al. (2010, March 1). Diagnosis, prevention, and treatment of catheter-associated infection in adults: 2009 international clinical practice guidelines from the Infectious Diseases Society of America. *Clinical Infectious Diseases, 50*(5), 625–663.

Hunter, K. F., Moore, K. N., Cody, D. J., et al. (2007). Conservative management for postprostatectomy urinary. *Cochrane Database of Systematic Reviews*, Issue 2. Art. No.: CD001843. DOI: 10.1002/14651858.CD001843.pub3. Retrieved December 11, 2009.

Institute of Medicine (IOM). (2004). *Dietary reference intakes for electrolytes and water*. Washington, DC: National Academies Press. Retrieved December 10, 2009, from http://www.iom.edu/en/Activities/Nutrition/DRIElectrolytes.aspx

Jahn, P., Preuss, M., Kernig, A., et al. (2007). Types of indwelling urinary catheters for long-term bladder drainage in adults. *Cochrane Database of Systematic Reviews*, Issue 3. Art. No.: CD004997. DOI: 10.1002/14651858.CD004997.pub2. Retrieved December 10, 2009, from http://www.cochrane.org/reviews/en/ab004997.html

Jirovec, M. M., & Templin, T. (2001). Predicting success using individualized scheduled toileting for memory-impaired elders at home. *Research in Nursing & Health, 24*(1), 1–8.

The Joanna Briggs Institute. (2006). Removal of short-term indwelling urethral catheters. *Best Practice, 10*(3), 1–4.

Johansson, I., Athlin, E., Frykholm, L., et al. (2002). Intermittent versus indwelling catheters for older patients with hip fractures. *Journal of Clinical Nursing, 11*(5), 651–656.

Kelleher, M. M. B. (2002). Removal of urinary catheters: Midnight vs. 0600 hours. *British Journal of Nursing, 11*, 84, 86, 88–90.

Kiel, R. J., & Nashelsky, J. (2003, February). Does cranberry juice prevent or treat urinary tract infection? *Journal of Family Practice*. Retrieved February 23, 2010, from http://www.jfponline.com/pages.asp?aid=1391&UID=

Krause, K., Mowassee, M., & Auerhahn, C. (2008). Urinary tract infections in the elderly: Symptomatology and prevention. *The American Journal for Nurse Practitioners, 12*(9), 57–63.

Landefeld, C. S., Bowers, B. J., Feld, A. D., et al. (2008, March). National Institutes of Health state-of-the-science conference statement: Prevention of fecal and urinary incontinence in adults. *Annals of Internal Medicine, 148*(6), 449–458.

Lekan-Rutledge, D. (2000). Diffusion of innovation: A model for implementation of prompted voiding in long-term care settings. *Journal of Gerontological Nursing, 26*(4), 25–33.

Lewis, L. (2003). Managing incontinence at home. *American Journal of Nursing, 3*(Supplement), 41.

Lo, E., Nicolle, L., Classen, D., et al. (2008). Strategies to prevent catheter-associated urinary tract infections in acute care hospitals. *Infection Control Hospital Epidemiology*, Supplement 1, 41–50. The Cochrane Library. Chichester, UK: John Wiley & Sons.

Madigan, E., & Neff, D. (2003). Care of patients with long-term indwelling urinary catheters. *Online Journal of Issues in Nursing, 8*(3). Retrieved May 11, 2009, from http://www.nursingworld.org/MainMenuCategories/ANAMarketplace/ANAPeriodicals/OJIN/TableofContents/Volume82003/No3Sept2003/HirshArticle/CareofPatientswithLongTermIndwellingUrinaryCatheters.aspx

Massachusetts Healthcare-Associated Infections Expert Panel. (2008, January 31). Prevention of catheter-associated urinary tract infections. In: Betsy Lehman Center for Patient Safety and Medical Error Reduction, JSI Research and Training Institute, Inc. Prevention and control of healthcare-associated infections in Massachusetts. Part 1: final recommendations of the Expert Panel. Boston (MA): Massachusetts Department of Public Health, 83-9. Retrieved February 22, 2010, from http://www.guideline.gov/summary/summary.aspx?doc_id=12923&nbr=006637&string=urinary+AND+tract+AND+infection

McConnell, E. A. (2001). Clinical do's and don'ts: Applying a condom catheter. *Nursing, 31*(1), 70.

Moore, K. N., Fader, M., & Getliffe, K. (2007). Long-term bladder management by intermittent catheterisation in adults and children. *Cochrane Database of Systematic Reviews*, Issue 4. Art. No. CD006008. Retrieved December 7, 2009, from http://www.cochrane.org/reviews/en/ab006008.html

NANDA International. (2009). *Nursing diagnoses: Definitions and classification 2009–2011*. Philadelphia: Author.

National Collaborating Centre for Women's and Children's Health. (2006, October). Urinary incontinence: the management of urinary incontinence in women. London (UK): *Royal College of Obstetricians and Gynaecologists* (RCOG, 221). National Guideline Clearinghouse Summary. Retrieved May 12, 2009, from http://www.guideline.gov/summary/summary.aspx?view_id=1&doc_id=9926

National Institute for Health and Clinical Excellence (NICE). (2006). Urinary incontinence. The management of urinary incontinence in women. Quick reference guide. National Collaborating Centre for Women's and Children's Health. Retrieved May 12, 2009, from http://www.nice.org.uk/nicemedia/pdf/word/CG40quickrefguide1006.pdf

National Institutes of Health (NIH), U.S. National Library of Medicine. (2008, November 17). *Unified medical language system*. Retrieved December 3, 2009, from http://www.diseasesdatabase.com/umlsdef.asp?glngUserChoice=23641

National Institutes of Health (NIH), Warren Grant Magnuson Clinical Center. (1999, last updated 2009, March 31) 24–hour urine collection. *Procedures/Diagnostic Tests*. Retrieved April 29, 2009, from http://clinicalcenter.nih.gov/ccc/patient_education/procdiag/24hr.pdf

The National Kidney and Urologic Diseases Information Clearinghouse (NKUDIC). (2005). Urinary tract infection in adults. Retrieved February 22, 2010, from http://kidney.niddk.nih.gov/Kudiseases/pubs/utiadult/

Nazarko, L. (2008). Reducing the risk of catheter-related urinary tract infection. *British Journal of Nursing*, 17(16), 1002–1010.

Newman, D. K. (2004). Incontinence products and devices for the elderly. *Urologic Nursing*, 24(4), 316–334.

Newman, D. K. (2007). The indwelling urinary catheter: Principles for best practice. *Journal of Wound, Ostomy and Continence Nursing*, 34(6), 655–661.

Newman, D. K., & Giovanni, D. (2002). The overactive bladder: A nursing perspective. *American Journal of Nursing*, 102(6), 36–46.

Newman, D. K., & Palmer, M. H. (Eds.). (2003). State of the science on urinary incontinence. *American Journal of Nursing*, 3(Supplement), 1–5.

Niël-Weise, B. S., & van den Broek, P. J. [amended 2006, May] (2005). Urinary catheter policies for short-term bladder drainage in adults. *Cochrane Database of Systematic Reviews*, Issue 3. Art. No.: CD004203. DOI: 10.1002/14651858.CD004203.pub2. Retrieved on December 6, 2009, from http://www.ncbi.nlm.nih.gov/pubmed/16034973

Niël-Weise, B. S., & van den Broek, P. J. [amended 2008, May] (2005). Antibiotic policies for short-term catheter bladder drainage in adults. *Cochrane Database of Systematic Reviews*, Issue 3. Art. No.: CD005428. DOI: 10.1002/14651858.CD005428.

Ord, J., Lunn, D., & Reynard, J. (2003). Bladder management and risk of bladder stone formation in spinal cord injured patients. *Journal of Urology*, 170(5), 1734–1737.

Palmer, M. H. (2004). Physiologic and psychologic age-related changes that affect urologic clients. *Urologic Nursing*, 24(4), 247–252, 257.

Pilloni, S., Krhut, J., Mair, D., et al. (2005). Intermittent catheterisation in older people: A valuable alternative to indwelling catheterization. *Age and Ageing*, 34, 57–60.

Rhoads, J., & Meeker, B. J. (2008). *Davis's guide to clinical nursing skills*. Philadelphia: F.A. Davis.

Saint Jude's Children's Research Hospital. (2004). Collecting urine cultures from infant girls. *Do You Know... An Educational Series for Patients and Their Families*. Retrieved May 2, 2009, from http://www.stjude.org/SJFile/sedation_collecting_urine_cultures_infant_girls.pdf

Sampselle, C. M., Wyman, J. G., Thomas, K. K., et al. (2006). Evidence-based clinical practice guideline: Continence for women. *Journal of Obstetric and Neonatal Nurses*, 29(1), 18–26.

Scanlon, V. C., & Sanders, T. (2007). *Essentials of anatomy and physiology*. Philadelphia: F. A. Davis.

Schumm, K., & Lam, T. B. (2008). Types of urethral catheters for management of short-term voiding problems in hospitalised adults. *Cochrane Database of Systematic Reviews*, 16(2), Art. No.: CD004013. Retrieved December 8, 2009, from http://www.cochrane.org/reviews/en/ab004013.html

Selius, B. A., & Subedi, R. (2009, updated.). Urinary retention in adults: diagnosis and initial management. *American Family Physician*, 77, 643–650. Retrieved December 7, 2009, from http://www.nlm.nih.gov/medlineplus/ency/article/003972.htm

Seymour, C. (2006). Audit of catheter-associated UTI using silver alloy-coated Foley catheters. *British Journal of Nursing*, 15(11), 598–603.

Shamliyan, T., Wyman, J., Blissm, D. Z., et al. (2007, December). Prevention of Fecal and Urinary Incontinence in Adults. Evidence Report/Technology Assessment No. 161 (Prepared by the Minnesota Evidence-based Practice Center under Contract No. 290-02-0009). AHRQ Publication No. 08–E003. Rockville, MD. Agency for Healthcare Research and Quality. Retrieved February 25, 2009, from http://www.ahrq.gov/downloads/pub/evidence/pdf/fuiad/fuiad.pdf

Singapore Ministry of Health. (2005, August 24). Nursing management of patients with urinary incontinence. Retrieved December 7, 2009, from http://www.guideline.gov/summary/summary.aspx?doc_id=7154

State of the Science on Urinary Incontinence. (2003a, March). State of the science on urinary incontinence: Executive summary. *American Journal of Nursing*, 3(Supplement), 4–8.

State of the Science on Urinary Incontinence. (2003b, March). Discussion and recommendations: Overcoming barriers to nursing care of people with urinary incontinence. *American Journal of Nursing*, 3(Supplement), 47–53.

Stuempfle, K. J., & Drury, D. G. (2003). Comparison of 3 methods to compare urine specific gravity in college athletes. *Journal of Athletic Training*, 38(4), 315–319.

Thiedke, C. C. (2003). Nocturnal enuresis. *American Family Physician*, 67(7), 1499–1506. Retrieved May 20, 2009, from http://www.aafp.org/afp/20030401/1499.html

Thompson, J., & Manore, M. (2008). *Nutrition and health: An applied approach* (2nd ed.). San Francisco: Benjamin Cummings.

Urinary Continence Guideline Panel (UCGP). (1996). *Urinary incontinence in adults: Clinical practice update*. Rockville, MD: Agency for Healthcare Policy and Research, Public Health Service, U.S. Department of Health and Human Services. Retrieved December 8, 2009, from http://www.ahrq.gov/clinic/uiovervw.htm

U.S. Department of Health and Human Services (USDHHS), Centers for Medicare and Medicaid Services. (2007). Nursing home data compendium. Retrieved May 19, 2009, from http://www.cms.hhs.gov/certificationandcomplianc/12_nhs.asp

VanKampen, M., DeWeerdt, W., VanPoppel, H., et al. (2000, January 8). Effect of pelvic-floor re-education on duration and degree of incontinence after radical prostatectomy: A randomised controlled trial. *The Lancet*, 355, 98–102.

Van Leeuwen, A., Kranpitz, T., & Smith, L. (2006). *Davis's comprehensive handbook of laboratory and diagnostic tests with nursing implications*. Philadelphia: F. A. Davis.

Watson, N. M., Brink, C. A., Zimmer, J. G., et al. (2003). Use of the agency for health care policy and research urinary incontinence guideline in nursing homes. *Journal of the American Geriatric Society*, 51(12), 1810–1812.

Weber, B. A., Roberts, B. L., Chumbler, N. R., et al. (2007). Urinary, sexual, and bowel dysfunction and bother after radical prostatectomy. *Urologic Nursing*, 27(6), 527–533.

Weiss, B. D., & Newman, D. K. (2002). New insight into urinary stress incontinence: Advice for the primary care clinician. Retrieved September 2, 2009, from http://www.medscape.com/viewprogram/1961

Wilde, M. H., & Getliffe, K. (2006). Urinary catheter care for older adults. *Annals of long-term Care: Clinical Care and Aging*, 8(14), Retrieved May 11, 2009, from http://www.annalsoflongtermcare.com/article/6051

Wong, E. S. (1981, updated 2005). Guideline for prevention of catheter-associated urinary tract infections. *Centers for Disease Control and Prevention (CDC)*. Retrieved December 10. 2009, from http://www.cdc.gov/ncidod/dhqp/gl_catheter_assoc.html

Wound, Ostomy and Continence Nurses Society. (2003). Identifying and treating reversible causes of urinary incontinence. *Ostomy and Wound Management*, 49(12), 28–33.

Wound, Ostomy and Continence Nurses Society. (2008). Catheter associated urinary tract infections (CAUTI): Fact sheet. Retrieved February

23, 2010, from http://www.google.com/search?sourceid=navclient&ie=UTF-8&rlz=1T4SKPB_enUS268US268&q=wilde+urinary+tract+infection+antibiotic

Wyman, J. F. (2003). Treatment of urinary incontinence in men and older women. *American Journal of Nursing, 103*(3), Supplement, 26–35.

Chapter 28

Addison, R., Ness, W., Abulafi, M., & Swift, I. (2000). How to administer enemas and suppositories. *Nursing Times, 96*(6), 3–4.

Allison, J. (2005). Colon cancer screening guideline: The fecal occult blood test has become a better fit. *Gastroenterology, 129*(2), 745–748.

The American Cancer Society (n.d., last revised February 4, 2008). Colostomy guide. Retrieved February 2, 2009, from http://www.cancer.org/docroot/CRI/content/CRI_2_6x_Colostomy.asp?sitearea=&level

The American Cancer Society. (2008). Detailed guide: Colon and rectum cancer. Revised April 21, 2008. Retrieved February 3, 2009, from http://www.cancer.org/docroot/CRI/content/CRI_2_4_7x_CRC_Colorectal_Cancer_PDF.asp

The American Cancer Society. (2009a). Cancer facts and figures 2009. Retrieved October 3, 2009, from http://www.cancer.org/downloads/STT/500809web.pdf

The American Cancer Society. (2009b). Cancer statistics for 2009. A presentation from the American Cancer Society. Retrieved October 3, 2009, from http://www.cancer.org/docroot/PRO/content/PRO_1_1_Cancer_Statistics_2009_Presentation.asp

American Gastroenterological Association. (2007). Brochure. Understanding constipation. Retrieved January 31, 2009, from http://www.gastro.org/user-assets/Documents/09_Patient_Center/brochures/brochure_Constipation.pdf

Annells, M., & Koch, T. (2002). Faecal impaction: Older people's experiences and nursing practice. *British Journal of Community Nursing, 7*(3), 118, 120–122, 124–126.

Atkins, D. (2008). The periodic health examination. In: L. Goldman & D. Ausiello (Eds.), *Cecil medicine* (23rd ed., Chapter 13). Philadelphia: Saunders Elsevier.

Ayello, E., & Sibbald, R. (2008). Preventing pressure ulcers and skin tears. In: E. Capezuti, D. Zwicker, M. Mezey, et al. (Eds.), *Evidence-based geriatric nursing protocols for best practice* (3rd ed., pp. 403–429). New York: Springer. Retrieved November 5, 2008, from http://www.guideline.gov/summary/summary.aspx?doc_id=12262&nbr=006346&string=Bedpan

Balas, M., Casey, C., & Happ, M. (2008). Comprehensive assessment and management of the critically ill. In: E. Capezuti, D. Zwicker, M. Mezey, et al. (Eds.). *Evidence-based geriatric nursing protocols for best practice* (3rd ed., pp. 565–593). New York: Springer. Retrieved November 5, 2008, from http://www.guideline.gov/summary/summary.aspx?doc_id=12253&nbr=006337&string=Bedpan

Baldwin, C., Grant, M., Wendel, C., et al. (2008). Influence of intestinal stoma on spiritual quality of life of U.S. veterans. *Journal of Holistic Nursing, 26*(3), 185–194. Retrieved February 2, 2009, from http://jhn.sagepub.com/cgi/content/abstract/26/3/185

Beltz, J. (2006). Fecal incontinence in acutely and critically ill patients: Options in management. *Ostomy Wound Management, 52*(12), 56–58, 60, 62–66.

Benoit R., & Watts, C. (2007). The effect of a pressure ulcer prevention program and the bowel management system in reducing pressure ulcer prevalence in an ICU setting. *Journal of Wound, Ostomy, & Continence Nursing, 34*(2), 163–175.

Black, P. (2008). Peristomal skin care: An overview of available products. *British Journal of Nursing, 16*, 1048–1056.

Brandt, L., Prather, C., Quigley, E., et al. (2005). Systematic review on the management of chronic constipation in North America. *American Journal of Gastroenterology, 100*(Supplement 1), S5–S21.

Bulechek, F., Butcher, H., & Dochterman, J. (2008). *Nursing interventions classification (NIC).* (5th ed.). St. Louis, MO: C. V. Mosby.

Burch, J., & Sica, J. (2008). Common peristomal skin problems and potential treatment options. *British Journal of Nursing, 17*, S4–11.

Chapman, J., Bernstein, L., Lee, R., et al. (Eds.). (2006). Food allergy: A practice parameter. *Annals of Allergy, Asthma & Immunology, 96*, S1–S68.

Christer, R., Robinson, L., & Bird, C. (2003). Constipation: Causes and cures. *Nursing Times, 99*(25), 26–27.

Colorectal Cancer Health Center, WebMD. (2000–2004). Colostomy irrigation. Retrieved August 16, 2008, from http://www.webmd.com/content/article/45/1811_50433.htm

(2007, September). The constipation conundrum: What now in chronic constipation and IBS-C. A Self-Study Supplement to *Clinician Reviews*, 2–12.

Creason, N., & Sparks, D. (2000). Fecal impaction: A review. *Nursing Diagnosis, 11*(15), 15–23.

Cronin, E. (2008). Colostomies and the use of colostomy appliances. *British Journal of Nursing, 17*, S12–16.

Davis, R., Rao, S., Pallentino, J., et al. (2007, September). Managing the chronically constipated adult: Emerging approaches to diagnosis and treatment. *Clinical Advisor* (Supplement), 3–15.

Erwin-Toth, P. (2003). Ostomy pearls: A concise guide to stoma siting, pouching systems, patient education & more. *Advanced Skin Wound Care, 16*(3), 146–152.

Foran, M., Petersen, J., & Llewandrowski, K. (2006). Occult blood. In: *Laboratory medicine practice guidelines: Evidence-based practice for point-of-care testing* (pp. 95–104). Washington, DC: National Academy of Clinical Biochemistry (NACB). Retrieved April 20, 2009, from http://www.guideline.gov/summary/summary.aspx?doc_id=10819&nbr=005644&string=fecal+AND+occult+AND+blood

Gallagher, P., O'Mahony, D., & Quigley, E. (2008). Management of chronic constipation in the elderly. *Drugs & Aging, 25*(10), 807 822.

Ginsberg, D., Phillips, S., Wallace, J., et al. (2007). Evaluating and managing constipation in the elderly. *Urologic Nursing, 27*(3), 191–200.

Gomella L., & Haist, S. (n.d.). Laboratory diagnosis: Chemistry, immunology, serology. *Clinician's pocket reference: The scut monkey* (11th ed., Chapter 4). New York: McGraw-Hill Professional.

Goodheart, C. R., & Leavitt, S. B. (2006). Managing opioid-induced constipation in ambulatory care patients. Retrieved April 16, 2009, from http://pain-topics.org/pdf/Managing_Opioid-Induced_Constipation.pdf

Gray-Micelli, D. (2008). Preventing falls in acute care. In: E. Capezuti, D. Zwicker, M. Mezey, et al. (Eds.), *Evidence-based geriatric nursing protocols for best practice* (3rd ed., pp. 161–198). New York: Springer. Retrieved November 5, 2008, from http://www.guideline.gov/summary/summary.aspx?doc_id=12265&nbr=006349&string=Bedpan

Guiandalini, S., Frye, R. E., & Tamer, M. A. (2009). Diarrhea treatment and management. *eMedicine*. Retrieved April 26, 2009, from http://emedicine.medscape.com/article/928598–overview

He, J., Streiffer, R. H., Muntner, P., et al. (2005). Effect of dietary fiber intake on blood pressure: A metaanalysis of randomized, double-blind, controlled trials. *Journal of Hypertension, 23*(3), 475–481.

Hinrichs, M. D., & Huseboe, J. (2001). Research-based protocol: Management of constipation. *Journal of Gerontological Nursing, 27*(2), 17–28.

Hyland, J. (2002). The basics of ostomies. *Gastroenterology Nursing, 25*(6), 241–244.

Institute for Clinical Systems Improvement (ICSI) (2008). Colorectal cancer screening. Bloomington, MN: Institute for Clinical Systems Improvement (ICSI). In: Brief Summary. National Guidelines Clearinghouse (NGC). Retrieved February 3, 2009, from http://www.guideline.gov/summary/summary.aspx?doc_id=12692&nbr=006580&string=colorectal+AND+cancer+AND+screening

The Joanna Briggs Institute. (2008). Management of constipation in older adults. *Best Practice, 12*(7), 33–36.

Johnson, M., Bulechek, G., Dochterman, J., et al. (2005). *Nursing diagnoses, outcomes, and interventions: NANDA, NOC, and NIC linkages* (2nd ed.). St. Louis, MO: C. V. Mosby.

The Joint Commission Accreditation Program. (2008). Critical Access Hospital National Patient Safety Goals 2009. Retrieved January 13, 2009, from http://www.jointcommission.org/NR/rdonlyres/4BAD7889-79DE-493F-A6FD-CEB9F003434D/0/CAH_NPSG.pdf

Kaiser Permanente Care Management Institute. (2006). Colorectal screening clinical practice guideline. Oakland, CA: Kaiser Permanente Care Management Institute. In: Brief Summary. National Guidelines Clearinghouse (NGC) [Web site]. Retrieved November 5, 2008, from http://www.guideline.gov/summary/summary.aspx?doc_id=10847&nbr=005662&string=fecal+AND+occult+AND+blood

Karadag, A., Mentex, B., & Ayaz, S. (2005). Colostomy irrigation: results of 25 cases with particular reference to quality of life. *Journal of Clinical Nursing, 14*(4), 479–485.

Kenny, K. A., & Skelly, J. M. (2001). Dietary fiber for constipation in older adults: A systematic review. *Clinical Effectiveness in Nursing, 5*(3), 120–128.

Kent, M. (2008). Changing an ostomy pouching system. *Nursing2008, 38*(12), 50–54.

Keshava, A., Renwick, A., Stewart, P., et al. (2007). A nonsurgical means of fecal diversion: The Zassi bowel management system. *Diseases of the Colon & Rectum, 50*, 1017–1022.

Korzenik, J. (2008). Diverticulitis: New frontiers for an old country: Risk factors and pathogenesis. *Journal of Clinical Gastroenterology, 42*(10), 1128–1129.

Kranpitz, T., & Smith, L. (2006). *Davis's comprehensive handbook of laboratory and diagnostic tests with nursing implications* (2nd ed.). Philadelphia: F. A. Davis.

Landefeld, C., Bowers, B., Feld, A., et al. (2008). National Institutes of Health State-of-the-Science conference statement: Prevention of fecal and urinary incontinence in adults. *Annals of Internal Medicine, 148*(6), 449–458. Retrieved February 23, 2009, from http://consensus.nih.gov/2007/2007IncontinenceSOS030Statement.pdf

Lembo, A. (n.d.). Chronic constipation. Retrieved from the American Gastroenterological Association [Web site], January 31, 2009, at http://www.gastro.org/user-assets/Documents/08_Publications/06_GIHep_Annual_Review/Articles/Lembo.pdf

Lembo, A., & Camilleri, M. (2003). Chronic constipation. *New England Journal of Medicine, 349*(14), 1360–1368.

Medline Plus. Fecal impaction. Retrieved January 29, 2009, from http://www.nlm.nih.gov/medlineplus/ency/article/000230.htm

Merchant, M. (2003). Laxatives should be the last resort in constipation. *Nursing Times, 99*(37), 35.

Moorhead, S., Johnson, M., & Maas, M., et al. (Eds.). (2007). *Nursing outcomes classification (NOC)* (4th ed.). St. Louis, MO: C. V. Mosby.

Müeller-Lissner, S., Kamm, M., Scarpignato, C., et al. (2005). Myths and misconceptions about chronic constipation. *American Journal of Gastroenterology, 100*, 232–242.

NANDA International. (2009). *NANDA nursing diagnoses: Definitions and classification 2009–2011.* Ames, IA: Wiley-Blackwell.

National Guideline Clearinghouse (NGC) (n.d.). Brief guideline summary: Evaluation and treatment of constipation in infants and children: Recommendations of the North American Society for Pediatric Gastroenterology, Hepatology and Nutrition (2006). National Guideline Clearinghouse (NGC) [Web site]. Rockville, MD. Retrieved February 8, 2009, from http://www.guideline.gov/summary/summary.aspx?doc_id=9792&nbr=005245&string=fecal+AND+impaction

National Guideline Clearinghouse (NGC). (n.d., updated 2009). Brief guideline summary: Screening for colorectal cancer: U.S. Preventive Services Task Force recommendation statement. In: National Guideline Clearinghouse (NGC) [Web site]. Rockville (MD). Retrieved February 23, 2009, from http://www.guideline.gov/summary/summary.aspx?view_id=1&doc_id=13133

National Institute of Allergy and Infectious Diseases (NIAID). (2001, June). Food allergy and intolerances: NIAID fact sheet: NIAID. Retrieved January 29, 2009, from http://www.wrongdiagnosis.com/artic/food_allergy_and_intolerances_niaid_fact_sheet_niaid.htm

Norton, C., & Chelvanayagam, S. (2000). A nursing assessment tool for adults with fecal incontinence. *Journal of Wound, Ostomy and Continence Nursing, 27*, 279–291.

Norton, W. (2008). An overview of bowel incontinence: What can go wrong? *The Exceptional Parent, 38*(9), 67–70.

Padmanabhan, A., Stern, M., Wishin, J., et al. (2007). Clinical evaluation of a flexible fecal incontinence management system. *American Journal of Critical Care, 16*(4), 384–393.

Peate, I. (2003). Nursing role in the management of constipation: Use of laxatives. *British Journal of Nursing, 12*(19), 1130–1136.

Pillitteri, A. (2006). *Maternal & child health nursing: Care of the childbearing & childrearing family* (5th ed.). Philadelphia: Lippincott Williams & Wilkins.

Pullen, R. (2006). Teaching your patient to irrigate a colostomy. *Nursing2006, 36*(4), 22.

Richbourg, L., Fellows, J., & Arroyave, W. (2008). Ostomy pouch wear time in the United States. *Journal of Wound, Ostomy and Continence Nursing, 35*(5), 504–508.

Rudoni, C. (2008). A service evaluation of the use of silicone-based adhesive remover. *British Journal of Nursing.* Stoma Care Supplement, S4–S9.

Rushing, J. (2003). Administering an enema to an adult. *Nursing2003, 33*(11), 28.

Scarlett, Y. (2004). Medical management of fecal incontinence. *Gastroenterology, 126*, S55–S63.

Schmelzer, M., Case, P., Chappell, S. M., & Wright, K. B. (2000). Colonic cleansing, fluid absorption, and discomfort following tap water and soapsuds enemas. *Applied Nursing Research, 13*, 83–91.

Schnell, Z. B., Smith, L., Leeuwen, A., et al. (2006). *Davis's comprehensive handbook of laboratory and diagnostic tests with nursing implications* (2nd ed.). Philadelphia: F. A. Davis.

Schnelle, J. F., & Leung, F. W. (2004). Urinary and fecal incontinence in nursing homes. *Gastroenterology, 126*(1 Supplement 2), S41–S47.

Seidel, E., & Long, M. (2005). *Crash course: Gastrointestinal system.* St. Louis, MO: C. V. Mosby.

Shakil, A., Church, R., & Rao, S. (2008). Gastrointestinal complications of diabetes. *American Family Physician, 77*(12), 1697–1703.

Siegel, J., Rhinehart, E., Jackson, M., et al. and the Healthcare Infection Control Practices Advisory Committee (2007). Guideline for isolation precautions: Preventing transmission of infectious agents in healthcare settings, 2007. Centers for Disease Control and Prevention (CDC). Retrieved February 4, 2009, from http://www.cdc.gov/ncidod/dhqp/pdf/guidelines/Isolation2007.pdf

Simmons, K., Smith, J., Bobb, K-A, et al. (2007). Adjustment to colostomy: Stoma acceptance, stoma care self-efficacy and interpersonal relationships. *Journal of Advanced Nursing, 60*(6), 627–635.

SweetHaven Publishing Services. (2006). Nursing care related to the gastrointestinal system. Lesson 45. Colostomy irrigation. Retrieved February 2, 2009, from http://www.free-ed.net/sweethaven/MedTech/NurseCare/GastroNurse01.asp?iNum=45

United Ostomy Associations of America. (2005). Ostomates food reference chart; in *Diet & Nutrition Guide.* Retrieved February 1, 2009, from http://www.uoaa.org/ostomy_info/pubs/uoa_diet_nutrition_en.pdf

University of Pittsburgh Medical Center (2004). Colostomy care. Retrieved April 16, 2009, from http://patienteducation.upmc.com/Pdf/Colostomy.pdf

Van Leeuwen, A., Kranpitz, T., & Smith, L. (2006). *Davis's comprehensive handbook of laboratory and diagnostic tests with nursing implications* (2nd ed.). Philadelphia: F. A. Davis.

Wilkinson, J. (2009). *Nursing diagnosis handbook with NIC interventions and NOC outcomes* (9th ed.). Upper Saddle River, NJ: Prentice-Hall.

Wilson, L. (2005). Understanding bowel problems in older people. Part I. *Nursing Older People, 17*(8), 25–29.

Winawer, S., Fletcher, R., Rex, D., et al. Gastrointestinal Consortium Panel (2003). Colorectal cancer screening and surveillance: Clinical guidelines and rationale. Update based on new evidence. *Gastroenterology, 124*(2), 544–560.

Wishin, J., Gallagher, T., & McCann, E. (2008). Emerging options for the management of fecal incontinence in hospitalized patients. *Journal of Wound, Ostomy and Continence Nursing, 35*(1), 104–110.

Wound, Ostomy and Continence Nurses Society. (2003). *Guideline for prevention and management of pressure ulcers.* Glenview, IL: Author.

Yuan, C. (Ed). (2005). *Handbook of opioid bowel dysfunction.* New York: Haworth Reference Press.

Chapter 29

American Association of Neuroscience Nurses. (2007). *Care of the patient with seizures.* Glenview, IL: Author. Retrieved April 24, 2009, from http://www.aann.org/pubs/cpg/seizures.pdf

American Optometric Association (AOA). (2005). Comprehensive adult eye and vision examination. St. Louis, MO: AOA. National Guideline Clearinghouse (NGC). Complete Summary. Rockville, MD. Retrieved April 28, 2009, from http://www.guideline.gov/summary/summary.aspx?ss=15&doc_id=8464&nbr=4725

Bonder, B., Haas, V., & Wagner, M. (2009). *Functional performance in older adults* (3rd ed.). Philadelphia: F. A. Davis.

Borson, S., Scanlan, J., Brush, M., et al. (2000). The Mini-Cog: A cognitive "vital signs" measure for dementia screening in multi-lingual elderly. *International Journal of Geriatric Psychiatry, 15*(11), 1021–1027.

Braun, C., Stangler, T., Narveson, J., et al. (2009). Animal-assisted therapy as a pain relief intervention for children. *Complementary Therapies in Clinical Practice, 15*(2), 105–109.

Buckle J. (2001). The role of aromatherapy in nursing care. *Nursing Clinics of North America, 36*(1), 57–72.

Bulechek, G., Butcher, H., & Dochterman, J. (2007). *Nursing interventions classification (NIC).* (5th ed.). St. Louis, MO: C. V. Mosby.

Burtin, M., & Doree, C. (2009). Ear drops for the removal of ear wax. *Cochrane Database of Systematic Reviews,* Issue 1. Art. No.: CD004326. DOI: 10.1002/14651858.CD004326.pub2. Retrieved May 2, 2009, from http://www.mrw.interscience.wiley.com/cochrane/clsysrev/articles/CD004326/frame.html

Cheetham, C., Hammond, M., Edwards, C., et al. (2007). Sensory experience alters cortical connectivity and synaptic function site specifically. *The Journal of Neuroscience, 27*(13), 3456–3465.

Deglin, J., & Vallerand, A. (2009). *Davis's drug guide for nurses* (11th ed.). Philadelphia: F. A. Davis.

Demers, K. (2007). Hearing screening in older adults: A brief hearing loss screener. *Try this: Best practices in nursing care to older adults,* Issue No. 12. The Hartford Institute for Geriatric Nursing, New York University, College of Nursing. Retrieved April 29, 2009, from http://consultgerirn.org/uploads/File/trythis/issue_12.pdf

Epilepsy Foundation of America. (n.d.). About epilepsy. Retrieved May 6, 2009, from http://www.epilepsyfoundation.org/about/

Espmark, A., Rosenhall, U., Erlandsson, S., et al. (2002). The two faces of presbycusis: Hearing impairment and psychosocial consequences. *International Journal of Audiology, 41*(2), 125–135.

Fenech, A., & Baker, M. (2008). Casual leisure and the sensory diet: A concept for improving quality of life in neuropalliative conditions. *NeuroRehabilitation, 23*(4), 369–376.

The Foundation of the American Academy of Ophthalmology. (2007). Eye exams: What to expect. Retrieved April 26, 2009, from eyecareAmerica, http://www.eyecareamerica.org/eyecare/treatment/eye-exams.cfm

Gleeson, M., & Higgins, A. (2009). Touch in mental health nursing: An exploratory study of nurses' views and perceptions. *Journal of Psychiatric & Mental Health Nursing, 16*(4), 382–389.

Gleeson, M., & Timmins, F. (2005). A review of the use and clinical effectiveness of touch as a nursing intervention. *Clinical Effectiveness in Nursing, 9*(1–2), 69–77.

Graf, C. (2006). Functional decline in hospitalized older adults. *American Journal of Nursing, 106*(1), a58–67, quiz 67–68.

Guyton, A., & Hall, J. (2006). *Textbook of medical physiology* (11th ed.). Philadelphia: W. B. Saunders.

Gwinner, N. (n.d.). Your VA hearing aid. VA Healthcare Network Upstate New York Communications; U.S. Department of Veterans Affairs. Retrieved April 26, 2008, from http://www.ncrar.research.va.gov/ForVets/documents/HearingAidbook.pdf

Harkin, H. (2008). Guidance document in ear care. The Primary Ear Care Centre. Retrieved May 2, 2009, from http://www.earcarecentre.com/protocols.htm

Herz, R. S. (2004). A naturalistic analysis of autobiographical memories triggered by olfactory visual and auditory stimuli. *Chemical Senses, 29*(3), 217–224.

Hicks-Moore, S. (2008). Favorite music and hand massage. *Dementia, 7*(1), 95–108.

Hockenberry, M., & Wilson, D. (2007). *Wong's nursing care of infants and children* (8th ed.). Philadelphia: F. A. Davis.

Hooker, S. D., Freeman, L. H., & Stewart, P. (2002). Pet therapy research: A historical review. *Holistic Nursing Practice, 17*(1), 17–23.

Hopper, P., & Williams, L. (2007). *Understanding medical surgical nursing* (3rd ed.). Philadelphia: F. A. Davis.

Huntley, A. (2008). Documenting level of consciousness. *Nursing2008, 38*(8), 63–64.

Johnson, M., Bulechek, G., Butcher, H., et al. (2006). *NANDA, NOC, and NIC linkages.* St. Louis, MO: C. V. Mosby.

The Joint Commission (TJC). (2008). *2008 hospital accreditation standards.* Oakbrook Terrace, IL: Author.

Kennedy-Malone, L., Fletcher, K., & Plank, L. (2004). *Management guidelines for nurse practitioners working with older adults* (2nd ed.). Philadelphia: F. A. Davis.

Lin, S., Cermak, S., Coster, W., et al. (2005). The relation between length of institutionalization and sensory integration in children adopted from Eastern Europe. *The American Journal of Occupational Therapy, 59*(2), 139–147.

Luggen, A. (2009). Epileptic seizures in older adult patients. *The Clinical Advisor, 12*(5), 26–28, 32–35.

McElligott, D., Holz, M. B., Carollo, L., et al. (2003). A pilot feasibility study of the effects of touch therapy on nurses. *Journal of the New York State Nurses Association, 34*(1), 16–24.

Moorhead, S., Johnson, M., Maas, M., et al. (2007). *Nursing outcomes classification (NOC)* (4th ed.). St. Louis, MO: C. V. Mosby.

Moss, M., Cook, J., Wesnes, K., et al. (2003). Aromas of rosemary and lavender essential oils differentially affect cognition and mood in healthy adults. *International Journal of Neuroscience, 113*(1), 15–38.

NANDA International. (2009). *Nursing diagnoses: Definitions and classification 2009–2011.* Ames, IA: Wiley-Blackwell.

National Guideline Clearinghouse (NGC). (n.d., last modified April 20, 2009). Guideline summary: Clinical practice guideline: Cerumen impaction. In: National Guideline Clearinghouse (NGC) [Web site]. Rockville, MD. Retrieved April 27, 2009, from http://www.guideline.gov/summary/summary.aspx?view_id=1&doc_id=13402

Nightingale, F. (1866/1932). *Notes on nursing.* London: Camelot Press.

Polan, E., & Taylor, D. (2007). *Journey across the life span: Human development and health promotion* (3rd ed.). Philadelphia: F. A. Davis.

Scanlon, V., & Sanders, T. (2007). *Essentials of anatomy and physiology* (5th ed.). Philadelphia: F. A. Davis.

Stanley, M., Blair, K., & Beare, P. (2005). *Gerontological nursing: Promoting successful aging with older adults* (3rd ed.). Philadelphia: F. A. Davis.

Valentijn, S., van Boxtel, M., van Hooren, S., et al. (2005). Change in sensory functioning predicts change in cognitive functioning: Results from a 6-year follow-up in the Maastricht aging study. *Journal of the American Geriatrics Society, 53*(3), 374–380.

Van Rompaey, B., Schuurmans, M., Shortridge-Baggett, L., et al. (2008). Risk factors for intensive care delirim: A systematic review. *Intensive and Critical Care Nursing, 24*(2), 98–107.

Venes, D. (2009). *Taber's cyclopedic medical dictionary* (21st ed.). Philadelphia: F. A. Davis.

Wåhlin, I., Ek, A., & Idvall, E. (2006). Patient empowerment in intensive care—An interview study. *Intensive and Critical Care Nursing, 22*(6), 370–377.

Whiteside, M., Wallhagen, M., & Pettengill, E. (2006). Sensory impairment in older adults: Part 2: Vision loss. *American Journal of Nursing, 106*(11), 52–62.

Wiegand, L. (2005). *AACN procedure manual for critical care*. Philadelphia: W. B. Saunders.

Wilkinson, J., & Ahern, N. (2009). *Prentice-Hall nursing diagnosis handbook* (9th ed.). Upper Saddle River, NJ: Prentice-Hall Health.

Zervakis, J., & Schiffman, S. (2004). Adverse taste side effects of cardiovascular medications. *Geriatric Times, 5*(1), 405–413.

Chapter 30

Agency for Healthcare Policy and Research, Public Health Service, U.S. Department of Health and Human Services. (2009). Comparative effectiveness of pain management interventions for hip fracture – Research protocol document. Retrieved on March 6, 2010, from http://www.effectivehealthcare.ahrq.gov/index.cfm/search-for-guides-reviews-and-reports/?pageaction=displayproduct&productid=368

Agency for Healthcare Policy and Research, Public Health Service, U.S. Department of Health and Human Services. (2009). Comparative effectiveness of pain management interventions for hip fracture – Research protocol document. Retrieved March 6, 2010, from http://www.effectivehealthcare.ahrq.gov/index.cfm/search-for-guides-reviews-and-reports/?pageaction=displayproduct&productid=368

American Academy of Pain Management. (2008). *19th Annual Meeting of the American Academy of Pain Management* (AAPM), held September 8–11, 2008 at the Gaylord Opryland Resort & Convention Center in Nashville, TN.

American Academy of Pediatrics (AAP), Committee on Psychological Aspects of Child and Family Health and American Task Force on Pain in Infants, Children, and Adolescents. (2001a). The assessment and management of acute pain in infants, children and adolescents. *Pediatrics, 118*(5), 2231–2241.

American Academy of Pediatrics (AAP), Committee on Psychological Aspects of Child and Family Health and American Task Force on Pain in Infants, Children, and Adolescents. (2001b). The assessment and management of acute pain in infants, children and adolescents. *Pediatrics, 108*(3), 793–797.

American Geriatrics Society, Panel on Persistent Pain in Older Persons. (2002). The management of persistent pain in older persons. *Journal of the American Geriatric Society, 50*(6 Supplement), S205–224.

American Geriatrics Society, Panel on Persistent Pain in Older Persons. (2009). Pharmacological management of persistent pain in older persons. *Journal of the American Geriatrics Society, 57*(8), 1331–1346.

American Pain Society. (1994). Part III: Pain terms, a current list with definitions and notes on usage. In: H. Merskey, N. Bogduk, & IASP Task Force on Taxonomy (Eds.), *Classification of chronic pain* (2nd ed.). Seattle: IASP Press.

American Pain Society. (2008). *Principles of analgesic use in the treatment of acute pain and cancer pain* (6th ed.). Shobie, IL: Author.

Arcidonco, P. (2006). Using a spinal cord stimulator to ease chronic pain. *Nursing2006, 36*(8), 18–20.

Ballantyne, J. C., & LeForge, K. S. (2007). Opioid dependence and addiction during opioid treatment of chronic pain. *Pain, 129*(3), 235–255.

Barnes, P. M., Bloom, B., & Nahin, R. L. (2008). Complementary and alternative medicine use among adults and children: United States, 2007. *National Health Statistics Reports;* No. 12. Hyattsville, MD: National Center for Health Statistics.

Berdine, H. J. (2002). The fifth vital sign: Cornerstone of a new pain management strategy. *Disease and Management Outcomes, 10*(3), 155–156.

Best practices: Evidence-based nursing procedures (2008). (pp. 117–124). Philadelphia: Lippincott Williams & Wilkins.

Bishop, F. L., Yardley. L., & Lewith, G. T. (2008). Treat or treatment: a qualitative study analyzing patients' use of complementary and alternative medicine. *American Journal of Public Health, 98*(9), 1700–1705.

Bjoro, K., Bergen, K., & Herr, K. (2008). Tools for pain assessment in older adults with end-stage dementia. *American Academy of Hospice and Palliative Medicine Bulletin, 9*(3), 1–4.

Bouhassira D., Lanteri-Minet, M., Attal, N., et al. (2008, June). Prevalence of chronic pain with neuropathic characteristics in the general population. *Pain, 136*(3), 380–387.

Bringager, B. C., Friis, A. H., Husebye, H. T., et al. (2008). A long-term follow-up study of chest pain patients: Effect of panic disorder on mortality, morbidity, and quality of life. *Cardiology, 110*(1), 8–14.

Bulechek, G., Butcher, G., & Dochterman, J. (Eds.). (2007). *Nursing interventions classification (NIC)* (5th ed.). St. Louis, MO: C. V. Mosby.

Cassileth, B., Trevisan, C., & Jyothirmai, G. (2007). Complementary therapies for cancer pain. *Current Pain & Headache Reports, 11*(4), 265–269.

Centers for Disease Control and Prevention (CDC). (2008, December 16). National Center for Health Statistics. Health Data Interactive. *Trends in healthcare and aging.* Retrieved February 1, 2009, from http://www.cdc.gov/nchs/hdi.htm

Chou, R., Fanciullo, G., Fine, P., et al. (2009, February). Opioids for chronic noncancer pain: Prediction and identification of aberrant drug-related behaviors: A review of the evidence for an American Pain Society and American Academy of Pain Medicine Clinical Practice Guideline. *The Journal of Pain, 10*(2), 131–146.

Christo, P. J. (2009). Clinical concepts in pain and aging. American Academy of Pain Management. 20th Annual Meeting of the American Academy of Pain Management (AAPM), held January 31, 2009 Honolulu.

Cohen, M. R., Weber, R. J., & Moss, J. (2006, April 1). Patient-controlled analgesia: Making it safer for patients. Institute for Safe Medicine Practice (ISMP). Retrieved January 24, 2009, from http://www.ismp.org/CE/Default.asp

Cousins, M. J., Bridenbaugh, P. O., Carr, B., et al. (Eds.) (2008, December 1). *Cousins and Bridenbaugh's neural blockade in clinical anesthesia and pain medicine.* Philadelphia: Lippincott Williams & Wilkins.

Crook, R., Rideout, E., & Browne, G. (1984). The prevalence of pain complaints in a general population. *Pain, 18,* 299–314.

D'Arcy, Y. (2008a, January). Keep your patient safe during PCA. *Nursing, 38*(1), 50–55.

D'Arcy, Y. (2008b, February). What you need to know about opioids. *Nursing, 38*(2), 26–28.

Deglin, J. H., & Vallerand, A. H. (2009). *Davis's drug guide for nurses* (11th ed.). Philadelphia: F. A. Davis.

Donovan, M., & Miaskowski, C. (1992). Striving for a standard of pain relief. *American Journal of Nursing, 92*(3), 106–107.

Elkins, G., Jensen, M., & Patterson, D. R. (2007). Hypnotherapy for the management of chronic pain. *International Journal of Clinical and Experimental Hypnosis, 55*(3), 275–287.

Ernst, E. (2008). *Complementary therapies for pain management: An evidence-based approach.* St. Louis, MO: Elsevier.

Evans, D. (2002). The effectiveness of music as an intervention for hospital patients: A systematic review. *Journal of Advanced Nursing, 37*(1), 8–18.

Evans, F. J. (1974). The placebo response in pain reduction. *Advances in Neurology, 4,* 289–296.

Flaherty, E. (2007). Pain assessment in older adults. *Try this: Best practices in nursing care to older adults.* The Hartford Institute for Geriatric Nursing, 7, 1–2.

Gregoire, M. C., & Frager, G. (2006). Ensuring pain relief for children at the end of life. *Pain Research & Management, 11*(3), 163–171.

Hagle, M., Lehr, V., Brubakken, K., & Shippee, A. (2004). Respiratory depression in adult patients with intravenous patient-controlled analgesia. *Orthopedic Nursing, 28*(1), 18–25.

Hart, J. (2008, April 1). Complementary therapies for chronic pain management. *Alternative and Complementary Therapies, 14*(2), 64–68.

Heidrich, D. (2002). The Indiana State Nurses Association by special arrangements with the Ohio Nurses Foundation presents: The physiological basis for pain medications: Independent study. *Indiana State Nurses Association Bulletin, 28*(3), 23–27.

Herr, K. (2002). Pain assessment in cognitively impaired older adults. *American Journal of Nursing, 102*(12), 65–66, 68.

Herr, K. (2004). Evidence-based assessment of acute pain in older adults: current nursing practices and perceived barriers. *Clinical Journal of Pain, 20,* 331–340.

Herr, K., Bjoro, K., & Decker S. (2006). Tools for assessment of pain in nonverbal older adults with dementia: A state-of-the-science review. *Journal of Pain Symptom Management, 31*(2), 170–192.

Horgas, A. L. (2007). Assessing pain in older adults with dementia. *Try this: Best practices for nursing care for hospitalized older adults.* The Hartford Institute for Geriatric Nursing and the Alzheimer's Association, D2, 1–2.

Idvall, E., Holm, C., & Runeson, I. (2005). Pain experiences and non-pharmacological strategies for pain management after tonsillectomy: A qualitative interview. *Journal of Child Health, 9*(3), 196–207.

Institute for Clinical Systems Improvement. (2008, March). *Health care guideline: Assessment and management of acute pain* (6th ed.). Retrieved December 5, 2009, from http://www.icsi.org/pain_acute/pain__acute__assessment_and_management_of__3.html

Institute for Safe Medicine Practice (ISMP). (2002, May 29). More on avoiding opiate toxicity with PCA by proxy: Too much of a good thing. *ISMP Medication.*

Institute for Safe Medicine Practice (ISMP). (2002, July 24). Pain scales don't weigh every risk. *ISMP Medication.* Retrieved September 12, 2010, from http://www.ismp.org/newsletters/acutecare/articles/20020724.asp?ptr=y

Jansen, M. (2008, March). *Managing pain in the older adult.* New York: Springer.

Jensen, M., & Patterson, D. R. (2006). Managing pain in the older adult. *Journal of Behavioral Medicine, 29*(1), 95–124.

The Joint Commission (TJC). (2004, December 20). Patient controlled analgesia by proxy. Sentinel event alert. Retrieved December 5, 2009, from http://www.jointcommission.org/sentinelevents/sentineleventalert/sea_33.htm

Katz, N. P., McCarberg, B. H., & Reisner, L. (2007). *Managing chronic pain with opioids in primary care.* Newton, MA: Inflexxion, Inc.

Kortesluoma, R. L., & Nikkonen M. (2004). 'I had this horrible pain': The sources and causes of pain experiences in 4- to 11-year-old hospitalized children. *Journal of Child Health, 8*(3), 210.

Krieger, D. (1993). *Accepting your power to heal: The personal practice of therapeutic touch.* Sante Fe, NM: Bear and Co.

Ladak, S. S., Chan, V. W., Easty, T., et al. (2007, December). Right medication, right dose, right patient, right time, and right route: How do we select the right patient-controlled analgesia. *Pain Management Nursing, 8*(4), 140–145.

Lewandowski, C. S., Good, M., & Draucker, C. B. (2005). Changes in the meaning of pain with the use of guided imagery. *Pain Management Nursing, 6*(2), 58–67.

Li, J. M. (2008). Pain management in the hospitalized patient. *Medical Clinics of North America, 92*(2), 371–385, ix.

Mailis-Gagnon, A. F., Sandoval, J. A., & Taylor, R. S. (2004; reviewed 2009). Spinal cord stimulation for chronic pain. *Cochrane Database of Systematic Reviews,* Issue 3. Art. No.: CD003783. DOI: 10.1002/14651858.CD003783.pub2. Retrieved December 8, 2009, from http://www.cochrane.org/reviews/en/ab003783.html

Marders, J. (2004). PCA by proxy: Too much of a good thing. *Nursing2004, 34*(4), 24.

Mayer, D., Torma, L., Byock, I., et al. (2001). Speaking the language of pain. *American Journal of Nursing, 101*(2), 44–50.

McCaffery, M. (2003). Pain control: Switching from IV to PO. *American Journal of Nursing, 103*(5), 62–63.

McCaffery, M., Latham, J., & Beebe, A. (1994). *Pain: Clinical manual for nursing practice.* St. Louis, MO: C. V. Mosby.

McCaffery, M., & Pasero, C. (1999). *Pain clinical manual* (2nd ed.). St. Louis, MO: C. V. Mosby.

McCreaddie, M., & Davidson, S. (2002). Pain management in drug users. *Nursing Standard, 16*(19), 20.

McMahon, S., & Koltzenburg, M. (Eds.) (2005). *Wall and Melzack's textbook of pain* (5th ed.). New York: Churchill Livingstone.

Melzack, R., & Wall, P. (1965). Pain mechanisms: A new theory. *Science, 150,* 971–979.

Melzack, R., & Wall, P. (1996). *The challenge of pain* (2nd ed.). London: Penguin.

Mersky, H., & Bogduk, N. (Eds.). (1994). *Classification of chronic pain* (2nd ed.). Seattle, WA: International Association for the Study of Pain.

Middleton, C. (2006, April). Epidural analgesia in acute pain management. London: Whurr Publishers Limited (a subsidiary of John Wiley & Sons).

Molony, S. L., Kobayashi, M., Holleran, E. A., et al. (2005, March). Assessing pain as a fifth vital sign in long-term care facilities: Recommendations from the field. *Journal of Gerontological Nursing, 31*(3), 16–24.

Montal, E., Fujimoto, K., Kiyohara, E., et al. (2008, April). Screening for discomfort as the fifth vital sign using an electronic medical recording system: a feasibility study. *Journal of Pain and Symptom Management, 35*(4), 430–436.

Muller, U., Tanzler, K., Burger, A., et al. (2008, May). A pain assessment scale for population-based studies: Development and validation of the pain module of the Standard Evaluation Questionnaire. *Pain, 136*(1–2), 62–74.

National Guideline Clearinghouse (NGC). (2003; updated 2005, May 13). Assessment and management of pain. In: National Guideline Clearinghouse (NGC) [Web site]. Rockville, MD. Retrieved December 5, 2009, from http://www.guideline.gov/summary/summary.aspx?doc_id=11507&nbr=005960&string=assessment+and+%22Management+of+pain%22

National Institutes of Health (NIH), National Institute on Drug Abuse. (2005, revised.). Research report series: Prescription drugs abuse and addiction. Retrieved November 28, 2009, from http://www.nida.nih.gov/ResearchReports/Prescription/prescription.html

Ness, J., Cirillo, D. J., Weir, D. R., et al. (2005). Use of complementary medicine in older Americans: Results from the health and retirement study. *The Gerontologist, 45,* 516–524.

Nichols, R. (2003). Pain management in patients with addictive disease. *American Journal of Nursing, 103*(3), 87–88.

O'Mathuna, D. (2000). Evidence-based practice and reviews of therapeutic touch. *Journal of Nursing Scholarship, 32*(3), 279–285.

O'Rourke, D. (2004). The measurement of pain in infants, children, and adolescents: From policy to practice. *Physical Therapy, 84*(6), 560–570.

Panke, J. (2002). Difficulties in managing pain at the end of life. *American Journal of Nursing, 102*(7), 26–34.

Papagallo, M. (2005). *The neurological basis of pain.* New York: McGraw-Hill.

Pasero, C. (1997). Pain ratings: The fifth vital sign. *American Journal of Nursing, 97*(2), 15–16.

Pasero, C., Manworren, R. C. B., & McCaffery, M. (2008). IV opioid range orders for acute pain management. *American Journal of Nursing, 107*(2), 52–60.

Patterson, C. (2008). Six myths about opioid use. *Nursing2008, 38*(11), 60–61.

Puntillo, K., Neighbor, M., O'Neill, N., et al. (2003). Accuracy of emergency nurses in assessment of patients' pain. *Pain Management Nursing, 4*(4), 171–175.

Quinn, T. E. (n.d.). Pain assessment in the difficult-to-assess patient. Retrieved November 29, 2009, from http://www2.massgeneral.org/painrelief/Pain%20Topics/Pain_Assessment_in_the_Difficult_Rev2_7.06.pdf

Reiff, P., & Niziolek, M. (2001). Trouble-shooting tips for PCA. *RN, 64*(4), 33–37.

Richards, T., Johnson, J., Sparks, A., et al. (2007). The effect of music therapy on patients' perception and manifestation of pain, anxiety and patient satisfaction. *MedSurg Nursing, 16*(1), 7–14.

Rieman, M. T., Gordon, M., & Marvin, J. M. (2007). Pediatric nurses knowledge and attitudes survey regarding pain: A competency tool modification. *Pediatric Nursing, 33*(4).

Robinson, M. (2008). Pain management and assessment at the end of life. *Journal of the South Dakota State Medical Association.* Special edition, 44–46.

Schneider, J. P. (2006–2007, Winter). Opioids, pain management, and addiction. *Pain Practitioner, 16,* 17–24.

Schoefield, P. (2007, May). *The management of pain in older people.* Hoboken, NJ: John Wiley & Sons.

Sheehan, S. (2008, December 1). Study: Patient harm more common with patient-controlled pain medication. The Joint Commission

News Entry. Retrieved December 5, 2009 at http://www.jcrinc.com/News/2008/12/1/Study-Patient-Harm-More-Common-with-Patient-Controlled-Pain-Medication/

Simons, J., & McDonald, L. M. (2006). Changing practice: Implementing validated paedriatric pain assessment tools. *Journal of Child Health*, 10(2), 160–176.

Slater, R., Cantarella, A., Fanck, L., et al. (2008, June 24th). How well do clinical pain assessment tools reflect pain in infants? *PLoS Medicine*, 5(6), e129. Retrieved March 5, 2010, from http://www.asianhhm.com/Knowledge_bank/research_insights/clinical_pain_assessment_tools_reflect_pain.htm

Slaughter, A., Pasero, C., & Manworren, R. (2002). Unacceptable pain levels: Approaches to pain relief. *American Journal of Nursing*, 102(5), 75–77.

Smith, C. A., Collins, C. T., Cyna, A. M., et al. (2006). Complementary and alternative therapies for pain management in labour. *Cochrane Database of Systematic Reviews*, Issue 4. Retrieved March 5, 2010, from http://www.cochrane.org/reviews/en/ab003521.html

Snidvongs S., Nagaratnam, M., & Stephens, R. (2008). Assessment and treatment of pain in children. *British Journal of Hospital Medicine*, 69(4), 211–213.

Soderhamn, O., & Idvall, E. (2003). Nurses' influence on quality of care in postoperative pain management: A phenomenological study. *International Journal of Nursing Practice*, 9(1), 26–32.

Spies, C., Rehberg, B., Schug, S. A., et al. (2009). *Pocket guide pain management*. New York: Springer.

Spragud, L. J., Piira, T., & Baeyer, C. L. (2003). Children's self-report of pain intensity. *American Journal of Nursing*, 103(12), 62–64.

Stanfield, C. L. (2010). *Principles of human physiology* (4th ed.). San Francisco: Benjamin Cummings.

Sterpina, V. S., & Frenkel, M. A. (2005). Acupuncture: A clinical review. *Southern Medical Journal*, 98(3), 330–337.

Taddio, A., Katz, J., Hersich, A., et al. (1997). Effects of neonatal circumcision on pain response during subsequent routine vaccination. *The Lancet*, 349, 599–603.

Turk, D. C., Swanson, K. S., & Tunks, E. R. (April, 2008). Psychological approaches in the treatment of chronic pain patients—when pills, scalpels, and needles are not enough. *Canadian Journal of Psychiatry*, 53(4), 213–223.

U.S. Department of Health and Human Services (USDHHS), Public Health Service Agency for Health Care Policy and Research, Cancer Pain Guideline Panel. (2007). Management of cancer pain: Adults. *Journal of the American Academy of Nurse Practitioners*, 7(4), 171–187.

Valente, S. M. (2006). Hypnosis for pain management. *Journal of Psychological Nursing and Mental Health Services*, 44(2), 22–30.

Vissers, K. C. (2006, March 30). The clinical challenge of chronic neuropathic pain. *Disability and Rehabilitation*, 28, 343–349.

Vitale A. (2007). An integrative review of Reiki touch therapy research. *Holistic nursing practice: The science of health and healing*, 21(4), 167–179.

Wardell, D. W., & Weymouth, K. F. (2004). Review of studies of healing touch. *Journal of Nursing Scholarship*, 36(2), 147–154.

Warfield, C. A., & Bajwha, Z. H. (2004). *Principles and practice of pain: Management* (2nd ed.). Columbus, OH: McGraw-Hill.

Warren, D. (1996). Practical use of rectal medications in palliative care. *Journal of Pain Symptom Management*, 11(6), 378–387.

Webster, L. R., & Webster, R. M. (2005). Predicting aberrant behaviors in opioid-treated patients: Preliminary validation of the Opioid Risk Tool. *Pain Medicine*, 6(6), 432–442.

Ying, K. N., & White, A. (2007, August). Pain relief in osteoarthritis and rheumatoid arthritis: TENS. *British Journal of Community Nursing*, 12(8), 364–371.

Zacharaff, K. L., Zeis, J., Krayjo, K., et al. (2009). *Cross-cultural pain management: Effective treatment of pain in the Hispanic population*. Newton, MA: Inflexxion Inc.

Zwakhalen, S. M., Hamers, J. P., Abu-Saad, H. H., et al. (2006). Pain in elderly people with severe dementia: A systematic review of behavioural pain assessment tools. *BMC Geriatrics*, 6, 3. Retrieved January 21, 2009, from http://www.biomedcentral.com/1471–2318/6/3

Chapter 31

American College of Sports Medicine. (2009, February). Appropriate physical activity intervention strategies for weight loss and prevention of weight regain for adults. Position Stand. *Medicine & Science in Sports & Exercise*, 41(12). Retrieved February 13, 2009, from http://www.acsm-msse.org/pt/pt-core/template-journal/msse/media/0209.pdf

American Nurses Association (ANA). (2006). Preventing back injuries: Safe patient handling and movement. Retrieved March 1, 2009, from http://www.nursingworld.org/MainMenuCategories/OccupationalandEnvironmental/occupationalhealth/OccupationalResources/PreventingBackInjuries.aspx

Astrand, P. O. (2003). *Textbook of work physiology: Physiological basis of exercise* (4th ed.). Stockholm, Sweden: Human Kinetics.

Binks, M., & Housle, B. (2009). Commentary. How much should my patient exercise? *The Clinical Advisor*, 12(1), 75.

Blair, S. N., Cheng, Y., & Holder, J. S. (2002). Exercise adherence and 10-year mortality in chronically ill older adults. *Journal of the American Geriatric Society*, 50(12), 1929–1933.

Brain Injury Resource Foundation. (2000, updated 2009, March 6). Functional independence measure. The Center for Outcome Measurement in Brain Injury. Retrieved May 12, 2009, from http://www.birf.info/home/bi-tools/tests/fam.html

Bulechek, G., Butcher, H., & Dochterman, J. (2007). *Nursing interventions classification (NIC)*. (5th ed.). St. Louis, MO: C. V. Mosby.

Borg, G. (1998). *Borg's perceived exertion and pain scales*. Stockholm, Sweden: Human Kinetics.

Centers for Disease Control and Prevention (CDC). (2008, updated December 17). Physical activity for everyone. Retrieved February 22, 2009, from http://www.cdc.gov/physicalactivity/everyone/guidelines/olderadults.html

Converso, A., & Murphy, C. (2004). Winning the battle against back injuries. *RN*, 67(2), 52–57.

de Castro, A. B. (2004, September). Handle With Care®: The American Nurses Association's campaign to address work-related musculoskeletal disorders. *Online Journal of Issues in Nursing*, 9(3), Manuscript 2. Retrieved April 1, 2009, from http://www.nursingworld.org/MainMenuCategories/ANAMarketplace/ANAPeriodicals/OJIN/TableofContents/Volume92004/No3Sept04/HandleWithCare.aspx

Fletcher, G. F., Balady, G. J., & Amsterdam, E. A. (2001). Exercise standards for testing and training: A statement for healthcare professionals from the American Heart Association. *Circulation*, 106(14), 1694–1740.

Forman, D. E., & Farquhar, W. (2002). Cardiac rehabilitation and secondary prevention programs for elderly cardiac patients. *Clinics in Geriatric Medicine*, 16(3), 619–629.

Foster, C. (2004). "Talk test" measures exercise intensity. *Medicine & Science in Sports & Exercise*, 36(9), 1632–1636.

Frimel, T. N., Sinacore, D. R., & Villareal, D. T. (2008, July). Exercise attenuates the weight-loss induced reduction in muscle mass in frail obese older adults. *Medicine & Science in Sport & Exercise*, 40(7), 1213–1219.

Gillis, A., & MacDonald, B. (2005, June). Deconditioning in the hospitalized elderly. *Canadian Nurse*, 101(6), 16–20.

Gregg, E. W., Gerzoff, R. B., Caspersen, C. J., et al. (2003). Relationship of walking to mortality among U.S. adults with diabetes. *Archives of Internal Medicine*, 163(12), 1440–1447.

Haskell, W. L., Lee, I. M., Pate, R. R., et al. (2007). Physical activity and public health updated recommendation for adults from the American College of Sports Medicine and the American Heart Association. *Circulation*, 116, 1081–1093. Retrieved May 11, 2009, from http://circ.ahajournals.org/cgi/reprint/CIRCULATIONAHA.107.185649

Jakicic, J. M., Marcus, B. H., Gallagher, K. I., et al. (2003). Effect of exercise duration and intensity on weight loss in overweight, sedentary women: A randomized trial. *JAMA*, 290(10), 1323–1330.

Jitramontree, N. (2007). Evidence-based practice guideline. Exercise promotion: Walking in elders. Iowa City (IA): University of Iowa

Gerontological Nursing Interventions Research Center, Research Dissemination Core; 2007 June, p. 57. Retrieved April 1, 2009, from http://www.guideline.gov/summary/summary.aspx?ss=15&doc_id=10948&nbr=5728

Lee, I. M., Sesso, H. D., Oguma, Y., et al. (2003). Relative intensity of physical activity and risk of coronary heart disease. *Circulation, 107*(8), 1110–1116.

Maddalozzo, G. F., & Snow, C. M. (2000). High intensity resistance training: Effects on bone in older men and women. *Calcified Tissue International, 66*, 399–404.

Manson, J. E., & Bassuk, S. S. (2003). Obesity in the United States: A fresh look at its high toll. *JAMA, 289*(2), 229–230.

Manson, J. E., Greenland, P., LaCroix, A. Z., et al. (2002, September). Walking compared with vigorous exercise for the prevention of cardiovascular events in women. *New England Journal of Medicine, 347*(10), 716–725.

Metules, T. J. (2001). Occupational hazards. Watch your back! *RN, 64*(6), 65–66, 82.

Moorhead, S., Johnson, M., Maas, M., et al. (2007). *Nursing outcomes classification (NOC)* (4th ed.). St. Louis, MO: C. V. Mosby.

Nelson, A., & Baptiste, A. (2004, September 30). Evidence-based practices for safe patient handling and movement. *Online Journal of Issues in Nursing, 9*(3). Retrieved April 1, 2009, from http://www.nursingworld.org/MainMenuCategories/ANAMarketplace/ANAPeriodicals/OJIN/TableofContents/Volume92004/No3Sept04/EvidenceBasedPractices.aspx

Nelson, A., Fragala, G., & Menzel, N. (2003). Myths and facts about back injuries in nursing. *American Journal of Nursing, 103*(2), 32–40.

Nelson, A., Lloyd, J. D., Menzel, N., et al. (2003). Preventing nursing back injuries. *American Association of Occupational Health Nursing Journal, 51*(3), 126–134.

Nelson, M. E., Rejeski, W. J., Blair, S. N., et al. (2007). Physical activity and public health in older adults: Recommendation from the American College of Sports Medicine and the American Heart Association. *Circulation, 116*(9), 1094–1105.

Noakes, T. (2006, March). Exercise in the heat: Old ideas, new dogmas. *International Sports Medicine Journal, 7*(1), 58–74.

Noakes, T. (2007, February 15). Hydration in the marathon: using thirst to gauge safe fluid replacement. *Sports Medicine, 37*(4–5), 463–466.

Simkin, B. S., & Simkin, M. A. (2002). Maximizing the benefits of exercise in the elderly. *Family Practice Recertification, 24*(1), 38–40.

Simoes, E. J., Kobau, R., Waterman, B., et al. (2006, December). Associations of physical activity and body mass index with activities of daily living in older adults. *Journal of Community Health, 31*(6), 453–467.

Swann, J. (2007). Rheumatoid arthritis: When the body rebels against itself. *Nursing & Residential Care, 9*(5), 222–224.

U.S. Department of Health and Human Services (USDHHS). (2001). *Overweight and obesity: What you can do. Being physically active can help you attain a healthy weight.* Washington, DC: Author.

U.S. Department of Health and Human Services (USDHHS). (2004). *Healthy People 2010:* Understanding and improving health. Retrieved April, 2005, from http://www.healthypeople.gov

U.S. Department of Health and Human Services (USDHHS). (2008). 2008 physical activity guidelines for Americans. Retrieved February, 2009, from http://www.health.gov/paguidelines

Chapter 32

Alan Guttmacher Institute. (2002, updated 2006, December). Sexual and reproductive health: Women and men. In: *Facts in brief.* Washington, DC: Author.

American Academy of Pediatrics (AAP), Committee on Adolescents. (2001). Care of the adolescent sexual assault victim. *Pediatrics, 107*(6), 1476–1479. Retrieved April 19, 2009, from http://pediatrics.aappublications.org/cgi/content/full/107/6/1476

American Geriatrics Society Foundation for Health in Aging. (n.d.). Aging in the know. Sexual problems. Retrieved April 22, 2009, from http://www.healthinaging.org/agingintheknow/chapters_print_ch_trial.asp?ch=51

American Psychiatric Association (APA). (2000). *Diagnostic and statistical manual of mental disorders* (4th ed.), text revision. Washington, DC: Author.

Annon, J. (1974). *The behavioral treatment of sexual problems.* Honolulu: Enabling Systems.

Arena, J. M., & Wallace, M. (2008). Sexuality issues in aging: Nursing standard of practice protocol sexuality in older adults. Hartford Institute for Geriatric Nursing. Retrieved April 23, 2009, from http://www.consultgerirn.org/topics/sexuality_issues_in_aging/want_to_know_more

Basson, R. (2001). Using a different model for female sexual response to address women's problematic low sexual desire. *Journal of Sex and Marital Therapy, 27*, 395–403.

Beach, E. K., Maloney, B. H., Plocica, A. R., et al. (1992). The spouse: A factor in recovery after acute myocardial infarction. *Heart & Lung, 21*(1), 30–38.

Beckman, N., Waern, M., & Gustafson, D. (2008). Secular trends in self reported sexual activity and satisfaction in Swedish 70 year olds: Cross sectional survey of four populations, 1971–2001. *BMJ, 337,* A279.

Brown, J., O'Brien, P. M. S., Marjoribanks, J., et al. (2002, updated April 29, 2008). Selective serotonin reuptake inhibitors for premenstrual syndrome. *Cochrane Database of Systematic Reviews,* Issue 3. Art. No.: CD001396. DOI: 10.1002/14651858.CD001396. Retrieved December 8, 2009, from http://www.cochrane.org/reviews/en/ab001396.html

Bulechek, G., Butcher, H., & Dochterman, J. (2008). *Nursing interventions classification (NIC)* (5th ed.). St. Louis, MO: C. V. Mosby.

Centers for Disease Control and Prevention (CDC). (2007a). National Center for Health Statistics Health, 2007 with chartbook trends on the health of Americans. Hyattsville, MD: U.S. Department of Health and Human Services. Retrieved April 19, 2009, from http://www.cdc.gov/nchs/data/hus/hus07.pdf#051

Centers for Disease Control and Prevention (CDC). (2007b). National Center for Health Statistics Sexually Transmitted Diseases Surveillance, 2007. Hyattsville, MD: U.S. Department of Health and Human Services. Retrieved April 19, 2009, from http://www.cdc.gov/std/stats07/natoverview.htm

Cooper, A., Skinner, J., Nherera, L., et al. (2007). Clinical guidelines and evidence review for post myocardial infarction: Secondary prevention in primary and secondary care for patients following a myocardial infarction. London: National Collaborating Centre for Primary Care and Royal College of General Practitioners.

Davidson, M. R. (2004). Sexually transmitted infections: Screening and counseling. *Clinician Reviews, 14*(6), 56–62.

DeBusk, R., Drory, Y., Goldstein, I., et al. (2000). Management of sexual dysfunction in patients with cardiovascular disease: Recommendations of the Princeton consensus panel. *American Journal of Cardiology, 86*(2), 175–181.

EngenderHealth. (2007). Sexual response and sexual practices: Normal changes in response with aging. *Sexuality and Sexual Health: An Online MiniCourse.* Retrieved April 22, 2009, from http://www.engenderhealth.org/res/onc/sexuality/response/miw/pg5.html

Frankel, D. (1994). U.S. surgeon general forced to retire. *Lancet, 34,* 1695.

Friedman, S. (2000). Cardiac disease, anxiety and sexual functioning. *American Journal of Cardiology, 86* (Supplement) (2A), 46F–50F.

Hyde, J. S., & Delamater, J. D. (2008). *Understanding human sexuality* (10th ed). Columbus OH: McGraw-Hill.

Iannacchione, M. A. (2004). The vagina dialogues: Do you douche? *American Journal of Nursing, 104*(1), 40–46.

Johns Hopkins Children's Center. (2004). *Syndromes of abnormal sex differentiation: A guide for patients and their families.* Baltimore: Johns Hopkins University Press.

Kaufman, J., & American Academy of Pediatrics, Committee on Adolescence. (2008). Care of the adolescent sexual assault victim. *Pediatrics, 122*(2), 462–470.

King, B. M. (2009). *Human sexuality today* (6th ed.). Upper Saddle River, NJ: Prentice-Hall.

Klein, M. J., & Merritt, L. (2008). Sexuality and disability. eMedicine. Retrieved April 25, 2009, from http://emedicine.medscape.com/article/319119–overview

Kleinplatz, P. J. (2008). Sexuality and older people. *BMJ, 337,* a239.

Laumann, E. O., Paik, A., Glasser, D. B., et al. (2006). A cross-national study of subjective sexual well-being among older women and men: Findings from the Global Study of Sexual Attitudes and Behaviors. *Archives of Sexual Behavior, 35,* 145–161.

Lindau, S. T., Schumm, P., Laumann, E. O., et al. (2007). A study of sexuality and health among older adults in the United States. *New England Journal of Medicine, 357*(8), 762–774. Retreived April 22, 2009, from http://nejm.highwire.org/cgi/content/full/357/8/762

Masters, W. H., & Johnson, V. E. (1966). *Human sexual response.* Philadelphia. Lippincott Williams & Wilkins.

Miner, M. M. (2006). Sexual activity after myocardial infarction: When to resume the use of erectogenic drugs. *Current Sexual Health Reports, 3*(1), 30–34.

Moorhead, S., Johnson, M., Maas, M., et al. (Eds.). (2008). *Nursing outcomes classification (NOC)* (4th ed.). St. Louis, MO: C. V. Mosby.

Moser, D. K. (2007). The rust of life: Impact of anxiety on cardiac patients. *American Journal of Critical Care, 16*(4), 361–369.

Muller, J. E. (2000). Triggering of cardiac events by sexual activity: Findings from a case-crossover analysis. *American Journal of Cardiology, 86* (Supplement) (2A), 14F–18F.

Parashar, S., Rumsfeld, J. S., Reid, K. J., et al. (2008). Impact of depression on sex differences in outcome after myocardial infarction. *Circulation: Cardiovascular Quality and Outcomes, 2,* 33–40.

Penhollow, T. M., & Young, M. (2008, October 15). Predictors of sexual satisfaction: The role of body image and fitness. *Electronic Journal of Human Sexuality, 11.* Retrieved April 11, 2009, from http://www.ejhs.org/volume11/Penhollow.htm

Penhollow, T. M., Young, M., & Denny, G. (2009, January/February). Predictors of quality of life, sexual intercourse, and sexual satisfaction in older adults. *American Journal of Health Education, 40*(1), 13–22.

Reaume, C., & Mitty, E. (2008, October). Sexuality and intimacy in older adults. *Geriatric Nursing, 29*(5), 342–349.

Rennison, C. M., & Rand, M. R. (2008). Crime victimization, 2007: Findings from the National Crime Victimization Survey. Washington, DC: Bureau of Justice Statistics, U.S. Department of Justice. Retrieved December 7, 2009, from http://ojp.usdoj.gov/bjs/cvictgen.htm

Rodgers, J. E. (2003). *Sex: A natural history.* New York: Times Books.

Rowland, D. L., & Incrocci, L. (2007). *Handbook of sexual and gender identity.* Hoboken, NJ: John Wiley & Sons.

Salaman, M. (2008). Sex after a heart attack—for men: Be careful with performance enhancing drugs. About.com: Heart Disease. Retrieved on May 5, 2009, from http://heartdisease.about.com/lw/Health-Medicine/Conditions-and-diseases/Sex-after-a-Heart-Attack-for-Men.htm

Stehle, B. F. (1985). *Incurably romantic.* Philadelphia: Temple University Press.

Steinke, E. E. (2000). Sexual counseling after myocardial infarction. *American Journal of Nursing, 100*(12), 38–43.

Steinke, E. E. (2002). A videotape intervention for sexual counseling after myocardial infarction. *Heart & Lung, 31*(5), 348–354.

Steinke, E. E., & Patterson-Midgley, P. (1996). Sexual counseling of MI patients: Nurses' comfort, responsibility, and practice. *Dimensions of Critical Care Nursing, 15*(4), 216–223.

Taylor, B., & Davis, S. (2006). Using the extended PLISSIT model to address sexual healthcare needs. *Nursing Standard, 21*(11), 35–40.

U.S. Department of Health and Human Services, Centers for Disease Control and Prevention, National Center for Health Statistics. (2008, October 15). Recent trends in teenage pregnancy in the United States, 1990–2002. Retrieved May 1, 2009, from http://www.cdc.gov/nchs/data/infosheets/infosheet_teen_preg.htm

Wallace, M. A. (2008). Assessment of sexual health in older adults. *American Journal of Nursing, 108*(7), 52–60.

Wallace, M. A. (revised 2007). Sexuality assessment for older adults. In: *Try this: Best practices in nursing care of older adults.* The Hartford Institute for Geriatric Nursing. Retrieved April 20, 2009, from http://consultgerirn.org/uploads/File/trythis/issue10.pdf

Wilkinson, J. M. (2009). *Nursing diagnosis handbook with NIC interventions and NOC outcomes* (9th ed.). Upper Saddle River, NJ: Prentice-Hall Health.

Women's Health Initiative Steering Committee (2004). Effects of conjugated equine estrogen in postmenopausal women with hysterectomy. *JAMA, 291*(14), 1701–1712.

World Health Organization (WHO). (2002). Gender and reproductive rights. WHO draft working definition, October 2002. Retrieved December 8, 2009, from http://www.who.int/reproductive-health/gender/glossary.html

World Health Organization (WHO). (2008, May). Female genital mutilation. WHO Fact Sheet #241. Retrieved April 22, 2009, from http://www.who.int/mediacentre/factsheets/fs241/en/print.html

World Health Organization (WHO). (n.d.). Sexual health. Retrieved April 20, 2009, from http://who.int/topics/sexual_health/en

Zucker, K. J. (2000). Gender identity disorder. In A. J. Sameroff, M. Lewis, & S. M. Miller (Eds.), *Handbook of developmental psychopathology* (2nd ed., pp. 671–686). New York: Plenum Publishers.

Chapter 33

American Sleep Apnea Association. (2007, December). Treatment options for adults with obstructive sleep apnea. American Sleep Apnea Association. Retrieved June 1, 2009, from http://www.sleepapnea.org/resources/pubs/treatment.html

American Sleep Apnea Association. (2008). Sleep apnea fact sheet. Retrieved June 1, 2009, from http://www.sleepapnea.org/info/media/factsheet.html

Ball, E., & Caivano, C. K. (2008). Internal medicine: Guidance to the diagnosis and management of restless legs syndrome. *Southern Medical Journal, 101*(6), 631–634.

Beecroft, J. M., Ward, M., Younes, M., et al. (2008). Sleep monitoring in the intensive care unit: Comparison of nurse assessment, actigraphy and polysomnography. *Intensive Care Medicine, 34,* 2076–2083.

Birath, J. B., & Martin, J. L. (2007). Common sleep problems affecting older adults. *Annals of Long-Term Care, 12.* Retrieved June 6, 2009, from http://www.annalsoflongtermcare.com/article/8100

Bulechek, G., Butcher, H., & Dochterman, J. (Eds.). (2008). *Nursing interventions classification (NIC)* (5th ed.). St. Louis, MO: C. V. Mosby.

Chee, M. W., & Chuah, L. Y. (2008). Functional neuroimaging insights into how sleep and sleep deprivation affect memory and cognition. *Current Opinion in Neurology, 21*(4), 417–423.

Cmiel, C., Karr, D., Gasser, O., et al. (2004). Noise control: A nursing team's approach to sleep promotion. *American Journal of Nursing, 104*(2), 40–48.

Cohen, G. (2004). *American Academy of Pediatrics Guide to your child's sleep.* New York: Villard Books.

Cohen, S., Doyle, W. J., Alper, C. M., et al. (2009). Sleep habits and susceptibility to the common cold. *Annals of Family Medicine, 169*(1), 62–67.

Colten, H. R., & Altevogt, B. M. (2006). *Sleep disorders and sleep deprivation: An unmet public health problem,* Committee on Sleep Research. Washington, DC: National Academies Press.

Eguchi, K. (2008). Short sleep duration as an independent predictor of cardiovascular events in Japanese patients with hypertension. *Archives of Internal Medicine, 168*(20), 2225–2231.

Eliopoulos, C. (2004). *Gerontological nursing.* Philadelphia: Lippincott Williams & Wilkins.

Germann, W. J., & Stanfield, C. L. (2008). *Principles of human physiology* (3rd ed.). San Francisco: Benjamin Cummings.

Haesler, E. J. (2004). Effectiveness of strategies to manage sleep in residents of aged care facilities. *Joanna Briggs Institute Reports, 2*(4), 115–183. Retrieved May 28, 2009, from http://www.joannabriggs.edu.au/pubs/best_practice.php

Hening, W. A. (2007). Current guidelines and standards of practice for restless legs syndrome. *American Journal of Medicine*, 230(Supplement 1), S22–27.

Holcomb, S. S. (2006). Recommendations for assessing insomnia. *Nurse Practitioner*, 31(2), 55–60.

Holcomb, S. S. (2007). Putting insomnia to rest. *Nurse Practitioner*, 32(4), 28–34.

Hui, L., Hua, F., Diandong, H., et al. (2007). Effects of sleep and sleep deprivation on immunoglobulins and complement in humans. *Brain, Behavior, & Immunity*, 21(3), 308–310.

The Joanna Briggs Institute. (2004). Strategies to manage sleep in residents of aged care facilities. *Best Practice*, 8(3), 1–4.

Johnson, M., Bulechek, G., Butcher, H., et al. (2006). *NANDA, NOC, and NIC linkages* (2nd ed.). St. Louis, MO: C. V. Mosby.

Kazuo, E., Pickering, T. J., Phil, D., et al. (2008). Short sleep duration as an independent predictor of cardiovascular events in Japanese patients with hypertension. *Archives of Internal Medicine*, 168, 2225–2231.

Kryger, M. H., Roth, T., & Dement, W. C. (2005). *Principles and practice of sleep medicine* (4th ed.). Philadelphia: W. B. Saunders.

Lee-Chiong, T. (2008). *Sleep medicine: Essentials and review*. New York: Oxford University Press.

Lockley, S. W., Barger, L. K., Ayas, N. T., et al. (2007). Effects of health care provider work hours and sleep deprivation on safety and performance. *Joint Commission Journal on Quality & Patient Safety*, 33(11 Supplement), 7–18.

Marshall, N. S., Glazier, N., & Grunstein, R. R. (2008). Is sleep duration related to obesity? A critical review of the epidemiological evidence. *Sleep Medicine Review*, 12(4), 299–302.

McCance, K. L., & Huether, S. E. (2005). *Pathophysiology: The biologic basis for disease in adults and children* (5th ed.). St. Louis, MO: C. V. Mosby.

Moorhead, S., Johnson, M., & Maas, M., et al. (Eds.). (2008). *Nursing outcomes classification (NOC)* (4th ed.). St. Louis, MO: C. V. Mosby.

Mulcahy, N. (2009). Poor sleep before rhinovirus exposure linked to lower resistance to illness. *Medscape*. Retrieved May 12, 2009, from http://cme.medscape.com/viewarticle/586677

National Institutes of Health (NIH). (2007, December). Lack of sleep disrupts emotional controls. *NIH News in Health*. Retrieved June 2, 2009, from http://newsinhealth.nih.gov/pdf/NIHNiH%20December07.pdf

National Institutes of Health (NIH). (2009). Headaches and migraines. Retrieved May 29, 2009, from http://health.nih.gov/topic/HeadacheandMigraine

National Institute of Neurological Disorders and Stroke (NINDS). (2009). Narcolepsy fact sheet. National Institutes of Health. Retrieved May 29, 2009, from http://www.ninds.nih.gov/disorders/narcolepsy/detail_narcolepsy.htm

National Sleep Foundation. (n.d.). Restless leg syndrome (RLS) and sleep. Retrieved June 4, 2009, from http://www.sleepfoundation.org/article/sleep-related-problems/restless-legs-syndrome-rls-and-sleep

National Sleep Foundation. (n.d.). Shift work and sleep. Retrieved June 1, 2009, from http://www.sleepfoundation.org/article/sleep-topics/shift-work-and-sleep

National Sleep Foundation. (n.d.). Sleep studies. Retrieved December 8, 2009, from http://www.sleepfoundation.org/article/sleep-topics/sleep-studies

National Sleep Foundation. (2006). Sleep-wake cycle: Its physiology and impact on health. http://www.sleepfoundation.org/atf/cf/%7BF6BF2668–A1B4–4FE8–8D1A–A5D39340D9CB%7D/Sleep-Wake_Cycle.pdf

National Sleep Foundation. (2008). 2008 Sleep in America poll: Summary of findings. Retrieved June 1, 2009, from http://www.sleepfoundation.org/article/press-release/sleep-america-poll-summary-findings

Neubauer, D. N., & Roc, A. (2009). Pathophysiology and slow wave sleep. *Medscape*. Retrieved May 29, 2009, from http://cme.medscape.com/viewprogram/19011

Ong, J. C., Stepanski, E. J., & Gramling, S. E. (2009, February 15). Pain coping strategies for tension-type headache: Possible implications for insomnia. *Journal of Clinical Sleep Medicine*, 5(1), 52–56.

Oswald, I. (1984). Good, poor, and disordered sleep. In: R. G. Priest (Ed.), *Sleep: An international monograph*. London: Update Books.

Pizzorno, J. E., Murray, M. T., & Joiner-Bay, H. (2007). *The clinician's handbook of natural medicine*. St. Louis, MO: Elsevier.

Polan, E., & Taylor, D. (2007). *Journey across the life span* (2nd ed.). Philadelphia: F. A. Davis.

Ranjbaran, Z., Keefer, L., Stepanski, E., et al. (2007). The relevance of sleep abnormalities to chronic inflammatory conditions. *Inflammatory Resource*, 56, 51–57.

Roth, T., Roehrs, T., & Pies, R. (2007). Insomnia: Pathophysiology and implications for treatment. *Sleep Medicine Reviews*, 11(1), 71–79.

Smyth, C. A. (2008). Evaluating sleep quality in older adults. *American Journal of Nursing*, 108(5), 42–50.

Sorrentino, S. A., & Kelly, R. T. (2007). *Mosby's textbook for nursing assistants* (7th ed.). St. Louis, MO: C. V. Mosby.

Tuller, D. (2004, March 30). Poll finds even babies don't get enough rest. *New York Times*.

Chapter 34

3M. (2004, December). 3M surgical tapes and adhesive skin closures. Retrieved February 5, 2009, from http://solutions.3m.com/wps/portal/3M/en_US/wound-care/skin/

Agency for Healthcare Research and Quality. (2009, July). On-Time Pressure Ulcer Healing Project. Agency for Healthcare Research and Quality, Rockville, MD. Retrieved September 1, 2009, from http://www.ahrq.gov/research/pressurulcerhealing/

Armstrong, D. G., Attinger, C. E., Boulton, A. J., et al. (2004). Guidelines regarding negative pressure wound therapy (NPWT) in the diabetic foot: Results of the Tucson expert consensus Conference (TECC) on V.A.C. therapy. *Ostomy Wound Management*, 50(4 Supplement B), 3S-27S.

Armstrong, D. G., Ayello, E. A., Capitulo, K. L., et al. (2008). New opportunities to improve pressure ulcer prevention and treatment: Implications of the CMS inpatient hospital care present on admission indicators/hospital-acquired conditions policy—a consensus paper from the International Expert Wound Care Advisory Panel. *Advances in Skin Wound Care*, 21, 469–70, 472–478. Retrieved July 19, 2009, from http://www.medline.com/OpportunitiestoImprovePressureUlcerPreventionandTreatment.pdf

Association of periOperative Registered Nurses (AORN). (2008). Perioperative standards and recommended practices. Denver: AORN.

Atiyeh, B. S., & Hayek, S. N. (2004). An update on management of acute and chronic open wounds: The importance of moist environment on optimal wound healing. *Medicinal Chemistry Reviews*, 1, 111–121.

Autio, L., & Olsen, K. K. (2002). The four S's of wound management: Staples, sutures, steri-strips, and sticky stuff. *Holistic Nursing Practice*, 16(2), 80–88.

Ayello, E. A. (2007). Predicting pressure ulcer risk. *Try this: Best practices in nursing care of older adults*. The Hartford Institute for Geriatric Nursing, 5, 1–2.

Ayello, E. A., & Braden, B. (2002). How and why to do a pressure ulcer risk assessment. *Advances in Skin & Wound Care*, 15(3), 125–131.

Ayello, E. A., Cuddigan, J., & Kerstein, M. D. (2002). Skip the knife: Debriding wounds without surgery. *Nursing*, 32(9), 58–64.

Ayello, E. A., & Lyder, C. H. (2008). A new era of pressure ulcer accountability in acute care. *Advances in Skin & Wound Care*, 21(3), 134–140.

Ayello, E. A, & Sibbald, R. G. (2008, January). Preventing pressure ulcers and skin tears. In: E. Capezuti, D. Zwicker, M. Mezey, & T. Fulmer (Eds.), *Evidence-based geriatric nursing protocols for best practice* (3rd ed., pp. 403–429). New York: Springer.

Baranoski, S. (2008). Choosing a wound dressing, part 2. *Nursing2008*, 38(2), 14–15.

Bates-Jensen, B. M. (2007). Quality indicators for the care of pressure ulcers in vulnerable elders. *Journal of the American Geriatrics Society* (Supplement 2), S409–416.

Beam, J. W. (2006). Wound cleansing: water or saline? *Journal of Athletic Training, 41*(2), 196–197.

Bergeron, J. D., Bizjak, G., Le Badour, G., et al. (2009). *First responder* (8th ed.). Upper Saddle River, NJ: Prentice-Hall.

Bergstrom, N., Bennett, M. A., Carlson, C., et al. (1994). Treatment of pressure ulcers. Clinical practice guideline, No 15. Rockville, MD: U.S. Department of Health and Human Services, Public Health Service, Agency for Health Care Policy and Research. AHCPR Pub. No. 95–0622.

Bergstrom, N., Braden, B. J., Laguzza, A., et al. (1987). The Braden-scale for predicting pressure sore risk. *Nursing Research, 87*(36), 205–210.

Best practices: Evidence-based nursing procedures (2nd ed., pp. 59–62). Philadelphia: Lippincott Williams & Wilkins.

Bill, T. J., Ratliff, C. R., Donovan, A. M., et al. (2001). Quantitative swab culture versus tissue biopsy: A comparison in chronic wounds. *Ostomy Wound Management, 47*(1), 34–37.

Black, J., Baharestani, M., Cuddigan, J., et al. (2007a). National Pressure Ulcer Advisory Panel's Updated Pressure Ulcer Staging System. *Dermatology Nursing, 19*(4), 343–349.

Black, J., Baharestani, M., Cuddigan, J., et al. (2007b). National Pressure Ulcer Advisory Panel's Updated Pressure Ulcer Staging System. *Advances in Skin and Wound Care, 20*(5), 269–274.

Branom, R. (2002). Is this wound infected? *Critical Care Nursing Quarterly, 25*(1), 55–62.

Brown, G. (2003). Long-term outcomes of full-thickness pressure ulcers: Healing and mortality. *Ostomy Wound Management, 49*(10), 42–50.

Bryant, R. A., & Nix, D. P. (2006). *Acute and chronic wounds: Current management concepts,* (3rd ed., pp. 100–129). St. Louis, MO: C. V. Mosby Year Book.

Bulechek, F., Butcher, H., & Dochterman, J. (2008). *Nursing interventions classification (NIC).* (5th ed.). St. Louis, MO: C. V. Mosby.

Buss, I. C., Halfens, R. J. G., & Abu-Saad, H. H. (2002). The most effective time interval for repositioning subjects at risk of pressure sore development: A literature review. *Rehabilitation Nursing, 27*(2), 59–63.

Campbell, P. E., Smith, G. S., & Smith, J. M. (2008). Retrospective clinical evaluation of gauze-based negative pressure wound therapy. *International Wound Journal, 5,* 280–286.

Campton-Johnston, S. M., & Wilson, J. A. (2001). Infected wound management: Advanced technologies, moisture-retentive dressings, and die-hard methods. *Critical Care Nursing Quarterly, 24*(2), 64–77.

Centers for Medicare & Medicaid Services. (2004, November 14). Guidance to surveyors for long term care facilities. *CMS Manual System.* Department of Health and Human Services.

Chariker, M. (2009). Moisture balance: Exploring options in negative pressure wound therapy. *Skin and Wound Care, 22*(Supplement 1), 10–12.

Clay, K. S. (2008). *Evidenced-based pressure ulcer prevention: A study guide for nurses* (2nd ed.). Marblehead, MA: HCPro.

Cutting, K. F., & White, R. J. (2005, January). Criteria for identifying wound infection—revised. *Ostomy Wound Management, 51*(1), 28–34.

Dunaway, E., & Goldrick, B. A. (2007, July/August). Sternal wound infections: What every nurse should know. *OR Nurse Online,* 28–34.

Earthy, A. (2007). Updating current skin care practices. *Canadian Nursing Home, 18*(2), 4–7, 9–12.

European Pressure Ulcer Advisory Panel and National Pressure Ulcer Advisory Panel. (2009). Treatment of pressure ulcers: Quick reference guide. Washington, DC: National Pressure Ulcer Advisory Panel.

Fernandez, R., & Griffiths, R. (2007, November 2). Water for wound cleansing. *Cochrane Database of Systematic Reviews,* Issue 1. Art. No.: CD003861. DOI: 10.1002/14651858.CD003861.pub2. Retrieved June 11, 2009, from http://www.cochrane.org/reviews/en/ab003861.html

Fletcher, R. K. (1999). Physical and laboratory assessment. In: J. T. Stone, J. F. Wyman, & S. A. Salisbury (Eds.), *Clinical gerontological nursing: A guide to advanced practice* (2nd ed., pp. 85–128). Philadelphia: W. B. Saunders.

Franz, R. A. (2008). Identifying infection in chronic wounds. *Nursing2008, 37*(7), 73.

Gardner, S. E., & Frantz, R. A. (2004). Wound bioburden. In: S. Baranoski & E. A. Ayello (Eds.), *Wound care essentials: Practice principles.* (pp. 91–116). Springhouse, PA: Lippincott Williams & Wilkins.

Gardner, S. E., Frantz, R. A., Saltzman, C. L., et al. (2006). Diagnostic validity of three swab techniques for identifying chronic wound infection. *Wound Repair Regeneration, 14*(5), 548–557.

Gibson, M. C., Keast, D., Woodbury, M. G., et al. (2004). Educational intervention in the management of acute procedure-related wound pain: A pilot study. *Journal of Wound Care, 13*(5), 187–190.

Goldberg, M. T., & Tomaselli, N. L. (2006). Management of pressure ulcers and fungating wounds. In: A. Berger, R. K. Portenoy, & D. E. Weissman (Eds.), *Principles and practice of palliative care and supportive oncology* (periodicals) (3rd ed.). Philadelphia: Lippincott Williams & Wilkins.

Graff, M. K., Bryant, J., & Beinlich, N. (2000). Preventing heel breakdown. *Orthopedic Nursing, 19*(5), 63–69.

Gray, M., Ratliff, C., & Donovan, A. (2002). Perineal skin care for the incontinent patient. *Advances in Skin & Wound Care, 15*(4), 120–175.

Gupta, S. (2004). Guidelines for managing pressure ulcers with negative pressure wound therapy. *Advances in Skin and Wound Care, 17*(Supplement 2), 1–16.

Hanson, D. S., Langemo, D., Anderson, J., et al. (2005). Can pressure mapping prevent ulcers? *Nursing 2009, 29*(6), 50–51.

Harding, K. G., Morris, H. L., & Patel, G. K. (2002). Healing chronic wounds. *BMJ, 324*(7330), 160–163.

Hess, C. T. (2007). *Clinical guide: Skin and wound care.* Philadelphia: Lippincott, Williams & Wilkins.

Hess, C. T. (2008). Managing tissue loads. *Advances in Skin & Wound Care, 21*(3), 144.

Horrocks, A. (2006). Prontosan wound irrigation and gel: Management of chronic wounds. *British Journal of Nursing, 15*(22), 1222–1229.

Howard-Ruben, J. (2002). People who pierce—and the nurses who care for (and about) them. *American Journal of Nursing, 3*(8), 29–30.

Immunization Action Coaltition. (2007, reviewed 2009, February). Tetanus vaccine questions and answers. Reviewed by Centers for Disease Control and Prevention (CDC). Retrieved July 23, 2009, from http://www.vaccineinformation.org/tetanus/qandavax.asp

Institute for Clinical Systems Improvement (ICSI). (2007, March 31). Skin safety protocol: risk assessment and prevention of pressure ulcers. Health care protocol. Bloomington (MN): Institute for Clinical Systems Improvement (ICSI). Retrieved August 25, 2009, from http://www.guideline.gov/summary/summary.aspx?doc_id=13699&nbr=007033&string=skin+AND+safety+AND+protocol%3a

Institute for Clinical Systems Improvement (ICSI). (2008, January 28). Pressure ulcer treatment. Health care protocol. Bloomington (MN): Institute for Clinical Systems Improvement (ICSI). Retrieved August 25, 2009, from http://www.guideline.gov/summary/summary.aspx?view_id=1&doc_id=13698

The Joanna Briggs Institute. (2006). Solutions, techniques and pressure in wound cleansing. *Best Practice, 10*(2), 1–4.

The Joanna Briggs Institute. (2007). Topical skin care in aged care facilities. *Best Practice, 11*(3), 1–4.

The Joanna Briggs Institute. (2008a). Pressure ulcers: Management of pressure-related tissue damage. *Best Practice, 12*(3), 1–4.

The Joanna Briggs Institute. (2008b). Pressure ulcers: Prevention of pressure-related damage. *Best Practice, 12*(2), 1–4.

Jones, K. R., Fennie, K., & Lenihan, A. (2007). Evidence-based management of chronic wounds. *Advances in Skin and Wound Care, 20*(11), 591–600.

Junkin, J., & Selekof, J. (2008). Beyond "diaper rash": Incontinence-associated dermatitis. Does it have you seeing RED? *Nursing2008, 38*(11), 2–11.

Kaya, A. Z., Turani, N., & Akyuz, M. (2005). The effectiveness of a hydrogel dressing compared with standard management of pressure ulcers. *Journal of Wound Care, 14*(1), 42–44.

Kinetic Concepts Incorporated. (2007). *V.A.C. therapy clinical guidelines: A reference source for clinicians.* San Antonio, TX: KCI.

Kinetic Concepts Incorporated. (2008). *Basic V.A.C. dressing application pocket guide.* Retrieved February 10, 2009, from http://www.kci1.com/Pocket_Guide.pdf

Krapfl, L. A., & Gray, M. (2008). Does regular repositioning prevent pressure ulcers? *Journal of Wound Ostomy Continence Nursing, 35*(6), 572–577.

Krasner, D. L., Shapshak, D., & Hopf, H. W. (2007). Managing wound pain. In: R. A. Bryant & D. P. Nix (Eds.), *Acute and chronic wounds: Current management concepts* (3rd ed., pp. 539–565). St. Louis, MO: C. V. Mosby/Elsevier.

Kravitz, S. R., McGuire, J., & Shanahan, S. D. (2003). Physical assessment of the diabetic foot. *Advances in Skin & Wound Care, 16*(2), 68–75.

LaMorte, W. W. (2003). Basics of wound closure and healing. *Boston University School of Medicine.* Retrieved July 21, 2009, from http://www.bumc.bu.edu/generalsurgery/technical-training/suturing-basics/

Landis, S. J. (2008, November). Advances in skin and wound care. *The Journal for Prevention and Healing, 21*(11), 531–540.

Langemo, D., Anderson, J., Hanson, D., et al. (2008). Measuring wound length, width, and area: Which technique? *Advances in Skin and Wound Care, 21*(1), 42–45.

Leininger, S. M. (2002). The role of nutrition in wound healing. *Critical Care Nursing Quarterly, 25*(1), 13–21.

McGuckin, M., Goldman, R., Bolton, L., et al. (2003). The clinical relevance of microbiology in acute and chronic wounds. *Advances in Skin & Wound Care, 16*(1), 12–23.

Medica-Rents Co. (2008). *Prospera PRO-I: Negative pressure wound therapy.* Fort Worth, TX: Medica-Rents.

Meehan, M. (2009). Pressure ulcers: The stakes just got higher. *Nursing2009, 39*(10), 45–47.

Monahan, F. D., Sands, J. K., Marek, J. F., et al. (2006). *Phipps's Medical-surgical nursing: Health and illness perspectives* (8th ed.). St. Louis, MO: C. V. Mosby.

Moore, Z., & Cowman, S. (2007). Effective wound management: Identifying criteria for infection. *Nursing Standard, 21*, 24, 68–76.

Moorhead, S., Johnson, M., & Maas, M., et al. (Eds.). (2008). *Nursing outcomes classification (NOC)* (4th ed.). St. Louis, MO: C. V. Mosby.

Morykwas, M. J. (1997). Vacuum-assisted closure: A new method for wound control and treatment: Animal studies and basic foundation. *Annals of Plastic Therapy, 38*(6), 553–562.

Myer, J. S. (1997). Diabetes and wound healing. *Critical Care Nursing in North America, 8*(2), 195–201.

Myers, B. A. (2008). *Wound management: principles and practice* (2nd ed.). Upper Saddle River, NJ: Pearson Education.

NANDA International. (2009). *Nursing diagnoses: Definitions and classification 2009–2011.* Philadelphia: Author.

National Guideline Clearinghouse (NGC). (2006; revised December 2008). Guideline synthesis: Management and treatment of pressure ulcers. National Guideline Clearinghouse (NGC) [Web site]. Rockville, MD. Retrieved July 20, 2009, from http://www.guideline.gov/summary/summary.aspx?doc_id=11013&nbr=005793&string=Management+and+%22treatment+of+pressure+ulcers%22

National Pressure Ulcer Advisory Panel (NPUAP). (2002). PUSH Tool. Retrieved June 16, 2009, from http://www.npuap.org/pushins.htm

National Pressure Ulcer Advisory Panel (NPUAP). (2007a). NPUAP recommendation on measurement of wound area. *Inside the NPUAP,* Volume 21. Retrieved December 9, 2009, from http://www.npuap.org/Fall07.pdf

National Pressure Ulcer Advisory Panel (NPUAP). (2007b). Pressure ulcer stages revised by NPUAP. Retrieved June 16, 2009, from http://www.npuap.org/pr2.htm

National Pressure Ulcer Advisory Panel (NPUAP). (2007c). Terms and definitions related to support surfaces. Retrieved December 9, 2009, from http://www.npuap.org/NPUAP_S3I_TD.pdf

National Pressure Ulcer Advisory Panel (NPUAP). (2007d). Frequently asked questions. Retrieved December 9, 2009, from http://www.npuap.org/faq.htm

National Pressure Ulcer Advisory Panel (NPUAP). (2007e). Updated staging systems. Retrieved July 19, 2009, from http://www.npuap.org/pr2.htm

National Quality Forum. (2009). Pressure ulcer framework. Retrieved on March 22, 2010, from http://www.qualityforum.org/Projects/n-r/Pressure_Ulcer/Pressure_Ulcers.aspx

Nelson, D. B., & Dilloway, M. A. (2002). Principles, products, and practical aspects of wound care. *Critical Care Nursing Quarterly, 25*(1), 33–54.

Nix, D. P. (2007). *Patient assessment and evaluation of healing.* In: R. A. Bryant & D. P. Nix (Eds.), *Acute and chronic wounds: Current management concepts* (3rd ed., pp. 130–148). St. Louis, MO: C. V. Mosby/Elsevier.

Ovington, L. G. (2002). Hanging wet-to-dry dressings out to dry. *Advances in Skin & Wound Care, 15*(2), 79–84.

Pancorbo-Hidalgo, P. L. (2006). Risk assessment scales for pressure ulcer prevention: a systematic review. *Journal of Advanced Nursing, 54*(1), 94–110.

Panel for the Prediction and Prevention of Pressure Ulcers in Adults. (1992, May). *Pressure ulcers in adults: Prediction and prevention. Clinical Practice Guideline, No. 3.* AHRQ Pub. No. 92–0047. Rockville, MD: Agency for Health Care Policy and Research, Public Health Service, U.S. Department of Health and Human Services.

Park-Lee, E., Caffrey, C., & Division of Health Care Statistics. (2009, February). Pressure ulcers among nursing home residents: United States, 2004. Centers for Disease Control and Prevention (CDC). *HCHS Data Brief, 14.* Retrieved June 17, 2009, from http://www.cdc.gov/nchs/data/databriefs/db14.htm

Pervical, S. L., & Bowler, P. M. (2004). Biofilms and their potential role in wound healing. *Wounds, 16*(7). Retrieved July 16, 2009, from http://www.woundsresearch.com/article/2870

Pieper, B., Langemo, D., & Cuddigan, J. (2009). Pressure Ulcer Pain: A Systematic Literature Review and National Pressure Ulcer Advisory Panel White Paper. *Ostomy Wound Management, 55*(2). Retrieved February 11, 2009, from http://www.o-wm.com/content/pressure-ulcer-pain-a-systematic-literature-review-and-national-pressure-ulcer-advisory-panel

Pierce, G. F., Mustoe, T. A., Altrock, B. W., et al. (1991). Role of platelet-derived growth factor in wound healing. *Journal of Cell Biochemistry, 45*(4), 319–326.

Porth, C. M. (2004). *Pathophysiology: Concepts of altered health states* (7th ed.). Philadelphia: Lippincott Williams & Wilkins.

Registered Nurses Association of Ontario (RNAO). (2002, revised March, 2005). Risk assessment & prevention of pressure ulcers. Toronto (ON): Registered Nurses Association of Ontario (RNAO), 1–80.

Rolstad, B. S., & Ovington, L. G. (2007). Principles of wound management. In: R. A. Bryant & D. P. Nix (Eds.), *Acute and chronic wounds: Current management concepts* (3rd ed., pp. 391–426). St. Louis, MO: C. V. Mosby Elsevier.

Romanelli, M., Gaggio, G., Piaggesi, A., et al. (2002). Technological advances in wound bed measurements. *Wounds, 14*(2), 58–66.

Rosenberg, C. J. (2002). New checklist for pressure ulcer prevention. *Journal of Gerontological Nursing, 28*(8), 7–12.

Rosenthal, M. B. (2007). Nonpayment for performance? Medicare's new reimbursement rule. *New England Journal of Medicine, 357*(16), 1573–1575.

Rudolph, D. M. (2002). Why won't this wound heal? Understanding the causes of and interventions for chronic wounds. *American Journal of Nursing, 102*(2), 24dd–24hh.

Russo, C. A., Steiner, C., & Spector, W. (2008). Hospitalizations related to pressure ulcers among adults 18 and older, 2006. *HCUP Statistical Brief #64.* Rockville, MD: Agency for Healthcare Research and Quality. Retrieved July 20, 2009, from http://www.hcup-us.ahrq.gov/reports/statbriefs/sb64.pdf

Samson, D., Lefevre, F., & Aronson, N. (2004). Wound-Healing Technologies: Low-Level Laser and Vacuum-Assisted Closure. Summary, Evidence Report/Technology Assessment: Number 111. AHRQ Publication Number 05-E005-1, December 2004. Agency for Healthcare Research and Quality, Rockville, MD. Retrieved December 9, 2009, from http://www.ahrq.gov/clinic/epcsums/woundsum.htm

Sherman, R. A. (2002). Maggot therapy for foot and leg wounds. *The International Journal of Lower Extremity Wounds, 1*(2), 135–142.

Retrieved February 11, 2009, from http://ijl.sagepub.com/cgi/content/abstract/1/2/135

Shore, J. T., Gabriel, A., & Gupta, S. (2007). Skin substitutes and alternatives: A review. *Advances in Skin & Wound Care, 20*(9), 493–508.

Sibbald, R. G., Orsted, H. L., Coutts, P. M., et al. (2007). Best practice recommendations for preparing the wound bed: Update 2006. *Advances in Skin and Wound Care, 20*(7), 390–407.

Siegel, J. D., Rhinehart, E., Jackson, M., et al., & the Healthcare Infection Control Practices Advisory Committee. (2007, June). 2007 Guideline for isolation precautions: preventing transmission of infectious agents in healthcare settings, Retrieved July 15, 2009, from http://www.cdc.gov/ncidod/dhqp/gl_isolation.html

Silverstein, P. (1992). Smoking and wound healing. *American Journal of Medicine, 93*(1A), 22S–24S.

Slatchta, P. A. (2008, July). Caring for chronic wounds: A knowledge update. *American Nurse Today, 3*(7), 27–32.

Stotts, N. A., & Gunningberg, L. (2007). Predicting pressure ulcer risk, using the Braden scale with hospitalized older adults; the evidence supports it. *American Journal of Nursing, 107*(11), 40–49.

Sullivan, N., Snyder, D. L., Tipton, K., et al. (2009, May 26). Negative pressure wound therapy devices: Technology assessment report. Agency for Healthcare Research and Quality, Rockville, MD: U.S. Department of Health and Human Services. Retrieved July 21, 2009, from http://www.ahrq.gov/clinic/ta/negpresswtd/negpresswtd.pdf

Sussman, C., & Bates-Jensen, B. M. (2007). *Wound care: A collaborative practice manual for health care professionals* (3rd ed.). Gaithersburg, MD: Aspen.

U.S. Department of Health and Human Services. (2010). Healthy People 2020 public meetings: 2009 draft objectives. Retrieved March 29, 2010, from http://www.healthypeople.gov/HP2020/

U.S. Department of Health and Human Services (USDHHS). (2000). *Healthy people 2010: Understanding and improving health* (conference edition), Volume 1. Washington, DC: U.S. Government Printing Office.

VanRijswijk, L. (2009, August). Pressure ulcer prevention updates. *American Journal of Nursing, 109*(8), 56.

Whitney, J. D., & Heitkemper, M. M. (1999). Modifying perfusion, nutrition, and stress to promote wound healing in patients with acute wounds. *Heart and Lung, 28*(2), 123–133.

Wooten, M. K., Hawkins, K., for the WOCN Council and the APIC 2000 Guidelines Committee. (updated 2005). WOCN position statement clean versus sterile: Management of chronic wounds. Wound, Ostomy and Continence Nurses Society and the Association for Professionals in Infection Control and Epidemiology. Retrieved July, 22, 2009, from http://www.wocn.org/pdfs/WOCN_Library/Position_Statements/clvst.pdf

Wound, Ostomy and Continence Nurses Society (WOCN). (2007). Position statement: Pressure ulcer staging. Mount Laurel, NJ: Wound, Ostomy and Continence Nurses Society (WOCN), 52.

Wright, K., & O'Connor, A. D. (2007). Causes and risks of pressure sores. *Nursing in Residential Care, 16*(11), 518, 520–523.

Wysocki, A. B. (2002). Evaluating and managing open skin wounds: Colonization versus infection. AACN Clinical Issues: *Advanced Practice in Acute Critical Care, 13*(3), 383–397.

Zulkowski, K., & Gray-Leach, K. (2009). Staging pressure ulcers: What's the buzz in wound care? *American Journal of Nursing, 109*(1), 27–28.

Chapter 35

American Academy of Pediatrics Committee on Infectious Diseases, (2008). Prevention of influenza. Recommendations for influenza immunizations of children 2008–2009. *Pediatrics* 2008, *122*(5), 1135–1141. National Guideline Clearinghouse (NGC) [Web site]. Rockville, MD. Retrieved May 19, 2009, from http://www.guide-line.gov/summary/summary.aspx?view_id=1&doc_id=13435

American Association of Critical-Care Nurses (AACN). (2005). *AACN procedure manual for critical care* (5th ed.). Philadelphia: W. B. Saunders.

American Association of Critical-Care Nurses (AACN). (2007). AACN practice alert. Oral care in the critically ill. Retrieved December 18, 2008, from http://classic.aacn.org/AACN/practiceAlert.nsf/Files/OC/$file/Oral%20Care%20in%20the%20Critically%20Ill%20.pdf

American Association of Critical-Care Nurses (AACN). (2008a). AACN practice alert. Ventilator associated pneumonia. Retrieved May 19, 2009, from http://www.aacn.org/WD/Practice/Docs/Ventilator_Associated_Pneumonia_1–2008.pdf

American Association of Critical-Care Nurses (AACN). (2008b). AACN practice alert. Dysrhythmia monitoring. Retrieved May 19, 2009, from http://www.aacn.org/WD/Practice/Docs/Dysrhythmia_Monitoring_04–2008.pdf

American Association for Respiratory Care. (2004a). AARC clinical practice guideline. Nasotracheal suctioning—2004 revision and update, 2004. Retrieved June 1, 2009, from http://www.rcjournal.com/cpgs/pdf/09.04.1080.pdf

American Association for Respiratory Care. (2004b). AARC clinical practice guideline: Resuscitation and defibrillation in the health care setting. *Respiratory Care, 49*(9), 1085–1099.

American Cancer Society (2009). American Cancer Society guidelines for the early detection of cancer. Retrieved December 13, 2009, from http://www.cancer.org/docroot/PED/content/PED_2_3X_ACS_Cancer_Detection_Guidelines_36.asp?sitearea=PED

American Heart Association (AHA). (2005). 2005 American Heart Association guidelines for cardiopulmonary resuscitation and emergency cardiovascular care: International consensus on science. Part 3: Overview of CPR; Part 4: Adult basic life support; Part 5: Electrical therapies: automated external defibrillators, defibrillation, cardioversion, and pacing; Part 7.1: *Circulation 112*(24 Supplement): IV-12–57. Retrieved June 9, 2009, from http://circ.aha-journals.org/content/vol112/24_Supplement/

American Heart Association (AHA). (2008). Hands Only™ CPR. Retrieved May 22, 2009, from http://handsonlycpr.eisenberginc.com/

American Heart Association (AHA). (2009a). Cigarette smoking and cardiovascular diseases. Retrieved May 20, 2009, from http://www.americanheart.org/presenter.jhtml?identifier=4545

American Heart Association (AHA). (2009b). Medications commonly used to treat heart failure. Retrieved May 23, 2009, from http://www.americanheart.org/presenter.jhtml?identifier=118

American Lung Association (ALA). (2009a). Quit smoking. Smoking and teens fact sheet. Retrieved May 5, 2009, from http://www.lungusa.org/site/c.dvLUK9O0E/b.39871/

American Lung Association (ALA). (2009b). Secondhand smoke fact sheet. Retrieved May 23, 2009, from http://www.lungusa.org/site/c.dvLUK9O0E/b.35422/k.7D0B/Secondhand_Smoke_Fact_Sheet.htm

American Lung Association (ALA). (2008a). Tobacco use. Retrieved May 5, 2009, from http://www.lungusa.org/atf/cf/{7a8d42c2–fcca-4604–8ade-7f5d5e762256}/ALA_LDD08_TOBUSE_FINAL.PDF

American Lung Association (ALA). (2008b). Asthma & Allergy: Peak flow meters. Retrieved May 21, 2009, from http://www.lungusa.org/site/pp.asp?c=dvLUK9O0E&b=22586

American Lung Association (ALA). (2002a). The asthma handbook. Retrieved July 4, 2009, from http://www.alaw.org/asthma/asthma_management/asthma_handbook

American Thoracic Society (n.d.). Care of the child with a chronic tracheostomy: Components of tracheostomy care: Suctioning. Retrieved May 28, 2009, from http://www.thoracic.org/sections/education/care-of-the-child-with-a-chronic-tracheostomy/components-of-tracheostomy-care/suctioning.html

American Thoracic Society and the Infectious Diseases Society of America. (2005). Guidelines for the management of adults with hospital-acquired, ventilator-associated, and healthcare-associated pneumonia. *American Journal of Respiratory and Critical Care Medicine, 171*, 388–416.

Barnett, M. (2005). Tracheostomy management and care. *Journal of Community Nursing, 19*(1), 4–8.

(2007). *Best practices: Evidence-based nursing procedures* (2nd ed., pp. 59–62). Philadelphia: Lippincott Williams & Wilkins.

Birmingham East and North Primary Care Trust. (2006). Oral and tracheostomy suctioning policy. Retrieved May 28, 2009, from http://www.bpcssa.nhs.uk/policies/_ben%5Cpolicies%5C607.pdf

Booker, R. (2008). Pulse oximetry. *Nursing Standard, 22*(30), 39–41.

Bozyk, P., & Hyzy, R. (2008). Modes of mechanical ventilation. *UpToDate for Patients.* [web site] Retrieved June 5, 2009, from http://www.uptodate.com/patients/content/topic.do?topicKey=~yKvPqf2EgC44W#1

Bulechek, G., Butcher, H., & Dochterman, J. (2008). *Nursing interventions classification (NIC)* (5th ed.). St. Louis, MO: C. V. Mosby.

California Department of Public Health. (2007). Guidelines for collecting and shipping specimens for influenza A (H5N1) Diagnostics. Retrieved May 23, 2009, from http://www.co.fresno.ca.us/uploadedFiles/Departments/Public_Health/Divisions/CH/content/CD/content/Diseases/Avian_Flu/H5N1specimencollectionguidelines08.13.07%5B1%5D.pdf

Centers for Disease Control and Prevention (CDC). (2009a). CDC estimates of 2009 H1N1 influenza cases, hospitalizations and deaths in the United States, April–November 14, 2009. Retrieved December 17, 2009, from http://www.cdc.gov/h1n1flu/estimates_2009_h1n1.htm

Centers for Disease Control and Prevention (CDC). (2009b). 2009 H1N1 and seasonal flu: What you should know about flu antiviral drugs. Retrieved December 17, 2009, from http://www.cdc.gov/H1N1flu/antivirals/geninfo.htm#box

Centers for Disease Control and Prevention (CDC)/NCHS. (2008). Health, United States, 2008. In: FastStats, Centers for Disease Control and Prevention (CDC), U.S. Department of Health and Human Services. Retrieved May 5, 2009, from http://www.cdc.gov/nchs/fastats/smoking.htm

Centers for Disease Control and Prevention (CDC). (2009). Recommended adult immunization schedule—United States, 2009. QuickGuide. *MMWR, 57*(53), Q1–Q4. Retrieved May 9, 2009, from http://www.cdc.gov/mmwr/PDF/wk/mm5753-Immunization.pdf

Centers for Disease Control and Prevention (CDC). (2008a). Cold and cough medicines: Information for parents. Atlanta, GA. Retrieved May 20, 2009, from http://www.cdc.gov/features/pediatric-ColdMeds/

Centers for Disease Control and Prevention (CDC). (2008b). Respiratory syncytial virus infection (RSV). Infection and incidence. Retrieved July 2, 2009, from http://www.cdc.gov/rsv/about/infection.html

Centers for Disease Control and Prevention (CDC). (2004). Guidelines for preventing health-care-associated pneumonia, 2003. *MMWR, 53*, 1–36.

Clark, A., Giuliano, K., & Chen, H. (2006). Pulse oximetry revisited: "But his O_2 sat was normal!" *Clinical Nurse Specialist, 20*(6), 268–262.

Cleveland Clinic. (2005). Tracheal suction guidelines. Retrieved May 28, 2009, from http://my.clevelandclinic.org/services/tracheostomy/hic_tracheal_suction_guidelines.aspx

Coffin, W., Klompas, M., Classen, D., et al. & the Healthcare-Associated Infections Task Force. (2008). Guideline Summary: Strategies to prevent ventilator-associated pneumonia in acute care hospitals. *Infection Control and Hospital Epidemiology, 29*(Supplement 1), S31–S40. National Guideline Clearinghouse (NGC) [Web site]. Rockville, MD. Retrieved May 19, 2009, from http://www.guideline.gov/summary/summary.aspx?ss=15&doc_id=13396&nbr=&string=

D'Arcy, Y. (2007). Eyeing capnography to improve PCA safety. *Nursing2007, 37*(9), 18–19.

Dawood, N., Vaccarino, V., Reid, K., et al. (2008). Predictors of smoking cessation after a myocardial infarction. The role of institutional smoking cessation programs in improving success. *Archives of Internal Medicine, 168*(18), 1961–1967. Retrieved May 16, 2009, from http://archinte.ama-assn.org/cgi/content/short/168/18/1961

Dennis-Rouse, M. D., & Davidson, J. E. (2008). An evidence-based evaluation of tracheostomy care practices. *Critical Care Nursing Quarterly, 31*(2), 150–160.

Devereaux, T., & Nativio, D. (2007). Smoking cessation. A protocol for adolescents. *Advance for Nurse Practitioners, 15*(7), 35–36, 41–44.

Dillon, P. (2007). *Nursing health assessment: A critical thinking, case studies approach* (2nd ed.). Philadelphia: F. A. Davis.

Dufault, M., Davis, B., Garman, D., et al. (2008). Translating best practices in assessing capillary refill. *Worldviews on Evidence-Based Nursing, 5*(1), 36–44.

Eisner, M. (2009). Passive smoking and cognitive impairment. *BMJ, 338*, a3070. Retrieved May 16, 2009, from http://www.bmj.com/cgi/content/extract/338/feb12_2/a3070

Fiore, A., Shay, D., Broder, K., et al. (2008). Prevention and control of influenza. Recommendations of the Advisory Committee on Immunization Practices (ACIP), 2008. *Morbidity and Mortality Weekly Report, 57*(RR07), 1–60. Retrieved May 9, 2009, from http://www.cdc.gov/mmwr/preview/mmwrhtml/rr57e717a1.htm

Fiore, M., Jaén, C., Baker, T., et al. (2008). Treating tobacco use and dependence: 2008 update. Clinical Practice Guideline. Rockville, MD: U.S. Department of Health and Human Services. Public Health Service. Retrieved May 16, 2009, from http://www.surgeongeneral.gov/tobacco/treating_tobacco_use08.pdf

Garza, A., Gratton, M., Salomone, J., et al. (2009). Improved patient survival using a modified resuscitation protocol for out-of-hospital cardiac arrest. *Circulation.* DOI: 10.1161/CIRCULATIONAHA.108/815621. Retrieved May 22, 2009, from http://circ.ahajournals.org

Goodrich, C. (2006). Continuous central venous oximetry monitoring. *Critical Care Nursing Clinics of North America, 18*(2), 203–209.

Green, C. (2000). *Critical thinking in nursing: Case studies across the curriculum.* Upper Saddle River, NJ: Prentice-Hall Health.

Gulanick, M., Myers, J. L., Klopp, A., et al. (2003). *Nursing care plans: Nursing diagnosis and intervention* (5th ed.). St. Louis, MO: C. V. Mosby.

Guyton, A. C., & Hall, J. E. (2006). *Textbook of medical physiology* (11th ed.). New York: Saunders.

Hazinski, M. F., Nadkarni, V. M., Hickey, R. W., et al. (2005). Major changes in the 2005 AHA guidelines for CPR and ECC: reaching the tipping point for change. *Circulation, 112*, IV-206-IV-211. [online] http://circ.ahajournals.org/cgi/content/full/112/24_Supplement/IV-206

Hemilä, H., Chalker, E., Treacy, B., et al. (2007). Vitamin C for preventing and treating the common cold. *Cochrane Database of Systematic Reviews*, Issue 3. Art. No.: CD000980. DOI: 10.1002/14651858CD000980.pub3. Retrieved May 18, 2009, from http://www.mrw.interscience.wiley.com/cochrane/clsysrev/articles/CD000980/frame.html

Herbal solution hastens resolution of common cold. (2008). Evidence-based medicine. *The Clinical Advisor, 11*(5), 110.

Hess, D. (2005). Tracheostomy tubes and related appliances. *Respiratory Care, 50*(4), 497–510.

Hill, E., & Stoneham, M. (2000). Practical applications of pulse oximetry. *Update in Anaesthesia, 11*(4). Retrieved June 15, 2009, from http://www.nda.ox.ac.uk/wfsa/html/u11/u1104_01.htm

Hockenberry, M., & Wilson, D. (2007). *Wong's nursing care of infants and children* (8th ed.). St. Louis, MO: C. V. Mosby.

Hunt, S. A., Baker, D. W., Chin, M. H., et al. (2005). ACC/AHA 2005 guidelines for the diagnosis and management of chronic heart failure in the adult. A report of the American College of Cardiology/American Heart Association Task Force on Practice Guidelines (Writing Committee to update the 2001 guidelines for the Evaluation and Management of Heart Failure). *Journal of the American College of Cardiology, 46*, e1–e82. Retrieved May 23, 2009, from http://content.onlinejacc.org/cgi/reprint/46/6/e1.pdf

Jarvis, C. (2007). *Physical examination and health assessment* (5th ed.). Philadelphia: W. B. Saunders.

The Joanna Briggs Institute. (2008). Evidence based information sheets for health professionals. Smoking cessation interventions and strategies. *Best Practice, 12*(8), 1–4.

The Joanna Briggs Institute. (2000). Tracheal suctioning of adults with an artificial airway. *Best Practice, 4*(4), 1–6.

Johnston, J., Davis, S., & Sherman, J. (n.d.). Care of the child with a chronic tracheostomy. In: American Thoracic Society [Web site]. Retrieved May 27, 2009, from http://www.thoracic.org/sections/education/care-of-the-child-with-a-chronic-tracheostomy/index.html

Kellum, M., Kennedy, K., & Ewy, G. (2006). Cardiocerebral resuscitation improves survival of patients with out-of-hospital cardiac arrest. *American Journal of Medicine, 119*, 335–340.

Kennedy, S. (2007). Detecting changes in the respiratory status of ward patients. *Nursing Standard, 21*(40), 42–46.

Kidd, P. S., & Wagner, K. D. (2005). *High acuity nursing* (4th ed.). Upper Saddle River, NJ: Prentice-Hall.

Kligfield, P., Leonard, S. G., Bailey, J. J., et al. (2007). Recommendations for the standardization and interpretation of the electrocardiogram. Part I: The Electrocardiogram and its technology. *Circulation, 115*, 1306–1324 [online] http://circ.ahajournals.org/cgi/content/full/115/10/1306?maxtoshow=&HITS=10&hits=10&RESULTFORMAT=&fulltext=EKG+placement+in+the+clinical+setting&searchid=1&FIRSTINDEX=0&resourcetype=HWCIT

Kuriakose, A. (2008). Using the synergy model as best practice in endotracheal tube suctioning of critically ill patients. *Dimensions of Critical Care Nursing, 27*(1), 10–15.

Kuriyama, S., Shimazu, T., Ohmori, K., et al. (2007). Green tea consumption and mortality due to cardiovascular disease, cancer, and all causes in Japan: The Ohsaki study. *JAMA, 296*(10), 1255–1265.

Lackner, T. E., Hamilton, G., Hill, J., et al. (2003). Pneumococcal polysaccharide revaccination: Immunoglobulin G seroconversion, persistence, and safety in frail, chronically ill older subjects. *Journal of the American Geriatric Society, 51*(2), 240–245.

Lazzara, D. (2002). Eliminate the air of mystery from chest tubes. *Nursing2002, 32*(6), 36–45.

Lehne, R. A. (2006). *Pharmacology for nursing care* (5th ed.). New York: W. B. Saunders.

Lewarski, J. (2005). Long-term care of the patient with a tracheostomy. *Respiratory Care, 50*(4), 534–537.

Lewis, S. M., Heitkemper, M. M., Dirksen, S. R., et al. (2007). *Medical surgical nursing: Assessment and management of clinical problems* (7th ed.). St. Louis, MO: C. V. Mosby.

Lilley, L. L., & Aucker, R. S. (2007). *Pharmacology and the nursing process* (5th ed.). St. Louis, MO: C. V. Mosby.

Linde, K., Barrett, B., Bauer, R., et al. (2006). Echinacea for preventing and treating the common cold. *Cochrane Database of Systematic Reviews*, Issue 1. Art. No.: CD000530. DOI: 10.1002/14651858.CD000530.pub2.

Lipkus, I. M., McBride, C. M., Pollak, K. I., et al. (2004). A randomized trial comparing the effects of self-help materials and proactive telephone counseling on teen smoking cessation. *Health Psychology, 23*(4), 397–406.

Llewellyn, D., Lang, I., Langa, K., et al. (2009). Exposure to second-hand smoke and cognitive impairment in non-smokers: National cross-sectional study with cotinine measurement. *BMJ, 338*, b462. Retrieved May 16, 2009, from http://www.bmj.com/cgi/content/abstract/338/feb12_2/b462

McCance, K. L., & Huether, S. E. (2006). *Pathophysiology: The biologic basis for disease in adults and children* (5th ed.). St. Louis, MO: C. V. Mosby.

Moorhead, S., Johnson, M., Maas, M., et al. (2008). *Nursing outcomes classification (NOC)* (4th ed.). St. Louis, MO: C. V. Mosby.

Morrow, B., & Argent, A. (2008). A comprehensive review of pediatric endotracheal suctioning: Effects, indications, and clinical practice. *Pediatric Critical Care Medicine, 9*(5), 465–477.

Moser, D. (2007). "The rust of life": Impact of anxiety on cardiac patients. *American Journal of Critical Care, 16*, 361–369.

Munro, C., Grap, M., Jones, D., et al. (2009). Chlorhexidine, toothbrushing, and preventing ventilator-associated pneumonia in critically ill adults. *American Journal of Critical Care, 18*, 425–437.

Murry, R. B., Zentner, J. P., & Yakimo, R. (2009). *Health promotion strategies through the life span* (8th ed.). Upper Saddle River, NJ: Prentice-Hall.

Mutchner, L. (2007). The ABCs of CPR again. *American Journal of Nursing, 107*(1), 60–70.

Nagao, K. (2007). Cardiopulmonary resuscitation by bystanders with chest compression only (SOS-KANTOL): An observational study. *The Lancet, 369*, 920–926.

Nainggolan, L., & Bega, C. (2008). Smoking cessation must not be an afterthought, new studies say. Medical News. Medscape CME. Retrieved May 30, 2009, from http://cme.medscape.com/viewarticle/582058

NANDA International. (2009). *NANDA nursing diagnoses: Definitions and classifications 2009–2011.* Ames, IA: Wiley-Blackwell.

National Guideline Clearinghouse (NGC). (2008). Guideline synthesis: Tobacco use cessation and prevention. In: National Guideline Clearinghouse (NGC) [Web site]. Rockville, MD. 2001 July 29 (revised October 2008). Retrieved May 16, 2009, from http://www.guideline.gov/Compare/comparison.aspx?file5TOBACCO9.inc

National Institutes of Health Panel. (2001). Third report of the National Cholesterol Education Program (NCEP) Expert Panel on Detection, Evaluation, and Treatment of High Cholesterol in Adults (Adult Treatment Panel III). NIH Publication No. 01–3670. Bethesda, MD: National Institutes of Health.

National Institutes of Health (NIH). (2000). Critical Care Therapy and Respiratory Care Section: Airway suctioning and the use of the Ballard closed tracheal suctioning system. Bethesda, MD: National Institutes of Health, Critical Care Medicine Department. Retrieved May 31, 2009, from http://www.cc.nih.gov/ccmd/cctrcs/pdf_docs/Airway%20Management/01–airway-suctioning-bal.pdf

Ontario Agency for Health Protection and Promotion. (2008). Specimen collection guide – Specimen collection details. Public Health Laboratories. Retrieved May 23, 2009, from http://www.health.gov.on.ca/english/providers/pub/labs/specimen_guide/specimen_collection_details.pdf

Paul, I., Beiler, J., McMonagle, A., et al. (2007). Effect of honey, dextromethorphan, and no treatment on nocturnal cough and sleep quality for coughing children and their parents. *Archives of Pediatrics & Adolescent Medicine, 161*(12), 1140–1146.

Pease, P. (2006). Oxygen administration: Is practice based on evidence? *Paediatric Nursing, 18*(8), 14-8.

Pierson, D., Epstein, S., Durbin, C. Jr., et al. (2005). Symposium: Tracheostomy from A to Z. *Respiratory Care, 50*(4), 473–559.

Porth, C. M. (2008). *Pathophysiology: Concepts of altered states* (8th ed.). New York: Lippincott Williams & Wilkins.

Rajkumar, A., Karmarkar, A., & Knott, J. (2006). Pulse oximetry: An overview. *Journal of Perioperative Practice, 16*(10), 502–504.

Ramsay, J., & Hoffmann, A. (2004). Smoking cessation and relapse prevention among undergraduate students: A pilot demonstration project. *Journal of American College Health, 53*(1), 11–18.

Rauen, C., Chulay, M., Bridges, E., et al. (2008). Seven evidence-based practice habits: Putting some sacred cows out to pasture. *Critical Care Nurse, 28*(2), 98–124.

Rice, V., & Stead, L. (2008). Nursing interventions for smoking cessation. *Cochrane Database of Systematic Reviews*, Issue 1. Art. No.: CD001188. DOI: 10.1002/14651858.CD001188.pub3. Retrieved May 16, 2009, from http://www.cochrane.org/reviews/en/ab001188.html

Rigotti, N., Munafo, M., & Stead, L. (2008). Smoking cessation interventions for hospitalized smokers. A systematic review. *Archives of Internal Medicine, 168*(18), 1950–1960.

Roberts, J. (2004). *Clinical procedures in emergency medicine* (4th ed.). St. Louis, MO: W. B. Saunders.

Roberts, K., Whalley, H., & Bleetman, A. (2005). The nasopharyngeal airway: dispelling myths and establishing the facts. *Emergency Medicine Journal, 22*, 394–396.

Rodden, A., Spicer, L., Diaz, V., et al. (2007). Does fingernail polish affect pulse oximeter readings? *Intensive & Critical Care Nursing, 23*(1), 51–55.

Roman, M., & Mercado, D. (2006). Review of chest tube use. *MedSurg Nursing, 15*(1), 41–43.

Rushing, J. (2007). Managing a water-seal chest drainage unit. *Nursing2006, 37*(12), 12.

Sayre, M., Berg, R., Cave, D., et al. (2008). Hands-only (compression-only) cardiopulmonary resuscitation: A call to action for bystander response to adults who experience out-of-hospital sudden cardiac arrest: A science advisory for the public from the American Heart Association Emergency Cardiovascular Care Committee. *Circulation, 117*, 2162–2167. Retrieved June 11, 2009, from http://circ.ahajournals.org/cgi/reprint/CIRCULATIONAHA.107.189380

Scanlon, V. C., & Sanders, T. (2007). *Essentials of anatomy and physiology* (5th ed.). Philadelphia: F. A. Davis.

Schick, S., & Glantz, S. (2005). Philip Morris toxicological experiments with fresh sidestream smoke: More toxic than mainstream smoke. *Tobacco Control, 14*(6), 396–404. Retrieved May 5, 2009, from http://www.pubmedcentral.nih.gov/articlerender.fcgi?artid=1748121

Shiao, S-Y. & Ou, C-N. (2007). Validation of oxygen saturation monitoring in neonates. *American Journal of Critical Care, 16*(5), 428–429.

Shields, M., Bush, A., Everard, M., et al. (2008). BTS guidelines: Recommendations for the assessment and management of cough in children. *Thorax, 63*(Supplement 3), iii1 – iii15.

Siegel, J., Rhinehart, E., Jackson, M., et al. and the Healthcare Infection Control Practices Advisory Committee. (2007). 2007 Guideline for isolation precautions: Preventing transmission of infectious agents in healthcare settings. Retrieved May 27, 2009, from http://www.cdc.gov/ncidod/dhqp/pdf/guidelines/Isolation2007.pdf

Sierpina, V. S. (2001). *Integrative health care: Complementary and alternative therapies for the whole person.* Philadelphia: F. A. Davis.

Smith, G., Vijaykrishna, D., Bahl, J., et al. (2009). Origins and evolutionary genomics of the 2009 swine-origin H1N1 influenza A epidemic. *Nature, 459*, 1122–1125.

Stich, J., & Cassella, D. (2009). Getting inspired about oxygen delivery devices. *Nursing2009, 39*(9), 51–54.

Tablan, O., Anderson, L., Besser, R., et al. (2004). Guidelines for preventing healthcare-associated pneumonia, 2003. Recommendations of CDC and the Healthcare Infection Control Practices Advisory Committee. *MMWR, 53*(RR03), 1–36. Retrieved May 19, 2009, from http://www.cdc.gov/mmwr/preview/mmwrhtml/rr5303a1.htm

Texas Department of State Health Services. Laboratory Services Section Home (2009). Guidelines for specimen collection and submission: Mycobacteriology (AFB) collection, transport, and storage. Retrieved May 23, 2009, from http://www.dshs.state.tx.us/LAB/myco_guidelines.shtm

Thille, A., Rodriguez, P., Cabello, B., et al. (2006). Patient-ventilatory asynchrony during assisted mechanical ventilation. *Intensive Care Medicine, 32*(10), 1515–1522.

Thompson, L. (2000). Suctioning adults with an artificial airway. The Joanna Briggs Institute for Evidence Based Nursing and Midwifery. Systematic Review No. 9, 4(4), 1–6. ISSN 1329–1874.

United States Department of Health and Human Services. (2000). *Healthy People 2010* (conference edition in two volumes). Washington, DC: U.S. Government Printing Office.

U.S. Food and Drug Administration/Consumer Health Information. (2008). Using over-the-counter cough and cold products in children. Retrieved May 20, 2009, from http://www.fda.gov/z consumer/updates/coughcold102208.pdf

Vandenberg, J., Lutz, R., & Vinson, D. (1999). Large-diameter suction system reduces oropharyngeal evacuation time. *The Journal of Emergency Medicine, 17*(6), 941–944.

Vandenberg, J., & Vinson, D. (1999). The inadequacies of contemporary oropharyngeal suction. *American Journal of Emergency Medicine, 17*(6), 611–613.

Walters, T. (2007). Pulse oximetry knowledge and its effects on clinical practice. *British Journal of Nursing, 16*(21), 1332–1340.

Wong, D. L., Perry, S. E., Hockenberry M. F., et al. (2006). *Maternal-child nursing care* (3rd ed.). St. Louis, MO: C. V. Mosby.

Zimmerman, P. (2008). Minimally interrupted cardiac resuscitation. *American Journal of Nursing, 108*(10), 73–74.

Chapter 36

AABB. (2004). Facts about blood and blood banking. Retrieved April 25, 2009, from http://www.aabb.org/Content/About_Blood/Facts_About_Blood_and_Blood_Banking/fablood.htm

AABB. (2008a). FAQ. Retrieved February 28, 2009, from http://www.aabb.org/Content/About_Blood/FAQ/bloodfaq.htm

AABB. (2008b). Blood Management: Options for Better Patient Care. MD: AABB.

Ainsman, S. (2008, October 2). *Emergency clinical guide: ABGs.* Retrieved April 25, 2009, from http://www.anisman.com/ecg/index.asp?mainpage=abg.htm

American Medical Directors Association (AMDA). (2001, reviewed 2007). Guideline: Dehydration and fluid maintenance. American Medical Directors Association. Retrieved January 2, 2009, from http://www.guidelines.gov

Anderson, K. (2008). Clinical uses of brain naturetic peptide in diagnosing and managing heart failure. *Journal of the American Academy of Nurse Practitioners, 20*(6), 305–310.

The Association of periOperative Registered Nurses (AORN). (2009). *Safe environment of care, Recommendation XVI, Perioperative standards and recommended practices* (pp. 431–432). Denver, CO: Author.

Ayers, P., & Warrington, L. (2008). Diagnosis and treatment of simple acid-base disorders. *Nutrition in Clinical Practice, 23*(2), 122–127.

Betsy Lehman Center for Patient Safety and Medical Error Reduction, JSI Research and Training Institute, Inc. Prevention and control of healthcare-associated infections in Massachusetts. Part 1: Final recommendations of the Expert Panel. Boston, MA: Massachusetts Department of Public Health, 2008 January 31, pp. 69–82. National Guideline Clearinghouse Brief Summary. Prevention of bloodstream infections. Retrieved March 2, 2009, from http://www.guideline.gov/summary/summary.aspx?doc_id=12922&nbr=006636&string=intravenous+AND+administration

Blest, A., Roberts, M., Murdock, J., et al. (2007). How often should a red blood cell administration set be changed while a patient is being transfused? A commentary and review of the literature. *Transfusion Medicine, 18*, 121–133.

Bulechek, G., Butcher, H., & Dochterman, J. (Eds.). (2008). *Nursing interventions classification (NIC)* (5th ed.). St. Louis, MO: C. V. Mosby.

Centers for Disease Control and Prevention (CDC). (2002). Guidelines for the prevention of intravascular catheter-related infections. *Morbidity and Mortality Weekly Report, 51*(RR10), 1–26. Retrieved March 2, 2009, from http://www.cdc.gov/mmwr/preview/mmwrhtml/rr5110a1.htm

Cook, L. (2007). Choosing the right intravenous catheter. *Home Healthcare Nurse, 25*(8), 523–531.

Delahanty, K. M., & Myers, F. E. (2007). Nursing2007 infection control survey report. *Nursing2007, 37*(6), 28–38.

Finnish Medical Society Duodecim. (2008). Guidelines: Blood transfusion: indications and administration. Retrieved January 12, 2009, from http://www.guidelines.gov/summary/summary.aspx?doc_id=12787&nbr=006589&string

Fischback, F., & Dunning, M. (2005). *Nurse's quick reference to common laboratory and diagnostic tests.* Philadelphia: Lippincott Williams & Wilkins.

Freu, A., & Schears, G. (2006). Why are we stuck on tape and suture? A review of catheter securement devices. *Journal of Infusion Nursing, 29*(1), 34–38.

Gillies, D., Wallen, M., Morrison, A., et al. (2005). Optimal timing for intravenous administration set replacement. *Cochrane Database of Systematic Reviews*, Issue 4, Art. No: CD003588.

Gorski, L. (2007a). Infusion nursing standards of practice: Standard 43: catheter stabilization. *Journal of Infusion Nursing, 30*(1), 20–21.

Green, J. (2008). Care and management of patients with skin-tunnelled catheters. *Nursing Standard, 22*(42), 41–48.

Guthrie, D., Dreher, D., & Munson, M. (2007a). What you need to know about PICCS, part 1. *Nursing 2007, 37*(8), 18.

Guthrie, D., Dreher, D., & Munson, M. (2007b). What you need to know about PICCS, part 2. *Nursing2007, 37*(9), 14–15.

Hadaway, L. (2006). Technology of flushing vascular access devices. *Journal of Infusion Nursing, 29*(3), 137–145.

Hadaway, L. (2007). Infiltration and extravasation. *American Journal of Nursing, 107*(8), 64–72.

Hadaway, L. (2010). Don't disconnect IV administration sets. Lynn Hadaway Associates, Inc. (blog). Retrieved June 27, 2010, from http://hadawayassociates.blogspot.com/2010/03/don't-disconnect-iv-administration-sets.html

Harnage, S. (2008a). A PICC team ends CRBSIs. *RN, 71*(5), 34–36, 38–39.

Harnage, S. (2008b). Innovative bundle wipes out catheter-related bloodstream infections. *Nursing2008, 38*(10), 17–18.

Hertzog, D., & Waybill, P. (2008). Complications and controversies associated with peripherally inserted central catheters. *Journal of Infusion Nursing, 31*(3), 159–163.

Holcomb, S. (2008). Third-spacing: When body fluid shifts. *Nursing2008, 38*(7), 50–53.

Houck, D., & Whiteford, J. (2007). Transfusion with infusion pump for peripherally inserted central catheters and other vascular access devices. *Journal of Infusion Nursing, 30*(6), 341–344.

Hunt, S., Abraham, W., Chin, M., et al. (2005). American College of Cardiology/American Heart Association Practice Guidelines: Heart Failure. Retrieved January 12, 2009, from http://www.acc.org/qualityandscience/clinical/guidelines/failure/index.pdf

Infusion Nurses Society (INS). (2006a). *Policies and procedures for infusion nurses* (3rd ed.). Infusion Nurses Society Clinical Practice Committee. Norwood, MA: Author.

Infusion Nurses Society (INS). (2006b). Infusion nursing standards of practice. *Journal of Infusion Nursing, 29*(1S), S1–S92. Norwood, MA: Author.

Institute for Healthcare Improvement (n.d.). Implement the central line bundle. IHI.org [Web site]. Retrieved March 26, 2009, from http://www.ihi.org/IHI/Topics/CriticalCare/IntensiveCare/Changes/ImplementtheCentralLineBundle.htm

Institute of Medicine (IOM). (2004). *Dietary reference intakes for electrolytes and water.* Washington, DC: National Academies Press.

International Council of Nurses. (n.d.). *ICN on Selecting Safer Needle Devices.* Retrieved January 20, 2009, from http://www.icn.ch/matters_saferneedles.htm

The Joanna Briggs Institute. (2008). Management of peripheral intravascular devices. *Best Practice, 12*(5). Retrieved March 3, 2009, from http://www.joannabriggs.edu.au/pdf/BP_Book_Vol12_5.pdf

The Joint Commission (TJC). (2009). The Joint Commission Accreditation Program: Hospital national patient safety goals. Retrieved March 20, 2009, from http://www.jointcommission.org/NR/rdonlyres/31666E86–E7F4–423E-9BE8–F05BD1CB0AA8/0/09_NPSG_HAP.pdf

Kee, J., Paulanka, B., & Polek, C. (2008). *Fluid and electrolytes with clinical applications* (8th ed.). Clifton Park, NY: Delmar Cengage Learning.

Langley, D., & Moran, M. (2008). Intraosseous needles: They're not just for kids anymore. *Journal of Emergency Nursing, 34*(4), 318–319.

Lapides, J., Bourne, R., & Maclean, L. (1965). Clinical signs of dehydration and extracellular fluid loss. *JAMA, 191*, 413–415.

Lavery, I., & Smith, E. (2007). Peripheral vascular access devices: Risk prevention and management. *British Journal of Nursing, 16*(22), 1378–1383.

LeDuc, K. (1997). Efficacy of normal saline solution versus heparin solution for maintaining patency of peripheral intravenous catheters in children. *Journal of Emergency Nursing, 23*(4), 306–309.

Lockhart, A. (Ed.). (2007). *Best practices: Evidence-based nursing procedures.* Philadelphia: Lippincott Williams & Wilkins.

Ludeman, K. (2007). Choosing the right vascular access device. *Nursing2007, 37*(9), 38–41.

Macklin, D. (2003). Phlebitis. *American Journal of Nursing, 103*(2), 55–60.

Marschall, J., Mermel, L., Classen, D., et al. (2008). Guideline Summary. Strategies to prevent central line-associated bloodstream infections in acute care hospitals. *Infection Control and Hospital Epidemiology, 29*(Supplement1), S22–S30. National Guideline Clearinghouse (NGC) [Web site]. Rockville, MD. Retrieved May 19, 2009, from http://www.guideline.gov/summary/summary.aspx?view_id=1&doc_id=13395

Masoorli, S. (2007). Nerve injuries related to vascular access insertion and assessment. *Journal of Infusion Nursing, 30*(6), 346–350.

Mentes, J. (2008). Managing oral hydration. In: E. Capezuti, D. Zwicker, M. Mezey, et al. (Eds.). *Evidence-based geriatric nursing protocols for best practice* (3rd ed.). New York: Springer. Retrieved February 27, 2009, from http://www.guideline.gov/summary/summary.aspx?doc_id=12256&nbr=6340&ss=6&xl=999

Metheney, N., & Snively, W. Jr. (1978). Perioperative fluids and electrolytes. *The American Journal of Nursing, 78*(5), 840–845.

Miller, Y., Bachowski, G., Benjamin, R., et al. (2007). *Practice guidelines for blood transfusion* (2nd ed.). American National Red Cross. Retrieved March 1, 2009, from http://www.redcross.org/www-files/Documents/WorkingWiththeRedCross/practiceguidelinesforbloodtrans.pdf

Mok, E., Kwong, T., & Chan, M. (2007). A randomized controlled trial for maintaining peripheral intravenous lock in children. *International Journal of Nursing Practice, 13*(1), 33–45.

Moorhead, S., Johnson, M., Maas, M., et al. (Eds.). (2008). *Nursing outcomes classification (NOC)* (4th ed.). St. Louis, MO: C. V. Mosby.

Moureau, N. (2008). Tips for inserting an I.V. device in an older adult. *Nursing2008, 38*(12), 12.

NANDA International. (2009). *Nursing diagnoses: Definitions and classifications 2010–2011.* Ames, IA: Wiley-Blackwell.

National Guideline Clearinghouse (NGC). (2008). Guideline summary: Prevention of bloodstream infections. In: Prevention and control of healthcare-associated infections in Massachusetts. In: National Guideline Clearinghouse (NGC) [Web site]. Rockville, MD. Retrieved February 27, 2009, from http://www.guideline.gov/summary/summary.aspx?doc_id=12922

National Guideline Clearinghouse (NGC) (2009, April). Guideline summary: Screening for osteoporosis in the adult U.S. population: ACPM Position statement on preventive practice. In: National Guideline Clearinghouse (NGC) [Web site]. Rockville, MD. Retrieved September 18, 2010, from http://www.guideline.gov/summary/summary.aspx?view_id=1&doc_id=15270

National Institutes of Health (NIH). (2007). Osteoporosis. Retrieved January 1, 2009, from http://www.niams.nih.gov/Health_Info/Bone/Osteoporosis/default.asp

National Osteoporosis Foundation. (2008). *Clinician's guide to the prevention and treatment of osteoporosis.* Washington, DC: National Osteoporosis Foundation. Retrieved October 25, 2008, from http://www.nof.org/professionals/NOF_Clinicians_Guide.pdf

Negoianu, D., & Goldfarb, S. (2008). Editorial: Just add water. *Journal of the American Society of Nephrology, 19*, 1041–1043.

Nichols, I., & Humphrey, J. (2008). The efficacy of upper arm placement of peripherally inserted central catheters using bedside ultrasound and microintroducer technique. *Journal of Infusion Nursing, 31*(3), 165–176.

Niesen, K. M., Harris, D. Y., Parkin, L. S., et al. (2003). The effects of heparin versus normal saline for maintenance of peripheral intravenous locks in pregnant women. *Journal of Obstetrics, Gynecology, & Neonatal Nursing, 32*(4), 503–508.

Oncology Nursing Society (ONS). (2004). *Access device guidelines: Recommendations for nursing practice and education* (2nd ed.). Pittsburgh, PA: Oncology Nursing Society (ONS). Updated, 2006 and 2008. Retrieved April 25, 2009, from http://www.guidelines.gov/summary/summary.aspx?doc_id=8338&nbr=004666&string=prevention+AND+intravascular+AND+catheter-related+AND+infections

Palmer, B. (2008). Approach to fluid and electrolyte disorders and acid-base problems. *Primary Care: Clinics in Office Practice, 35*(2), 195–213.

Pflaum, S. (1979). Investigation of intake-output as a means of assessing body fluid balance. *Heart & Lung: Journal of Acute & Critical Care, 8*(3), 495–498.

Pflaum, S. (2000). Evaluating the reliability and utility of cumulative intake and output. *Journal of Nursing Care Quality, 14*(3), 37–42.

Pflaum, S. (2006). Evaluating the reliability of recorded fluid balance to approximate body weight change in patients undergoing cardiac surgery. *Heart & Lung: Journal of Acute & Critical Care, 35*(1), 27–33.

Phillips, L. (2005). *Manual of IV therapeutics* (4th ed.). Philadelphia: F. A. Davis.

Polovich, M., White, J., & Kelleher, L. (Eds.) (2006). Chemotherapy and biotherapy guidelines and recommendations for practice, *Journal of Infusion Nursing*, 29(1 Supplement), S1–S92.

Powell, J., Tarnow, K., & Perucca, R. (2008). The relationship between peripheral intravenous catheter indwell time and the incidence of phlebitis. *Journal of Infusion Nursing*, 31(1), 39–45.

Preston, R. A. (2002). *Acid-base, fluids, and electrolytes made ridiculously simple*. Miami: Medmaster.

Pronovost, P., Needham, D., Berenholtz, S., et al. (2006). An intervention to decrease catheter-related bloodstream infections in the ICU. *New England Journal of Medicine*, 355, 2725–2732.

Pronovost, P., Goeschel, C., Colantuoni, E., et al. (2010). Sustaining reductions in catheter related bloodstream infections in Michigan intensive care units: Observational study. *BMJ*, 340, c309. Retrieved March 22, 2010, from http://www.bmj.com/cgi/content/full/340/feb04_1/c309

Randolph, A., Cook, D., Gonzales, C., et al. (1998). Benefit of heparin in peripheral venous and arterial catheters: Systematic review and meta-analysis of randomized controlled trials. *British Medical Journal*, 316, 969–975.

Rauen, C. (2008). Blood transfusion in the intensive care unit. *Critical Care Nurse*, 28(3), 78–80.

Rhoads, J., & Meeker, B. (2008). *Davis's guide to clinical nursing skills*. Philadelphia: F. A. Davis.

Riley, M-S. (n.d.). CE476. A lurking danger: A 'bundle' of safety measures available to fight central line infections. Nurse. com [Web site]. Retrieved March 26, 2009, from http://www.nurse.com/ce/course.html?CCID=4507&PageNum=3&Begin=9339

Roman, M., Thimothee, S., & Vidal, J. (2008). Arterial blood gases. *MedSurg Nursing*, 17(4), 268–269.

Rowlands, A., Ingledew, D., Powell, S., et al. (2004). Interactive effects of habitual physical activity and calcium intake on bone density in boys and girls. *Journal of Applied Physiology*, 97(4), 1203–1208.

Rutal, W., Weber, D., & the Healthcare Infection Control Practices Advisory Committee (HICPAC). (2008). Guideline for disinfection and sterilization in healthcare facilities, 2008. Retrieved March 11, 2009, from http://www.cdc.gov/ncidod/dhqp/pdf/guidelines/Disinfection_Nov_2008.pdf

Saladin, K. (2008). *Anatomy and physiology: The unity of form and function* (4th ed.). New York: McGraw-Hill.

Sandler, S., & Johnson, V. (2008). *Transfusion Reactions*. Emedicine. Retrieved January 12, 2009, from http://emedicine.medscape.com/article/206885–print

Scales, K., & Pilsworth, J. (2008). The importance of fluid balance in clinical practice. *Nursing Standard*, 22(47), 50–57.

Scanlon, V. C., & Sanders, T. (2006). *Essentials of anatomy and physiology* (5th ed.). Philadelphia: F. A. Davis.

Siegel, J., Rhinehart, E., Jackson, M., et al. and the Healthcare Infection Control Practices Advisory Committee. (2007). *Guideline for isolation precautions: Preventing transmission of infectious agents in healthcare settings 2007*. Centers for Disease Control and Prevention (CDC). Retrieved March 3, 2009, from http://www.cdc.gov/ncidod/dhqp/pdf/guidelines/Isolation2007.pdf

Smeltzer, S., Bare, B., Hinkle, J., et al. (2008). *Brunner & Suddarth's textbook of medical-surgical nursing*. Philadelphia: Lippincott Williams & Wilkins.

Smith, B., & Royer, T. (2007). New standards for improving peripheral IV catheter securement. *Nursing2007*, 37(3), 72–74.

The Society for Healthcare Epidemiology of America. (2008). Supplement article: SHEA/IDSA practice recommendation. Strategies to prevent central line-associated bloodstream infections in acute care hospitals. *Infection Control & Hospital Epidemiology*, 29, S22–S30. Retrieved March 6, 2009, from http://www.journals.uchicago.edu/doi/pdf/10.1086/591059

Springhouse Corporation. (2008). *Nursing 2009 drug handbook with Web Toolkit (Nursing drug handbook*, 29th ed.). Philadelphia: Lippincott Williams & Wilkins.

Thibodeau, S., Riley, J., & Rouse, K. (2007). Effectiveness of a new flushing and maintenance policy using peripherally inserted central catheters for adults: Best practice. *Journal of Infusion Nursing*, 30(5), 287–292.

Thompson, C., Edwards, C., & Stout, L. (2008). Blood transfusions. 2: signs and symptoms of acute reactions. *Nursing Times*, 104(3), 28–29.

Timsit, J-F, Schwebel, C., Boudma, L., et al. (2009). Chlorhexidine-impregnated sponges and less frequent dressing changes for prevention of catheter-related infections in critically ill adults: A randomized controlled trial. *JAMA*, 301(12), 1231–1241, 1285–1287.

Treas, L., & Latinis-Bridges, B. (1992). Efficacy of heparin in peripheral venous infusion in neonates. *Journal of Obstetric, Gynecologic, and Neonatal Nursing*, 21, 214–219.

Tripathi, S., Kaushik, V., & Sing, V. (2007). Peripheral IVs: Factors affecting complications and patency – a randomized controlled trial. *Journal of Infusion Nursing*, 31(3), 182–188.

U.S. Department of Agriculture (USDA). (n.d.). Dietary supplement fact sheet: Calcium. Retrieved January 28, 2009, from http://ods.od.nih.gov/factsheets/calcium.asp

U.S. Department of Agriculture (USDA). (2004). Dietary Reference Intakes: Recommended Intakes for Individuals. National Academy of Sciences. Retrieved January 29, 2010, from http://www.iom.edu/Global/News%20Announcements/~/media/48FAAA2FD9E74D95BBDA2236E7387B49.ashx

U.S. Department of Health and Human Services (USDHHS). (updated, 2009). *Osteoporosis*. NIH Publication No. 07–5158. Bethesda, MD: National Institute of Arthritis and Musculoskeletal and Skin Diseases, NIAMS/National Institutes of Health. Retrieved from http://www.niams.nih.gov/Health_Info/Bone/Osteoporosis/default.asp

Uslusoy, E., & Mete, S. (2008). Predisposing factors to phlebitis in patients with peripheral intravenous catheters: A descriptive study. *Journal of the American Academy of Nurse Practitioners*, 20(4), 172–180.

Van Leeuwen, A., & Poelhuls-Leth, D. (2009). *Davis's comprehensive handbook of laboratory and diagnostic tests with nursing implications* (3rd ed.). Philadelphia: F. A. Davis.

Venes, D. (2009). *Taber's cyclopedic medical dictionary* (21st ed.). Philadelphia: F. A. Davis.

Watson, D., Murdock, J., Doree, C., et al. (2008). Blood transfusion administration – one- or two-person checks: Which is the safest method? *Transfusion*, 48, 783–789.

Wenzel, R., & Edmond, M. (2006). Team-based prevention of catheter-related infections. *New England Journal of Medicine*, 355, 2781–2783.

Younger, G., & Khan, M. (2008). Setting up and priming an intravenous infusion. *Nursing Standard*, 22(4), 40–44.

Zarate, L., Mandleco, B., Wilshaw, R., et al. (2008). Peripheral intravenous catheters started in prehospital and emergency department settings. *Journal of Trauma Nursing*, 15(2), 47–52.

Chapter 37

Agency for Healthcare Research and Quality (AHRQ). (2003). Efforts to reduce medical errors: AHRQ's response to Senate Committee on Appropriations questions. *AHRQ's patient safety initiative: Building foundations, reducing risk* (Chapter 2). Interim report to the Senate Committee on Appropriations. Retrieved July 1, 2009, from http://www.ahrq.gov/qual/pscongrpt/

Agency for Healthcare Research and Quality (AHRQ). (2008). Press release: New AHRQ study finds surgical errors cost nearly $1.5 billion annually. Retrieved July 10, 2009, from http://www.ahrq.gov/news/press/pr2008/surgerrpr.htm

Allied Healthcare Products, Inc. (n.d.). Gomco® mobile pump constant and intermittent models 6036 & 6037 operation, maintenance and service manual. Retrieved July 15, 2009, from http://www.alliedhpi.com/images/zs168–274–001.pdf

American Association of Critical-Care Nurses (AACN). (2005). AACN practice alert. Deep vein thrombosis prevention. Retrieved July 3, 2009, from http://www.aacn.org/WD/Practice/Docs/DVT_Prevention_12–2005.pdf

American Association of Nurse Anesthetists (AANA). (2008). Questions and answers: A career in nurse anesthesia. Retrieved September 27, 2009, from http://www.aana.com/BecomingCRNA.aspx?ucNavMenu_TSMenuTargetID=103&ucNavMenu_TSMenuTargetType=4&ucNavMenu_TSMenuID=6&id=110

American Society of PeriAnesthesia Nurses (2009a). ASPAN's evidence-based clinical practice guideline for the promotion of perioperative normothermia. Retrieved March 24, 2010, from https://www.aspan.org/Portals/6/docs/ClinicalPractice/Guidelines/Normothermia_Guideline_10-09_JoPAN.pdf

Association of periOperative Registered Nurses (AORN). (2007). *Perioperative nursing data set* (rev. 2nd ed.). Denver, CO: Author.

Association of periOperative Registered Nurses (AORN). (2009b). *Perioperative standards and recommended practices.* Denver, CO: Author.

Baker, J. (2005). Specialty nomenclature. A worthwhile challenge. *Gastroenterology Nursing, 28*(1), 52–55.

Bartley, M. (2006). Keep venous thromboembolism at bay. *Nursing 2006, 36*(10), 36–43.

Berliner, E., Ozbilgin, B., & Zarin, D. (2003). A systematic review of pneumatic compression for treatment of chronic venous insufficiency and venous ulcers. *Journal of Vascular Surgery, 37*(3), 539–544.

Bernier, M. J., Sanares, D. C., Owen, S. V., et al. (2003). Preoperative teaching received and valued in a day surgery setting. *AORN Journal, 77*(3), 563–572, 575–578, 581–582.

Boyce, J., & Pittet, D. (2002). Guideline for hand hygiene in health-care settings. Recommendations of the Healthcare Infection Control Practices Advisory Committee and the HICPAC/SHEA/APIC/IDSA Hand Hygiene Task Force. *MMWR, 51*(RR16), 1–44. Retrieved July 15, 2009, from http://www.cdc.gov/mmwr/tpreview/mmwrhtml/rr5116a1.htm

Bulecheck, G. M., Dochterman, J. M., Butcher, H. K., et al. (Eds.). (2007). *Nursing interventions classification (NIC)* (5th ed.). St. Louis, MO: C. V. Mosby.

Bulechek, G. M., Butcher, H. K., & Dochterman, J. M. (Eds.). (2008). *Nursing interventions classification (NIC)* (5th ed.). St. Louis, MO: C. V. Mosby

Centers for Diseases Control and Prevention (CDC). (2001). *CDC's 7 healthcare safety challenges.* Retrieved July 10, 2009, from http://www.cdc.gov/ncidod/dhqp/about_challenges.html

Centers for Disease Control (CDC) National Center for Health Statistics. (2009). U.S. outpatient surgeries on the rise. NCHS press room. Retrieved July 15, 2009, from http://www.cdc.gov/nchs/pressroom/09newsreleases/outpatientsurgeries.htm

Centers for Medicare & Medicaid Services. (2006). Press Release. Eliminating serious, preventable, and costly medical errors — never events. Department of Health & Human Services. Retrieved July 20, 2009, from http://www.cms.hhs.gov/apps/media/press/release.asp?Counter=1863

Centers for Medicare and Medicaid Services. (2008). Press release. Medicare and Medicaid move aggressively to encourage greater patient safety in hospitals and reduce never events. CMS Office of Public Affairs, July 31, 2009. Retrieved October 20, 2008, from http://www.cms.hhs.gov/apps/media/press/release.asp?Counter=3219&intNumPerPage=10&checkDate=&checkKey=&srchType=1&numDays=3500&srchOpt=0&srchData=&keywordType=All&chkNewsType=1%2C+2%2C+3%2C+4%2C+5&intPage=&showAll=&pYear=&year=&desc=&cboOrder=date

Cohen, A., Tapson, V., Bergman, J-F., et al. (2008). Venous thromboembolism risk and prophylaxis in the acute hospital care setting (ENDORSE study): A multinational cross-sectional study. *The Lancet, 371*(9610), 387–394.

Crowe, L., Chang, A., Fraser, J., et al. (2008). Systematic review of the effectiveness of nursing interventions in reducing or relieving post-operative pain. *International Journal of Evidence-Based Healthcare, 6*(4), 396–430.

Dale, A., Rothrock, J., & McEwen, D. (Eds.). (2003). *Alexander's care of the patient in surgery* (12th ed.). St. Louis, MO: C. V. Mosby.

Deysine, M. (2006). Infection control in a hernia clinic: 24-year results of aseptic and antiseptic measure implementation in 4,620 "clean cases." *Hernia, 10*(1), 25–29.

Digison, M. (2007). A review of antiseptic agents for pre-operative skin preparation. *Plastic Surgical Nursing, 27*(4), 185–189.

Duchene, P. (2007). Perioperative concerns in older adults. *Advance for Nurse Practitioners, 17*(9), 39–42, 44.

Editorial Board Palliative Care. (2006). *Practice guidelines. Nausea and vomiting.* Utrecht, The Netherlands. Association of Comprehensive Cancer Centres (AACC). In: National Guideline Clearinghouse (NGC). (2009). Complete summary: Nausea and vomiting. Retrieved July 19, 2009, from http://www.guideline.gov/summary/summary.aspx?ss=15&doc_id=11793&nbr=&string=

Gilmartin, J. (2004). Day surgery: Patients' perceptions of a nurse-led preadmission clinic. *Journal of Clinical Nursing, 13*(2), 243–250.

Green, S., Harris, C., & Singer, J. (2008). Gastrointestinal decontamination of the poisoned patient. *Pediatric Emergency Care, 24,* 176–178.

Haynes, A., Weiser, T., Berry, W., et al. (2009). A surgical safety checklist to reduce morbidity and mortality in a global population. *New England Journal of Medicine, 360*(5), 491–499.

Hendrickson, S., Wadhera, R., & ElBardissi, A. (2008). Development and pilot evaluation of a preoperative briefing protocol for cardiovascular surgery. *Journal of the American College of Surgeons, 208*(6), 1115–1123.

Institute for Healthcare Improvement. (n.d.). Overview of the 100,000 lives campaign. Retrieved July 10, 2009, from http://www.ihi.org/IHI/Programs/Campaign/100kCampaignOverviewArchive.htm.

The Joanna Briggs Institute. (2007). Pre-operative hair removal to reduce surgical site infection. *Best practice, 11*(4).

The Joanna Briggs Institute. (2008a). Graduated compression stockings for the prevention of post-operative venous thromboembolism. *Best practice, 12*(4).

The Joanna Briggs Institute. (2008b). Preoperative fasting for preventing perioperative complications in children. *Best practice, 12*(1), 29–32.

Johnson, T. K., Holm, C. D., & Godshall, S. D. (2000). Next-generation strategies for physicians and hospitals. *Healthcare Financial Management, 54*(1), 48–51.

Johnston, J., & Davis, M. (2008). When sequential-compression devices cause falls. *American Journal of Nursing, 108*(4), 37–38.

The Joint Commission (TJC). (2008). *National patient safety goals for 2009.* Retrieved September 27, 2009 at http://www.jointcommission.org/PatientSafety/NationalPatientSafetyGoals/

Kleinbeck, S., & Dopp, A. (2005, July). The perioperative nursing data set—A new language for documenting care. *AORN Journal.* Home study program. Retrieved July 10, 2009, from http://findarticles.com/p/articles/mi_m0FSL/is_1_82/ai_n15394472/?tag=content;col1

Kohn, M. L. (Ed.) (2003). *Berry and Kohn's operating room technique* (10th ed.). St. Louis, MO: C. V. Mosby.

Larry, C. (Ed.) (2003). Applying anti-embolism stockings. Retrieved September 27, 2009, from http://www.newlook.com.sg/info.asp?key=TED%20ApplyTh

Makary, M., Mukherjee, A., Sexton, J., et al. (2007). Operating room briefings and wrong-site surgery. *Journal of the American College of Surgeons, 204*(2), 236–243.

Mangram, A., Horan, T., Pearson, M., et al. (1999). The Hospital Infection Control Practices Advisory Committee. Guideline for prevention of surgical site infection, 1999. *Infection Control and Hospital Epidemiology, 20*(4), 247–278. Centers for Disease Control and Prevention (CDC) [Web site]. Atlanta, GA. Retrieved July 1, 2009, from http://www.cdc.gov/ncidod/dhqp/pdf/guidelines/SSI.pdf

Markel, D., & Morris, G. (2002). Effect of external sequential compression devices on femoral venous blood flow. *Journal of the Southern Orthopaedic Association, 11*(1), 2–9.

Moorhead, S., Johnson, M., Maas, M., et al. (Eds.). (2008). *Nursing outcomes classification (NOC)* (4th ed.). St. Louis, MO: C. V. Mosby.

NANDA International. (2009). *Nursing diagnoses: Definitions and classification 2009–2011.* Philadelphia: Author.

National Guideline Clearinghouse (NGC). (2008). Guideline summary: Guideline for the management of postoperative nausea and vomiting. National Guideline Clearinghouse (NGC) [Web site]. Rockville, MD. Retrieved July 15, 2009, from http://www.guideline.gov/summary/summary.aspx?view_id=1&doc_id=13386

National Guideline Clearinghouse (NGC). (2009). Guideline summary: Strategies to prevent surgical site infections in acute care hospitals. National Guideline Clearinghouse (NGC) [Web site]. Rockville, MD. Author. Retrieved July 15, 2009, from http://www.guideline.gov/summary/summary.aspx?view_id=1&doc_id=13399

National Institute for Health and Clinical Excellence (NICE). (2007). *Venous thromblism. Reducing the risk in surgical inpatients. Methods, evidence & guidance.* London: National Collaborating Centre for Acute Care.

National Institute for Health and Clinical Excellence (NICE). (2008). Surgical site infection: Prevention and treatment of surgical site infection. NICE clinical guideline 74. Retrieved July 25, 2009, from http://www.nice.org.uk/CG74

National Priorities Partnership. (2008). *National priorities and goals: Aligning our efforts to transform America's healthcare.* Washington, DC: National Quality Forum.

Quinn, D. M., & Schick, L. (2004). *Perianesthesia nursing core curriculum* (4th ed.). Philadelphia: W. B. Saunders.

Ridge, R. (2008). Doing right to prevent wrong-site surgery. *Nursing2008, 38*(3), 24–25.

Rothrock, J. C. (Ed.). (2006). *Alexander's care of the patient in surgery* (13th ed.). St. Louis, MO: C. V. Mosby.

Sarasota Memorial Hospital. (reviewed 2008). Nursing procedure: Gastric suction—GOMCO. SMH Nursing Procedures. Retrieved July 15, 2009, from http://www.smh.com/sections/services-procedures/medlib/nursing/Procedures/Suction/suc04_gastric_041408.pdf

Siegel, J., Rhinehart, E., Jackson, M., et al. & the Healthcare Infection Control Practices Advisory Committee. (2007). *2007 Guideline for isolation precautions: Preventing transmission of infectious agents in healthcare settings.* Retrieved July 15, 2009, from http://www.cdc.gov/ncidod/dhqp/pdf/guidelines/isolation2007.pdf

Tsay, S-L., Chen, H-L., Chen, S-C., et al. (2008). Effects of reflexotherapy on acute postoperative pain and anxiety among patients with digestive cancer. *Cancer Nursing, 31*(2), 109–115.

Winslow, E., & Brosz, D. (2008). Graduated compression stockings in hospitalized postoperative patients: Correctness of usage and size. *American Journal of Nursing, 108*(9), 40–51.

World Health Organization (WHO). (2008). Surgical safety checklist (1st ed.). Retrieved July 1, 2009, from http://www.who.int/patientsafety/safesurgery/tools_resources/SSSL_Checklist_final-Jun08.pdf

Chapter 38

American Association of Colleges of Nursing (AACN). (2005). Faculty shortages in baccalaureate and graduate nursing programs: Scope of the problem and strategies for expanding the Supplementy. Retrieved August 2, 2009, from http://www.aacn.nche.edu/publications/whitepapers/facultyshortages.htm

American Nurses Association (ANA). (2002). *Position statements: Registered nurse utilization of unlicensed assistive personnel.* Washington, DC: Author.

American Nurses Association (ANA). (2007). *Position statements: Registered nurses' utilization of nursing assistive personnel in all settings.* Washington, DC: Author.

American Nurses Association (ANA). (2010). *Nursing: Scope and standards of practice* (2nd ed.). Public comment draft, January 2010. Silver Spring, MD: Nursebooks.org Retrieved February 1, 2010, from http://www.nursingworld.org/DocumentVault/NursingPractice/Draft-Nursing-Scope-Standards-2nd-Ed.aspx

American Nurses Credentialing Center. (2009). Magnet Recognition Program. Retrieved May 15, 2009, from http://www.nursecredentialing.org

Anderzén, K., & Arnetz, B. (2005). The impact of a prospective survey-based workplace intervention program on employee health, biologic stress markers, and organizational productivity. *Journal of Occupational and Environmental Medicine, 47*(7), 671–682.

Arnold, E., & Boggs, K. (2007). *Interpersonal relationships* (5th ed.). Philadelphia: W. B. Saunders.

Baggett, M., & Baggett, F. (2005). Move from management to high-level leadership. *Nursing Management, 36*(7), 12.

Baldwin, F. D. (2002, March). Making do with less. *Healthcare Informatics,* 1–7.

Barker, A. M. (1992). *Transformational nursing leadership: A vision for the future.* New York: National League for Nursing.

Barker, A. M., Sullivan, D. T., & Emery, M. J. (2006). *Leadership competencies for clinical managers: The renaissance of transformational leadership.* Sudbury, MA: Jones and Bartlett

Barraclough, R. A., & Stewart, R. A. (1992). Power and control: Social science perspectives. In: V. P. Richmond & J. C. McCroskey (Eds.), *Power in the classroom: Communication, control and concern.* Hillsdale, NJ: Lawrence Erlbaum.

Bass, B. M., & Avolio, B. J. (1993). Transformational leadership: A response to critique. In: M. M. Chemers & R. Ayman (Eds.), *Leadership theory and research: Perspectives and directions.* San Diego: Academic Press.

Bennis, W., Spreitzer, G., & Cummings, T. G. (2001). *The future of leadership.* San Francisco: Jossey-Bass.

Blais, K. B., Hayes, J. S., & Kozier, B. (2006). *Professional nursing practice: Concepts and perspectives* (5th ed.). Upper Saddle River, NJ: Prentice-Hall.

Blake, R. R., Mouton, J. S., & Tapper, M. (1981). *Grid approaches for managerial leadership in nursing.* St. Louis, MO: C. V. Mosby.

Browne, M. M., & Kelley, S. M. (2010). *Asking the right questions: A guide to critical thinking* (9th ed.). Upper Saddle River, NJ: Prentice-Hall.

Buerhaus, P., Auerbach, D., & Staiger, D. (2007). Recent trends in the registered nurse labor market in the US: Recent changes in employment and earnings growth in the nurse labor market in the United States. *Nursing Economics, 25*(2), 59–66.

The Center for Health Design. (2009). Pebble Project® Data Summary. Retrieved August 2, 2009, from http://www.healthdesign.org/research/pebble/data.php

Christmas, K. (2009). 2009: The year of positive leadership. *Nursing Economic$, 27*(2), 128–129, 133

Dantley, M. E. (2005). Moral leadership: Shifting the management paradigm. In: F. W. English (Ed.), *The Sage handbook of educational leadership* (pp. 34–46). Thousand Oaks, CA: Sage Publications.

Dent, H. S. (1995). *Job shock: Four new principles transforming our work and business.* New York: St. Martin's Press.

Drath, W. (2001). *The deep blue sea.* San Francisco: Jossey-Bass.

Ellis, M. (1999). Self-assessment: Discovering yourself and making the best choices for you! *Black Collegian, 30*(1), 30, 3p, 1c.

Farrell, K., & Broude, C. (1987). *Winning the change game: How to implement information systems with fewer headaches and bigger paybacks.* Los Angeles: Breakthrough Enterprises.

Felman, D. A. (2002). *Critical thinking: Strategies for decision making.* Menlo Park, CA: Crisp Publications.

First Consulting Group for the American Hospital Association. (2001). The healthcare workforce shortage and its implications for America's hospitals. Retrieved August 1, 2009, from http://www.aha.org/aha/content/2002/pdf/FcgWorkforceReport.pdf

Fitton, R. A. (1997). *Leadership: Quotations from the world's greatest motivators.* Boulder, CO: Westview Press.

Fralic, M. F. (2000). What is leadership? *Journal of Nursing Administration, 30*(7/8), 340–341.

Greenleaf, R. K. (2004). Who is the servant-leader? In: L. Spears & M. Lawrence (Eds.), *Practicing servant-leadership.* San Francisco: Jossey-Bass.

Grossman, S. C., & Valiga, T. M. (2009). *The new leadership challenge: Creating the future of nursing* (3rd ed.). Philadelphia: F. A. Davis.

Halloran, L. (2008). Time management: Ten commandments for reshaping your schedule. *Advance for Nurse Practitioners, 16*(12), 74.

Haslan, S. A. (2001). *Psychology in organizations*. Thousand Oaks, CA: Sage.

Heifetz, R. A., & Linsky, M. (2002, June). A survival guide for leaders. *Harvard Business Review*, 65–74.

Heller, R. (1998). *Managing change*. New York: DK Publishing.

Hendrich, A., Chow, M., Sklerczynski, B., et al. (2008). A 36–hospital time and motion study. How do medical-surgical nurses spend their time? *Permanence Journal*, 12, 25–34.

Holman, L. (1995). *Eleven lessons in self-leadership: Insights for personal and professional success*. Lexington, KY: A Lessons in Leadership Book.

Hunter, J. C. (2004). *The world's most powerful leadership principle*. New York: Crown Business.

Jones, R. D., & Rudd, R. D. (2007). Transactional, transformational, or laissez-faire: An assessment of college of agriculture academic program leaders (deans) leadership styles. *Proceedings of the 2007 AAAE Research Conference*, 34, 520–530.

Kellerman, B. (2008). *Followership: How followers are creating change and changing leaders*. Boston: Harvard Business Press.

Kleinman, C. S. (2004). Leadership: A key strategy in staff nurse retention. *The Journal of Continuing Education in Nursing*, 35(3), 128–132.

Kotter, J. P. (1999). Leading change: The eight steps to transformation. In: J. A. Conger, G. M. Spreitzer, & E. E. Lawler (Eds.), *The leader's change handbook*. San Francisco: Jossey-Bass.

Lansdale, B. M. (2002). *Cultivating inspired leaders: Making participatory management work*. West Hartford, CT: Kumarian Press.

Lapp, J. (2002, May). Thriving on change. *CARING Magazine*, 40–43.

Leach, L. S. (2005). Nurse executive transformational leadership and organizational commitment. *Journal of Nursing Administration*, 35(5), 228–237.

Lee, J. A. (1980). *The gold and the garbage in management theories and prescriptions*. Athens, OH: Ohio University Press.

Lewin, K. (1951). *Field theory in social science: Selected theoretical papers*. New York: Harper & Row.

Locke, E. A. (1982). The ideas of Frederick Taylor: An evaluation. *Academy of Management Review*, 7(1), 14.

Lukes, S. (1986). *Power*. New York: New York University Press.

Mander, A., Gomes, A., & Castle, D. (2002). The management of change in a community mental health team. *Australian Health Review*, 25(2), 115–121.

Maslow, A. H. (1970). *Motivation and personality*. New York: Harper & Row.

McGregor, D. (1960). *The human side of enterprise*. New York: McGraw-Hill.

McNichol, E. (2000). How to be a model leader. *Nursing Standard*, 14(45), 24.

Mintzberg, H. (1989). *Mintzberg on management: Inside our strange world of organizations*. New York: Free Press.

Mondros, J. B., & Wilson, S. M. (1994). *Organizing for power and empowerment*. New York: Columbia University Press.

Mulholland, J. (1991). *The language of negotiation: A handbook of practical strategies*. London: Rutledge.

National Council of State Boards of Nursing (NCSBN). (2009). Joint statement on delegation. American Nurses Association and National Council State Boards of Nursing. Retrieved May 15, 2009 https://www.ncsbn.org/Joint_statement.pdf

Navuluri, R. B. (2001). Our time management in patient care. *Research for Nursing Practice*, 3(1). Retrieved August 1, 2005, from http://www.graduateresearch.com/NavuTime.htm

Nelson, M. (2002, May 31). Educating for professional nursing practice: Looking backward into the future. *Online Journal of Issues in Nursing*. Retrieved August 2, 2009, from http://www.nursingworld.org/ojin/topic18/tpc18_3.htm

Pavitt, C. (1999). Theorizing about the group communication-leadership relationship. In: L. R. Frey (Ed.), *The handbook of group communication theory and research*. Thousand Oaks, CA: Sage Publications.

Porter-O'Grady, T. (2003). A different age for leadership. Part II. *Journal of Nursing Administration*, 33(2), 105–110.

Riggio, R., Chaleff, I., & Lipman-Blumen, J. (2008). *The art of followership: How great followers create great leaders and organizations*. San Francisco: Jossey-Bass (John Wiley & Sons).

Ritter-Teitel, J. (2002). The impact of restructuring on professional nursing practice. *Journal of Nursing Administration*, 32(1), 31–41.

Robert Wood Johnson Foundation. (2009). Charting nursing's future. Addressing the quality and safety gap—Part I: Case studies in transforming hospital nursing and building cultures of safety. Retrieved August 3, 2009, from http://www.rwjf.org/humancapital/product.jsp?id=45629

Ruskin, J. (2007). Followership. Retrieved August 12, 2009, from http://www.union.uiuc.edu/involvement/rso/leader_readers/followership.htm

Shingleton, J. (1994). The job market for '94 grads. In: *College Placement Council* (Ed.), *Planning job choices* (pp. 19–26). Philadelphia: College Placement Council.

Simonetti, J., & Ariss, S. (1999). Through the top with mentoring. *Business Horizons*, 42(6), 56–62.

Smith-Trudeau, P. (2009). The future of nursing is here now! Do you have what it takes to lead? *Vermont Nurse Connection*, 12(1), 4.

Spears, L. C., & Lawrence, M. (2004). *Practicing servant-leadership*. San Francisco: Jossey-Bass.

Sportsman, S. (2005). Build a framework for conflict assessment. *Nursing Management*, 36(4), 32–40.

Spreitzer, G., & Quinn, R. (2001). *A company of leaders: Five disciplines for unleashing the power in your workforce*. San Francisco: Jossey-Bass.

Stavros, J., Cooperrider, D., & Kelley, L. (2007). SOAR: A new approach to strategic planning. *Fast Fundamentals. The BK Whitepaper Series*. Retrieved July 31, 2009, from http://www.scribd.com/doc/17330716/SOAR-A-New-Approach-to-Strategic-Planning-by-Jackie-Stavros-David-Cooperrider-and-D-Lynn-Kelley. Excerpted from *The change handbook* (2nd ed.), San Francisco: Berrett-Koehler.

Thomas, D. O. (1995). Speak up! We need good followers too. *Medical Economics*, 58(9), 72.

Thompson, L., & Fox, C. R. (2001). Negotiation within and between groups in organizations: Levels of analysis. In: M. E. Turner (Ed.), *Groups at work* (pp. 221–266). Mahwah, NJ: Lawrence Erlbaum.

Trofino, J. (1995). Transformational leadership in health care. *Nursing Management*, 26(8), 42–27.

Tzeng, H., & Yin, C. (2009). Historical trends in human resource issues of hospital nursing in the past generation. *Nursing Economic$*, 27(1), 19–25.

Upenieks, V. (2002). What constitutes successful nurse leadership? *Journal of Nursing Administration*, 32(12), 622–632.

U.S. Department of Health and Human Services (USDHHS), Health Resources and Service Administration, Bureau of Health Professions Division of Nursing. (2006). The registered nurse population, March 2004. Findings from the national sample survey of registered nurses. Retrieved May 15, 2009, from ftp://ftp.hrsa.gov/bhpr/workforce/0306rnss.pdf

Villarreal, J. (2002). What employers want: The measure of importance of various skills for registered nurses. *Applied Research Projects*. Paper 60. Retrieved July 31, 2009, from http://ecommons.txstate.edu/arp/60

White, R., & Lippitt, R. (1960). *Autocracy and democracy: An experimental inquiry*. New York: Harper & Row.

Whitehead, D., Weiss, S., & Tappen, R. (2007). *Essentials of nursing leadership and management* (4th ed.). Philadelphia: F. A. Davis.

Chapter 39

Agency for Healthcare Research and Quality. (2010, March 10, updated). Enabling patient-centered care through health IT, systematic review protocol. Rockville, MD: Agency for Healthcare Research and Quality. Accessed April 1, 2010, from http://www.ahrq.gov/clinic/tp/pcchittp.htm

American Nurses Association (ANA). (2007, April). *Scope and standards of nursing informatics practice*. ANA Pub. #NIP21. Washington, DC: American Nurses Publishing/American Nurses Foundation.

American Nurses Association (ANA). (2008). *Nursing informatics nursing scope and standards of practice*. Silver Spring, MD: American Nurses Publishing.

Ash, J. S., Sittig, D. F., Dykstra, R., et al. (2009). The unintended consequences of computerized provider order entry: Findings from a mixed methods exploration. *International Journal of Medical Informatics, 78S*, S69–S76.

Baln, J. W. (2009, July). Addressing the quality and safety gap—part II: How nurses are shaping, and being shaped by health information technologies. Robert Wood Johnson Foundation. *Charting Nursing's Future, 11*, 1–8.

Banner, L., & Olney, C. (2009). Automated clinical documentation—does it allow nurses more time for patient care? *Computers, Informatics, Nursing, 27*(2), 75–81.

Bell, M. M. (2009, May). Bar code point of care systems: Benefits and pitfalls. *Pennsylvania Nurse*, 9–10.

Beyea, S. (2000, May). Standardized nursing vocabularies and the perioperative nursing data set: Making clinical practice count. *CIN Plus, 3*(2), 1, 5, 6.

Blanchet, K. D. (2008). Remote patient monitoring. *Telemedicine and e-HEALTH, 14*(2), 127–130.

Cadmus, E., Van Wynen, E., Chamberlain, B., et al. (2008). Nurses' skill level and access to evidence-based practice. *Journal of Nursing Administration, 38*(11), 494–503.

Cannon-Diehl, M. R. (2009). Simulation in healthcare and nursing. *Critical Care Nursing Quarterly, 32*(2), 128–136.

Chaudry, B., Wang, J., Wu, S., et al. (2006). Systematic review: Impact of health information technology on quality, efficiency, and costs of medical care. *Annals of Internal Medicine, 144*(10), 742–752.

Checklist to evaluating web sites. (2003). University Libraries, University of Maryland, College Park, MD. Retrieved March 3, 2003, from http://www.lib.umd.edu/UES/webcheck.html

Ciesielka, D. (2008). Using a wiki to meet graduate nursing education competencies in collaboration and community health. *Educational Innovations, 47*(10), 473–476.

Davis, M. (2007). Stage 6 Hospitals: The journey and the accomplishments. Retrieved June 1, 2009, from http://www.himssanalytics.org

DeLong, D. (2009). The TIGER Initiative: Collaborating to integrate evidence and informatics into nursing practice and education: An executive summary, pp. 1–30. Retrieved May 20, 2009, from http://www.tigersummit.com

Donovan, S., & Bernardo, L. M. (2009). The role of collaborative web publishing tools in evidence-based practice. *Journal of Emergency Nursing, 35*(2), 149–150.

Doyle, C. S. (1992). Final report to National Forum on Information Literacy. University of Calgary. Information Literacy Group, 1998. Retrieved October 27, 2009, from http://www.asla.org.au/pubs/ws/accommat5.htm

Enrado, P. (2009, May 1). Tele-nurses help with 911 calls as cities cope with tight budgets. Retrieved June 20, 2009, from http://www.healthcareitnews.com/news/tele-nurses-help-911-calls-cities-cope-tight-budgets

Federal Health IT Strategic Plan. (2009). Why health IT? Retrieved June 15, 2009, from http://healthit.hhs.gov/portal/server.pt

Ford, E. W., Menachemi, N., Peterson, L. T., et al. (2009). Resistance is futile: But it is slowing the pace of EHR adoption nonetheless. *Journal of the American Medical Informatics Association, 16*(3), 274–281.

Fowler, S. B., Sohler, P., & Zarillo, D. F. (2009). Bar-code technology for dedication administration: Medication errors and nurse satisfaction. *MedSurg Nursing, 18*(2), 103–109.

Graves, J., & Corcoran, S. (1989). The study of nursing informatics. *Image: The Journal of Nursing Scholarship, 21*(4), 227–230.

Hart, M. D. (2008). Informatics competency and development within the US nursing population workforce. *Computers, Informatics, Nursing, 26*(6), 320–329.

Hood, G., & Scherger, J. E. (2009, August 5). No, don't buy an EMR now! Yes, buy an EMR now! *Medscape for Nurses*. Retrieved August, 9, 2009, from http://www.medscape.com/viewarticle/706725

Hook, J. M., Pearlstein, J., Samarth, A., et al. (2009). Using barcode medication administration to improve quality and safety. Findings from the AHRQ Health IT Portfolio. Retrieved May 20, 2009, from http://healthit.ahrq.gov/images/dec08bcmareport/bcma_issue_paper.htm

Information Literacy Standards, from Council of Australian University Librarians (2001). Canberra. Retrieved October 27, 2009, from http://ilp.anu.edu.au/Infolit_standards_2001.html

Institute of Medicine. (2000). *To err is human: Building a safer health system*. Washington, DC: National Academy of Sciences.

Koppel, R. (2008). Workarounds to barcode medication. Administration systems: Their occurrences, causes, and threats to patient safety. *Journal of the American Medical Informatics Association, 15*(4), 408–423.

Kossman, S. P., & Scheidenhelm, S. L. (2008). Nurses' perceptions of the impact of electronic health records on work and patient outcomes. *Computers, Informatics, Nursing, 26*(2), 69–77.

Krumsieg, K., & Baehr, M. (2000). *Foundations of learning* (3rd ed.). Corvallis, OR: Pacific Crest.

Kuhns, K. A. (2009, May). Do you know what your patients are learning online? *Pennsylvania Nurse*, 4–7.

Mador, R. L., & Shaw, N. T. (2009). The impact of a critical care information system on time spent charting and in direct patient care by staff in the ICU: A review of the literature. *International Journal of Medical Informatics, 78*, 435–445.

McGonigle, D. (2009). *Nursing informatics: A foundation of knowledge*. Sudbury, MA: Jones and Bartlett.

Moniz, B. (2009). Examining the unintended consequences of computerized provider order entry system implementation. *Online Journal of Nursing Informatics, 13*(1), 1–12.

National Institutes of Health (NIH). (2009). The National Library of Medicine fact sheet. Retrieved July 31, 2009, from http://www.nlm.nih.gov/pubs/factsheets/nlm.html

Nelson, R., & Joos, I. (1989, Fall). On language in nursing: From data to wisdom. *PLN Visions, 6*, 7.

Newhouse, R. P. (2007). Diffusing confusion among evidence-based practice, Quality Improvement, and Research. *Journal of Nursing Administration, 37*(10), 432–435.

Ozbolt, J. G., & Saba, V. K. (2008). A brief history of nursing informatics in the United States. *Nursing Outlook, 56*(5), 199–205.

Pipe, T. B., Cisar, N. S., Caruso, E., et al. (2008). Leadership strategies: Inspiring evidence-based practice at the individual, unit, and organizational levels. *Journal of Nursing Care Quality, 23*(5), 265–271.

Priyan, S. (2009). Hospital information systems market in Europe: Trends in 2009. Retrieved June 15, 2009, from http://www.frost.com/prod/servlet/market-insight-top.pag?docid=163558230

Ralston, J. D., Hirsch, I. B., Hoath, J., et al. (2009). Web-based collaborative care for type 2 diabetes. *Diabetes Care, 32*(2), 234–239.

Reti, S. R., Feldman, H. J., & Safran, C. (2009). Governance for personal health records. *Journal of the American Informatics Association, 16*(1), 14–17.

Rogers, E. M. (1964). *Diffusion of innovations*. New York: Free Press.

Rogers, E. M. (2005). *Diffusion of innovations*. New York: Free Press.

Sittig, D. F., & Singh, H. (2009). Eight rights of safe electronic health record use. *JAMA, 302*, 1111–1113.

Skiba, D. J. (2008). Nursing Education 2.0: Social networking for professionals. *Nursing Education Perspectives, 29*(6), 370–371.

Taylor, H. (2008). Number of "cyberchondriacs" adults going online for health information has plateaued or declined. *Healthcare News, 8*(8), 1–6.

Thede, L. (2009). Informatics: Electronic personal health records: Nursing's role. *Online Journal of Issues in Nursing, 14*(1), 1–5.

Turisco, F., & Rhoads, J. (2008). Equipped for efficiency: Improving nursing care through technology. Retrieved May 31, 2009, from http://www.chcf.org

U.S. Department of Health and Human Services (USDHHS). (2003). The Health Insurance Portability and Accountability Act of 1996 (HIPAA) Privacy Rule. Retrieved August 7, 2009, from http://www.hhs.gov/ocr/privacy/index.html

White, K., & Brown, J. (2009). "Present on admission" impacts everyone's practice. *Nursing Management, 40*(Supplement, 6), 2–6.

Chapter 40

American Heart Association (AHA). (2009). Questions and answers about chelation therapy. Retrieved August 27, 2004, from http://www.americanheart.org/presenter.jhtml?identifier=3000843

American Music Therapy Association, Inc. (n.d.). What is music therapy? Retrieved August 11, 2009, from http://www.musictherapy.org/

Assefi, N., Bogart, A., Goldberg, J., et al. (2008). Reiki for the treatment of fibromyalgia: A randomized controlled trial. *Journal of Alternative and Complementary Medicine, 14*(9), 1115–1122.

Astin, J. A. (1998). Why patients use alternative medicine: Results of a national study. *JAMA, 279*(19), 1548–1553.

Astin, J. (2004). Mind-body therapies for the management of pain. *Clinical Journal of Pain, 20*(1), 27–32.

Baldwin, A., & Schwartz, G. (2006). Personal interaction with a Reiki practitioner decreases noise-induced microvascular damage in an animal model. *Journal of Alternative and Complementary Medicine, 12*(1), 15–22.

Baldwin, A., Wagers, C., & Schwartz, G. (2008). Reiki improves heart rate homeostasis in laboratory rats. *Journal of Alternative and Complementary Medicine, 14*(4), 417–422.

Barclay, L., & Murata, P. (2008). AAP addresses use of complementary and alternative medicine. Medscape Medical News, Medscape-CME. Retrieved August 8, 2009, from http://cme.medscape.com/viewarticle/584824

Barnes, P., Bloom, B., & Nahin, R. (2008). Complementary and alternative medicine use among adults and children: United States, 2007. *National health statistics reports* (12). Hyattsville, MD: National Center for Health Statistics. Retrieved August 9, 2009, from http://nccam.nih.gov/news/2008/nhsr12.pdf

Barrett, B., Marchand, L., Scheder, J., et al. (2004). What complementary and alternative medicine practitioners say about health and health care. *Annals of Family Medicine, 2*(3), 253–259.

Bendit, L. J., & Bendit, P. D. (1977). *The etheric body of man: The bridge of consciousness.* Wheaton, IL: Quest.

Benjamin, P. (2010). *Tappan's Handbook of Healing Massage Techniques* (5th ed.). Upper Saddle River, NJ: Pearson, Prentice-Hall.

Bohm, D. (1980). *Wholeness and the implicate order.* New York: Routledge.

Bright, M. A. (2002). *Holistic health and healing.* Philadelphia: F. A. Davis.

Broom, A., & Adams, J. (2007). Current issues and future directions in complementary and alternative medicine (CAM) research. *Complementary Therapies in Medicine, 15*(3), 217–220.

Buckle, J. (2002). Clinical aromatherapy: Therapeutic uses for essential oils. *Advances in Nursing Practice, 10*(5), 67–68, 88.

Bulechek, G., Butcher, H., & Dochterman, J. (2008). *Nursing interventions classification (NIC)* (5th ed.). St. Louis, MO: C. V. Mosby.

Carson, R. (1994). *Silent spring.* Boston: Houghton Mifflin.

Carter, R., Hall, T., Aspy, C., et al. (2002). The effectiveness of magnet therapy for treatment of wrist pain attributed to carpal tunnel syndrome. *Journal of Family Practice, 51*(1), 38–40.

Cassidy, C. M. (1994). Unraveling the ball of string: Reality, paradigms, and the study of alternative medicine. *Advances: The Journal of Mind-Body Health, 10*(6), 58–92.

Cepeda, M. S., Carr, D. B., Sarquis, T., et al. (2007). Static magnetic therapy does not decrease pain or opioid requirements: A randomized double-blind trial. *Anesthesia and Analgesia, 104*(2), 290–294.

Chao, M., & Wade, C. (2008). Socioeconomic factors and women's use of complementary and alternative medicine in four racial/ethnic groups. *Ethnicity & Disease, 18*(1), 65–71.

Chiarioni, B., Whitehead, W., Pezza, V., et al. (2006). Biofeedback is superior to laxatives for normal transit constipation due to pelvic floor dyssynergia. *Gastroenterology, 130*(3), 930.

Cho, Z., Son, Y., Han, J., et al. (2002). fMRI neurophysiological evidence of acupuncture mechanisms. *Medical Acupuncture, 14*(1), 16–22. Retrieved August 8, 2009, from http://www.medicalacupuncture.org/aama_marf/journal/vol14_1/article1.html

Chou, R., & Huffman, L. (2007). Nonpharmacologic therapies for acute and chronic low back pain: A review of the evidence for an American Pain Society/American College of Physicians clinical practice guideline. *Annals of Internal Medicine, 147*(7), 492–504.

Cohen, S., Doyle, W., Turner, R., et al. (2003). Emotional style and susceptibility to the common cold. *Psychosomatic Medicine, 65*(4), 652–657.

Coppa, D. (2008). The internal process of Therapeutic Touch. *Journal of Holistic Nursing, 26*(1), 17–24.

Coulter, I., Hardy, M., Shekelle, P., et al. (2003). Effect of the supplemental use of antioxidants vitamin C, vitamin E, and the coenzyme Q10 for the prevention and treatment of cancer. Summary, Evidence Report/Technology Assessment: Number 75. AHRQ Publication Number 04-E002, October 2003. Agency for Healthcare Research and Quality, Rockville, MD. Retrieved August 29, 2009, from http://www.ahrq.gov/clinic/epcsums/aoxcansum.htm

Cousins, N. (1979). *Anatomy of an illness.* New York: Bantam Books.

Dannemann, K., Hecker, W., Haberland, H., et al. (2008). Use of complementary and alternative medicine in children with Type 1 diabetes mellitus—prevalence, patterns of use, and costs. *Pediatric Diabetes, 9*(3 Pt.1), 228–235.

Dekosky, S., Williamson, J., Fitzpatrick, A., et al. (2008). *Ginkgo biloba* for prevention of dementia. *JAMA, 300*(19), 2253–2262.

Denison, B. (2004). Touch the pain away: New research on the therapeutic touch and persons with fibromyalgia syndrome. *Holistic Nursing Practice, 28*(3), 142–151.

Di Martino, P., Agniel, R., David, K., et al. (2006). Reduction of *Escherichia coli* adherence to uroepithelial bladder cells after consumption of cranberry juice: A double-blind randomized placebo-controlled cross-over trial. *World Journal of Urology, 24*(1), 21–27.

Dossey, B. M., & Keegan, L. (2008). *Holistic nursing: A handbook for practice* (5th ed.). Boston: Jones and Bartlett.

Engebretson, J., & Wardell, D. (2007). Energy-based modalities. *Journal of Midwifery & Women's Health, 42*(2), 243–259.

Ernst, R. (2000). Chelation therapy for coronary heart disease: An overview of all clinical investigations. *American Heart Journal, 140*(1), 139–141.

Figueroa, L., Davis, B., Baker, S., et al. (2006). The influence of spirituality on health care-seeking behaviors among African Americans. *ABNF Journal, 17*(2), 82–88.

Flannery, M. (n.d.). An integrative approach to complementary and alternative medicine in primary care settings. *Docstoc* [web site]. Retrieved August 23, 2009, from http://www.docstoc.com/docs/4020483/An-Integrative-Approach-to-Complementary-and-Alternative-Medicine-

Friel, P. (2007). EEG biofeedback in the treatment of attention deficit/hyperactivity disorder. *Alternative Medicine Review, 12*(2), 146–151.

Furlan, A., Imamura, M., Dryden, T., et al. (2000, updated 2008). Massage for low-back pain. *Cochrane Database of Systematic Reviews,* Issue 3. Art. No.: CD001929. DOI: 10.1002/14651858.CD001929.pub2. Retrieved August 15, 2009, from http://www.cochrane.org/reviews/en/ab001929.html

Gansler, T., Kaw, C., Crammer, C., et al. (2008). A population-based study of prevalence of complementary methods used by cancer survivors. *Cancer, 113*(5), 1048–1057.

Gardiner, P., Graham, R., Legedza, A., et al. (2007). Factors associated with herbal therapy use by adults in the United States. *Alternative Therapies in Health & Medicine, 13*(2), 22–29.

Gardner, M., & Hunter, B. C. (2006). Using music therapy for patient symptom management. *Sigma Theta Tau 2006 Conference.* Retrieved August 28, 2009, from http://www.nursinglibrary.org/Portal/main.aspx?pageid=4024&pid=15702

German Federal Institute for Drugs and Medical Devices. (1998). *Complete German Commission E monographs: The therapeutic guide to herbal medicines.* Boston: Integrative Medical Communications.

Graham, R., Ahn, A., Davis, R., et al. (2005). Use of complementary and alternative medical therapies among racial and ethnic minority adults: Results from the 2002 National Health Interview Survey. *Journal of the National Medical Association, 97*(4), 535–545.

Han, A., Judd, M., Welch, V., et al. (2004). Tai chi for treating rheumatoid arthritis. *Cochrane Database of Systematic Reviews,* Issue 3. Art. No.: CD004849. DOI:1002/14651858.CD004849. Retrieved August 21, 2009, from http://www.cochrane.org/reviews/en/ab004849.html

Hansen, N., Jorgensen, T., & Ortenblad, L. (2006). Massage and touch for dementia. *Cochrane Database of Systematic Reviews,* Issue 4. Art. No: CD004989. DOI: 10.1002/14651858.CD004989.pub2, Retrieved August 15, 2009, from http://www.cochrane.org/reviews/en/ab004989.html

Harding, S., Flannelly, K., Galek, K., et al. (2008). Spiritual care, pastoral care, and chaplains: Trends in health care literature. *Journal of Health Care Chaplaincy, 14*(2), 99–117.

Hart, J. (2008). Complementary therapies for chronic pain management. *Alternative & Complementary Therapies, 14*(2), 64–68.

Herxheimer, A., & Petrie, K. (2002). Melatonin for the prevention and treatment of jet lag. *Cochrane Database of Systematic Reviews,* Issue 2. Retrieved August 15, 2009, from http://www.mrw.inter-science.wiley.com/cochrane/clsysrev/articles/CD001520/frame.html

Hickson, M., D'Souza, A., Muthu, N., et al. (2007). Use of probiotic *Lactobacillus* preparation to prevent diarrhoea associated with antibiotics: Randomised double blind placebo controlled trial. *BMJ, 335,* 407–408. Retrieved August 14, 2009, from http://www.bmj.com/cgi/content/full/335/7610/80

Hulisz, D. (2008). Top herbal products: Efficacy and safety concerns. *MedscapeCME,* January 4, 2008. Retrieved August 21, 2009, from http://cme.medscape.com/viewarticle/568235.

Hypericum Depression Trial Study Group. (2002). Effect of *Hypericum perforatum* (St. John's wort) in major depressive disorder: A randomized controlled trial. *JAMA, 287*(14), 1807–1814.

Iqbal, N., Cardillo, S., Volger, S., et al. (2009). Chromium picolinate does not improve key features of metabolic syndrome in obese nondiabetic adults. *Metabolic Syndrome and Related Disorders, 7*(2), 143–150.

Irwin, M., Olmstead, R., & Oxman, M. (2007). Augmenting immune responses to varicella zoster virus in older adults: A randomized, controlled trial of tia chi. *Journal of the American Geriatrics Society, 55*(4), 511–517.

Jansen, S., Forbes, D., Duncan, V., et al. (2006). Melatonin for cognitive impairment. *Cochrane Database of Systematic Reviews,* Issue 3, 2009 (status in this issue: Unchanged.). Retrieved August 15, from http://www.mrw.interscience.wiley.com/cochrane/clsysrev/articles/CD003802/frame.html

Jensen, M., & Patterson, D. (2006). Hypnotic treatment of chronic pain. *Journal of Behavioral Medicine, 29*(1), 95–124.

Johnson, P. (2002). The use of humor and its influences on spirituality and coping in breast cancer survivors. *Oncology Nursing Forum, 29*(4), 691–695.

Kabat-Zinn, J. (1994). *Wherever you go, you are there: Mindfulness meditation in everyday life.* New York: Hyperion.

Kreiger, D. (1993). *Accepting your power to heal: The personal practice of therapeutic touch.* Santa Fe: Bear & Company.

Lake, K. (2007). Commentary. Beware of bioidentical hormones! *The Clinical Advisor, 10*(9), 121.

Lang, E., Berbaum, K., Faintuch, S., et al. (2006). Adjunctive self-hypnotic relaxation for outpatient medical procedures: A prospective randomized trial with women undergoing large core breast biopsy. *Pain 126*(1–3), 155–164.

Larden, C. (2004). Efficacy of Therapeutic Touch in treating pregnant inpatients who have a chemical dependency. *Journal of Holistic Nursing, 22*(4), 320–332.

Levine, S. (1984). *Healing into life and death.* New York: Doubleday.

Li, X-M., & Brown, L. (2009). Efficacy and mechanisms of action of traditional Chinese medicines for treating asthma and allergy. *Journal of Allergy and Clinical Immunology, 123*(2), 297–306.

Mackay, N., Hansen, S., & McFarlane, O. (2004). Autonomic nervous system changes during Reiki treatment: A preliminary study. *The Journal of Alternative and Complementary Medicine, 10*(6), 1077–1081.

Macy, J., & Young, M. Y. (1998). *Coming back to life: Practices to reconnect ourselves, our world.* Stony Creek, CT: New Society.

Magill, L., & Berenson, S. (2008). The conjoining use of music therapy and reflexology with hospitalized advanced stage cancer patients and their families. *Palliative and Supportive Care, 6*(3), 289–296.

Mayo Clinic. (2007). Hypnosis: Another way to manage pain, kick bad habits. MayoClinic.com reprint. Retrieved August 11, 2009, from http://www.mayoclinic.com/print/hypnosis/SA00084/METHOD=print

Mayo Clinic. (2008). Omega-3 fatty acids, fish oil, alpha-linolenic acid. MayoClinic.com. Retrieved August 15, 2009, from http://www.mayoclinic.com/health/fish-oil/NS_patient-fishoil

McCaffrey, A., Eisenberg, D., Legedza, A., et al. (2004). Prayer for health concerns: Results of a national survey on prevalence and patterns of use. *Archives of Internal Medicine, 164*(8), 858–862.

McSherry, W. (2006). The principal components model: A model for advancing spirituality and spiritual care within nursing and health care practice. *Journal of Clinical Nursing, 15*(7), 905–917.

MedlinePlus. (updated 2009). Complementary and alternative medicine. U.S. National Library of Medicine and the National Institutes of Health. Retrieved August 7, 2009, from http://www.nlm.nih.gov/medlineplus/complementaryandalternativemedicine.html

Meeks, T., Wetherell, J., Irwin, M., et al. (2007). Complementary and alternative treatments for late-life depression, anxiety, and sleep disturbance: A review of randomized controlled trials. *Journal of Clinical Psychiatry, 56*(10), 1461–1471.

Memorial Sloan-Kettering Cancer Center. (n.d.). Cancer information. About herbs. Melatonin. Retrieved August 14, 2009, from http://www.mskcc.org/mskcc/html/69298.cfm

Memorial Sloan-Kettering Cancer Center. (updated 2009). Cancer information. About herbs. Aloe vera. Retrieved August 14, 2009, from http://www.mskcc.org/mskcc/html/69116.cfm

Moorhead, S., Johnson, M., Maas, M., et al. (2008). *Nursing outcomes classification (NOC)* (4th ed.). St. Louis, MO: C. V. Mosby.

Movaffaghi, A., Hasanpoor, M., Farsi, M., et al. (2006). Effects of Therapeutic Touch on blood hemoglobin and hematocrit level. *Journal of Holistic Nursing, 24*(1), 41–48.

Nahin, R., Pecha, M., Welmerink, D., et al. (2009). Concomitant use of prescription drugs and dietary supplementements in ambulatory elderly people. *Journal of the American Geriatric Society, 57*(7), 1197–1205.

NANDA International. (2009). *Nursing diagnoses: Definitions and classification 2009–2011.* Philadelphia: Author.

National Cancer Institute. (last updated May 23, 2008). Aromatherapy and essential oils (PDQ®). Retrieved August 12, 2009, from http://www.cancer.gov/cancertopics/pdq/cam/aromatherapy/

National Center for Complementary and Alternative Medicine (n.d., updated 2007). Energy medicine: An overview. Retrieved August 16, 2009, from http://nccam.nih.gov/health/whatiscam/energy/energymed.htm#ref19

National Center for Complementary and Alternative Medicine. (2004a). More than one-third of U.S. adults use complementary and alternative medicine, according to new government survey. NIH News Advisory. Retrieved August 8, 2009, from http://nccam/nih.gov/news/2004/052704.htm

National Center for Complementary and Alternative Medicine. (2004b). What Is CAM? Retrieved August 8, 2009, from http://nccam.nih.gov/health/whatiscam/overview.htm#

National Center for Complementary and Alternative Medicine. (2004c). Research reports. Questions and answers about using magnets to treat pain. Retrieved August 22, 2009, from http://nccam.nih.gov/health/magnet/magnetq-and-a.htm

National Center for Complementary and Alternative Medicine. (2005). Prayer and spirituality in health: Ancient practices, modern science. *CAM at the NIH, XII*(1). Retrieved August 8, 2009, from http://nccam.nih.gov/news/newsletter/2005_winter/prayer.htm

National Center for Complementary and Alternative Medicine. (2006a). Herbs at a glance. Saw palmetto. Retrieved August 12, 2009, from http://nccam.nih.gov/health/palmetto/

National Center for Complementary and Alternative Medicine. (2006b). Herbs at a glance. Flaxseed and flaxseed oil. Retrieved August 12, 2009, from http://nccam.nih.gov/health/flaxseed/

National Center for Complementary and Alternative Medicine. (2006c). Herbs at a glance. Aloe vera. Retrieved August 14, 2009, from http://nccam.nih.gov/health/aloevera/D333_Herbs.pdf

National Center for Complementary and Alternative Medicine. (2006d). Massage therapy: An introduction. Retrieved August 14, 2009, from http://nccam.nih.gov/health/massage/

National Center for Complementary and Alternative Medicine. (2006e). Reiki: An introduction. NCCAM Publication No. D315, updated July 2008. Retrieved August 21, 2009, from http://nccam.nih.gov/health/reiki/

National Center for Complementary and Alternative Medicine. (2007a). Biologically based practices: An overview. NCCAM Publication No. D237. Updated March, 2007. Retrieved August 11, 2009, from http://nccam.nih.gov/health/whatiscam/biological/biobasedprac.htm

National Center for Complementary and Alternative Medicine. (2008a). Consumer advisory. Vitamin E supplements. Retrieved August 9, 2009, from http://nccam.nih.gov/news/alerts/vitamine/vitamine.htm

National Center for Complementary and Alternative Medicine. (2008b). Get the facts. Spinal Manipulation for Low-Back Pain. Retrieved August 15, 2009, from http://nccam.nih.gov/health/pain/spinemanipulation.htm

National Center for Complementary and Alternative Medicine. (2008c). Get the facts. Magnets for pain. Retrieved August 15, 2009, from http://nccam.nih.gov/health/magnet/magnetsforpain.htm#studies

National Center for Complementary and Alternative Medicine. (2009a). Statistics on CAM Costs. 2007 National health interview survey. Retrieved August 6, 2009, from http://nccam.nih.gov/news/camstats/costs/

National Center for Complementary and Alternative Medicine. (2009b). Americans spend billions on alternative medicine. News. MedlinePlus. Retrieved August 9, 2009, from http://www.nlm.nih.gov/medlineplus/news/fullstory_87552.html

National Center for Complementary and Alternative Medicine. (2009c). Tai chi: An introduction. Retrieved August 20, 2009, from http://nccam.nih.gov/health/taichi/

National Institutes of Health (NIH). (n.d.). Acupuncture (PDQ®). National Cancer Institute. Retrieved August 8, 2009, from http://www.cancer.gov/cancertopics/pdq/cam/acupuncture/Patient/page1

National Institutes of Health (NIH). (1997). Acupuncture. National Institutes of Health consensus statement 1997 November 3–5, 15(5), 1–34. Retrieved August 8, 2009, from http://consensus.nih.gov/1997/1997Acupuncture107html.htm

National Institutes of Health (NIH). (2009). Fact sheet. Mind-body medicine practices in complementary and alternative medicine. Retrieved August 11, 2009, from http://www.nih.gov/about/researchresultsforthepublic/mind-body.pdf

Ness, J., Cirillo, D., Weir, D., et al. (2005). Use of complementary medicine in older Americans: Results from the health and retirement study. Gerontologist, 45(4), 516–524.

The North American Menopause Society (NAMS). (2007). Understanding the controversy: Hormone testing and bioidentical hormones. Proceedings from the Postgraduate Course presented prior to the 17th Annual Meeting of The North American Menopause Society, October 11, 2006, Nashville, TN. James A. Simon, Course Director and Moderator.

O'Connor, D., Marshall, S., & Massy-Westropp, N. (2003). Nonsurgical treatment (other than steroid injection) for carpal tunnel syndrome. Cochrane Database of Systematic Reviews, Issue 1. Art. No.: CD003219. DOI: 10.1002/14651858.CD003219. Retrieved August 22, 2009, from http://www.cochrane.org/reviews/en/ab003219.html.

O'Mathuna, D., & Ashford, R. (2007). Therapeutic touch for healing acute wounds. Cochrane Database of Systematic Reviews, Issue 4. Art. No.: CD002766. DOI: 10.1002/14651858.CD002766. Retrieved August 16, 2009, from http://www.cochrane.org/reviews/en/ab002766.html

Ospina, M., Bond, T., Karkhaneh, M., et al. (2007). Meditation Practices for Health: State of the Research, Structured Abstract. Evidence Report/Technology Assessment No. 155. (Prepared by the University of Alberta Evidence-based Practice Center under Contract No. 290-02-0023.) AHRQ Publication No. 07-E010, June 2007. Agency for Healthcare Research and Quality, Rockville, MD. Retrieved August 29, 2009, from http://www.ahrq.gov/clinic/tp/medittp.htm

Paul, I., Beiler, J., McMonagle, A., et al. (2007). Effect of honey, dextromethorphan, and no treatment on nocturnal cough and sleep quality for coughing children and their parents. Archives of Pediatrics & Adolescent Medicine, 161(12), 1140–1146.

Perry, R., & Dowrick, C. F. (2000). Complementary medicine and general practice: An urban perspective. Complementary Therapies & Medicine, 8(2), 71–75.

Phipps, S. (2002). Reduction of distress associated with paediatric bone marrow transplant: Complementary health promotion interventions. Pediatric Rehabilitation, 5(4), 223–234.

Prasad, A., Beck, F., Bao, B., et al. Zinc lozenges ameliorate cold symptoms. Journal of Infectious Diseases, 197(6), 795–802.

Pumpkin Hollow Farm. (2004). Therapeutic touch. Retrieved August 20, 2009, from http://www.therapeutictouch.org/what_is_tt.html

Qato, D., & Jacobs, L. (2008). Use of prescription and over-the-counter medications and dietary supplements among older adults in the United States. JAMA, 300(24), 2867–2878.

Radzyminski, S. (2007). Legal parameters of alternative-complementary modalities in nursing practice. Nursing Clinics of North America, 42(2), 189–212, v-vi.

Ratterman, R., Secrest, J., Norwood, B., et al. (2002). Magnet therapy: What's the attraction? Journal of the American Academy of Nurse Practitioners, 14(8), 347–353.

Richardson, J. (2004). What patients expect from complementary therapy: A qualitative study. American Journal of Public Health, 94(6), 1049–1053.

Robinson, J., Biley, F., & Dolk, H. (2007). Therapeutic touch for anxiety disorders. Cochrane Database of Systematic Reviews, Issue 3. Art. No.: CD00620. DOI: 10.1002/14651858.CD006240.pub2. Retrieved August 16, 2009, from http://www.cochrane.org/reviews/en/ab006240.html

Sancier, K., & Holman, D. (2004). Commentary: Multifaceted health benefits of medical qigong. The Journal of Alternative and Complementary Medicine, 10(1), 163–165.

Santaguida, P., Gross, A., Busse, J., et al. (2009). Evidence Report on Complementary and Alternative Medicine in Back Pain Utilization Report. Evidence Report/Technology Assessment No. 177. (Prepared by the McMaster University Evidence-based Practice Center, under Contract No. 290-02-0020.) AHRQ Publication No.09-E006). Rockville, MD. Agency for Healthcare Research and Quality.

Saper, R., Kales, S., Paquin, J., et al. (2004). Heavy metal content of Ayurvedic herbal medicine products. JAMA, 292(23), 2868–2873.

Saper, R., Phillips, R., Sehgal, A., et al. (2008). Lead, mercury, and arsenic in US- and Indian-manufacturered Ayurvedic medicines sold via the Internet. JAMA, 300(8), 915–923

Sawitzke, A., Shi, H., Finco, M., et al. (2008). The effect of glucosamine and/or chondroitin sulfate on the progression of knee osteoarthritis: A report from the Glucosamine/Chondroitin Arthritis Intervention Trial. Arthritis & Rheumatism, 58(10), 3183–3191.

Sego, S. (2007). Alternative meds update. Coenzyme Q10. The Clinical Advisor, 10(10), 126, 128.

Sego, S. (2008). Alternative meds update. Aloe vera. The Clinical Advisor, 11(3), 134, 137.

Sherman, K., Cherkin, D., Erro, J., et al. (2005). Comparing yoga, exercise and a self-care book for chronic low back pain. Annals of Internal Medicine, 143, 849–856.

Sloman, R. (1995). Relaxation and the relief of cancer pain. *Nursing Clinics of North America, 30,* 697–709.

Smania, N., Corato, E., Fiaschi, A., et al. (2003). Therapeutic effects of peripheral repetitive magnetic stimulation on myofascial pain syndrome. *Clinical Neurophysiology, 114*(2), 350–358.

Smith, A., & Nicholson, K. (2001). Psychosocial factors, respiratory viruses and exacerbation of asthma. *Psychoneuroendocrinology, 26*(4), 411–420.

So, P., Jiang, Y., & Qin, Y. (2008). Touch therapies for pain relief in adults. *Cochrane Database of Systematic Reviews,* Issue 4. Art. No.: CD006535. DOI: 10.1002/14651858.CD006535.pub2. Retrieved August 16, 2009, from http://www2.cochrane.org/reviews/en/ab006535.html

Steinberg, E. M. (2001). *The balance within: The science of connecting health and emotions.* New York: W. H. Freeman.

Stirling, L., Raab, G., Alder, E., et al. (2007). Randomized trial of essential oils to reduce perioperative patient anxiety: Feasibility study. *Journal of Advanced Nursing, 60*(5), 494–501.

Stothers, L. (2002). A randomized trial to evaluate effectiveness and cost effectiveness of naturopathic cranberry products as prophylaxis against urinary tract infection in women. *Canadian Journal of Urology, 9*(3), 1558–1562.

Sun, Y., & Gan, T. (2008). Acupuncture for the management of chronic headache: A systematic review. *Anesthesia & Analgesia, 107,* 2038–2047. Retrieved August 8, 2009, from http://www.anesthesia-analgesia.org/cgi/content/abstract/107/6/2038

Swenson, R. (2003). Therapeutic modalities in the management of nonspecific neck pain. *Physical Medicine and Rehabilitation Clinics of North America, 14*(3), 605–627.

Tindle, H., Wolsko, P., Davis, R., et al. (2005). Factors associated with the use of mind body therapies among United States adults with musculoskeletal pain. *Complementary Therapies in Medicine, 13*(3), 155–164.

Turner, R., & Bauer, R. (2005). An evaluation of Echinacea angustifolis in experimental rhinovirus infections. *New England Journal of Medicine, 353*(4), 341–348.

U.S. Food and Drug Administration (FDA). (2002). Status of certain additional over-the-counter drug category II and III active ingredients. Retrieved August 14, 2009, from http://www.fda.gov/ohrms/dockets/98fr/050902a.htm

Vickers, A., Ohlsson, A., Lacy, J., et al. (1998, updated 2004). Massage for promoting growth and development of preterm and/or low birth-weight infants. *Cochrane Database of Systematic Reviews,* Issue 1. Art. No.: CD000390. DOI: 10.1002/14651858.CD000390.pub2. Retrieved August 15, 2009, from http://www.cochrane.org/reviews/en/ab000390.html

Vitale, A. (2007). An integrative review of Reiki touch therapy research. *Holistic Nursing Practice, 21*(4), 167–179.

Vitale, A., & O'Connor, P. (2006). The effect of Reiki on pain and anxiety in women with abdominal hysterectomies: A quasi-experimental pilot study. *Holistic Nursing Practice, 20*(6), 263–272.

Vogler, B., & Ernst, E. (1999). Aloe vera. A systematic review of its clinical effectiveness. *British Journal of General Practice, 49,* 823–828.

Wardell, D., & Weymouth, K. (2004). Review of studies of healing touch. *Journal of Nursing Scholarship, 36*(2), 147–154.

Wardell, D., & Engebretson, J. (2008). Biological correlates of Reiki Touch(sm) healing. *Journal of Advanced Nursing, 33*(4), 439–445.

Winstead-Fry, P., & Kijek, J. (1999). An integrative review and meta-analysis of therapeutic touch research. *Alternative Therapies in Health and Medicine, 5*(6), 58–67.

Wolsko, P., Eisenberg, D., Davis, R., et al. (2002). Insurance coverage, medical conditions, and visits to alternative medicine providers: Results of a national survey. *Archives of Internal Medicine, 162,* 281–287.

Wolsko, P., Eisenberg, D., Davis, R., et al. (2004). Use of mind-body medical therapies. *Journal of General Internal Medicine, 19*(1), 43–50.

Wolsko, P., Eisenberg, D., Simon, L., et al. (2004). Double-blind placebo-controlled trial of static magnets for the treatment of osteoarthritis of the knee: Results of a pilot study. *Alternative Therapies in Health & Medicine, 10*(2), 36–43.

Woolard, A., Tatham, K., Barker, S., et al. (2007). Randomized trial of essential oils to reduce perioperative patient anxiety: Feasibility study. *Journal of Advanced Nursing, 60*(5), 494–501.

Wooldrige, S. (2005). The effect of an alternative therapy (music therapy) on adults with chronic low back pain. *Midwest Nursing Research Society.* Retrieved August 29, 2009, from http://www.nursinglibrary.org/Portal/main.aspx?pageid=4024&pid=12170

Yagci, S., Kibar, Y., Akay, O., et al. (2005). The effect of biofeedback treatment on voiding and urodynamic parameters in children with voiding dysfunction. *The Journal of Urology, 174*(5), 1994–1998.

Yeh, G., Wang, C., Wayne, P., et al. (2008). The effect of tai chi exercise on blood pressure: A systematic review. *Preventive Cardiology, 11*(2), 82–89.

Chapter 41

Abbott, A. (2002). Health care challenges created by substance abuse: The whole is definitely bigger than the sum of its parts. *Health & Social Work, 27*(3), 162–165.

Agency for Healthcare Research and Quality. (2009a). Preventive services. Retrieved October 5, 2009, from http://www.ahrq.gov/clinic/prevenix.htm

Agency for Healthcare Research and Quality. (2009b). The guide to clinical preventive services 2009: Recommendations of the U.S. Preventive Services Task Force. Retrieved October 5, 2009, from http://www.ahrq.gov/clinic/pocketgd09/pocketgd09.pdf

American Academy of Family Physicians (AAFP). (2009, April 15). Summary of recommendations for clinical preventive services. Revision 6.8. Leawood, KS: American Academy of Family Physicians (AAFP).

American Cancer Society. (2009a). Skin cancer prevention and early detection. Atlanta, GA: American Cancer Society. Retrieved August 25, 2009, from http://www.cancer.org/docroot/PED/content/ped_7_1_Skin_Cancer_Detection_What_You_Can_Do.asp

American Cancer Society. (2009b). Cancer facts and figures 2009. Atlanta, GA: American Cancer Society. Retrieved on December 8, 2009, from http://www.cancer.org/downloads/STT/500809web.pdf

American Cancer Society. (2009c). Detailed guide. Breast cancer: Can breast cancer be found early? Atlanta, GA: American Cancer Society. Retrieved September 2, 2009, from http://www.cancer.org/docroot/CRI/content/CRI_2_4_3X_Can_breast_cancer_be_found_early_5.asp

American Cancer Society. (2009d). American Cancer Society guidelines for the early detection of cancer. Atlanta, GA: American Cancer Society. Retrieved September 12, 2009, from http://www.cancer.org/docroot/ped/content/ped_2_3x_acs_cancer_detection_guidelines_36.asp

American Cancer Society. (2009e). Detailed guide: Can testicular cancer be found early? Atlanta, GA: American Cancer Society. Retrieved September 12, 2009, from http://www.cancer.org/docroot/CRI/content/CRI_2_4_3X_Can_Testicular_Cancer_Be_Found_Early_41.asp?sitearea=

American College of Sports Medicine (ACSM). (2009). *ACSM'S guidelines for exercise testing and prescription* (8th ed.). New York: Lippincott Williams & Wilkins.

American Heart Association (AHA). (n.d.). How do I know if I have high blood pressure? Retrieved December 7, 2009, from http://www.americanheart.org/presenter.jhtml?identifier=219

Blechek, G., Butcher, H., & Dochterman, J. (2008). *Nursing interventions classification (NIC)* (5th ed.). St. Louis, MO: C. V. Mosby.

Centers for Disease Control and Prevention (CDC). (2009a). Smoking-attributable mortality, years of potential life lost, and productivity losses—United States, 2000–2004. *JAMA, 301*(6), 593–594.

Centers for Disease Control and Prevention (CDC). (2009b). *National Vital Statistics Reports, 58*(1). Retrieved August 30, 2009, from http://www.cdc.gov/nchs/products/nvsr.htm#vol58

Daniels, S. R., & Greer, F. R. (2009). Lipid screening and cardiovascular health in childhood. *Pediatrics, 122*(1), 198–208. Retrieved September 9, 2009, from http://pediatrics.aappublications.org/cgi/content/full/122/1/198

DiClemente, R., & Cobb, B. (1999). Adolescent health promotion and disease prevention. In: J. M. Raczynski & R. J. DiClemente (Eds.), *Handbook of health promotion and disease prevention* (pp. 491–520). New York: Kluwer Academic/Plenum.

Engle, M., & Kratt, P. (1999). Health promotion in health care settings. In: J. M. Raczynski & R. J. DiClemente (Eds.), *Handbook of health promotion and disease prevention* (pp. 443–457). New York: Kluwer Academic/Plenum.

Erikson, E. (1963). *Childhood and society* (2nd ed.), New York: W. W. Norton.

Ford, E. S., van Dam, R. M., & Fonarow, G. C. (2009). Trends in the prevalence of low risk factor burden for cardiovascular disease among United States adults. *Circulation*, online. Retrieved September 19, 2009, from http://circ.ahajournals.org/cgi/content/abstract/CIRCULATIONAHA.108.835728v1

Halls, C., & Rhodes, J. (2002, September). Employee wellness and beyond at Appleton Papers Inc. *Athletic Therapy Today*, 46–47.

Hettler, W. (1984). Wellness: Encouraging a lifetime pursuit of excellence. *Health Values: Achieving High Level Wellness*, 8, 13–17.

Janssen, I., Katzmarzyk, P. T., & Ross R. (2004, March). Waist circumference and not body mass index explains obesity related health risk. *American Journal of Clinical Nutrition*, 79(3), 379–384.

Kobasa, S. (1979). Stressful life events, personality, and health: An inquiry into hardiness. *Journal of Personality and Social Psychology*, 37(1), 1–11.

Kodali, V., Kodavanti, M., Tripuraribhatla, P., et al. (1999). Dietary factors as determinants of hypertension: A case control study in an urban Indian population. *Asia Pacific Journal of Clinical Nutrition*, 8(3), 184–189.

Kosaka, M. (1996). Relationship between hardiness and psychological stress response. *Journal of Performance Studies*, 3, 35–40.

Kösters, J., & Gøtzsche, P. (2003, updated October 9, 2007). Regular self-examination or clinical examination for early detection of breast cancer. *Cochrane Database of Systematic Reviews*, Issue 4. Art. No.: CD003373. Retrieved December 7, 2009, from http://www.cochrane.org/reviews/en/ab003373.html

Lazarus, R. S. (1966). *Psychological stress and the coping process*. New York: McGraw-Hill.

Leavell, H., & Clark, E. (1965). *Preventive medicine for doctors in the community*. New York: McGraw-Hill.

Levy, S. B. (2006). Sunscreens and Photoprotection. *eMedicine*. Retrieved December 7, 2009, from http://www.emedicine.com/derm/topic510.htm

Linn, H. H., Ezzati, M., Chang, H. Y., et al. (2009). Association between tobacco smoking and and active tuberculosis in Taiwan: prospective cohort study. *Journal of Respiratory Critical Care Medicine*, 180(5), 475–480.

Maddi, S. R., Koshaba, D. M., Fazel, M., et al. (2009, July 1). The personality construct of hardiness, IV. *Journal of Humanistic Psychology*, 49(3), 292–305.

Mandic, S., Myers, J. N., Oliviera, R. B., et al. (2009). Characterizing differences in mortality at the low end of the fitness spectrum. *Medicine & Science in Sports & Exercise*, 41(8), 1573–1579.

Marma, A. K., & Lloyd-Jones, D. M. (2009). Systematic examination of the updated Framingham Heart Study General Risk Profile. *Circulation*, 120, 383–390.

McGinnis, J. M. (1992). The public health burden of a sedentary lifestyle. *Medicine, Science, Sports, and Exercise*, 24(6 Supplement), S196–200.

McGinnis, J. M., & Foege, W. H. (1994). Actual causes of death in the United States. *JAMA*, 270, 2207–2211.

Meadows M. (2003). Don't be in the dark about tanning. *FDA Consumer*, 37, 16–17.

Moorhead, S., Johnson, M., Maas, M., et al. (2008). *Nursing outcomes classification (NOC)* (4th ed.). St. Louis, MO: C. V. Mosby.

Morey, M. C. (2009). Diet and exercise intervention helps older, overweight cancer survivors reduce functional decline. *JAMA*, 301(18), 1883–1891.

Myers, J., Sweeney, T., & Witmer, J. (2000). The wheel of wellness counseling for wellness: A holistic model for treatment planning. *Journal of Counseling & Development*, 78(3), 251–267.

NANDA International. (2009). *Nursing diagnosis: Definitions and classifications 2009–2011*. Philadelphia: Author.

National Cancer Institute. (2009a, March 18). Prostate-Specific Antigen (PSA) Test. Retrieved September 3, 2009, from http://cancertrials.nci.nih.gov/cancertopics/factsheet/Detection/PSA

National Center for Health Statistics, United States, 2008 with chartbook. (2009b). Hyattsville, MD. Retrieved September 1, 2009, from http://www.cdc.gov/nchs/hus/updatedtables.htm

National Institutes of Health (NIH). (2004). Third report of the National Cholesterol Education Program (NCEP) expert panel on detection, evaluation, and treatment of high blood cholesterol in adults (adult treatment panel III). NIH Publication No. 01–3670. Washington, DC: Author. Retrieved September 1, 2009, from http://www.nhlbi.nih.gov/guidelines/cholesterol/index.htm

National Safety Council. (2004). Preventing slips and falls in the home. Retrieved August 27, 2009, from http://www.nasdonline.org/document/208/d000006/preventing-injuries-from-slips-trips-and-falls.html

Naylor, M. F., & Rigel, D. S. (2005). Current concepts in sunscreens and usage. In: D. S. Rigel, R. J. Friedman, L. M. Dzubow, et al. (Eds.), *Cancer of the skin* (pp. 71–83). Philadelphia: Elsevier/Saunders.

Neuman, B. (1995). *The Neuman systems model* (3rd ed.). Stamford, CT: Appleton & Lange.

Olson, M. B., Krantz, D. S., Kelsey, S. F., et al. (2005, July-August). Hostility scores are associated with increased risk of cardiovascular events in women undergoing coronary angiography: A report from the NHLBI-Sponsored WISE Study. *Psychosomatic Medicine*, 67(4), 546–552.

Parra, E. K., & Stevens, J. A. (2000). Fall prevention programs for seniors: Selected programs using home assessment and home modification. Atlanta, GA: Centers for Disease Control and Prevention, National Center for Injury Prevention and Control. Retrieved August 28, 2009, from http://www.cdc.gov/ncipc/falls/default.htm#PDF

Pender, N. J., Murdaugh, C. L., & Parsons, M. A. (2006). *Health promotion in nursing practice* (5th ed.). Upper Saddle River, NJ: Prentice-Hall.

Pope, M. A., Burnett, R. T., Krewski, D., et al. (2009). Cardiovascular mortality and exposure to airborne fine particulate matter and cigarette smoke. Shape of the exposure-response relationship. *Circulation*, 120(6), 941–948. Retrieved September 17, 2009, from http://circ.ahajournals.org/cgi/content/abstract/120/11/941

Prochaska, J., & DiClemente, C. (1982). Transtheoretical therapy: Toward a more integrative model of change. *Psychotherapy: Theory, research and practice*, 19(3), 276–288.

Qureshi, N., Wilson, B., Santaguida, P., et al. (2009, August). NIH State-of-the-Science Conference: Family history and improving health. *Evidence Report/Technology Assessment No. 186*. (Prepared by the McMaster University Evidence-based Practice Center, under Contract No. 290-2007-10060-I.) AHRQ Publication No. 09–E016. Rockville, MD: Agency for Healthcare Research and Quality. Retrieved September 17, 2009, from http://www.ahrq.gov/clinic/tp/famhimptp.htm

Rahe, R. (1974). Life change and subsequent illness reports. In: E. K. Gunderson & R. H. Rahe (Eds.), *Life stress and illness*. Springfield, IL: Charles C Thomas.

Reynolds, K., Pass, M., Galvin, M., et al. (1999). Schools as a setting for health promotion and disease prevention. In: J. M. Raczynski & R. J. DiClemente (Eds.), *Handbook of health promotion and disease prevention*. New York: Kluwer Academic/Plenum Publishers.

Selye, H. (1976). *The stress of life*. New York: McGraw-Hill.

Sinha, V. (2009). Immunological role of hardiness on depression. *Indian Journal of Psychological Medicine*, 31(1), 39–44. Retrieved on September 21, 2009, from http://www.ijpm.info/article.asp?issn=0253-7176;year=2009;volume=31;issue=1;spage=39;epage=44;aulast=Sinha

Soinio, M., Laakso, M., Lehto, S., et al. (2003). Dietary fat predicts coronary heart disease events in subjects with type 2 diabetes. *Diabetes Care*, 26(3), 619–624.

Spector, R. (2009). *Cultural diversity in health and illness* (7th ed.). Upper Saddle River, NJ: Prentice-Hall.

Task Force on Community Preventive Services. (2005a). Recommendations to increase physical activity in communities. *American Journal of Preventive Medicine*, 22(4S), 67–72. Retrieved September 1, 2009, from http://www.thecommunityguide.org/pa/pa-ajpm-recs.pdf

Task Force on Community Preventive Services. (2005b). *The Guide to Community Preventive Services: What Works to Promote Health?* New York: Oxford University Press.

Tindle, H. A., Chang, Y. F., Kuller, L. H., et al. (2009, August 10). Optimism, cynical hostility, and incident coronary heart disease and mortality in the Women's Health Initiative. *Circulation*, 120(8), 656. Retrieved from http://circ.ahajournals.org/cgi/content/abstract/CIRCULATIONAHA.108.827642v1

U.S. Department of Agriculture (USDA). (2009, last updated.). MyPyramid: Steps to a healthier you. Retrieved September 19, 2009, from http://www.mypyramid.gov/

U.S. Department of Health and Human Services (USDHHS). (2005). Dietary guidelines for Americans. Retrieved September 4, 2009, from http://www.health.gov/dietaryguidelines/dga2005/document/default.htm

U.S. Department of Health and Human Services (USDHHS). The Secretary's Advisory Committee on National Health Promotion and Disease Prevention. *Developing healthy people 2020*. (2008a). Phase I report: Recommendations for the framework and format of *Healthy People 2020*. Objectives for 2020. Retrieved December 12, 2009, from http://www.healthypeople.gov/hp2020/advisory/PhaseI/default.htm

U.S. Department of Health and Human Services (USDHHS). (2008b). 2008 physical activity guidelines for Americans. Retrieved September, 3, 2009, from http://www.health.gov/paguidelines/

U.S. Department of Health and Human Services (USDHHS), Office of Disease Prevention & Health Promotion and Human Services. (2009, October 30, revised). Proposed *Healthy People 2020* objectives. Retrieved April 2, 2010, from http://www.healthypeople.gov/hp2020/Objectives/TopicAreas.aspx

U.S. Food and Drug Administration (FDA). (2006). Sunless tanners and bronzers. Retrieved August 22, 2009, from http://www.fda.gov/Cosmetics/ProductandIngredientSafety/ProductInformation/ucm134064.htm

U.S. Food and Drug Administration (FDA). (2007). FDA proposes new rule for sunscreen products. Retrieved August 22, 2009, from http://www.fda.gov/bbs/topics/NEWS/2007/NEW01687.html

U.S. Food and Drug Administration (FDA). (2009a, November 30). Indoor tanning: The risks of Ultraviolet Rays. *FDA Consumer Updates*. Retrieved December 7, 2009, from http://www.fda.gov/ForConsumers/ConsumerUpdates/ucm186687.htm

U.S. Food and Drug Administration (FDA). (2009a, November 30). Sun safety: Save your skin. *FDA Consumer Updates*. Retrieved December 7, 2009, from http://www.fda.gov/ForConsumers/ConsumerUpdates/ucm049090.htm

United Health Foundation. (2008, December). America's health rankings: A call to action for individuals & their communities. Retrieved September 2, 2009, from http://www.americashealthrankings.org/

Wallston, K. A., Wallston, B. S., & DeVellis, R. (1978, last modified June 15, 2007). Development of the multidimensional health locus of control (MHLC) scales. *Health Education Monographs*, 6, 160–170. (MHLC scales available at Vanderbilt University, Multidimensional health locus of control scales). Retrieved September 1, 2009, from http://www.vanderbilt.edu/nursing/kwallston/mhlcscales.htm

Watson, J. (1979). *Nursing: The philosophy and science of caring*. Boston: Little, Brown.

Witmer, J., & Sweeney, T. (1992). A holistic model for wellness and prevention over the life span. *Journal of Counseling & Development*, 71, 140–148.

World Health Organization (WHO). (1948). Preamble to the constitution of the World Health Organization as adopted by the International Health Conference, New York, June 19–22, 1946; signed on July 22, 1946 by the representatives of 61 states (Official Records of the World Health Organization, No. 2, p. 100) and entered into force on 7 April 1948.

World Health Organization (WHO). (1986). Ottawa charter for health promotion. First International Conference on Health Promotion, Ottawa, November 21, 1986. Retrieved August 25, 2009, from http://www.who.int/hpr/NPH/docs/ottawa_charter_hp.pdf

Chapter 42

Allender, J. A., Rector, C., & Warner, K. (2010). *Community health nursing: Promoting and protecting the public's health* (7th ed.). New York: Wolters Kluwer Health, Lippincott Williams & Wilkins.

American Nurses Association (ANA). (1986). *Standards of community health nursing practice*. Washington, DC: American Nurses Association Publishing.

American Nurses Association (ANA). (2001a). *Nursing bill of rights*. Washington, DC: American Nurses Association Publishing.

American Nurses Association (ANA). (2001b). *Revised code of ethics of the American Nurses Association (ANA)*. Washington, DC: American Nurses Association Publishing.

American Nurses Association and the Health Ministries Association. (2005). *Faith Community Nursing: Scope and standards of practice*. Silver Spring, MD: Author.

American Nurses Association (ANA) and the National Association of School Nurses (NASN). (2005). *School nursing: Scope and standards of practice*. Silver Spring, MD: Author.

American Nurses Association (ANA). (2007a). *Corrections nursing: Scope and standards of practice*. Silver Spring, MD: Author.

American Nurses Association (ANA). (2007b). *Public health nursing: Scope and standards of practice*. Silver Spring, MD: Author.

Berberich, F. R., & Landman, Z. (2009). Reducing immunization discomfort in 4- to 6-year-old children: a randomized clinical trial. *Pediatrics*, 124(2), e203.

Bodenheimer, T. S., & Grumbach, K. (2009). *Understanding health policy: A clinical approach* (5th ed.). New York: Lange/McGraw-Hill.

Broadway, R. L. (2002, July). Anthrax threat intensifies focus on disaster preparedness. *Healthcare Financial Management*, 28–31.

Centers for Disease Control and Prevention (CDC). (2007). Practical methods: Direct observations and windshield surveys. Retrieved October 25, 2009, from http://www.cdc.gov/dhdsp/library/seh_handbook/chapter_five.htm

Centers for Disease Control and Prevention (CDC). (2009, June). Interim guidance for clinicians on identifying and caring for patients with swine-origin influenza A (H1N1) virus infection. Retrieved October 1, 2009, from http://www.cdc.gov/h1n1flu/identifying-patients.htm

Centers for Disease Control and Prevention (CDC). (2009a). Recommended adult immunization schedule—United States, 2009. *MMWR Morbidity and Mortality Weekly Report*, 57:Q1–Q4. Retrieved October 12, 2009, from http://www.cdc.gov/mmwr/preview/mmwrhtml/mm5753a6.htm

Centers for Disease Control and Prevention (CDC). (2009b). 2009 H1N1 flu (swine flu). Retrieved October 14, 2009, from http://www.cdc.gov/h1n1flu/

Clark, M. J. (2008). *Community health nursing: Advocacy for population health* (5th ed.). Upper Saddle River, NJ: Prentice-Hall.

Dawood, F. S., Jain, S., Finelli, L., et al. (2009). Emergence of a novel swine-origin influenza A (H1N1) virus in humans. *New England Journal of Medicine*, 360, 2605–2615.

Greene, J. (2002, October). JCAHO's approach to disaster. *Material Management in Health Care*, 14–15.

Hicks, P., Tarr, G. M., & Hicks, X. P. (2007). Reminder cards and immunization rates among Latinos and the rural poor in northeast Colorado. *Journal of the American Board of Family Medicine*, 20(6), 581–586.

Larsson, L. S., & Butterfield, P. (2002). Mapping the future of environmental health and nursing: Strategies for integrating national competencies into nursing practice. *Public Health Nursing*, 19(9), 301–308.

Martin, K. S. (2005). *The Omaha System: A key to practice, documentation, and management* (2nd ed.). New York: Elsevier.

Martin, K. S., & Norris, J. (1996). The Omaha system: A model for describing practice. *Holistic Nursing Practice, 11*(1), 75–83.

Martin, K. S., & Scheet, N. J. (1992). *The Omaha system: Applications for community health nursing.* Philadelphia: W. B. Saunders. Retrieved October 11, 2009, from http://www.omahasystem.org/interventionscheme.html

Martin, K., & Scheet, N. (1995). The Omaha system: Nursing diagnoses interventions and outcomes. In: N. Lang (Ed.), *Nursing data systems: The emerging framework.* Washington, DC: American Nurses Association Publishing.

Maslow, A. H. (1970). *Motivation and personality* (2nd ed.). New York: Harper and Row.

Moore, M. L., & Parker, A. L. (2006). Influenza vaccine compliance among pediatric asthma patients: What is the better method of notification? *Pediatric Asthma and Allergy Immunology, 19*(4), 200–204.

Nightingale, F. (1860/1969). *Notes on nursing: What it is, and what it is not.* New York: Dover Publications.

Pope, A. M., Snyder, M. A., & Mood, L. H. (Eds.). (1995). *Nursing, health and environment.* Washington, DC: Institute of Medicine, National Academies Press.

Pryor, E. (1987). *Clara Barton: Professional angel.* Philadelphia: University of Pennsylvania Press.

Rowan, J. (1999). Ascent and descent in Maslow's theory. *Journal of Humanistic Psychology, 39*(3), 125–133.

RTI International–University of North Carolina Evidence-based Practice Center. (2009, June). *Outcomes of Community Health Worker Interventions,* Agency for Healthcare Research and Quality, Rockville, MD. Retrieved October 14, 2009, from http://www.ahrq.gov/clinic/tp/comhworktp.htm

Siegel, B. (1983). *Lillian Wald of Henry Street.* New York: Macmillan.

Substance Abuse and Mental Health Services Administration. (1999). *Mental health: A report of the surgeon general.* Rockville, MD: U.S. Department of Health and Human Services, National Institutes of Health.

U.S. Bureau of the Census. (2002). United States census 2000 facts. [Available online.] Retrieved October 13, 2009, from http://www.census.gov/main/www/cen2000.html

U.S. Department of Health and Human Services (USDHHS). (1999a). Achievements in public health, 1900–1999: Family planning. *Morbidity and Mortality Weekly Report, 48*(47), 1073–1080.

U.S. Department of Health and Human Services (USDHHS). (1999b). Ten great public health achievements—United States, 1900–1999. *Morbidity and Mortality Weekly Report, 48*(50), 1141–1146.

U.S. Department of Health and Human Services (USDHHS). (2008). *Healthy People 2020* public meetings: 2009 draft objectives. [Available online.] Retrieved March 29, 2010, from http://www.healthypeople.gov/HP2020/

U.S. Department of Health and Human Services (USDHHS). (2010). *Healthy People 2020* fact sheet. Retrieved October 24, 2009, from http://www.healthypeople.gov/About/hpfact.htm

Veenema, T. G. (Ed.) (2007). *Disaster nursing and emergency preparedness for chemical, biological, and radiological terrorism and other hazards* (2nd ed.). New York: Springer.

West Virginia Department of Military Affairs and Public Safety. (2004). *Getting ready: A family emergency guide.* West Virginia Office of Emergency Services. Retrieved October 15, 2009, from http://www.wvdhsem.gov/g_ready1.htm

Chapter 43

111th Congress, first session (2010). *H.R.3962, the Affordable Health Care for America Act.* Retrieved July 23, 2010, from http://docs.house.gov/rules/health/111_ahcaa.pdf

American Nurses Association (ANA). (2008). *Home health nursing. Scope and standards of practice.* Silver Spring, MD: Author.

Borger, C., Smith, S., Truffer, C., et al. (2006). Health spending projections through 2015: Changes on the horizon. *Health Affairs, 25,* w61–w72, published online February 22, 2006. Retrieved September 3, 2009, from http://www.commed.vcu.edu/IntroPH/Introduction/percentgdp2015hamar06.pdf

Bradway, C., & Hirshman, K. B. (2008, October). Working with families of hospitalized older adults with dementia. *American Journal of Nursing, 108*(10), 52–60.

Buhler-Wilkerson, K. (2003). *No place like home: A history of nursing and home care in the United States.* Baltimore and London: Johns Hopkins University Press.

Bulechek, G., Butcher, H., & Dochterman, J. (Eds). (2008). *Nursing interventions classification (NIC)* (5th ed.). St. Louis, MO: C. V. Mosby.

Centers for Disease Control and Prevention (CDC). (modified 2008). Guidelines for infection control in home care settings. Atlanta, GA: CDC. Retrieved September 5, 2009, from http://www.cdc.gov/ncidod/dhqp/gl_home_care.html

Centers for Medicare & Medicaid Services. (2007). Medicare and home health care. CMS Publication No. 10969. Baltimore, MD: U.S. Department of Health and Human Services. Retrieved September 4, 2009, from http://www.medicare.gov/Publications/Pubs/pdf/10969.pdf

Centers for Medicare & Medicaid Services. (2009). OASIS C. Home Health Quality Initiatives. Baltimore, MD: U.S. Department of Health and Human Services. Retrieved September 5, 2009, from http://www.cms.hhs.gov/HomeHealthQualityInits/06_OASISC.asp#TopOfPage

Collopy, B., Dubler, N., & Zuckerman, C. (1990). The ethics of home care: Autonomy and accommodation. *Hastings Center Report, 20*(2), S1–16.

Dyck, I., Kontos, P., Angus, J., et al. (2004). The home as a site for long-term care: Meanings and management of bodies and spaces. *Health & Place, 11*(2), 173–185.

Egan, M., & Kadushin, G. (2005). Managed care in home health: Social work practice and unmet client needs. *Social Work in Health Care, 41*(2), 1–18.

Feldman, P., Murtaugh, C., Pezzin, L., et al. (1999). Just-in-time evidence-based e-mail "reminders" in home health care: Patient impact. *HSR: Health Services Research, 40*(3), 865–885.

Fialova, D., Topinkova, E., Gambassi, G., et al. (2005). Potentially inappropriate medication use among elderly home care patients in Europe. *JAMA, 293*(11), 1348–1358.

Gershon, R., Pogorzelska, M., Qureshi, K., et al. (2008). Home health care registered nurses and the risk of percutaneous injuries: A pilot study. *AJIC: American Journal of Infection Control, 36*(3), 165–172.

Gingerich, B. (2007). *The 36-hour day.* Baltimore, MD: Johns Hopkins University Press. www.press.jhu.edu

Hall, G. H., & Maslow, K. (2007). Working with families of hospitalized older adults with dementia. *Try this: Best practices for older adults with dementia, D10.* John A. Hartford Institute for Geriatric Nursing, College of Nursing, New York University, New York.

Head, B., Maas, M., & Johnson, M. (1997). Outcomes for home and community nursing in integrated delivery systems. *Caring, 16*(1), 50–56.

Hokenstad, A. (2006). Closing the home care case: Home health aides' perspectives on family caregiving. *Home Health Care Management & Practice, 18*(4), 306–314.

Humphrey, C. (2007). *Home care nursing handbook* (4th ed.). Boston: Jones & Bartlett.

Huynh-Hohnbaum, A-L., Villa, V., Aranda, M., et al. (2008). Evaluating a multicomponent caregiver intervention. *Home Health Care Services Quarterly, 27*(4), 299–325.

Inglis, S., Pearson, S., Treen, S., et al. (2006). Extending the horizon in chronic heart failure: Effects of multidisciplinary, home-based intervention relative to usual care. *Circulation, 114*(23), 2466–2473.

Jansen, L., Forbes, D., Markle-Reid, M., et al. (2009). Formal care providers' perceptions of home- and community-based services: Informing dementia care quality. *Home Health Care Services Quarterly, 28*(1), 1–23.

The Joint Commission (TJC). (2008). Accreditation: Home Care National Patient Safety Goals. Retrieved September 5, 2009, from http://www.jointcommission.org/PatientSafety/NationalPatientSafetyGoals/09_ome_npsgs.htm

Kitchener, M., Ng, T., & Harrington, C. (2007). State Medicaid home care policies: Inside the black box. *Home Health Care Services Quarterly, 26*(3), 23–38.

Koch, S. (2005). Home telehealth—Current state and future trends. *International Journal of Medical Informatics, 75*(8), 565–576.

Lander, F., Onder, G., Cesari, M., et al. (2006). Functional decline in frail community-dwelling stroke patients. *European Journal of Neurology, 13*(1), 17–23.

Lescure, F-X, Locher, G., Eveillard, M., et al. (2009). Community-acquired infection with healthcare-associated methicillin-resistant *Staphylococcus aureus*: The role of home nursing care. *Infection Control & Hospital Epidemiology, 27,* 1213–1218. Retrieved September 5, 2009, from http://www.journals.uchicago.edu/doi/pdf/10.1086/507920

Leutz, W., Capitman, J., Ruwe, M. (2002). Caregiver education and support: Results of a multi-site pilot in an HMO. *Home Health Care Services Quarterly, 21*(2), 49–72.

Levine, C., Albert, S., Hokenstad, A., et al. (2006). "This case is closed": Family caregivers and the termination of home health care services for stroke patients. *Milbank Quarterly, 84*(2), 305–331.

Martin, S. (2006). Infection control matters in home healthcare. *Home Healthcare Nurse, 24*(8), 485–486.

Moorhead, S., Johnson, M., & Maas, M., et al. (Eds.). (2008). *Nursing outcomes classification (NOC)* (4th ed.). St. Louis, MO: C. V. Mosby.

Mosocco, D. (2009). Introducing the PACE concept: Managed care for the frail older adult. *Home Healthcare Nurse, 27*(7), 423–428.

MyMedicare.gov (n.d.). Glossary. (Updated 2008, March 7). Retrieved September 4, 2009, from http://www.medicare.gov/Glossary/Search.as

National Association for Home Care (NAHC). (n.d.). What is home care? Retrieved September 6, 2009, from http://www.nahc.org/consumer/FAQs/whatis.html

National Association for Home Care & Hospice (NAHC). (updated 2008). Basic statistics about home care. Retrieved September 3, 2009, from http://www.nahc.org/facts/08HC_Stats.pdf

Pande, A., Laditka, S., Laditka, J., et al. (2007). Aging in place? Evidence that a state Medicaid waiver program helps frail older persons avoid institutionalization. *Home Health Care Services Quarterly, 26*(3), 39–60.

Polzien, G. (2007). Promoting safety and security at home. *Home Healthcare Nurse, 25*(3), 218–222.

Rehm, S., Campion, M., Katz, D., et al. (2009). Community-based outpatient parenteral antimicrobial therapy (CoPAT) for *Staphylococcus aureus* bacteraemia with or without infective endocarditis: Analysis of the randomized trial comparing daptomycin with standard therapy. *Journal of Antimicrobial Chemotherapy, 63*(5), 1034–1042.

Rhinehart, E. (2001). Infection control in the home. *Emerging Infectious Diseases, 7*(2), 1–12. Retrieved September 6, 2009, from http://www.cdc.gov/ncidod/eid/vol7no2/rhinehart.htm#21

Rhinehart, E., & McGoldrick, M. (2006). *Infection control in home care and hospice* (2nd ed.). Boston: Jones and Bartlett.

Saba, V. K. (n.d.). About. Clinical Care Classification System. Retrieved September 6, 2009, from http://sabacare.com/About/

Saba, V. (2002). Home health care classification system (HHCC): An overview. *Online Journal of Issues in Nursing, 7*(3). Retrieved September 6, 2009, from http://www.nursingworld.org/MainMenuCategories/ANAMarketplace/ANAPeriodicals/OJIN/TableofContents/Volume72002/No3Sept2002/ArticlesPreviousTopic/HHCCAnOverview.aspx

Saba, V. (2007). *Clinical care classification (CCC) system manual: A guide to nursing documentation.* New York: Springer.

Scherr, D., Kastner, P., Kollman, A., et al. and the MOBITEL investigators. (2009) Original paper: Effect of home-based telemonitoring using mobile phone technology on the outcome of heart failure patients after an episode of acute decompensation: Randomized control trial. *Journal of Medical Internet Research, 11*(3), e34. Retrieved September 5, 2009, from http://www.jmir.org/2009/3/e34

Shannon, G., Yip, J., & Wilber, K. (2004). Does payment structure influence change in physical functioning after rehabilitation therapy? *Home Health Care Services Quarterly, 23*(1), 63–78.

Sharkey, J. (2004). Variations in nutritional risk among Mexican American and non-Mexican American homebound elders who receive home-delivered meals. *Journal of Nutrition for the Elderly, 23*(4), 1–19.

Skarupski, K., McCann, J., Bienias, J., et al. (2008). Use of home-based formal services by adult day care clients with Alzheimer's disease. *Home Health Care Services Quarterly, 27*(3), 217–239.

Stocker, J. (2004). Evaluating home health care nursing outcomes with OASIS and NOC. *Abstracts of the Academy Health Meeting (2004: San Diego, CA). 21*(abstract. 1714). Retrieved September 6, 2009, from http://gateway.nlm.nih.gov/MeetingAbstracts/ma?f=103624748.html

Tullai-McGuinness, S., Madigan, E., & Fortinsky, R. (2009). Validity testing the Outcomes and Assessment Information Set (OASIS). *Home Health Care Services Quarterly, 28*(1), 45–57.

Vasquez, M. (2008). Down to the fundamentals of telehealth and home healthcare nursing. *Home Healthcare Nurse, 26*(5), 280–287.

Visiting Nurse Associations of America. (n.d.). Home healthcare. Retrieved September 4, 2009, from http://vnaa.org/vnaa/g/?h=html/homehealthcareoverview.html

Warrington, D., Cholowski, K., & Peters, D. (2003). Effectiveness of home-based cardiac rehabilitation for special needs patients. *Journal of Advanced Nursing, 41*(2), 121–129.

Chapter 44

Abma, T., Widdershoven, G., Frederiks, B., et al. (2008). Dialogical nursing ethics: The quality of freedom restrictions. *Nursing Ethics, 15*(6), 789–802.

Ahern, K., & McDonald, S. (2002). The beliefs of nurses who were involved in a whistleblowing event. *Journal of Advanced Nursing, 38*(3), 303–309.

Aiken, T. (2008). *Legal and ethical issues in health occupations* (2nd ed.). Philadelphia: W. B. Saunders.

Alister, B. (2008). The Institute of Medicine on non-heart-beating organ transplantation. *Cambridge Quarterly of Healthcare Ethics, 17*(1), 75–86.

Alister, B., & Bill, S. (2006). Advance directives in Canada. *Cambridge Quarterly of Healthcare Ethics, 15*(3), 256–260.

Altun, I. (2002). Burnout and nurses' personal and professional values. *Nursing Ethics, 9*(3), 269–278.

American Colleges of Nursing Association (AACN). (2008). *The essentials of baccalaureate education for professional nursing practice.* Washington, DC: Author. Retrieved September 12, 2009, from http://www.aacn.nche.edu/Education/pdf/BaccEssentials08.pdf

American Hospital Association. (2003). *Patient care partnership: Understanding expectations, rights and responsibilities.* Retrieved September 15, 2009, from http://www.aha.org/aha/issues/Communicating-With-Patients/pt-care-partnership.html

American Nurses Association (ANA). (1988a). *Nursing and the human immunodeficiency virus: A guide for nursing's response to AIDS.* Kansas City, MO: Author.

American Nurses Association (ANA). (1988b). *Ethics in nursing: Position statements and guidelines.* Kansas City, MO: Author.

American Nurses Association (ANA). (1991). American Nurses Association: Position statement on HIV testing. Retrieved June 25, 2009, from http://www.nursingworld.org/BloodborneandAirborneDiseases

American Nurses Association (ANA). (1992). *Ethics and human rights position statements: Foregoing nutrition and hydration.* Retrieved June 25, 2008, from http://www.nursingworld.org/EthicsHumanRights

American Nurses Association (ANA). (1994a). Ethics and human rights position statements: Assisted suicide. Retrieved September 18, 2009, from http://www.nursingworld.org/EthicsHumanRights

American Nurses Association (ANA). (1994b). Ethics and human rights position statements: Background information: Active euthanasia. Retrieved September 18, 2009, from http://www.nursingworld.org/EthicsHumanRights

American Nurses Association (ANA). (1994c). American Nurses Association: Position statement on assisted suicide. *Health Care & Ethics, 10*(1–2), 125–127.

American Nurses Association (ANA). (2001). *Code of ethics for nurses with interpretive statements.* Washington, DC: American Nurses Publishing. Retrieved September 10, 2009, from http://nursingworld.org/ethics/code/protected_nwcoe813.htm

American Nurses Association (ANA). (2002). The profession's response to the problems of addictions and psychiatric disorders in nursing. Resolution by the House of Delegates. Retrieved September 12, 2009, from http://www.nursingworld.org/MainMenuCategories/ThePracticeofProftessionalNursing/workplace/ImpairedNurse/Response.aspx

American Nurses Association (ANA). (2003). *Position statement on nursing care and do-not-resuscitate (DNR) decisions.* Retrieved June 30, 2008, from http://www.nursingworld.org/EthicsHumanRights

American Nurses Association (ANA). (2010). *Nursing: Scope and standards of practice* (2nd ed.). Public Comment draft, January 2010. Silver Spring, MD: Nursebooks.org Retrieved February 1, 2010, from http://www.nursingworld.org/DocumentVault/NursingPractice/Draft-Nursing-Scope-Standards-2nd-Ed.aspx

American Nurses Association (ANA) & Association of Nurses in AIDS Care (ANAC). (2007). HIV/AIDS nursing: Scope and standards of practice. Silver Spring, MD: ANA.

Amnon, G. (2005). Disease, illness, and ethics. *Cambridge Quarterly of Healthcare Ethics, 13*(3), 256–260.

Arries, E. (2005). Virtue ethics: An approach to moral dilemmas in nursing. *Curationis, 28*(3), 64–72.

Association of periOperative Registered Nurses (AORN). (2004). *AORN position statement: Perioperative care of patients with do not resuscitate (DNR) orders.* Retrieved September 20, 2009, from http://www.aorn.org/PracticeResources/AORNPositionStatements/Position_DoNotResuscitate

Attree, M. (2007). Factors influencing nurses' decisions to raise concerns about care quality. *Journal of Nursing Management, 15*(4), 392–402.

Austin, W. (2008). Ethics in a time of contagion: A relational perspective. *Canadian Journal of Nursing Research, 40*(4), 10–24.

Austin, W., Kelecevic, J., Goble, E., et al. (2009). An overview of moral distress and the paediatric intensive care team. *Nursing Ethics, 16*(1), 57–68.

Balch, S. (2006). The dubious value of value neutrality. *Academic Questions, 19*(4), 44–48.

Bandman, E., & Bandman, B. (2002). *Nursing ethics through the life span* (4th ed.). Upper Saddle River, NJ: Prentice-Hall.

Barnes, M., & Brannelly, T. (2008). Achieving care and social justice for people with dementia. *Nursing Ethics, 15*(3), 384–395.

Bayles, M. (1984). *Reproductive ethics.* Englewood Cliffs, NJ: Prentice-Hall.

Beauchamp, T. L., & Childress, J. F. (2008). *Principles of biomedical ethics* (6th ed.). New York: Oxford University Press.

Beckwith, F. J., & Peppin, J. F. (2000). Physician value neutrality: A critique. *Journal of Law, Medicine, and Ethics, 28*(1), 67–75.

Bell, J., & Breslin, M. (2008). Healthcare provider moral distress as a leadership challenge. *JONA'S Healthcare Law, Ethics, and Regulation, 10*(4), 94–97.

Benner, P. (1997). A dialogue between virtue ethics and care ethics. *Theoretical Medicine, 18,* 47–61.

Benner, P. (2000). The roles of embodiment, emotion, and lifeworld for rationality and agency in nursing practice. *Nursing Philosophy 1,* 5–19.

Benner, P. (2002). Creating compassionate institutions that foster agency and respect. *American Journal of Critical Care, 11*(2), 164–167.

Berry, P., & Planalp, S. (2008). Ethical issues for hospice volunteers. *American Journal of Hospice & Palliative Care, 25*(6), 458–462.

Beumer, C. (2008). Innovative solutions: The effect of a workshop on reducing the experience of moral distress in an intensive care unit setting. *Dimensions of Critical Care Nursing, 27*(6), 263–267.

Bolmsjo, I., & Hermeren, G. (2003). Conflicts of interest: Experiences of close relatives of patients suffering from amyotrophic lateral sclerosis. *Nursing Ethics, 10*(2), 186–198.

Brier-Mackie, S. (2001). Patient autonomy and medical paternity: Can nurses help doctors to listen to patients? *Nursing Ethics, 8*(6), 510–521.

Brock, D. W. (2006). Is a consensus possible on stem cell research? Moral and political obstacles. *Journal of Medical Ethics, 32,* 36–42.

Browne, A. (2008). The Institute of Medicine on non-heart-beating organ transplantation. *Cambridge Quarterly of Healthcare Ethics, 17,* 75–86.

Brownsey, D. (2001). Nurses and their right to whistle blow. *AORN Journal, 73*(3), 693–697.

Bruce, N. W., & Robyn, A. R. (2008). Informed consent: Good medicine, dangerous side effects. *Cambridge Quarterly of Healthcare Ethics, 17*(10), 66–74.

Burkhardt, M., & Nathaniel, A. (2008). *Ethics and issues in contemporary nursing* (3rd ed.). Clifton Park, NY: Thomson Delmar Learning.

Butts, J., & Rich, K. (2008). *Nursing ethics: Across the curriculum and into practice* (2nd ed.). Boston: Jones and Bartlett.

Cahn, M. T. (1987). The nurse as moral hero: A case for required dissent. *Dissertation Abstracts International, 50*(3). (University Microfilms International No. 88–22134).

Cameron, B. (2004). Ethical moments in practice: The nursing "how are you" revisited. *Nursing Ethics, 11*(1), 53–62.

Cameron, M., Schaffer, M., & Park, H. (2001). Nursing students' experience of ethical problems and use of ethical decision-making models. *Nursing Ethics, 8*(5), 432–447.

Canadian Nurses Association (CNA). (1998). *Advance directives: The nurse's role.* Ottawa: Author. Retrieved June 2, 2008, from http://www.cna-aiic.ca/cna/practice/ethics/inpractice/default_e.aspx

Canadian Nurses Association (CNA). (1999). I see and I am silent/I see and speak out: The ethical dilemma of whistleblowing. Ottawa: Author. Retrieved June 4, 2008, from http://www.cna-aiic.ca/cna/practice/ethics/inpractice/default_e.aspx

Canadian Nurses Association (CNA). (2000).*Working with limited resources: Nurses' moral constraints.* Ottawa: Author. Retrieved June 4, 2008, from http://www.cna-aiic.ca/cna/practice/ethics/inpractice/default_e.aspx

Canadian Nurses Association (CNA). (2001). Futility presents many challenges for nurses. Ottawa: Author. Retrieved September 20, 2009, from http://www.cna-aiic.ca/cna/documents/pdf/publications/Ethics_Pract_Futility_challenges_May_2001_e.pdf

Canadian Nurses Association (CNA). (2003). *Ethical distress in health care environments.* Ottawa: Author. Retrieved June 4, 2008, from http://www.cna-aiic.ca/cna/practice/ethics/inpractice/default_e.aspx

Canadian Nurses Association (CNA). (2008a). *Code of ethics for registered nurses.* Retrieved September 15, 2009, from http://www.cna-nurses.ca/CNA/practice/ethics/code/default_e.aspx

Castledine, G. (2009). Haywood case is a lesson for nurses and managers. *British Journal of Nursing, 18*(2), 583.

Catalano, J. T. (2008). *Nursing now!* (5th ed.). Philadelphia: F. A. Davis.

Catlin, A., & Volat, D. (2009). When the fetus is alive but the mother is not: Critical care somatic support as an accepted model of care in the twenty-first century? *Critical Care Nursing Clinics of North America, 21*(2), 267–276.

Catlin, A., Volat, D., Hadley, M., et al. (2008). Conscientious objection: A potential neonatal nursing response to care orders that cause suffering at the end of life? Study of a concept. *Neonatal Network®: The Journal of Neonatal Nursing, 27*(2), 101–108.

Clark, C. (2006). Moral character in social work. *The British Journal of Social Work, 36*(1), 75–89.

Cochran, M. (1999). The real meaning of patient-nurse confidentiality. *Critical Care Quarterly, 22*(1), 42–49.

Collis, S. P. (2006). The importance of truth-telling in health care. *Nursing Standard, 20*(17), 41–45.

Corley, M. C. (2002). Nurse moral distress: A proposed theory and research agenda. *Nursing Ethics, 9*(6), 636–650.

Corley, M. C., & Minick, P. (2002). Moral distress or moral comfort. *Bioethics Forum, 18*(1–2), 7–14.

Corley, M., Minick, P., Elswick, R., et al. (2005). Nurse moral distress and ethical work environment. *Nursing Ethics, 12*(4), 381–390.

Cortis, J. D., & Kendrick, K. (2003). Nursing ethics, caring and culture. *Nursing Ethics, 10*(1), 636–650.

Crawford, D., & Way, C. (2009). Just because we can, should we? A discussion of treatment withdrawal. *Paediatric Nursing, 21*(1), 22–25.

Crigger, N. J. (2008). Towards a viable and just global nursing ethics. *Nursing Ethics, 15*(1), 17–27.

Curtin, L., & Flaherty, J. (1982). *Nursing ethics: Theories and pragmatics.* Bowie, MD: Robert J. Brady.

Dahnke, M. (2009). The role of the American Nurses Association Code in ethical decision making. *Holistic Nursing Practice, 23*(2), 112–119.

DePalma, J., Ozanich, E., Miller, S., et al. (1999). "Slow" code: Perspectives of a physician and critical care nurse. *Critical Care Quarterly, 22*(3), 89–96.

DeVita, M. A., Snyder, J. V., Arnold, R. M., et al. (2002). Observations of withdrawal of life-sustaining treatment from patients who became non-heart-beating organ donors. *Critical Care Medicine, 28*(6), 1709–1712.

Dierckx de Casterlé, B., Izumi, S., Godfrey, N., et al. (2008). Nurses' responses to ethical dilemmas in nursing practice: Meta-analysis. *Journal of Advanced Nursing, 63*(6), 540–549.

Donahue, M. P. (2000). Nursing values: A look back, a view forward. *Creative Nursing, 6*(3), 5–10.

Drew, M., & Garrahan, K. (2005). Whistleblower protection for nurses and other health care professionals. *Journal of Nursing Law, 10*(2), 79–87.

Duchscher, J., & Myrick, F. (2008). The prevailing winds of oppression: Understanding the new graduate experience in acute care. *Nursing Forum, 43*(4), 191–206.

Eby, M. (2000). Withdrawing or withholding artificial hydration and nutrition. *Nursing Ethics, 7*(5), 374–375.

Effa-Heap, G. (2009). Blood transfusion: Implications of treating a Jehovah's Witness patient. *British Journal of Nursing, 18*(3), 174–177.

Ellis, J., & Hartley, C. (2008). *Nursing in today's world: Trends, issues, and management* (9th ed.). Philadelphia: Lippincott Williams & Wilkins.

Emmanuel, L., Ferris, F., von Gunten, C., et al. (Eds.). (2005). *EPEC™-O: Education in palliative and end-of-life care for oncology (Module 11: Withdrawing nutrition, hydration).* Copyright The EPEC™ Project, Chicago, IL. Produced by the EPEC™ Project, with major funding provided by the National Cancer Institute, and with supplemental funding provided by the Lance Armstrong Foundation.

Erlen, J. (2001). Moral distress: A pervasive problem. *Orthopaedic Nursing, 20*(2), 76–82.

Erlen, J. (2002). When there are limits on health care resources. *Orthopaedic Nursing, 21*(4), 69–74.

Erlen, J. (2008). How confidential is confidential? *Orthopaedic Nursing, 27*(6), 357–360.

Eycheson, C. (2008). Contemporary ethical challenges in healthcare. *Minnesota Nursing Accent, 80*(1), 14–16.

Fenton, M. T. (1987). Ethical issues in critical care: A perceptual study of nurses' attitudes, beliefs and ability to cope. Unpublished master's thesis, University of Manitoba, Winnipeg.

Fenton, M. T. (1988). Moral distress in clinical practice: Implications for the nurse administrator. *Canadian Journal of Nursing Administration, 1*(3), 8–11.

Fowler, M. (2008). *Guide to the code of ethics for nurses: Interpretation and application.* Silver Spring, MD: American Nurses Association.

Fredrikson, L., & Eriksson, K. (2003). The ethics of the caring conversation. *Nursing Ethics, 10*(2), 138–149.

Freysteinson, W. (2009). The twins: A case study in ethical deliberation. *Nursing Ethics, 16*(1), 127–130.

Fry, S. (2008). *Ethics in nursing practice: A guide to ethical decision making* (3rd ed.). Malden, MA: Wiley-Blackwell.

Fry, S., & Veatch, R. (2005). *Case studies in nursing ethics* (3rd ed.). Sudbury, MA: Jones and Bartlett.

Gastmans, C. (1999). Care as a moral attitude in nursing. *Nursing Ethics, 6*(3), 214–223.

Georges, J. J., & Grypdonck, M. (2002). Moral problems experienced by nurses when caring for terminally ill people: A literature review. *Nursing Ethics, 9*(2), 155–178.

Gibbs, J. (2009). *Moral development & reality: Beyond the theories of Kohlberg and Hoffman.* Upper Saddle River, NJ: Pearson Education (Allyn & Bacon).

Gielen, J., van den Branden, S., & Broeckaert, B. (2009). Religion and nurses' attitudes to euthanasia and physician assisted suicide. *Nursing Ethics, 16*(3), 303–318.

Gilligan, C. (1993). *In a different voice.* Cambridge, MA: Harvard University Press.

Gilligan, C. (1995). Hearing the difference: Theorizing connection. *Hypatia, 10*(2), 120–127.

Glasberg, A-L, Eriksson, S., & Norberg, A. (2008). Factors associated with "stress of conscience" in healthcare. *Scandinavian Journal of Caring Sciences, 22*(2), 249–258.

Glass, E., & Cluxton, D. (2004). Truth-telling: Ethical issues in clinical practice. *Journal of Hospice and Palliative Nursing, 6*(4), 232–235.

Goldenberg, M. (2005). On evidence and evidence-based medicine: Lessons from the philosophy of science. *Social Science & Medicine, 62*(11), 2621–2632.

Gray, M. T. (2008). Nursing leaders' experiences with the ethical dimensions of nursing education. *Nursing Ethics, 15*(2), 174–185.

Guido, G. W. (2005). *Legal and ethical issues in nursing* (5th ed.). Upper Saddle River, NJ: Prentice-Hall.

Gunnarsson, B., & Warrén Stomberg, M. (2009). Factors influencing decision making among ambulance nurses in emergency care situations. *International Emergency Nursing, 17*(2), 83–89.

Gutierrez, K. M. (2005). Critical care nurses' perceptions of and responses to moral distress. *Dimensions of Critical Care Nursing, 24*, 229–241.

Halvorsen, K., Førde, R., & Nortvedt, P. (2008). Professional challenges of bedside rationing in intensive care. *Nursing Ethics, 15*(6), 715–728.

Hamric, A., & Blackhall, L. (2007). Nurse-physician perspectives on the care of dying patients in intensive care units: Collaboration, moral distress, and ethical climate. *Critical Care Medicine, 35*(2), 1–8.

Hamric, A., Davis, W. S., & Childress, M. D. (2006). Moral distress in health care professionals. *Pharos of Alpha Omega Alpha Honor Medical Society, 69*(1), 16–23.

Hanna, D. R. (2004). Moral distress: The state of the science. *Research and Theory for Nursing Practice, 18*(1), 73–93.

Hart, T. J. (2009, September 2). Moral distress in a non-acute continuing care setting: The experience of registered nurses. Thesis (Master, Nursing). Queen's University, Kingston, Ont., Canada. Retrieved September 12, 2009, from https://qspace.library.queensu.ca/bitstream/1974/5115/1/Hart_Thomas_J_200908_MSc+.pdf

Helft, P., Bledsoe, P., Hancock, M., et al. (2009). Facilitated ethics conversations: A novel program for managing moral distress in bedside nursing staff. *JONA'S Healthcare Law, Ethics, and Regulation, 11*(1), 27–33.

Hodkinson, K. (2008). How should a nurse approach truth-telling? A virtue ethics perspective. *Nursing Philosophy, 9*(4), 248–256.

Hoffman, M. (2000). *Empathy and moral development: Implications for caring and justice.* Cambridge, UK: Cambridge University Press.

Hunnibell, L., Reed, P., Quinn-Griffin, M., et al. (2008). Self-transcendence and burnout in hospice and oncology nurses. *Journal of Hospice & Palliative Nursing, 10*(3), 172–179.

Husted, J., & Husted, G. (2008). *Ethical decision making in nursing and healthcare* (4th ed.). New York: Springer.

Hyland, D. (2002). An exploration of the relationship between patient autonomy and patient advocacy: Implications for nursing practice. *Nursing Ethics, 9*(5), 472–482.

International Council of Nurses (ICN). (2006). The ICN code of ethics for nurses. Geneva, Switzerland: Author. Retrieved September 14, 2009, from http://www.icn.ch/icncode.pdf

James, F. K. (2005). Developments in bioethics from the perspective of HIV/AIDS. *Cambridge Quarterly of Healthcare Ethics, 14*(4), 416–423.

Jameton, A. (1984). *Nursing practice: The ethical issues.* Englewood Cliffs, NJ: Prentice-Hall.

Jeffrey, D. (2006). *Patient-centered ethics and communication at the end of life.* Oxford; Seattle: Radcliffe.

Jensen, A., & Lidell, E. (2009). The influence of conscience in nursing. *Nursing Ethics, 16*(1), 31–42.

Johnstone, M. (2004). *Bioethics: A nursing perspective* (4th ed.). New York: Elsevier.

The Joint Commission (TJC). (2008). *2008 Hospital accreditation standards.* Oakbrook Terrace, IL: The Joint Commission on Accreditation of Healthcare Organizations.

Juping, Y. (2008). The ethics of care and empathy. *Nursing Ethics, 15*(4), 562–563.

Keenan, J. F. (2005). Developments in bioethics from the perspective of HIV/AIDS. *Cambridge Quarterly of Healthcare Ethics, 14,* 416–423.

Kenny, G. (2002). The importance of nursing values in interprofessional collaboration. *British Journal of Nursing, 11*(1), 65–68.

Klein, S. (2009). Moral distress in pediatric palliative care: A case study. *Journal of Pain and Symptom Management, 38*(1), 157–160.

Kohlberg, L. (1968). Moral development. In: *International encyclopedia of social science.* New York: Macmillan.

Kohlberg, L. (1981). *Essays on moral development.* Volumes 1–3. San Francisco: Harper & Row.

Kothai, S., & Kirschner, K. (2006). Abandoning the Golden Rule: The problem with "putting ourselves in the patient's place." *Topics in Stroke Rehabilitation, 13*(4), 68–73.

Kuhse, H. (1997). *Caring: Nurses, women, and ethics.* Malden, MA: Blackwell.

Lachman, V. (2008). Making ethical choices: Weighing obligations and virtues. *Nursing2008, 38*(10), 42–46.

Lachman, V. (2009). Practical use of the nursing code of ethics: Part I. *MedSurg Nursing, 18*(1), 55–57.

Lagana, K. (2000). The "right" to a caring relationship: The law and ethic of care. *Journal of Perinatal and Neonatal Nursing, 14*(2), 12–25.

Laskowski-Jones, L. (2007). Should families be present during resuscitation? *Nursing2007, 37*(5), 44–47.

LeDuc, K., & Kotzer, A. (2009). Bridging the gap: A comparison of the professional nursing values of students, new graduates, and seasoned professionals. *Nursing Education Perspectives, 30*(5), 279–284.

Leininger, M. (1988). Leininger's theory of nursing: Cultural care diversity and universality, *Nursing Science Quarterly, 1*(4), 150–152.

Leininger, M. (2002). Culture care theory: A major contribution to advance transcultural nursing knowledge and practice. *Journal of Transcultural Nursing, 13*(3), 189–192.

Levine, M. E. (1989). Beyond dilemma. *Seminars in Oncology Nursing, 5*(2), 124–128.

Lewenson, S., & Truglio-Londrigan, M. (2008). *Decision-making in nursing: Thoughtful approaches for practices.* Boston: Jones and Bartlett.

Lipp, A., & Fothergill, A. (2009). Nurses in abortion care: Identifying and managing stress. *Contemporary Nurse, 31*(2), 108–120.

Lundqvist, A., & Nilstun, T. (2009). Noddings's caring ethics theory applied in a paediatric setting. *Nursing Philosophy, 10*(2), 113–123.

Matheny, M. (1999). Nursing's 21st century values. *Creative Nursing, 5*(3), 5–6.

Mathes, M. M. (2001). Withholding and withdrawing nutrition and hydration by medical means: Ethical perspective. *MedSurg Nursing, 10*(2), 96–102.

McCarthy, J., & Deady, R. (2008). Moral distress reconsidered. *Nursing Ethics, 15*(2), 254–262.

Meddings, F., & Haith-Cooper, M. (2008). Culture and communication in ethically appropriate care. *Nursing Ethics, 15*(1), 52–61.

Meyers, J. L. (1994). Working in the grey zone: The moral suffering of critical care nurses. Unpublished master's thesis, Gonzaga University, Spokane, WA.

Milton, C. (2001). Institutional ethics committees: A nursing perspective. *Nursing Science Quarterly, 14*(1), 22–23.

Milton, C. (2002). Ethical implications for acting faithfully in the nurse-person relationship. *Nursing Science Quarterly, 15*(1), 21–24.

Milton, C. L. (2008a). Boundaries: Ethical implications for what it means to be therapeutic in the nurse-person relationship. *Nursing Science Quarterly, 21*(2), 115–118.

Milton, C. L. (2008b). Ethical implications for living with adversity: The ever-present experience in the global nursing community. *Nursing Science Quarterly, 21*(2), 115–118

Miola, J. (2006). The need for informed consent: Lessons from the ancient Greeks. *Cambridge Quarterly of Healthcare Ethics, 15*(2), 152–160.

Mitty, E., & Ramsey, G. (2008). Advance directives. In: E. Capezuti, D. Zwicker, M. Mezey, et al. (Eds.), *Evidence-based geriatric nursing protocols for best practice* (3rd ed., pp. 539–563). New York: Springer.

Mohammed, S., & Peter, E. (2009). Rituals, death and the moral practice of medical futility. *Nursing Ethics, 16*(3), 292–302.

Mula, C. (2002). The dilemmas of resource allocation. *International Journal of Palliative Nursing, 8*(4), 160.

Murphy, N., Canales, M., Norton, S., et al. (2005). Striving for congruence: The interconnection between values, practice, and political action. *Policy, Politics, and Nursing Practice, 6*(1), 20–29.

Myhrvold, T. (2006). The different other-towards an including ethics of care. *Nursing Philosophy, 7*(3), 125–136.

National Conference of Commissioners on Uniform State Laws. (2006). *Revised Uniform Anatomical Gift Act.* Retrieved September 18, 2009, from http://www.anatomicalgiftact.org/desktopdefault.aspx

National League for Nursing. (2007). *Core values.* Retrieved October 11, 2009, from http://www.nln.org/aboutnln/corevalues.htm

National Student Nurses Association (NSNA). (2001). *Code of academic and clinical conduct.* National Student Nurses Association. Retrieved July 16, 2008, from http://www.nsna.org/pubs/resources/academic_clinical_conduct.asp

Neades, B. (2009). Presumed consent to organ donation in three European countries. *Nursing Ethics, 16*(3), 267–282.

Noddings, N. (2003). *Caring: A feminine approach to ethics and moral education* (2nd ed.). Berkeley, CA: University of California Press.

O'Keefe, M. E. (Ed.). (2000). *Nursing practice and the law: Avoiding malpractice and other legal risks.* Philadelphia: F. A. Davis.

Olsen, D. (2007). Ethical issues. Unwanted treatment: What are the ethical implications. *American Journal of Nursing, 107*(9), 51–53.

O'Mathúna, D., & Lang, K. (2008). Medicine vs. prayer: The case of Kara Neumann. *Pediatric Nursing, 34*(5), 413–416.

O'Neil, J. A. (2002). What is a moral dilemma and what would you do if you were faced with one? *Journal of Pediatric Oncology Nursing, 19*(4), 145–147.

Parkes, N., & Jukes, M. (2008). Professional boundaries in a person-centered paradigm. *British Journal of Nursing, 17*(21), 1358–1364.

Pask, E. (2003). Moral agency in nursing: Seeing value in the work and believing that I make a difference. *Nursing Ethics, 10*(2), 165–174.

Pauly, B., MacKinnon, K., & Varcoe, C. (2009). Revisiting "Who gets care?": Health equity as an arena for nursing action. *ANS Advances in Nursing Science, 32*(2), 118–127.

Payne, J., & Thornlow, D. (2008). Clinical perspectives on portable do-not-resuscitate orders. *Journal of Gerontological Nursing, 34*(10), 11–16.

Pellegrino, E. D. (2000). Commentary: Value neutrality, moral integrity, and the physician. *Journal of Law, Medicine, and Ethics, 28*(1), 78–81.

Peternelj-Taylor, C. (2003). Whistleblowing and boundary violations: Exposing a colleague in the forensic milieu. *Nursing Ethics, 10*(5), 526–540.

Pfrimmer, D. (2009). Duty to care. *Journal of Continuing Education in Nursing, 40*(2), 53–54.

Piaget, J. (1932). *The moral development of a child.* New York: Free Press.

Pijl-Zieber, E., Hagen, B., Armstrong-Esther, C., et al. (2008). Moral distress: An emerging problem for nurses in long-term care? *Quality in Ageing, 9*(2), 39–48.

Pinquart, M., & Silbereisen, R. K. (2004). Transmission of values from adolescents to their parents: The role of value content and authoritative parenting. *Adolescence, 39*(153), 83–100.

Power, F., Higgins, A., & Kohlberg, L. (1989). *Lawrence Kohlberg's approach to moral education.* New York: Columbia University Press.

Purnell, M. (2009). Gleaning wisdom in the research on caring. *Nursing Science Quarterly, 22*(2), 109–115.

Purtilo, R. (2005). *Ethical dimensions in the health professions* (4th ed.). Philadelphia: W. B. Saunders.

Rabetoy, C. P., & Bair, B. C. (2007). Nephrology nurses' perspectives on difficult ethical issues and practice guidelines for shared decision making. *Nephrology Nursing Journal, 34*(6), 599–629.

Raines, D. (1994). Moral agency in nursing. *Nursing Forum, 29*(1), 5–11.

Raths, L., Harmin, M., & Simon, S. (1978). *Values and teaching.* Columbus, OH: Merrill.

Ray, S. (2006). Whistleblowing and organizational ethics. *Nursing Ethics*, 13(4), 438–445.

Redman, B. (2008). When is patient education unethical? *Nursing Ethics*, 15(6), 813–820.

Resnick, H., Schuur, J., Heineman, J., et al. (2008). Advance directives in nursing home residents aged > or =65 years: United States 2004. *American Journal of Hospice and Palliative Care*, 25(6), 476–482.

Rodney, P., & Starzomski, R. (1993). Constraints on the moral agency of nurses. *The Canadian Nurse*, 89(9), 23–26.

Rodney, P. A., Storch, J. L., & Starzomski, R. (2004). *Toward a moral horizon: Nursing ethics in leadership and practice.* Toronto: Pearson Prentice-Hall.

Roe v. Wade, 410 U.S. 133 (1973). Retrieved July 1, 2008, from http://caselaw.lp.findlaw.com/scripts/getcase.pl?court=us&vol=410&invol=113

Ross, L. F. (2004). Informed consent in pediatric research. *Cambridge Quarterly of Healthcare Ethics*, 13(4), 346–358.

Sahraian, A., Fazelzadeh, A., Mehdizadeh, A., et al. (2008). Burnout in hospital nurses: A comparison of internal, surgery, psychiatry, and burns wards. *International Nursing Review*, 55(1), 62–67.

Salladay, S. A. (2002). Ethics committee. *Nursing*, 32(8), 76–77.

Salter, B., & Salter, C. (2007). Bioethics and the global moral economy. The cultural politics of human embryonic stem cell science. *Science, Technology, & Human Values*, 32(5), 554–581.

Sayers, K. L. (2008). A concept development of 'being sensitive' in nursing. *Nursing Ethics*, 15(3), 289–303.

Schluter, J., Winch, S., Holzhauser, K., et al. (2008). Nurses' moral sensitivity and hospital ethical climate: A literature review. *Nursing Ethics*, 15(3), 304–321.

Schmidlin, E. (2008). Artificial hydration: The role of the nurse in addressing patient and family needs. *International Journal of Palliative Nursing*, 14(10), 485–489.

Schroeder, D. (2005). Human rights and their role in global bioethics. *Cambridge Quarterly of Healthcare Ethics*, 14(2), 221–223.

Schroeter, K. (2002). *Practical ethics for nurses and nursing students: A short reference manual.* Hagerstown, MD: University Publishing Group.

Schwarz, J. (2009). Stopping eating and drinking. *American Journal of Nursing*, 109(9), 53–62.

Schwenzer, K., & Wang, L. (2006). Assessing moral distress in respiratory care practitioners. *Critical Care Medicine*, 34(12), 2967–2973.

Scott, R. S. (1985). When it isn't life or death. *American Journal of Nursing*, 85(1), 19–20.

Seroka, A. M. (1994). Values clarification and ethical decision making. *Seminars for Nurse Managers*, 2(1), 8–15.

Shaw, H., & Degazon, C. (2008). Integrating the core professional values of nursing: A profession, not just a career. *Journal of Cultural Diversity*, 15(2), 44–50.

Sloan, A. J. (1999). Whistleblowing: There are risks! *RN*, 62(7), 65–66.

Sowney, M., & Barr, O. (2007). The challenges for nurses communicating with and gaining valid consent from adults with intellectual disabilities within the accident and emergency care service. *Journal of Clinical Nursing*, 16(9), 1678–1686.

Steele, S. M., & Harmon, V. M. (1979). *Values clarification in nursing.* New York: Appleton-Crofts.

Steele, S. M., & Harmon, V. M. (1983). *Values clarification in nursing* (2nd ed.). New York: Appleton-Lange.

Storch, J., Rodney, P., Pauly, B., et al. (2009). Enhancing ethical climates in work environments. *Canadian Nurse*, 105(3), 20–25.

Sumner, J., & Fisher, W., Jr. (2008). The moral construct of caring in nursing as communicative action: The theory and practice of a caring science. *ANS Advances in Nursing Science*, 31(4), E19–36.

Tariman, J. D. (2007). When should you blow the whistle for ethical reasons? *ONS Connect*, 22(2), 22–23.

Tepehan, S., Ozkara, E., & Yavuz, M. (2009). Attitudes to euthanasia in ICUs and other hospital departments. *Nursing Ethics*, 16(3), 319–327.

Thacker, K. (2008). Nurses' advocacy behaviors in end-of-life nursing care. *Nursing Ethics*, 15(2), 174–185.

Thiroux, J. (1977). *Ethics, theory and practice.* Philadelphia: MacMillan.

Thompson, I., Melia, K., Boyd, K., et al. (2006). *Nursing ethics* (5th ed.). London: Churchill-Livingstone Elsevier.

Tong, R. (1997). *Feminist approaches to bioethics: Theoretical reflection and practical applications.* Boulder, CO: Westview Press.

Trobec, I., Herbst, M., & Zvanut, B. (2009). Differentiating between rights-based and relational ethical approaches. *Nursing Ethics*, 16(3), 283–291.

Tschundin, V. (2003). *Ethics in nursing: The caring relationship* (3rd ed.). New York: Butterworth-Heinemann.

U.S. Department of Health and Human Services (USDHHS). (2002). Modifications to the standards for privacy of individually identifiable health information—Final rule. Retrieved September 20, 2009, from http://www.hhs.gov/news/press/2002pres/20020809.html

Vaartio, H., & Leino-Kilpi, H. (2005). Nursing advocacy—A review of the empirical research 1990–2003. *International Journal of Nursing Studies*, 42(6), 705–714.

Vaartio, H., Leino-Kilpi, H., Suominen, T., et al. (2009). Nursing advocacy in procedural pain care. *Nursing Ethics*, 16(3), 340–362.

Van Hooft, S. (1990). Moral education for nursing decisions. *Journal of Advanced Nursing*, 15, 210–215.

Van Hooft, S. (1999). Acting from the virtue of caring in nursing. *Nursing Ethics*, 6(3), 189–201.

Volbrecht, R. M. (2002). *Nursing ethics: Communities in dialogues* (3rd ed.). Upper Saddle River, NJ: Prentice-Hall.

Wadensten, B., Wenneberg, S., Silén, M., et al. (2008). A cross-cultural comparison of nurses' ethical concerns. *Nursing Ethics*, 15(6), 745–760.

Wainwright, P., & Gallagher, A. (2007). Ethical aspects of withdrawing and withholding treatment. *Nursing Standard*, 21(33), 46–50.

Watson, J. (1981, Summer). Socialization of the nursing student in a professional nursing education programme. *Nursing Papers*, 13, 19–24.

Watson, J. (2005). *Caring science as scared science.* Philadelphia: F. A. Davis.

Watson, J. (2007). *Nursing: Human science and human care. A theory of nursing.* Sudbury, MA: Jones and Bartlett.

Waugh, D. (1978). Moral development: Theory and process. In: *Teaching and Evaluating the Affective Domain in Nursing Programs* (pp. 17–30). New York: Charles B. Slack.

Webster, G. C., & Baylis, F. E. (2000). Moral residue. In: S. B. Rubin & L. Zoloth (Eds.), *Margin of error: The ethics of mistakes in the practice of medicine* (pp. 217–230). Hagerstown, MD: University Publishing Group.

Westrick, S., & McCormack, K. (2009). *Essentials of nursing law & ethics.* Boston: Jones and Bartlett.

White, G. B. (1983). Philosophical ethics and nursing: A word of caution. In: P. L. Chinn (Ed.), *Advances in nursing theory development.* Rockville, MD: Aspen Systems.

Wilkinson, J. M. (1987/88). Moral distress in nursing practice: Experience and effect. *Nursing Forum*, 23, 16–29.

Wilkinson, J. M. (1997). Toward a context-sensitive theory of nursing ethics: Classification and comparison of nurses' narratives from four time periods (1934, 1979, 1989 & 1995). Doctoral dissertation, University of Kansas, Kansas City, KS.

Wilmot, S. (2000). Nurses and whistleblowing: The ethical issues. *Journal of Advanced Nursing*, 32(5), 1051–1057.

Woods, S. (2007). *Death's dominion: Ethics at the end of life.* Columbus: McGraw Hill Open University Press.

Yoder-Wise, P. (2007). *Leading and managing in nursing* (4th ed.). St. Louis, MO: C. V. Mosby.

Zuzelo, P. R. (2007). Exploring the moral distress of registered nurses. *Nursing Ethics*, 14, 344–359.

Chapter 45

Aiken, T. D. (2004). *Legal, ethical, and political issues in nursing* (2nd ed.). Philadelphia: F. A. Davis.

American Hospital Association. (1992). *A patient's bill of rights.* Chicago: Author.

American Nurses Association (ANA). (n.d.). The impaired nurse resource center. Retrieved September 7, 2009, from http://www.nursingworld.org/MainMenuCategories/ThePracticeofProfessionalNursing/workplace/ImpairedNurse.aspx

American Nurses Association (ANA). (1991). Ethics and human rights position statements: Nursing and the patient self-determination acts. Retrieved September 8, 2009, from http://www.nursingworld.org/MainMenuCategories/HealthcareandPolicyIssues/ANAPositionStatements/EthicsandHumanRights.aspx

American Nurses Association (ANA). (2001). Code of ethics for nurses with interpretive statements. Washington, DC: American Nurses Publishing. Retrieved March 19, 2004, from http://www.nursingworld.org/MainMenuCategories/EthicsStandards/CodeofEthicsforNurses.aspx

American Nurses Association (ANA). (2002, September 24). Statement of the American Nurses Association for the Institute of Medicine's Committee on Work Environment for Nurses and Patient Safety. Washington, DC: ANA, 1–8. Retrieved August 20, 2009, from http://nursingworld.org/FunctionalMenuCategories/MediaResources/PressReleases/2006_1/ANAonWorkEnvironment.aspx

American Nurses Association (ANA). (2005). Code of ethics. Retrieved August 18, 2009, from http://www.nursingworld.org/MainMenuCategories/ThePracticeofProfessionalNursing/EthicsStandards/CodeofEthics.aspx

American Nurses Association (ANA). (2006). Ethics and human rights: Risk and responsibility in providing nursing care. Retrieved August 22, 2009, from http://www.nursingworld.org/EthicsHumanRights

American Nurses Association (ANA). (2007). Position statement: Registered nurse utilization of nursing assistive personnel. Washington, DC: Author. Retrieved August 18, 2009, from http://www.nursingworld.org/MainMenuCategories/HealthcareandPolicyIssues/ANAPositionStatements/uap.aspx

American Nurses Association (ANA). (2009). Nurses' Bill of Rights FAQs. Retrieved August 18, 2009, from http://nursingworld.org/EspeciallyForYou/staffnurses/FAQs.aspx

American Nurses Association (ANA). (2010). Nursing: Scope and standards of practice (2nd ed.). Draft for public comment, January 2010. Silver Spring, MD: Nursebooks.org Retrieved February 1, 2010, from http://www.nursingworld.org/DocumentVault/NursingPractice/Draft-Nursing-Scope-Standards-2nd-Ed.aspx

Americans with Disabilities Act (ADA) of 1990, Pub.L. 101-336, 104 Stat. 327, enacted July 26, 1990, codified at 42 U.S.C. § 12101 et seq. Retrieved September 10, 2009, from http://www.ada.gov/statute.html

Ashley, R. C. (2005). Weighing the evidence in your favor. Critical Care Nurse, 25(1), 60–61.

Austin, S. (2008). 7 tips for safe nursing practice. Nursing2008, 28(3), 34–39.

Ballard, K. (2003, September 30). Patient safety: A shared responsibility. Online Journal of Issues in Nursing, 8(3), Manuscript 4. Available: http://www.nursingworld.org/MainMenuCategories/ANAMarketplace/ANAPeriodicals/OJIN/TableofContents/Volume82003/No3Sept2003/PatientSafety.aspx

Canadian Nurses Association (CNA). (2002). Code of ethics for registered nurse: 2008 Centennial edition. Ottawa, Ontario: Author. [Online] Retrieved September 11, 2009, from http://www.cna-aiic.ca/CNA/practice/ethics/code/default_e.aspx

Equal Employment Opportunity Commission. (1992). A technical assistance manual on the employment provisions (title I) of the Americans with Disabilities Act. Retrieved August 16, 2009, from http://www.jan.wvu.edu/links/ADAtam1.html

Equal Employment Opportunity Commission. (2002, modified March 11, 2009). Guidelines on discrimination because of sex. (Section 1604.11, Sexual harassment. Code of Federal Regulations, Title 29, Vol. 4). Retrieved September 11, 2009, from http://www.access.gpo.gov/nara/cfr/waisidx_06/29cfr1604_06.html

Fedorka, P., & Resnick, L. K. (2001). Defining nursing practice. In: M. O'Keefe (Ed.), Nursing practice and the law: Avoiding malpractice and other legal risks (pp. 97–117). Philadelphia: F. A. Davis.

Ferrell, K. G. (2007). Documentation, part 2: The best evidence of care. Complete and accurate charting can be crucial to exonerating nurses in civil lawsuits. American Journal of Nursing, 107(7), 61–64.

Flores, J., & Dodier, A. (2005, May 31). HIPAA: Past, Present and Future Implications for Nurses. Online Journal of Issues in Nursing, 10(2), Manuscript 4. Retrieved August 19, 2009, from http://www.nursingworld.org/MainMenuCategories/ANAMarketplace/ANAPeriodicals/OJIN/TableofContents/Volume102005/No2May05/tpc27_416020.aspx

Frew, S. A. (2006, November). Nurse charged with felony in medication error death. Retrieved April 6, 2010, from http://www.medlaw.com/healthlaw/MEDMAL/nurse-charged-with-felony.shtml

Georgia Nurses Association. (n.d.). Nurse Advocate Program. The impaired nurse: Checklist for detecting potential chemical dependence in an employee. Retrieved August 17, 2009, from http://www.georgianurses.org/impaired_nurse.htm#pabi

Hall, J. K. (2001). Vicarious liability for nursing negligence. In: M. O'Keefe (Ed.), Nursing practice and the law: Avoiding malpractice and other legal risks (pp. 150–162). Philadelphia: F. A. Davis.

Hall, J. K., & Hall, D. (2001). Negligence specific to nursing. In: M. O'Keefe (Ed.), Nursing practice and the law: Avoiding malpractice and other legal risks (pp 132–149). Philadelphia: F. A. Davis.

Health Insurance Portability and Accountability Act (HIPAA), 29 U.S.C.A Section 1181 et seq.

Holloway, R. (2001). Patient rights. In: M. O'Keefe (Ed.), Nursing practice and the law: Avoiding malpractice and other legal risks (pp. 189–198). Philadelphia: F. A. Davis.

Iver, P. W., & Levin, B. J. (2007). Nursing malpractice (3rd ed.). Tucson, AZ: Lawyers and Judges Publishing Company.

Job Accommodation Network. (2006, June 22). Office of Disability Employment Policy, Accommodation and Compliance Series: Nurses with Disabilities. Morgantown, WV: Job Accommodation Network. Retrieved August 20, 2009, from http://www.jan.wvu.edu/media/nurses.html

Kansas State Board of Nursing, Unprofessional Conduct. (1993, last amended April 20, 2007). Retrieved December 8, 2009, from http://www.ksbn.org/npa/pages/60-7-106.pdf

Lunsford vs. Board of Nurse Examiners, 648 S.W. 2nd. 391 (Tex. App.—Austin 1983). Retrieved December 8, 2009, from http://www.bne.state.tx.us/practice/position.html

Marchand, D. V. (2001). American jurisprudence. In: M. O'Keefe (Ed.), Nursing practice and the law: Avoiding malpractice and other legal risks (pp. 3–22). Philadelphia: F. A. Davis.

Mathews, M. D. (2001). In: M. O'Keefe (Ed.), Nursing practice and the law: Avoiding malpractice and other legal risks (pp. 42–57). Philadelphia: F. A. Davis.

Meyer, G., & Lavin, M. A. (2005, June 23). Vigilance: The Essence of Nursing. Online Journal of Issues in Nursing, 10(1). Retrieved August 20, 2009, from http://www.nursingworld.org/MainMenuCategories/ANAMarketplace/ANAPeriodicals/OJIN/TableofContents/Volume102005/No3Sept05/ArticlePreviousTopic/VigilanceTheEssenceofNursing.aspx

Missouri Nurse Practice Acts (NPA). (n.d.). Nursing Practice Act & Code of State Regulations. Retrieved August 19, 2009, from http://www.dhss.mo.gov/LPHA/PHNursing/PracticeAct_Code_R_04.htm

Monarch, K. (2007). Documentation, part 1: Principles for self-protection: Preserve the medical record and defend yourself. American Journal of Nursing, 107(7), 58–60.

National Council of State Boards of Nursing (NCSBN). (n.d.). Professional boundaries: A nurse's guide to the importance of appropriate professional boundaries. Retrieved August 18, 2009, from https://www.ncsbn.org/ProfessionalBoundariesbrochure.pdf

National Council of State Boards of Nursing (NCSBN). (2005). Working with others: A position paper. Retrieved April 6, 2010 from https://www.ncsbn.org/314.htm

Nurses Service Organization (NSO). (2008, June). Legal case study. Retrieved April 6, 2010 from http://www.nso.com/case-studies/article/237.jsp

Nurses Service Organization (NSO). (2008, August). Legal Case Study. Retrieved August 22, 2009, from: http://www.nso.com/case-studies/casestudy-article/240.jsp

Nurses Service Organization (NSO). (2009). CNA Healthpro nurse claims study: An analysis of claims with risk management recommendations 1997–2007. Hatboro, PA: Nurse Service Organization. Retrieved September 8, 2009, from http://www.nso.com/rnclaimstudy

Nursing 2009. (2009). Legal liability: New study alerts RNs to daily practice risks. *Nursing 2009, 39*(9), 21–23.

O'Keefe, M. E. (Ed.). (2001). *Nursing practice and the law: Avoiding malpractice and other legal risks*. Philadelphia: F. A. Davis.

(1991). Patient Self Determination Act of 1991, Sections 4206 and 4751 of Omnibus Reconciliation Act of 1990, Pub L No. 101-508. Retrieved December 7, 2009, from http://www.nvcc.edu/home/bhays/dogwood/selfdeterminationact.htm

Pozzi, C. (2001). Violence in nursing. In: M. O'Keefe (Ed.), *Nursing practice and the law: Avoiding malpractice and other legal risks* (pp. 431–457). Philadelphia: F. A. Davis.

Quill, T. E. (2005). Terry Schiavo—A tragedy compounded. *New England Journal of Medicine, 352*(16), 1630–1633.

Sidlinger, L., & Hornberger, C. (2008). Current characteristics of the investigated impaired nurse in Kansas. *The Kansas Nurse, 83*(1), 3–5.

Strango v. Hammond, 2008 WL 501322 (S.D. Tex., February 21, 2008). *The Free Library*, 2008.

Synder, E. K. (n.d.). Emergency Medical Treatment and Active Labor Act: What every healthcare negligence lawyer should know. *Legal Eagle Eye Newsletter for the Nursing Profession*. Retrieved August, 15, 2009, from http://www.nursinglaw.com/EMTALA022306.htm#_ednref13

Texas Secretary of State. (2008). Texas Administrative Code, Safe Harbor Review for Nurses and Whistleblower Protection, Title 22, Chapter 217, Rule Section 217–20. Retrieved on August 20, 2009, from http://info.sos.state.tx.us/pls/pub/readtac$ext.TacPage?sl=R&app=9&p_dir=&p_rloc=&p_tloc=&p_ploc=&pg=1&p_tac=&ti=22&pt=11&ch=217&rl=20

The Water Buffalo Press (2007). Rochester nurse guilty of Medicaid fraud. Retrieved August 19, 2009, from http://waterbuffalopress.blogspot.com/2007/03/rochester-nurse-guilty-of-medicaid.html

UMKC. (2009). The right of privacy. Retrieved August 14, 2009, from http://www.law.umkc.edu/faculty/projects/ftrials/conlaw/rightofprivacy.html

U.S. Department of Health and Human Services (USDHHS). (2001). Standards for privacy of individually identifiable health information. [45 CFR Parts 160 and 164]. Retrieved December 8, 2009, from http://www.hhs.gov/ocr/hipaa/

U.S. Department of Health and Human Services (USDHHS), Centers for Medicare and Medicaid Services (2003). Emergency Medical Treatment & Labor Act (EMTALA) resource. Retrieved August 20, 2009, from http://www.cms.hhs.gov/emtala/

Vaughn, C. (1998, May 1). Accused of failure to report suspected abuse by colleague—Charges filed against 2 Fort Worth educators. *Star-Telegram*. Retrieved August 20, 2009, from http://www.nospank.net/n-c38.htm

Chapter 46

Advisory Committee on Health Human Resources. (2000). *The nursing strategy for Canada*. Ottawa: Health Canada.

Advisory Committee on Health Human Resources. (2002). *Our health, our future: Creating quality workplaces for Canadian nurses. Final report of the Canadian Nursing Advisory Committee*. Ottawa: Health Canada.

Advisory Committee on Population Health. (1996). *The report on the health of Canadians*. Ottawa: Health Canada.

Advisory Committee on Population Health. (1999). *Toward a healthy future: Second report on the health of Canadians*. Ottawa: Health Canada.

Alberta to Scratch Health Premiums. (2008). *Health Edition—Canada's Health Newsweekly, 12*(5), 2. Retrieved December 8, 2009, from http://www.healthedition.com/viewarticle.cfm?id=6228

Association of Canadian Academic Healthcare Organizations, et al. (2007). *The health care in Canada survey*. Toronto: Merck Frosst Canada.

Australian Government. (2008a). *International information on the safety and quality of health care*. Retrieved April 14, 2009, from http://www.aihw.gov.au/safequalityhealth/international_stats_20080916.cfm

Australian Government. (2008b). *Safety and quality of health care*. Retrieved April 14, 2009, from http://www.aihw.gov.au/safequalityhealth/index.cfm

Bramley, D., Hebert, P., Jackson, R., et al. (2005). Indigenous disparities in disease-specific mortality, a cross-country comparison: New Zealand, Australia, Canada, and the United States. *Journal of the New Zealand Medical Association, 117*(1207). Retrieved from http://www.nzma.org.nz/journal/117–1207/1215/

Broughton, H. (2001). *Nursing leadership: Unleashing the power*. Ottawa: Canadian Nurses Association (CNA).

Browne, G. (2001). Key findings from the system-linked research unit on health and social service utilization. Presented to the Advisory Committee on Health Human Resources Working Group on Nursing and Unregulated Healthcare Workers. Ottawa, October 24, 2001. Retrieved December 8, 2009, from http://fhs.mcmaster.ca/slru/paper/wp0101.htm

Browne, G., Roberts, J., Byrne, C., et al. (2001). Translating research—The costs and effects of addressing the needs of vulnerable populations: Results of 10 years of research. *Canadian Journal of Nursing Research, 33*(1), 65–76.

Buresh, B., & Gordon, S. (2000). *From silence to voice: What nurses know and must communicate to the public*. Ottawa: Canadian Nurses Association (CNA).

Butler, D. (2008). The identity of this frightful scourge? Depression. *OttawaCitizen.com*. January 12, 2008. Retrieved from http://www.canada.com/ottawacitizen/news/observer/story.html?id=5ea55e99–9050–4aeb-9744–f311504cac39

Campaign 2000. (2009). *It takes a nation to raise a generation: time for a national poverty reduction strategy*. Retrieved November 25, 2009, from http://www.campaign2000.ca/

Canadian Association of Occupational Therapists. (2009). 2008 annual report. Retrieved December 9, 2009, from http://www.caot.ca/pdfs/AR_2007–8.pdf

Canadian Federation of Nurses Unions (CFNU). (1991). *Funding health care*. Ottawa: Canadian Federation of Nurses Unions.

Canadian Federation of Nurses Unions (CFNU). (1993). *Human rights*. Ottawa: Canadian Federation of Nurses Unions.

Canadian Federation of Nurses Unions (CFNU). (1998). *Privatization of health care position statement*. Ottawa: Canadian Federation of Nurses Unions.

Canadian Federation of Nurses Unions (CFNU). (2008). *A renewed call for action: A synthesis report on the nursing shortage in Canada*. Retrieved April 17, 2009, from http://www.nursesunions.ca

Canadian Federation of Nurses Unions (CFNU). (2009). Mission statement. Retrieved November 24, 2009, from http://www.nursesunions.ca/content.php?sec=1

Canadian Institute for Health Information (CIHI). (2001). *Canada's health care providers*. Ottawa: Author.

Canadian Institute for Health Information (CIHI). (2002a). *Health indicators*. Ottawa: Author.

Canadian Institute for Health Information (CIHI). (2003). *Health care in Canada*. Ottawa: Author.

Canadian Institute for Health Information (CIHI). (2005a). *Exploring the 70/30 split: how Canada's health system is financed*. Ottawa: Author.

Canadian Institute for Health Information (CIHI). (2006a). *2005 national survey of the work and health of nurses*. Ottawa: Author.

Canadian Institute for Health Information (CIHI). (2006b). *Facility-based continuing care in Canada, 2004–2005*. Ottawa: Author.

Canadian Institute for Health Information (CIHI). (2007a). *Canada's health care providers*. Ottawa: Author.

Canadian Institute for Health Information (CIHI). (2007b). *Workforce trends of registered nurses in Canada, 2006*. Ottawa: Author.

Canadian Institute for Health Information (CIHI). (2007c). *Workforce trends of registered psychiatric nurses in Canada, 2006*. Ottawa: Author.

Canadian Institute for Health Information (CIHI). (2007d). *Workforce trends of licensed practical nurses in Canada, 2006*. Ottawa: Author.

Canadian Institute for Health Information (CIHI). (2007e). *Public-sector expenditures and utilization of home care services in Canada: Exploring the data, 2007*. Ottawa: Author.

Canadian Institute for Health Information (CIHI). (2008a). *National health expenditure trends, 1975–2008*. Ottawa: Author.

Canadian Institute for Health Information (CIHI). (2008b). *Health care in Canada*. Ottawa: Author.

Canadian Institute for Health Information (CIHI). (2008c). *An up-close look at seven major health professions*. Ottawa: Author.

Canadian Institute for Health Information (CIHI). (2008d). *Regulated Nurses: Trends, 2003 to 2007*. Ottawa: Author.

Canadian Nurse. (2000). Nursing policy: Making the talk matter. Interview with Judith Shamian. *Canadian Nurse, 96*(10), 16–20.

Canadian Nurses Association (CNA). (1998). *The quiet crisis in health care: A submission to the House of Commons Standing Committee on Finance and the Minister of Finance*. Ottawa: Author.

Canadian Nurses Association (CNA). (2000a). *The environment is a determinant of health*. Ottawa: Author.

Canadian Nurses Association (CNA). (2000b). *Framework for Canada's health system*. Ottawa: Author.

Canadian Nurses Association (CNA). (2000c). *International trade and labour mobility*. Ottawa: Author.

Canadian Nurses Association (CNA). (2000d). *The primary health care approach*. Ottawa: Author.

Canadian Nurses Association (CNA). (2001a). *Financing Canada's health system*. Ottawa: Author.

Canadian Nurses Association (CNA). (2001b). *Reducing the use of tobacco products*. Ottawa: Author.

Canadian Nurses Association (CNA). (2002a). *2001 annual report*. Ottawa: Canadian Nurses Association (CNA).

Canadian Nurses Association (CNA). (2002b). *Framework for Canada's health system*. Ottawa: Author.

Canadian Nurses Association (CNA). (2002c). *The primary health care approach*. Ottawa: Author.

Canadian Nurses Association (CNA). (2002d). *Supporting self-care: A shared initiative, 1999–2002*. Ottawa: Author.

Canadian Nurses Association (CNA). (2003a). *Clinical nurse specialist*. Ottawa: Author.

Canadian Nurses Association (CNA). (2003b). *Peace and security*. Ottawa: Author.

Canadian Nurses Association (CNA). (2006a). *E-Nursing strategy for Canada*. Ottawa: Author.

Canadian Nurses Association (CNA). (2006b). *Trends in illness and absenteeism and overtime among publically employed registered nurses*. Ottawa: Author. Retrieved November 28, 2009, from http://www.caccn.ca/files/trends_illness_injury_report.pdf

Canadian Nurses Association (CNA). (2006c). *Towards 2002: Visions for nursing*. Ottawa: Author. Retrieved April 6, 2010, from http://www.cna-nurses.ca/CNA/documents/pdf/publications/Towards_2020_Snapshot_e.pdf

Canadian Nurses Association (CNA). (2007). Understanding Self-Regulation. *Nursing Now: Issues and Trends in Canadian Nursing*. February (No. 21). Ottawa: Author.

Canadian Nurses Association (CNA). (2008a). *Signposts for Nursing: The Canadian Nurses Association Looks Ahead*. Ottawa: Author.

Canadian Nurses Association (CNA). (2008b). *CNA's preferred future: health for all*. Ottawa: Author.

Canadian Nurses Association (CNA). (2009). *About CNA*. Retrieved March 26, 2009, from http://www.cna-nurses.ca/CNA/about/default_e.aspx

Canadian Nurses Association & Canadian Medical Association. (2000). *Joint CNA/CMA position statement on environmentally responsible activity in the health sector*. Ottawa: Canadian Nurses Association (CNA).

Canadian Nurses Association & College of Family Physicians of Canada. (2001). *Joint CFPC/CNA position statement on physical activity*. Ottawa: Canadian Nurses Association (CNA).

Canadian Occupational Health Nurses Association. (2009). *About us*. Retrieved April 17, 2009, from http://www.cohna-aciist.ca/pages/content.asp?catID=2

Canadian Physiotherapy Association. (2009). *2008–2009 annual report*. Retrieved November 26, 2009, from http://www.physiotherapy.ca/public.asp?WCE=C=47%7CK=222584%7CRefreshT=223377%7CRefreshS=LeftNav%7CRefreshD=2233775

CBC News World. (2008). Desperately seeking doctors. Aired January 19, 2008. Retrieved April 14, 2009, from http://www.cbc.ca/doczone/desperatelyseekingdoctors.html

Cetron, M., & Davies, O. (2003). Trends shaping the future: Technological, workplace, management, and institutional trends. *The Futurist, 37*(2), 30–44.

Clarke, H. (2003). Health and nursing policy: A matter of politics, power, and professionalism. In: M. McIntyre & E. Thomlinson (Eds.), *Realities of Canadian nursing: Professional, practice, and power issues* (pp. 60–82). Philadelphia: Lippincott Williams & Wilkins.

Clarke, H., Lashinger, H. S., Giovannetti, P., et al. (2001). Nursing shortages: Workplace environments are essential to the solution. *Hospital Quarterly, 4*(4), 50–57.

Commission on the Future of Health Care in Canada. (2002). *Building on values: The future of healthcare in Canada—Final report*. [Commissioner Roy. J. Romanow]. Saskatoon, SK: Author.

Coster, G., & Buetow, S. (2001). *Quality in the New Zealand health system: Background paper to the National Health Committee*. Auckland, NZ: National Health Committee.

Council of the Federation. (2008). *Labour Market: Meeting the Requirements of the 21st Century*. Retrieved November 25, 2009, from http://www.councilofthefederation.ca/pdfs/COMMUNIQUE_EN_Labour_marketJuly13clean.pdf

Davis, E. (2005). Dory, rainbow and inukshuk: The journey to a strong health system in Canada. Paper presented at the Canadian Health Services Research Foundation 7th annual workshop – Leveraging knowledge: Tools & strategies for action, Montreal. Retrieved December 8, 2009, from http://ppn.sagepub.com/cgi/content/abstract/9/4/334

Department of Justice Canada. (2003a). Canada Health Act. Retrieved June 7, 2004, from http://laws.justice.gc.ca/en/C-6/15995.htm

Department of Justice Canada. (2003b). Indian Act. Retrieved June 7, 2004, from http://laws.justice.gc.ca/en/I-5/73349.html

Duncan, S., Hyndman, K., Estabrooks, C., et al. (2003). Nurses' experiences of violence in Alberta and British Columbia hospitals. *Canadian Journal of Nursing Research, 32*(4), 57–78.

EKOS Research Associates. (2002). *Report on the future of health care in Canada: General public survey*. Ottawa: Author. Retrieved December 8, 2009, from http://www.mapleleafweb.com/features/romanow-commission-future-health-care-findings-and-recommendations

First Ministers' Meeting. (2002). *Provinces pave the way for the future of health care*. Provincial-territorial premiers' meeting, January 24–25, Vancouver. Ottawa: Canadian Intergovernmental Conference Secretariat. Retrieved December 8, 2009, from http://www.scics.gc.ca/cinfo02/850085004_e.html

Fletcher, M. (2003). Be vigilant, nurses warned. *Canadian Nurse, 99*(4), 21.

Fooks, C., & Lewis, S. (2002). *Romanow and beyond: A primer on health reform issues in Canada*. Discussion Paper No. H/05. Ottawa: Canadian Policy Research Network.

Government of Alberta. (2001). *A framework for reform. Report of the Premier's Advisory Council on Health*. [D. Mazankowski, Chair]. Edmonton, AB: Premier's Advisory Council on Health. Retrieved December 8, 2009, from http://www.assembly.ab.ca/lao/library/egovdocs/alpm/2001/132279.pdf

Government of Alberta. (2006). *Alberta's Cancer Prevention Legacy Act*. Retrieved April 6, 2009, from http://www.international.alberta.ca/documents/Trade/France-UkraineMissionReport-June06_000.pdf

Government of British Columbia. (2003). Health Authorities Act, 1996. Retrieved September 16, 2005, from http://www.gov.bc.ca

Government of Canada. (1986). *Achieving health for all: A framework for health promotion*. Ottawa: Health and Welfare Canada.

Government of Canada. (2002). *The health of Canadians—The federal role. Final report on the state of the health care system in Canada. Volume six: Recommendations for reform*. [M. J. L. Kirby, Chair]. Ottawa: Standing Senate Committee on Social Affairs, Science and Technology. Retrieved December 8, 2009, from http://www.parl.gc.ca/37/2/parl-bus/commbus/senate/Com-e/soci-e/rep-e/repoct02vol6-e.htm

Government of Manitoba. (2009a). Manitoba's New Public Health Act, 2009. Retrieved April 6, 2009, from http://www.gov.mb.ca/health/publichealth/act.html

Government of Manitoba. (2009b). The Regulated Health Professions Act, 2009. Retrieved April 6, 2009, from http://www.health.gov.on.ca/english/public/legislation/regulated/regulated_health_professions.html

Government of New Brunswick. (2002). *Health renewal by the Premier's Health Quality Council, Province of New Brunswick, 2000–2002.* Fredericton, NB: Government of New Brunswick. Retrieved December 8, 2009, from http://www.health.alberta.ca/initiatives/health-initiatives-past.html

Government of New Brunswick. (2003). Mental Health Act. Retrieved September 16, 2009, from http://www.gnb.ca/0062/regs/m-10reg.htm

Government of Saskatchewan. (2001a). *Healthy people, a healthy province: An action plan for health in Saskatchewan.* Regina, SK: Author. Retrieved December 8, 2009, from http://www.health.gov.sk.ca/

Government of Saskatchewan. (2001b). *SchoolPlus: A vision for children and youth.* Final Report of the Task Force and Public Dialogue on the Role of the School. Regina, SK: Government of Saskatchewan. Retrieved December 8, 2009, from http://www.education.gov.sk.ca/SchoolPLUS

Government of Saskatchewan. (2003). Vital Statistics Act, 1995. Retrieved September 16, 2009, from http://publications.gov.sk.ca/details.cfm?p=931&cl=7

Grant, T. (2008). Filipinos find work faster. *The Globe and Mail,* February 13, 2008.

Grinspun, D., Virani, T., & Bajnok, I. (2001–2002). Nursing best practice guidelines: The RNAO (Registered Nurses Association of Ontario) project. *Hospital Quarterly,* Winter, 5(2), 56–60.

Haley, L. (2003). Students take on native recruitment. *Medical Post,* 39(20).

Hall, E. M. (1964). Royal Commission on Health Services. Ottawa: Government of Canada.

Hall, E. M. (1980). *Canada's national-provincial health program for the 1980's: A commitment for renewal.* Justice E. M. Hall, Special Commissioner. Ottawa: Department of National Health and Welfare.

Hart Wasekeesikaw, F. (2003). Challenges for the new millennium: Nursing in First Nations communities. In: M. McIntyre & E. Thomlinson (Eds.), *Realities of Canadian nursing: Professional, practice, and power issues* (pp. 447–469). Philadelphia: Lippincott Williams & Wilkins.

Health Canada. (2001). *Tactical plan for a pan-Canadian health infostructure. 2001 Update.* Federal-Provincial-Territorial Advisory Committee on Health Infostructure. Ottawa: Office of Health and the Information Highway. Retrieved September 16, 2009, from http://www.hc-sc.gc.ca/hcs-sss/pubs/ehealth-esante/2001–plan-tact/index-eng.php

Health Canada. (2003). Canada Health Act. Retrieved December 9, 2009, from http://www.hc-sc.gc.ca/hcs-sss/medi-assur/index-eng.php

Health Canada. (2004). Public Health Agency of Canada. Retrieved August 9, 2009, from http://www.phac-aspc.gc.ca/index-eng.php

Health Canada. (2005). *Canada's Health Care System.* Ottawa: Author.

Health Canada. (2006a). *About Health Canada: Legislation and Guidelines.* Retrieved March 20, 2009, from http://www.hc-sc.gc.ca/ahc-asc/legislation/index-eng.php

Health Canada. (2006b). 2003 First Ministers' Accord on Health Care Renewal. Retrieved November 23, 2009, from http://www.hc-sc.gc.ca/hcs-sss/delivery-prestation/fptcollab/2003accord/index-eng.php

Health Canada. (2006c). First Minister's Meeting on the Future of Health Care, 2004. *A 10–year plan to strengthen health care.* Retrieved November 23, 2009, from http://www.hc-sc.gc.ca/hcs-sss/delivery-prestation/fptcollab/2004–fmm-rpm/index-eng.php

Health Canada. (2006d). First Ministers' Meeting with Leaders of National Aboriginal Organizations, November 24–25, 2005. Retrieved April 13, 2009, from http://www.hc-sc.gc.ca/hcs-sss/delivery-prestation/fptcollab/2005–fmm-rpm-abor-auto/index-eng.php

Health Canada. (2007). *First Nations, Inuit and Aboriginal health: Aboriginal diabetes initiative.* Retrieved from http://www.hc-sc.gc.ca/fniah-spnia/diseases-maladies/diabete/index-eng.php#a7

Health Canada. (2008a). Introduction to assisted human reproduction (AHR). Retrieved April 6, 2009, from http://www.hc-sc.gc.ca/hl-vs/reprod/hc-sc/index-eng.php

Health Canada. (2008b). *Canada Health Act Annual Report 2007–2008.* Ottawa: Author.

Health Canada. (2008c). *2008–2009 Report on Plans and Priorities.* Ottawa: Author.

Health Canada. (2009). *Health care system.* Health Canada. Retrieved November 25, 2009, from http://www.hc-sc.gc.ca/hcs-sss/index-eng.php

Health Council of Canada (2008). *Fixing the foundations: an update on primary health care and home care renewal in Canada, 2008.* Toronto: Health Council. http://www.healthcouncilcanada.ca/en/index.php?option=com_content&task=view&id=214&Itemid=10

Health Services Restructuring Commission. (1999). *Primary health care strategy.* Toronto: Health Services Restructuring Commission.

Indian and Northern Affairs Canada. (2009). Aboriginal Peoples and Communities. Retrieved April 17, 2009, from http://www.ainc-inac.gc.ca/ap/index-eng.asp

Institute of Medicine, Committee on Quality of Health Care in America. (2001). *Crossing the quality chasm: A new health system for the 21st century.* Washington, DC: National Academies Press.

International Council of Nurses. (2009, May). Nurses in the workplace: Expectations and needs. Retrieved October 19, 2009, from http://www.icn.ch/Workplace/survey/index.html

International Council of Nurses and World Health Organization (WHO). (2005). *Nursing regulation: A futures perspective.* Geneva, Switzerland: Author.

Kohn, L. T., Corrigan, J. M., & Donaldson, M. S. (Eds.) (2000). *To err is human: Building a safer health system.* Institute of Medicine. Washington, DC: National Academies Press. Retrieved December 9, 2009, from http://www.nap.edu/openbook.php?isbn=0309068371

Kouri, D., Chessie, K., & Lewis, S. (2002). *Regionalization: Where has all the power gone? A survey of Canadian decision makers in health care regionalization.* Saskatoon, SK: Canadian Centre for Analysis of Regionalization and Health. Retrieved April 6, 2010 from http://www.longwoods.com/product.php?productid=16847

Kouri, D., & Lewis, S. (2004). Regionalization: Making sense of the Canadian experience. *Healthcare Papers,* 5(1), 12–31.

Krotz, L. (2008). Poaching foreign doctors. *The Walrus,* 5(5), 38–45. Retrieved December 9, 2009, from http://www.walrusmagazine.com/articles/2008.06–canada-poaching-foreign-international-immigrant-doctors-larry-krotz/

Lalonde, M. (1974). *The Lalonde Report.* Ottawa: Health and Welfare Canada.

Laschinger, H., Finegan, J., Shamian, J., et al. (2001). Testing Karasek's demands control model in restructured health care settings: Effects of job strain on staff nurses. *Nursing Administration,* 31(5), 233–243.

Lemire Rodger, G. (2003). Canadian Nurses Association (CNA). In: M. McIntyre & E. Thomlinson (Eds.), *Realities of Canadian nursing: Professional, practice, and power issues* (pp. 124–142). Philadelphia: Lippincott Williams & Wilkins.

Margoshes, D. (1999). *Tommy Douglas: Building the new society.* Montreal: XYZ Publishing.

Maxwell, J. (2002). Medicare reform: Bringing values into health care reform. *Canadian Medical Association Journal,* 166(12), 1543–1544.

McIntyre, M. (2003). The workplace environment. In: M. McIntyre & E. Thomlinson (Eds.), *Realities of Canadian nursing: Professional, practice, and power issues* (pp. 304–321). Philadelphia: Lippincott Williams & Wilkins.

McIntyre, M., & McDonald, C. (2003). Unionisation: Collective bargaining in nursing. In: M. McIntyre & E. Thomlinson (Eds.), *Realities of Canadian nursing: Professional, practice, and power issues* (pp. 322–337). Philadelphia: Lippincott Williams & Wilkins.

McIntyre, M., & Thomlison, E. (2003). Introduction to nursing issues: Implications for the nursing profession. In: M. McIntyre & E. Thomlinson (Eds.), *Realities of Canadian nursing: Professional, practice, and power issues* (pp. 2–16). Philadelphia: Lippincott Williams & Wilkins.

Metis National Council. (2003). Who Are the Metis? Retrieved December 8, 2009, from http://www.metisnation.ca/who/index.html

Ministry of Advanced Education and Labour Market Development, British Columbia. (2008). Health Care Assistant Program: Provincial Curriculum Guide.

Mowat, D., & Butler-Jones, D. (2007). Public Health in Canada: A difficult history. *Health Care Papers, 7*(3), 31–36.

National Association of Pharmacy Regulating Authorities. (2009). Available at http://www.napra.org

National Forum on Health Care. (1997). *Canada health action: Building on the legacy. Final report of the National Forum on Health.* Ottawa: Health Canada.

National Steering Committee on Patient Safety. (2002). *Building a safer system: A national integrated strategy for improving patient safety in Canadian health care.* Ottawa: National Steering Committee on Patient Safety.

National Task Force on Recruitment and Retention Strategies. (2002). *Against the odds: Aboriginal nursing.* Ottawa: Health Canada. Retrieved December 9, 2009, from http://findarticles.com/p/articles/mi_qa3911/is_200212/ai_n9161452/

Nurses for Medicare. (2009). *Medicare 101.* Retrieved March 20, 2009, from http://www.nursesformedicare.ca/medicare/default_e.aspx

Nursing Sector Study Corporation. (2006). *Building the Future: an integrated strategy for nursing human resources in Canada: Phase II final report.* Retrieved October 24, 2009, from http://www.hrhresourcecenter.org/node/1204

Ontario Health Services Restructuring Commission. (2000). *Looking back, looking forward: A legacy report from the Ontario Health Services Restructuring Commission, 1996–2000.* Toronto: Author. Retrieved December 8, 2009, from http://www.health.gov.on.ca/hsrc/HSRC.pdf

Public Health Agency of Canada. (2007). *Strategic plan, 2007–2012.* Ottawa: Author. Retreived on December 8, 2009, from http://www.phac-aspc.gc.ca/publicat/2007/sp-ps/FLA-Placemat-eng.php

Quebec Commission d'etude sure les services de sante et les service sociaux. (2001). *Emerging solutions: Report and recommendations.* [M. Clair, Chairman]. Quebec: Ministere de la Sante et des Services Sociaux. Retrieved December 8, 2009, from http://msssa4.msss.gouv.qc.ca/en/document/publication.nsf/b640b2b84246d64785256b1e00640d74/978c5d86bea2903e8525753c00650c1c?OpenDocument

Registered Psychiatric Nurses Association of Saskatchewan, Saskatchewan Association of Licensed Practical Nurses, & Saskatchewan Registered Nurses Association. (2000). *Nursing in collaborative environments.* Regina, SK: Saskatchewan Health.

Sanmartin, C., & Ross, N. (2006). Experiencing difficulties accessing first-contact health services in Canada. *Healthcare Policy, 1*(2), 103–119.

Saskatchewan Commission on Medicare. (2001). *Caring for Medicare: Sustaining a quality system.* [K. J. Fyke, Commissioner]. Regina, SK: Saskatchewan Health.

Saskatchewan Health Quality Council. (2003). *Room for improvement: Setting priorities for making Saskatchewan health care better.* Saskatoon, SK: Author. Retrieved December 8, 2009, from http://www.health.gov.sk.ca/health-care-action-plan

Shamian, J., Skelton-Green, J., & Villeneuve, M. (2003). Policy is the lever for effecting change. In: M. McIntyre & E. Thomlinson (Eds.), *Realities of Canadian nursing: Professional, practice, and power issues* (pp. 83–104). Philadelphia: Lippincott Williams & Wilkins.

Statistics Canada. (2005). Canada's Aboriginal population in 2017. *The Daily.* June 28, 2005. Retrieved April 8, 2009, from http://www.statcan.gc.ca/daily-quotidien/050628/dq050628d-eng.htm

Storch, J. (2003). The Canadian health care system and Canadian nurses. In: M. McIntyre & E. Thomlinson (Eds.), *Realities of Canadian nursing: Professional, practice, and power issues* (pp. 34–59). Philadelphia: Lippincott Williams & Wilkins.

Sutherland, K., & Coyle, N. (2009). *Quality of healthcare in England, Wales, Scotland, Northern Ireland: an intra-UK chartbook.* Retrieved April 14, 2009, from http://www.health.org.uk/publications/research_reports/intrauk_chartbook.html

Villeneuve, M., & MacDonald, J. (2006). *Toward 2020: Visions for Nursing.* Ottawa: Canadian Nurses Association (CNA).

Woolhandler, S., & Himmelstein, D. U. (2002). Paying for national health insurance—and not getting it. *Health Affairs, 21*(4), 88–98.

World Health Organization (WHO). (1978). *Declaration of Alma-Ata.* International Conference on Primary Health Care, Alma-Ata, USSR, 6–12 September.

World Health Organization (WHO). (1986). *Ottawa charter for health promotion: An international conference on health promotion.* November 17–21, 1986.

World Health Organization (WHO). (2002). *The world health report.* Geneva, Switzerland: Author.

World Health Organization Regional Office for Southeast Asia. (2008). *Mental health and substance abuse.* Retrieved December 9, 2009, from http://www.searo.who.int/en/Section1174/Section1199/Section1567/Section1826_8096.htm

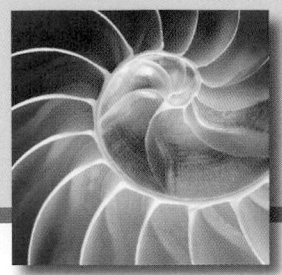

Index

Note: Page numbers followed by *f* refer to figures; page numbers followed by *t* refer to tables; page numbers followed by *b* refer to boxes; page numbers followed by *p* refer to procedures.

A

A-delta fibers, *(V1) 728–729, (V1) 729f, (V1) 730f*
Abbreviations
  do-not-use list of, *(V1) 299*
  for documentation, *(V1) 298–299, (V2) 183–184*
  for drug names, *(V2) 520–521*
  for medications, *(V1) 515, (V2) 518–522*
ABCcodes, *(V2) 1000*
ABCDE assessment, *(V2) 242–243*
Abdellah, Faye, G., nursing theory of, *(V1) 143t*
Abdomen
  assessment of, *(V1) 396–397, (V2) 288p–294p*
    for bowel elimination, *(V1) 686*
    critical aspects of, *(V1) 406–407, (V2) 288*
    documentation of, *(V1) 405*
    for urinary incontinence, *(V2) 640*
  auscultation of, *(V1) 397, (V2) 290p–291p*
  bimanual palpation of, *(V2) 292p*
  circumference of, *(V1) 625*
  color of, *(V2) 289*
  dilated veins of, *(V2) 289*
  inspection of, *(V1) 396–397, (V1) 397f, (V2) 289p*
  one-handed palpation of, *(V2) 292p*
  pain in, *(V2) 294*
  palpation of, *(V1) 397, (V2) 292p–293p*
  percussion of, *(V1) 397, (V2) 291p*
  postoperative distention of, *(V1) 973t*
  pulsations in, *(V2) 290*
  quadrants of, *(V1) 396, (V1) 396f*
  radiography of, *(V1) 686, (V2) 678*
  respiration-related movement of, *(V1) 339*
  striae of, *(V1) 382, (V2) 289*
  tightening of, *(V1) 690–691*
Abdominal binder, *(V1) 860, (V1) 861, (V2) 803p–804p, (V2) 805p*
  critical aspects of, *(V1) 863, (V2) 803*
Abducens nerve (CN VI), assessment of, *(V1) 400t, (V1) 401f, (V2) 306p*
Abduction, *(V2) 299*
Ablative surgery, *(V1) 952*
ABO blood groups, *(V1) 946, (V1) 947t*
Abrasion, *(V1) 472, (V1) 835t*
Abscess, *(V1) 835t. See also* Infection
Absorbent products
  for fecal incontinence, *(V1) 697*
  for urinary incontinence, *(V1) 670*
Absorption, drug. *See* Drug(s), absorption of
Abstinence, *(V2) 753*

Abuse
  assessment of, *(V1) 164, (V2) 79p–83p*
    critical aspects of, *(V1) 163, (V2) 79*
  child, *(V1) 215*
    assessment of, *(V2) 78, (V2) 79p–83p*
  documentation of, *(V2) 83*
  domestic, *(V1) 215, (V1) 798*
  flow chart for, *(V2) 78*
  older adult, *(V2) 83*
  psychological, *(V2) 80, (V2) 82*
  report of, *(V1) 1128–1129*
  sexual, *(V1) 798–799*
    assessment for, *(V2) 80p–83p*
  substance. *See* Substance abuse
Abusive head trauma, *(V2) 80*
A1c testing, *(V1) 114*
Acceptance, communication and, *(V1) 177–178*
Accessory muscles, during inspiration, *(V1) 878*
Accessory nerve (CN XI), assessment of, *(V1) 400t, (V1) 401f, (V2) 308p*
Accidents, *(V1) 436–437. See also* Hazards
  assessment for, *(V1) 446–448*
  developmental factors and, *(V1) 436–437*
  equipment-related, *(V1) 443*
  motor vehicle, *(V1) 436, (V1) 436t, (V1) 437, (V1) 440, (V1) 451, (V1) 455, (V2) 1021*
  needlestick, *(V1) 445, (V1) 532–533, (V1) 532f, (V2) 374*
  prevention of. *See* Safety
  risk factors for, *(V1) 436–437, (V1) 438t*
Accommodation
  cognitive, *(V1) 162*
  pupillary, *(V1) 385*
Accountability, *(V1) 103*
Accreditation, *(V1) 1117*
Acculturation, *(V1) 224–225*
Acetaminophen, *(V1) 739, (V1) 740, (V1) 746*
Acetone odor, *(V1) 377*
Achilles reflex, *(V2) 312p*
Achondroplasia, *(V1) 762*
Acid-base balance
  assessment of, *(V2) 941–943*
  critical thinking about, *(V2) 949–952*
  disorders of, *(V1) 925–928, (V1) 926t, (V1) 927t, (V2) 936*
    nursing interventions for, *(V2) 946–947*
    nursing outcomes for, *(V2) 945*
  full-spectrum nursing and, *(V2) 949–950*
  knowledge map for, *(V2) 953*
  proteins in, *(V1) 607*
  regulation of, *(V1) 921–922*

Acidosis, *(V1) 922, (V1) 925–928, (V1) 926t, (V2) 936*
  metabolic, *(V1) 926, (V1) 927t*
  respiratory, *(V1) 926, (V1) 927t*
Acne, *(V1) 472, (V2) 245*
Acrochordons, *(V2) 242*
Acromegaly, *(V1) 384*
Activated partial thromboplastin time, *(V2) 825*
Active euthanasia, *(V1) 275*
Active immunity, *(V1) 419*
Active listening, *(V1) 258–259, (V1) 365, (V2) 21*
Active range of motion, *(V1) 398, (V1) 754. See also* Range of motion
  for mobility, *(V1) 776–777*
Active transport, *(V1) 915, (V1) 916–917, (V1) 917f, (V1) 917t*
Activities of daily living (ADLs), *(V1) 465*
  for ambulation conditioning, *(V1) 778, (V2) 732*
  assessment of, *(V1) 43–44, (V1) 44b*
  hygiene self-care and, *(V1) 465–467*
    assessment for, *(V1) 467, (V1) 468b*
    nursing diagnosis for, *(V1) 467–468*
    nursing interventions for, *(V1) 468–469*
    nursing outcomes for, *(V1) 468*
Activity. *See* Exercise(s); Mobility; Physical activity
Activity intolerance, *(V2) 743, (V2) 895*
  exercise and, *(V1) 767, (V2) 737*
  postoperative, *(V2) 981*
  sexuality and, *(V1) 801*
Actual nursing diagnosis, *(V1) 60, (V1) 61f, (V1) 64. See also* Nursing diagnosis
  intervention and, *(V1) 107t*
Acupressure, for pain, *(V1) 736*
Acupuncture, *(V1) 1024, (V1) 1024f*
  for pain, *(V1) 736*
  for stress, *(V1) 594*
  for urinary incontinence, *(V2) 636*
Acute confusion, *(V2) 695, (V2) 696*
Acute illness, *(V1) 173, (V1) 175*
Acute infection, *(V1) 413*
Acute pain, *(V1) 727, (V1) 735, (V2) 709*
Acute renal failure, *(V1) 655b*
Acute wound, *(V1) 834–835*
Adaptation, *(V1) 162, (V1) 576*
  in leadership, *(V1) 983–984*
  sensory, *(V1) 707, (V1) 708*
  stress. *See* Stress, adaptation to
Addendum care plan, *(V1) 90*
Addiction, *(V1) 740, (V1) 746. See also* Substance abuse

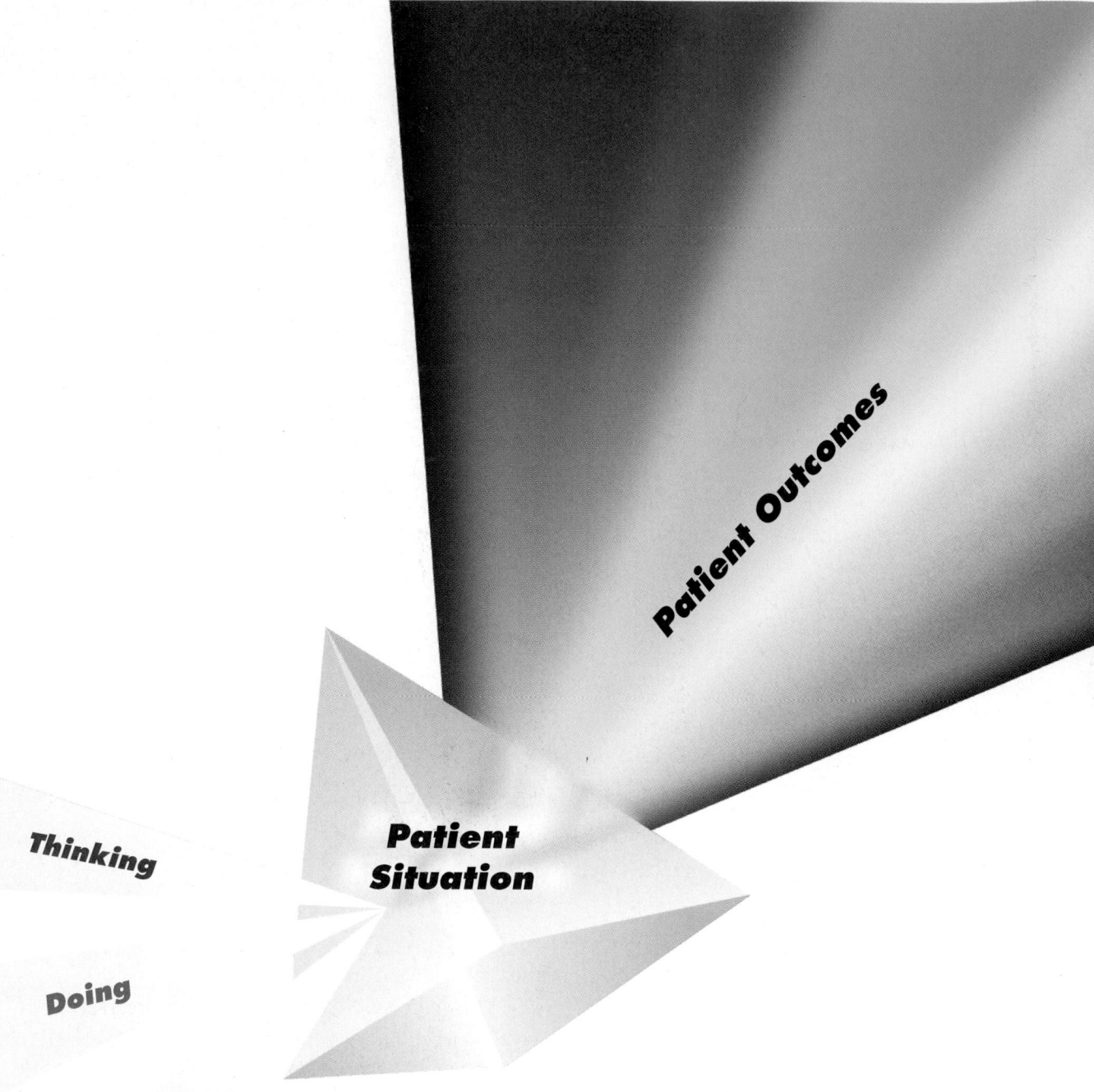

This illustration depicts the full-spectrum model of nursing used throughout this learning package. A full-spectrum nurse uses critical thinking and the nursing process to apply various types of knowledge (theoretical, practical, ethical, and self-knowledge) to the patient situation to bring about desired health outcomes. Truly, thinking and doing.